Neurology in Clinical Practice

Volume I

Neurology in Clinical Practice

Principles of Diagnosis and Management

Second Edition

Edited by Walter G. Bradley, D.M., F.R.C.P.
Professor and Chairman, Department of Neurology,
University of Miami School of Medicine, Miami, Florida
Chief, Department of Neurology,
Jackson Memorial Hospital, Miami, Florida

Robert B. Daroff, M.D.
Professor of Neurology and Associate Dean,
Case Western Reserve University School of Medicine, Cleveland, Ohio;
Chief of Staff and Senior Vice President for Medical Affairs,
University Hospitals of Cleveland, Cleveland, Ohio

Gerald M. Fenichel, M.D.
Professor of Neurology and Pediatrics and Chairman, Department of
Neurology, Vanderbilt University Medical Center, Nashville, Tennessee

C. David Marsden, D.Sc., F.R.C.P., F.R.S.
Professor of Neurology, University Department of Neurology,
National Hospital for Neurology and Neurosurgery, London, England

Associate Editors Nadir E. Bharucha, M.D., M.N.A.M.S., F.R.C.P.
Michael E. Cohen, M.D.
Owen B. Evans, M.D.

With 137 contributing authors

Butterworth–Heinemann

Boston Oxford Singapore Melbourne
Toronto Munich Tokyo New Delhi

Every effort has been made to ensure that the drug dosage schedules within this text are accurate and conform to standards accepted at time of publication. However, as treatment recommendations vary in the light of continuing research and clinical experience, the reader is advised to verify drug dosage schedules herein with information found on product information sheets. This is especially true in cases of new or infrequently used drugs.

Recognizing the importance of preserving what has been written, Butterworth–Heinemann prints its books on acid-free paper whenever possible.

Library of Congress Cataloging-in-Publication Data

Neurology in clinical practice : principles of diagnosis and management / edited by Walter G. Bradley ... [et al.].--2nd ed.
p. cm.
Includes bibliographical references and index.
ISBN 0-7506-9477-7 (set). ISBN 0-7506-9742-3 (v. 1 : alk. paper).--ISBN 0-7506-9743-1 (v. 2 : alk. paper)
1. Neurology. 2. Nervous system--Diseases. I. Bradley, W. G. (Walter George)
[DNLM: 1. Nervous System Diseases. WL 140 N493 1995]
RC346.N4535 1995
616.8--dc20
DNLM/DLC
for Library of Congress 94-41095
CIP

British Library Cataloguing-in-Publication Data

A catalog record for this book is available from the British Library.

The publisher offers discounts on bulk orders of this book.
For information, please write:

Manager of Special Sales
Butterworth–Heinemann
313 Washington Street
Newton, MA 02158–1626

10 9 8 7 6 5 4 3 2 1

Printed in the United States of America

Contents

Volume II The Neurological Disorders

Contributing Authors

Harold P. Adams, Jr., M.D.
Professor of Neurology, University of Iowa College of Medicine, Iowa City; Attending Neurologist and Director, Acute Stroke Care and Monitoring Unit, Department of Neurology, University of Iowa Hospitals and Clinics, Iowa City
58A. Vascular Diseases of the Nervous System: Ischemic Cerebrovascular Disease

Mazen Al-Hakim, M.D.
Assistant Clinical Professor of Neurology, Wayne State University School of Medicine, Detroit; Staff Neurologist, William Beaumont Hospital, Royal Oak, Michigan
78. Disorders of Bones, Joints, Ligaments, Cartilage, and Meninges

Michael J. Aminoff, M.D., F.R.C.P.
Professor of Neurology, University of California, San Francisco, School of Medicine, San Francisco; Attending Neurologist, The Medical Center at the University of California, San Francisco
56A. Neurological Complications of Systemic Disease: In Adults

Jack P. Antel, M.D., Ph.D.
Professor and Chairman, Department of Neurology and Neurosurgery, McGill University Faculty of Medicine, Montreal; Neurologist-in-Chief, Department of Neurology, Montreal Neurological Hospital, Montreal, Quebec, Canada
61. Inflammatory Demyelinating Diseases of the Central Nervous System

Ram Ayyar, M.D.
Professor of Neurology, University of Miami School of Medicine, Miami; Attending Neurologist and Director, EMG Laboratory, Department of Neurology, Jackson Memorial Hospital, Miami
65D. Effect of Toxins and Physical Agents on the Nervous System: Marine Toxins

Alberto O. Barroso, M.D., F.A.C.P.
Clinical Associate Professor of Medicine, Gastroenterology Section, Department of Internal Medicine, Baylor College of Medicine, Houston; Associate Attending Active Staff, Gastroenterology Section, Department of Internal Medicine, Methodist Hospital, Houston
13. Difficulties with Speech and Swallowing

Roy W. Beck, M.D., Ph.D.
Director, Jaeb Center for Health Research, Tampa, Florida
15. Abnormalities of the Optic Nerve and Retina

D. Frank Benson, M.D.
The Augustus S. Rose Professor of Neurology, University of California, Los Angeles, UCLA School of Medicine, Los Angeles
7. Approaches to Intellectual and Memory Impairments

Alan R. Berger, M.D.
Vice-Chairman and Chief-of-Service, Department of Neurology, Albert Einstein College of Medicine of Yeshiva University, Bronx, New York; Director, Clinical EMG Laboratory, Department of Neurology, Montefiore Medical Center, Bronx, New York
65A. Effect of Toxins and Physical Agents on the Nervous System: Effects of Occupational and Environmental Agents on the Nervous System

Joseph R. Berger, M.D.
Professor and Chairman, Department of Neurology, University of Kentucky College of Medicine, Lexington; Staff Physician, Department of Neurology, University of Kentucky Hospital, Lexington
5. Clinical Approach to Stupor and Coma; 60D. Infections of the Nervous System: The Neurological Manifestations of Human Immunodeficiency Virus Infection; 60E. Infections of the Nervous System: Central Nervous System Diseases Caused by Unconventional Transmissible Agents and Chronic Viral Infections

Sorab K. Bhabha, M.D., D.M.
Consultant Neurologist, Department of Clinical Neurosciences, The Hinduja Hospital and Medical Research Centre, Bombay, India
60A. Infections of the Nervous System: Bacterial Infections; 60B. Infections of the Nervous System: Fungal and Parasitic Infections; 60C. Infections of the Nervous System: Viral Infections

Eddie P. Bharucha, M.D., F.A.M.S.
Emeritus Professor of Neurology, Seth G.S. Medical College and K.E.M. Hospital, Bombay; Neurologist, Department of Neurology and Neuroepidemiology, Bombay Hospital Institute of Medical Sciences and Medical Research Centre, Bombay, India
60A. Infections of the Nervous System: Bacterial Infections; 60B. Infections of the Nervous System: Fungal and Parasitic Infections; 60C. Infections of the Nervous System: Viral Infections

Nadir E. Bharucha, M.D., M.N.A.M.S., F.R.C.P.
Associate Professor of Neurology and Head, Department of Neuroepidemiology, Bombay Hospital Institute of Medical Sciences and Medical Research Centre, Bombay; Neurologist, Department of Neurology and Epidemiology, Bombay Institute of Medical Sciences and Medical Research Centre, Bombay, India
60A. Infections of the Nervous System: Bacterial Infections; 60B. Infections of the Nervous System: Fungal and Parasitic Infections; 60C. Infections of the Nervous System: Viral Infections

José Biller, M.D., F.A.C.P.
Professor and Chairman, Department of Neurology, Indiana University School of Medicine, Indianapolis; Chief, Neurology Services, Department of Neurology, Indiana University Medical Center, Indianapolis
58A. Vascular Diseases of the Nervous System: Ischemic Cerebrovascular Disease

Thomas D. Bird, M.D.
Professor of Neurology, University of Washington School of Medicine, Seattle; Chief, Department of Neurology, Veterans Affairs Medical Center, Seattle
47. Clinical Neurogenetics

Hans-Georg O. Bock, M.D., Ph.D.
Associate Professor, Pediatric Attending Physician, and Medical Geneticist, Department of Preventive Medicine, University of Mississippi Medical Center, Jackson
69. Inborn Errors of Metabolism of the Nervous System

E. Peter Bosch, M.D., F.A.C.P.
Professor of Neurology, Mayo Medical School, Rochester, Minnesota; Consultant, Department of Neurology, Mayo Clinic Scottsdale, Scottsdale, Arizona
81. Disorders of Peripheral Nerves

Walter G. Bradley, D.M., F.R.C.P.
Professor and Chairman, Department of Neurology, University of Miami School of Medicine, Miami, Florida; Chief, Department of Neurology, Jackson Memorial Hospital, Miami, Florida
1. Approach to the Diagnosis of Neurological Disease; 35. Low Back and Lower-Limb Pain; 36. The Place of Laboratory Investigations in Diagnosis and Management of Neurological Disease; 51. General Principles in the Management of Neurological Disease; 78. Disorders of Bones, Joints, Ligaments, Cartilage, and Meninges

Michael H. Brooke, M.B., B.Ch., F.R.C.P.(C).
Professor and Head, Division of Neurology, University of Alberta Faculty of Medicine, Edmonton, Alberta, Canada
29. Proximal, Distal, and Generalized Weakness; 84. Disorders of Skeletal Muscle

Joseph Bruni, M.D., F.R.C.P.(C).
Associate Professor of Medicine, University of Toronto Faculty of Medicine, Toronto; Head, Division of Neurology, The Wellesley Hospital, Toronto, Ontario, Canada
2. Episodic Impairment of Consciousness

Thomas N. Byrne, M.D.
Clinical Professor of Neurology and Medicine, Yale University School of Medicine, New Haven; Assistant Chief, Department of Neurology, Yale-New Haven Hospital, New Haven, Connecticut
28. Paraplegia and Spinal Cord Syndromes

J. Keith Campbell, M.D., F.R.C.P. (Ed.)
Emeritus Professor of Neurology, Mayo Medical School and Mayo Clinic, Rochester, Minnesota
74. Headache and Other Craniofacial Pain

Niall E. F. Cartlidge, M.B.B.S., F.R.C.P.
Consultant Neurologist and Senior Lecturer in Neurology, Division of Clinical Neuroscience, The Medical School, University of Newcastle Upon Tyne, Framlington Place, Newcastle; Consultant Neurologist, Royal Victoria Infirmary, Newcastle Upon Tyne, England
78. Disorders of Bones, Joints, Ligaments, Cartilage, and Meninges

Richard J. Caselli, M.D.
Associate Professor of Neurology, Mayo Medical School, Rochester, Minnesota; Consultant, Department of Neurology, Mayo Clinic Scottsdale, Scottsdale, Arizona
74. Headache and Other Craniofacial Pain

David A. Chad, M.D.
Professor of Neurology and Attending Neurologist, University of Massachusetts Medical Center, Worcester
80. Disorders of Nerve Roots and Plexuses

Michael E. Cohen, M.D.
Professor of Neurology and Pediatrics and Chairman, Department of Neurology, State University of New York at Buffalo School of Medicine and Biomedical Sciences, Buffalo
59D. Primary and Secondary Tumors of the Central Nervous System: Molecular Biology of Nervous System Tumors; 59E. Primary and Secondary Tumors of the Central Nervous System: Clinical Presentation and Therapy of Nervous System Tumors; 59F. Primary and Secondary Tumors of the Central Nervous System: Clinical Presentation and Therapy of Spinal Tumors; 59G. Primary and Secondary Tumors of the Central Nervous System: Clinical Presentation and Therapy of Peripheral Nerve Tumors; 59I. Primary and Secondary Tumors of the Central Nervous System: Quality of Life and Late Effects of Treatment

Paul E. Cooper, M.D.
Associate Professor of Clinical Neurological Sciences, Department of Medicine, University of Western Ontario Faculty of Medicine, London; Chief of Clinical Neurological Sciences and Vice-President of Medical Affairs, St. Joseph's Health Centre, London, Ontario, Canada
50. Neuroendocrinology

Terry A. Cox, M.D.
Assistant Consulting Professor of Ophthalmology, Duke University Hospital, Durham, North Carolina
17. Pupillary and Eyelid Abnormalities

Valerie A. Cwik, M.D.
Assistant Professor of Neurology, Department of Medicine, University of Alberta Faculty of Medicine, Edmonton, Alberta, Canada
29. Proximal, Distal, and Generalized Weakness; 84. Disorders of Skeletal Muscle

Antonio R. Damasio, M.D., Ph.D.
Professor of Neurology, University of Iowa College of Medicine, Iowa City; Head, Department of Neurology, University of Iowa Hospitals and Clinics, Iowa City
11. Agnosias and Apraxias

Robert B. Daroff, M.D.
Professor of Neurology and Associate Dean, Case Western Reserve University School of Medicine, Cleveland; Chief of Staff and Senior Vice President for Medical Affairs, University Hospitals of Cleveland, Cleveland, Ohio
1. Approach to the Diagnosis of Neurological Disease; 3. Falls and Drop Attacks; 17. Pupillary and Eyelid Abnormalities; 36. The Place of Laboratory Investigations in Diagnosis and Management of Neurological Disease; 51. General Principles in the Management of Neurological Disease

James O. Donaldson, M.D.
Professor of Neurology, University of Connecticut School of Medicine, Farmington
86. Neurological Problems of Pregnancy

Patricia K. Duffner, M.D.
Professor of Neurology and Pediatrics, Department of Neurology, State University of New York at Buffalo School of Medicine and Biomedical Sciences, Buffalo; Attending Physician, Department of Child Neurology, Children's Hospital of Buffalo, Buffalo
59E. Primary and Secondary Tumors of the Central Nervous System: Clinical Presentation and Therapy of Nervous System Tumors; 59I. Primary and Secondary Tumors of the Central Nervous System: Quality of Life and Late Effects of Treatment

Pierre Duquette, M.D., F.R.C.P.
Professor of Medicine, University of Montreal Faculty of Medicine, Montreal; Head, Division of Neurology, Department of Medicine, Notre-Dame Hospital, Montreal, Quebec, Canada
61. Inflammatory Demyelinating Diseases of the Central Nervous System

Ronald G. Emerson, M.D.
Associate Professor of Neurology, Columbia University College of Physicians and Surgeons, New York; Associate Attending Physician, Department of Neurology, Presbyterian Hospital in the City of New York, New York
37A. Clinical Neurophysiology: Electroencephalography and Evoked Potentials

Owen B. Evans, M.D.
Professor and Chairman, Department of Pediatrics, University of Mississippi Medical Center, Jackson; Attending Physician, Department of Pediatrics, University Hospitals and Clinics, Jackson
69. Inborn Errors of Metabolism of the Nervous System

Gerald M. Fenichel, M.D.
Professor of Neurology and Pediatrics and Chairman, Department of Neurology, Vanderbilt University Medical Center, Nashville, Tennessee
1. Approach to the Diagnosis of Neurological Disease; 8. Developmental Delay and Regression in Infants; 31. The Hypotonic Infant; 36. The Place of Laboratory Investigations in Diagnosis and Management of Neurological Disease; 51. General Principles in the Management of Neurological Disease

Pasquale F. Finelli, M.D.
Associate Professor of Neurology, University of Connecticut School of Medicine; Attending Physician, Department of Neurology, Hartford Hospital, Hartford
20. Disturbances of Taste and Smell

Daniel W. Fort, M.D.
Assistant Professor of Pediatrics, University of Virginia School of Medicine, Charlottesville; Assistant Professor, Department of Pediatric Hematology and Oncology, University of Virginia Medical Center, Charlottesville
59C. Primary and Secondary Tumors of the Central Nervous System: Chemotherapy for Nervous System Tumors

Clare J. Fowler, M.B.B.S., M.Sc., F.R.C.P.
Consultant, Department of Uro-Neurology, National Hospital for Neurology and Neurosurgery, London, England
45. Neuro-Urology

Richard S. J. Frackowiak, M.A., F.R.C.P.
Professor of Neurology, Wellcome Department of Cognitive Neurology, Institute of Neurology, London; Consultant Neurologist, National Hospital for Neurology and Neurosurgery, London, England
40. Functional Neuroimaging

Gordon S. Francis, M.D.
Associate Professor, Department of Neurology and Neurosurgery, McGill University Faculty of Medicine, Montreal; Director, Multiple Sclerosis Clinic, Department of Neurology, Montreal Neurological Hospital, Montreal, Quebec, Canada
61. Inflammatory Demyelinating Diseases of the Central Nervous System

Frank R. Freemon, M.D., Ph.D.
Professor of Neurology, Vanderbilt University School of Medicine, Nashville; Chief of Neurology, Veterans Administration Medical Center, Nashville, Tennessee
27. Hemiplegia and Monoplegia

David G. Gadian, D.Phil.
Head, RCS Unit of Biophysics, Institute of Child Health, London; Head, Department of Radiology and Physics, Great Ormond Street Hospital for Children NHS Trust, London, England
40. Functional Neuroimaging

David S. Geldmacher, M.D.
Assistant Professor of Neurology, Case Western Reserve University School of Medicine, Cleveland; Clinical Director, Alzheimer Center, University Hospitals of Cleveland, Cleveland, Ohio
58F. Vascular Diseases of the Nervous System: Spinal Cord Vascular Disease

Gerald S. Golden, M.D.
Adjunct Professor of Neurology, University of Pennsylvania School of Medicine, Philadelphia; Vice President, Division of Exam Support Services and Medical School Liaison, National Board of Medical Examiners, Philadelphia
68. Developmental Disabilities

Jonathan M. Goldstein, M.D.
Assistant Professor of Neurology, Yale University School of Medicine, New Haven; Attending Physician and Director, Neuromuscular Division, Department of Neurology, Yale-New Haven Hospital, New Haven, Connecticut
32. Sensory Abnormalities of the Limbs and Trunk

Manuel R. Gomez, M.D.
Emeritus Professor of Pediatric Neurology, Department of Neurology, Mayo Medical School and Mayo Clinic, Rochester; Consultant, Department of Pediatric Neurology, Mayo Clinic and St. Mary's Hospital, Rochester, Minnesota
70. Neurocutaneous Diseases

Thomas R. Gordon, M.D.
Affiliate Associate Professor, Biomedical Program, University of Alaska, Anchorage; Neurologist, Department of Medicine, Providence Alaska Medical Center and Alaska Regional Hospitals, Anchorage
32. Sensory Abnormalities of the Limbs and Trunk

Steven J. Greenberg, M.D.
Assistant Professor of Neurology, State University of New York at Buffalo School of Medicine and Biomedical Sciences, Buffalo; Chief, Department of Neurology and Head, Laboratory of Neuroimmunology and Neurovirology, Roswell Park Memorial Cancer Institute, Buffalo
59D. Primary and Secondary Tumors of the Central Nervous System: Molecular Biology of Nervous System Tumors

Richard Haas, M.B., BChir., M.R.C.P.
Associate Professor, Department of Neurosciences and Pediatrics, University of California, San Diego, School of Medicine, La Jolla; Attending Physician, Department of Neurosciences and Pediatrics, University of California, San Diego, Medical Center, San Diego
69. Inborn Errors of Metabolism of the Nervous System

Robert W. Hamill, M.D.
Professor and Chairman, Department of Neurology, University of Vermont College of Medicine, Burlington; Physician Leader, Department of Neurology, Fletcher Allen Health Care, Burlington
87. Geriatric Neurology

Maurice R. Hanson, M.D.
Staff Neurologist, Department of Neurology, Cleveland Clinic Hospital, Fort Lauderdale, Florida
21. Disturbances of Lower Cranial Nerves; 75. The Cranial Neuropathies

Richard J. Hardie, T.D., M.D., F.R.C.P.
Consultant Neurologist, Royal Devon and Exeter Hospital (Wonford), Exeter, England
55. The Principles of Neurological Rehabilitation

Anita E. Harding, M.D., F.R.C.P.
Professor of Clinical Neurology, Institute of Neurology, London; Consultant Neurologist, National Hospital for Neurology and Neurosurgery, London, England
24. Ataxic Disorders; 77. Cerebellar and Spinocerebellar Disorders

Reid R. Heffner, Jr., M.D.
Professor and Associate Chairman, Department of Pathology, State University of New York at Buffalo School of Medicine and Biomedical Sciences, Buffalo
59A. Primary and Secondary Tumors of the Central Nervous System: Pathology of Nervous System Tumors

Albert Hijdra, M.D.
Staff Neurologist, Department of Neurology, Academisch Medisch Centrum, Amsterdam, The Netherlands
71C. The Dementias: Vascular Dementia

Alan Hill, M.D., Ph.D.
Professor and Head, Department of Neurology, University

of British Columbia Faculty of Medicine, Vancouver; Head, Department of Neurology, British Columbia Children's Hospital, Vancouver, British Columbia, Canada
85. Neurological Problems of the Newborn

James F. Howard, Jr., M.D.
Professor of Neurology, University of North Carolina at Chapel Hill School of Medicine, Chapel Hill
83. Disorders of Neuromuscular Transmission

Kurt A. Jaeckle, M.D.
Professor of Medicine and Associate Neurologist, Department of Neuro-Oncology, University of Texas M.D. Anderson Cancer Center, Houston
59E. Primary and Secondary Tumors of the Central Nervous System: Clinical Presentation and Therapy of Nervous System Tumors

Luke D. Kartsounis, M.Sc., Ph.D.
Honorary Lecturer, Institute of Neurology, London; Clinical Neuropsychologist, Department of Clinical Neuropsychology, National Hospital for Neurology and Neurosurgery, London, England
41. Neuropsychology

Carlos S. Kase, M.D.
Professor of Neurology, Boston University School of Medicine, Boston; Visiting Neurologist, Department of Neurology, Boston University Medical Center Hospital, Boston
58B. Vascular Diseases of the Nervous System: Intracerebral Hemorrhage

Roger E. Kelley, M.D.
Professor and Chairman, Department of Neurology, and Chief of Neurology Service, Louisiana State University Hospital-Shreveport, Shreveport
38. Noninvasive Craniovascular Studies

Jun Kimura, M.D.
Professor and Chairman, Department of Neurology, Kyoto University Hospitals, Kyoto, Japan
37B.Clinical Neurophysiology: Electrodiagnosis of Neuromuscular Disorders

Howard S. Kirshner, M.D.
Professor and Vice-Chairman, Department of Neurology, Vanderbilt University School of Medicine, Nashville; Director, Adult Neurology Service, Department of Neurology, Vanderbilt University Hospital, Nashville, Tennessee
12A. Language Disorders: Aphasia

David G. Kline, M.D.
Professor and Chairman, Department of Neurosurgery, Louisiana State University School of Medicine in New Orleans, New Orleans; Visiting Surgeon, Medical Center of Louisiana at Charity Hospital; Staff Neurosurgeon, Ochsner Foundation Hospital, Baptist-Mercy Hospitals, and Touro Infirmary, Nashville, Tennessee
57C. Trauma of the Nervous System: Peripheral Nerve Trauma

John F. Kurtzke, M.D.
Professor of Neurology and Community and Family Medicine, Georgetown University School of Medicine, Washington, D.C.; Chief, Neurology Service, Veterans Administration Hospital, Washington, D.C.
46. Neuroepidemiology

Anthony E. Lang, M.D., F.R.C.P. (C)
Professor of Neurology, Department of Medicine, University of Toronto Faculty of Medicine, Toronto; Director, Movement Disorders Centre, Department of Medicine, Toronto Hospital, Toronto, Ontario, Canada
25. Movement Disorder Symptomatology; 76. Movement Disorders

Patrick J. M. Lavin, M.D.
Associate Professor of Neurology and Ophthalmology, Vanderbilt University Hospital, Nashville, Tennessee
16. Eye Movement Disorders and Diplopia; 42. Neuro-Ophthalmology

Robert B. Layzer, M.D.
Professor of Neurology, University of California, San Francisco, School of Medicine, San Francisco
30. Muscle Pains and Cramps

Ronald P. Lesser, M.D.
Professor of Neurology and Neurosurgery, Johns Hopkins University School of Medicine, Baltimore; Professor of Neurology and Neurosurgery, Johns Hopkins Hospital, Baltimore, Maryland
72. The Epilepsies

Alan H. Lockwood, M.D.
Professor, Department of Neurology and Nuclear Medicine, State University of New York at Buffalo School of Medicine and Biomedical Sciences, Buffalo; Department of Veterans Affairs Medical Center, Buffalo
63. Toxic and Metabolic Encephalopathies

Robert Mair, Ph.D.
Professor of Psychology, University of New Hampshire, Durham
20. Disturbances of Taste and Smell

C. David Marsden, D.Sc., F.R.C.P., F.R.S.
Professor of Neurology, University Department of Neurology, National Hospital for Neurology and Neurosurgery, London, England
1. Approach to the Diagnosis of Neurological Disease; 26. Walking Disorders; 36. The Place of Laboratory Inves-

tigations in Diagnosis and Management of Neurological Disease; 51. General Principles in the Management of Neurological Disease

Christopher J. Mathias, M.B.B.S., D.Phil., F.R.C.P.
Professor of Neurovascular Medicine, Institute of Neurology and St. Mary's Hospital Medical School and Imperial College of Science, Technology, and Medicine, London; Consultant Physician, Autonomic Unit, National Hospital for Neurology and Neurosurgery and the Cardiovascular Medicine Unit, St. Mary's Hospital, London, England
82. Disorders of the Autonomic Nervous System

Justin C. McArthur, M.B.B.S., M.P.H.
Associate Professor, Departments of Neurology and Epidemiology, Johns Hopkins University School of Medicine, Baltimore; Department of Neurology, Johns Hopkins Hospital, Baltimore, Maryland
60D. Infections of the Nervous System: The Neurological Manifestations of Human Immunodeficiency Virus Infection

Micheline McCarthy, M.D., Ph.D.
Assistant Professor of Neurology, University of Miami School of Medicine, Miami; Associate Chief, Department of Neurology, Veterans Administration Medical Center, Miami, Florida
49. Neurovirology; 60E. Infections of the Nervous System: Central Nervous System Diseases Caused by Unconventional Transmissible Agents and Chronic Viral Infections

Michael J. McLean, M.D., Ph.D.
Associate Professor, Departments of Neurology, Pharmacology, and Psychiatry, Vanderbilt University Hospital and Department of Veterans Affairs Medical Center, Nashville, Tennessee
52. Principles of Neuropharmacology and Therapeutics

Laszlo Mechtler, M.D.
Assistant Professor of Neurology and Neuro-Oncology, Roswell Park Memorial Cancer Institute, Dent Neurologic Institute, and State University of New York at Buffalo School of Medicine and Biomedical Sciences, Buffalo; Head of Neuro-Oncology, Department of Neurology, Roswell Park Memorial Cancer Institute, Buffalo
59F. Primary and Secondary Tumors of the Central Nervous System: Clinical Presentation and Therapy of Spinal Tumors; 59G. Primary and Secondary Tumors of the Central Nervous System: Clinical Presentation and Therapy of Peripheral Nerve Tumors

Mario F. Mendez, M.D., Ph.D.
Associate Professor of Neurology, University of California, Los Angeles, UCLA School of Medicine, Los Angeles; Director, Neurobehavior Unit, Veterans Affairs Medical Center, West Los Angeles
4. Delirium

Hiroshi Mitsumoto, M.D., D.Sc.
Associate Professor of Neurology, Ohio State University College of Medicine, Columbus; Head, Neuromuscular/EMG Section, Department of Neurology, Cleveland Clinic Foundation, Cleveland, Ohio
81. Disorders of Peripheral Nerves

Paul L. Moots, M.D.
Assistant Professor of Neurology, Vanderbilt University Hospital, Nashville, Tennessee
53. Principles of Pain Management

Hugo Moser, M.D.
University Professor, Department of Neurology and Pediatrics, Johns Hopkins University School of Medicine, Baltimore; Director, Center for Research on Mental Retardation, Kennedy Krieger Institute, Baltimore, Maryland
69. Inborn Errors of Metabolism of the Nervous System

Sakkubai Naidu, M.D.
Neurologist, Department of Neurogenetics, Kennedy Krieger Institute, Baltimore; Neurologist, Departments of Neurology and Pediatrics, Johns Hopkins Hospital, Baltimore, Maryland
69. Inborn Errors of Metabolism of the Nervous System

Ruth Nass, M.D.
Associate Professor of Neurology, New York University Medical Center, New York
12B. Language Disorders: Developmental Language Disorders

David Neary, M.D., F.R.C.P.
Professor of Neurology, University of Manchester, Manchester; Consultant Neurologist, Manchester Royal Infirmary, Manchester, England
71D. The Dementias: Progressive Focal Cortical Syndromes

Trevor Owens, Ph.D.
Associate Professor, Department of Neurology and Neurosurgery, McGill University Faculty of Medicine, Montreal, Quebec, Canada
48. Neuroimmunology

Colette Parker, M.D.
Former Clinical Associate, Developmental and Metabolic Neurology Branch, National Institute of Neurological Disorders and Stroke, Bethesda, Maryland
69. Inborn Errors of Metabolism of the Nervous System

J. David Parkes, M.D., F.R.C.P.
Professor of Clinical Neurology, University Department of Neurology, Kings College Hospital School of Medicine and Institute of Psychiatry, London, England; Consultant Neu-

rologist, Kings Healthcare and Maudsley Hospitals, London
6. Excessive Daytime Sleepiness; 73. Disorders of Sleep

Timothy A. Pedley, M.D.
Professor and Vice Chairman, Department of Neurology, Columbia University College of Physicians and Surgeons, New York; Director, Comprehensive Epilepsy Center and Associate Director, Neurology Service, Columbia-Presbyterian Medical Center, New York
37A. Clinical Neurophysiology: Electroencephalography and Evoked Potentials

David Pilgrim, M.D.
Clinical Instructor, Department of Neurology, Harvard Medical School, Boston; Neurologist, Harvard Community Health Plan, Boston; Neurologist, Hebrew Rehabilitation Center for the Aged, Boston; Associate in Medicine, Department of Medicine, Brigham and Women's Hospital, Boston
87. Geriatric Neurology

Jerome B. Posner, M.D.
Professor of Neurology and Neuroscience, Cornell University Medical College, New York; Chairman, Department of Neurology, Memorial Sloan-Kettering Cancer Center, New York
59H. Primary and Secondary Tumors of the Central Nervous System: Paraneoplastic Syndromes

Robert M. Quencer, M.D.
Professor and Chairman, Department of Radiology, University of Miami School of Medicine, Miami; Chief of Service, Department of Radiology, Jackson Memorial Hospital, Miami, Florida
39. Neuroimaging

Robert A. Ratcheson, M.D.
Harvey Huntington Brown, Jr., Professor and Chairman, Department of Neurological Surgery, Case Western Reserve University School of Medicine, Cleveland; Director, Department of Neurological Surgery, University Hospitals of Cleveland, Cleveland, Ohio
58C. Vascular Diseases of the Nervous System: Intracranial Aneurysms; 58D. Vascular Diseases of the Nervous System: Arteriovenous Malformations

Bernd F. Remler, M.D.
Assistant Professor of Neurology and Ophthalmology, Case Western Reserve University School of Medicine, Cleveland; Staff Member, Departments of Neurology and Ophthalmology, University Hospitals of Cleveland and Veterans Affairs Medical Center, Cleveland, Ohio
3. Falls and Drop Attacks

David E. Riley, M.D.
Assistant Professor of Neurology, Case Western Reserve University School of Medicine, Cleveland; Director, Movement Disorder Center, Department of Neurology, Mount Sinai Medical Center, Cleveland, Ohio
76. Movement Disorders

Gustavo C. Román, M.D., F.A.C.P.
Clinical Professor of Neurology, University of Texas Medical School at San Antonio, San Antonio
88. Tropical Neurology

David B. Rosenfield, M.D.
Professor of Speech and Director, Stuttering Center Speech Motor Control Laboratory, Departments of Neurology and Otorhinolaryngology and Communicative Sciences, Baylor College of Medicine, Houston; Attending Physician, Department of Neurology, The Methodist Hospital, Houston
13. Difficulties with Speech and Swallowing

Martin N. Rossor, M.A., M.D., F.R.C.P.
Senior Lecturer, Department of Neurology, Institute of Neurology, London; Consultant Neurologist, Department of Neurology, National Hospital for Neurology and Neurosurgery, London, England
71A. The Dementias: Primary Degenerative Dementia; 71B. The Dementias: Dementia as Part of Other Degenerative Diseases; 71E. The Dementias: Other Causes of Dementia

David N. Rushton, M.D., F.R.C.P.
Professor, Department of Rehabilitation, London Hospital Medical College, London; Head of Service, Department of Rehabilitation, Tower Hamlets Healthcare Trust, London, England
33. Sexual and Sphincter Dysfunction

Juan R. Sanchez-Ramos, Ph.D., M.D.
Associate Professor of Neurology, University of Miami School of Medicine, Miami; Neurologist, Geriatric Research and Education Clinical Center, Veterans Administration Medical Center, Miami, Florida
65B. Effect of Toxins and Physical Agents on the Nervous System: Effects of Drugs of Abuse on the Nervous System

Donald B. Sanders, M.D.
Professor of Medicine, Division of Neurology, Duke University School of Medicine, Durham, North Carolina
83. Disorders of Neuromuscular Transmission

Harvey B. Sarnat, M.D., F.R.C.P. (C)
Professor, Departments of Neurology, Pediatrics, and Pathology, University of Washington School of Medicine, Seattle; Head, Division of Pediatric Neurology, Departments of Neurology and Pediatrics, Children's Hospital and Medical Center, Seattle
67. Developmental Disorders of the Nervous System

Herbert H. Schaumburg, M.D.
Professor and Chairman, Department of Neurology and Di-

rector, Residency Training Program, Albert Einstein College of Medicine of Yeshiva University, Bronx, New York; Professor and Chairman, Department of Neurology, Montefiore Medical Center, Bronx, New York
65A. Effect of Toxins and Physical Agents on the Nervous System: Effects of Occupational and Ennvironmental Agents on the Nervous System

James W. Schmidley, M.D.
Associate Professor of Neurology, Case Western Reserve University School of Medicine, Cleveland; Chair, MetroHealth Campus, Department of Neurology, MetroHealth Medical Center, Cleveland, Ohio
58G. Vascular Diseases of the Nervous System: Central Nervous System Vasculitis

S. Clifford Schold, Jr., M.D.
Professor and Chair, Department of Neurology, University of Texas Southwestern Medical Center at Dallas Southwestern Medical School, Dallas
59C. Primary and Secondary Tumors of the Central Nervous System: Chemotherapy for Nervous System Tumors

Warren R. Selman, M.D.
Professor of Surgery, Department of Neurological Surgery, Case Western Reserve University School of Medicine, Cleveland; Vice Chairman, Department of Neurological Surgery, University Hospitals of Cleveland, Cleveland, Ohio
58C. Vascular Diseases of the Nervous System: Intracranial Aneurysms; 58D. Vascular Diseases of the Nervous System: Arteriovenous Malformations

Kapil D. Sethi, M.D., M.R.C.P.
Associate Professor of Neurology, Medical College of Georgia School of Medicine, Augusta; Physician, Department of Neurology, Medical College of Georgia Hospital and Clinics and Veterans Administration Medical Center, Augusta
34. Arm and Neck Pain

Kyu H. Shin, M.D., F.R.C.P. (C)
Chairman and Professor, Department of Radiation Oncology, State University of New York at Buffalo School of Medicine and Biomedical Sciences, Buffalo; Chairman, Department of Radiation Medicine, Roswell Park Memorial Cancer Institute, Buffalo
59B. Primary and Secondary Tumors of the Central Nervous System: The Role of Radiation Therapy in the Management of Tumors of the Central Nervous System

Roger P. Simon, M.D.
Professor and Chairman, Department of Neurology, University of Pittsburgh School of Medicine, Pittsburgh, Pennsylvania
64. Deficiency Diseases of the Nervous System

Evelyn M. L. Sklar, M.D.
Associate Professor of Clinical Radiology and Neurological Surgery, University of Miami School of Medicine, Miami; Attending Staff Radiologist, Department of Radiology, Jackson Memorial Hospital, Miami, Florida
39. Neuroimaging

J. S. Snowden, Ph.D.
Neuropsychologist, Department of Neurology, University of Manchester, Manchester; Neuropsychologist, Department of Neurology, Manchester Royal Infirmary, Manchester, England
71D. The Dementias: Progressive Focal Cortical Syndromes

Bruce D. Snyder, M.D.
Clinical Professor of Neurology, University of Minnesota Medical School-Minneapolis; Staff Neurologist, Department of Internal Medicine, Riverside Medical Center, and Neurologist, Minneapolis Clinic of Neurology, Minneapolis
62. Anoxic and Ischemic Encephalopathies

Yuen T. So, M.D., Ph.D.
Associate Professor of Neurology, Oregon Health Sciences University School of Medicine, Portland; Director, EMG Laboratory, University Hospital, Portland
64. Deficiency Diseases of the Nervous System

Subramaniam Sriram, M.B.B.S.
Professor of Neurology, Vanderbilt University Medical Center, Nashville, Tennessee
48. Neuroimmunology

Bennett M. Stein, M.D.
Chairman, Department of Neurological Surgery, Columbia University College of Physicians and Surgeons, New York; Director of Service, Department of Neurological Surgery, Presbyterian Hospital in the City of New York, New York
54. Principles of Neurosurgery

Jerry W. Swanson, M.D.
Associate Professor of Neurology, Mayo Medical School, Rochester; Consultant, Department of Neurology, Mayo Clinic, Rochester, Minnesota
22. Cranial and Facial Pain

Patrick J. Sweeney, M.D., F.A.C.P.
Director, Neurology Residency Program, Cleveland Clinic Foundation, Cleveland; Clinical Associate Professor of Neurology, Case Western Reserve University School of Medicine, Cleveland, and Ohio State University College of Medicine, Columbus, Ohio
21. Disturbances of Lower Cranial Nerves; 75. The Cranial Neuropathies

Thomas R. Swift, M.D.
Professor and Chairman, Department of Neurology, Medical College of Georgia School of Medicine, Augusta
34. Arm and Neck Pain

Rup Tandan, M.D., M.R.C.P.
Associate Professor of Neurology, University of Vermont College of Medicine, Burlington; Attending Neurologist, Medical Center Hospital of Vermont, Fletcher Allen Health Care, Burlington
79. Disorders of the Upper and Lower Motor Neurons

Philip D. Thompson, M.B., Ph.D., F.R.A.C.P.
Associate Professor of Medicine, University Department of Medicine, University of Adelaide, Adelaide; Associate Professor of Medicine and Senior Visiting Neurologist, Departments of Medicine and Neurology, Royal Adelaide Hospital, Adelaide, South Australia, Australia
26. Walking Disorders

Robert L. Tiel, M.D.
Assistant Professor of Neurosurgery, Louisiana State University School of Medicine in New Orleans, New Orleans
57C. Trauma of the Nervous System: Peripheral Nerve Trauma

Robert L. Tomsak, M.D., Ph.D.
Clinical Associate Professor of Ophthalmology and Neurology, Case Western Reserve University School of Medicine, Cleveland; Head, Section of Neuro-Ophthalmology, Division of Ophthalmology, Mount Sinai Medical Center, Cleveland, Ohio
14. Visual Loss; 43. The Afferent Visual System

Daniel Tranel, Ph.D.
Professor of Neurology, University of Iowa College of Medicine, Iowa City; Chief, Benton Neuropsychology Laboratory, Department of Neurology, University of Iowa Hospitals and Clinics, Iowa City
11. Agnosias and Apraxias

William H. Trescher, M.D.
Assistant Professor of Neurology, Johns Hopkins University School of Medicine, Baltimore; Neurologist, Department of Neuroscience, Kennedy Krieger Institute, Baltimore, Maryland
72. The Epilepsies

Michael R. Trimble, M.D., F.R.C.P., F.R.C.Psych.
Professor of Behavioral Neurology, Department of Neurology, Institute of Neurology, London; Consultant Physician, Department of Psychological Medicine, National Hospital for Neurology and Neurosurgery, London, England
9. Behavior and Personality Disturbances; 10. Depression and Psychosis in Neurological Practice

B. Todd Troost, M.D.
Professor and Chairman, Department of Neurology, Bowman Gray School of Medicine of Wake Forest University, Winston-Salem, North Carolina
18. Dizziness and Vertigo; 19. Hearing Loss and Tinnitus Without Dizziness or Vertigo; 44. Neuro-Otology

John W. Tulloch, M.D.
Assistant Professor of Neurology, University of Minnesota Medical School-Minneapolis; Head, Neurodiagnostic Laboratory, Department of Neurology, Saint Paul-Ramsey Medical Center, St. Paul
62. Anoxic and Ischemic Encephalopathies

James R. van Dellen, M.B.B.Ch., F.R.C.S. (Edin.), Ph.D. (Med.)
Neurosurgeon, Dean, and Professor, Department of Neurosurgery, University of Natal Medical School, Durban; Consultant Neurosurgeon, Wentworth Hospital, Durban, Natal, South Africa
57A. Trauma of the Nervous System: Craniocerebral Trauma; 57B. Trauma of the Nervous System: Spinal Cord Trauma

Ashok Verma, M.D., D.M.
Instructor, Department of Neurology, University of Miami School of Medicine, Miami, Florida
65C. Effect of Toxins and Physical Agents on the Nervous System: Neurotoxins of Animals and Plants; 65E. Effect of Toxins and Physical Agents on the Nervous System: Effects of Physical Agents on the Nervous System

Joseph J. Volpe, M.D.
Bronson Crothers Professor of Neurology, Harvard Medical School, Boston; Neurologist-in-Chief, Department of Neurology, Children's Hospital, Boston
85. Neurological Problems of the Newborn

Steven L. Wald, M.D.
Associate Professor, Department of Neurosurgery, University of Vermont College of Medicine, Burlington; Associate Professor, Department of Neurosurgery, Medical Center Hospital of Vermont, Burlington
66. Disorders of Cerebrospinal Fluid Circulation and Brain Edema

Michael Wall, M.D.
Associate Professor, Departments of Neurology and Ophthalmology, University of Iowa College of Medicine, Iowa City; Attending Physician, Department of Neurology, University of Iowa Hospitals and Clinics and Veterans Affairs Medical Center, Iowa City
23. Brain Stem Syndromes

Melissa A. Waller, M.S.
Clinical Audiologist, Department of Otolaryngology, University of Texas Southwestern Medical Center at Dallas, Dallas
19. Hearing Loss and Tinnitus Without Dizziness or Vertigo; 44. Neuro-Otology

Elizabeth K. Warrington, D.Sc, F.R.S.
Institute of Neurology, London; Head of Neuropsychology,

National Hospital for Neurology and Neurosurgery, London, England
41. Neuropsychology

Stephen G. Waxman, M.D., Ph.D.
Professor and Chairman, Department of Neurology, Yale University School of Medicine, New Haven; Neurologist and Chief, Department of Neurology, Yale-New Haven Hospital, New Haven, Connecticut
28. Paraplegia and Spinal Cord Syndromes; 32. Sensory Abnormalities of the Limbs and Trunk

Thomas Weber, M.D.
Associate Professor of Neurology, University Hospital, Lower Saxony (Niedersachsen); Consultant Neurologist, University Hospital, Lower Saxony, Germany
60E. Infections of the Nervous System: Central Nervous System Diseases Caused by Unconventional Transmissible Agents and Chronic Viral Infections

Barbara Weissman, M.D.
Associate Professor, Department of Pediatrics (Neurology), Emory University School of Medicine, Atlanta; Medical Director, Department of Rehabilitation Services, Egleston Children's Hospital at Emory University, Atlanta, Georgia
42. Neuro-Ophthalmology

Charles Wood, Ph.D.
Associate Professor of Neurology, University of Miami School of Medicine, Miami, Florida
49. Neurovirology

Richard S. K. Young, M.D., M.P.H.
Associate Clinical Professor of Pediatrics and Neurology, Yale University School of Medicine, New Haven; Chair, Department of Pediatrics, Hospital of St. Raphael, New Haven, Connecticut
58E. Vascular Diseases of the Nervous System: Stroke in Childhood

Donald P. Younkin, M.D.
Associate Professor, Departments of Neurology and Pediatrics, University of Pennsylvania School of Medicine, Philadelphia; Senior Physician, Department of Pediatrics, Children's Hospital of Philadelphia, Philadelphia
56B. Neurological Complications of Systemic Disease: In Children

Preface to the Second Edition

In the five years since we published the first edition of *Neurology in Clinical Practice*, it has become established as one of the most frequently read textbooks of neurology. We have been gratified by the favorable reviews of the first edition, by its being chosen as the Most Outstanding Book published in 1991 by the Professional and Scholarly Publishing Division of the Association of American Publishers, and by the response of our readers.

The Congress of the United States of America declaration of the 1990s as the Decade of the Brain has been endorsed by the World Federation of Neurology and many major national neurological societies. The rapid expansion of knowledge in the basic and clinical neurosciences more than justifies this declaration. The new knowledge and techniques that have appeared since the publication of the first edition in 1991 necessitates the updating of the vast amount of information in this book.

The preparation for the second edition prompted a complete review of the material included in the first edition. To this end, we invited one external authority and one of the other contributors to examine critically each chapter in the first edition. We are grateful to all who took part in this exercise for their helpful suggestions. We provided these comments, along with our own, to the authors, who completely revised every chapter. Many chapters have been completely rewritten. We added a number of new authors, whose expertise broadens and strengthens the book. We introduced a number of new chapters that enhance the coverage in such areas as clinical diagnosis, pediatric neurology, neuroimaging, molecular neurogenetics, and the effects of toxic and physical agents on the nervous system. We rearranged the chapters to improve the logical progression of development of knowledge for those who read the book from beginning to end. We have simplified the organization into three main sections: Part I, The Approach to Common Neurological Problems, which is the clinical guide to diagnosis; Part II, The Neurological Investigations and Related Clinical Neurosciences, which provides a practical review of the subspecialty disciplines the practicing neurologist needs to understand; and Part III, The Neurological Diseases.

Although this second edition has been completely revised, the basic structure remains unchanged. Our goal remains to provide the reader with a multidimensional learning and teaching tool. In this book, neurological knowledge can be approached from the perspectives of the clinical history and signs, from disease categories, and from the subspecialty disciplines and investigational methodologies. We believe that the successful acquisition of knowledge requires multiple presentations. The success of the first edition and the comments of students and peers have reinforced our belief in the soundness of this goal.

In preparing the second edition, we imposed strict guidelines concerning references on our contributors. If we had encouraged complete referencing of the text, the size would have been significantly increased. We also believe that it is difficult to read text broken by multiple references. We have tried to limit these references to publications since 1988, and to no more than two per page. These references are primarily to provide a recent publication on each topic, through which the reader can access key material and the earlier literature. Hence, they may not be the most influential original publications. This limitation of the number of references allows more space for text and, as editors, we take responsibility for these guidelines.

The second edition would not have been possible without the selfless work of many people. We particularly want to thank our many authors for their forbearance at the demands we put upon them, and for their superb contributions. This second edition is a tribute to the innovation and continuing support provided by Susan Pioli, the Director of Medical Publishing of Butterworth-Heinemann. Karen Oberheim, Associate Editor, has worked hard and long on the manuscript and ensured a consistent standard throughout the production. We could not have even attempted the second edition without the help of our hard-working and ever efficient administrative assistants and secretaries, Janice Setney, Donna Pesch, Nelda Tilley, and Beth Howell-Hughes.

Walter G. Bradley
Robert B. Daroff
Gerald M. Fenichel
C. David Marsden

Part I

Approach to Common Neurological Problems

Chapter 1
Approach to the Diagnosis of Neurological Disease

Walter G. Bradley, Robert B. Daroff, Gerald M. Fenichel, and C. David Marsden

Neurologists should take no satisfaction in stumbling on a diagnosis by having ordered a diagnostic test. A considerable menu of laboratory tests has become available in the last two decades. They are a powerful aid to diagnosis and when properly used serve as an extension of a careful history and examination. But when diagnostic tests are substituted for clinical judgment, the results are often misleading and we may end up treating abnormal laboratory values instead of patient complaints. This rush to embrace technology at the expense of doctor-patient interactions needlessly increases the cost of medical care and at the same time degrades its quality.

The patient's history is the key to determining the nature of the disease process, and the neurological examination is required to determine its localization. The two are sometimes interwoven, as when the patient's responses indicate a disturbance of speech or thought, or when the patient's appearance is diagnostic, as in some movement disorders and some mental retardation syndromes. Neither history nor examination is useful unless the neurologist first has a firm understanding of the anatomy, development, physiology, and biochemistry of the nervous system.

Drawing on our knowledge of neurological disease, we use the history and physical examination to develop a list of diseases that could be responsible for the symptoms and signs (Figure 1.1). This chapter reviews each part of the diagnostic process and highlights how that process must be modified when dealing with children and incompetent patients.

THE HISTORY

The classic advice is to begin by asking the patient's chief complaint, but perhaps before that, it is advisable to start a new patient encounter by having patients define why they have come. "How can I help you?" is a productive opening statement that defines the relationship and allows patients to express their expectations for the consultation. Patients are often surprised to learn that the doctor is there to provide a service; they may pause before answering. Many consultations are requested to prove that something is *not* present (the headache is not caused by brain tumor), or because a form needs to be filled out to do or not do some activity, or because other doctors "never tell me anything" (which sometimes means that the patient does not listen).

After determining the patient's expectation, the interview portion of the consultation begins. It consists of recording the patient's chief complaint, history of present illness, developmental milestones (in children), review of systems, history of other illnesses, personal profile, and family history. At the end of the history-taking, the physician should have analyzed the features of the patient's description that are most relevant, synthesized them into the possible anatomical localization of the lesion or the neuronal systems involved, and reached a preliminary conclusion about the mechanism of disease. These working hypotheses may need revision based on the neurological examination and laboratory investigations, but conceptualizing the disease process on the basis of the history is necessary to focus the examination. A diagnosis is unlikely to be achieved if the neurologist has not formulated a working hypothesis before commencing the neurological examination.

Personal Profile

Some neurologists like to begin collecting information about the patient's personal profile at the beginning of the interview. What are the patient's age, handedness, and occupation? Usually more information is needed, and it is common to have to return to an earlier line of questioning later in the consultation after earning the patient's confidence. Is the patient or other person giving the history reli-

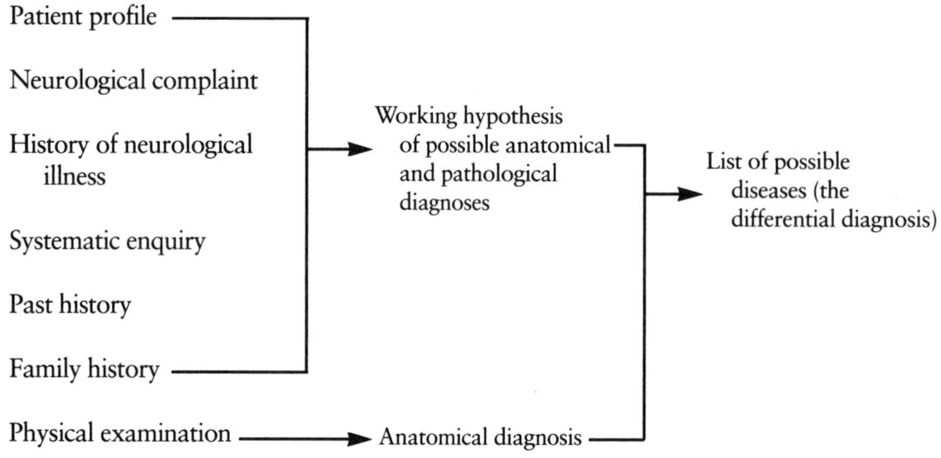

FIGURE 1.1 The approach to the neurological diagnosis.

able? Reliability depends on intelligence, memory, language function, educational and social status, and secondary gain from symptoms. What are the patient's occupation and environment? Exposure to toxins may occur not only in the workplace but in the home and by the use of alcohol, tobacco, and substances of abuse. Is there excessive stress at home, in school, or in the workplace? Abuse and neglect of children and spouses are worst cases, but divorce, loss of job, and loss of a loved one cause symptoms in children and adults. Is the patient homosexual, heterosexual, or bisexual? Sexual preference cannot be ignored at a time when sexually transmitted diseases are reaching epidemic proportions throughout the world. Children and adolescents must be questioned separately from their parents to learn about sexual activity and substance abuse.

Chief Complaint

The chief complaint is the starting point of the diagnostic thought process. An example might be the triad of headaches, dizziness, and double vision. Words used to define symptoms may have very different meanings for physicians and patients, and sometimes even among physicians. Therefore the complaints must not be accepted at face value. They serve to focus the neurologist's attention on the questions that need to be addressed during the history of present illness and provide the first clues to diagnosis and localization.

History of Present Illness

The tradition that patients should be allowed to describe their symptoms in their own words is valid up to a point. Some guidance is always needed. One should quickly assess the competence of the patient or caregiver to provide a history and be prepared to direct the discussion. Information from an observer other than the patient is helpful to diagnose many neurological conditions, such as seizure and dementia. Directed questioning must be balanced against the risk of having the patient answer "yes" to every question. One should suspect a somatiform disorder in any patient who claims to have every symptom. History-taking from children is further complicated by shyness with strangers, a different sense of time, and a restricted vocabulary; hence the history is almost always the composite perception of the child and the parent. Patients and physicians may use the same word to refer to different things, and the exact meaning of a word used to describe a symptom must be ascertained. For instance, patients often describe a limb as being "numb" or "stiff" when it is actually weak or paralyzed. "Dizziness" and "tiredness" are sometimes used to refer to generalized weakness. A patient may describe vision as "blurred" when further questioning reveals diplopia. "Blackouts" may be loss of consciousness, loss of vision, or simply a sense of detachment. "Pounding" headaches may not necessarily be pulsating.

Temporal sequence, clustering of symptoms, and severity of illness are critical elements of the history leading to the diagnosis. The physician must understand fully the onset, duration, and periodicity of each symptom, and the temporal relationship of one symptom to another. Are symptoms getting better, staying the same, or getting worse? What relieves them and what makes them worse? In infants and young children, temporal sequence also includes the timing of developmental milestones; failure to achieve is as important as loss of achievement.

An example will make clear how the history can make the diagnosis. A 28-year-old woman with a 10-year history of recurrent headaches associated with her menses is likely to have migraine. The unilaterality of pain in some attacks, and the association with flashing lights in front of the eyes, nausea, and vomiting confirm the diagnosis.

Clustering of symptoms is expected in most disease states. Both the absence of expected features and the presence of unexpected features direct attention to or away from the consideration of a specific diagnosis. Backache and loss of sphincter control are unlikely to be seen in a peripheral neuropathy but instead suggest a spinal cord or cauda equina lesion.

It has become customary for patients to arrive for neurological consultation with neuroimaging studies and a folder of prior laboratory tests in hand. Patients often dwell on these tests and their interpretation by other physicians. Obviously, these test results and opinions were not fully satisfying or further opinions would not be needed. Be wary of previous test results and opinions. They are part of the history of present illness and can be useful in formulating the differential diagnosis, but the shrewd neurologist avoids accepting the previous diagnosis and makes a new formulation based on all of the features of the history, examination, and investigations.

One must take into account the patient's or caregiver's response to symptoms. The child who was not brought to the hospital despite hours of seizures is likely to be a victim of child abuse, or at least neglect. A nighttime visit to the emergency room for a new-onset headache should not be dismissed without investigation.

Review of Systems

The review of systems should also include a complete overview of nervous system function that did not surface in the history of present illness. At a minimum, the physician should inquire about the following: cognition, personality change, seizures and other impairments of consciousness, headaches, special senses, speech and language function, swallowing, coordination and strength, gait, sensation, pain, and sphincter control.

A positive finding may help clarify a diagnosis. For instance, admission of unilateral deafness in a patient complaining of ataxia and hemiparesis may suggest an acoustic neuroma, while the occurrence of headaches in a patient with paraparesis leads to the consideration of a parasagittal meningioma rather than a spinal cord lesion. Developmental history must be assessed for children and may also be of value in adults whose illness may have started during childhood, especially with some slowly progressive neuromuscular disorders.

The review should include other organs. Neurological function is adversely affected by dysfunction of liver, kidney, gastrointestinal tract, and heart, among others. Several neurological diseases are characterized by multiorgan involvement, such as mitochondrial disorders and storage diseases.

History of Previous Illnesses

The relevance of items in the patient's prior medical and surgical history to the present complaint may not be immediately apparent. However, all such items must be considered to determine if a single diagnosis can account for past and present symptoms. For instance, previous seizures in a patient complaining of worsening headaches suggest a brain tumor. Chronic low-back pain in a patient complaining of exertional pain and weakness in the legs suggests lumbar canal stenosis. The record should include dates and details of all surgical procedures, significant injuries including head trauma and fractures, hospitalizations, and conditions requiring medical consultation and medications. For pediatric patients, information concerning the pregnancy and delivery should be recorded.

Some features in the history should always alert the physician to the possibility of neurological complications. Gastric surgery may lead to vitamin B_{12} deficiency. Sarcoidosis may cause Bell's palsy, diabetes insipidus, ophthalmoplegia, and peripheral neuropathy. Disorders of the liver, kidney, and small bowel can be associated with a wide variety of neurological disorders. Systemic malignancy or its treatment can cause direct and indirect (paraneoplastic) neurological problems. A patient's memory of past medical events may be surprisingly poor. An abdominal scar may be found on a patient who has only minutes before denied any past surgical procedures.

Medications are often the cause of neurological disturbances. Lithium carbonate can be toxic to neurons in the brain stem and cerebellum. Neuroleptics produce a myriad of movement disorders. Unfortunately, most patients do not think of substances such as vitamins, oral contraceptives, nonprescription analgesics, and herbal compounds as medications. Specific questions are often needed to compile a complete list of medications.

Family History

Many neurological disorders are hereditary, and a history of consanguinity or of similar disease in family members is of diagnostic importance. However, the expression of a gene abnormality may be quite different in other family members, with respect not only to the severity of neurological dysfunction but to organ system involvement. Myotonic dystrophy exemplifies both points. Because of DNA amplification, gene expression may become increasingly severe in each successive generation. The first generation may have only cataracts and the second only mild muscle weakness, but the third may be a child who is profoundly weak at birth, requiring ventilatory support. Similarly, Charcot-Marie-Tooth's disease may be suggested in a patient with a peripheral neuropathy who has relatives with pes cavus.

Some conditions, such as epilepsy, may still be considered "family secrets." Parents may not know that they or their siblings had seizures during infancy. Therefore, one should be cautious in accepting a patient's assertion that there is no family history of a similar disorder. Where possible, it is helpful to obtain information from parents and grandparents and to examine as many as possible of the relatives at risk. Minimum data should include age (currently or at death), cause of death, and any significant neurological or systemic diseases.

THE EXAMINATION

Neurological Examination

Detailed descriptions of the neurological examination may be found in several excellent texts (see references) and are not presented here. The *complete neurological examination* in which every muscle, sensory modality, and reflex is tested is a theoretical exercise and never performed. Nevertheless, the medical student and resident need to learn every aspect of the neurological examination to have it available when needed. The primary purpose of the neurological examination is to reveal functional disturbances that localize abnormalities. It is less effective when used to monitor the course of a disease or its temporal response to treatment. Measuring change over time often requires special quantitative tests and scoring systems.

A *focused examination* is one that is concentrated to confirm, refute, or alter the initial hypotheses of disease causation derived from the history. Both the presence and absence of abnormalities are diagnostically relevant. For instance, if a patient's symptoms suggest right cerebral hemisphere dysfunction, the examiner searches carefully for a hemianopia and for evidence that the blink or smile is slowed on the left side of the face, that rapid repetitive movements are impaired in the left limbs, that the tendon reflexes are brisker on the left than the right, that the left abdominal reflexes are depressed, and that the left plantar response is extensor. Along with testing the primary modalities of sensation on the left side, the examination should include the higher integrative aspects of sensation, such as graphesthesia, stereognosis, and sensory extinction with double simultaneous stimuli.

When the history does not permit a focused examination, as in a patient whose only symptom is headache or fatigue, a *screening examination* is conducted (Table 1.1). Here the emphasis is on functional testing of the limbs and gait and the examination of cranial nerves, mental status, and tendon reflexes. Highly coordinated activities are tested first; if these are performed well, component functions are assumed to be normal. The patient who can walk heel to toe (tandem gait) with eyes closed does not have a disturbance of the cerebellum, the spinal cord, or the peripheral nerves. Similarly, the patient who can do a pushup, rise from the floor without using the hands, and walk on toes and heels has normal limb strength.

The screening examination may miss unexpected neurological abnormalities. For instance, a bitemporal field defect may not be detected when the visual fields are tested simultaneously rather than separately. Similarly, a parietal lobe syndrome may not be uncovered unless visuospatial function is assessed.

It is sometimes difficult to decide whether a physical finding is normal or abnormal, and only experience prevents physicians from mistaking normal variation as supposed disease. Every person has some degree of facial and limb asymmetry, and what is normal at one age is not normal at another. Children cannot detect the distal stimuli when the hand and face are simultaneously touched on the same side of the body until they are 7 years old. Loss of the Achilles reflex and of vibration sense at the big toes are common findings after 60 years of age.

Table 1.1: Outline of the screening neurological examination

Mental status: Partially assessed while recording the history
Cranial nerves:
I: Not tested
II: Gross visual acuity each eye:
Visual fields by confrontation, including double simultaneous stimuli
Funduscopy
III, IV, VI: Lateral and vertical eye movements
Pupillary response to light
V: Pinprick sensation on face
VII: Close eyes, show teeth
VIII: Whispered voice each ear
IX, X: Palate lifts in midline, gag reflex present
XI: Shrug shoulders
XII: Protrude tongue
Each limb separately:
Tone
Power of main muscle groups
Coordination, finger to nose and heel to shin
Tendon reflexes
Plantar responses
Pinprick and light touch on hands and feet
Double simultaneous stimuli on hands and feet
Joint position sense in hallux and index finger
Vibration sense at ankle and wrist
Gait
Romberg's test

The normal range of neurological function in different individuals must also be understood. The beginner frequently records mild impairment of a number of different functions, such as deviation of the tongue to one side, impaired triceps reflexes, and inconstant sensory abnormalities. Such *soft signs* are suspicious but not diagnostic unless they are consistent with other parts of the history and examination. On the other hand, subtle neurological signs can sometimes be sufficient for the expert to confirm the diagnosis.

If an abnormality is identified, all associated functions should be examined, since some aspects of the neurological examination may be misleading. For instance, a hemiparetic or deafferented limb may appear ataxic. Thus, a patient with ataxia on finger-to-nose testing should be examined for abnormal rapid alternating movements (dysdiadochokinesis), ataxia of the lower limbs and gait, nystagmus, and ocular dysmetria, as well as for joint position sense, strength, and reflexes.

At the end of the neurological examination, the abnormal physical signs should be classified as definitely abnormal (*hard signs*) or mildly or equivocally abnormal (*soft signs*). The hard signs, when combined with symptoms from the history, provide the basis for a hypothesis about the anatomical site of the lesion or the neurological systems involved

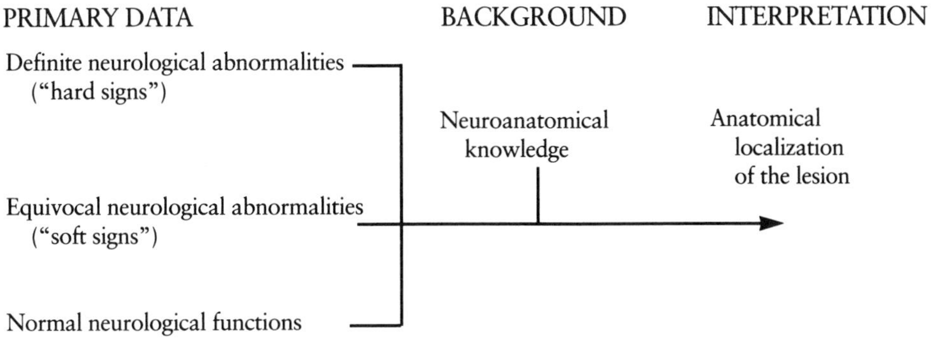

FIGURE 1.2 Logical pathway for the identification of the anatomical location of the neurological lesion.

(Figure 1.2). The soft signs can then be reviewed to determine if they conflict with or support the initial conclusion.

General Physical Examination

A focused general physical examination of other body systems is needed in most patients. Some diseases affect the brain as well as other organs, such as mitochondrial disorders and storage diseases. Moreover, systemic diseases may have adverse affects on the nervous system. Valvular heart disease or an atrial septal defect may cause embolic infarction of the nervous system. Hypertension increases the risk for all types of stroke. Signs of malignancy raise the possibility of metastatic lesions of the nervous system or paraneoplastic syndromes such as cerebellar degeneration or progressive multifocal leukoencephalopathy.

The Differential Diagnosis

After completing the examination, the neurologist must analyze all the information gleaned from the history and examination and must synthesize this into a unified hypothesis that will explain the anatomical localization or the neuronal systems involved, and hence the pathophysiology of the disorder. The list of diseases that may be responsible for a patient's symptoms and signs is termed the *differential diagnosis*. Such a list, by necessity, can only contain one correct diagnosis, with several incorrect diagnoses. It is cost-effective to prioritize the list to reduce the time spent on the incorrect diagnoses. Prioritization requires knowledge of neurological diseases, the parts of the nervous system affected by each disease, the types of clinical presentation, and the relative frequency of each disease.

Anatomical Localization

Experience proves that attempts at anatomical localization should precede determination of cause. The initial question is whether the disease is located in the brain, spinal cord, peripheral nerves, or muscles. Then, is the disease focal or multifocal? A few examples will clarify this point.

A patient complaining of tingling and numbness in the limbs might be thought to have a peripheral neuropathy. However, if examination shows hyperreflexia, nystagmus, and optic atrophy, the disease is clearly localized to the central nervous system, and the many causes of peripheral neuropathy can be dropped from consideration. Another example would be a patient with weakness of the left arm and leg. Many intracranial diseases, such as stroke or tumor, can cause hemiparesis. However, if the neurological examination shows abnormal signs only below the neck and no involvement of the cranial nerves, then the cervical spinal cord is the likely site of the lesion. Probable causes include spinal cord tumor, cervical spondylotic myelopathy, and multiple sclerosis.

The first step in arriving at the anatomical localization is to translate the patient's symptoms and signs into abnormalities of a nucleus, tract, or system. For instance, loss of pain and temperature sensation on one half of the body excluding the face indicates a lesion of the contralateral spinothalamic tract in the high cervical region. A left sixth nerve palsy, with weakness of left face and right limbs, right-sided hyperreflexia, and an extensor right plantar response point to a left pontomedullary lesion. A left homonymous hemianopia indicates a lesion in the right optic tract, optic radiations, or occipital cortex.

After determining anatomical localization, the next step is to decide if dysfunction involving different neurological systems could all arise from one focal lesion. The principle of parsimony, or Occam's razor, should be applied. The differential diagnosis will be quite different if all the neurological defects can be explained by a single focal lesion rather than by two or more lesions. Thus, a patient complaining of loss of vision to the left and left-sided weakness affecting the limbs and face is likely to have a lesion in the right cerebral hemisphere, possibly caused by stroke or tumor. On the other hand, if the visual difficulty is due to a central scotoma in the left eye and the weakness affects the left limbs but spares the face, then there must be two lesions, one in the left optic nerve and one in the left corticospinal tract below the medulla; multiple sclerosis is the likely diagnosis.

The synthesis of symptoms and signs into the anatomical localization of a lesion requires a working knowledge of neuroanatomy, including the location of all major tracts in the nervous system and their interrelationships at different levels. It is particularly helpful to have diagrams available that show transverse sections of the spinal cord, medulla, pons, and midbrain, the brachial and lumbosacral plexuses, the dermatomes, and myotomes. Knowledge of the functional anatomy of the cerebral cortex and the blood supply of the brain and spinal cord is also essential. Even the expert may find it useful to make an anatomical drawing showing the suspected location to determine whether a single lesion can explain all of the clinical features.

Symptoms and signs may arise not only from disturbances caused at the focus of an abnormality but also at a distance. An example is the injury resulting from shifting of intracranial contents due to an expanding tumor, producing a third or sixth nerve palsy. Clinical features caused by damage away from the primary site of abnormality are called *false localizing signs*. The term derives from an era when clinical examination was the major means of lesion localization for neurosurgery. In fact, they are not "false" but alert the clinician to the full extent of disease.

The principle of parsimony requires that a single locus be sought to explain a patient's symptoms and signs. However, if several levels of the nervous system are considered possible sites for the lesion, each should be investigated for evidence of damage. The complex vascular anatomy of the brain can often explain multifocal lesions. For instance, a patient with a midbrain lesion, a hemianopia, and an amnesic syndrome may have suffered a thrombosis or embolism of the basilar and posterior cerebral arteries. Lesions that cannot be explained by a single anatomical site or blood supply suggest disorders such as multiple sclerosis, multiple metastases, or embolic infarctions.

Pathology and Etiology

Once the likely site of disease is identified, the cause of the lesion must be determined. Occasionally, only a single disease can be incriminated, but more commonly there are several candidates in the differential diagnosis. The list of possibilities should take into account both the temporal features of the patient's symptoms and the pathological processes known to affect the relevant area of the nervous system. For example, in a patient with signs indicating a lesion of the internal capsule, the cause is likely to be stroke if the hemiplegia had a sudden onset, whereas progression over weeks or months suggests an expanding tumor. Another example is a patient with signs of multifocal lesions. If symptoms have relapsed and remitted over several years, the diagnosis is likely to be multiple sclerosis or multiple strokes; if symptoms have appeared recently and progressed, then multiple metastases should be considered.

Usually, the patient's history and the site of the lesion suggest a pathological process that can be caused by several diseases. Thus, a clinical diagnosis of intracranial neoplasm generates a list of the types of tumors that can affect the brain. Similarly, hemorrhage, infarction, vascular spasm, embolism, and thrombosis may underlie the clinical diagnosis of a stroke. The physician should begin the list of diagnostic possibilities with the most likely and end with rare entities, remembering that unusual presentations of common diseases are more frequent than common presentations of rare diseases.

Again, the principle of parsimony should be applied when constructing the differential diagnostic list. Consider a patient with a 3-week history of a progressive spinal cord lesion who suddenly becomes dysphasic. Perhaps he had a tumor compressing the spinal cord and has fortuitously developed a small stroke, but parsimony would suggest a single disease, probably cancer with multiple metastases. Another example is a patient with progressive atrophy of the small muscles of the hands for 6 months prior to the appearance of a pseudobulbar palsy. She could have bilateral ulnar nerve lesions and recent bilateral strokes, but amyotrophic lateral sclerosis is more likely.

The skilled diagnostician is justly proud of placing the correct diagnosis at the top of the list, but if a disease is not considered, it is unlikely to be diagnosed. Treatable diseases, even those with low probability, should always be considered, especially when they mimic more common incurable neurological disorders such as Alzheimer's disease or amyotrophic lateral sclerosis.

When the differential diagnostic list is complete, the beginner should read more about each disease to determine if the list needs revision. The differential diagnosis determines the investigations needed to establish the final diagnosis.

LABORATORY INVESTIGATIONS

Laboratory tests should be ordered with a clear objective in mind and with thought to the cost-benefit and risk-benefit ratios. "Routine investigations" are not justified. A complete blood count, blood urea nitrogen, and electrolytes are appropriate in a patient admitted with an acute stroke because there may be hematological and metabolic complications; such studies, however, would not be warranted in a patient with migraine or Bell's palsy.

Some investigations, notably myelography, angiography, and electromyography, are painful and potentially risky. The physician should carefully weigh the risks and potential benefits before recommending the test, and must explain the risk-benefit analysis to the patient.

Another problem with ordering unjustified tests is that they sometimes turn up a seemingly abnormal result that distracts attention from the correct diagnosis. The finding might actually be a laboratory error, or the result of an inconsequential intercurrent condition, or simply an instance of the occasional normal value that falls outside the laboratory's definition of the normal range. Avoiding unnecessary tests is considered more fully in Chapter 36.

The first tests to order are those that are least invasive and yield the most information. One should begin with hematological and biochemical blood studies, then proceed when necessary to neuroimaging (Chapter 39) and neurophysiological testing (Chapter 37), before considering organ biopsy to obtain pathological, bacteriological, or virological confirmation. Thus, discovering macrocytosis on the blood count and a low vitamin B_{12} level in the blood will spare a patient with subacute combined degeneration of the spinal cord from undergoing extensive imaging tests for a myelopathy.

The neurologist requesting a neurophysiological, neuroimaging, or neuropathological study must provide the laboratory specialist with complete clinical details to allow accurate evaluation of the results. Still, the clinician has the best knowledge of the likely location and cause of a lesion and should not rely solely on the report of someone who has not examined the patient, unless the interpretation is clear. For instance, the neuroradiologist might interpret a computed tomography (CT) scan in the first 2 days of a presumed left middle cerebral artery infarction as normal. Review by the neurologist may show slight obliteration of the sulci and reduced density of part of the left cerebral hemisphere sufficient to support the clinical diagnosis.

THE FINAL DIAGNOSIS

The test results may establish a final diagnosis and allow the cause, prognosis, treatment, and management of the disorder to be discussed fully with the patient (Figure 1.3).

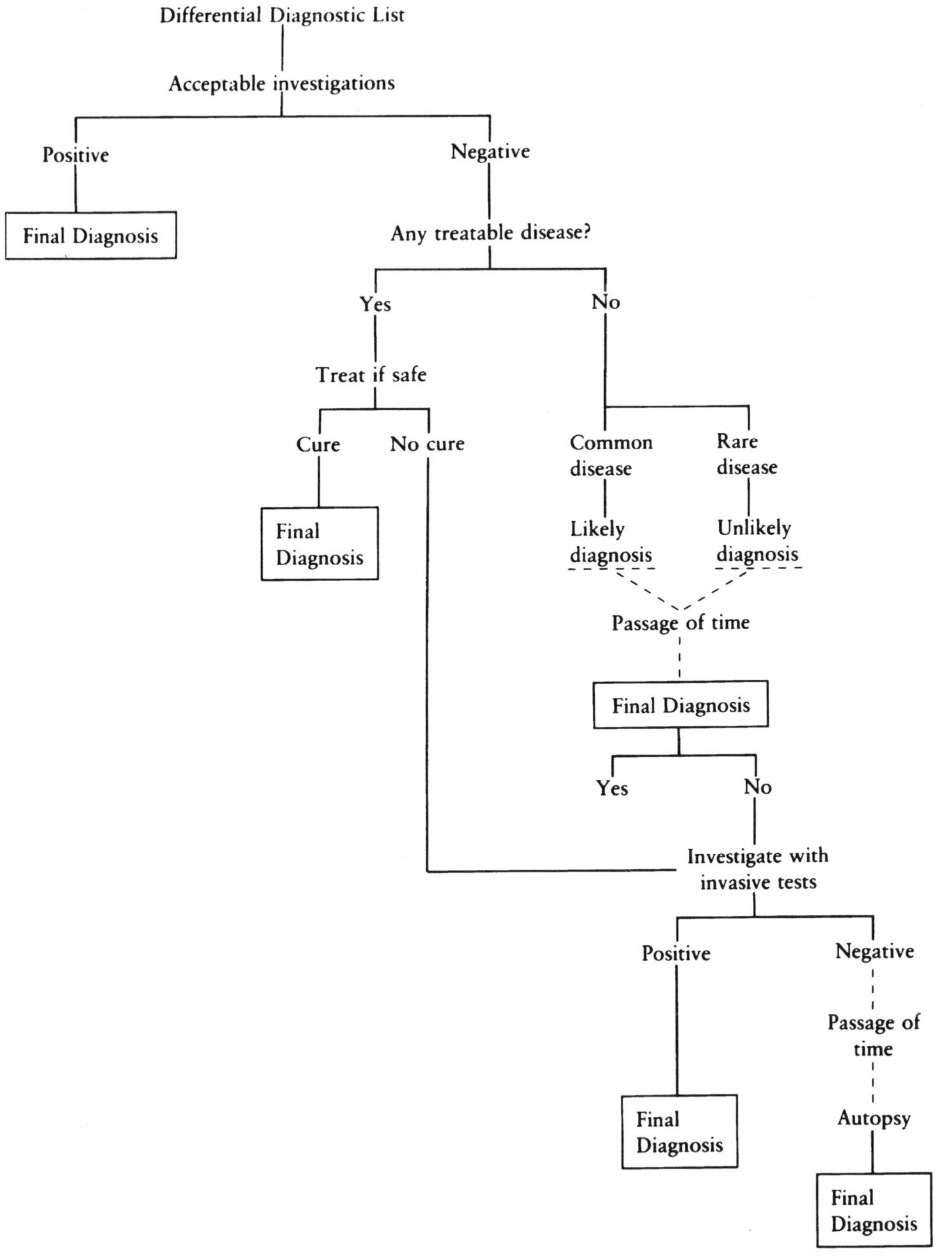

FIGURE 1.3 Diagnostic pathway from the differential diagnostic list to the final diagnosis.

Occasionally, however, the results are inconclusive or the definitive investigation, such as a brain biopsy, may not be justified. Management in this situation is difficult, and the matter must be fully discussed with the patient and relatives. These issues are considered in Chapter 51.

In some cases, the differential diagnosis includes one disorder that is treatable and others for which there is no known therapy. If the therapy is not hazardous, a therapeutic trial is justified to see if the patient improves. Thus, a patient with known human immunodeficiency virus infection whose CT scan shows multiple enhancing lesions in the cerebral hemispheres may have multiple tumors, toxoplasmosis, or bacterial abscesses. A reasonable approach is to give therapy against toxoplasmosis for 2–3 weeks to see if the symptoms and CT changes resolve before considering surgical exploration for an abscess or multiple tumors such as lymphomas. In other cases, the passage of time and serial evaluations may eventually reveal the nature of the underlying disease.

THE EXPERIENCED NEUROLOGIST'S APPROACH TO COMMON NEUROLOGICAL PROBLEMS

The skills of a good neurologist must be learned. Seeing many cases of a disease teaches which symptoms and signs should be present, and, just as important, which should not. Although there is no substitute for experience, the trainee can be acquainted with many of the clues used by the seasoned practitioner to achieve the diagnosis. Part I of this book covers most of the usual symptoms and signs of neurological disease. Each chapter in Part I describes how an experienced neurologist approaches a particular presenting feature in a patient, such as a movement disorder, gait disturbance, or dizziness and vertigo. These accounts are replete with the clinical wisdom that should be valuable to the less-experienced physician.

REFERENCES

Bickerstaff ER. Neurological Examination in Clinical Practice (4th ed). Oxford, England: Blackwell, 1980.

DeJong RN. The Neurological Examination (5th ed). New York: Harper & Row, 1992.

Fenichel GM. The neurological examination of the newborn. Brain Develop 1993;15:403–410.

Mayo Clinic. Clinical Examination in Neurology (5th ed). Philadelphia: Saunders, 1981.

Munsat TL. Quantification of Neurologic Deficits. Boston: Butterworth, 1989.

Paine RS, Oppe TE. Neurological Examination of Children (2nd ed). London: Heinemann, 1971.

Plum F, Posner JB. The Diagnosis of Stupor and Coma (3rd ed). Philadelphia: FA Davis, 1980.

Spillane JD, Spillane JA. An Atlas of Clinical Neurology (3rd ed). Oxford, England: Oxford University Press, 1982.

Swaiman KF. Pediatric Neurology: Principles and Practices (2nd ed). St. Louis: Mosby, 1994.

Van Allen MW, Rodnitsky RL. Pictorial Manual of Neurologic Tests (2nd ed). Chicago: Year Book, 1984.

Chapter 2
Episodic Impairment of Consciousness

Joseph Bruni

Temporary loss of consciousness may be related to impaired cerebral perfusion (syncope, fainting), cerebral ischemia due to cerebrovascular disease or migraine, epileptic seizures, metabolic disturbances, sudden increases in intracranial pressure, or sleep disorders. Anxiety attacks, psychogenic seizures, and malingering may be difficult to distinguish diagnostically from these conditions; at times, the diagnosis may not be obvious until detailed laboratory examinations and prolonged periods of observation have been carried out.

Syncope may result from diseases that interfere with cardiac output. A reduced cardiac output may be related to cardiac arrhythmias, outflow obstruction, hypovolemia, orthostatic hypotension, or decreased venous return. Cerebrovascular disturbances from either transient ischemic attacks of the posterior or anterior cerebral circulations or cerebral vasospasm from migraine, subarachnoid hemorrhage, or hypertensive encephalopathy may result in temporary loss of consciousness. Metabolic disturbances due to hypoxia, anemia, and hypoglycemia may result in frank syncope or, more frequently, may present with the sensation of an impending faint.

Generalized absence seizures, tonic-clonic seizures, and complex partial seizures are associated with alterations of consciousness and in most cases can be easily distinguished from syncope. Epileptic seizures may be more difficult to distinguish from pseudoseizures (psychogenic seizures) and malingering. In children, breath-holding spells may cause transient alteration of consciousness and have to be distinguished from epileptic seizures.

Although sudden increases of intracranial pressure, which may result from intermittent hydrocephalus, severe head trauma, brain tumors, intracerebral hemorrhage, and Reye's syndrome, may produce sudden loss of consciousness, these patients frequently have other neurological symptoms that lead one to suspect this diagnosis.

In patients with episodic impairment of consciousness, a diagnosis relies heavily on the clinical history as described by the patient and observers. Laboratory investigations, however, may provide useful information that frequently aids in the diagnosis. In a small number of patients, a cause for the loss of consciousness may not be established, and these patients may require longer periods of observation. Table 2.1 compares the clinical features of syncope and seizures.

SYNCOPE

The pathophysiological basis of syncope is the gradual failure of the cerebral circulation with a reduction in cerebral oxygen utilization. *Syncope* refers to a symptom complex characterized by lightheadedness, generalized muscle weakness, giddiness, visual blurring, tinnitus, and gastrointestinal symptoms. The patient may appear pale or ashen in color and may feel cold and sweaty. The onset of loss of consciousness is generally gradual but may be rapid if re-

Table 2.1: Comparison of clinical features of syncope and seizures

Features	*Syncope*	*Seizure*
Relation to posture	Common	No
Time of day	Diurnal	Diurnal or nocturnal
Skin color	Pallor	Cyanosis or normal
Aura or premonitory symptoms	Long	Brief
Convulsion	Rare	Common
Injury	Rare	Common (with convulsive seizures)
Urinary incontinence	Rare	Common
Postictal confusion	Rare	Common
Postictal headache	No	Common
Focal neurological signs	No	Occasional
Cardiovascular signs	Common (cardiac syncope)	No
Abnormal electroencephalogram	Rare	Common

lated to certain conditions, such as a cardiac arrhythmia. The gradual onset may allow the patient to protect himself or herself against falling and injury. A simple faint is usually precipitated by emotional upset, unpleasant visual stimuli, prolonged standing, or pain.

Although the duration of unconsciousness is brief, it may vary from seconds to minutes. During the faint, the patient may be motionless or display myoclonic jerks (Lempert et al. 1994). Urinary incontinence is rare. The pulse is weak and may be barely perceptible. Breathing may be shallow and the blood pressure barely obtainable. As the fainting episode corrects itself (for instance, by the patient becoming horizontal), the color returns, breathing becomes more regular, and the pulse and blood pressure return to normal. After the faint there is some residual weakness, but unlike in seizures, confusion, headaches, and drowsiness are uncommon sequelae. Nausea may be noted when the patient regains consciousness. Once it is established that the patient experienced a syncopal episode, a differential diagnosis has to be considered. Syncope is generally classified according to the pathophysiological mechanism involved. The final common pathway is cerebral hypoperfusion.

History and Physical Examination

The history and physical examination are the most important parts of the initial evaluation of syncope. There are significant age and sex differences in the incidence of the various types of syncope. Syncope occurring in children and young adults is most frequently due to hyperventilation or vasovagal attacks and less frequently due to congenital heart disease. Fainting associated with benign tachycardias without underlying organic heart disease may also appear in the younger age groups. Syncope due to basilar migraine is more commonly seen in young females. When repeated syncope begins in later life, organic disease of the cerebral circulation or cardiovascular system is most frequently responsible.

In establishing the cause of syncope, the most important step is a careful history. Frequently, the diagnosis can be made from the patient's description. The general features of the syncopal episode have been described above, and certain clues in the history may help establish the cause. The physician should always obtain as full a description as possible of the first faint. The clinical features should be established, with emphasis on the precipitating factors, the posture of the patient, the type of onset of the faint, whether it was abrupt or gradual, the position of the head and neck, the presence and duration of preceding and associated symptoms, the duration of the loss of consciousness, and the rate of recovery and sequelae. If possible, an observer should be questioned for observations on clonic movements, color changes, diaphoresis, pulse, respiration, urinary incontinence, and the nature of recovery.

Clues in the history that suggest cardiac syncope include a history of palpitations or a fluttering sensation in the chest prior to losing consciousness. These symptoms are common in arrhythmias. In vasodepressor syncope and orthostatic hypotension, preceding symptoms of lightheadedness may be common. Episodes of cardiac syncope are generally briefer than vasodepressor syncope, and the onset is usually rapid. Episodes due to cardiac arrhythmias occur independent of position, whereas in vasodepressor syncope and syncope due to orthostatic hypotension, the patient is usually standing.

Attacks of syncope precipitated by exertion suggest cardiac syncope. Exercise may induce arrhythmic syncope or syncope due to decreased cardiac output secondary to blood flow obstruction, such as may occur with aortic or subaortic stenosis. Syncope accentuated by exercise may also be due to cerebrovascular disease, aortic arch disease, congenital heart disease, pulseless disease (Takayasu's disease), pulmonary hypertension, anemia, hypoxia, and hypoglycemia. A family history of sudden cardiac death, especially in females, might suggest the long QT interval syndrome. Since many drugs can induce orthostatic hypotension or produce cardiac arrhythmias, a careful and complete medical and medication history is mandatory.

The neurologist should make a careful inquiry concerning the frequency of the attacks of loss of consciousness and the presence of cerebrovascular or cardiovascular symptoms between the repeated episodes. The patient should be questioned as to whether all the episodes are similar, since some patients experience more than one type of attack.

With an accurate description of the attacks and with familiarity with the clinical features of the various types of syncope, the physician should be able to correctly diagnose the majority of patients. Differential features distinguishing syncope from seizures and other alterations of consciousness are discussed later in this chapter.

After a complete history, the physical examination is of next importance. Examination during the episode is very informative but frequently impossible unless syncope can be reproduced by maneuvers such as carotid sinus massage or by reproducing the circumstances of the attack, such as by position change. The physical findings on examination can be considered significant only when they reproduce symptoms similar to the clinical features of the attack.

In the patient with suspected cardiac syncope, particular attention should be paid to the vital signs and determination of supine and erect blood pressure. Normally, with standing, the systolic blood pressure rises and the pulse rate may increase. An orthostatic drop in blood pressure of greater than 15 mm Hg may suggest autonomic dysfunction. Blood pressure should be assessed in both arms if cerebrovascular disease, subclavian steal, or Takayasu's arteritis is suspected.

During syncope due to a cardiac arrhythmia, a heart rate faster than 140 beats per minute usually indicates an ectopic cardiac rhythm, while a marked bradycardia of less than 40 beats per minute suggests complete atrioventricular block. A supraventricular tachycardia may be terminated abruptly by carotid sinus massage, while a ventricular tachycardia shows no response. Stokes-Adams attacks may be of longer duration and may be associated with audible atrial contraction and a variable first heart sound.

The patient should undergo cardiac auscultation and should be carefully evaluated for the presence of cardiac murmurs and abnormalities of the heart sounds. There may be the murmur of aortic stenosis, subaortic stenosis, or mitral valve disease. An intermittent posture-related murmur may be heard in the presence of an atrial myxoma. A systolic click in a young person suggests mitral valve prolapse. A pericardial rub suggests pericarditis.

All patients should undergo observation of the carotid pulse and auscultation of the neck. The degree of aortic stenosis may at times be reflected in a delayed carotid upstroke. Carotid, ophthalmic, and supraclavicular bruits suggest underlying cerebrovascular disease. Carotid artery massage is not without risk and should be carried out under electrocardiographic monitoring, with simultaneous monitoring of blood pressure to diagnose the vasodepressor type of response.

Causes of Syncope

Cardiac Arrhythmias

Both bradyarrhythmias and tachyarrhythmias may result in syncope, and abnormalities of cardiac rhythm due to dysfunction from the sinoatrial node to Purkinje's network may be involved. Arrhythmias are a common cause of syncope and must be considered in all cases in which an obvious mechanism is not known. Syncope due to cardiac arrhythmias generally occurs more quickly than syncope from other causes. Cardiac syncope may occur in any position, may occasionally be exercise-induced, and may occur in both congenital and acquired heart disease.

Although some patients experience palpitations during some arrhythmias, other patients are not aware of any cardiac symptoms. Syncopal episodes secondary to cardiac arrhythmias may be more prolonged than those with benign causes.

The most common arrhythmias causing syncope are atrioventricular (AV) block, sinoatrial (SA) block, and paroxysmal supra- and infraventricular tachyarrhythmias. *AV block* is used to describe disturbances of conduction occurring in the AV conducting system, which includes the AV node to the bundle of His and Purkinje's network. *SA block* is the term used to describe a failure of consistent pacemaker function of the SA node. *Paroxysmal tachycardia* refers to a cardiac rhythm disturbance that results in a rapid heart rate secondary to an ectopic focus outside the SA node; this may be either supra- or intraventricular.

Atrioventricular Block

Atrioventricular block is probably the most common cause of arrhythmic cardiac syncope. The term *Stokes-Adams attack* is frequently used to describe disturbances of consciousness occurring in association with AV block.

Complete AV block is seen primarily in elderly patients. The onset of a Stokes-Adams attack is generally sudden, although a number of visual, sensory, and perceptual premonitory symptoms may be experienced. During the syncopal attack, the pulse disappears and no heart sounds are audible. The patient is pale and, if standing, may fall, with resultant injury. If the attack is sufficiently prolonged, respiration may be labored and urinary incontinence and clonic muscle jerks may be noted. Prolonged confusion and neurological signs of cerebral ischemia may be noted. Regaining of consciousness is generally rapid.

The clinical features of complete AV block include a slow-collapsing pulse and elevation of the jugular venous pressure, sometimes with cannon waves. The first heart sound is of variable intensity, and heart sounds related to atrial contractions may be audible. The diagnosis is confirmed by electrocardiography (ECG), which demonstrates the independence of atrial P waves and ventricular QRS complexes. During Stokes-Adams attacks, the ECG generally shows ventricular standstill, but ventricular fibrillation or tachycardia may also occur.

Sinoatrial Block

Sinoatrial block may result in dizziness, lightheadedness, and syncope. It is most frequently seen in the elderly. Palpitations are common, and the patient appears pale. Patients with SA node dysfunction frequently have other conduction disturbances, and certain drugs, such as verapamil, digoxin, and beta blockers, may further impair SA node function.

On examination, the patient's pulse may be regular between attacks. During an attack, the pulse may be slow or irregular, and a number of rhythmic disturbances may be noted.

Paroxysmal Tachycardia

Supraventricular tachycardias include atrial fibrillation with a rapid ventricular response, atrial flutter, or the Wolff-Parkinson-White syndrome. These arrhythmias may suddenly reduce cardiac output sufficiently to cause syncope.

Ventricular tachycardia or ventricular fibrillation may result in syncope if the heart rate is sufficiently fast and if the arrhythmia lasts longer than a few seconds. Patients are generally elderly and usually have evidence of underlying cardiac disease. The arrhythmias may be preceded by ventricular premature beats and may result in the more serious ventricular fibrillation that causes syncope.

Ventricular fibrillation may be seen as part of the long QT syndrome in association with congenital deafness in children. In most patients with the long QT syndrome, episodes begin in the first decade of life, but onset may be much later. Exercise may precipitate an episode of cardiac syncope. Long QT syndromes may be acquired and present in adults as epilepsy (Pacia et al. 1994). Acquired causes include cardiac ischemia, mitral valve prolapse, myocarditis, drugs, and electrolyte disturbances.

Reflex Cardiac Arrhythmias

A hypersensitive carotid sinus may be a cause of syncope in the elderly, most frequently in men. Syncope may result from a reflex sinus bradycardia, sinus arrest, or AV block, from peripheral vasodilatation with a fall in arterial pressure, or from a combination of these two mechanisms. It is important to note that although 10% of the population over the age of 60 years may have a hypersensitive carotid sinus, not all such patients experience syncope. Accordingly, this diagnosis should be considered only when the clinical history is compatible. Carotid sinus syncope may be initiated by a tight collar or by carotid sinus massage on clinical examination. When syncope occurs, the patient is usually upright, and the duration of the loss of consciousness is generally a few minutes. When consciousness is regained, the patient is mentally clear. Unfortunately, there are no accepted diagnostic criteria for carotid sinus syncope and many cases are overdiagnosed (Landau 1994).

It should be remembered that syncope induced by unilateral carotid massage or compression may also be caused by partial occlusion, usually atherosclerotic, of the contralateral carotid or a vertebral artery, or it may be due to the release of atheromatous emboli. The rare syndrome of glossopharyngeal reflex syncope is characterized by intense paroxysmal pain in the throat and neck and is accompanied by bradycardia or asystole, severe hypotension, and, if prolonged, seizures (Barbash et al. 1986). Episodes of pain may be initiated by swallowing but also by chewing, speaking, laughing, coughing, shouting, sneezing, yawning, or talking. The episodes of pain always precede the loss of consciousness.

Rarely, cardiac syncope may be due to vagus nerve irritation, producing bradyarrhythmias. Esophageal diverticuli, tumors and aneurysms in the region of the carotid sinus, mediastinal masses, and gallbladder disease may produce such irritation.

Decreased Cardiac Output

Syncope may occur as a result of a sudden and marked decrease in cardiac output. Both congenital and acquired conditions have to be considered. Tetralogy of Fallot is the most common congenital malformation causing syncope; it does so by producing hypoxia due to the right-to-left shunting. Other congenital conditions associated with cyanotic heart disease may also cause syncope. Ischemic heart disease and myocardial infarction, aortic stenosis, idiopathic hypertrophic subaortic stenosis, pulmonary hypertension, and other causes of obstruction to pulmonary outflow, atrial myxoma, and cardiac tamponade may sufficiently impair cardiac output to cause syncope. Exercise-induced or effort syncope may be seen in aortic or subaortic stenosis and other states in which there is reduced cardiac output and associated peripheral vasodilatation induced by the exercise. Exercise-induced cardiac syncope may also be related to exercise-induced cardiac arrhythmias; this may be an independent or accentuating cause of syncope.

In patients with valvular heart disease, syncope may be related to arrhythmias. Syncope may also be due to reduced cardiac output secondary to myocardial failure, to mechanical prosthetic valve malfunction, or to thrombus formation. Mitral valve prolapse is generally a benign condition but rarely cardiac arrhythmias can occur. The most significant arrhythmias are ventricular.

In atrial myxoma or with massive pulmonary embolism, a sudden drop in left ventricular output may occur. In atrial myxoma, syncope is frequently positional and occurs when the tumor falls into the atrioventricular valve opening during a change in position of the patient, thereby causing obstruction to the left ventricular inflow.

A decreased cardiac output may also be secondary to conditions that result in inflow obstruction or reduced venous return. These include superior and inferior vena cava obstruction, tension pneumothorax, constrictive cardiomyopathies, constrictive pericarditis, and cardiac tamponade. Syncope associated with aortic dissection may be due to cardiac tamponade but may also be secondary to hypotension, obstruction of cerebral circulation, or a cardiac arrhythmia.

Hypovolemia

Acute blood loss, usually due to gastrointestinal tract bleeding, may cause weakness and faintness and occasionally syncope if sufficient blood is lost. A history of peptic ulcer disease or esophageal varices may be obtained in some of these patients. A history of the passage of black stools suggests upper gastrointestinal tract blood loss. Blood volume depletion by dehydration may cause faintness and weakness, but true syncope is less common, unless the dehydration is combined with exercise.

Hypotension

A number of conditions cause syncope by producing a fall in arterial pressure. The cardiac causes are discussed above. The common faint (vasovagal attack) is the most frequent cause of a transient fall in blood pressure resulting in syncope. It is frequently recurrent and tends to occur in relation to emotional stimuli. It may affect 20–25% of young people. Less commonly, it is seen in older patients with cardiovascular disease. The term *vasovagal* or *vasodepressor syncope* is frequently employed.

The common faint may or may not be associated with bradycardia. There is impairment of consciousness, with loss of postural tone. Signs of autonomic hyperactivity such as pallor, diaphoresis, nausea, and dilated pupils are common. After recovery, the patient may have persistent pallor, sweating, and nausea; if the patient gets up too quickly, he or she may black out again.

The common faint may be preceded by lethargy and fatigue, nausea, weakness, a sensation of an impending faint, and yawning. It is more likely to occur in certain circumstances, such as a hot crowded room, especially if the person is tired or hungry. The episode of fainting may be brought on by venipuncture, the sight of blood, or a sudden painful or traumatic experience. The patient is usually upright or sitting.

When the patient regains consciousness, there usually is no confusion or headache, although weakness is frequently described. As in other causes of syncope, if the period of cerebral hypoperfusion is sufficiently prolonged, urinary incontinence and a few clonic movements may be observed (convulsive syncope).

Orthostatic syncope occurs when autonomic factors that compensate for the upright posture are inadequate. This can result from a variety of clinical disorders. Blood volume depletion or venous pooling may result in syncope when the individual assumes an upright posture. Orthostatic hypotension resulting in syncope may also occur with drugs that impair sympathetic nervous system function. Diuretics, antihypertensive medications, nitrates, arterial vasodilators, calcium channel blockers, phenothiazines, levodopa, alcohol, and tricyclic antidepressants may all result in orthostatic hypotension.

Autonomic nervous system dysfunction resulting in syncope due to orthostatic hypotension may be a result of primary autonomic failure due to the Shy-Drager syndrome or the Riley-Day syndrome. Neuropathies that affect the autonomic nervous system include those of diabetes mellitus, amyloidosis, the Guillain-Barré syndrome, alcoholic neuropathy, hepatic porphyria, and beriberi. Rarely, subacute combined degeneration, syringomyelia, and other spinal cord lesions may damage the descending sympathetic pathways, producing orthostatic hypotension.

Cerebrovascular Ischemia

Syncope may be observed occasionally as a result of reduction of cerebral blood flow in either the carotid or vertebrobasilar system. Most frequently, the underlying condition is atherosclerosis of the cerebral vessels, but reduction of cerebral blood flow due to cerebral embolism, mechanical factors in the neck such as severe osteoarthritis, and arteritis such as Takayasu's disease or cranial arteritis may be responsible. In the subclavian steal syndrome, impairment of consciousness is associated with upper-extremity exercise and results from diversion of cerebral blood flow to the peripheral circulation. Occasionally, cerebral vasospasm secondary to basilar migraine or subarachnoid hemorrhage may be responsible. Insufficiency of the cerebral circulation frequently causes other neurological symptoms, depending on the circulation involved, and many patients have other symptoms of transient cerebral ischemia.

Reduction in blood flow in the carotid circulation may lead to loss of consciousness, but lightheadedness, giddiness, and a sensation of an impending faint are more common.

Reduction in blood flow in the vertebrobasilar system may also lead to loss of consciousness, but dizziness, lightheadedness, drop attacks without loss of consciousness, and bilateral motor and sensory symptoms are more common. Dizziness and lightheadedness alone, however, should not be considered as symptoms of vertebrobasilar insufficiency. Syncope due to compression of the vertebral artery during certain head and neck movements may be associated with episodes of vertigo, disequilibrium, or drop attacks. Patients may describe blackouts when they look upward suddenly or when they turn their heads quickly to one side. Generally, symptoms persist for several seconds after the movement is terminated.

In Takayasu's disease, there may be major occlusion of blood flow in the carotid and vertebrobasilar systems; in addition to fainting, other neurological symptoms are frequent. Pulsations in the neck and arm vessels are usually absent, and blood pressure in the arms is unobtainable. The syncopal episodes characteristically occur with mild or moderate exercise and with certain head movements.

Cerebral vasospasm may result in syncope, particularly if the posterior circulation is involved. In basilar artery migraine, usually seen in young women and children, a variety of brain stem symptoms may also be observed, and a vascular headache is frequent. The loss of consciousness is usually gradual, but a confusional state may last for hours.

Metabolic Disorders

A number of metabolic disturbances, including hypoglycemia, anoxia, and hyperventilation-induced alkalosis, may predispose to syncope. Most frequently, however, the symptoms of lightheadedness and dizziness are observed. The abruptness of onset of the loss of consciousness depends on the acuteness and reversibility of the metabolic disturbances. Syncope due to hypoglycemia generally develops gradually. The patient experiences a sensation of hunger, there is a relationship to fasting, there may be a history of diabetes mellitus, and there is a prompt response to ingestion of food. Symptoms are unrelated to posture but may be aggravated by exercise. During the syncopal attack, there is no significant change in blood pressure or pulse. Anoxia may produce syncope because of the lack of oxygen or through the production of a vasodepressor type of syncope. Symptoms of lightheadedness are common, but true syncope is less common. Patients with underlying cardiac or pulmonary disease are susceptible. In patients with chronic anemia or certain hemoglobinopathies that impair oxygen transport, similar symptoms may be experienced. Syncopal symptoms may be more prominent with exercise or physical activity.

Hyperventilation-induced syncope is most frequently psychogenic in origin. During hyperventilation, the patient may experience paresthesia of the face, hands, and feet; a buzzing sensation in the head; lightheadedness; giddiness; blurring of vision; dryness of the mouth; and occasionally tetany. The patient may complain of a tightness in the chest and may experience a sense of panic. Symptoms can occur in the supine or erect positions and are gradual in onset. The symptoms of hyperventilation may be helped by having the patient rebreathe into a paper bag. During hyperventilation, a tachycardia may be noted, but blood pressure generally remains normal.

Miscellaneous Causes of Syncope

As already discussed, in certain types of syncope, more than one mechanism may be responsible for the loss of consciousness. In the common faint, both vasodepressor and cardioinhibitory factors may be operational. In cardiac syncope, a reduction of cardiac output may be due to a single cause, such as obstruction to inflow or outflow or a cardiac arrhythmia, but multiple factors are frequently responsible.

Cough or tussive syncope and micturition syncope represent special cases of reflex syncope for which the mechanisms are poorly understood and probably multifactorial. In cough syncope, loss of consciousness occurs following a paroxysm of severe coughing. This is most likely to occur in obese males, usually smokers or patients with chronic bronchitis. The syncopal episodes occur suddenly, generally after repeated coughing but occasionally after a single cough. Before losing consciousness, the patient may feel lightheaded. The individual's face often becomes congested and then pale. Diaphoresis may be observed. There may be loss of muscle tone. Syncope is generally brief, lasting only seconds, and recovery is rapid (DeMaria et al. 1984). Several factors are probably operational in causing syncope. The most significant is the blockage of venous return by the raised intrathoracic pressure.

Micturition syncope is most often seen in men during or after micturition, usually after arising from bed to urinate in the middle of the night. There may be a history of drinking alcohol before going to bed. It has been suggested that syncope results from sudden peripheral vasodilatation caused by the release of intravesicular pressure and bradycardia. The relative peripheral vasodilatation from recent alcohol use and a supine sleeping position is contributory, since blood pressure is lowest in the middle of the night. Syncope may also occur in association with fever, particularly when the man arises in the middle of the night to urinate. Rarely micturition syncope may result from a pheochromocytoma in the bladder wall. Defecation syncope is uncommon, but it probably shares the underlying pathophysiological mechanisms responsible for micturition syncope. Convulsive syncope is an episode of syncope sufficiently prolonged to result in a few clonic jerks. The other features are those of syncope and these should not be confused with epileptic seizures.

Investigations of Patients with Syncope

In the investigation of the patient with episodic impairment of consciousness, the diagnostic tests performed depend on the neurologist's initial differential diagnosis. Investigations should be individualized, but certain investigations, such as measurement of the hematocrit and blood glucose and routine ECG, are indicated in most patients. A resting ECG may reveal an abnormality of cardiac rhythm or the presence of underlying ischemic or congenital heart disease.

In the patient suspected of cardiac syncope, a chest x-ray may show evidence of cardiac hypertrophy, valvular heart disease, or pulmonary hypertension. Cardiac fluoroscopy may be useful in assessing valve dysfunction. Other noninvasive investigations include radionucleotide cardiac scanning, echocardiography, and prolonged Holter monitoring for the detection of cardiac arrhythmias. Echocardiography is useful in the diagnosis of valvular heart disease, cardiomyopathy, atrial myxoma, prosthetic valve dysfunction, pericardial effusion, aortic dissection, and congenital heart disease. Prolonged Holter monitoring detects twice as many electrocardiographic abnormalities as a routine ECG and may detect an arrhythmia at the time of a syncopal episode. Holter monitoring is frequently performed for 24-hour periods, although longer periods of recording may be required.

Exercise testing and electrophysiological studies are carried out in a select group of patients (Sra et al. 1993). Exercise testing may be useful in detecting coronary artery disease and exercise-related syncopal events. Electrophysiological studies using intracardiac recordings may help localize the site of conduction disturbances.

In patients suspected of syncope due to cerebrovascular causes, noninvasive diagnostic studies, including Doppler flow studies of the cerebral vessels, cervical spine x-rays, and computed tomographic studies, may provide useful information. Occasionally, cerebral angiography is indicated, usually in patients who have other associated neurological symptoms of cerebral ischemia.

Electroencephalography (EEG) is useful in differentiating syncope from epileptic seizure disorders, which is discussed below. The EEG should only be performed when a seizure disorder is suspected. Table 2.2 presents the classification of syncope discussed in this section.

SEIZURES

Sudden, unexplained loss of consciousness in a child or adult may be caused by an epileptic seizure disorder, and a distinction from syncope has to be made. An epileptic seizure is defined as a transient neurological dysfunction resulting from an excessive abnormal electrical discharge of cerebral neurons. The clinical manifestations are numerous, including disturbances of consciousness, changes in emotions, changes in sensation, abnormal movements, and changes in visceral

Table 2.2: Classification of syncope

Cardiac
Arrhythmias
Bradyarrhythmias
Tachyarrhythmias
Reflex arrhythmias
Decreased cardiac output
Outflow obstruction
Inflow obstruction
Cardiomyopathy
Hypovolemic
Hypotensive
Vasovagal attack
Drugs
Dysautonomia
Cerebrovascular
Carotid disease
Vertebrobasilar disease
Vasospasm
Takayasu's arteritis
Metabolic
Hypoglycemia
Anemia
Anoxia
Hyperventilation
Multifactorial
Vasovagal attack
Cardiac syncope
Cough, micturition

functions or behavior. In the evaluation of a patient with an alteration of consciousness, the neurologist should try to establish whether the patient suffered from an epileptic seizure as opposed to syncope or other conditions that can result in an alteration of consciousness. Epileptic seizures may be classified according to clinical manifestations and EEG findings. (The classification of different types of seizures can be found in Chapter 72.) This section discusses only seizures associated with an alteration of consciousness.

Both generalized seizures (absence and tonic-clonic) and complex partial seizures have an alteration of consciousness as part of their clinical manifestations. In most patients, a correct diagnosis can be made on the basis of the history, the physical examination, and EEG findings. Myoclonic seizures or sudden startle-induced episodes may produce motor manifestations, but generally there is no alteration of consciousness.

History and Physical Examination

The most definitive way to diagnose epilepsy and the type of seizure is clinical observation of the seizure, although this is frequently not possible except in the case of very frequent seizures. The history, as obtained from the patient and an observer, is of paramount importance. The neurologist should obtain a family history and should inquire about birth complications, central nervous system infections, head trauma, and previous febrile seizures, since they may all be responsible factors.

The neurologist should obtain a complete description of the event and should inquire whether the patient had any warning prior to the event. An inquiry should be made concerning possible precipitating events. Does the patient have other neurological symptoms to suggest an underlying structural cause?

Data should be obtained about the age of onset, frequency, and diurnal variation of the patient's clinical events. Seizures are generally brief and have stereotyped patterns, as described earlier. With complex partial seizures and tonic clonic seizures, a period of postictal confusion is highly characteristic. Unlike some types of attacks that cause transient loss of consciousness, seizures are unrelated to posture and generally last longer. In a tonic-clonic seizure, cyanosis is frequently present, pallor is uncommon, and breathing may be stertorous.

Absence seizures have an age of onset between 5 and 15 years in the majority of patients, and a family history of seizures is noted in 20–40% of patients. Tonic-clonic and complex partial seizures may begin at any age from infancy to late adulthood, although young infants may not demonstrate the typical features because of incomplete development of the nervous system.

The neurological examination may reveal an underlying structural disturbance responsible for the seizure disorder. Birth-related trauma may result in asymmetries of physical development; cranial bruits may indicate an arteriovenous malformation; and space-occupying lesions may result in papilledema or in focal motor, sensory, or reflex changes. In the pediatric age groups, mental retardation may be found in association with birth injury or metabolic defects. The skin should be examined for abnormal pigment changes and other dysmorphic features seen in some of the neurodegenerative disorders.

If absence seizures are suspected, the diagnosis can frequently be made in the office by having the patient hyperventilate for 3–4 minutes. Hyperventilation induces an absence seizure in many such patients. If the patient is examined immediately after a suspected tonic-clonic seizure, the physician should search for abnormal focal neurological signs, such as focal motor weakness and reflex asymmetry, and for the presence of pathological reflexes, such as Babinski's reflex.

Absence Seizures

The absence seizure is a well-defined clinical and electroencephalographic event. The essential feature is an abrupt, brief episode of decreased awareness without any warning or aura or postictal symptoms. At the onset of the absence seizure, there is an interruption of activity. A simple absence seizure is characterized only by an alteration of consciousness. A complex absence seizure is characterized by an alteration of consciousness and other symptoms, such as minor motor automatisms. During a simple absence seizure, the patient remains immobile, breathing is normal, no color changes are observed, there is no loss of postural tone, and there are no motor manifestations. After the seizure, the patient immediately resumes the previous activities and may be unaware of the attack. An absence seizure generally lasts 10–15 seconds, but it may be shorter or as long as 40 seconds.

Complex absence seizures have additional symptoms, such as diminution of postural tone, which may cause the patient to fall; an increase in postural tone; minor clonic movements of the face or extremities; minor face or extremity automatisms; or autonomic phenomena such as pallor, flushing, tachycardia, piloerection, mydriasis, or urinary incontinence.

Tonic-Clonic Seizures

The tonic-clonic seizure is the most dramatic manifestation of epilepsy and is characterized by motor activity and loss of consciousness. Tonic-clonic seizures may be the only manifestation of epilepsy or may be associated with other seizure types. In a primary generalized tonic-clonic seizure, the patient generally has no warning or aura, although some patients may experience a few myoclonic jerks. The seizure begins with a tonic phase, during which there is sustained muscle contraction lasting 10–20 seconds. This phase is followed by a clonic phase that lasts approximately 30 seconds and is characterized by recurrent muscle contractions. During a tonic-clonic seizure, a number of autonomic changes can be observed, including an increase in blood pressure and heart rate, apnea, mydriasis, urinary or fecal incontinence, piloerection, cyanosis, and diaphoresis. Injury may result from a fall or tongue biting.

In the postictal period, consciousness is regained slowly. The patient may remain lethargic and confused for a variable period. Abnormal extensor plantar responses may be elicited.

Some generalized motor seizures with transient alteration of consciousness may have only tonic or only clonic components. Tonic seizures consist of an increase in muscle tone, and alteration of consciousness is generally brief. Clonic seizures are characterized by a brief impairment of consciousness and bilateral clonic movements. Recovery may be rapid, but if the seizure is more prolonged, a postictal period of confusion may be noted.

Complex Partial Seizures

In a complex partial seizure, the first manifestation of the seizure may be an alteration of consciousness, but frequently the patient experiences an aura or warning. The seizure may have a simple partial onset, which may include motor, sensory, visceral, or psychic symptoms. The patient may initially experience hallucinations or illusions; affective symptoms, such as fear or depression; cognitive symptoms, such as a sense of depersonalization or unreality; or dysphasic symptoms.

The complex partial seizure generally lasts 1–3 minutes but may occasionally be shorter or longer. A complex partial seizure may become generalized and evolve into a tonic-clonic convulsion. During a complex partial seizure, automatisms, generally more complex than those observed in absence seizures, may be noted. The automatisms may involve continuation of the patient's activity prior to the onset of the seizure or they may be new motor acts. The automatisms are varied but frequently consist of chewing or swallowing movements, lip smacking, grimacing, or automatisms of the extremities, including fumbling with objects, walking, or trying to stand up.

The duration of the postictal period after a complex partial seizure is variable, with a gradual return to normal consciousness and normal response to external stimuli. Table 2.3 provides a comparison of absence seizures and complex partial seizures.

Investigations of Seizures

In the initial investigations of the patient with tonic-clonic seizures or complex partial seizures, a complete blood count, urinalysis, biochemical screening, blood glucose level, serum calcium concentration, and serological test for syphilis should be obtained. Laboratory investigations generally are not helpful in establishing a diagnosis of absence seizures. In infants and children, biochemical screening for amino acid disorders should be considered.

Computed tomographic (CT) scans can reveal tumors, cerebral atrophy, hydrocephalus, cerebral hemorrhage, infarction, subdural hematoma, cystic lesions, and vascular malformations. Although children with absence seizures may have some abnormalities on CT scans, this procedure is generally not required for diagnosis or management. Magnetic resonance imaging is the imaging modality of choice for the investigation of patients with suspected seizures. It is superior to CT scanning and increases the yield of focal structural disturbances.

Cerebrospinal fluid examination is not necessary in every patient with a seizure disorder and should be reserved for the patient whose recent seizure may be related to an acute central nervous system infection.

The role of the EEG is to provide laboratory support for a clinical impression and to help classify the type of seizure (Sato and Rose 1986). Epilepsy is a clinical diagnosis; therefore, EEG cannot produce a diagnosis with certainty unless the patient has a clinical event during the recording. It is important to realize that a normal EEG does not exclude epilepsy and that minor nonspecific abnormalities do not confirm epilepsy. Some patients with clinically documented seizures show no abnormality even after serial EEG recordings, sleep recordings, and special activation

Table 2.3: Comparison of absence and complex partial seizures

Feature	*Absence Seizure*	*Complex Partial Seizure*
Age of onset	Childhood	Any age
Aura or warning	No	Frequent
Onset	Abrupt	Gradual
Duration	Seconds	Up to minutes
Automatisms	Simple	More complex
Termination	Abrupt	Gradual
Frequency	Possibly multiple seizures per day	Occasional
Postictal phase	No	Confusion, fatigue
Electroencephalogram	Generalized spike and wave	Focal epileptic discharges or nonspecific lesions
Neuroimaging	Usually normal	May demonstrate focal lesions

techniques. The EEG is most frequently helpful in the diagnosis of absence seizures (Holmes et al. 1987). EEG evaluation can be supplemented with simultaneous video monitoring for the documentation of ictal events allowing for a strict correlation between EEG changes and clinical manifestations. Simultaneous EEG and video monitoring is also useful in distinguishing seizures from nonepileptic phenomena (Leis et al. 1993).

Although an accurate diagnosis can be made in the majority of patients on the basis of the clinical history and the foregoing investigations, some patients present a diagnostic dilemma. A more definite diagnosis of a seizure versus a nonepileptic phenomenon or a clearer classification of the specific type of seizure can be made through the use of a 24-hour ambulatory EEG recording as suggested by Ebersole (1986).

Psychogenic or Pseudoseizures (Nonepileptic Seizures)

Pseudoepileptic seizures are paroxysmal episodes of altered behavior that superficially resemble epileptic seizures but lack the expected EEG epileptic changes. It is important to note, however, that approximately 40% of patients with pseudo- or nonepileptic seizures also suffer from true epileptic seizures.

It is frequently difficult to establish a diagnosis based on initial history alone. Often, a correct diagnosis can be made only after witnessing the patient's clinical episodes. Nonepileptic seizures may occur in both children and adults and are more common in females. Most frequently, they superficially resemble tonic-clonic seizures. They generally are abrupt in onset, occur in the presence of others, and do not occur during sleep. Motor activity is uncoordinated, but urinary incontinence is rare and physical injury is uncommon. They tend to be more prolonged than true tonic-clonic seizures. Pelvic thrusting is clinically associated with pseudoseizures. During and immediately following the seizure, the patient may not be responsive to verbal or painful stimuli. Cyanosis is not observed. Postictally, no focal neurological signs or abnormal plantar responses are noted.

In the patient with known epilepsy, the diagnosis of nonepileptic seizures should be considered when seizures that previously had been under good control become medically refractory. For the diagnosis of nonepileptic seizures, the patient should have a psychological assessment, since the majority of such patients have a high incidence of emotional and other psychiatric disturbances. In this patient group, there is a high incidence of hysteria, depression, and personality disturbances. At times, a secondary gain can be identified. In some patients with psychogenic seizures, the clinical episodes can frequently be precipitated by suggestion and by certain clinical tests, such as intravenous saline infusion or tactile (vibration) stimulation. Proposed methods to precipitate pseudoseizures include intravenous administration of saline, suggestion, and nose-pinching to induce apnea.

The interictal EEG in patients with pseudoseizures is normal and remains normal during the clinical episode, demonstrating no evidence of a cerebral dysrhythmia. With the introduction of long-term ambulatory EEG monitoring, the episodic behavior of a patient can be correlated with EEG changes; thus, psychogenic seizures can be distinguished from true epileptic seizures. Table 2.4 summarizes the features of psychogenic seizures as compared to those of epileptic seizures.

As an auxiliary investigation of suspected psychogenic seizures, plasma prolactin concentrations may provide additional supportive data. Plasma prolactin concentrations have been shown to be frequently elevated following tonic clonic seizures and less frequently so following complex partial seizures (Fisher et al. 1991). Serum prolactin levels are normal following psychogenic seizures, although such a finding does not exclude the diagnosis of true epileptic seizures.

MISCELLANEOUS CAUSES OF ALTERED CONSCIOUSNESS

In children, alterations of consciousness may be observed in breath-holding spells and metabolic disturbances. Breath-holding spells are common in infants and young children and have to be distinguished from epilepsy. Most spells start at 6–28 months of age, but they may occur as early as the first month of life and usually disappear by 5 or 6 years

Table 2.4: Comparison of psychogenic and epileptic seizures

Feature	*Psychogenic Seizure*	*Epileptic Seizure*
Stereotypy of attack	May be variable	Usually stereotyped
Diurnal variation	Daytime	Nocturnal or daytime
Injury	Rare	Can occur with tonic-clonic seizures
Tongue biting	Rare	Can occur with tonic-clonic seizures
Urinary incontinence	Rare	Frequent
Motor activity	Prolonged, uncoordinated; pelvic thrusting	Automatisms or coordinated tonic-clonic
Postictal confusion	Rare	Common
Relation to medication changes	Unrelated	Usually related
Interictal EEG	Normal	Frequently abnormal
Ictal EEG	Normal	Abnormal
Presence of secondary gain	Common	Uncommon
Psychiatric disturbances	Common	Uncommon

EEG = electroencephalogram.

of age. Breath-holding spells may occur several times per day. There are both cyanotic and pallid syncope subgroups.

In cyanotic breath-holding spells, loss of consciousness is triggered by a sudden injury or fright, anger, or frustration. The child is initially provoked, cries vigorously for a few breaths, then holds his or her breath in expiration and cyanosis develops. Consciousness is lost because of hypoxia. Although stiffening, a few clonic movements, and urinary incontinence are occasionally observed, these episodes can be clearly distinguished from epileptic seizures on the basis of the history of provocation and by noting that the apnea and cyanosis occur before any alteration of consciousness. In these children, the neurological examination and EEG are normal.

Rather than developing cyanosis, some of these children develop pallor before losing consciousness. These episodes generally are provoked by a mild painful injury or a startle. The infant cries initially, then becomes pale and loses consciousness. As in the cyanotic type, stiffening, clonic movements, and urinary incontinence may be observed. In the pallid infant syncope syndrome, loss of consciousness is secondary to excessive vagal tone, resulting in bradycardia and subsequent cerebral ischemia; this is similar to a vasovagal attack.

A number of pediatric metabolic disorders may have clinical manifestations of alterations of consciousness, lethargy, or seizures. These include disorders of amino acid metabolism, such as phenylketonuria, Hartnup's disease, and maple syrup urine disease; the various disorders of the urea cycle; and miscellaneous metabolic disorders such as hyperglycinemia and disorders of pyruvate metabolism. Neurological abnormalities in these patients may be seen at birth or later in infancy and childhood. Metabolic screening of urine and blood should be considered in an infant who presents with neurological disorders early in life. Examination of the urine for the detection of amino aciduria, excess urinary ketones, and urea excretion should be considered. Biochemical screening of the serum for these disorders should also be considered for the infant or child who presents with transient lethargy, apneic episodes, syncope, or seizures.

Increased intracranial pressure may result from a number of causes, including periodic obstruction of the circulation of cerebrospinal fluid, as in aqueductal stenosis of colloid cysts of the third ventricle. These patients are subject to paroxysmal increases of intracranial pressure that may last up to 20 minutes. These episodes may occur spontaneously or may be related to postural changes or Valsalva's maneuver. If sufficient to impair cerebral perfusion, the plateau waves of Lundberg may result in sudden, severe headaches, which may be followed by loss of consciousness. Occasionally, this is accompanied by opisthotonos and clonic movements. In intermittent obstruction to cerebrospinal fluid circulation, leg buckling, and atonic episodes may occur with changes in head position. Tinnitus is a frequent accompanying symptom under these circumstances.

In the patient who presents with an apparent loss of consciousness, the neurologist must also consider the possibility of malingering or some other underlying psychogenic cause. However, it is always important to exclude organic causes first. The neurologist should also distinguish sleep disorders such as cataplexy and other causes of drop attacks from alterations of consciousness. These nonsyncopal spells include drop attacks of the elderly, narcolepsy, systemic mastocytosis, carcinoid syndrome, and pheochromocytoma. Systemic mastocytosis, carcinoid syndrome, and pheochromocytoma may also cause true syncope secondary to rapid changes in blood pressure (see Chapter 3.)

REFERENCES

Barbash GI, Keren G, Korozyn AD et al. Mechanisms of syncope in glossopharyngeal neuralgia. Electroencephalogr Clin Neurophysiol 1986;63:321–325.

DeMaria AA, Westmoreland BF, Sharbrough FW. EEG in cough syncope. Neurology 1984;34:371–374.

Ebersole JS. Ambulatory EEG: Telemetered and Cassette-Recorded. In RJ Gumnit (ed), Advances in Neurology. Vol. 46. Intensive Neurodiagnostic Monitoring. New York: Raven, 1986:139–155.

Fisher RS, Chan DW, Bare M et al. Capillary prolactin measurements for diagnosis of seizures. *Ann Neurol* 1991;29:187–190.

Holmes GL, McKeever M, Adamson M. Absence seizures in children: clinical and electroencephalographic features. *Ann Neurol* 1987;21:268–273.

Landau WM. Clinical neuromythology XIII. Neuroskepticism: sovereign remedy for the carotid sinus syndrome. *Neurology* 1994;44:1570–1576.

Leis AA, Ross MA, Summers AK. Psychogenic seizures: characteristics and diagnostics pitfalls. *Neurology* 1992;42:95–99.

Lempert T, Bauer M, Schmidt D. Syncope: a videometric analysis of 56 episodes of transient cerebral hypoxia. *Ann Neurol* 1994;36:233–237.

Pacia S, Luciano D, Vazquez B et al. The prolonged QT syndrome presenting as epilepsy. A report of two cases and literature review. *Neurology* 1994;44:1408–1410.

Sato S, Rose DF. The electroencephalogram in the evaluation of the patient with epilepsy. *Neurol Clin* 1986;4:509–529.

Sra JS, Jazayer MR, Dhala A et al. Neurocardiogenic syncope. Diagnosis, mechanisms, and treatment. *Cardiol Clin* 1993;11:183–191.

Chapter 3
Falls and Drop Attacks

Bernd F. Remler and Robert B. Daroff

Everyone occasionally loses balance and, infrequently, falls. When falls occur repeatedly or if falling is unassociated with a prior sense of imbalance, the patient may have a neurological problem. Various disease states and neurological impairments cause falls and drops. Associated loss of consciousness implies syncope or seizures (see Chapter 2). *Transient ischemic attacks* (TIAs) in the posterior circulation or the anterior cerebral artery distribution cause monosymptomatic drops. Third-ventricular or posterior fossa tumors may also cause abrupt drops. Patients with lower-extremity weakness, spasticity, rigidity, sensory loss, or ataxia frequently fall. Narcoleptics experience cataplexy, and patients with Ménière's disease occasionally fall as a result of otolithic dysfunction. Middle-aged women may fall with no discernible cause. Finally, the elderly, with their inevitable infirmities, fall frequently. These associations permit a classification of falls and drops as presented in Table 3.1. We use the words *falls* and *drops* interchangeably but use the phrase *drop attacks* specifically to describe sudden falls occurring without warning, when secondary to either TIA or intracranial tumors in the third ventricle or posterior fossa.

The medical history is essential in evaluating patients with falls and drops. The situational and environmental circumstances of the events must be ascertained. On the basis of the causes listed in Table 3.1, basic questions must be asked of the patient. Was there loss of consciousness? If so, for how long? Was there preceding lightheadedness or palpitations? Is there a history of a seizure disorder? Were there previous symptoms suggestive of TIA? Does the patient have headaches? Are there symptoms of distal sensory loss, limb weakness, or stiffness? Has the patient had excessive daytime sleepiness, and are the falls precipitated by elation or laughter? Is there a history of visual impairment, hearing loss, vertigo, and tinnitus? Given the tendency for middle-aged women and for elderly men and women to fall, the patient's age and sex are important to the evaluation.

The neurological examination is particularly relevant in ascertaining that falling might be related to motor or sensory involvement of the lower limbs. Does the patient have the rigidity, spasticity, or tremor of Parkinson's disease (PD); the ophthalmoparesis of progressive supranuclear palsy; lower limb weakness, ataxia, sensory loss, or spasticity; or signs compatible with multiple sclerosis? Patients who frequently experience near-falls without injuries may have a psychogenic disorder of station and gait (Lempert et al. 1991). Patients with normal neurological examinations and no history of associated neurological symptoms should be examined periodically. If the falling persists, magnetic resonance imaging might be considered to rule out an otherwise silent midline cerebral neoplasm or malformation.

LOSS OF CONSCIOUSNESS

Syncope

The manifestations and causes of syncope are described in Chapter 2. Severe ventricular arrhythmias and hypotension lead to cephalic ischemia, loss of consciousness, and falling. If there is a sudden third-degree heart block (Stokes-Adams attack), the patient loses consciousness and falls without warning. Less severe causes of decreased cardiac output, such as bradyarrhythmias or tachyarrhythmias, are associated with a prodromal sensation of faintness before the loss of consciousness. Hypotension is always associated with a presyncopal syndrome of progressive lightheadedness, dimming of vision, roaring in the ears, and rubbery legs, before consciousness is lost.

Table 3.1: Causes and types of falls and drops

Loss of consciousness
Syncope
Seizures
Transient ischemia attacks (drop attacks)
Vertebrobasilar
Anterior cerebral
Third ventricular and posterior fossa tumors (drop attacks)
Motor and sensory impairment of lower limbs
Basal ganglia disorders
Parkinson's disease
Progressive supranuclear palsy
Neuromuscular disorders (myopathy and neuropathy)
Myelopathy
Cerebral or cerebellar disorders
Cataplexy
Vestibular disorders
Cryptogenic falls in middle-aged women
Aged state

The workup for cardiogenic syncope may require the assistance of a cardiologist and invariably involves Holter monitoring, echocardiography, and possibly cardiac catheterization. Proper recognition of benign recurrent vasovagal syncope ("neurocardiogenic syncope") may spare patients excessive expense and risk. The basic workup includes an electrocardiogram, complete blood count (to rule out anemia), electrolytes, and blood pressure measurements in the supine and standing positions.

Seizures

Falls and drop attacks in patients with seizures range from the initial tonic axial destabilization of a primary generalized tonic-clonic seizure (see Chapter 2), through the varied muscular manifestations of infantile spasms, to "temporal lobe drop attacks" (Gambardella et al. 1994). Temporal lobe drop attacks are commonly associated with prolonged impairment of consciousness. Arrhythmogenic seizures mimicking cardiogenic syncope have also been described (Gilchrist 1985). Drop attacks of presumed epileptic origin, without associated disturbances of consciousness, are unusual. Electroencephalographic (EEG) monitoring by closed-circuit television of epileptic patients with falls has identified distinct motor phenomena causing loss of posture: tonic axial and hip flexor spasms, as well as axial myoclonic, myoclonic-atonic, and atonic events (Ikeno et al. 1985; Egli et al. 1985). For the clinician, however, the precise nature of these events is less important than establishing a diagnosis of seizures. This is often simple in patients with long-standing epilepsy, but falls in patients with poststroke hemiparesis may be falsely attributed to motor weakness rather than to new-onset seizures. Further confusion may result from the difficulties involved in differentiating the destabilizing extensor spasms of spasticity from focal seizures.

A challenging differential diagnosis in the border zone of syncope and epilepsy is posed by the patient who faints (cardiogenic or hypotensive) and then exhibits tonic or clonic movements. Referred to as "convulsive syncope," this phenomenon is nonepileptic, and its motor manifestations probably reflect brain stem release due to loss of inhibitory cortical influences. EEG recordings in patients with cardiogenic syncope (Aminoff et al. 1988) demonstrate large-amplitude irregular slowing or transient flattening during the period of unconsciousness and convulsive movements. Breath-holding spells in children, long QT syndromes, blood donation, and glossopharyngeal neuralgia are other causes of convulsive syncope.

TRANSIENT ISCHEMIC ATTACKS

Drop attacks secondary to TIAs are sudden falls occurring without warning or obvious explanation (such as tripping) while walking or standing. There is no, or only momentary, loss of consciousness; the sensorium and lower limb strength are intact immediately or shortly after the patient hits the ground. Neurological examination should not reveal lower-limb motor or sensory dysfunction between episodes. If such abnormalities are present, it might be impossible to distinguish drop attacks from the falls associated with motor or sensory impairment of the lower limbs. The vascular distributions of drop attacks from TIA are the posterior circulation (vertebrobasilar insufficiency) and the anterior cerebral artery.

Vertebrobasilar Insufficiency

Drop attacks due to posterior circulation insufficiency result from transient ischemia to the corticospinal tracts or the paramedian reticular formation. These drop attacks rarely occur in isolation; most patients have a history of other occasions of the more usual symptoms of vertebrobasilar insufficiency, such as vertigo, diplopia, ataxia, weakness, and hemisensory loss. Occasionally, a drop attack may herald progressive thrombosis of the basilar artery, hours before major and permanent neurological signs evolve.

Anterior Cerebral Artery Ischemia

Anterior cerebral artery ischemia results in drop attacks by impairing perfusion of the parasagittal premotor and motor cortex controlling the lower extremities (Meisner et al. 1986). Derivation of both anterior cerebral arteries from the same internal carotid artery (a common vascular anomaly, with an approximate prevalence of 20%) is anatomically predisposing to this syndrome. In such patients, an embolus may lodge in the single anterior cerebral artery and produce bilateral parasagittal ischemia with a consequent drop attack.

THIRD VENTRICULAR AND POSTERIOR FOSSA TUMORS

Drop attacks can be manifestations of colloid cysts of the third ventricle or mass lesions within the posterior fossa (Lee et al. 1994). With colloid cysts, unprovoked falling is the second most common symptom, next to positionally induced headaches. This history may be the only clinical clue to the diagnosis, as the neurological examination may be entirely normal. Abrupt neck flexion may precipitate drop attacks in otherwise asymptomatic patients who are harboring posterior fossa tumors. Other intracranial mass lesions, such as parasagittal meningiomas, foramen magnum tumors, or subdural hematomas, are usually associated with baseline abnormalities of gait and motor functions, and falling occurs consequent to these impairments (see Table 3.1) rather than to true drop attacks.

MOTOR AND SENSORY IMPAIRMENT OF THE LOWER LIMBS

A wide variety of neurological disorders impair motor functions, coordination, and balance. Such conditions are frequent causes of falls and drop attacks.

Disorders of the Basal Ganglia

Parkinson's Disease

Patients with PD frequently fall, particularly if they are bradykinetic and rigid. They have marked postural instability and are readily retropulsed. Although they often fall backward, they may also, without warning, drop directly to the ground. This is most common in patients with dopamine-induced motor fluctuations, particularly from peak dose dyskinesias and during off periods (see Chapter 76). PD patients shift their center of gravity forward (explaining, in part, their flexed axial posture) and have difficulty regaining balance when their center of gravity is altered. Impaired righting reflexes are, in part, due to muscular rigidity and bradykinesia, which prevent rapid corrective muscle activation and weight shifts.

Progressive Supranuclear Palsy

Patients with progressive supranuclear palsy (see Chapter 76) are characterized by parkinsonian features, axial rigidity, nuchal dystonic rigidity, spasticity, and ophthalmoparesis. They are more likely to fall than PD patients, even with equivalent functional impairment, in part because they frequently are unable to look down and thereby avoid obstacles during ambulation.

Neuromuscular Disorders (Myopathy and Neuropathy)

Myopathies characteristically involve proximal muscles and increase the tendency to fall. The multiple causes of myopathy and neuropathy (genetically determined or acquired) are discussed in Chapters 81 and 84. Most neuropathies are mixed (motor and sensory) in type. Regardless of cause, neuropathies predispose the patient to falling because of lower-limb weakness and impairment of afferent sensations from feet, joints, and muscles. Sensory neuropathies delay or reduce the relay of sensory signals to the central nervous system, which retards modification of lower-limb motor function and hence allows falling when postural imbalance occurs. Falling may herald the onset of acute polyneuropathies such as the Guillain-Barré syndrome; this neuropathy has a typical predilection for nerves to proximal muscles, which increases the likelihood of falling.

Myelopathy

Patients with spinal cord disease (see Chapter 28) are at particular risk of falling because all the descending major motor and ascending sensory tracts traverse the cord. These patients develop weakness and spasticity, impaired somatosensory and proprioceptive input from the lower limbs, and vestibulospinal disruption that precludes adequate peripheral and central (including cerebellar) corrections for shifts in the center of gravity.

Cerebral or Cerebellar Disorders

Weakness, spasticity, sensory loss, and vestibular dysfunction may occur in isolation or in any combination in patients with cerebral disease (neoplasm, infarction, hemorrhage, demyelination, and trauma). Patients with acute basal ganglia lesions may show a slow contralateral tilting movement causing falls (Labodie et al. 1989). Metabolic encephalopathies cause characteristic transient loss of the postural tone (asterixis). If this is extensive and involves the axial musculature, episodic loss of the upright posture may mimic drop attacks in chronic uremic patients (Massey et al. 1988). Cerebellar disease causes gait ataxia, a prime cause of postural instability and falling. Moreover, patients with cerebellar disease, particularly of the degenerative variety (see Chapter 77) or due to multiple sclerosis (see Chapter 61), usually have coexisting brain stem, spinal cord, or cerebral involvement.

CATAPLEXY

Cataplexy, the sudden loss of lower-limb tone, is a part of the tetrad of narcolepsy that also includes excessive daytime sleepiness, hypnagogic hallucinations, and sleep paralysis (see Chapter 73). Consciousness is preserved during a cataplectic attack, which varies from slight lower-limb weakness to complete flaccid paralysis and abrupt falling. Once on the ground, the patient is unable to move but continues breathing. The attacks usually last less than a minute and only rarely exceed several minutes. Cataplectic attacks are provoked by laughter, anger, surprise, and startle. Occasionally, they interrupt or follow sexual orgasm. Electromyographic silence in antigravity muscles occurs during the attacks, and deep tendon reflexes and the H-reflex (see Chapter 37B) are unelicitable.

Cataplexy occurs in the absence of narcolepsy only when it is associated with structural cerebral disease (symptomatic cataplexy). Rare causes are Niemann-Pick's disease and hypothalamic or brain stem lesions (D'Cruz et al. 1994; Fernandez et al. 1995).

VESTIBULAR DISORDERS (OTOLITHIC CRISIS)

During attacks of vertigo, patients often lose balance and fall (see Chapter 18). By contrast, Ménière's disease (see Chapter 44) is complicated by drop attacks unassociated with preceding or accompanying vertigo. These have been called Tumarkin's otolithic crisis (Baloh et al. 1990). Presumably, stimulation of otolithic receptors in the saccule triggers inappropriate reflex postural adjustments, via vestibulospinal pathways, leading to the falls. The patients, without warning, feel as if they are being thrown to the ground. They may fall straight down or be propelled in any direction. Indeed, one of us (RBD) had a patient who suddenly saw and felt her legs moving forward in front of her as she had a spontaneous back-flip secondary to an otolithic crisis. This condition occurs only in patients with Ménière's disease and is associated with sensorineural hearing loss, tinnitus, and attacks of vertigo. Tulio's phenomenon, which is also commonly associated with Ménière's disease, refers to the induction of dizziness by noise. Low-frequency sound induces inappropriate stimulation of the vestibular end organ (Ishizaki et al. 1991).

CRYPTOGENIC FALLS IN MIDDLE-AGED WOMEN

Enigmatically, women over the age of 40 have a tendency to fall. The fall is usually forward and occurs, without warning, while walking. There is no loss of consciousness, dizziness, or even a sense of imbalance. The patients are convinced that they have not tripped but that their legs suddenly gave way. As soon as they get to their feet, walking continues normally. Stevens and Mathews (1973) elicited a history of falling in 3.5% of 200 consecutive women visiting a gynecological clinic; no men among 100, interviewed prior to elective surgery, gave a history of unexplained falling.

About 75% of these women develop the disorder after the age of 40. About one-third were aware of female relatives with a similar condition. Twenty percent have at least one close relative (mother, aunt, or sister) with the condition, and one of Stevens and Mathews's patients had a mother, maternal grandmother, and maternal aunt similarly afflicted. The falling frequency is quite variable. Most patients fall between 2 and 12 times per year. Only one-fourth fall more than once a month or have clusters of frequent falls with prolonged asymptomatic intervals. None of the patients interviewed were aware of male relatives with the problem.

These women often scrape their hands and knees during the fall. Wrist, rib, and nose fractures occasionally occur. Rarely, head trauma and significant intercranial injury results (Rapoport 1986).

Causal factors for this strictly female condition have been elusive. Footwear, specifically high heels, is not the cause: Most patients fall while wearing low-heeled shoes or walking barefoot. Occasional patients date the onset of the disorder to early in a pregnancy, before abdominal distention would be expected to alter postural stability. When falls begin during pregnancy, the women invariably continue falling even after delivery. The perimenstrual period makes some women with this condition more vulnerable. There is no relationship between the falling and body weight. The most reasonable explanatory postulate is a prolonged long-loop (transcortical) reflex in women that delays the generation of sufficient quadriceps tension to decelerate a falling trunk (Greenwood and Hopkins 1982).

The diagnosis is made in a middle-aged woman with inexplicable falls, a normal neurological examination, and no evidence of any other known cause of falling (see Table 3.1). There is no pharmacological therapy. All that can be done is to reassure the patient, and the patient may prevent injury by using protective knee and elbow padding. Some women, fearing falls, tend to become agoraphobic; this should be countered with behavioral intervention.

THE AGED STATE

Most patients presenting to neurologists with a chief complaint of falling are elderly and chronically impaired. As the chance of falling increases with age, so does the severity of injury and the number of chronic disabilities predisposing to falls. This is well summarized by Wolfson (1992) and Black et al. (1993). Next to fractures, falls are the single most disabling condition leading to nursing home admission; as would be expected, the institutionalized elderly have the highest prevalence of falls. In the very old, falls constitute the leading source of injury-related deaths.

The normal aging process is associated with a decline in multiple physiological functions (see Chapter 87), diminishing the ability to compensate for external stressors that challenge the upright posture. Decreased proprioception, loss of muscle bulk, arthritis of the knee and ankle joints, cardiovascular disturbances, deteriorating vision and ocular motor functions (Paige 1994), cognitive impairment, and failing postural reflexes ("presbyastasis"—Norre et al. 1987) summate and increase the risk of falling. Although the healthy elderly may show normal balance on posturographic testing (Wolfson et al. 1992), there is excessive head movement during locomotion in old age (Hirasaki et al. 1993).

Most of the falling elderly have one, or more commonly several, pathological predisposing conditions, and the chance of falling increases markedly with the number of identified risk factors (Tinetti et al. 1994). A large proportion of these falls in predisposed patients are accidental, reflecting an interaction between a debilitated patient and potential environmental hazards. This should be contrasted with endogenous falls related to loss of consciousness, which are consistently less frequent. Among the important conditions associated with falls are dementia, metabolic and toxic encephalopathies, depression, cerebral infarcts, parkinsonism, neuropathy, arthritis, and gait disorders (see Chapter 26). The prevalence of gait disorders increases dramatically with age and may be found in nearly 50% of nursing home residents (Sudarsky 1990). Older adults with cognitive impairment have an even higher rate of falling (Alexander et al. 1995). Compared to the healthy elderly, patients with Alzheimer's disease have slower walking speed and more difficulty clearing obstacles.

The clinical evaluation should aim at identifying the predisposing conditions and differentiating accidental from endogenous falls. A detailed medication history is essential. Commonly used drugs such as antihypertensives, antidepressants, and tranquilizers all increase the risk of falls. Finally, a description of contributing environmental factors should be obtained either from the patients or from others familiar with their living circumstances. Poorly lit staircases with variable step height, loose carpeting, cluttered room arrangements, and lack of sturdy furniture or hand rails for support are but a few examples of environmental hazards.

Therapeutic and risk reduction intervention for the falling elderly patient requires the following (Tinetti et al. 1994): (1) treatment of correctable conditions, (2) provision of rehabilitative services and assistive devices, and (3) prevention by controlling environmental hazards. Pacemakers, supportive stockings, and medications may be helpful for patients suffering from autonomic dysfunction, cardiac dysrhythmias, and pharmacologically treatable movement disorders. Proper spectacle lenses and orthotic and other assistive devices such as walkers, canes, and crutches can return a progressively immobilized falling patient to a safer and more independent life-style. A variety of exercise programs, particularly those stressing balance components, significantly reduce the risk of falls. In addition, their beneficial effect can persist for prolonged periods of time beyond cessation of exercise (Province et al. 1995). Intensive rehabilitative efforts are indicated in patients who, after a few falls, develop a postfall syndrome consisting of phobic avoidance and restrictive behavior. This approach is indicated not only for those living independently but also for the hospitalized or institutionalized patients who make up a large proportion of the falling population.

SUMMARY

A careful history and physical examination should, in most cases, uncover the cause of falls and drops. Unfortunately, with middle-aged women and the elderly, the cause may be merely a function of sex or age. Patients with fixed motor or sensory impairments must be advised honestly about their almost unavoidable proneness to falling. Nevertheless, even without specific treatment of an underlying condition, reassurance that there is no serious neurological condition, environmental adjustments, and protective devices reduce injuries related to falls and drops.

REFERENCES

Alexander NB, Mollo JM, Giordani B et al. Maintenance of balance, gait patterns, and obstacle clearance in Alzheimer's disease. Neurology 1995;45:908–914.

Aminoff JM, Scheinman MM, Griffin JC, Herre JM. Electrocerebral accompaniments of syncope associated with malignant ventricular arrhythmias. Ann Intern Med 1988;108:791–796.

Baloh RW, Jacobson K, Winder T. Drop attacks with Ménière's syndrome. Ann Neurol 1990;28:384–387.

Black SE, Maki BE, Fernie GR. Aging, Imbalance and Falls. In JA Sharpe, HO Barber (eds), The Vestibulo-Ocular Reflex and Vertigo. New York: Raven, 1993.

D'Cruz OF, Vaughn BV, Gold SH, Greenwood RS. Symptomatic cataplexy in ponto-medullary lesions. Neurology 1994;44:2189–2191.

Egli M, Mothersill I, O'Kane M, O'Kane F. The axial spasm—the predominant type of drop seizure in patients with secondary generalized epilepsy. Epilepsia 1985;26:401–415.

Fernandez JM, Salaba F, Villaverde FJ et al. Cataplexy associated with midbrain lesion. Neurology 1995;45:393–394.

Gambardella A, Reutens DC, Anderman NF et al. Late-onset drop attacks in temporal lobe epilepsy: a reevaluation of the concept of temporal lobe syncope. Neurology 1994;44:1074–1078.

Gilchrist JW. Arrhythmogenic seizures: diagnosis by simultaneous EEG/ECG recording. Neurology 1985;35:1503–1506.

Greenwood R, Hopkins A. An attempt to explain the mechanism of drop attacks. J Neurol Sci 1982;57:203–208.

Haan J, Jansen EM, Oostrom J, Roos RA. Falling spells in normal pressure hydrocephalus: a favorable prognostic sign? Eur Neurol 1987;27:216–220.

Hirasaki E, Kubo T, Nozawa S et al. Analysis of head and body movements of elderly people during locomotion. Acta Otolaryngol Suppl (Stockh) 1993;501:25–30.

Ikeno T, Shigematsu H, Miyakoshi M et al. An analytic study of epileptic falls. Epilepsia 1985;26:612–621.

Ishizaki H, Pyykko I, Aalto H, Starck J. The Tulio phenomenon in patients with Ménière's disease as revealed with posturography. Acta Otolaryngol Suppl (Stockh) 1991;481:593–595.

Labodie EL, Awerbuch GI, Hamilton RH, Rapesak SZ. Falling and postural deficits due to acute unilateral basal ganglia lesions. Arch Neurol 1989;46:492–496.

Lee MS, Choi YC, Heo JH, Choi IS. "Drop attacks" with stiffening of the right leg associated with posterior fossa arachnoid cyst. Movement Disorders 1994;9:377–378.

Lempert T, Brandt T, Dieterich M, Huppert D. How to identify psychogenic disorders of stance and gait. J Neurol 1991;238:140–146.

Massey EW, Bowman MH, Rozear MP. Asterixis mimicking drop attacks in chronic renal failure. Neurology 1988;38:663.

Meisner I, Wiebers DO, Swanson JW, O'Fallon WM. The natural history of drop attacks. Neurology 1986;36:1029–1034.

Norre ME, Forrez G, Beckers A. Vestibular dysfunction causing instability in aged patients. Acta Otolaryngol Suppl (Stockh) 1987;104:50–55.

Paige GD. Senescence of human visual-vestibular interactions: smooth pursuit, optokinetic, and vestibular control of eye movements with aging. Exp Brain Res 1994;98:355–372.

Province MA, Hadley EC, Hornbook MC et al. for the FICSIT group. The effects of exercise on falls in elderly patients. A preplanned meta-analysis of the FICSIT trials. JAMA 1995;273:1341–1347.

Rapoport S. The management of drop attacks. DM 1986;32:122–162.

Stevens DL, Mathews WB. Cryptogenic drop attacks: an affliction of women. Br Med J 1973;1:439–442.

Sudarsky L. Geriatrics: gait disorders in the elderly. N Engl J Med 1990;322:1441–1445.

Tinetti ME, Baker DI, McAvay G et al. A multifactorial intervention to reduce the risk of falling among elderly people living in the community. N Engl J Med 1994;331:821–827.

Wolfson L. Falls and Gait. In R Katzman, JW Rowe (eds). Principles of Geriatric Neurology. Philadelphia: FA Davis, 1992.

Wolfson L, Whipple R, Derby CA et al. A dynamic posturographic study in healthy elderly. Neurology 1992;42:2069–2075.

Chapter 4
Delirium

Mario F. Mendez

Delirium is a neurobehavioral disorder characterized by an acute onset and fluctuating course of abnormal attention, disorganized thinking, an altered level of consciousness, and other cognitive and behavioral disturbances. Delirium is the most common neurobehavioral disorder seen in general hospitals (Lipowski 1990; Taylor and Lewis 1993). Among hospitalized patients, delirium occurs in about 5–15% of those on medical surgical wards, 18–30% of those in surgical intensive care units, and 2–20% of those in coronary care units (Lipowski 1990). Delirium is especially a disorder of the elderly. Among hospitalized patients who are 65 and older, 14–56% have delirium and more than half of these cases begin after admission.

Physicians have known about this disorder since antiquity (Lipowski 1990). Hippocrates referred to it as *phrenitis*, the origin of our word *frenzy*. In the first century A.D., Celsus introduced the term *delirium* from the Latin for "out of furrow," meaning derailment of the mind, and Galen observed that delirium was frequently due to physical diseases that affected the mind "sympathetically." In the nineteenth century, Gowers recognized that these patients could be either lethargic or delirious. Finally, Bonhoffer, in his classification of organic behavioral disorders, established that delerium is associated with clouding of consciousness.

Despite this long history, delirium has generated little interest or research. Delirium is frequently missed more from lack of recognition than from misdiagnosis. The lack of familiarity with the topic is reflected in the many terms used to describe this disorder: acute brain failure, acute brain syndrome, acute cerebral insufficiency, acute confusional states, acute organic syndrome, delirium, exogenous psychosis, metabolic encephalopathy, organic psychosis, toxic encephalopathy, toxic psychosis, and others.

Because much of the terminology has been borrowed from the lay language, we must first define the terms used with these disorders. *Attention* is the ability to focus on specific stimuli, to the exclusion of others. *Arousal*, a basic prerequisite for attention, indicates responsivity or excitability into action. *Coma, stupor, wakefulness,* and *alertness* are states of arousal. *Consciousness*, a product of arousal, means clarity of awareness of the environment.

CLINICAL CHARACTERISTICS

Delirium can be caused by a large number of physical illnesses. Among the American Psychiatric Association's criteria (DSM-IV, 1994) for these disorders are an acute onset with fluctuations over the course of a day, reduced ability to focus and sustain attention, disorganized thinking, and evidence of a neurological or medical cause. Furthermore, delirious patients have disorganized thinking and altered level of consciousness, perceptual disturbances, disturbance of the sleep-wake cycle, increased or decreased psychomotor activity, disorientation, and memory impairment. Other cognitive, behavioral, and emotional disturbances may also occur as part of the spectrum of delirium.

Acute Onset with Fluctuating Course

Delirium develops rapidly over hours or days, but rarely over more than a week, and fluctuations in the course occur throughout the day. Gross swings in attention, arousal, or both occur unpredictably and irregularly and become worse at night. Because of potential lucid intervals, with improved attention and awareness, medical personnel may be misled unless the patients are evaluated over time.

Attentional Deficits

A disturbance of attention is the cardinal symptom of delirium. Patients are distractable, and stimuli may gain attention indiscriminately, trivial ones often getting more attention than important ones. All components of attention are disturbed, including selectivity, sustainability, processing capacity, ease of mobilization, monitoring of the environment, and the ability to shift attention when necessary. Despite the fact that many of the same illnesses result in a spectrum of disturbances from mild inattentiveness to coma, delirium is not the same as disturbance of arousal.

Disorganized Thinking

The stream of thought is disturbed in delirium. There are multiple intrusions of competing thoughts and sensations, and patients are unable to order symbols, carry out sequenced activity, and organize goal-directed behavior. *Confusion* refers to this inability to maintain the stream of thought with the accustomed clarity, coherence, and speed.

The patient's speech reflects this jumbled thinking. Speech shifts from subject to subject and is rambling, tangential, and circumlocutory, with hesitations, repetitions, and perseverations. Decreased relevance of the speech content and decreased reading comprehension are characteristic of delirium. Confused speech is further characterized by an abnormal rate, frequent dysarthria, and nonaphasic misnaming, particularly of words related to stress or illness, such as those referable to hospitalization.

Altered Level of Consciousness

Consciousness or clarity of awareness may be disturbed. Most patients have lethargy and decreased arousal. Others, like those with delirium tremens, are hyper-alert and easily aroused. In hyper-alert patients, the extreme arousal does not preclude attentional deficits because patients are indiscriminate in their alertness, are easily distracted by irrelevant stimuli, and cannot sustain attention. The two extremes of consciousness may overlap or alternate in the same patient or may occur from the same causative factor.

Perceptual Disturbances

The most common perceptual disturbance is decreased perceptions per unit of time; patients miss things going on around them. Illusions and other misperceptions result from abnormal sensory discrimination. Perceptions may be multiple, changing, or abnormal in size or location. Hallucinations also occur, particularly in younger patients and in those in the delirium subtype. They are most frequent in the visual sphere and are often vivid, three-dimensional, and in full color. Patients may see lilliputian animals or people that appear to move about. Hallucinations are generally unpleasant, and some patients attempt to fight them or run away with fear. Some hallucinatory experiences may be release phenomena, with intrusions into wakefulness of dreams or of visual imagery. Psychotic auditory hallucinations, with voices commenting on the patient's behavior, are unusual.

Disturbed Sleep-Wake Cycle

Disruption of the day-night cycle causes excessive daytime drowsiness and reversal of the normal diurnal rhythm. "Sundowning"—with restlessness and confusion during the night—is frequent, and delirium may be manifest only at night. Nocturnal peregrinations can result in a serious problem when the delirious patient, partially clothed in a hospital gown, has to be retrieved from the hospital lobby or from the street in the middle of the night. This is one of the least specific symptoms and also occurs in dementia, depression, and other behavioral conditions. In delirium, however, disruption of circadian sleep cycles may result in rapid eye movement or dream state overflow into waking (Lipowski 1990).

Altered Psychomotor Activity

There are two subtypes of delirium, based on changes in psychomotor activity (Liptzin and Levkoff 1992). The *hypoactive subtype* is characterized by psychomotor retardation. These are the patients with lethargy and decreased arousal. The *hyperactive subtype* is usually hyper-alert and agitated and has prominent overactivity of the autonomic nervous system. Moreover, the hyperactive type is more likely to have delusions and perceptual disorders such as hallucinations. About half of delirium patients are mixed with elements of both subtypes or fluctuating between the two (Liptzin and Levkoff 1992). Only about 15% are strictly hyperactive. In addition to being younger, the hyperactive subtype has more drug-related causes, a shorter hospital stay, and a better prognosis.

Disorientation and Memory Impairment

Disturbances in orientation and memory are related. Patients are disoriented first to time of day, followed by other aspects of time, and then to place. They may have an abnormal juxtapositioning of events or places. Disorientation to person—in the sense of loss of personal identity—is rare. Disorientation is not specific for delirium; it also occurs in dementia and amnesia and can reflect disturbances in both memory and attention. Moreover, recent memory is disrupted in large part by the decreased registration caused by attentional problems.

In delirium, *reduplicative paramnesia*, a specific memory-related disorder, results from decreased integration or recent observations with past memories. Persons or places are "replaced" in this condition. In general, delirious patients tend to mistake the unfamiliar for the familiar. For example, they tend to relocate the hospital closer to their homes. In a form of reduplicative paramnesia known as *Capgras's syndrome*, however, a familiar person is mistakenly thought to be an unfamiliar imposter.

Other Cognitive Deficits

Disturbances occur in visuospatial abilities and in writing. Higher visual processing deficits include difficulties in visual object recognition, environmental orientation, and organization of drawings and other constructions.

Writing disturbance is the most sensitive language abnormality in delirium. The most salient characteristics are abnormalities in the mechanics of writing: the formation of letters and words is indistinct, and words and sentences are sprawled in different directions (Figure 4.1). Sometimes there are perseverations of loops. Spelling and syntax are also disturbed, with spelling errors particularly involving consonants, small grammatical words, and the last letters of words. Writing is easily disrupted in these disorders, possibly because it depends on multiple components and is the least-used language function.

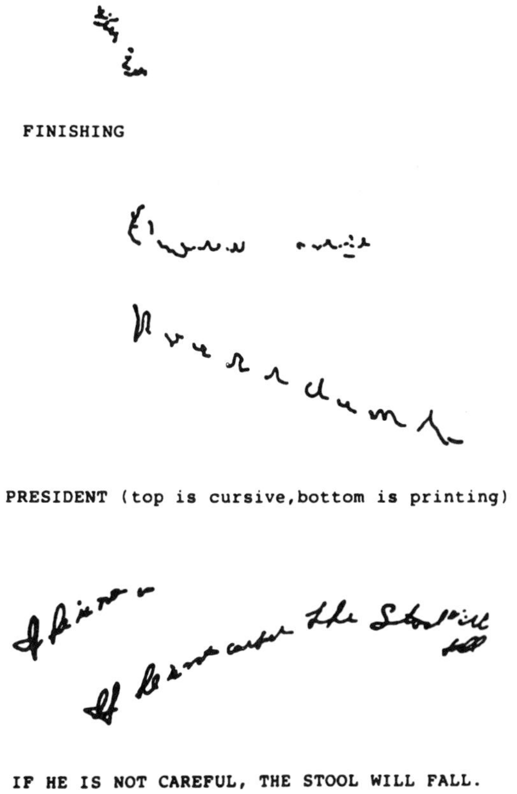

FINISHING
PRESIDENT (top is cursive,bottom is printing)
IF HE IS NOT CAREFUL, THE STOOL WILL FALL.

FIGURE 4.1 Writing disturbances in delirium. The patients were asked to write the indicated words to dictation. (Reprinted with permission from J Chédru, N Geschwind. Writing disturbance in acute confusional states. Neuropsychologia 1972;10:343–353.)

Behavioral and Emotional Abnormalities

Behavioral changes include poorly systematized delusions, often with persecutory and other paranoid ideation, and personality alterations. Delusions, like hallucinations, are probably release phenomena and are generally fleeting, changing, and readily affected by sensory input. Some patients have been described as exhibiting facetious humor and playful behavior, unconcern about their illness, poor insight, and impaired judgment.

There can be marked emotional lability. Sometimes patients are agitated and fearful; sometimes they are depressed; and sometimes they are quite apathetic. Dysphoric (unpleasant) emotional states are the more common, and emotions are not sustained. Mood changes are congruent with delusions, impaired perceptions, and hallucinations and are probably due to direct effects of the confusional state on the limbic system and its regulation of emotions.

Finally, more elementary behavioral changes may be the principal symptoms of delirium. This is especially the case in the elderly, in whom decreased activities of daily living, urinary incontinence, and frequent falls are among the major manifestations of this disorder.

PATHOPHYSIOLOGY

The pathophysiology of delirium is not entirely understood. It depends on a widely distributed neurological substrate. Normal attention requires both the ascending reticular activating system (ARAS) in the upper brain stem and polymodal association areas of the cortex. Stimulation of the ARAS elicits arousal, and lesions of the ARAS may result in sleep, coma, or akinetic mutism, rather than attentional problems or delirium (see Chapters 5 and 73). The ARAS primes the cortex for stimulus reception, while the polymodal association cortex controls and focuses this arousal energy for attention. The prefrontal cortex is involved in maintaining the attention system, and the parietal cortex

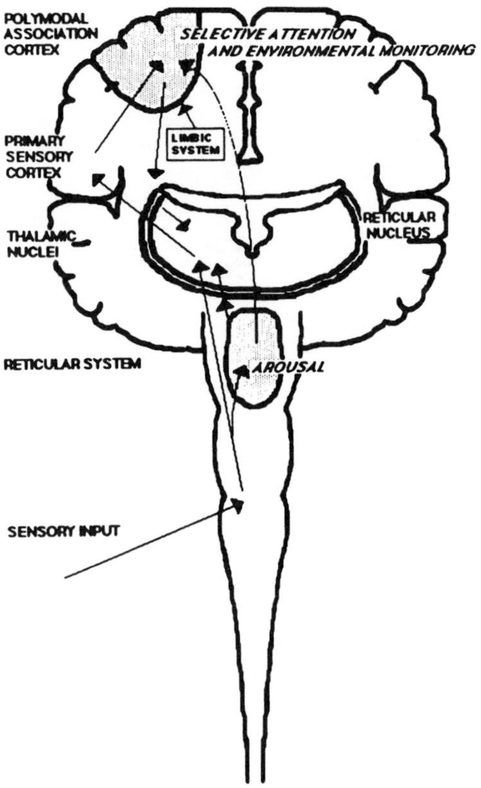

FIGURE 4.2 Pathways of the attention system. Sensory input is relayed from the thalamus to the primary sensory areas where selective attention occurs. These cortical areas have connections with other structures that affect attention, such as the limbic system and the basal ganglia. The important polymodal areas are the prefrontal cortex and the posterior parietal cortex, particularly in the right hemisphere. Environmental monitoring and the "gate" function of attention may occur through feedback from these areas to the nucleus reticularis of the thalamus, a modulator of sensory input.

may play a role in shifting attention. Cortical blood flow studies suggest that these polymodal cortical areas and their limbic connections are the "attentional gate" for sensory input through feedback to the reticular nucleus of the thalamus (Figure 4.2). In addition, there is evidence that the right hemisphere is dominant for attention, although split brain studies clearly point out the need for bihemispheric cooperation in maintaining attention.

A second explanation for delirium is alterations in neurotransmitters, particularly the cholinergic system (Francis 1992). Anticholinergic agents can induce delirium, which is reversible with the administration of anticholinergic medications such as physostigmine. Moreover, cholinergic neurons project to the cortex from the pons and the basal forebrain and make cortical neurons more responsive to other inputs. A decrease in acetylcholine results in decreased perfusion in the frontal cortex. Furthermore, hypoglycemia, hypoxia, and other metabolic changes may differentially affect acetylcholine-mediated functions.

Any explanation of delirium must take into account not only specific structural lesions and neurotransmitter changes but also the diffuse metabolic causes that can result in the same disturbances of attention. The diffuse causes, the universal susceptibility to developing delirium, and the minimal or nonspecific pathological changes suggest an impairment of some common metabolic pathways in nerve cells. Metabolic pathways involving the ARAS and the polymodal cortex may be more vulnerable because these two areas have the most polysynaptic chains.

DIAGNOSIS OF DELIRIUM

Diagnosis is a two-step process. The first step is the recognition of delirium, which requires a thorough history, a bedside mental status examination focusing on attention, and a review of established diagnostic scales or criteria for delirium. The second step is identifying the cause from a large number of potential diagnoses. Since the clinical manifestations offer few clues to the cause, the differential diagnosis relies primarily on the general history, the physical examination, and the laboratory assessment.

History

Although a patient may state that he or she cannot think straight or concentrate, a family member or other good historian should be available to describe the patient's behavior and past medical history. The observer may have noted early symptoms of delirium, such as inability to perform at a usual level, decreased awareness of complex details, insomnia, and frightening or vivid dreams. Furthermore, it is crucial to obtain accurate information about systemic illnesses, drug use, recent trauma, occupational and environmental exposures, malnutrition, allergies, and any preceding symptoms leading up to a confusional state.

The patient's risk factors for delirium should be assessed. The most important risk factor is dementia (Inouye et al. 1993; Levkoff et al. 1992). As many as one-half of hospitalized patients with delirium have an underlying dementia, and many of the rest have some baseline cognitive impairment. Advanced age itself seems to be an independent risk factor, especially for those over age 80 (Schor et al. 1992). Many of these elderly patients predisposed to delirium have cerebral atrophy or white matter and basal ganglia ischemic changes on neuroimaging. A third factor is the severity of the illness and the degree of physical impairment (Inouye et al. 1993). Additional risk factors include visual impairment (less than 20/70 binocular); hip and other bone fractures; dehydration, serum sodium changes, and azotemia; infections and fevers; and the use of psychoactive drugs and narcotics. Particularly noteworthy are the presence of a multiple drug regimen and the use of drugs with anticholinergic properties. The predisposing factors are additive, each new factor increasing the risk considerably.

Sensory overstimulation or understimulation facilitates confusional behavior, probably because optimal attention requires an optimal amount of sensory input. Novel situations and unfamiliar surroundings contribute to sensory overstimulation in the elderly, and sensory overload may be a factor in producing "ICU psychosis" in intensive care units. Immobilization, with decreased kinesthetic inputs, contributes to sensory deprivation. Going several days without sleep may cause confusion; however, it is not the decreased total amount of sleep that predisposes to delirium but the resulting disruption of circadian sleep cycles.

Mental Status Examination

Initial general behavioral observations are an important part of the neurological mental status examination. The most important are observations of attentiveness and arousability. Attention may wander so much that it must constantly be brought back to the subject at hand. General behavior may range from falling asleep during the interview to agitation and combativeness. The examiner may note slow and loosely connected thinking and speech, with irrelevancies, perseverations, repetitions, and intrusions. Patients may propagate their errors in thinking and perception by elaboration and by bringing other observations into agreement with them. Finally, the examiner should evaluate the patient's general appearance and grooming, motor activity and spontaneity, mood and affect, and propriety and witticisms, and the presence of any special preoccupations or inaccurate perceptions.

Bedside tests of attention can be divided into serial recitation tasks, continuous performance tasks, and alternate response tasks. The digit span test is a serial recitation task in which a series of digits is presented, one digit per second, and the patient is asked to repeat the entire sequence immediately after presentation. Perceptual clumping is avoided by the use of random digits and a regular rhythm of presentation. Recitation of seven (plus or minus two) digits correctly is considered normal. The serial reversal test is a form of recitation task in which the patient recites backward a digit span, the spelling of a word such as *world*, or the results of counting by ones, threes, or sevens from a predetermined number. Continuous performance tasks include the A vigilance test, in which the patient must indicate whenever he or she hears the letter A among random letters presented one per second. This can also be done by asking the patient to cross out every instance of a particular letter in a magazine or newspaper paragraph. Alternate response tasks are exemplified by the repetition of a three-step motor sequence (palm-side-fist), which is also a test of frontal functions. These attentional tests are not overly specific, and they can be affected by the patient's educational background, the degree of effort, or the presence of other cognitive deficits. In sum, the best assessment of attention may be the general behavioral observations; the tests should be used to help document and confirm the initial impression of an acute confusional state.

Attentional or arousal deficits may preclude the opportunity to pursue the mental status examination much further, but the examiner should attempt to assess orientation and other areas of cognition. Patients who are off 3 days on the date, 2 days on the day of the week, or 4 hours on the time of day may be significantly disoriented to time. The examiner should inquire whether the patient knows where he or she is, what kind of a place it is, and under what circumstances he or she is there. Disturbed recent memory is demonstrated by asking the patient to retain the examiner's name or three words for 5 minutes. A language examination should distinguish between the language of confusion and that of a primary aphasia (see discussion of special problems in diagnosis below). Attempts at simple constructions, such as copying a cube, may be unsuccessful. Hallucinations can sometimes be brought out by holding a white piece of paper or an imaginary string between the fingers and asking the patient to describe what he or she sees.

Diagnostic Scales and Criteria

The clinical criteria for the diagnosis of delirium vary greatly (Liptzin et al. 1993). Moreover, the usual mental status scales and tests may not help in differentiating delirium from dementia and other cognitive disturbances. Because of the variability in diagnosis, specific scales and criteria have been developed for the diagnosis of delirium. Foremost among these are the DSM-IV criteria for delirium. Investigators have criticized these criteria because of the required disturbance of consciousness and the broadness of the criteria of a "change in cognition." Among more recent structured interviews for delirium, the Confusion Assessment Method relies on the presence of an acute onset with a fluctuating course, attentional deficits, and either disorganized thinking or alteration in consciousness (Inouye et al. 1990). The diagnosis of delirium is facilitated by the use of this interview, along with the history from collateral sources such as family and nursing notes and a mental status examination focusing on attention.

Physical Examination

The physical examination should elicit any signs of systemic illness, focal neurological abnormalities, meningism, increased intracranial pressure, extracranial cerebrovascular disease, or head trauma. In acute confusional states, less specific findings include an action or sustention tremor of high frequency at about 8–10 Hz, asterixis or brief lapses in tonic posture especially at the wrist, multifocal myoclonus or shocklike jerks from diverse sites, choreiform movements, dysarthria, and gait instability. Patients may manifest agitation or psychomotor retardation, apathy, waxy flexibility, catatonia, or carphologia ("lint-picking" behavior). The presence of hyperactivity of the autonomic nervous system may be life-threatening because of possible dehydration, electrolyte disturbances, or tachyarrhythmias.

Laboratory Tests

Electroencephalographic (EEG) changes virtually always accompany delirium when the EEGs are followed serially over time (see Chapter 37A). Disorganization of the usual cerebral rhythms and generalized slowing are the most common changes (Taylor and Lewis 1993). The mean EEG frequency or degree of slowing correlates with the degree of delirium. Both hypoactive and hyperactive subtypes of delirium have similar EEG slowing; however, predominant low-voltage fast activity is also present on withdrawal from sedative drugs or alcohol. Additional EEG patterns from intracranial causes of delirium include focal slowing, asymmetrical delta activity, and paroxysmal discharges (spikes, sharp waves, spike and wave complexes). Periodic complexes, such as triphasic waves, and periodic lateralizing epileptiform discharges (PLEDs) may help in the differential diagnosis (see Chapter 37A). In sum, EEGs are of value in deciding whether confusional behavior may be due to an intracranial cause, in making the diagnosis of delirium in patients with unclear behavior, in evaluating demented patients who might have a superimposed delirium, in differentiating delirium from schizophrenia and other primary psychiatric states, and in following the course of delirium over time (Figure 4.3).

Other essential laboratory tests include a complete blood count; measurements of glucose, electrolytes, blood urea nitrogen, creatinine, transaminase, and ammonia levels; thyroid function tests; arterial blood gas studies; chest x-ray films; electrocardiogram; urinalysis; and urine drug screening. Although nonspecific, evoked potential studies often show prolonged latencies. The need for a lumbar puncture deserves special comment. This valuable test, which is often neglected in the evaluation of patients with confusional states, should be performed as part of the workup when the cause is uncertain. The lumbar puncture should be preceded by a computed tomographic or magnetic resonance imaging scan of the brain if there are focal neurological findings or suspicions of increased intracranial pressure, a space-occupying lesion, or head trauma.

DIFFERENTIAL DIAGNOSIS

The following discussion is a selective commentary that illustrates some basic principles and helps organize the approach to working through the large differential diagnosis. Almost any sufficiently severe medical or surgical illness can cause delirium, and the best advice is to follow all available diagnostic leads. For further discussion of individual entities, the reader should refer to corresponding chapters in this book. The confusion-inducing effects of these disturbances are additive, and there may be more than one causal factor, the individual contribution of which cannot be elucidated. Nearly one-half of elderly patients with delirium have more than one cause for their disorder. Of the following eight categories of causes for delirium, the most common among the elderly are metabolic disturbances, infection, stroke, and drugs, particularly anticholinergic and narcotic medications (Lipowski 1990). The most common causes among the young are drug abuse and alcohol withdrawal.

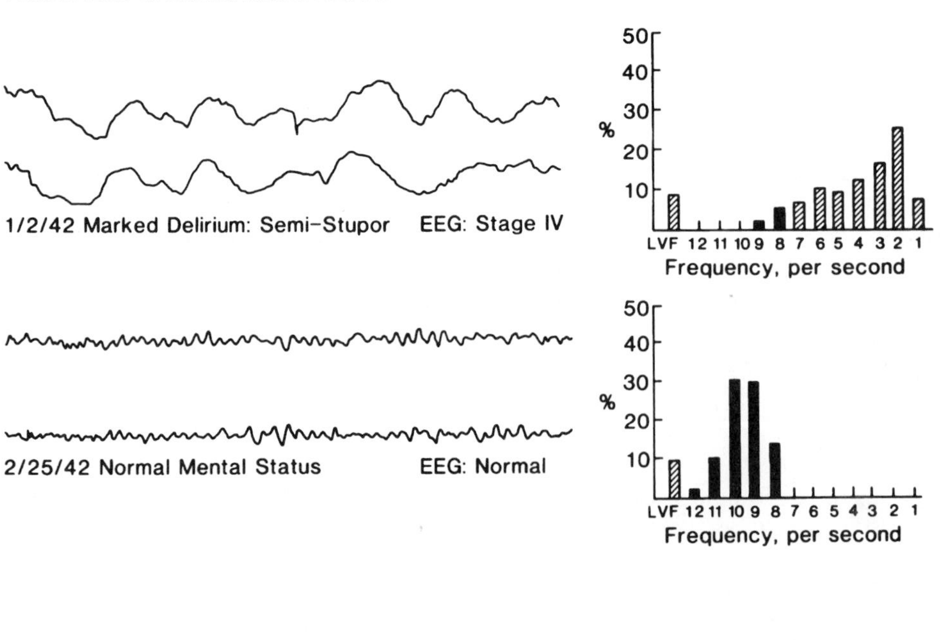

FIGURE 4.3 Electroencephalogram showing changes due to delirium. (Reprinted with permission from J Romano, GL Engel. Delirium. 1. EEG data. Arch Neurol Psychiatry 1944;51:356. Copyright ® 1944, American Medical Association.)

Metabolic Disturbances

Metabolic disturbances are the most common causes of delirium (see Chapters 56, 62, 63, 64). Fortunately, the examination and routine laboratory tests outlined above screen for most acquired metabolic disturbances that might be encountered. Because of the potential for life-threatening or permanent damage, some of these conditions—particularly hypoxia and hypoglycemia—must be considered immediately. Also consider dehydration, fluid and electrolyte disorders, and disturbances of calcium and magnesium. The rapidity of change in an electrolyte level may be just as important a factor as its absolute value for the development of delirium. For example, some people tolerate chronic sodium levels of 115 mEq/liter or less, but a rapid fall to this level can precipitate delirium, seizures, or even central pontine myelinolysis. Hypoperfusion from low cardiac output or heart failure is another common cause of delirium. Also consider other major organ failures, such as liver and kidney failure, including the possibility of unusual causes, such as undetected portocaval shunting or acute pancreatitis with the release of lipases. Delirium caused by endocrine dysfunction often has prominent affective symptoms, such as hyperthyroidism and Cushing's syndrome. Delirium occasionally results from toxins including industrial agents, pollutants, and heavy metals such as arsenic, bismuth, gold, lead, mercury, thallium, and zinc. Other considerations are inborn errors of metabolism such as acute intermittent porphyria. Finally, it is particularly important to consider the thiamine deficiency state. In alcoholics and others at risk, thiamine must be given immediately to avoid precipitating Wernicke's encephalopathy with the administration of glucose.

Drugs

Drug intoxication and drug withdrawal are among the most common causes of delirium. Drug effects are additive, and delirium may occur especially with drugs that have anticholinergic properties, including many over-the-counter cold preparations, antihistamines, antidepressants, and neuroleptics. Patients with anticholinergic intoxication present "hot as a hare, blind as a bat, dry as a bone, red as a beet, mad as a hatter," reflecting fever, dilated pupils, dry mouth, flushing, and a confusional state. Other important groups of drugs associated with delirium, especially in the elderly, are sedative-hypnotics, narcotic analgesics, and histamine-2 receptor blockers (Francis 1992). Antiparkinsonian drugs result in confusion, with prominent hallucinations and delusions in patients with Parkinson's disease, who are particularly susceptible. Corticosteroid psychosis has to be considered in those who develop delirium on the equivalent of 40 mg/day or more of prednisone. The behavioral effects of corticosteroids often begin with euphoria and hypomania and proceed to a hyperactive delirium. Any drug, such as metrizamide, that is administered intrathecally is prone to induce confusional behavior. Drug withdrawal syndromes can be caused by many agents, including barbiturates and other minor tranquilizers, sedative-hypnotics, amphetamines, cocaine or "crack," and, of course, alcohol. Delirium tremens begins 72–96 hours after alcohol withdrawal, with profound agitation, tremulousness, diaphoresis, tachycardia, fever, and frightening visual hallucinations.

Infections

Infections and fevers frequently produce delirium. The main offenders are urinary tract infections, pneumonias, and septicemia. In a sporadic encephalitis or meningoencephalitis, important causal considerations are herpes simplex virus, Lyme disease, and acquired immune deficiency syndrome (AIDS) (see Chapter 60). Patients with AIDS may be delirious because of the causative virus itself or because of an opportunistic infection. Immunocompromised patients are at greater risk of infection, and any suspicion of infection should prompt urine, sputum, blood, and cerebrospinal fluid cultures.

Strokes

Delirium can be the nonspecific consequence of any acute stroke, but postinfarct confusion usually resolves in 24–48 hours (see Chapter 58). Sustained delirium can result from specific strokes including right middle cerebral artery infarcts affecting frontal and posterior parietal areas (Mori and Yamadori 1987) and posterior cerebral artery infarcts resulting in either bilateral or left-sided occipitotemporal lesions (fusiform gyrus). The latter lesions usually involve the left hemisphere, may be slowly progressive, and can lead to agitation, visual field changes, and even Anton's syndrome (Devinsky et al. 1988). Delirium may also follow occlusion of the anterior cerebral artery or rupture of the anterior communicating artery with involvement of the anterior cingulate gyrus and septal region.

Other cerebrovascular conditions include high-grade bilateral carotid stenosis, hypertensive encephalopathy, subarachnoid hemorrhage, and central nervous system vasculitides such as systemic lupus erythematosus, temporal arteritis, and Behçet's syndrome. Migraine can present with delirium, particularly in children. It must be emphasized that the incidence of delirium in transient ischemic attacks, even in vertebrobasilar insufficiency, is low; such attacks should not be considered the cause of delirium unless there are other neurological signs and an appropriate time course.

Epilepsy

Abnormal brain electrical activity is associated with delirium in four conditions: (1) ictally, with absence status, partial complex status, tonic status without convulsions, or PLEDs (Terzano et al. 1986); (2) postictally, after partial complex or generalized tonic-clonic seizures (see Chapter 72); (3) interictally, including epileptic delirium, manifested as increasing irritability, agitation, and affective symptoms associated with impending seizures; and (4) from cognitive effects of anticonvulsant medications.

Perioperative Causes

The cause of delirium in perioperative patients is multifactorial. Perioperative factors include residual anesthetic and drug effects, especially following premedication with anticholinergic drugs; postoperative hypoxia; perioperative hypotension; electrolyte imbalances; infections; psychological stress; and multiple awakenings with fragmented sleep. Postoperative delirium may start at any time but often becomes evident about the third day and abates by the seventh, but may last considerably longer. Patients over 60 years of age who are undergoing cardiac or eye surgery are at special risk. Delirium occurs in 30% of patients after open heart or coronary artery bypass surgery (Smith and Dimsdale 1989). Additional factors are decreased postoperative cardiac output and length of time on cardiopulmonary bypass, with its added risk for microemboli. Cataract surgery is associated with a 7% incidence of acute confusional states, possibly because of sensory deprivation. Prostate surgery patients may develop water intoxication due to absorption of irrigation water from the bladder.

Other Neurological Causes

In a sporadic encephalitis or meningoencephalitis, important causal considerations are herpes simplex virus; *Borrelia burgdorferi*, the organism for Lyme disease; and human immunodeficiency virus, the organism for AIDS (see Chapter 60E). Patients with AIDS may be in a confusional state because of the causative virus itself or because of an opportunistic infection. Other central nervous system disturbances predispose to delirium. In general, patients with dementia, Lewy body disease, Parkinson's disease, and atrophy or subcortical ischemic changes on neuroimaging are particularly susceptible. Electroconvulsive therapy in these patients often produces a delirium of a week or more. Head trauma can result in delirium as a consequence of brain concussion, brain contusion, intracranial hematoma, or subarachnoid hemorrhage. Moreover, subdural hematomas can occur in the elderly with little or no history of head injury. Rapidly growing tumors in the supratentorial region are especially likely to cause delirium with increased intracranial pressure. Paraneoplastic processes produce limbic encephalitis and multifocal leukoencephalitis. Delirium can result from acute demyelinating diseases and other diffuse multifocal lesions and from communicating or noncommunicating hydrocephalus. In transient global amnesia, there is initial delirium, disproportionate anterograde amnesia, some retrograde amnesia for the preceding hours, and improvement within 24 hours. In Wernicke's encephalopathy, there is delirium accompanied by oculomotor paresis, nystagmus, ataxia, and, frequently, residual amnesia (Korsakoff's psychosis).

Miscellaneous Causes

A variety of other disturbances can produce delirium. Bone fractures are associated with delirium in the elderly, and about 50% of those admitted with a hip fracture have delirium (Schor et al. 1992). In orthopedic cases, the possibility of fat emboli requires evaluation of urine, sputum, or cerebrospinal fluid for fat (Jacobson et al. 1986). ICU psychosis is associated with sleep deprivation, immobilization, unfamiliarity, fear, and frightening sensory overstimulation or sensory deprivation. Delirium results from blood dyscrasias, including anemia, thrombocytopenia, and disseminated intravascular coagulopathy. Finally, physical factors such as heatstroke, electrocution, and hypthermia should be considered.

SPECIAL PROBLEMS IN DIFFERENTIAL DIAGNOSIS

Delirium must be distinguished from dementia, Wernicke's aphasia, and psychiatric conditions (see Chapters 7, 9, 12, and 71). The usual cognitive scales used in dementia screening may not reliably distinguish between dementia and delirium. The main differentiating features of dementia are the longer time course and the absence of prominent fluctuating attentional and perceptual deficits. Chronic confusional states lasting 6 months or more are a form of dementia. Patients with delirium that becomes chronic tend to settle into a lethargic state that is not as inattentive or fluctuating throughout the day, and they have fewer perceptual problems and less disruption of the day-night cycle. In addition, delirium and dementia often overlap, because demented patients have an increased susceptibility for developing a superimposed delirium. Demented patients who suddenly get worse should always be evaluated for delirium.

The language examination should distinguish Wernicke's aphasia from the language of delirium. Aphasics have prominent paraphasias of all types, including neologisms, and they have relatively preserved axial or whole body commands. Their agraphia is also empty of content and paragraphic, as compared to the mechanical and other writing disturbances previously described for patients with delirium.

Psychiatric conditions that may be mistaken for delirium include schizophrenia, depression, mania, attention deficit disorder, autism, dissociative states, and Ganser's syndrome,

Table 4.1: Special problems in the differential diagnosis of delirium*

Clinical Feature	*Delirium*	*Progressive Dementias*	*Stroke with Wernicke's Aphasia*	*Schizophrenia*
Course	Acute onset; hours, days, or more	Insidious onset; months or years; progressive	Sudden onset; chronic, stable deficit	Insidious onset, 6 months or more; acute psychotic phases
Attention	Markedly impaired attention and arousal	Normal early; impairment later	Normal	Normal to mild impairment
Fluctuation	Prominent in attention arousal; disturbed day-night cycle	Prominent fluctuations absent; lesser disturbances in day-night cycle	Absent	Absent
Perception	Misperceptions; hallucinations, usually visual, fleeting; paramnesia	Perceptual abnormalities much less prominent; paramnesia	Normal	Hallucinations, auditory with personal reference
Speech and language	Abnormal clarity; speed and coherence; disjointed and dysarthric; misnaming; characteristic dysgraphia	Early anomia; empty speech; abnormal comprehension	Prominent paraphasias and neologisms; empty speech; abnormal comprehension	Disorganized, with a bizarre theme
Other cognition	Disorientation to time, place; recent memory and visuospatial abnormalities	Disorientation to time, place; multiple other higher cognitive deficits	No other necessary deficits	Disorientation to person; concrete interpretations
Behavior	Lethargy or delirium; nonsystematized delusions; emotional lability	Disinterested; disengaged; disinhibited; delusions and other psychiatric symptoms	Paranoia may ensue	Systematized delusions; paranoia; bizarre behavior
Electroencephalogram	Diffuse slowing; low-voltage fast activity; specific patterns	Normal early; mild slowing later	Normal	Normal

* The characteristics listed are the relative and usual ones and are not exclusive.

which is characterized by ludicrous or approximate responses. In general, patients with psychiatric conditions lack the fluctuating attentional and related deficits described for those with delirium. Schizophrenic patients may have a very disturbed verbal output, but their speech often has an underlying bizarre theme. Schizophrenic hallucinations are more often consistent persecutory voices rather than fleeting visual images, and their delusions are more systematized and have personal reference. Conversely, delirious hallucinations are usually visual, and their delusions are more transitory and fragmented. Mood disorders may also be mistaken for delirium, particularly if there is an acute, agitated depression or a predominantly irritable mania. Finally, a general rule is that psychiatric behaviors may be due to delirium, especially if they occur in someone who is 40 or older without a prior psychiatric history.

Table 4.1 outlines the special problems that must be considered in the differential diagnosis of acute confusional states.

MANAGEMENT

Like its diagnosis, the management of delirium is a two-step process. First, attention is aimed at finding the cause and eliminating it. Second, the delirium is managed with symptomatic measures. These measures involve attention to fluid and electrolyte balance, nutritional status, and early treatment of infections. One should also maintain a moderate sensory balance in the patient by avoiding sensory overstimulation or deprivation. It is desirable to limit ambient noise and the number of visits from strangers and to provide a radio or a television set, eyeglasses and hearing aids, and a night-light. The environment should be structured to reduce unfamiliarity by providing a calendar, a clock, family pictures, and personal objects and by promoting social support, including frequent family visits and a full-time attendant. The patient should receive emotional support and provisions for frequent reorientation to place, time, and situation. As much as possible, everything should be explained. Delusions and hallucinations should be neither endorsed nor challenged. Other symptomatic measures include providing soft music and warm baths and allowing the patient to take walks when possible.

In general, it is best to avoid the use of drugs in confused patients, because they further cloud the picture and may worsen the delirium. All the patient's medications should be reviewed, and any unnecessary drugs should be discontinued. When medication is needed, these patients should receive the lowest possible dose and should not get drugs such as phenobarbital, which can cause a paradoxical reaction. Many patients benefit from regulation of the sleep-wake cycle and from a good night's sleep, provided by hypnotics such as chloral hydrate or temazepam. Medication may be necessary if the patient's behavior is potentially dangerous, interferes with medical care, or causes the patient profound distress. Drug treatment can be directed at anxiety, fear, paranoia, hallucinations, delusions, agitation, and aggression. The most commonly used drugs are haloperidol (starting at 0.5 mg daily), and lorazepam (starting at 0.5–0.1 mg daily). The issue of whether these chemical restraints are better than physical restraint is controversial. One form of restraint may work better than the other in individual patients; however, physical restraints should be avoided as much as possible and a sitter used instead.

PROGNOSIS

If the causative factor is corrected, the prognosis is good in most cases, though not in all. The average duration of a confused state is a few days to 2 weeks; however, this duration is longer in the elderly. Older patients may not recover back to baseline (Francis and Kapoor 1992; Levkoff et al. 1992). A partial delirium, which meets some but not all criteria, occurs in about one-third of postdelirium elderly, and less than 20% have returned to their baseline by 6 months. Moreover, after delirium, elderly patients often have a decline in activities of daily living and increased likelihood of nursing home placement. Delirium is also associated with increased mortality, but this is due to underlying dementia, advanced age, and severity of illness. In the elderly, delirium may unmask dementia and impaired brain reserve, or alternatively, may include neurological damage.

Children may also show residual deficits, with regression and persistence of mild perceptual motor abnormalities and learning difficulties. In general, improved prognosis should follow an increased awareness of delirium, with more rapid diagnosis of the causative factor and better overall management. One final reason for the vigorous management of delirium is that delirium itself is a stressor that may lead to depression or posttraumatic stress disorder.

REFERENCES

Chédru J, Geschwind N. Writing disturbance in acute confusional states. Neuropsychologia 1972;10:343–353.

Devinsky O, Bear D, Volpe BT. Confusional states following posterior cerebral artery infarction. Arch Neurol 1988;45:160–163.

Diagnostic and Statistical Manual of Mental Disorders (4th ed) (DSM-IV). Washington, DC: American Psychiatric Association, 1994.

Francis J. Delirium in older patients. J Am Geriatr Soc 1992;40:829–838.

Francis J, Kapoor WN. Prognosis after hospital discharge of older medical patients with delirium. J Am Geriatr Soc 1992;40:601–606.

Inouye SK, van Dyck CH, Alessi CA et al. Clarifying confusion: the confusion assessment method (a new method for detection of delirium). Ann Intern Med 1990;113:941–948.

Inouye SK, Viscoli CM, Horwitz RI et al. A predictive model for delirium in hospitalized elderly medical patients based on admission characteristics. Ann Intern Med 1993;119:474–481.

Jacobson DM, Terrence CF, Reinmuth OM. The neurological manifestations of fat embolism. Neurology 1986;36:847–851.

Levkoff SE, Evans DA, Liptzin B et al. Delirium: the occurrence and persistence of symptoms among elderly hospitalized patients. Arch Intern Med 1992;152:334–340.

Lipowski ZJ. Delirium: Acute Confusional States. New York: Oxford University Press, 1990.

Liptzin B, Levkoff SE. An empirical study of delirium subtypes. Br J Psychiatry 1992;161:843–845.

Liptzin B, Levkoff SE, Gottlieb GL, Johnson JC. Delirium. J Neuropsychiatry Clin Neurosci 1993;5:154–160.

Mori E, Yamadori A. Acute confusional state and acute agitated delirium: occurrence after infarction in the right middle cerebral artery territory. Arch Neurol 1987;44:1139–1143.

Romano J, Engel GL. Delirium: 1. EEG data. Arch Neurol Psychiatry 1944;51:356.

Schor JD, Levkoff SE, Lipsitz LA et al. Risk factors for delirium in hospitalized elderly. JAMA 1992;267:827–831.

Smith LW, Dimsdale JE. Postcardiotomy delirium: conclusions after 25 years? Am J Psychiatry 1989;146:452–458.

Taylor D, Lewis S. Delirium. J Neurol Neurosurg Psychiatry 1993;56:742–751.

Terzano MG, Parrino L, Mazzucchi A, Moretti G. Confusional states with periodic lateralized epileptiform discharges (PLEDs). Epilepsia 1986;27:446–457.

Chapter 5
Clinical Approach to Stupor and Coma

Joseph R. Berger

DEFINITIONS

Consciousness may be defined as a state of awareness of self and surroundings. Alterations in consciousness are conceptualized into two types. One, which affects arousal, is the subject of this chapter. The other involves cognitive and affective mental function, sometimes referred to as the "content" of mental function. Examples of the latter type of alteration in consciousness include dementia (see Chapter 7), delusions, confusion, and inattention (see Chapter 9). These altered states of consciousness, with the exception of advanced dementia, do not affect the level of arousal. Sleep, the only normal form of altered consciousness, is discussed in Chapter 6.

The term *delirium* describes a clouding of consciousness with reduced ability to sustain attention to environmental stimuli (Taylor and Lewis 1993). Diagnostic criteria for delirium from the DSM-III-R include at least two of the following: (1) perceptual disturbance (misinterpretations, illusions, or hallucinations), (2) incoherent speech at times, (3) disturbance of sleep-wake cycle, and (4) increased or decreased psychomotor activity (DSM-III-R 1987). Delirium is a good example of a confusional state in which a mild decline in arousal may be clinically difficult to separate from a change in cognitive or affective mental function. In clinical practice, the exact boundary between different forms of altered consciousness may be vague.

Alterations in arousal, though often referred to as levels of consciousness, do not actually form discrete levels but rather are made up of a continuum of subtly changing behavioral states that range from alert to comatose. It is clinically important to note that these states are dynamic and thus may change with time. Four points on the continuum of arousal are often used in describing the clinical state of a patient: alert, lethargic, stuporous, and comatose. *Alert* refers to a perfectly normal state of arousal. *Stupor* is defined as "unresponsiveness from which the subject can be aroused only by vigorous and repeated stimuli." *Coma* is "unarousable unresponsiveness," in which the patient lies with the eyes closed (Plum and Posner 1980). *Lethargy* lies between alertness and stupor. The terms *lethargy* and *stupor* cover a broad area on the continuum of behavioral states and thus are subject to misinterpretation by subsequent observers of a patient when used without further qualification. In clinical practice, where relatively slight changes in arousal may be significant, only the terms *alert* and *comatose* (the endpoints of the continuum) have enough precision to be used without further qualification.

Table 5.1: Behavioral states confused with coma

Behavioral State	*Definition*	*Lesion*	*Comments*
Locked-in syndrome	Alert and aware, quadriplegic with lower cranial nerve palsy	Bilateral anterior pontine	A similar state may be seen with severe polyneuropathies, myasthenia gravis, and neuromuscular blocking agents.
Persistent vegetative state	Absent cognitive function but retained "vegetative" components	Extensive cortical gray or subcortical white matter with relative preservation of brain stem	Synonyms include apallic syndrome, coma vigile, cerebral cortical death.
Abulia	Severe apathy, patient neither speaks nor moves spontaneously	Bilateral frontal medial	Severe cases resemble akinetic mutism, but patient is alert and aware.
Catatonia	Mute, with marked decrease in motor activity	Usually psychiatric	May be mimicked by frontal lobe dysfunction or drugs.
Pseudocoma	Feigned coma		

BEHAVIORAL STATES CONFUSED WITH COMA

Several different behavioral states may appear similar to coma or may be confused with it (Table 5.1). Moreover, patients who survive initial coma may progress to certain of these syndromes after varying lengths of time. Once sleep-wake cycles occur, true coma is no longer present. Differentiation of these states from true coma is important to administer appropriate therapy and to help determine prognosis.

In the *locked-in syndrome (de-efferented state),* patients are alert and aware of their environment but are quadriplegic, with lower cranial nerve palsies because of bilateral ventral pontine lesions that involve the corticospinal, corticopontine, and corticobulbar tracts. The patients are awake and alert but voluntarily able only to move their eyes vertically, to blink, or both. The locked-in syndrome is most often observed as a consequence of pontine infarction accompanying basilar artery thrombosis. Other causes include central pontine myelinolysis and brain stem mass lesions. A state similar to the locked-in syndrome may also be seen with severe polyneuropathy—in particular, acute inflammatory demyelinating polyradiculoneuropathy, myasthenia gravis, and neuromuscular blocking agents.

In the *persistent vegetative state*, patients have lost cognitive neurological function but retain vegetative or noncognitive neurological function such as cardiac action, respiration, and maintenance of blood pressure (ANA Committee on Ethical Affairs 1993). This state follows coma and is characterized by the absence of cognitive function or awareness of the environment, despite a preserved sleep-wake cycle. Spontaneous movements may occur and the eyes may open in response to external stimuli, but the patient does not speak or obey commands. A number of poorly defined syndromes have been used synonymously with persistent vegetative state, including *apallic syndrome* or *state, akinetic mutism, coma vigil, alpha coma, neocortical death*, and *permanent unconsciousness*. These terms, used variously by different authors, are probably best avoided because of their lack of precision (ANA Committee on Ethical Affairs 1993). The diagnosis of persistent vegetative state should be made cautiously and only after extended periods of observation (Childs et al. 1993).

Abulia is a severe apathy in which patients have blunting of feeling, drive, mentation, and behavior such that they neither speak nor move spontaneously (Mesulam 1986). Severe cases resemble akinetic mutism, except that the patients remain alert and aware of their environment.

Catatonia may result in a state of muteness, with dramatically decreased motor activity. The maintenance of body posture, with preserved ability to sit or stand, distinguishes it from organic pathological stupor. It is generally a psychiatric manifestation but may be mimicked by frontal lobe dysfunction or drug effect.

Pseudocoma is the term for patients who appear comatose (that is, unresponsive, unarousable, or both) but have no structural, metabolic, toxic, or psychiatric disorder.

APPROACH TO COMA

The initial clinical approach to stupor and coma is based on the principle that *all* alterations in arousal are acute, life-threatening emergencies until vital functions such as blood pressure and oxygenation are stabilized, potentially reversible causes of coma are treated, and the underlying cause of the alteration in arousal is understood. Urgent steps may be necessary to avoid or minimize permanent brain damage from reversible causes. In view of the urgency of this situation, every physician should develop a diagnostic and therapeutic routine to use with a patient with an alteration in consciousness. A basic understanding of the mechanisms that lead to impairment in arousal is necessary to develop this routine. The anatomical and physiological bases for alterations in arousal are discussed in Chapter 73.

Although one should keep in mind the concept of a spectrum of arousal, for the sake of simplicity and brevity we use only the term *coma* in the rest of this chapter. Table 5.2 lists many of the common causes of coma. More than half of all cases of coma are due to diffuse and metabolic brain dysfunction. In Plum and Posner's study (1995) of 500 patients initially diagnosed as having coma of unknown cause (in whom the diagnosis was ultimately established), 326 patients had diffuse and metabolic brain dysfunction. Almost half of these had drug poisonings. Of the remaining patients, 101 had supratentorial mass lesions, including 77 hemorrhagic lesions and nine infarctions; 65 had subtentorial lesions, mainly brain stem infarctions; and eight had psychiatric coma.

A logical decision tree often used in searching for the cause of coma divides the categories of diseases that cause coma into three groups: structural lesions, which may be above or below the tentorium; metabolic and toxic causes; and psychiatric causes. The history and physical examination determine the presence or absence of a structural le-

Table 5.2: Causes of coma

I. Symmetrical-nonstructural		
		Infections
Toxins	Metabolic	Bacterial meningitis
Lead	Hypoxia	Viral encephalitis
Thallium	Hypercapnia	Postinfectious encephalomyelitis
Mushrooms	Hypernatremia	Syphilis
Cyanide	Hyponatremia[a]	Sepsis
Methanol	Hypoglycemia[a]	Typhoid fever
Ethylene glycol	Hyperglycemic nonketotic coma	Malaria
Carbon monoxide	Diabetic ketoacidosis	Waterhouse–Friderichsen syndrome
Drugs	Lactic acidosis	Psychiatric
Sedatives	Hypercalcemia	Catonia
Barbiturates[a]	Hypocalcemia	Other
Other hypnotics	Hypermagnesemia	Postictal[a]
Tranquilizers	Hyperthermia	Diffuse ischemia (myocardial infarction, congestive heart failure, arrhythmia)
Bromides	Hypothermia	
Alcohol	Reye's encephalopathy	
Opiates	Aminoacidemia	Hypotension
Paraldehyde	Wernicke's encephalopathy	Fat embolism[a]
Salicylate	Porphyria	Hypertensive encephalopathy
Psychotropics	Hepatic encephalopathy[a]	Hypothyroidism
Anticholinergics	Uremia	
Amphetamines	Dialysis encephalopathy	
Lithium	Addisonian crisis	
Phencyclidine		
Monoamine oxidase inhibitors		
II. Symmetrical-structural		
Supratentorial	Subarachnoid hemorrhage	Infratentorial
Bilateral internal carotid occlusion	Thalamic hemorrhage[a]	Basilar occlusion[a]
Bilateral anterior cerebral artery occlusion	Trauma—contusion, concussion[a]	Midline brain stem tumor
	Hydrocephalus	Pontine hemorrhage[a]
III. Asymmetrical-structural		
Supratentorial	Subdural hemorrhage bilateral subdurals (may be symmetrical)	Subdural empyema
Thrombotic thrombocytopenic purpura[b]	Intracerebral bleed	Thrombophlebitis[b]
Disseminated intravascular coagulation	Pituitary apoplexy[b]	Multiple sclerosis
Nonbacterial thrombotic endocarditis (marantic endocarditis)	Massive or bilateral supratentorial infarction	Leukoencephalopathy associated with chemotherapy
Subacute bacterial endocarditis	Multifocal leukoencephalopathy	Acute disseminated encephalomyelitis
Fat emboli	Creutzfeldt–Jakob disease	Infratentorial
Unilateral hemispheric mass (tumor, bleed) with herniation	Adrenal leukodystrophy	Brain stem infarction
	Cerebral vasculitis	Brain stem hemorrhage
	Cerebral abscess	

[a]Relatively common asymmetrical presentation.
[b]Relatively symmetrical.
Source: Data from F Plum, JB Posner. The Diagnosis of Stupor and Coma (4th ed). Philadelphia: FA Davis, 1995; and CM Fisher. The neurological evaluation of the comatose patient. Acta Neurol Scand 1969;45 [Suppl. 36].

sion and quickly differentiate the general categories to decide what further diagnostic tests are needed or to allow for immediate intervention if necessary.

Serial examinations are needed, with precise description of the behavioral state at different points in time, to determine if the patient is improving or, more ominously, worsening and to decide if a change in therapy or further diagnostic tests are necessary. Subtle declines in the intermediate states of arousal may herald precipitous changes in brain stem function, which may affect regulation of vital functions such as respiration or blood pressure. The dynamic quality of alterations of consciousness and the need for accurate documentation at different points in time cannot be overemphasized.

RAPID INITIAL EXAMINATION AND EMERGENCY THERAPY

A relatively quick initial assessment of the comatose patient is important to make sure the patient is medically and neurologically stable before a more detailed assessment is made. One must be sure that the patient is not in immediate need of medical or surgical intervention.

Urgent and sometimes empirical therapy is given to prevent further brain damage. Potential immediate metabolic needs of the brain are supplied by empirical use of supplemental oxygen, thiamine (at least 100 mg), and intravenous 50% dextrose in water (25 g). A baseline serum glucose level should be obtained before glucose administration.

The use of intravenous glucose in patients with ischemic or anoxic brain damage is controversial. Extra glucose may augment local lactic acid production by anaerobic glycolysis and may worsen ischemic or anoxic damage. Clinically, however, we currently recommend empirical glucose administration when the cause of coma is unknown. There are two reasons for our approach: the frequent occurrence of alterations in arousal due to hypoglycemia and the relatively good prognosis for coma due to hypoglycemia when it is treated expeditiously and the potentially permanent consequences if it is not treated. In comparison, the prognosis for anoxic or ischemic coma is generally poor and probably will remain poor regardless of glucose supplementation.

Thiamine must always be given in conjunction with glucose to prevent precipitation of polioencephalitis haemorrhagica superior (Wernicke's encephalopathy). Naloxone hydrochloride may be given parenterally, preferably intravenously, in doses of 0.4–2.0 mg if opiate overdose is the suspected cause of coma. An abrupt and complete reversal of narcotic effect may precipitate an acute abstinence syndrome in individuals who are physically dependent on opiates.

An initial examination should include a check of general appearance, blood pressure, pulse, temperature, respiratory rate and breath sounds, best response to stimulation, pupil size and responsiveness, and posturing or adventitious movements.

The neck should be stabilized in all instances of trauma until cervical spine fracture or subluxation can be ruled out. The airway is protected in all comatose patients and an intravenous line is placed.

Abdominal rigidity is a feature of peritonitis or perforated viscus. In coma, however, the classic signs of an acute condition in the abdomen may be subtle or nonexistent. In addition, the diagnosis of blunt abdominal trauma is difficult in patients with a change in mental status. Therefore, in unconscious patients with a history of trauma, peritoneal lavage by an experienced surgeon may be warranted.

Hypotension, marked hypertension, bradycardia, arrhythmias causing depression of blood pressure, marked hyperthermia, and signs of herniation mandate immediate therapeutic intervention.

Hyperthermia or meningismus leads to consideration of urgent lumbar puncture. *A computed tomography (CT) scan of the brain should be performed prior to lumbar puncture in any comatose patient.* Although the only absolute contraindication to lumbar puncture is the presence of an infection over the site of puncture, medicolegal considerations make a CT scan mandatory before lumbar puncture. To avoid a delay in therapy required to perform a CT scan, some authorities recommend initiating antibiotics immediately when acute bacterial meningitis is strongly suspected. If there is an inordinate delay in obtaining an emergency CT scan, lumbar puncture may have to be performed before the CT to allow the administration of antibiotics.

The risk of herniation from a lumbar puncture in patients with evidence of increased intracerebral pressure is difficult to ascertain from the literature; estimates range from 1–12%, depending on the series (Plum and Posner 1995). One must always keep in mind that both central and tonsillar herniation may increase neck tone.

Despite an elevated intracranial pressure, sufficient cerebrospinal fluid should always be obtained to perform the necessary studies. The performance of bacterial culture and cell count, essential in cases of suspected bacterial meningitis, requires but a few milliliters of fluid. Intravenous access and intravenous mannitol should be ready in case unexpected herniation begins after the lumbar puncture. When the cerebrospinal fluid pressure is greater than 500 mm H_20, some authorities recommend leaving the needle in place to monitor the pressure and administering intravenous mannitol to lower the pressure. If focal signs develop during or after the lumbar puncture, immediate intubation and hyperventilation may also be necessary to reduce intracerebral pressure urgently until more definitive therapy is available.

Ecchymosis, petechiae, or evidence of easy bleeding on general examination may indicate coagulation abnormality or thrombocytopenia. This increases the risk of epidural hematoma, which may cause devastating spinal cord compression. Measurements of prothrombin time, partial thromboplastin time, and platelet count should precede lumbar puncture in these cases, and the coagulation abnormality or thrombocytopenia should be corrected prior to lumbar puncture.

COMMON PRESENTATIONS

Coma usually presents in one of three ways. Most commonly, it occurs as an expected or predictable progression of an underlying illness. Examples of this are focal brain stem infarction with extension; the patient with chronic obstructive pulmonary disease who is given too high a concentration of oxygen, decreasing the patient's respiratory drive and resulting in carbon dioxide narcosis; and the patient with known barbiturate overdose when the ingested drug cannot be fully removed and begins to cause unresponsiveness. Second, coma occurs as an unpredictable event in a patient whose prior medical conditions are known to the physician. The coma may be a complication of an underlying medical illness, such as in a patient with arrhythmia who suffers anoxia after a cardiac arrest. Or an unrelated event may occur, such as sepsis from an intravenous line in a cardiac patient or a stroke in a hypothyroid patient. Finally, coma can occur in a patient who is totally unknown to the physician. Sometimes this type of presentation is associated with a known probable cause, such as head trauma following a motor vehicle accident, but often the unknown comatose patient presents to the physician without an obvious associated cause. Although the patient without an obvious cause of coma may seem most challenging, thorough objective systematic assessment must be applied to every comatose patient. Special care must be taken not to be lulled or misled by an apparently predictable progression of an underlying illness or other obvious cause of coma.

HISTORY

Once the patient is relatively stable, clues to the cause of the coma should be sought by briefly interviewing relatives, friends, bystanders, or medical personnel who may have observed the patient before or during the decrease in consciousness. Telephone calls to family members may be helpful. The patient's wallet or purse should be examined for lists of medications, a physician's card, or other information.

Attempts should be made to ascertain the patient's social background and prior medical history and the circumstances in which the patient was found. The presence of drug paraphernalia or empty medicine bottles suggests a drug overdose. Oral hypoglycemic agents or insulin in the medicine cabinet or refrigerator imply possible hypoglycemia. Antiarrhythmic agents such as procainamide or quinidine suggest existing coronary artery disease with possible myocardial infarction or warn that an unwitnessed arrhythmia may have caused cerebral hypoperfusion, with resulting anoxic encephalopathy. Warfarin is given to patients with deep venous thrombosis or pulmonary embolism, those at risk of cerebral emboli, and those with a history of prior brain stem or cerebral ischemia. Its use may be complicated by massive intracerebral bleeding. Patients found to be unresponsive at the scene of an accident, such as a motor vehicle accident, may be unresponsive because of trauma that occurred in the accident; alternatively, sudden loss of consciousness may have precipitated the accident.

The neurologist is often called when patients do not awaken following surgery or when coma supervenes following a surgical procedure. Postoperative causes of coma include many of those mentioned in Table 5.2. In addition, the physician must also have a high index of suspicion for certain neurological conditions that occur in this setting, including fat embolism, addisonian crisis, or hypothyroid coma (precipitated by acute illness or surgical stress); Wernicke's encephalopathy from carbohydrate loading without adequate thiamine stores; and iatrogenic overdose of a narcotic analgesic.

Attempts should be made to ascertain if the patient complained of symptoms prior to coma. Common symptoms include headache prior to subarachnoid hemorrhage, chest pain with aortic dissection or myocardial infarction, shortness of breath from hypoxia, stiff neck in meningoencephalitis, or vertigo in brain stem cerebrovascular accident. Nausea and vomiting are common in poisonings. Coma may also be due to increased intracranial pressure. Observers may have noted head trauma, drug abuse, seizures, or hemiparesis. Descriptions of falling to one side, dysarthria or aphasia, ptosis, pupillary dilation, or disconjugate gaze may help localize structural lesions. The time course of the disease as noted by family or friends may help differentiate the often relatively slow, progressive course of toxic-metabolic or infectious causes from abrupt, catastrophic changes that are seen most commonly with vascular events.

Finally, family members or friends may be invaluable in identifying psychiatric causes of unresponsiveness. The family may describe a long history of psychiatric disease, previous similar episodes from which the patient recovered, current social stresses on the patient, or the patient's unusual, idiosyncratic response to stress. Special care must be taken with psychiatric patients because of the often biased approach to these patients, which may lead to incomplete evaluation. Psychiatric patients are subject to all the causes of coma listed in Table 5.2.

GENERAL EXAMINATION

A systematic, detailed general examination is especially helpful in the approach to the comatose patient who is unable to describe his or her prior or current medical problems. This examination was begun in the initial rapid examination, with evaluation of blood pressure, pulse, respiratory rate, and temperature.

Blood Pressure Evaluation

Hypotension

Cerebral hypoperfusion secondary to hypotension may result in coma if the mean arterial pressure falls below the value for which the brain is able to autoregulate (normally 60 mm Hg). This value is substantially higher in chronically hypertensive individuals, as the cerebral blood flow-mean arterial pressure curve is shifted to the right. Among the causes of hypotension are hypovolemia, massive external or internal hemorrhage, myocardial infarction, cardiac tamponade, dissecting aortic aneurysm, intoxication with alcohol or other drugs (especially barbiturates), toxins, Wernicke's encephalopathy, Addison's disease, and sepsis. Although most patients with hypotension are cold because of peripheral vasoconstriction, patients with Addison's disease or sepsis may have warm shock due to peripheral vasodilation. Medullary damage may also result in hypotension because of damage to the pressor center.

Hypertension

Hypertension is the cause of alterations in arousal in hypertensive crisis and is seen secondarily as a response to cerebral infarction, in subarachnoid hemorrhage, with certain brain stem infarctions, and with increased intracerebral pressure. The Kocher-Cushing (or Claude Bernard) reflex is hypertension associated with bradycardia and respiratory irregularity due to increased intracranial pressure. This response occurs more commonly in the setting of a posterior fossa lesion and in children. It results from compression or ischemia of the pressor area lying beneath the floor of the fourth ventricle. Hypertension is a common condition and thus may be present but unrelated to the cause of coma.

Heart Rate

In addition to the Kocher-Cushing reflex, bradycardia can result from myocardial conduction blocks, certain poisonings, and drugs such as the beta blockers. Tachycardia is a result of hypovolemia, hyperthyroidism, fever, anemia, and certain toxins and drugs, including cocaine, atropine, and other anticholinergic medications.

Respiration

The most common causes of decreased respiratory rate are metabolic or toxic, such as carbon dioxide narcosis or drug overdose with central nervous system (CNS) depressants. Increased respiratory rate can result from hypoxia, hypercapnia, acidosis, hyperthermia, hepatic disease, toxins or drugs (especially those that produce a metabolic acidosis, such as methanol, ethylene glycol, paraldehyde, and salicylates), sepsis, pulmonary emboli (including fat emboli), and sometimes psychogenic unresponsiveness. Brain stem lesions causing hypopnea or hyperpnea are discussed below. Changes in respiratory rate or rhythm in a comatose patient may be deceiving, because a metabolic disorder may coexist with a CNS lesion.

Temperature

Core temperature must be measured with a rectal probe in a comatose patient, because oral or axillary temperatures are unreliable. Pyrexia is most often a sign of infection. Thus, any evidence of fever in a comatose patient warrants strong consideration of lumbar puncture. Absence of an elevated temperature does not rule out infection. Immunosuppressed patients, elderly patients, and patients with metabolic or endocrine abnormalities such as uremia or hypothyroidism may not have increased temperature in response to overwhelming infection. Pure neurogenic hyperthermia is rare and is usually due to subarachnoid hemorrhage or diencephalic (hypothalamus) lesions. A clue to brain stem origin is shivering without sweating. Shivering in the absence of sweating, particularly when unilateral in nature, may also be observed with a deep intracerebral hemorrhage. Other causes of increased temperature associated with coma are heatstroke, thyrotoxic crisis, and drug toxicity. (Atropine and other anticholinergics elevate core temperature but decrease diaphoresis, resulting in a warm, dry patient with dilated pupils and diminished bowel sounds.)

Except in heatstroke and malignant hyperthermia, fever does not result in stupor or coma by itself. Conversely, hypothermia, regardless of cause, is anticipated to lead to altered consciousness. Hypothermia causes diminished cerebral metabolism and, if the temperature is sufficiently low, may result in an isoelectric electroencephalogram. Hypothermia is usually metabolic or environmental in cause; however, it is also seen with hypotension accompanied by vasoconstriction and may occur with sepsis. Other causes of hypothermia associated with coma are hypothyroid coma, hypopituitarism, Wernicke's encephalopathy, cold exposure, drugs (barbiturates), and other poisonings. Central lesions causing hypothermia are found in the posterior hypothalamus. The absence of shivering or vasoconstriction or the presence of sweating is a clue to the central origin of these lesions.

General Appearance

The general appearance of the patient may provide further clues to the diagnosis. Torn or dishevelled clothing may indicate prior assault. Vomitus may be a sign of increased intracranial pressure, drug overdose, or metabolic or other toxic cause. Urinary or fecal incontinence indicates an epileptic seizure or may result from a generalized autonomic discharge resulting from the same cause as the coma. Examination of body habitus may reveal a cushingoid patient at risk for an acute addisonian crisis with abrupt withdrawal of his or her medications or additional stress from intercurrent illness. Cachexia suggests cancer, chronic inflammatory disorders, Addison's disease, hypothyroid coma, or hyperthyroid crisis. The cachectic patient is also subject to Wernicke's encephalopathy in association with carbohydrate loading. Gynecomastia, spider nevi, testicular atrophy, and decreased axillary and pubic hair are common in the alcoholic with cirrhosis.

Head and Neck Examination

The head and neck must be carefully examined for signs of trauma. Palpation for depressed skull fractures and edema should be attempted, though it is not very sensitive. Laceration or edema of the scalp is indicative of head trauma. The term *raccoon eyes* refers to orbital ecchymosis due to anterior basal skull fracture. *Battle sign* is a hematoma overlying the mastoid, originating from basilar skull fracture extending into the mastoid portion of the temporal bone. The ecchymotic lesions are typically not apparent until 2–3 days after the traumatic event.

Meningismus

The slightest degree of neck stiffness may be a sign of infectious or carcinomatous meningitis, subarachnoid hemorrhage, or central or tonsillar herniation. Neck stiffness is absent in coma from any cause but may be present in less severe alterations in arousal. Scars on the neck may be from endarterectomy, implying vascular disease, or from thyroidectomy or parathyroidectomy, suggesting concomitant hypothyroidism, hypoparathyroidism, or both. Goiter may be found with hypothyroidism or hyperthyroidism.

Eye Examination

Examination of the eyes includes observation of the cornea, conjunctiva, sclera, iris, lens, and eyelids. Edema of the conjunctiva and eyelids may occur in congestive heart failure and nephrotic syndrome. Congestion and inflammation of the conjunctiva often occur in the comatose patient as a result of exposure. Enophthalmos indicates dehydration. Scleralicterus is seen with liver disease, and yellowish discoloration of the skin without scleral involvement may be due to drugs such as rifampin. Band keratopathy is caused by hypercalcemia, whereas hypocalcemia is associated with cataracts. Kayser-Fleischer rings are seen in progressive lenticular degeneration (Wilson's disease). Arcus senilis is seen in normal aging but also in hyperlipidemia. Fat embolism may cause petechiae in conjunctiva and eye grounds.

Funduscopic Examination

Funduscopic examination demonstrates evidence of hypertension or diabetes. Grayish deposits surrounding the disc have been reported in lead poisoning. The retina is congested and edematous in methyl alcohol poisoning, and the disc margin may be blurred. Subhyloid hemorrhage appears occasionally as a consequence of a rapid increase in intracranial pressure due to subarachnoid hemorrhage. Papilledema results from increased intracranial pressure and may be indicative of an intracranial mass lesion or hypertensive encephalopathy.

Otoscopic Examination

Otoscopic examination should rule out hemotympanum or otorrhea from a basilar skull fracture involving the petrous ridge as well as infection of the middle ear. Infections of the middle ear, mastoid, and paranasal sinuses are the most common sources of underlying infection in brain abscess (Osenbach and Loftus 1992). Rhinorrhea, which appears as clear fluid from the nose, may depend on head position. The presence of glucose in this watery discharge is virtually diagnostic, though false-positives may be observed.

Oral Examination

Alcohol intoxication, diabetic ketoacidosis (acetone odor), uremia, and hepatic encephalopathy (musty odor of cholemia or fetor hepaticus) may be suspected from the odor of the breath. Arsenic poisoning produces the odor of garlic. Poor oral hygiene or oral abscesses may be a source of sepsis or severe pulmonary infection with associated hypoxemia. Pustules on the nose or upper lip may seed the cavernous sinus with bacteria by way of the angular vein. Lacerations on the tongue, whether old or new, suggest seizure disorder. Thin, blue-black pigmentation along the gingival margin may be seen in certain heavy-metal poisonings (bismuth, mercury, and lead).

Integument Examination

Systematic examination of the integument includes inspection of the skin, nails, and mucous membranes. A great deal of information can be gained by a brief examination of the skin (Table 5.3). Hot, dry skin is a feature of heatstroke. Sweaty skin is seen with hypotension or hypoglycemia. Drugs may cause macular-papular, vesicular, or petechial-purpuric rashes or bullous skin lesions. Bullous skin lesions are most often a result of barbiturates but also may be caused by imipramine, meprobamate, glutethimide, phenothiazine, and carbon monoxide. Kaposi's sarcoma, anogenital herpetic lesions, or oral candidiasis should suggest the acquired immune deficiency syndrome (AIDS), with its plethora of CNS abnormalities.

Table 5.3: Skin lesions and rashes in coma

Lesion or Rash	*Possible Cause*
Antecubital needle marks	Opiate drug abuse
Pale skin	Anemia or hemorrhage
Sallow, puffy appearance	Hypopituitarism
Hypermelanosis (increased pigment)	Porphyria, Addison's disease, chronic nutritional deficiency, disseminated malignant melanoma, chemotherapy
Generalized cyanosis	Hypoxemia or carbon dioxide poisoning
Grayish-blue cyanosis	Methemoglobin (aniline or nitrobenzene) intoxication
Localized cyanosis	Arterial emboli or vasculitis
Cherry-red skin	Carbon monoxide poisoning
Icterus	Hepatic dysfunction or hemolytic anemia
Petechiae	Disseminated intravascular coagulation, thrombotic thrombocytopenic purpura, drugs
Ecchymosis	Trauma, corticosteroid use, abnormal coagulation from liver disease or anticoagulants
Telangiectasia	Chronic alcoholism, occasionally vascular malformations of the brain
Vesicular rash	Herpes simplex Varicella Behçet's disease Drugs
Petechial-purpuric rash	Meningococcemia Other bacterial sepsis (rarely) Gonococcemia Staphylococcemia *Pseudomonas* ubacute bacterial endocarditis Allergic vasculitis Purpura fulminans Rocky Mountain spotted fever Typhus Fat emboli

Macular-papular rash	Typhus
	Candida
	Cryptococcus
	Toxoplasmosis
	Subacute bacterial endocarditis
	Staphylococcal toxic shock
	Typhoid
	Leptospirosis
	Pseudomonas sepsis
	Immunological disorders
	  Systemic lupus erythematosus
	  Dermatomyositis
	  Serum sickness

Other skin lesions	
Ecthyma gangrenosum	Necrotic eschar often seen in the anogenital or axillary area in *Pseudomonas* sepsis
Splinter hemorrhages	Linear hemorrhages under the nail, seen in subacute bacterial endocarditis, anemia, leukemia, and sepsis
Osler's nodes	Purplish or erythematous painful, tender nodules on palms and soles, seen in subacute bacterial endocarditis
Gangrene of digits' extremities	Emboli to larger peripheral or arteries

Source: Data on diseases associated with rashes from L Corey, P Kirby. Rash and Fever. In E Braunwald, KJ Isselbacher, RG Petersdorf (eds), Harrison's Principles of Internal Medicine (11th ed). New York: McGraw-Hill. 1987:240–244.

Examination of Lymph Nodes

Generalized lymphadenopathy is nonspecific, as it may be seen with neoplasm, infection (including AIDS), collagen vascular disease, sarcoid, hyperthyroidism, Addison's disease, and drug reaction (especially due to phenytoin). Local lymph node enlargement or inflammation, however, may provide clues to a primary tumor site or source of infection.

Cardiac Examination

Cardiac auscultation will confirm the presence of arrhythmias such as atrial fibrillation, with its inherent increased risk of emboli. Changing mitral murmurs are heard with atrial myxomas and papillary muscle ischemia, which is seen with current or impending myocardial infarction. Constant murmurs indicate valvular heart disease and may be heard with the valvular vegetation of bacterial endocarditis.

Abdominal Examination

Possibly helpful findings on abdominal examination include abnormal bowel sounds, organomegaly, masses, or ascites. Bowel sounds are absent in an acute abdominal condition as well as with anticholinergic poisoning. Hyperactive bowel sounds may be a consequence of increased gastrointestinal motility from exposure to acetylcholinesterase inhibitor (a common pesticide ingredient). The liver may be enlarged as a result of right heart failure or tumor infiltration. Nodules or a rock-hard liver may be due to hepatoma or metastatic disease. The liver may be small and hard in cirrhosis.

Splenomegaly is caused by portal hypertension, hematological malignancies, infection, and collagen vascular diseases. Intraabdominal masses may indicate carcinoma. Ascites occurs with liver disease, right heart failure, neoplasms with metastasis to liver, or ovarian cancer.

Miscellaneous Examinations

Examination of the breasts in the female and the testicles in the male and rectal examination may reveal common primary tumors. Stool from a rectal examination that tests positive for blood is consistent with gastrointestinal bleeding and, possibly, bowel carcinoma. Blood in the gastrointestinal tract may be sufficient to incite hepatic encephalopathy in the patient with cirrhosis.

NEUROLOGICAL EXAMINATION

Neurological signs may show every degree of change along a continuum, and they may be partial or incomplete. For example, the patient may have a partial third nerve palsy with pupillary dilation rather than a complete absence of all third nerve function, or muscle tone may be decreased but not absent. This concept is especially important in the examination of the stuporous or comatose patient, as the level of arousal may also influence the expression of neurological signs. In the stuporous or comatose patient, findings that are not completely normal should not be dismissed as unimportant. These findings should be carefully considered until their pattern or meaning is understood.

The neurological examination of a comatose patient serves three purposes: (1) to aid in determining the cause of coma, (2) to provide a baseline, and (3) to help determine the prognosis of coma. For prognosis and localization of a structural lesion, certain parts of the examination have been found to be most helpful: (1) state of consciousness, (2) respiratory pattern, (3) pupillary size and response to light, (4) spontaneous and reflex eye movements, and (5) skeletal muscle motor response.

State of Consciousness

The importance of a detailed description of the state of consciousness has been stressed above. It is imperative that the exact stimulus and the patient's specific response be recorded. Several modes of stimulation should be used, including auditory, visual, and noxious. Stimuli of progressively increasing intensity should be applied to the patient, with the maximal state of arousal noted and the stimuli, site of stimulation, and patient's exact response described. One should start with verbal stimuli, softly and then more loudly calling the patient's name or giving simple instructions to open his or her eyes. If there is no significant response, more threatening stimuli, such as taking the patient's hand and advancing it toward the patient's face, are applied. Finally, painful stimuli may be needed to arouse the patient. All patients in apparent coma should be asked to open their eyes and look up and down, thus avoiding the possibility of mistaking the locked-in syndrome, in which these voluntary movements are preserved, for coma.

Supraorbital pressure evokes a response in patients who may have lost afferent pain pathways as a result of peripheral neuropathy or spinal cord or some brain stem lesions. Pinching the chest or extremities may help localize a lesion. Care must be taken to avoid soft-tissue damage. Purposeful movements indicate a milder alteration in consciousness. Vocalization to pain in the early hours of a coma, even if only a grunt, indicates relatively light alteration in consciousness. Later, primitive vocalization may be a feature of the vegetative state. Asymmetry in response from either side of the face or body may localize structural lesions.

The Glasgow Coma Scale (Table 5.4) is used widely to assess the initial severity of traumatic brain injury. This battery assesses three separate aspects of a patient's behavior: the stimulus required to induce eye opening, the best motor response, and the best verbal response. Degrees of increasing dysfunction are scored. Its reproducibility and simplicity make the Glasgow Coma Scale an ideal method of assessment for nonneurologists involved in the care of comatose patients, such as neurological intensive care nurses. However, its failure to assess other essential neurological parameters limits its utility.

Respiration

Normal breathing is quiet and unlabored. The presence of any respiratory noise implies airway obstruction, which must be dealt with immediately to prevent hypoxia. Normal respiration depends on two components: a brain stem mechanism, located between the midpons and cervical medullary junction, that regulates metabolic needs, and

Table 5.4: The Glasgow Coma Scale

Best motor response	
Obeys	M6
Localizes	5
Withdraws	4
Abnormal flexion	3
Extensor response	2
Nil	1
Verbal response	
Oriented	V5
Confused conversation	4
Inappropriate words	3
Incomprehensible sounds	2
Nil	1
Eye opening	
Spontaneous	E4
To speech	3
To pain	2
Nil	1

forebrain influences that subserve behavioral needs such as speech production. The organization and function of brain stem mechanisms responsible for respiratory rhythm generation as well as forebrain influences are complex and beyond the scope of this chapter. For an excellent review of this subject, the reader is referred to Long and Duffin (1986). Neuropathological correlates of respiration are presented in Figure 5.1.

Respiratory patterns that are helpful in localizing level of involvement include Cheyne-Stokes respiration, central neurogenic hyperventilation, apneustic breathing, cluster breathing, and ataxic respiration. *Cheyne-Stokes respiration* is a respiratory pattern that slowly oscillates between hyperventilation and hypoventilation. Cheyne in 1818 described his patient in the following manner: "For several days his breathing was irregular; it would entirely cease for a quarter of a minute, then it would become perceptible, though very low, then by degrees it became heaving and quick and then it would gradually cease again. This revolution in the state of his breathing occupied about a minute during which there were about 30 acts of respiration." Cheyne-Stokes respiration is associated with bilateral hemispheric or diencephalic insults, but it may occur as a result of bilateral damage anywhere along the descending pathway between the forebrain and upper pons. It also is seen with cardiac disorders that prolong circulation time. Alertness, pupillary size, and heart rhythm may vary during Cheyne-Stokes respiration (Plum and Posner 1995). Patients are more alert during the waxing portion of breathing.

A stable pattern of Cheyne-Stokes respiration is a relatively good prognostic sign, usually implying that permanent brain stem damage has not occurred. However, the emergence of Cheyne-Stokes respiration in a patient with a unilateral mass lesion may be an early sign of herniation. A change in pattern from Cheyne-Stokes respiration to the respiratory patterns described below is ominous.

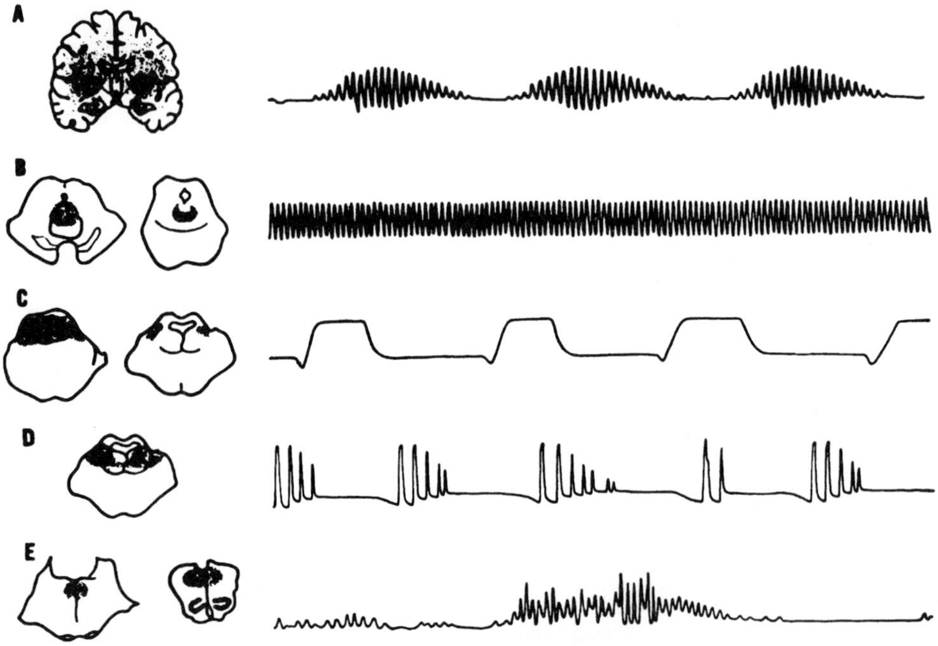

FIGURE 5.1 Abnormal respiratory patterns associated with pathological lesions (shaded areas) at various levels of the brain. Tracings by chest-abdomen pneumograph; inspiration reads up. A. Cheyne-Stokes respiration—diffuse forebrain damage. B. Central neurogenic hyperventilation—lesion of low midbrain ventral to aqueduct of Sylvius and of upper pons ventral to the fourth ventricle. C. Apneusis— dorsolateral tegmental lesion of the mid- and caudal pons. D. Cluster breathing—lower pontine tegmental lesion. E. Ataxic breathing—lesion of the reticular formation of the dorsomedial part of the medulla. (Reprinted with permission from F Plum, JB Posner. The Diagnosis of Stupor and Coma [4th ed]. Philadelphia: FA Davis, 1995.)

Two breathing patterns similar to Cheyne-Stokes respiration should not be confused with it. *Short-cycle periodic breathing* is a respiratory pattern with a shorter cycle (faster rhythm) than Cheyne-Stokes respiration, with one or two waxing breaths, followed by two to four rapid breaths, then one or two waning breaths. It is seen with increased intracranial pressure, lower pontine lesions, or expanding lesions in the posterior fossa (Plum and Posner 1995). A similar type of respiration, in which there are short bursts of seven to ten rapid breaths, then apnea without a waning and waxing prodrome, has been erroneously referred to as Biot's breathing. Biot, in fact, described an ataxic respiratory pattern.

Central neurogenic respiration refers to rapid breathing, from 40–70 breaths per minute, usually due to central tegmental pontine lesions just ventral to the aqueduct or fourth ventricle (Plum and Posner 1995). This type of breathing is rare and must be differentiated from reactive hyperventilation due to metabolic abnormalities of hypoxemia secondary to pulmonary involvement. Large CNS lesions may cause neurogenic pulmonary edema, with associated hypoxemia and increased respiratory rate. Increased intracerebral pressure causes spontaneous hyperpnea. Hyperpnea cannot be ascribed to a CNS lesion when arterial oxygen pressure is less than 70–80 mm Hg or carbon dioxide pressure is greater than 40 mm Hg.

Kussmaul breathing is a deep, regular respiration observed with metabolic acidosis. *Apneustic breathing* is a prolonged inspiratory gasp with a pause at full inspiration. It is caused by lesions of the dorsolateral lower half of the pons (Plum and Posner 1995). *Cluster breathing*, which results from high medullary damage, involves periodic respirations that are irregular in frequency and amplitude, with variable pauses between clusters of breaths.

Ataxic breathing is irregular in rate and rhythm and is usually due to medullary lesions. Ataxic respiration and bilateral sixth nerve palsy may be a warning sign of brain stem compression from an expanding lesion in the posterior fossa. This is an important sign, because brain stem compression due to tonsillar herniation (or other causes) may result in abrupt loss of respiration or blood pressure. Ataxic and gasping respiration are signs of lower brain stem damage and are often preterminal respiratory patterns.

Pupil Size and Reactivity

Normal pupil size in the comatose patient depends on the level of illumination and the state of autonomic innervation. The sympathetic efferent innervation consists of a three-neuron arc. The first-order neuron arises in the hypothalamus and travels ipsilaterally through the posterolateral tegmentum to the ciliospinal center of Budge at the level of T1 spinal cord. The second-order neuron leaves this center and synapses in the superior cervical sympathetic ganglion. The third-order neuron travels along the internal carotid artery and then through the ciliary ganglion to the pupillodilator muscles. The parasympathetic efferent innervation of the pupil arises in the Edinger-Westphal nucleus and travels in the oculomotor nerve to the ciliary ganglion, from which it innervates the pupillosphincter muscle (Figure 5.2).

Afferent input depends on the integrity of the optic nerve, optic chiasm, optic tract, and projections into the midbrain tectum and efferent fibers through the Edinger-Westphal nucleus and oculomotor nerve. Abnormalities in pupil size and reactivity help delineate structural damage between the thalamus and pons (Figure 5.3), act as a warning sign heralding brain stem herniation, and help differentiate structural causes of coma from metabolic causes.

Thalamic lesions cause small, reactive pupils, which are often referred to as *diencephalic pupils*. Similar pupillary findings are noted in many toxic-metabolic conditions resulting in coma. Hypothalamic lesions or lesions elsewhere along the sympathetic pathway result in *Horner's syndrome*. Midbrain lesions produce three types of pupillary abnormality, depending on where the lesion occurs. Dorsal tectal lesions interrupt the pupillary light reflex, resulting in *midposition eyes*, which are fixed to light but react to accommodation, though the reaction is impossible to test in the comatose patient. Spontaneous fluctuations in size occur, and the ciliospinal reflex is preserved. Nuclear midbrain lesions usually affect both sympathetic and parasympathetic pathways, resulting in *fixed, irregular midposition pupils*, which may be unequal. Lesions of the third nerve in the brain stem or after the nerve has left the brain stem parenchyma cause *wide pupillary dilation*, unresponsive to light. Pontine lesions interrupt sympathetic pathways only to cause small, so-called *pinpoint pupils*, which remain reactive, though magnification may be needed to observe this. Lesions above the thalamus and below the pons should leave pupillary function intact, except for Horner's syndrome in medullary or cervical spinal cord lesions. The pathophysiology of pupillary response is discussed further in Chapters 16 and 42.

Asymmetry in pupillary size or reactivity, even of minor degree, is important. Asymmetry of pupil size may be due to dilation (mydriasis) of one pupil, such as with third nerve palsy, or contraction (miosis) of the other, as in Horner's syndrome. These may be differentiated by associated neurological deficits. A dilated pupil due to a partial third nerve palsy is less reactive and may also be associated with extraocular muscle involvement. The pupil in Horner's syndrome is reactive and, if it results from a lesion in the CNS, may be associated with anhidrosis of the entire ipsilateral body. Cervical sympathetic lesions produce anhidrosis only of face, neck, and arm. A partial or complete third nerve palsy causing a dilated pupil may result from an intramedullary lesion, most commonly in the midbrain, such as an intramedullary glioma or infarction; uncal herniation compressing the third nerve; or a posterior communicating artery aneurysm. A sluggishly reactive pupil may be one of the first signs of uncal herniation, soon to be followed by dilation of that pupil and, later, complete third nerve paralysis.

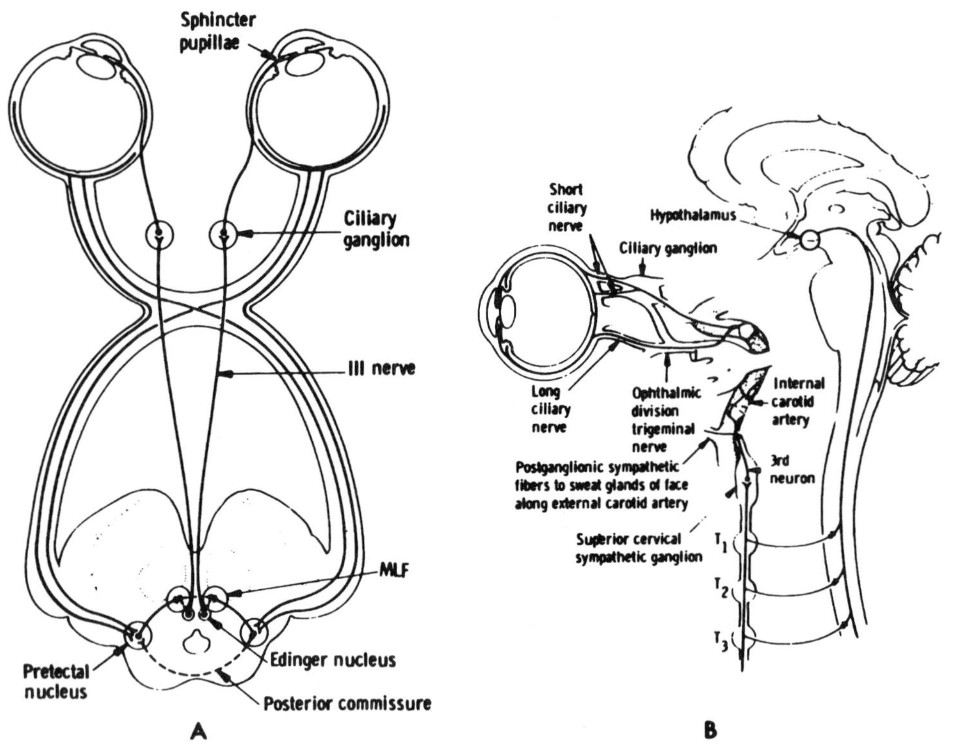

FIGURE 5.2 A. The parasympathetic pupilloconstrictor pathway. B. The sympathetic pupillodilator pathway. (Reprinted with permission from F Plum, JB Posner. The Diagnosis of Stupor and Coma [4th ed]. Philadelphia: FA Davis, 1995.)

Several caveats are important when examining the pupil or pupillary reflexes. A common mistake is the use of insufficient illumination. The otoscope may be useful in this regard, as it provides both adequate illumination and magnification. Rarely, preexisting ocular or neurological injury may fix the pupils or result in pupillary asymmetry. Seizures may cause transient anisocoria. Local and systemic medications may affect pupillary function. Topical ophthalmological preparations containing acetylcholinesterase inhibitor, used in the treatment of glaucoma, result in miosis. The effect of a mydriatic agent placed by the patient or a prior observer may wear off unevenly, resulting in pupillary asymmetry. Some common misleading causes of a unilateral dilated pupil include prior mydriatic administration, old ocular trauma or ophthalmic surgery, and, more rarely, carotid insufficiency.

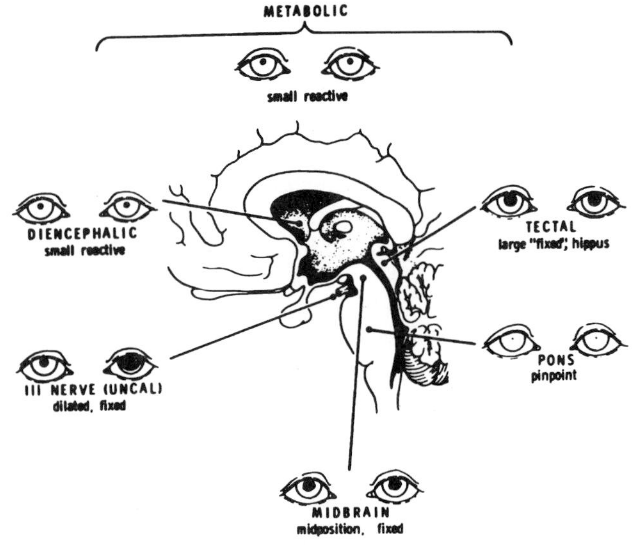

FIGURE 5.3 Pupils in comatose patients. (Reprinted with permission from F Plum, JB Posner. The Diagnosis of Stupor and Coma [4th ed]. Philadelphia: FA Davis, 1995.)

Ocular Motility

Normal ocular motility depends on the integrity of a large portion of the cerebrum, cerebellum, and brain stem. Preservation of normal ocular motility implies that a large portion of the brain stem from the vestibular nuclei at the pontomedullary junction to the oculomotor nucleus in the midbrain is intact. Voluntary ocular motility cannot be judged in the comatose patient, so one must rely on reflex eye movements that allow for assessment of the oculomotor system. The eyes normally are conjugate and in the midposition in the alert person. Sleep or obtundation alone may unmask a latent vertical or horizontal strabismus, resulting in disconjugate gaze; therefore, patients must be examined when maximally aroused. The eyes return to the midposition in brain-dead patients.

Evaluation of ocular motility consists of three main elements: (1) observation of the resting position of the eyes, including eye deviation; (2) notation of spontaneous eye movements; and (3) testing of reflex ocular movements.

Abnormalities in Resting Position

Careful attention must be paid to the resting position of the eyes. Even a small discrepancy in eye position may represent a partial extraocular nerve palsy. Partial nerve palsies or combined nerve palsies predictably result in a more complex picture on examination. Unilateral third nerve palsy from either an intramedullary midbrain lesion or extramedullary compression causes the affected eye to be displaced downward and laterally. A sixth nerve palsy produces inward deviation. Isolated sixth nerve palsy, however, is a poor localizer because of its extensive course and because nonspecific increases in intracranial pressure may cause a sixth nerve palsy, presumably from stretching of the extramedullary portion of the nerve. A fourth nerve palsy is difficult to assess in the comatose patient because of the subtle nature of the deficit in ocular motility. Extraocular nerve palsies often become more apparent with the "doll's eye maneuver" or cold caloric testing in the comatose patient.

Eye Deviation

Spontaneous eye deviation may be conjugate or dysconjugate. Conjugate lateral eye deviation is usually due to an ipsilateral lesion in the frontal eye fields but may be due to a lesion anywhere in the pathway from the ipsilateral eye fields to the contralateral parapontine reticular formation (lateral gaze center). Dysconjugate lateral eye movement may result from a sixth nerve palsy in the abducting eye, a third nerve palsy in the adducting eye, or an internuclear ophthalmoplegia. An internuclear ophthalmoplegia may be differentiated from a third nerve palsy by the preservation of vertical eye movements.

Downward deviation of the eyes below the horizontal meridian is usually due to brain stem lesions (most often from tectal compression); however, it may also be seen in metabolic disorders such as hepatic coma. Thalamic and subthalamic lesions produce downward and inward deviation of the eyes. Patients with these lesions appear to be looking at the tips of their noses. Sleep, seizure, syncope, apnea of Cheyne-Stokes respiration, hemorrhage into the vermis, and brain stem ischemia or encephalitis cause upward eye deviation, making it a poor localizing sign. Skew deviation is a maintained deviation of one eye above the other (hypertropia) that is not due to a peripheral neuromuscular lesion or a local extracranial problem in the orbit. It usually indicates a posterior fossa lesion (brain stem or cerebellar) (Leigh and Zee 1991). Dysconjugate vertical eye position may sometimes occur in the absence of a brain stem lesion in the obtunded patient.

Spontaneous Eye Movements

Spontaneous eye movements are of many types. Purposeful-appearing eye movements in a patient who otherwise seems unresponsive lead to consideration of the locked-in syndrome, catatonia, pseudocoma, or the persistent vegetative state. *Roving eye movements* are slow, conjugate, lateral to-and-fro movements. For roving eye movements to be present, the oculomotor nuclei and their connections must be intact. Generally, when roving eye movements are present, the brain stem is relatively intact and coma is due to a metabolic or toxic cause or bilateral lesions above the brain stem. Roving eye movements may be complicated by ocular palsies or internuclear ophthalmoplegia. These superimposed lesions produce relatively predictable patterns but often obscure the essential roving nature of the movement for the inexperienced observer.

Nystagmus occurring in comatose patients suggests an irritative or epileptogenic supratentorial focus. An epileptogenic focus in one frontal eye field causes contralateral conjugate eye deviation. Nystagmus due to an irritative focus may rarely occur alone, without other motor manifestations of seizures. In addition, inconspicuous movements of the eye, eyelid, face, jaw, or tongue may be associated with electroencephalographic status epilepticus. An electroencephalogram may be required to ascertain this condition.

Spontaneous conjugate vertical eye movements are separated into different types according to the relative velocities of their downward and upward phases. In *ocular bobbing*, there are rapid downward jerks of both eyes, followed by a slow return to the midposition (Leigh and Zee 1991). In the typical form, there is associated paralysis of both reflex and spontaneous horizontal eye movements. *Monocular* or *paretic bobbing* occurs when a coexisting ocular motor palsy alters the appearance of typical bobbing. The term *atypical bobbing* refers to all other variations of bobbing that cannot be explained by an ocular palsy superimposed on typical bobbing. Most commonly, the term is used to describe ocular bobbing when lateral eye movements are preserved. *Typical ocular bobbing* is specific but not pathognomonic for acute pontine lesions. Atypical ocular bobbing occurs with anoxia and is nonlocalizing. *Ocular dipping*, also known as *inverse ocular bobbing*, refers to spontaneous eye movements in which an initial slow downward phase is followed by a relatively rapid return. Reflex horizontal eye movements are preserved. It is usually associated with diffuse cerebral damage. In *reverse ocular bobbing* there is a slow initial downward phase, followed by a rapid return that carries the eyes past the midposition into full upward gaze. Then the eyes slowly return to the midposition. It is nonlocalizing.

Vertical nystagmus, due to an abnormal pursuit or vestibular system, is slow deviation of the eyes from the primary position, with a rapid, immediate return to the primary position. It is differentiated from bobbing because there is no latency between the corrective saccade and the next slow deviation. *Ocular-palatal myoclonus* occurs after damage to the lower brain stem involving the Guillain-Mollaret triangle, which extends between the cerebellar dentate nucleus, red nucleus, and inferior olive. Ocular movements, which may be rotatory or circular, move with the same beat

Table 5.5: Oculocephalic reflex (to be performed only after neck stability has been ascertained)

Method	*Response*	*Interpretation*
Lateral: rotation of the head	Eyes remain conjugate, move in direction opposite to head movement (appear to maintain fixation)	Normal
	No movement in either eye on rotating head to left or right	Brain stem lesion Bilateral labyrinth dysfunction Drugs Anesthesia
	Eyes move appropriately when head is rotated in one direction but do not move when head is rotated in opposite direction	Unilateral lesion in lateral gaze center (PPRF)
	One eye abducts, the other eye does not adduct	Third nerve palsy Intranuclear ophthalmoplegia
	One eye abducts, the other does not adduct	Fourth nerve palsy
Vertical: flexion and extension of the head	Eyes remain conjugate, move in direction opposite to head movement	Normal
	No movement in either eye	Same as above with no movement on lateral head rotation
	Only one eye moves	Third nerve palsy
	Bilateral symmetrical limitation of upgaze	Aging

as palatal movements. Ocular flutter is back-to-back saccades in the horizontal plane and may be a feature of cerebellar disease.

Reflex Ocular Movements

Examination of ocular movement is not complete in the comatose patient without assessment of reflex ocular movements, including the oculocephalic reflex ("doll's eye phenomenon") and, if necessary, the vestibulooculogyric reflex, by caloric (thermal) testing. In practice, the terms *doll's eye phenomenon* and *doll's eye maneuver* are used synonymously to refer to the oculocephalic reflex, but these terms are often confusing to the nonneurologist. It is better to use the term *oculocephalic reflex*, followed by a description of the response. This reflex is tested by sudden passive rotation of the head in both directions laterally and flexion and extension of the neck while observing the motion of the eyes. When supranuclear influences on the oculomotor nerve are removed, the eyes appear to retain their fixation on a point in the distance when the head is turned. *This maneuver should not be performed on any patient until the stability of the neck has been adequately assessed.* If there is any question of neck stability, a neck brace should be applied and caloric testing substituted. In the normal oculocephalic reflex (normal or positive doll's eye phenomenon), the eyes move conjugately in a direction opposite to the direction of movement of the head. Cranial nerve palsies predictably alter the response to this maneuver (Table 5.5).

Clinical caloric testing (as distinct from quantitative calorics, used to assess vestibular end organ disorders) is commonly done by applying cold water to the tympanic membrane. It is done with the head tilted backward 60 degrees from the horizontal to allow maximal stimulation of the lateral semicircular canal, which is most responsible for reflex lateral eye movements. After carefully checking to make sure that the ear canal is patent and the tympanic membrane is free of defect, 10 ml of ice-cold water are slowly injected into one ear canal. For purposes of the neurological examination, irrigation of each ear with 10 ml of ice water is generally sufficient.

Cold water applied to the tympanic membrane causes currents to be set up in the endolymph of the semicircular canal. This results in a change in the baseline firing of the vestibular nerve and slow (tonic) conjugate deviation of the eyes toward the stimulated ear. In an awake person, the eye deviation is corrected with a resulting nystagmoid jerking of the eye toward the midline (fast phase). Warm-water irrigation produces reversal of flow of the endolymph, which causes conjugate eye deviation with a slow phase away from the stimulated ear and a normal corrective phase toward the ear. By tradition, the nystagmus is named by the direction of the fast phase. The mnemonic COWS (*c*old *o*pposite, *w*arm *s*ame) refers to the fast phases. Simultaneous bilateral cold water application results in slow downward deviation, whereas simultaneous bilateral warm water application causes upward deviation.

Oculocephalic or caloric testing may elicit subtle or unsuspected ocular palsies. Abnormal dysconjugate responses occur with cranial nerve palsies, intranuclear ophthalmoplegia, or restrictive eye disease. Movements may be hyperactive, sluggish, or absent. Sometimes reinforcement of cold caloric testing with superimposed passive head turning after injection of cold water into the ear may reveal eye movement when either test alone shows none.

False-negative or misleading responses on caloric testing occur with preexisting inner ear disease, vestibulopathy like that due to ototoxic drugs such as streptomycin, vestibular paresis caused by illnesses such as Wernicke's encephalopathy, and drug effects. There is no response when the labyrinth

Table 5.6: Caloric testing

Method	*Response*	*Interpretation*
Cold water instilled in right ear	Slow phase to right, fast (corrective) phase to the left	Normal
	No response (make sure canal is patent, apply warm-water stimulus to opposite ear)	Obstructed ear canal, "dead" labyrinth, eighth nerve or nuclear dysfunction, false negative (see text)
	Slow phase to right, no fast phase	Toxic-metabolic disorder, drugs, structural lesion above brain stem
	Downbeating nystagmus	Horizontal gaze palsy
Cold water instilled in left ear		Responses should be opposite to above
Warm water instilled in left ear after no response from cold water in right ear	Slow phase to right, fast phase to left	Peripheral eighth nerve or labyrinth disorder on right (assuming canal right is patent)

is destroyed; however, partial lesions of the labyrinth may increase or decrease the response. Lesions of the vestibular nerve cause a decreased or absent response. Drugs that suppress either vestibular or oculomotor function, or both, include sedatives, anticholinergics, anticonvulsants, tricyclic antidepressants, and neuromuscular blocking agents. If the response from one ear is indeterminate, both cold- and warm-water stimuli should be applied to the other ear. If the test remains equivocal, superimposition of the doll's eye maneuver is recommended. The interpretation of abnormal cold caloric responses is summarized in Table 5.6.

Motor System

Examination of the motor system of a stuporous or comatose patient begins with a description of the resting posture and adventitious movements. Purposeful and nonpurposeful movements are noted and the two sides of the body compared. Head and eye deviation to one side, with contralateral hemiparesis, suggests a supratentorial lesion, whereas ipsilateral paralysis indicates a probable brain stem lesion. External rotation of the lower limb is a sign of hemiplegia or hip fracture.

Decerebrate posturing is bilateral extensor posture, with extension of the lower extremities and adduction and internal rotation of the shoulders and extension at the elbows and wrist. Bilateral midbrain or pontine lesions are usually responsible for decerebrate posturing. Less commonly, deep metabolic encephalopathies or bilateral supratentorial lesions involving the motor pathways may produce a similar pattern.

Decorticate posturing is bilateral flexion at the elbows and wrists, with shoulder adduction and extension of the lower extremities. It is a much poorer localizing posture, as it may result from lesions in many locations, though usually above the brain stem. Decorticate posture is not as ominous a sign as decerebrate posture because the former occurs with many relatively reversible lesions.

Unilateral decerebrate or decorticate postures are also less ominous. Lesions causing unilateral posturing may be anywhere in the motor system from cortex to brain stem. Unilateral extensor posturing is common immediately after a cerebrovascular accident, followed in time by a flexor response.

Posturing may occur spontaneously or in response to external stimuli such as pain, or may even be set off by such minimal events as the patient's own breathing. These postures, though common, may also be variable in their expression because of other associated brain stem or more rostral brain damage. Special attention should be given to posturing because it often signals a brain stem herniation syndrome. Emergency room personnel and inexperienced physicians may mistake these abnormal postures for convulsions (seizures) and institute anticonvulsant therapy, resulting in an unfortunate delay of appropriate therapy for these patients.

Adventitious movements in the comatose patient may be helpful in separating metabolic from structural lesions. Tonic-clonic or other stereotyped movements signal seizure as the probable cause of decreased alertness. *Myoclonic jerking*, nonrhythmic jerking movements in single or multiple muscle groups, is seen with anoxic encephalopathy or other metabolic comas, such as hepatic encephalopathy. *Rhythmic myoclonus*, which must be differentiated from epileptic movements, is usually a sign of brain stem injury. Tetany occurs with hypocalcemia. *Cerebellar fits* result from intermittent tonsillar herniation. They are characterized by a deterioration of level of arousal, opisthotonos, respiratory rate slowing and irregularity, and pupillary dilation.

The motor response to painful stimuli should be tested, though it should be noted that the pattern of response may vary depending on the site stimulated. Purposeful responses may be difficult to discern from more primitive reflexes. Flexion, extension, and adduction may be either voluntary or reflex in nature. In general, abduction is most reliably voluntary, with shoulder abduction stated to be the only definite nonreflex reaction. This is tested by pinching the medial aspect of the upper arm.

Reflex flexor response to pain in the upper extremity consists of adduction of the shoulder, flexion of the elbow, and pronation of the arm. The *triple flexion response* in the lower extremities refers to reflex withdrawal, with flexion at the hip and knee and dorsiflexion at the ankle, in response to painful stimulation on the foot or lower extremity. Such reflexes are seldom helpful in localizing a lesion.

Spinal reflexes are reflexes mediated at the level of the spinal cord and do not depend on the functional integrity of the brain or brain stem. Most patients with absent cortical or brain stem function have some form of spinal reflex.

The *plantar reflex* may be extensor in coma from any cause, including drug overdoses and postictal states. It becomes flexor on recovery of consciousness if there is no underlying structural damage.

Muscle tone and asymmetry in muscle tone are helpful in localizing a focal structural lesion and may help differentiate metabolic from structural coma. Acute structural damage above the brain stem usually results in decreased or flaccid tone. In older lesions, tone is usually increased. Metabolic insults generally cause a symmetrical decrease in tone. Finally, one must remember that generalized flaccidity is ultimately seen after brain death.

BRAIN HERNIATION

Clinical Signs of Herniation

Herniation syndromes are explained in Chapter 57A. However, a knowledge of some of the clinical signs of herniation is especially important in the clinical approach to coma. Traditional signs of herniation due to supratentorial masses are usually variations of either an uncal or central pattern. Classically, in the former, there are early signs of third nerve and midbrain compression. The pupil initially dilates as a result of third nerve compression but later returns to the midposition with midbrain compression that involves the sympathetic as well as the parasympathetic tracts. In the central pattern, the earliest signs are mild impairment of consciousness, with poor concentration, drowsiness, or unexpected agitation; small but reactive pupils; loss of the fast component of cold caloric testing; poor or absent reflex vertical gaze; and bilateral corticospinal tract signs, including increased tone of the body ipsilateral to the hemispheric mass lesion responsible for herniation (Plum and Posner 1995).

Signs of herniation tend to progress generally in a rostrocaudal manner. An exception occurs when intraventricular bleeding extends to the fourth ventricle and produces a pressure wave compressing the area around the fourth ventricle. Also, when a lumbar puncture reduces cerebrospinal fluid pressure suddenly in the face of a mass lesion that produced increased intracranial pressure, sudden herniation of the cerebellar tonsils through the foramen magnum may result (Plum and Posner 1995). In both cases there may be sudden, unexpected failure of medullary functions that support respiration or blood pressure. The clinical examination of patients with herniation syndromes may be confusing because of changing signs or the expression of scattered, isolated signs of dysfunction in separate parts of the brain. In addition, certain signs may be more prominent than others.

Increased intracranial pressure invariably accompanies brain stem herniation and may be associated with increased systolic blood pressure, bradycardia, and sixth nerve palsies. These signs, however, as well as many of the traditional signs of herniation described above, actually occur relatively late. Earlier signs of potential herniation are decreasing level of arousal, slight change in depth or rate of respiration, or the appearance of a Babinski sign. It is important to suspect herniation early, because once midbrain signs develop, structural injury is likely to have occurred; subsequently there is less chance of reversal.

DIFFERENTIAL DIAGNOSIS

Differentiating Toxic-Metabolic Coma from Structural Coma

Many features of the history and physical examination help differentiate structural from metabolic and toxic causes of coma. Some have already been mentioned above. When the history is available, a patient's underlying illnesses and medications or the setting in which he or she is found often guide the physician to the appropriate cause. The time course of the illness resulting in coma can be helpful. Generally, structural lesions have a more abrupt onset, whereas metabolic or toxic causes are more slowly progressive. Multifocal structural diseases such as vasculitis or leukoencephalopathy are an exception to this rule, as they may exhibit slow progression, usually in a stepwise manner. Supratentorial or infratentorial tumors characterized by slow growth and surrounding edema may also mimic metabolic processes.

The response to initial emergency therapy may help differentiate metabolic or toxic causes of coma. The hypoglycemic patient usually awakens following administration of glucose, the hypoxic patient responds to oxygen, and the patient experiencing an opiate drug overdose responds to naloxone.

In general, structural lesions have focal features or at least notable asymmetry on neurological examination. Toxic, metabolic, and psychiatric diseases are characterized by their symmetry. Bilateral and often multilevel involvement is frequently seen with metabolic causes. Asymmetries may be observed but are generally of small degree and tend to fluctuate over time.

Many features of the neurological examination differentiate metabolic or toxic causes from structural lesions:

1. *State of consciousness.* Patients with metabolic problems often have milder alterations in arousal and tend to have waxing and waning of the behavioral state. Patients with acute structural lesions tend to stay at the same level of arousal or progressively deteriorate. Toxins may also cause progressive decline in level of arousal.
2. *Respiration.* Deep, frequent respiration is most commonly due to metabolic abnormalities, though rarely it is caused by pontine lesions or by neurogenic pulmonary edema secondary to acute structural lesions.

3. *Funduscopic examination.* Subhyaloid hemorrhage or papilledema are almost pathognomonic of structural lesions. Papilledema due to increased intracranial pressure may be indicative of an intracranial mass lesion or hypertensive encephalopathy. Papilledema does not occur in metabolic diseases except hypoparathyroidism, lead intoxication, and malignant hypertension.

4. *Pupil size.* The pupils are usually symmetrical in coma from toxic-metabolic causes. Patients with metabolic or toxic encephalopathies often have small pupils with preserved reactivity. Exceptions occur with methyl alcohol poisoning, which may produce dilated and unreactive pupils, or late in the course of toxic or metabolic coma if hypoxia or other permanent brain damage has occurred. In terminal asphyxia the pupils dilate initially and then become fixed at midposition within 30 minutes. The initial dilation is attributed to massive sympathetic discharge.

5. *Pupil reactivity.* Assessment of the pupillary reflex is one of the most useful means of differentiating metabolic from structural causes of coma. Pupillary reactivity is relatively resistant to metabolic insult and is usually spared in coma from drug intoxication or metabolic causes, even when other brain stem reflexes are absent. Hypothermia may fix pupils, as does severe barbiturate intoxication; neuromuscular blocking agents produce midposition or small pupils, and glutethimide and atropine dilate them.

6. *Ocular motility.* Asymmetry in oculomotor function is typically a feature of structural lesions.

7. *Spontaneous eye movements.* Roving eye movements with full excursion most often suggest metabolic or toxic abnormalities.

8. *Reflex eye movements.* Reflex eye movements are normally intact in toxic-metabolic coma, except rarely in phenobarbital or phenytoin intoxication or deep metabolic coma from other causes.

9. *Adventitious movement.* Coma punctuated by periods of motor restlessness, tremors, or spasm is often due to drugs or toxins such as chlorpromazine or lithium. Brain stem herniation or intermittent CNS ischemia may also produce unusual posturing movements. Myoclonic jerking is generally metabolic and often anoxic in origin.

10. *Muscle tone.* Muscle tone is usually symmetrical and normal or decreased in metabolic coma. Structural lesions cause asymmetrical muscle tone. Tone may be increased, normal, or decreased by structural lesions.

The examiner should be aware of common structural lesions that mimic toxic-metabolic causes and, conversely, toxic or metabolic causes of coma that may have focal findings on examination. Structural lesions that may mimic toxic-metabolic causes include subarachnoid hemorrhage, sinus vein thrombosis, chronic or bilateral subdural hemorrhage, and other diffuse or multifocal disorders, such as vasculitis, demyelinating diseases, or meningitis. Any toxic-metabolic cause of coma may be associated with focal findings; however, focal features are most often observed with barbiturate or lead poisoning, hypoglycemia, hepatic encephalopathy, and hyponatremia. Old structural lesions such as prior stroke may leave residual findings on neurological examination in a patient who is comatose from toxic or metabolic causes. Moreover, metabolic abnormalities such as hypoglycemia may unmask relatively silent structural abnormalities. Detailed descriptions of the toxic and metabolic encephalopathies are provided in Chapter 63.

Differentiating Psychiatric Coma and Pseudocoma from Metabolic or Structural Coma

The patient who appears unarousable as a result of psychiatric disease and the patient who is feigning unconsciousness for other reasons may be difficult to differentiate from each other. In these cases, the history, when available, and the physical examination may seem suspect to the physician, hinting that a nonphysiological mechanism is at work. Multiple inconsistencies are present on examination, and abnormalities that are found do not fit the pattern of usual neurological syndromes. Examinations of the eyelid, pupil, adventitious eye movements, and vestibulooculogyric reflex by cold caloric testing are especially useful to confirm the suspicion of pseudocoma.

Eyelid tone is difficult to alter voluntarily. In the patient with true stupor or coma, passive eyelid opening is easily performed and is followed by slow, gradual eyelid closure. The malingering or hysterical patient often gives active resistance to passive eye opening and may even hold his or her eyes tightly closed. It is nearly impossible for the psychiatric or malingering patient to mimic the slow, gradual eyelid closure. Blinking also increases in hysterical patients but decreases in true stupor.

The pupils normally constrict in sleep or (eyes-closed) coma but dilate with the eyes closed in the awake state. Passive eye opening in a sleeping person or a truly comatose patient (if pupillary reflexes are spared) results in pupillary dilation. Opening the eyes of an awake person produces constriction. This principle may help to differentiate a comatose patient from a patient with pseudocoma.

Roving eye movements cannot be mimicked and thus are also a good sign of true coma. Finally, if the fast phase of ocular movement is preserved on cold caloric testing, the diagnosis of coma is suspect. Cold caloric testing often serves as a sufficient stimulus to awaken the patient.

Laboratory Studies

Laboratory tests that are extremely helpful in evaluating the comatose patient are listed in Table 5.7. Arterial blood gas determinations rule out hypoxemia and carbon dioxide narcosis and help differentiate primary CNS problems from secondary respiratory problems. Liver disease, myopathy, or rhabdomyolysis elevate alanine aminotransferase and as-

Table 5.7: Laboratory tests helpful in coma

Laboratory Study	*Result*	*Associated Disorders*
Electrolytes (Na, K, Cl, CO_2)		See Chapters 56 and 63 for discussion of disorders associated with abnormalities of electrolytes, glucose, BUN, calcium, and magnesium
Glucose		
Blood urea nitrogen		
Creatinine		
Calcium		
Magnesium		
Complete blood count with differential	*Hematocrit:*	
	Increased	Volume depletion, underlying lung disorder, myeloproliferative disorder, cerebellar hemangioblastoma; may be associated with vascular sludging (hypoperfusion)
	Decreased	Anemia, hemorrhage
	White blood cell count:	
	Increased	Infection, acute stress reaction, steroid therapy, after epileptic fit, myeloproliferative disorder
	Decreased	Chemotherapy, immunotherapy, viral infection, sepsis
	Lymphocyte count:	
	Decreased	Viral infection, malnutrition, acquired immune deficiency syndrome
Platelet count	Decreased	Sepsis, disseminated intravascular coagulation, thrombotic thrombocytopenic purpura, idiopathic thrombocytopenic purpura, drugs; may be associated with intracranial hemorrhage
Prothrombin time	Increased	Coagulation factor deficiency, liver disease, anticoagulants, disseminated intravascular coagulation
Partial thrombo plastin time	Increased	Heparin therapy, lupus anticoagulant
Arterial blood gases		See text
Creatine phosphokinase		See text
Liver function studies		See text
Thyroid function studies		See text
Plasma cortisol level		See text
Drug and toxin screen		See text
Serum osmolality		See text

partate aminotransferase levels. Liver function tests may be misleading in end-stage liver disease, as they may be normal or only mildly elevated with markedly abnormal liver function. Although the blood ammonia level does not correlate well with the level of hepatic encephalopathy, it often may be markedly elevated and thus helpful in cases of suspected liver disease with relatively normal liver function studies. Hepatic encephalopathy may continue for up to 3 weeks after liver function studies return to normal.

Thyroid function studies are necessary to document hypothyroidism or hyperthyroidism. When addisonian crisis is suspected, a serum cortisol level should be obtained. A low or normal level in the stressful state of coma or illness strongly suggests adrenal insufficiency. Further testing of adrenal function should be performed as appropriate.

When the cause of coma is not absolutely certain, or in possible medicolegal cases, a blood alcohol level and a drug and toxin screen are mandatory. The results of these tests are not usually available immediately but may be invaluable later. Serum osmolality can usually be measured rapidly by the lab and may be used to estimate alcohol level, since alcohol is an osmotically active particle and increases the osmolar gap in proportion to its blood level. Serum osmolality can be calculated by the following:

$$\text{Serum osmolality} = 2\ Na^+(\text{mEq/liter}) + \text{BUN (mg/dl)}/2.8 + \text{glucose (mg/dl)}/18$$

The osmolar gap, which is the difference between the measured serum osmolality and the calculated serum osmolality, represents unmeasured osmotically active particles.

Creatine kinase levels should routinely be measured in comatose patients initially and then at least daily for the first several days because of the great risk of rhabdomyolysis and subsequent preventable acute tubular necrosis in these patients. Measuring creatine kinase MB isoenzyme levels every 8 hours for the first 24 hours helps rule out a myocardial infarction.

Other Studies

Electrocardiography

The electrocardiogram is useful to show myocardial infarction, arrhythmia, conduction blocks, bradycardia, or evidence of underlying hypertension or atherosclerotic coronary vascular disease. Hypocalcemia causes QT prolongation. Hypercalcemia shortens QT interval. The heart rate is slow in hypothyroid patients with low-voltage QRS, flat or inverted T waves, and flattened ST segments. Hyperthyroid patients are generally tachycardic.

Neuroradiological Imaging

Once the patient is treated and stabilized, the initial examination is complete, and necessary laboratory studies are ordered, the next test of choice is a CT scan of the brain, without contrast but with 5-mm cuts of the posterior fossa. Alternatively, magnetic resonance imaging (MRI) may be performed, depending on the clinical setting and the stability of the patient's condition. MRI provides superb visualization of the posterior fossa and its contents, an extremely useful feature when structural disease of the brain stem is suspected. However, MRI is not as specific for visualizing early intracranial hemorrhage as the CT scan is, and it is limited at present by the length of time required to perform the imaging, image degradation by even a slight movement of the patient, and the relative inaccessibility of the patient during the imaging process. The CT scan, when performed as described, is currently the most expedient imaging technique, giving the physician the most information about possible structural lesions with the least risk to the patient. Intravenous dye may later be necessary to better define lesions seen on the initial CT scan.

The value of the CT scan in demonstrating mass lesions and hemorrhage is undeniable. Furthermore, it may demonstrate features of brain herniation. Uncal herniation is characterized on CT scan by (1) displacement of the brain stem toward the contralateral side, with increase in width of subarachnoid space between the mass and ipsilateral free edge; (2) medial stretching of the posterior cerebral and posterior communicating arteries; (3) obliteration of the interpeduncular cistern; (4) occipital lobe infarction; and (5) distortion and elongation of the U-shaped tentorial incisura. The clinician should be aware that the CT scan may miss early infarction, encephalitis, and isodense subdural hemorrhage. Special caution must be taken in evaluating CT scans in comatose patients, especially prior to lumbar puncture, to rule out isodense subdural or bilateral subdural hemorrhage. Interpretation of CT scans is discussed in Chapter 39.

Electroencephalography

The electroencephalogram (EEG) is helpful in many situations, including confirming underlying cortical structural damage in patients too unstable to travel to a CT scan; postictal states in patients slow to wake after a presumed seizure; partial complex seizures; electroencephalographic or nonconvulsive status epilepticus, such as seen in comatose patients following anoxic ischemic damage; and toxic-metabolic. With metabolic disorders, the earliest EEG changes are typically a decrease in the frequency of background rhythms and the appearance of diffuse theta activity that progresses to more advanced slowing in association with a decrease in the level of consciousness. In hepatic encephalopathy, bilaterally synchronous and symmetric, medium- to high-amplitude, broad triphasic waves, often with a frontal predominance, may be observed. Herpes simplex encephalitis may be suggested by the presence of unilateral or bilateral periodic sharp waves with a temporal preponderance. The EEG also helps confirm the clinical impression of catatonia, pseudocoma, the locked-in syndrome, the persistent vegetative state, and brain death. Electroencephalograms are discussed further in Chapter 37A.

Evoked Potentials

Evoked potentials may help in evaluating brain stem integrity and in assessing prognosis for comatose patients. Brunko and Zegers de Beyl (1987) studied 50 hemodynamically stable patients remaining in coma 4 hours after resuscitation from cardiopulmonary arrest with short latency somatosensory evoked potentials within 8 hours after arrest. They found that none of the 30 patients without cortical potentials recovered cognition. Five of the 20 patients with cortical potentials recovered. Forty percent of their patients who did not recover had preserved brain stem reflexes, allowing some evaluation of prognosis in a group of patients in whom prognosis is difficult to assess by other means.

CLINICAL APPROACH TO PROGNOSIS

Given our current state of knowledge, one cannot reliably predict outcome in any comatose patient with 100% certainty unless that patient meets the criteria for brain death, as described below. Available studies do not allow us to say definitely that any single non-brain-dead patient will not recover from coma, nor do they allow us to prognosticate on how much recovery may occur in specific cases. However, general statistics on the outcome of coma based on serial exams at various times after the onset of coma have been compiled (Levy et al. 1981; Torner 1992) and give the examiner a general idea of how patients may do.

The natural history of coma can be considered in terms of three subcategories: drug-induced, nontraumatic, and traumatic coma. Drug-induced coma is usually reversible unless the patient has not had appropriate systemic support while comatose and has sustained secondary injury from hypoperfusion, hypoxia, or lack of other necessary metabolic substrates.

Nontraumatic Coma

Only about 15% of patients in nontraumatic coma make a satisfactory recovery. Functional recovery is related to the cause of coma. Diseases causing structural damage, such as cerebrovascular disease including subarachnoid hemorrhage, have the worst prognosis; coma from hypoxia-ischemia due to such causes as cardiac arrest has an intermediate prognosis; coma due to hepatic encephalopathy and other metabolic causes has the best ultimate outcome. Age does not appear to be predictive of recovery. The longer a coma lasts, the less likely the patient is to regain independent functioning (Levy et al. 1981).

In the early days after the onset of nontraumatic coma, it is not possible to predict with certainty which patients will ultimately enter or remain in a persistent vegetative state. Although rare cases have been reported of patients awakening after prolonged vegetative states, patients with nontraumatic coma who have not regained awareness by the end of 1 month are unlikely to regain consciousness. Even if they do regain consciousness, they have practically no chance of achieving an independent existence. Clinical experience must be combined with data from studies such as this one to aid the individual physician in prognosticating about each individual patient who is comatose from nontraumatic causes but not clinically brain dead.

Traumatic Coma

The prognosis for traumatic coma differs from that for nontraumatic coma in many ways. First, many patients with head trauma are young. Second, prolonged coma of up to several months does not preclude a satisfactory outcome in traumatic coma. Third, in relationship to their initial degree of neurological abnormality, traumatic coma patients do better than nontraumatic coma patients (Levy et al. 1981).

The prognosis for coma from head trauma may be considered in terms of survival; however, because many more patients survive traumatic coma than nontraumatic coma, it is equally important to consider the ultimate disabilities of the survivors, since many who survive are left with profound disabilities.

The Glasgow Outcome Scale is a practical system for describing outcome in traumatic coma. As originally proposed, there are five categories in this scale: (1) death; (2) persistent vegetative state; (3) severe disability (conscious but disabled and dependent on others for activities of daily living); (4) moderate disability (disabled but independent); and (5) good recovery (resumption of normal life even though there may be minor neurological and psychiatric deficits).

Jennett et al. (1979) studied 1,000 patients in coma longer than 6 hours from severe head trauma: 49% of these patients died, 3% remained vegetative, 10% survived with severe disability, 17% survived with moderate disability, and 22% had good recovery. Depth of coma, as evaluated by the Glasgow Coma Scale, pupil reaction, eye movements, and motor response in the first week after injury, and patient's age were found to be the most reliable predictors of outcome 6 months later.

In summary, early predictors of the outcome of posttraumatic coma include patient's age, motor response, pupillary reactivity, eye movements, and depth and duration of coma. The prognosis worsens with increasing age. The cause of injury, skull fracture, lateralization of damage to one hemisphere, and extracranial injury appear to have little influence on the outcome.

Clinical Approach to Brain Death

A thorough knowledge of the criteria for brain death is essential for the physician whose responsibilities include evaluation of comatose patients. Despite differences in state laws, the criteria for the establishment of brain death are fairly standard within the medical community. These criteria include the following:

1. *Coma.* The patient should exhibit an unarousable unresponsiveness. There should be no meaningful response to noxious, externally applied stimuli. The patient should not obey commands or demonstrate any verbal response, either reflexively or spontaneously. Spinal reflexes, however, may be retained.
2. *No spontaneous respirations.* The patient should be removed from ventilatory assistance and carbon dioxide should be allowed to build up because of the respiratory drive that hypercapnia produces. The diagnosis of absolute apnea requires the absence of spontaneous respiration at a carbon dioxide tension of at least 60 mm Hg. A safe means of obtaining this degree of carbon dioxide retention involves the technique of apneic oxygenation, in which 100% oxygen is delivered endotracheally through a thin sterile catheter for 10 minutes. Arterial blood gas levels should be obtained to confirm the arterial carbon dioxide pressure.
3. *Absence of brain stem reflexes.* Pupillary, oculocephalic, vestibulooculogyric on cold calorics, corneal, and gag reflexes must all be absent.
4. *Electrocerebral silence.* An isoelectric EEG should denote the absence of cerebrocortical function. Some authorities do not regard the performance of an EEG as mandatory in assessing brain death, and instances of preserved cortical function, despite irreversible and complete brain stem disruption, have been reported.
5. *Absence of cerebral blood flow.* Cerebral contrast angiography or radionuclide angiography can substantiate the absence of cerebral blood flow, which is expected in brain death. These tests are considered confirmatory rather than mandatory. On rare occasions in the presence of supratentorial lesions with preserved blood flow to the brain stem and cerebellum, cerebral angioscintigraphy may be misleading.
6. *Absence of any potentially reversible causes of marked CNS depression.* This includes hypothermia (temperature 32°C or less), drug intoxication (particularly barbiturate overdose), and severe metabolic disturbance.

REFERENCES

ANA Committee on Ethical Affairs. Persistent vegetative state: report of the American Neurological Association Committee on Ethical Affairs. Ann Neurol 1993;33:386–390.

Brunko E, Zegers de Beyl D. Prognostic value of early cortical somatosensory evoked potentials after resuscitation from cardiac arrest. Electroencephalogr Clin Neurophysiol 1987;66:15–24.

Childs NL, Mercer WN, Childs HW. Accuracy of diagnosis of persistent vegetative state. Neurology 1993;43:1465–1467.

Corey L, Kirby P. Rash and Fever. In E Braunwald, KJ Isselbacher, RG Petersdorf et al. (eds), Harrison's Principles of Internal Medicine (11th ed). New York: McGraw-Hill, 1987:240–244.

Diagnostic and Statistical Manual of Mental Disorders (3rd ed, revised) (DSM-III-R). Washington, DC: American Psychiatric Association, 1987.

Fisher, CM. The neurological evaluation of the comatose patient. Acta Neurol Scand 1969;45 [Suppl. 36].

Jennett B, Teasdale G, Braakman R et al. Prognosis of patients with severe head injury. Neurosurgery 1979;4:283–289.

Leigh RJ, Zee DS. The Neurology of Eye Movements (2nd ed). Philadelphia: FA Davis, 1991.

Levy DE, Bates D, Coronna JJ et al. Prognosis in nontraumatic coma. Ann Intern Med 1981;94:293.

Long S, Duffin J. The neuronal determinants of respiratory rhythm. Prog Neurobiol 1986;27:101–182.

Mesulam MM. Editorial: frontal cortex and behavior. Ann Neurol 1986;19:320–324.

Osenbach RK, Loftus CM. Diagnosis and management of brain abscess. In SJ Haines, WA Hall (eds), Neurosurg Clin North Am 1992;3:403–420.

Plum F, Posner JB. The Diagnosis of Stupor and Coma (4th ed). Philadelphia: FA Davis, 1980.

Taylor D, Lewis S. Delirium (review). J Neurol Neurosurg Psychiatry 1993;56:742–751.

Torner JC. Outcome evaluation in acute neurological injury (review). Curr Opinions Neurol Neurosurg 1992;5:831–839.

SUGGESTED READING

Berger AJ, Mitchell RA, Severinghaus JW. Regulation of respiration. N Engl J Med 1977;297:92–97, 138–143, 194–201.

Finney LA, Walker AE. Transtentorial Herniation. Springfield, IL: Charles C Thomas, 1962.

Moruzzi G, Magoun HW. Brain stem reticular formation and activation of the EEG. Electroencephalogr Clin Neurophysiol 1949;1:455–473.

The Multi-Society Task Force on PVS. Medical aspects of the persistent vegetative state. N Engl J Med 1994;330:1499–1508, 1572–1579.

Chapter 6
Excessive Daytime Sleepiness

J. David Parkes

In humans there are major changes in the sleep-wake pattern from infancy to old age. In the 30-week-old fetus there are regular cycles of sleeping and waking or at least rest and activity. At birth most of life is spent asleep and about half of this sleep time is occupied by the active phase of sleep, the neonatal equivalent of adult rapid eye movement (REM) sleep. With development, the percentage of each 24-hour cycle spent asleep as well as the percentage of time in active sleep declines.

In adults, the time spent asleep depends on ethnic, environmental, psychological, psychiatric, and disease factors and also on the day of the week, the nature of employment, the personality of the subject, the subject's prevalent mood, and the time of year. On average, agricultural workers in Oxfordshire, England, spend about one-third of their lives asleep and one-tenth dreaming (Taub 1982). However, normal values vary considerably. A few normal adult subjects sleep for only 2–3 hours each 24 hours, while others spend 10–12 hours asleep.

In old age sleep usually deteriorates, although a few 80-year-old subjects sleep as well as young adults. With increasing age, the time taken to fall asleep (sleep latency) increases, total sleep time becomes shorter, and night arousals are more frequent. Sleep has a less refreshing quality and sleep disorders, in particular insomnia, sleep apnea, and sleep myoclonus (periodic movements in sleep), are more frequent with increasing age.

Deaths at night are more common than deaths during the day, with a peak between 4 and 6 A.M. The likelihood of suffering a heart attack is greatest between 6 and 10 A.M. (Mitler et al. 1988). A common reason for the elderly dying painlessly and peacefully during their sleep is probably sleep apnea. Diseases of many body systems may present during sleep rather than wakefulness, as occurs with ulcer pain, paroxysmal nocturnal hemoglobinuria, cluster headache, and some forms of epilepsy.

Much of our knowledge of sleep mechanisms derives from animal studies. Sleep-wake patterns show great diversity in different species depending on age, environment, metabolic rate, and body size. The largest living terrestrial animals, elephants, are, like humans, awake during the day and asleep at night. Elephants' total sleep time is a little less than that of humans, and they show a greater difference between winter and summer sleep. Most mammalian species show cycles of REM and non-rapid eye movement (NREM) sleep. However, REM sleep has not been identified in either the primitive species of echidna (the spiny anteater) or advanced dolphin species. A few animals hibernate, including hedgehogs, brown bats, hamsters, and bears, perhaps as an adaptation to conserve energy. Hibernation starts with a high proportion of NREM sleep followed by a dramatic decline in body temperature, heart rate, and respiratory rate lasting a few hours to several weeks, with eventual return to euthermia. In all animal species that have been studied there is a greater prevalence of sleep in the young than in the old.

NORMAL SLEEP

The Normal Sleep-Wake Cycle

In adults sleep is usually consolidated in one single episode during each day-night cycle (with the exception of the Mediterranean siesta, which is usually taken at the lowest point of waking vigilance, commonly around 3 P.M.). Night sleep consists of two main phases, NREM and REM sleep. As stated above, in infancy the equivalents of these phases are known as quiet and active sleep.

In adults sleep usually starts with NREM activity. However, sleep may start with REM activity in infancy and in a number of pathological states, including the narcoleptic syndrome, alcoholism, depressive illness, and recovery from metabolic coma, and also following head injury and sleep deprivation. Sleep-onset REM activity is defined as occurring within 20 minutes of sleep onset.

NREM sleep is conventionally divided into four stages characterized by a progressive increase in sleep depth and an increase in the strength of stimulus necessary to cause arousal. The occurrence of sleep spindles signals stage 2 sleep onset. Together with the two or three initial REM periods, stages 3 (slow-wave sleep) and 4 (delta sleep) constitute the "core sleep" of the early night. A variety of models, notably those of Hobson et al. (1975) and Borbély et al. (1983), have been developed to explain the brain processes that regulate these aspects of sleep homeostasis.

In normal adults NREM sleep stages occupy the first 60–90 minutes of sleep and are followed by the first REM sleep cycle of the night. During each complete nocturnal sleep cycle there are about four to six NREM-REM cycles. Stages 3 and 4 NREM sleep are most intense during early sleep cycles. In contrast, REM stages in the second half of the night last longer than those in the first half. Thus there is more REM activity in late than in early sleep, and REM-linked sleep disorders may be more prominent in late sleep.

In NREM sleep, electroencephalographic cyclic alternating patterns express the organized complexity of arousal-related phasic events. Frequent arousals, many or all of which may not be recalled on final waking, are particularly disruptive to sleep and may result in severe excessive daytime sleepiness.

The Rechtschaffen and Kales (1968) score system is the standard for sleep studies. Such scoring is accurate and reproducible but time-consuming. It forms the basis for a number of different systems of automatic analysis that give a clinically valuable overview of sleep architecture. The system is being increasingly supplemented by additional physiological studies investigating, for example, motor activity or phasic events during sleep. Thus, it may be important in the study of obstructive sleep apnea to analyze changes in the QT interval, to determine the effects of sleep posture, and to study anatomical changes in the upper airway during sleep.

Anatomy of Sleeping and Waking

The control of sleeping and waking involves many brain structures, including the basal forebrain area, the massa intermedia, the intralaminar thalamic nuclei, the mesencephalic and pontine reticular formation and raphe system nuclei, and the locus coeruleus. In the 1950s most researchers focused their attention on the brain stem. The reticular theory, which viewed sleep as a passive phenomenon, held a dominant position. Since then the neuroanatomy of sleep has been understood to be highly complex and incompatible with a single "sleep center" notion.

From the time of Von Economo, who observed patients with encephalitis lethargica from 1917–1927, it has been known that patients who died in a state of insomnia consistently had inflammatory lesions of the anterior hypothalamus, whereas posterior hypothalamic lesions caused hypersomnia. From this work arose the idea that the brain had two separate systems to control sleep and waking. The experiments of Moruzzi and Magoun suggested there was a reticular formation in the brain stem that influenced the cortex through an activating system, which then induced an arousal state. This system was called the ascending activating reticular system. The system was recognized to be more complicated when it was observed that electrical stimulation of the basal forebrain induced electroencephalograph (EEG) synchronization or sleep. The paramedian preoptic areas that receive serotoninergic terminals originating from raphe neurons are responsible for the induction of synchronized and desynchronized sleep. One major problem at present is to understand how specific structures ascending from the brain stem, locus coeruleus, and raphe modulate thalamic activity and hence EEG synchronization and sleep.

Various studies support the theory that sleep mechanisms, particularly REM sleep mechanisms, are localized in the brain stem but are subjected to complex monitoring by hypothalamic and thalamic structures. The thalamus is the diencephalic structure most closely involved with the control of the sleep-wake cycle, although it might not be indispensable to the organization of sleep-wake rhythms. Clinical studies of progressive fatal insomnia, in which there is massive bilateral degeneration of the nucleus medialis dorsalis as well as anterior thalamic nuclei, have stressed the importance of these regions for sleep control. Experimental investigations in animals suggest that the nucleus medialis dorsalis rather than the anterior thalamic nucleus is most closely involved.

EEG synchronization represents a transfer to the cerebral cortex of excitatory-inhibitory thalamic synaptic sequences. Although this thalamocortical synchronization cannot be considered equivalent in all cases to behavioral sleep, this oscillatory phenomena must be important in sleep-wake control.

The participation of the hypothalamus is central to the organization of sleep. This area links the suprachiasmatic nucleus (SCN) central time clock mechanisms, thermoregulation control, gene transcription sleeping and waking in the brain, and anterior forebrain mechanisms of sleep.

Physiological Changes During Sleep

At the start of sleep, the polysomnogram changes from that of relaxed wakefulness to stage 1 NREM sleep. Slow, rolling eye movements occur, and respiration may become periodic or regular and slow. Heart rate, cardiac output, and blood pressure fall. Body movements and muscle tone are reduced. With the change in motor tone at sleep onset, a single (or less commonly multiple) leg or whole body hypnic jerk may occur. With increasing depth of NREM sleep the degree of muscle atonia increases.

During REM sleep periodic rapid vertical, oblique, and horizontal as well as rolling eye movements occur. There is marked variability in respiration, heart rate, and blood pressure, with usually the highest and lowest blood pressure of the night. Thermoregulation is lost for brief periods. Muscle tone is markedly reduced although the diaphragm and, to a lesser extent, other respiratory muscles are largely spared. Obstructive sleep apnea-associated with atonia of upper airway muscles in the presence of an anatomically narrow upper airway, resulting in periodic airway occlusion, is usually of greater severity during REM than NREM sleep. Penile tumescence lasts an average of 100–200 minutes throughout the night during REM sleep in young adult males.

Dream recall is more frequent in awakenings from REM than from NREM sleep. The false idea has arisen that mental activity in NREM sleep is somehow second rate in comparison to that in REM. There are some qualitative differences in the reported dream mentation in the two sleep phases. REM sleep dreams are usually considered to be vivid and egocentric with frequent scene changes, little or no auditory component, and an overall bizarre quality. NREM sleep dreams are considered to be more vague, less distinct, and less graphic. However, these differences are largely artificial, perhaps byproducts of differences in the dream length and the level of arousal at the time of dream recall. Dream reports differ between home and laboratory environment. Although normal subjects dream with every sleep period, the average recall of dreams in adults is limited to around two to five times a week. A few subjects report many dreams each night, particularly at times of high anxiety or with frequent sleep disturbance. In neurological disorders such as pontine lesions, progressive supranuclear palsy, and some forms of olivopontocerebellar atrophy, which disrupt both REMs during sleep and saccadic eye movements in wakefulness, both REM sleep and dream recall may be reduced or lost.

Several attempts have been made to link dreams with REM sleep physiology and with the motor as well as the autonomic changes that occur during this sleep phase. Ideas about the function of dreams are legion, but there is little or no evidence for the now outdated view of Freud that dreams are "a royal road to the unconscious." Occasionally dreams have been considered to be a source of new ideas and creative thinking. The importance of dreams to the clinical neurologist lies more in their timing than in their nature and may allow the correlation of clinical symptoms with REM-related activity such as occurs in cluster headache, painful nocturnal erections, and REM-linked epileptic phenomena.

The function of sleep is unknown. It is probably necessary for every aspect of human life. The high prevalence of sleep and REM sleep in the young of all species indicates an important role in brain development and the establishment of learning and memory. Many biological systems show marked changes in activity with sleeping and waking. From the behavioral viewpoint, Horne (1988) has distinguished two forms of sleep: core sleep (NREM stages 3 and 4 sleep and the first two to three cycles of REM sleep), deprivation of which results in impairment of many aspects of cerebral function; and optional sleep (the remainder of sleep), loss of which results in subsequent impairment of waking motivation.

Neuropharmacology of Sleeping and Waking

The idea that sleep is regulated by humeral mechanisms is more than two millennia old and was first suggested by Aristotle. The scientific investigation of this idea began this century with the isolation of hypnogenic substances from the brain and cerebrospinal fluid in a number of laboratories. In 1967, Krueger, Pappenheimer, and their colleagues described a transmissible sleep chemical, identified as a muramyl peptide in 1978, thought to act as a sleep factor via the leukocyte cytokine interleukin-1 (Krueger et al. 1978). This finding has been linked to the occurrence of excessive sleepiness with infectious disease and immune-dependent release of cytokines in the brain. Further cytokine sleep factors were identified by Hayaishi (1989), who discovered that prostaglandin D2 was present in anterior hypothalamic preoptic sleep centers of the brain and induced physiological sleep in rats.

Jouvet's discovery of the mechanisms of REM sleep marked the beginning of the neurochemical era and greatly added to our understanding of the complexity of the sleep process (Jouvet 1972). The importance of this work was to show that in the brain stem, along with the classical nonspecific reticular regions, specific structures (such as the raphe nuclei and the locus coeruleus) with specific neurotransmitters (5HT and noradrenaline) played a critical role in sleep mechanisms.

Many animal studies have suggested a major role for 5HT in sleep mechanisms, the regulation of REM sleep, and the maintenance of sleep atonia. However, reports of the action of the 5HT precursors L-tryptophan and 5-HTP on sleep in humans are conflicting. Drugs that alter the storage, release, and reuptake of 5HT in the brain have only minor effects on sleep duration and sleep architecture in humans. The 5HT2 antagonist ritanserin doubles NREM stages 3-4 sleep, and in some insomniac subjects with hypothalamic tumors, this compound restores normal sleep duration.

The importance of cholinergic mechanisms in the generation of REM sleep has been discussed since the 1960s (Hobson et al. 1986). In many species there appears to be an endogenous cholinergic drive for REM sleep originating in cholinergic cell groups of the pontine tegmentum. This system is probably gated by local aminergic and peptidergic neurons.

Sleeping with and without noradrenaline and dopamine has been studied in dopamine beta hydroxylase deficiency and the different forms of parkinsonism. The effects of the dopamine precursor L-dihydroxyphenylalanine and the noradrenaline precursor L-dihydroxyphenylserine have been determined. No major alteration of sleep is found in either disorder, nor do the catecholamine precursors greatly affect sleep architecture.

The effects of alerting a sleeping person with sleep-preventing drugs such as amphetamines and hypnotic drugs such as benzodiazepines have been attributed to central actions on catecholamine and GABA systems, respectively. Amphetamines increase the availability of noradrenaline and dopamine and increase regional cerebral blood flow and glucose oxidative metabolism. The alerting effect may be primarily due to noradrenergic alpha-1 stimulation. Amphetamines reduce total sleep time and also REM sleep. Most hypnotics promote sleep onset, reduce deep NREM and REM sleep, and inhibit motor activity during sleep.

Circadian Organization of Sleep-Wake Cycles

Under normal light-dark, day-night conditions, the sleep-wake cycle occurs regularly every 24 hours, but in the absence of external time cues (e.g., the morning alarm clock, the daily routine of fixed meal times, the alternation between light and dark), the cycle lengthens to approximately 25 hours. Cycle length is slightly greater in males than in females (Moore-Ede et al. 1983).

There is considerable evidence that most if not all of the body circadian rhythms are determined by an internal pacemaker or body clock. One such clock has been localized in the SCN where lesions in animals impair circadian rhythmicity with disruption of rest-activity cycles. The evidence for a functional SCN system in humans is based on the results of hypothalamic lesions, which occasionally alter temperature rhythmicity, and also on studies in subjects blind from birth, in whom retinal-SCN connections may not develop and who sometimes lack definite 24-hour sleep-wake cycles. The retinal-SCN system determines the light-dark rhythmicity of pineal melatonin synthesis and release. The integrity of this system can be tested in humans. A 300-lux light pulse for 30 minutes, given at the time of peak melatonin release (in the dark period, normally 2–4 A.M.) inhibits melatonin synthesis or release in normally sighted subjects.

In animals melatonin, in addition to acting as a chronobiological marker of day length, acts as a stimulus for seasonal breeding with changing day length between summer and winter. Although melatonin levels rise at puberty, a reproductive role for this hormone is not established in humans.

The internal clock of humans is very stable; it is difficult to disrupt normal 24-hour sleep-wake patterns. The internal clock can, however, be reset by external stimuli and, in particular, light. The response is determined by the specific phase at which the stimulus is given during the day-night cycle. The degree of internal adjustment to external time markers is usually quite small—about 1–2 hours forward or backward in each 25-hour intrinsic cycle. This allows for adjustment to a 23.5- to 26.5-hour day-night cycle, a possible explanation for the greater tolerance of east-west than west-east transmeridinal travel.

Body temperature falls after sleep onset due to a combination of circadian and sleep-related factors. Because of its consistency and relative ease of measurement, the temperature rhythm is the most frequently used marker of the circadian oscillator in humans.

DAYTIME SLEEPINESS

Complaints of daytime sleepiness (excessive daytime sleepiness, sleep attacks) are very common. These complaints may result from a *primary disturbance* of circadian or sleep-wake mechanisms in the brain but are more commonly *secondary* to medical, psychiatric, or psychological problems. In many of these cases physical signs are lacking, neuroimaging shows a normal brain, and EEG findings are nonspecific. Despite these problems the clinical discipline of sleep disorder medicine has advanced greatly in the last 25 years with the accumulation of clinical and laboratory data as well as a clinically orientated classification of sleep disorders (International Classification of Sleep Disorders 1990).

The *patient's* view of his or her own sleep problem is often that of a very disabling illness causing marked difficulties with education, work, and social and family life. At least 10% of all subjects who complain of persistent daytime sleepiness or poor sleep are chronically discontent, often with an unsatisfactory life-style and sometimes with false expectations of sleep and a history of many years of chronic invalidism.

The *physician's* view of daytime sleepiness is usually different. Daytime sleepiness (and also insomnia) may appear to be a relatively unimportant symptom in comparison with conditions such as epilepsy, motor disorders, or blindness. However, the narcoleptic syndrome can be at least as disabling as epilepsy, sleep apnea may result in fatal pulmonary hypertension, and some parasomnias may be lethal. Failure of diagnosis and nonrecognition of sleep disorders are common, and undertreatment of daytime sleepiness is frequent, as, for example, in the narcoleptic syndrome.

The need to consider psychological and social as well as medical factors in the diagnosis and management of sleep disorders requires a holistic medical approach.

Excessive daytime sleepiness is sometimes intermittent. Subjects with seasonal affective disorder may be more sleepy in winter than in summer. In the Kleine-Levin syndrome, sleep attacks usually last 3–10 days, separated by several months of normal alertness. Hypersomnolence is occasionally linked to the menstrual cycle.

Terminology

The terminology applied to daytime sleepiness and related symptomatology is often inexact or misleading.

A *circadian disorder* is a disorder of the 24-hour rhythmic timing mechanism—for example, of the sleep-wake, rest-activity, or hormonal rhythm.

The word *narcolepsy* (i.e., sleep seizure, sleep attack) is not synonymous with the term *narcoleptic syndrome*, in which sleep attacks are only one of several features including cataplexy, sleep paralysis, and disturbed nocturnal sleep. However, historical usage has established the word "narcolepsy" as referring to both daytime sleepiness and the narcoleptic syndrome. To avoid confusion, "narcolepsy" should not be used to describe sleep episodes of uncertain cause.

Cataplexy is the sudden onset of paralysis and loss of muscle tone but has other essential components including the presence of a trigger factor, in particular laughter, and the occurrence of phasic jerking of the facial musculature during an attack. The latter feature is of clinical diagnostic value, particularly if an attack is observed. *Catatonia* is an entirely separate condition, not related to any sleep disorder, and is characterized by muscular rigidity, not atonia, and fixed abnormal postures.

Hypnagogic hallucinations, which occur at sleep onset, are different in nature from REM sleep dreams. They are uncommon and incorporate visual patterns with waking mentation but lack any true dreamlike quality. Applying the term *hypnagogic hallucinations* to the presleep dreams of subjects with the narcoleptic syndrome is incorrect, since these take the form of typical REM dreams and are accompanied by REM sleep activity in the polysomnogram. *Hypnopompic hallucinations* (dreams on waking) are normal phenomena, usually derived from characteristic REM dream material. *Sleep paralysis* is a motor paralysis with preserved awareness, occurring at the start or end of sleep.

Hypersomnia, or daytime sleepiness, refers to sleep periods during normal wakefulness. Perhaps the term is best applied to the condition of *idiopathic ("essential") hypersomnia*, in which the propensity to excessive sleepiness is present throughout the complete 24-hour cycle with both prolonged night sleep and daytime sleepiness. *Parasomnia* is a motor or autonomic event occurring around or during sleep or at the junction between sleeping and waking.

Excessive daytime sleepiness, napping, and *dozing* are similar terms that embrace day sleep attacks, subwakefulness, and automatic behavior. *Subalertness*, with reduced awareness of self and environment, failure of self-monitoring, and occasional automatic behavior with subsequent partial or complete amnesia, is a common accompaniment to many forms of excessive daytime sleepiness.

It is important to separate daytime sleepiness from less specific symptoms such as *tiredness* or *excess fatigue*. The complaint of physical tiredness may not be accompanied by any increase in sleep.

Terms used by patients to describe tiredness, fatigue, and sleepiness include the following:

Tired
Feel sleepy
Poor concentration
Fatigued
Poor memory
Exhausted
Can't stay awake
Irritable
Muscle aching
Always half awake
Sad
Lie down to recover
Do not have to go to bed to sleep
Look sleepy
Little interest
Weak
Sleep anywhere
Jaded
No energy
Always dozing
Cannot get out of bed

Subjects with excessive daytime sleepiness have a high propensity to fall asleep quickly with any monotonous activity and, in particular, while lying down in the afternoon when circumstances permit. However, they also fall asleep under unusual circumstances, such as while standing up, talking, or driving. Cognitive and motor performance may be decreased, with unavoidable napping. There is sometimes, but not always, an increase in total 24-hour sleep and occasional difficulty in achieving full arousal on awakening—so-called sleep drunkenness with defocusing, slurred speech, and impaired motor control.

Prevalence of Daytime Sleepiness

Excessive daytime sleepiness is a common yet often neglected symptom. Population surveys and reports from sleep laboratories indicate that 0.3–4.0% of the adult population complain of excessive daytime sleepiness and 14–35% of all adults complain of insomnia. In an investigation of 8,000 subjects presenting with sleep-wake disorders, however, Coleman (1983) found that hypersomnia was a more common complaint than insomnia.

Sleep apnea is the most common cause of excessive daytime sleepiness, although the reported prevalence varies widely. A representative figure is that of Lavie (1981), who found the prevalence of sleep apnea to be 1.1% in all Israeli industrial workers. However, sleep apnea is not always symptomatic. The reported prevalence of the *narcoleptic syndrome* varies from 0.5 to 16.0 per 10,000 (Lavie and Peled 1987; Honda 1979). *Parasomnias*, which are more frequent in children than adults, are an occasional cause of daytime sleepiness. *Psychiatric disorders* (with the exception of endogenous depression) rarely produce daytime sleepiness. Persistent daytime sleepiness is a feature of many *neurological illnesses*. It may, for example, follow head injury or viral infection, or accompany type 2 diabetes, neuromuscular disorders including myotonic dystrophy, and developmental disorders such as the Prader-Willi syndrome. Daytime sleepiness is sometimes secondary to insomnia or results from long-term treatment with *sedative drugs*. Other causes of daytime sleepiness are less common. They include the *delayed sleep phase syndrome*, which has a reported prevalence in Norway of 0.17% (Schrader et al. 1993).

Problems Associated with Daytime Sleepiness

Daytime sleepiness causes considerable and sometimes life-long disability comparable in the narcoleptic syndrome to that of people with epilepsy (Broughton and Ghanem 1976). Many subjects with excessive daytime sleepiness are wrongly considered to be dull, lazy, work-shy, or stupid. If they need treatment they may be viewed as stimulant drug addicts. Work, social, and marital problems due to daytime sleepiness or sleepiness are often considerable. Daytime sleepiness contributes to traffic accidents, particularly rear-end collisions, and is an important cause of accidents at work.

Despite an increasing awareness of sleep disorders by both patients and physicians, a long interval between symptom presentation and disease diagnosis is common. Guilleminault and Dement (1978) suggested, however, that the cause of persistent daytime sleepiness could be successfully established in over 90% of their subjects if detailed investigative facilities were available.

DIAGNOSIS OF DAYTIME SLEEPINESS

Diagnosis depends on a careful history, physical findings, and appropriate investigation including objective and subjective measures of daytime sleepiness such as the multiple sleep latency test (MSLT; Thorpy 1992), the Stanford Sleepiness Scale (SSS), the Epworth Sleepiness Scale (ESS; Johns 1992), and the Maintenance of Wakefulness Test. The SSS and ESS are subjective scales designed to determine the propensity for or level of sleepiness. Subjective ESS scores correlate quite closely with objective MSLT results. The MSLT is the best clinical laboratory measure of excessive sleepiness. The test measures the latency in a 20-minute window to stage 1, stage 2, or REM sleep on five occasions at 120-minute intervals during the day under standard conditions. For reliable results the duration of sleep during the previous night must be known, and the patient must abstain from drugs, alcohol, and coffee before the test. A median latency of less than 7 minutes on three or more tests is considered abnormal, but a few apparently normal subjects do fail the test.

Clinical criteria and major investigative findings for different types of excessive daytime sleepiness are given in Table 6.1.

The Sleep History

The in-depth sleep history should review the patient's activities over an entire 24-hour period; in addition, a standardized questionnaire is useful (Table 6.2). Information taken from other family members can be essential, particularly for revealing events during sleep of which the patient may not be aware. The sleep history must often be supplemented by a clear knowledge of the patient's general physical health in addition to psychological testing with the Minnesota Multiphasic Personality Inventory and other psychometric instruments to measure depression and anxiety. Where indicated, a thorough psychiatric evaluation should also be done. A sleep-wake log, kept over a minimum 2- to 4-week period, is a valuable supplement to the history.

In many cases the cause of daytime sleepiness can be elicited from a careful history supplemented by watching the patient sleep. A number of principles help diagnosis (Tables 6.3 and 6.4). Important diagnostic features include episodes of sleep (rather than just sleepiness during the day); the inability to stay awake; and the propensity to fall asleep anywhere, not just in bed. Most subjects with the narcoleptic syndrome have a very short sleep latency at night, within seconds or minutes of going to bed, although their sleep may then be interrupted.

Fatigue, exhaustion, and tiredness should be differentiated where possible from excessive daytime sleepiness. However, a major problem in the historical diagnosis of sleep disorders is to separate these from fatigue syndromes. In many illnesses, both fatigue and daytime sleepiness may be present.

It is important to distinguish between daytime sleep attacks and other causes of altered awareness such as epilepsy, hypoglycemia, orthostatic hypotension, cardiac disease, and a variety of psychologically triggered events. It is sometimes difficult to differentiate between atonic seizures and cataplectic attacks during wakefulness, and between so-called paroxysmal hypnogenic dystonia and seizures during sleep. Many behavioral problems in childhood may be associated with daytime sleepiness; in adults, hypochondriasis, personality disorders, depression, and possibly schizophrenia may cause similar symptoms.

The *narcoleptic syndrome* is indicated by a history of daytime sleepiness, often starting at school or during the young adult years, although in a few instances the syndrome does not present until late in life. Most, if not all, subjects report a high propensity to fall asleep in any monotonous circumstance but also are unable to stay awake when sustained attention is required. The occurrence of definite cataplexy is necessary for unequivocal clinical diagnosis. Additional features include a short sleep latency, disturbed nocturnal sleep, and a high frequency of motor parasomnias such as sleepwalking, talking, movement during sleep, and sleep paralysis. The pattern of day sleep attacks—short or long, refreshing or nonrefreshing, resistible or irresistible—is not of value in clinical diagnosis. Reports of presleep dream timing may be of little or no diagnostic value. An affected first-degree relative is found in 5–10% of subjects. In a subject with daytime sleepiness but without cataplexy, alternative diagnoses to that of the narcoleptic syndrome must be considered.

The major pointers to the diagnosis of *obstructive sleep apnea* as the cause of excessive daytime sleepiness include a history of loud snoring and frequent witnessed respiratory arrest during sleep. These episodes may be terminated by a sudden inspiratory gasp and are accompanied by sleep rest-

Table 6.1: Common causes of persistent daytime sleepiness

Condition	*Main Clinical Features*	*Investigative Findings*
Obstructive sleep apnea	Children (often with tonsil-adenoid enlargement)	Frequent sleep hypoxia Greater than 3–4% drop in SaO_2
	Highest prevalence in adult males	
	Night sleep snoring, apnea, sometimes sleep restlessness	Imaging shows upper airway narrowing
	Anatomical cause for upper airway obstruction	Polysomnography aids diagnosis and management
	Associated factors including obesity, alcoholism, ENT problems, hypnotics	
The narcoleptic syndrome	Brief (under 60 minutes) day sleep attacks with monotony and under unusual circumstances	Short sleep latency on MSLT SOREMs present
	Cataplexy: triggered (e.g., laughter, also anger, excitement, sport, emotion) atonia with facial muscle quivering	HLA status DR2-DQw1–positive (99% white subjects, 66% black)
	Additional features include short night sleep latency, motor parasomnias, insomnia, sleep paralysis, and presleep dreams	
Idiopathic hypersomnolence	Unrefreshing daytime sleepiness, long naps, prolonged night sleep, difficulty in morning arousal; no cataplexy, sleep paralysis, or sleep apnea	Short sleep latency on MSLT NREM sleep onset Prolonged 24-hour total sleep time
Sleep-related motor disorders	Hypnic jerks, sleep myoclonus, akathisia, bruxism Frequent sleep arousals	Abnormal sleep EMG, video-visual observation
Postviral	History of mononucleosis, other viral illnesses; sleep, tiredness, and fatigue may be long-term consequences	Epstein-Barr virus IgG- and IgM-positive
Post–head injury	Daytime sleepiness may persist for long periods after any head injury	Check for subdural hematoma
Depressive illness	20% of depressed subjects with a sleep disturbance have hypersomnia, not insomnia; particularly bipolar depression	Hypersomnia may respond to antidepressant drug treatment
Familial, genetic	Familial clustering of long sleep duration in idiopathic hypersomnia, Prader-Willi syndrome, myotonic dystrophy	
Metabolic, toxic, endocrine	Sleepiness with left ventricular failure, severe anemia, hypoglycemia, in type 2 diabetes, hepatic encephalopathy, uremia	Endocrine studies, LFTs, check for sleep apnea in thyroid disease, acromegaly
Drugs, alcohol	Alcohol, benzodiazepine, and other hypnotic drugs may cause daytime sleepiness. Many other drugs disrupt the sleep-wake cycle—e.g., sympathomimetic amines, beta blockers	Plasma or urinary drug screen
Neurodegenerative disorders	Alzheimer's disease, diffuse cerebrovascular disease	Neuroimaging
Structural	Brain tumors, encephalitis, multiple sclerosis	Neuroimaging
Cyclical	Kleine-Levin syndrome	EEG slow activity prevalent during sleep episodes
Circadian disorders	Delayed sleep phase syndrome	Circadian monitoring, actimetry

ENT = ear, nose, and throat; EMG = electromyogram; LFT = liver function test; MSLT = multiple sleep latency test; SOREM = sleep-onset REM activity; HLA = human leukocyte antigen (DR = D-related); NREM = non–rapid eye movement; SaO_2 = arterial blood oxygen saturation.

Table 6.2: Checklist for a sleep history (to help define etiological factors)

1. **General:** pain, weight, appetite, work, and environment
2. **Familial and genetic:** Some disorders result in sleep apnea (e.g., nemaline myopathy, Prader-Willi syndrome). Familial or genetic sleep-wake disorders include narcoleptic syndrome, sleepwalking, delayed sleep phase syndrome, sleep paralysis, fatal familial insomnia, idiopathic hypersomnolence, and familial insomnia.
3. **Neurological, psychiatric, and psychological:** These include depressive illness, Parkinson's disease, Alzheimer's disease, and high arousal with anxiety.
4. **Metabolic:** Myxedema and acromegaly can cause sleep apnea.
5. **Cyclical:** Includes menstrual excessive daytime sleepiness and Kleine-Levin syndrome
6. **Drug-related:** Many drugs disrupt the sleep-wake cycle, particularly alcohol, sympathomimetic amines, beta blockers, and hypnotics

Source: Reprinted with permission from JD Parkes. Daytime Sleepiness. In CM Shapiro (ed), ABC of Sleep Disorders. London: British Medical Journal Publishing Group, 1993;15–19.

Table 6.3: Basic principles in clinical diagnosis of excessive daytime sleepiness

1. Daytime sleepiness is usually the result of organic disease. In contrast, insomnia is usually the result of functional or psychiatric disorders (there are many exceptions, however).
2. Clinical diagnosis depends on a careful, detailed 24-hour sleep-wake history, witnessed accounts, and sleep logs as well as evaluation of medical factors. The examination is usually normal with the exception of sleep apnea.
3. Psychological and psychiatric assessment is often of great value in the evaluation of daytime sleepiness.
4. Be alert for uncommon associations with daytime sleepiness—e.g., multisystem atrophy, myotonic dystrophy, acid maltase deficiency.
5. Consider drug-related and circadian factors in any subject presenting with excessive daytime sleepiness.
6. Sleep videotape–sleep oximetry may be cost-effective in preliminary screening for sleep apnea.
7. Consider HLA typing. HLA DR2–negative status almost entirely excludes diagnosis of the narcoleptic syndrome. However, DR2 positivity is not confirmatory.
8. The MSLT is of value in establishing the presence and degree of excessive daytime sleepiness. PSG may be necessary to evaluate the severity and management of sleep apnea. However, laboratory investigation rarely discloses a hidden cause for daytime sleepiness that cannot be established by history and sleep observation.

MSLT = multiple sleep latency test; PSG = polysomnogram.

Table 6.4: Checklist to help categorize the sleep-wake problem

1. Bedtime
2. Sleep onset time
3. Wake time
4. Get up time
5. Owl or lark? What is peak time of waking performance and alertness?
6. Arousals from sleep. If yes, what time, how many, and why?
7. Sleep quality (rate from extremely poor to excellent)
8. Excessive daytime sleepiness—if yes, what time, how severe, under what circumstances?
9. Sleep-related motor events:
   a. Sleep onset (hypnic) motor jerks?
   b. Increased motor activity during sleep including leg restlessness or kicking?
   c. Epilepsy?
   d. Sleep talking, bruxism, sleepwalking?
10. Sleep-atonia related events:
    a. Sleep paralysis (at sleep onset or on waking)?
    b. Cataplexy (stimulus-provoked paralysis and atonia during wakefulness—a clinical diagnostic feature of the narcoleptic syndrome)?
11. Sleep-related autonomic events:
    a. Sweating
    b. Piloerection
    c. Tachycardia in night terrors
    d. Respiratory abnormality (apnea, other respiratory irregularity, choking?)
    e. Nocturnal enuresis
12. Sleep-related cortical-subcortical activity
    a. Dream frequency
    b. Dream timing (sleep-onset dreams, equivalent to sleep-onset REM activity, may occur in depression, following sleep deprivation, or in the narcoleptic syndrome)

Source: Reprinted with permission from JD Parkes. Daytime Sleepiness. In CM Shapiro (ed), ABC of Sleep Disorders. London: British Medical Journal Publishing Group, 1993;15–19.

lessness. Obstructive sleep apnea may occur at any age including childhood, but the condition is most common in the middle-aged or elderly and sometimes in overweight males (60% of subjects). Cataplexy and sleep paralysis do not occur (unless an obese subject with the narcoleptic syndrome also develops sleep apnea). Associated features that result in a narrow upper airway, such as skeletal, mandibular, neuromuscular, and cervical problems, may be obvious. Autonomic failure in multiple system atrophy may present with obstructive sleep apnea, which is present in up to one-third of all children and adolescents with the Prader-Willi syndrome. Assessments of ear, nose and throat, dental, drug, autonomic, alcohol, respiratory, and cardiovascular factors are all necessary.

The reported pattern of daytime sleepiness is of no value in the distinction between the narcoleptic syndrome and obstructive sleep apnea. Sleepiness in subjects with the narcoleptic syndrome, as determined by the ESS and MSLT, is overall a little more severe than with obstructive sleep apnea and may be more severe in the evening than in the morning, but this is not invariable. Irresistible sleep attacks, and also occasional prolonged sleep periods with difficulty in arousal lasting 1–2 days, may occur in both conditions. The pattern of night sleep, not the pattern of day sleep, gives the important clue to diagnosis.

While obstructive sleep apnea and the narcoleptic syndrome account for two-thirds of all patients with daytime sleepiness, it is important to consider other causes. Patients should be questioned regarding a history of virus infection, in particular infectious mononucleosis, which may be followed by both fatigue and hypersomnia; a history of drug use and abuse; alcohol intake; seizure disorders; depression; and rhythmic kicking during sleep suggesting the diagnosis of sleep myoclonus (periodic movements during sleep). Sleep myoclonus and also presleep leg akathisia are common in subjects with daytime sleepiness, but the exact relationship between motor hyperactivity and sleep disturbance is sometimes difficult to establish.

The familial history may be of value in a number of familial or genetic sleep-wake disorders, including, in addition to the narcoleptic syndrome, sleepwalking, sleep paralysis, the delayed sleep phase syndrome, familial insomnia, fatal familial insomnia, and idiopathic hypersomnolence.

Daytime sleepiness is common among elderly patients and may indicate the development of circadian as well as sleep-wake disorders in degenerative brain disease. Particularly important in the elderly is chronic insomnia as a result of physical or psychiatric illness, resulting in secondary daytime sleepiness. In all subjects, circadian factors need to be evaluated in the sleep-wake history, and both daytime sleepiness and parasomnias such as sleep paralysis may be secondary to shift work and other causes of disturbed circadian timing.

Physical Examination

In many patients who complain of excessive daytime sleepiness the results of physical examination are normal. In obstructive sleep apnea, however, it is essential to evaluate obesity, a neck circumference greater than 45 cm, macroglossia, shape of the palate, crowding of pharyngeal structures, pulmonary hypertension, accentuation of the second sound, and peripheral edema.

The possibility of neuromuscular, skeletal, autonomic, metabolic, or endocrinological disease should be considered. The combination of the narcoleptic syndrome with multiple sclerosis is well documented. One-third of subjects with myotonic dystrophy complain of extreme daytime sleepiness, and many neuromuscular disorders—in particular, those that affect the diaphragm, such as acid maltase deficiency—may be associated with severe sleep apnea early in the evolution of the illness.

Laboratory Investigations

The sleep history and clinical examination should determine the direction of sleep laboratory investigation. Laboratory studies, centering on the polysomnogram (PSG), are sometimes essential. Where facilities are available and with enough evidence of a significant sleep disturbance, it is often helpful to document this by PSG. However, PSG does not always give clinically useful information beyond that obtained outside the laboratory.

Polysomnography in sleep disorder centers (SDCs) allows the simultaneous monitoring and recording of the different physiological processes that occur during sleep onset, sleep, and on arousal. SDCs include quiet sleeping rooms equipped with low light or infrared video monitor and recording instruments, polygraphs with multichannel capability for recording the electroencephalogram, electrooculogram and electromyogram with respiratory monitoring, electrocardiogram recording, and, as appropriate, recording of esophageal pressure, blood oxygenation, and pH and rectal temperature. Most laboratories also do MSLTs. Two nights of recording are done in many evaluations, although longer study periods may be necessary to allow the assessment of internight variability.

It is generally agreed that the sleep laboratory approach is useful for the diagnostic evaluation and treatment of patients with sleep-related breathing disorders. It may also be helpful in evaluating suspected cases of the narcoleptic syndrome where other findings are inconclusive or contradictory, and it is sometimes indicated in cases of parasomnia and suspected epilepsy where the distinction between seizure activity and other forms of sleep disturbance is uncertain (Agency for Health Care Policy and Research 1991).

In addition to PSG studies, brain imaging may be indicated if a structural lesion is suspected. Sleep oximetry and video and motor activity monitoring (Cole et al. 1992) can all be used in both the home and laboratory environment and may be more applicable than laboratory-based PSG studies for initial patient screening in sleep apnea and daytime sleepiness.

Over 99% of white subjects with the narcoleptic syndrome are positive for human leukocyte antigen (HLA) DR2-DQw1 (new terminology: DR15 DQ6; susceptibility marker HLA DQB1 0602). The percentage is a little lower in black subjects. The finding of DR2 negativity almost completely excludes a possible diagnosis of the narcoleptic syndrome. However, only 1 in 500 subjects positive for DR2 DQw1 has the narcoleptic syndrome, so a positive finding does not necessarily indicate this condition.

Specialized investigations in sleep apnea are considered in Chapter 73. Tests of autonomic and neuromuscular function, as well as the determination of thyroid status, may be relevant. Determination of Epstein-Barr virus and immunoglobulin G and M may give evidence of previously unsuspected infectious mononucleosis, but this is a common finding in many population studies, and the relevance to the complaint of persistent daytime sleepiness is often uncertain. Stimulant drug abusers sometimes complain of daytime sleepiness to obtain amphetamines and related compounds. In suspicious cases a plasma or urinary amphetamine screen should be done.

REFERENCES

Agency for Health Care Policy and Research. Polysomnography and Sleep Disorder Centers Health Technology Assessment Reports, No. 4. AHCPR Publication No. 92-0027. Rockville, MD: US Department of Health and Human Services, 1991.

Borbély AA, Tobler I, Croos G. Sleep Homeostasis and the Circadian Sleep-Wake Rhythm. In M Chase, ED Weitzmann (eds), Sleep Disorders: Basic and Clinical Research. Lancaster, England: MTP Press, 1983:227–244.

Broughton R, Ghanem Q. The Impact of Compound Narcolepsy on the Life of the Patient. In C Guilleminault, WC Dement, P Passouant (eds), Narcolepsy: Advances in Sleep Research. Vol. III. New York: Spectrum, 1976;201–220.

Cole RJ, Kripke DF, Gruen W et al. Automatic sleep/wake identification from wrist activity. Sleep 1992;15:461–469.

Coleman RM. Diagnosis, Treatment and Follow-up of About 8000 Sleep/Wake Disorder Patients. In C Guilleminault, E. Lugaresi (eds), Sleep/Wake Disorders: Natural History, Epidemiology and Long-Term Evolution. New York: Raven, 1983:87–97.

Hayaishi O. Prostaglandin D2 and sleep. Ann N Y Acad Sci 1989;559:374–381.

Hobson JA, McCarley RW, Wyzinski PW. Sleep cycle oscillations: reciprocal discharge by two brain stem neuronal groups. Science 1975;18:55–58.

Hobson JA, Lydic R, Baghdoyan HA. Evolving concepts of sleep cycle generation: from brain centers to the neuronal populations. Behav Brain Sci 1986;9:371–448.

Honda Y. Census of narcolepsy, cataplexy and sleep life amongst teenagers in Fujisawa city. Sleep Res 1979;8:191.

Horne J. Why We Sleep. Oxford, England: Oxford University Press, 1988.

International Classification of Sleep Disorders. Diagnostic and Coding Manual. American Sleep Disorders Association, 1990.

Johns MW. Reliability and factor analysis of the Epworth Sleepiness Scale. Sleep 1992;15:287–390.

Jouvet M. The role of monoamines and acetylcholine-containing neurons in the regulation of sleep-wake cycle. Ergeb Physiol 1972;64:166–307.

Krueger JM, Pappenheimer JR, Karnovsky ML. Sleep promoting factor S purification and properties. Proc Natl Acad Sci USA 1978;75:5235–5238.

Lavie P, Peled P. Narcolepsy is a rare disease in Israel. Sleep 1987;10:608–609.

Lavie P. Sleep habits and sleep disturbances in industry workers in Israel: main findings and some characteristics of workers complaining of excessive daytime sleepiness. Sleep 1981;4:147–158.

Mitler MM, Carskadon M, Czeisler CA et al. Catastrophes, sleep and public policy: consensus report. Sleep 1988;11:100–109.

Moore-Ede MC, Czeisler CA, Richardson GS. Circadian timekeeping in health and disease. N Engl J Med 1983;309: 469–476.

Parkes JD. Daytime Sleepiness. In CM Shapiro (ed), ABC of Sleep Disorders. London: British Medical Journal Publishing Group, 1993:15–19.

Rechtschaffen A, Kales A. A Manual of Standardized Terminology, Techniques and Scoring System for Sleep Stages of Human Subjects. Los Angeles: University of California at Los Angeles Brain Information Service/Brain Research Institute, 1968.

Schrader H, Bovim G, Sand T. The prevalence of delayed and advanced sleep phase syndromes. J Sleep Res 1993;2:51–55.

Taub JM. Effects of scheduled afternoon naps and bedrest on daytime alertness. Int J Neurosci 1982;16;107–127.

Thorpy MJ. The clinical use of the Multiple Sleep Latency Test. Sleep 1992;15:268–276.

Chapter 7
Approaches to Intellectual and Memory Impairments

D. Frank Benson

Intellect—the cognitive processes that carry out thinking—and one fundamental constituent of intellect, *memory*—the individual's fund of knowledge—are crucial elements in human existence. Intellect and memory are brain functions, and their operations and impairments are legitimate concerns for the neurologist and neuroscientist. Establishing a neural basis for intellect and memory has proved difficult, however; the neurological basis of these high-level cognitive functions remains far behind the understanding of most other aspects of nervous system function. This chapter proposes a neural structure for "higher cortical function" and, from this base, presents approaches to the assessment of intellect and memory.

NEURAL BASIS OF HIGHER CORTICAL FUNCTION

The human cerebral cortex, the thin layer of neurons wrapped over the surfaces of the brain hemispheres, is well described by anatomists (Carpenter 1991). The human cortex is vast; Nauta and Feirtag (1986) estimate that it contains 70% of all of the neurons in the human central nervous system. They also suggest that 75% of all cortical neurons in the human brain are located in the association cortex. Almost all operations that can be defined as "higher cortical functions" are carried out by the association cortex.

In recent decades, three novel approaches to the understanding of higher cortical function have been developed and actively pursued. One, which probes the differences between right- and left-hemisphere functions, has received major emphasis from the study of subjects who have undergone section of the corpus callosum for seizure control. A second approach borrows principles from information processing theory and its offspring, artificial intelligence, to produce theories of brain function based on complex distributed neural networks (Goldman-Rakic and Friedman 1991; Mesulam 1990). A third approach has concentrated on the role played by the prefrontal cortex in higher mental control (Fuster 1989). To provide a background for higher cognitive functions, four functional subdivisions of the human cortex are proposed and two operational hierarchies of higher cortical function are suggested. The proposed functional subdivisions of the cortex, along with the primary operational characteristic of each, are listed in Table 7.1.

The *primary cortex* (visual, auditory, somesthetic, and motor) is relatively well-known and readily identified by both anatomical and operational characteristics. Each primary cortex receives and processes information from a single (exteroceptive) modality and has cortical-cortical connections only to an adjacent area of association cortex, the *unimodal association cortex*, which is also dedicated to that modality. The primary cortex is relatively limited in size in the human, and each primary area is anatomically distinct. In contrast, the surrounding unimodal association cortex is large and relatively indistinct in cytoarchitectural features. It is the task of the various unimodal association areas to process information from the primary input into unimodal information (percepts).

Table 7.1: Functional subdivisions of cortex

Cortical Area	*Operation*
Primary cortex	Receive and transfer primary exteroceptive sensory (and motor) stimuli
Unimodal association cortex	Formation of unimodal percept
Heteromodal association cortex	
Posterior	Cross-modal associations
Anterior	Sequential associations
Supramodal association cortex	Receive and transfer interoceptive sensory information

The third subdivision of the cortex in the human, the *heteromodal association cortex*, can be subdivided further into two anatomically and operationally separate units. The first, the *posterior heteromodal association cortex*, centers in the region of the angular gyrus and appears essential for cross-modal association, the ability to combine percepts derived from multiple modalities. The second, the *anterior heteromodal association cortex*, occupies the lateral (dorsal) aspect of the prefrontal cortex and is essential for maintaining serially presented information over time (Fuster 1989). The two heteromodal association cortex regions, although separate in both location and function, are interconnected so intimately in their operations that they are difficult to separate.

Each major region (visual, auditory, and somesthetic) of sensory unimodal association cortex abuts, and is linked directly to, the posterior heteromodal association cortex; each also is connected to the anterior heteromodal association cortex and to homotopical areas of the opposite hemisphere via long white-matter fasciculi. Unimodal and heteromodal association cortices, plus their massive and complex connections, provide the neural substrate (distributed neural networks) for higher cortical functions.

A fourth important subdivision of the human cortex, the *supramodal association cortex*, has strong connections to both unimodal and heteromodal association areas but operates independently. Located in the anterior, medial, and orbital prefrontal regions and possibly the temporal poles, the supramodal association cortex has strong links to limbic structures. This cortical area receives almost all cortical input from the visceral, autonomic, and emotional systems (interoceptive functions). It is through the supramodal association cortex connections that these homeostatic structures most robustly interact with the exteroceptive (sensorimotor) system.

Subcortical inputs to the cortex are distinct and separate. Each primary cortex region receives input from an individual sensory system directly via the sensory thalamus; the unimodal and the heteromodal association cortices do not receive significant direct exteroceptive input. The supramodal association cortex receives major input both from the limbic cortex and from many other subcortical structures such as the reticular system, the hypothalamus, and the medial (limbic) thalamus. In addition, subcortical motor structures (particularly the basal ganglia), via connections in the motor thalamus, have strong links to the anterior heteromodal association cortex and possibly some connections to the supramodal association cortex.

In summary, higher cortical functions are performed in two areas of the cortex: the relatively massive unimodal association cortices and the far smaller but crucial heteromodal association cortices. These areas receive almost all of their input from two cortical sources: primary sensory input from the primary cortex, and homeostatic and limbic input from the supramodal association cortex. *Thought processing* (intellect) is the product of the combined unimodal and heteromodal association cortex system, which is influenced constantly by inputs from the primary and the supramodal association cortices. Thus, higher cortical functions are produced by the interaction of two separate neural systems: exteroceptive and interoceptive. Memory and intellect are two processes of higher cortical function.

MEMORY

Fundamental to human intellectual function is the ability to receive, process, maintain, and later retrieve information—the mental operation called *memory*. Memory is a multifaceted function, not a single unitary act, and the need to subdivide memory functions has produced a bewildering number of subclassifications. Twenty different bipartite divisions of memory (e.g., long-term/short-term) and seven examples of tripartite divisions (e.g., immediate, recent, short-term), plus additional classifications containing four, five, and even more separations of memory function have been presented since 1985 (Benson 1994). For the clinician, however, this bewildering memory nosology is circumvented readily. Clinicians have long recognized three major variations of memory function that they monitor in a routine mental status evaluation. For this chapter these three memory functions will be termed: (1) *immediate recall*; (2) *learning ability*; and (3) *retrieval*. Although often intermixed, pure disorders of each can be identified by appropriate test procedures and each of the three appears to have a distinct neuroanatomical basis.

Immediate Recall

Immediate recall, also called immediate, short-term, or primary memory, refers to the ability to maintain a small amount of information with total accuracy over a brief period of time. Although it is not truly a memory function (the information is not necessarily maintained), intact immediate recall is essential for all subsequent memory activities.

Disorder of immediate recall produces a well-known clinical condition called *confusion* (clinically termed acute confusional state, delirium, or metabolic or toxic encephalopathy). This brain disorder, which often indicates serious medical dysfunction, is described in Chapter 4. The full syndrome includes disturbed attention (inability to maintain attention, distractibility, stimulus-bound status); inability to maintain coherent thought; lethargy (may or may not be present); dysfunctional cognition and learning; hallucinations or delusions, or both; and a disturbed sleep-wake cycle. The most prominent disturbance is the difficulty maintaining attention; disordered immediate recall is a defining element of acute confusion.

The basic evaluation for immediate recall is observation of the subject's distractibility and the incoherent nature of his or her conversation and thinking. A simple formal test is the digit

Table 7.2: Clinical features of amnesia

Immediate recall	Normal
Learning	Impaired to absent
Retrieval	Normal (except for long retrograde amnesia)
Cognition and personality	Basically normal

span. A normal individual should have a digit span of five or more. Patients with immediate recall disorders often (but not always) show significant limitation (two to four). Mental control tests (e.g., counting backwards from 20; the serial sevens exercise; reciting the months in reverse) are more challenging and often are failed by the confused individual. Each test must be analyzed with caution, however, as it can be failed because of other disturbances (e.g., acalculia, aphasia).

Learning Ability

Impaired ability to learn new information is the prime constituent of amnesia. In relatively pure examples of amnesia (e.g., Korsakoff's syndrome, status post-herpes encephalitis), the individual will have normal immediate recall, normal ability to recall old, overlearned information (except for an extended period of retrograde amnesia), and relative retention of cognitive competency and personality characteristics. The clinical findings that characterize amnesia are recorded in Table 7.2.

Bedside tests of learning ability challenge the ability to maintain newly presented information over a finite period of time that is filled with supervening distractions. One common test offers the patient three or four unrelated words or a name, address, and flower (three bits of information) with instructions to retain them for a period of 5–10 minutes, during which time other testing is performed. More formal bedside tests probe the ability to learn 8- or 10-item supraspan word lists, the Babcock sentence ("For a nation to be rich and powerful, it must have a strong, secure supply of wood"), or similar supraspan material.

Impaired learning (amnesia) with little or no other problem in higher mental function is present in only a few disease processes. Table 7.3 lists the disorders that can cause relatively pure amnesia and the recognized neuroanatomical loci of pathology for some of the disorders. Medial temporal lobe damage is the most common but not the only cause of amnesia (Squire and Zola-Morgan 1991). By far the most common cause of amnesia is trauma, but posttraumatic amnesia almost routinely is associated with other, confounding neurobehavioral abnormalities. Korsakoff's psychosis, amnesic stroke (based on posterior cerebral artery occlusion), and the amnesias secondary to cerebral tumors, cerebral infections, hypoglycemia, hypoxia, or the postconvulsion state are less common. One striking disorder, *transient global amnesia* (TGA), is a short-lived amnesic state that may follow some physical stress or alteration of body temperature (Caplan 1985). Although TGA produces a dramatic disability, the amnesia is transient, most often occurs only once, and leaves no residuals. Psychogenic amnesia, although often described in literature and the lay press, is seen rarely in clinical practice. Psychogenic amnesia does not fit the characterization outlined in Table 7.2, as the individual can learn new material but shows a selective disorder of information retrieval. Specifically, the information that cannot be retrieved in psychogenic amnesia is highly overlearned personal history, whereas less personal information such as the names of presidents, recent news events, and so on may be recalled.

Amnesia (learning disability) often coexists with other cognitive disorders and is considered a prime indicator of dementia (American Psychiatric Association 1994). Tests to demonstrate amnesia also can demonstrate the memory disorder of dementia but, almost as a rule, other concurrent cognitive disorders of dementia will obscure the clinical findings of amnesia. Many (possibly most) causes of dementia produce a retrieval deficit in addition to, or in place of, the learning disorder of amnesia (see Chapter 41).

Retrieval

The ability to retrieve information learned in the past represents an essential component of human thought processing. The amount of information that can be stored by the

Table 7.3: Etiologies of amnesia

Disorder	*Site of Major Pathology*
Thiamine deficiency (Korsakoff's disease)	Diencephalon (mamillary bodies)
Traumatic brain injury	Widespread, predominantly medial temporal
Cerebrovascular disease (most often posterior cerebral artery occlusion)	Medial temporal
Cerebral infection (most often herpes simplex encephalitis)	Limbic, medial temporal
Surgical lobectomy (bilateral temporal lobectomy)	Medial temporal
Neoplasm	Medial temporal, fornix, thalamus
Epilepsy/electroconvulsive therapy	
Anoxia	
Transient global amnesia	
Psychogenic amnesia	

Source: Adapted from DF Benson. The Neurology of Thinking. New York: Oxford University Press, 1994.

Table 7.4: The UCLA Memory Test

Registration	*(1)*	*(2)*	*(3)*	*(4)*	*Recall*	*Category Clue*	*Multiple Choice*
Cabbage	_____	_____	_____	_____	_____	Vegetable _____	_____
Table	_____	_____	_____	_____	_____	Furniture _____	_____
Dog	_____	_____	_____	_____	_____	Animal _____	_____
Baseball	_____	_____	_____	_____	_____	Sport _____	_____
Chevrolet	_____	_____	_____	_____	_____	Car _____	_____
Rose	_____	_____	_____	_____	_____	Flower _____	_____
Belt	_____	_____	_____	_____	_____	Clothing _____	_____
Blue	_____	_____	_____	_____	_____	Color _____	_____
TOTAL							

normal human brain for later retrieval is prodigious; the accuracy of retrieved information, however, is far from exact. A disorder of information retrieval often coexists with disordered learning (as in Alzheimer's disease), but retrieval disorder is the primary memory disorder in many disease states and is a normal phenomenon that increases with age (Cummings and Benson 1992).

Testing retrieval competency is considerably more difficult than testing either immediate recall or learning ability, primarily because the examiner cannot know the patient's fund of knowledge. Standard information questions such as the names of national leaders, both past and present; information concerning dramatic news events (e.g., the Kennedy assassination, the Gulf War, recent earthquakes or wars) or standard knowledge (e.g., the capital of France) depend on the patient's interests and level of education. Retrieval ability can be evaluated, but failures demand cautious interpretation by the examiner.

The memory disorders associated with subcortical cognitive disorders (e.g., the dementia of Huntington's disease or progressive supranuclear palsy and the relatively common causes of vascular dementia such as Binswanger's disease and multi-infarct dementia) produce disproportionate difficulties of retrieval. Disordered information retrieval is a cardinal finding of some "frontal disorders," particularly those that involve orbital and midline structures, and often is complicated by posttraumatic amnesia.

The UCLA Memory Test

Table 7.4 presents, in outline form, a short and efficient test that can be administered in the clinic or at the bedside to assess the three varieties of memory. Although longer, more rigidly administered, and far better validated memory tests can be administered by the neuropsychologist (see Chapter 41), the UCLA Memory Test quickly provides the clinician with much information. It consists of eight unrelated words that are recited by the examiner four times. After each recitation the patient repeats as many of the words (in any order) as possible. Over the four presentations a learning curve (or lack of one) can be established. After approximately 10 minutes, with distractions by other tests, the patient is asked to recall as many of the eight words as possible. The first test score records spontaneous recall. For those words that cannot be recalled, two types of cues are offered in sequence: a category cue and then selection from a multiple-choice list (three related items including the original).

Immediate recall can be gauged from the learning curve. Patients with disordered immediate recall will show a relatively flat curve (e.g., 3-3-4-3), whereas normal subjects and many patients with amnesia or retrieval disturbance will show improving performance (e.g., 4-5-7-8). After the delay, normal subjects will retrieve most of the eight words spontaneously (5-8, somewhat dependent on the intelligence of the subject) and most normal subjects will produce confidently the words that they missed when given a category cue or a multiple-choice selection. Normal subjects seldom show confabulatory responses or intrusions.

Patients with amnesia perform poorly on spontaneous recall, as expected, and show little better than chance-level results in response to cues. Intrusions (incorrect words presented during spontaneous recall) and confabulatory presentations (wrong guesses following cueing) are common in amnesic patients.

Patients with retrieval disturbance often perform just as poorly on spontaneous recall as the amnesic patients but improve considerably with prompting, identifying most or all remaining words from one or the other type of cueing. In addition, their degree of confidence in their selection and the lack of confabulatory or intrusive responses helps separate the subject with retrieval disorder from the true amnesic patient.

INTELLECT

Intellect comprises the cognitive processes of thinking, relating, and judging, as "the power or faculty of knowing as distinguished from the power to feel and to will" (Webster's Third New International Dictionary of the English Language 1986). Sternberg (1987) simply states: "The intellect is associated with cortical brain function." These definitions, although broadly acceptable, are notably nonspecific. More exact delineation demands recognition of the individual constituents of intellect and their interactions, which lead to the processing of thought (Benson 1994). The three fundamental aspects of intellect are the fund of knowledge, cognition, and executive (cognitive) control.

The Fund of Knowledge

Crucial to all intellectual functions is the availability of a vast storehouse of previously learned information, the accumulated product of the memory apparatus. This information can be subdivided into three major categories: *verbal*, *nonverbal* (primarily visual), and *homeostatic*. Current conceptions (Damasio 1989; Zola-Morgan and Squire 1990) suggest that long-term storage of information occurs through sizable interconnected networks of neuronal aggregates located in the (unimodal and heteromodal) association cortices of both hemispheres. The networks are vast, with entry available through several individual neurons that provide access to large quantities of stored knowledge. Although the fund of knowledge is constantly growing, it also decays and alters, decreasing the accuracy of individual memories.

Cognition

The ability to manipulate the body of knowledge stored as memory is an indispensable factor of human intellectual competency. Cognition, defined in this restricted sense, includes the ability to compare, use, and combine newly received or stored material to produce new information (Benson 1994). The reformulation of information derived from multiple sources to produce new information vastly increases the breadth, complexity, and utility of the intellectual process. Although performed to a limited degree by some higher primates, the ability to manipulate information from multiple modalities is so vastly superior that it is unique to humans.

Executive (Cognitive) Control

A third critical component of intellect is the ability to monitor, anticipate, inhibit, and thus control mental processing. Control of higher-level mental functions, known as executive control (Fuster 1989), is achieved through multiple monitoring processes and the inhibition of most simultaneously activated neural channels. Executive control function includes the ability to carry out retrospective analyses and to formulate plans for the future, using both newly realized information and material from the fund of knowledge. Both retrospective analyses and plan formulation processes provide breadth and novelty to cognitive processing, well beyond the stimulus-response instrumentality of basic behavior. Daydreaming and fantasy are everyday examples of this future-thought capability; human creativity is a crowning glory of the executive control function.

Although material processed through the unimodal sensory system provides the most obvious ingredients of intellect, all three aspects of cognitive processing are acted on by powerful supramodal (homeostatic) inputs. A personal, emotional motivation influences almost every activity of the intellect. Supramodal input to cognitive processing is both integral and powerful.

Neural Basis of Intellect

Each primary sensory cortex (visual, auditory, and somesthetic) receives information from external sources that has been partially processed (selected and categorized) by the time the material reaches the cortex. The primary sensory cortex further categorizes the information by transferring it to selected regions of the surrounding unimodal association cortex. The primary motor cortex carries out a similar, relatively specific, function by accepting processed data from the surrounding unimodal motor association cortex for transfer to external effectors.

The sensory unimodal association cortex processes single modality information into single modality percepts by further categorizing and discriminating the new stimuli and comparing and contrasting this product with previous stimuli of a similar nature. Essential for this matching process is a vast store of previously processed stimuli for comparison. The stored memories used to assemble unimodal percepts represent a significant core of the fund of knowledge. Unimodal percept formation, based on the comparison with previously experienced stimuli, is a complex task that demands a vast cortical expanse (Jerison 1991). Most long-term memories are stored in the interconnected neuronal ensembles scattered throughout the unimodal association cortex.

The supramodal association cortex influences cognitive processing in a manner analogous to the primary cortex/unimodal association cortex operations that provide homeostatic percepts. The supramodal association cortex, which is located in the anterior cerebral regions, occupies vast areas of the medial, polar, and orbital frontal cortex and anterior temporal cortex. Through these anterior cortical regions, almost all information concerning intrinsic (bodily) functions is received, processed, and transferred. Information processed by the supramodal association cortex enters the neural networks formed within the heteromodal and unimodal association cortices of both hemispheres. Through these connections, autonomic, visceral, and emotional factors influence cognitive processing.

The heteromodal association cortex carries out two distinct operations in two separate cortical areas. The posterior heteromodal association cortex, centering around the angular gyrus, interrelates unimodal percepts, blending and integrating information from multiple modalities. The resultant cross-modal associations allow unimodal percepts to be more fully recognized and identified. Simple cognitive processes such as provision of a phonated name to a visualized object are performed so rapidly and (apparently) automatically that only through the demonstration of unusual clinical cases can the initial step, the formation of the unimodal percept, be demonstrated. Although occurring to a limited degree in some advanced primates, cross-modal associations are established to a far greater degree in the human brain; this operation, carried out through the posterior heteromodal association cortex, is fundamental to the cognitive processing of the intellect.

A second function performed by the heteromodal association cortex occurs in a more anterior location—the dorsal lateral prefrontal lobes (centering on Brodmann's area 46). Ingenious investigations (Fuster 1989; Goldman-Rakic and Friedman 1991) have demonstrated that this region of the primate cortex is needed to maintain sequences of information over short periods of time, a temporal factor critical for advanced cognitive processing. The collection and management of information bits over time demands numerous interconnections with the posterior heteromodal association cortex and with each unimodal association area. The result is a richly integrated matrix of neural elements capable of manipulating complex arrays of information.

Strong supramodal association cortex input (primarily to inhibit multiple, simultaneously activated polymodal circuits) provides a major control mechanism for anterior heteromodal functions. The anterior heteromodal association cortex provides monitoring and inhibitory controls that are crucial to higher mental processing.

Mechanisms of Intellect

In addition to the two major subcortical inputs to the cortex—the direct thalamocortical relays and the indirect, multisynaptic homeostatic relays to the supramodal association cortex—significant connections link established neural structures of the basal ganglia and thalamus to various prefrontal sites. These connections evidently monitor and control the motor responses of cognitive processing (Goldberg 1987). High-level cognitive functions such as language, calculation, visual-constructive processes, and others apparently are performed entirely by cortical structures, primarily by the consortiums of unimodal and heteromodal association neurons that receive and process exteroceptive and interoceptive inputs. A vast number of neural networks, readily accessed through multiple neural sites and operating simultaneously across interrelated circuits, produce both the competence and the rich variety that characterize human intellect.

Tests of Intellect

Traditionally, intelligence (combining the fund of knowledge and cognitive processing) has been tested by formal intelligence tests such as the Wechsler Adult Intelligence Scale (Wechsler 1958). The components and interpretations of these tests, which are administered by psychologists, are discussed in Chapter 41. The clinical neurologist, however, must determine, at least to a limited degree, the patient's mental competency on an ongoing basis that defies formal psychological evaluation. Many short mental status evaluations have been developed but even these tests are too time consuming for many clinical purposes. Simple, selective, and broadly informative evaluations are needed for routine patient management.

Language

A few informal, bedside clinical evaluations of language function should be in the armamentarium of all practicing neurologists. Basic evaluations—of the characteristics of conversational speech and the ability to comprehend spoken language, as well as tests of competency in repetition, naming, reading, and writing—can be performed quickly and provide valuable information.

A simple dichotomy of conversational speech—nonfluent versus fluent-paraphasic—indicate, respectively, an anterior or posterior language area lesion. A similar separation of aphasic subjects, into those who cannot repeat easily and those who can, indicates perisylvian (inability to repeat) or extrasylvian (ability to repeat) damage (Benson and Geschwind 1971). Comprehension of spoken language is more difficult to test and to interpret. Whether the patient can point to objects when the examiner presents the name (both individually and in sequences) provides one crude gauge of language comprehension. Yes-no questions and requests to carry out simple commands may provide additional data. All tests of comprehension can be failed because of other factors (e.g., apraxia), however, and caution is needed for interpretation.

One sensitive (easily disturbed) language function is word-finding. The patient's failure to name objects, parts of objects, body parts, or colors often indicates aphasia. Monitoring the subject's ability to produce a list of words in a category suggested by the examiner (e.g., animals, articles of clothing, words beginning with the letter *R*) provides a different, diagnostically significant evaluation of lexical competency.

The patient's abilities to read aloud and to comprehend written material may be disordered independently and should be evaluated separately. In a similar vein, writing may be disordered on a mechanical or on an aphasic basis.

The basic interpretation of language abnormality need not be complicated. The presence of aphasia (acquired impairment of language) almost always indicates left-hemisphere dysfunction; further division of the language problem into fluent or nonfluent combined with assessment of the patient's ability to repeat provides valuable anatomical information. Figure 7.1 presents a useful algorithm for determining aphasia types; this information suggests the basic localization of the cortical area damaged.

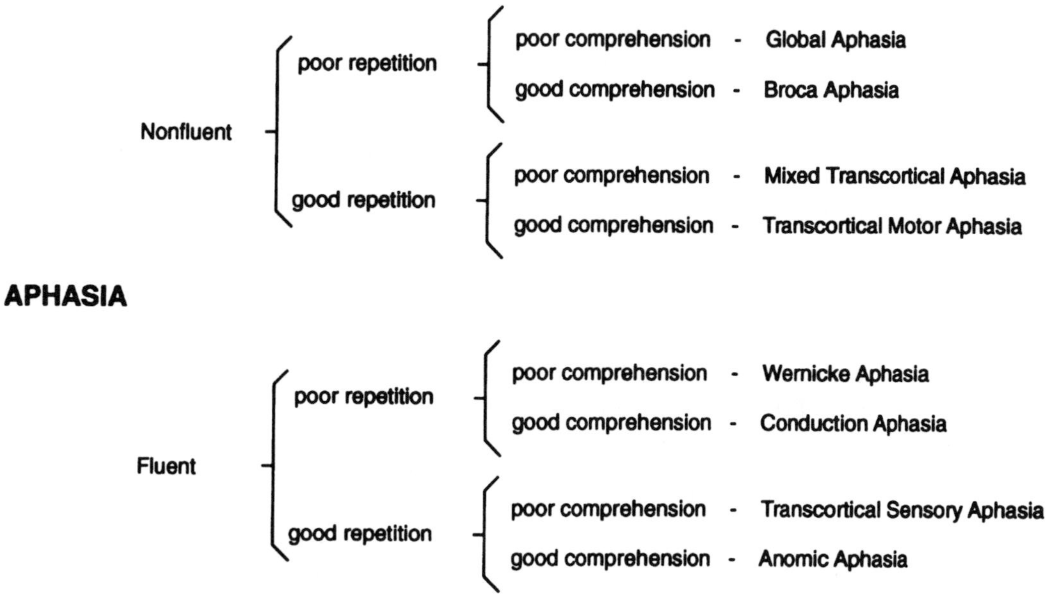

FIGURE 7.1 Algorithm used to determine the basic aphasia syndromes.

Visual-Spatial Skill

Just as essential to cognitive function as language but considerably more difficult to evaluate and even harder to interpret is competency in visual-spatial skills. One simple probe of visual-spatial competency for use in the clinic is to request that the patient copy simple two-dimensional and three-dimensional line drawings. Figure 7.2 illustrates several drawings of the type that can be used with almost all subjects.

Disordered drawing skill can follow either a right- or left-hemisphere disorder. Right-hemisphere damage produces disordered discrimination of the visualized object as it lies in space, whereas left-hemisphere damage interferes with the executive (motor) skills needed to reproduce the image. Although representing a strong indication of brain dysfunction, the copy-drawing test provides limited localizing data; more specific determination of visual-spatial competency usually demands specialized testing.

Data from the patient's history and several simple bedside tasks can provide valuable information. The clinician can suspect a visual-spatial disorder if the patient easily gets lost (environmental agnosia); cannot read maps

FIGURE 7.2 Two- and three-dimensional line drawings that can be used to test a patient's visual-spatial competency.

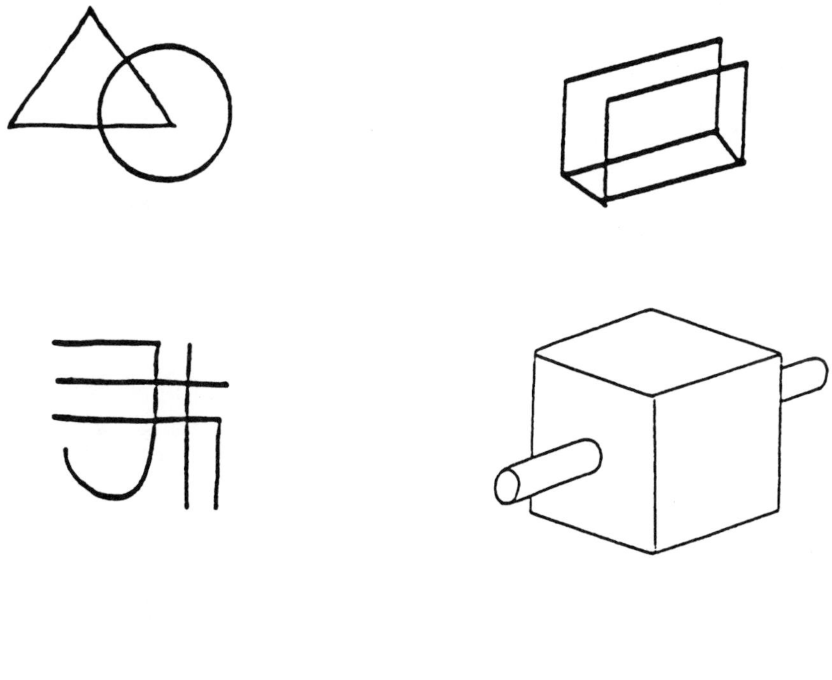

(topographagnosia); cannot recognize familiar faces (prosopagnosia); cannot identify colors (color agnosia); cannot recognize or identify visually presented objects (visual agnosia); or has another visually oriented dysfunction. Grüsser and Landis (1991) provide an excellent review of higher visual dysfunction as demonstrated in the clinic. The neural basis of visual skills has been analyzed actively (Poggio and Edelman 1990; Tanaka 1993) but is difficult to evaluate in the clinic.

Cognition (Manipulation of Knowledge)

Cognition is tested readily in a clinical setting. One elementary probe of the patient's ability to manipulate knowledge is to test simple mathematics. Many elementary arithmetic facts (e.g., 8 + 5=___; 13 − 6=___; 6 × 7=___) are held as rote memories. In contrast, the ability to solve computations of more complex numbers (e.g., 39 + 17=___; 52 − 24=___) demands combination of the previously learned data and provides a relatively pure reflection of cognitive (manipulative) skill. More complex tests such as word problems (e.g., "If you place 18 books on 2 shelves so that twice as many books are on one shelf as the other, how many books go on each shelf?") (Luria 1966) demand manipulation of knowledge, but language competency becomes a more pertinent factor. Educational level is of significance but, for most patients, simple arithmetic problems provide an easily analyzed indicator of cognitive ability.

Competency at recognizing similarities and differences and the ability to understand the metaphors needed for proverb interpretation provide additional gauges of cognitive skill. Both similarities and differences and idioms and proverbs can be categorized, at least roughly, as simple, moderate, or difficult. Most subjects should be able to define simple similarities (e.g., "How are an apple and an orange similar?") or interpret simple idioms (e.g., "What is meant when you say that two persons see eye to eye?"), but the level of difficulty at which failure occurs can vary greatly among subjects. Even more than with arithmetic, an educational influence must be acknowledged. With minimal experience, however, a clinician can interpret the results of these tests sufficiently to provide a useful gauge of the patient's cognitive competency.

Basic Frontal Control Functions

Clinical correlation studies have demonstrated a variety of "frontal" dysfunctions that influence cognitive behavior (Damasio and Anderson 1993). Competency in the evaluation and interpretation of tests of frontal functions (whether performed by the clinician or the neuropsychologist) remains unsatisfactory. Several subdivisions of frontal lobe function have been proposed (Petrides 1991) with the recognition that frontal lobe damage may hinder operations in one or several of these components to provide a complex, difficult-to-interpret set of findings. Three basic divisions of frontal lobe function are sequencing, drive, and executive control.

Sequencing. The ability to maintain sequences of information against interference (distraction) represents one prime function performed by the prefrontal cortex. Often termed *working memory* (Baddeley 1992; Goldman-Rakic and Friedman 1991), this ability is tested easily and is thus the object of most formal psychological tests of frontal lobe function (such as Consonant Trigrams, the Stroop Test, Trails B, and the Wisconsin Card Sorting Test).

At a less formal level, the clinician can test the patient's ability to imitate tapped rhythms, to learn sequences of motor activities (e.g., the three-step hand sequence of Luria—"slap/fist/cut"), to maintain digit or word sequences, and to continue lines of alternating figures or multiple loops (Figure 7.3) to probe the patient's ability to handle serial activities in the face of distraction. Inability to maintain sequences most often indicates dorsal lateral frontal dysfunction. Some degree of right-hemisphere/left-hemisphere differentiation can be read into results based on differences in verbal and nonverbal proficiency in these tests.

Drive. A second attribute of frontal lobe function, strongly but not exclusively influenced by frontal damage, is the patient's ability to carry out activities; disorder is most often recognized as decreased drive (apathy), poor motivation, or both. Almost invariably, altered drive indi-

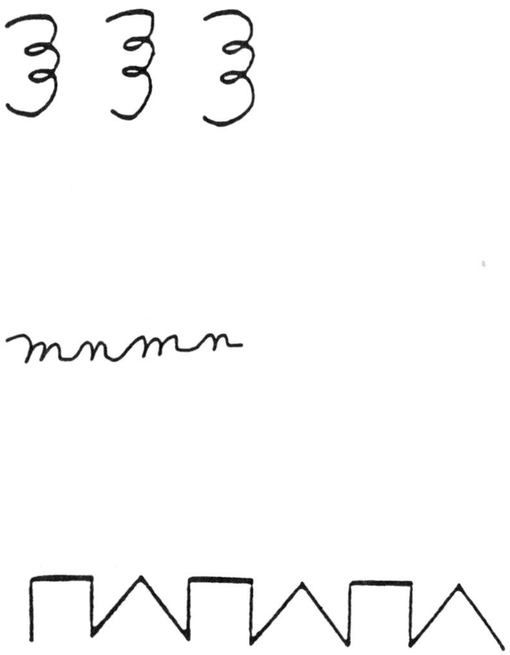

FIGURE 7.3 Alternating figures and multiple loops for evaluation of a patient's ability to maintain simple sequences.

cates midline frontal dysfunction. The opposite behavior, however, a hyperkinetic, manic behavior, also can be associated with midline frontal disorder, particularly when right medial structures are involved. Apathy and mania are best determined by observing the patient. Indications that these disorders are present can come from neuropsychological test data, but interpretations from this material must be confirmed by appropriate observation and correlation to be acceptable. Drive is a fundamental cognitive process that is determined primarily by the clinician's observation.

Executive Control. Executive control is another prime attribute of human frontal function and is even more difficult to quantify than sequencing or drive. The observer can note disordered monitoring and poor control of verbal or physical activities, or both, but these observations can prove difficult to confirm with specific tests. An abnormal, almost jarring frankness (lack of self-concern) in conversation (called verbal dysdecorum by Alexander and Benson 1991), evidence of impulsivity and distractibility, and problems in maintaining or selective changing of requested activities (sets) can be interpreted as evidence of executive control dysfunction.

Certain personal behavior disturbances such as lack of foresight, poor planning, inability to foresee the consequences of impulsive behavior, and similar problems strongly suggest prefrontal brain dysfunction. Most often classed as "frontal personality disorders," these difficulties are often severely disabling but difficult to quantify. (See Chapter 9 for additional discussion of the personality aberrations observed following frontal damage.)

Absolute demonstration of prefrontal abnormality is always difficult. All tests of prefrontal function must use cognitive and behavioral activities such as language or visual-spatial skills that may be disordered by damage to the nonfrontal cortex. Thus, any damage to more posterior or basal brain areas is likely to contaminate and confound results of frontal lobe testing. Careful evaluation of the symptom cluster or neighborhood findings, or both, however, often allows the clinician to distinguish between the posterior-basal or the frontal locus of a lesion that is producing abnormal cognitive behavior. The difference is often important for the diagnosis of behavioral problems and can be crucial for the management of the aphasias and related disorders, the various causes of dementia, and the frontal behavioral disorders. Investigation of frontal dysfunction can be augmented by appropriate neuropsychological tests, but in most situations it is the clinician's observations that provide the strongest evidence for the appropriate diagnosis and implications for management.

Disorders Affecting Intellect

Interpretation of the abnormalities of intellectual function that can be demonstrated in tests such as those outlined above has always proved difficult. Unlike memory, in which the number of potential disorders is relatively finite, disorders that can alter intellectual function appear almost infinite. To date, no absolute, positive approach to the disorders of higher cortical function can be presented.

One relatively elementary approach to interpreting impairment of higher cortical function, introduced in the 1980s, is division into predominantly cortical and predominantly subcortical symptom clusters. Originally suggested to distinguish types of dementia (Benson 1983; Cummings and Benson 1984), the basic principle can be used across a broad spectrum. Unfortunately, many disorders that involve higher cortical function have a mixture of cortical and subcortical characteristics. Nonetheless, the basic division can prove helpful in the interpretation of mental disorders.

Relatively pure examples of subcortical and cortical impairments are readily distinguished. Subcortical disorders show a slowness of response, often of striking degree, that represents a true psychomotor retardation (Albert et al. 1974). In addition, subcortical dementia features a disturbance of memory best described as forgetfulness, a disorder of retrieval. The combination of slow processing and impaired memory retrieval produces a cognitive dysfunction that has been characterized as dilapidated (McHugh and Folstein 1975). Individuals with subcortical impairments can perform cognitive manipulations but are both slow and incompetent. Verbal output is often pathological and can best be described as a speech disorder (hypophonia; poor articulation; altered melody, inflection, and rhythm) with little or no true language defect (aphasia). Finally, most individuals with significant subcortical disease suffer an abnormality of affect, with apathy and depression as the most prominent findings.

In sharp distinction, patients with cortical disorders show a memory disorder that can be characterized as a learning defect (amnesia). They tend to have a language disorder (e.g., aphasia, alexia, agraphia) but little or no speech abnormality and may show ideomotor apraxia, acalculia, or other evidence of higher cortical dysfunction. Almost invariably, impaired or entirely lost cognitive competency will be prominent. The affect tends to be indifferent, in some cases almost to the degree of anosognosia. All of the above features may be present if there is a widespread cortical disorder. More common is a focal impairment producing some but not all of the above findings.

The picture becomes much less precise when the primary involvement impairs frontal function. Subcortical disorders tend to involve (disrupt) frontal functions and can be considered the cause of the so-called frontal system disorders. In contrast, several disease processes produce a purely cortical abnormality that involves the frontal cortex (Brun 1993). The frontal cortical disorders produce a clinical picture distinctly different from the subcortical disorders. Table 7.5 presents some characteristics that distinguish the subcortical from the cortical frontal disorders.

Table 7.5: Frontal dysfunction

Characteristic	*Cortical Involvement*	*Subcortical Involvement*
Language disorder	+++	±
Speech disorder	±	+++
Motor dysfunction	±	+++
Psychomotor retardation	±	+++
Disinhibition	+++	++
Klüver-Bucy signs	+++	±
Altered mood		
Depression	±	+++
Indifference	+++	±

+++ = strong involvement; + and ± = weak involvement.
Source: DF Benson. Progressive frontal dysfunction. Dementia 1993;4:149–153. With permission of S. Karger AG, Basel.

Many brain disorders produce a combination of cortical and subcortical dysfunctions; the intellectual impairments in these cases will be a mixture of findings that cannot be portrayed cleanly as either cortical or subcortical.

Clinical examples can help illustrate the distinction between subcortical and cortical disturbances. Classic examples of a subcortical disorder include the confusional state (see Chapter 4) and most toxic and metabolic disorders (see Chapter 63). Subcortical alterations in higher cognitive functions often are found in patients with the movement disorders (e.g., Parkinson's disease, Huntington's disease, Wilson's disease, progressive supranuclear palsy, thalamic dysfunction) (see Chapters 25 and 76). Many vascular insults, particularly lacunar disorder and Binswanger's disease, produce a subcortical type of altered higher mental function. Infectious disorders that involve the brain tend to produce subcortical dysfunction. One prime example is the AIDS-dementia complex, in which subcortical pathology produces a subcortical alteration of mental function, unless altered by an opportunistic infection that involves cortical structures.

Examples of relatively pure cortical dysfunction are also numerous. The most distinct examples are the "cortical" dementias such as Alzheimer's disease, Pick's disease, frontal degenerative dementia, and progressive aphasia (see Chapters 12, 41, and 71). These disorders produce some or all of the dysfunctions described as cortical cognitive disorder. Many cerebrovascular abnormalities impair higher cortical function directly. In particular, infarction in the middle cerebral artery often produces focal cortical dysfunction, and some embolic infarcts can produce almost pure cortical dysfunction. Many intracerebral neoplasms are first noted when they produce higher cortical dysfunction. In retrospect, however, it is often evident that the growing neoplasm had produced symptoms that were not recognized until cortical dysfunction appeared.

Finally, several brain disorders produce combinations of cortical and subcortical dysfunction. Thus, many vascular insults to the brain involve both cortical and subcortical structures and produce a mixed clinical picture. Traumatic brain injury almost invariably produces a mixture of cortical and subcortical cognitive dysfunctions and, as noted above, many neoplasms present with a mixed picture.

SUMMARY

The evaluation and interpretation of findings leading to the diagnosis and management of disordered intellect or memory, or both, remain among the most difficult problems confronting the neurologist. Intellect, including both cognitive and memory processes, is a brain function; it is thus axiomatic that acquired disorders of intellect represent brain disorder and fall within the realm of the neurologist or neuropsychiatrist. Significant advances have been made toward understanding the higher cognitive processes and their dysfunctions, but these studies are still in very early stages. Much remains to be learned before either intellect or memory can be confidently explained as neural processes.

REFERENCES

Albert ML, Feldman RG, Willis AL. The subcortical dementia of progressive supranuclear palsy. J Neurol Neurosurg Psychiatry 37:121–130, 1974.

Alexander MP, Benson DF. The Aphasias and Related Disturbances. In RJ Joynt (ed), Clinical Neurology. Vol. 1. Philadelphia: Lippincott, 1991.

American Psychiatric Association. Diagnostic and Statistical Manual of Mental Disorders (4th ed). Washington, DC: American Psychiatric Association, 1994.

Baddeley A. Working memory. Science 1992;255:556–559.

Benson DF. Subcortical Dementia: A Clinical Approach. In R Mayeux, WG Rosen (eds), Advances in Neurology. Vol. 38. The Dementias. New York: Raven, 1983:185–194.

Benson DF. Progressive frontal dysfunction. Dementia 1993;4:149–153.

Benson DF. The Neurology of Thinking. New York: Oxford University Press, 1994.

Benson DF, Geschwind N. The Aphasias and Related Disturbances. In AB Baker, LH Baker (eds), Clinical Neurology. Vol. 1. New York: Harper & Row, 1971.

Brun A. Frontal lobe degeneration of the non-Alzheimer type revisited. Dementia 1993;4:126–131.

Caplan LR. Transient Global Amnesia. In JAM Frederiks (ed). Handbook of Clinical Neurology. Vol. 45. Clinical Neuropsychology. Amsterdam: Elsevier, 1985:205–218.

Carpenter MB. Core Text of Neuroanatomy. Baltimore: Williams & Wilkins, 1991.

Cummings JL, Benson DF. Subcortical dementia. Arch Neurol 1984; 41:874–879.

Cummings JL, Benson DF. Dementia: A Clinical Approach (2nd ed). Boston: Butterworth-Heinemann, 1992.

Damasio AR. Time-locked multiregional retroactivation: a system-level proposal for the neural substrates of recall and recognition. Cognition 1989;33:25–62.

Damasio AR, Anderson SW. The frontal lobes. In KM Heilman, E Valenstein (eds). Clinical Neuropsychology (3rd ed). New York: Oxford University Press, 1993:409–460.

Fuster JM. The Prefrontal Cortex: Anatomy, Physiology, and Neuropsychology of the Frontal Lobe. New York: Raven, 1989.

Goldberg G. From Intent to Action: Evolution and Function of the Premotor Systems of the Frontal Lobe. In E Perecman (ed), The Frontal Lobes Revisited. New York: IRBN Press, 1987:273–306.

Goldman-Rakic PS, Friedman HR. The Circuitry of Working Memory Revealed by Anatomy and Metabolic Imaging. In HS Levin, HM Eisenberg, AL Benton (eds), Frontal Lobe Function and Dysfunction. New York: Oxford University Press, 1991:72–91.

Grüsser O-J, Landis T. Visual Agnosias and Other Disturbances of Visual Perception and Cognition. London: Macmillan, 1991.

Jerison HJ. Brain Size and the Evolution of Mind. New York: American Museum of Natural History, 1991.

Luria AR. Higher Cortical Functions in Man. New York: Basic Books, 1966.

McHugh PR, Folstein MF. Psychiatric Syndromes of Huntington's Chorea: A Clinical and Phenomenologic Study. In DF Benson, D Blumer (eds), Psychiatric Aspects of Neurologic Disease. New York: Grune & Stratton, 1975:267–286.

Mesulam M-M. Large scale neurocognitive networks and distributed processing for attention, language and memory. Ann Neurol 1990; 28:597–613.

Nauta WJH, Feirtag M. Fundamental Neuroanatomy. New York: W.H. Freeman, 1986.

Petrides M. Learning Impairments Following Excisions of the Primate Frontal Cortex. In HS Levin, HM Eisenberg, AL Benton (eds). Frontal Lobe Function and Dysfunction. New York: Oxford University Press, 1991:256–272.

Poggio T, Edelman S. A network that learns to recognize three-dimensional objects. Nature 1990;343:263–266.

Squire LR, Zola-Morgan S. The medial temporal lobe memory system. Science 1991;253:1380–1386.

Sternberg RJ. Intellect. In RL Gregory (ed). The Oxford Companion. New York: Oxford University Press, 1987:375.

Tanaka K. Neuronal mechanisms of object recognition. Science 1993;262:685–688.

Webster's Third New International Dictionary of the English Language, Unabridged. Springfield, MA: Merriam-Webster, 1986.

Wechsler D. The Measurement and Appraisal of Adult Intelligence. Baltimore: Williams & Wilkins, 1958.

Zola-Morgan S, Squire LR. The neuropsychology of memory: parallel findings in human and non-human primates. Ann N Y Acad Sci 1990;608:434–450.

SUGGESTED READING

Benson DF, Blumer D (eds). Psychiatric Aspects of Neurologic Disease. New York: Grune & Stratton, 1975.

Benson DF, Blumer D (eds). Psychiatric Aspects of Neurologic Disease. Vol. 2. New York: Grune & Stratton, 1982.

Brun A, Englund B, Gustafson L et al. Consensus statement: clinical and neuropathological criteria for frontotemporal dementia. J Neurol Neurosurg Psychiatry 57:416–418, 1994.

Cummings JL. Clinical Neuropsychiatry. Orlando: Grune & Stratton, 1985.

Frederiks JAM (ed). Handbook of Clinical Neurology. Vol. 45. Clinical Neuropsychology. Amsterdam: Elsevier, 1985.

Frederiks JAM (ed). Handbook of Clinical Neurology. Vol. 46. Neurobehavioral Disorders. Amsterdam: Elsevier, 1985.

Fuster JM. The prefrontal cortex, mediator of cross-temporal contingencies. Human Neurobiology 1985;4:169–179.

Heilman KM, Valenstein E. Clinical Neuropsychology (3rd ed). New York: Oxford University Press, 1993.

Lishman WA. Organic Psychiatry (2nd ed). Oxford: Blackwell, 1987.

Mesulam M-M. Principles of Behavioral Neurology. Philadelphia: FA Davis, 1985.

Squire LR. Memory and Brain. New York: Oxford University Press, 1987.

Stuss DT, Benson DF. The Frontal Lobes. New York: Raven, 1986.

Trimble M. Neuropsychiatry. New York: Wiley, 1981.

Yudofsky SC, Hales RE (eds). The American Psychiatric Press Textbook of Neuropsychiatry (2nd ed). Washington, DC: American Psychiatric Press, 1992.

Chapter 8
Developmental Delay and Regression in Infants

Gerald M. Fenichel

Slow progress in the attainment of developmental milestones (*developmental delay*) may be caused by static or progressive disorders of the brain. In contrast, the loss of previously attained developmental milestones (*developmental regression*) is almost always caused by progressive diseases of the nervous system. Distinguishing delay from regression is critical for formulating an approach to diagnosis. Therefore, the important first question is "Has the child lost skills that were previously attained?" If the answer is "yes," the family should be pressed for specifics; it should be certain that the child's performance has truly declined. New symptoms such as involuntary movements and seizures do not necessarily indicate progressive disease. If the answer is "no," the child probably has developmental delay.

DEVELOPMENTAL DELAY

The evaluation of developmental delay begins with the determination of whether the delay is global or restricted (Table 8.1). The Denver Developmental Screening Test (DDST) is an efficient and reliable method for assessing development in the physician's office. It rapidly assesses four components of development: personal-social, fine-motor adaptive, language, and gross motor. The results can be amplified by several psychometric tests, but the DDST in combination with neurological assessment provides sufficient information to initiate further diagnostic studies.

Language Delay

Normal infants and children have a remarkable facility for acquiring language and will learn two languages concurrently if both are spoken in the household. Table 8.2 shows the sequence of language development expected in 75% of normal children. Many infants begin articulating consonants, usually M, D, and B, at 6 months of age. These first consonants are automatic and sometimes occur even in deaf children. Parents translate these automatic sounds as "mama," "dada," and "bottle" and reinforce these meanings. Failure to develop further speech then is misinterpreted as the loss of speech that was attained previously; this suggests developmental regression when the problem is really developmental delay.

Receptive skills always appear more highly developed to parents than expressive skills (language must be decoded before it can be encoded). "He understands everything," is a common response of a mother whose child has language delay. However, expressive skills keep pace with speech understanding in normal children. By 2 years of age, most children understand simple commands and point to body parts, but their speech is not understandable by strangers and only in part by family members.

Table 8.1: Diagnosis of developmental delay: No regression

Predominant speech delay
Hearing loss
Infantile autism
Predominant motor delay
Cerebral palsy
Cerebral hypotonia
Clumsiness
Neuromuscular disorders
Normal variation
Orthopedic disturbances
Toe walking
Global delay
Cerebral malformations
Chromosomal disturbances
Intrauterine infection
Perinatal disorders
Progressive encephalopathies (see Table 8.7)

Table 8.2: Normal speech acquisition (75th percentile)

2 months	"Ooo/Ah"
3 months	Laughs and squeals
6–7 months	Imitates speech sounds, single syllables
8–9 months	"Da/ma/ba," jabbers
11 months	"Dada/mama" specific
13 months	One-word vocabulary
19 months	Six-word vocabulary
22 months	Combines words
24 months	250-word vocabulary

Table 8.3: Causes of hearing impairment and deafness

Congenital problems
Aplasia of the inner ear
Chromosome disorders
Trisomy 13
Trisomy 18
18q-syndrome
Genetic disorders
Isolated deafness
Pendred's syndrome
Usher syndrome
Intrauterine viral infection
Maternal drug use
Drugs
Antibiotics
Beta blockers
Chemotherapeutic agents
Genetic neurological disorders
Infantile Refsum disease
Pontobulbar palsy with deafness
Infectious diseases
Bacterial meningitis
Otitis media
Viral encephalitis
Viral exanthems
Skeletal disorders
Apert syndrome (acrocephalosyndactyly)
Cleidocranial dysostosis
Craniofacial dysostosis (Crouzon's disease)
Craniometaphyseal dysplasia (Pyle's disease)
Klippel-Feil syndrome
Mandibulofacial dysostosis (Treacher Collins syndrome)
Osteogenesis imperfecta
Osteopetrosis (Albers-Schönberg disease)

Hearing Impairment

Hearing impairment is the major cause of isolated speech delay (see Table 8.1). A limited impairment, such as high-frequency loss, may cause profound impairment in the use of consonants. For this reason, all infants with isolated delay in speech development should be tested by audiometry. Crude testing in the office by slamming objects and ringing bells is inadequate. Hearing loss should be suspected in children who use gesture excessively or stare at the lips of people who are talking, and in children with mental retardation who fail to imitate sounds or have a disorder that ordinarily causes both mental retardation and hearing loss (e.g., intrauterine viral infection, neonatal meningitis, several genetic disorders) (Table 8.3).

Infantile Autism

Infantile autism is a behavioral disorder caused by abnormal brain development (Minshew and Payton 1988a, 1988b). The major diagnostic criteria are failure of language development, severe impairment of interpersonal relationships, a restricted repertoire of activities, and onset of symptoms before 3 years of age. All children with autism are mentally retarded; failure to develop language by age 5 years predicts severe mental retardation. Autistic children show little affection to their parents or other care providers but treat people as if they were inanimate objects. Some children show a morbid preoccupation with spinning objects, stereotyped behavior such as rocking and spinning, and relative insensitivity to pain.

Some aspects of the severely aberrant behavior can be improved by behavior modification techniques. Despite the best program of treatment, however, these children function in a moderately to severely retarded range.

Delayed and Variant Motor Development

Table 8.4 shows the sequence of motor development expected in 75% of normal children. Four-point reciprocal crawling with belly off the floor is the optimal method of prewalking ambulation. Infants who do this effectively will walk. Less optimal means of prewalking ambulation are persistent creeping (belly on floor) and scooting or bottom shuffling (moving in the sitting position). Many infants who only creep and most infants who only scoot will have neurological abnormalities.

Hypotonic infants with delayed gross-motor development but normal language and social skills may have a neuromuscular disease (see Chapters 31 and 84). Isolated delay in motor function can also occur in some forms of cerebral palsy, sufficient to delay the achievement of motor milestones but not severe enough to cause a recognizable dis-

Table 8.4: Motor development in 75% of normal infants

2 months	Hold head up 45 degrees
4 months	Grasp objects, bear weight on legs
6 months	Pass objects hand to hand, sit with minimal support
8 months	Crawl on all fours, sit without support
9 months	Thumb-finger grasp, pull to standing, get to sitting
12 months	Stand alone
13 months	Walk alone, stoop and recover
18 months	Walk up steps
24 months	Throw ball overhead

Table 8.5: Indications for further evaluation of children with developmental delay

Absent tendon reflexes
AIDS risk factors
Coarse facial features
Cutaneous abnormalities
Dysmorphic features
Family member with similar disease
Macrocephaly
Parental consanguinity

turbance of cognitive function during infancy (see Chapter 67); this developmental pattern is often seen in children with infantile hemiplegia.

The Clumsy Child

In the normal biological spectrum of motor coordination there should be one clumsy child for each Wimbledon finalist. Both are on opposite ends of a normal distribution curve; the lower end of the curve is no more a sign of neurological dysfunction than the upper end. Some authorities would argue that clumsy children are dyspraxic, but the distinction between clumsy and dyspraxia in children is more semantic than real and only serves to label the child as neurologically abnormal.

Clumsy children, usually boys, are often referred to neurologists by school authorities because of poor handwriting or failure in physical education. One parent, usually the father, has often had a similar school experience. Developmental history is generally normal except that hand dominance was established late (after 2 years), and the child is described as ambidextrous, although "ambiclumsy" is closer to the mark. The neurological examination is normal.

High-technology investigations are not cost-effective in such children and only reinforce the perception that the child is "abnormal." Further, medical consultation should be discouraged and instead the child should be directed to activities with the possibility of success (such as karate and running).

Toe Walking

Some children begin walking with their heels off the ground and never attain a normal heel-toe gait. The tendency for toe walking increases with time. At first, the foot can be passively moved to a neutral position but later the ankle tendon becomes tight. The differential diagnosis of persistent toe walking includes abnormalities of the lumbar-sacral spinal cord, infantile autism, muscular dystrophy, and cerebral palsy. However, these diagnoses are unlikely if neurological development and examination are otherwise normal. It is reasonable to measure the concentration of serum creatine kinase (CK) and obtain a magnetic resonance image (MRI) of the lumbar-sacral cord before concluding that the child has idiopathic shortening of the ankle tendon and recommending surgical correction.

Global Developmental Delay

Global developmental delay usually indicates a static encephalopathy caused by an antenatal or perinatal disturbance. Every child with global developmental delay deserves at least a head MRI in the hope of establishing a definitive diagnosis. The birth of a retarded child engenders considerable guilt in parents; failure to diagnose the underlying cause reinforces the parental belief that their child is defective because of something they did. In addition, some diagnoses have genetic implications for future pregnancies.

An exhaustive search to determine the underlying cause in every infant who is developing slowly is not cost-effective. Table 8.5 lists factors in children with global delay that indicate the need for further investigation.

Chromosomal Disturbances

Abnormalities in chromosome structure or number are responsible for one-third of all cases of severe mental retardation. The fragile X syndrome is the most common chromosomal cause of mental retardation and should be considered in every male with mental retardation of unknown cause. The name derives from a constriction at the Xq 27.3 site at the distal end of the long arm of the X chromosome that breaks during karyotype preparation (Tarleton and Saul 1993).

All children with autosomal chromosome disorders are hypotonic at birth. In addition, there are usually multiple minor face and limb abnormalities, which in themselves are not unusual but assume diagnostic significance in combination. Clinical features that suggest chromosomal aberrations are summarized in Table 8.6, and the major chromosome syndromes are discussed in Chapter 67.

Cerebral Malformations

Cerebral malformations may be primary (genetic) or secondary to intrauterine diseases (see Chapter 66). The exposure of an embryo to infectious or toxic agents during the first weeks after conception can disorganize the delicate sequencing of neural development. Alcohol, environmental toxins, prescription drugs, and substances of abuse all have been implicated in causing cerebral malformations, although cause-and-effect relationships are difficult to establish in individual cases. Maternal cocaine use is an important consideration in fetuses who have suffered vas-

Table 8.6: Clinical indications for chromosome analysis

Genitourinary	
	Ambiguous genitalia
	Polycystic kidney
Head and neck	
	High nasal bridge
	Hypertelorism or hypotelorism
	Microphthalmia
	Mongoloid slant (in non-Asian child)
	Occipital scalp defect
	Small mandible
	Small or fish mouth (hard to open)
	Small or low-set ears
	Upward slant of eyes
	Webbed neck
Limbs	
	Abnormal dermatoglyphics
	Low-set thumb
	Overlapping fingers
	Polydactyly
	Radial hypoplasia
	Rocker-bottom feet

Source: GM Fenichel. Clinical Pediatric Neurology: A Signs and Symptoms Approach (2nd ed). Philadelphia: Saunders, 1993.

cular insufficiency and infarction of organs, including the brain (Dominguez et al. 1991).

Cerebral malformations should be suspected in any retarded child who is dysmorphic, has malformations of other organs, has an abnormal head size and shape, or an intractable seizure disorder. In such children, MRI may be helpful in identifying even minor malformations such as heterotopia.

Intrauterine Infections

The two most common organisms that cause intrauterine infections are *cytomegalovirus* (CMV) and *Toxoplasma gondii* (see Chapter 60). The typical clinical presentation of neonatal CMV infection includes skin rash, hepatosplenomegaly, jaundice, chorioretinitis, and microcephaly with cerebral calcification. Hearing loss may be an isolated sequelae of intrauterine infection.

Toxoplasma gondii is a protozoan estimated to infect 1 per 1,000 live births in the United States each year. Transplacental transmission of toxoplasmosis is possible only if primary maternal infection occurs during pregnancy. About 25% of infected newborns have multisystem involvement (fever, rash, hepatosplenomegaly, jaundice, and thrombocytopenia) at birth. Neurological dysfunction is manifested as seizures, altered states of consciousness, and increased intracranial pressure. The triad of hydrocephalus, chorioretinitis, and intracranial calcification is the hallmark of congenital toxoplasmosis in older children.

Congenital syphilis had declined steadily as a cause of intrauterine infection until 1988, when an increase occurred because of an actual increase in cases and a broadening of the case definition. All stillbirths and live children born to women with a history of untreated or inadequately treated syphilis are considered to have congenital syphilis (Ikeda and Jensen 1990). The common features in symptomatic newborns and infants are condylomata lata, periostitis or osteochondritis, persistent rhinorrhea, and maculopapular rash. The onset of neurological disturbances is usually after age 2 and includes mental retardation, nerve deafness, and mental retardation. The combination of nerve deafness, interstitial keratitis, and peg-shaped upper incisors is the *Hutchinson triad*.

Rubella embryopathy may cause developmental delay. However, the last major epidemic of rubella was in 1964–1965. Mass immunization had almost eliminated rubella embryopathy, but it quickly reemerges when immunization rates decline. Rubella embryopathy is a multisystem disease characterized by intrauterine growth retardation, cataracts, chorioretinitis, congenital heart disease, sensorineural deafness, hepatosplenomegaly, jaundice, anemia, thrombocytopenia, and rash. Neurological dysfunction is manifested as lethargy, hypotonia, and seizures that may be delayed until 3 months of age.

Postnatal Disorders

Infection, asphyxia, and trauma are the major events occurring in newborns and infants that cause psychomotor retardation (see Chapter 85). The important infectious diseases are bacterial meningitis and viral encephalitis (see Chapter 60). The neurological sequelae are mental and motor disabilities, hydrocephalus, epilepsy, deafness, and visual loss. Psychomotor retardation may be the only or the most prominent sequela, and progressive mental deterioration can occur if meningitis causes a secondary hydrocephalus.

Perinatal asphyxia, when it causes brain damage, always causes a motor impairment (cerebral palsy). Chronic brain damage syndromes such as mental retardation and epilepsy cannot be attributed to perinatal asphyxia unless the child also has cerebral palsy. However, most cases of cerebral palsy, even when associated with mental retardation and epilepsy, are caused by prenatal events and not by perinatal asphyxia.

Child abuse is the most common cause of traumatic brain injury in infants and continues to be an important cause of brain damage throughout childhood. More than 1 million cases of child abuse and neglect are reported annually in the United States, and more than 100,000 deaths are attributed to it each year. This national epidemic that exceeds acquired immune deficiency disease (AIDS) as a cause of morbidity and mortality in the United States. Child abuse must be suspected in every infant with an injury and in every case of sudden infant death syndrome (SIDS).

Table 8.7: Progressive encephalopathy: Onset before age 2

Acquired immunodeficiency syndrome encephalopathy
Aminoacidurias
Homocystinuria
Maple syrup urine disease (MSUD)
Phenylketonuria
Hypothyroidism
Lysosomal enzyme disorders
Glycoprotein degradation disorders
Mucolipidoses
Mucopolysaccharidoses
Sphingolipidoses
Mitochondrial disorders
Mitochondrial myopathy, encephalopathy, lactic acidosis, and stroke (MELAS)
Progressive infantile poliodystrophy (Alper's disease)
Subacute necrotizing encephalomyelopathy (Leigh disease)
Trichopoliodystrophy (Menkes' disease)
Neurocutaneous syndromes
Chédiak-Higashi syndrome
Neurofibromatosis
Tuberous sclerosis
Other genetic disorders of gray matter
Infantile ceroid lipofuscinosis (Santavuori
Infantile neuroaxonal dystrophy
Lesch-Nyhan syndrome
Rett syndrome
Other genetic disorders of white matter
Alexander's disease
Classic galactosemia (transferase deficiency)
Neonatal adrenoleukodystrophy
Pelizaeus-Merzbacher disease
Spongy degeneration of infancy (Canavan-van Bogaert-Bertrand disease)
Progressive hydrocephalus

Table 8.8: Progressive encephalopathy: Onset after age 2

Infectious diseases
Congenital syphilis
Subacute sclerosing panencephalitis
Lysosomal enzyme disorders
Glycoprotein degradation disorders
Mucopolysaccharidoses types II and VII
Sphingolipidoses
Other genetic disorders of gray matter
Ceroid lipofuscinosis
Heller syndrome
Huntington's disease
Mitochondrial disorders
Xeroderma pigmentosum
Other genetic disorders of white matter
Adrenoleukodystrophy
Alexander's disease
Cerebrotendinous xanthomatosis

DEVELOPMENTAL REGRESSION

Children who lose developmental milestones that were previously attained are probably suffering from a progressive disease of the nervous system. Developmental regression is an intimidating complaint for many physicians because the differential diagnosis is considerable and includes many esoteric disorders. The wrong response is a shotgun of diagnostic tests, because it is not cost-effective and often misses the mark.

A complete family history is the first step in constructing a differential diagnosis. Establishing that there is a mode of genetic transmission (mendelian or maternal) immediately limits the diagnostic possibilities (see Chapter 47). A complete family history requires contact with both parents and both sets of grandparents, either by the physician or through a parent. One more unhappy consequence of the high divorce rate and mobility of Western families is the difficulty in accessing important family members for medical information. Families must be questioned, not only about similar symptoms but also alternate phenotypic expressions, which are especially important in the diagnosis of mitochondrial disorders.

Next, the age at symptom onset should be established. The causes of developmental regression are somewhat different in infants (younger than 2 years) than in children 2 years and older (Tables 8.7 and 8.8). The long lists of possible causes then can be further refined by answering the following three questions: (1) Does the disease affect only the nervous system or are other organs involved? (2) Does the disease affect the peripheral nervous system as well as the central nervous system? (3) Does the disease affect primarily the gray matter or the white matter?

Organ Involvement Other Than Brain

The skin, eyes, and abdominal viscera, either alone or in combination, are the organs most often affected concurrently with the brain in disorders that cause developmental regression. Neurocutaneous syndromes are readily recognized by inspection and examination should always begin with the questions "Does the child have any birthmarks?" "Do other family members have birthmarks?" (see Chapter 70).

Nonparalytic strabismus is often a nonspecific accompaniment of brain dysfunction because of faulty fusion or control of conjugate gaze mechanisms by the abnormal brain. Progressive paralytic strabismus and retinal degenerations are usually specific signs of associated progressive brain disorders, whereas malformations of the optic nerve and globe indicate brain malformations that cause developmental delay. Tapetoretinal degeneration, "the cherry-red spot" at the macula, was once thought to be a specific sign of Tay-Sachs' disease but is now recognized as a feature of several metabolic disorders (Table 8.9).

The most recognizable syndrome of multiorgan involvement is the Hurler phenotype (Table 8.10). It occurs fully or partially in infants with mucopolysaccharidoses (types I and III), glycoprotein degradation disorders (mannosidosis, sialidosis, and fucosidosis), mucolipidosis type II (I-cell dis-

Table 8.9: Lysosomal enzyme disorders with a cherry-red spot

Cherry-red spot myoclonus
Farber's lipogranulomatosis
GM_1 gangliosidosis
GM_2 gangliosidosis
Multiple sulfatase deficiency
Niemann-Pick disease
Sialidosis type III

Table 8.10: The Hurler phenotype

Abdominal hernia
Coarse facial features
Corneal opacity
Deafness
Dysostosis multiplex
Mental retardation
Stiff joints
Visceromegaly

ease), GM_1 gangliosidosis, and multiple sulfatase deficiency (see Chapter 69).

Peripheral Nervous System Involvement

Absence of ankle tendon reflexes is an early clinical feature of peripheral neuropathy and indicates the need for electrophysiological studies to determine its type. Combined disease of the central and peripheral nervous systems usually indicates either a lysosomal disorder with storage of an abnormal metabolic product, such as metachromatic leukodystrophy, or a mitochondrial disorder. Mitochondrial disorders are also a cause of multiorgan abnormalities. Combined cerebral and peripheral nerve dysfunction also occurs in some immune-mediated demyelinating diseases. Such cases are characterized by a rapid progression of symptoms.

Gray Matter Versus White Matter Disease

Some diseases first affect the gray matter and others the white matter, though both are eventually affected. The initial clinical features are most helpful in differentiating gray matter from white matter diseases. Gray matter diseases begin as personality change, seizures, and dementia. The electroencephalogram (EEG) is abnormal early in the course; epileptiform activity is often present, the background is disorganized, and the posterior rhythm slowed. MRI is initially normal but later shows enlargement of the ventricles and the subarachnoid space.

The initial features of white matter disease are usually corticospinal tract dysfunction, blindness, and focal neurological deficits. MRI, especially T2-weighted images, shows cerebral demyelination. Visual-evoked responses and motor conduction velocities are often useful to document subclinical demyelination in the optic and peripheral nerves, respectively.

THE DIAGNOSIS OF DEVELOPMENTAL DISORDERS

The identification of specific causes of developmental delay and regression has improved considerably in the past 30 years. The probability of identifying the cause of developmental regression has increased from perhaps 10% to 90% (Table 8.11). This improvement was achieved in part by better diagnostic technology but also because of a better understanding of the disease processes that affect infants. Chapter 69 presents a new classification of metabolic diseases based on the abnormal cellular organelle rather than the abnormal metabolic product.

Most global developmental delay (see Chapter 67) is caused by events occurring during pregnancy that adversely affect the developing brain. Some events can be identified, but most cannot. MRI may show that the brain is poorly developed but rarely explains the cause. More often than not the MRI is normal and the neurologist must explain to a mother that her child is mentally retarded despite the normal appearance of the brain. The invariable response is "What did I do that caused this to happen?"

The birth of a normal child is a miracle that has come to be expected. When the miracle does not happen there is anger, always directed inward and often at the messenger. Assisting the parents to adjust to this tragedy requires knowledge, concern, and patience. The goal of telling parents that their child will be mentally retarded is not to soften the blow—that is not possible—but to be certain that they hear what you are saying. People must be prepared to accept bad news; do not tell them more than they are ready to accept. Too often, parents bring their child for a second or third opinion because previous doctors "didn't tell us anything." In fact, they said too much too fast and were tuned out.

My goal for the first visit is that parents know that the child is not normal (not a normal developmental variation) and that something is wrong with the brain. Unfortunately, the mother often comes without the father for this critical visit, and she must later restate your comments to the doubting father and grandparents. Most parents cannot handle more information than "the child is not normal" at the first consultation and further discussion is saved for a later visit. However, probing questions should always be answered fully. Parents must never lose confidence in the neurologist's willingness to be forthright. The timing of the next visit depends on the age of the child and the severity of the retardation. The more the child falls behind in reaching developmental milestones, the more ready parents will be to accept the diagnosis of mental retardation.

When the time comes that you tell a mother that her child is retarded, she will cry. If she does not cry, she has

Table 8.11: Evaluation of developmental regression

A. No clues from history or examination
   1. Magnetic resonance image (MRI) of brain: Distinguishes white matter disease from gray matter disease; especially useful for demyelination; also shows ventricular size and has characteristic features in ceratin metabolic disorders (e.g., subacute necrotizing encephalopathy).
   2. Electroencephalogram (EEG): Shows seizure activity; especially useful when subclinical seizures are contributing to dementia.
   3. Blood lactate, organic acid, and amino acid concentrations: Order when MRI and EEG suggest gray matter disease.
   4. Electromyography and nerve conduction: Order when tendon reflexes are absent or when MRI indicates demyelinating disease.
   5. Serum very long-chain fatty acid concentrations, enzyme activity of galactosylceramidase, arylsulfatase A, and sphingomyelinase: Order when MRI or nerve conduction studies indicate a demyelinating disease.

B. Coarse facial features and/or visceromegaly
   1. MRI and EEG: Same reasons as above
   2. Thyroid function tests
   3. Urine mucopolysaccharide and oligosaccharide concentrations
   4. Examination of lymphocytes for vacuolar change: Suggests some ceroid lipofuscinoses, mucopolysaccharidoses, glycoprotein degradation disorders, and gangliosidoses.
   5. Enzyme analysis in leukocytes: As suggested by initial screening tests.

C. Ataxia and/or involuntary movement disorder
   1. MRI and EEG: Same reasons as above
   2. Blood smear for acanthocytes: Abetaliproteinemia, neurological acanthocytosis
   3. Blood immunoglobulins, alpha-fetoprotein, lactate, liver function tests, ceruloplasmin: Ataxia-telangiectasia, mitochondrial disorders, hepatolenticular degeneration
   4. Urine concentrations of glutaric acid: Glutaric aciduria

not heard what you were saying or understood its implications and you have failed to communicate effectively. It is not helpful to describe mental retardation as mild, moderate, or severe. Parents want to know what the child will do: will he walk? need special schools? live alone? The next question is "What can I do to help my child?" Parents must do something and should be directed to programs that provide developmental specialists and other parents who can help them learn how to live with a chronic handicapping disorder and to gain access to community resources (see Chapter 67).

REFERENCES

Dominguez R, Vila-Coro AA, Slopis JM et al. Brain and ocular abnormalities in infants with in utero exposure to cocaine and other street drugs. Am J Dis Child 1991;145:688–695.

Fenichel GM. Clinical Pediatric Neurology: A Signs and Symptoms Approach (2nd ed). Philadelphia: Saunders, 1993.

Ikeda MK, Jensen HB. Evaluation and treatment of congenital syphilis. J Pediatr 1990;117:843–852.

Minshew NJ, Payton JB. New perspectives in autism. I. The clinical spectrum of autism. Curr Probl Pediatr 1988a;18:561–610.

Minshew NJ, Payton JB. New perspectives in autism. II. The differential diagnosis and neurobiology of autism. Curr Probl Pediatr 1988b;18:615–634.

Tarleton JC, Saul RA. Molecular genetic advances in fragile X syndrome. J Pediatr 1993;122:169–185.

Chapter 9
Behavior and Personality Disturbances

Michael R. Trimble

DEFINITIONS

The *Oxford English Dictionary* gives several interrelated meanings to the word *behavior.* It refers to "a manner of conducting oneself in the external relations of life, demeanor, deportment, bearing, manners." It relates to "conduct, general practice, course of life; course of action towards or to others, treatment of others." Behavior problems thus relate to alterations of these aspects of an individual's existence, and in many cases, these changes are observed by a third party rather than by the person so affected. The brain is the central organ that regulates behavior, so it is hardly surprising that behavior disturbances are reflected in brain changes and, conversely, that the brain changes will, in many cases, be accompanied by observable alterations of the behavioral repertoire. Traditional neurology, dealing as it does mainly with motor and sensory abnormalities, has been concerned primarily with the alteration of behavior of isolated body parts; this focus has stemmed in part from the success of localization of cerebral abnormalities from clinical examination. However, the individual has the propensity to undergo a change, reflected in an alteration of behavior as defined above, that is often profound, influencing the sensory, motor, conative, emotional, and cognitive aspects of the individual's life.

Disturbances of the brain that account for such integral and complete behavioral manifestations may be regarded as either structural or functional—*functional* here being used in the true meaning of the word, emphasizing disturbance of brain function. Neurologists interested in behavioral disorders have concentrated on patients with lesions that cause structural changes, whereas psychiatrists have dealt more with the consequences of disturbances of function, where underlying structural lesions have been more difficult to discern.

Behavioral neurology has become a popular epithet in recent years. The origins of the term are difficult to discover, although inquiries usually lead back to the influential writings of the late Professor Norman Geschwind. The discipline itself may be traced to the elegant and important writings of the late nineteenth-century neuropsychiatrists, such as Wernicke, Liepmann, and Dejerine. Behavioral neurology emphasizes the consequences of certain cerebral lesions for disturbance of higher cognitive function, and central to its development has been the description and analysis of such conditions as aphasia, alexia, and agraphia. However, the scope of behavioral neurology in recent years has extended to embrace organic mental disorders, including dementia and delirium, and the behavioral consequences of both frontal and temporal lobe dysfunction. Behavioral neurology partially overlaps the older discipline of neuropsychiatry, which takes a more holistic view of the relationship of brain to behavior, and seeks to explore the neurological underpinnings of psychiatric syndromes. A variety of behavioral problems are seen in a neurological setting; this chapter discusses personality disorders and the neuroses.

PERSONALITY CHANGE

A useful starting point is the work of Jaspers, who in 1963 made a clear distinction between psychogenic development and organic process—in other words, between personality and illness. He said: "We differentiate abnormal personality types that are anlage variants, from sick personalities in the narrower sense, where the change has been brought on by a process." The change in the patient's habitual patterns of behavior indicates that a process has taken place, and that process may relate to underlying structural or functional changes within the central nervous system (CNS).

The various forms of personality disorder are described in such manuals as the *Diagnostic and Statistical Manual of*

Mental Disorders (DSM-III-R [1987] and DSM-IV [1994]). For this chapter, two points must be clarified. First, the kinds of personality changes seen with neurological disease do not necessarily conform to the personality disorders of diagnostic manuals of psychiatrists. Second, the personality change reported is usually a combination of both an exacerbation of the premorbid personality and, particularly if the burden of pathological change is falling on the frontal or temporal lobes, some new and distinctive feature that provides a clue to the possible cerebral localization of the underlying process.

Clinical Spectrum

The following personality types are frequently encountered in the neurological clinic.

Psychopathic Personality (ICD 10—Dissocial; DSM-IV—Antisocial)

The term *psychopathic personality* implies antisocial personality traits. *Sociopathy, sociopathic personality,* and *antisocial personality* are alternative terms. This personality type is characterized by a disregard for social obligations, a lack of feeling for others, and impetuous violence or callous unconcern. It becomes apparent in early life, often initially presenting with conduct disturbance at school, or possibly even earlier, with hyperactivity during childhood. There is a continuing history of poor interpersonal relationships, a poor work record, and continuing marital difficulties. Drug abuse, alcoholism, pathological lying, and prison convictions all may be recorded, and sociopaths tend to display more than accepted sexual deviation, somatization (the tendency to present with physical signs and symptoms in the absence of accompanying comparable disease), and outbursts of physical violence. A characteristic feature of the psychopathic personality is the tendency to remit over time, generally in early adulthood. The onset of the psychopathic personality in midlife almost inevitably implies the development of an underlying process.

Obsessional Personality (ICD 10—Anancastic; DSM-IV—Obsessive-Compulsive)

The obsessional personality is characterized by a lifelong tendency to meticulousness and punctuality. Patients have difficulty in expressing their emotions and check and recheck their actions. To avoid confusion with the full-blown obsessive-compulsive disorder, this type of personality is best referred to as an anancastic personality. Many patients attending neurological clinics who present with neurological symptoms but do not have accompanying neurological disease have this type of personality. Williams in 1975 referred to these patients as having "a common rigidity of attitude...[which]...may range from reasonable but evident self-discipline to marked obsessionality; but in some degree they have the hallmarks of the obsessive." The patient's meticulous circumstantiality may make history-taking a remarkably tedious and laborious process, and the inexperienced clinician may find it difficult to obtain adequate information from the obsessional patient.

Hysterical Personality (ICD 10—Histrionic; DSM-IV—Histrionic)

The hysterical personality is another personality style frequently encountered in the neurological setting. It is similar to the antisocial personality and may be contrasted with the anancastic personality. The characteristic traits are excessive dependence; shallow, labile affects; impulsiveness; verbal exaggeration and excessive gestural display; seductiveness; and self-dramatization. There is a tendency to take overdoses of medication or make other attempts at self-harm, and there is an association with somatization. The verbal exaggeration, combined with the impulsive cognitive style, again leads to difficulties in taking accurate histories from patients; this trait, combined with the tendency to somatization, makes interpretation of patients' symptoms difficult. Although antisocial personalities tend to be male, hysterical personalities are more common in women.

Paranoid Personality (ICD 10—Paranoid; DSM-IV—Paranoid)

The paranoid personality is distinguished by continued suspiciousness and mistrust and excessive sensitivity. Jealousy, transient ideas of reference, litigiousness, and a tendency to avoid intimacy are all features, and individuals often take up minor concerns or causes with tenacious vigor, collecting vast amounts of documentary evidence to support their cause.

Schizoid Personality (ICD 10—Schizoid; DSM-IV—Schizoid)

People with the schizoid personality have little affective or social contact and have a tendency to detachment and eccentricity. They are often socially rather reclusive, hypersensitive individuals who display oddities of behavior, thinking, and perception; these complaints may lead them to neurologists.

Neurasthenic Personality (ICD 10—Neurasthenia)

Patients with the neurasthenic personality show what Jaspers referred to as "irritable weakness." They have both an increased sensitivity and an easy fatigability, and they often complain of exhaustion and minor aches and pains.

Borderline Personality (ICD 10—Borderline; DSM-IV—Borderline)

The borderline personality was introduced into DSM-III (1980) and is now included in ICD 10. Such patients have unstable personal relationships, impulsivity that often leads to self-harm or outbursts of intense anger, affective instability, and possibly transient paranoid episodes. They are susceptible to dissociative episodes, and in a neurological setting may present with pseudoseizures.

Anxious Personality (ICD 10—Anxious; DSM-IV—Avoidant)

The anxious personality type defines people who display lifelong anxiety and who, under stress, readily develop anxiety or panic disorders. In a neurological setting, these patients may present with fleeting neurological symptoms, and a panic disorder is frequently confused with a seizure disorder (see section on Pseudoseizures).

Explosive Personality (ICD 10—Emotionally Unstable Personality Disorder)

The explosive personality style occurs in patients who are liable to intemperate outbursts of anger but who do not otherwise appear prone to antisocial behavior. This type of personality is related to the episodic dyscontrol condition and paroxysmal outbursts of rage (see sections on General and Neurological Examination and Investigations).

Personality Changes Secondary to Neurological Disease

The foregoing personality styles are often encountered in the neurological clinic and may lead to difficulties both in physician-patient relationships and in the appropriate gathering of clinical information. These styles are not the direct result of neurological disease, although any one of these profiles may be exaggerated by neuropathology. There are certain personality changes, however, that are commonly associated with underlying neurological change, especially of the temporal and frontal lobes.

Organic Personality Change (ICD 10—Organic Personality Change)

After head trauma, changes of personality are associated with three different variables. First, an exacerbation of premorbid personality traits is common—for example, anancasts turning into rigid obsessive-compulsive patients; patients with preexisting anxious personalities developing anxiety neurosis, with excessive worry about small matters and panic attacks; and patients with explosive personalities becoming dangerous, with outbursts of violence.

Second, any brain lesion may disrupt the personality, provoking what may be called an organic personality change. This change includes irritability and restlessness, lassitude, poor concentration and attention, loss of initiative, and excessive emotionality. There may be poor tolerance for environmental change; increasing insecurity, with anxiety and loss of confidence; and a tendency to withdraw from everyday events. The patient becomes more irritable with relatives and friends, finds even slight overcrowding intolerable, and may complain of an inability to tolerate sensory stimuli such as noise from the radio or television. With more severe damage, extremes of this profile are seen, with social disorganization, loss of interest in the self, explosive irritability, shallowness of affect, and blunting of emotional responses.

These symptoms may become intertwined at one level with a related symptom pattern, sometimes referred to as a posttraumatic neurosis. This overlaps with posttraumatic stress disorder (see below). Patients display an increase in emotionality; the development of anxieties and phobias; disturbed affect with depressive overtones; a tendency to withdraw from company; somatic complaints of headache, dizziness, and visual disturbances; poor memory and concentration; irritability; and aggression. Posttraumatic neurosis, however, is more often seen following slighter head injuries, which result in limited posttraumatic amnesia and a greater contribution of the premorbid personality. Although it may appear frequently in the setting of compensation, it is important to recognize this constellation of symptoms, because it may reflect subtle neuronal damage that occurs during a head injury, especially when the constitutional liability to neurosis is slight; identical clinical pictures are seen in patients for whom compensation is not an issue.

The third type of personality change relates to more recognized syndromes that occur following damage to the frontal lobes and the temporal lobes.

Frontal Lobe Damage

Although there are extensive reviews of frontal lobe syndromes (Stuss and Benson 1986), frontal lobe damage often goes unnoticed, and its manifestations, particularly after head injury, are often not sought. This oversight is because the subtle and polymorphous expressions of frontal lobe damage are not recognized or understood.

Various pathological conditions lead to frontal lobe damage, including tumors, cerebrovascular accidents, infections, and some degenerative diseases, particularly lobar atrophy (Pick's disease) and other forms of frontal dementia. Damage to both the anterior and middle cerebral arteries also can injure the frontal lobes, because the middle cerebral artery supplies the lateral parts of the orbital gyri and the inferior and middle frontal gyri.

One of the main consequences of frontal lobe damage is alteration of attention; patients present with distractibility, poor memory, and what has been referred to as "forgetting to remember." Thinking in frontal lobe patients tends to be concrete, and they may show perseveration, with an inability to switch from one line of thinking to another. This inability leads to difficulties in arithmetical calculations, such as serial 7s and subtractions, and stereotypy of responses. An aphasia is seen, but it is different from both cortical sensory (Wernicke's) and Broca's aphasia. In 1973, Luria referred to this

Table 9.1: Clinical characteristics of the three principal frontal lobe syndromes

Orbitofrontal syndrome (disinhibited)
Disinhibited, impulsive behavior (pseudopsychopathic)
Inappropriate jocular affect, euphoria
Emotional lability
Poor judgment and insight
Distractibility
Frontal convexity syndrome (apathetic)
Apathy (occasional, brief angry or aggressive outbursts are common)
Indifference
Psychomotor retardation
Motor perseveration and impersistence
Loss of behavioral set
Stimulus boundedness
Discrepant motor and verbal behavior
Motor programming deficits:
Three-step hand sequence
Alternating programs
Reciprocal programs
Rhythm tapping
Multiple loops
Poor word-list generation
Poor abstraction and categorization
Segmented approach to visuospatial analysis
Medial frontal syndrome (akinetic)
Paucity of spontaneous movement and gesture
Sparse verbal output (repetition may be preserved)
Lower-extremity weakness and loss of sensation
Incontinence

Source: Data from J Cummings. Clinical Neuropsychiatry. Orlando, FL: Grune & Stratton, 1985; and MR Trimble. Biological Psychiatry (2nd ed). Chichester, England: Wiley, 1996.

aphasia as dynamic aphasia, noting that patients have well-preserved motor speech and no anomia, and repetition is intact. However, they show marked difficulty of propositioning, and active speech is severely disturbed. This syndrome is similar to that referred to as transcortical motor aphasia.

Other features of frontal lobe syndromes include reduced activity, particularly diminution of spontaneous activity; lack of drive; inability to plan ahead; and lack of concern. Sometimes associated with this damage are bouts of restlessness and aimless, uncoordinated behavior. The affect is often disturbed, with patients showing apathy, emotional blunting, and an indifference to the world around them. Clinically, this condition can resemble a major affective disorder with psychomotor retardation. In marked contrast, on other occasions, euphoria and disinhibition are described. The euphoria is not that of a manic condition, however; it has an empty quality to it, lacking conviction. The disinhibition can lead to markedly abnormal behavior, which is sometimes associated with outbursts of irritability and aggression.

L'hermitte and colleagues (1986) have described utilization and imitation behaviors as variants of environmental dependency syndromes. In these syndromes there is excessive control over behavior by environmental stimuli. In imitation behavior, patients imitate gestures and movements

Table 9.2: Useful tests of frontal lobe function

Word fluency test (word-list generation)
Abstract thinking test ("If I have 18 books and two bookshelves, and I want twice as many books on one shelf as the other, how many books go on each shelf?")
Proverb and metaphor interpretation
Wisconsin Card Sorting Test
Other sorting tasks
Block design
Trail-making test
Porteus maze test
Hand position test and other motor programming defects
Copying tasks
Rhythm tapping tasks
Cognitive estimates

of an examiner when not asked to do so. In utilization behavior, patients use objects placed before them inappropriately, a classic example being the patient, who, on being shown a pair of glasses, will take them and put them on, in spite of already wearing a pair. The inferior half and mediobasal areas of the frontal lobes usually are affected. These behaviors are probably related to a lack of inhibition of parietal activity (L'hermitte et al. 1986).

Some authors have distinguished between lesions of the lateral frontal cortex (most closely linked to motor structures of the brain), which lead to disturbances of movement and action with perseveration and inertia, and lesions of the orbital frontal cortex interlinked with limbic and reticular areas, which lead to disinhibition and changes of affective life. A third syndrome, the medial frontal syndrome, is marked by akinesia and is associated with mutism, gait disturbances, and incontinence. The clinical characteristics of these three principal frontal lobe syndromes are shown in Table 9.1, and some useful tests of frontal lobe function are shown in Table 9.2; in reality, an admixture of features is found in many cases. In some patients, short-lived paroxysmal behavior disorders are recorded, which include episodes of confusion and occasionally hallucinations. These are thought to reflect transient disturbances of the frontolimbic connections. Finally, following massive frontal lobe lesions, the so-called apathetico-akinetico-abulic syndrome may occur, in which patients lie around passively, unaroused and unable to complete tasks or listen to commands.

Temporal Lobe Syndromes

The temporal lobes contain vital limbic system structures that are closely involved in the modulation of emotional behavior. It is hardly surprising, therefore, that pathological conditions that affect the temporal lobes, particularly the hippocampus and the amygdala, commonly are associated with changes of personality and other psychopathological conditions. A condition seen with increasing frequency is herpes simplex encephalitis, which previously was referred to as acute necrotizing encephalitis. This condition is caused by the herpes simplex virus (HSV)-1. Among survivors, the subsequent psychopathological effect is severe; it may be noted during recovery and continue thereafter. Patients may display amnestic syndrome, hypermetamorphosis (a persistent overattention to external stimuli), a tendency to explore objects orally, agnosias, eating and drinking problems, and inappropriate sexual displays. Irritability, easy distractibility, aggressive outbursts, emotional blunting, periods of apathy and depression, and episodes of restlessness and overactivity are seen in many patients. Some survivors exhibit part or the whole of the Klüver-Bucy syndrome, the features of which are loss of fear and aggression, hypersexuality, excessive oral exploration of the environment, and visual agnosia. Elements of this syndrome incidentally can be seen in several other conditions in which the amygdala is affected bilaterally, such as Pick's disease, or after head injury.

Mild forms of herpes encephalitis may occur that, while generally having a good prognosis, lead to personality changes. An increase in HSV-1 neutralizing antibody has been reported in aggressive psychopaths and in patients with schizophrenia, psychotic depression, and other psychiatric conditions that include personality disorders. Case histories describe patients with markedly disturbed behavior who, at some point in their illness, had received a psychiatric label but which turned out to be due to a subacute or chronic encephalitis, commonly of the limbic system. The term *limbic encephalitis* is applied to this type of illness, and herpes simplex, measles, and rabies viruses have been implicated.

One of the most common conditions affecting the temporal lobes seen in neurological practice is *epilepsy*, particularly localization-related or focal epilepsy, in which the brunt of the disease falls on medial temporal structures. The association between epilepsy deriving from the temporal lobe and personality disorders has been an issue of constant debate and confusion, but the concept that there may be an interictal temporal lobe syndrome has been advocated most strongly by Geschwind and his colleagues. They defined the interictal behavior syndrome of temporal lobe epilepsy, emphasizing alterations in sexual behavior, hyperreligiosity, and hypergraphia—a tendency toward extensive and often compulsive writing. They suggested that in some patients, the syndrome appeared before any seizures; when present, even in the absence of further evidence, these features suggest dysfunction at this specific anatomical site. They contrasted this picture both with the frontal lobe syndrome and with the Klüver-Bucy syndrome, identifying some characteristics almost opposite to those of the latter syndrome. The religiosity may be seen as sudden religious conversion or as a growing interest in mystical and religious themes, often with behavior out of keeping with the patient's normal pattern. There may be compulsive church attendance, repetitive Bible reading, or obsessive attachment to some unorthodox religious group. Alternatively, there may be merely an interest in the cosmic and supernatural or the conviction that the person has some special significance in the world or some messianic mission.

Meticulous attention to detail and continual working over of an idea are other features of temporal lobe syndromes. Circumstantiality of speech and verbosity also are seen, with prolonged and tortuous explanations often being given for trivial events. This tendency may be reflected in hypergraphia, with detailed and meticulous accounts of events being recorded, often with a moral or religious theme.

The disturbed sexuality of temporal lobe syndromes usually is referred to as hyposexuality, with indifference to sexual contacts. In other patients, however, it may manifest as a plasticity of responses, with development of unusual proclivities. The symptoms and signs that are associated with this syndrome are not necessarily maladaptive; some patients display remarkable talents and are productive and valuable members of society.

One interpretation of these findings was that an epileptic focus somehow leads to enhanced associations between affects and stimuli, a so-called functional hyperconnection between neocortical and limbic structures; this hyperconnection possibly inhibits events that normally prevent fortuitous sensory and affective connections from developing. This tendency is the opposite of the Kluver-Bucy syndrome, in which limbic dysfunction leads to failure to attribute the appropriate emotional significance to stimuli, resulting in emotional blunting, diminished fear and aggression, inappropriate sexual behavior, and hypermetamorphosis—a limbic agnosia.

The personality changes associated with temporal lobe epilepsy often are not detected clinically unless they are specifically inquired about. Such features as hyperreligiosity, obsessionality, and circumstantiality are hardly the things that relatives or patients complain about to doctors. However, another feature of temporal lobe epilepsy, again quite controversial, is the association with aggressive behavior. This behavior is a common complaint in neurological clinics. Although ictal violence has been recorded clearly by videotelemetry, the problem of recording and quantifying interictal aggressive behavior has led to considerable variability of results from clinical investigations. The main arguments revolve around whether epilepsy deriving from the temporal lobes is more likely than other forms of epilepsy to provoke interictal aggression or whether the aggression is a nonspecific manifestation of brain damage, low socioeconomic status, and poor environmental upbringing.

Fenwick (1986) noted the evidence from intracranial-implanted electrode studies in humans, which suggests that the amygdala is involved in the mediation of aggression in humans and, further, that amygdalectomy improves patients' aggressive behavior. In addition, patients who undergo temporal lobectomy for epilepsy show improvement in their seizures and in their behavior (most notably aggression). His conclusion was that there is a relationship between seizure discharges and aggressive behavior, but in interictal states, findings were better explained as a manifestation of brain damage leading to poor impulse control rather than to a seizure-related process.

An associated condition is the episodic dyscontrol syndrome, in which there are sudden, short-lived episodes of spontaneously released aggression, often with minimal provocation. These episodes may be provoked by the ingestion of small amounts of alcohol; after the event, patients feel remorse.

Typically, the dysphoric and irritable personality changes of epilepsy start shortly after the onset of the seizure disorder, particularly if it occurs in late adolescence or early adulthood, and usually coincide with the initiation of anticonvulsant medication. The drugs themselves, however, are not necessarily implicated, although the older barbiturate drugs and excessive polytherapy are related to similar behavior problems (Trimble and Thompson 1986).

Examination and Investigations

History

To unravel some of these complex behavioral problems, it is important to obtain an accurate history from the patient and from a third party who knows the patient well. As emphasized earlier, personality relates to the enduring traits by which we come to know an individual, and any marked change in personality, particularly if it occurs over a short period of time, implies the onset of some process. Careful inquiry is therefore necessary regarding the patient's premorbid pattern of life, and certain indicators from the history are helpful in attempting to understand the development of any personality change. The family history may reveal evidence suggestive of a genetic propensity to personality disturbance, such as alcoholism, sociopathy, or clearly hysterical traits in the parents. As a child, the patient may have shown behavior disturbances early on, reflected in excessive temper tantrums, an inability to get along with peers, a tendency to be shy and lonely, or one of the numerous anxiety-related neurotic traits of childhood. These traits, though individually having little meaning, when clustered may be of value in helping suggest a susceptibility to the later onset of neurotic illness. They include such behaviors as nail biting; sleepwalking; early childhood phobias, such as fear of the dark; food faddism; enuresis; school refusal; and stammering, tics, or mannerisms.

Physical and sexual abuse are important in the history of patients who later develop conversion disorder, especially pseudoseizures. This subject can be difficult to inquire about, and indeed usually is not revealed until much later in a patient's treatment (e.g., in psychotherapy).

Early childhood hyperactivity and a tendency toward truculence, frequent fighting, truancy, and delinquency in the school years hint at the continued development of a sociopathic personality disorder in later life. This disorder may be reflected in a poor work record, with the patient holding numerous jobs for short periods of time and often being fired. Interpersonal relationships may be continuously disrupted, with poor peer relationships, failure of marriage, and failure at work. Alcoholism may become a problem, perhaps preceded by adolescent drug taking.

With an adequate history, an understanding of the patient's behavior problems often becomes clear. Thus, the late development of an explosive personality or a pattern similar to the episodic dyscontrol syndrome, when it occurs after the onset of epilepsy or after a head injury and in the absence of these other indicators of earlier personality disturbance, would suggest that the behavior is related to underlying neurological change. The flowering of a posttraumatic neurosis following a relatively trivial head injury may again, in the absence of obvious premorbid indicators, reflect subtle neurological damage, which has allowed latent premorbid personality traits to flourish.

General and Neurological Examination

Clinical examination is important, particularly when minimal or subtle brain dysfunction is suspected. So-called soft neurological signs always should be looked for. These signs refer to release or primitive reflexes such as the grasp reflex, the sucking reflex, the snout reflex, the palmomental reflex, and the glabellar tap. The grasp reflex is elicited by firmly stroking the palm and fingers of the patient's hands in an outward direction; it involves a reflex grasping of the examiner's hand. The grasp tends to persist, and the more force exerted, the greater the intensity of the grasp. Unlike a normal grasp, the thumb usually remains extended. This reflex is associated with disease of the contralateral frontal lobe, and its presence is highly suggestive of an underlying neurological process. The snout reflex is a reflex protrusion of the lips in response to a gentle tap, and the palmomental reflex is produced by firm stroking of the palm in the radial direction from the thenar eminence to the opposite index finger; it is accompanied by contraction of the ipsilateral mentalis muscle. Although the palmomental reflex and the snout reflex occur in normal persons, their presence suggests underlying subtle neurological damage, especially if they are grouped with other abnormal reflexes. In particular, sustained presentation of these reflexes on repetition is of clinical importance. The jaw jerk, elicited by tapping the chin when the mouth is opened and the jaw relaxed, is another reflex that, when exaggerated, is of clinical significance.

Other soft signs include clumsiness, awkwardness, and poor coordination when carrying out tasks such as finger-to-nose testing, dysdiadochokinesia, and complex fine-motor activities such as repetitive tapping. Also included are dysgraphesthesia (the inability to detect symbols traced on the palm or surface of the hand while the eyes are closed); astereognosis (the incorrect identification of three-dimensional objects placed in the outstretched hand); subtle gait disturbances; and movement abnormalities reminiscent of, but not necessarily corresponding to, recognized movement disorders such as tics, chorea, or athetosis.

Several reports (see Trimble and Rogers 1987) emphasize that patients with psychiatric disorders show an increased frequency of these signs, and their presence in early childhood suggests a susceptibility to the later development of psychiatric illness. Their designation "soft" should not be misunderstood; it has arisen because in most cases these signs have no specific localizing value and do not lead to the detection of recognizable neurological disease. However, their presence does imply some CNS factor that may substantiate the neurological underpinnings of the behavioral syndrome; the localization, if it need be sought, would have to be seen in the context of subcortical and frontolimbic abnormalities.

Detecting frontal lobe damage can be difficult, especially with only traditional methods of testing. With frontal lobe damage, the whole of the patient's motoric and psychic life is influenced, and the behavior disturbance itself reflects the disease. Standard neurological examination is often normal, and the results of standard psychological tests, such as the Wechsler Adult Intelligence Scale (WAIS), may not reveal changes.

Patients may display sensory inattention in the contralateral sensory field, abnormalities of visual searching, echo phenomena such as echolalia and echopraxia, confabulation, various changes in cognitive function, and imitation or utilization behavior. Orbitofrontal lesions are associated with anosmia. The more the lesions extend posteriorly, the more such neurological signs as obvious aphasia, paralyses, grasp reflexes, and oculomotor abnormalities become apparent.

Table 9.2 lists various clinical tasks that can be used to detect frontal lobe damage. However, not all patients with frontal lobe damage show these abnormalities on testing, and not all of these tests are exclusively abnormal in frontal lobe disease. Cognitive tests include the word fluency test, in which the patient is asked to generate in 1 minute as many words as possible that begin with a particular letter (the normal number is around 15). The patient's proverb or metaphor interpretation may be remarkably concrete. Problem solving (e.g., doing carry-over additions or subtractions) can be tested by simple questioning; serial 7s may be difficult to perform. Cognitive estimates can be a useful way of detecting frontal damage. The patient is asked such questions as "How fast does a race horse run?" or "How high is the Empire State Building?" The answers can reveal a total lack of insight.

Laboratory-based tests of abstract reasoning include the Wisconsin Card Sorting Test and other sorting tasks. The essential nature of these tests is to arrange a variety of objects into groups according to one abstract common property, such as a color. The property then is changed, for example to shape. Patients with frontal lobe damage poorly overcome previously established responses and therefore show a high frequency of errors. These deficits are most likely with lateral lesions of the dominant hemisphere.

Patients with frontal lobe lesions also do badly on maze learning tasks (for example, the Porteus maze test), the category test, and block design. They show perseveration of motor tasks and difficulty carrying out sequences of motor action. Skilled movements are no longer performed smoothly, and previously automated actions such as handwriting or playing musical instruments are often impaired. The patient's ability to follow a succession of hand positions (with the hand first placed flat, then on the side, and then as a fist on a flat surface) or to tap aloud a complex rhythm (for example, two loud and three soft beats) is impaired. Perseveration, which is especially prominent with deeper lesions in which the modulating function of the premotor cortex on the motor structures of the basal ganglia is lost, may be tested by asking the patient to draw a circle, for example, or to copy a complex diagram with recurring shapes in it that alternate with one another. The patient may continue to draw circle upon circle, not stopping after one revolution, or may miss the pattern of recurring shapes (Figure 9.1). Patients with suspected frontal or temporal lobe disease should be referred for neuropsychological testing, with a specific request that tasks with a frontal lobe emphasis be examined.

Investigations

The electroencephalogram (EEG) is revealing in patients with epilepsy, especially if a seizure can be captured by videotelemetry, by ambulatory monitoring, or by chance during a routine EEG procedure. If a localization-related epilepsy in the temporal lobes is suspected but the routine investigation is equivocal, then sleep or sleep deprivation recordings and, ultimately, nasopharyngeal or sphenoidal investigations should be requested.

In many cases, particularly in association with psychopathic personality disorders and aggression, nonspecific findings are reported. Abnormalities on the EEG in such patients have been observed since the introduction of the EEG, particularly bilateral theta activity in temporal and central regions. A far higher incidence of abnormal EEGs has been reported in aggressive psychopaths than in individuals selected for personality stability, such as flying personnel. Patients suffering from the episodic dyscontrol syndrome commonly have EEG abnormalities, mainly within the temporal lobes. These data suggest links between cerebral dysrhythmia (particularly posterior, often bilateral, temporal paroxysmal discharges) and certain personality features, and the emphasis is on impulsive, aggressive behavior. The cause of these dysrhythmias is unclear, but they may reflect maturational factors, possibly genetically determined; earlier brain damage; or later structural or functional disturbances of the brain stem-limbic system structures. Clinically, such abnormalities are often seen in association with paroxysmal behavior disorders and do not imply a diagnosis of epilepsy. Their presence in aggressive and psychopathic patients should be seen as a reflection of underlying limbic system dysfunction, which may be related to the behavior disturbance; in the absence of a clear history of seizures, however, the diagnosis of epilepsy should be avoided.

A computed tomographic (CT) scan is mandatory in patients who have undergone a clear personality change that cannot be understood in terms of the development of their premorbid personality. Cases in which meningioma or cerebral tumors have been detected on CT scan, often after many years of complaints of behavior changes, are well known clinically. Frontotemporal lobar atrophy may in-

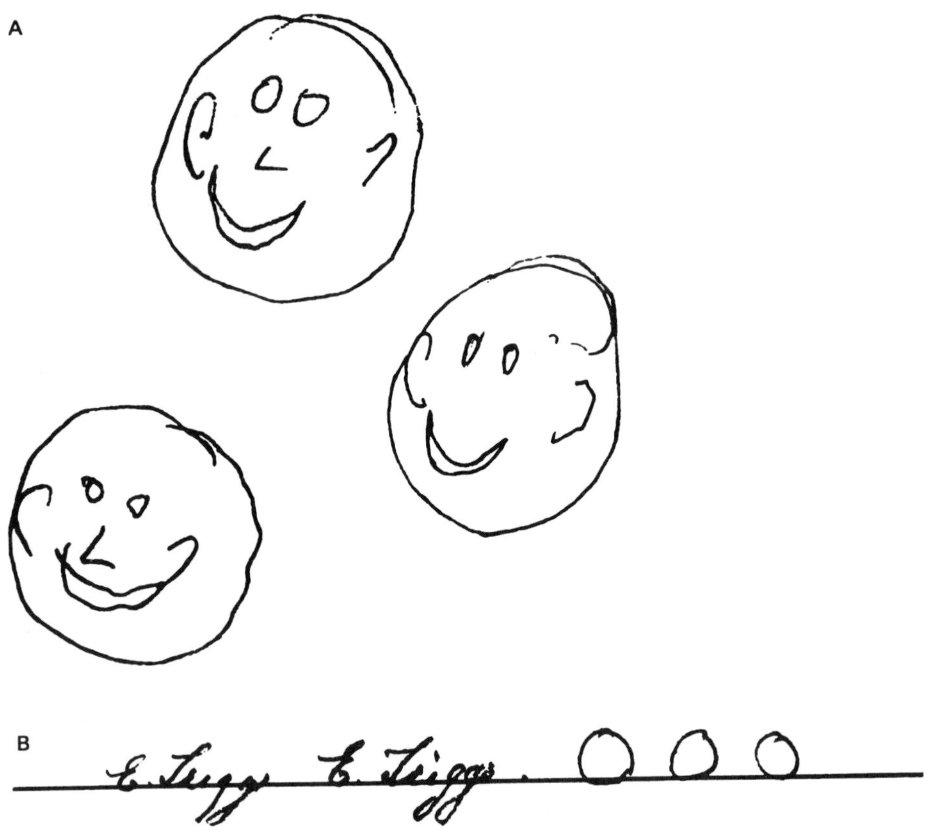

FIGURE 9.1 Some consequences of frontal lobe disease. A. The patient was asked to draw a circle but produced three faces. B. The patient was asked to write her name and to draw a circle.

crease the suspicion of the development of Pick's disease, and temporal lobe destruction may be observed in severe cases of limbic encephalitis.

Magnetic resonance imaging (MRI) may reveal intra-cerebral demyelinating plaques of multiple sclerosis, and their periventricular or temporal lobe location may explain some of the behavioral features of this disorder. MRI also may reveal extensive structural damage to the frontal and temporal lobes following head injury; this damage may not have been detected on conventional CT scanning and perhaps was unsuspected from clinical and neuropsychological investigations. MRI also is required to show subtle temporal lobe lesions in epilepsy, especially amygdala and hippocampal sclerosis.

ANXIETY DISORDERS

The hallmark of anxiety disorders is anxiety itself, not associated with another psychiatric condition. ICD 10 and DSM-IV have broadly similar categories, the most important of which are panic disorder (with or without agoraphobia), generalized anxiety disorder, specific phobias, posttraumatic stress disorder, and obsessive-compulsive disorder. In neurological clinical practice, the anxiety states are most commonly seen, including generalized anxiety disorders and panic disorders.

In generalized anxiety, the patient has anxiety of at least a month's duration without associated phobic symptoms or panic attacks. The manifestations of anxiety are multiple and affect every body system. Further, because anxiety is so common and many of the symptoms are somatic, patients with anxiety disorders are often referred for unnecessary investigations, misdiagnosed, and treated inappropriately. Common symptoms include palpitations, sometimes associated with anterior chest pain over the heart; dyspnea and a sense of choking or a feeling of not being able to take in sufficient breath; dry mouth, with unpleasant, often metallic tastes; abdominal tension, sometimes associated with nausea or actual vomiting; constipation or diarrhea; retention of urine or frequency of urination; poor concentration and memory difficulties; dizziness, vertigo, faint feelings, and, on occasion, blackouts that resemble epileptic seizures; increased muscle tone, with pain and tremor; fatigue and loss of energy; and sensory symptoms such as tingling (especially of the hands), diminished vision, or a generalized hyperesthesia in which sounds are distorted or magnified. This hyperestheisa is sometimes accompanied by photophobia.

In *panic disorder*, relatively frequent, discrete episodes of panic are associated with apprehension and fear. The paroxysmal nature and sudden onset of these episodes and the common absence of any obvious precipitating factor may lead to a diagnosis of complex partial seizures. The DSM-IV (1994) criteria for panic disorder are shown in Table 9.3.

A variant of this disorder is the phobic-anxiety depersonalization syndrome, in which depersonalization or derealization form a prominent part of the picture. This can be a much more pervasive disorder, with generalized anxiety, affective symptoms, and a danger of death by suicide.

Table 9.3: Diagnostic criteria for panic disorder

A discrete period of intense fear or discomfort in which at least four of the following symptoms develop abruptly and reach a peak within 10 minutes:

1. Palpitations, pounding heart, or accelerated heart rate
2. Sweating
3. Trembling or shaking
4. Sensations of shortness of breath or smothering
5. Feeling of choking
6. Chest pain or discomfort
7. Nausea or abdominal distress
8. Feeling dizzy, unsteady, lightheaded, or faint
9. Derealization (feelings of unreality) or depersonalization (being detached from oneself)
10. Feeling of losing control or going crazy
11. Fear of dying
12. Paresthesias (numbness or tingling sensations)
13. Chills or hot flushes

In some patients, the depersonalization may persist between the more extreme manifestations. Patients may feel like automatons and may complain occasionally that they have left their bodies, sometimes with autoscopy.

In neurological clinical practice, patients may present with panic attacks and many of the other symptoms of anxiety, leading the unwary physician into alternative diagnoses. Anxiety states are misinterpreted as epilepsy, vestibular neuronitis, benign essential tremor, multiple sclerosis, and even dementia. The protean and often paroxysmal nature of anxiety symptoms leads to such misinterpretations; only familiarity with the multiple presentations of anxiety disorders, and accurate history taking can aid in diagnosis.

Hyperventilation is a symptom that is commonly met in neurological practice. Although this symptom may be secondary to brain stem pathology, the most common cause is anxiety. Usually the hyperventilation is just one of a group of anxiety symptoms, often leading to a full-blown panic attack; thus, the full spectrum of associated features should be sought. Patients are often unaware that they hyperventilate, especially if the problem is one of increased volume of air intake as opposed to increased rate of respiration. The hyperventilation physiologically leads to a fall in the pCO_2 in the peripheral blood, with an increase of pH. There will be associated vasoconstriction and cerebral hypoxia. The exact relationship of these changes to the patients symptoms is unclear, but the latter may be induced by getting patients to overbreathe for approximately 3 minutes. Helping the patient to control breathing by behavior modification is of value in management. In some patients hyperventilation may lead to a seizure, confusing the differential diagnosis.

Posttraumatic stress disorder (PTSD) is a variant of posttraumatic neurosis, which is sometimes incorrectly referred to as accident neurosis or compensation neurosis. The clinical criteria for PTSD require a specific stress, and the disorder presents with a combination of anxiety and depressive symptoms. Special emphasis is given to reexperiencing the trauma in flashbacks or nightmares; the former may be triggered by stimuli, such as the noise of screeching tires following a car accident; in practice, searching for these experiences is of utmost importance, as it often holds the key to the diagnosis. The other symptom groups are related to the development of avoidance of stimuli that remind a victim of or symbolize the psychological trauma, and a numbing of emotional responses. Patients typically do not talk about what happened, avoid the scene of an accident, and switch off television programs that provoke unpleasant recollections. There are also signs of increased autonomic arousal. An interesting feature is an increased startle response, which is sometimes so severe that it can be mistaken for a tic disorder such as the Gilles de la Tourette's syndrome, or even startle epilepsy. The full DSM-IV criteria are given in Table 9.4.

The reporting of some of these symptoms (e.g., sleeplessness, nightmares, and avoidance) in the immediate aftermath of a psychological trauma represents a normal human reaction. In some patients, however, the symptoms become protracted, and over time, especially if interlinked with a chronic pain syndrome attributable to associated physical trauma, depressive symptoms emerge. Furthermore, PTSD must be distinguished from bereavement, with its specific anguish over a lost loved one and rituals of grief, which are natural human reactions to loss.

On examination, patients with anxiety states often show sweating but have cold extremities and may be flushed. The resting pulse, respiration rate, and blood pressure may be elevated, and increased central body movement or restless hand movements, with tremor, may be seen. There may be startle to a sudden, unexpected noise. It is customary to examine thyroid function; occasionally, thyrotoxicosis and severe anxiety states are allomorphic. If there is a suspicion of a pheochromocytoma, urinary monoamine metabolites should be measured, but the EEG and CT scan are usually unrewarding.

In the differential diagnosis of pseudoseizures (see below), many patients (up to 75% according to Kloster [1993]) have nonspecific EEG changes, and some show paroxysms of theta activity and sometimes focal temporal spike or sharp waves. Videotelemetry is of great value in the diagnosis of these attacks. In such settings, a postictal prolactin assessment can be of help. In pseudoseizures there is never the substantial rise in prolactin (>1,000 IU/liter) 10–20 minutes after the attack, which returns to baseline after 1 hour, that is seen in generalized tonic-clonic attacks. The rise is less substantial with complex partial seizures, and no rise is seen with simple partial seizures, pseudoseizures, frontal seizures, and status epilepticus.

FATIGUE, WEAKNESS, AND NEURASTHENIA

Fatigue is a common complaint in a neurological setting, but curiously, it has been little studied. The term *neurasthenia* was coined by Beard in the nineteenth century to define a condition that he thought was peculiarly American

Table 9.4: Diagnostic criteria for posttraumatic stress disorder

I. The person has been exposed to a traumatic event in which both of the following have been present:
   A. The person has experienced, witnessed, or been confronted with an event or events that involve actual or threatened death or serious injury, or a threat to the physical integrity of oneself or others.
   B. The person's response involved intense fear, helplessness, or horror. In children, the response may be expressed instead by disorganized or agitated behavior.

II. The traumatic event is reexperienced persistently in at least one of the following ways:
   A. Recurrent and intrusive distressing recollections of the event, including images, thoughts, or perceptions. In young children, repetitive play may occur in which themes or aspects of the trauma are expressed.
   B. Recurrent distressing dreams of the event. In children, there may be frightening dreams without recognizable content.
   C. Acting or feeling as if the traumatic event were recurring (includes a sense of reliving the experience, illusions, hallucinations, and dissociative flashback episodes, including those that occur upon awakening or when intoxicated). Note: in young children, trauma-specific reenactment may occur.
   D. Intensive psychological distress at exposure to internal or external cues that symbolize or resemble an aspect of the traumatic event.
   E. Physiological reactivity on exposure to internal or external cues that symbolize or resemble an aspect of the traumatic event.

III. The person persistently avoids stimuli associated with the trauma and experiences numbing of general responsiveness (not present before the trauma), as indicated by at least three of the following:
   A. Efforts to avoid thoughts, feelings, or conversations associated with the trauma.
   B. Efforts to avoid activities, places, or people that arouse recollections of the trauma.
   C. Inability to recall an important aspect of the trauma.
   D. Markedly diminished interest or participation in significant activities.
   E. Feeling of detachment or estrangement from others.
   F. Restricted range of affect (e.g., unable to have loving feelings).
   G. Sense of a foreshortened future (e.g., does not expect to have a career, marriage, children, or a normal life span).

IV. The person experiences persistent symptoms of increased arousal (not present before the trauma), as indicated by at least two of the following:
   A. Difficulty falling or staying asleep.
   B. Irritability or outbursts of anger.
   C. Difficulty concentrating.
   D. Hypervigilance.
   E. Exaggerated startle response.

V. The duration of the disturbance (symptoms in II, III, and IV) is more than 1 month.

VI. The disturbance causes clinically significant distress or impairment in social, occupational, or other important areas of functioning.

Source: Reprinted with permission from the *Diagnostic and Statistical Manual of Mental Disorders, Fourth Edition.* Copyright 1994 American Psychiatric Association.

and caused by nervous exhaustion. The symptoms were varied, including tenderness of the scalp, headaches, heaviness in the back of the head, eye irritations, noises in the ears, poor concentration, irritability, hopelessness, fears and hypochondriasis, insomnia, drowsiness, dyspepsia, sweating, heaviness in the limbs, pain in the feet, muscle spasms, convulsive movements on falling asleep, numbness, pruritus, and many other small complaints. Many cases once diagnosed as neurasthenia now would be categorized as anxiety or affective disorders, but the heaviness of limbs, hyperirritability, and fatigue form a group of symptoms frequently seen by neurologists. Patients complain of lassitude and lack motivation to carry out everyday tasks; the heaviness of their limbs is accompanied by a similar reduced capacity for mental effort, and any new activity produces rapid tiring.

The term *myalgic encephalomyelitis* (ME) was misleading, because it suggested that patients with the above constellation of symptoms had contracted some identifiable CNS pathology attributable to infection. However, the search for specific neuromuscular pathology, viruses, or immunological abnormalities has failed. The term *chronic fatigue syndrome* (CFS) is preferred.

Wessely (1991) re-emphasized that most patients with CFS who are seen in specialist centers have a recognizable psychiatric illness, especially depression, anxiety, or a somatization disorder. Such patients often do not accept a line of psychological inquiry, and assessment depends on picking up subtle clues of psychopathology, changes of sleep and appetite patterns, diurnal variation of mood and symptoms, tearfulness, irritability, loss of libido, and perhaps associated suicidal thoughts. The tenacity with which patients hold to a neurological explanation for their symptoms is sometimes itself revealing of *abnormal illness behavior*—the persistence of an inappropriate mode of perceiving, evaluating, and acting in relation to one's state of health. There is a discrepancy between the degree of objective somatic pathology revealed and the patient's reaction to it.

Fatigue is a common symptom of underlying anxiety; it may be reported both by patients with major affective disorders and by some psychotic patients who may have a delusional interpretation of what has happened to their energy. Prominent complaints of fatigue are noted in the postviral syndrome (a potential variant of ME)—a diagnosis of an often disputed entity that occurs especially following infectious mononucleosis but may be a sequel to many infections, including influenza. The fatigue often emerges several weeks after the illness itself, and some patients remain so weak that they can hardly get out of bed. A full neurasthenic picture may develop, often with a poor prognosis; as time passes, a major affective disorder may become apparent.

The fatigue of these patients should be distinguished from that of myasthenia gravis, in which patients complain excessively of fatigue from ordinary activities; symptoms disappear with short periods of rest, as they usually do in other forms of neuromuscular incapacity. Patients with arthritis, neuritis, and polyneuritis also may complain of fatigue, particularly when they use specific muscle groups that may be affected by the condition. Fatigue is common in patients with multiple sclerosis, although here, as with other neurological conditions, the quality of the presentation is different from that of the patient with a neurosis, who commonly has other associated complaints and may have, in the background, evidence of an underlying personality disorder.

Treatment of CFS is problematic, especially if the patient is somatically orientated and rigidly insists on a neurological explanation of his or her symptoms. Psychotropic drugs, especially antidepressants, are often helpful, and occasionally electroconvulsive therapy is needed. For most patients a combination of physical rehabilitation and cognitive-behavior therapy appears to be most appropriate (Denman 1990).

OBSESSIVE-COMPULSIVE DISORDER (ICD 10—OBSESSIVE COMPULSIVE DISORDER; DSM-IV—OBSESSIVE COMPULSIVE DISORDER)

Of all the neuroses, obsessive-compulsive disorder (OCD) is perhaps the most neurological in flavor; in many cases, the intensity of the symptoms and the imperative way in which compulsions are carried out raises questions as to whether OCD should be considered a neurosis at all.

Tuke was one of the earliest writers to recognize the cerebral underpinnings of this condition; he quoted the ideas of Laycock and Hughlings Jackson with approval. The encephalitis pandemics of the early part of this century led to a rich variety of neuropsychiatric symptoms, which were well described by Von Economo in 1931. The symptoms included obsessive and compulsive behaviors. Many patients developed postencephalitic Parkinson's disease, and in some cases the compulsive behavior was "awakened" by L-dopa therapy. The association between Parkinson's disease and obsessive-compulsive traits has been mentioned frequently, in terms of either rigid, moralistic, and inhibited premorbid personality profiles or the development of obsessive-compulsive symptoms in association with the motor manifestations of the disease. Obsessional slowness—the excessive time required by some patients to carry out acts—has been likened to a failure of executive motor planning, possibly similar to that underlying Parkinson's disease itself.

The findings (on positron-emission tomography) of increased activity in frontal orbital and caudate structures substantiate these ideas (Baxter et al. 1987). Although the findings are not yet completely in concordance, there is increasing agreement that frontal-basal ganglia-thalamic neuronal circuits are involved in this condition (Cummings 1993).

Gilles de la Tourette's syndrome is characterized by multiple tics, including vocal tics, which usually manifest before the age of 15 years. Although the tics wax and wane with time, the condition, once established, appears lifelong. The richness of this disorder, however, extends far beyond the tics, and the motor symptoms include a great variety of complicated movements, many of which have a compulsive quality. Furthermore, some 30–50% of patients have obsessive-compulsive phenomena, equivalent in severity to OCD as defined by the DSM-III-R (Trimble and Robertson 1987). These symptoms are linked closely with some of the central features of the disease, such as coprolalia and echo phenomena; these features suggest a close biological link between the motoric and psychological phenomena. Recent genetic research has emphasized that if Gilles de la Tourette's syndrome, OCD, and chronic motor tics are taken as phenotypes, then a pattern of autosomal-dominant inheritance is found. Men tend to express more motor disorders and women tend to express more obsessive-compulsive behaviors (Robertson and Gourdie 1990).

There is a long history of an association between epilepsy and obsessional forms of thinking, sometimes reflected in hypergraphia, and EEG studies of obsessive-compulsive patients reveal significant cerebral abnormalities in 6–60% of cases.

The obsessive-compulsive phenomena found in association with some of these neurological conditions are important in terms of management. In many cases, it is the behavior disorder that leads to the most profound social handicaps, and effective remedies may be available for the behavior disorder in the absence of useful treatments for the associated neurological phenomena.

FUGUE STATES

A *fugue state* is a condition in which a person, with clouding of consciousness, wanders away from his or her normal surroundings. During the fugue, the patient maintains good contact with his or her surroundings and rarely draws attention to himself or herself, but is amnesic regarding events that have occurred. In a typical case history, the patient takes a train or walks many miles and is discovered by some third party; often a complete failure of personal identity is noted. On other occasions a false identity may be given, which may be associated with a retrograde amnesia for the patient's whole life. After discovery, new learning is possible; patients rapidly find their way around their new surroundings.

There are several associations with fugues, and one of the strongest is recurrent depressive illness. There may be a tendency to compulsive lying, head injury with associated concussion at some earlier time, and a history of epilepsy.

Related conditions include epileptic automatisms, which are briefer and in which patients are unable to manipulate their environment successfully; the accompanying confusional state is usually obvious. Poiromania is a prolonged fugue state supposedly associated with nonconvulsive status epilepticus. In transient global amnesia, there is a sudden onset of global amnesia associated with clouding of consciousness, but personal identity is retained, significant persons are recognized, and motor skills are unimpaired. Patients continually seek reassurance about their environment, are perplexed, and are repetitive in their questions.

Transient global amnesia may last up to 24 hours; when memory returns, there is an amnesic gap for the period of the episode. There is usually an associated retrograde amnesia, which may extend several years previously but usually shrinks quickly after recovery. The cause of this condition is unclear, although epilepsy and cerebrovascular accidents have been implicated in a few cases, and the EEG is abnormal during the attack.

Patients with multiple personalities possess one or more altered personalities, with different sets of behaviors from the primary personality; each claims various degrees of amnesia for the other. Although associations with epilepsy have been claimed, many authors consider this condition to be a form of hysteria with dissociation. A related state is somnambulism, in which, shortly after falling asleep, the patient will get up and wander in a semipurposeful way; there is usually complete amnesia for the event. These patients commonly have a history of sleepwalking earlier in life, and the onset of somnambulism in adult life should raise a clinical suspicion of a significant stress and a diagnosis of a conversion disorder.

Investigation of these states mainly involves careful dissection of the patient's psychiatric history and, particularly for patients with fugue states, a search for some intolerable circumstance from which the patient is fleeing. An EEG should be taken when there is any suspicion of underlying epilepsy, although in many settings the EEG shows nonspecific abnormalities.

SEXUAL DISORDERS

Sexual disorders can be described in terms of altered drive, altered performance, or alteration of the object of sexual gratification (paraphilia). In neurological practice, diminished libido and failure of performance (impotence, premature ejaculation, or anorgasmy) are common complaints, although excessive libido and paraphilia are occasionally problematic.

Disorders of the peripheral nerves that affect the genital area may partially or totally impair the sexual response, and diabetes may present with impotence. Multiple sclerosis may be an unsuspected cause of performance failure, as can other diseases of the spinal cord.

CNS disorders, again primarily of the frontal or temporal lobes, commonly give rise to sexual symptoms. Depressive illness is the most common cause of loss of libido, and anxiety states often impair performance. Hypothalamic disorders, by alteration of the output of androgens, will impair arousal and performance in men, and posterior hypothalamic and mamillary body disease may give rise to precocious puberty. Hypersexuality in adults is reported with temporal and limbic disease, as part of the Klüver-Bucy syndrome, in frontal lobe disease, and with mania.

The relationship of epilepsy to sexual behavior has been well documented. Impotence is associated with temporal lobe epilepsy, although a peri-ictal hypersexuality, often related to postictal automatism, is well recorded. Interictal impotence is occasionally accompanied by a complete lack of libido and lifelong sexual disinterest. In male epileptic patients, free testosterone levels may be low, although they rarely fall outside the normal range, and the relationship of this factor to the behavior is unclear. It probably reflects chronic liver enzyme induction by anticonvulsant drugs.

Plasticity of sexual response, as part of the interictal syndrome of Geschwind, includes paraphilias and gender dysphorias (for example, transsexualism). Many transsexuals show EEG abnormalities.

Drugs are a common cause of impotence and delayed ejaculation; the clinician always should inquire whether the patient has taken antihypertensives, antidepressants, major tranquilizers, or excessive alcohol. Administration of L-dopa has been associated with increased libido and paraphilia, and trazodone may lead to priapism and to increased libido in women.

HYSTERIA (ICD 10—DISSOCIATIVE [CONVERSION] DISORDER; DSM-IV—CONVERSION DISORDER)

A chapter on behavior disturbances would not be complete without reference to hysteria. The interested reader is referred to other reviews (Trimble 1989). As a diagnosis, hysteria generally is considered a psychiatric problem, yet the historical and contemporary associations are largely neurological. Definitions tend to emphasize the patient's motivation in the development of symptoms, the hallmark being the presence of somatic symptoms in the absence of an associated neurological disease that could explain the symptoms in their entirety. The hysterical personality, as defined earlier, should be distinguished from hysteria in the sense of conversion or dissociative symptoms. The current DSM-IV classification of these disorders is given in Table 9.5. It is pragmatic to accept these symptoms as clinical realities and not attempt to discern psychodynamic principles for their presence. Although there is a relationship between the hysterical personality and conversion symptoms, it is not strong; patients of all personality predispositions may develop symptoms of hysteria.

An important consideration is the relationship of neurological disease to conversion phenomena, because several investigators have noted a high frequency of neurological disease associated with hysteria. Epilepsy is frequently noted, particularly in relationship to nonepileptic (pseudo)seizures, and other investigators have highlighted a relationship with multiple sclerosis. Since there is a high frequency of the later development of organic disease, "the diagnosis of hysteria may be a disguise for ignorance and a fertile source of clinical error."

There are many ways that a conversion disorder can present, from a monosymptomatic pseudoparalysis to a polysymptomatic Briquet's hysteria or syndrome (see section on Hysteria and Psychiatric Disorders). Sometimes the onset is with trauma, physical or psychological, and factors such as

Table 9.5: Classification of somatoform disorders (DSM-IV).

1. Somatization disorder (Briquet's syndrome): Many physical complaints, beginning before age 30, patients usually female.
2. Conversion disorder: One or more symptoms or deficits affecting motor or sensory function, not fully explained by a general or medical condition.
3. Hypochondriasis: Preoccupation and fears of having a serious disease in spite of appropriate medical evaluation and reassurance.
4. Body dysmorphic disorder: Preoccupation with an imagined defect in appearance.
5. Pain disorder: Pain is the predominant focus of the clinical presentation, and psychological factors are judged to have the important role of maintaining it.
6. Undifferentiated somatoform disorder: One or more physical complaints that are unexplained by a known medical condition, leading to considerable impairment in social functioning; or when related to a known medical condition, there is social impairment grossly in excess of what would be expected from the physical findings.
7. Somatoform disorder not otherwise specified: Those that do not fit the above. Includes fatigue, pseudocyesis.

bereavement always should be sought. Although any CNS symptom can be reported, motor loss of function and paresthesias or anaesthesias are the most frequent. In neurological practice, florid presentations are still seen; these presentations are reminiscent of the cases described by Charcot. Although motor disorders, such as the dystonias, are no longer ascribed to hysteria, presentation with abnormal movements is still common. Typical is the patient who, after a relatively trivial injury to an arm or leg, goes on to develop complete loss of function, sometimes with pain, but usually with an associated anesthesia. Over time the problem appears to get worse, not better, and there may be spread to another limb. Dystonia as a conversion disorder is still seen, often as a variant of spasmodic torticollis. This diagnosis should be included in the differential diagnosis of unusual gaits, atypical tics, and chaotic choreas.

Diagnosis is difficult and rests on the demonstration of positive neurological criteria, positive psychiatric criteria, and abnormal illness behavior. The former result from a discrepancy between the patient's symptoms and the signs on neurological examination. The presence of hemianesthesia, or of the anesthetic patches, not conforming to known patterns of sensory loss in neurological disease is important. The hemianesthesia is often well demarcated, on the body and face up to the midline. These sensory findings are overrepresented on the left side (for review, see Trimble 1989), may affect all modalities, and may be associated with diminished taste, smell, and hearing. The motor reflexes may be diminished on the side of the lesion. Other signs include normal tone and reflexes and the absence of wasting in paralyzed limbs, contraction of antagonist muscles following demonstration by special maneuvers that they are not paralyzed, and spiral or concentric patterns on visual field testing.

The psychiatric criteria depend on identifying present or past psychopathology, or both, including personality disorders and past episodes of conversion. The abnormal illness behavior is reflected both in a long history of complaints, investigations, and operations, and in current expressions of denial (sometimes a classic *belle indifférence*), anger, or dogmatic assertion of illness with adherence to the "sick role."

PSEUDOSEIZURES

In recent years the importance of pseudoseizures in neurological practice has been realized. Eight to 20% of patients attending an epilepsy clinic for intractable seizures have nonepileptic seizures. The term *pseudoseizures* is unsatisfactory, because the seizures are not "pseudo"; they are, if anything, pseudo-epileptic. Alternative names are psychogenic attacks, nonepileptic attack disorder, hysterical seizures, functional attacks, and (the least disturbing) nonepileptic seizures.

There are several underlying pathogeneses of these episodes, which in many patients are diagnosable only after a complete neurological and psychiatric clinical evaluation with full anamnesis. It is not acceptable to simply take the patient's description of attacks at face value; this can be misleading, as can eyewitness reports. Over time, with repeated telling, both tend to conform to that expected for a diagnosis of epilepsy. Videotelemetry is usually necessary to properly evaluate these seizures.

The most common underlying psychiatric conditions are anxiety (especially panic disorder and states of derealization or depersonalization), depression, and personality disorders. The histrionic and borderline types are overrepresented. Such underlying causes must be sought, as some are readily treatable, and they do not require anticonvulsant therapy.

Pseudo-pseudo seizures also are recognized, namely frontal seizures with rapid onset and seizure spread, short duration with a full return of consciousness immediately after the attack, with associated, often bizarre and extravagant movements that have been misdiagnosed as pseudoseizures. The ictal EEG may remain normal, and prolactin levels do not rise postictally.

PSYCHOGENIC AMNESIAS

Psychogenic amnesia is classified in DSM-IV as *dissociative amnesia*, under the dissociative disorders, separate from somatoform disorders. Psychogenic amnesia refers to an episode of "inability to recall important personal information, usually of a traumatic or stressful nature, that is too extensive to be explained by ordinary forgetfulness." The ability to comprehend environmental information and to perform complex learned skills is preserved. Dissociation and repression are commonly held underlying mechanisms.

Table 9.6: Varieties of psychogenic amnesias

Situational amnesia
Posttraumatic stress disorder[a]
Ganser syndrome[b]
Psychogenic fugue
Hysterical pseudodementia
Depressive dementia
Multiple personality disorder[b]
Histrionic personality disorder[a]

[a]Amnesia not invariably present.
[b]The nosological validity of these syndromes is least certain.
Source: Reprinted with permission from C Mace, MR Trimble. Psychogenic Amnesias. In T Yanagihara, RC Petersen (eds), Memory Disorders. New York: Decker, 1991;429–456.

Psychogenic amnesia often occurs in the setting of a neurological illness. A list of psychogenic amnesias, in approximate order of the length of the episode, is given in Table 9.6.

Situational amnesia may occur in isolation, associated with a psychologically significant or traumatic event, or as part of PTSD. Fugues are episodes of wandering, with amnesia. Patients remain in good contact with their surroundings, and when they emerge from the fugue they have an amnesic gap, loss of their identity, and sometimes amnesia for their whole life.

The Ganser syndrome is a complex of hallucinations, cognitive disorientation, conversion disorders, and the symptom of approximate answers (vorbeireden). It has been described in many settings and associated with head injury, depression, schizophrenia, epilepsy, chronic neurological disorders, and malingering. Vorbeireden is the inability to answer even simple questions correctly; even though the nature of the questions is known, approximate answers are given. The absurd nature of the latter is striking.

Pseudodementia includes such conditions as the cognitive and memory impairments of depression, the Ganser syndrome, and hysterical dementia. In the latter, a bizarre memory loss, associated with variable results on psychological testing, is seen, often associated with other conversion phenomena. It may be acute or chronic and may be precipitated by a head injury. Ganser syndromes may be brief, whereas hysterical dementia may be chronic and relapsing.

A marked cognitive impairment accompanies depressive illness, and patients' complaints of poor memory, impaired concentration, difficulty with planning and decision making, and poor abstracting abilities are common. The term pseudodementia has been used to specify this impairment, but it may be better referred to as a reversible dementia and categorized as subcortical (Trimble 1988). The presentation can so resemble dementia that many patients are misdiagnosed as having Alzheimer's disease and are left untreated. Of the causes of pseudodementia, that associated with depression is the most common, and some degree of cognitive impairment is found in most cases of affective disorder. Important clues that help distinguish pseudodementia from dementia include a history of affective disorder; a relatively acute onset, with little evidence of decline before the development of affective symptoms; the patient's distress and complaints about cognitive function (as opposed to the lack of insight often seen in dementia); the patient's responses to questions in the mental state examination (patients often use "don't know" as an answer, whereas in dementia the answers are more evasive, skirting the correct, but lost, answer); and performance on more structured psychological tests, which does not reveal the focal deficits of Alzheimer's disease but indicates patchy and inconsistent impairments.

No clear pattern of cognitive change emerges, but often the patient's subjective complaints are worse than the performance on objective tests. When patients with depressive illness are compared with controls on cognitive test batteries, they tend to show impairments of attention, a decrease in the speed of mental processing, poor attention to detail, difficulty in abstraction, and memory difficulties, especially on tasks that require effort, motivation, and active processing.

HYSTERIA AND PSYCHIATRIC DISORDERS

In clinical practice, patients with conversion symptoms fall into one of several categories. There are those with obvious psychiatric disorders—the main one being a major affective disorder with somatization—in whom there is little or no evidence of any underlying neurological illness, although neurological signs may be present. These signs may relate to the cognitive changes of pseudodementia or to the presence of anesthetic patches, often a total hemianesthesia, that are not in keeping with an underlying neurological lesion.

Anxiety states often present with neurological symptoms. Hyperventilation may provoke some somatic symptoms, and this mechanism may be involved in the provocation of both epileptic and nonepileptic seizures. In contrast to the persistent anxious preoccupation with illness referred to as hypochondriasis, patients with hysteria are less concerned with their apparent fate, although the classic *belle indifférence* is not always encountered. Psychotic conditions, particularly schizophrenia, rarely present to the neurologist with conversion phenomena. Of these associated psychopathological conditions, the most important to recognize is depressive illness. Not only is it a readily treatable condition, but also suicide is a potential outcome in these patients.

One form of psychopathological condition with which all neurologists should be acquainted is Briquet's syndrome, a form of stable hysteria also referred to as *somatization disorder*. This polysymptomatic disorder begins early in life and almost invariably affects females. It is characterized by recurrent multiple somatic complaints, often described dramatically, which are unexplained by known clinical disorders. The symptoms are legion, and patients repeatedly visit physicians and hospitals, use many medications, and have usually had several surgical procedures, particularly gynecological ones.

The importance of recognizing this condition is that it is an intractable disorder. Further invasive procedures should not be carried out, and patients should not be prescribed addictive medications. This diagnosis should be considered in difficult patients who present with problems such as seizures, faints, amnesia, reports of loss of consciousness, visual symptoms, weakness, headaches, chronic pain, anesthesias, and paralyses; a misdiagnosis of multiple sclerosis is common. Briquet's syndrome should be viewed as a severe form of personality disorder, and strict limits should be set for patients regarding what is and is not medically acceptable.

MUNCHAUSEN'S SYNDROME AND MALINGERING

Munchausen's syndrome is a pattern of behavior in which patients present to hospitals with various complaints that are manifestly factitious. On confrontation, or on being referred to a psychiatrist, they soon discharge themselves, only to reappear at another hospital at a later date with usually the same symptoms. Unlike patients with hysteria, the patients present themselves mostly through an emergency department, rather than being referred by another doctor. They are usually males who are seeking narcotic drugs.

A variant is *Munchausen's by proxy*. In this condition, one or both parents or guardians will keep presenting a child to physicians and report physical problems. Seizures are commonly used as the symptom, and the involved persons may administer substances such as insulin to the child to provoke signs and symptoms.

Malingering is a sociological comment on the behavior of some people who fabricate symptoms for an overt gain, usually financial. In neurological practice it is mostly seen in medicolegal practice and can be difficult to detect. The distinction between symptoms of hysteria and malingering has always caused argument, especially over the dubious suggestion that in hysteria symptoms are unconscious, whereas in malingering they are conscious. Over the course of time, patients' awareness of their symptoms vary, as do their motivations. Factitious disorder sits uncomfortably between the two, because it is a condition in which the symptoms and signs are clearly factitious, but the extrinsic incentives appear lacking, and the psychopathology is more obvious.

HYSTERIA AND NEUROLOGICAL DISORDERS

Patients with neurological illness who present with conversion symptoms are generally of three sorts. First, there are those whose "threshold for neuroticism" is decreased in a nonspecific way by cerebral lesions and who are thus more likely to present with a neurotic illness in the setting of stress. This important fact may reflect one reason for the high association of underlying neurological illness in patients with conversion phenomena, particularly illnesses that involve the CNS, such as multiple sclerosis, epilepsy, cerebrovascular accidents, and early dementia. Second, there are patients whose conversion symptoms replicate their existing neurological illness—for example, nonepileptic seizures in a patient with epilepsy or extreme motor weakness in a patient with mild multiple sclerosis, the onset of which may relate to an intercurrent life stress, an underlying affective disorder, or an alternative psychiatric problem.

Finally, there are patients with undiagnosed neurological disease for whom the diagnosis of hysteria is given. It is because of this group that the diagnosis of hysteria should be made only on positive grounds. Secondary gain alone is insufficient to make a diagnosis of hysteria; in many settings it is purely in the eye of the beholder. When there is no clear evidence of a psychopathological cause for the symptoms, it is better to wait awhile before committing the patient to a diagnosis of hysteria, which may have unfortunate consequences.

Management

Management of conversion disorders depends on the symptoms, the chronicity of the illness, and the presence of underlying diagnoses. Acute disorders often respond to anxiety management techniques, including behavior therapy, hypnosis, and in some settings abreaction with amylobarbital. Any underlying depression should be treated vigorously, as should agoraphobia and panic disorder.

The personality disorders and patients with more chronic presentations, especially those involved in compensation (litigation), can be difficult to manage. In fact, the prognosis for chronic somatoform disorders is not good, and for Briquet's syndrome it is bad. Confrontation and endless arguing over the cause of symptoms ("Are you saying it is all in my mind?") are rarely rewarding. Motor symptoms, with loss of function, often respond to vigorous physiotherapy from a sympathetic therapist. Pseudoseizures can be alleviated with behavior therapy if there is an obvious anxiety component. Psychotherapy can be rewarding, especially with pseudoseizures, although candidates should be chosen carefully and the therapist should be experienced in dealing with the traumas of earlier sexual or physical abuse.

REFERENCES

Baxter LR, Phelps ME, Mazziotta JC, Guze BH, Schwartz JM, Selin CE. Local cerebral glucose metabolic rates in obsessive-compulsive disorder. Arch Gen Psychiatry 1987;44:211–218.

Cummings J. Clinical Neuropsychiatry. Orlando, FL: Grune & Stratton, 1985.

Cummings J. Frontal-subcortical circuits and human behaviour. Arch Neurol 1993;50:873–880.

Denman A. The chronic fatigue syndrome: A return to common sense. Postgrad Med 1990;66:499–501.

Diagnostic and Statistical Manual of Mental Disorders (3rd ed, revised) (DSM-III-R). Washington, DC: American Psychiatric Association, 1980.

Diagnostic and Statistical Manual of Mental Disorders (DSM-IV draft criteria). Washington, DC: American Psychiatric Association, 1994.

Fenwick P. Aggression and Epilepsy. In MR Trimble, T Bolwig (eds), Aspects of Epilepsy and Psychiatry. Bristol, England: Wiley, 1986:31–60.

International Classification of Diseases 10 (ICD 10); Classification of Mental and Behavioural Disorders. Geneva: WHO, 1992.

Kloster R. Pseudo-Epileptic and Epileptic Seizures. In L Gram (ed), Pseudo-Epileptic Seizures. Petersfield, UK: Wrightson Biomedical Publishing Ltd., 1993;3–16.

L'hermitte F, Pillon B, Serdane M. Human autonomy and the frontal lobes. Ann Neurol 1986;19:326–334.

Mace C, Trimble MR. Psychogenic Amnesias. In T Yanagihara, RC Petersen (eds), Memory Disorders. New York: Decker, 1991;429–456.

Robertson MM, Gourdie A. Familial Tourette's syndrome in a large British pedigree. Br J Psychiatry 1990;156:515–521.

Stuss DT, Benson F. The frontal lobes. New York: Raven, 1986.

Trimble MR. Biological Psychiatry (2nd ed). Chichester, England: Wiley, 1996.

Trimble MR. Hysteria. In EH Reynolds, MR Trimble (eds), The Bridge Between Neurology and Psychiatry. Edinburgh: Churchill Livingstone, 1989:159–176.

Trimble MR, Robertson MM. The Psychopathology of Tics. In CD Marsden, S Fahn (eds), Movement Disorders. Vol. 2. London: Butterworth, 1987:406–437.

Trimble MR, Rogers DJ. The Neurology of Schizophrenia. In L Dilisi, F Henn (eds), Handbook of Schizophrenia. Vol. 2. Amsterdam: Elsevier, 1987:439–465.

Trimble MR, Thompson PJ. Neuropsychological Aspects of Epilepsy. In LGrant, KM Adams (eds), Neuropsychological Assessment of Neuropsychiatric Disorders. New York: Oxford University Press, 1986:321–346.

Wessely S. Chronic fatigue syndrome. J Neurol Neurosurg Psychiatry 1991;54:699–671.

Chapter 10
Depression and Psychosis in Neurological Practice

Michael R. Trimble

The personality disorders, neuroses, and related conditions that are of most importance to neurological practice are discussed in Chapter 9. Everyone has a personality style, which may or may not relate to the categories diagnosed in clinical practice; the latter tend to be the more exaggerated forms of stereotypes recognized by clinicians. Personality develops over years, maturing in early adulthood, and thereafter it tends to remain stable as an enduring set of characteristics by which we come to know a person.

Personality can be altered by neurological disease or injury. Neurological illness, however, also can give a personality an entirely new dimension—an added psychopathological illness—that in many settings resembles or closely resembles primary psychiatric illness. Many patients with more severe psychiatric illness thus will reveal brain pathology if it is looked for. The distinction between organic and nonorganic psychoses (or psychiatric illness), an artificial Cartesian dichotomy that has hindered logical thinking in these areas for generations, is outmoded by contemporary knowledge.

Although there are often some differences between the psychopathologies associated with gross structural disease and primary psychiatric illness, these differences have been overemphasized in theoretical discussion. Somehow it is thought that to make a distinction between "organic" and "functional" allows a greater understanding of the former, although at the expense of the latter. Furthermore, if a patient presents with a psychosis that is diagnosed as schizophrenia and it is later discovered that the patient has a condition such as epilepsy or Wilson's disease, the diagnosis is changed to the latter with an assumption that the former classification was incorrect and misguided. In fact, all that has happened is that an etiology for the psychosis has been found, and in reality the latter depends only on knowledge, the sophistication of the investigation techniques, and the examining physician. Such a step does not mean that the psychosis is any the less "psychiatric," or that the neurological lesion explains the development or the pathogenesis of the psychotic state.

The *Diagnostic and Statistical Manual of Mental Disorders* (4th edition) (DSM-IV) (1994) has been helpful in this regard. Instead of classifying the problems discussed here under "organic mental disorders" as was the case in DSM-III (1980), it does away with the term *organic* altogether. It has a category under "mood disorders" for "mood disorders attributable to a general medical condition" and a similar one for psychoses. In ICD 10, the category is "other mental disorders attributable to brain damage and dysfunction and to physical disease," which falls within the penumbra of "organic mental disorders."

In this chapter the affective disorders and the psychoses are described. The term *affective* generally refers to conditions in which an alteration of mood is the central feature. Psychosis is used as in ICD 10 (1992) to express a disorder with the presence of "hallucinations, delusions, or a limited number of severe abnormalities of behavior, such as gross excitement and overactivity, marked psychomotor retardation, and catatonic behavior."

AFFECTIVE DISORDERS

Disorders of affect, particularly depression, are frequently encountered in neurological practice. In psychiatric liaison practice, approximately 30% of referrals are for patients with depression, although an even higher percentage of neurological inpatients suffer from some kind of emotional disorder and most are discharged without psychiatric consultation.

This raises two important questions regarding the quality of the depressive symptoms reported by these patients and the relationship of any change of affect to underlying central nervous system (CNS) disease. Thus, in clinical practice, a common but important error is to confuse depression

Table 10.1: Criteria for a major depressive episode

I. Five (or more) of the following symptoms have been present during the same 2-week period and represent a change from previous functioning; at least one of the symptoms is either (A) depressed mood or (B) loss of interest or pleasure.
Note: Do not include symptoms that are clearly due to a general medical condition or mood-congruent delusions or hallucinations.
- A. Depressed mood most of the day, nearly every day, as indicated by either subjective report (e.g., feels sad or empty) or observation made by others (e.g., appears tearful). Note: In children and adolescents, the mood can be irritable.
- B. Markedly diminished interest or pleasure in all, or almost all, activities of the day, nearly every day (as indicated by either subjective account or observation made by others).
- C. Significant weight loss when not dieting or weight gain (e.g., a change of more than 5% of body weight in a month), or decrease or increase in appetite nearly every day. Note: In children, consider failure to make expected weight gains.
- D. Insomnia or hypersomnia nearly every day.
- E. Psychomotor agitation or retardation nearly every day (observable by others, not merely subjective feelings of restlessness or being slowed down).
- F. Fatigue or loss of energy nearly every day.
- G. Feelings of worthlessness or excessive or inappropriate guilt (which may be delusional) nearly every day (not merely self-reproach or guilt about being sick).
- H. Diminished ability to think or concentrate, or indecisiveness, nearly every day (either by subjective account or as observed by others).
- I. Recurrent thoughts of death (not just fear of dying), recurrent suicidal ideation without a specific plan, or a suicide attempt or a specific plan for committing suicide.

II. The symptoms do not meet criteria for a mixed episode.

III. The symptoms cause clinically significant distress or impairment in social, occupational, or other important areas of functioning.

IV. The symptoms are not due to the direct physiological effects of a substance (e.g., a drug of abuse, a medication) or a general medical condition (e.g., hypothyroidism).

V. The symptoms are not better accounted for by bereavement (i.e., after the loss of a loved one, the symptoms persist for longer than 2 months or are characterized by marked functional impairment, morbid preoccupation with worthlessness, suicidal ideation, psychotic symptoms, or psychomotor retardation).

Source: Reprinted with permission from the *Diagnostic and Statistical Manual of Mental Disorders, Fourth Edition.* Copyright 1994 American Psychiatric Association.

as an illness with depressive symptoms as a reaction or as an ordinary state of misery. The essential criterion of a depressive illness is disturbance of mood, which moreover must be prolonged and continuous. Episodes of a more transient mood change or chronic mild changes of mood are referred to as *dysthymic disorder*. The DSM-IV criteria for major depressive disorder and dysthymic disorder are shown in Tables 10.1 and 10.2.

In the assessment of depressive symptoms, personality factors, particularly premorbid neuroticism, are often insufficiently taken into account. Many patients suffering from dysphoric symptoms and complaining of depression in fact have long-standing personality disorders and tolerate life's stresses poorly. These patients are best not diagnosed as having depressive illness and are not helped much by the prescription of psychotropic medication.

The change of mood in depressive illness is associated with loss of vitality; the patient ceases to enjoy life and admits to a loss of emotional well-being. Concentration difficulties, with complaints of poor memory; increased apathy, with diminution of movements; and changes of appetite, food intake, and sleep patterns are found. Patients lose their appetite, complain that food is tasteless, and often lose weight. Their sleep may be disturbed in a variety of ways, the most common being nocturnal restlessness with periodic waking or the more typical early morning waking with morbid ruminations and inability to get to sleep again.

Feelings of anxiety and tension are invariably present, and sometimes, in contrast to psychomotor retardation, agitation with indecision and excessive motor activity occurs. In the extreme form of depression, intense, aimless pacing is noted. Loss of energy, fatigability, and tiredness are reported, and diurnal variation is common, with symptoms improving as the day passes.

Some patients do not report, or underreport, mood changes and present with somatic symptoms. These symptoms, referable to any system in the body, easily become the focus of attention for both the patient and the physician and may lead them to a multitude of investigations, which usually have negative results.

Suicidal thoughts and preoccupations are frequent, and the physician should inquire about them. Thoughts of worthlessness, guilt, and letting people down are typical; crying is often not reported but always should be asked about, especially in men. Increased irritability, hostility, and aggressive episodes, especially within the family setting, are troublesome, and libido is diminished.

These mental states should be distinguished from lability of mood, with rapid oscillations between one mood state and another, and the excessive laughing and crying of a pseudobulbar palsy, which occur without the equivalent underlying mood changes.

Mania is another mood disorder often associated with depression in a bipolar affective (DSM-IV bipolar disorder,

Table 10.2: Diagnostic criteria for a dysthymic disorder

I. Depressed mood for most of the day, for more days than not, as indicated by either subjective account or observation by others, for at least 2 years. Note: In children and adolescents, the mood can be irritable and the duration must be at least 1 year.
II. Presence, while depressed, of two (or more) of the following:
  A. Poor appetite or overeating
  B. Insomnia or hypersomnia
  C. Low energy or fatigue
  D. Low self-esteem
  E. Poor concentration or difficulty making decisions
III. During the 2-year period (1 year for children or adolescents) of the disturbance, the person has never been without the symptoms in criteria I and II for more than 2 months at a time.
IV. No major depressive episode (see Table 10.1) has been present during the first 2 years of the disturbance (1 year for children and adolescents); i.e., the disturbance is not better accounted for by chronic major depressive disorder or major depressive disorder in partial remission.
Note: There may have been a previous major depressive episode provided there was a full remission (no significant signs or symptoms for 2 months) before development of the dysthymic disorder. In addition, after the initial 2 years (1 year in children or adolescents) of dysthymic disorder, there may be superimposed episodes of major depressive disorder, in which case both diagnoses may be given when the criteria are met for a major depressive episode.
V. There has never been a manic episode (see Table 10.3), a mixed episode, or a hypomanic episode, and criteria have never been met for a cyclothymic disorder.
VI. The disturbance does not occur extensively during the course of a chronic psychotic disorder, such as schizophrenia or a delusional disorder.
VII. The symptoms are not due to the direct physiological effects of a substance (e.g., a drug of abuse, a medication) or a general medical condition (e.g., hypothyroidism).
VIII. The symptoms cause clinically significant distress or impairment in social, occupational, or other important areas of functioning.
Specify:
  Early onset: if onset is before age 21 years
  Late onset: if onset is age 21 years or older
Specify (for most recent 2 years of dysthymic disorder):
  With **atypical features.**

Source: Reprinted with permission from the *Diagnostic and Statistical Manual of Mental Disorders, Fourth Edition.* Copyright 1994 American Psychiatric Association.

often referred to as manic depressive) illness. The DSM-IV criteria are given in Table 10.3. Here the mood is associated with an increased sense of well-being and euphoria. Again, the process is pervasive and affects the patient's thoughts, with pressure of speech, flight of ideas, and motor activity with excessive pace. Concentration is poor, patients are distractible and irritable, sleep is often brief, and appetite is usually increased. In extreme forms of mania, patients are restless and show disordered speech, with rhyming, punning, and word play; their mood is no longer euphoric but is clearly dysphoric.

When strictly applied, the diagnosis of major depressive disorder occurs in a relatively small percentage of patients, and the diagnosis of mania is rarer. Usually, depression is diagnosed in patients who are actually suffering from more long-standing personality disturbances or understandable dysphoric reactions to neurological disability.

Depressive Illness and Neurological Disorders

There are patients in whom depression is more than just an accompaniment of chronic illness; it is related directly to underlying neuropsychiatric disorders, touching on the biochemical and neurological underpinnings of affective expression. The approximate frequency of reporting of depressive illness in several important neurological illnesses is given in Table 10.4.

In head injury, some patients develop a posttraumatic depression that may be associated with a posttraumatic stress disorder (PTSD). It often does not arise immediately but comes on several months after injury, often in the course of recovery of neurological disability. An association between left anterior lesions and subsequent depression has been suggested (Fedoroff et al. 1992).

The occurrence of depression in dementia is perhaps less frequent than is generally supposed, because it is more common in early disease before the inevitable loss of insight occurs. In some patients, the dementia is heralded by the onset of a depressive illness.

With regard to tumors, meningiomas, especially frontal lobe meningiomas, are notoriously liable to induce a picture typical of a major depressive disorder, and diencephalic tumors have lead to an affective disorder with hypomanic swings.

The association between basal ganglia disorders and depression is of particular interest. Approximately 30–60% of patients with Parkinson's disease have a depressive illness that is not entirely explained by the limitations of the chronic disability. In some patients there is a clear history of a mood disorder before the onset of any motor symptoms.

Table 10.3: Criteria for a manic episode

I. A distinct period of abnormally and persistently elevated, expansive, or irritable mood, lasting at least 1 week (or any duration if hospitalization is necessary).
II. During the period of mood disturbance, three or more of the following symptoms have persisted (four if the mood is only irritable) and have been present to a significant degree.
  A. Inflated self-esteem or grandiosity.
  B. Decreased need for sleep (e.g., feels rested after only 3 hours of sleep).
  C. More talkative than usual or feels pressure to keep talking.
  D. Flight of ideas or subjective experience that thoughts are racing.
  E. Distractibility (i.e., attention too easily drawn to unimportant or irrelevant external stimuli).
  F. Increase in goal-directed activity (either socially, at work or school, or sexually) or psychomotor agitation.
  G. Excessive involvement in pleasurable activities that have a high potential for painful consequences (e.g., engaging in unrestrained buying sprees, sexual indiscretions, or foolish business investments).
III. The symptoms do not meet criteria for a mixed episode.
IV. The mood disturbance is sufficiently severe to cause marked impairment in occupational functioning or in usual social activities or relationships with others, or to necessitate hospitalization to prevent harm to self or others, or there are psychotic features.
V. The symptoms are not due to the direct physiological effects of a substance (e.g., a drug of abuse, a medication, or other treatment) or a general medical condition (e.g., hyperthyroidism).
  Note: Manic-like episodes that are clearly caused by somatic antidepressant treatment (e.g., medication, electroconvulsive therapy, light therapy) should not count toward a diagnosis of bipolar I disorder.

Source: Reprinted with permission from the *Diagnostic and Statistical Manual of Mental Disorders, Fourth Edition*. Copyright 1994 American Psychiatric Association.

The clinical presentation is often atypical, with a high frequency of anxiety symptoms (Schiffer et al. 1988), and is most common in patients with a younger age of onset (Starkstein et al. 1989).

There are several interesting associations between depression and biological findings, including a link to initial right-sided motor impairment (Starkstein et al. 1989), to low levels of serotonin metabolites in the cerebrospinal fluid (CSF) (Mayeux et al. 1986), and to decreased cerebral blood flow in specific regions of the frontal cortex (Ring et al. 1994).

Patients with chronic (Huntington's) chorea also present with disorders of affect, including psychotic depressive and hypomanic disorders. Again, the affective disorders can be dissociated from the motor disability and may be seen before the onset or diagnosis of the chorea. Furthermore, a high incidence of suicide is reported in these patients, even in those with no knowledge of their diagnosis. The Huntington's disease patients showed twice the incidence and frequency of major affective disorders as those with Alzheimer's disease. Other basal ganglia disorders that have been associated with affective changes, either depressive or euphoric, include progressive lenticular degeneration (Wilson's disease), chorea minor (Sydenham's chorea), and the blepharospasm-oromandibular dystonia syndrome (Meige's disease).

Cerebrovascular accidents regularly leave neuropsychiatric sequelae, and depression is common. In a series of studies, Robinson and colleagues examined post-stroke depression (Starkstein and Robinson 1993). They found that the phenomenology of the depression is similar to that of depression in the absence of stroke, although slowness and psychomotor retardation are more common in the former and concentration problems worse in the latter. The depression can last at least 1 year, although it tends to be shorter in those patients with cerebellar or brain stem lesions. Lesions in the anterior left hemisphere appear important; this controversial finding has had some replication (Eastwood et al. 1989).

Subcortical lesions provide similar findings—namely, left anterior, mainly basal ganglia lesions, being most strongly correlated with post-stroke depression.

Starkstein and Robinson (1989) emphasized the importance of recognizing the accompanying depression in a patient with a stroke, because it delays recovery.

In these studies, no association with aphasia was found. However, others have reported that depression is more frequent with Broca's aphasia, and the affective expression of patients with a Wernicke's aphasia is often inappropriate, with a hint of expansiveness and jocularity that lacks the conviction of hypomania.

In epilepsy, although no clear associations to the site or side of the focus have been found, left-sided lesions may be overrepresented (Robertson et al. 1987). Other associations are with polytherapy, especially with barbiturate anticonvulsants, and low folate levels in the serum or red blood cells.

Table 10.4: Frequency of depression in various neurological diseases reported in the literature

Disease	*(%)*
Alzheimer's disease	10–20
Cerebrovascular disease	30–50
Epilepsy	22
Head trauma	25–50
Huntington's chorea	38
Multi-infarct dementia	25
Multiple sclerosis	27–54
Parkinson's disease	41

Table 10.5: Neurological causes of secondary mania

Cerebrovascular accidents
Epilepsy
Parkinson's disease with dopamine agonist therapy
Idiopathic basal ganglia calcification (Fahr's disease)
Huntington's disease
Traumatic brain injury
Multiple sclerosis
Frontal lobe degenerations
Cerebral syphilis

Source: Reprinted with permission from J Cummings, MR Trimble. A Concise Guide to Behavioral Neurology and Neuropsychiatry. Washington, DC: American Psychiatric Association Press, 1995.

Secondary Mania

Several conditions have been associated with mania and hypomania (Table 10.5). The most common associations are with lesions of the right hemisphere and involve the orbitofrontal cortex, caudate nuclei, thalamus or perithalamic regions, and the basotemporal area.

In one study of a small group of patients with bipolar disorder after stroke, in all with subcortical right-sided lesions, there was an increased association with both a family history of affective disorder and subcortical atrophy with enlarged ventricular-to-brain ratios. In epilepsy, hypomania is seen most often periictally, secondarily to clusters of right-sided temporal lobe seizures.

Investigations

Results of psychometric testing can be abnormal in patients with affective disorders, and neuropsychological testing in cases of suspected pseudodementia (see Chapter 9) is important. Specific intellectual functions such as reading, repetition, naming, mathematical skills, and motor praxis tend to be spared; the tasks that are impaired are those that relate to attention, speed of mental processing, spontaneous problem solving, and analysis of detail. Proverb interpretation may be concrete, and performance on memory tasks is patchy; this reflects ineffective initial acquisition of information and poor retrieval.

A low-dose (1 mg) dexamethasone suppression test may be of value (Table 10.6); failure of suppression is related to a psychopathological condition (in the absence of other causes; see Trimble 1996), especially depression.

The EEG can be deceptive in affective disorders, because two waveforms have been associated with affective symptoms that are occasionally misinterpreted as being related to epilepsy. Six-per-second rhythmic waves, also referred to as rhythmic midtemporal discharges, are associated with a generalized increased risk for a psychopathological condition, including hypochondriasis and depression. Small sharp waves—brief-duration, small-amplitude waves that are sometimes exclusively temporal in location and occur in drowsy states or light sleep—have been associated with neurovegetative symptoms, affective disorders, and a tendency to suicide. Furthermore, 43% of patients with bipolar affective disorder have been reported as showing small sharp waves, which may be significantly related to a family

Table 10.6: Schedule for the low-dose dexamethasone (DEX) test

Schedule:			
Day 1		*Day 2*	
2300 hours	*0800 hours*	*1600 hours*	*2300 hours*
DEX 1 mg oral		Cortisol determinations	
		Nonsuppression >5 μg/dl (138 n/mol/liter)	
False-positives seen with			
Medications		Benzodiazepines	
		Barbiturates	
		Hepatic enzyme–inducing anticonvulsants	
		Methadone; morphine	
		Indomethacin	
Recreational drugs		Alcohol; excess caffeine	
Disease		Diabetes mellitus	
		Dementia	
		Cerebral tumor	
		Cardiac failure	
		Cushing's disease	
Metabolic conditions		Dehydration	
Other		Pregnancy	
		Acute trauma	

history of affective disorder. Patients with affective disorders, presenting with paroxysmal episodes of poor concentration and coordination—sometimes, if prolonged, extending to a fugue state—may be thought to be suffering from symptoms of complex partial seizures, and their EEGs may be abnormal. However, close attention to the rest of the clinical picture and to the family history and patient's history will reveal the appropriate diagnosis.

The CT scan may be of value in detecting unsuspected tumors, particularly meningiomas, and there is a subgroup of patients with affective disorders who show atrophy on CT scan. This atrophy is mainly ventricular dilation, and elderly patients presenting with depressive illness and enlarged ventricles have a greater than expected mortality.

If available, MRI is the imaging technique of choice. Studies confirm the high frequency of ventricular dilation and cortical atrophy in elderly patients with affective disorder and also reveal an association with subcortical hyperintensities, especially in the deep white matter and the periventricular regions. The latter appear to be associated with risk factors for vascular disease, although the relevance of these findings for the pathogenesis of the affective disorder is still unclear (Coffey et al. 1990).

Treatment of Affective Disorder in Neurological Patients

Generally, the treatment of depression in these settings is the same as depression in the absence of associated neurological illness. Not all patients need antidepressants, and for many, explanation of their problems, dealing with their worries, doubts, and fantasies about their illness, and psychosocial rehabilitation are all that is required. Sometimes, more formal psychotherapy is indicated.

If antidepressants are used, they should be given in realistic dosages. Often patients are given small dosages and remain on such amounts, even though they do not respond for a long time. The dosage should be low to start with, and then should be increased gradually until side effects intervene or a clinical response is obtained. One drug at the right dose is preferable to two at the wrong dose. Patients with neurological disease tend to have a lowered seizure threshold, and most antidepressants are proconvulsant. It appears likely that the newer, selective 5-HT uptake inhibitors (SSRIs) are less likely to have this problem, are less sedative, and have no anticholinergic side effects. Anticholinergic side effects are problematic for the elderly and those with autonomic instability. The most proconvulsant antidepressants are maprotiline, mianserin, bupropion (in higher dosages), and clomipramine.

The value of some anticonvulsants for the treatment of affective disorder is recognized in psychiatric practice, especially carbamazepine and valproic acid. Although mainly used in bipolar affective disorders, they sometimes are used in cyclical depression and can be of good value in patients with depression with neurological illness. Sometimes they are combined with lithium.

Electroconvulsive therapy (ECT) is an effective treatment for a severe depressive illness and is often necessary for disturbed patients with suicidal ideas. It is not contraindicated in neurological disease, with the exception of patients with suspected raised intracranial pressure.

HALLUCINATIONS, DELUSIONS, AND SCHIZOPHRENIA-LIKE PSYCHOSES

In contrast to neurotic conditions and major affective disorders, psychotic conditions are not seen often in neurological practice; when they are present, they usually reflect an underlying neurological disturbance. In other words, the CNS, ontogenically, must allow the individual to interpret the world in a logical way, which is sufficient for the individual to adapt to environmental circumstances. Hallucinations and delusions, the hallmark of psychosis, suggest some deviant neurological processing, underlying which are usually structural but sometimes solely functional alterations of activity. Although hallucinations and delusions may be experienced in certain settings for which patients have clear insight, in most cases insight is lacking and the condition is truly psychotic.

A hallucination is a perception in the absence of an adequate peripheral stimulus; it must be distinguished from an illusion, which is a misinterpretation of a perception. Illusions occur in normal people, especially when they are tired, inattentive, or in states of high expectation. In clinical practice, they occur in patients with delirium but are also reported in patients with severe affective disorder and schizophrenia. Pseudohallucinations are hallucinatory experiences that occur in subjective space, are less clearly delineated, and lack objectivity when compared to true hallucinations. They thus depend on the person creating them, and the images readily dissipate and have to be recreated. In true hallucinations, the experiences are constant, occur in objective space, have concrete reality, and are substantial. They usually are retained unaltered, and there is usually absence of insight.

Delusions are unshakable convictions that are manifestly incorrect. They should be interpreted within the patient's cultural setting, but it is the tenacity with which the patient will sustain his or her belief against all logic that is crucial to the diagnosis. Delusions should be distinguished from overvalued ideas, which, while being strongly held, are not incorrigible. Delusions are the hallmarks of a paranoid illness but occur in a spectrum of psychiatric disorders from paranoia to schizophrenia. In the latter condition they are associated with certain characteristic symptoms, such as specific types of auditory hallucinations. These are referred to as Schneiderian first-rank symptoms (Table 10.7). Although still somewhat controversial, these symptoms do have clinical value. In the setting of clear consciousness they usually signify schizophrenia. They are, however, sometimes seen in mania and delirium, and a diagnosis of schizophre-

Table 10.7: The first-rank symptoms of Schneider

The hearing of one's thoughts being spoken aloud in one's head
The hearing of voices commenting on what one is doing at the time
Voices arguing in the third person
Experiences of bodily influence
Thought withdrawal and other forms of thought interference
Thought diffusion
Delusional perception*
Everything in the spheres of feeling, drive, and volition that the patient experiences as being imposed on him or her or influenced by others

*An abnormal significance attached to a real perception without any cause that is understandable in rational or emotional terms.

nia can be made in their absence. They have similar significance for the psychiatrist that a Babinski sign has for a neurologist. They have good objective reliability and probably signify disruption of temporal lobe–limbic mechanisms (Trimble 1990).

Delusions are either mood congruent, as in a morbid depressive delusion, or mood incongruent. The latter delusions are simply not understandable and seem bizarre. Such delusions are typical for schizophrenia.

The content of delusions varies considerably. Typical are persecutory, jealous, erotomaniac, somatic, and grandiose delusions. In the Capgras syndrome, a significant person in a patient's life is replaced by a supposed identical double, and in the Fregoli syndrome, a supposed persecutor can change his or her appearance and appear as other people. Another variant of such misidentification syndromes is reduplicative paramnesia, with misidentification of places. There is some evidence that these syndromes are associated with right hemisphere dysfunction (Collins et al. 1990).

Table 10.8: Differential diagnosis of visual hallucinations

1. Ocular
   - Macular degeneration
   - Cataracts
   - Enucleation
2. Sensory deprivation
3. Optic nerve and tract; midbrain; geniocularcalcarine radiation
   - Multiple sclerosis
   - Ischemia
   - Compression
   - Stroke
   - Tumors
4. Occipital or temporal cortex
   - Stroke
   - Tumors
   - Seizures
5. Other
   - Migraine
   - Narcolepsy
   - Alzheimer's disease
   - Diffuse Lewy body disease
   - Parkinson's disease with dopaminergic treatment
   - Drug intoxication or withdrawal
   - Metabolic encephalopathies (delirium)
   - Schizophrenia
   - Depression or mania (mood congruent)

Source: Reprinted with permission from J Cummings, MR Trimble. A Concise Guide to Behavioral Neurology and Neuropsychiatry. Washington, DC: American Psychiatric Association Press, 1995.

Nature and Causes of Hallucinations and Delusions

Hallucinations may occur in association with strong affective disturbances such as depression, in which case they take on a morbid tone. The patient may say that his or her body odor is offensive and that he or she can smell the body rotting away. In organic brain syndromes, both acute and chronic, hallucinations may be florid and frightening; complete scenes may be reported of animals, gremlins, or human persecutors, coming in multitudes to take revenge on the suffering patient. Hypnogogic and hypnopompic hallucinations occur as patients are falling asleep and waking, respectively; they occur in normal people, but they are also a cardinal feature of Gélineau's syndrome of narcolepsy. These hallucinations may be auditory, visual, or tactile, and they can be frightening.

Hallucinations that occur with clear consciousness for which there is no insight and that are mood-incongruent are highly suggestive of schizophrenia. In this condition, the hallucinations are usually auditory, although patients may experience them in more than one sensory modality. The voices reported are of family, friends, God, or persecutors, and the main feature is that people argue or talk about the patient in the third person. This is one of the so-called first-rank symptoms of Schneider. This, and other hallucinations, such as when a patient hears his or her own thoughts spoken aloud or hears a commentary on his or her actions, which is often critical, are characteristic of schizophrenia.

Visual hallucinations are less frequent in schizophrenia than auditory ones, but when they are present, they often occur in association with other hallucinations. Visual hallucinations of small animals are noted in delirium, especially delirium tremens, and formication, the sensation that animals are crawling under the skin or over the body, has been associated with cocaine psychosis. A differential diagnosis of visual hallucinations is given in Table 10.8. Essentially, visual hallucinations caused by neurological disease can be attributable to lesions anywhere in the visual system from the retinal to the occipital lobe, and they sometimes reflect sensory deprivation.

Olfactory hallucinations are often reported in schizophrenia but are usually noted in complex partial seizures of the uncinate variety. In schizophrenia, these hallucinations are bizarre and prolonged, whereas in uncinate seizures they are typically brief, extremely unpleasant, and hard to characterize. Furthermore, they are consistent in their appearance—the same smell appearing over and over again—whereas in schizophrenia the smells tend to differ with time.

Somatic hallucinations, which may be misinterpreted as sensory neurological symptoms, occur in schizophrenia. Often the patient interprets them as being brought about by some external agency (so-called passivity experiences), which obviously leads one immediately to the diagnosis of a psychosis. In cenesthesic hallucinations, the body or part of the body may feel distorted or changed, often in quite fantastic ways. These hallucinations occur in many psychotic states but also occur in migraine and following cerebrovascular accidents. Several body image disturbances may be grouped under this category, including reduplicative phenomena involving limbs or parts of limbs and macro- and microsomatognosia, all of which may be associated with a variety of cerebral pathological conditions.

Hallucinations are common in epilepsy that arises from the temporal lobes. As with the olfactory hallucinations, the stereotypical repetition of the hallucinations, their paroxysmal nature, and their florid descriptions are important in the diagnosis; schizophrenic hallucinations are rarely short-lived, whereas drug-induced hallucinations, which may have a similar quality, will be associated with drug ingestion and are not likely to be so overtly paroxysmal. In some patients, however—particularly those with complex partial seizure status—hallucinations, often associated with paranoid delusions, may continue for a considerable time. In these patients, careful testing will reveal subtle changes of cognitive function and will identify the underlying confusional state.

Some patients with epilepsy that arises from the temporal lobes develop an interictal psychosis, which in many cases resembles schizophrenia. These patients usually have a seizure disorder that began in mid-childhood, around puberty, and the disorder has been poorly controlled by a variety of antiseizure medications. They continue to have complex partial seizures, which occasionally or often secondarily generalize, and their psychosis may begin with discrete bouts of a periictal disorder, which gradually becomes more and more persistent. Alternatively, the psychosis may emerge gradually, often in the setting of decreased seizure frequency, first presenting to the clinician several years after the onset of seizures.

An alternative expression of psychosis may be a paranoid state, with vigilance, overt hostility, suspiciousness, and oversensitivity to the environment. Delusions of persecution may be present, and there is often coexistence of marked affective symptoms, with suicidal thoughts and occasionally actions. In one variety of ictally related psychosis, the patient, usually after a bout of generalized seizures followed by a lucid interval of 24–48 hours, presents with an intense disturbance of affect with paranoia or elation and dysphoria, sometimes with religious delusions and illusions or hallucinations of a religious content. Mild clouding of consciousness may be seen, and the state may last for several days, if not weeks, occasionally slowly resolving into a chronic psychotic state.

The onset of a delusional illness, with schizophrenic-type features and bizarre hallucinations within a short period of time after the onset of seizures, should raise the possibility of progressive underlying disease such as a neurostorage disorder. The differential diagnosis of delusions is given in Table 10.9.

The acute presentation of a psychosis following the sudden cessation of seizures, either spontaneously or with administration of anticonvulsant drugs, raises the possibility of forced normalization, a state of affairs more commonly encountered in clinical practice than recorded in the literature. The EEG will be less abnormal or show no spike and wave discharges during the time of the behavior problems, and will revert to its previous abnormal state with resolution of the psychosis.

Patients with schizophrenia often are referred to a neurological clinic when they have had a seizure or some form of paroxysmal behavior disorder that has led to the question of an underlying diagnosis of epilepsy. The DSM-IV criteria for the diagnosis of schizophrenia are shown in Table 10.10 and for delusional disorder in Table 10.11. Generally, patients with established schizophrenia rarely go on to develop epilepsy, although isolated seizures are reported. These seizures may occur spontaneously, particularly in patients with catatonia, but are more likely to be precipitated by administration of epileptogenic neuroleptic drugs. Paroxysmal behavior disorders, with or without associated release of aggression, have been recorded often as part of the clinical picture of schizophrenia and should not be confused with epileptic phenomena.

A characteristic feature of schizophrenia is disturbance of language. This disturbance may vary from subtle flattening of expression and concrete thinking, to the florid schizophasia. In the latter, neologisms (paraphasias), loose connections between thoughts, tangential thinking, and intrusive delusional content can lead to an unintelligible word

Table 10.9: Differential diagnosis of delusions

Schizophrenia
Delirium
Epilepsy (especially temporal lobe)
Alzheimer's disease
Frontal-temporal degenerations (e.g., Pick's disease)
Diffuse Lewy body disease
Huntington's chorea
Parkinson's disease with dopamine agonists
Idiopathic basal ganglia calcification (Fahr's disease)
Posttraumatic encephalopathy
Viral encephalitis
Creutzfeldt-Jakob disease
Cerebrovascular accident and vascular dementia
Metachromatic leukodystrophy
Adrenoleukodystrophy
Cerebral (especially temporal) tumors
Vitamin B_{12} deficiency
GM_2 gangliosidosis
Neuronal ceroid lipofuscinosis
Mitochondrial encephalopathy

Source: Reprinted with permission from J Cummings, MR Trimble. A Concise Guide to Behavioral Neurology and Neuropsychiatry. Washington, DC: American Psychiatric Association Press, 1995.

Table 10.10: DSM-IV criteria for schizophrenia

I. Characteristic symptoms: At least two of the following, each present for a significant portion of time during a 1-month period (or less if successfully treated):
   A. Delusions
   B. Hallucinations
   C. Disorganized speech (e.g., frequent derailment or incoherence)
   D. Grossly disorganized or catatonic behavior
   E. Negative symptoms (i.e., affective flattening, alogia, or avolition)
   Note: Only one category I symptom is required if delusions are bizarre or hallucinations consist of a voice keeping up a running commentary on a person's behavior or thoughts, or two or more voices conversing with each other.

II. Social/occupational dysfunction: For a significant portion of the time since the onset of the disturbance, one or more major areas of functioning such as work, interpersonal relations, or self-care is markedly below the level achieved prior to the onset (or when the onset is in childhood or adolescence, failure to achieve expected level of interpersonal, academic, or occupational achievement).

III. Duration: Continuous signs of the disturbance persist for at least 6 months. This 6-month period must include at least 1 month of symptoms that meet criterion I (i.e., active phase symptoms) and may include periods of prodromal or residual symptoms. During these prodromal or residual periods, the signs of the disturbance may be manifested by only negative symptoms or two or more symptoms listed in criterion I present in an attenuated form (e.g., odd beliefs, unusual perceptual experiences).

IV. Schizoaffective and mood disorder exclusion: Schizoaffective disorder and mood disorder with psychotic features have been ruled out because either (1) no major depressive or manic episodes have occurred concurrently with the active phase symptoms or (2) if mood episodes have occurred during active phase symptoms, their total duration has been brief relative to the duration of the active and residual periods.

V. Substance/general medical condition exclusion: The disturbance is not due to the direct effects of a substance (e.g., drugs of abuse, medication) or a general medical condition.

Source: Reprinted with permission from the *Diagnostic and Statistical Manual of Mental Disorders, Fourth Edition.* Copyright 1994 American Psychiatric Association.

Table 10.11: DSM-IV criteria for delusional disorder

I. Nonbizarre delusions (i.e., involving situations that occur in real life, such as being followed, poisoned, infected, loved at a distance, having a disease, or being deceived by one's spouse or lover) of at least 1 month's duration.

II. Has never met criterion I for schizophrenia (i.e., none of the following for more than a few hours: hallucinations, disorganized speech, grossly disorganized or catatonic behavior); or negative symptoms (i.e., affective flattening, alogia, or avolition). Note: Tactile or olfactory hallucinations are not excluded if related to the delusional theme.

III. Apart from the impact of the delusion(s) or its ramifications, functioning is not markedly impaired or behavior is not obviously odd or bizarre.

IV. If mood episodes have occurred concurrently with delusions, their total duration has been brief relative to the duration of the delusional periods.

V. Not due to the direct effects of a substance (e.g., drugs of abuse, medication) or a general medical condition.

Source: Reprinted with permission from the *Diagnostic and Statistical Manual of Mental Disorders, Fourth Edition.* Copyright 1994 American Psychiatric Association.

salad that resembles Wernicke's aphasia. In the absence of a history, careful neurological testing and an EEG usually will resolve the diagnosis.

The most comprehensive survey of the relationship of psychotic disorders, particularly schizophrenia-like psychosis, to neurological conditions was that of Davison and Bagley in 1969. They reported a higher than expected incidence of epilepsy, Huntington's chorea, narcolepsy, cerebrovascular disease, cerebral gliomas, and pituitary adenomas in patients with schizophrenia-like psychosis. A lower than expected incidence has been found in patients with Parkinson's disease, although psychoses are frequently seen with Lewy body dementia.

Schizophrenia-like and paranoid conditions have been described in patients with Huntington's chorea. These conditions often emerge before the onset of a movement disorder. Other basal ganglia conditions that have been associated with a schizophreniform psychosis include Wilson's disease, Sydenham's chorea, and idiopathic calcification of the basal ganglia.

More transitory psychotic phenomena may emerge at any stage in a dementia, especially multi-infarct dementia, and schizophrenia-like states have been reported occasionally in some white matter disorders such as multiple sclerosis, adrenoleukodystrophy, and more commonly in metachromatic leukodystrophy. Isolated hallucinoses, with or without a paranoid flavor, are seen in a variety of conditions, including middle and inner ear disease, Parkinson's disease, and chronic alcoholism.

Tumors that are most likely to lead to a psychosis are those located in the temporal lobes and diencephalon (for review, see Trimble 1996). Following head injury, the most severe psychopathological conditions, particularly psychoses, are more likely to occur with left-sided injuries affecting the temporal lobes.

Table 10.12: Differential diagnosis of catatonia

Psychiatric disorders
Depression
Mania
Schizophrenia
Neurological disorders
Cerebrovascular disease (basilar artery thrombosis; bilateral anterior cingulate infarcts; thalamic infarction; bilateral temporal lobe hemorrhage)
Tumors (especially third ventricle and periventricular, and corpus callosum)
Head trauma
Encephalitis (herpes and subacute sclerosing panencephalomyelitis)
Cerebral syphilis
Basal ganglia disease (Parkinson's disease, globus pallidus lesions)
Epilepsy
Systemic disease
Hyperthyroidism
Addison's disease
Cushing's disease
Uremia
Diabetic ketoacidosis
Hypercalcemia
Hepatic encephalopathy
Systemic lupus erythematosus
Neuroleptic malignant syndrome
Drug-induced states (phencyclidine, amphetamine, sedative, hypnotic withdrawal)

In most patients in whom a neurological condition is associated with the onset of psychosis, the psychosis occurs several years after the onset of the CNS disorder. Premorbid schizoid personality and a family history of schizophrenia are not usually found in these patients, which suggests that the neurological disorder itself directly provokes the psychotic state.

Catatonia

The catatonia syndrome is characterized by mutism, psychosis, and bizarre motor activity that ranges from outbursts of agitated excitement to stupor. Sustained postures and waxy flexibility are often present. Associated features are negativism, echolalia and echopraxia, stereotypies, mannerisms, and automatic obedience. The differential diagnosis is given in Table 10.12. The paroxysms of excitement with sudden onset can be mistaken for some kind of epilepsy-related behavior, but the most common cause is an affective disorder. Intravenous barbiturates or benzodiazepines can help to temporarily melt the catatonic stupor and reveal an underlying psychiatric illness. ECT remains a treatment of choice.

Lethal catatonia is a rare disorder of psychosis, catatonia, and intense autonomic output with fever; this condition has links to the neuroleptic malignant syndrome but was observed in the preneuroleptic era.

Investigations

In the investigation of psychotic patients, it is important to rule out metabolic disturbances; if alcoholism is suspected, estimation of red-cell transketolase activity may be of value. A drug screen should be performed if the patient is suspected of having taken drugs. Careful cognitive testing at the bedside may be sufficient to detect the confusion of an underlying delirium, which may be missed if the fluctuating course of the disorder with lucid intervals is not appreciated.

Rarely, psychosis is secondary to cerebral systemic lupus erythematosus (SLE), in which case tests for lupus erythematosus cells and antinuclear factors will be required; where a storage disorder is suspected, screening for known conditions should be performed. Testing for porphyrins still occasionally yields rewarding results when porphyria is suspected, and it is still wise to test syphilis serology. Human immunodeficiency virus status also may require evaluation in high-risk subjects.

The EEG is extremely helpful in distinguishing psychotic conditions secondary to delirium from schizophrenia. The generalized slowing of background rhythms associated with delirium contrast with the more regular rhythms of interictal states and of schizophrenia. However, abnormal EEGs are noted often in schizophrenia. Thus, EEGs suggestive of epilepsy have been reported with catatonia, and generalized nonparoxysmal dysrhythmias and paroxysmal phenomena are noted often in schizophrenia. Slow-wave asymmetries, slow bursts, spikes, or sharp waves are the recorded changes; their presence, in the setting of paroxysmal behavior disorders associated with a chronic psychotic disorder, should not lead to a diagnosis of epilepsy. In patients in whom epileptic psychosis is suspected, the EEG will most often reveal a temporal lobe focus; in schizophreniform presentations with Schneiderian auditory hallucinations, the dominant hemisphere is often affected. In some patients, the temporal lobe origin for the focus does not become clear until sleep or sphenoidal recording has been performed or, occasionally, only when a seizure itself is captured using ambulatory monitoring or videotelemetry.

There are many reports of patients with schizophrenia having ventricular enlargement on CT or MRI scan (for review, see Trimble 1996). Patients with cerebral atrophy have a poorer premorbid adjustment, show a poorer response to therapy, display more minor soft neurological signs, and have more abnormal EEGs than those with normal scans. They generally show more cognitive decline, apathy, and withdrawal. Other investigators have reported the presence of third and fourth ventricular dilation, cerebellar atrophy, and occasionally aqueduct stenosis in relationship to the schizophrenia.

Few investigators doubt that schizophrenia is a neurological illness, in the sense of being associated with identifiable neuropathology in many cases. Studies of brain structure have emphasized changes, especially neuron loss or disarray in the hippocampal and parahippocampal cortex, although other sites, notably in the basal ganglia, frontal cortex, and cerebellum also may be affected. Functional changes, as identified with positron emission tomography (PET), include frontal hypometabolism, which has been reported in several studies. Schizophrenia is viewed as a neurodevelopmental disorder, with probable genetic causation (Carpenter and Buchanan 1994).

When patients with schizophrenia are examined, soft neurological signs are often seen. Offspring of schizophrenic parents—a high-risk group for later development of the disorder—show increased evidence of soft neurological signs, poor motor coordination, and perceptual deficits (Marcus et al. 1985). Up to 60% of patients diagnosed as schizophrenic show abnormal neurological signs on routine testing. These include potential frontal lobe signs, such as the grasp and palmomental reflexes, and perseveration. Abnormal face-hand tests; graphesthesia; minor motor and sensory disturbances; more recognizable choreoathetoid, dystonic, and tic-like presentations; gait disturbances; difficulties with coordination and smooth performance of motor activities; reflex changes (increased or decreased); mirror movements, and variable Babinski's responses all have been reported.

Schizophrenic patients have an increased incidence of sinistrality and also show abnormal patterns of eye blinking, disturbed eye tracking with abnormal smooth pursuit, and abnormal saccades.

Treatment of Psychoses in Neurological Patients

As for depression, the guidelines for treatment of psychoses in neurological patients are essentially as for psychotic illness in the absence of neurological illness. All neuroleptics lower the seizure threshold, chlorpromazine more so than the butyrophenones, haloperidol and pimozide. Sulpiride may have some advantages in not being so sedative and being less likely to provoke movement disorders. Other atypical neuroleptics, with even less potential for such side effects, such as clozapine, represent an advantage in the treatment of the psychoses of Parkinson's disease, although clozapine is proconvulsant and requires the patient to have regular hematological monitoring. In some patients with epilepsy, in whom a psychosis emerges in the setting of a diminution of seizure frequency, a proconvulsant agent may be preferred and a course of ECT may be necessary. Intramuscular preparations are not contraindicated and are of value in chronic psychosis.

BEHAVIORAL NEUROLOGY

This chapter and Chapter 9 have considered interrelationships between psychiatry and neurology, with particular reference to behavioral problems encountered by neurologists. In many cases, after adequate examination and investigation, it might be concluded that no neurological disease is discernible and therefore that the problem is "purely psychiatric." However, as is becoming clear—particularly as we investigate the major psychoses further—the distinction between what is "functional" and what is "organic," based on an old-fashioned dichotomy relating one to psychogenesis and the other to neurogenesis, can no longer be upheld. It also appears that in many psychiatric disorders that yield neurological findings, their discovery does not lead to the designation of a recognized neurological syndrome. There is a neurology of psychiatry, which often reflects neurological change in subcortical and limbic system structures of the brain, of either a functional or a structural nature. This change does not produce classic neurological signs on examination, and its main influence relates to a change in the behavior of the organism as a whole.

As these chapters also show, there is a psychiatry of neurology; in other words, many patients with neurological disorders present with behavior problems that often require methods of treatment familiar to psychiatrists. Again, the areas of the brain that tend to be affected reflect limbic system structures, and the importance of the frontal and temporal lobes in personality change, affective disorders, and psychosis has been pointed out. The existence of so many patients displaying the neurology of psychiatry or the psychiatry of neurology has led to the development of such disciplines as behavioral neurology and neuropsychiatry, which attempt—from clinical, intellectual, and research points of view—to understand the complex and subtle interrelationships between the brain and behavior.

REFERENCES

Carpenter WT, Buchanan RW. Schizophrenia. N Engl J Med 1994;330:681–690.

Coffey CE, Figiel GS, Djang WT, Weiner RD. Subcortical hyperintensity on MRI: A comparison of normal and depressed elderly subjects. Am J Psychiatry 1990;147:187–189.

Collins M, Hawthorne M, Gribbin N, Jacobson R. Capgras syndrome with organic disorders. Postgrad Med 1990;66: 1064–1067.

Cummings J, Trimble MR. A Concise Guide to Behavioral Neurology and Neuropsychiatry. Washington, DC: American Psychiatric Association Press, 1995.

Davidson K, Bagley CR. Schizophrenia-like psychoses associated with organic disorders of the CNS. R Herrington (ed), Current Problems in Neuropsychiatry. Kent, England: Headley Brothers, 1969;133–184.

Diagnostic and Statistical Manual of Mental Disorders (3rd ed, revised) (DSM-III-R). Washington, DC: American Psychiatric Association, 1980.

Diagnostic and Statistical Manual of Mental Disorders (4th ed) (DSM-IV) Draft criteria. Washington, DC: American Psychiatric Association, 1994.

Eastwood MR, Rifat SL, Nobbs H, Ruderman J. Mood disorder following cerebrovascular accident. Br J Psychiatry 1989; 154:195–200.

Fedoroff JP, Starkstein SE, Forrester AW et al. Depression in patients with acute traumatic brain injury. Am J Psychiatry 1992;149:918–923.

International Classification of Diseases 10. Classification of Mental and Behavioral Disorders. Geneva: World Health Organization, 1992.

Marcus J, Hans SL, Mednick SA et al. Neurological dysfunctioning in offspring of schizophrenics in Israel and Denmark. Arch Gen Psychiatry 1985;42:753–761.

Mayeux R, Stern Y, Williams JBW et al. Clinical and biochemical features of depression in Parkinson's disease. Am J Psychiatry 1986;143:756–759.

Ring HA, Bench CJ, Trimble MR et al. Depression in Parkinson's disease: A PET study. Br J Psychiatry 1994;165:333–340.

Robertson MM, Trimble MR, Townsend H. Phenomenology of depression in epilepsy. Epilepsia 1987;28:364–372.

Schiffer RB, Kurian R, Rubin A, Boer S. Evidence for atypical depression in Parkinson's disease. Am J Psychiatry 1988;145: 1020–1022.

Starkstein SE, Berthier ML, Bolduc PL et al. Depression in patients with early -v- late-onset Parkinson's disease. Neurology 1989; 39:1441–1445.

Starkstein SE, Robinson RG. Affective disorders and cerebrovascular disease. Br J Psychiatry 1989;154:170–182.

Starkstein SE, Robinson RG. Depression in Cerebrovascular Disease. In SE Starkstein, RG Robinson (eds), Depression in Neurologic Disease. Baltimore: Johns Hopkins University Press, 1993;28–49.

Trimble MR. Biological Psychiatry (2nd ed). Chichester, England: Wiley, 1996.

Trimble MR. First rank symptoms of Schneider, a new perspective. Br J Psychiatry 1990;156:195–200.

Chapter 11
Agnosias and Apraxias

Daniel Tranel and Antonio R. Damasio

A THEORETICAL FRAMEWORK

Before we review current thinking on the neurology of the agnosias and apraxias, it is necessary to explain, however briefly, the theoretical framework we will use as a reference. That framework specifies a *relative functional compartmentalization* in the human brain. One large set of systems, in early sensory cortices and motor cortices, explicitly represents "sense" and "action" knowledge. Another set of systems, in higher-order cortices and in subcortical nuclei such as the basal ganglia and amygdala, orchestrates the construction of those explicit representations in sensory-motor cortices. Those systems promote activity in separate brain areas and establish temporal correspondences among those separate areas. Yet another set of systems ensures the attentional enhancement required for the concerted operation of the others. All these systems operate under the influence of internal preferences and biases, as expressed in brain core networks concerned with enacting survival-related biological drives and instincts (Damasio and Damasio 1994).

The reconstruction of explicit representations of an object, face, or action is accomplished in separate "early sensory" regions by means of long-range cortico-cortical feedback projections that mediate relatively synchronous excitatory activation. The time scale of the large-scale synchronization paced from higher-order cortices is on the order of several thousand milliseconds, the scale required for meaningful cognition. At more local levels, the scale is smaller, on the order of tens of milliseconds.

In this framework, the neural device from which reconstructions are conducted is known as a *convergence zone* (Damasio 1989a, 1989b). A convergence zone is an ensemble of neurons within which many feedforward/feedback loops make contact. A convergence zone (1) receives feedforward projections from cortical regions located in the connectional level immediately below; (2) sends reciprocal feedback projections to the originating cortices; (3) sends feedforward projections to cortical regions in the next connectional level; and (4) receives projections from heterarchically placed cortices and from subcortical nuclei in the thalamus, basal forebrain, and brain stem.

Knowledge retrieval is based on relatively simultaneous, attended activity in many early cortical regions, engendered over several recurrences in such a system. The result of such recurrences is a *topographically organized* representation. In other words, concepts are represented dispositionally along a series of neural processing stations, and meaning is arrived at by multiple recurrences and iterations within such a system.

Knowledge can be retrieved at different *levels* of complexity, ranging from very specific (subordinate) to very broad (superordinate). Consider the following example. Knowledge about the unique horse "Hawk" is specific and unique, and is classified as "subordinate level"; less specific and unique knowledge about "horses" (of which Hawk is an example) is classified as "basic object level"; and even less specific knowledge concerning "living entities" (of which horses and Hawk are examples) is classified as "superordinate level."

The level at which knowledge is retrieved depends on the scope of multiregional activation, which in turn depends on the level of convergence zone that is activated. Low-level convergence zones bind signals relative to entity categories (e.g., color, shape), and are placed in association cortices located immediately beyond ("downstream" from) the cortices, whose activity defines featural representations. Higher-level convergence zones bind signals relative to more complex combinations and are placed at a higher level in the cortico-cortical hierarchy. The convergence zones capable of binding entities into events and describing their categorization are located at the "top" of the hierarchical streams, in anterior temporal and frontal regions.

The *dispositional* representations embodied in a convergence zone are the result of previous learning, during which feedforward projections and reciprocating feedback projections were simultaneously active. Both during learning and retrieval, the neurons in a convergence zone are under the control of a variety of cortical and noncortical projections. These include projections from the thalamus, nonspecific neurotransmitter nuclei, and other cortical projections from convergence zones in prefrontal cortices; cortices located higher up in the feedforward hierarchy; homologous cortices of the opposite hemisphere; and heterarchical cortices of parallel hierarchical streams.

In short, the structures and processes required to store and access dispositional representations must be distinguished from the structures and processes needed for on-line topographically organized representations. In the framework used here, activation of neuron assemblies in the anterior temporal region does *not* produce, within the assembly itself, a topographically organized representation. As a consequence, we cannot be made conscious of the activity within the anterior temporal cortex itself. Instead, when the neuron assemblies that hold dispositional representations are activated and lead in turn to the activation of early sensory cortices, they cause topographically organized representations to be formed in those cortices. Eventually, we experience typographically organized representations as images. The quality of those images is less vivid than the quality of images produced during perception, but the essential nature is no different.

We turn now to a discussion of the agnosias and apraxias, with a particular focus on the neural basis of knowledge representation and retrieval..

THE AGNOSIAS

The term *agnosia* signifies lack of knowledge and is virtually synonymous with an impairment of recognition. In the traditional literature, two types of agnosia were commonly described. One, termed *associative agnosia*, referred to a failure of recognition that results from defective activation of information pertinent to a given stimulus. The other, termed *apperceptive agnosia*, referred to a disturbance of the integration of otherwise normally perceived components of a stimulus.

Teuber in 1968 gave a narrower definition, in which agnosia was synonymous with having normal percepts stripped of their meaning. In this sense, agnosia is conceptualized as a disorder of memory, not as a disorder of perception, and only associative agnosia truly qualifies for this stricter definition. In practical terms, however, it has been useful to retain the concept of apperceptive agnosia and to maintain a distinction between apperceptive and associative agnosia. In both conditions, recognition is disturbed. In the apperceptive variety, the problem can be traced, at least in part, to faulty perception, usually in reference to aspects of higher-order perceptual capacities (it is not appropriate to use the term *agnosia* for conditions in which perceptual problems are severe and obviously preclude the patient's apprehension of meaningful information). In associative agnosia, perception is largely intact and the recognition defect is strictly or primarily a disorder of memory.

The difficulties of trying to separate apperceptive and associative forms of agnosia underscore the fact that the processes of perception and memory are not discrete. Rather, those processes operate on a physiological and psychological continuum, and demarcation of a clear separation point at which perceptual processes end and memory processes begin is simply not possible (Damasio et al. 1990a). Many patients with recognition defects have elements of both conditions (i.e., high-level perceptual problems and disturbances of memory). Some defects, however, can be classified unequivocally into one type or the other. We thus prefer to use the following operational definitions. *Associative agnosia* is a modality-specific impairment of the ability to recognize previously known stimuli (or new stimuli for which learning would normally have occurred), that occurs in the absence of disturbances of perception, intellect, or language, and is the result of acquired cerebral damage. The designation *apperceptive agnosia* applies when the patient meets the above definition in all respects except that perception is altered.

The term *agnosia* should be restricted to situations in which recognition impairments are confined to one sensory modality, such as vision, audition, or touch. When recognition defects extend across two or more modalities, the appropriate designation is *amnesia*. As noted earlier, the term agnosia should not be used for patients in whom recognition defects develop in connection with major disturbances of basic perception, nor should the term be applied to patients with major impairments of intellect. The term *agnosia* should be reserved for conditions that develop suddenly, following the onset of acquired cerebral dysfunction.

One other important distinction is between *recognition* and *naming*. The two capacities are often confused. Recognition of an entity, under normal circumstances, is frequently indicated by naming (e.g., that's a "groundhog" or that's "Aunt Mabel"). Recent studies of brain-injured subjects, however, have shown that recognition and naming are dissociable capacities, and the two terms should not be used interchangeably (Damasio et al. 1990b). Brain damage in the left inferotemporal region, for example, can render a patient incapable of naming a wide variety of stimuli, while leaving unaffected the patient's ability to recognize those stimuli (Damasio and Tranel 1993). For the two examples above, for example, the patient may produce the descriptions of "that's a roly-poly animal that digs holes under barns and hibernates in the winter," and "that's my aunt who lives on the east side of town in our old house," both of which indicate unequivocal *recognition* of the specific entities, even if their names are never produced. In short, it is important to maintain a distinction between recognition, which can be indicated by any number of responses signifying that the patient understands the meaning of a partic-

Table 11.1: Principal agnosic conditions

Modality/Capacity	*Subtypes*	*Neuroanatomical Correlates*
Vision	Visual object agnosia	Bilateral occipitotemporal; left occipitotemporal
	Associative prosopagnosia	Bilateral occipitotemporal
	Apperceptive prosopagnosia	Right occipitotemporal and occipitoparietal
Audition	Environmental sound agnosia	Bilateral posterior superior temporal
	Phonagnosia	Right inferior parietal
	Amusia	Right posterior temporal, inferior parietal
Somatosensory	Tactile object agnosia (complete)	Right and left parietal operculum; posterior insula; S_2
	Tactile object agnosia (nonmanipulable stimuli)	Right superior mesial parietal
Perception of disease	Anosognosia	Right parietal; bilateral ventromedial frontal

ular stimulus, and naming, which may not, and need not, accompany accurate recognition.

In principle, agnosia can occur in any sensory modality, relative to any type of entity or event. In practice, however, some types of agnosia are the most frequent. *Visual agnosia*, especially agnosia for faces (*prosopagnosia*), is the most commonly encountered form of recognition disturbance affecting a primary sensory modality. The condition of *auditory agnosia* is rarer, followed by the even less frequent *tactile agnosia*. A frequently encountered condition that also conforms to the designation of agnosia is a disturbance in the *recognition of illness*, or what has been termed *anosognosia*. A summary of these conditions is provided in Table 11.1.

Accurate detection and diagnosis of agnosia are important on several accounts. Both visual and auditory agnosia are strongly associated with the presence of bilateral cerebral disease. Thus, the presence of one of these conditions can be a useful clue in the localization of brain dysfunction. This clue can be especially helpful in the early stages of acquired cerebral dysfunction, when even modern neuroimaging procedures may fail to detect a lesion. Such conditions furnish additional diagnostic clues because they are associated typically with cerebrovascular disease affecting the territories of the posterior or middle cerebral arteries. To avoid misdiagnosis, note that the complaints or behaviors of patients with agnosia can appear so bizarre as to raise questions about their veracity. Clinicians once doubted whether such conditions existed at all. That agnosic conditions do occur is no longer a contentious issue; nonetheless, clinicians may be skeptical of a patient who suddenly claims an inability to recognize familiar faces, despite normal vision, or of a patient who suddenly behaves as though all auditory information has lost its meaning.

Despite their relative rarity, agnosias are important "experiments of nature," and they have assisted with the investigation of the neural bases of human perception, learning, and memory. Careful study of agnosic patients over the past couple of decades, facilitated by the advent of modern neuroimaging techniques (computed tomography [CT], magnetic resonance imaging [MRI]) and by the development of sophisticated experimental neuropsychological procedures, has yielded important new insights into the manner in which the human brain acquires, maintains, and retrieves various types of knowledge.

Visual Agnosia

Description and Examination

Visual agnosia is a disorder of recognition confined to the visual realm, in which a patient cannot arrive at the meaning of some or all categories of previously known nonverbal visual stimuli, despite normal or near-normal visual perception and intact alertness, attention, intelligence, and language. Most patients manifest a comparable defect in the anterograde compartment; that is, they cannot recognize new nonverbal, visual stimuli that would normally have been learned after adequate exposure.

Patients with visual agnosia often have some type of visual field defect, most frequently a superior quadrantanopia or a hemianopia, or both. Often, however, one-half or even three-fourths of central vision remains intact. In all cases, careful neuro-ophthalmological assessment is crucial. Visual acuity should be normal, and there should be no gross distortion of contrast sensitivity or texture perception. When patients complain that their vision is blurry or foggy, or that the stimuli in the visual field are jumbled or quavery, a basic perceptual impairment is indicated and the diagnosis of visual agnosia should be excluded.

Perception should be assessed also with several detailed probes that can be conducted at the bedside or in the neuropsychological laboratory. For example, the examiner should ask the patient to describe a variety of different stimuli presented in the intact portion of the visual field. These things might include objects, faces, colors, meaningful and meaningless geometric forms, and signs and symbols. Static as well as moving stimuli should be shown. Accurate descriptions by the patient of shape, number, and position of stimuli are evidence that visual perception is sufficient for recognition. If it can be established that a patient comprehends the entire shape of a stimulus, and yet fails to recognize it, the traditional classification of *associative visual agnosia* applies. When the patient has sufficient form perception but can only comprehend fragments of a stimulus and cannot analyze the whole entity, the term *apperceptive visual agnosia* can be applied. The neural processes involved in higher-level perception overlap considerably with processes involved in memory.

Perception can be investigated in considerable detail with several standard neuropsychological techniques (Tranel 1994), including tests such as the Facial Recognition Test and Judgment of Line Orientation Test (Benton et al. 1983) and the Hooper Visual Organization Test (Hooper 1983). The Facial Recognition Test is *not* a test of face recognition but rather a test of face matching. It is an excellent measure of visuo-perceptual discrimination, but it does not measure memory for faces. Drawing tests are also helpful in determining the visual processing capacities of a patient, and the examiner should include both copying procedures (e.g., the copy administration of the Complex Figure Test; Lezak 1983) and drawing to dictation (e.g., "draw-a-clock" and "draw-a-person"). Not all patients with visual agnosia will pass all of these procedures, but most can perform most of the tasks within normal or near-normal limits. When a patient fails badly on all of these types of procedures, the integrity of visual perception is clearly not sufficient for the diagnosis of agnosia to apply.

One potentially problematic differential diagnosis that arises with some regularity in the investigation of visual agnosia is the condition known as *Balint's syndrome* (Damasio 1985). Balint's syndrome involves an inability to attend to more than a very limited sector of the visual field at any given time (visual disorientation), with inability to look voluntarily into different parts of the visual field (ocular apraxia) and defective visual guidance of reaching behavior and mislocalization when pointing to targets (optic ataxia). The problem of attending simultaneously to different parts of the visual field, which is the core feature of Balint's syndrome, has been called "*simultanagnosia,*" which is unfortunate because the behavior is not a *recognition* disturbance and thus does not conform to a true condition of agnosia. Balint's syndrome is associated with dysfunction of visual association cortices, but unlike visual agnosia, Balint's syndrome results from damage to *superior* portions of the region (superior occipital and occipitoparietal), rather than inferior parts of this sector (the damage of which causes visual agnosia). Patients with Balint's syndrome can recognize various visual stimuli, including objects and faces, even if they have trouble locating them in space. One curious problem in many Balint's patients is a defect in motion detection and recognition. Patients may be unable to detect direction and velocity of moving stimuli and may fail to grasp the meaning of certain stereotyped movements (e.g., dance steps, sporting-related behaviors, or familiar gaits and strides). The defect in motion recognition may actually conform more appropriately to the concept of agnosia than does the better-known manifestation of simultanagnosia.

Subtypes

Category-Specific Visual Agnosia. Visual object agnosia rarely affects all types of visual stimuli with equal magnitude (e.g., Damasio et al. 1990a; Damasio et al. 1990b). In one common profile of visual recognition impairment, there is a major defect in categories of living things, especially animals, with relative or even complete sparing of categories of manufactured things (e.g., tools and utensils). We have also observed the reverse pattern—defective recognition of manufactured things and normal recognition of living things—although it is much rarer. Together, the two patterns constitute a *double dissociation.* At first glance, these types of dissociations may seem bizarre or arbitrary, but the patterns simply reflect the fact that different types of stimuli are mapped by different neural systems. Factors such as shape similarity (visual "ambiguity") and manipulability (whether the entity is learned and operated purely through vision, or through both vision and touch) have been identified as important determinants of whether or not recognition of a certain class of stimuli will be disrupted by a particular brain lesion.

Dissociations between different classes of visual stimuli can be remarkably complete. For example, a patient may manifest a severe defect for animals and yet have entirely preserved recognition of tools and utensils. It is thus important that investigation of visual recognition capacities cover, in sufficient depth, a variety of different categories of entities. Many standardized procedures (e.g., the Visual Naming subtest of the Multilingual Aphasia Examination [MAE]; the Boston Naming Test) provide inadequate coverage of some types of stimuli. Neither the Visual Naming nor the Boston Naming tests, for example, provides good coverage of living, animate entities, such as animals and fruits and vegetables. This lack can lead to erroneous conclusions regarding the status of visual recognition. For instance, a patient with a defect for animals may be misdiagnosed as normal based on successful performances on the MAE Visual Naming and Boston Naming tests, or category-specific recognition defects may be missed if the patient is not provided the opportunity to attempt stimuli from varied classes of objects.

Prosopagnosia. The inability to recognize familiar faces is known as *prosopagnosia* or *face agnosia*, and it is the most frequent and well established of the visual agnosias (Damasio et al. 1990c). The phenomenon has been noted since the turn of the century, and it has been the focus of a good deal of scientific inquiry. The fascination with prosopagnosia stems from the oddity of the disorder, along with the opportunity it provides to investigate perception, learning, and recall of complex and unique knowledge. The condition is also important from a clinical standpoint, given its devastating effect on its victims, accurate diagnosis and management of the condition are essential. Investigation of prosopagnosia has been marked by controversy regarding the relative importance of *perceptual* versus *mnestic* factors in the development of the condition and a dispute about whether prosopagnosia requires *bilateral* lesions or can be caused by *unilateral* damage.

Neuropsychological and Neuroanatomical Correlates of Prosopagnosia. The face recognition defect in prosopagnosia typically covers both the retrograde and anterograde compartments. Patients can no longer recognize the faces of previously known individuals and are unable to learn new ones. They are unable to recognize the faces of family members, close friends, and, in the most paradigmatic instances, even their own face in a mirror. On seeing those faces, the patients experience no sense of familiarity, no inkling that those faces are *known* to them; that is, they fail to conjure up consciously any pertinent information that would trigger recognition. As with agnosia in general, prosopagnosia must be distinguished from disorders of *naming*—that is, it is *not* an inability to name faces of persons who are otherwise recognized as familiar. There are numerous examples of face-naming failure, from both brain-injured populations and from the realm of normal everyday experience, but in such instances, the unnamed face is invariably detected as familiar, and the precise identity of the possessor of the face is usually apprehended accurately. In prosopagnosia, however, the defect sets in at the level of recognition. The patients will also manifest a face-naming impairment (they will not name faces they cannot recognize), but this is artifactual and not a true naming defect. Several major types of prosopagnosia can be distinguished.

"Pure Associative" Prosopagnosia. In this variety of prosopagnosia, the recognition impairment is relatively pure, in that it is confined to the visual modality, and occurs in the setting of normal or near-normal visual perception. Associative prosopagnosia largely conforms to the strict definition of agnosia—that is, "a normal percept stripped of its meaning." The patients perform normally on standard neuropsychological tests of visuo-perceptual discrimination and visual-spatial judgment (such as the Facial Recognition Test and Judgment of Line Orientation Test). Recognition via other modalities is unaffected. Thus, on hearing the voices of individuals whose faces go unrecognized, the patients will recognize instantly the identities of those individuals. Even within the visual modality, the defect is highly circumscribed. For instance, patients may be able to recognize individuals on the basis of a distinctive feature (e.g., hairstyle) or gait or posture.

Most patients with pure associative prosopagnosia also have achromatopsia, an acquired impairment of color perception. The combination of the defects is due to the contiguity of the neural processing systems for form and color, and their sweeping damage by one lesion (see below). The color perception defect per se, however, does not account for the face recognition impairment, as normal individuals can recognize faces easily in black and white. The ability to read may or may not be affected in prosopagnosic patients, depending on the location of the lesion in the left occipital region. When the lesion encompasses both the left occipitotemporal region and the left periventricular region (the white matter beside, beneath, and behind the occipital horn), reading impairment (alexia) coexists with prosopagnosia.

Pure associative prosopagnosia is caused by bilateral damage in inferior occipital and temporal visual association cortices—that is, in the inferior component of cytoarchitectonic areas 18 and 19, and part of the nearby cytoarchitectonic area 37. Most cases are attributable to cerebral infarctions caused by occlusion in posterior cerebral artery branches. Head injury and cerebral tumors, especially gliomas originating in one occipital lobe and traversing into the opposite hemisphere via the splenium of the corpus callosum, also can produce prosopagnosia. Prosopagnosia in connection with lesions (bilateral or unilateral) located exclusively above the calcarine fissure, in superior visual association cortices, has never been reported, although there are cases of face agnosia in which the inferior lesions extend upward above the calcarine fissure on one or both sides.

"Apperceptive" Prosopagnosia. Face agnosia in the setting of significant visuo-perceptual disturbance has been termed "apperceptive" prosopagnosia. Apperceptive face agnosics have defects in basic visual perception, demonstrable on neuropsychological testing, that compromise abilities such as matching of unfamiliar faces, judgment of line orientations, and mental manipulation of pictures and picture fragments. Such defects, however, are not so severe as to compromise most aspects of basic form vision; thus, the condition conforms in a broad sense to the definition of agnosia. Perceptual processes and recognition/recall processes cannot be rigidly compartmentalized. Even in "pure" cases of associative prosopagnosia, there may be fairly subtle, albeit important, disturbances of high-level integrative abilities, which cannot be detected by available probes. Any explanation of face agnosia tied to perceptual factors must reconcile the fact that most patients with visual perceptual defects, even severe ones, do not lose their ability to recognize faces; that is, visuo-perceptual disturbance as detected by neuropsychological or perimetric probes does not necessarily cause face agnosia.

Apperceptive face agnosia is most often associated with damage in right visual association cortices within the occipital and parietal regions. It appears that the damage must involve both the inferior and superior components of posterior visual association cortices (areas 18 and 19), mesially and laterally, for severe and lasting face agnosia to develop. In most cases, parts of areas 39 and 37 on the right also will be damaged.

"Developmental" Prosopagnosia. Some individuals never developed a normal capacity for learning faces. They have a lifelong deficiency in learning and recognizing faces that ought to have been readily mastered, and because the problem begins in childhood, it is appropriate to call it developmental prosopagnosia. No neural correlates for this condition have been identified. Developmental prosopagnosia has not been widely reported or studied, but it may be far more frequent than suspected, its apparent rarity being due to the fact that affected persons tend either to not recognize or to conceal their disability. It is probably associated with learning disability for other classes of visual stimuli which, like faces, require individual identification and have many similar exemplars.

Other Aspects of Face Processing

Nature and Extent of the Defect. In prosopagnosia, the recognition impairment occurs at the most *subordinate* taxonomic level—that is, at the level of identification of unique faces. Prosopagnosics are fully capable of recognizing faces as faces; that is, performance is normal at the *superordinate* taxonomic level. Also, most prosopagnosics can recognize facial expressions and can make accurate determinations of gender and age based on face information (Tranel et al. 1988). These dissociations highlight the fact that recognizing faces at the level of unique identity is a highly demanding task that requires the brain to distinguish between numerous different exemplars that highly resemble one another.

Although face agnosics will recognize any number of visual entities at *basic object level* (e.g., cars as cars, buildings as buildings, dogs as dogs), they often will fail to recognize these items at the subordinate level of unique identity. Thus, as with faces, they are unable to recognize the specific identity of a particular car or building. These recognition impairments are common in prosopagnosia and underscore the notion that the core defect in face agnosia is the inability to disambiguate fully individual visual stimuli.

Prosopagnosic patients often can recognize identity from movement. This means not only that their perception of movement is intact but also that they can evoke appropriate memories from the perception of unique patterns of movement. The recovery of identity from motion can be impaired by lesions in superior occipitoparietal regions that usually are spared in prosopagnosia.

Nonconscious Discrimination of Familiar Faces. Recent evidence has revealed that many prosopagnosic patients show accurate covert or nonconscious discrimination of familiar faces, despite their complete inability to recognize those faces at an overt level, based on self-report or verbal ratings of familiarity. For example, prosopagnosics generate large, discriminatory electrodermal responses to familiar faces that are otherwise unrecognized (Tranel and Damasio 1988). Preserved covert face discrimination has been demonstrated in other experimental paradigms, such as reaction time tasks and forced choice procedures. In the electrodermal paradigm, covert face discrimination has even been demonstrated for faces from the anterograde compartment, which indicates that the brain can continue to learn new visual information even without conscious influence.

Adaptation and Recovery. Prosopagnosic patients often become quite adroit at using nonface information to recognize the persons around them. For example, they rely on voice, gait, or a distinctive visual feature. It is often helpful to add a distinctive visual feature in situations in which recognition is highly demanded but difficult. At a crowded social gathering, for example, the patient might have his or her spouse wear a special hat or other article of clothing, which would facilitate rapid and accurate identification. The earlier in the course of recovery that compensatory strategies such as these can be taught, the better the chances for healthy adaptation to the disability.

Auditory Agnosia

Description and Examination

Auditory agnosia is a disorder of recognition confined to the auditory realm in which a patient cannot arrive at the meaning of some or all categories of previously known auditory stimuli, despite normal or near-normal auditory perception and intact alertness, attention, and intelligence. Unfortunately, the term auditory agnosia has been variously applied to patients in whom there is a recognition defect for all auditory stimuli (verbal and nonverbal), or only verbal or nonverbal ones. In our view, the term should be reserved for an inability to recognize nonverbal sounds, such as environmental sounds, melodies, and timbres, and the term *aphasia* should apply to the verbal component of an auditory agnosia.

Auditory agnosia often coexists with Wernicke's aphasia, and patients with both will be unable to recognize speech and nonspeech sounds. Other related terms include *word deafness* (essentially equivalent to Wernicke's aphasia) and *pure word deafness*, the latter designating those rare instances in which patients fail to comprehend and repeat words but are able to produce normal, nonparaphasic speech—that is, they are not aphasic. The term *cortical deafness* can be applied to patients who demonstrate a striking unawareness of auditory stimuli of any kind, and such patients typically have defects in basic aspects of auditory perception (e.g., audiometric pure-tone thresholds are markedly abnormal).

Unlike the situation with visual agnosia, the presence of language impairment is not an exclusionary criterion for the diagnosis of auditory agnosia. Most patients with auditory agnosia have bilateral lesions of auditory cortex, and some degree of aphasia (related typically to the left temporal lobe lesion) is virtually always present. Many of these patients have preserved language capacities via the visual modality, however, and they remain capable of reading and writing. Thus, it is important to test auditory agnosic patients by allowing the patient to read the examiner's questions and attempt to write the answers. Many auditory agnosics can give a satisfactory oral account of their nonverbal experiences, in spite of some degree of aphasia.

As with visual agnosia, auditory agnosia starts acutely. The patient suddenly becomes entirely or almost entirely deaf. Such patients frequently also become speechless, perhaps failing to realize, because of the sudden loss of auditory feedback, that they can speak normally. Either orally or by writing, the patient complains of complete or near-complete loss of hearing. The appropriate label at this point actually is *cortical deafness*. Although this condition evolves rapidly and within a few days or weeks, the patient reports being able to hear sounds, and audiometry may become normal. At this juncture, when the audiometric pattern normalizes and the patient continues to report an inability to recognize sounds, the diagnosis of auditory agnosia can be applied.

In the acute phase, it is common for auditory agnosic patients to manifest severe behavioral disturbances, including anxiety, agitation, and even disorderly behavior. Undoubtedly, these behavioral features are attributable to the sudden and seemingly inexplicable deprivation of auditory feedback. It is very important to understand the reasons for the patient's behavior and to provide continual reassurance and support. These behaviors may prompt a psychiatric evaluation, but a psychiatric approach to the condition will prove frustrating for both the patient and the examiner.

To establish the diagnosis of auditory agnosia, it is essential to decide on the patency of the auditory channel. At the bedside, the clinician should instruct the patient in written notes to raise his or her hand when hearing a sound produced outside the field of vision. The clinician can be located behind the patient and can snap the fingers or clap hands on different sides of the patient's head. Patients should be asked to repeat finger-tapping patterns on a tabletop, given without visual or vibratory cues. Correct detection of sounds or correct finger tapping indicates that the patient is hearing. Pure-tone audiometry is needed to quantify formally the basic auditory perceptual capacities of the patient. Auditory-evoked potentials should also be obtained when available.

Subtypes

Environmental Sound Agnosia. The most common manifestation of auditory agnosia is a defect in the recognition of common environmental sounds. The patient will not be capable of determining the meaning of sounds such as knocking on the door, a telephone ringing, a baby crying, or a bird chirping. We have not observed category-related specificity of these defects (e.g., a patient whose defect was confined to sounds made by living things, but not sounds made by manufactured things), but this has not been studied in sufficient detail. As in the case of visual agnosia, the defect is modality-specific; hence, the patient will have normal recognition of entities presented visually, even though the sounds of those stimuli go unrecognized.

This presentation is strongly associated with bilateral lesions to the posterior one-third of the superior temporal gyrus. The damage involves auditory association cortices (posterior area 22) while sparing, at least to some extent, the primary auditory cortices (areas 41 and 42). Invariably, such lesions are caused by stroke. A staged presentation of this condition has been observed, whereby the patient suffers a unilateral lesion (e.g., on the right) that may fail to produce noticeable, permanent defects, and then sustains a second lesion on the other side. The combined lesions produce the full-blown unfolding of cortical deafness evolving into auditory agnosia. It is rare for unilateral lesions in either the left or right auditory cortex to produce auditory agnosia for environmental sounds.

Agnosia for Familiar Voices. There have been a few reports of patients who lost the ability to recognize familiar voices, a condition termed *phonagnosia* (Van Lancker et al. 1989). The condition is analogous to prosopagnosia, in that the recognition defect sets in at the level of identification of unique stimuli. Thus, the patient loses the capacity to recognize the identity of a speaker, based on hearing the voice. Available evidence suggests that phonagnosia is associated with right inferior parietal lesions, but this relationship has not been studied in detail. There are reports of patients with environmental sound agnosia who do not lose their ability to recognize familiar voices, but again, this profile has not been investigated in enough detail to draw firm conclusions.

Amusia. Auditory amusia, in which a patient loses the ability to recognize the unique timbre of a singing voice as well as the identity of familiar melodies, is another rare condition that can occur with or without other components of auditory agnosia. The condition is manifestly difficult to evaluate in patients who lack a musical education or regular musical activities. In the few cases that have been reported, the evidence suggests that the condition is caused by a right inferior parietal or posterior temporal lesion that disconnects right auditory association cortices from other important parts of the auditory processing system, including portions of the temporal and parietal lobes on the right and homologous areas on the left. A person with auditory amusia has showed covert discrimination of familiar singing voices, demonstrated by large-amplitude skin conductance responses, in a manner analogous to the covert recognition of familiar faces in prosopagnosics.

Tactile Agnosia

Description and Examination

There has been considerable controversy surrounding the notion of tactile agnosia, which refers to an impairment of recognition of entities presented in the somatosensory (tactile) channel, not attributable to defective perception or to alterations of intellect, language, or attention. The principal source of disagreement stems from the fact that most patients with so-called tactile object agnosia turn out to have major impairments of somatosensory perception, making rather questionable the application of the term *agnosia*. Several studies using careful methodology have established, however, that there are some patients who have tactile recognition defects that conform to the formal definition of agnosia (Caselli 1991; Damasio et al. 1992).

Unlike visual agnosia and, to a lesser extent, auditory agnosia, the concept of tactile agnosia cannot be applied with much meaning to identification of unique stimuli, simply because there are very few entities that are learned and recognized tactually at a unique level (Tranel 1991). Thus, there is really nothing comparable to familiar faces or voices in the tactile channel. Hence, tactile agnosia is more or less tantamount to the notion of tactile object agnosia, referring to defective recognition of objects such as tools, utensils, musical instruments, fruits, vegetables, and animals. The defect is restricted to the tactile modality, and patients can easily recognize these stimuli when they are presented visually. The condition has been associated with damage to temporoparietal cortices, especially in and near the region of the inferior parietal operculum and posterior insula, possibly including the second somatosensory cortex, in either hemisphere (Caselli 1991). A restricted form of tactile object agnosia, in which the patient could not recognize nonmanipulable entities (i.e., stimuli that are learned and operated exclusively via the visual modality, such as large animals, buildings, and vehicles) but was capable of recognizing manipulable entities (e.g., tools and utensils), has been described in connection with a mesial superior parietal lesion in the right hemisphere (Damasio et al. 1992). The most frequent neuropathological factor is cerebral infarction, followed by a few cases attributable to tumor, head injury, or herpes simplex encephalitis.

The principal challenge in establishing tactile object agnosia is to demonstrate that perceptual defects cannot explain the patient's poor performance. Caselli (1991) has outlined a detailed series of procedures that can be used to determine the patency of basic (e.g., touch, pain, temperature, vibration, and proprioception) and intermediate (e.g., weight, texture, size, shape, and substance) somatosensory functions. If such tasks are performed normally or near normally and the patient has significant recognition defects for various entities, then the diagnosis of tactile object agnosia can be applied.

Other Considerations

Several conditions that clearly do not conform to the concept of agnosia but that have been labeled in such a way as to imply a kind of agnosic manifestation include *astereognosis, amorphognosis*, and *ahylognosis*. All these descriptors refer to conditions in which there are major alterations of perception and thus none of them conforms, even in a broad sense, to the notion of a "normal percept stripped of its meaning."

Tactile object agnosia is a far more subtle condition than visual agnosia or auditory agnosia, and it may go entirely unnoticed (and unreported) by the patient. Outside of those occasions when we may rummage through our pockets or purse in search of a particular object, there are few situations in which pure tactile object recognition (i.e., unaccompanied by visual input) is called for. Thus, the condition may actually be more common than believed, if clinicians were careful to investigate thoroughly for its presence. There is little question, though, that tactile object agnosia is considerably less disabling than agnosic disorders involving vision or audition.

Anosognosia

Description and Examination

The term *anosognosia* denotes a condition in which patients lose the ability to recognize disease states in themselves. In the most extreme and paradigmatic examples, patients fail to recognize major disabilities such as a complete hemiplegia or hemianesthesia; sphincter dysfunction or marked pain may be ignored; and the gravity of heart disease, stroke, or cancer may go entirely unacknowledged. Anosognosia also can occur in relation to cognitive and behavioral deficits and, in fact, such a manifestation is common. Patients give no sign of understanding that their cognition and behavior are compromised and fail to appreciate the ramifications of their disabilities.

Our operational definition of anosognosia parallels the definitions we have given for other modality-specific recognition impairments: Anosognosia is a disorder of recognition in which a patient cannot arrive at the meaning of certain types of stimulus input, despite normal or near-normal capacity to perceive those stimuli. Investigation and measurement of anosognosia are difficult, but in general, the term can be applied whenever there is a significant discrepancy between the patient's report of his or her disabilities and the objective evidence regarding his or her level of functioning.

The "stimulus input" in this situation comprises a set of signals hailing from various parts of intra- and extrapersonal space. These include signals from visceral and musculoskeletal systems from both sides of the body, as well as extrapersonal signals pertinent to the current status of the body. Normally, these signals find a comprehensive meeting ground in a group of right-hemisphere cortices, which includes the primary somatosensory region (areas 3, 1, and 2 in the parietal lobe), somatosensory association cortices in the insula, and a secondary somatosensory region known as S2 in the depth of the sylvian fissure. In anosognosia, such signals fail to trigger appropriate neural records. For example, the somatic signals that would denote the presence of a paralyzed arm do not activate the pertinent neural regions that would allow the patient to become conscious of this perception. Physiologically, then, anosognosia corresponds to the inability of somatosensory percepts to activate pertinently linked memories that would give them appropriate meaning. There is a disruption of the continually updated representation of normal somatic and psychological states and their placement in autobiographical context.

Anosognosia is strongly associated with damage to the right somatosensory cortices in the parietal and insular regions. It is rarely observed in connection with left-hemisphere dysfunction, producing an arrangement that mirrors the situation regarding language (where there is an overwhelming dominance by the left hemisphere). This reflects the fact that the right hemisphere has a relative specialization for the processing of somatic information, in keeping with its relative specialization in emotional and affective processing.

The ventromedial frontal region, including the orbital and lower mesial frontal cortices, is another frequent neural correlate of anosognosia (Damasio et al. 1990d). Damage to this area is commonly produced by head injury, rupture of anterior cerebral or anterior communicating artery aneurysms, or tumors. Such patients frequently manifest severe agnosognosia for acquired defects in social conduct and decision making. For example, patients manifest a striking unawareness of the fact that their poor decisions have produced a steady record of personal catastrophes in terms of interpersonal relationships, social rank, and occupational endeavors. The patients demonstrate little insight into the relationship between their own behavior and the responses of those around them.

Related Conditions

Anosognosia should be distinguished from several closely related conditions. One is *anosodiaphoria*, a condition in which a patient acknowledges but fails to appreciate the significance of acquired impairments in physical or psychological function. Although anosodiaphoria is not a true form of agnosia, in practice there is a certain degree of overlap between anosodiaphoria and anosognosia. In fact, it is common to observe that blatant forms of anosognosia, such as denial of hemiplegia, tend to evolve over time, as the patient recovers, into various degrees of anosodiaphoria. Anosognosia and anosodiaphoria are both associated with left-sided neglect, especially visual neglect. Another condition is psychological denial of illness, which should be reserved for situations in which patients under severe stress are making an adaptive psychological response that permits them to cope with the calamitous consequences of disease.

Another condition refers to a disorder of body schema (Benton and Sivan 1993). Body schema disturbances are conditions in which patients become unable to localize various parts of their bodies. The most common manifestations are *autotopagnosia*, *finger agnosia*, and *right-left disorientation* (the latter two being essentially partial forms of the first). Autotopagnosia is a condition in which the patient loses the ability to identify parts of the body, either to verbal command or by imitation. In its most severe form, the disorder affects virtually all body parts; however, this is rare, and it is far more common to observe partial forms of the condition, including deficits in finger localization (finger agnosia) and right-left discrimination.

THE APRAXIAS

Apraxia is a broad term that has been used to refer to a wide variety of conditions in which patients lose the ability to execute skilled or learned movements as a consequence of acquired brain disease. The term has been used in conjunction with various neuropsychological disabilities such as constructional apraxia, dressing apraxia, gait apraxia, gaze apraxia, apraxic agraphia, and verbal (speech) apraxia. The essence of the concept, however, refers to an acquired disability in the execution of a learned and skilled motor action on command that cannot be accounted for by basic defects in motor or sensory functions. In principle, such a condition could occur in relationship to virtually any skilled movement, but in practice, there are only a few types of apraxia that occur with some regularity and that have been properly studied. The current discussion will focus on the better-understood manifestations of apraxia, including limb-kinetic, ideomotor, ideational, and buccofacial.

Limb-Kinetic Apraxia

Definition and Examination

Limb-kinetic apraxia involves a specific motor disability of one limb, usually an arm, in the absence of gross weakness or ataxia. The most common manifestation is difficulty in the manipulation of small objects and with fine finger movements, despite normal or near-normal hand and arm strength. For example, the patient will be unable to pick up a dime off a flat surface and will have to slide the coin to the edge of the table and let it fall into the hand. Limb-kinetic apraxia is hard to quantify, and its neuroanatomical correlates are poorly understood. There is some disagreement as to whether this should even be considered a true form of apraxia, and many modern neurologists believe that this type of disability reflects mild pyramidal or corticospinal tract dysfunction or an elementary motor deficit.

Ideomotor Apraxia

Definition and Examination

Ideomotor apraxia constitutes the most frequent and best-understood form of apraxia. It is the type most clinicians are referring to when they simply describe a patient as having "apraxia." It refers to the condition in which a patient becomes unable to carry out a motor command, despite adequate comprehension of the command and adequate motor and sensory functions to perform the command. Ideomotor apraxia is distinguished from *ideational apraxia*, which refers to conditions in which patients fail to execute commands because they have lost the *idea* of the motor program; that is, the basic concept of the movement is lacking. In ideomotor apraxia, the concept is normal (or near normal) but the execution is deficient.

Praxis can be assessed by asking the patient to perform a variety of skilled movements, including symbolic gestures (e.g., saluting, waving) and pantomiming the use of tools (e.g., hammering, sawing). Reviews of this topic provide good sources for comprehensive testing procedures for praxis (Heilman and Rothi 1993; Kirshner 1991). It is important to test the patient in two basic paradigms: *verbal command*, in which the patient is asked verbally to produce a movement (e.g., "show me how to use a scissors"), and *imitation*, in which the patient is asked to imitate a movement produced by the examiner. If both of these tests are failed, the examiner should determine whether the patient can perform actions when allowed to use actual objects. This assessment will help establish whether the patient actually does conjure up the concepts of various actions and fails to perform them (which conforms to ideomotor apraxia), or whether there is a more fundamental defect in the conjuring up of motor concepts (ideational apraxia). Also, most investigators recommend using stimuli that vary in (1) whether or not an object is usually involved (e.g., waving versus hammering), (2) whether the action is proximal or distal, and (3) the principal muscle groups involved (fingers, hand, arm).

In cases in which there is hemiparesis or hemianesthesia, testing of praxis is most meaningful in the ipsilesional limb, because defects in the contralesional (sensorimotor impaired) limb are not of interest with regard to the diagnosis of apraxia. The patient with ideomotor apraxia will have difficulty especially in the proper execution of the spatial components of a movement. For example, the patient will not orient make-believe scissors correctly when asked to cut paper or will not maintain the correct orientation of a make-believe knife when asked to slice bread. Sequencing and timing errors, as well as perseveration, are also common in apraxic patients. Typically, errors are more pronounced for stimuli that involve a pretend object (e.g., "Pretend you are using a hammer"), and the patient will perform relatively better at symbolic gestures (e.g., "How do you wave goodbye?") or when allowed to perform an action while actually holding the implement (as opposed to pantomiming).

Neuroanatomical Correlates

Ideomotor apraxia is strongly associated with damage to the left hemisphere, and it is a frequent, although not invariable, accompaniment of aphasia. Apraxia in right-handers is nearly always associated with left hemisphere lesions. The most common area of damage is the parietal region, especially the inferior parietal lobule (areas 40 and 39). Left-sided lesions to the basal ganglia and supplementary motor area also can cause ideomotor apraxia. The strong association between left hemisphere lesions and apraxia is in keeping with the specialization of left hemisphere structures in most individuals for the execution of skilled, learned motor movements (which are strongly correlated with hand preference).

There is an intriguing, albeit rare, condition in which apraxia develops in the left limbs, following damage to the anterior corpus callosum (so-called *callosal apraxia*). This presentation has been explained as a result of disconnection between the left and right supplementary motor areas. Anterior callosal damage prevents the right supplementary motor area (and adjacent motor cortex) from receiving motor program information from homologous regions on the left (which are specialized for such processing), leading to ideomotor apraxia of the left limbs.

Ideational Apraxia

Definition and Examination

Ideational apraxia is a term applied to conditions in which patients are apraxic because they have lost the *concepts* (ideas) behind skilled movements. As in ideomotor apraxia, the patient loses the capacity to pantomime the use of an object or to execute symbolic gestures. In *ideational apraxia*, however, the patient cannot indicate by any means a basic understanding of the concept behind the action. Thus, patients will fail even when presented with the actual object. In a paradigmatic case, the patient will name and define an object (e.g., "that's a hammer, used for pounding nails in") but not know how to manipulate the object when it is placed in the hand.

In the early descriptions of ideational apraxia, emphasis was placed on the inability to perform a sequence of actions in which the order is critical (e.g., filling, lighting, and smoking a pipe). Recent authors presented somewhat different definitions of the term and, for example, emphasized the defective execution of actions even when the actual object was provided or the complete inability to perform a motor response when given a verbal command (Heilman and Rothi 1993). The net result has been enormous confusion about what the term actually means, and now it is difficult to find even roughly equivalent definitions of the concept from one source to another. Kirshner (1991) advocated abandoning the term altogether and suggested it be replaced by terms such as *apraxia for sequential acts* or *apraxia for actual objects.*

Neuroanatomical Correlates

Traditionally, ideational apraxia has been associated with lesions in the left parieto-occipital junction, situated slightly posteriorly to those that produce ideomotor apraxia. Pure cases of ideational apraxia, however, are exceedingly rare, and the localizing value of the condition has been repeatedly questioned. Full-blown ideational apraxia is associated with bilateral parieto-occipital lesions. Such lesions, of course, are rare, and thus the condition appears infrequently. Perhaps the most common neuropathological conditions to cause lesions of this type are degenerative, such as Alzheimer's disease and perhaps Pick's disease. To the extent that this is true, ideational apraxia as an isolated symptom is rare in the extreme.

Buccofacial Apraxia

Definition, Examination, and Neuroanatomical Correlates

In *buccofacial (oral) apraxia,* the patient cannot perform learned skilled movements of the mouth, lips, cheeks, tongue, and throat, but the disorder cannot be attributed to paresis or other elementary motor impairments. For example, when asked to perform actions such as "blow out a match," "whistle," "blow a kiss," or "suck a straw," the patient will be unable to pantomime the action. Typically, the patient also fails when asked to imitate the examiner's pantomiming of such actions, leading to the conclusion that the defect cannot be attributed to defective language comprehension. Patients usually improve their performance if they are allowed to use the actual object (e.g., blowing out a real match).

Buccofacial apraxia has been considered a special form of ideomotor apraxia, but in fact, the two conditions can be dissociated. Thus, a patient may have buccofacial but not ideomotor apraxia, or vice versa. Also, studies have demonstrated different lesion correlates for the two conditions. Ideomotor apraxia is more marked and frequent following damage to the left inferior parietal operculum. Buccofacial apraxia, by contrast, is more strongly associated with damage to the frontal operculum, and also with lesions in the central operculum and anterior insula.

Buccofacial apraxia is distinct from *apraxia of speech*, the latter being an increasingly popular term used to refer to the phonological selection and sequencing defects observed in nonfluent aphasia. There is, in fact, a high incidence of buccofacial apraxia in nonfluent aphasics, but the term apraxia of speech should be reserved for the speech-related component of defective articulation, leaving buccofacial apraxia as the term to be applied to disorders of nonverbal facial gesture. Whether the two conditions might actually share a common underlying mechanism remains unclear, but the fact that they can be dissociated implies that the mechanism is not necessarily the same.

REFERENCES

Benton AL, Hamsher K, Varney NR, Spreen O. Contributions to Neuropsychological Assessment. New York: Oxford University Press, 1983.

Benton AL, Sivan AB. Disturbances of Body Schema. In KM Heilman, E Valenstein (eds), Clinical Neuropsychology (3rd ed). New York: Oxford University Press, 1993:123–140.

Caselli RJ. Rediscovering tactile agnosia. Mayo Clin Proc 1991;66:129–142.

Damasio AR. Disorders of Complex Visual Processing: Agnosias, Achromatopsia, Balint's Syndrome, and Related Difficulties of Orientation and Construction. In M-M Mesulam (ed), Principles of Behavioral Neurology. Philadelphia: FA Davis, 1985;259–288.

Damasio AR. Time-locked multiregional retroactivation: A systems level proposal for the neural substrates of recall and recognition. Cognition 1989a;33:25–62.

Damasio AR. The brain binds entities and events by multiregional activation from convergence zones. Neural Computation 1989b;1:123–132.

Damasio AR, Damasio H. Cortical Systems for Retrieval of Concrete Knowledge: The Convergence Zone Framework. In C Koch, JL Davis (eds), Large-Scale Neuronal Theories of the Brain. Cambridge, MA: MIT Press, 1994;61–74.

Damasio AR, Damasio H, Tranel D. Impairments of Visual Recognition as Clues to the Processes of Categorization and Memory. In GM Edelman, WE Gall, WM Cowan (eds), Signal and Sense: Local and Global Order in Perceptual Maps. New York: Wiley-Liss, 1990a;451–473.

Damasio AR, Damasio H, Tranel D, Brandt JP. Neural regionalization of knowledge access: Preliminary evidence. Symposia on Quantitative Biology, Vol. 55. Cold Spring Harbor Laboratory Press, 1990b: 1039–104.

Damasio AR, Tranel D. Nouns and verbs are retrieved with differently distributed neural systems. Proc Natl Acad Sci USA 1993;90:4957–4960.

Damasio AR, Tranel D, Bellugi U et al. Selective impairment of concept retrieval through a tactile channel. Society for Neuroscience Abstracts 1992;18:1207.

Damasio AR, Tranel D, Damasio H. Face agnosia and the neural substrates of memory. Annu Rev Neurosci 1990c;13:89–109.

Damasio AR, Tranel D, Damasio H. Individuals with sociopathic behavior caused by frontal damage fail to respond autonomically to social stimuli. Behav Brain Res 1990d;40:193–200.

Heilman KM, Rothi LJ. Apraxia. In KM Heilman, E Valenstein (eds), Clinical Neuropsychology (3rd ed). New York: Oxford University Press, 1993;141–163.

Hooper HE. Hooper Visual Organization Test. Los Angeles: Western Psychological Services, 1983.

Kirshner HS. The Apraxias. In WG Bradley, RB Daroff, GM Fenichel, CD Marsden (eds), Neurology in Clinical Practice, Vol. 1. Boston: Butterworth-Heinemann, 1991;117–122.

Lezak M. Neuropsychological Assessment (2nd ed). New York: Oxford University Press, 1983.

Tranel D. What has been rediscovered in "Rediscovering tactile agnosia"? Mayo Clin Proc 1991;66:210–214.

Tranel D, Damasio AR. Nonconscious face recognition in patients with face agnosia. Behav Brain Res 1988;30:235–249.

Tranel D. Assessment of higher-order visual function. Curr Opinion Ophthalmol 1994;5:29–37.

Tranel D, Damasio AR, Damasio H. Intact recognition of facial expression, gender, and age in patients with impaired recognition of face identity. Neurology 1988;38:690–696.

Van Lancker D, Kreiman J, Cummings J. Voice perception deficits: Neuroanatomical correlates of phonagnosia. J Clin Exp Neuropsychol 1989;11:665–674.

SUGGESTED READING

Damasio AR. Concepts in the brain. Mind Lang 1989;4:24–28.

Damasio AR. Category-related recognition defects as a clue to the neural substrates of knowledge. TINS 1990;13:95–98.

Damasio AR, Damasio H. Cortical Systems Underlying Knowledge Retrieval: Evidence from Human Lesion Studies. In TA Poggio, DA Glaser (eds), Exploring Brain Functions: Models in Neuroscience. New York: Wiley, 1993;233–248.

Damasio AR, Tranel D, Damasio H. Similarity of structure and the profile of visual recognition defects: a comment on Gaffan and Heywood. J Cogn Neurosci 1993;5:371–372.

Chapter 12
Language Disorders

A. APHASIA

Howard S. Kirshner

The study of language disorders involves the analysis of that most human of attributes, the ability to communicate through common symbols. Symbolic communication provided the foundation of human civilization and learning, and so has been the province of philosophers as well as of physicians. The study of language, however, also has a practical use in neurological diagnosis. Language was the first higher cortical function to be correlated with specific sites of brain damage, and it still serves as a model for the practical use of a cognitive function in the localization of brain lesions and for the understanding of human cortical processes in general.

Aphasia is defined as a disorder of language, acquired secondary to brain damage. This definition, adapted from that of Alexander and Benson (1992), separates aphasia from several related disorders. First, aphasia is distinguished from congenital or developmental language disorders, called *dysphasias*. It is recommended that the term *dysphasia* be used for developmental language disorders rather than for partial or incomplete aphasia.

Second, aphasia is a disorder of language, rather than of speech. Speech refers to the articulation and phonation of language sounds; language is a complex system of communication symbols and rules for their use. Aphasia is distinguished from motor speech disorders, which include dysarthria, dysphonia (voice disorders), stuttering, and speech apraxia. Dysarthrias are disorders of articulation of single sounds. Dysarthria may result from mechanical disturbance of the tongue or larynx or from neurological disorders including dysfunction of the muscles, neuromuscular junction, cranial nerves, bulbar anterior horn cells, corticobulbar tracts, cerebellar connections, or basal ganglia. Apraxia of speech is a syndrome in which series of single sounds (*phonemes*) cannot be articulated properly, in the absence of the consistent abnormal articulation of phonemes that characterizes dysarthria. In theory, the disorder is an apraxia because there is no primary motor deficit in articulation of individual phonemes. Clinically, speech-apraxic patients produce inconsistent errors of phoneme substitution and omission. Apraxia of speech, so defined, is commonly involved in speech production difficulty in the aphasias.

Third, aphasia is distinguished from disorders of thought. Thought involves the mental processing of images, memories, and perceptions, usually but not necessarily involving language symbols. Psychiatric disorders derange thought and alter the content of speech, without affecting its linguistic structure. Schizophrenic patients, for example, may manifest bizarre and individualistic word choices, with loose associations and a loss of organization in discourse (Benson 1989). Such psychiatric disorders are not considered aphasias. Language disorders associated with diffuse brain diseases, such as encephalopathies and dementias, are disorders of language, but the involvement of other cognitive functions distinguishes them from aphasia secondary to focal brain lesions.

An understanding of language disorders requires an elementary review of linguistic components. These include

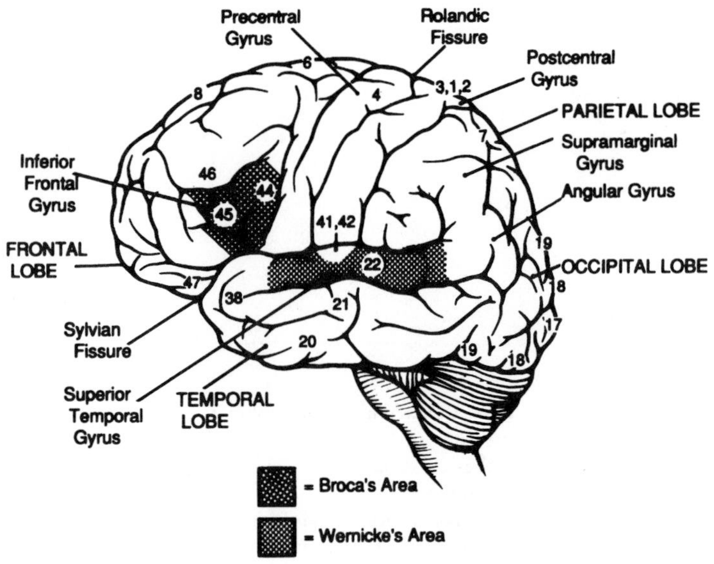

FIGURE 12A.1 Diagram of the lateral surface of the left hemisphere, showing a simplified gyral anatomy and the relationships between Wernicke's area and Broca's area. Not shown is the arcuate fasciculus, which connects the two cortical speech centers in the deep, subcortical white matter.

phonemes, the smallest meaning-carrying sounds; morphology, the use of appropriate word endings and connector words for tenses, possessives, and singular versus plural; semantics, or word meanings; lexicon, the internal dictionary; syntax, the grammatical construction of phrases and sentences; and discourse, the use of these elements to create organized and logical expression. Specific language disorders affect one or more of these elements.

Language processes have a clear neuroanatomic basis. In simplest terms, reception of spoken language is processed by the auditory system, beginning with the cochlea and proceeding through a series of way stations to the auditory cortex, *Heschl's gyrus*, in each superior temporal gyrus. The decoding of sounds into linguistic information involves the posterior part of the left superior temporal gyrus, *Wernicke's area* or *Brodmann area 22*, which in turn accesses a network of cortical associations to assign word meanings. For both repetition and spontaneous speech, auditory information is transmitted to *Broca's area* in the posterior inferior frontal gyrus. This area of cortex "programs" neurons in the adjacent motor cortex subserving the mouth and larynx, from which descending axons travel to the brain stem cranial nerve nuclei. These anatomic relationships are shown in Figures 12A.1 and 12A.2. Reading requires the perception of visual language stimuli by the occipital cortex, followed by correlation with auditory language information, via the intermodality association cortex of the angular gyrus. Writing involves the activation of motor neurons projecting to the arm and hand.

These pathways, and doubtless others, constitute the cortical circuitry for language comprehension and expression. In addition, other cortical centers involved in cognitive processes project into the primary language cortex, influencing the content of language. Finally, subcortical structures play increasingly recognized roles in language functions. The thalamus, a relay for the reticular activating system, appears to alert the language cortex, and lesions of the dominant thalamus frequently produce language disorders. Nuclei of the basal ganglia involved in motor functions, especially the caudate nucleus and putamen, participate in expressive speech. No wonder, then, that language disorders are seen in a wide variety of left hemisphere lesions and are important in practical neurological diagnosis and localization.

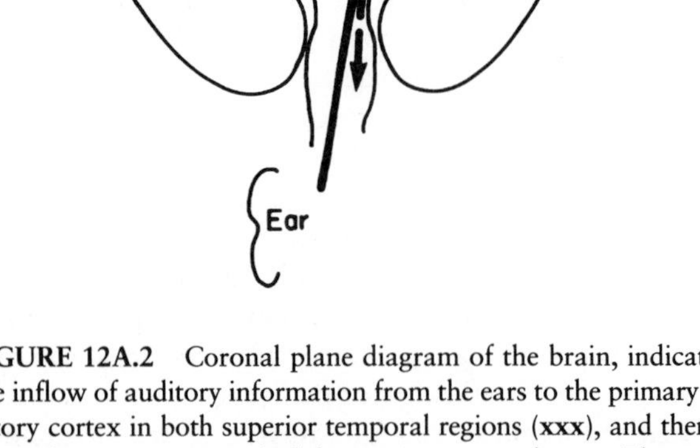

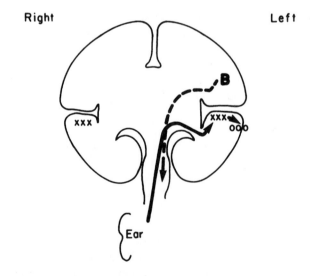

FIGURE 12A.2 Coronal plane diagram of the brain, indicating the inflow of auditory information from the ears to the primary auditory cortex in both superior temporal regions (**xxx**), and then to Wernicke's area (**ooo**) in the left superior temporal gyrus. The motor outflow of speech descends from Broca's area (B) to the cranial nerve nuclei of the brain stem via the corticobulbar tract (dashed arrow). In actuality, Broca's area is anterior to Wernicke's area, and the two areas would not appear in the same coronal section.

In right-handed people, and in a majority of left-handers as well, the left hemisphere is dominant for language functions. Most clinical syndromes of aphasia result from left hemisphere lesions. Language functions may be less rigidly localized in left-handed persons, such that a lesion of either hemisphere may produce language dysfunction; some left-handed persons may have a "Broca's area" in the right hemisphere but a "Wernicke's area" in the left hemisphere, or vice-versa. Recovery from aphasia also may be better in left-handers than right-handers, although one series has found only minor differences between matched left- and right-handed patients with aphasia.

SYMPTOMS AND DIFFERENTIAL DIAGNOSIS OF DISORDERED LANGUAGE

Muteness, a total loss of speech, may represent severe aphasia (see section on Aphemia). Muteness can also be a sign of dysarthria, frontal lobe dysfunction with akinetic mutism, severe extrapyramidal system dysfunction as in Parkinson's disease, nonneurological disorders of the larynx and pharynx, or even psychogenic syndromes such as catatonia. Caution must therefore be taken in diagnosing the mute patient as aphasic. A good rule of thumb is that if the patient can write or type, and the language form and content are normal, the disorder is probably not aphasic in origin. If the patient cannot speak or write but makes apparent effort to vocalize, and if there is also evidence of deficient comprehension, aphasic muteness is likely. Associated signs of a left hemisphere injury, such as right hemiparesis, also aid in diagnosis. Finally, if the patient gradually begins to make sounds containing paraphasic errors, aphasia can be identified with confidence.

Hesitant speech is likewise a symptom of aphasia but also of motor speech disorders such as dysarthria or stuttering. A second rule of thumb is that if one can transcribe the utterances of a hesitant speaker into normal language, the patient is not aphasic. Hesitancy occurs in many aphasia syndromes for varying reasons, including difficulty in speech initiation, imprecise articulation of phonemes, deficient syntax, or word-finding difficulty.

Anomia, or inability to produce a specific name, is generally a reliable indicator of language disorder, though it may also reflect memory loss. Anomia is manifest in aphasic speech by word-finding pauses and circumlocutions, or use of a phrase where a single word would suffice.

Paraphasic speech refers to the presence of errors in the patient's speech output. Paraphasic errors are divided into "literal" or "phonemic" errors, involving substitution of an incorrect sound (e.g., "shoon" for "spoon"); and "verbal" or "semantic" errors, involving substitution of an incorrect word (e.g., "fork" for "spoon"). A related language symptom is *perseveration*, the inappropriate repetition of a previous response. Occasionally, aphasic utterances involve nonexistent word forms called *neologisms*. When paraphasic errors and neologisms so contaminate speech that the meaning cannot be discerned, the pattern is called *jargon speech*.

Another cardinal symptom of aphasia is the failure to comprehend the speech of others. Most aphasic patients also have difficulty with comprehension and production of written language, or reading and writing.

Fluent, paraphasic speech usually makes an aphasic disorder obvious. The chief differential diagnosis here is between aphasia, acute encephalopathy or delirium, and dementia. Aphasic patients are usually not confused or inappropriate in behavior; they do not act agitated or misuse objects, with occasional exceptions such as acute Wernicke's or global aphasia. In addition, most psychotic patients speak in an easily understood, grammatically appropriate manner, although their behavior and speech content are abnormal. Only rarely do schizophrenics speak in "clang association" or "word salad" speech. Sudden onset of fluent, paraphasic speech in a middle-aged or elderly patient should always be suspected to represent a left hemisphere lesion with aphasia.

Patients with acute encephalopathies may manifest paraphasic speech and "higher" language disorders such as inability to write, but the grammatical expression of language is less disturbed than its content. These language symptoms, moreover, are less prominent than accompanying behavioral disturbances such as agitation, hallucinations, drowsiness, or excitement, and cognitive difficulties such as disorientation, memory loss, and delusional thinking.

Chronic encephalopathies, or dementias, pose a more difficult diagnostic problem, since involvement of the language cortex produces readily detectable language deficits, especially involving naming, reading, and writing. These language disorders, which will be discussed later, differ from aphasia secondary to focal lesions mainly by the involvement of other cognitive functions, such as memory and visuospatial processes.

BEDSIDE LANGUAGE EXAMINATION

The first part of any bedside examination of language is the observation of the patient's speech and comprehension during the clinical interview. Considerable information about language function can be obtained, if the examiner pays deliberate attention to the patient's speech patterns and responses to questions.

Benson and Geschwind popularized a bedside language examination of six parts, updated by Alexander and Benson (1992); see Table 12A.1. This examination provides useful localizing information about brain dysfunction and is well worth the few minutes it takes.

The first part of the examination is a description of *spontaneous speech*. A speech sample may be elicited by asking the patient to describe the weather or the reason for coming to the doctor. If speech is sparse or absent, recitation of lists, such as counting or listing days of the week, may be

Table 12A.1: Bedside language examination

1. Spontaneous speech
a. Informal interview
b. Structured task
c. Automatic sequences
2. Naming
3. Auditory comprehension
4. Repetition
5. Reading
a. Reading aloud
b. Reading comprehension
6. Writing
a. Spontaneous sentences
b. Writing to dictation
c. Copying

helpful. The most important variable in spontaneous speech is fluency: Fluent speech flows rapidly and effortlessly, while nonfluent speech is uttered in single words or short phrases, with frequent pauses and hesitations. Attention should first be paid to such elementary characteristics as initiation difficulty, articulation, phonation or voice volume, rate of speech, prosody or melodic intonation of speech, and phrase length. Second, the content of speech utterances should be analyzed in terms of the presence of word-finding pauses, circumlocutions, and errors such as literal and verbal paraphasias and neologisms.

Naming, the second part of the bedside examination, is tested by asking the patient to name objects, object parts, pictures, colors, or body parts to confrontation. A few items from each category should be tested, since anomia can be specific to word classes. The ability to say proper names of persons is often affected severely, as assessed using pictures of famous people. The examiner should ask questions to be sure that the patient recognizes the items or persons that he or she cannot name.

Auditory comprehension is tested first by asking the patient to follow a series of commands of one, two, and three steps. An example of a one-step command is "stick out your tongue"; a two-step command is "hold up your left thumb and close your eyes." Successful following of commands ensures adequate comprehension, at least at this simple level, but failure to follow commands does not automatically establish a loss of comprehension. The patient must hear the command, speak the same language as the examiner, and possess the motor ability to execute it, including absence of apraxia. Apraxia is discussed in Chapter 11 but is defined operationally as the inability to carry out a motor command despite normal comprehension and normal ability to carry out the motor act in another context, such as to imitation or with use of a real object. Since apraxia is difficult to exclude with confidence, it is advisable to test comprehension by tasks that do not require a motor act, such as yes-no questions, or by commands that require only a pointing response. The responses to nonsense questions such as "Do you vomit every day?" quickly establish whether the patient is comprehending. Nonsense questions often produce surprising results, given the tendency of some aphasics to cover up comprehension difficulty with social chatter.

Repetition of words and phrases should be deliberately tested. Dysarthric patients have difficulty with rapid sequences of consonants, such as "Methodist Episcopal," whereas aphasics have special difficulty with grammatically complex sentences. The phrase "no ifs, ands, or buts" is especially challenging for aphasics. Aphasics can often repeat familiar or "high probability" phrases much better than unfamiliar ones.

Reading should be tested both aloud and for comprehension. The examiner should carry a few printed commands, to facilitate a rapid comparison of auditory versus reading comprehension. Of course, the examiner must have some idea of the patient's premorbid reading ability.

Writing, the element of the bedside examination most often omitted, not only provides a further sample of expressive language but also allows an analysis of spelling, which is not possible with spoken language. A writing specimen may be the most sensitive indicator of mild aphasia, and it provides a permanent record for future comparison. Spontaneous writing, such as a sentence describing why the patient has come for examination, is especially sensitive for the detection of language difficulty. When this fails, writing to dictation and copying should be tested as well.

Finally, the neurologist combines the results of the bedside language examination with those of the rest of the mental status examination and of the neurological examination in general. These "associated signs" help both in the classification of the type of aphasia and in the localization of the responsible brain lesion.

DIFFERENTIAL DIAGNOSIS OF APHASIC SYNDROMES

Broca's Aphasia

In 1861, the French physician Broca described two patients, thus establishing the aphasic syndrome that now bears his name. The speech pattern is nonfluent; on bedside examination, the patient speaks hesitantly, often producing the principal, meaning-containing nouns and verbs but omitting the small grammatical words and morphemes. This pattern is called *agrammatism* or *telegraphic speech*. An example is "wife come hospital." Patients with acute Broca's aphasia may be mute or may produce only single words, often with dysarthria and apraxia of speech. They make many phonemic errors, inconsistent from utterance to utterance, but with substitution of phonemes differing only slightly from the correct target (e.g., "p" for "b") (Blumstein 1991). Naming is deficient, but the patient often manifests a "tip of the tongue" phenomenon, getting out the first letter or phoneme of the correct name. Paraphasic errors in naming

Table 12A.2: Bedside features of Broca's aphasia

Feature	*Syndrome*
Spontaneous speech	Nonfluent: mute or telegraphic, usually dysarthric
Naming	Impaired
Comprehension	"Intact" (mild difficulty with complex grammatical phrases)
Repetition	Impaired
Reading	Often impaired ("third alexia")
Writing	Impaired (dysmorphic, dysgrammatic)
Associated signs	Right hemiparesis
	Right hemisensory loss
	± Apraxia of left limbs

are more frequently of literal than verbal type. Auditory comprehension seems intact, but detailed testing usually reveals some deficiency, particularly in the comprehension of complex syntax. For example, sentences with embedded clauses involving prepositional relationships cause difficulty for Broca's aphasics in comprehension as well as in expression. Repetition is hesitant in these patients, resembling their spontaneous speech. Reading is often impaired, despite relatively preserved auditory comprehension. Benson in 1977 termed this reading difficulty of Broca's aphasics the "third alexia," in distinction to the two classical types of alexia to be discussed later. Broca's aphasics may have difficulty with syntax in reading, just as in auditory comprehension and speech. Writing is virtually always deficient in Broca's aphasics. Most patients have a right hemiparesis, necessitating use of the nondominant, left hand for writing, but this left-handed writing is far more abnormal than the awkward renditions of a normal, right-handed subject. Many patients can scrawl only a few letters.

Associated neurological deficits of Broca's aphasics include right hemiparesis, hemisensory loss, and apraxia of the oral apparatus and of the nonparalyzed left limbs. Apraxia in response to motor commands is important to recognize, since it may be mistaken for comprehension disturbance. Therefore comprehension should be tested by responses to yes-no questions or commands to point to an object. The common features of Broca's aphasia are listed in Table 12A.2.

An important clinical feature of Broca's aphasia is its frequent association with depression (Benson and Ardila 1993). Patients with Broca's aphasia are typically aware of and frustrated by their deficits. At times they become withdrawn and refuse help or therapy. Usually, the depression lifts as the deficit recovers, though it may be a limiting factor in rehabilitation.

The lesions responsible for Broca's aphasia usually include the traditional Broca's area in the posterior part of the inferior frontal gyrus, along with damage to adjacent cortex and subcortical white matter. Most patients with lasting Broca's aphasia, including Broca's original cases, have much larger left frontoparietal lesions, including most of the territory of the upper division of the left middle cerebral artery. Such patients typically evolve from global to Broca's aphasia over weeks to months. Patients who manifest Broca's aphasia immediately after their strokes, by contrast, have smaller lesions of the inferior frontal region, and their deficits generally resolve quickly. In computed tomography (CT) scan analyses by the group at the Boston Veterans Administration Medical Center (Alexander et al. 1990), lesions restricted to the lower precentral gyrus produced only dysarthria and mild expressive disturbance; those involving the traditional Broca's area (Brodmann areas 44 and 45) resulted in difficulty initiating speech; and lesions combining Broca's area, the lower precentral gyrus, and subcortical white matter yielded the full syndrome of Broca's aphasia. Damage to two subcortical white matter sites—the rostral subcallosal fasciculus deep to Broca's area and the periventricular white matter adjacent to the body of the left lateral ventricle—are required to cause permanent nonfluency. Figure 12A.3 shows a magnetic resonance imaging (MRI) scan from a case of Broca's aphasia.

Aphemia

A rare variant of Broca's aphasia is *aphemia*, a nonfluent syndrome in which the patient is initially mute, then able to speak with phoneme substitutions and pauses. All other language functions are intact, including writing. This rare and usually transitory syndrome results from small lesions of Broca's area or its subcortical white matter or of the inferior precentral gyrus. Since written expression and auditory comprehension are normal, aphemia is not a true language disorder; aphemia may be equivalent to pure apraxia of speech.

Wernicke's Aphasia

Wernicke's aphasia may be considered a syndrome opposite to Broca's aphasia, in that expressive speech is fluent but comprehension is impaired. The speech pattern is effortless and sometimes even excessively fluent ("*logorrhea*"). A speaker of a foreign language notices nothing amiss, but a listener who shares the patient's language detects speech empty of meaning, containing verbal paraphasias, neologisms, and jargon productions. Neurolinguists refer to this pattern as *paragrammatism*. In milder cases, the intended meaning of an utterance may be discerned, but the sentence goes awry with paraphasic substitutions. Naming in Wernicke's aphasia is deficient, often with bizarre, paraphasic substitutions for the correct name. Auditory comprehension is impaired, sometimes even for simple nonsense questions. Auditory perception of phonemes is deficient in Wernicke's aphasia, but deficient semantics is the major cause of the compre-

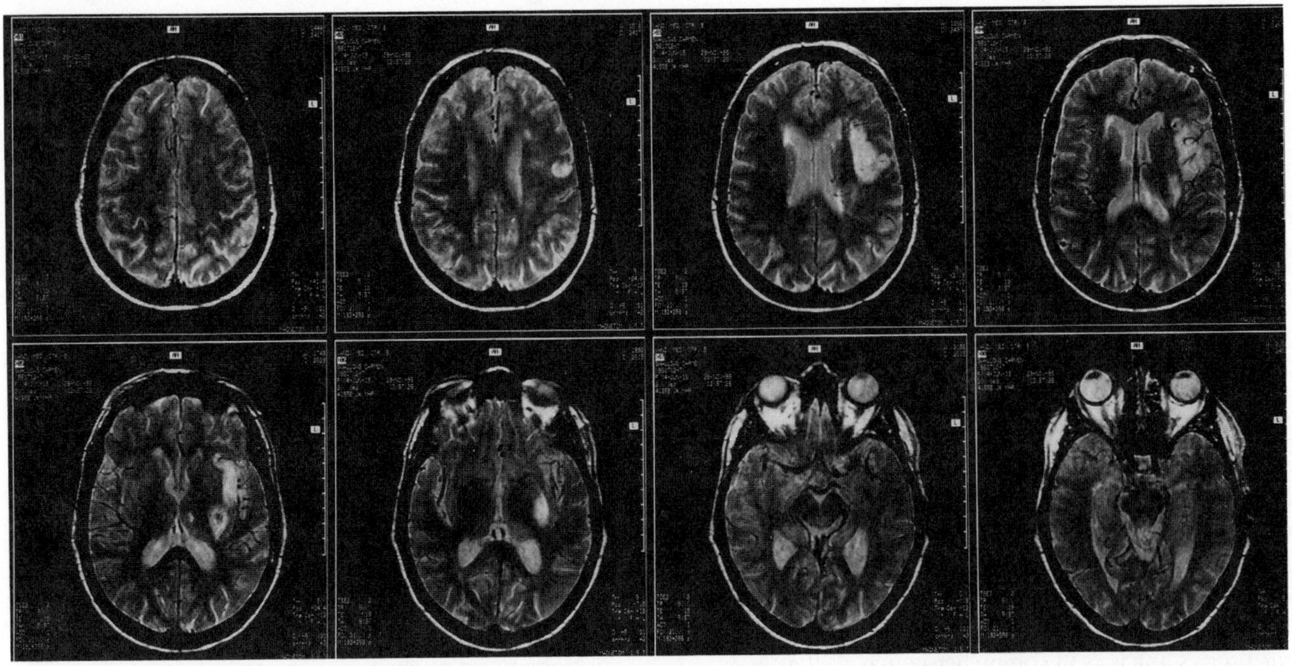

FIGURE 12A.3 MRI scan from a patient with Broca's aphasia. The cortical Broca's area, subcortical white matter, and insula were all involved in the infarction. The patient made a good recovery.

hension disturbance (Blumstein 1991); disturbed access to semantics and to the internal lexicon is central to the deficit of Wernicke's aphasia. Repetition is impaired; whispering a phrase in the patient's ear, as in a hearing test, may help cue the patient to attempt repetition. Reading comprehension is usually affected similarly to auditory comprehension, but occasional patients show greater deficit in one modality. The discovery of spared reading ability in Wernicke's aphasics is important in allowing these patients to communicate and also in refining neurolinguistic theories of reading, which must include access of visual language images to semantic interpretation, even in the absence of auditory comprehension (Margolin 1991). Writing is also impaired, but in a manner quite different from that of the Broca's aphasic.

Table 12A.3: Bedside features of Wernicke's aphasia

Feature	*Syndrome*
Spontaneous speech	Fluent, with paraphasic errors Usually not dysarthric Sometimes logorrheic
Naming	Impaired (often bizarre paraphasic misnamings)
Comprehension	Impaired
Repetition	Impaired
Reading	Impaired for comprehension, reading aloud
Writing	Well-formed, paragraphic
Associated signs	± Right hemianopsia Motor, sensory signs usually absent

The patient usually has no hemiparesis and can grasp the pen and write easily. Written productions are even more abnormal than oral ones, however, in that errors in spelling are also evident. Writing samples are especially useful in the detection of mild Wernicke's aphasia.

Associated signs are limited in Wernicke's aphasia; most patients have no elementary motor or sensory deficits, though a partial or complete right homonymous hemianopsia may be present. The characteristic bedside examination findings in Wernicke's aphasia are summarized in Table 12A.3.

The psychiatric manifestations of Wernicke's aphasia are quite different from those of Broca's aphasia. Depression is much less common; many Wernicke's aphasics seem unaware of or unconcerned about their communicative deficits. With time, some patients become angry or paranoid about the inability of family members and medical staff to understand them. This behavior, like depression, may hinder rehabilitative efforts.

The lesions of patients with Wernicke's aphasia are usually in the posterior portion of the superior temporal gyrus, sometimes extending into the inferior parietal lobule. Figure 12A.4 shows a typical example. The exact confines of Wernicke's area have been controversial. Damage to Wernicke's area (Brodmann area 22) has been reported to correlate most closely with persistent loss of comprehension of single words, though others (Kertesz et al. 1993) have found only larger temporoparietal lesions in patients with lasting Wernicke's aphasia. Electrical stimulation of Wernicke's area produces consistent interruption

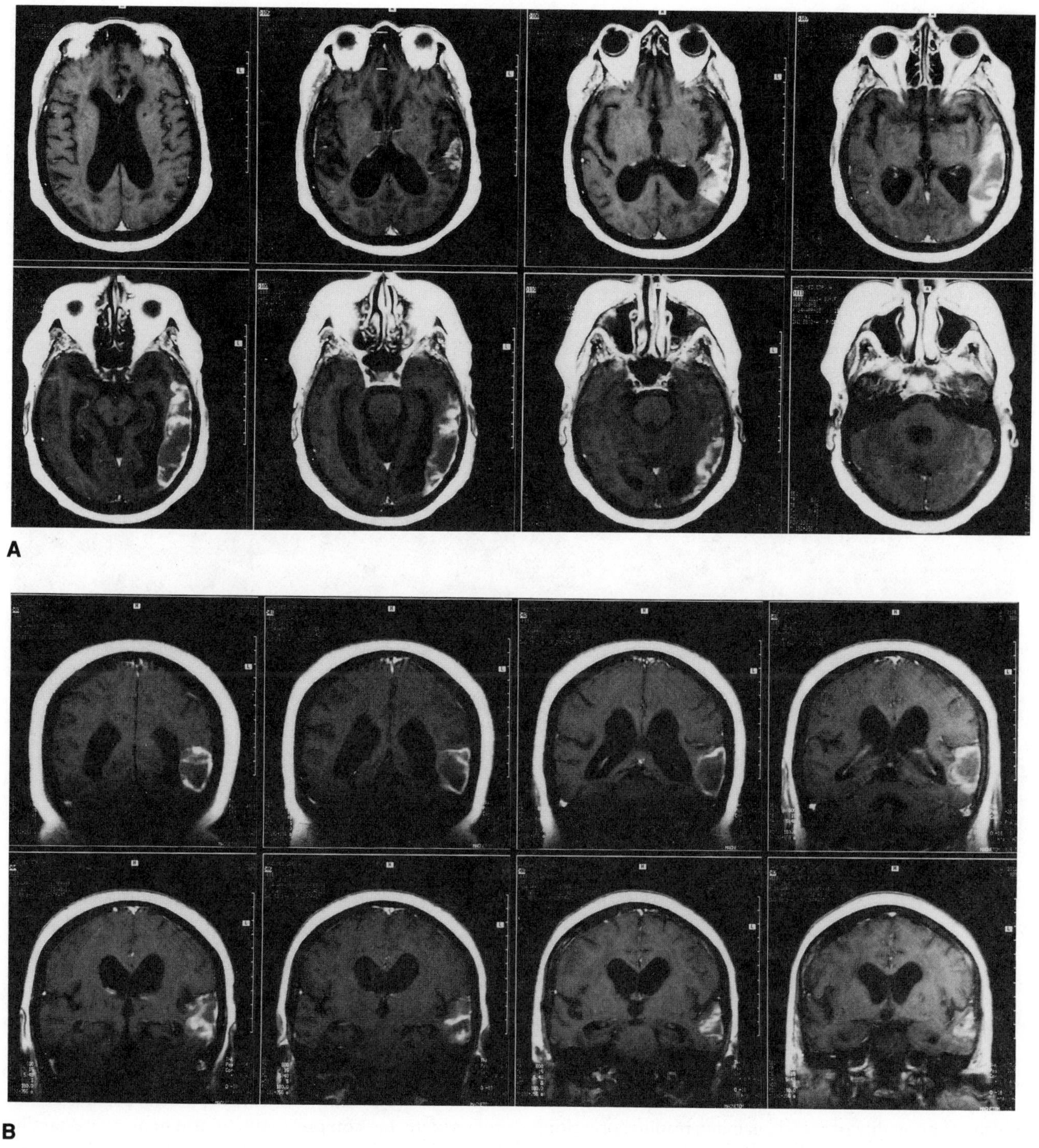

FIGURE 12A.4 Axial and coronal MRI slices (A and B) and an axial PET scan (C) (page 138) view of an elderly woman with Wernicke's aphasia. There is a large left, superior temporal lobe lesion. The onset of the deficit was not clear, and the PET scan was useful in showing that the lesion had reduced metabolism, favoring a stroke over a tumor.

of auditory comprehension, supporting the importance of this region for decoding of auditory language. A receptive speech area in the left inferior temporal gyrus has also been suggested by electrical stimulation studies, but aphasia has not been recognized with destructive lesions of this area. Extension of the lesion into the inferior parietal region may predict greater involvement of reading comprehension. In terms of vascular anatomy, Wernicke's area lies within the territory of the inferior division of the left middle cerebral artery.

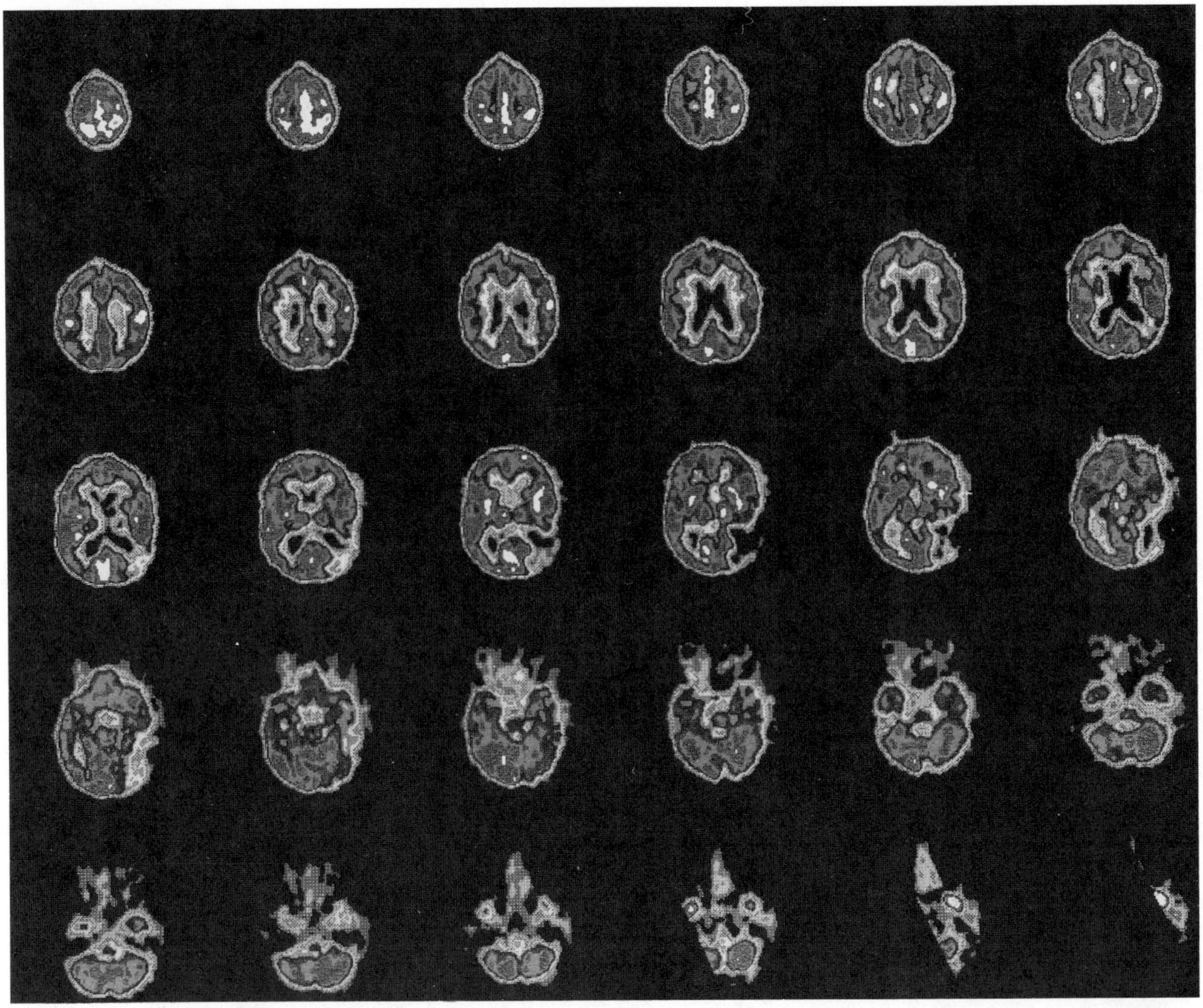

C

FIGURE 12A.4 *(continued)*

Pure Word Deafness

Pure word deafness is a rare but striking syndrome of isolated loss of auditory comprehension and repetition, without any abnormality of speech, naming, reading, or writing. Hearing for pure tones and for nonverbal noises such as animal cries is intact. Most cases have mild aphasic deficits, especially paraphasic speech. Classically, the causative lesion is a bilateral lesion, isolating Wernicke's area from input from both Heschl's gyri. Pure word deafness is thus an example of a "disconnection syndrome," in which the deficit results from loss of white matter connections rather than of gray matter language centers. Some cases of pure word deafness, however, have unilateral, left temporal lesions (Takahashi et al. 1992). These cases closely resemble Wernicke's aphasia with greater impairment of auditory comprehension than of reading.

Global Aphasia

Global aphasia may be thought of as a summation of the deficits of Broca's and Wernicke's aphasia. Speech is nonfluent or mute, but comprehension is also poor, as are naming, repetition, reading, and writing. Most patients have dense right hemiparesis, hemisensory loss, and often hemianopsia, although occasional patients have little hemiparesis. Milder aphasic syndromes in which all modalities of language are affected are often called "mixed" aphasias. The lesions of patients with global aphasia are usually large, involving both the inferior frontal and superior temporal regions, and often much of the parietal lobe in between. This lesion represents most of the territory of the left middle cerebral artery. Patients in whom the superior temporal gyrus is spared tend to recover their auditory comprehension and to evolve toward the syndrome of Broca's aphasia (Naeser et al. 1990).

Table 12A.4: Bedside features of global aphasia

Feature	*Syndrome*
Spontaneous speech	Mute or nonfluent
Naming	Impaired
Comprehension	Impaired
Repetition	Impaired
Reading	Impaired
Writing	Impaired
Associated signs	Right hemiparesis
	Right hemisensory loss
	Right hemianopsia

Table 12A.5: Bedside features of conduction aphasia

Feature	*Syndrome*
Spontaneous speech	Fluent, some hesitancy, literal paraphasic errors
Naming	May be moderately impaired
Comprehension	Intact
Repetition	Severely impaired
Reading	± Inability to read aloud; some reading comprehension
Writing	Variable deficits
Associated signs	± Apraxia of left limbs
	± Right hemiparesis, usually mild
	± Right hemisensory loss
	± Right hemianopsia

Recovery in global aphasia may be prolonged; global aphasics may recover more during the second than the first 6 months after a stroke. Characteristics of global aphasia are presented in Table 12A.4.

Conduction Aphasia

Conduction aphasia is an uncommon but theoretically important syndrome that can be remembered by its striking deficit of repetition. Most patients have relatively normal spontaneous speech, though some make literal paraphasic errors and hesitate frequently for self-correction. Naming may be impaired, but auditory comprehension is preserved. Repetition may be disturbed to seemingly ridiculous extremes, such that a patient who can express himself or herself at a sentence level and comprehend conversation may be unable to repeat even single words. One such patient could not repeat the word "boy" but said "I like girls better." Reading and writing are somewhat variable, but reading aloud may share some of the same difficulty as repeating. Associated deficits include hemianopia in some patients; right-sided sensory loss may be present, but right hemiparesis is usually mild or absent. Some patients have limb apraxia, creating a misimpression that comprehension is impaired. Bedside examination findings in conduction aphasia are summarized in Table 12A.5.

The lesions of conduction aphasia are usually in either the superior temporal or inferior parietal regions. Benson and associates in 1973 suggested that patients with limb apraxia have parietal lesions, while those without apraxia have temporal lesions. Conduction aphasia may represent a stage of recovery in patients with Wernicke's aphasia in whom the damage to the superior temporal gyrus is not complete.

Conduction aphasia has been advanced as a classical disconnection syndrome. Wernicke originally postulated that a lesion disconnecting Wernicke's and Broca's area would produce this syndrome; Geschwind later pointed to the arcuate fasciculus, a white matter tract traveling from the deep temporal lobe, around the sylvian fissure to the frontal lobe, as the site of disconnection. Anatomic involvement of the arcuate fasciculus is present in most if not all cases of conduction aphasia, but there is usually also cortical involvement of the supramarginal gyrus or temporal lobe. Others have pointed out that lesions of the arcuate fasciculus do not always produce conduction aphasia. Another theory of conduction aphasia has involved a defect in auditory verbal short-term memory (Shallice and Warrington, 1977).

Anomic Aphasia

Anomic aphasia refers to aphasic syndromes in which naming, or access to the internal lexicon, is the principal deficit. Spontaneous speech is normal except for the pauses and circumlocutions produced by the inability to name. Comprehension, repetition, reading, and writing are intact, except for the same word-finding difficulty in written productions. Anomic aphasia is common but less specific in localization than other aphasic syndromes. Isolated, severe anomia may indicate focal left hemisphere pathology. Alexander and Benson (1992) refer to the angular gyrus as the site of lesions producing anomic aphasia, but lesions there usually produce other deficits as well, including alexia and the four elements of the Gerstmann syndrome: agraphia, right-left disorientation, acalculia, and finger agnosia, or inability to identify fingers. Isolated lesions of the temporal lobe can produce pure anomia (Damasio, 1992), and positron emission tomography (PET) studies of naming in normal subjects have also shown consistent activation of the superior temporal lobe (Frith et al. 1991). Anomia is also seen with mass lesions elsewhere in the brain, however, and in diffuse, degenerative disorders such as Alzheimer's disease. Anomic aphasia is also a common stage in the recovery of many aphasic syndromes. Anomic aphasia thus serves as an indicator of left hemisphere or diffuse brain disease, but it has only limited localizing value. The typical features of anomic aphasia are presented in Table 12A.6.

Transcortical Aphasias

The transcortical aphasias are syndromes in which repetition is normal, presumably because the causative lesions do not disrupt the perisylvian language circuit

Table 12A.6: Bedside features of anomic aphasia

Feature	*Syndrome*
Spontaneous speech	Fluent, some word-finding pauses, circumlocutions
Naming	Impaired
Comprehension	Intact
Repetition	Intact
Reading	Intact
Writing	Intact, except for anomia
Associated signs	Inconsistent

from Wernicke's area through the arcuate fasciculus to Broca's area. Instead, these lesions disrupt connections from other cortical centers into the language circuit (hence the name *transcortical*). The transcortical syndromes are easiest to think of as analogues of the syndromes of global, Broca's, and Wernicke's aphasia, with intact repetition. Thus *mixed transcortical aphasia*, or the syndrome of the isolation of the speech area, is a global aphasia in which the patient repeats, often echolalically, but has no propositional speech or comprehension. This syndrome is rare, occurring predominantly in large, watershed infarctions of the left or both hemispheres, sparing the perisylvian cortex, or in advanced dementias. *Transcortical motor aphasia* is an analogue of Broca's aphasia in which speech is hesitant or telegraphic, comprehension is relatively spared, but repetition is fluent. This syndrome occurs with lesions in the frontal lobe, anterior to Broca's area, and hence within the territory of the anterior cerebral artery. Disruption of the supplementary motor area or disconnection of this area from Broca's area by subcortical frontal white matter lesions may produce the syndrome. The occurrence of transcortical motor aphasia in an arterial territory other than the middle cerebral artery separates this syndrome from the many middle cerebral artery syndromes discussed previously. The third transcortical syndrome, *transcortical sensory aphasia*, is an analogue of Wernicke's aphasia in which fluent, paraphasic speech, paraphasic naming, impaired auditory and reading comprehension, and abnormal writing coexist with normal repetition. This syndrome is relatively uncommon, occurring in strokes of the left temporo-occipital area and in dementias. Bedside examination findings in the transcortical aphasias are summarized in Table 12A.7.

Subcortical Aphasias

A current area of interest in aphasia research involves the "subcortical" aphasias. While all of the syndromes discussed up to now have been defined by behavioral characteristics that can be diagnosed on the bedside examination, the subcortical aphasias are defined by lesion localization in the basal ganglia or deep cerebral white matter. As knowledge about subcortical aphasia has accumulated, a division has developed between aphasia with thalamic lesions and aphasia with lesions of the subcortical white matter and basal ganglia.

Left thalamic hemorrhages frequently produce a Wernicke-like fluent aphasia, with better comprehension than cortical Wernicke's aphasia. A fluctuating or "dichotomous" state has been described, alternating between an alert state with nearly normal language and a drowsy state in which the patient mumbles paraphasically and comprehends poorly. Luria has called this a "quasi-aphasic" abnormality of vigilance, in that the thalamus plays a role in alerting the language cortex. Thalamic aphasia can occur even with a right thalamic lesion in a left-handed patient, indicating that hemispheric language dominance extends to the thalamic level. A debate has continued as to whether thalamic aphasia is truly the result of specific damage to the thalamus and its connections, or of mass effect on cortical language areas. Thalamic aphasia has been described with small ischemic lesions, especially those involving the paramedian thalamus or anterior thalamus, in the territory of the tuberothalamic artery (Bogousslavsky et al. 1988). Since these lesions produce little or no mass effect, such cases indicate that the thalamus and its connections play a definite role in language function.

Hemorrhages in the vicinity of the left basal ganglia, especially involving the putamen, the most common site of hypertensive intracerebral hemorrhage, often produce aphasia. Here the aphasic syndromes are more variable, depending on the size of the hemorrhage, but most commonly involving global or Wernicke-like aphasia. As in thalamic lesions, ischemic strokes have provided better localizing information. The most common lesion is an infarct involving the anterior putamen, caudate nucleus, and anterior limb of the internal capsule. Patients with this lesion have an "anterior subcortical syndrome" involving dysarthria, decreased fluency, mildly impaired repetition as compared with Broca's aphasia, and mild comprehension disturbance

Table 12A.7: Bedside features of transcortical aphasias

Feature	*Isolation Syndrome*	*Transcortical Motor*	*Transcortical Sensory*
Speech	Fluent, echolalic	Nonfluent	Fluent, echolalic
Naming	Impaired	Impaired	Impaired
Comprehension	Impaired	Intact	Impaired
Repetition	Intact	Intact	Intact
Reading	Impaired	± Spared	Impaired
Writing	Impaired	± Spared	Impaired

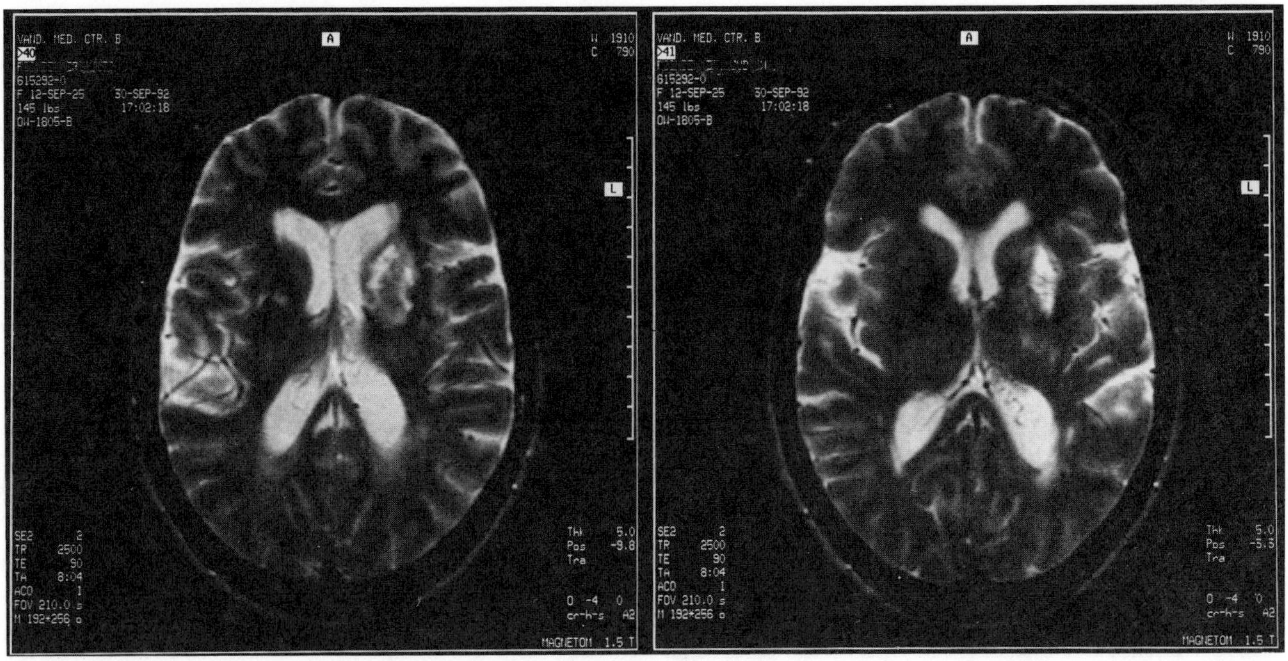

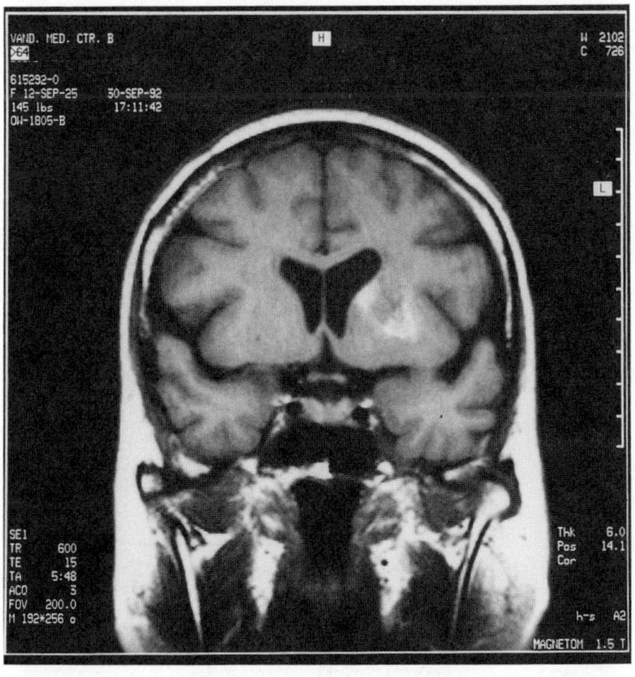

FIGURE 12A.5 MRI scan slices in the axial, coronal, and sagittal planes from a patient with subcortical aphasia. The lesion is an infarction involving the anterior caudate, putamen, and the anterior limb of the left internal capsule. The patient had dysarthria and mild, nonfluent aphasia with anomia, with good comprehension. The advantage of MRI in permitting visualization of the lesion in all three planes is apparent. (See continuation of figure on page 142.)

(Mega and Alexander 1994). Figure 12A.5 is an example of this syndrome. More restricted lesions of the anterior putamen, head of caudate, and periventricular white matter produce hesitancy or slow initiation of speech but little true language disturbance. More posterior lesions involving the putamen and deep temporal white matter referred to as the "temporal isthmus" are associated with fluent, paraphasic speech resembling Wernicke's aphasia. Small lesions in the posterior limb of the internal capsule and adjacent putamen cause mainly dysarthria, but mild aphasic deficits may occasionally occur. Finally, larger subcortical lesions involving both the anterior and posterior lesion sites produce global aphasia. Crosson (1985) proposed a model of subcortical involvement in language processes, based on the known motor functions and fiber connections of the basal ganglia. Evidence from PET suggests that basal ganglia lesions affect language both directly and indirectly, via decreased activation of cortical language areas.

In clinical terms, subcortical lesions do produce aphasia, though less commonly than cortical lesions, and the language characteristics of subcortical aphasias are often atypical. The presentation of a difficult-to-classify aphasic syndrome, in the presence of dysarthria and right hemiparesis, should lead to suspicion of a subcortical lesion.

Pure Alexia Without Agraphia

Alexia, or acquired inability to read, is a form of aphasia by the definition given at the beginning of this chapter. The first syndrome, pure alexia without agraphia, was described by the French neurologist Dejerine in 1892. This syndrome may be thought of as a linguistic blindfolding; the patient can

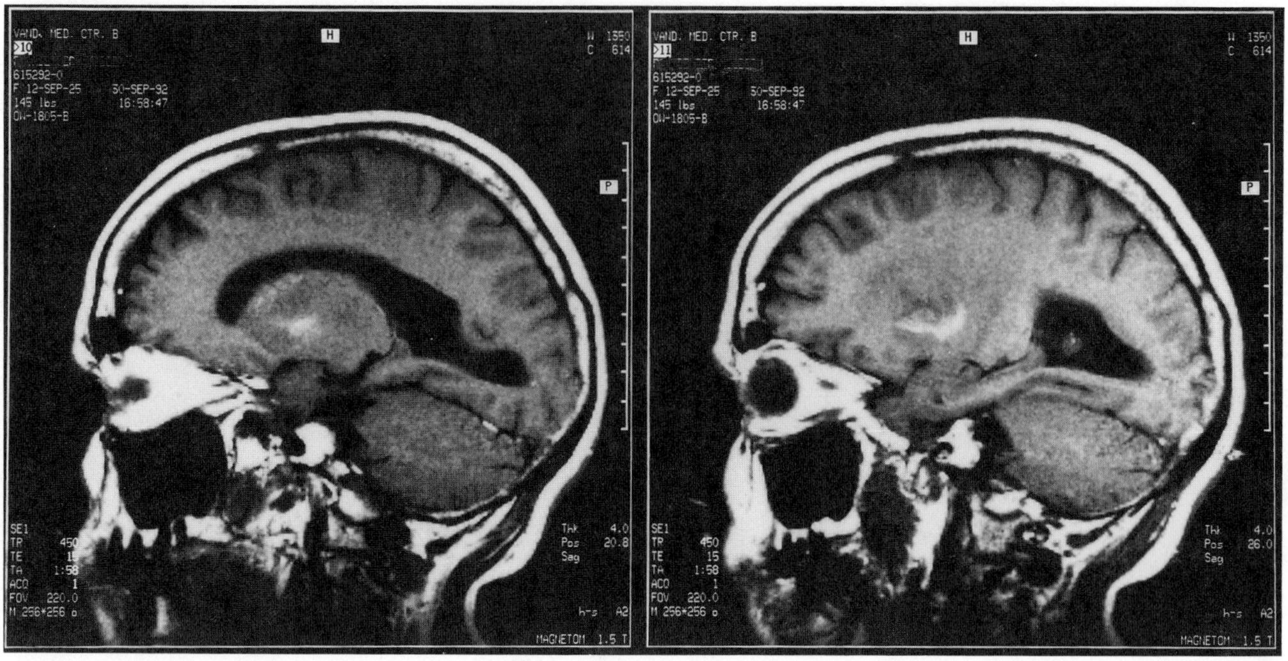

FIGURE 12A.5 *(continued)*

write but cannot read his or her own written productions. On the bedside examination, speech, auditory comprehension, and repetition are normal. Naming may be deficient, especially for colors. Patients initially cannot read at all; as they recover, they learn to read letter by letter, spelling out words in laborious fashion. They cannot read words at a glance, as normal readers do. By contrast, they quickly understand words spelled orally to them, and they can spell normally. Some patients can match words to pictures, indicating that there is some subconscious awareness of the word, perhaps in the right hemisphere. Associated deficits include a right hemianopsia or right upper quadrant defect in nearly all patients, and frequently a deficit of short-term memory. There is usually no hemiparesis or sensory loss.

The causative lesion in pure alexia is nearly always a stroke in the territory of the left posterior cerebral artery, with infarction of the medial occipital lobe, the splenium of the corpus callosum, and often the medial temporal lobe. Dejerine postulated a disconnection between the intact right visual cortex and left hemisphere language centers, particularly the angular gyrus. (Figure 12A.6 is an adaptation of Dejerine's original diagram.) Geschwind later rediscovered this disconnection hypothesis. While Damasio and Damasio (1983) found splenial involvement in only 2 of 16 cases, they postulated a disconnection within the deep white matter of the left occipital lobe. As in the disconnection hypothesis for conduction aphasia, the theory fails to explain all of the behavioral phenomena, such as the sparing of single letters. A deficit in short-term memory for visual language elements, or an inability to perceive multiple letters at once, can also

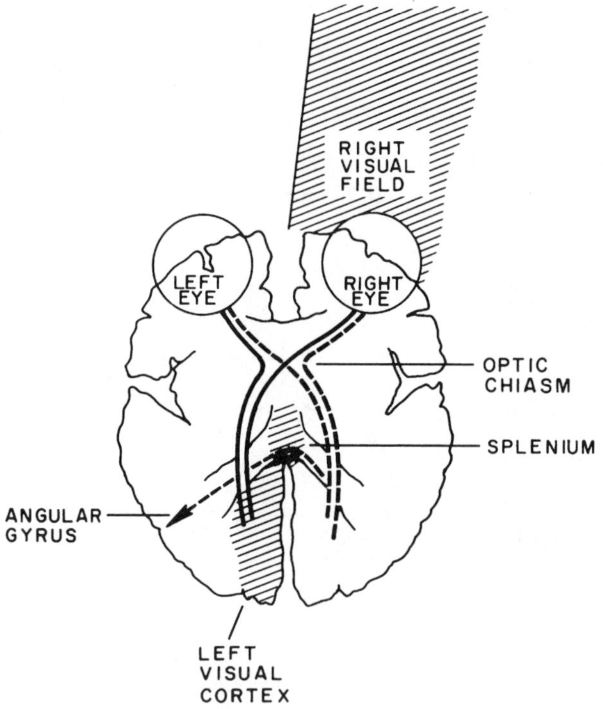

FIGURE 12A.6 Horizontal brain diagram of pure alexia without agraphia. Visual information from the left visual field reaches the right occipital cortex but is "disconnected" from the left hemisphere language centers by the lesion in the splenium of the corpus callosum. (Adapted from Dejerine, 1892.)

explain many features of the syndrome. Typical findings of pure alexia without agraphia are presented in Table 12A.8.

Alexia with Agraphia

The other classical alexia syndrome, alexia with agraphia, described by Dejerine in 1891, may be thought of as an acquired illiteracy, in which a previously educated patient is rendered unable to read or write. The oral language modalities of speech, naming, auditory comprehension, and repetition are largely intact, though many cases manifest a fluent, paraphasic speech pattern with impaired naming. This syndrome thus overlaps with Wernicke's aphasia, especially with those cases in which reading is more impaired than auditory comprehension. Associated deficits include right hemianopsia and elements of the Gerstmann syndrome: agraphia, acalculia, right-left disorientation, and finger agnosia. The lesions are typically in the inferior parietal lobule, especially the angular gyrus. Etiologies include strokes in the territory of the angular branch of the left middle cerebral artery or mass lesions in the same region. Characteristic features of the syndrome of alexia with agraphia are summarized in Table 12A.9.

Aphasic Alexia

In addition to the two classical alexia syndromes, many patients with aphasia have associated reading disturbance. Examples already cited are the *third alexia* syndrome of Broca's aphasia and the reading deficit of Wernicke's aphasia. Neurolinguists and cognitive psychologists have divided alexias according to breakdowns in specific stages of the reading process. The linguistic concepts of *surface* structure versus the *deep* meanings of words have been instrumental in these new classifications. Four patterns of alexia (or *dyslexia*, as English authors call it) have been recognized: *letter-by-letter, deep, phonological,* and *surface* dyslexia. Figure 12A.7 diagrams the steps in the reading process and the points of breakdown in the four syndromes. *Letter-by-letter dyslexia* is equivalent to pure alexia without agraphia. *Deep dyslexia* is a severe reading disorder in which patients recognize and read aloud only familiar words, and especially concrete, imageable nouns and verbs. They make semantic or visual errors in reading and fail completely in reading nonsense syllables or nonwords. Word reading is not affected by word length or by regularity of spelling; one patient, for example, could read "ambulance" but not "am." Most cases have severe aphasia, with extensive left frontoparietal damage.

Phonological dyslexia is similar to deep dyslexia, with poor reading of nonwords, but single nouns and verbs are read in a nearly normal fashion, and semantic errors are rare. Patients appear to read words without access to meaning. The fourth type, *surface dyslexia*, involves spared ability to read laboriously by grapheme-phoneme conversion, but inability to recognize words at a glance. These patients can read nonsense syllables but not words of irregular spelling, such as "colonel." Their errors tend to be phonological rather than semantic or visual; an example would be to pronounce "rough" and "though" alike.

Table 12A.8: Bedside features of pure alexia without agraphia

Feature	*Syndrome*
Spontaneous speech	Intact
Naming	± Impaired, especially colors
Comprehension	Intact
Repetition	Intact
Reading	Impaired (some sparing of single letters)
Writing	Intact
Associated signs	Right hemianopsia or superior quadrantanopsia
	Motor, sensory signs usually absent

Table 12A.9: Bedside features of alexia with agraphia

Feature	*Syndrome*
Spontaneous speech	Fluent, often some paraphasia
Naming	± Impaired
Comprehension	Intact, or less impaired than reading
Repetition	Intact
Reading	Severely impaired
Writing	Severely impaired
Associated signs	Right hemianopsia
	Motor, sensory signs usually absent

Agraphia

Like reading, writing may be affected either in isolation (*pure agraphia*) or in association with aphasia (*aphasic agraphia*). In addition, writing can be impaired by motor disorders, by apraxia, and by visuospatial deficits. Isolated agraphia has been described with left frontal or parietal lesions. Agraphias can be analyzed in the same way as the alexias (Figure 12A.8). Thus, *phonological agraphia* involves the inability to convert phonemes into graphemes or write pronounceable nonsense syllables, in the presence of ability to write familiar words.

Deep dysgraphia is similar to phonological agraphia, but with a marked superiority of nouns and verbs over other word types. In *lexical* or *surface dysgraphia*, patients can write regularly spelled words and pronounceable nonsense words but not irregularly spelled words. These patients have intact phoneme-grapheme conversion but cannot write by a whole word or "lexical" strategy.

Language in Right Hemisphere Disorders

Language and communication disorders are important even in patients with right hemisphere disease. First, left-handed

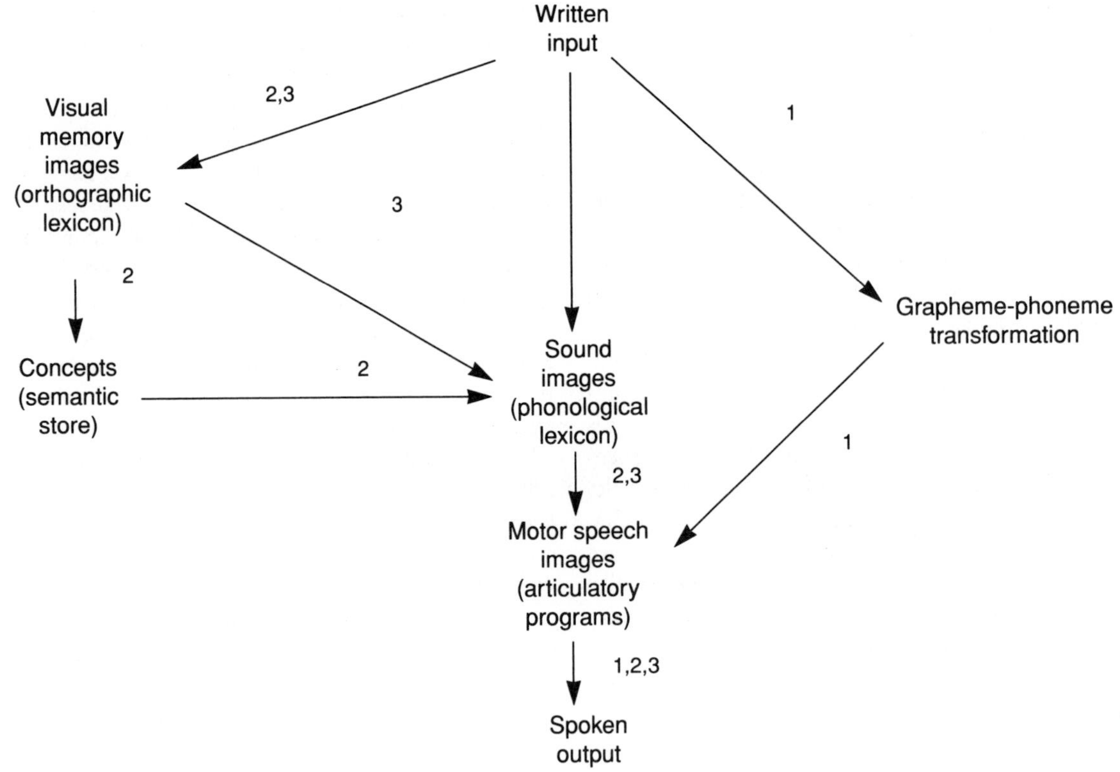

FIGURE 12A.7 Neurolinguistic model of the reading process. According to evidence from the alexias, there are three separate routes to reading: 1 is the phonological (or grapheme-phoneme conversion) route, 2 the semantic (or lexical-semantic-phonological) route, and 3 the nonlexical phonological route. In deep dyslexia, only route 2 can operate; in phonological dyslexia, 3 is the principal pathway; in surface dyslexia, only 1 is functional. (Adapted from DI Margolin. Cognitive neuropsychology. Resolving enigmas about Wernicke's aphasia and other higher cortical disorders. *Arch Neurol* 1991;48:751–765.)

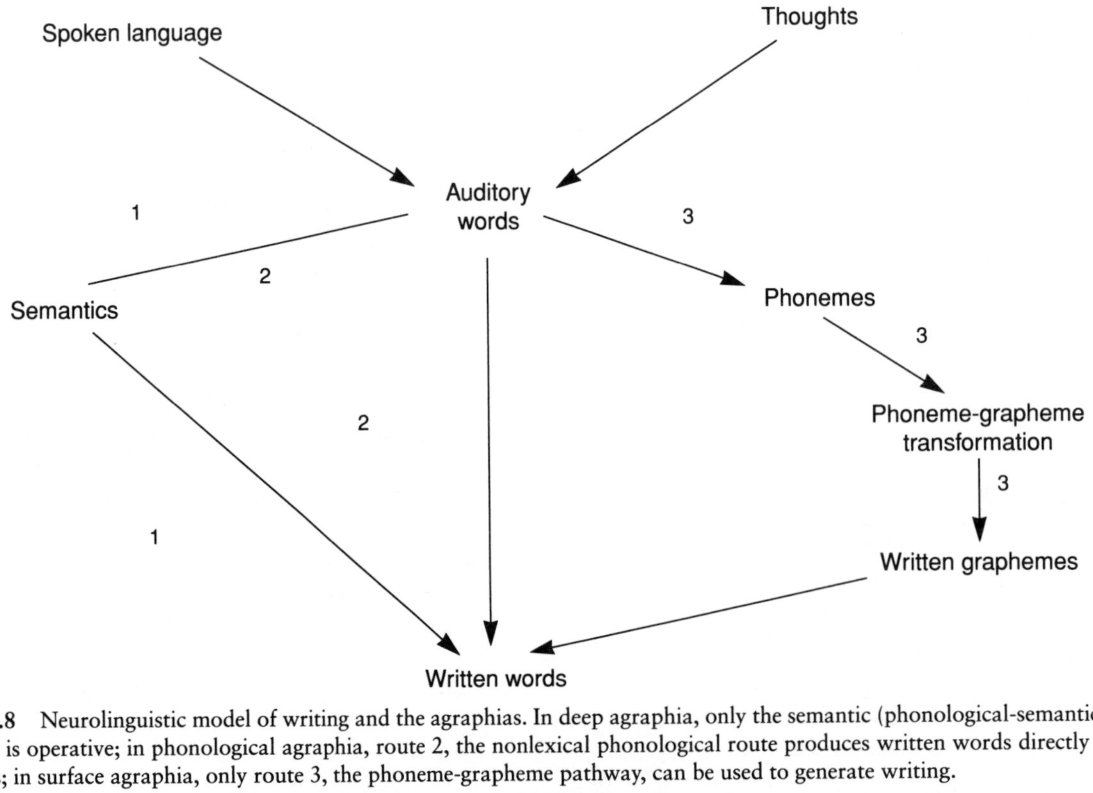

FIGURE 12A.8 Neurolinguistic model of writing and the agraphias. In deep agraphia, only the semantic (phonological-semantic-lexical) route (1) is operative; in phonological agraphia, route 2, the nonlexical phonological route produces written words directly from spoken words; in surface agraphia, only route 3, the phoneme-grapheme pathway, can be used to generate writing.

patients may have right hemisphere language dominance and may develop aphasic syndromes from right hemisphere lesions. Second, right-handed patients occasionally become aphasic after right hemisphere strokes, a phenomenon called "crossed aphasia in dextrals." These patients presumably have crossed or mixed dominance, more like that of left-handed patients. Third, even right-handed persons with typical left hemisphere dominance for language suffer subtle alterations in language function after right hemisphere damage. Such patients are not aphasic, in that the fundamental mechanisms of speech production, repetition, and comprehension are undisturbed. Affective aspects of language are impaired, however, such that the speech sounds flat and unemotional; the normal "prosody," or emotional intonation, of speech is lost. Syndromes of loss of emotional aspects of speech are termed *aprosodias*; for example, *motor aprosodia* involves loss of expressive emotion with preservation of emotional comprehension, whereas *sensory aprosodia* involves loss of comprehension of affective language. Stress and emphasis within a sentence are also affected by right hemisphere disease. Gardner and others have shown that metaphor, humor, sarcasm, irony, and related aspects of language that transcend the literal meaning of words are especially sensitive to right hemisphere disease. Such higher-level language deficits are related to the right hemisphere disorders of inattention and neglect, discussed in Chapters 4 and 41.

Language in Dementing Diseases

As mentioned previously, language impairment is commonly seen in patients with dementia. Despite considerable variability from patient to patient, two patterns of language dissolution can be described. The first, the common presentation of Alzheimer's disease, involves early loss of memory and general cognitive deterioration. In these patients, mental status examinations are most remarkable for deficits in short-term memory, insight, and judgment, but language impairments can be found in naming and in discourse, with impoverished language content and loss of abstraction and metaphor. The mechanics of language—grammatical construction of sentences, receptive vocabulary, auditory comprehension, repetition, and oral reading—tend to remain preserved until later stages. By aphasia testing, these patients have anomic aphasia. In later stages, language functions become more obviously impaired. Reading and writing, the last learned language functions, are among the first to deteriorate. Auditory comprehension later becomes deficient, while repetition and articulation remain normal. The language profile may then resemble that of transcortical sensory or Wernicke's aphasia. In terminal stages, speech becomes reduced to the expression of simple biological wants; eventually, even muteness can develop. By this time, most patients are institutionalized or bedridden.

The second pattern of language dissolution in dementia, considerably less common than the first, involves the gradual onset of a progressive aphasia, often without other cognitive deterioration. Auditory comprehension is involved early in the illness, and specific aphasic symptoms such as paraphasic or even nonfluent speech, misnamings, and errors of repetition are evident. These deficits worsen gradually, mimicking the course of a brain tumor or mass lesion rather than a typical dementia (Karbe et al. 1993). CT scans may show focal atrophy in the left perisylvian region, while electroencephalograph (EEG) studies may show focal slowing. PET has shown prominent areas of decreased metabolism in the left temporal region and adjacent cortical areas. The pathology underlying primary progressive aphasia is varied (Kertesz et al. 1994). Some cases show the frontotemporal, lobar atrophy of Pick's disease, while others may show a localized spongiform degeneration. Cases of isolated aphasia secondary to Creutzfeldt-Jakob disease and corticobasal degeneration have also been reported. Finally, a few patients with pathologically proved Alzheimer's disease have presented with focal involvement of the language cortex.

INVESTIGATION OF THE APHASIC PATIENT

Clinical Tests

The bedside language examination is useful in forming a preliminary impression of the type of aphasia and the localization of the causative lesion. Follow-up examinations are also helpful; as in all neurological diagnosis, the evolution of a neurological deficit over time is the most important clue to the specific disease process. For example, an embolic stroke and a brain tumor might both produce Wernicke's aphasia, but strokes occur suddenly, with improvement thereafter, whereas tumors produce gradually worsening aphasia.

In addition to the bedside examination, a large number of standardized aphasia test batteries have been published. The physician should think of these tests as more detailed extensions of the bedside examination. They have the advantage of quantitation and standardization, permitting comparison over time, and in some cases even a diagnosis of the specific aphasia syndrome. Research on aphasia depends on these standardized tests. For neurologists, the most helpful battery is the Boston Diagnostic Aphasia Examination (BDAE), or its Canadian adaptation, the Western Aphasia Battery (WAB). The BDAE and WAB provide subtest information analogous to the bedside examination and therefore meaningful to neurologists, as well as aphasia syndrome classification. The Porch Index of Communicative Ability quantitates performance in a number of specific functions, allowing comparison over time. Other aphasia tests are designed to evaluate specific language areas. For example, the Boston Naming Test evaluates a wide variety of naming stimuli, while the Token Test evaluates higher-level comprehension deficits. Further information on neuropsychological tests can be found in Chapter 41.

Further diagnosis of the aphasic patient rests on the confirmation of a brain lesion by neuroimaging. The CT brain scan, discussed in Chapter 39, revolutionized the localization of aphasia by permitting "real-time" delineation of a focal lesion in a living patient; previously, the physician had to outlive his or her patient to obtain a clinical-pathological correlation at autopsy. MRI scanning provides better resolution of areas difficult to see on CT, such as the temporal cortex adjacent to the petrous bones, and more sensitive detection of tissue pathology such as early changes of infarction. The anatomic distinction of cortical from subcortical aphasia is best made by MRI.

The EEG is helpful in aphasia in localizing seizure discharges, interictal spikes, and slowing seen after destructive lesions such as traumatic contusions and infarctions. The EEG can provide evidence that aphasia is an ictal or postictal phenomenon and can furnish early clues to aphasia secondary to mass lesions or to herpes simplex encephalitis.

Cerebral arteriography is useful in the diagnosis of aneurysms, arteriovenous malformations (AVMs), arterial occlusions, vasculitis, and venous outflow obstructions.

Single photon emission computed tomography (SPECT) and PET, discussed in Chapter 39, are contributing greatly to the study of language. Patterns of normal brain activation in response to language stimuli have been recorded (Posner et al. 1988), and the localizations of metabolic as well as structural changes in the brains of patients with aphasia secondary to stroke have been mapped. Subcortical contributions to aphasia and language in degenerative conditions have been studied with PET. These techniques provide the best correlation between brain structure and function currently available and should help advance our understanding of language disorders and their recovery.

Differential Diagnosis

Vascular lesions, especially ischemic strokes, are the most common causes of aphasia. Historically, most research studies in aphasia have used stroke patients, since stroke is an "experiment" of nature in which one area of the brain is damaged, while the rest remains theoretically intact. Strokes are characterized by the abrupt onset of a neurological deficit in a patient with vascular risk factors. The precise temporal profile is important; most embolic strokes are sudden and maximal at onset, whereas thrombotic strokes typically wax and wane or increase in steps. The bedside aphasia examination is helpful in delineating the vascular territory affected. For example, the sudden onset of Wernicke's aphasia nearly always indicates an embolus to the inferior division of the left middle cerebral artery. Global aphasia may be caused by an embolus to the middle cerebral artery stem, thrombosis of the internal carotid artery, or even a hemorrhage into the deep basal ganglia. Whereas most of aphasic syndromes involve the territory of the left middle cerebral artery, transcortical motor aphasia is specific to the anterior cerebral territory, pure alexia without agraphia to the posterior cerebral artery territory. The clinical features of the aphasia are thus of crucial importance to the vascular diagnosis.

Hemorrhagic strokes are also an important cause of aphasia, most commonly the basal ganglionic hemorrhages associated with hypertension. The deficits tend to worsen gradually over minutes to hours, in contrast to the sudden or stepwise onset of ischemic strokes. Headache, vomiting, and obtundation are more common in hemorrhages. Since hemorrhages compress cerebral tissue without necessarily destroying it, the ultimate recovery from aphasia is often better in hemorrhages than in ischemic strokes, though hemorrhages are more often fatal. Other etiologies of intracerebral hemorrhage include anticoagulants, head injury, blood dyscrasias, thrombocytopenia, vasculitis, and bleeding into structural lesions such as infarctions, tumors, AVMs, and aneurysms. Hemorrhages from AVMs mimic strokes, with abrupt onset of focal neurological deficit. Ruptured aneurysms, on the other hand, present with severe headache and stiff neck or with coma; most have no focal deficits, but delayed deficits such as aphasia may develop secondary to vasospasm. Lobar hemorrhages may occur in elderly patients without hypertension. These hemorrhages occur near the cortical surface, sometimes extending into the subarachnoid space, and they may be recurrent. Pathological studies have shown amyloid deposition in small arterioles, or amyloid angiopathy. A final vascular cause of aphasia is cerebral vasculitis, discussed in Chapter 56.

Traumatic brain injury is a common cause of aphasia. Cerebral contusions, depressed skull fractures, and hematomas of the intracerebral, subdural, and epidural spaces all cause aphasia when they disrupt or compress left hemisphere language structures. Trauma tends to be less localized than ischemic stroke, and thus aphasia is often admixed with the general effects of the head injury, such as depressed consciousness, encephalopathy or delirium, amnesia, and other deficits. Head injuries in young people may be associated with severe deficits yet excellent long-term recovery. Language deficits, especially involving discourse organization, can be found in most cases of significant closed head injury (Chapman et al. 1992). Gunshot wounds produce focal aphasic syndromes, which rival stroke as a source of clinical-anatomic correlation. Subdural hematomas are infamous for mimicking other neurological syndromes. Aphasia is occasionally associated with subdural hematomas overlying the left hemisphere, though it may be mild and may be overlooked because of the patient's more severe complaints of headache, memory loss, and drowsiness.

Tumors of the left hemisphere frequently present with aphasia. The onset of the aphasia is gradual, and other cognitive deficits may be associated because of edema and mass effect. Aphasia secondary to an enlarging tumor may thus be difficult to distinguish from a diffuse encephalopathy or early dementia. Therefore, any syndrome of abnormal language function should be investigated for a focal, dominant hemisphere lesion.

Infections of the nervous system may also cause aphasia. Brain abscesses can mimic tumors in every respect, and those in the left hemisphere can present with a slowly progressive aphasia. Chronic infections, such as tuberculosis or syphilis, can result in focal abnormalities that run the entire gamut of central nervous system symptoms and signs. Herpes simplex encephalitis has a predilection for the temporal lobe and orbital frontal cortex, and aphasia can be an early symptom, along with headache, confusion, fever, and seizures. Aphasia is often a permanent sequela in survivors of herpes encephalitis. Acquired immune deficiency syndrome (AIDS) is rapidly becoming a common cause of language disorders. Opportunistic infections can cause focal lesions anywhere in the brain, and the neurotropic human immunodeficiency virus (HIV) agent itself produces a dementia, in which language deficits play a part.

Aphasia is frequently caused by the degenerative central nervous system diseases. Reference has already been made to the focal, progressive aphasia in patients with Pick's disease and spongiform degenerations, as compared to the more diffuse cognitive deterioration characteristic of Alzheimer's disease. Language dysfunction in Alzheimer's disease may be more common in familial cases and may predict poor prognosis. Cognitive deterioration in patients with Parkinson's disease may also include language deterioration similar to that of Alzheimer's disease, though there tends to be more fluctuation in orientation and more tendency to active hallucinations and delusions in Parkinson's disease. A striking abnormality of speech with initial stuttering followed by true aphasia and dementia has been described in the dialysis dementia syndrome. This disorder may be associated with spongiform degeneration of the frontotemporal cortex, similar to Creutzfeldt-Jakob's disease. Paraphasic substitutions and nonsense speech are also occasionally encountered in acute encephalopathies such as hyponatremia or lithium toxicity.

A final etiology of aphasia is seizures, which can be associated with aphasia in children as part of the Landau-Kleffner syndrome or in adults as either an ictal or postictal *Todd's phenomenon*. This *epileptic aphasia* is important to recognize, in that anticonvulsant drug therapy can prevent the episodes, and unnecessary investigation or treatment for a new lesion such as a stroke can be avoided.

RECOVERY AND REHABILITATION OF APHASIA

Patients with aphasia from acute disorders such as stroke generally show spontaneous improvement over the first several months. In general, the greatest recovery occurs during the first 3 months, but improvement may continue over a prolonged period, especially in young patients and in global aphasics. The aphasia type often changes during recovery; global aphasia evolves into Broca's aphasia, Wernicke's aphasia into conduction or anomic aphasia (Pashek and Holland, 1988). Language recovery may be mediated by shifting of functions to the right hemisphere or to adjacent left hemisphere regions. Studies of activation of language areas by PET and SPECT scanning techniques promise to advance our understanding of the neuroanatomy of language recovery (Heiss et al. 1993).

Speech therapy, provided by speech-language pathologists, attempts to facilitate language recovery by a variety of techniques and to help the patient compensate for lost functions (see Chapter 55). Repeated practice in articulation and comprehension tasks has traditionally been used to stimulate improvement. Other techniques include melodic intonation therapy, which uses melody to involve the right hemisphere in speech production; visual action therapy, which uses gestural expression; treatment of aphasic perseveration program, which aims to reduce repetitive utterances; functional communication therapy, which takes advantage of extralinguistic communication; and cVIC or "Lingraphica," a computer program originally developed for primate communication. Patients who cannot speak can learn to produce simple sentences via computer. Augmentative devices make language expression possible through use of printers or voice simulators (Kratt, 1990). Speech therapy has remained controversial; while some studies have suggested that briefly trained volunteers can induce as much improvement as speech language pathologists, large, randomized trials have clearly indicated that patients who undergo formal speech therapy recover better than untreated patients.

Another approach to language rehabilitation is the use of pharmacologic agents to improve speech. Albert and colleagues (1988) reported that the dopaminergic drug bromocriptine promotes spontaneous speech output in transcortical motor aphasia. As new information accumulates on the neurochemistry of cognitive functions, other drug therapies may be forthcoming.

REFERENCES

Albert ML, Bachman DL, Morgan A, Helm-Estabrooks N. Pharmacotherapy for aphasia. Neurology 1988;38:877–879.

Alexander MP, Benson DF. The Aphasias and Related Disturbances. In RJ Joynt (ed), Clinical Neurology. Vol. 1. Philadelphia: Lippincott, 1992:1–58.

Alexander MP, Naeser MA, Palumbo C. Broca's area aphasias: aphasia after lesions including the frontal operculum. Neurology 1990;40:353–362.

Benson DF. Disorders of Verbal Expansion in Neuropsychiatry. In EH Reynolds, MR Trimble (eds), The Bridge Between Neurology and Psychiatry. London: Churchill Livingstone, 1989;88–105.

Benson DF, Ardila A. Depression in Aphasia. In SE Starkstein, RG Robinson (eds), Depression in Neurologic Disorders. Baltimore: Johns Hopkins University Press, 1993;152–164.

Blumstein SE. Phonological Aspects of Aphasia. In MT Sarno (ed), Acquired Aphasia (2nd ed). San Diego: Academic, 1991:151–180.

Bogousslavsky J, Regli F, Uske A. Thalamic infarcts: clinical syndromes, etiology, and prognosis. Neurology 1988;38:837–848.

Chapman SB, Culhane KA, Levin HS et al. Narrative discourse after closed head injury in children and adolescents. Brain Lang 1992;43:42–65.

Crosson B. Subcortical functions in language: a working model. Brain Lang 1985;25:257–292.
Damasio AR. Aphasia. N Engl J Med 1992;326:531–539.
Damasio AR, Damasio H. The anatomic basis of pure alexia. Neurology 1983;33:1,573–1,583.
Frith CD, Friston KJ, Liddle PF, Frackowiak RSJ. A PET study of word finding. Neuropsychologia 1991;29:1137–1148.
Heiss W-D, Kessler J, Karbe H et al. Cerebral glucose metabolism as a predictor of recovery from aphasia in ischemic stroke. Arch Neurol 1993;50:958–964.
Karbe H, Kertesz A, Polk M. Profiles of language impairment in primary progressive aphasia. Arch Neurol 1993;50:193–201.
Kertesz A, Hudson L, Mackenzie IRA, Munoz DG. The pathology and nosology of primary progressive aphasia. Neurology 1994;44:2065–2072.
Kertesz A, Lau WK, Polk M. The structural determinants of recovery in Wernicke's aphasia. Brain Lang 1993;44:153–164.
Kratt AW. Augmentative and alternative communication (AAC): does it have a future in aphasia rehabilitation? Aphasiology 1990;4:321–338.
Margolin DI. Cognitive neuropsychology. Resolving enigmas about Wernicke's aphasia and other higher cortical disorders. Arch Neurol 1991;48:751–765.
Mega MS, Alexander MP. Subcortical aphasia: the core profile of capsulostriatal infarction. Neurology 1994;44:1824–1829.
Naeser MA, Gaddie P, Palumbo CL, Stiassny Eder D. Late recovery of auditory comprehension in global aphasia. Improved recovery observed with subcortical temporal isthmus lesion versus Wernicke's cortical area lesion. Arch Neurol 1990;47:425–432.
Pashek GV, Holland AL. Evolution of aphasia in the first year post-onset. Cortex 1988;24:411–423.
Posner MI, Petersen SE, Fox PT, Raichle ME. Localization of cognitive operations in the human brain. Science 1988;240: 1627–1631.
Shallice T, Warrington EK. Auditory-verbal short-term memory impairment and conduction aphasia. Brain Lang 1977;4:479–491.
Takahashi N, Kawamura M, Shinotou H et al. Pure word deafness due to left hemisphere damage. Cortex 1992;28:295-303.

SUGGESTED READING

Kirshner HS (ed). Handbook of Neurological Speech and Language Disorders. New York: Marcel-Dekker, 1995.
Sarno MT (ed). Acquired Aphasia (2nd ed). San Diego: Academic, 1991.

B. DEVELOPMENTAL LANGUAGE DISORDERS

Ruth Nass

THE DIAGNOSIS OF DEVELOPMENTAL LANGUAGE DISORDERS

Developmental language disorder (DLD) is defined as the failure to develop normal language in a child with adequate intelligence. The extant accepted discrepancy criteria for identifying children with developmental language disorders have several shortcomings. For example, only 40–60% of children diagnosed with DLD by trained clinicians were identified using the Stanford Binet IQ test versus the Test of Language Development Discrepancy Scores. By contrast, using a standard deviation of 1, the Wechsler Performance IQ (a nonverbal test) versus the Peabody Picture Vocabulary Test (a specific language test) identified one-third of very low birth weight 7-year-olds and almost half of controls as having a DLD. A 2–standard deviation discrepancy criterion yielded 14% and 19% frequencies in these two groups. Therefore, both over- and underdiagnosis occur even when the best available and most commonly used criteria are applied (Aram et al. 1992). The difficulty in applying strict discrepancy criteria is caused, in part, by the large individual variability in rates of language acquisition. This variability makes it difficult to distinguish DLD from initial idiosyncratic language delay in children who will eventually speak normally, and probably accounts for the range of 1–25% in the reported prevalence of DLD in preschool children. The National Collaborative Perinatal Project identified low birth weight, prematurity, and parental mental retardation as risk factors for DLD. The strongest predictors of future language deficits were failure to vocalize to social stimuli and failure to vocalize two syllables at 8 months. Another important risk factor is a family history of DLD.

Overdiagnosis and treatment of young children with delayed speech is better than underdiagnosis. Hearing should be evaluated by audiological assessment in all children with isolated language delay. The availability of brain stem evoked responses, as well as behavioral audiometry, makes possible the assessment of even uncooperative young children. An electroencephalogram (EEG), including a sleep record, is appropriate in many children with isolated language delay to rule out subclinical seizures (Tuchman 1994).

SUBTYPES OF DEVELOPMENTAL LANGUAGE DISORDERS

The characteristic features, causes, prognosis, and treatment response of DLDs depend on their subtype. The subtypes defined by Rapin and colleagues (1991) focus on psycholinguistic features that approximate adult aphasias (Table 12B.1).

Articulation and Fluency Disorders

Pure Articulation Disorders

Articulatory skills improve with age, and the degree of normal variability is considerable. Sixty-nine percent of children speak intelligibly by 2 years, and only 16% of children are unintelligible by 3 years. However, even at 4 years, 50% of children have minor articulation problems, such as the defective use of [th] and/or [r], or have intelligible speech with some consonant substitutions other than, or in addition to, [th] and/or [r]. One-third of children continue to have minor to mild articulation defects at age 5 years, but speech is unintelligible in only 4%.

Stuttering

Stuttering is a disorder in the rhythm of speech. The speaker knows what to say but is unable to say it because of an involuntary, repetitive prolongation or cessation of a sound. Some degree of dysfluency is common as language skills evolve during the preschool years, particularly between 3 and 4 years, when the mean length of utterance reaches 6–8 words. However, stuttering, in contrast to developmental dysfluencies, is probably a language disorder rather than a speech disorder. It occurs more frequently in children with other types of developmental language disorders (Nippold 1990).

The cause of developmental stuttering is unknown. Genetic predisposition exists, and the main theoretical mechanisms are anomalous dominance, abnormalities of interhemispheric connections, or both. Supporting the theory

Table 12B.1: Developmental language disorders

	Verbal-Auditory Agnosia	*Semantic-Pragmatic*	*Phonolgic-Syntactic*	*Lexical-Syntactic*	*Verbal Dyspraxia*	*Phonological Programming*
Comprehension-receptive						
Phonology	↓↓	*	↓	*	*	*
Syntax	↓↓	*	↓	*	*	*
Semantics	↓↓	↓↓	?	↓	*	*
Production-expressive						
Semantics	↓↓	↓↓	↓	Nl or ↓	*	*
Syntax	↓↓	*	↓	↓	?	?
Phonology	↓↓	*	↓	*	↓	↓
Fluency	↓↓	Nl or ↓ or ↑	↓	↓	Nl or ↓	Nl or ↓
Pragmatics	Nl or ↓	↓↓	Nl or ↓	↓	*	*

↓↓ = very impaired; ↓ = impaired; ↑ = logorrhea; nl = normal; * = generally not affected; ? = not clear whether affected.

that faulty interhemispheric communication causes stuttering are several experimental psychological studies showing that stutterers, more often than controls, have difficulty performing complex bimanual tasks.

Phonological Programming Disorder

Children with phonological programming disorder have relatively fluent speech and their utterance length is nearly normal, but intelligibility is poor (Rapin et al. 1991). Serviceable speech is usually achieved, and language comprehension is preserved. This disorder may be a severe articulation problem or a milder form of verbal apraxia.

Verbal Apraxia ("Dilapidated Speech")

Children with verbal apraxia are extremely dysfluent. Their utterances are short and effortful. The phonological impairment includes inconsistent omissions, substitutions, and distortions of speech sounds. Syntactic skills are difficult to assess in view of the dysfluency. Language comprehension is relatively preserved. Children with verbal apraxia who do not have intelligible speech by 6 years are unlikely to acquire speech and may need prolonged speech and language therapy.

The frequency of concurrent nonverbal apraxic deficits, such as oral apraxia for nonspeech movements (the struggle to position muscles of articulation), and generalized apraxia or clumsiness in this disorder is controversial. The presence or absence of generalized apraxia has significant therapeutic implications, since children with verbal apraxia are dependent on their signing and writing skills for communication.

The cause of verbal apraxia is unknown. The excess of males and a familial tendency suggest a genetic basis. One patient with a similar speech disorder and features of suprabulbar palsy was found to have hypoplasia of the motor tract running from the Rolandic region to cranial nerve nuclei X and XII. Decreased blood flow to the frontal lobes and failure of verbal activation to increase perfusion to Broca's area is found in some patients. Rapin and Allen (1988) suggest that the disorder most resembles the adult aphasia, aphemia.

Disorders Predominately of Expressive Language

Phonological Syntactic Syndrome

Phonological syntactic syndrome is probably the most common DLD (Rapin et al. 1991). It is also called *mixed receptive expressive disorder*, *expressive disorder*, and *nonspecific formulation-repetition deficit*. The phonological disturbances are omissions, substitutions, and distortions of consonants and consonant clusters in all word positions. The sounds produced are unpredictable as well as unrecognizable, often making the child impossible to understand. Syntactic impairment is usually evidenced by the absence of small grammatical words (and, but) and appropriate inflected endings (ed, ing). The deficit is not just a developmental lag; while normal young children may say "baby cry" or "a baby crying," children with the phonological syntactic syndrome create deviant constructions like "the baby is cry." Telegraphic speech is common. Disturbances in other language areas are variable. Comprehension is relatively spared, and semantic skills are usually intact. Repetition, pragmatics, and prosody may be affected. Autistic children with the phonological syntactic syndrome tend to produce a significant amount of jargon.

Neurological dysfunction is especially common. Sucking, swallowing, and chewing difficulties make feeding problems common, and drooling is often persistent. Neurological examination may show features of pseudobulbar palsy, oromotor apraxia, hypertonia, and incoordination. Bilateral anterior and posterior perisylvian hypoperfusion has been shown in some children. The phonological syntactic syndrome most resembles Broca's aphasia (Rapin and Allen, 1988).

Lexical Syntactic Syndrome

In the lexical syntactic syndrome, speech is dysfluent with many hesitancies and false starts, even to the point of stuttering, because of word-finding difficulties and poor syntactic skills. Both literal and semantic paraphasias are common. Syntax is immature, not deviant. Phonology is normal and speech is intelligible. Repetition is generally better than spontaneous speech. In conversation, overlearned language is better than spontaneous speech. Pragmatics may be impaired, particularly in autistic children. Comprehension is generally acceptable, although complex questions and other linguistic forms that tax higher-level receptive syntactic skills are often deficient (Rapin et al. 1991).

Although the lexical syntactic syndrome is rarely reported as a specific entity, it was diagnosed in 14% of 104 preschool children with expressive developmental language disorders. This syndrome has no similar counterpart among the acquired aphasias of adulthood but shows similarities to anomic, conduction, and transcortical aphasias (Rapin and Allen, 1988).

Disorders Predominately of Language Comprehension

Semantic Pragmatic Syndrome

Children with the semantic pragmatic syndrome speak fluently and may be verbose. Vocabulary is often large and somewhat formal. Parents are often fooled and believe that the child's large vocabulary indicates superior verbal and cognitive skills. In fact, such children fall short in the basic semantic skills required for meaningful conversation and informative exchange of ideas. They talk to talk. Phonological and syntactic skills are generally intact, but comprehension is impaired. For example, they may answer a different "wh" question from the one being asked. Further, they lack pragmatic skills and have not learned the rules that govern the use of language in conversation: turn taking, topic maintenance, varying style when talking to a peer versus a younger child or an adult, knowledge of the appropriate timing of interruptions, repetitions as contrasted with echoing, gaze direction, and appropriate physical contact. Finally, children with the semantic pragmatic syndrome often show deficits in prosody. Their speech has a monotonous, mechanical, or singsong quality that prevents them from conveying the additional pragmatic intentions that prosody affords, like speaking with the proper emotion or indicating by tone of voice that they are asking a question.

The syndrome has been referred to as "repetition strength and comprehension deficit" or as "language without cognition." This syndrome is often seen in the higher-functioning, more verbal autistic child and is also called the *cocktail party syndrome* in children with hydrocephalus, particularly those with meningomyeloceles.

The neuroanatomical basis of this disorder is unknown. Repetition strength in the setting of fluent speech with impaired comprehension characterizes the adult aphasia syndrome of transcortical sensory aphasia (Rapin and Allen, 1988). A form of disconnection is suggested by the fact that hydrocephalics have a thin corpus callosum and by the cases with agenesis of the corpus callosum. Difficulties with prosody and pragmatics suggest right, as well as left, hemisphere dysfunction.

Verbal Auditory Agnosia

Children with verbal auditory agnosia cannot understand meaningful language despite intact hearing. It occurs on a congenital-developmental and an acquired basis. The developmental form is also called *generalized low performance* and *global dysfunction*.

The acquired form of verbal auditory agnosia is called the Landau-Kleffner syndrome (LKS). It is an acquired aphasia associated with a convulsive disorder. A previously normal, usually male child, between the ages of 3 and 7 years, loses the ability to understand language over days to weeks. Parents often think that the child is becoming deaf, but hearing is intact as measured clinically and by laboratory methods. The progressive verbal auditory agnosia is followed by the insidious loss of language fluency, sometimes to the point of mutism. Paraphasias and neologistic jargon may occur. Some children with LKS are able to access language visually; they gesture, learn sign, read, and write. Except for their language impairment, children with LKS are intellectually normal but may have behavioral disturbances such as hyperactivity or even frank psychosis, presumably secondary to their impaired ability to speak. Verbal auditory agnosia and paroxysmal EEG findings with or without seizures are also reported in autistic children both on a developmental and acquired basis (Perez et al. 1993).

A paroxysmal EEG is required for the diagnosis of LKS. Most have bilateral EEG abnormalities that are bitemporal, generalized, or multifocal. Ten percent have unilateral paroxysmal abnormalities. All clinical seizure types are reported. Seizures may occur before, during, or after recovery from the aphasia. The seizures are usually easy to control. The extent of correlation between the presence and severity of the EEG abnormalities and the aphasic disorder is controversial. Some children with fluctuating aphasia have a fluctuating EEG abnormality, but longitudinal case studies fail to demonstrate a parallel between the EEG and clinical status (Paquier et al. 1992). The relationship between EEG abnormalities and clinical language deficits is further confounded because children with DLD of all types may have paroxysmal abnormalities on EEG.

The outcome of developmental verbal auditory agnosia is not established. The outcome of the acquired form is better characterized but is variable. About one-third of patients with classic LKS eventually have normal language, one-third have mildly impaired language, and one-third have severely impaired language. Many suggest anticonvulsant treatment, even to the point of treating the EEG in the absence of clinical seizures. Yet no consistent parallel between treatment course and language outcome has been demonstrated. Nonetheless, EEG assessment, including a sleep recording, and a limited trial of anticonvulsants when the EEG shows paroxysmal abnormalities, even in the absence of clinical seizures, is warranted in children with isolated developmental or acquired language disorder (Paquier et al. 1992).

The etiology of congenital and acquired verbal auditory verbal agnosia is unknown. The belief that the acquired form is a chronic focal encephalitis is not supported by biopsies and epilepsy surgery specimens. Several patients with left temporal lesions have responded to surgery (Nass et al. 1993).

Neuropsychological data also support a focal origin for LKS. Recovery of language, when it occurs, compromises functions ordinarily mediated by the right hemisphere. This suggests the transfer of recovered language from the left to the right hemisphere. Teuber's term *crowding* is used to explain such a recovery pattern when it occurs after early structural left brain damage. However, recovery from this syndrome is significantly less frequent than after acquired aphasia in childhood from structural left brain injury. MRI volumetrics may show bilateral reduced posterior temporal volume in patients with verbal auditory agnosia. Positron emission tomography studies and xenon inhalation flow studies in children with LKS show focal pathology in some and diffuse pathology in others. Asymmetrical temporoparietal perfusion on single photo emission computed tomography (SPECT) scanning may be characteristic of LKS as compared to other DLD (O'Tuama et al. 1992).

FOLLOW-UP OF THE DEVELOPMENTAL LANGUAGE DISORDERS

DLDs are very likely to affect later educational achievement, emotional state, social adjustment, and vocational status. Preschool nonverbal intelligence is the best single predictor of long-term outcome, expressive syntactic abilities are the best predictor of adolescent language skills, and preschool language skills are the best single predictor of later reading ability. Children presenting with speech and language difficulties are at risk and should be screened and followed for learning disabilities and psychiatric disturbance.

ACQUIRED SPEECH AND LANGUAGE DISORDERS IN CHILDHOOD

Acquired Stuttering

As with the aphasias, the neuroanatomical basis of developmental stuttering may be extrapolated from acquired stuttering. Acquired stuttering from brain injury is relatively uncommon in the adult and is rare in children (Aram 1990). Children with acquired brain injury of either hemisphere have increased stuttering-like nonfluencies, but neither the location nor the size predicts dysfluent speech. The report of a child with acquired stuttering in the setting of subcortical pathology (Nass et al. 1994) supports the view that damage to collosal pathways coordinating the activity of both hemispheres during speech may underlie stuttering.

Childhood Aphasia

Left Hemisphere Lesions Causing Childhood Aphasia

Recent studies in which patients with bilateral disease were excluded and which specify handedness and emphasize good anatomical localization show that children, like adults, develop aphasia almost exclusively after left hemisphere injuries. Left subcortical and thalamic injury also cause aphasia in children (Aram 1990).

Recovery Is Excellent But Not Complete

While complete recovery from acquired childhood aphasia was thought to be the rule, recent studies show that many children do poorly in school and that higher-level language functions, particularly reading and writing, are permanently impaired. Those whose injuries occurred before age 5 years are no better than those whose injuries occurred later. Left hemisphere injury, even prior to language acquisition, interferes with the development of completely normal language (Thal et al. 1991).

Greater plasticity of the central nervous system rather than a lesser degree of specialization of the left hemisphere for language may be a factor that accounts for better recovery from aphasia in children than adults. The better prognosis for complete language recovery after head trauma (a more common etiology for aphasia in children) than after stroke, for example, may favorably bias recovery statistics in children.

Types of Acquired Aphasia in Childhood and Intrahemispheric Specialization for Language

The relatively high frequency of nonfluent aphasia with spared comprehension during childhood led to the suggestion that language is not well localized in the left hemisphere until adolescence. However, children with traditional fluent aphasias are being recognized more frequently (Martins et al. 1991). Fluency criteria for children are probably different from those for adults. Nonfluency in adults is characterized by a reduced speech rate, mean length of utterance, and articulatory agility, as well as excessive pauses, marked effort, agrammatism, and dysprosody. In contrast, children who produce sentences that are reduced in length, speech rate, or both, but that are well articulated, effortless, and with normal prosody can still be considered fluent. Seeming nonfluency in children may really reflect word-finding difficulties with pauses preceding content words, overall articulatory slowing, and hypospontaneity of emotional origin, present even in some with jargonaphasia (Van Dongen and Paquier 1991). The timing of the examination may also contribute to the findings vis-à-vis fluency; in some patients, paraphasias characteristic of fluent aphasia are only briefly present on recovery from coma. Intrahemispheric localization of language deficits paralleling those in adults has been documented in some cases (i.e., mutism associated with anterior lesions, comprehension problems with posterior lesions, and conduction aphasia with an arcuate fasciculus lesion). The view of fully spared comprehension in childhood aphasia also must be reconsidered, because even nonfluent aphasia in young children may show the same semantic-syntactic comprehension dissociation as seen in adults with Broca's aphasia. The age-aphasia–type dichotomy in the adult, with young adults more frequently developing nonfluent aphasias, may reflect a difference in lesion location resulting from the causes of brain injury in this age group rather than differences in degrees of intrahemispheric specialization. This could bias studies of childhood aphasia types as well. More lesion localization data comparable to that now available for adults are obviously needed.

Language lateralization may be incomplete in the child, but the concept of an innate asymmetry does not preclude increasing specialization of the left hemisphere for language. Nor does innate hemispheric specialization preclude neuroplasticity; it just redefines its limits. When dominance is transferred to the right hemisphere, language as such is not the same, nor does the innate specialization of the left hemisphere for language argument deny a right hemisphere role in the development of verbal cognition (Thal et al. 1991). Rather, it denies that the right hemisphere is ever equipped completely like the left hemisphere to mediate language. While plasticity minimizes the effects of early focal injury on all cognitive systems, innate specialization limits the ultimate efficacy of plasticity.

REFERENCES

Aram D. Acquired Aphasia in Children. In M Sarno (ed), Acquired Aphasia (2nd ed). New York: Academic, 1990;61–69.

Aram DM, Morris R, Hall NE. The validity of discrepancy criteria for identifying children with developmental language disorders. J Learn Dis 1992;25:549–554.

Martins IP, Castro-Caldas A, van Dongen HR, van Hout A (eds). Acquired Aphasia in Children. Dordrecht, the Netherlands: Kluwer Academic Publishers, 1991.

Nass R, Heier L, Schreter B. Acquired stuttering in a two year old after a second stroke. Dev Med Child Neurol 1994:36:73–78.

Nass R, Heier L, Walker R. Acquired aphasia with convulsive disorder due to tumor responding to surgery. Pediatr Neurol 1993:9:303–308.

Nippold M. Concomitant speech and language disorders in stuttering children. J Speech Hear Dis 1990;55:51–60.

O'Tuama LA, Urion DK, Janicek MJ et al. Regional cerebral perfusion in Landau-Kleffner syndrome and related childhood aphasias. J Nucl Med 1992;33:1758–1765.

Paquier P, Van Dongen H, Loonen C. The LKS or "acquired aphasia with convulsive disorder." Arch Neurol 1992;49:354–359.

Perez ER, Davidoff V, Despland P-A, Deonna T. Mental and behavioral deterioration of children with epilepsy and CSWS: acquired epileptic frontal syndrome. Dev Med Child Neurol 1993:35:661–674.

Rapin I, Allen D. Syndromes in Developmental Dysphasia and Adult Aphasia. In F Plum (ed), Language, Communication and the Brain. New York: Raven, 1988.

Rapin I, Allen D, Dunn M. Developmental Language Disorders. In S Segalowitz, E Rapin (eds), Handbook of Neuropsychology. Vol. 7, Child Psychology. Amsterdam: Elsevier, 1991:111–137.

Thal D, Marchman V, Stiles J et al. Early lexical development in children with focal brain injury. Brain Lang 1991;40:491–527.

Tuchman R. Epilepsy, language and behavior. J Child Neurol 1994;9:95–102.

Van Dongen HR, Paquier P. Fluent Aphasias in Children. In IP Martins, A Castro-Caldas, HR van Dongen, A van Hout (eds), Acquired Aphasia in Children. Dordrecht, the Netherlands: Kluwer Academic Publishers, 1991:125–142.

Chapter 13
Difficulties with Speech and Swallowing

David B. Rosenfield and Alberto O. Barroso

Communication through language includes semantics (e.g., the meaning of sounds and words), syntax (e.g., grammar), and phonology (e.g., actual sounds). Disruption of these elements can result in language disorders (the *aphasias,* described in Chapters 12A and 12B). Disturbance purely of the sound input, sparing semantics and syntax, can result in *dysarthria* and *dystonia,* both of which are major subjects of this chapter. We also discuss disorders of fluent production of sound output, especially stuttering. Further, because there is considerable overlap between the neuromotor control of speech and swallowing, we address disorders of swallowing (*dysphagia*).

Speech is, a priori, motor output. The central nervous system (CNS) regulates the activity of the respiratory and laryngeal muscles to produce sound, which is subsequently altered by supralaryngeal articulators to produce meaningful components of language. The vocal folds (vocal cords) consist of striated muscles and articulatory joints that are under neural control. Several vocal fold muscles, all but one of which are adductors, influence vocal fold movement. Contraction of each individual muscle has a particular effect on the edge of the vocal fold and the distribution of muscle mass within that fold. These factors alter the nature of the sound waves produced (Titze 1993; Bordon et al. 1994).

The production of sound (*phonation*) requires appropriate stiffness or slackness of laryngeal vocal folds, an appropriate opening between the vocal folds, and a specified volume and velocity of air moving through that opening. The volume and velocity are altered by changes in subglottic (below the vocal folds) pressure and by supraglottic contractions, such as those caused by movements of the pharynx and supralaryngeal articulators. There is a narrow but specific range of values for these three variables to produce phonation. Compromise of any of them can alter sound output (Rosen and Howell 1991; Titze 1993).

The sound waves produced by the larynx are filtered through rostral air passages and are altered by changes in the shape of this cavity. Compromise in the sound source can produce *dysphonia*, and articulator compromise can produce slurred speech. The term *dysarthria*, though implying a problem of articulation only, is often used to refer to defects in phonation as well as in resonation. Patients who have dysarthria in association with a language disturbance—that is, altered grammar, semantics, and comprehension—usually have a nonfluent aphasia. This chapter addresses only motor disturbances of speech output, without association with aphasia.

Clinicians frequently view dysphonia as resulting from focal, mechanical disruption of the laryngeal sound source and view dysarthria as resulting from neurologic compromise of the articulators. Although one can separately address signs, symptoms, and differential diagnosis of dysphonia, one must remember that dysphonia is a dysarthria and that either can reflect neurological compromise. This chapter does not emphasize actual diseases causing the dysarthrias, but the accompanying tables do provide the differential diagnosis of signs and symptoms of speech-motor compromise.

DYSARTHRIA

Patients may have altered speech as a result of compromise in sound output or the supralaryngeal articulators (lips, tongue, jaw, and palate). Too frequently, physicians comment on slurred speech without describing the exact changes in the patient's speech. An improved understanding of the analysis of sound production helps promote diagnostic expertise and aids the physician in following disease progression and response to therapy.

Symptoms

Patients with dysarthric symptoms can have multiple complaints, including weak, slurred, or indistinct speech. Organically induced speech motor disturbances usually have a gradual onset, unless they result from a stroke. Psychogenic disturbances usually present with an abrupt onset. Further, neurological disturbances involving speech motor production are rarely associated with periods of true normality. Patients may say that at times their speech is normal, but on more detailed inquiry they note that although their speech becomes more normal at times, it is never totally normal. Individuals with abnormal speech who truly have intermittent periods of normal speech usually have psychogenic disturbance. However, myasthenia gravis can also be associated with periods of normality in otherwise continuous dysarthria (Rosenfield 1994).

A motor disturbance in speech, whether neurological or functional in origin, usually worsens in situations of emotional stress, because the finely controlled motor system of speech output is sensitive to the person's emotional status. This is similar to what occurs in patients with other disturbances in neuromotor control, such as those with Parkinson's disease, who have more tremor when under stress. The greater severity of speech disturbance in patients under stress is not a helpful clue in differentiating organic from nonorganic disease.

Most speech motor disruptions are not associated with laryngeal pain. When pain is present, one should consider focal laryngeal pathology or acid reflux involving the vocal folds. This reflux may be only nocturnal and may be associated with speech improvement following antireflux therapy. If pain is present as well as dysphagia, oropharyngeal tumor, infection, or inflammation should be suspected. When patients complain of strain or a strangled sensation, with or without pain, spasmodic dysphonia should be considered. The sensation of tightness and strain may reflect the patient's coping strategy in dealing with the underlying sound production deficit; it does not necessarily imply that a focal cervical and laryngeal dystonia is the cause of the discomfort. Thus, if vocal fold tremor causes difficulty in producing appropriate oscillation, the patient may apply increased tone to the laryngeal and extralaryngeal neuromuscular system, resulting in strain. If the patient tries to speak without these manuevers, there may be multiple staccato catches (*glottal stops*) and obvious phonation tremor.

Many patients with neurolaryngeal motor control difficulty can speak at one pitch but not at another, because they have less interference from the movement disturbance at some pitches. This can result in speaking at a higher pitch, which in turn can cause strain. Singing is normally performed at a pitch higher than the pitch for normal speech, and therefore may be spared in some speech motor disturbances. Intactness of singing does not necessarily imply a psychogenic disturbance.

The subglottic pressure and laryngeal muscle tension required for sound production in laughter and crying are different from those required for normal speech output. The presence of normal laughter and crying, in the setting of abnormal speech production, is seen in functional aphonia, voice abuse, and voice misuse, but is also seen in spasmodic dysphonia (Rosenfield 1994).

Sometimes associated systemic dystonic features aid in the diagnosis of a speech disorder. Complaints of photophobia and excessive need for sunglasses have many ocular and systemic causes. In the context of a speech or swallowing disorder, photophobia may raise the suspicion of blepharospasm, which can be associated with dystonia elsewhere. If the patient complains of cramping in the hands when opening a jar or writing, an underlying dystonia may also be affecting speech-related structures.

Speech improvement following consumption of a mild to moderate amount of alcohol suggests that the vocal fold tremor is part of the syndrome of benign essential tremor. The speech improvement reflects the direct effects of alcohol on the tremor more than the effects of alcohol on anxiety.

Some individuals complain of a weak voice and tremor when anxious. This is probably due to accentuation of physiological tremor. This can even cause cessation of speech output and probably accounts for the expression "scared speechless." The person is not scared speechless but, rather, scared *voiceless*. The tremor results in transglottal aerodynamic changes such that appropriate oscillation does not occur. The literature suggests that the majority of people who maintain their aphonia have it for functional reasons. Patients with psychogenic aphonia may not complain of strain or strangle and are usually able to cough and laugh appropriately. It should be borne in mind that normal coughing and laughing involve different tone of the vocal folds, and thus that aphonia with preserved cough and laugh does not connote a psychogenic disorder. To make a definitive diagnosis of functional aphonia, one needs evidence of a conversion reaction; in this setting, these patients should be seen by a psychiatrist as well as a speech-language pathologist (Rosenfield 1994).

Some patients complain of hoarseness and a raspy voice without strain or strangle. Although this may reflect vocal abuse, such as screaming at a sports event, it often reflects voice misuse. Both frequently improve with voice rest. The patient with voice misuse should be counseled by a speech clinician on appropriate speaking habits.

If the patient complains of tremor, dystonic activity, or any other movement disorder activity in non–speech-related organs, a movement disorder should be suspected, especially if there is a family history of movement disorders.

Examination

The examiner should carefully listen to the patient's speech while taking the history and then proceed with the neurologic examination, including formal assessment of speech output. The resting posture of the head and neck should be evaluated for tremor. Tremor of the thyroid cartilage often suggests associated vocal fold tremor. If the head turns to one side, spasmodic torticollis should be considered. Tremor and torticollis are both associated with spasmodic dysphonia. Vocal fold tremor can produce phonatory tremor, result in compensatory straining, or both, such that a non–tremor-type speech pattern is heard, with marked strain and strangle.

When a patient sits on the edge of an examining table with eyes closed and arms outstretched and pronated, orofacial dyskinesias as well as dyskinesias of the limbs may appear, suggesting an underlying movement disturbance affecting speech-motor output. When finger-to-nose movements reveal cerebellar tremor, vocal fold tremor may also be present.

The rate of blinking should be evaluated. Most patients blink fewer than 17 times per minute. If this figure is increased, the physician should suspect cranial dystonia syndrome.

Impairment of the gag reflex frequently does not indicate a lesion of the glossopharyngeal nerve, since tonsillectomy frequently causes an asymmetrical response. An increased gag reflex may suggest bilateral corticobulbar tract lesions. Chronic difficulty in deglutition may cause habituation and the impairment of the gag reflex.

The palate should elevate normally and symmetrically. The soft palate may oscillate in synchrony with essential tremor. Myoclonic movements of the soft palate at rest and during phonation occur in palatal myoclonus.

When there is a question of soft palate weakness, a mirror held under the nares while the patient repeats nonnasal sounds (nasal sounds are */m/*, */n/*, and */ng/*) should not fog. Normally, the soft palate and pharynx close off the nasal passages during nonnasal sounds, and the mirror demonstrates no sign of nasal airway leak. When these words are uttered in the presence of velopharyngeal insufficiency, air leaks through the nasal airway and clouds the mirror.

The most common cause of hypernasal speech and nasal air emission is vagal damage at or above the level of the pharyngeal branches. Unilateral damage produces mild hypernasality; bilateral damage produces more pronounced hypernasal symptoms. Also, persons with myasthenia can have palate weakness resulting in hypernasal speech, as can patients with myopathy. The second most common cause is bilateral upper motor neuron corticobulbar damage. In this situation, velopharyngeal closure is not flaccid and paralyzed, as it is in lower motor neuron compromise. Rather, spasticity slows the movement of the soft palate and pharynx and interferes with their synchrony during speech. The velum appears symmetric, and the gag reflex may be hyperactive, although, as noted earlier, chronic difficulty with deglutition can cause habituation of the gag reflex.

Patients with hyponasal speech (*/m/* becomes */b/*; */n/* becomes */d/*; */ng/* becomes */g/*) seldom have CNS disease. Common causes include enlarged adenoids, deviated nasal septum, rhinitis, and nasopharyngeal tumor.

The tongue should be strong and capable of applying good pressure against the interior of the cheek, as demonstrated by pushing against the examiner's externally applied digit. Fasciculations, atrophy, and anteroposterior furrows suggest lower motor neuron damage. When the lesion is unilateral, attempted tongue protrusion produces deviation toward the defective side. Unilateral tongue paralysis seldom affects speech severely, but bilateral involvement causes marked dysarthria, with virtually all lingual consonants (*/l/*, */r/*) being distorted.

The lips should pucker well and, together with the muscles of the cheeks, should be able to apply air pressure against pursed lips. Unilateral lower motor neuron facial weakness causes the mouth to droop and the cheek to bulge when plosive sounds (*/p/*, */b/*) are produced. The intact opposite side usually provides sufficient compression of the lips, so that the deficit is mild. If facial nerve damage is bilateral, the lips bulge considerably with plosive sound production and the deficit is more pronounced. Patients may bite the lower lip because they are unable to turn it inward, resulting in additional compromise of labiodental fricatives (*/f/*, */v/*).

The power of the jaw can be assessed by asking the patient to open against resistance. A lesion of the motor division of the fifth nerve causes mandibular weakness, compromising tongue and lower lip approximation to the upper lip, teeth, and hard palate. Unilateral lesions that cause the mandible to deviate to the side of the lesion when the jaw is opened still permit the contralateral masseter, temporalis, and pterygoid to close the mouth. Speech is not normally compromised with unilateral lesions, but with bilateral weakness of these muscles, all speech sounds are severely distorted and virtually unintelligible. An increased jaw jerk suggests bilateral upper motor neuron compromise, above the pons.

The patient's contextual speech provides information on respiration, phonation, resonance, articulation, and prosody. Compromise of the recurrent laryngeal nerve, a branch of the vagus, produces short phrases, decreased volume, and mild inhalation stridor. Sometimes the voice is hoarse. A higher vagal lesion, compromising palate function, adds a component of hypernasality to speech. Multiple lower motor neuron cranial nerve lesions result in breathiness, decreased volume, hypernasality, nasal emission of air, inhalation stridor, short phrases, imprecise consonants, monopitch, and monoloudness.

Bilateral corticobulbar tract lesions cause spasticity, slowing the rate of speech, producing a harsh, strained, or strangled output. Consonants are imprecise, pitch may be low (many patients strain, in which case pitch may be high) and monotonous, and phrases are short with altered stress, mono-volume, breathiness, distorted vowels, effortful grunts at the end of phrases, hypernasality, and pitch breaks.

Cerebellar lesions can cause abnormalities in contextual speech such that there are irregular random breaks in articulation, vowel distortions, excesses in stress, prolongation of sounds, increased intervals between words, variable harshness, and decreased rate.

Hypokinetic dysarthria, as seen in Parkinson's disease, results in short rushes of speech, increased rate, monopitch, decreased volume, monoloudness, altered stress, breathiness, imprecise consonants, harshness, low pitch, variations in rate, inappropriate silences, and palilalia.

Hyperkinetic dysarthria (Table 13.1) is dysarthria associated with hyperkinetic movement disturbance. It is associated with different findings, depending on the underlying cause. The more common findings are variable rate, inappropriate silences, imprecise consonants, irregular articulatory breakdowns, distorted vowels, harshness, strain or strangle, and monopitch.

It is often difficult for the neurologist to have a precise understanding of contextual speech alteration. In this setting, the repetitive utterance of the individual sounds */pa/*, */ta/*, and */ka/* provides a good indication of the speech deficit. The */p/* sound depends on good orbicularis oris power (seventh nerve). The crispness of the */ta/* sound depends on adequate power in the tip of the tongue (twelfth nerve), and the clarity of T */ka/* depends on appropriate power and tone in the posterior part of the tongue as well as the palate (ninth, tenth, and twelfth nerves). Furthermore, all sounds depend on appropriate mandibular power. The sounds should be crisp, with normal volume, and the rate should be regular and fast. A slow but rhythmic rate implies bilateral upper motor neuron lesions. An irregularly irregular rhythm implies cerebellar dysfunction. Air wastage through the nares implies palate weakness. The speech motor system is further assessed by evaluating laryngeal and velopharyngeal dysfunction (see Table 13.1).

Examination of the larynx by a laryngologist is important whenever patients complain of laryngeal pain, phonation is defective, or neurological disease has not been clearly implicated. Laryngologists frequently concentrate on the presence or absence of a mass, while also making certain that the vocal folds are not paralyzed. The neurologist's need to determine the presence of tremor, dystonia, or dyskinesia, both at rest and during phonation, should be emphasized when requesting the consultation.

One can best observe laryngeal movements with a nasopharyngeal fiberoptoscope, which permits examination of the vocal folds at rest and during speech. Videotaping provides consultants as well as the patient with an opportunity to examine the deficits and see whether aberrant or nonproductive vocal strategies are present.

Unilateral or bilateral vagus nerve damage (Tables 13.2 and 13.3) causes visible displacement of vocal folds to the paramedian (abducted) position. Vagal lesions above the takeoff of the superior laryngeal nerve result in the paralysis of vocal folds in a more abducted position, resulting in turn in a wider glottis than is seen with the lower lesions affecting only the recurrent laryngeal branch. Consequently, dysphonia is worse when the vagus lesion is above the superior laryngeal nerve than when it is not. Bilateral vocal cord paralysis results in a greater dysphonia than does unilateral vocal cord paralysis. Bilateral lesions above the takeoff of the superior laryngeal nerve, at the brain stem level, make the patient virtually aphonic. An even higher lesion of the vagus nerve, in the brain stem, above the takeoff of the pharyngeal branch, causes soft palate paralysis in addition to vocal fold paralysis, producing hypernasality and nasal emission. Thus, soft palate paralysis in addition to laryngeal compromise should lead the physician to suspect a high vagal or brain stem lesion, affecting vagus lower motor neuron output.

Asking the patient to sustain the vowel */a/* as long as possible permits assessment of phonation (see Table 13.1). The sound should be clear and steady, with appropriate volume. Flaccid laryngeal muscles produce a breathy voice with decreased volume. Unilateral vocal fold paralysis produces a voice less breathy but hoarser than does bilateral vocal fold paralysis. *Diplophonia* (two tones produced simultaneously) is common in unilateral vocal cord paralysis because there are different vibration frequencies for each vocal fold. Some patients with bilateral recurrent laryngeal nerve disease develop paralysis of the vocal folds in the midline. When this occurs, the voice may be deceptively normal, but abductor vocal cord paralysis prevents the opening of the glottis during inhalation, resulting in inspiratory stridor.

Strained and strangled hoarseness with vowel prolongation may indicate hyperadduction of the vocal folds. This can result from increased tone (upper motor neuron lesions or dystonia) or may reflect the patient's coping strategy for dealing with underlying tremor, intermittent movement disturbance, or mild weakness. The presence of a pseudobulbar cry clearly implies bilateral upper motor neuron tract damage (Rosenfield 1994).

Tremor on vowel prolongation suggests essential phonatory tremor. Nonlaryngeal muscles are usually also involved in this disturbance, but they need not be. Vocal fold tremor can usually be seen on indirect laryngoscopy and may be present only during phonation. Sometimes, the tremor cycle is accompanied by voice arrest (glottal stop). This is more frequently seen in patients with symptoms of spasmodic dysphonia (Rosenfield 1994).

Interruption of vowel prolongation is also observed in palatal-pharyngeal-laryngeal myoclonus. These interruptions, as opposed to those seen with essential phonatory tremor, are not usually associated with a rise and fall in pitch during contextual speech. Rather, the tone is steady between interruptions. Also, the rate of volume prolongation interruptions is usually one to four per second, as opposed to four to eight per second for essential tremor. More important, laryngeal myoclonic movements are seen at rest as movements of the larynx under the skin of the neck, as well as with indirect laryngoscopy.

When a patient's cough is a weak explosive sound, vocal fold adductor weakness may be present. The cough sound is

Table 13.1: Differential diagnosis of dysarthria

Disease	*Laryngeal (Phonatory)*	*Velopharyngeal*	*Oral*
Myopathy, myositis	Hoarse, breathy, diplophonia, low volume	Hypernasal, nasal emission	All vowels and consonants may be compromised, depending on which muscles are involved
Myasthenia gravis	Similar to above but may be intermittent; improves with rest	Similar to above but may be intermittent; improves with rest	Similar to above but may be intermittent; improves with rest
Twelfth nerve lesion	Normal	Normal	Weak tongue, atrophy, fasciculations; drooling; imprecise vowels and lingual consonants
Tenth nerve lesion	Hoarse, breathy, low volume, diplophonia	Hypernasal, nasal emission, if lesion is above pharyngeal branch	Normal
Seventh nerve lesion	Normal	Normal	Weak orbicularis oris; imprecise vowels and labial consonants
Fifth nerve lesion	Normal	Normal	Weak mandibular muscles; imprecise vowels and consonants
Multiple cranial nerves	Breathiness, decreased volume, inhalation stridor, monopitch	Hypernasal, nasal emission	Imprecise vowels and consonants
Bilateral corticobulbar tract	Vocal fold hyperadduction, strained, strangled, harsh, variable pitch, monopitch	Hypernasal	Imprecise consonants, slow rate, increased gag, drooling
Amyotrophic lateral sclerosis	Strained, harsh, wet, gurgly quality; flutter during vowel prolongation	Hypernasal, nasal emission	Slow articulation, imprecise consonants, short phrases, vowel distortion
Parkinson's disease	Weak, monopitch, low volume, hoarse	Normal	Accelerated rate, repetitive dysfluencies, imprecise consonants
Cerebellar disease	Tremor, variations of loudness, or near normal	Normal	Irregular articulatory breakdowns, imprecise consonants, sometimes excessive and equal stress on all syllables of words
Hyperkinetic dysarthria-chorea	Sudden pitch and loudness alterations, phonatory arrest, strained harshness	Normal	Sudden alternations in precision of vowels and consonants
Hyperkinetic dysarthria–dystonia	Slow alterations of pitch and loudness, phonatory arrest, strained harshness	Normal	Slow alterations in consonant and vowel precision
Hyperkinetic dysarthria-palatal-pharyngeal-laryngeal myoclonus	Rhythmic contractions of instrinsic–extrinsic pharyngeal muscles (1–4 per second)	Rhythmic contractions (1–4 per second)	Normal or imprecise vowels and consonants
Hyperkinetic dysarthria–phonatory tremor	Rhythmic alterations of pitch and loudness, adductor phonatory arrests, compensatory strain or strangle	Normal	Near normal
Hyperkinetic dysarthria–Gilles de la Tourette syndrome	Grunt, bark, squeaks, throat clearing, gurgling, moaning	Snorting, sniffing	Whistling, clicking, lip smacking, spitting, unintelligible sounds, echolalia, coprolalia; can have dysfluencies

Source: Adapted from AE Aronson. Motor Speech Signs of Neurologic Disease. In OK Darby (ed), Speech Evaluation in Medicine. New York: Grune & Stratton, 1981:159–180.

usually mildly compromised in unilateral vocal cord paralysis from recurrent laryngeal nerve damage, but is very much reduced with a higher unilateral vagal lesion above the takeoff of the superior laryngeal nerve. Bilateral vagal lesions at this level cause an extremely defective or absent cough and are often associated with aspiration. CNS (upper motor neuron) lesions seldom cause major cough compromise.

The diseases that cause bilateral damage to lower motor neurons affecting speech output usually have a poor prognosis. The diseases that cause bilateral upper motor neuron

Table 13.2: Causes of bilateral abductor vocal cord paralysis in adults

Thyroidectomy (58%)	
Neck malignancy (6%)	
Primary neurological disease (22%)	
	Poliomyelitis
	Parkinson's disease (?)
	Brain stem stroke
	Guillain-Barré syndrome
	Multiple sclerosis
	Central nervous system neoplasm
	Central nervous system infection
	Charcot-Marie-Tooth disease
Miscellaneous (14%)	
	Foreign bodies
	Bilateral neck dissection
	Neck infection
	Congenital
	Head or neck trauma
	Substernal thyroid
	Idiopathic

Source: Adapted from LD Holinger, PC Holinger, PH Holinger. Etiology of bilateral abductor vocal cord paralysis—a review of 389 cases. Ann Otol 1976;85:428–436.

corticobulbar lesions usually produce a permanent deficit, although the patient may experience some improvement after the ictus in those with an acute onset. Unilateral upper motor neuron corticobulbar damage due to a stroke can produce acute speech motor compromise, as well as possible associated swallowing difficulty. This usually improves considerably in 6 weeks to 6 months, as some degree of recovery occurs and as the intact side takes over some of the lost function, as a result of the bilateral innervation.

The physician should have patients produce a prolonged */a/* sound and repetitive */pa/*, */ta/*, and */ka/* sounds. The */a/* vocalization provides a good assessment of laryngeal phonation. Careful listening to repetitive utterance of */pa/*, */ta/*, and */ka/* provides good assessment of articulator function, as well as hypernasality and hyponasality. Just as rapid finger tapping provides evidence of cerebellar dysfunction (irregular tapping) and upper motor neuron dysfunction (slow rate), so does the repetitive utterance of these speech sounds, with irregular rate and slow rate, respectively. These sounds, the examination of which is more completely delineated in Table 13.1, provide information on speech motor dysfunction.

The patient should be asked to repeat individually */pa/*, */ta/*, and */ka/*, at slow as well as rapid rates. The rapid rate can fatigue the muscles, whereas the slow rate may not. Patients with weak palate muscles may substitute */ba/* for */pa/*, proceeding to produce */ma/*. Likewise, weak palate muscles can cause */ta/* to become */da/* then */na/*, and */ka/* becomes */ga/* and then */nga/*. This pattern of change (e.g., */pa/* > */ba/* > */ma/*; */ta/* > */da/* > */na/*; */ka/* > */ga/* > */nga/*) is aerodynamically induced. It reflects an inability to maintain zero transglottal pressure (i.e., no pressure differential across the rostral and inferior portions of the laryngeal opening). This

Table 13.3: Causes of recurrent laryngeal nerve paralysis

Inflammation	
Pulmonary tuberculosis	
	Coccidiomycosis
	Collagen vascular disease
	Viral
	Polyneuropathy (especially diabetes and alcohol)
Trauma	
	Congestive heart failure
	Intubation
	Thyroid enlargement
	Chronic obstructive pulmonary disease
	Neck trauma
	Head trauma
	Mediastinoscopy
	Radical neck dissection
	Carotid endarterectomy
	Cardiovascular surgery
	Thyroidectomy
	Esophageal resection for carcinoma
Neoplasm	
	Primary of lung
	Metastatic to lung
	Cervical neoplasm
	Esophagus
	Thyroid
	Glomus jugulare
	Cervical lymph node metastasis
	Tongue
	Multiple myeloma
	Lymphatic leukemia
	Lymphoma
	Syringomyelia
	Parkinson's disease (?)
	Stroke (brain stem)
	Multiple sclerosis (?)
Miscellaneous	
	Pancytopenia
	Hemolytic anemia
	Thrombophlebitis
	Idiopathic

Source: Adapted from LL Titch. Causes of recurrent laryngeal nerve paralysis. Arch Otolaryngol 1976;102:259–261.

"unintended" lessened transglottal pressure difference results from weak velopharyngeal muscle (levator palatini), producing air leakage through the nares. The airflow through the laryngeal opening creates the Bernoulli phenomenon, which, in turn, prematurely approximates the vocal folds. This reduces the voice onset time, producing laryngeal-induced phonation earlier than intended. Thus, what are known as *voiced cognates* (e.g., the sound substitutions described above) occur. As the patient continues to repeat, further tiring the levator palatini muscle, the velopharyngeal opening now becomes appropriate for nasal sound substitution (technically, the nasal consonant is produced with the same place of articulation as for the voiceless plosive) (Rosenfield et al. 1992).

Investigation

Most dysarthric patients require a detailed investigation to ascertain the cause of their disturbance. The history and examination help the physician determine the type of dysfunction, whether it is due to brain, nerve, neuromuscular junction, or muscle compromise (see Table 13.1). Individuals with speech compromise of the type seen with muscle dysfunction should have a complete evaluation for possible myositis, myopathy, and dystrophy. The most frequent causes of abnormality include polymyositis and hypothyroidism. Myasthenia gravis produces the signs and symptoms noted earlier. If a nerve lesion is present, the patient should be fully evaluated for underlying diseases including collagen vascular diseases, toxic neuropathies, and tumors and neoplasms compressing the nerve. If lower motor neuron vagal dysfunction is present, a chest x-ray and a computed tomographic (CT) scan from the base of the skull through lower portions of the thyroid gland are required to exclude tumor. If signs of CNS dysfunction are found, full neuroimaging studies may be needed (see Tables 13.2 and 13.3).

SPASMODIC DYSPHONIA

Spasmodic dysphonia (SD) is a chronic phonatory disorder of unknown cause that usually appears in adulthood. Increased interest in this disorder has revealed that many SD patients have dystonia, although the exact cause of the abnormal speech is not known. There are two main types of SD—adductor and abductor. The *adductor* type is characterized by jerky or choppy breaks in phonation; staccato catches; strain, strangle, or harsh voice quality; and monopitch. Phonation is frequently associated with jerky, effortful, strained sounds, and is frequently associated with laryngeal discomfort (Blitzer and Brin 1992; Rosenfield 1994). The *abductor* type of SD is characterized by a breathy, often effortful, voice quality with sudden cessation of voicing, resulting in aphonic whispered speech segments. It is not known whether these patients have too little tone in laryngeal adductors or excessive tone in laryngeal abductors (posterior cricoarytenoid). Some patients have a mixture of both types (Blitzer and Brin 1992; Rosenfield 1994).

Interruptions of phonatory airflow in SD presumably result from intermittent spasmodic hyperadduction of the vocal folds, although indirect laryngoscopy is usually said to be normal. Careful examination for a movement disorder of the limbs (dystonia, tremor, dyskinesia) often reveals abnormalities (Blitzer and Brin 1992; Rosenfield 1994).

Symptoms

The diagnosis is not certain unless the patient complains of sensation of strain or strangle during speech production. If these symptoms are absent, the physician should suspect voice misuse or abuse, disturbances that may relate to poor voice habits and vocal hygiene (Blitzer and Brin 1992).

Many SD patients state that they had a sore throat before the onset of symptoms. This aspect of the history may be unreliable, in that the upper respiratory symptoms are often recognized after the onset of the SD symptoms. Also, SD patients may interpret their initial complaint as a sore throat, especially if they strained their vocal folds to accomplish adequate voicing, resulting in laryngeal discomfort. It is possible, however, that focal trauma, such as that resulting from laryngitis, voice abuse, or strain during excessive speaking, might precipitate a focal dystonia, just as peripheral trauma elsewhere can produce focal dystonia (Rosenfield 1994).

Patients referred to a neurologist for SD symptoms may constitute a different population than those referred to a speech pathologist. Usually, by the time they see a neurologist, they have seen several speech pathologists as well as an otolaryngologist. Approximately two-thirds of SD patients who see a neurologist have evidence of movement disturbance manifested elsewhere. The primary differential diagnosis consists of benign essential tremor, Meige's syndrome, hypothyroidism, and possible focal dystonia. Approximately one-third have a totally normal examination apart from the speech abnormality; it is not known whether their disturbance is functional or represents focal dystonia (Rosenfield 1994).

Investigation

After obtaining a careful history and physical examination, the neurologist must decide what studies are appropriate for investigating each individual SD patient. The studies should reflect the postulated cause. Thus, if an SD patient has tremor, an investigation to delineate the underlying cause is warranted. If dystonia is suspected, especially in the presence of Meige's syndrome, a full dystonia evaluation is warranted.

If no particular etiology is found on clinical examination, an initial laboratory investigation is usually not warranted, but these patients, as well as others, should be seen by a speech-language pathologist. Some patients respond well to speech therapy, especially in conjunction with the pharmacological therapy given for the underlying disorder. Botulinum toxin injection into the disordered laryngeal muscles is effective therapy (Ludlow et al. 1994). Pharmacologic intervention, using beta blockers or carbamazepine for underlying tremor, or trihexiphendyl or baclofen for underlying dystonia, can also be effective in stopping strain and strangle, as well as the intermittent cessation of sound output (glottal stops).

DYSFLUENCY

Stuttering

Stuttering is a disturbance of human speech manifested as repetitions, lengthening, and inappropriate pauses in the

Table 13.4: Dysfluency

Feature	*Developmental Stuttering*	*Acquired Stuttering*	*Cluttering*	*Palilalia*
Locus of lesion	Unknown	Usually cortical, but subcortical cases reported	Unknown	Basal ganglia; bilateral frontal cortex
Cause	Unknown	Vascular, metabolic, tumor	Unknown	Parkinson's disease, postencephalitis, syphilis
Duration	80% of children outgrow, adults have worse prognosis	Unilateral: good prognosis; bilateral: poor prognosis	Varies	Progressive
Locus of dysfluency	Beginning of sentence or phrase	Frequently scattered through sentence	Varies	Throughout sentence
Volume	Normal	Normal	Normal	Decreases at end of phrase
Response to singing	Fluent	Many improved somewhat, but not totally fluent	Varies	No change
Onset	Subacute	Subacute or acute	Gradual	Gradual
Adaptation effect	Promotes fluency	No effect	Varies	No effect
Reaction to dysfluencies	Anxious	Not anxious	Not concerned	Sometimes anxious
Metronome pacing	Promotes fluency	Little effect	Usually promotes fluency	Transiently promotes fluency

generation of consonants, vowels, and words. These pauses, lengthenings, and repetitions, which give a choppy quality to the stutterer's speech, are commonly referred to as *dysfluencies*. Pauses associated with muscular tension in the lips, face, and jaw are often referred to as *stuttering blocks*.

The stutterer's speech consists of sounds that are improperly patterned in time. It is difficult to pinpoint the exact location of the abnormality. When a stutterer says, "s-s-s sound," where is the actual dysfluency? At one time it was contended that the dysfluency was on the *s*. Most investigators now concur that the deficit is on the transition from one sound to the next. Indeed, the stutterer is able to say the *s* but not the *ound*. The stutterer's coping mechanism is such that he or she repeats the *s* until the transition into the following *ound* is secured (Bloodstein 1995).

As stutterers struggle to produce the intended sound, their muscle contractions and distorted movements can appear dystonic. However, not only can they stop these aberrant movements by cessation of talking, they can often use speech therapy techniques to eradicate these movements. These distorted movements (e.g., marked eye closure, pronounced lip puckering, tongue thrusting) associated with their speech production are referred to as secondary characteristics of speech and do not represent a true dystonia (Rosenfield 1994; Bloodstein 1995).

Stuttering occurs in all cultures, all civilizations, and all languages. One percent of the world's adult population stutters. There is a higher concordance of stuttering among identical and fraternal twins, suggesting a strong genetic component. Stuttering is two to four times more common among males than among females (Bloodstein 1995).

Stutterers have difficulty appropriately controlling their laryngeal sound source. Indeed, stutterers who undergo laryngectomy for laryngeal cancer become fluent when they use an electronic larynx. The electromyographic relationship between laryngeal abductor and adductor muscles is abnormal during moments of a stutterer's dysfluency. Voice onset time and voice termination time, indices of neurolaryngeal control, are likewise abnormal in stutterers (Bloodstein 1995). Nudelman et al. (1992) model stuttering as a momentary instability in a complex multiloop control system.

The location of stuttered dysfluencies is not random (Table 13.4). Stutterers' dysfluencies occur where fluent speakers' occasional dysfluencies also occur, at the beginning of sentences and phrases. One seldom hears a stutterer say, "Go to the hospital-l-l." Rather, "G-G-Go to the hospital." Stuttering is worse under stress, although stuttering has never been shown to be a psychogenic disturbance. Psychotherapy does not cure stuttering (Bloodstein 1995).

Several maneuvers evoke fluency in stutterers. The most potent is singing. Others include speaking in cadence with a metronome, oral reading, white noise, broad-band noise, delayed auditory feedback, speaking while inhaling, and repetition of the same passage (adaptation effect) (Bloodstein 1995).

Although it is rare for an individual to become a stutterer de novo, there are a number of reports of fluent individuals who became nonaphasic stutterers following a cerebral insult. This can result from cortical or subcortical damage in either hemisphere, which is usually mild but can be severe. Causes include vascular stroke, mild head trauma, electrical injury, and psychogenic factors. Their dysfluencies differ from those of developmental stutterers. Whereas the latter have difficulty in achieving the target sound (e.g., ba-ba-ba-book), the acquired stutterers achieve the target but repeat

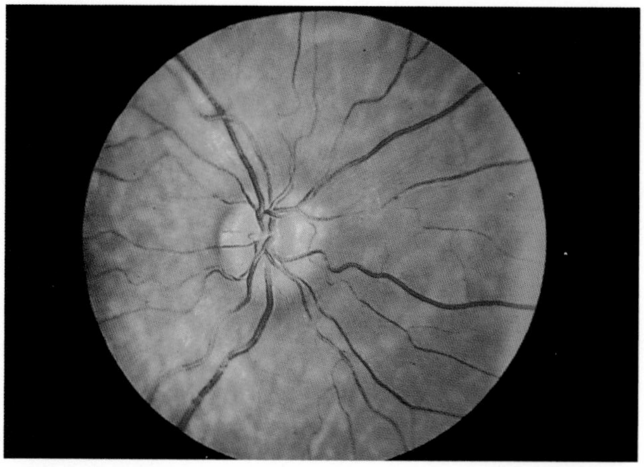

PLATE 15.I Pseudopapilledema in a 14-year-old boy. Note that the disc margins are blurred but the nerve fiber layer appears clear. No drusen are evident on the surface. The fellow eye appeared similar. (From RW Beck, CH Smith. Neuro-ophthalmology: A Problem-Oriented Approach. Boston: Little, Brown, 1988. Reprinted with permission of the author and publisher.)

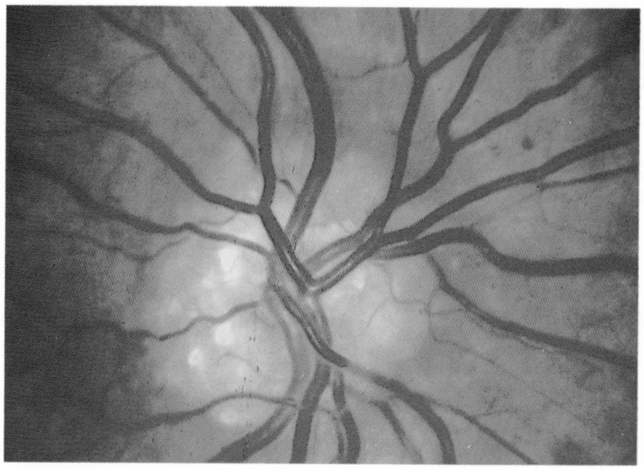

PLATE 15.II Optic disc drusen in a 50-year-old man. (From RW Beck, CH Smith. Neuro-ophthalmology: A Problem-Oriented Approach. Boston: Little, Brown, 1988. Reprinted with permission of the author and publisher.)

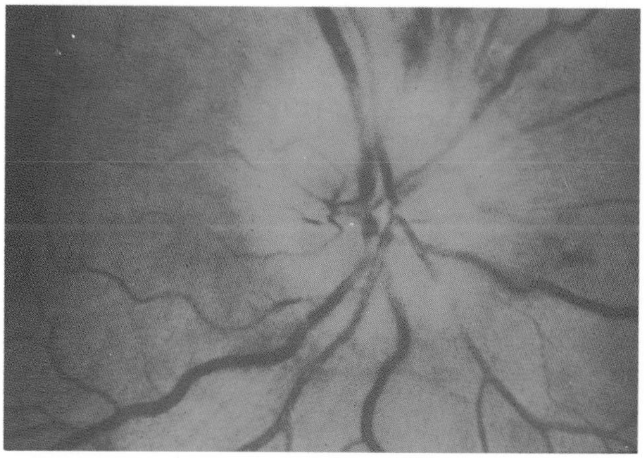

PLATE 15.III Anterior ischemic optic neuropathy in a 52-year-old woman.

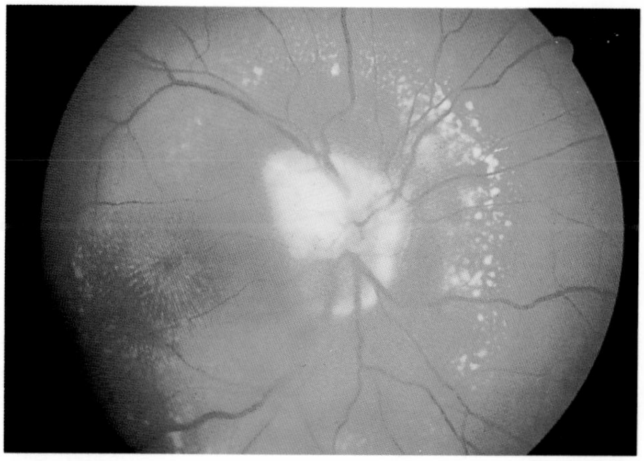

PLATE 15.IV Neuroretinitis in a 6-year-old boy. Although exudates of this type are usually not present in optic neuritis, when present, they indicate an inflammatory cause for the disc edema. (From RW Beck, CH Smith. Neuro-ophthalmology: A Problem-Oriented Approach. Boston: Little, Brown, 1988. Reprinted with permission of the author and publisher.)

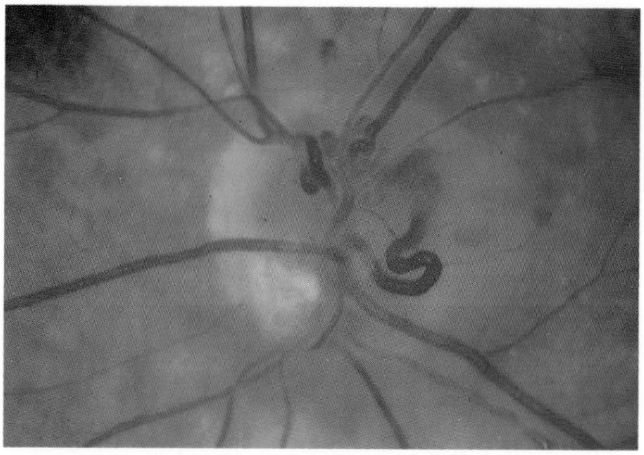

PLATE 15.V Optic disc swelling and optociliary shunt vessels in a 44-year-old woman with a sphenoid meningioma. (From RW Beck, CH Smith. Neuro-ophthalmology: A Problem-Oriented Approach. Boston: Little, Brown, 1988. Reprinted with permission of the author and publisher.)

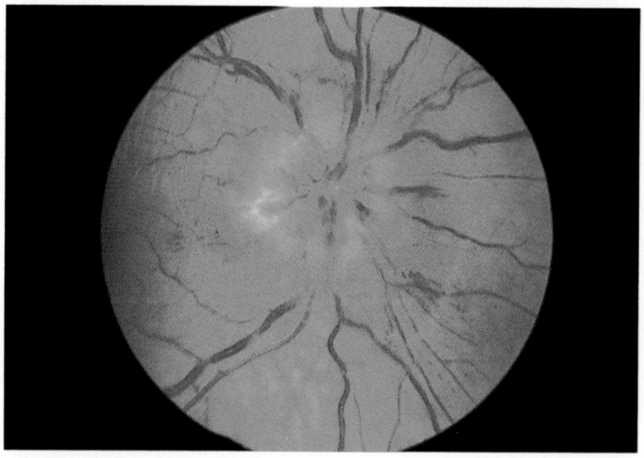

PLATE 15.VI Papillophlebitis in a 23-year-old woman. (From RW Beck, CH Smith. Neuro-ophthalmology: A Problem-Oriented Approach. Boston: Little, Brown, 1988. Reprinted with permission of the author and publisher.)

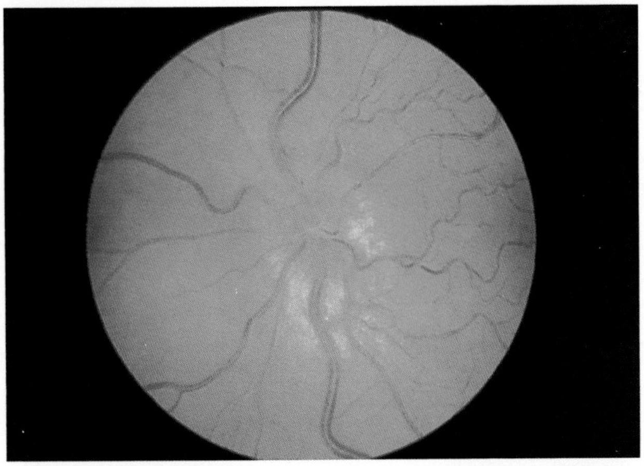

PLATE 15.VII Optic disc edema and hyperemia from central retinal vein occlusion in a 55-year-old asymptomatic woman. (From RW Beck, CH Smith. Neuro-ophthalmology: A Problem-Oriented Approach. Boston: Little, Brown, 1988. Reprinted with permission of the author and publisher.)

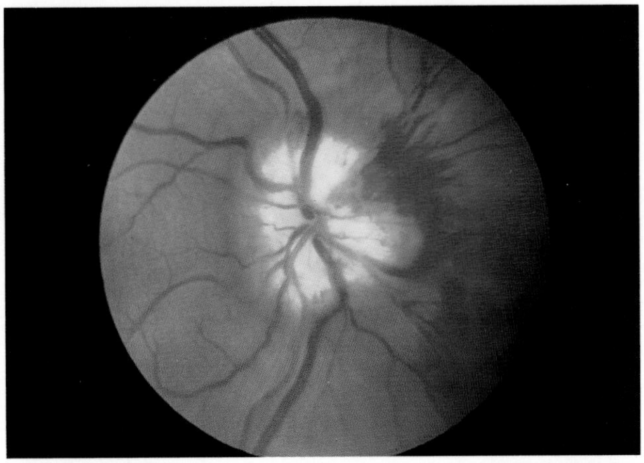

PLATE 15.VIII Optic disc swelling, hemorrhage, and infiltration in sarcoidosis in a 30-year-old man. (From RW Beck, CH Smith. Neuro-ophthalmology: A Problem-Oriented Approach. Boston: Little, Brown, 1988. Reprinted with permission of the author and publisher.)

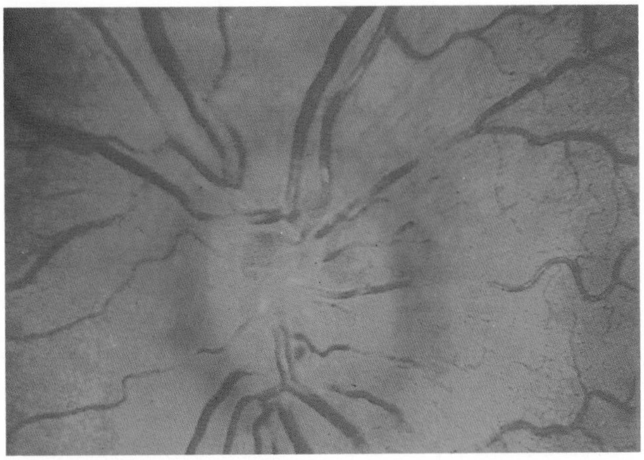

PLATE 15.IX Hyperemic disc with telangiectatic vessels in the peripapillary nerve fiber layer in a 26-year-old man with Leber's optic neuropathy. (From RW Beck, CH Smith. Neuro-ophthalmology: A Problem-Oriented Approach. Boston: Little, Brown, 1988. Reprinted with permission of the author and publisher.)

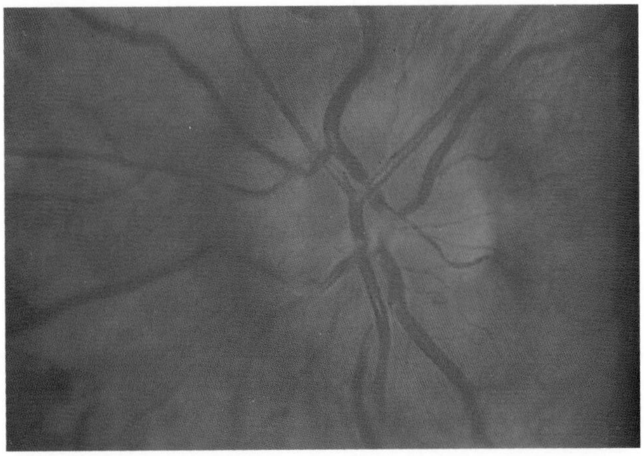

PLATE 15.X Swollen optic disc in early papilledema. Note that the swelling is more prominent superiorly and inferiorly than it is temporally. (From RW Beck, CH Smith. Neuro-ophthalmology: A Problem-Oriented Approach. Boston: Little, Brown, 1988. Reprinted with permission of the author and publisher.)

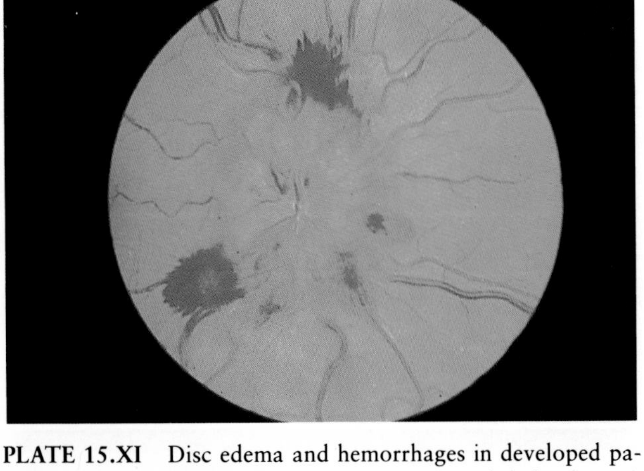

PLATE 15.XI Disc edema and hemorrhages in developed papilledema. (From RW Beck, CH Smith. Neuro-ophthalmology: A Problem-Oriented Approach. Boston: Little, Brown, 1988. Reprinted with permission of the author and publisher.)

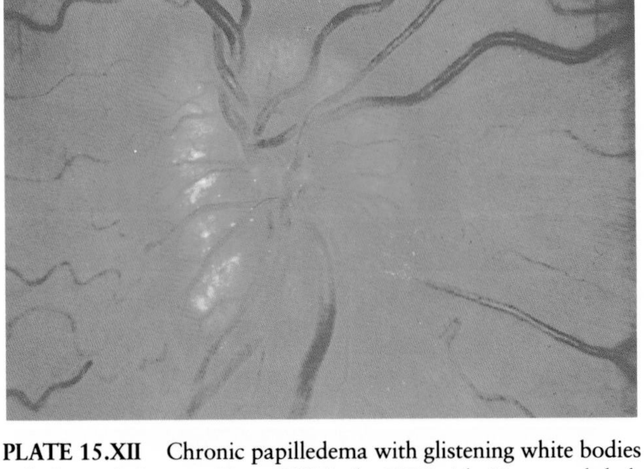

PLATE 15.XII Chronic papilledema with glistening white bodies called pseudodrusen. (From RW Beck, CH Smith. Neuro-ophthalmology: A Problem-Oriented Approach. Boston: Little, Brown, 1988. Reprinted with permission of the author and publisher.)

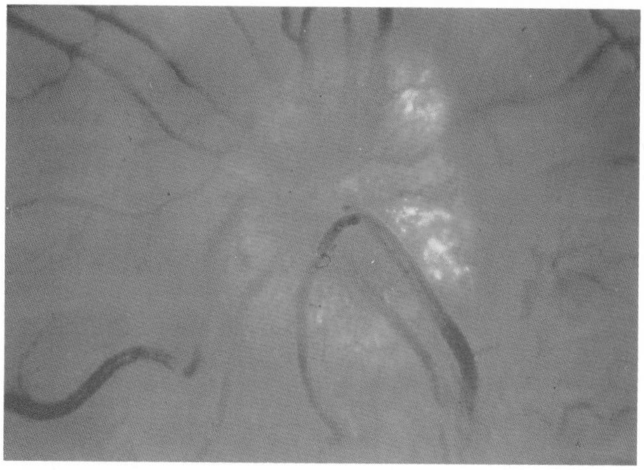

PLATE 15.XIII Chronic papilledema with marked disc elevation and gliotic appearance to disc surface. Note that hemorrhages are not present.

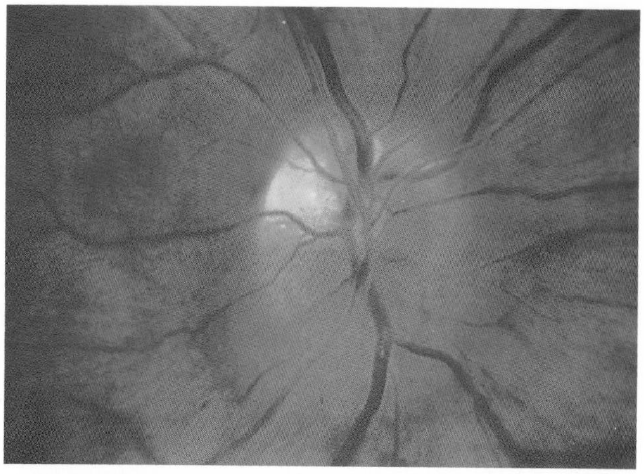

PLATE 15.XIV Chronic papilledema with optic atrophy. Note that the superior portion of the optic disc is pale and not swollen as a result of damaged axons. (From RW Beck, CH Smith. Neuro-ophthalmology: A Problem-Oriented Approach. Boston: Little, Brown, 1988. Reprinted with permission of the author and publisher.)

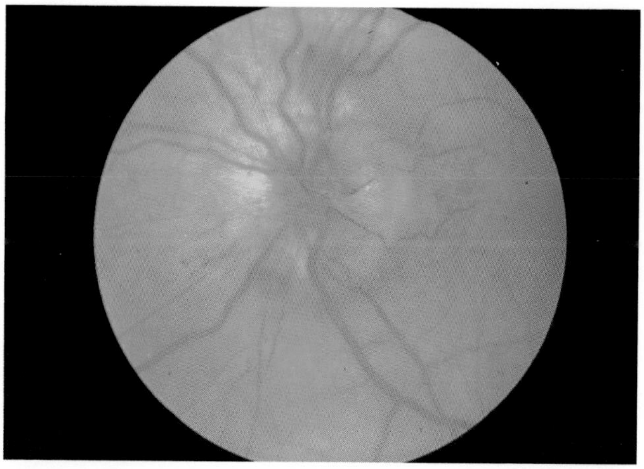

PLATE 15.XV Swollen optic disc from malignant hypertension. The fellow disc appeared similar. (From RW Beck, CH Smith. Neuro-ophthalmology: A Problem-Oriented Approach. Boston: Little, Brown, 1988. Reprinted with permission of the author and publisher.)

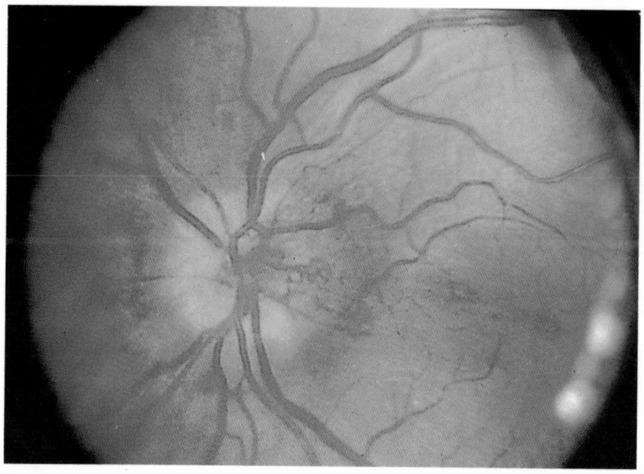

PLATE 15.XVI Diabetic papillopathy in a 17-year-old girl. Note the telangiectatic vessels on the disc surface. (From RW Beck, CH Smith. Neuro-ophthalmology: A Problem-Oriented Approach. Boston: Little, Brown, 1988. Reprinted with permission of the author and publisher.)

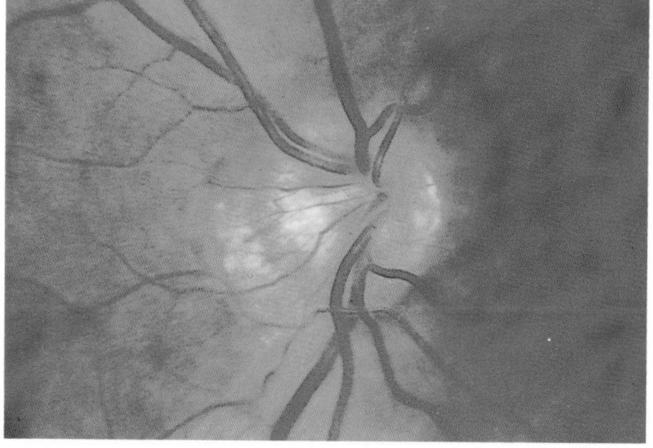

PLATE 15.XVII Tilted optic disc. The fellow eye appeared similar.

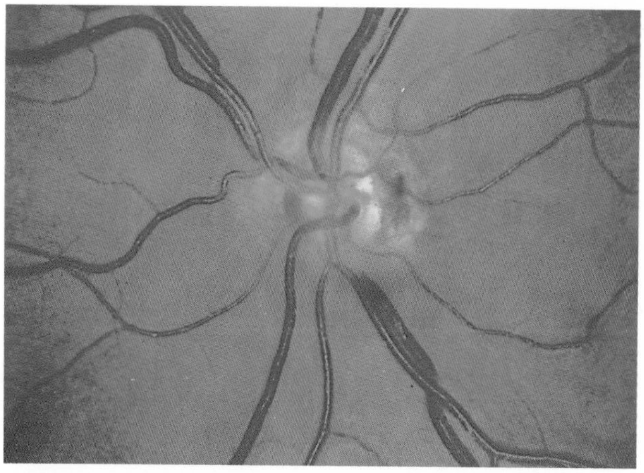

PLATE 15.XVIII Optic nerve hypoplasia. (From RW Beck, CH Smith. Neuro-ophthalmology: A Problem-Oriented Approach. Boston: Little, Brown, 1988. Reprinted with permission of the author and publisher.)

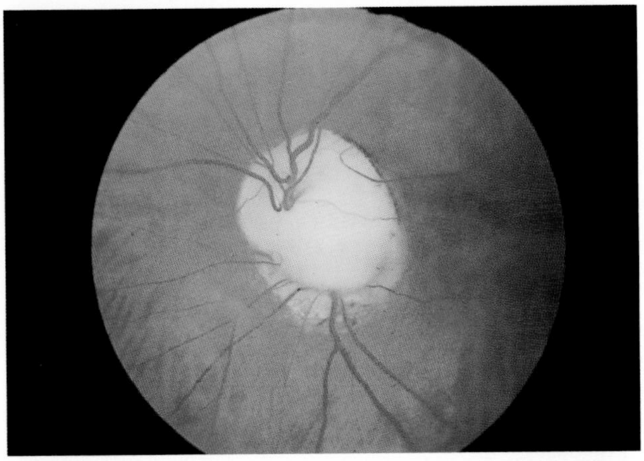

PLATE 15.XIX Optic disc coloboma. (From RW Beck, CH Smith. Neuro-ophthalmology: A Problem-Oriented Approach. Boston: Little, Brown, 1988. Reprinted with permission of the author and publisher.)

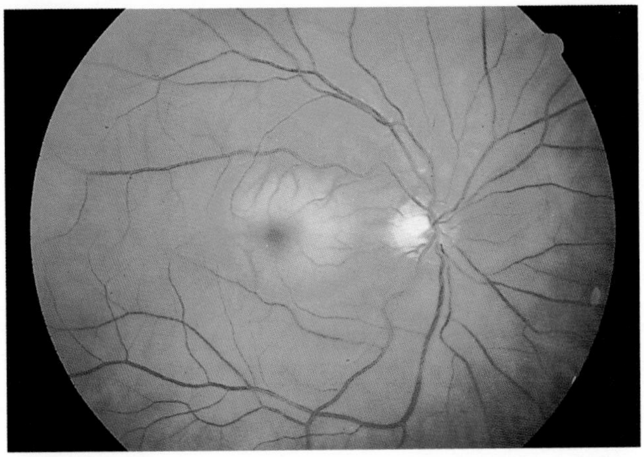

PLATE 15.XX Central retinal artery occlusion. Note the cherry-red spot in the center of the fovea, with surrounding whitening of the retina.

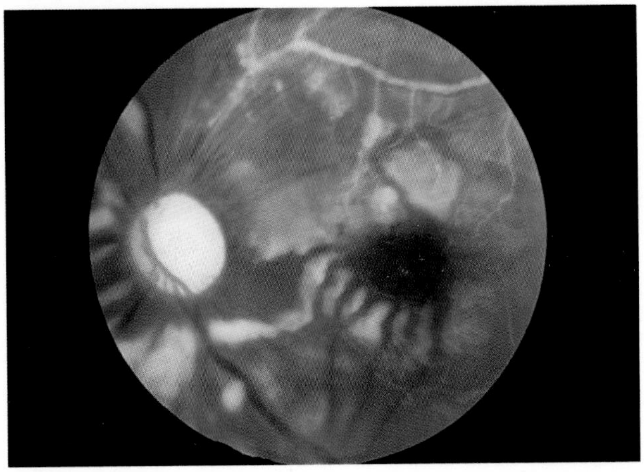

PLATE 15.XXI Multiple cotton wool spots in a patient with lupus.

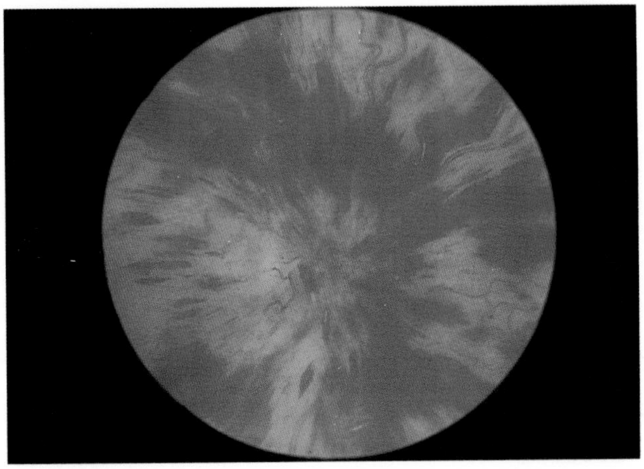

PLATE 15.XXII Central retinal vein occlusion.

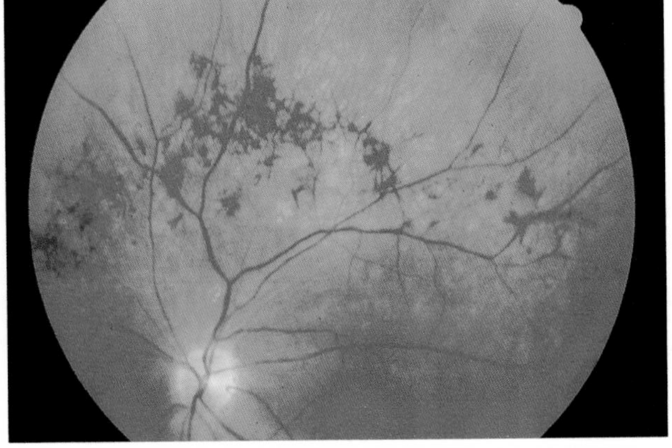

PLATE 15.XXIII Retinitis pigmentosa.

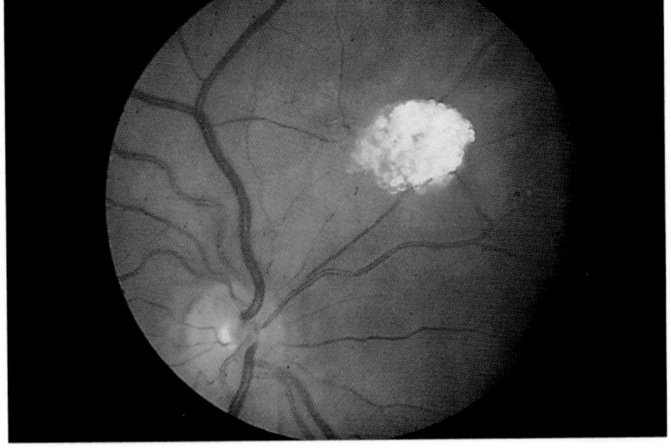

PLATE 15.XXIV Astrocytic hamartoma in a patient with tuberous sclerosis.

it (e.g., boo-boo-book). This difference is often clinically perceptible at the bedside and further underlines the possibility of psychogenic factors in some acquired dysfluents: If they usually achieve the target, why do they repeat it? These patients are also distinguished from developmental stutterers in that acquired stutterers have dysfluencies scattered throughout the sentence, and that fluency-evoking maneuvers are ineffective. Further, unlike developmental stutterers, they are usually not distraught over their altered output (Rosenfield et al. 1991).

Cluttering

Clutterers produce abnormal speech characterized by excessive speed, repetitions, drawling, interjections, disturbed prosody, monotony, and sometimes inconsistent articulatory disturbances (see Table 13.4). Some authors contend that they have grammatical difficulties, hyperactivity, poor concentration, and poorly integrated thought processes, although this has never been proved (Hardcastle 1989).

There may be omission of sounds, syllables, and whole words, as well as inversion of the orders of sounds, or repetition of the initial sounds, and a tendency to prolong several syllables of the word. Although the rate of speech may not always be markedly increased, the listener usually has a sensation that it is. As opposed to developmental stutterers, clutterers are frequently unconcerned about their speech deficit and often become irritated when someone points it out to them (Hardcastle 1989).

Palilalia

Palilalics compulsively repeat phrases or words with reiteration at increasing speed and a frequent decrescendo of phonatory volume (see Table 13.4). Often, the volume begins near normal and then decreases markedly, creating difficulty in hearing the patient and distinguishing speech sounds. As opposed to developmental stutterers, they seldom repeat phonemes but do repeat whole words and phrases, sometimes even whole sentences. This phenomenon is usually seen in postencephalitic Parkinson's disease, pseudobulbar palsy, and idiopathic Parkinson's disease. In the past, it was frequently associated with syphilis (Rosenfield 1994).

Examination and Investigation

Stutterers and clutterers usually have a normal neurological examination. Palilalics may have stigmata of parkinsonism. Acquired stutterers can have any type of neurological deficit; this disturbance has been associated with lesions just about anywhere in the nervous system above the level of the brain stem.

Psychiatric evaluation seldom proves fruitful in ascertaining the cause of developmental stuttering. It may, however, be useful in determining why the patient with a long-standing speech defect has only now decided to see a physician about the problem.

All dysfluent individuals who see a neurologist (see Table 13.4) should also be referred to a speech-language pathologist for evaluation and therapy. Stutterers and clutterers with no other complaints do not require any particular neurological investigations. The evaluation for acquired stuttering should involve investigation for an underlying organic cause, including neuroimaging of the brain, electroencephalogram (EEG), and other studies relating to acquired dysfunction, concentrating on tumor, vascular disease, and toxic and metabolic disturbances. Palilalics should have a thorough examination for basal ganglia disturbance, possible stroke, and tumor. Clutterers frequently warrant neuropsychological assessment to rule out any underlying learning disturbance.

DYSPHAGIA

Dysphagia, or difficulty in swallowing, is a subjective symptom, as opposed to an objective sign, until there is documentation of delay or disruption in the swallowing mechanism. If no objective evidence of dysphagia can be documented, globus hystericus should be considered. *Odynophagia*, or deglutition-induced pain, can coexist with dysphagia, although the two also can occur independently. Dysphagia may be due to mechanical factors that physically narrow the oropharyngeal lumen and obstruct food passage, or to neuromotor diseases that cause inadequate food bolus propulsion into the stomach. Dysphagia almost invariably leads to reduction of oral nutrition intake and may lead to severe malnutrition, independent of the underlying primary disease.

There are three stages of swallowing (Logemann 1991). The first, or oral preparatory stage, refers to food passing from the mouth into the pharynx. The swallow reflex mediates the first stage into the second, or pharyngeal transfer stage, in which food passes through the pharynx, over the larynx, and into the esophagus. The third (esophageal) stage involves food transport from the proximal esophagus, the upper one-third of which contains striated muscle, down through the lower two-thirds (smooth muscle) and across the lower esophageal sphincter into the stomach.

The oral preparatory stage of deglutition involves a complex series of motions within the oral cavity: lip closure, tension within the buccinator muscles, downward movement of the soft palate (allowing breathing while masticating), and actual chewing of the food. The final step in the oral preparatory stage is positioning of the adequately mixed food bolus on the mid-dorsum of the tongue, which subsequently sweeps against the hard palate, pushing the bolus toward the posterior tongue surface and into the oropharynx.

The swallow reflex consists of several movements. The soft palate moves upward (velar elevation), closing the passageway between the oral and nasal cavity; the pharyngeal muscles contract (pharyngeal peristalsis), the larynx elevates, and there is posterior flexion of the epiglottis, closing the airway to the trachea. Vocal cord closure occurs, followed by relaxation of the cricopharyngeus muscle, the upper esophageal sphincter.

The pharyngeal stage of swallowing is initiated in response to the swallow reflex. Pharyngeal contraction generates high pressure behind the food bolus, pushing it toward the upper esophageal sphincter. The upper sphincter opens, with associated contraction of muscles that elevate the larynx. After passage of the bolus, the upper sphincter contracts and closes firmly. This mechanism generates a high pressure gradient between the pharyngeal area rostral to the upper sphincter (approximately 45 mm Hg) and the intrathoracic esophagus (–6 mm Hg). This results in powerful transport of the food bolus into the thoracic esophagus. Coordinated peristaltic waves transport the food bolus into the stomach following lower esophageal sphincter relaxation.

The vagus nerve supplies motor fibers to the striated muscle of the esophagus. Thus, a serious consequence of damaging the vagus at the origin of the main esophageal branches is dysphagia. A high vagotomy permanently paralyzes the striated muscle of the upper one-third of the esophagus. Peristalsis in the lower two-thirds of the esophagus is an automatic function, mediated by the intrinsic myoenteric plexuses and smooth muscle (Richter 1993).

Symptoms

Patients with preserved mental status usually distinguish the stage of swallowing at which their problem occurs. It is first necessary to differentiate the level of dysphagia, oropharyngeal or esophageal, and whether the cause is mechanical or neuromotor. A meticulous history often allows a precise diagnosis without expensive and time-consuming investigations.

Symptoms related to oropharyngeal dysphagia (mechanical or neuromotor) typically occur immediately on swallowing and include the sensation of food sticking in the neck, odynophagia, nasal regurgitating of fluids or foods, and coughing or choking due to aspiration. Nasal regurgitation can occur from soft palate weakness, usually reflecting damage to vagus output. Tracheobronchial aspiration can reflect dysfunction of oropharyngeal swallowing coordination or tracheoesophageal fistula and occurs in esophageal dysphagia. Patients with oropharyngeal dysphagia usually locate discomfort to the midneck area, as opposed to the retrosternal or suprasternal notch discomfort seen in esophageal dysphagia.

Symptoms related to mechanical (oropharyngeal or esophageal) dysphagia are usually caused by difficulty in swallowing solid foods, progressing to difficulty in swallowing liquids. At advanced stages, patients cannot even swallow their own salivary secretions. Symptoms can occur immediately or seconds or minutes after swallowing, depending on the level and chronicity of the underlying process. More rostral levels of dysfunction cause earlier symptoms. Slowly developing diseases allow for physiological accommodation to the dysfunction, delaying the onset of symptoms.

Transient dysphagia, commonly associated with odynophagia, suggests an inflammatory process such as peptic esophagitis or monilial esophagitis. Chronic episodic dysphagia suggests a benign process such as a motility disorder or a lower esophageal muscular ring.

A long history of gastroesophageal reflux symptoms (heartburn), followed by the appearance of dysphagia, suggests peptic stricture complicating chronic esophagitis. Severe weight loss in association with dysphagia suggests esophageal carcinoma. Laryngeal involvement can occur from compression of the laryngeal nerve by an esophageal tumor. In this setting, hoarseness usually follows dysphagia. Hoarseness preceding dysphagia suggests a primary laryngeal lesion.

Benign tumors of the esophagus rarely cause dysphagia because of the mobility of the esophagus within the thorax. Malignant tumors fix the esophagus by invading local structures, causing dysphagia at an earlier stage. Rarely, congenital vascular rings may compress the thoracic portion of the esophagus. For instance, abnormal origin of the right subclavian artery may cause the classic syndrome of *dysphagia lusoria*, in which the esophagus is caught between the abnormal artery originating from the distal aortic arch and the aorta, thoracic spine, or sternum.

Neuromotor disturbance of esophageal motility often presents with dysphagia for liquids, solids, or both. In this setting, dysphagia for solids is proportionally more consistent in both standing and supine positions. Dysphagia may occur in both positions for liquids as well, but it is usually much less severe when the patient is standing. Radiological and esophageal endoscopic examination, together with manometry, usually provide the diagnosis.

Neuromotor dysphagia (oropharyngeal or esophageal) is more frequently precipitated by fluids than by solids. Solid meals usually maintain integrity of the food bolus, as opposed to liquid meals, which tend to spill over the laryngeal structures into the airway. Patients with neuromotor dysphagia due to oropharyngeal compromise have fewer symptoms with semisolid foods such as scrambled eggs, yogurt, or mashed potatoes.

Neuromotor dysphagia usually has an insidious onset, although a sudden onset can occur following trauma or stroke. Mechanical dysphagia usually has an insidious onset. Hot or cold liquids can trigger dysphagia due to esophageal motility disorders, such as diffuse esophageal spasm or symptomatic esophageal peristalsis.

Examination

Oral motor examination includes careful evaluation of power and movement of the lips, tongue, and soft palate. The patient should maintain lip closure during chewing and swallowing in various head postures. Lingual movements should demonstrate normal anterior and posterior function. Anterior function is tested by asking the patient to move the tongue up, down, and sideways while touching the lips. Posterior function is assessed by asking the patient to hold the sound */ka/*. The tongue should touch the soft palate. The soft palate is assessed by having the patient say a long */a/* syllable. The palate should elevate symmetrically. The sound */ka/* and the word *Coca-Cola* should be crisp and not hypernasal.

The palatal reflex is evaluated by mechanically stimulating the junction of the hard and soft palates, observing bilateral elevation of the soft palate but no gag reflex. The gag reflex is elicited by mechanically stimulating the base of the tongue or the posterior pharyngeal wall. Again, elevation should be bilaterally symmetrical. If the patient has had multiple aspirations and food trauma to that area, it may be markedly diminished (Logemann 1991).

Oral examination enables the physician to diagnose the presence of dysfunction in the oral stage of dysphagia. Ancillary radiological examinations, such as the modified barium swallow and the cine-esophagram, may delineate details of the muscular dysfunction (Logemann 1991).

Complete physical examination provides additional evidence for the underlying disorder. Signs of neurological diseases that can cause oropharyngeal dysphagia, such as multiple sclerosis, basal ganglia disorders, and stroke, should be sought.

Physical examination is most helpful in revealing the cause in dysphagia of oropharyngeal origin. Examination seldom produces a diagnosis in esophageal dysphagia, unless systemic disease is also present. Systemic diseases with neuromotor involvement, such as dermatomyositis, polymyositis, diabetes mellitus, scleroderma, and amyloidosis, are diagnosed by the other manifestations of these disturbances. Dysphagia is usually a late secondary symptom in such disorders.

Investigation

Esophageal manometry is indispensable in all cases in which dysphagia is identified as being in the esophageal stage and an obvious mechanical cause is absent. It is invaluable for assessing manometric phenomena below the upper esophageal sphincter. However, this procedure is not very helpful in assessing oropharyngeal dysphagia because the upper swallowing events occur too fast for adequate detection.

Computerized solid-state circumferential transducers have been successfully used in evaluating manometric events of the pharynx and upper esophageal sphincter (Castell et al. 1993). This technology makes possible accurate recording of intraluminal pharyngeal pressure changes during swallowing. Although still investigational, this technique offers exciting perspectives in understanding the dynamics of oropharyngeal swallowing.

Esophageal manometry measures the intraluminal pressures during swallowing, through a multilumen catheter passed nasally into the esophagus. Each lumen is infused with water by a low-compliance infusing system with constant pressure generated by a pneumohydraulic pump. A transducer transmits the pressures to a polygraph, which then records them on paper running at constant speed. An examination of this recording permits determination of the amplitude and duration of esophageal contractions, as well as the characteristics of the peristalsis. The lower esophageal spincter is examined, and its baseline pressure gradient (compared to intragastric pressure) is measured, as is its ability to relax immediately following a swallow. The absence of esophageal peristalsis, associated with an increased pressure gradient at the lower esophageal sphincter along with incomplete relaxation of the lower sphincter after the swallow, is virtually diagnostic of achalasia. Absence of peristalsis with no detectable lower sphincter pressure suggests scleroderma.

Esophagoscopy allows detection of mucosal lesions, such as early neoplasms of the upper gastrointestinal tract, inflammatory changes of the mucosa, assessment of the benign or malignant nature of strictures, and the presence of epithelial metaplasia and gastroesophageal reflux disease (Barrett's esophagus). It is not a sensitive test for detecting motility disorders of the esophagus or extrinsic compression. Aside from the ability to collect samples for microbiological and pathological examinations, endoscopy also allows for still photography and video recording of the pathological findings.

Gastrointestinal endoscopy is of little value in neuromotor oropharyngeal dysphagia, other than to substantiate the absence of organic disease. This may be necessary if barium studies are not possible because of the risk of aspiration. Gastrointestinal endoscopy is necessary in evaluating esophageal dysphagia of any origin, as it has diagnostic and therapeutic capability (biopsy, dilation, coagulation of obstructive lesions).

Conventional barium swallow (esophagram) studies are of little help in oropharyngeal dysphagia. Barium swallow roentgenographic investigation demonstrates the contour of esophageal movements, documenting mucosal lesions such as ulcers, tumors, strictures, extrinsic compression, and intramural lesions. Severe motility disorders can also be noted on barium swallow. The first and second stages of swallowing occur too rapidly for adequate documentation of the events. This is a valuable exam in mechanical esophageal dysphagia and also in the particular case of achalasia, in which esophageal dilation with the typical pencil-shaped distal esophagus is well shown. A barium-impregnated marshmallow tablet of predetermined size may be helpful in demonstrating mechanical narrowing of the esophageal lumen, which might not otherwise be seen.

The barium swallow with cine-esophagram is often of great help in any patient with dysphagia. The cine-esophagram is a barium swallow recorded on videotape, permitting careful slow-motion examination of the different stages of swallowing. Motor incoordination of oral and pharyngeal muscles, nasal regurgitation, and aspiration of the dye are all well delineated with this technique. The ability to freeze motion of the pharyngeal stage and to analyze it in a frame-by-frame mode permits identification of dysmotility of that segment. This is the most important radiological examination for oropharyngeal dysphagia. Further, cine-esophagrams better demonstrate esophageal peristalsis. A variety of neuromotor disorders can be identified, including achalasia, diffuse esophageal spasm, and scleroderma.

The modified barium swallow, a modification of the cine-esophagram, permits assessment of oropharyngeal transit while swallowing three boluses of different consistencies (liquid, paste, and solid). It is also called the "cookie swallow test" because the solid swallow consists of a barium-impregnated cookie. It differs from the traditional barium swallow in that the former is designed to fill the pharynx with barium, outlining lesions and anatomic deformities. Although the modified test may not be essential for diagnosis, it provides information on dysphagia dynamics that facilitates the design of an appropriate dietary program.

In most cases, barium swallow with cine-esophagram establishes the level of dysphagia and the type, whether mechanical or neuromotor. If the dysphagia is esophageal, endoscopic examination is usually required.

In cases of oropharyngeal neuromotor dysphagia, little diagnostic information is attained by investigation beyond barium swallow with cine-esophagram. The underlying disorder is usually diagnosed by careful clinical evaluation. In esophageal neuromotor dysphagia, the absence of tumor must be confirmed by endoscopy. Additional diagnostic data obtained through esophageal manometry helps differentiate among various esophageal neuromotor motility disorders.

Simultaneous, synchronized videoradiology and computerized solid-state manometry are being investigated for the study of oropharyngeal dysphagia. This technology makes possible accurate measurements of intraluminal pharyngeal pressure changes during swallowing and correlates them precisely with radiologically observed events recorded on videotape (Castell et al. 1993).

Differential Diagnosis

Neurological disturbances can produce oropharyngeal weakness affecting the first and second stages of swallowing. Dysphagia due to stroke, syringomyelia, amyotrophic lateral sclerosis, and demyelinating disease may be due to bilateral corticobulbar tract damage, lower motor neuron damage, or both. If the disturbance is upper motor neuron and predominantly unilateral, symptoms frequently disappear after several months as a result of the bilateral innervation of the lower bulbar structures. If the disturbance is upper motor neuron and bilateral, symptoms may be permanent. If the disease produces unilateral lower motor neuron damage, symptoms persist but are much less severe than if the disease is bilateral (Tables 13.5 and 13.6).

Myopathy, neuromuscular junction disturbances, and neuropathy can alter deglutition. Diseases such as dermatomyositis and polymyositis can cause weak pharyngeal muscles with consequent dysphagia, aspiration, and nasal regurgitation, and can compromise skeletal muscle in the proximal esophagus. Disorders such as scleroderma involve preferentially the lower two-thirds of the esophagus and cause esophageal dysphagia. Diphtheria is sometimes followed by palatial and pharyngeal paralysis.

Autonomic nervous system involvement such as that seen in the Shy-Drager syndrome (idiopathic orthostatic hy-

Table 13.5: Causes of mechanical dysphagia

Oropharyngeal	*Esophageal*
Oropharyngeal tumor	Esophageal carcinoma
Zenker's diverticulum	Metastatic disease to esophagus (hematogenous, lymphatic, or contiguous spread)
Cervical anterior osteophytes	Benign esophageal tumor
Dislocation of temporomandibular joint	Postinflammatory strictures of the esophagus: peptic esophagitis, postsclerotherapy lye ingestion (caustic esophagitis), radiation-induced esophagitis
Macroglossia	Pill dysphagia (tetracycline, quinidine, potassium)
Congenital anomalies	Pancreatitis with pseudocysts
Tight circumoral tissue due to scleroderma or burns	Pancreatic tumors
Neck surgery	Postvagotomy hematoma or fibrosis
Retropharyngeal mass	Dysphagia lusoria (abnormal origin of right subclavian artery)
Large goiter	Thoracic aortic aneurysm
Right-sided aorta	Posterior mediastinal mass
	Fundal plication (antireflux surgery)
	Large hiatal hernia
	Large epiphrenic esophageal diverticulum

Table 13.6: Causes of neuromotor dysphagia

Oropharyngeal	*Esophageal*
Amyotrophic lateral sclerosis	Scleroderma
Brain tumor	Achalasia
Stroke (corticobulbar upper motor neuron, or lower motor neuron)	Diffuse esophageal spasm
Neuropathy (includes mechanical nerve injury)	Polymyositis and dermatomyositis (usually oropharyngeal)
Demyelinating disease (especially multiple sclerosis)	Idiopathic autonomic dysfunction
Degenerative diseases (especially spinocerebellar)	Postvagotomy dysphagia
Syringobulbia	Neuropathy (vagal disease, especially diabetes)
Arnold-Chiari malformation	Amyloidosis (primary or secondary)
Poliomyelitis	Symptomatic esophageal peristalsis ("nutcracker esophagus")
Neuromuscular junction abnormalities (myasthenia gravis)	
Myopathy, including oculopharyngeal muscular dystrophy, hyperthyroidism, polymyositis, and dermatomyositis	
Parkinson's disease	
Cerebral palsy	
Drug-induced (tardive) dyskinesia	
Cricopharyngeal achalasia	
Xerostomia (dry mouth) and Sjögren's syndrome	
Scleroderma	

potension and multiple system atrophy) as well as neuropathies (especially diabetes) can interfere with the esophageal (third) stage of swallowing. Destruction of the ganglion cells and intrinsic nervous plexuses of the esophagus, as is seen in Chagas' disease, interferes with the motility of the body of the esophagus and inhibits the relaxation of the lower esophageal sphincter, causing potentially serious dysphagia.

Diffuse esophageal spasm and symptomatic esophageal peristalsis (so-called nutcracker esophagus) are frequent causes of esophageal dysphagia. The former is characterized by prolonged, forceful, painful contraction of long segments of the distal esophagus, often precipitated by very cold or very hot fluids. Contractions are nonpropulsive by definition and are perceived by the patient either as episodes of chest pain or as dysphagia for liquids. Symptomatic esophageal peristalsis is a similar disorder, wherein the peristaltic contractions are very forceful and painful but over short segments of the esophagus and with the characteristic of peristaltic waves. Both disorders are of unknown cause.

REFERENCES

Aronson AE. Motor Speech Signs of Neurologic Disease. In DK Darby (ed), Speech Evaluation in Medicine. New York: Grune & Stratton, 1981;159–180.

Blitzer A, Brin M. The dystonic larynx. J Voice 1992;6:294–297.

Bloodstein O. A Handbook on Stuttering (5th ed). San Diego: Singular Publishing Group, 1995.

Borden GJ, Harris KS, Raphael LJ. Speech Science Primer: Physiology, Acoustics, and Perception of Speech. Baltimore: Williams & Wilkins, 1994.

Castell JO, Olsson R, Castell DO, Ekberg O. Simultaneous video radiography and manometry in dysphagia patients with normal barium swallows. Am J Gastroenterol 1993;88:1,483.

Hardcastle D. Disorders of Fluency. London: Whurr Publishers, 1989;120–128.

Logemann J. Evaluation and Treatment of Swallowing Disorders. San Diego: Pro-Ed, 1991.

Ludlow CL, Rhew K, Nash EA. Botulinum Toxin Injection for Adductor Spasmodic Dysphonia. In J Jankovic, M Hallett (eds), Therapy with Botulinum Toxin. New York: Marcel Dekker, 1994;437–451.

Nudelman HB, Herbrich KE, Hess KR et al. A model of the phonatory response time of stutterers and fluent speakers to frequency-modulated tones. J Acoust Soc Am 1992;92: 1882–1888.

Richter JE. Heartburn, Dysphagia, Odynophagia, and Other Esophageal Symptoms. In MH Sleisenger, JS Fordtran (eds), Gastrointestinal Disease. Philadelphia: Saunders, 1993;331–340.

Rosen S, Howell P. Signals and Symptoms for Speech and Hearing. London: Academic Press, 1991;259–281.

Rosenfield DB. Clinical Aspects of Speech Motor Compromise. In J Jankovic, M Hallett M (eds), Therapy with Botulinum Toxin. New York: Marcel Dekker, 1994;397–420.

Rosenfield DB, Viswanath NS, Callis-Landrum L et al. Patients with Acquired Aysfluencies: What They Tell Us About Developmental Stuttering. In HFM Peters, W Hulstijn, CW Starkkweather (eds), Speech Motor Control and Stuttering. Amsterdam: Excerpta Medica 1991;277–284.

Rosenfield DB, Viswanath N, Herbrich KE, Nudelman HB. Evaluation of the speech motor control system in amyotrophic lateral sclerosis. J Voice 1992;5:224–230.

Titze I. Vocal Fold Physiology: Frontiers in Basic Science. San Diego: Singular Publishing Group, 1993.

SUGGESTED READING

Gates GA. Guest editor for spasmodic dysphonia. J Voice 1992;6:293–400.

Netsell R. A Neurobiologic View of Speech Production and the Dysarthrias. San Diego: College-Hill, 1985.

Sonies BC, Baum BJ. Evaluation of swallowing pathophysiology. Otorhinolaryngol Clin North Am 1988;21:637–648.

Chapter 14
Visual Loss

Robert L. Tomsak

Visual loss frequently accompanies neurological illness and is one of the most disturbing symptoms a patient experiences. Loss of vision is often due to a benign or treatable process, but it may be the first sign of blinding or life-threatening disease. Common ocular causes of impaired vision or visual loss include uncorrected refractive errors, corneal problems, cataracts, glaucoma, retinal and choroidal diseases, strabismus, and amblyopia. At times, however, ocular causes of loss of vision are not apparent to the nonophthalmologist. Conversely, neurological causes of visual deterioration frequently confuse ophthalmologists. Thus, the approach to evaluating visual loss must be systematic and methodical so that important causes are not missed and simple causes are not evaluated to the extreme. This chapter deals mainly with the symptoms of visual loss; examination techniques are discussed in Chapter 42, and the appearance of specific funduscopic abnormalities is covered in Chapter 15.

TYPE AND SEVERITY OF VISUAL LOSS

Central Visual Field Loss

Any defect in the field of vision is called a *scotoma,* from the Greek word meaning "darkness." Loss of central vision, resulting in a central, or centrocecal, scotoma, is usually quickly noticed and reported. Peripheral visual field defects like homonymous hemianopia may be asymptomatic, or they may be referred to the eye with the larger homonymous visual field (Figure 14.1). If a central or centrocecal scotoma is present, it is usually due to disease involving the central retina or optic nerve anywhere along its intraocular, intraorbital, intracanalicular, or intracranial course. In the case of predominantly one-sided involvement of the optic chiasm, a central scotoma may be associated with a contralateral silent temporal hemianopia (Figure 14.2). Therefore, it is imperative that visual function of each eye be assessed separately in history taking as well as during the examination.

In general, scotomas due to macular disease are positive, meaning that they are perceived as a black or gray spot in the visual field. Patients with macular visual loss may also complain of distortion of images, so that straight edges or geometric figures appear crooked or distorted. This symptom, called *metamorphopsia,* is almost always caused by a retinal problem; only rarely does metamorphopsia represent a disorder of higher cortical function.

Optic nerve lesions characteristically produce negative scotomas, or areas of absent vision not otherwise perceptible, often in conjunction with decreased appreciation of color and light brightness. On occasion, paradoxical photophobia or glare is a prominent symptom of optic nerve damage (Glaser 1990). *Photopsias* (light flashes) may be perceived with retinal or optic nerve disease and imply an active or irritative cause; they may also be a result of migrainous cortical phenomena and are therefore nonlocalizing unless they are clearly correlated with eye movement, which implicates the retina or optic nerve.

Aside from ocular diseases, deficits of bilateral central visual function can also be produced by chiasmal lesions or by bilateral lesions in the macular visual cortex; the possibility of feigned or hysterical visual loss must also be considered (see Chapter 42). The importance of carefully examining the visual field in cases of visual loss cannot be overemphasized.

Patterns of Visual Field Loss

For simplicity, visual field defects can be classified in one of three groups: prechiasmal, chiasmal, or retrochiasmal. Unilateral prechiasmal lesions affect the visual field in one eye only; chiasmal lesions affect the fields of both eyes in a nonhomonymous fashion; and retrochiasmal lesions cause homonymous field defeats with variable degrees of congruity depending on their location (Figure 14.3) (Glaser 1990). See Chapter 42 for additional discussion of patterns of visual field loss.

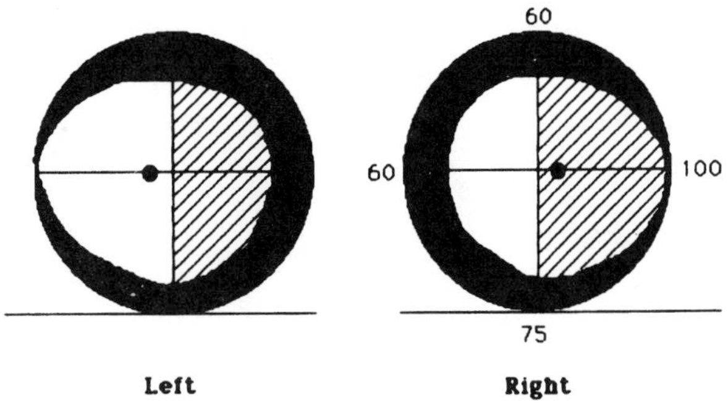

FIGURE 14.1 Right homonymous hemianopia. Visual loss may be referred to the right eye because the temporal visual field is larger than the nasal visual field. Numbers refer to normal extent of visual field in degrees.

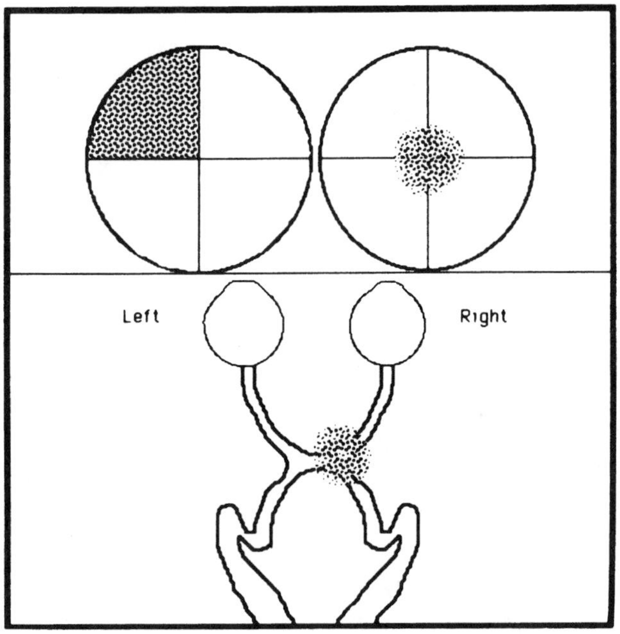

FIGURE 14.2 Junction scotoma with chiasmal lesion. The right optic nerve is primarily involved, leading to centrocecal scotoma. Crossing fibers are also affected, resulting in an upper temporal visual field defect; this is often asymptomatic and must be carefully searched for (see Chapter 42).

TEMPORAL PROFILE OF VISUAL LOSS

Visual Loss of Sudden Onset

Visual loss of sudden onset can be divided into three temporal patterns: transient, nonprogressive, or progressive.

Unilateral Transient Visual Loss (Table 14.1)

Amaurosis Fugax. The term *amaurosis fugax* is commonly reserved for transient monocular blindness (TMB) due to emboli to the retinal circulation from carotid vessels or from the heart (Winterkorn et al. 1993). Typically, these attacks are sudden in onset, last 5–15 minutes, and are usually accompanied by scotomas that sometimes are described as a shade or curtain being pulled in front of the eye (usually downward) (Wray 1995). Only rarely do attacks of TMB from carotid disease cause photopsias (Gautier 1993). The visual loss may also be quadrantic or total. Ipsilateral hemispheric symptoms may or may not be present.

Table 14.1: Causes of transient monocular blindness

1. Embolic cerebrovascular disease
2. Migraine (vasospasm)
3. Hypoperfusion (hypotension, hyperviscosity, hypercoagulability)
4. Ocular (intermittent angle closure glaucoma, hyphema, optic disc edema, partial retinal vein occlusion)
5. Vasculitis (e.g., giant cell arteritis)
6. Other (Uhthoff's phenomenon,* idiopathic, psychogenic)

*Temporary decrease in acuity consequent to exercise or other causes of increased body temperature, in patients with demyelinating optic neuropathy.

Retinal Migraine. TMB can be caused by retinal migraine, presumably a vasospastic event. Patients with migrainous monocular visual loss tend to be younger and do not have risk factors for embolic or atherosclerotic disease, although increased platelet aggregability may play a role. Retinal migraine is usually longer lasting than embolic fleeting blindness and may be accompanied by positive visual phenomena such as white-outs or sparklers. The visual loss often begins as concentric constriction of the visual field indicative of generalized ocular hypoperfusion. It may be brought on by postural change or exercise, and an aching sensation around the eye is often mentioned by those affected (Wray 1995).

Angle Closure Glaucoma. Subacute attacks of angle closure glaucoma should also be considered in the differential diagnosis of intermittent monocular visual loss, especially if the patient complains of halos around lights. This symptom results from corneal edema related to rapid elevations of intraocular pressure and may not be associated with eye pain or redness.

Visual Loss in Bright Light. Some patients with severe impairment of blood flow to the eye also lose vision in bright light, presumably as a result of impaired regeneration of photopigments by ocular ischemia. This symptom can be thought of as a pathological variant of the *macular photostress phenomenon* (see Chapter 42) and is usually seen in the setting of complete internal carotid artery occlusion. Other retinal diseases, like cone dystrophy, also cause evanescent visual worsening in bright light, otherwise known as *hemeralopia* or day blindness.

Uhthoff's Phenomenon. Temporary loss of vision with elevation of body temperature (Uhthoff's phenomenon) is most often seen in the setting of optic neuritis associated

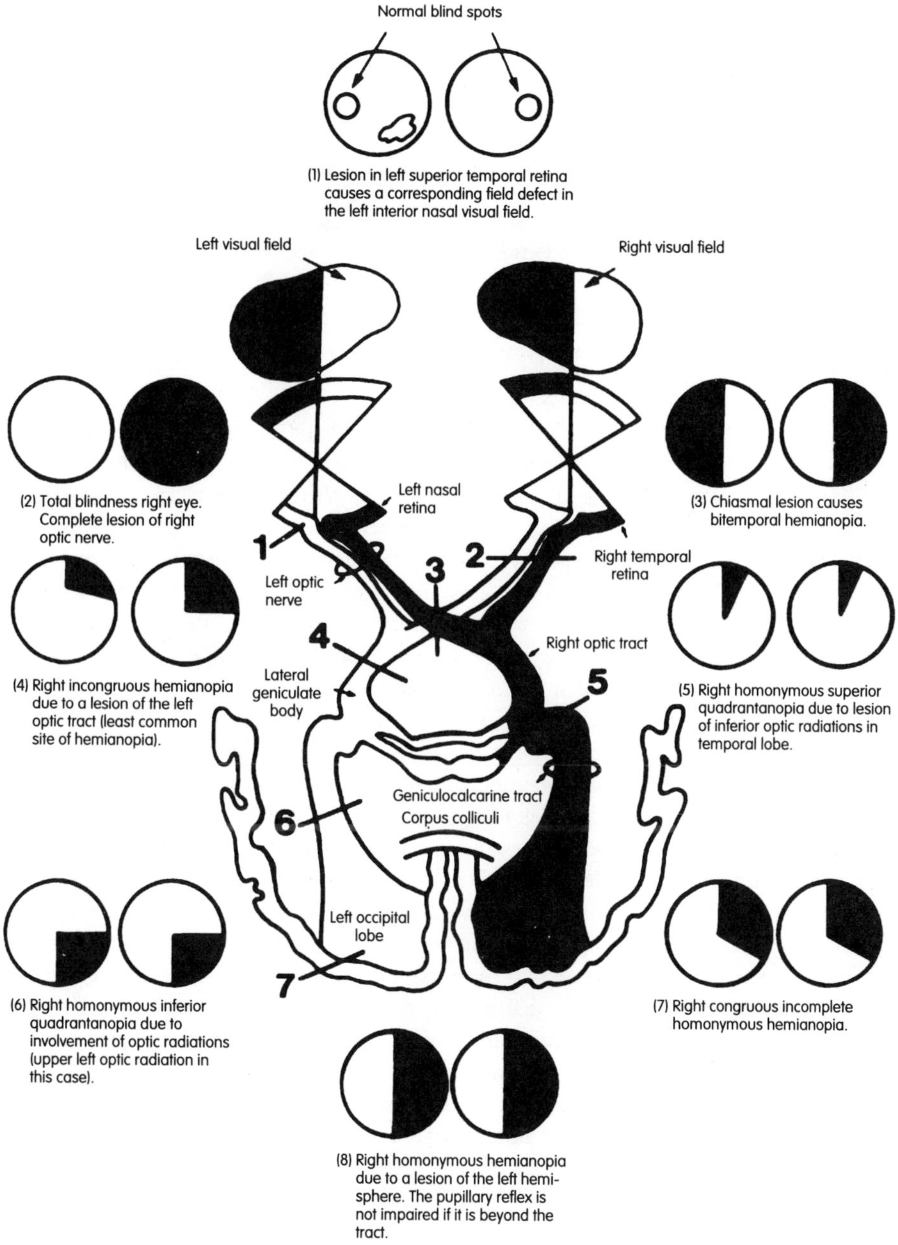
Normal blind spots
(1) Lesion in left superior temporal retina causes a corresponding field defect in the left interior nasal visual field.
Left visual field
Right visual field
(2) Total blindness right eye. Complete lesion of right optic nerve.
(3) Chiasmal lesion causes bitemporal hemianopia.
Left nasal retina
Right temporal retina
Left optic nerve
Right optic tract
Lateral geniculate body
(4) Right incongruous hemianopia due to a lesion of the left optic tract (least common site of hemianopia).
(5) Right homonymous superior quadrantanopia due to lesion of inferior optic radiations in temporal lobe.
Geniculocalcarine tract
Corpus colliculi
Left occipital lobe
(6) Right homonymous inferior quadrantanopia due to involvement of optic radiations (upper left optic radiation in this case).
(7) Right congruous incomplete homonymous hemianopia.
(8) Right homonymous hemianopia due to a lesion of the left hemisphere. The pupillary reflex is not impaired if it is beyond the tract.

FIGURE 14.3 Topographic diagnosis of visual field defects. (Reprinted with permission from C Vaughn, T Asbury, and KF Tabbara. General Ophthalmology [12th ed]. Norwalk, CT: Appleton & Lange, 1989: 244.)

with demyelinating disease but may also occur in other conditions such as Leber's optic neuropathy, Friedreich's ataxia, and suprasellar tumor.

Transient Visual Obscurations. Visual loss (unilateral or bilateral) lasting seconds in patients with chronic swelling of the optic discs is called a *transient visual obscuration*; the visual disturbance may be described as a gray-out and is often brought on by postural change or straining. This symptom is thought to represent transient hypoperfusion of the swollen nerve or nerves. Transient visual obscurations that are gaze-evoked are a hallmark of orbital tumors; they may also occur with systemic hypotension, temporal arteritis, or retinal venous stasis.

Other Remitting Visual Loss. Recurrent remitting visual loss has also been described with cystic tumors like sphenoid sinus mucocele, craniopharyngioma, and pituitary tumor (Wray 1995).

Bilateral Transient Visual Loss (Table 14.2)

Other than transient visual obscurations in patients with bilateral optic disc swelling, simultaneous complete or in-

Table 14.2: Causes of bilateral transient visual loss

1. Migraine
2. Cerebral hypoperfusion
   a. Thromboembolism
   b. Systemic hypotension
   c. Hyperviscosity
   d. Vascular compression
3. Epilepsy
4. Papilledema (transient visual obscurations)

Table 14.3: Causes of unilateral sudden visual loss—nonprogressive

1. Branch or central retinal artery occlusion
2. Anterior ischemic optic neuropathy—arteritic or nonarteritic
3. Branch or central retinal vein occlusion
4. Traumatic optic neuropathy
5. Central serous choroidopathy
6. Retinal detachment
7. Vitreous hemorrhage
8. Functional (psychogenic) visual loss

complete loss of vision in both eyes is virtually always evidence of transient visual cortex dysfunction. This symptom is usually due to decreased cerebral perfusion resulting from vasospasm, thromboembolism, systemic hypotension, hyperviscosity, or vascular compression (Glaser 1990). Transient posttraumatic blindness may occur, especially in children, and may represent a variant of migraine (Eldridge and Punt 1988). Hysteria or malingering may also be causes (see Chapter 42). Blindness as an epileptic phenomenon is extremely rare.

In most neuro-ophthalmological practices, visual migraine accompaniments are the most common cause of bilateral transient visual disturbances, especially when they occur in patients younger than 40. Fisher (1986) believes that similar migraine accompaniments occur in older people as well. Some criteria that support the diagnosis of late-life migrainous variants include the presence of scintillating scotomas with migration and expansion; headache; stereotyped recurrences; duration of 15–25 minutes; no permanent sequelae; and the absence of systemic risk factors. However, the diagnosis of a migraine accompaniment should be made only after other causes are excluded.

Nonprogressive Unilateral Sudden Visual Loss (Table 14.3)

Ischemic events affecting the optic nerve or retina are characteristically of sudden onset and are usually nonprogressive, although rarely a stuttering or step-by-step decline in vision may occur.

Anterior ischemic optic neuropathy presents mostly as infarction of the optic disc and is readily observable with the direct ophthalmoscope. In patients under age 60, it is usually due to atherosclerosis affecting the microcirculation to the optic nerve head. Congenital structural features of optic disc anatomy may also play a role. In people over 60, the possibility of cranial arteritis needs to be considered. Retrobulbar optic nerve infarction, also termed *posterior ischemic optic neuropathy*, is far less common but may occur in the setting of severe perioperative hypotension. Optic nerve infarction of embolic cause, or related to migraine, is exceptionally rare.

By contrast, branch or central retinal artery occlusions are mostly embolic or thrombotic in cause; opacification of the retinal nerve fiber layer with a cherry-red spot at the macula is the classic ophthalmoscopic presentation (see Chapter 15). Altitudinal, quadrantal, or complete visual field losses may occur with retinal arterial occlusions.

Occlusion of the central retinal vein presents as sudden visual loss with a characteristic hemorrhagic retinopathy; it usually occurs in adults with systemic hypertension or diabetes and results from venous thrombosis at the level of the lamina cribrosa of the sclera. A dense central scotoma with spared peripheral visual field is characteristic.

Idiopathic central serous chorioretinopathy can present as the sudden onset of a positive scotoma, often with symptoms of metamorphopsia or micropsia and a positive photo-stress test (see Chapter 42). This condition results from leakage of fluid into the subretinal space and occurs most often in males in the 20- to 45-year age range. The diagnosis may be difficult to make without the aid of fluorescein angiography. Spontaneous recovery usually occurs within a period of weeks to months, but occasionally laser photo-coagulation is needed to seal leaking vessels (Gass 1987).

Seemingly mild periocular contusion injuries can result in permanent optic nerve dysfunction. The mechanisms for traumatic optic neuropathy include contusion or laceration of the optic nerve in its canal, or shearing of nutrient vessels with subsequent ischemia.

Nonprogressive Bilateral Sudden Visual Loss (Table 14.4)

Sudden, permanent visual loss affecting bilateral vision, if not caused by trauma, is usually the result of an infarct in the visual radiations resulting in a homonymous hemianopia (Glaser 1990). In patients who are otherwise neurologically asymptomatic, the site of the insult is commonly the occipital lobe. Bilateral occipital lobe infarcts can result in tubular visual fields, checkerboard visual fields (see Fig-

Table 14.4: Causes of bilateral sudden visual loss—nonprogressive

1. Occipital lobe infarctions
2. Pituitary apoplexy
3. Functional (psychogenic) visual loss
4. Leber's hereditary optic neuropathy
5. Head trauma

Table 14.5: Causes of progressive visual loss

1. Anterior visual pathway inflammation
   a. Optic neuritis
   b. Sarcoidosis
   c. Meningitis
2. Anterior visual pathway compression
   a. Tumors
   b. Aneurysms
   c. Dysthyroid optic neuropathy
3. Hereditary optic neuropathies
4. Optic nerve drusen
5. Low-tension glaucoma
6. Chronic papilledema
7. Toxic and nutritional optic neuropathies
8. Drugs (e.g., ethambutol)
9. Radiation damage to anterior visual pathways
10. Paraneoplastic retinopathy or optic neuropathy

ure 14.3), or total cortical blindness. Cortical blindness from bilateral occipitoparietal lobe infarcts may be accompanied by denial of the visual defect and confabulation, also known as *Anton's syndrome*.

Sudden, bilateral loss of vision may also accompany pituitary apoplexy. This condition is usually associated with severe headache, diplopia, and alteration of mental status (Glaser 1990).

Leber's hereditary optic neuropathy is a maternally transmitted disease associated with mitochondrial DNA mutations in the genes encoding subunits of respiratory chain complex I. Mutations have been identified at positions 11,778, 3,460, 15,257, and 14,484 (Newman 1995) (see Chapter 42). This condition presents as rapid, often permanent, loss of central vision, usually in men during early adulthood. Most often, both eyes are affected within 1 year, sometimes simultaneously. In the acute phase, the triad of findings includes circumpapillary telangiectatic microangiopathy, nonedematous elevation of the optic disc (pseudoedema), and absence of fluorescein leakage during angiography. Arteriolar narrowing can be marked, and vascular tortuosity is often a clue early in the disease. Although Leber's hereditary optic neuropathy may cause loss of vision in women, it tends to be less severe than in men.

Visual Loss of Sudden Onset with Progression (Table 14.5)

Visual loss that appears suddenly and progressively worsens is often due to optic nerve demyelination (optic neuritis). The usual period for worsening is hours to days, but almost never longer than 2 weeks. An unusual presentation of bilateral optic neuritis combined with transverse myelitis is called *Devic's disease* (neuromyelitis optica). Less often, long-standing visual loss may be suddenly discovered and misinterpreted as being of sudden onset; in these cases, the examiner should beware of a chronic compressive problem.

Visual Loss of Gradual Onset (see Table 14.5)

Gradual onset is the hallmark of a compressive lesion affecting the prechiasmal or chiasmal visual pathways. Common causes include pituitary tumors, aneurysms, craniopharyngiomas, meningiomas, and gliomas (Glaser 1990). Granulomatous involvement of the optic nerve from sarcoidosis or tuberculosis can cause chronic progressive visual loss. Compression of the optic nerve at the orbital apex from ocular dysthyroidism may occur with minimal periocular signs of ocular motility disturbance (Glaser 1990). As noted previously, the visual loss may be so insidious as to go unnoticed until it is fortuitously discovered by the patient or during a routine examination.

Hereditary or degenerative diseases of the optic nerve or retina also need to be included in the differential diagnosis. For example, the familial optic atrophies are bilateral and are usually discovered in the first two decades of life (Glaser 1990). Visual loss may range from mild to severe and can be asymmetrical. Central and centrocecal scotomas with sparing of the peripheral fields is the rule. Temporal pallor of the discs sometimes occurs in association with a focal area of cupping. Color vision is usually abnormal, with red-green and blue-yellow defects predominating. Nystagmus as well as other neurological and endocrine abnormalities may be present.

Drusen of the optic nerve, a common form of pseudopapilledema, are often associated with visual field defects (see Chapter 15). Approximately 75% of patients have some form of visual field loss, which may include arcuate defects, sectoral scotomas, enlargement of the blind spot, and generalized visual field constriction. Loss of central visual acuity is unusual and is most commonly the result of a subretinal neovascular membrane forming with subsequent hemorrhage into the macula. If loss of central visual acuity occurs with optic disc drusen without obvious retinal pathology, a search for a retrobulbar compressive lesion should be undertaken. Drusen are thought to form from the extracellular deposition of plasma proteins and a variety of inorganic materials that act to compress optic nerve axons near the surface of the nerve head.

Low-tension glaucoma, often confused with a compressive optic neuropathy, is a condition in which glaucomatous disc and field changes develop in the presence of normal levels of intraocular pressure. Low-tension glaucoma is bilateral in 70% of patients. The average age is 66 years. Women are affected about twice as frequently as men. Small disc hemorrhages are seen in approximately 10% of patients. Diastolic hypertension and a history of sudden visual loss are present in about 20% of cases. A prior history of cardiovascular shock is acknowledged by about 5% of patients. The disease may be either progressive or static (Glaser 1990).

Chronic papilledema from pseudotumor cerebri can become a bilateral progressive optic neuropathy (Wall 1991). It is characterized by the development of a milky gray color to the discs, with pseudodrusen. Often, sheathing of retinal vessels occurs. Visual fields tend to become constricted, with nasal defects progressing to involve fixation. Optociliary shunt vessels can develop, as can sudden visual loss from ischemic optic neuropathy in rare cases. On occasion, optic atrophy progresses despite the relief of elevated intracranial pressure.

Toxic and nutritional amblyopias also are bilateral and usually progressive (Glaser 1990). This subject is controversial, and the disease is difficult to define. Its nutritional form is characterized by a history of a poor diet, gradual painless onset of visual impairment over weeks to months, impairment of color vision, centrocecal scotomas, and development of optic atrophy late in the disease. The current thought is that most cases of tobacco-alcohol amblyopia are related to vitamin B deficiencies. Other conditions that lead to nutritional deficiency states, such as jejunoileal bypass and ketogenic diet, have also been associated with bilateral optic neuropathy.

Medications that have definitely been shown to be toxic to the optic nerve in certain situations include ethambutol, isoniazid, chloramphenicol, and diiodohydroxyquin. Retinal toxins include chloroquin and phenothiazines.

Slowly progressive visual loss from radiation damage to the anterior visual pathways, especially the retina, may follow direct radiotherapy to the eye for primary ocular tumors or metastases, or after periocular irradiation for basal cell carcinoma, sinus carcinoma, and related malignancies (Guy and Schatz 1995). It may also occur after whole brain irradiation for metastases of gliomas or after parasellar radiotherapy for pituitary tumors or other neoplasms in this region (Capo and Kupersmith 1991). Radiation retinopathy becomes clinically apparent after a variable latent period of 3 months to a few years following radiotherapy and is usually irreversible. Its incidence is directly related to fraction size, total dose of radiation, and the use of concomitant chemotherapy (Guy and Schatz 1995). Radiation-induced retinal capillary endothelial cell damage is the initial event that triggers a retinopathy usually indistinguishable from diabetic retinopathy. Laser photo-coagulation is used for proliferative retinopathy and macular edema.

A rapidly progressive paraneoplastic retinopathy (cancer-associated retinopathy [CAR] syndrome) causes bilateral visual loss in some patients with cancer over a period of weeks to months. Small-cell carcinoma of the lung is the most often associated malignancy. The visual loss often precedes the diagnosis of cancer and is associated with a circulating antibody directed at the tumor and retinal and optic nerve antigens (Thirkill et al. 1989). Retinitis pigmentosa–like signs and symptoms are present including night blindness, constricted visual fields, and a subnormal to extinguished electroretinogram. No effective treatment is available. Paraneoplastic optic neuropathies have also been described (Malik et al. 1992).

REFERENCES

Capo H, Kupersmith MJ. Efficacy and complications of radiotherapy of anterior visual pathway tumors. Neurol Clin North Am 1991;9:179–204.

Eldridge PR, Punt JAG. Transient traumatic cortical blindness in children. Lancet 1988;1:815–816.

Fisher CM. Late-life migraine accompaniments: further experience. Stroke 1986;17:1033–1042.

Gass JDM. Stereoscopic Atlas of Macular Diseases (3rd ed). Vol. 1. St. Louis: Mosby, 1987;46–58.

Gautier J-C. Amaurosis fugax. N Engl J Med 1993;329:426–428.

Glaser JS. Neuro-ophthalmology (2nd ed.) Philadelphia: Lippincott, 1990.

Guy J, Schatz NJ. Radiation-induced Optic Neuropathy. In RJ Tusa, SA Newman (eds), Neuro-ophthalmological Disorders: Diagnostic Work-Up and Management. New York: Marcel Dekker, 1995;437–450.

Malik S, Furlan AJ, Sweeney PJ, et al. Optic neuropathy: a rare paraneoplastic syndrome. J Clin Neuro-ophthalmol 1992;12: 137–141.

Newman NJ. Hereditary Optic Neuropathies. In RJ Tusa, SA Newman (eds), Neuro-ophthalmological Disorders: Diagnostic Work-Up and Management. New York: Marcel Dekker, 1995;143–152.

Thirkill CE, FitzGerald P, Sergott RC et al.Cancer-associated retinopathy (CAR syndrome) with antibodies reacting with retinal, optic nerve and cancer cells. N Engl J Med 1989;321: 1589–1594.

Wall M. Idiopathic intracranial hypertension. Neurol Clin North Am 1991;9:73–96.

Winterkorn JMS, Kupersmith MJ, Wirtschaften SD, Forman S. Brief report: treatment of vasospastic amaurosis fugax with calcium-channel blockers. N Engl J Med 1993;329:396–398.

Wray SH. Amaurosis Fugax. In RJ Tusa, SA Newman (eds), Neuro-ophthalmological Disorders: Diagnostic Work-Up and Management. New York: Marcel Dekker, 1995;3–26.

Chapter 15
Abnormalities of the Optic Nerve and Retina

Roy W. Beck

A visual disturbance to the optic nerve can almost always be localized on the basis of visual acuity, color vision, pupillary reaction, and visual field. A differential diagnosis for the cause of the optic neuropathy in a given patient can be established by categorizing the patient on the basis of the history of the visual loss, whether one or both eyes are involved, the pattern of visual field loss, and the appearance of the optic disc. Chapter 14 describes the various patterns of visual field loss and history typically elicited in specific optic nerve disorders. This chapter presents the differential diagnosis of optic neuropathies based on the optic disc appearance. Many of the entities described here are discussed in more detail in Chapter 42.

Acquired optic neuropathies can be classified according to whether the optic disc appears normal, swollen, or pale. Table 15.1 provides a differential diagnosis based on the appearance of the optic disc.

SWOLLEN OPTIC DISC

In assessing an elevated optic disc, the physician must first determine whether there is acquired disc edema or whether the disc appearance is that of pseudopapilledema.

Pseudopapilledema

Pseudopapilledema can be present with or without visible drusen (hyaline bodies) (Plates 15.I and 15.II). Even when drusen are not apparent, the distinction between true and pseudopapilledema can almost always be made on the basis of the ophthalmoscopic findings (Table 15.2). Whether the nerve fiber layer is hazy, obscuring the underlying retinal vessels, as it is with edema, or whether the nerve fiber layer seems normal, as is usual in pseudopapilledema, is an important distinguishing feature. The evaluation for the presence of spontaneous venous pulsations is almost never of value because pseudopapilledematous discs usually do not show spontaneous venous pulsations. Hemorrhages are also not a completely differentiating feature, as they may be present in both conditions.

Optic disc drusen may be inherited in an autosomal dominant pattern. The prevalence is approximately 2% of the population. Drusen are much more commonly present in whites than in blacks. The pathogenesis of drusen has been postulated to be related to axonal degeneration from altered axoplasmic flow. In children, drusen tend to be buried, whereas in adults they are more often on the surface; the progression from buried to surface drusen in a given individual has been well documented.

Optic disc drusen generally do not produce visual symptoms, although rarely a patient may experience transient visual obscurations similar to those with increased intracranial pressure. Visual field defects are common, however, occurring in about 70% of eyes with visible drusen and in 35% of those with pseudopapilledema but no visible drusen. The visual field defects are generally in a nerve fiber bundle distribution, with inferior nasal visual field loss being the most common. An enlargement of the blind spot and generalized field constriction are also possible. Progression of visual field defects is well documented, but it is rare for visual acuity to be decreased as a result of drusen. If decreased visual acuity is present in a patient with drusen, an evaluation for an alternative cause should be performed.

Visual loss from drusen can also occur secondary to he-

Table 15.1: Causes of unilateral and bilateral optic neuropathy categorized by appearance of the optic disc

Edematous		*Normal-Appearing*		*Atrophic*	
Unilateral	*Bilateral*	*Unilateral*	*Bilateral*	*Cupped*	*Not Cupped*
Optic neuritis Ischemic optic neuropathy Orbital tumor Other: papillophlebitis, central retinal vein occlusion, infiltrative disorders	Papilledema (increased intracranial pressure) Malignant hypertension Diabetic papillopathy Any of the unilateral causes	Retrobulbar neuritis Compressive lesion Infiltration: granulomatous, carcinomatous, lymphomatous Any of the unilateral causes	Tobacco–alcohol Nutritional Drugs Toxins Hereditary*	Glaucoma Giant-cell arteritis	Any optic neuropathy

*Optic disc may appear swollen acutely in Leber's optic neuropathy.
Source: RW Beck, CH Smith. Neuro-Ophthalmology: A Problem-Oriented Approach. Boston: Little, Brown, 1988. Reprinted with permission of the author and publisher.

Table 15.2: Differentiation of early papilledema and pseudopapilledema

Feature	*Papilledema*	*Pseudopapilledema*
Disc color	Hyperemic	Pink, yellowish-pink
Disc margins	Indistinct early at superior and inferior poles, later entire margin	Irregularly blurred, may be lumpy
Disc elevation	Minimal	Minimal to marked; center of disc most elevated
Vessels	Normal distribution, slight fullness; spontaneous venous pulsations absent	Emanate from center, frequent anomalous pattern, ±spontaneous venous pulsations
Nerve fiber layer	Dull as a result of edema, which may obscure blood vessels	No edema; may glisten with circumpapillary halo of feathery light reflections
Hemorrhages	Splinter	Subretinal, retinal, vitreous

Source: RW Beck, CH Smith. Neuro-Ophthalmology: A Problem-Oriented Approach. Boston: Little Brown, 1988. Reprinted with permission of the author and publisher.

morrhage or to an associated retinal degeneration. Approximately 2% of patients with retinitis pigmentosa also have optic disc drusen. The clinician must be sure not to make the incorrect diagnosis of papilledema with visual loss, when in fact the diagnosis is optic disc drusen with visual loss secondary to retinitis pigmentosa.

Unilateral Optic Disc Edema

If true disc edema is determined to be present, it is useful to separate cases into unilateral and bilateral categories and further subdivide them as to whether optic nerve function is normal or impaired.

The most common causes of unilateral optic disc edema are optic neuritis, anterior ischemic optic neuropathy (AION), and orbital compressive lesions. As a rule, optic nerve function is abnormal in each. The optic disc appearance may be indistinguishable in these entities; however, certain features of the disc appearance, if present, may be more suggestive of a specific diagnosis. Disc hemorrhages, for example, are much more common in AION than in optic neuritis or compressive lesions (Plate 15.III). A cellular reaction in the vitreous overlying the optic disc or retinal exudates is highly suggestive of optic neuritis (Plate 15.IV). Both optociliary shunt vessels and glistening white bodies on the disc surface (these have been called "pseudodrusen" and indicate chronic disc swelling) can be seen with compressive disc edema (Plate 15.V) but would not be expected with optic neuritis or AION. Optociliary shunt vessels represent communications between the ciliary and retinal venous circulations. In addition to orbital tumors, these vessels can be seen in retinal vein occlusions, glaucoma, malignant hypertension, and chronic papilledema, and as a congenital variant.

Although differentiation among optic neuritis, AION, and compressive lesions may not be possible on the basis of optic disc appearance, diagnosis can usually be made based on the history of visual loss and the pattern of the visual field deficit. Visual loss is generally slowly progressive in patients with compressive lesions, is sudden with subsequent improvement in those with optic neuritis, and is sudden without improvement in those with AION. Both optic neuritis and compressive lesions generally produce some form of central scotoma, whereas AION typically produces a nerve fiber bundle–type of visual field defect. Chapter 14 describes these features in further detail.

In about 25% of cases, AION consecutively affects the two eyes. When the second eye is affected, a picture of optic atrophy in one eye and disc edema in the fellow eye occurs (pseudo–Foster Kennedy syndrome) (Figure 15.1). A true Foster Kennedy syndrome is produced by a tumor that causes optic atrophy in one eye due to compression and disc edema in the fellow eye from increased intracranial pressure.

Compressive lesions producing disc edema almost always affect the intraorbital portion of the optic nerve. Meningiomas of the optic nerve sheath or sphenoid wing are common causes of compressive disc edema (see Plate 15.V). Canalicular (within the optic canal) and intracranial compressive lesions only rarely produce disc edema, unless they are large enough to raise intracranial pres-

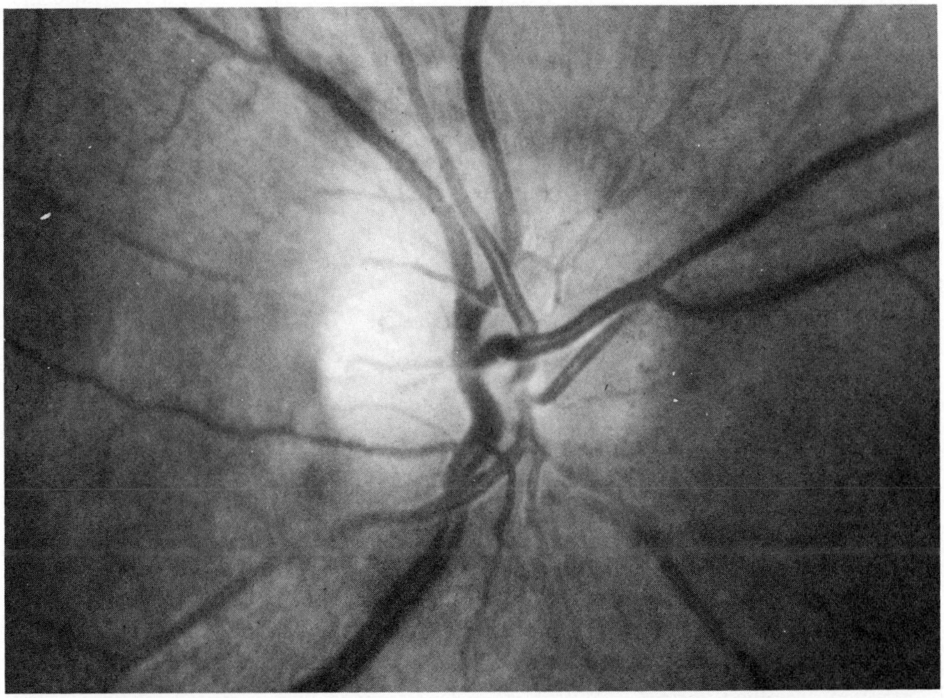

A

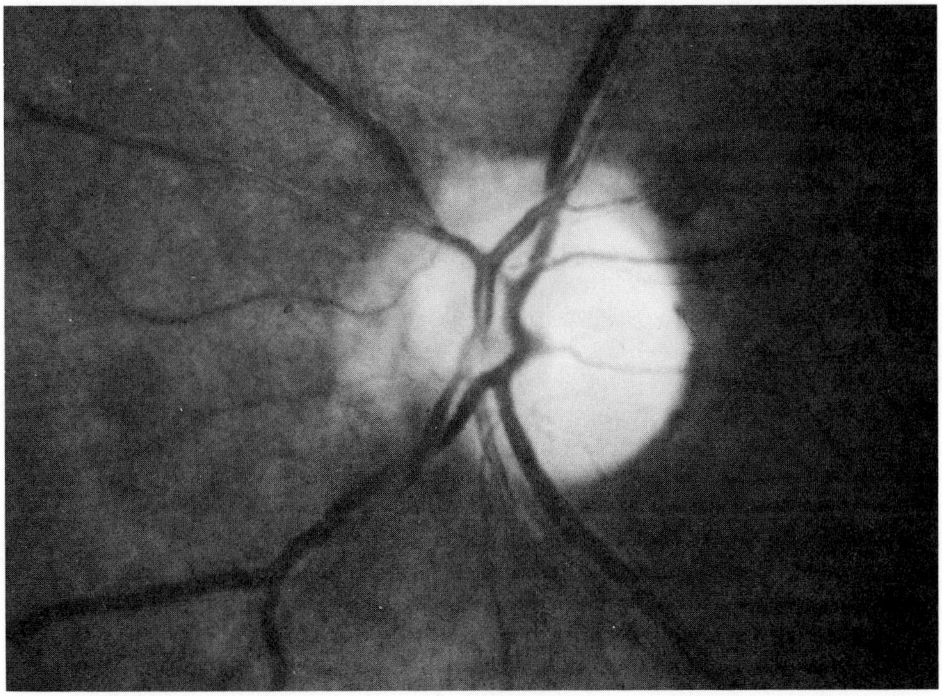

B

FIGURE 15.1 Pseudo–Foster Kennedy syndrome from (A) acute ischemic optic neuropathy in the right eye (disc edema) and from (B) previous ischemic optic neuropathy in the left eye (optic atrophy) in a 53-year-old man. (From RW Beck, CH Smith. Neuro-Ophthalmology: A Problem-Oriented Approach. Boston: Little, Brown, 1988. Reprinted with permission of the author and publisher.)

sure. A nontumor cause of disc edema is Graves' ophthalmopathy.

When optic neuritis is associated with macular exudates, often in a star pattern, the condition is termed *neuroretinitis*. The importance of recognizing such exudates is that the etiology of the condition is likely to be viral and the possibility of multiple sclerosis as the cause is remote.

Uncommon Causes of Unilateral Disc Edema

Less common causes of unilateral optic disc edema include obstruction of the central retinal vein and infiltrative disorders.

Retinal vein obstruction is occasionally manifested primarily as optic disc edema with minimal or no retinal hemorrhages. *Papillophlebitis* is a syndrome of presumed retinal vein inflammation producing optic disc edema in young adults (Plate 15.VI). The disc elevation is often marked, and the retinal veins are generally dilated. Other than enlargement of the blind spot, the visual field is usually normal. This condition tends to resolve without residual visual loss. In older patients, retinal vein obstruction may be due to compression of the vein by an atherosclerotic artery. The disc typically appears extremely hyperemic, but edema is usually mild (Plate 15.VII). Optociliary shunt vessels may be present. As with papillophlebitis, visual function is usually not affected, but unlike papillophlebitis, the disc edema tends to be present chronically.

Infiltration of the optic nerve can occur with carcinomatous, lymphoreticular, and granulomatous processes. One or both optic nerves may be affected. Involved optic nerves may have swollen or normal-appearing optic discs. Occasionally, optic nerve infiltration produces optic disc edema without an effect on visual function, but more often there is a decrease in visual acuity and visual field loss. Almost any carcinoma can metastasize to infiltrate the optic nerve; breast and lung carcinoma are the most common. Carcinomatous meningitis is frequently associated. Lymphomas and leukemias also can involve the optic nerve. Sarcoidosis frequently gives a characteristic disc appearance of swelling with whitish nodules on the disc surface (Plate 15.VIII).

Optic neuropathy as a delayed effect of radiation can occur with or without disc edema. When this rare complication occurs, it usually follows the radiation by 6–24 months.

There are a number of other causes of unilateral optic disc edema. Some of the entities to be described in the section on bilateral disc edema, such as diabetic papillopathy, occasionally produce only unilateral edema. (Syphilis can affect the prelaminar or retrobulbar optic nerves.) Increased intracranial pressure may produce solely unilateral papilledema in rare cases. Leber's optic neuropathy is an uncommon hereditary optic nerve disorder predominantly affecting males. Though not a cause of true disc edema, in the acute phase the optic disc affected in this condition may appear hyperemic and mildly swollen (Plate 15.IX). If fluorescein angiography is performed, however, there is no leakage from the disc. Telangiectatic vessels, which are frequently present in the peripapillary nerve fiber layer, are another clue to the diagnosis. These funduscopic changes may also be noted in presymptomatic eyes. Thus, a patient may present with symptoms of involvement of only one eye and be diagnosed as having Leber's neuropathy because the characteristic disc changes are present in both eyes.

Bilateral Optic Disc Edema

Papilledema

Bilateral optic disc edema is commonly due to increased intracranial pressure. In this setting, it is called *papilledema*. In the acute phase, optic nerve function and visual acuity are generally normal, and visual field testing shows only an enlarged blind spot. Papilledema results from blockage of axoplasmic flow in nerve fibers, with a consequent increase in the volume of axoplasm in the optic disc. Papilledema can be divided into early, fully developed, chronic, and atrophic stages.

In early papilledema, edema is most prominent at the superior and inferior poles of the optic disc (Plate 15.X). The retinal veins may be slightly distended, and the disc may appear mildly hyperemic. Spontaneous venous pulsations are usually absent.

With further development, edema more uniformly covers the disc surface, and disc elevation increases. The physiological cup may become increasingly obscured, and retinal vein dilation becomes more prominent. Splinter hemorrhages may develop on the disc and at its margin (Plate 15.XI). As papilledema becomes chronic, usually after several months or longer, the disc appearance changes. The nerve fiber layer may take on a gliotic appearance. Hemorrhages are less prominent, and small glistening white bodies (pseudodrusen) may be noted (Plate 15.XII). With further chronicity champagne cork appearance may develop (Plate 15.XIII).

With prolonged increased intracranial pressure and papilledema, optic nerve fibers may be damaged and visual field loss develops. At this stage, optic disc edema lessens and disc edema develops (Plate 15.XIV). Disc edema decreases because axoplasmic flow diminishes in damaged axons. Therefore, when a large number of nerve fibers are damaged, there is less axoplasmic flow within the nerve, and hence less obstipation of axoplasm and less edema. With end-stage damage, the nerve appears atrophic without edema.

Malignant Hypertension

A marked elevation in blood pressure may produce bilateral optic disc edema that is indistinguishable from papilledema (Plate 15.XV). Encephalopathic signs are usually but not always present. Disc edema tends to develop at a lower blood pressure in patients with renal failure than in those without renal disease.

Diabetic Papillopathy

A rare entity consists of the development of bilateral, or sometimes unilateral, optic disc edema in juvenile diabetes. This entity is distinct from AION in that it is frequently bilateral simultaneously, and there is often no visual field loss except for an enlarged blind spot. There is disc edema accompanied by marked telangiectasia of capillaries overlying the disc surface (Plate 15.XVI). Measurement of cerebrospinal fluid (CSF) pressure after full neuroimaging to rule out intracranial mass lesions may be necessary to distinguish this condition from papilledema due to increased intracranial pressure. In many cases, optic disc edema resolves without residual visual deficit.

Other Causes

Other causes of bilateral disc edema include anemia, hyperviscosity syndromes, Pickwickian syndrome, hypotension, and blood loss. The clinical setting generally provides clues to diagnosis. Any of the entities described under unilateral optic disc edema can occur bilaterally, especially the infiltrative disorders. Optic neuritis is frequently bilateral in children. Bilateral AION suggests a diagnosis of giant-cell arteritis in the elderly. Although most toxic optic neuropathies present with normal-appearing optic discs, disc edema is characteristic of methanol poisoning and may occur with ethambutol toxicity.

OPTIC NEUROPATHIES WITH NORMAL-APPEARING OPTIC DISCS

In many optic nerve disorders, the optic disc may appear completely normal. Such a disorder would be classified as a *retrobulbar optic neuropathy*. Differential diagnosis varies for unilateral and bilateral cases.

Unilateral Cases

In unilateral retrobulbar optic neuropathies, a compressive lesion or retrobulbar neuritis is the most likely cause. The time course of visual loss is usually helpful in distinguishing the two entities. There is no definite way to distinguish these disorders on examination, but the detection of a superior temporal field defect in the fellow eye would be highly suggestive of a compressive lesion affecting the optic chiasm. Retrobulbar ischemic optic neuropathy is an extremely rare condition that has been documented only in giant-cell arteritis and other vasculitides. For practical purposes, there is no retrobulbar correlate to nonarteritic AION.

Bilateral Cases

Bilateral optic neuropathies in which the optic discs appear normal are nutritional optic neuropathy (including tobacco-alcohol amblyopia), vitamin B_{12} or folate deficiencies, toxic neuropathy (heavy metals), drug-related neuropathy (chloramphenicol, isoniazid, ethambutol, placidyl, chlorpropamide, and others), and inherited optic neuropathies. When these conditions are chronic, optic atrophy may ensue. Other diagnostic considerations in this category include bilateral compressive lesions and bilateral retrobulbar neuritis.

OPTIC ATROPHY

Any optic neuropathy that produces damage to the optic nerve may result in optic atrophy. At this stage, the optic disc appearance frequently is not helpful in determining the underlying cause. The presence of gliotic changes suggests that the disc was previously swollen. Disc cupping is, of course, typical of glaucoma, but it is also common after AION as a result of giant-cell arteritis. Dominantly inherited optic atrophy often has a characteristic disc appearance, with pallor and excavation of the temporal portion of the disc. Rarely, disc cupping is acquired with intracranial compressive lesions of the optic nerve.

Optic atrophy is also a possible consequence of lesions in the retina, optic chiasm, and optic tract. With an optic tract lesion, a specific pattern of disc pallor may be noted, with temporal pallor of the ipsilateral disc and both nasal and temporal pallor of the contralateral disc. Acquired geniculocalcarine lesions never produce disc pallor, but congenital lesions in this area may do so.

CONGENITAL OPTIC DISC ANOMALIES

Optic disc drusen were discussed earlier in this chapter. Other congenital optic nerve anomalies include the tilted optic disc and optic nerve dysplasia.

Tilted Optic Disc

A tilted optic disc is usually easily recognized on ophthalmoscopy. The disc may appear foreshortened on one side, and one portion may appear elevated with the opposite end depressed (Plate 15.XVII). Often, the retinal vessels run in an oblique direction. Tilted optic discs are of neurological importance in that they are usually bilateral and may be associated with temporal field loss, thus mimicking a chiasmal syndrome. Differentiation from chiasmal disease is virtually always possible based on the pattern of visual field loss. With a tilted optic disc, the visual field defect generally extends to the blind spot and not to the vertical meridian as it does in a chiasmal lesion.

Optic Nerve Dysplasia

There are several types of optic nerve dysplasia. Optic nerve hypoplasia is the most common and, for the neurologist, the most important because of frequent associated neurological anomalies. In this condition, the optic disc appears small, and the nerve substance is surrounded by choroid and retinal pigment changes that often resemble a double ring (Plate 15.XVIII). The abnormality may be unilateral or bilateral. In most cases a specific cause cannot be identified. The prevalence appears to be increased in children of mothers with diabetes mellitus or mothers who ingested antiepileptic drugs, quinine, or lysergic acid diethylamide (LSD) during pregnancy. Endocrine abnormalities and midline craniofacial anomalies may be associated, particularly in bilateral cases. De Morsier's syndrome (septo-optic dysplasia) consists of bilateral optic nerve hypoplasia, absent septum pellucidum, and pituitary gland dysfunction (classical growth hormone deficiency). Nystagmus is frequently present when visual loss is severe. Optic nerve aplasia is extremely rare.

Optic nerve coloboma is more common and results from incomplete closure of the fetal fissure (Plate 15.XIX). It may be an isolated finding or may be part of a congenital disorder such as Aicardi's syndrome, trisomy 13, or Goldenhar's syndrome. Another type of congenital anomaly, an optic pit, is manifested as a small grayish area, usually located in the inferior temporal portion of the optic disc.

In some optic nerve dysplasias, the disc appears enlarged. This is true of the so-called morning glory disc, in which there is a large whitish concavity surrounded by pigmentation that is said to resemble a morning glory flower. This condition may be associated with a basal encephalocele.

RETINAL DISORDERS

This section deals with retinal disorders that have some relevance to neurology. The reader is referred to ophthalmology texts for more detailed descriptions.

Retinal Arterial Disease

Retinal arterial disease can present as a central or branch retinal artery occlusion or amaurosis fugax. Carotid disease is the most frequent association. The workup and treatment of these conditions is similar to that for cerebrovascular disease in general (see Chapter 58). In acute artery occlusions, the retina appears whitish as a result of edema. This is usually more prominent in the posterior pole than it is in the periphery (Plate 15.XX). A marked narrowing of the retinal arterioles is often noted. The edema occurs in the ganglion cell layer of the retina. Because there are no ganglion cells in the fovea (the center of the retina), this portion retains its normal reddish-orange color. Thus, the so-called cherry-red spot in the macula is noted. The retinal edema usually recovers fairly rapidly over days to weeks. Following resolution, the retinal appearance typically returns to normal, although the vision generally does not recover.

When present, retinal emboli are most often located at arteriole bifurcations (Figure 15.2). They appear glistening and whitish and can be noted on or near the optic disc or in the periphery. With impaired blood flow following a central retinal artery occlusion, a portion of a retinal arteriole may take on a whitish appearance. This does not represent an embolus but, rather, either stagnant lipid in the blood or, more than likely, changes in the arteriole wall.

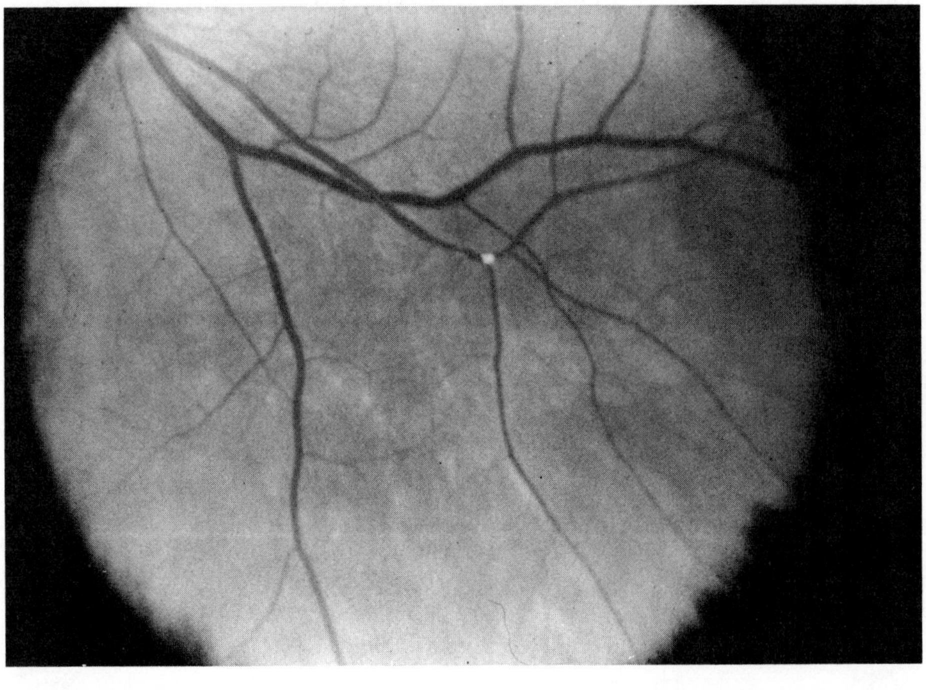

FIGURE 15.2 Hollenhorst plaque at a retinal arteriole bifurcation. (From RW Beck, CH Smith. Neuro-Ophthalmology: A Problem-Oriented Approach. Boston: Little, Brown, 1988. Reprinted with permission of the author and publisher.)

Vasculitis

In vasculitis, focal areas of retinal infarction develop. These areas, known as "cotton wool spots," are usually bilateral and may be extensive (Plate 15.XXI).

Branch Retinal Artery Occlusions and Encephalopathy

Branch retinal artery occlusions and encephalopathy is an unusual disorder of unknown cause that is characterized by multiple branch retinal artery occlusions and neurological dysfunction (Susac 1994). The disorder most commonly affects women between the ages of 20 and 40 years. A viral syndrome may precede the development of the ocular and neurological signs. The most prominent neurological manifestations are impaired mentation and sensorineural hearing loss, although many other neurological signs are possible. The CSF generally shows a mild pleocytosis (mostly lymphocytes) and elevation of the protein. Antinuclear antibody testing and cerebral arteriography are generally normal, but the magnetic resonance imaging scan of the head shows multiple areas of high signal on T2-weighted images that resemble multiple sclerosis.

Ocular Ischemic Syndrome

Generalized ocular ischemia indicates impairment of both the retinal and ciliary circulations in the eye. Signs of optic nerve and retinal ischemia may be present as well as evidence of anterior segment ischemia with iris atrophy, loss of pupil reactivity, cataract formation, and rubeosis iridis. Carotid occlusion and giant-cell arteritis are possible causes.

Retinal Vein Occlusion

Central or branch retinal vein occlusions rarely occur in patients younger than 50 years. Diagnosis is established on funduscopy by the presence of diffuse (central retinal vein occlusion) or focal (branch retinal vein occlusion) retinal hemorrhages (Plate 15.XXII). Disc edema is also possible and, in some cases, is the predominant feature (see earlier discussion). There are no direct correlations between retinal vein occlusions and carotid disease. Patients should be evaluated for risk factors for vascular disease, but a specific carotid investigation is generally not indicated. Bilateral cases should be evaluated for hyperviscosity syndromes.

NEUROLOGICAL DISEASES WITH RETINAL FINDINGS

Retinal Degenerations

There are a multitude of retinal degenerations, some of which may have neurological associations. Retinitis pigmentosa is a degeneration of the retinal rods and cones. Rods are predominantly affected early, and thus night vision is impaired. Visual field loss occurs first in the midperiphery and, when advanced, results in severe field constriction. Pigmentary changes in the retina appear like bony spicules and are the hallmark of the diagnosis (Plate 15.XXIII). In some cases, however, pigment changes are not prominent. In these cases, the diagnosis may be missed, and the visual field loss may mistakenly be considered to have a neurological basis. This may result in unnecessary testing and sometimes even unnecessary treatment (Heidemann and Beck 1987). Even without bone spicule–type changes, the diagnosis is usually obvious to the astute observer because of the thinning of the retina, narrowing of retinal arterioles, and waxy pallor of the optic disc. Regardless of the degree of pigment change, electroretinography is diagnostic.

Retinitis pigmentosa usually appears without systemic findings. However, a retinal degeneration of this type may be seen in Kearns-Sayre's syndrome, aberalipoproteinemia (Bassen-Kornsweig's disease), Laurence-Moon-Bardet-Biedl's syndrome, Friedreich's ataxia, Marie's ataxia, Cockayne's syndrome, Refsum's syndrome, Batten's disease, and Hallervorden-Spatz's disease.

A retinal photoreceptor degeneration can occur as a remote effect of cancer. This entity has been described most often with small-cell carcinoma of the lung. Arteriolar narrowing is a consistent finding, but pigment changes in the fundus are variable. An electroretinogram (ERG) is markedly abnormal (showing reduced to extinguished rod and cone components), and antiphotoreceptor antibodies are often identified in the serum.

A progressive cone dystrophy can develop most commonly through autosomal dominant inheritance. Typically visual loss develops in both eyes beginning in the teens and worsens over several years. Early, the fundus may appear normal, but with time pigment changes develop in the macula and ERG demonstrates a characteristic loss of the photopic response.

Uveoretinal Meningoencephalitis Syndromes

Certain disorders have the tendency to produce inflammatory changes in both the eye and the central nervous system. Vogt-Koyanagi-Harada's syndrome, the most common uveomeningoencephalitis syndrome, is marked by exudative retinal detachments. Table 15.3 lists some of the causes of ocular and central nervous system inflammation.

Phakomatoses

Certain of the phakomatoses have characteristic retinal findings. Neurological features are described in Chapter 70. In tuberous sclerosis, retinal astrocytic hamartomas may occur (Plate 15.XXIV). These are usually multiple and may

Table 15.3: Causes of uveoretinal meningoencephalitis syndromes

Infectious	*Inflammatory*	*Malignant*
Syphilis	Vogt-Koyanagi-Harada's syndrome	Reticulum cell sarcoma
Fungus	Sarcoidosis	Lymphoma
Tuberculosis	Multiple sclerosis	Leukemia
Cytomegalovirus	Behçet's disease	Metastatic carcinoma
Herpes simplex	Systemic lupus erythematosus	
Herpes zoster	Inflammatory bowel disease	
Subacute sclerosing panencephalitis	Acute posterior multifocal placoid pigment epitheliopathy	
Miscellaneous viruses		
Toxoplasmosis		
Whipple's disease		
Acquired immune deficiency syndrome		

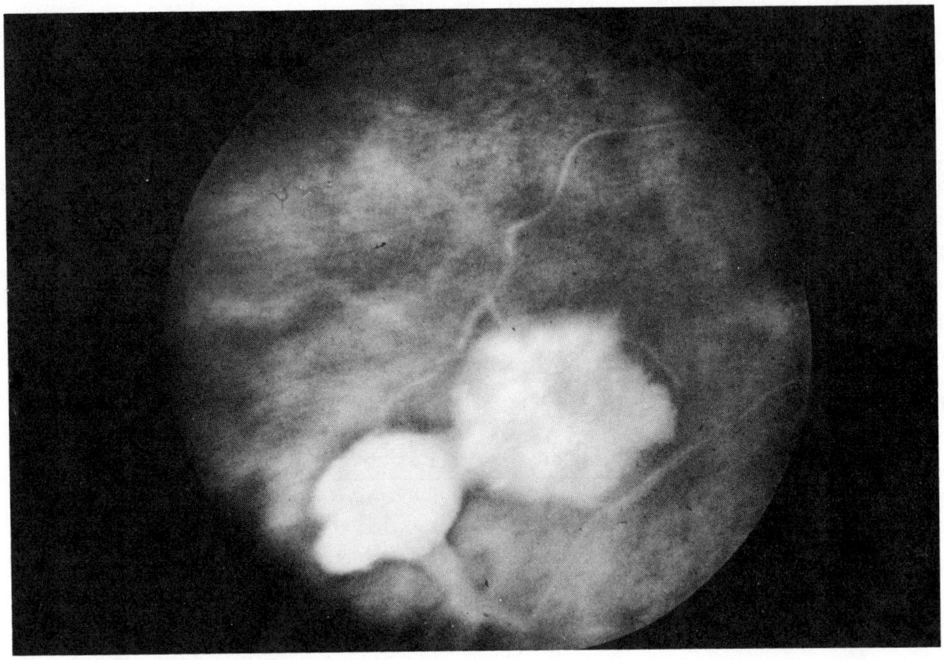

FIGURE 15.3 Retinal angioma in a patient with von Hippel-Lindau disease.

appear either as a fullness in the nerve fiber layer of the retina or as a nodular refractile lesion (mulberry type). Von Hippel-Lindau's disease is characterized by one or more retinal angiomas, which appear as a reddish mass with a feeding artery and a draining vein (Figure 15.3). Wyburn-Mason disease is characterized by a racemose arteriovenous malformation in the retina (Figure 15.4).

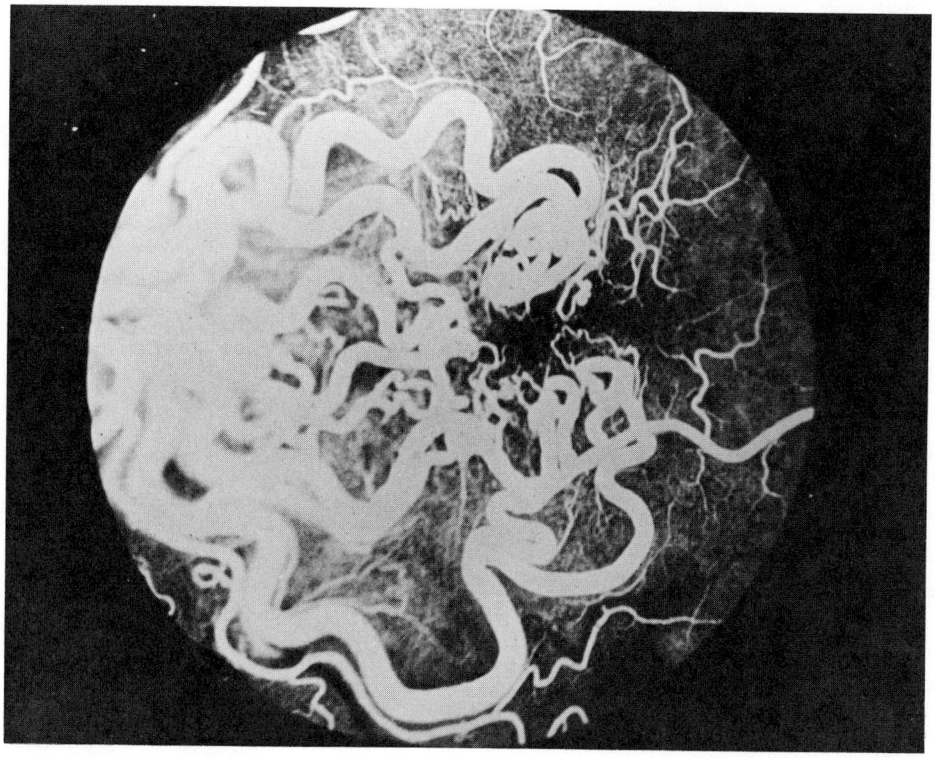

FIGURE 15.4 Fluorescein angiogram of a racemose arteriovenous malformation in the retina in a patient with Wyburn-Mason disease.

REFERENCES

Beck RW, Smith CH. Neuro-Ophthalmology: A Problem-Oriented Approach. Boston: Little, Brown, 1988.

Heidemann DG, Beck RW. Retinitis pigmentosa: a mimic of neurologic disease. Surv Ophthalmol 1987;32:45–51.

Susac JO. Susac's syndrome. Neurology 1994;44:591–593.

SUGGESTED READINGS

Glaser JS. Neuro-Ophthalmology (2nd ed). Philadelphia: Lippincott, 1990.

Miller NR. Walsh and Hoyt's Clinical Neuro-Ophthalmology (4th ed). Vol 1. Baltimore: Williams & Wilkins, 1982.

Chapter 16
Eye Movement Disorders and Diplopia

Patrick J. M. Lavin

This chapter discusses disorders of extraocular muscle function that cause diplopia, strabismus, nystagmus, ocular flutter, opsoclonus, and ocular intrusions. A brief outline of the anatomy, physiology, and innervation of the extraocular muscles is followed by a discussion of the mechanisms of nystagmus. The reader is guided through the clinical assessment of a patient with an ocular motility disorder, from analysis of symptoms to specialized clinical tests used in evaluating eye movement abnormalities. Therapeutic strategies are discussed at appropriate points throughout the chapter. The development and supranuclear control of the ocular motor system, supranuclear gaze disorders, and oculographic recording techniques are discussed in Chapter 42.

The human fovea is a highly sensitive part of the retina capable of resolving angles of less than 100 seconds of arc. The ocular motor system places images of objects of regard on the fovea and maintains foveation if the object, or head, moves. Each eye has six extraocular muscles (Table 16.1), yoked in pairs (Table 16.2), that move the eyes conjugately (versions) to maintain alignment of the visual axes (Figure 16.1). The actions of the medial and lateral recti are confined to the horizontal plane. The actions of the superior and inferior recti are solely vertical when the eye is abducted 23 degrees; the oblique muscles, the main cyclotortors, also act as pure vertical movers when the eye is adducted 51 degrees (Figure 16.2). For practical purposes, the vertical actions may be tested at 30 degrees of adduction and abduction. According to Hering's law of dual innervation, yoked muscles receive equal and simultaneous innervation, while, at the same time, their antagonists are inhibited (Sherrington's law of reciprocal inhibition), allowing the eyes to move conjugately and with great precision.

Images of the same target must fall on corresponding points of each retina to maintain binocular single vision (fusion) (Figure 16.3). Misalignment of the visual axes as a result of dysconjugate positioning of the eyes causes diplopia because images of the target fall on noncorresponding (disparate) points of each retina (Figure 16.4). The image from the nonfixing paretic eye is the *false image* and is displaced in the direction of action of the weak muscle. Thus, a patient with esotropia has uncrossed diplopia (see Figure 16.4A), and one with exotropia has crossed diplopia (see Figure 16.4B). After a variable period of time, the patient learns to ignore or suppress one image. If suppression occurs early in life (up to 9 years of age) and persists, the child fails to develop fully central connections in the afferent visual system. This failure leads to permanently impaired visual acuity (developmental amblyopia) in the weaker eye.

HETEROPHORIAS AND HETEROTROPIAS

When the degree of misalignment—that is, the angle of deviation—of the visual axes is constant, the patient has a *comitant strabismus (heterotropia)*. When it varies with gaze direction, however, the patient has a *noncomitant (paralytic* or *restrictive) strabismus*. In general, comitant strabismus is ophthalmological (congenital) in origin, whereas noncomitant strabismus is neurological (acquired). Three to four percent of preschool children have some form of ocular misalignment. Most people have a latent tendency for

Table 16.1: Actions of extraocular muscles

Muscle	*Primary*	*Secondary*	*Tertiary*
Medial rectus	Adduction	—	—
Lateral rectus	Abduction	—	—
Superior rectus	Elevation (sursumduction)	Intorsion	Adduction
Inferior rectus	Depression (deorsumduction)	Extorsion	Adduction
Superior oblique	Intorsion (incycloduction)	Depression	Abduction
Inferior oblique	Extorsion (excycloduction)	Elevation	Abduction

Table 16.2: Yoked muscle pairs

Ipsilateral	*Contralateral*
Medial rectus	Lateral rectus
Superior rectus	Inferior oblique
Inferior rectus	Superior oblique

ocular misalignment, *heterophoria,* which may be manifested as a heterotropia under conditions of stress, such as fatigue, bright sunlight, ingestion of alcohol, anticonvulsants, or sedative medications. Divergent eyes are designated *exotropia* and convergent eyes *esotropia;* vertical misalignment of the visual axes, which is less common, is termed *hypertropia* (determined by the higher eye, irrespective of which eye is paretic; that is, right eye higher is right hypertropia). When stress unmasks such a latent tendency for the visual axes to deviate, the diplopia is present in all directions of gaze (comitant).

Asymptomatic hypertropia on lateral gaze is often a congenital or "physiologic hyperdeviation."

Comitant Strabismus

Comitant strabismus occurs early in life; the degree of misalignment (deviation) is constant in all directions of gaze, and each eye has a full range of movement (ductions). The central synchronizing mechanism fails to keep the eyes aligned during attempted conjugate eye movements (versions). Infantile (congenital) esotropia may be associated with maldevelopment of the afferent visual system including the visual cortex. Because early surgical correction of esotropia during the first few months of life can result in high-grade stereo acuity (Wright et al. 1994), it is uncertain whether infantile esotropia is a cause or effect of these abnormalities. Those cases of esotropia that present in the third year of life are caused by hyperopia resulting in accommodative esotropia. Occasionally children with posterior fossa tumors may present with isolated acute esotropia before developing other symptoms or signs. Acquired esotropia in adults may occasionally result from a Chiari malformation or acute thalamic hemorrhage.

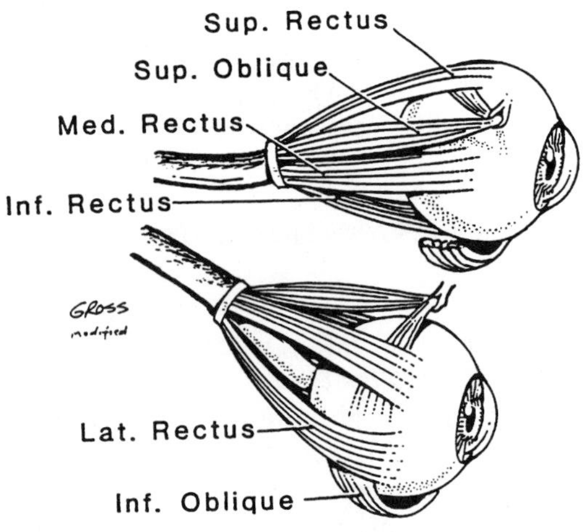

FIGURE 16.1 Each eye has six extraocular muscles, which are yoked in pairs.

Noncomitant Strabismus

Noncomitant strabismus occurs when the degree of misalignment of the visual axes varies with the direction of gaze as a result of weakness of one, or asymmetrical weakness of more than one, extraocular muscle. When a patient with paralytic strabismus fixates on an object and the paretic eye is covered, the angle of misalignment is referred to as *primary deviation;* if the patient then fixes with the paretic eye while the nonparetic eye is covered, the angle of misalignment is referred to as *secondary deviation.* Secondary deviation is always greater than primary deviation in noncomitant strabismus because of Hering's law of dual innervation and may mislead the examiner to believe that the eye with the greater deviation is the weak one (Figure 16.5).

DIPLOPIA (TABLE 16.3)

Theoretically, the onset of double vision should be abrupt. In practice, however, the onset may be vague either because the patient does not realize that blurring is subtle diplopia unless one eye is covered, either inadvertently or intentionally, or because the diplopia initially is intermittent and of small amplitude, as may be the case in congenital superior oblique palsy or ocular myasthenia.

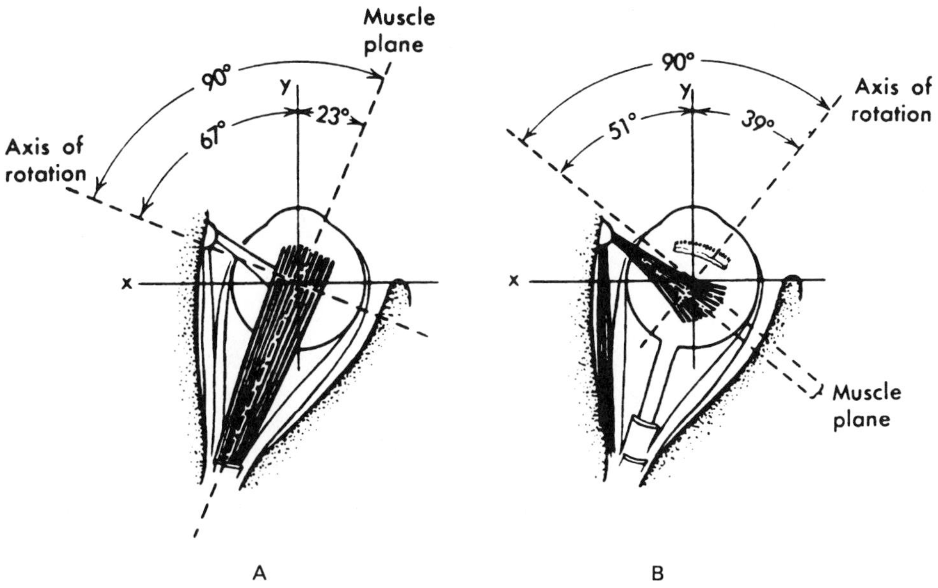

FIGURE 16.2 A. Relationship of muscle plane of vertical rectus muscles to X and Y axes. B. Relationship of muscle plane of oblique muscles to X and Y axes. (Reprinted with permission from GK Von Noorden. Burian-Von Noorden's Binocular Vision and Ocular Motility [3rd ed]. St. Louis: Mosby, 1985.)

Patients with heterotropia may complain of frank double vision, blurred vision, ghosting of images, visual confusion, dizziness, or eyestrain. If the images are close together, the patient may not be aware of frank diplopia but may merely perceive blurring or strain. Others may be aware of overlapping images (ghosting). Occasionally, if one image is not suppressed, visual confusion occurs because the patient views a different object with each fovea at the same time and perceives two objects in the same place (Figure 16.6).

Anxious or histrionic subjects may misinterpret physiological diplopia as a pathological symptom. Physiological diplopia occurs in normal subjects. It may be demonstrated by having the subject select an object in the foreground and then select another object that is farther away but in the same direction. While the subject fixates on the far object, the near object appears double, and vice versa, because the nonfixated object is seen by noncorresponding parts of each retina and is perceived by the mind's cyclopian eye as double (Figure 16.7).

Isolated vertical diplopia (Table 16.4) is most frequently caused by a superior oblique muscle palsy (90%); if the palsy is acquired, the false image is virtually always tilted, an infrequent finding when the palsy is congenital. If recently acquired diplopia is worse in upgaze, the weak muscle is an elevator; if worse in downgaze, it is a depressor. *Spread of comitance*—that is, the tendency for the ocular deviation to "spread" to all fields of gaze—occurs in longstanding cases; the diplopia then no longer obeys the usual rules. If one image is tilted, then the weak muscle is more likely an oblique than a vertically acting rectus.

If double vision persists when one eye is covered, the patient has *monocular diplopia,* which may be bilateral. The most common cause of monocular diplopia is optical aberration (Table 16.5). Less commonly, monocular diplopia is psychogenic; occasionally, it can be attributed to dysfunction of the retina or the cerebral cortex. The *pinhole test*

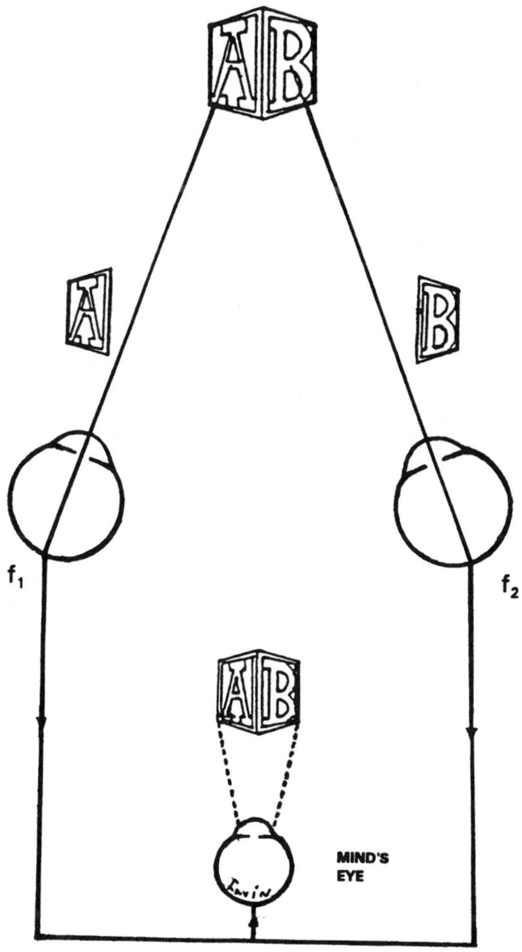

FIGURE 16.3 Each eye views the target AB from a different angle. The fovea of the left eye (f_1) views the "A" side of the target; the fovea of the right eye (f_2) views the "B" side of the target. The occipital cortex, the cyclopian (mind's) eye, integrates the disparate images so that a three-dimensional image (AB) of the target is perceived. This phenomenon is called *sensory fusion.*

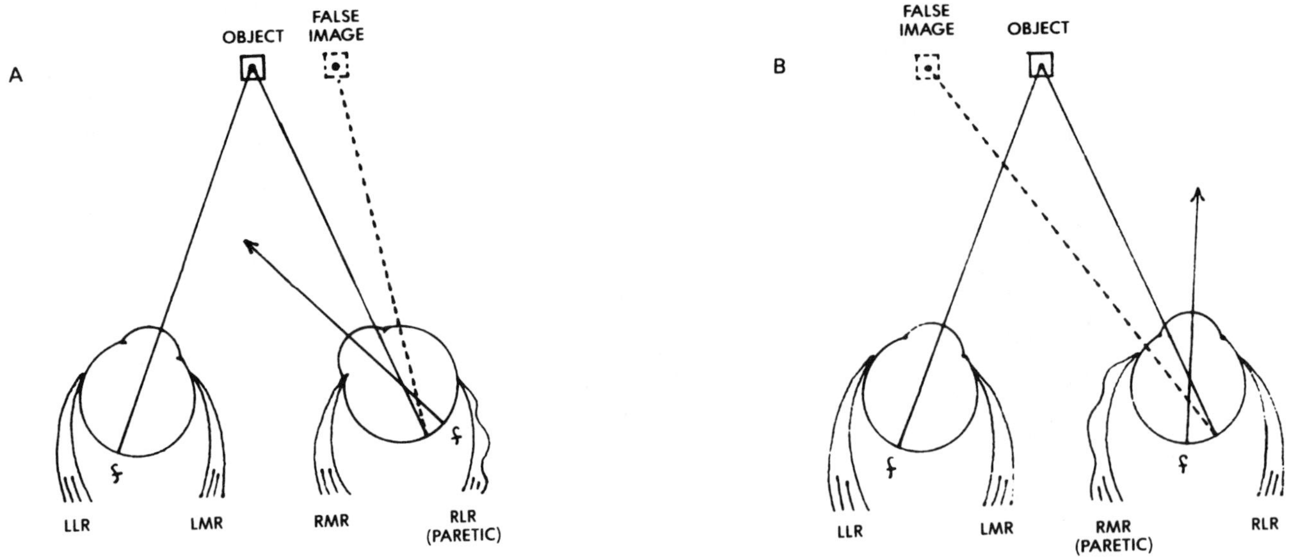

FIGURE 16.4 Misalignment of the visual axes. A. Esotropia caused by a right lateral rectus (RLR) palsy results in the right eye turning inward so that the image falls on the retina nasal to the fovea and is projected, by the mind's eye, to the temporal field; that is, the false image is projected in the direction of action of the paretic muscle, causing uncrossed (homonymous) diplopia. B. Exotropia caused by a paretic right medial rectus muscle (RMR) results in the image falling on the retina temporal to the fovea with projection to the nasal field, in the direction of the action of the paretic RMR, causing crossed (heteronymous) diplopia.

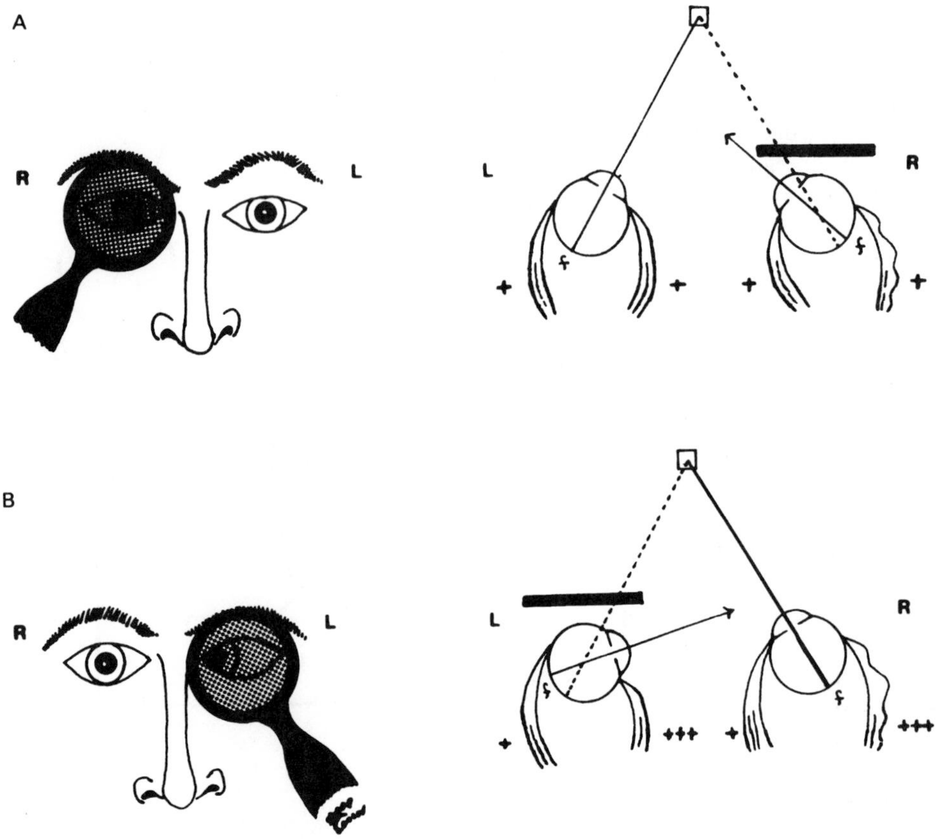

FIGURE 16.5 Primary and secondary deviation with a palsy of the right lateral rectus muscle. A. The right eye is covered with an occluder while the left eye fixates on the target. A small right esotropia (primary deviation) is demonstrated. (The opaque occluder is shown here to be partly transparent to allow the reader to observe the position of the covered eye.) B. The left eye is covered while the right eye fixates on the target. The right eye can fixate on the target despite the weak right lateral rectus muscle because that muscle is overdriven by the central nervous system. The normal left medial rectus muscle is also overdriven (Hering's law of dual innervation), resulting in a large esotropia (secondary deviation).

Table 16.3: Diplopia rules

1. *Head tilt*: When the weak extraocular muscle is unable to move the eye, the head moves the eye. Therefore the head tilts and turns in the direction of action of the weak muscle (see Figure 16.8).
2. *The image from the nonfixing eye is the false image* and is displaced in the direction of action of the paretic muscle (see Figure 16.4), except when the patient fixes with the paretic eye.
3. *The false image is the most peripheral image* and is displaced in the direction of action of the weak muscle, except when the patient fixes with the paretic eye.
   When the lateral rectus is paralyzed, the eyes are *esotropic* (crossed), but the images are uncrossed (see Figure 16.4A). The diplopia is worse at a distance and on looking to the side of the weak muscle.
   When the medial rectus is paralyzed, the eyes are *exotropic* (wall-eyed), but the images are crossed (see Figure 16.4B). The diplopia is worse at near and on looking to the opposite side.
4. *The images are most widely separated when an attempt is made to look in the direction of the paretic muscle.*
5. *Secondary deviation* (the angle of ocular misalignment when the paretic eye is fixating) is always greater than primary deviation (when the good eye is fixating) (see Figure 16.5).
   Patients who fixate with the paretic eye may appear to have intracranial disease.
6. *Comitance*: With a *comitant strabismus*, the angle of ocular misalignment is relatively constant in all directions of gaze. With a *noncomitant (paralytic) strabismus*, the angle of misalignment varies with the direction of gaze.

quickly settles the matter. The patient is asked to look through a pinhole. If the cause is refractive, the diplopia abates because the optical distortion is eliminated. Occasionally, oscillopsia may be misinterpreted as diplopia.

Clinical Assessment

History

Table 16.6 shows the procedure for assessment of the patient with diplopia. First, whether there are any associated symptoms, such as headache, dizziness, vertigo, or weakness, should be determined. The following points should be clarified, if the information has not been volunteered. Is diplopia relieved by covering either eye (if not, it is monocular diplopia) (see Table 16.5)? Is it worse in the morning or in the evening? Is it affected by fatigue? Are the images separated horizontally, vertically, or obliquely? If obliquely, is the horizontal or vertical component more obvious? Does the distance between images vary with direction of gaze? Is the diplopia worse for near vision or for distance? Is one image tilted? Do the eyelids droop? Is the diplopia influenced by head posture? Has this condition remained stable, improved, or deteriorated? Are there any general health problems? What medications are taken? Is there a family history of ocular or neurological disease? Has the patient had previous eye muscle surgery?

For example, lateral rectus muscle weakness causes diplopia that is worse at distance than near and is worse on looking to the side of the weak muscle. Superior oblique weakness causes diplopia that is worse on looking downward to the side opposite the weak muscle and causes difficulty with tasks such as reading, watching television in bed, going down a staircase, and walking on uneven ground. Medial rectus muscle weakness causes diplopia that is worse for near than for distance vision and is worse to the contralateral side.

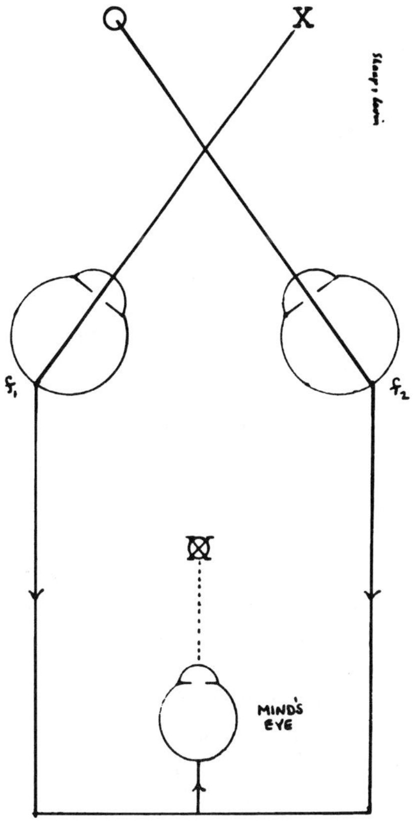

FIGURE 16.6 Visual confusion. Each fovea views a different object, which is projected to the visual cortex—the cyclopian eye—and perceived in the same place at the same time, causing visual confusion (rare).

General Inspection

Ptosis that fatigues suggests myasthenia gravis. Ptosis associated with a dilated pupil suggests an oculomotor nerve palsy. Lid lag suggests thyroid orbitopathy or myotonia. Lid

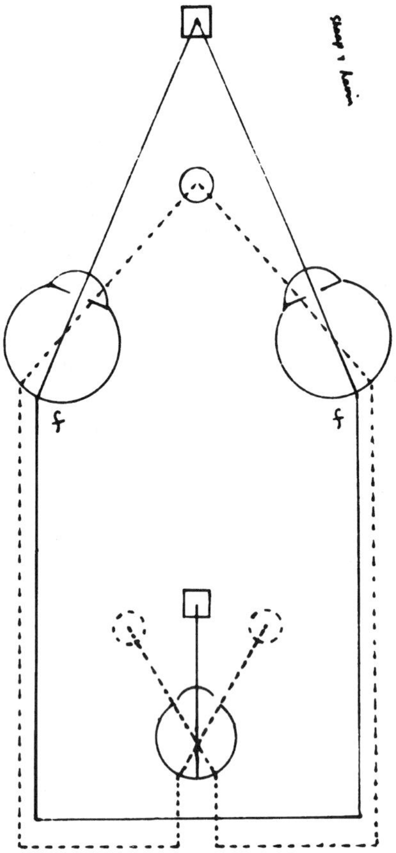

FIGURE 16.7 Physiological diplopia. The cyclopian eye views the target (the square) as a single object because each fovea fixates it. The images of a nonfixated target (the circle) fall on noncorresponding points of each retina and so appear as a double image.

retraction suggests thyroid orbitopathy, aberrant reinnervation following a third nerve palsy, a cyclic third nerve palsy (see Chapter 42), a dorsal midbrain lesion, hypokalemic periodic paralysis, or chronic corticosteroid use. Proptosis suggests an orbital lesion and, if associated with conjunctival injection and periorbital swelling, an inflammatory disorder such as orbital pseudotumor or lymphoma, dural shunt fistula, or infection.

Head Posture

Because the weak extraocular muscle cannot move the eye fully, patients compensate by tilting or turning the head in the direction of action of the weak muscle. For example, with a right lateral rectus palsy, the head turn is slightly to the right; on attempted right gaze, the patient turns the head further to the right (Figure 16.8A). With a right superior oblique palsy, the head is tilted forward and to the left (Figure 16.8B). The rule is as follows: *The head is turned or tilted in the direction of action of the weak muscle.*

Table 16.4: Causes of vertical diplopia

Common causes
Superior oblique palsy
Dysthyroid orbitopathy (muscle infiltration)
Myasthenia
Skew deviation (brain stem, cerebellar, hydrocephalus)
Less common causes
Orbital inflammation (myositis, pseudotumor)
Orbital infiltration (lymphoma, metastases, amyloid)
Primary orbital tumor
Entrapment (blowout fracture)
Third nerve palsy
Superior division third nerve palsy
Atypical third nerve (partial nuclear lesion)
Aberrant third nerve reinnervation
Brown's syndrome (congenital, acquired)
Congenital extraocular muscle fibrosis, or muscle absence
Other causes
Chronic progressive external ophthalmoplegia
Fisher's syndrome
Botulism
Monocular supranuclear gaze palsy
Vertical nystagmus (oscillopsia)
Superior oblique myokymia
Dissociated vertical deviation
Wernicke's encephalopathy
Vertical one-and-a-half syndrome
Monocular vertical diplopia (see Table 16.5)

Sensory Visual Function

Visual acuity, color vision, and confrontation visual fields should be checked in each eye, separately.

Stability of Fixation

Fixation and stability of the gaze-holding mechanism should be checked by having the patient look at a target and then observing for spontaneous eye movements such as saccadic intrusions, drift, microtremor, nystagmus, opsoclonus, ocular myokymia, or ocular myoclonus.

Table 16.5: Causes of monocular diplopia

Corneal disease such as astigmatism or keratoconus
Iris abnormalities
Lens: multirefractile (combined cortical and nuclear) cataracts, subluxation
Foreign body in aqueous or vitreous media
Retinal disease (rarely)
Corrected long-standing tropia (eccentric fixation)
Following surgery for long-standing tropia (eccentric fixation)
Monocular oscillopsia (nystagmus, superior oblique myokymia, eyelid twitching)
Occipital cortex: migraine, epilepsy, stroke, tumor, trauma (palinopsia, polyopia)
Equipment failure (defective contact lens, ill-fitting bifocals in patient with dementia)
Psychogenic

Table 16.6: Assessment of a patient with diplopia

History
Define symptoms
Effect of covering either eye?
Horizontal or vertical separation of the images?
Monocular?
Effect of distance of target (worse at near or far)?
Effect of gaze direction?
Tilting of one image?
Observation
Head tilt or turn? ("FAT scan")
Ptosis (fatigue)?
Pupil size?
Proptosis?
Spontaneous eye movements?
Examination
Visual acuity (each eye separately)
Versions (pursuit, saccades, and muscle overaction)
Convergence (does miosis occur?)
Ductions
Ocular alignment (muscle balance) in the "forced primary position"
Pupils
Lids (examine palpebral fissures, levator function, fatigue)
Vestibulo-ocular reflexes (doll's eyes)
Bell's phenomenon
Prism measurements
Stereopsis (Titmus stereo test)
Optokinetic nystagmus
General neurological examination
Bruits
Forced ductions
Edrophonium (Tensilon) test

FAT = family album tomography—that is, review of old photographs for head tilt, pupil size, lids, ocular alignment, etc. For magnification use ophthalmoscope, glass, slit lamp, etc.

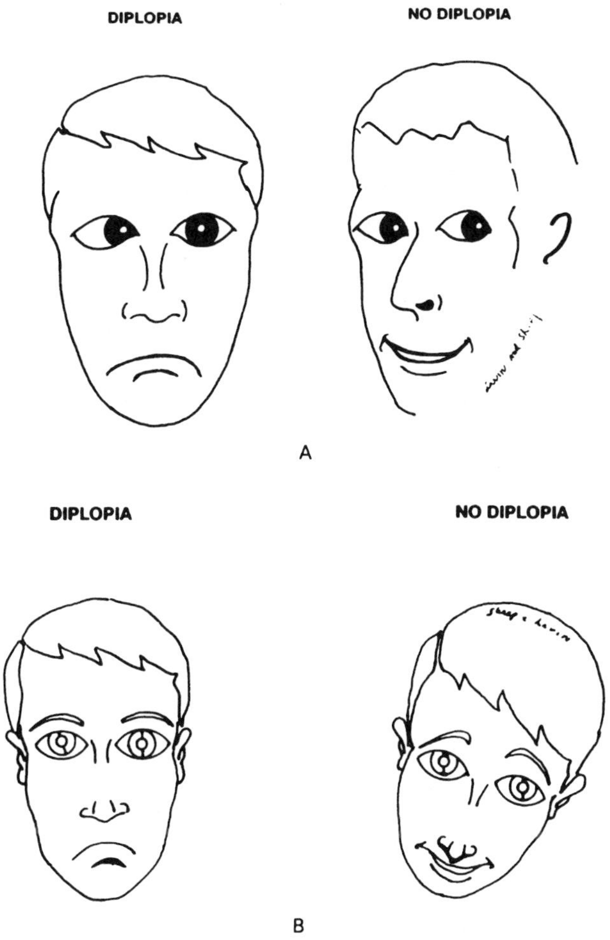

FIGURE 16.8 A. Right lateral rectus palsy. A right esotropia is present in primary gaze; however, by turning the head to the right (in the direction of action of the weak right lateral rectus muscle), the patient can maintain both eyes on target (orthotropia) and thus have binocular single vision. B. Right superior oblique muscle palsy. The right eye extorts (excycloduction) because of the unopposed action of the right inferior oblique muscle. By tilting the head to the left and forward (in the direction of action of the weak muscle), the right eye is passively intorted while the left eye actively intorts to compensate and maintain binocular single vision. The head also tilts forward to compensate for the depressor action of the weak right superior oblique.

Versions (Pursuit, Saccades, and Ocular Muscle Overaction)

Pursuit movements are tested by asking the patient to fixate on and follow (track) a moving target in all directions (Figure 16.9A). This test determines the range of eye movement and provides an opportunity to observe for gaze-evoked nystagmus. If spontaneous primary-position nystagmus is present, the effects of the direction of gaze and convergence on the nystagmus may be determined. Pursuit movements should be smooth and full. Cog wheel (saccadic) pursuit is a nonspecific finding and normal in infants; when it is present in only one direction, however, it suggests a defect of the ipsilateral pursuit system (see Chapter 42).

Saccades (rapid conjugate eye movements) are tested by asking the patient to look from one target to another—for example, from the examiner's nose to a pen—while observing for a delay in initiating the movement (latency) as well as the movement's speed and accuracy. If a specific muscle, particularly an oblique, is under- or overacting, that can be observed in eccentric gaze before testing *ductions* in each eye separately as shown in Figure 16.9B. Assessment of disorders of conjugate (supranuclear) gaze is discussed in more detail in Chapter 42.

Convergence

Convergence is tested by asking the patient to fixate on a target moving toward the nasium while observing the alignment of the eyes and constriction of the pupils. Miosis confirms an appropriate effort and its absence suggests less than optimal effort (see Chapter 42).

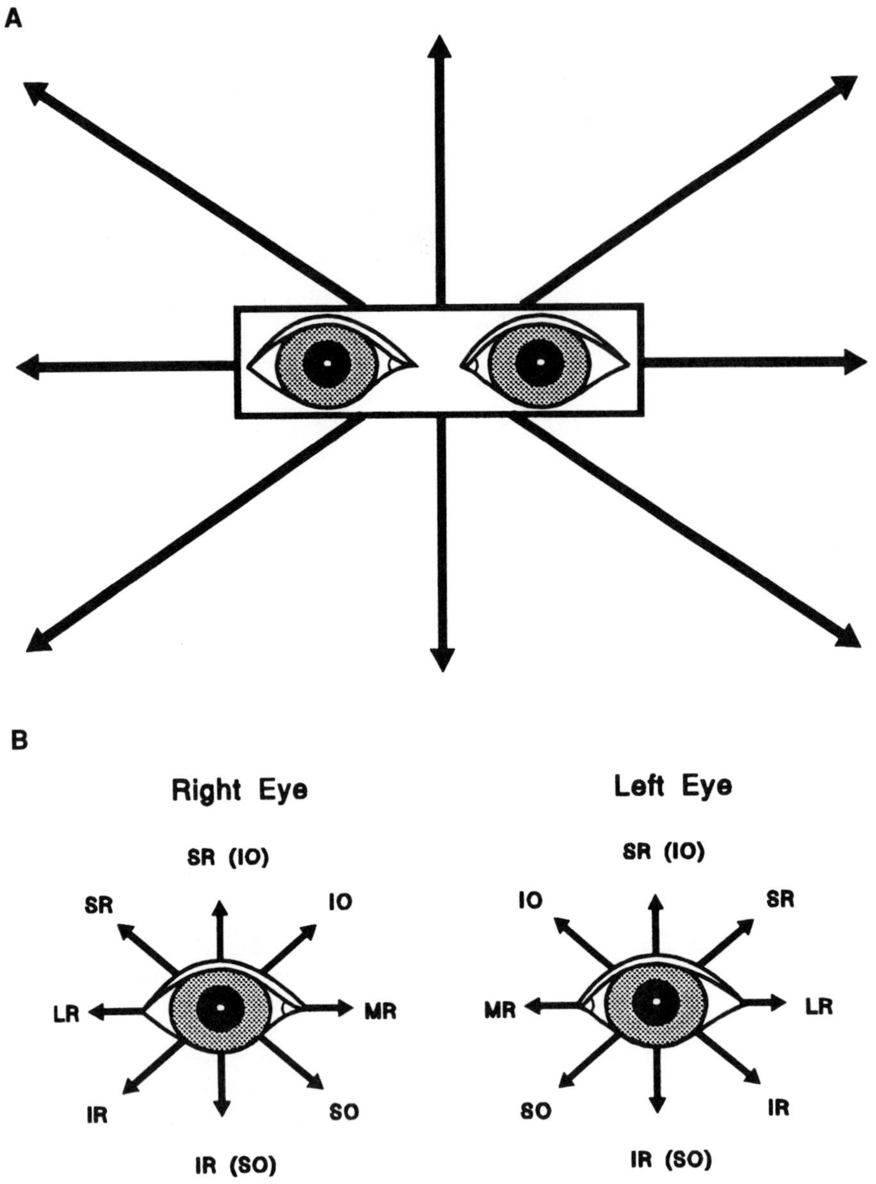

FIGURE 16.9 A. The nine diagnostic positions of gaze, used for testing versions (saccades and pursuit). B. Ductions, used to test the isolated action of each of the six muscles of each eye (assuming the other five muscles are functioning normally). Pure elevation (supraduction) and depression (infraduction) of the eyes are predominantly functions of the superior and inferior rectus muscles, respectively, with some help from the oblique muscles; that is, the eyes are rotated directly upward primarily by the superior rectus with some help from the inferior oblique; the eyes are rotated directly downward primarily by the inferior rectus with some help from the superior oblique.

Ductions

Ductions are tested monocularly by having the patient cover one eye and checking the range of movements of the other eye (see Figure 16.9B). If ductions are not full, then the physician should check for restrictive limitation by moving the eye forcibly (see the section on forced ductions).

Ocular Alignment and Muscle Balance

Before determining ocular alignment, the examiner must first neutralize a head tilt or turn by placing the patient in the "forced primary position"; otherwise, the misalignment may go undetected because of the compensating head posture. Subjective tests of ocular alignment include the red glass, Maddox rod, Lancaster red-green, and Hess screen.

With the *red glass test*, the patient views a penlight while a red filter or glass is placed, by convention, over the right eye. This allows easier identification of each image; the right eye views a red light and the left a white light. The addition of a green filter over the left eye, using red-green glasses, further simplifies the test for younger or less cooperative patients. The target light is shown to the patient in the nine diagnostic positions of gaze (see Figure 16.9A). As the light moves into the field of action of a paretic muscle, the images separate. The patient is asked to signify where the images are most widely separated and also to describe their relative positions. Interpretation of the results is summarized in Figure 16.10.

The *Maddox rod* uses the same principle as the red glass test but completely dissociates the images by changing the point of light seen through the rod, which is a series of half

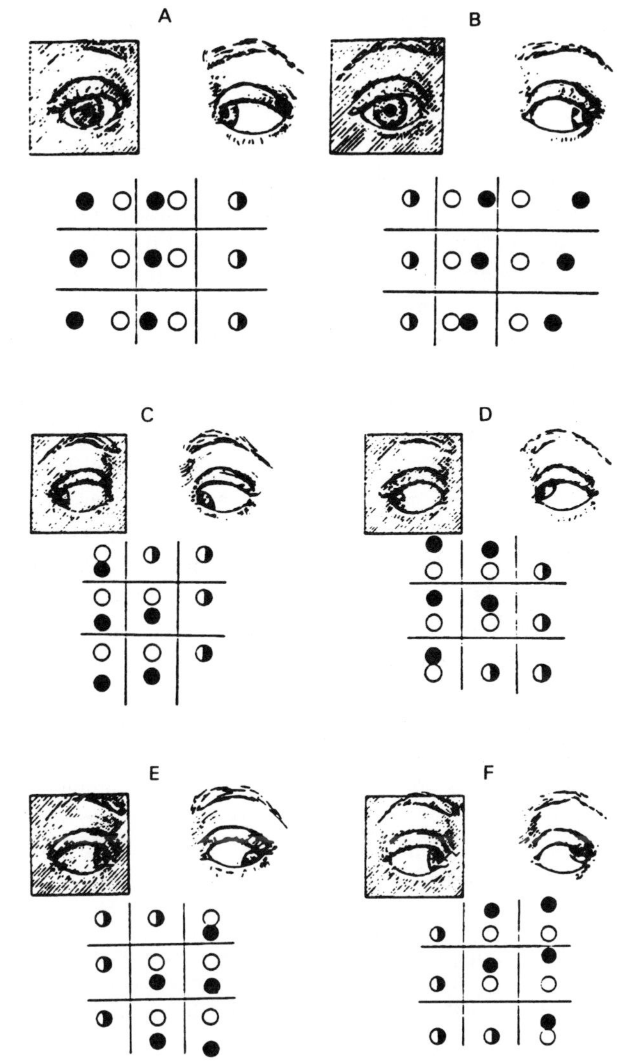

FIGURE 16.10 The red glass test. Diplopia fields for each individual muscle paralysis are shown. By convention, the red glass is placed over the right eye. The charts below each case are displayed as the subject, facing the examiner, indicates the position of the red (dark circle) and the white (white circle) images in the nine diagnostic positions of gaze. A. Right lateral rectus palsy. B. Right medial rectus palsy. C. Right inferior rectus palsy. D. Right superior rectus palsy. E. Right superior oblique palsy. F. Right inferior oblique palsy. (From DG Cogan. Neurology of the Ocular Muscles (2nd ed). Springfield, IL: Charles C Thomas, 1956. Courtesy of Charles C. Thomas, Publisher, Springfield, Illinois.)

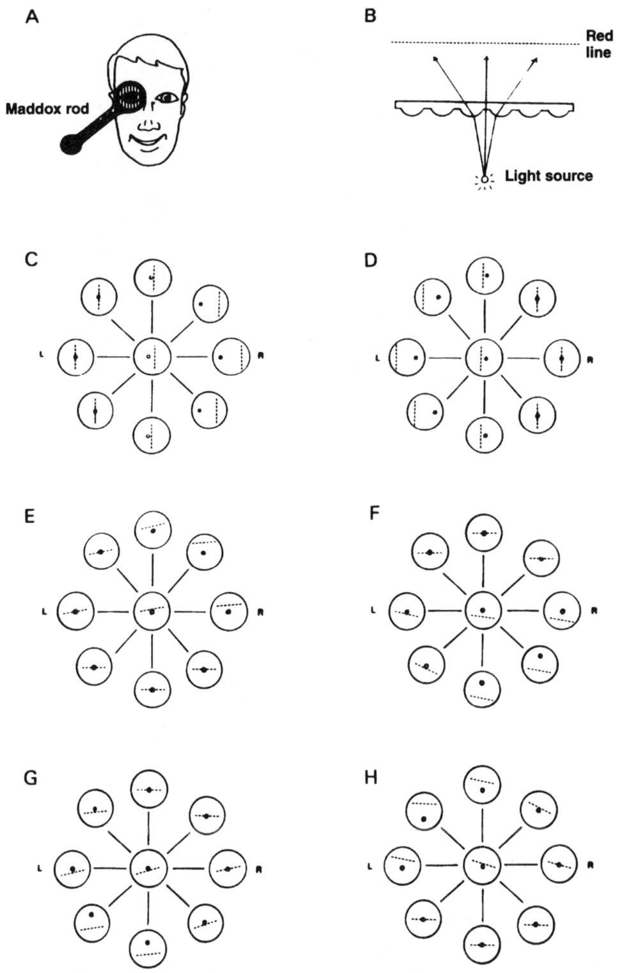

FIGURE 16.11 The Maddox rod test. (Unlike in Figure 16.10, the images are displayed as the patient perceives them.) A. By convention, the right eye is covered by the Maddox rod, which may be adjusted so that the patient sees a red line, at right angles to the cylinders, in the horizontal or vertical plane, as desired (red image seen by the right eye; light source seen by the left eye). B. The Maddox rod is composed of a series of cylinders that diffract a point of light to form a line. C. Right lateral rectus palsy. D. Right medial rectus palsy. E. Right superior rectus palsy. F. Right inferior rectus palsy. G. Right superior oblique palsy. H. Right inferior oblique palsy.

cylinders, to a straight line perpendicular to the cylinders (Figure 16.11). This dissociation of images (a point of light and a line) breaks fusion, allowing detection of heterophorias as well as heterotropias. Cyclotorsion may be detected by asking if the image of the line is tilted (see Figure 16.11). The Maddox rod can be positioned to produce a horizontal, vertical, or oblique line.

A further extension of these tests includes the *Lancaster red-green* and *Hess screen tests*, which use similar principles. Each eye views a different target (a red light through the red filter and a green light through the green filter). The relative positions of the targets are plotted on a grid screen and analyzed to determine the paretic muscle. These haploscopic tests are used mainly by ophthalmologists when quantitatively following patients with motility disorders.

The *Hirschberg test*, an objective method of determining ocular deviation in young or uncooperative patients, is performed by observing the point of reflection of a penlight held about 30 cm from the patient (Figure 16.12); 1 mm of decentration is equal to 7 degrees of ocular deviation. One de-

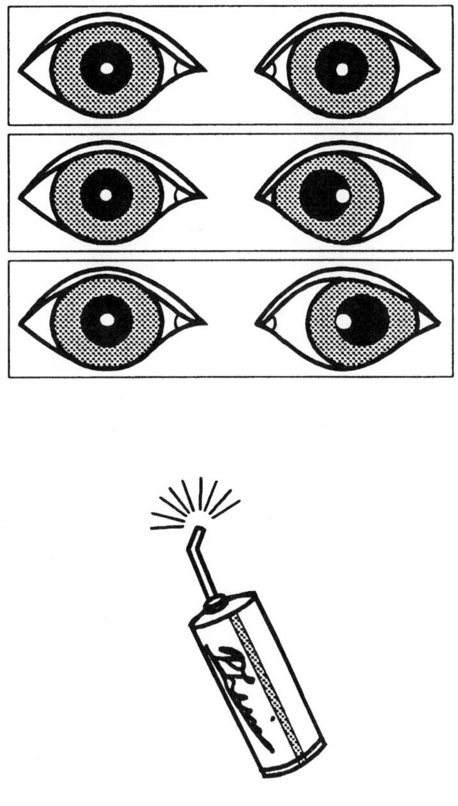

FIGURE 16.12 Hirschberg's method to estimate the amount of ocular deviation. The displacement of the corneal light reflex of the deviating eye varies with the amount of ocular misalignment. One millimeter is equivalent to about 7 degrees of ocular deviation, and one degree equals approximately two prism diopters. A. No deviation (orthotropic). B. Left esotropia. C. Left exotropia.

gree is equal to approximately two prism diopters. One prism diopter is the power required to deviate (diffract) a ray of light by one centimeter at a distance of 1 m (Figure 16.13).

The *cover-uncover test* is determined for both distance (6 m) and near (33 cm) vision. The patient is asked to fixate an object held at the appropriate distance. The left eye is covered while the patient maintains fixation on the target. If the right eye was fixating, it remains on target, but if the left eye was fixating, the right eye moves onto the target. If the uncovered right eye moves in (adducts), the patient has a right exotropia; if it moves out, the deviation is an esotropia; if it moves down, a right hypertropia; if it moves up, a left hypertropia.* *The physician should always observe the uncovered eye.* The cover should be removed and the test repeated by covering the other eye. If the patient has a tropia, then the physician must determine whether it is comitant or noncomitant by checking the degree of deviation in the nine diagnostic positions of gaze (see Figure 16.9A). With a lateral rectus palsy, the esotropia increases on looking to the side of the weak muscle and disappears on looking to the opposite side (see Figure 16.10A). Similarly, with a medial rectus weakness, the patient has an exotropia that increases on looking in the direction of action of that muscle (see Figure 16.10B). Prisms are used, mainly by ophthalmologists, to measure the degree of ocular deviation. If diplopia is due to breakdown of a long-standing (congenital) deviation, then prism measurement can detect supranormal fusional amplitudes (large fusional reserve). If no manifest deviation of the visual axes is found using the

* By convention, the vertical imbalance is always described in terms of one hypertropic (higher) eye irrespective of which eye is weak. Thus, if the right eye moves up with the cover test, the patient has a left hypertropia and not a right hypotropia.

FIGURE 16.13 A prism with the power of one diopter can defract a ray of light 1 cm at 1 m.

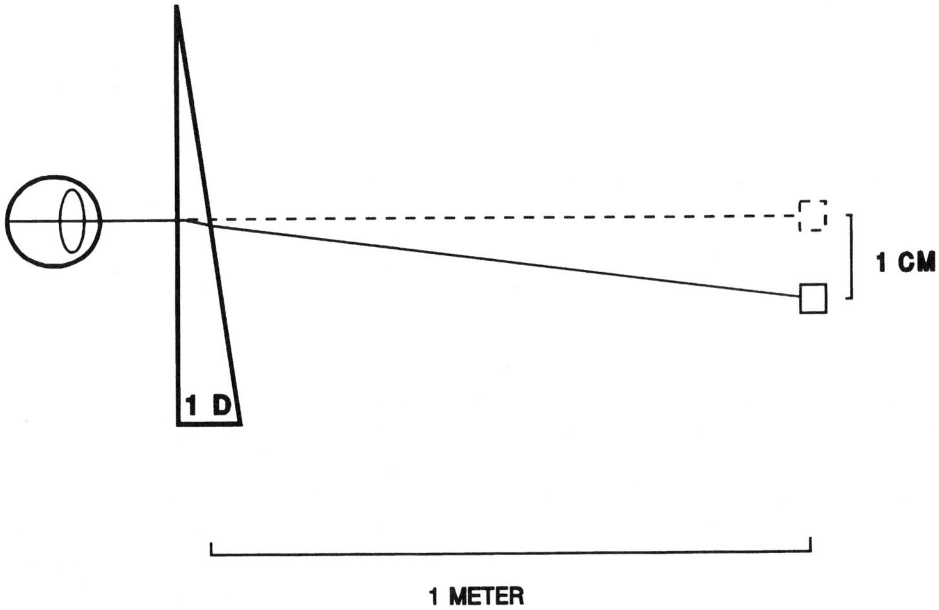

cover-uncover test, the patient is orthotropic. The physician should then perform the cross-cover test.

With the cross-cover (alternate cover test), the patient is asked to fixate on a target, and one eye is covered; again, the examiner should observe the uncovered eye. If the patient is orthotropic, the uncovered eye does not move, but the covered eye loses fixation and assumes its position of rest—latent deviation (heterophoria, also called phoria). In that case (usually exophoric), when the covered eye is uncovered, it refixates by moving inward; the uncovered eye is immediately covered and loses fixation. The cross-cover test prevents binocular viewing and thus foveal fusion by always keeping one eye covered. Unlike the cover-uncover test, the cross-cover test detects a heterophoria.

Dissociated vertical deviation (DVD) is an asymptomatic congenital anomaly that is usually discovered during the cover test. While the patient fixates a target, one eye is covered. The covered eye loses fixation and rises; the uncovered eye maintains fixation, but may intort. This congenital ocular motility phenomenon is usually bilateral, though frequently asymmetrical, and may often be associated with amblyopia, esotropia, and latent nystagmus. Whether there is an excessive number of axons decussating in the chiasm, suggested by evoked potential studies, remains controversial. DVD has no other clinical significance.

The Three-Step Test for Vertical Diplopia

Eight muscles are involved in vertical eye movements: four elevators and four depressors. If vertical diplopia is caused by one faulty muscle, then it should be possible to identify which one using the three-step test (Figure 16.14). Using the cover-uncover test, which is objective, or one of the subjective tests such as the red glass test, the physician can apply the three-step test. It is important to remember that the hypertrophic eye views the lower image.

The first step is to determine which eye is higher (hypertrophic) in primary position. The patient's head may have to be repositioned (forced primary position) because of a tilt. If the right eye is higher, then the weak muscle is either one of the two depressors of the right eye (inferior rectus or superior oblique) or one of the two elevators of the left eye (superior rectus or inferior oblique).

Step 2 involves observing whether the hypertropia increases on left gaze. If so, then the weak muscle is either the depressor in the right eye that acts best in adduction (i.e., the superior oblique) or the elevator in the left eye that acts best in abduction (i.e., the superior rectus).

With step 3, the physician should observe whether the ocular deviation is increased by tilting the head to the left. If so, then the weak muscle must be an intortor of the left eye (superior rectus); if it is worse on head tilt right, then it must be an intortor of the right eye (superior oblique).

With step 4 (optional), the physician should observe whether the deviation is worse on upgaze. If so, then the weak muscle is likely to be an elevator; if the deviation is greater on downgaze, then the weak muscle is a depressor. The fourth step is helpful in the acute situation, but because of spread of comitance, it does not always follow the rule predictably and may be misleading in patients with a long-standing palsy, especially if the third step is omitted.

The examiner should be aware of the *pitfalls of the three-step test,* where the rules break down and may be misleading. These include restrictive ocular myopathies (Table 16.7), long-standing strabismus, skew deviation (see Chapter 42), and disorders where more than one muscle is involved.

Fatigability

Once the weak muscle is identified, the physician should determine whether it fatigues by testing both its rapid (saccadic) action repetitively and its ability to sustain eccentric eye position without drift.

Forced Ductions

If the weak muscle does not fatigue, the physician should determine whether it is restricted by performing forced ductions. The use of phenylephrine hydrochloride eye drops beforehand reduces the risk of subconjunctival hemorrhage. Although this test falls into the realm of the ophthalmologist, it may be performed in the office using topical anesthesia and soft cotton swabs, but great care must be taken to avoid injuring the cornea. The causes of restrictive myopathy are listed in Table 16.7; however, any cause of prolonged extraocular muscle paresis results in contracture of its antagonist.

Signs Associated with Diplopia

Extraocular muscle or lid fatigue suggests myasthenia gravis, as does Cogan's lid twitch sign. Weakness of other muscles (for example, orbicularis oculi, other facial muscles, neck flexors, or bulbar muscles) may be found in oculopharyngeal dystrophy and myasthenia gravis (see Chapters 29 and 84). Narrowing of the palpebral fissure and retraction of the globe on adduction with an abduction deficit suggest Duane's retraction syndrome (see Chapter 75).

Paradoxical elevation of the upper lid on attempted adduction or downgaze occurs with aberrant reinnervation of the third cranial nerve, virtually always a result of trauma or compression caused by tumor or aneurysm (see Chapter 75); the pupil may also constrict on adduction and downgaze. Miosis accompanying apparent bilateral sixth nerve palsy occurs with spasm of the near reflex (see Chapter 42). Horner's syndrome, ophthalmoplegia, and impaired sensation in the distribution of the first division of the trigeminal nerve occur with superior orbital fissure/anterior cavernous sinus lesions.

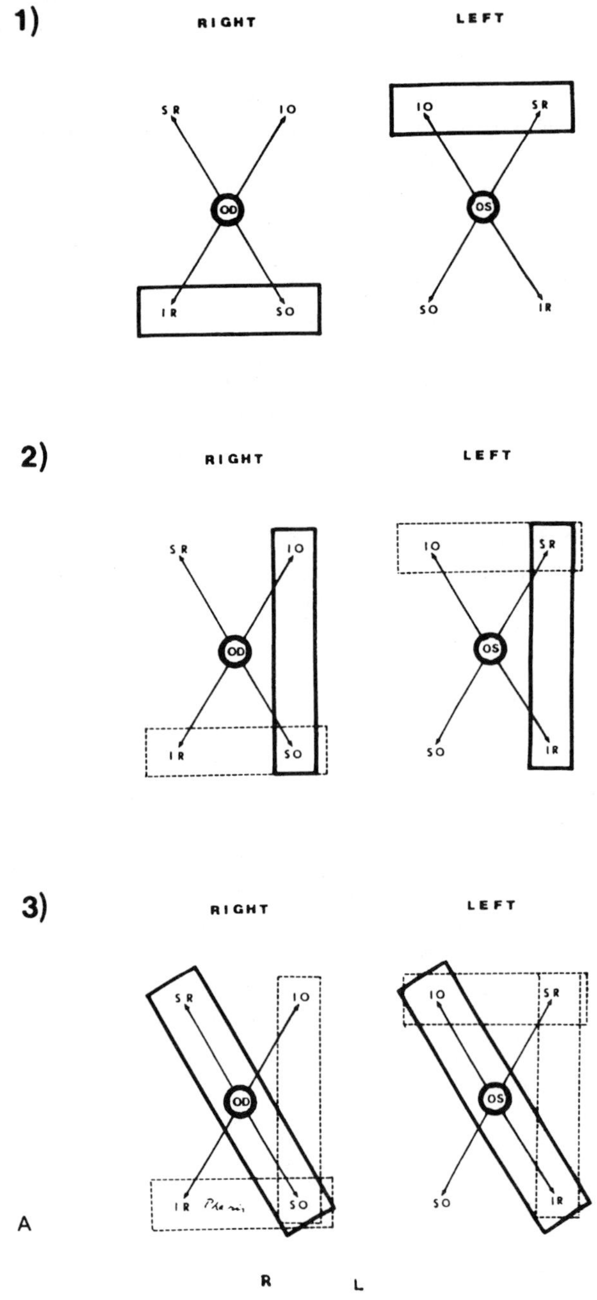

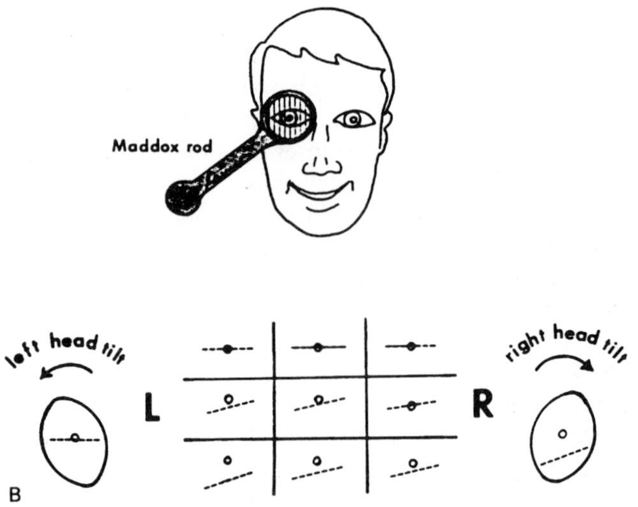

FIGURE 16.14 Example of the three-step test in a patient with an acute right superior oblique palsy. A. In a patient with hypertropia, one of eight muscles may be responsible for the vertical ocular deviation. Identifying the higher eye eliminates four muscles. (1) With a right hypertropia, the weak muscle is either one of the two depressors of the right eye (IR or SO) or one of the two elevators of the left eye (IO or SR) (enclosed by the solid line). (2) If the deviation (or displacement of images) is greater on left gaze, then one of the muscles acting in left gaze (enclosed by the solid line) must be responsible, in this case either the depressor in the right eye (SO) or the elevator in the left eye (SR). (3) If the deviation is greater on right head tilt, then one of the muscles acting during right head tilt, the incyclotortors of the right eye (SR and SO) or the excyclotortors of the left eye (IR and IO) (enclosed) must be responsible, in this case the right SO—that is, the muscle enclosed three times. If the deviation is greater on left head tilt, then the left SR would be responsible. (IO = inferior oblique; IR = inferior rectus; SO = superior oblique; SR = superior rectus.) B. The Maddox rod test (displayed as in Figure 16.11, as the subject perceives the images) in a patient with a right superior oblique palsy shows vertical diplopia that is worse in the direction of action of the weak muscle and demonstrates subjective tilting of the image from the right eye. When the head is tilted toward the left shoulder, the diplopia disappears, but when the head is tilted to the right shoulder, to the side of the weak muscle, the double vision is exacerbated (Bielschowsky's third step).

A third nerve palsy with pupillary involvement is most frequently caused by a compressive lesion.

Proptosis suggests an orbital lesion such as thyroid disease (bilateral), inflammatory or infiltrative orbital disease (tumor, pseudotumor, or amyloidosis), or carotid-cavernous fistula, which may be pulsatile. Ocular bruits, often heard by both patient and doctor, occur with carotid-cavernous or dural shunt fistulas. Other findings include entrapment (blowout fracture), which is a sign of periorbital and ocular injury, and nystagmus (see Chapter 42) seen with internuclear ophthalmoplegia. There may also be other cranial nerve deficits and various miscellaneous signs. Ophthalmoplegia, ataxia, nystagmus, and confusion suggest Wernicke's encephalopathy. Pyramidal and spinothalamic signs with crossed hemiparesis suggest brain stem syndromes (see Chapter 23). Facial pain, hearing loss, and ipsilateral lateral rectus weakness indicate Gradenigo's syndrome. Myotonia and retinitis pigmentosa suggest more widespread disorders.

The Edrophonium (Tensilon) Test

The edrophonium test is discussed in detail in Chapter 83, but the following points should be stressed here. There must be an objective end point such as ptosis, tropia, or

Table 16.7: Positive forced ductions (restrictive)

Thyroid ophthalmopathy
Duane's syndrome
Brown's syndrome
Congenital: short superior oblique tendon
Acquired: superior oblique tendinitis, myositis, or injury
Extraocular muscle fibrosis (congenital, postoperative)
Entrapment (blowout fracture)
Orbital infiltration: myositis, lymphoma, metastasis, amyloidosis, cysticercosis, trichinosis
Carotid-cavernous or dural shunt fistula
Long-standing muscle weakness

Table 16.8: Causes of acute bilateral ophthalmoplegia (in alphabetical order)[a]

Basilar meningitis, hypertrophic cranial pachymeningitis, or neoplastic infiltration[b]
Botulism
Brain stem encephalitis[b]
Brain stem stroke[b]
Carotid-cavernous or dural shunt fistula[b]
Cavernous sinus thrombosis (febrile, ill)[b]
Central herniation syndrome
Ciguatera poisoning
Diphtheria
Fisher's syndrome
AIDS encephalopathy
Intoxication (sedatives, tricyclics, organophosphates, anticonvulsants—consciousness impaired)
Leigh's disease (subacute necrotizing encephalomyelitis)
Multiple sclerosis
Myasthenia
Neuroleptic malignant syndrome (personal observation)
Orbital pseudotumor[b]
Paraneoplastic encephalomyelitis
Pituitary apoplexy[b]
Polyradiculopathy (associated with)
Psychogenic
Thallium poisoning
Tick paralysis
Tolosa-Hunt syndrome[b]
Trauma (impaired consciousness, signs of injury)[b]
Wernicke's encephalopathy

[a]All may be unilateral.
[b]Pain may be present. Painful ophthalmoplegia is discussed in Chapter 75.

limited ductions; the physician must observe an objective change. The edrophonium test will be negative if forced ductions are positive (restrictive myopathy) and will be difficult to interpret if the patient has no objective signs of extraocular muscle weakness or ptosis.

Optokinetic Nystagmus

Full visual field stimulation, either by rotating an image of the environment around the patient or by rotating the patient within the room in a rotating chair, is necessary to provoke true optokinetic nystagmus (OKN) (see Chapter 42). The OKN tape is useful at the bedside but only tests foveal pursuit and refixation saccades, which are helpful in the following circumstances: (1) in detecting a subtle internuclear ophthalmoplegia; (2) in provoking convergence-retraction nystagmus, where the tape is moved downward in an attempt to induce upward saccades; (3) in congenital nystagmus, where the direction of the fast phase may be paradoxical—that is, in the direction of the slowly moving tape or drum; (4) in patients feigning complete blindness or ophthalmoplegia; (5) in homonymous hemianopia caused by a large, deep-seated parietotemporooccipital lesion, where the OKN response will be depressed or absent as the tape moves toward the side of the lesion.

A large mirror may be used to induce optokinetic movements in patients with psychogenic ophthalmoplegia or psychogenic blindness. The examiner holds the mirror in front of the patient, whose eyes are open. The mirror is gently rocked so that the reflected environment (full visual field) moves; this compelling optokinetic stimulus forces reflex slow eye movements. The patient may close the eyes, look away, or converge in an attempt to avoid the reflex response. Care must be taken in diagnosing psychogenic ophthalmoplegia with this test in patients with supranuclear gaze palsies and ocular motor apraxia.

Vergence Disorders

Vergence disorders may cause diplopia (see Chapter 42).

Central Fusion Disruption

Central fusion disruption causes diplopia and is described in Chapter 42.

Acute Bilateral Ophthalmoplegia

The causes of acute bilateral ophthalmoplegia are outlined in Table 16.8.

Chronic Bilateral Ophthalmoplegia

The causes of chronic bilateral ophthalmoplegia are outlined in Table 16.9.

Treatment

Patching (occlusive) therapy is used mainly to eliminate one image. In children under age 9, each eye should be patched alternately to prevent developmental amblyopia. Such young patients should be followed by an experienced ophthalmologist. Adult patients may wear the patch over whichever eye is more comfortable, although some clinicians feel that alternating the patch reduces the incidence of contractures.

Table 16.9: Causes of chronic ophthalmoplegia

Myasthenia gravis
Dysthyroidism
Multiple sclerosis
Brain stem neoplasm
Chronic basal meningitis (infection, sarcoid, or carcinoma)
Myopathies e.g., mitochondrial, fiber-type disproportion (see Table 42.2)
Vitamin E deficiency
Congenital extraocular muscle fibrosis
Leigh's disease
Nuclear, paranuclear, and supranuclear gaze palsies (see Chapter 42)

Prisms are helpful in eliminating double vision if the deviation is not too great. A reasonable range of binocular single vision may be achieved with prisms, provided the patient's expectations are not too high and there is no significant cyclodeviation.

Botulinum toxin, a relatively new form of treatment for strabismus, has been used in patients with both comitant and noncomitant strabismus, with mixed success. It may be helpful in acute abducens palsies.

Extraocular muscle surgery can correct long-standing strabismus (comitant or noncomitant). Finally, *orthoptic exercises* are of use in patients with convergence insufficiency (see Chapter 42).

Related Disorders

Polyopia, the perception of multiple images, is frequently optical and can be determined by the pinhole test, discussed above. Polyopia may also be caused by cortical lesions (see Table 16.5).

Palinopia (also known as "palinopsia" or "paliopia"), the persistence or recurrence of visual images after the stimulus has been removed, may cause cerebral diplopia or polyopia. The images become more apparent and numerous when the target moves in front of the retina because it provokes persistent after-images (Figure 16.15). This visual perseveration occurs more frequently in patients with mild left homonymous visual field defects caused by right parieto-occipital lesions; it may be ictal and respond to anticonvulsant medication. It may also occur with metabolic disorders, carbon monoxide poisoning, mescaline, lysergic acid diethylamide (LSD), trazodone, and clomiphene (Purvin 1995).

Oscillopsia, an illusion of movement or oscillation of the environment, occurs with acquired nystagmus, superior oblique myokymia, other ocular oscillations, and disorders of the vestibuloocular reflex.

Superior oblique myokymia is a small, rapid, monocular torsional-vertical oscillation, discussed in more detail below.

Environmental tilting (*tortopia*), the illusion of tilting or even inversion of the visual environment for a period of seconds to minutes, may occur in patients with posterior fossa disease, most commonly vertebrobasilar ischemia. Tortopia may be associated with headache, dizziness, vertigo, and double vision and is presumed to be due to dysfunction of the vestibulo-otolithic system or its central connections.

Occasionally, after extremely prolonged monotonous visual and vestibular stimulation, as in interstate highway driving, the subject may observe the environment to be sloping downward when in fact it is flat ("interstate illusions" or "highway hallucinosis"). This type of vision is somewhat similar to the prolonged sensation of movement after a long sea voyage.

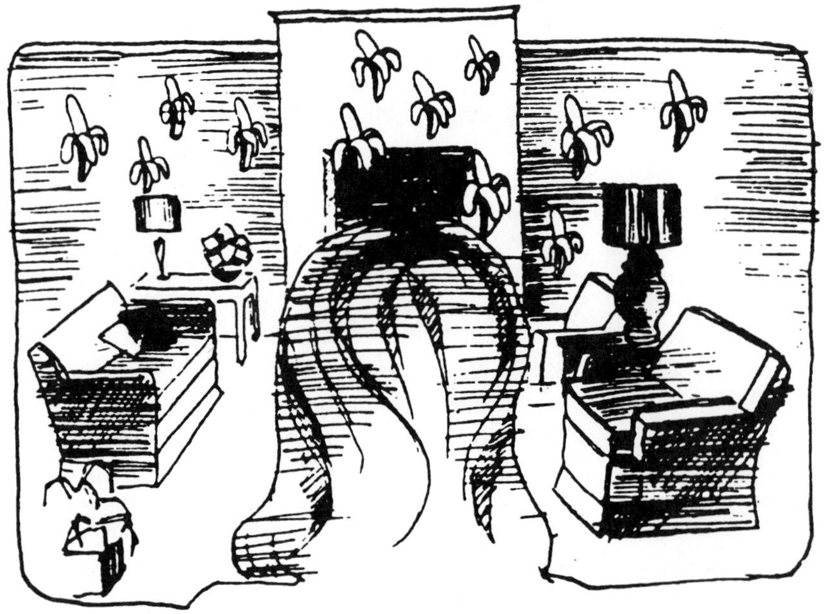

FIGURE 16.15 Palinopsia (cerebral polyopia). Visual images experienced by a patient moments after peeling a banana. (From EN Michel, BT Troost. Palinopsia: cerebral localization with computed tomography. Neurology 1980;30:887–889. Copyright © 1980. Reprinted by permission of the authors and publisher.)

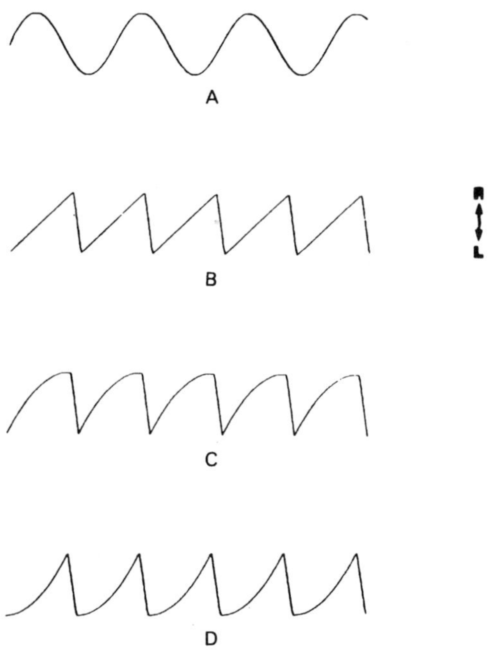

FIGURE 16.16 Oculographic diagrams of nystagmus waveforms. A. Pendular (sinusoidal nystagmus). B. Leftward-beating jerk nystagmus with a constant-velocity (linear) slow phase. C. Left-beating jerk nystagmus with a decreasing (exponential) velocity slow phase. D. Left-beating jerk nystagmus with an increasing (exponential) velocity slow phase.

Episodic blurring, watering, itching, diplopia, eyestrain, tiredness of the eyes or lids especially after reading, sleepiness, and photophobia are all features of *asthenopia* (neurasthenia of the eyes). Patients with this condition frequently exaggerate normal phenomena such as physiological diplopia, floaters, persistence of after-images, and difficulty in reading. Their symptoms may be associated with accommodative insufficiency, headache, and other asthenic complaints. Care must be taken to exclude true refractive errors, defective accommodation, convergence insufficiency, medication, and diabetes mellitus (Waltz and Lavin 1993). Although asthenopia is usually psychogenic, a cause for isolated accommodative insufficiency, such as parieto-occipital stroke, may be found. Management includes a thorough examination, recognition of real abnormalities, and confident and authoritative reassurance.

NYSTAGMUS

Nystagmus is an involuntary biphasic rhythmic ocular oscillation in which one or both phases are slow (Figure 16.16). The slow phase of jerk nystagmus is responsible for the initiation and generation of the nystagmus, whereas the fast (saccadic) phase is a corrective movement bringing the fovea back on target.

For clinical purposes, nystagmus may be divided into *pendular* and *jerk* forms. Either form may be horizontal or, less frequently, vertical. Jerk nystagmus is labeled conventionally by the direction of the fast phase and is divided into three types on the basis of the shape of the slow phase, detected by oculographic recordings (see Figure 16.16).

Mechanisms of Nystagmus

Nystagmus may result from dysfunction of the vestibular end organ, vestibular nerve, brain stem, cerebellum or cerebral centers for ocular pursuit (see Chapter 42). Pendular nystagmus (see Figure 16.16A) is central (brain stem or cerebellum) in origin (Averbuch-Heller et al. 1995a), whereas jerk nystagmus may be either central or peripheral. Jerk nystagmus with a linear (constant-velocity) slow phase (see Figure 16.16B) is caused by peripheral vestibular dysfunction (imbalance in vestibular input to the brain stem gaze centers). When the slow phase has a decreasing velocity exponential (see Figure 16.16C), the brain stem neural integrator (see Chapter 42) is at fault and is said to be leaky. The integrator is unable to maintain a constant output to the gaze center to hold the eyes in an eccentric position, resulting in *gaze-paretic nystagmus*. An increasing velocity exponential slow phase (see Figure 16.16D) in the horizontal plane is central in origin and is a form of congenital nystagmus. These mechanistic explanations for nystagmus waveforms are speculative.

Clinical Evaluation

The physician should determine whether the nystagmus has been present since birth or is acquired, and whether there is a family history. Congenital nystagmus is usually asymptomatic and rarely bothers the patient or causes oscillopsia. Symptoms such as headache, diplopia, impaired vision, oscillopsia, vertigo, or other neurological abnormalities must be taken into account. Examination should include a neurologist's ocular examination, with visual acuity, confrontation visual fields, pupil reflexes, observation for ocular albinism, and ophthalmoscopy. The latter may be used to detect subtle nystagmus not apparent to the naked eye. Ocular motility must also be assessed. The following features must be determined:

1. Is the nystagmus present in primary position or only with eccentric gaze (gaze-evoked)?
2. Is the nystagmus binocular and conjugate or is it dissociated?
3. Is the waveform pendular or jerk? If jerk, what is the direction of the fast phase?
4. Is there a latent component—that is, an increase in nystagmus intensity when one eye is covered?

5. Is there a torsional component?
6. Is there spontaneous alteration of direction, as with periodic alternating nystagmus, which must be distinguished from *rebound nystagmus* (discussed later in the chapter) and which requires observation for a period of time?
7. Is there a null zone (a direction of gaze where the nystagmus is minimal or absent)?
8. Does convergence damp the nystagmus or change its direction?
9. Is the nystagmus altered (accentuated or suppressed) by head positioning or posture, or by head shaking (as in spasmus nutans)?
10. What is the effect of optokinetic stimulation? (In congenital nystagmus, it is paradoxical.)
11. Are there associated rhythmic movements of other muscle groups, such as the face, tongue, ears, neck, palate (oculopalateal myoclonus), or limbs?

Nystagmus Syndromes

Congenital Nystagmus

Congenital nystagmus (CN) is usually present from birth but may not be noticed for the first few weeks, or occasionally even years, of life. It may be accompanied by severe visual impairment but is not the result of poor vision. It is sometimes associated with ocular albinism and head titubation. CN may be familial and is inherited in an autosomal recessive, X-linked dominant or recessive pattern.

CN is usually horizontal and may be either pendular or jerk in primary position. Pendular nystagmus often becomes jerk on lateral gaze. The patient often has good vision unless there is an associated afferent defect such as retinal disease or optic atrophy. CN damps with convergence; latent superimposition may be present (nystagmus amplitude increases with one eye covered). A null zone, where the nystagmus intensity is minimal, may be found; if this is to one side, the subject will have a head turn to improve vision. The head frequently oscillates as well. Both features—damping of nystagmus with convergence and a null zone—can be used in therapy by changing the direction of gaze with prisms or extraocular muscle surgery to improve head posture and visual acuity. Oculographic recordings (see Chapter 42) demonstrate either a sinusoidal (see Figure 16.16A) or slow phase with an increasing exponential waveform (see Figure 16.16D).

Rarely, CN may be pendular in the vertical plane or circumductory where the eyes move conjugately in a circular or cycloid pattern. Occasionally CN may be unilateral, occur later in the teens or adult life (Gresty et al. 1992), or become symptomatic if changes in the internal or external environment alter foveation stability and duration causing oscillopsia (Dell'Osso and Leigh 1992).

Latent Nystagmus and Manifest Latent Nystagmus

Latent nystagmus (LN) and manifest latent nystagmus (MLN) are both congenital forms of nystagmus (Gresty et al. 1992).

LN occurs with monocular fixation—that is, when one eye is covered. The slow phase is directed toward the covered eye. The amplitude of the oscillations increases on abduction of the fixating eye.

With MLN, the oscillation is present with both eyes open. However, only one eye is seeing; vision in the other is suppressed as a result of strabismus or amblyopia. The nystagmus waveform has a decreasing velocity slow phase (see Figure 16.16C), differing from true CN. Some patients with LN can suppress it at will (Kommerell and Zee 1993).

Spasmus Nutans

Spasmus nutans is transient, high-frequency, low-amplitude pendular nystagmus that occurs between the ages of 6 and 12 months and lasts about 2 years, though occasionally as long as 5 years. The direction of the oscillation may be horizontal, vertical, or torsional and is often dysconjugate, asymmetrical, and variable. It may be associated with torticollis and titubation (spasmus nutans triad). The titubation (head nodding) has a lower frequency than the nystagmus and is thus not compensatory. However, patients can improve vision by vigorously shaking the head, presumably to stimulate the vestibulo-ocular reflex and suppress or override the ocular oscillation. Some patients may have heterotropia. Although spasmus nutans is a benign and transient disorder, it must be distinguished from acquired nystagmus caused by structural lesions involving the anterior visual pathways; in the latter situation, a careful ophthalmological examination will reveal clinical evidence such as impaired vision, an afferent pupillary defect, or optic atrophy. Retinal disorders may also masquerade as spasmus nutans, but the electroretinogram will be abnormal (Lambert and Newman 1993).

Pendular Nystagmus

Pendular nystagmus (see Figure 16.16A) has a sinusoidal waveform and is usually horizontal. It may be either congenital or acquired. The most common cause of acquired pendular nystagmus is multiple sclerosis, followed by brain stem vascular disease, involving the deep cerebellar nuclei or their efferent connections. Barton and Cox (1993) found magnetic resonance imaging (MRI) changes in the dorsal pontine tegmentum in their patients and implicated the central tegmental tract, which is also affected in oculopalatal myoclonus (below). Pendular nystagmus may also occur in Cockayne's syndrome.

Convergent-divergent nystagmus, a rare variant of acquired pendular nystagmus, is dysconjugate (see below) and occurs in patients with demyelinating disease, brain stem stroke, Chiari malformations, cerebral Whipple's disease (see oculomasticatory myorhythmia below), and progressive ataxia (Averbuch-Heller et al. 1995a; Averbuch-Heller et al. 1995b). The eyes oscillate mainly horizontally in opposite directions simultaneously, although they sometimes form circular, elliptical, or oblique trajectories dependent on the phase relationship of the horizontal, vertical, and torsional vectors responsible for the oscillations. *Cycloverggent nystagmus*—that is, dysconjugate torsional nystagmus in which the upper poles of the eyes move in opposite directions—may be detected by scleral search coil oculography; on rare occations it may be observed clinically (Averbuch-Heller et al. 1995a).

Vertical pendular nystagmus closely resembles the vertical ocular oscillation associated with *palatal myoclonus* (the oculopalatal syndrome) (Deuschl et al. 1990) and may be a form of the same disorder, which also results from lesions of the deep cerebellar nuclei and their connections.

Elliptical pendular nystagmus with a larger vertical component and superimposed or interposed upbeat nystagmus, is characteristic of Pelizaeus-Merzbacher's disease (Trobe et al. 1991). This nystagmus can be difficult to detect with the naked eye. It is seen more easily with an ophthalmoscope, but oculography using scleral search coils may be necessary to detect it.

Pendular Pseudonystagmus

Patients with vestibular end organ damage and "essential" head tremor may develop *pendular pseudonystagmus* to compensate for an absent or defective vestibulo-ocular reflex (VOR) (see Chapter 42). In the absence of a normal VOR, head movements take the fovea off the target, causing blurred vision or oscillopsia. Eye movements, with longer latencies than normal VORs, are generated by alternative mechanisms (pursuit, cervico-ocular, and optokinetic movements) to maintain the fovea on target (Bronstein et al. 1992). This ocular oscillation, which is compensatory and not a sign of central nervous system disease, disappears when the patient's head is held still.

Oculomasticatory Myorhythmia. Oculomasticatory myorhythmia, described in patients with Whipple's disease and, to date, pathognomonic for that disorder, consists of continuous rhythmic jaw contractions synchronous with pendular vergence oscillations (dissociated). It may be associated with supranuclear vertical gaze palsy, altered mentation, somnolence, mild uveitis, or retinopathy (Knox et al. 1995).

Gaze-Paretic Nystagmus

Gaze-paretic nystagmus, the most common type of nystagmus, is usually symmetrical, with eccentric gaze to either side, but is absent in the primary position. It may be asymmetrical with asymmetrical disease such as myasthenia. Upward-beating nystagmus is frequently present on upgaze and downward-beating on downgaze. It has a jerk waveform with the fast phase in the direction of gaze. Oculographic recordings show a decreasing exponential slow phase (see Figure 16.16C). Gaze-paretic nystagmus results from dysfunction of the neural integrator (see Chapter 42), most frequently caused by alcohol or drug intoxication (anticonvulsants and tranquilizers).

Vestibular Nystagmus

Vestibular nystagmus has a linear slow phase (see Figure 16.16B) and results from damage to the labyrinth, the vestibular nerve, the vestibular nuclei, or their connections in the brain stem or cerebellum. Vestibular nystagmus may be divided into central and peripheral forms on the basis of the associated features outlined in Chapter 18. With central forms the slow phase may be variable. Peripheral vestibular nystagmus is usually associated with severe vegetative symptoms, including nausea, vomiting, perspiration, and diarrhea. On the other hand, with central vestibular nystagmus, vegetative symptoms are less severe, but other neurological features such as headache, dysconjugate gaze, and pyramidal tract signs may be present (see Chapter 23).

Caloric-Induced Nystagmus

Caloric-induced nystagmus is discussed in Chapters 18 and 44.

Physiological Nystagmus

Physiological (end-point) nystagmus is a jerk nystagmus observed on extreme lateral or upward gaze. If the bridge of the nose obstructs the view of the adducting eye, physiological nystagmus may be dysconjugate, the amplitude being greater in the abducting eye. A torsional component is sometimes seen. Physiological nystagmus is distinguished from pathological nystagmus by its symmetry on right and left gaze and by the absence of other neurological features; it is not present when the angle of gaze is less than 30 degrees from primary position. Oculographic recordings demonstrate primarily a linear slow phase (see Figure 16.16B) and may detect transient small-amplitude rebound nystagmus.

Dysconjugate and Monocular Nystagmus

Dysconjugate (dissociated) nystagmus occurs when the ocular oscillations are out of phase (different directions). It is seen with internuclear ophthalmoplegia (see Chapter 42), other brain stem lesions (see Convergent-Divergent Nystagmus), and spasmus nutans. Monocular nystagmus is also dysconjugate and may be associated with amblyopia (Table 16.10).

Table 16.10: Causes of monocular nystagmus (in alphabetical order)

Acquired monocular blindness (nystagmus in blind eye)
Amblyopia
Brain stem infarction (thalamus and upper midbrain)
Ictal nystagmus
Internuclear and pseudointernuclear ophthalmoplegia
Multiple sclerosis
Nystagmus with one eye absent
Nystagmus with monocular ophthalmoplegia
Spasmus nutans
Superior oblique myokymia
Pseudonystagmus (lid fasciculations)

Monocular nystagmus may be pendular or jerk and may also be horizontal, vertical, or oblique. Oculographic recordings may reveal small-amplitude oscillations in the fellow eye. Monocular nystagmus may occur in patients with amblyopia, strabismus, monocular blindness, spasmus nutans, marked internuclear ophthalmoplegia; rarely with seizures; and of course when the other eye is completely ophthalmoplegic or absent. Superior oblique myokymia may be mistaken for a monocular torsional or vertical nystagmus (see Table 16.10).

Upbeat Nystagmus

Upbeat nystagmus is a spontaneous jerk nystagmus with the fast phase upward while the eyes are in primary position. The amplitude and intensity of the nystagmus usually increase on upgaze. This finding strongly suggests structural disease of the brain stem, most commonly the pontomedullary and pontomescencephalic junctions or midline cerebellum (vermis). Rarely, upbeat nystagmus may be congenital or result from intoxication with anticonvulsants, organophosphates, lithium, or nicotine. In infants, upbeat nystagmus may be a sign of anterior visual pathway disease such as Leber's congenital amaurosis (see Chapter 43), optic nerve hypoplasia, aniridia, and cataracts (Good et al. 1990).

Downbeat Nystagmus

Downbeat nystagmus is a spontaneous downward-beating jerk nystagmus present in primary position. The amplitude of the oscillation increases if the eyes are directed downward and laterally (Daroff's sign). Downbeat nystagmus may be apparent only with changes in posture (positional downbeat nystagmus), particularly the head-hanging position, used as part of position testing in dizzy patients. Downbeat nystagmus occurs most frequently with structural lesions at the craniocervical junction. A thorough investigation for disorders such as Chiari malformations, basilar invagination, and foramen magnum tumors should be made (Schmidt, 1991). Currently, MRI of the foramen magnum region, in the sagittal plane, is the investigation of choice.

Downbeat nystagmus may also occur with cerebellar degeneration (alcoholic, familial, anoxic, and paraneoplastic); metabolic disorders, including intoxication with anticonvulsants, alcohol, lithium, meperidine (personal observation), and amiodarone; magnesium depletion; Wernicke's encephalopathy; brain stem encephalitis; multiple sclerosis; leukodystrophy; and vertebrobasilar ischemia. Downbeat nystagmus may be congenital or, rarely, occur as a transient ocular oscillation in normal neonates.

The treatment of downbeat nystagmus involves correction of the underlying cause where possible. When downbeat nystagmus damps on convergence, it may be treated successfully with base-out prisms, reducing the oscillopsia and improving the visual acuity.

Both upbeat and downbeat nystagmus may be altered, in amplitude and direction, by a variety of maneuvers, such as convergence, head tilting, and changes in posture.

Periodic Alternating Nystagmus

Periodic alternating nystagmus (PAN) is a horizontal jerk nystagmus in which the fast phase beats in one direction and then damps or stops for a few seconds before changing direction to the opposite side. A complete cycle takes about 3 minutes. PAN has the same clinical significance as downbeat nystagmus and may sometimes coexist. Attention should be focused at the craniocervical junction. PAN has been described in Creutzfeldt-Jakob disease (Grant et al. 1993). When PAN is congenital it may be associated with albinism (Abadi and Pascal 1994). Baclofen has been used successfully in the acquired form of the disease. PAN should be distinguished from rebound nystagmus, discussed below.

Rebound Nystagmus

Rebound nystagmus is a horizontal gaze–evoked jerk nystagmus in which the direction of the fast phase reverses with sustained lateral gaze. When the eyes return to primary position, the fast phase may beat transiently in the opposite direction (sometimes a physiologic finding). It is caused by dysfunction of the cerebellum or the perihypoglossal nuclei in the medulla (Halmagyi 1994).

Convergence-Evoked Nystagmus

Convergence-evoked nystagmus is an unusual ocular oscillation, usually pendular, induced by voluntary convergence (see Convergent-Divergent Nystagmus). The movements may be conjugate or dissociated. This condition may be congenital or acquired and has been described in patients with multiple sclerosis. A jerk form has been associated with a Chiari I malformation. Convergence-evoked vertical nystagmus (upbeat more common than downbeat) is a sign of posterior fossa disease. Convergence-evoked nystagmus should be distinguished from voluntary nystagmus and from convergence-retraction nystagmus (see below).

Seesaw Nystagmus

Seesaw nystagmus is a spectacular ocular oscillation in which one eye rises and intorts as the other eye falls and extorts. It occurs with lesions in the region of the mesodiencephalic junction, particularly the zona inserta and the interstitial nucleus of Cajal. The waveform appears pendular. Disordered control of the normal ocular tilt reflex is the most likely mechanism. Congenital seesaw nystagmus may be associated with a superimposed horizontal pendular nystagmus. The acquired form may be accompanied by a bitemporal hemianopia caused by an expanding lesion in the third ventricular region. If seesaw nystagmus damps with convergence, base-out prisms may be helpful.

Transient seesaw nystagmus may occur for a few seconds after a blink (Barton 1995).

A jerk-waveform seesaw nystagmus occurs with unilateral mesodienceophalic lesions, presumed to be due to selective unilateral inactivation of the torsional eye-velocity integrator in the interstitial nucleus of Cajal (see Chapter 42); during the fast (jerk) phases the upper poles of the eyes rotate toward the side of the lesion (Halmagyi et al. 1994).

Torsional (Rotary) Nystagmus

In torsional nystagmus (TN), the eye oscillates in a pure rotary or cyclorotational plane. TN may be present in primary position, or with either head positioning or gaze deviation, and is usually caused by lesions in the central vestibular connections (Lopez et al. 1992). Pure TN occurs only with central vestibular dysfunction, whereas mixed torsional-linear nystagmus may occur with peripheral vestibular disease. Skew deviation frequently coexists (see Chapter 42).

Ictal Nystagmus

Ictal nystagmus often accompanies adversive seizures and beats to the side opposite the focus. Tusa et al. (1990) implicated the pursuit pathways originating from the temporo-occipital cortex in a patient with ipsiversive ictal eye deviation. It may be associated with transient pupillary dilation of the abducting eye. Pupillary oscillations synchronous with the nystagmus may rarely occur.

Nystagmus as the only motor manifestation of a seizure is rare; there are reports, however, of isolated ictal nystagmus, such as occurs in patients with vivid ictal visual hallucinations. It is difficult to draw any conclusion, clinically, regarding the location of the seizure discharge in these patients, as seizure foci have been reported in occipital, parietal, temporal, and frontal areas. The nystagmus is usually horizontal, but there are occasional reports of vertical nystagmus, mainly in comatose patients. Periodic eye movements in comatose patients should alert the physician to the possibility of status epilepticus.

Lid Nystagmus

Lid nystagmus, characterized by rhythmic jerking movements of the upper eyelids, occurs in the following situations: (1) synchronous with vertical ocular nystagmus, (2) synchronous with the fast phase of gaze-evoked horizontal nystagmus in some patients with the lateral medullary syndrome, and (3) during voluntary convergence in some patients with disease of the rostral medulla (Dell'Osso et al. 1990).

Episodic (Periodic) Nystagmus

Episodic nystagmus is associated with a disorder in which the patient has paroxysmal episodes of vertigo, ataxia, and nystagmus lasting up to 24 hours. The nystagmus may be torsional, vertical, or dissociated. The frequency of attacks varies from once a day to only a few times per year. Such periodic ataxia occurs in patients with hereditary inborn errors of metabolism, in a familial form without any detectable metabolic defect, and in patients with basilar migraine or multiple sclerosis. Acetazolamide or valproic acid may alleviate or prevent attacks in the familial form.

Treatment

Acuity should be corrected with a good refraction if necessary. With the exception of CN, in which prisms, surgery, and contact lenses are helpful, the treatment of other forms of nystagmus is discouraging. Prisms are occasionally helpful in acquired nystagmus. Various pharmacological agents, including benzodiazepines, baclofen, isoniazid, trihexyphenidyl, tetrabenazine, prochlorperazine, carbamazepine, L-dopa, alcohol, and carisoprodol, have been tried. Barton's group (1994) found some success treating acquired pendular and downbeat nystagmus with the central muscarinic antagonists benztropine and scopolamine. Otherwise, with the exceptions of clonazepam, baclofen for acquired PAN and upbeat and downbeat nystagmus, and trihexyphenidyl for the pendular nystagmus of multiple sclerosis, there has been little success. For an extensive review, see Leigh et al. (1994).

NON-NYSTAGMUS OCULAR OSCILLATIONS

Voluntary "Nystagmus"

Voluntary "nystagmus" is not true nystagmus but, rather, ocular flutter under voluntary control. It consists of a series of fast (saccadic) back-to-back eye movements, without any interval or slow phase (Figure 16.17A). The oscillation is usually horizontal but may be vertical, torsional, or, rarely, cycloid (personal observation). The ability to induce flutter voluntarily tends to be familial. Subjects

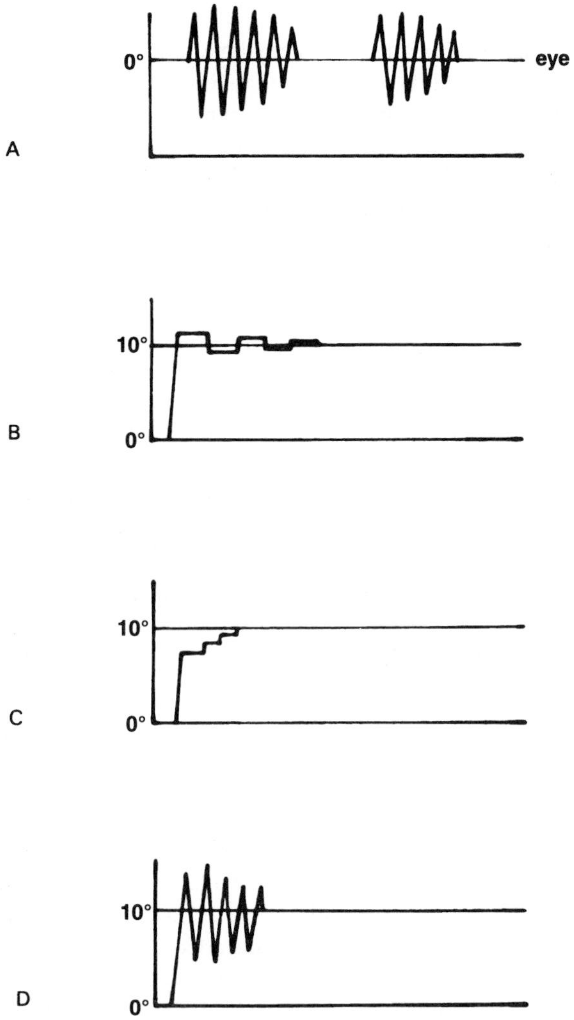

FIGURE 16.17 A. Spontaneous ocular flutter in primary position. B. Overshoot dysmetria (hypermetria). C. Undershoot dysmetria (hypometria). D. Flutter dysmetria exacerbated by refixation from 0–10 degrees.

usually converge to initiate the oscillation but are unable to sustain it for longer than 30 seconds or so. Occasionally, patients use this ability to feign acquired illness, but the phenomenon should be easily recognized.

Ocular Flutter

Ocular flutter (see Figure 16.17A) occurs with brain stem or cerebellar disease and consists of horizontal conjugate back-to-back saccades that occur spontaneously, in intermittent bursts. It is aggravated by attempts at fixation. Occasionally, it is triggered by a change in posture. Flutter is often associated with ocular dysmetria and may progress to opsoclonus.

Table 16.11: Causes of opsoclonus

Encephalitis (viral, pyogenic)
Postencephalitic
AIDS-related brain stem encephalitis or lymphoma
Paraneoplastic
Children: neuroblastoma (ACTH-responsive)
Adults: carcinoma (thiamine-responsive)
Multiple sclerosis
Drugs (amitriptyline, lithium, haloperidol, phencyclidine, thallium, chlordecone, phenytoin-diazepam, toluene, DDT, vidarabine, cocaine)
Hydrocephalus
Thalamic glioma
Thalamic hemorrhage
Pontine hemorrhage
Lipidoses
Hyperosmolar coma
Biotin-responsive multiple carboxylase deficiency
Transient phenomenon in healthy neonates

ACTH = adrenocorticotropic hormone.

Microsaccadic Flutter

Microsaccadic flutter, or microflutter, is a rare symptomatic ocular oscillation requiring magnification for detection (Ashe et al. 1991). Patients complain of episodes of "shimmering" vision. It has been associated with cerebellar degeneration and multiple sclerosis but in some patients may be a variant of voluntary "nystagmus."

Opsoclonus

Opsoclonus is a spontaneous chaotic multivectorial saccadic eye movement disorder that is virtually always conjugate. It is aggravated by attempts at fixation and may be associated with myoclonic jerks of the limbs and cerebellar ataxia (dancing eyes–dancing feet syndrome). It is caused by dysfunction of the pause cells in the pons (see Chapter 42) as a result of cerebellar or brain stem disease. The most frequent causes (Table 16.11) are viral or postviral encephalitis, as well as toxic, metabolic, and paraneoplastic disorders. The paraneoplastic opsoclonus-myoclonus-cerebellar syndrome that is a manifestation of neuroblastoma (7%), found in children, may be responsive to adrenocorticotropic hormone. In adults, opsoclonus may accompany paraneoplastic parenchymal cerebellar degeneration as a result of a remote carcinoma or lymphoma (Dropcho et al. 1993). It may also occur in hyperosmolar states and with many drugs (see Table 16.11).

Ocular Dysmetria

Ocular dysmetria occurs with refixation saccades that cause the eye either to overshoot (see Figure 16.17B) or to undershoot the target (see Figure 16.17C). It results from cerebellar dysfunction (dorsal vermis and fastigial nuclei). Normal subjects may show small-amplitude centrifugal saccadic undershoot dysmetria; this is particularly likely in older and tired patients. Sometimes, overshoot dysmetria is seen with small-amplitude centripetal downward saccades (Leigh and Zee 1991).

Flutter Dysmetria

Flutter dysmetria occurs immediately after the patient refixates on a target; the eye then briefly oscillates across the target for a few cycles (see Figure 16.17D). Both flutter and opsoclonus result from dysfunction of the pause cells in the paramedium pontine reticular formation (PPRF), which tonically suppress the burst cells (see Chapter 42). The pause cells have an input from the cerebellum; thus, cerebellar or brain stem dysfunction may result in flutter or opsoclonus.

Convergence Retraction "Nystagmus"

Convergence retraction "nystagmus" is not a true nystagmus but a rapid dysmetric horizontal eye movement induced by attempted upward saccades. It occurs as part of the dorsal midbrain (Parinaud's) syndrome. Clinically, rapid convergence with synchronous retraction of both globes caused by simultaneous co-contraction of the extraocular muscles, because of disruption of reciprocal inhibition, is followed by a slow divergent movement. Less commonly, if lateral rectus innervation is dominant, a rapid divergent movement occurs initially.

Ocular Bobbing

Ocular bobbing is a rapid downward movement of both eyes followed by a slow drift back to primary position. The oscillation recurs between 2 and 15 times per minute and is found in patients, usually comatose, with severe central pontine destruction and ophthalmoplegia. In *atypical bobbing*, horizontal eye movements are spared.

With *reverse bobbing*, the initial fast phase is upward, followed by a slow downward drift, whereas with *inverse bobbing (dipping)*, the initial deviation is a slow downward movement, followed by a rapid return to primary position. The latter two phenomena occur in patients with severe metabolic or structural damage involving the mesodiencephalic region. *Reverse dipping*, a slow upward movement followed by a fast downward movement, has been described in an obtunded patient with a seizure disorder and chronic meningitis. Bobbing may also be dysconjugate: Gaymard (1993) described an unconscious patient in whom one or the other or both eyes were variably involved.

Ocular Myoclonus

Ocular myoclonus is a vertical pendular oscillation, with a frequency of about 160 Hz, usually associated with similar oscillations of the soft palate and, sometimes, other muscles of the branchial origin as well (Deuschl et al. 1990). The latter condition, referred to as the "oculopalatal syndrome," occurs after brain stem infarction, particularly of the pons, involving the central tegmental tract. It also occurs with spinocerebellar degeneration. Dysfunction of the cerebellar nuclei or their connections (Guillain-Mollaret's triangle) is the most likely explanation for the oculopalatal syndrome, which is confined to the muscles of branchial origin.

Superior Oblique Myokmia

Superior oblique myokmia is a paroxysmal, rapid, small-amplitude monocular torsional-vertical oscillation caused by dysfunction of the superior oblique muscle. Patients may complain of monocular blurring, torsional or vertical oscillopia, torsional or vertical diplopia, or twitching of the eye. Oculography using magnetic search coils (see Chapter 42) has demonstrated both phasic and tonic contractions of intorsion, depression, and to a much lesser extent, abduction of the superior oblique muscle, not true myokymia (Leigh et al. 1991).

Superior oblique myokmia may be difficult to detect with the unaided eye and is more easily detected with a direct ophthalmoscope. It may be precipitated by activating the superior oblique muscle when the patient looks down in the direction of action of that muscle or tilts the head toward the affected eye. Superior oblique myokmia has a relapsing-remitting course in otherwise normal, healthy adults. It has been reported in adrenoleukodystrophy, lead poisoning, and cerebellar astrocytoma (Dehaene and Casselman 1993).

Superior oblique myokymia may respond dramatically to carbamazepine. Propanolol, in low dosage, amitriptyline, baclofen, phenytoin, benzodiazepines, and topical beta-blockers (used for glaucoma) may also be helpful. A base-down prism in front of the affected eye may alleviate the patient's symptoms, avoid potential side effects of long-term medication, and avert the need for surgery, which some advocate when the disorder is prolonged (Brazis et al. 1994). In resistant or protracted cases, the patient requires a superior oblique myotomy or tenotomy.

Saccadic Lateropulsion

See Chapter 42.

Saccadic Oscillations

Saccadic intrusions such as square wave jerks (see Chapter 42) are brief, unwanted, nonrepetitive saccadic interrup-

Table 16.12: Saccadic oscillations (see Chapter 42)

Flutter (voluntary, involuntary)
Flutter dysmetria
Microsaccadic flutter (variant of voluntary flutter?)
Opsoclonus
Macro square wave jerks
Ocular bobbing, reverse and inverse bobbing, dipping, and reverse dipping
Superior oblique myokymia
Convergence-retraction nystagmus
Abduction nystagmus with internuclear ophthalmoplegia
Tic-like ocular myoclonic jerks (eye tics)

tions of fixation (Table 16.12). Saccadic pulses (stepless saccades) interrupt fixation and are followed by a slow drift back on target (glissade). Other saccadic intrusions, including double saccadic pulses (fragment of flutter), dynamic overshoots, and ocular myoclonus (Dell'Osso 1988), are discussed briefly in Chapter 42.

REFERENCES

Abadi RV, Pascal E. Periodic alternating nystagmus in humans with albinism. Invest Ophthalmol Vis Sci 1994;35:4080–4086.

Ashe J, Hain TC, Zee DS, Schatz NJ. Microsaccadic flutter. Brain 1991;114:461–472.

Averbuch-Heller L, Zivotofsky AZ, Remler BF et al. Convergent-divergent nystagmus: possible role of the vergence system. Neurology 1995a;45:509–519.

Averbuch-Heller L, Zivotofsky AZ, Das VE et al. Investigations of the pathogenesis of acquired pendular nystagmus. Brain 1995b;118:369–378.

Barton JJS. Blink- and saccade-induced seesaw nystagmus. Neurology 1995;45:831–833.

Barton JJS, Cox TA. Acquired pendular nystagmus in multiple sclerosis: clinical observations and the role of optic neuropathy. J Neurol Neurosurg Psychiatry 1993;56:262–267.

Barton JS, Huaman AG, Sharpe JA. Muscarinic antagonists in the treatment of acquired pendular and downbeat nystagmus: a double blind, randomized trial of three intravenous drugs. Ann Neurol 1994;35:319–325.

Brazis PW, Miller NR, Henderer JD, Lee AG. The natural history and results of treatment of superior oblique myokymia. Arch Ophthalmol 1994;112:1063–1067.

Bronstein AM, Gresty MA, Mossman SS. Pendular pseudonystagmus arising as a combination of head tremor and vestibular failure. Neurology 1992;42:1527–1531.

Dehaene I, Casselman J. Left superior oblique myokymia and the right superior oblique paralysis due to a posterior fossa tumor. Neuro-ophthalmol 1993;13(1):13–16.

Dell'Osso LF. Nystagmus and Other Ocular Motor Oscillations and Intrusions. In S Lessells, JTW Van Dalen (eds), Current Neuro–Ophthalmology. Vol. 1. Chicago: Year-Book, 1988; 139–172.

Dell'Osso LF, Daroff RB, Troost BT. Nystagmus and Saccadic Intrusions and Oscillations. In TD Duane, EA Jaeger (eds), Clinical Ophthalmology. Vol. 2. New York: Harper & Row, 1990.

Dell'Osso LF, Leigh RJ. Ocular motor stability of foveation periods: required conditions for suppression of oscillopsia. Neuro-ophthalmol 1992;12:303–326.

Deuschl G, Mischke G, Schenck E et al. Symptomatic and essential rhythmic palateal myoclonus. Brain 1990;113:1645–1672.

Dropcho EJ, Kline LB, Riser J. Antineuronal (anti-Ri) antibodies in a patient with steroid-responsive opsoclonus-myoclonus. Neurology 1993;43:207–211.

Gaymard D. Disconjugate ocular bobbing. Neurology 1993; 43:2151.

Good WV, Brodsky MC, Hoyt CS, Ahn JC. Upbeating nystagmus in infants: a sign of anterior pathway disease. Binocular Vis Q 1990;5:13–18.

Grant MP, Cohen M, Petersen RB et al. Abnormal eye movements in Creutzfeldt-Jakob disease. Ann Neurol 1993;34:192–197.

Gresty MA, Metcalfe T, Timms C et al. Neurology of latent nystagmus. Brain 1992;115:1303–1321.

Halmagyi GM. Central Eye Movement Disorders. In DM Albert, FA Jakobiec (eds), Principles and Practice of Ophthalmology. Philadelphia: Saunders, 1994;2411–2444.

Halmagyi GM, Aw ST, Dahaene I et al. Jerk-waveform see-saw nystagmus due to unilateral meso-diencephalic lesion. Brain 1994;117:789–803.

Knox DL, Green WR, Troncosco JC et al. Cerebral ocular Whipple's disease. Neurology 1995;45:617–625.

Kommerell G, Zee DS. Latent nystagmus: release and suppression at will. Invest Ophthalmol Vis Sci 1993;34:1785–1792.

Lambert SR, Newman NJ. Retinal disease masquerading as spasmus nutans. Neurology 1993;43:1607–1609.

Leigh RJ, Averbuch-Heller L, Tomsak RL et al. Treatment of abnormal eye movements that impair vision: strategies based on current concepts of physiology and pharmacology. Ann Neurol 1994;36:129–141.

Leigh RJ, Tomsak RL, Seidman SH, Dell'Osso LF. Superior oblique myokymia: quantitative characteristics of eye movements in three patients. Arch Ophthalmol 1991;109:1710–1713.

Leigh RJ, Zee DS. The Neurology of Eye Movements. Philadelphia: FA Davis, 1991;79–114.

Lopez L, Bronctein AM, Gresty MA et al. Torsional nystagmus: a neuro-otological and MRI study of thirty-five cases. Brain 1992;115:1107–1124.

Purvin VA. Visual disturbance secondary to clomiphene citrate. Arch Ophthalmol 1995;113:482–484.

Schmidt D. Downbeat nystagmus: a review. Neuro-ophthalmol 1991;11:247–262.

Trobe JD, Sharpe JA, Hirsh DK, Gebarski SS. Nystagmus of Pelizaeus-Merzbacher disease: a magnetic search coil study. Arch Neurol 1991;48:87–91.

Tusa RJ, Kaplan PW, Hain TC, Naidu S. Ipsiversive eye deviation and epileptic nystagmus. Neurology 1990;40:662–665.

Waltz KL, Lavin PJM. Accommodative Insufficiency. In CE Margo, RN Mames, L Hamed (eds), Diagnostic Problems in Clinical Ophthalmology. Philadelphia: Saunders, 1993;862–866.

Wertenbaker C. Superior oblique myokymia. J Neuro-ophthalmol 1994;14(3)188.

Wright KW, Edelman PM, McVey JH et al. High-grade stereo acuity after early surgery for congenital esotropia. Arch Ophthalmol 1994;112:913–919.

SUGGESTED READING

Burde RM, Savino PJ, Trobe JD (eds). Clinical Decisions in Neuro-Ophthalmology (2nd ed). St. Louis: Mosby, 1992.
Fenichel GM. Clinical Pediatric Neurology: A Symptoms and Signs Approach (2nd ed). Philadelphia: Saunders, 1993.
Glaser JS. Neuro-Ophthalmology. In TD Duane, EA Jager (eds), Clinical Ophthalmology (2nd ed). Vol. 2. New York: Harper & Row, 1990.
Miller NR. Walsh and Hoyt's Clinical Neuro-Ophthalmology (4th ed). Vol. 2. Baltimore: Williams & Wilkins, 1985.
Van Noorden GK. Atlas of Strabismus (4th ed). St. Louis: Mosby, 1983.

Chapter 17
Pupillary and Eyelid Abnormalities

Terry A. Cox and Robert B. Daroff

ABNORMALITIES OF THE PUPILS

Clinical Presentation

The medical history of a patient rarely begins with the statement "I have unequal pupils." In fact, most patients with *anisocoria* (unequal pupils) first hear of it from their doctor, friend, or relative. Those who notice anisocoria themselves may confuse the diagnostician by giving a misleading account of the duration of the condition. Occasionally a patient has visual dysfunction caused solely by abnormal pupillary size. Photophobia and slow dark adaptation occur when a fixed, dilated pupil fails to protect the retina from increased illumination. Less often, a complaint of poor night vision (or dim daytime vision) may arise in patients with small, poorly reactive pupils; this symptom is caused by failure of the pupils to dilate normally, which decreases the light-gathering power of the eye in conditions of dim illumination.

Because pupillary disorders usually present as an abnormality on physical examination rather than a visual complaint, the following discussion is based on the different ways that abnormal pupils can be described by the clinician. Terms used include *anisocoria, poorly reactive pupils, light-near dissociation, pupillary irregularity,* and *hippus* (pupillary unrest); many pupillary disorders can be included in several of these categories. In her two-volume text, Loewenfeld (1993) provides detailed discussions of all aspects of every pupillary abnormality.

Anisocoria

Many unilateral and bilateral disorders affecting the iris or its innervation present as anisocoria, but there are only a few categories to consider in evaluating this sign: local disease of the eye, parasympathetic defects (affecting the third nerve or pupillary sphincter), sympathetic defects (affecting the iris dilator muscle or its innervation), and simple anisocoria (Slamovits and Glaser 1990).

A number of conditions affecting the iris can cause unequal pupils. Blunt trauma to the eye can damage the pupillary sphincter, causing mydriasis with poor pupillary constriction to both light and near stimuli. Immediately after injury, the pupil may be smaller than normal, but after a few minutes the pupil becomes dilated and poorly reactive. This course of events may simulate uncal herniation.

Syphilis causes a number of pupillary disorders, the best known being Argyll-Robertson pupils. A more common pupillary finding in syphilis, however, is anisocoria caused by degeneration of iris stroma.

Acute inflammatory disease of the eye (iritis) can cause mild pupillary constriction. If inflammation persists, adhesions between the iris and the anterior lens capsule may form, leading to pupillary irregularity and immobility. Usually the inflamed eye is red and the patient has a great deal of photophobia. However, some chronic forms of iritis (such as sarcoid) can cause iris adhesions without these symptoms.

Ischemia of the iris can cause mydriasis and poor pupillary reactivity. Two situations in which ischemia occurs are acute angle closure glaucoma and the ocular ischemic syndrome; in both disorders associated symptoms include poor vision and pain.

Some rare iris degenerations cause pupillary dilation, often with irregularity of the pupillary outline. These conditions include essential iris atrophy and Fuchs's heterochromic iridocyclitis.

Causes of parasympathetic defects include oculomotor (third) nerve palsy, tonic pupils, and pharmacological mydriasis. The pupil on the involved side is generally larger, but some long-standing tonic pupils are actually smaller than normal, though still poorly reactive. Third nerve palsies are discussed in Chapter 75. Usually pupillary involvement in third nerve palsies is accompanied by paresis of other extraocular muscles; isolated pupillary dilation occurs most commonly in the setting of early uncal herniation (Ropper 1990). Tonic pupils are caused most often by the Holmes-Adie syndrome (tonic pupils and diminished deep tendon reflexes) (Slamovits and Glaser 1990). Other causes include orbital trauma, herpes zoster ophthalmicus, syphilis, temporal arteritis, and various peripheral neuropathies.

Pharmacological mydriasis usually occurs after accidental or intentional instillation of atropinic agents. Accidental mydriasis usually occurs by hand-eye contact in individuals who have contact with atropinic agents; examples include use of a scopolamine skin patch for motion sickness and administration of eye drops to a family member with eye disease. Pharmacologically dilated pupils tend to be larger than the dilated pupil of third nerve palsy. Sympathomimetic agents such as phenylephrine cause mydriasis that is less extensive and prolonged than that caused by parasympathomimetics.

Sympathetic denervation causes pupillary miosis and ipsilateral ptosis (Horner's syndrome).

Simple (physiological, essential) anisocoria occurs in about 20% of the normal population. Usually, the difference in pupil size is small—rarely more than 0.6 mm. The amount of anisocoria may differ in a given individual at different times. Pharmacological testing (Thompson and Kardon 1991) or pupillography may be necessary to confirm the diagnosis.

Episodic Anisocoria

Anisocoria may be intermittent. As noted previously, simple anisocoria can vary from week to week and, occasionally, from hour to hour. Migraine headaches can cause unilateral mydriasis that may persist for several hours (Loewenfeld 1993). A rare condition known as "tadpole pupils" results from intermittent spasms of segments of the pupillary dilator muscle; often, these patients have an underlying Horner's syndrome. A related phenomenon is oculosympathetic spasm associated with lesions of the cervical spinal cord.

Cyclic oculomotor palsy is a rare condition in which periodic oculomotor spasms occur in a patient with a third nerve palsy. During the spasms, the eyelid rises, the exotropic eye moves to the midline, and the pupil constricts. In some cases, the spasms are limited to the pupil. Intermittent spasm of portions of the pupillary sphincter may occur in traumatic third nerve paralysis and with aberrant oculomotor regeneration. Unilateral pupillary dilation and other pupillary signs can occur during seizures (Rosenberg and Jabbari 1991).

Poorly Reactive Pupils Without Anisocoria

Large pupils that are poorly reactive but roughly equal in diameter can occur with hypothalamic (North et al. 1994) and midbrain lesions, syphilis, botulism, the Miller-Fisher variant of the Guillain-Barré syndrome, and autonomic neuropathy. Toxic and pharmacological causes should also be considered. Occasionally, bilateral mydriasis can be congenital. Anxious young adults and teenagers often have large, poorly reactive pupils.

Small, poorly reactive pupils, often combined with simple anisocoria, are common in the aging individual (sometimes prematurely so). Other acquired causes of this finding include syphilis, diabetes, and long-standing Holmes-Adie pupils. Glaucoma patients using drops containing pilocarpine have small pupils that do not react to light or near stimuli. Congenital miosis can be caused by Marfan's syndrome or congenital rubella infection, but this finding also occurs with no other physical abnormalities.

Light-Near Dissociation

The term *light-near dissociation* refers to pupils that have marked diminution of constriction to light, with a much better constriction to near stimuli. When the pupils are large, the differential diagnosis includes syphilis, tonic pupils, pretectal lesions, and bilateral afferent pupillary defects (for example, from bilateral optic atrophy). Small pupils with light-near dissociation can occur in patients with syphilis (Argyll-Robertson pupils), long-standing Holmes-Adie pupils, and diabetic neuropathy. In some patients with aberrant regeneration of the oculomotor nerve, the pupil constricts poorly to light and much better with eye movements such as adduction; this disorder could be mistaken for true light-near dissociation.

Irregular Pupils

Irregular pupils are usually caused by local iris disease. Conditions mentioned earlier that cause pupillary irregularity include syphilis, ischemia, posterior synechiae (adhesions of iris to lens), traumatic iridoplegia, degenerative disease of the iris, and Holmes-Adie syndrome. Infiltration of the iris by tumor or amyloid can also cause irregular pupils. Oval or eccentric pupils (corectopia) may occur with midbrain disease and increased intracranial pressure.

Hippus (Pupillary Unrest)

In most individuals with reactive pupils, shining a light in the eyes elicits spontaneous conjugate oscillations in pupillary diameter. These movements are probably a result of changes in retinal illumination induced by pupillary movements (the pupil constricts, causing the light to appear dimmer; then the pupil dilates, causing the light to appear brighter; then the pupil constricts, and so on), but oscillation in midbrain activity may play a role. Changes in the level of central nervous system (CNS) alertness also cause the pupil to change size; somnolent individuals have large-amplitude, low-frequency oscillations in pupillary diameter just before they fall asleep.

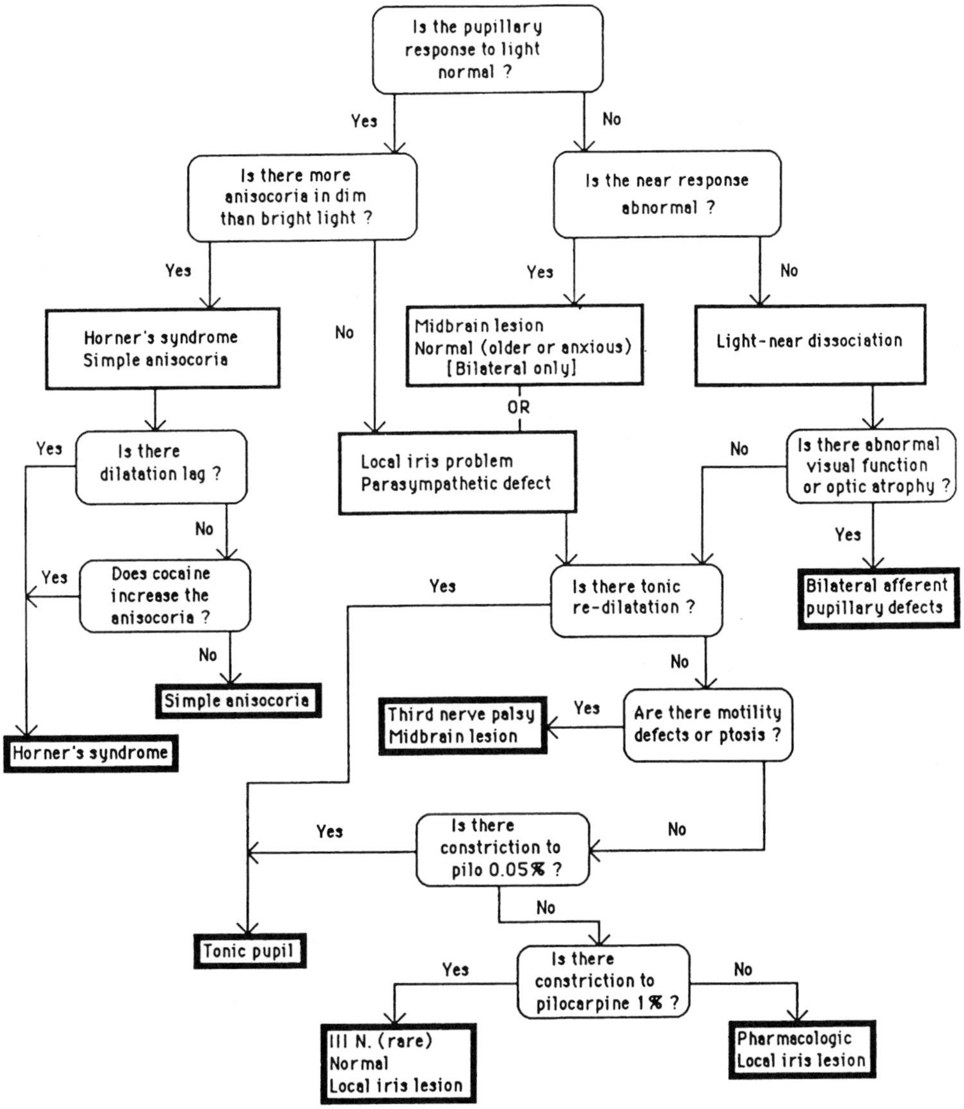

FIGURE 17.1 Flowchart for evaluation of anisocoria.

Examination

Figure 17.1 provides a systematic approach to the evaluation of the patient with anisocoria. First, the pupillary response to light should be checked. If both pupils constrict reasonably well when a light is shone in the eye, the next step is to assess pupillary diameter in both bright and dim light. Absence of anisocoria would be expected in normal individuals. If anisocoria is greater in bright light, the iris sphincter on the side of the larger pupil does not work well. The differential diagnosis would then include third nerve palsy, traumatic iridoplegia, and so forth. If the anisocoria is greater in dim light, the iris dilator muscle on the side of the smaller pupil works poorly, and both Horner's syndrome and simple anisocoria should be considered.

If the pupillary response to light is poor, the response to near should be assessed. Pupillary constriction to near effort that is much better than constriction to light indicates light-near dissociation. Poor constriction to both light and near usually implies a local iris problem, parasympathetic defects, or midbrain disease; however, both aging and anxiety should be considered.

If Horner's syndrome is a consideration, the pupils should be examined for dilatation lag. The smaller pupil of Horner's syndrome dilates more slowly in darkness than does the normal pupil. Therefore, anisocoria is maximal in these patients 3–5 seconds after the lights are turned off, as compared to anisocoria 15 seconds later (Figure 17.2). This sign is often difficult to elicit, particularly in brown-eyed individuals, because a certain amount of illumination of the pupils is necessary for the examiner to see. If there is any question about this finding, pharmacological testing should be done (Slamovits and Glaser 1990; Thompson and Kardon 1991).

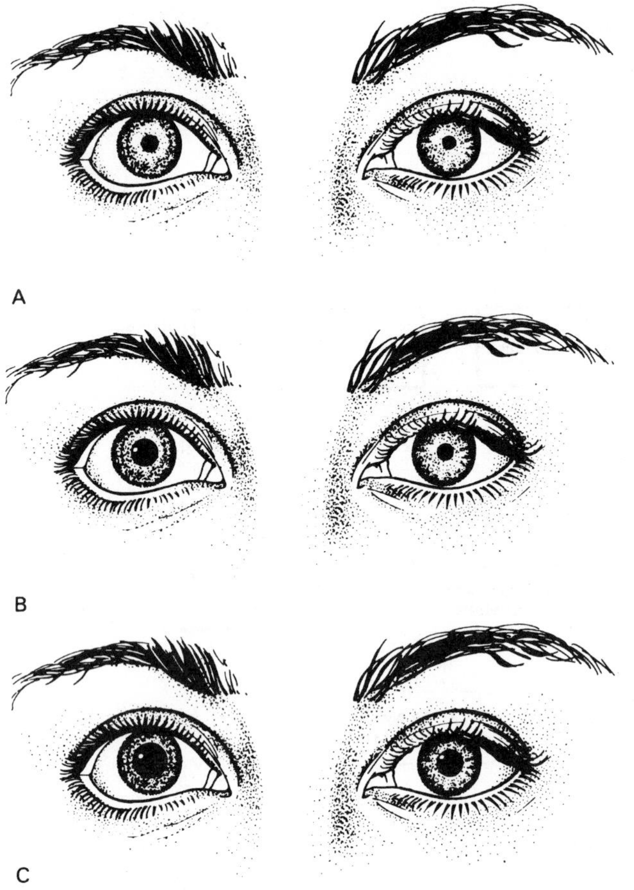

FIGURE 17.2 Horner's syndrome, left eye. A. Room light. Mild upper lid ptosis and lower lid elevation, simulating enophthalmos. B. Five seconds after lights off. Anisocoria increases. C. Fifteen seconds after lights off. Dilation lag manifested by more anisocoria in B than in C.

Any pupil with a parasympathetic defect should be assessed for tonic redilation, a sign that establishes the diagnosis of tonic pupil. If a patient with a large, unilateral tonic pupil has tonic redilation, the defective pupil can actually be transiently smaller than normal after near effort (Figure 17.3).

After initial categorization of the pupil defect, the examination proceeds with evaluation of visual function, eyelid position, ocular motility, and the ocular fundus.

Light-near dissociation that is caused by visual sensory deficits can be diagnosed by testing visual acuity and visual fields (confrontation techniques are adequate) and looking for optic atrophy or other fundus abnormalities.

As noted previously, both acute glaucoma and the ocular ischemic syndrome cause poor vision. Signs of acute glaucoma include corneal edema, ocular injection, and a pupil that is mid-dilated and unreactive. The ocular ischemia syndrome arises in patients with marked stenosis of an internal carotid artery, or narrowing of both internal and external carotid arteries on one side; associated eye findings include retinal neovascularization, rubeosis iridis, mild iritis, ocular hypotony, and corneal edema. Rubeosis iridis appears as a fine vascular network on the surface of the iris; its causes include diabetes, retinal vein occlusion, and other conditions associated with prolonged ocular ischemia.

Unilateral loss of accommodation often occurs in patients with parasympathetic denervation or pharmacological mydriasis; an eye with poor accommodation will have near vision that is greatly reduced in comparison to distance vision.

Patients with Horner's syndrome have ipsilateral ptosis, but this finding is not completely reliable in the diagnosis. The combined prevalence of simple anisocoria and mechanical ptosis (congenital or senile) is such that a small pupil and ptosis do not always imply sympathetic denervation.

Generally, a third nerve palsy can be diagnosed by associated findings of ptosis and limited ocular motility. Pretectal and other midbrain diseases that affect pupillary pathways cause abnormalities of ocular motility such as upgaze palsy and convergence-retraction nystagmus. Irregular pupils caused by midbrain disease can be diagnosed by the associated neurological findings. Local causes of irregular pupils cannot usually be distinguished without further investigation.

Assessment of deep tendon reflexes helps establish the diagnosis of Holmes-Adie syndrome, and examination of the neck, brachial plexus function, and sweating pattern helps to localize the lesion in Horner's syndrome.

Investigations

Further evaluation of pupillary abnormalities begins with examination using the slit-lamp biomicroscope. The Holmes-Adie pupil usually has segmental constriction to light. Similar segmental constrictions can be seen with eye movements in some patients with aberrant oculomotor regeneration. Eyes with traumatic iridoplegia often have tears at the pupillary margin. Iris transillumination defects are usually seen in eyes with the small pupils of congenital rubella or Marfan's syndrome, as well as in eyes affected by syphilis. Posterior synechiae can be seen easily with the slit lamp. Ischemic eyes usually have rubeosis of the iris. Neurologists without access to a slit lamp can diagnose tonic pupils by using dilute pilocarpine as described below.

Instillation of various drugs is often necessary to establish the cause of anisocoria (Thompson and Kardon 1991; Loewenfeld 1993). Cocaine acts by blocking reuptake of norepinephrine; in a 4–10% solution, cocaine dilates the normal pupil of simple anisocoria but not the sympathetically denervated pupil of Horner's syndrome. Hydroxyamphetamine 1% (no longer marketed in the United States but obtainable from Park Avenue Pharmacy, 1756 Park Avenue, San Jose, CA 95126) acts by releasing norepinephrine from the presynaptic terminal and can be used for pharmacological localization of Horner's syndrome. When the lesion causing sympathetic denervation affects the postsynaptic pathway originating in the superior cervical ganglion, the nerve terminal degenerates, and norepinephrine is not avail-

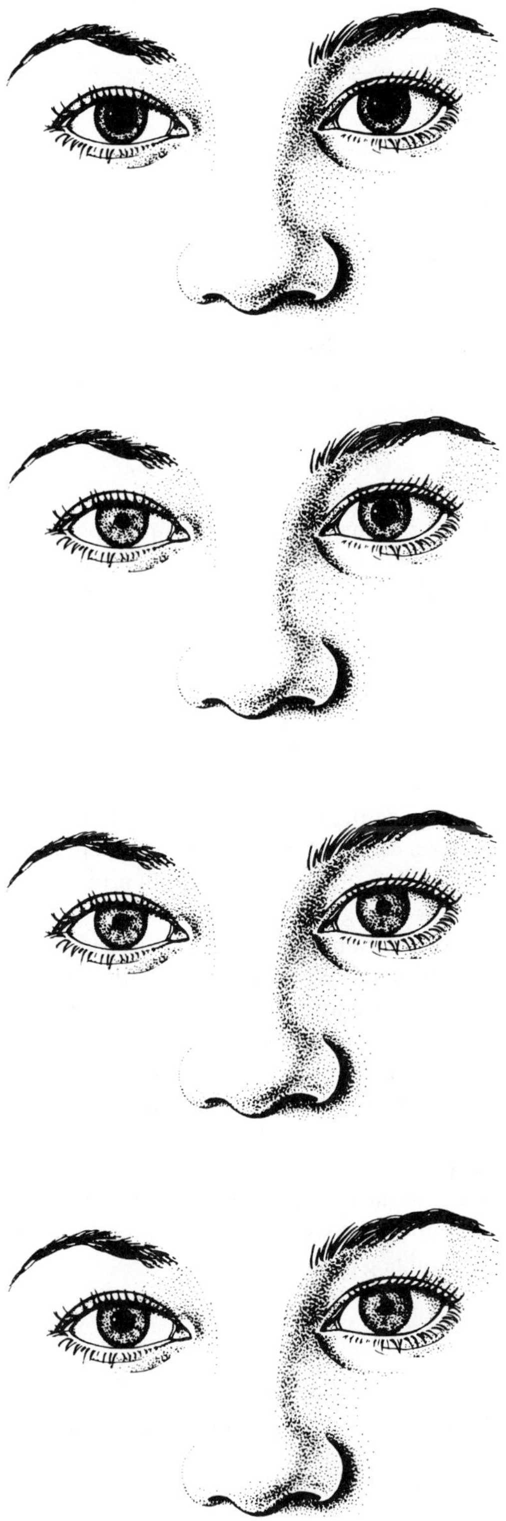

FIGURE 17.3 Tonic pupil, left eye. A. Darkness. Anisocoria is minimal. B. Bright light. C. Near, showing light-near dissociation. D. A few seconds after return of gaze to a distant target. Tonicity of redilation on the affected side has caused transient reversal of anisocoria.

able for release. Proximal lesions leave this neuron intact. Therefore, hydroxyamphetamine dilates normal pupils and those with preganglionic lesions, but not those with postganglionic sympathetic lesions.

Pilocarpine in a 0.05% solution is too dilute to cause pupillary constriction except in eyes with tonic pupils. Pilocarpine in a 1% solution causes marked pupillary constriction in normal individuals and in those with third nerve palsies, but not in pharmacological mydriasis. Eyes with local iris disease may or may not constrict in response to pilocarpine in a 1% solution, depending on the severity of involvement of the pupillary sphincter. Pilocarpine in a 0.05% solution is not commercially available and must be prepared by the clinician or pharmacist from stronger solutions, diluted with normal saline.

Examining old photographs (preferably with a magnifying glass) can help establish the length of time that a pupillary abnormality has been present. Horner's syndrome that has been present for 10 years has a better prognosis than Horner's syndrome that began in the past month, regardless of the localization. Old photographs may also help in establishing the diagnosis of episodic anisocoria.

Laboratory studies for tertiary syphilis (the fluorescent treponemal antibody absorption test, or the microhemagglutination assay for *Treponema pallidium*) should be done in any patient with bilateral tonic pupils, poorly reactive or irregular pupils, or pupils with light-near dissociation, if the cause remains uncertain after the foregoing evaluation. Because of the high frequency of false-negatives, the serum Venereal Disease Research Laboratories (VDRL) test should not be used for detecting tertiary disease in these cases.

Almost all stable pupillary conditions will have been diagnosed at this point. Further workup will depend on the specific diagnosis. Preganglionic Horner's syndrome may require a chest radiograph, computed tomography (CT) of the brachial plexus, or magnetic resonance imaging (MRI) of the head and cervical spine, depending on associated findings. Postganglionic Horner's syndrome of recent onset may require investigation for carotid dissection (Digre et al. 1992). Episodic conditions may not be well characterized after the initial exam. In these cases, repeat office evaluations or having the patient take pupil photos at home will be necessary.

ABNORMALITIES OF THE EYELIDS

Clinical Presentation

Lid abnormalities present as ptosis, lid retraction, insufficient eyelid closure, or excessive lid closure. Ptosis causes symptoms when the lid or lashes intrude on the visual axis; more often, the drooping lid is perceived as a cosmetic defect. Lid retraction usually causes no symptoms. Insufficient lid closure may result in exposure keratitis, causing the patient to complain of eye pain and blurred vision. Ble-

Table 17.1: Lid abnormalities associated with cerebral hemisphere lesions

Lid Abnormality	*Pathological Findings*
Unilateral ptosis	Contralateral hemisphere lesions; contralateral and ipsilateral hemisphere lesions
Bilateral ptosis	Bilateral frontal lobe lesions; unilateral and bilateral hemisphere lesions
Impairment of voluntary lid opening and closure	Dominant hemisphere or bilateral hemisphere lesions or basal ganglia disease
Impairment of voluntary and reflex lid opening (apraxia of lid opening)	Basal ganglia disease; bilateral hemisphere lesions; nondominant cerebral lesion
Difficulty maintaining lid closure (motor impersistence)	Nondominant hemisphere or bilateral hemisphere lesions
Difficulty maintaining lid opening (reflex blepharospasm)	Nondominant hemisphere or bilateral hemisphere lesions

Source: Modified from JG Nutt. Lid abnormality secondary to cerebral hemisphere lesions. Ann Neurol 1977;1:149–151; and JC Johnston, DM Rosenbaum, CM Picone, JC Grotta. Apraxia of eyelid opening secondary to right hemisphere infarction. Ann Neurol 1989;25:622–624.

pharospasm or inappropriate levator inhibition (apraxia of lid opening) may cause a functional disability equivalent to severe bilateral visual loss.

Ptosis

Congenital ptosis can be caused by abnormalities of the levator muscle or its innervation and can be either unilateral or bilateral (Siboney 1991). Muscular abnormalities include congenital maldevelopment and neonatal myasthenia. Congenital abnormalities of innervation (Glaser and Bachynski 1990) include trigeminal-levator synkinesis (the Marcus-Gunn jaw-winking phenomenon), Duane's syndrome, third nerve palsies, and Horner's syndrome. Trigeminal-levator synkinesis causes unilateral ptosis that varies in degree with movements of the jaw. This congenital condition can usually be diagnosed soon after birth; the affected infant has a drooping upper eyelid that twitches upward during bottle feeding or nursing. In older individuals, lid movements occur with opening the mouth, moving the jaw from side to side, or clenching the teeth. Duane's syndrome consists of paresis of abduction, adduction, or both, associated with globe retraction and ptosis on attempted adduction. In eyes affected by this congenital condition, the third nerve innervates the lateral rectus muscle, and the abducens nerve is absent.

One common cause of acquired ptosis is local disease of the eyelid, such as dehiscence of the levator aponeurosis (Siboney 1991). This condition occurs most often as an aging change (senile ptosis), but trauma can also be responsible. One traumatic cause to keep in mind is lid manipulation associated with contact lens wear. Ptosis can also occur when a lost contact lens becomes embedded in the conjunctiva of the upper lid. Other local lid diseases causing ptosis include inflammatory conditions such as chalazion or giant papillary conjunctivitis and infiltrative conditions such as amyloidosis or lymphoma.

Myopathic causes of acquired ptosis include myasthenia, botulism, myotonic dystrophy, and chronic progressive external ophthalmoplegia. In these cases, the associated systemic and ocular findings usually help the physician make the diagnosis. However, myasthenia is a frequent cause of acquired, isolated, painless, monocular ptosis.

Neuropathic causes of ptosis include Horner's syndrome, oculomotor paresis, Guillain-Barré syndrome, midbrain lesions, and facial paresis. Ptosis and a number of other eyelid abnormalities can be caused by diseases affecting the cerebral hemispheres (Table 17.1).

Pseudoptosis can be caused by blepharospasm, apraxia of lid opening, dermatochalasis, or contralateral lid retraction. The term *dermatochalasis* refers to redundancy of the skin of the eyelids, often associated with prolapse of orbital fat; treatment is surgical (blepharoplasty).

Lower lid elevation may accompany upper-lid ptosis. Elevation of the lower lid occurs in enophthalmos from, for example, orbital blowout fractures. The lower lid contains sympathetically innervated smooth muscle, and in Horner's syndrome this muscle is paretic, causing lid elevation that mimics enophthalmos. Other causes of lower-lid elevation are local edema, excessive lid closure (discussed below), and factitious ptosis.

Voluntary mimicking of ptosis by contraction of the orbicularis oculi causes lowering of the eyebrows and elevation and wrinkling of the lower lids.

Lid Retraction

Although an elevated upper eyelid may be a normal variant, lid retraction is most commonly caused by hyperthyroidism or Graves' ophthalmopathy. A number of other causes have been described (reviewed in Glaser 1990); the more common entities are discussed here.

In patients with thyroid disease, upper (and often lower) lid retraction may be present when the patient looks either straight ahead or down, and lid lag can be elicited by having the eyes pursue a target moving down (von Graefe's sign). Normally, the upper lid stays at the upper corneal limbus as the eyes move down; any visible sclera between lid and limbus during this movement is evidence of lid lag.

Patients with unilateral ptosis from, for instance, myasthenia may have lid retraction on the opposite side. When the ptotic lid is raised manually, the retracted lid falls (Lepore 1988). Generally these patients have contraction of forehead muscles as well. Patients with aberrant regeneration of the third nerve often have retraction of the eyelid with depression or adduction of the eye (pseudo–von Graefe's sign). In patients with trigeminal-levator synkinesis, the affected lid may elevate with jaw movements so that the palpebral fissure is transiently wider than normal. Upper lid retraction occasionally occurs as part of Parinaud's dorsal midbrain syndrome (Collier's sign) (Galetta et al. 1993). Usually there are also difficulties with conjugate upgaze, and lid retraction does not occur on looking down. Upper lid retraction has also been reported in hepatic disease (Summerskill's sign) and Guillain-Barré syndrome (Sibony 1991). In Horner's syndrome, the smooth muscle of the upper lid often develops denervation supersensitivity. In stressful situations, circulating catecholamines can cause transient lid retraction on the affected side. Failure of levator inhibition (spastic eyelids) may occur with brain stem disease; in these patients, the eyes may remain open during sleep.

Lower lid retraction may be congenital, but more often it is a sign of proptosis. Lower lid retraction can also be caused by conditions that contract or displace the lid, including lower lid tumor or chalazion, trauma with scarring, and aging (senile ectropion). The lower lid may appear to be retracted in three different situations: (1) when the contralateral lower lid is elevated (as in Horner's syndrome); (2) when the globe is elevated in conditions that cause hypertropia, such as fourth nerve palsy; and (3) when the lower lid is weak from myasthenia or seventh nerve palsy.

Insufficient Lid Closure

Poor eyelid closure does not usually pose a diagnostic dilemma, but this lid malfunction can cause serious ocular damage. Failure of the lids to cover the cornea during sleep, blinks, or forced eyelid closure results in exposure keratitis—corneal epithelial defects, eye pain, and conjunctival injection—with the risk of corneal ulceration or scarring.

Insufficient closure of the eye can result from marked proptosis, but the more usual cause is weakness of the orbicularis oculi muscle. Such weakness can be caused by myasthenia, chronic progressive external ophthalmoplegia, myotonic dystrophy, or seventh nerve palsy.

Another cause of insufficient lid closure with the threat of corneal damage is a reduced rate of blinking. This sign occurs frequently in patients with Parkinson's disease or progressive supranuclear palsy. In these disorders, blinks tend to be incomplete as well. Most normal blinks result in complete coverage of the cornea by the upper lid; incomplete or partial blinks cover only the superior cornea. Blinks in some normal individuals tend to be incomplete; these individuals are generally asymptomatic unless they try to wear contact lenses.

Table 17.2: Types of excessive eyelid closure

Blepharospasm
Apraxia of lid opening
Hemifacial spasm
Myokymia
Myotonia

Excessive Lid Closure (Table 17.2)

Blepharospasm consists of uncontrolled bilateral contraction of the orbicularis oculi causing eyelid closure (Figure 17.4). Ocular causes of photophobia and blepharospasm include conjunctival disorders (dry eyes), corneal disease (abrasion, keratitis), uveitis, pupillary dilation (for instance, after an eye examination), cataract, and meningitis. When there are no associated ocular or neurological abnormalities, the diagnosis is *benign essential blepharospasm.* When there are dystonic movements of the lower face, jaw, tongue, or neck, the designation is blepharospasm-oromandibular dystonia (Meige's syndrome) (Sibony 1991). In Parkinson's disease or other disorders of the basal ganglia, the condition is called *central blepharospasm.* When orbicularis contraction occurs only with lid manipulation or other stimulation, the term *reflex blepharospasm* is sometimes used; this finding has been reported in patients with lesions of the cerebral hemispheres and in one family with no other neurological disorder. Most patients with parkinsonism have reflex blepharospasm, and all types of blepharospasm are made worse by lid manipulation or conditions causing photophobia. Factitious (voluntary) blepharospasm is rare.

The term *apraxia of lid opening* (Johnston et al. 1989) is used to describe inappropriate inhibition of the levator palpebrae muscle that occurs in some patients with CNS disorders or bilateral or nondominant cerebral lesions or in association with benign essential blepharospasm. Rare patients have an isolated levodopa-responsive syndrome (Dewey and Maraganore 1994). *Hemifacial spasm* (Sibony 1991) is characterized by paroxysmal, involuntary, synchronous contraction of all muscles innervated by the

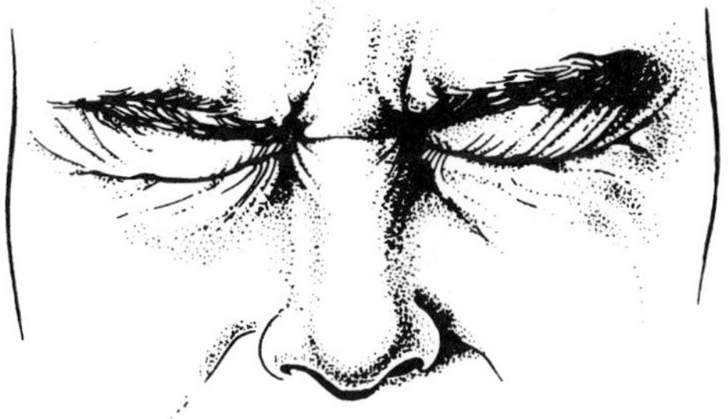

FIGURE 17.4 Blepharospasm. Bilateral contraction of the orbicularis oculi.

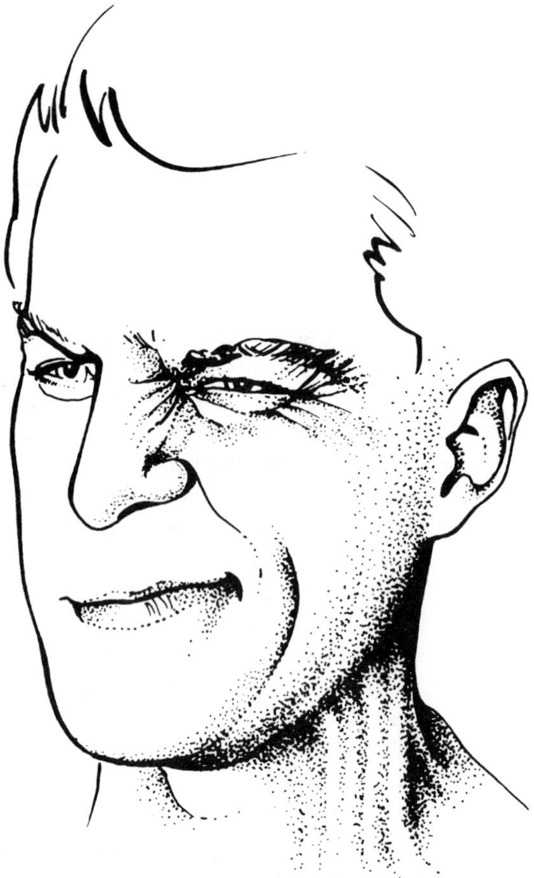

FIGURE 17.5 Hemifacial spasm. Synchronous contraction of muscles innervated by the left facial nerve, including platysma. Often, the orbicularis oculi muscles are involved as illustrated, but with less obvious contraction of other facial muscles.

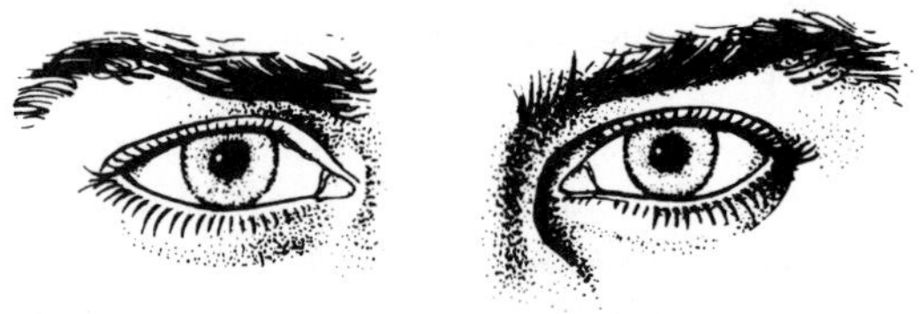

FIGURE 17.6 Normal eyelid position. The upper lid covers the upper 1–2 mm of the cornea. The lower lid just touches the lower limbus.

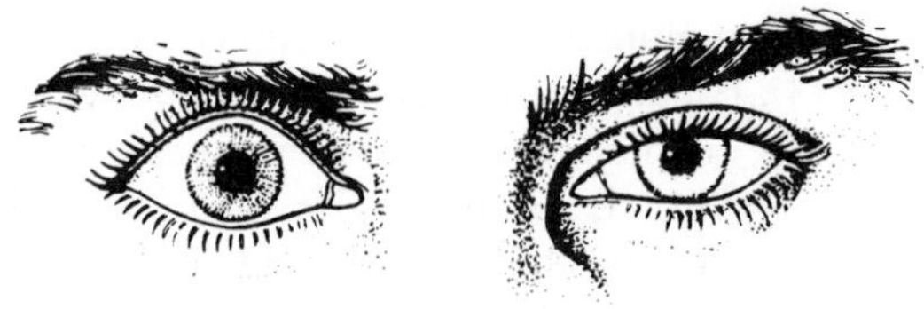

FIGURE 17.7 Lid retraction of the right eye and ptosis of the left upper lid.

facial nerve on one side (Figure 17.5) (see Chapter 75). Occasionally, the condition is bilateral; in these cases the paroxysms on each side are asynchronous.

Involuntary twitches of portions of the orbicularis muscle (orbicularis myokymia) are common in normal individuals. These fasciculations generally affect the lower eyelid; some patients describe oscillopsia when the twitches are strong enough to move the globe. In facial myokymia, these muscular contractions involve other facial muscles. Occasionally, facial myokymia is associated with spastic paretic facial contracture, a condition characterized by tonic contraction of facial muscles on one side with associated weakness of the same muscles. Facial myokymia may be unilateral or bilateral. This sign indicates brain stem disease; the most common causes are multiple sclerosis and brain stem neoplasm (usually gliomas). However, other disorders, including Guillain-Barré syndrome and extra-axial neoplasms, have been implicated (May and Galetta 1990).

Myotonia of lid closure may occur in myotonic dystrophy. Other conditions reported to cause myotonia include hypothyroidism and hyperkalemic familial periodic paralysis.

Table 17.3: Clinical examination of the eyelids

Observe for at least 1 minute
Look for proptosis and enophthalmos
Assess lid position in different gaze directions
Observe gentle and forced lid closure
Examine for pupillary and ocular motor abnormalities

Examination

The steps in the examination of the eyelids are summarized in Table 17.3. First, the eyelids and face should be observed and inspected and the blink rate measured. The upper eyelid normally covers the upper 1 or 2 mm of the cornea (Figure 17.6). The upper border of the lower lid normally just touches the lower border of the cornea. In an eye with mild upper lid retraction (Figure 17.7), the lid just touches the upper limbus of the cornea, or there is visible sclera between the cornea and the upper lid margin (superior scleral show); with lower lid retraction, there is visible sclera between the cornea and the lower lid margin (inferior scleral show). Patients with factitious (voluntary) ptosis have some contraction of both upper and lower lid orbicularis; the contraction of the lower orbicularis raises the eyelid and wrinkles the skin near the lid margin. Patients with bilateral ptosis often have associated frontalis contraction that elevates the eyebrows. In unilateral ptosis, the ptotic lid should be raised manually to determine if ptosis develops on the opposite side. Inspection of the lids is important to detect scarring or swelling caused by trauma, tumor, or inflammation. Lid changes from these causes are usually not difficult to detect. Normally, the blink rate during conversation is at least 18 per minute. Patients with parkinsonism and related disorders often have a greatly reduced rate of normal blinks. Subtle seventh nerve weakness may be manifested by incomplete spontaneous blinks on the affected side. In patients with excessive lid closure, the clinician should determine whether other facial muscles are involved, whether the contractions are synchronous in several different facial muscle groups, and whether the problem is unilateral or bilateral. In hemifacial spasm, facial muscle contractions are synchronous and, usually, unilateral. In blepharospasm, the orbicularis contractions are bilateral and synchronous. Myokymic contractions involve smaller muscle groups and are not synchronous. Facial synkinesis following seventh nerve paralysis can be evaluated by inspecting the lower face during spontaneous blinks; synkinetic mentalis or orbicularis ori contractions are most common.

Proptosis can be evaluated by inspecting globe position with respect to the orbital rim by looking tangentially across the orbital margin from above, from below, or laterally.

The next step is to assess lid position in different gaze directions. Lid retraction on gaze down suggests lid lag or aberrant regeneration of the third nerve. The latter condition also causes lid retraction on adduction. Ptosis on adduction occurs in Duane's syndrome. A variety of lid findings have been described with myasthenia. Ptosis often worsens with sustained upgaze; after looking down, ptosis often improves. When the eyes are returned to the primary position after looking down for several seconds, the eyelids often demonstrate transient elevation before settling down to the previous ptotic position (Cogan's lid twitch syndrome). Occasionally there will be several twitches before the lids stabilize. Transient elevation alone is not specific for myasthenia, but the twitches are virtually diagnostic for disease of the neuromuscular junction such as myasthenia or botulism.

The next step is to observe both gentle and forceful lid closure. Fatigue of gentle lid closure occurs in myasthenia and can be demonstrated by asking the patient to close the eyes gently as if he or she were sleeping; after a few seconds, the lids may open slightly. Poor lid closure is the rule in facial weakness from disorders such as facial nerve paralysis and chronic progressive external ophthalmoplegia. Weak orbicularis function in these cases can also be assessed by asking the patient to close his or her eyes forcefully (Figure 17.8). With forced eyelid closure, the eyelashes are normally buried by folds of skin; with even mild facial paresis, the lashes are more exposed. Forced lid closure with rapid reopening is an excellent technique for evaluating myokymia, hemifacial spasm, apraxia of lid opening, and blepharospasm, conditions that are often worsened by this maneuver.

Patients with apraxia of lid opening contract their forehead and elevate their brows after forced lid closure, but the eyes remain closed (Figure 17.9). Patients with blepharospasm have persistent orbicularis contraction after being asked to open their eyes.

A

B

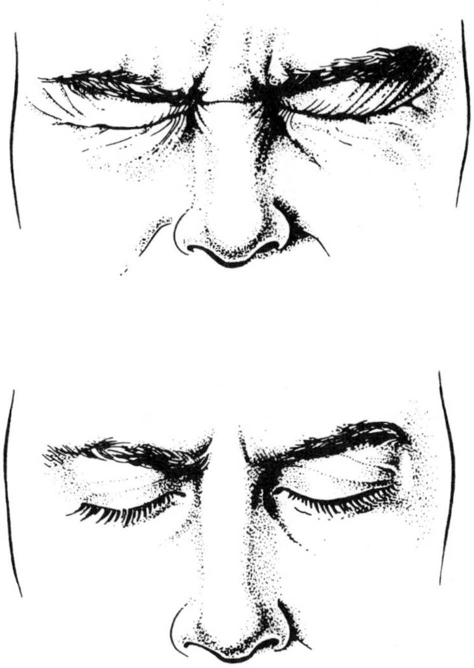

FIGURE 17.8 A. Normal forced eyelid closure. B. Weak eyelid closure. The lashes remain visible.

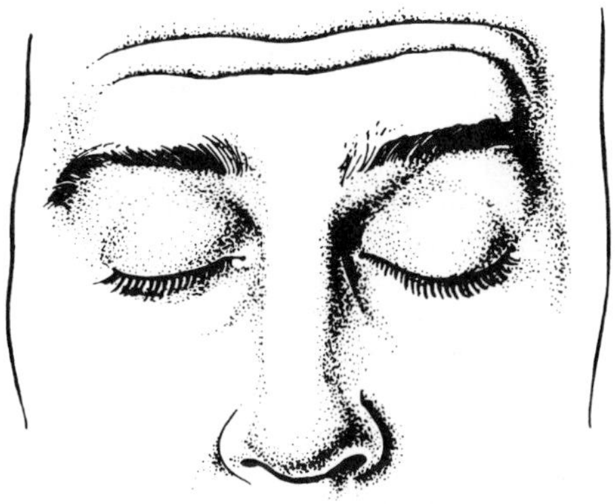

FIGURE 17.9 Apraxia of lid opening. Elevated eyebrows and forehead contraction with persistent eyelid closure.

The next step is to look for abnormalities of the pupil and ocular motility, suggesting Horner's syndrome, third nerve palsy, muscle disease, or congenital anomalies of innervation. Trigeminal-levator synkinesis can involve either external or internal pterygoid muscles (Glaser and Bachynski 1990). When the external pterygoid is involved, the eyelid rises with mouth opening or movement of the jaw to the opposite side. With internal pterygoid involvement, the lid elevates with clenching of the teeth. Babies with this form of congenital ptosis have movements of the involved eyelid when they suck.

In patients with eyelid disturbances associated with more generalized disease, the neurological examination provides essential diagnostic information.

Investigations

Ophthalmological examination should be done in most patients with lid abnormalities and should include exophthalmometry, tonometry in primary position and upgaze (an increase in intraocular pressure by 5 mm or more in upgaze suggests dysthyroid orbitopathy; low pressures occur in myotonic dystrophy), slit lamp examination for the lens opacities of myotonic dystrophy, and ophthalmoscopy to detect the pigmentary degeneration of the retina seen in some cases of chronic progressive external ophthalmoplegia and myotonic dystrophy. The edrophonium test is essential in the diagnosis of myasthenia. When available, quantitative orbital echography is a sensitive test for detecting dysthyroid orbitopathy. CT scanning of the orbit is the most useful single test for evaluation of proptosis and enophthalmos. MRI head scanning should be done in patients with blepharospasm, hemifacial spasm, and facial myokymia. Cardiac evaluation of patients with chronic progressive external ophthalmoplegia is important. Laboratory studies to consider include acetylcholine receptor antibodies and thyroid function studies.

REFERENCES

Dewey RB, Maraganore DM. Isolated eyelid opening apraxia: report of a new levodopa-responsive syndrome. Neurology 1994; 44:1752–1754.

Digre KB, Smoker WRK, Johnston P et al. Selective MR imaging approach for evaluation of patients with Horner's syndrome. AJNR 1992;13:223–227.

Galetta SL, Gray LG, Raps EC, Schatz NJ. Pretectal eyelid retraction and lag. Ann Neurol 1993;33:554–557.

Glaser JS. Neuro-ophthalmology (2nd ed). Philadelphia: Lippincott, 1990;437–457.

Glaser JS, Bachynski B. Congenital Motor and Sensory Anomalies. In JS Glaser (ed), Neuro-ophthalmology (2nd ed). Philadelphia: Lippincott, 1990;419–435.

Johnston JC, Rosenbaum DM, Picone CM, Grotta JC. Apraxia of eyelid opening secondary to right hemisphere infarction. Ann Neurol 1989;25:622–624.

Lepore FE. Unilateral ptosis and Hering's law. Neurology 1988;38:319–322.

Loewenfeld IE. The Pupil. Anatomy, Physiology, and Clinical Applications. Ames, IA: Iowa State University Press, 1993.

May M, Galetta S. The Facial Nerve and Related Disorders of the Face. In JS Glaser (ed), Neuro-opthalmology (2nd ed). Philadelphia: Lippincott, 1990:239–277.

North KN, Ouvrier RA, McLean CA, Hopkins IJ. Idiopathic hypothalamic dysfunction with dilated unresponsive pupils: report of two cases. J Child Neurol 1994;9:320–325.

Ropper AH. The opposite pupil in herniation. Neurology 1990;40:1707–1709.

Rosenberg ML, Jabbari B. Miosis and internal ophthalmoplegia as a manifestation of partial seizures. Neurology 1991;41:737–739.

Sibony PA. The Eyelid. In S Lessell, JTW van Dalen (eds), Current Neuro-ophthalmology. Vol. 3. St. Louis: Mosby, 1991;103–128.

Slamovits TL, Glaser JS. The Pupils and Accommodation. In JS Glaser (ed), Neuro-ophthalmology (2nd ed). Philadelphia: Lippincott, 1990;459–486.

Thompson HS, Kardon RH. The Pupil. In S Lessell, JTS van Dalen (eds), Current Neuro-ophthalmology. Vol. 3. St. Louis: Mosby, 1991;223–233.

SUGGESTED READING

Czarnecki JSC, Thompson HS. The iris sphincter in aberrant regeneration of the third nerve. Arch Ophthalmol 1978;96:1606–1610.

Kean JR. Spastic eyelids: failure of levator inhibition in unconscious states. Arch Neurol 1975;32:695–698.

Lam BL, Thompson HS, Corbett JJ. The prevalence of simple anisocoria. Am J Ophthalmol 1987;104:69–73.

Miller NR. Walsh and Hoyt's Clinical Neuro-ophthalmology (4th ed). Baltimore: Williams & Wilkins: 1985;932–995.

Thompson HS. Adie's syndrome: some new observations. Trans Am Ophthalmol Soc 1977;75:587–626.

Thompson HS, Zackon DH, Czarnecki JSC. Tadpole-shaped pupils caused by segmental spasm of the iris dilator muscle. Am J Ophthalmol 1983;96:467–477.

Chapter 18
Dizziness and Vertigo

B. Todd Troost

Dizziness, vertigo, and disequilibration are common complaints in patients referred for neurological evaluation. Because the entire physical examination and all diagnostic tests may be normal, the diagnosis depends primarily on the history. Vestibular tests described in Chapter 44 rarely provide an exact diagnosis; they should be used as confirmatory measures in an attempt to document abnormality in the peripheral or central vestibular system.

SYMPTOMS AND SIGNS

Vertigo, strictly defined, refers to a hallucination of movement. Although it is true that some patients experience a definite sense of environmental spin or self-rotation, the majority do not present solely with true vertigo as defined. The most common complaint is of *dizziness*, a term that represents an entire gamut of symptoms (Table 18.1). The first attempt should be to elicit an exact description of what the patient is experiencing. Is it a spinning sensation that could be characterized as vertigo, pointing to the peripheral vestibular apparatus? Is it a sensation of falling without rotation? Is it a sensation of unsteadiness or imbalance? Is there a particular direction in which the patient tends to fall? When the patient's complaint is actually of incoordination or clumsiness, the possibility of cerebellar dysfunction or peripheral neuropathy is raised. When the description is of lightheadedness or a swimming head, one thinks of presyncope or syncope and would, perhaps, lean more toward a consideration of systemic factors, including vasodepressor syncope, postural hypotension, or cardiac dysrhythmia.

After trying to define the true qualitative nature of the symptom complex, one must proceed to a consideration of temporal factors. Is the patient's experience a continuous one? Are there episodes of severe symptomatology with symptom-free intervals? If the symptoms are episodic, do they occur only when the patient is upright?

Patients reportedly have a great deal of difficulty describing their symptoms. Descriptions of visual disturbance in conditions that affect the neural or ophthalmic system are often more easily elicited from the patient. Initially, it is paramount that patients provide their own description before the physician biases the outcome by suggesting descriptive phrases. Often patients who are asked to describe their symptoms without using the word *dizziness* cannot further characterize the symptoms but revert to descriptions such as "I'm just dizzy all the time."

The signs that accompany vertigo and dizziness of course depend primarily on the cause. When it is an acute peripheral vestibulopathy, the patient will probably have a nystagmus with a fast phase beating away from the side of the involved ear. The patient may tend to fall toward the side of the involved ear during Romberg testing and past point in a similar direction. If the symptom is really lightheadedness and the cause is postural hypotension, this physical finding will be documented on examination and sought. Central neurologic causes of dizziness are almost always accompanied by other signs of central nervous system (CNS) dysfunction, such as gaze-evoked nystagmus, facial weakness, other cranial nerve abnormality, ataxia, hemisensory loss, or even paralysis.

If the cause is anxiety, the examiner may become aware of it by observation of other subtle signs of nervousness, such as increased tremulousness.

Table 18.1: Symptoms encompassed by the term *dizziness*

Vertigo
Unsteadiness
Imbalance
Spinning
Floating
Fainting
Lightheadedness
Swaying
Twisting
Blurring vision
Disorientation
Poor equilibrium
Bouncing
Falling
Swimming
Staggering
Weaving
Moving
Passing out
Tilting
Listing
Rocking
Oscillating
Rolling

ELUCIDATING THE HISTORY

In addition to determining whether the symptom complex is episodic, the history must define factors such as duration, length of symptoms, and any associated symptoms such as tinnitus, hearing loss, double vision, slurred speech, numbness, or paralysis. A history of episodic disequilibration accompanied by diplopia, slurred speech, perioral numbness, dimming of vision, and occasional drop attacks would suggest transient vertebrobasilar episodes. Are there associated symptoms such as headache, and have these occurred before? If the patient had experienced severe episodes of imbalance in early life, followed by occipital or generalized headaches, especially throbbing, the history would be very suggestive of basilar artery migraine. Did the dizziness follow head trauma, a systemic illness accompanied by aminoglycoside antibiotic therapy, or a mild upper respiratory infection? Episodic positional vertigo following head trauma is suggestive of cupulolithiasis, described below. Did the symptom complex occur following ear surgery or infection, deep-sea diving, or a concussive blow to the ear? Such a history, with or without hearing loss, would suggest a perilymph fistula.

In many large clinics dealing with balance disorders, there are a significant number of patients who experience anxiety. If the symptom of disequilibration or dizziness is of long duration, it is often difficult to tell whether the symptom complex is caused by anxiety or depression or whether the anxiety or depression are secondary to the dizziness. I believe that very few (less than 20%) patients with a clear movement sensation (vertigo) have a symptom complex caused solely by anxiety. One should be able to make a positive diagnosis of a neurosis or chronic anxiety disorder based on other symptomology and historical information. There may be a history of previous episodes of serious depression or anxiety attacks, and these should be elucidated before arriving at the conclusion that dizziness is secondary to anxiety.

Neurologists and neuro-otologists follow a large number of patients with chronic vertiginous sensations who remain undiagnosed. Such patients complain of constant or intermittent disequilibration, often aggravated by position change, as well as by visual stimuli such as moving traffic, patterned wallpaper, striped rugs or curtains, or passing food displays in supermarkets. Many of these patients have become agoraphobic; they hesitate to leave their homes and particularly fear driving a car that will be passed by other automobiles. Some of these persons have had a single attack of acute peripheral vestibulopathy but have never made appropriate central compensation or adapted to their peripheral abnormality. Although mechanisms for compensation remain unclear, the majority of patients, particularly those younger than 30, rapidly recover from an acute peripheral vestibulopathy. Elderly patients or patients with a previously existing intrinsic brain stem abnormality rarely make adequate compensation for an acute peripheral vestibulopathy. Such patients continue to complain of severe disequilibration. Symptoms may be exacerbated by a variety of visual inputs. This significant group of dizzy patients has chronic symptoms and often consults more than one physician. They often have completely normal examinations and vestibular tests.

Figures 18.1 and 18.2 diagramatically illustrate what might happen following an acute peripheral vestibular abnormality. Figure 18.1, as described in the legend, suggests that there is a different afferent input from one peripheral end organ versus the other during the act of normal head turning. The stylized drawing is not meant to represent true anatomy, but rather the concept of asymmetrical afferent input. The right panel of Figure 18.1 suggests that when there is a unilateral injury to one peripheral vestibular end organ, the result may be asymmetrical input to the CNS. This could be interpreted centrally as a sensation of turning or vertigo. In Figure 18.2, one assumes that there has been, as a result of CNS plasticity, some attempt to compensate for an injured peripheral vestibular system. In this situation, there may still be a difference in afferent input, but some adjustment has been made such that the patient no longer experiences a sensation of vertigo and there is no nystagmus. In some individuals, as diagrammed in the right panel of Figure 18.2, there is either lessened or no ability to compensate for peripheral abnormality. One possibility would be a congenital inability to make CNS compensation, but others include (1) an acquired central inability to compensate due to CNS lesion, as from multiple sclerosis or previous brain stem stroke; (2) a fluctuating peripheral vestibular problem, such as might occur in Ménière's disease; (3) rela-

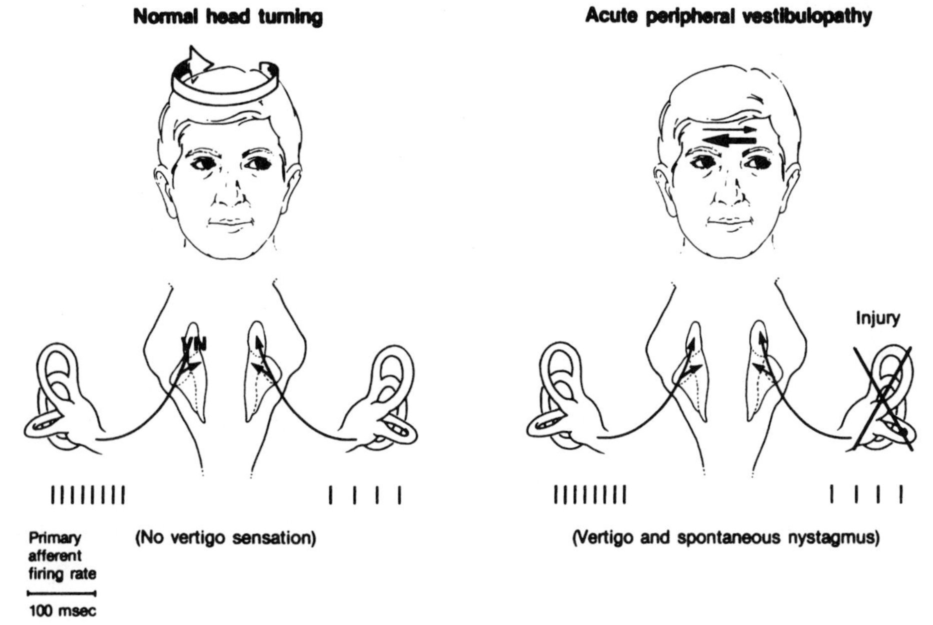

FIGURE 18.1 (Left) Vestibular afferent input during normal horizontal head rotation to the right. Increased firing rate from right peripheral vestibular apparatus. Ocular deviation shows slow-phase deviation to the left. (VN = vestibular nuclei.) (Adapted from RW Baloh, V Honrubia, K Jacobson. Benign positional vertigo: clinical and oculographic features in 240 cases. Neurology 1987;37:371–378; and RB Daroff. Evaluation of Dizziness and Vertigo. In JS Glaser (ed), Neuro-Ophthalmology. Vol. 9. St. Louis: Mosby, 1977:39–54.) (Right) Acute left peripheral vestibulopathy with resultant acute vertiginous sensation simulating head rotation to the right. Slow-phase ocular deviation to the left (small arrow) and fast phase of nystagmus to the right (bold arrow) and away from the side of the peripheral vestibular injury.

tive inactivity without much afferent input; and (4) a peripheral vestibular apparatus providing inaccurate, although nonfluctuating, afferent information. Careful history-taking may reveal childhood meningitis, a remote head injury, or particular susceptibility to motion sickness in childhood. An explicit search during history-taking should be made to define these possibilities.

DIFFERENTIAL DIAGNOSIS

Because ongoing or episodic conditions accompanied by vertigo, unsteadiness, or presyncope are produced by multiple and often subtle causes, it is not surprising that a significant number of patients cannot be readily diagnosed. A major differential diagnostic classification would include broad categories such as (1) peripheral vestibulopathy, (2) central neurological disorders, and (3) systemic conditions. There is some ambiguity in the use of the term *central*, which has been used by otolaryngologists to include causes that are central or proximal to the vestibular end organ and therefore include the vestibular portion of the eighth nerve. Neurologists, however, consider conditions that affect the vestibular nerve, such as tumors, as peripheral in location because they are on a cranial nerve and are extra-axial. Because masses or neoplasms can enlarge to involve other structures in the cerebellopontine angle, particularly the brain stem, conditions that affect the eighth nerve are discussed for convenience in the central category.

Peripheral Causes of Vertigo

Peripheral causes result from dysfunction of vestibular end organs (semicircular canals, utricle, and saccule) (Table 18.2).

Peripheral Vestibulopathy

Peripheral vestibulopathy encompasses terms such as *vestibular neuronitis*, *labyrinthitis*, and *viral neurolabyrinthitis*. Such terms imply an inflammatory mechanism, which is unproved. *Vestibular ne ronitis*, strictly speaking, is characterized by single or recurrent sudden episodes of true vertigo lasting from hours to days and often associated initially with vomiting. When the condition is associated with hearing loss, the entire labyrinth is assumed to be involved, and the term *labyrinthitis* is used. Despite this technical distinction, many neuro-otologists, otologists, and neurologists use the terms *vestibular neuronitis* and *labyrinthitis* interchangeably, whether or not auditory symptoms are present. In such patients the vertiginous sensation may be provoked by head movement, but not necessarily by a particular head position.

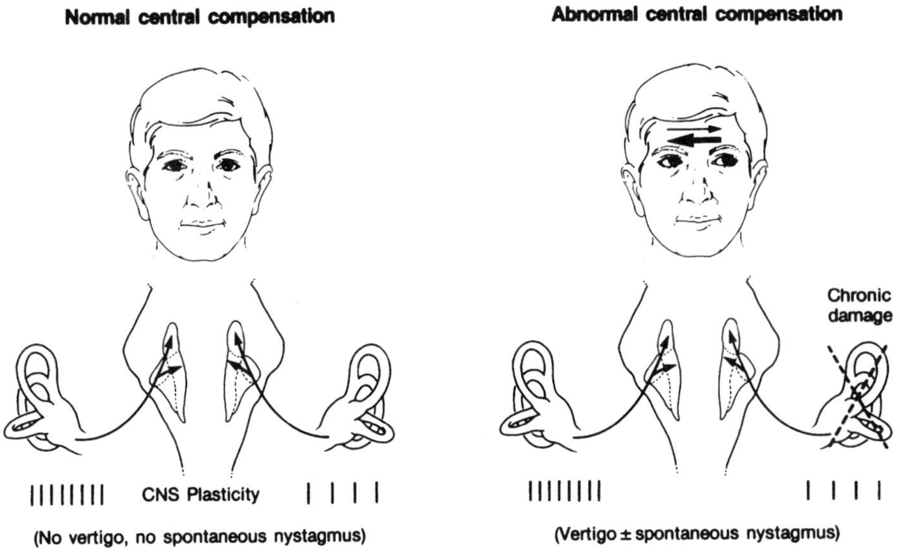

FIGURE 18.2 (Left) Normal adaptation for prior left peripheral vestibulopathy. Despite a reduced firing rate from the left side, the central nervous system has compensated for the disparity and there is no nystagmus or vertigo. (Right) Abnormal compensation for prior left peripheral vestibulopathy. The patient continues to experience vertiginous sensations and may have nystagmus with a fast phase to the right (solid arrow). (Adapted from RW Baloh, V Honrubia, K Jacobson. Benign positional vertigo: clinical and oculographic features in 240 cases. Neurology 1987;37:371–378; and RB Daroff. Evaluation of Dizziness and Vertigo. In JS Glaser (ed), Neuro-Ophthalmology. Vol. 9. St. Louis: Mosby, 1977:39–54.)

Whether isolated viral involvement of the vestibular nerves is a cause of acute or episodic vertigo is controversial. Many prefer the term *acute* or *recurrent peripheral vestibulopathy*. In the acute phase, many patients present with sudden severe vertigo, nausea, and vomiting without any hearing disturbance or facial weakness. The acute symptoms usually resolve in a few days to a week but may recur in weeks or months. If true vertigo is part of the symptom complex, the condition is most likely to be associated with some disorder of the peripheral end organ. However, patients with either acute peripheral vestibulopathy or, more commonly, recurrent attacks may experience only a sensation of lightheadedness or floating, or a feeling of "walking on tennis balls." Even if the patient has had hundreds of episodes, it is important to try to determine whether any of them were associated with spinning vertigo. Over time, the nature of the patient's symptom complex may change, even with peripheral vestibulopathy, from vertiginous sensations to those of pure unsteadiness or disequilibration.

Epidemic and seasonal outbreaks of acute vertigo have suggested an infectious origin due to viral disease, but this remains largely unproved. Viral labyrinthitis can also be part of a systemic viral infection such as mumps, measles, infectious mononucleosis, or upper respiratory tract viral infections. Isolated viral infections of the labyrinth are also believed to cause the sudden onset of hearing loss, vertigo, or both in both children and adults (Baloh 1984). Otitic herpes zoster is an infection characterized by pain in the ear, followed in 1–10 days by a vesicular eruption in the external ear. When the seventh and eighth nerves are affected, there is a combination of facial weakness, hearing loss, and vertigo known as the *Ramsay Hunt syndrome*. Whenever vertigo is associated with severe ear pain or facial pain, one must consider this possibility. A dysesthetic area of skin may precede, by many days, the appearance of the skin eruption.

Table 18.2: Peripheral causes of vertigo*

1. Peripheral vestibulopathy (includes labyrinthitis, vestibular neuronitis, acute and recurrent peripheral vestibulopathy)
2. Benign positional vertigo (includes benign positional nystagmus, benign paroxysmal vertigo)
3. Post-traumatic vertigo
4. Vestibulotoxic drug-induced vertigo
5. Ménière's syndrome
6. Other focal peripheral diseases (includes local bacterial infection, degeneration of hair cells, genetic anomalies of labyrinth, cupulolithiasis, tumor of eighth nerve, otosclerosis, fistula of labyrinth, and rarely focal ischemia and others)

*Hearing loss often.

Benign Positional Paroxysmal Vertigo

Benign positional paroxysmal vertigo (BPPV) is a symptom complex suggesting benign peripheral (end organ) disease (Troost and Patton 1992). Historical factors that should lead to the consideration of BPPV are the following: (1) symptoms associated with certain head positions; (2) rotational vertigo of brief duration and episodic in nature; (3) antecedent episode of severe rotary vertigo with or without nausea and vomiting associated with an upper respiratory infection that suggests prior viral neurolabyrinthitis; (4) history of head trauma before attacks of vertigo; (5) most severe symptomatology early in the day with lessening symptoms as the day progresses; and (6) relative absence of spontaneous symptoms without head movement or position change. These symptoms, differentiated from central neurological symptoms, are outlined in Table 18.3. The signs and symptoms of benign positional vertigo are transient and rarely last longer than 40 seconds. They frequently occur

Table 18.3: Characteristics of peripheral versus central positional vertigo

Symptom or Sign	*Peripheral*	*Central*
Latency (time to onset of vertigo or nystagmus)	0–40 seconds (mean 7.8*)	No latency Begins immediately
Duration	<1 minute	Symptoms may persist (signs and symptoms of single episode)
Fatigability (habituation) (lessening signs and symptoms with repetition of provocative maneuver)	Yes 87%*	No
Nystagmus direction	Direction fixed, torsional, up, upper pole of eyes toward ground	Direction changing, variable
Intensity of signs and symptoms	Severe vertigo, marked nystagmus, systemic symptoms such as nausea	Usually mild vertigo, less intense nystagmus, rare nausea
Reproducibility	Inconsistent	More consistent

*RW Baloh, V Honrubia, K Jacobson. Benign positional vertigo: clinical and oculographic features in 240 cases. Neurology 1987;37:371–378.

when a certain position is assumed, such as lying down or turning in bed. Depending on whether the symptom (vertigo) or sign (nystagmus) is being emphasized, this condition is also called "benign paroxysmal positional nystagmus" or "benign paroxysmal positional vertigo." Physical examination findings include (1) vertical-rotary benign positional paroxysmal nystagmus produced by provocative maneuvers (Figure 18.3), (2) latency to onset of symptoms once precipitating head position is achieved, (3) short-duration nystagmus (3–30 seconds), and (4) adaptation of nystagmus and symptoms—that is, disappearance with repeated maneuvers. The finding of the typical nystagmus on assumption of certain head positions is considered the single most important physical finding in making the diagnosis of BPPV (Figure 18.4). It is a major cause of vertigo. In the Baloh et al. study of 240 cases (1987), the average age of onset was 54 years, and the most common identifiable causes were head trauma (17%) and viral neurolabyrinthitis (15%).

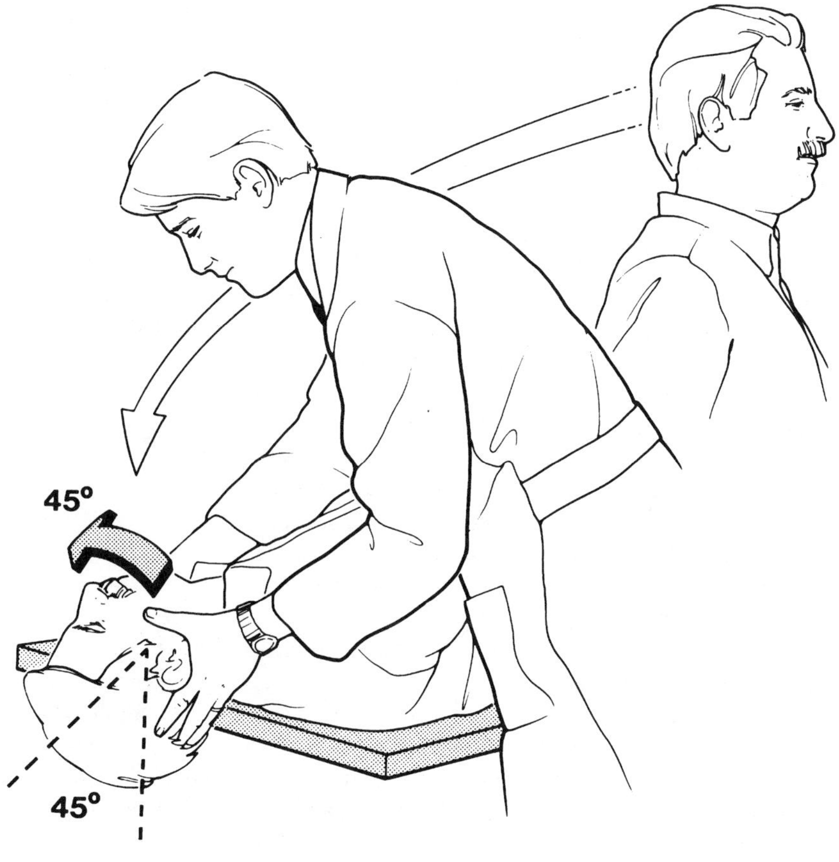

FIGURE 18.3 Provocative maneuvers for positional vertigo and nystagmus. The patient is abruptly moved from a seated position to one with the head hanging 45 degrees below the horizontal and rotated 45 degrees to one side. He or she is then observed for positional nystagmus. The maneuvers are repeated with the head straight back and turned to the other side.

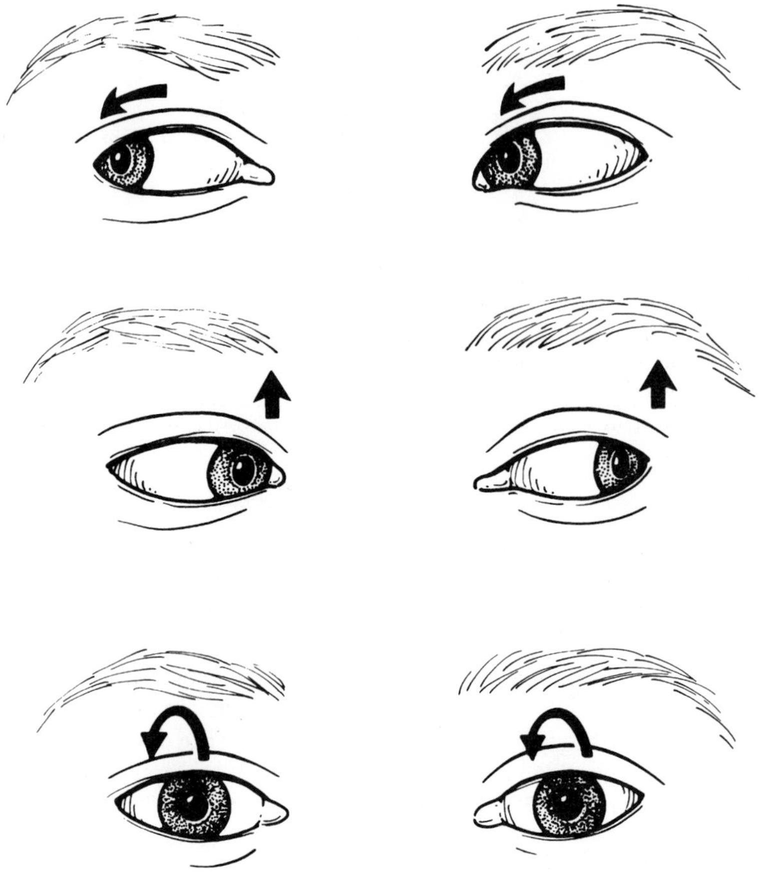

FIGURE 18.4 In benign paroxysmal positional nystagmus, the nystagmus fast phase is horizontal-rotary directed toward the undermost ear when gaze is directed toward the undermost ear (upper panel). The nystagmus fast phase is upward toward the forehead when gaze is directed to the uppermost ear (middle panel). With the eyes in the central orbital position, the nystagmus fast phase is vertical upward and rotary toward the down ear (bottom panel).

Posttraumatic Vertigo

Posttraumatic vertigo immediately follows head trauma in most cases. It implies end organ damage in the absence of other central nervous system signs and may be related to fracture of the temporal bone. The interval between injury and onset of symptoms can, however, be days or even weeks. The mechanism for the delay of symptoms is uncertain but may be hemorrhage into the labyrinth, with later development of serous labyrinthitis. Another mechanism for delayed posttraumatic positional vertigo is cupulolithiasis in which the calcareous deposits (otoconia) of a damaged organ of the labyrinth are displaced to a sensitive region of the posterior canal (Baloh et al. 1987), making it more susceptible to stimulation in certain head positions. Another mechanism posed is that there are three moving pathologic densities in the endolymph of the semicircular canal. This is known as the "canalith theory" (Epley 1992; Parnes and Price-Jones 1993). In posttraumatic vertigo, the symptoms may be those of general peripheral vestibulopathy or benign positional vertigo. Generally, the prognosis is good, with symptoms gradually resolving within weeks to months (Barber and Sharpe 1988). However, as pointed out by Baloh and colleagues (1987), disabling persistent positional vertigo, unresponsive to medical therapy, occurs more commonly than was previously recognized. Most patients respond to exercise therapy (Troost and Patton 1992), as described in Chapter 44 (Figure 18.5), and rarely need selective section of the nerve to the posterior semicircular canal.

Drug Toxicity

Patients with dizziness produced by vestibulotoxic drugs are presumed or documented to have persistent injury to the peripheral end organ. Among the agents causing such end organ injury are the aminoglycosides. Streptomycin and gentamicin have their greatest effect on the vestibular end organ; kanamycin, tobramycin, and neomycin cause more damage to the auditory end organ (Baloh and Honrubia 1990). Patients usually report progressive unsteadiness, particularly when visual input is diminished, as happens at night or in a darkened room. Vestibular testing documents a progressive bilateral loss of vestibular function. The aminoglycosides are concentrated in the endolymph and perilymph, so that the hair cells are exposed to high concentrations of the drugs. This type of end organ toxicity should be contrasted with that produced by the large group of drugs with widespread reversible central and peripheral nervous system effects (Table 18.4); the latter cause transient disequilibration, which subsides with cessation of the medication. Extreme caution should be used in patients with even mild renal disease because most of these agents are primarily eliminated by the kidney.

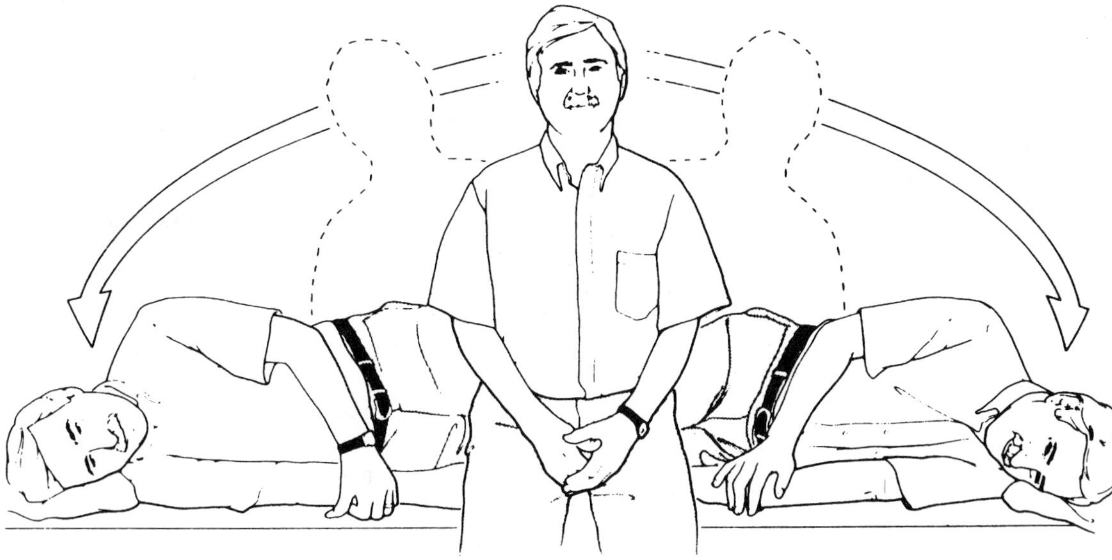

FIGURE 18.5 Exercise therapy. The patient begins in the seated position and then leans rapidly to the side, placing the head on the bed or table. The patient remains there until the vertigo subsides and then returns to the seated upright position, remaining there until all symptoms subside. The maneuver is repeated toward the opposite side, completing one full repetition. Ten to 20 repetitions should be performed three times a day.

Ménière's Syndrome

Ménière's syndrome is characterized by attacks of severe vertigo and vomiting, tinnitus, fluctuating hearing loss, ill-described aural sensations of fullness and pressure, and spontaneous recovery in hours to days. Usually the patient develops a sensation of fullness and pressure along with decreased hearing and tinnitus in a single ear. This is followed by severe vertigo, which reaches peak intensity within minutes and slowly subsides over hours, with a persistent sense of disequilibration for days after an acute episode. Occasionally, sufferers from Ménière's syndrome experience such severe attacks that they suddenly fall to the ground. Consciousness is not lost in such episodes, although awareness of surroundings may be altered by the intensity of the accompanying sensation and nausea. The most consistent pathological finding in Ménière's syndrome is an increase in the volume of the endolymphatic fluid and distention of the canals, hence the term *endolymphatic hydrops*. Although some specific causes such as bacterial, viral, and syphilitic infections may lead to the same pathological changes and symptoms, the majority of cases are idiopathic.

Table 18.4: Systemic causes of vertigo and dizziness

1. Drugs (including anticonvulsants, hypnotics, antihypertensives, alcohol, analgesics, tranquilizers)
2. Hypotension, presyncope (including primary cardiac causes and postural hypotension from a wide variety of causes)
3. Infectious diseases (including syphilis, viral and other bacterial meningitides, and systemic infection)
4. Endocrine diseases (including diabetes and hypothyroidism)
5. Vasculitis (including collagen-vascular disease, giant cell arteritis, and drug-induced vasculitis)
6. Other systemic conditions (including hematological disorders [polycythemia, anemia, and dysproteinemia], sarcoidosis, granulomatous disease, and systemic toxins)

Other Peripheral Vestibular Conditions

Many other disorders affect the peripheral labyrinth, including acute and chronic otitis media, hereditary degenerative disorders of the end organ, and local tumors. Conditions such as a vertebrobasilar transient ischemic attack (TIA) or focal ischemic stroke of the end organ, particularly in an elderly patient, are often cited as a cause of vertigo. Such isolated involvement is difficult to document, and vertebrobasilar insufficiency should not be diagnosed without associated brain stem symptoms and signs.

Central Causes of Vertigo

Central pathological causes of vertigo result from dysfunction of the vestibular portion of the eighth nerve, the vestibular nuclei within the brain stem, and their central connections (Table 18.5). Neural connections with the central vestibular nuclei include interaction with the vestibular portions of the cerebellum (primarily the cerebellar flocculus, nodulus, and uvula). Normal persons experience physiological vertiginous sensations when visual and

Table 18.5: Central neurological causes of vertigo*

1. Brain stem ischemia and infarction
2. Demyelinating disease: multiple sclerosis, postinfectious demyelination, remote effect of carcinoma
3. Cerebellopontine angle tumor; acoustic neuroma, meningioma, cholesteatoma, metastatic tumor, etc.
4. Cranial neuropathy; focal involvement of eighth nerve or in association with systemic disorders
5. Intrinsic brain stem lesions (tumor, arteriovenous malformation, trauma [rare])
6. Other posterior fossa lesions (primarily other intrinsic or extra-axial masses of the posterior fossa such as hematoma, metastatic tumor, and cerebellar infarction)
7. Seizure disorders (rare)
8. Heredofamilial disorders (such as spinocerebellar degeneration)
9. Malformations of the peripheral vestibular apparatus

*A hearing loss is rare except in the condition listed in no. 3.

vestibular inputs are in conflict or when they are initially exposed to heights (Brandt 1991).

Central pathological causes of vertigo are less common than either peripheral or systemic causes, the vertiginous symptoms are usually less prominent, and additional neurological signs are usually present on examination (Froehling et al. 1994).

Brain Stem Ischemia and Infarction

Vertigo, including brief episodes of isolated vertigo, is caused by postular circulary disturbances (Grad and Baloh 1989; Oas and Baloh 1992). The posterior circulation supplies blood to the brain stem, cerebellum, and peripheral vestibular apparatus, in addition to other structures. It is not surprising that vertibrobasilar insufficiency may be accompanied by vertigo. In general, brain stem TIAs should be accompanied by neurologic symptoms or signs in addition to vertigo or dizziness for a clear diagnosis to be entertained. However, it is clear that isolated episodes of vertigo lasting many minutes may be due to posterior circulation dysfunction. Symptoms include *transient* clumsiness, weakness, loss of vision, diplopia, perioral numbness, ataxia, drop attack, and dysarthria (Caplan 1993). Common signs of vertebrobasilar insufficiency include disorders of motor function such as weakness, clumsiness, or paralysis. A crossed defect (a motor or sensory deficit on one side of the face and the opposite side of the body) is good evidence of brain stem dysfunction. If the occipital lobes are the site of ischemia, transient visual loss in the form of complete or partial homonymous hemianopia occurs. Ataxia, imbalance, unsteadiness, or disequilibrium not necessarily associated with spinning vertigo may occur because of labyrinthine or cerebellar ischemia.

However, it is incorrect to believe that dizziness must be present before a TIA of the posterior circulation can be diagnosed. Isolated symptoms like those described may occur without dizziness. On the other hand, it has been overemphasized that such symptoms must *always* accompany dizziness, when the vertiginous symptoms are due to brain stem TIA. In elderly patients with no laboratory evidence of peripheral vestibulopathy or systemic disease, episodic disequilibration or dizziness may be due to vertebrobasilar disease (Grad and Baloh 1989).

Sudden hearing loss with moderate dizziness may be due to infarction in the distribution of the internal auditory artery. In isolation, this symptom complex is uncommon in elderly patients with atherosclerotic vertebrobasilar disease and is more suggestive of diseases affecting small- and intermediate-diameter arteries such as syphilis, systemic lupus erythematosus, or periarteritis nodosa. In the atherosclerotic patient, such symptoms are usually accompanied by other signs of brain stem or cerebellar dysfunction, which allow a more certain diagnosis. If actual brain stem infarction occurs, neurological signs are often present on examination. Such signs may not be obvious and should be carefully sought. They include nystagmus of the central type, hyperreflexia, internuclear ophthalmoplegia, homonymous visual field defects, dysarthria, vertebral bruits, and ataxia (Leigh and Zee 1991). Symptoms of dizziness are also quite common in proximal extracranial occlusion of the vertebral arteries (Caplan 1993) and in the subclavian steal syndrome.

Up to this point, the emphasis has been on the accompanying signs and symptoms that almost always occur with vertebrobasilar disease. It is noteworthy, however, that acute severe vertigo, mimicking labyrinthine disease, is an early symptom of acute cerebellar infarction in the distal territory of the posterior inferior cerebellar artery. To differentiate this condition from labyrinthine disease, particular attention is directed to the type of nystagmus that is present. Acute peripheral vestibulopathy usually causes *unidirectional* nystagmus, with the fast phase in the opposite direction. This is similar to the mnemonic COWS (Cold, Opposite, Warm, Same) for remembering the direction of the nystagmus fast phase during thermal irrigation of the ear. The fast phase is away from the side of the cold water irrigation. Cold water mimics a peripheral destructive lesion of the labyrinth, and almost all lesions are destructive. Therefore, with a peripheral labyrinthine disturbance, the nystagmus fast phase is in the opposite direction or away from the involved ear. The nystagmus increases during gaze in the direction of the phase or contralateral to the peripheral vestibulopathy. Swaying or falling occurs toward the side of the lesion (opposite the nystagmus fast phase). The nystagmus direction is said to be fixed in that it tends to be any direction, away from the side of the peripheral vestibulopathy, and tends to remain horizontal on upward gaze.

With incipient cerebellar infarction, the sway or fall is ipsilateral to the lesion and the nystagmus may be variable in direction but is most prominent ipsilateral to the lesion. In other words, with central lesions the fast phase of the nystagmus is in the direction of gaze (direction changing nystagmus) but becomes more prominent when gaze is directed ipsilateral to the lesion (Troost 1989; Oas and Baloh 1992). Ocular motor findings are often present in brain stem disease; conditions such as limitation of vertical gaze, upbeat or downbeat nystagmus, or disconjugate nystagmus are often present. However, in certain syndromes of the posterior circulation, the initial presentation can mimic acute vestibulopathy—in particular, the syndrome of the anterior cerebellar artery (Oas and Baloh 1992) and the syndrome of the distal posterior interior cerebellar artery.

Multiple Sclerosis

Multiple sclerosis should only be diagnosed following the documentation of disseminated CNS lesions such as optic neuritis, transverse myelitis, internuclear ophthalmoplegia or other brain stem signs, and magnetic resonance imaging (MRI) changes. Occasionally, signs and symptoms suggestive of multiple sclerosis, including disequilibration and dizziness, may be mimicked by an intrinsic brain stem tumor in a young patient.

Cerebellopontine Angle Tumors

Tumors of the cerebellopontine angle rarely present solely with episodic vertigo. The most common tumor in this location results from a proliferation of the Schwann cells, hence the name *schwannoma.* Most of these tumors arise on the vestibular portion of the eighth nerve within the internal auditory canal. They progressively enlarge, deforming the internal auditory meatus and compressing adjacent neural structures such as the acoustic portion of the eighth nerve, facial nerve, trigeminal nerve, brain stem, and cerebellum. Other tumors occurring in the cerebellopontine angle include meningiomas, epidermoids, and metastases.

The most common symptoms associated with eighth nerve tumors are progressive hearing loss and tinnitus. Vertigo occurs in approximately 20%, but a symptom of imbalance or disequilibration is more common, approaching 50%. All those with progressive unilateral hearing loss, and particularly those with any vestibular symptoms, should be carefully examined for additional neurological signs such as a depressed corneal reflex.

Cranial Neuropathy

Multiple or isolated cranial neuropathies occur in focal or systemic disease, including vasculitis, granulomatous disease, and meningeal carcinomatosis. Often, however, the cause is elusive. Evidence of systemic involvement is elicited by history, physical examination, and laboratory evaluation. Cogan's syndrome may be considered with cranial neuropathies. The condition is characterized by nonsyphilitic keratitis associated with vertigo, tinnitus, ataxia, nystagmus, rapidly progressive deafness, and systemic involvement (Vollertsen et al. 1986).

Posterior Fossa Lesions

Posterior fossa lesions in a variety of locations are unusual causes of isolated vertigo. The symptoms are usually positional vertigo of the central type (see Table 18.2). High-resolution computed tomography (CT) had a major impact in early diagnosis of such monosymptomatic posterior fossa disease. Of special note is the use of MRI with coronal and sagittal acquisitions, which permits identification of small tumors close to the tissue-bone interface, a region often blurred by bone artifact in CT scans.

Acquired disease of the brain stem and cerebellum produces a variety of types of nystagmus, which sometimes present as a complaint of oscillopsia, an illusion of environmental movement characterized by bouncing or jiggling of objects. Although *oscillopsia* is a common complaint with significant bilateral labyrinthine abnormality, the presence of vertical oscillopsia should alert the physician to look for primary position upbeat or downbeat nystagmus. These nystagmus types are reliable indicators of CNS abnormality due to structural intrinsic midline cerebellar disease or drugs (Troost 1989; Daroff et al. 1987).

Seizure Disorders

Seizure disorders, especially temporal lobe epilepsy, are rare causes of dizziness or vertigo. The history almost always reveals additional symptoms such as loss of awareness, automatic behavior, or generalized seizure activity following an aura of vertigo. However, some epileptics with psychomotor seizures, documented by additional history and electroencephalography (EEG), have isolated auras of the symptoms listed in Table 18.1.

Systemic Causes of Vertigo

Systemic causes have been given a separate category to include more widespread conditions that secondarily affect peripheral or central vestibular structures, or both, to produce vertigo (Table 18.4).

Drugs

Side effects of drug ingestion frequently cause dizziness in the broadest definition of the term. Vestibulotoxic drugs, as previously described, can produce true vertigo. The dizziness produced by other drugs is more a sense of weakness, disequilibration, or fuzzy-headedness. The agents listed in Table 18.4 are among the most common offenders. Every attempt should be made to determine the type and quantity of medication being taken by the dizzy patient. Frequently, the elimination or reduction of medication such as a mild tranquilizer produces a clear improvement. Unfortunately, the dizzy patient will have been treated with a variety of medications (to be discussed), which themselves may add to disequilibration or dizziness.

Hypotension

The multiple causes of *presyncope* or *postural hypotension* are often responsible for complaints of vertigo or dizziness. Again, careful historical review and documentation of physical findings such as postural hypotension or cardiac arrhythmia direct further investigation and therapy. Presyncope is described as lightheadedness and by other terms and is actually a common mechanism for dizziness or even vertiginous sensations. Postural hypotension is a common side effect of antihypertensive agents, diuretics, and dopaminergic agents. When the symptom is intermittent, a history of lightheadedness following change from recumbent or sitting posture to an erect position, but not the reverse, is more helpful than blood pressure measurements. In adolescents, a hyposensitive carotid sinus reflex during the growth spurt is not rare, and transient symptoms of postural dizziness might be explained by this mechanism.

Endocrine Disorders

Among the endocrinopathies that cause disorders of equilibration are diabetes and hypothyroidism. The mechanism in diabetes is probably the autonomic neuropathy and orthostatic hypotension that may accompany the disease. Though much less common as a specific cause, hypothyroidism should be considered when the symptoms of vertigo remain undiagnosed. Indeed, dizziness is not an infrequent presenting complaint in patients with thyroid deficiency. The remaining systemic conditions rarely present with isolated vertigo but are included as additional primary or secondary causes.

Multiple Afferent Sensory Loss

The vestibular system functions to provide (1) spatial orientation at rest or during acceleration, (2) visual fixation during head or body movement (the vestibulo-ocular reflex), and (3) feedback control of muscle tone to maintain posture. These functions and their control mechanisms are interconnected in complex fashion. Thus, the symptoms of episodic vertigo reflect disturbances in more than one system. The combination of multiple sensory deficits (Brandt 1991) can produce disorientation or disequilibration that is interpreted as dizziness or vertigo. This often occurs in the elderly, in whom vision (cataracts), hearing (presbycusis), and proprioception (peripheral neuropathy) may all be impaired. There is an entity known as "presbylibrium," or imbalances resulting from aging, that may be due to a selective progressive deterioration of the peripheral vestibular apparatus or a combination of sensory deficits.

Even a young, healthy person is easily confused by afferent sensory information, as exemplified by the sensation of spinning or true vertigo experienced during full-field optokinetic stimulation. Almost every individual, while quietly seated, will still experience a compelling illusion of rotation while viewing a moving environment of optokinetic stripes (the circular-vection illusion). Thus, it is not surprising that patients with subtle abnormalities of peripheral or central vestibular mechanisms experience momentary periods of disorientation while viewing a moving patterned environment. Some experience episodic vertigo during vehicular travel.

An age-related degeneration of vestibular receptors, analogous to presbycusis, contributes to vertigo. Although most younger patients readily compensate for unilateral peripheral vestibular damage, older patients frequently cannot, indicating either *bilateral* peripheral vestibular dysfunction or a separate central abnormality that decreases their ability to compensate.

Dizziness in Childhood

The most common causes of vertigo and dizziness in childhood and infancy are similar to those in the adult: acute peripheral vestibulopathy, trauma, and infection. Vertigo following air travel is more common in children than in adults because of the frequency of accompanying middle ear infection and effusion. Migraine is a significant cause of episodic dizziness or vertigo in childhood and should be considered even when the symptoms of headache are minimal.

Benign paroxysmal vertigo in childhood is a variety of vestibular neuronitis. Although unaccompanied by loss of consciousness, children may fall during the course of an attack. The episodes may last minutes to hours or recur for many weeks or even months, gradually decreasing in severity. The preservation of consciousness during an attack distinguishes the condition from temporal lobe seizures with a vestibular component and from vestibulogenic epilepsy in which an attack is triggered by labyrinthine stimulation. Congenital anomalies of the inner ear and brain stem are rare causes, as is vascular disease or tumor in childhood.

EXAMINATION OF THE DIZZY PATIENT

General Examination

Every patient with a disorder of equilibration or true vertigo should have a screening general physical examination. In particular, patients who exhibit symptoms suggesting presyncope or actual syncope must have particular attention paid to their cardiovascular system. Not only should patients have their blood pressure measured in the resting, sitting, and standing position, but they also should have their blood pressure measured 1, 2, 3, and 5 minutes after assuming the upright position, as delayed postural hypotension is not uncommon. Exercise-induced hypotension is an important observation and should lead to consideration of conditions such as the Shy-Drager syndrome, diabetic autonomic neuropathy, and cardiac defects such as aortic stenosis and obstructive cardiomyopathy. One should also pay careful attention to evaluation of the musculoskeletal system, as abnormalities adversely affect balance or the ability to recover successfully from a mild peripheral vestibular abnormality.

Whenever episodic symptomatology is associated with a question of alteration of consciousness or lightheadedness, particular attention should be paid to the possibility of cardiac dysrhythmia. Most patients with cardiac dysrhythmias do not report associated sensations of irregular heartbeat, thumping in the chest, or fluttering; however, examination may reveal an irregular cardiac rhythm or cardiac murmur (Dohrmann and Cheitlin 1986).

During the general examination, attention should be paid to systemic conditions that could give rise to a general feeling of malaise or weakness that may be interpreted by the patient as a disorder of balance. Conditions that may lead to sudden syncope may be revealed on the general physical examination. Patients with suspected extracranial vascular disease should not only have the head and neck auscultated for bruits but also should have a general examination of the peripheral vascular system, including the cranial and carotid pulses. The examiner should check for obstructive vascular disease by listening for bruits and should check for significant peripheral venous disease (varicose veins) that may lead to venous pooling and hypotensive episodes.

Neurological Examination

The neurological examination should be specifically determined by the patient's history. In patients with clear episodic vertigo, the neurological examination is usually normal with the exception of the ocular motor findings to be described. However, when the patient's symptom complex is more vaguely defined and includes disequilibration or unsteadiness, particular attention must be paid to examination of the motor system reflexes, sensation, and cerebellar function.

All patients with undiagnosed disorders of equilibration, however described, should have a complete neurological examination. The various parts of the neurological examination will be described only briefly, with each part followed by a suggestion of which entities might be discovered.

Mental Status Examination

Signs of diffuse alterations in consciousness may suggest overmedication, metabolic encephalopathy, or an acquired dementing process. Focal disturbances in intellectual function, such as a subtle aphasia, may lead to the consideration of a multi-infarction state (multi-infarct dementia) with accompanying brain stem infarctions, or of a mass lesion in the cranium.

Cranial Nerve Examination

Alterations in visual sensory function may be a primary or exacerbating cause of disequilibration. Even the recent addition of a new refractive correction, particularly lenses for presbyopia, may be an added or primary cause of imbalance. Visual field defects such as unsuspected bitemporal or homonymous field defects from tumors or infarcts may cause patients to run into objects or feel disoriented in space. The presence of papilledema or absent venous pulsations on fundoscopy should be an immediate clue to raised intracranial pressure. Altered corneal sensation may be the clue to a previously unsuspected cerebellopontine angle mass. Tuning fork tests (see Chapter 19) may confirm the patient's complaint of hearing loss and should lead to audiologic assessment. Abnormalities on examination of cranial nerves IX–XII raise the differential diagnosis of multiple cranial neuropathies such as collagen vascular disease, tumors of the base of the skull, and nasopharyngeal carcinoma.

Ocular Motor Examination

The presence of spontaneous or induced nystagmus is of crucial importance in making a diagnosis of peripheral, central, or systemic causes of imbalance. The patient should be evaluated for the presence of strabismus as this may be a relatively nonspecific cause of dizziness and intermittent diplopia. Some types of nystagmus that are of particular importance are described next. Failure of vertical gaze, particularly in a downward direction, may be the first sign of disequilibration due to progressive supranuclear palsy. The presence of asymmetrical slowing of the adducting eye may be a subtle but important clue to the presence of brain stem multiple sclerosis, brain stem infarction, or mass lesion of the posterior fossa.

Motor System Examination

Motor system examination may reveal focal or diffuse weakness indicative of CNS or neuromuscular disorders. A subtle hemiparesis may be the true cause of the patient's balance complaint. Diffuse hyperreflexia may reflect cerebral or spinal cord dysfunction and, in combination with cerebellar abnormality, may lead to the diagnosis of a spinocerebellar degeneration.

Sensory Examination

Sensory examination may reveal a significant peripheral neuropathy leading to a diagnosis of diabetes or toxic neuropathy. Selective loss of sensory modalities conveyed by the posterior column such as proprioception and vibration may indicate that the patient has vitamin B deficiency or early tabes dorsalis. Such patients may be relatively steady during the Romberg test with eyes open but rapidly lose balance and fall in any direction when visual compensation is eliminated by eye closure. Patients with symptomatic peripheral vestibulopathy tend to fall toward the side of the abnormality during eye closure with the head straight ahead.

Cerebellar System Examination

Clear limb or body ataxia should be an immediate clue to the CNS abnormality as the cause for the patient's imbalance. Unsteadiness during Romberg testing with eyes open and only slight exaggeration on eye closure indicates a cerebellar abnormality. It is usually accompanied by a definite abnormality during gait testing or even difficulty maintaining balance while seated. Unilateral limb ataxia is almost always an indicator of focal posterior fossa abnormality, such as infarct, demyelination, abscess, or tumor.

Directed Neuro-Otological Examination

A directed neuro-otological examination should be performed, particularly when there are abnormalities of the auditory, ocular motor, and vestibular systems. Audiometric testing is discussed in Chapter 19. During the neurological examination, there may be subtle signs of peripheral vestibular dysfunction indicated by nystagmus. During the funduscopic examination, particular attention should be paid to the movement of the optic disc. A rhythmical subtle horizontal slow and fast component is frequently present in patients with new peripheral vestibular dysfunction. This is brought out by reducing fixation during the funduscopic examination. For example, with the patient staring at a dimly lit target in the distance, the presence of a slow ocular drift to the left and a fast phase to the right of the optic disc should indicate to the examiner that the patient has a subtle left-beating nystagmus in the primary position. This indicates a right peripheral vestibular abnormality. One may also occlude the opposite eye during funduscopic examination to determine whether this brings out a subtle nystagmus in the absence of any fixation. Vertical drifts of the optic disc seen during funduscopy may signify the presence of vertical nystagmus, directing the examiner to search for the presence of nystagmus during upward, downward, and oblique gaze.

The need to search for the presence of any type of nystagmus during the directed neuro-otological examination cannot be overemphasized. All too often there is unnecessary dependence on the results of electronystagmographic testing. The directed neuro-otological examination should include a detailed otoscopic examination of the external auditory canal and the tympanic membrane. The presence of a retracted or scarred eardrum may be the clue to prior middle ear infection. The presence of a blue mass behind the tympanic membrane points to a glomus jugulare tumor.

The patient should be tested for balance during standing, walking, and turning, and for the presence of past-pointing—that is, a tendency for the repetitively elevated and lowered outstretched fingers to drift unidirectionally. Past-pointing is a clear indication of tonic imbalance in the vestibular system.

The physician may also clinically test for the presence of an intact vestibulo-ocular reflex (VOR) and may observe whether the patient is able to maintain steady ocular fixation during funduscopic examination as the head is gently rotated from side to side (Sharpe and Barber 1993). The patient with an intact VOR can still maintain fixation on distant objects during head turn. The absence of this ability produces an apparent nystagmus, most easily observed during funduscopic examination, which is good evidence for a defective VOR. A different test of vestibulo-ocular control is for the patient to fix on his or her own thumb while rotating the head in the same direction. During this maneuver, the patient must suppress the vestibulo-ocular response to permit combined head and eye tracking. The loss of this ability may be a subtle clue to cerebellar system dysfunction. The patient should also be examined for the presence of nystagmus when visual fixation is reduced by the wearing of Frenzel glasses, which blur the patient's vision and also magnify the eyes, thereby allowing the examiner to observe previously undetected nystagmus.

INVESTIGATIONS

Screening Tests

Patients with undiagnosed vertigo should have metabolic screening tests including blood count, electrolytes, glucose, erythrocyte sedimentation rate, thyroid function testing, and possibly a rheumatologic battery. Many physicians involved in the evaluation of dizzy patients also perform lipid screens for the presence of hypercholesterolemia or increased triglycerides. The laboratory investigation, like the physical examination, is directed particularly by the patient's history. If there is a history of presyncope or syncope, the patient must have a cardiac evaluation to include at least an electrocardiogram and rhythm strip. A more suggestive history would lead to a Holter 24-hour monitor or an event monitor, during which the patient wears a battery-powered apparatus that can be activated at times of symptoms. This device then records the cardiac rhythm. The presence of auditory symptoms requires complete audiometric tests as described in Chapter 19. Multiple or recurrent cranial neuropathy would lead to a variety of screening tests for collagen vascular disease or basal skull or meningitic processes.

Vestibular Tests

Vestibular testing may be divided into categories such as standard electronystagmographic testing, specific ocular

Table 18.6: Differential diagnosis of dizziness attacks

Single	*Recurrent*	*Chronic Disequilibration*
Acute peripheral vestibulopathy	Peripheral vestibulopathy	Uncompensated peripheral vestibulopathy
Trauma	Benign positional paroxysmal vertigo	Cerebellopontine tumor
Perilymph fistula	Ménière's syndrome	Multiple sclerosis
Air travel	Vertebrobasilar ischemia	Brain stem infarct
Ramsey Hunt syndrome	Migraine	Drugs
Syncope and presyncope	Complex partial seizure	Ototoxicity
	Familial periodic ataxia	Chronic otomastoiditis
		Autonomic neuropathy
		Multiple sensory deficits
		Arteritis
		Cogan's syndrome

motor testing, rotational tests, and posturography. Each test is reviewed briefly in Chapter 44.

DIAGNOSTIC FORMULATIONS

A set of symptoms, findings, and the results of investigations that would lead to a tentative diagnosis in each of the major categories of vestibular disorders presented here is briefly discussed below.

Peripheral Vestibulopathy

A patient who complains of episodic spinning vertigo, with or without auditory symptoms, whose neurological examination is entirely normal and who has evidence of reduced vestibular function in one ear on caloric testing, should initially be placed in this diagnostic category. Such patients often respond to vestibular suppressant medication early in the course and, thereafter, to vestibular exercises. Peripheral vestibulopathy of idiopathic, infectious, or post-traumatic origin is one of the most common causes of a single attack of vertigo (Table 18.6).

Central Vestibular Disorders

Patients with central vestibular disorders usually have vague descriptions of their symptomatology; they do not describe true spinning vertigo or symptoms evoked by position change (but see Table 18.3), and they have abnormalities such as nystagmus or hyper-reflexia on physical examination. These patients are candidates for additional neurological diagnostic investigations. If there is a history of alteration of consciousness, one may consider a rare presentation for temporal lobe seizures, and perform an EEG and MRI. The presence of progressive hearing loss or central auditory findings during audiometric testing leads to suspicion of a cerebellopontine angle tumor and the appropriate neuroradiological investigations. However, when faced with a patient with chronic vestibular symptoms, even including episodic imbalance, with failure to respond to medical therapy, neuroradiological investigation should be carried out even in the presence of a completely normal neurological examination. Such patients may have unsuspected multiple cerebral and brain stem infarctions or may be experiencing the late-life onset of multiple sclerosis. Central vestibular disorders, including uncompensated peripheral vestibulopathy, are among the most common causes of chronic dizziness. There is considerable overlap in the conditions causing single recurrent or chronic attacks of dizziness (see Table 18.6).

Systemic Conditions

Alteration in vestibular function may be suspected in patients taking multiple drugs used to lessen their vertiginous symptoms. In fact, the drugs often initially used to treat such patients, such as benzodiazepines, may later give rise to systemic effects, including imbalance. The patient's symptoms are usually much less clear, but often present as symptoms of disequilibration or imbalance rather than dizziness. The description of lightheadedness particularly suggests this category of disease and may prompt a more detailed search for postural hypotension occurring minutes after rising or a search for cardiac dysrhythmia as described earlier. Such patients deserve a complete metabolic workup and, frequently, repeated consultation with other specialists such as cardiologists. Syncope and presyncope are listed as a cause of a single attack of dizziness, but recurrent episodes are common.

REFERENCES

Baloh RW. Dizziness, Hearing Loss and Tinnitus: The Essentials of Neuro-Otology. Philadelphia: FA Davis, 1984.

Baloh RW, Honrubia V. Clinical Neurophysiology of the Vestibular System (2nd ed). Philadelphia: FA Davis, 1990.

Baloh RW, Honrubia V, Jacobson K. Benign positional vertigo: clinical and oculographic features in 240 cases. Neurology 1987;37:371–378.

Barber HO, Sharpe JA. Vestibular Disorders. Chicago: Year Book, 1988.

Brandt T. Vertigo: Its Multisensory Syndromes. London: Springer-Verlag, 1991.

Caplan LR. Stroke: A Clinical Approach (2nd ed). Boston: Butterworth-Heinemann, 1993.

Daroff RB, Troost BT, Dell'Osso LF. Nystagmus and Other Ocular Oscillations. In JS Glaser (ed), Neuro-Ophthalmology. Hagerstown, MD: Harper & Row, 1987;219–240.

Dohrmann ML, Cheitlin MD. Cardiogenic Syncope: Seizure Versus Syncope. In RJ Porter, WH Theodore (eds), Neurologic Clinics. Philadelphia: Saunders, 1986;549–562.

Epley JM. The canalith repositioning procedure: for treatment of benign paroxysmal positional vertigo. Otolaryngol Head Neck Surg 1992;107:399–404.

Froehling DA, Silverstein MD, Mohr DN, Beatty CW. Does this dizzy patient have a serious form of vertigo? JAMA 1994;271:385–388.

Grad A, Baloh RW. Vertigo of vascular origin. Clinical and electronystagmographic features in 84 patients. Arch Neurol 1989;46:281–284.

Leigh RJ, Zee DS. The Neurology of Eye Movements (2nd ed). Philadelphia: FA Davis, 1991.

Oas JG, Baloh RW. Vertigo and the anterior inferior cerebellar artery syndrome. Neurology 1992;42:2274–2279.

Parnes LS, Price-Jones RG. Particle repositioning maneuver for benign paroxysmal positional vertigo. Ann Otol Rhinol Laryngol 1993;102:325–331.

Sharpe JA, Barber HO. The Vestibulo-Ocular Reflex and Vertigo. New York: Raven, 1993.

Troost BT. Nystagmus: a clinical review. Rev Neurol (Paris) 1989;145:417–428.

Troost BT, Patton JM. Exercise therapy for positional vertigo. Neurology 1992;42:1441–1444.

Vollertsen RS, McDonald TJ, Younge BR et al. Cogan's syndrome: 18 cases and a review of the literature. Mayo Clin Proc 1986;61:344–361.

Chapter 19
Hearing Loss and Tinnitus Without Dizziness or Vertigo

B. Todd Troost and Melissa A. Waller

This chapter describes hearing loss and tinnitus *without* dizziness; dizziness *with* vertigo is described in Chapter 18.

The diagnosis and management of patients with hearing disorders is the responsibility of a variety of specialists, including the audiologist, the otolaryngologist, and occasionally the neurologist. Each may view the problem from a different perspective, but all should work in concert to increase the likelihood of the best possible care. Most neurologists' knowledge of hearing disorders is fragmentary. The purpose of this chapter is to provide basic information for the neurologist to gain an understanding of the approach to a patient with hearing loss or tinnitus.

HEARING LOSS

In the assessment of hearing impairment, one must remember that a dysfunction of the auditory system may be one manifestation of a systemic and possibly life-threatening disorder. Therefore, the examiner, in addition to obtaining a history of the past, present, and familial audiological and otologic complaints, must elicit a history of complaints referable to other systems. The first few minutes spent talking with the patient or relatives will help define the direction the inquiry should take and how detailed the history must be. The examination of the patient, the complaints, and the preliminary audiological findings determine how inclusive the examination must be and what subsequent tests must be ordered. Be aware that audiological tests do not always provide an exact diagnosis. Not only should the results from the audiological test battery be integrated, but these data should be used with the neurological, otoneurological, and radiological information for the maximum diagnostic accuracy.

Types of Hearing Loss

Hearing loss can result from a lesion anywhere within the auditory system (Nadol 1993). An abnormality within the outer or middle ear will create a *conductive* loss of hearing due to an inefficient transmission of sound to the inner ear system. When the loss of hearing is due to pathology in the cochlea or along the eighth cranial nerve from the inner ear to the brain stem, the loss is referred to as a *sensorineural* hearing loss. Patients may exhibit both conductive and sensorineural loss, which is referred to as a *mixed* hearing loss.

Central hearing loss (or central auditory dysfunction) is present when a lesion exists in the central auditory pathway beyond the eighth cranial nerve—for instance, in the cochlear nucleus in the pons or in the primary or association auditory cortex of the temporal lobe.

In addition to these organic types of hearing loss, one should also consider *functional hearing loss*. The diagnosis of functional hearing loss is made when an individual claims to have a hearing loss, but discrepancies in objective test measures or behavior suggest that the loss does not exist, or does not exist to the degree indicated by the test results.

Examination

A number of audiological tests provide differential information on the function of an auditory system. On this basis, various tests have been grouped to form test batteries. One such grouping can be used to differentiate conductive from sensorineural impairments and may further help in localizing a sensorineural loss to either the cochlea or the eighth cranial nerve. Other tests are used to examine auditory deficits of the central auditory system (Benjamin and Troost 1988). Still another set of tests is designed to detect functional or nonorganic hearing disorders. Although the results from these batteries may be helpful in establishing a diagnosis, differential auditory measures cannot be used to establish the *disease process* in auditory disorders. The findings from any audiological study must be integrated with the results from history-taking, physical examination, and laboratory tests.

Basic Office Examination of Hearing

Whether or not the patient's complaint is one of hearing loss, a basic assessment of auditory function should be part of the neurological examination. The external ear should be inspected with an otoscope to determine the patency of the external ear canal and the integrity of the tympanic membrane. If the external canal is occluded by cerumen, simple tests of hearing may be invalidated. The cerumen should be removed, if possible, with warm water lavage using a syringe with a 5- to 8-cm piece of rubber tubing affixed to the end to avoid injury to the ear. If water lavage has not removed impacted cerumen, a neurologist should refer the patient to an otolaryngologist for removal.

Assuming there is no cerumen in the external ear canal, the tympanic membrane should be inspected. The neurologist should be able to recognize an inflamed, bulging, or scarred drum, and should note whether there is perforation of the tympanic membrane; blood behind the eardrum; or a pulsating blue mass, which may be indicative of a glomus jugulare tumor. An excellent description of tympanic membrane findings may be found in modern texts of otology (Hughes 1985; Baloh 1984). At times it may be helpful to inspect the mobility of the eardrum by increasing pressure within the external canal, using a hand-held pneumatic bulb attached by tubing to an outlet in the otoscope. Little or no mobility of the tympanic membrane suggests fluid or a mass behind the drum, or a fixed ossicular chain.

The office examination of hearing loss may include tuning fork tests of air and bone conduction. Tuning forks at a frequency of 256 or 128 Hz should not be used due to the vibrations they produce by bone conduction, which the patient may mistake for sound; the 512 Hz is the lowest useful frequency. Two standard tuning fork tests are the Weber and Rinne tests.

Weber Test

The Weber test is based on the principle that the signal, when transmitted by bone conduction, will be localized to the better-hearing ear or the ear with the greatest conductive deficit. The test can determine the type of hearing impairment when the two ears are affected to different degrees. The stem of a vibrating tuning fork is placed on the skull in the midline, and the patient is asked to indicate in which ear the sound is heard. The usual location described is for placement on the forehead, but better locations are the nasal bones or teeth when a stronger bone conduction stimulus is required. In unilateral hearing losses, lateralization to the poorer-hearing ear indicates an element of conductive impairment in that ear. Lateralization to the better-hearing ear suggests that the problem in the opposite ear is sensorineural.

Rinne Test

The Rinne test is probably the most commonly used tuning fork test, but the name is usually mispronounced; the origination was German, not French, and the name is accentuated on the *first* syllable (Rin'neh). The Rinne test is a comparison of the patient's hearing sensitivity by bone conduction versus air conduction. A normal individual will perceive the air-conducted sound as louder or the same as bone-conducted sound. Proper placement of the tuning fork in each situation is important. When testing by bone conduction, the stem fork should be placed firmly on the mastoid, as near to the posterosuperior edge of the ear canal as possible. The stem should not touch the auricle of the external canal, which should be held to the side by the examiner's fingers. Touching the external ear itself could give false results due to vibration of the auricle. When testing by air conduction, the fork is held about 2.5 cm lateral to the tragus. In the Rinne test, when the conduction mechanism is normal in an ear (that is, in individuals with normal hearing and in those with sensorineural hearing impairment), air conduction will be heard better than bone conduction as it is a more efficient means of sound transmission. This finding is termed a *positive Rinne*. Bone conduction will be heard better than air conduction when there is a deficit in the conduction mechanism; this is referred to as a *negative Rinne*. A conductive deficit of more than 15 db reverses the tuning fork responses (that is, bone conduction is better than air conduction) at 512 Hz. When testing by bone conduction, the examiner should not forget to have the patient remove his or her eyeglasses: the earpiece can interfere with proper placement of the stem of the tuning fork or give inappropriate conduction or vibratory information. Although tuning fork tests allow the examiner to identify a conductive versus a sensorineural loss, and in some cases lateralize the symptomatic ear, it does not evaluate the degree of impairment or the effects of that impairment on speech understanding.

Audiological Assessment

An audiological assessment is comprised of pure-tone air and bone conduction testing, and speech threshold and word discrimination measures. The *threshold* is defined as the lowest intensity (measured in decibels) at which an individual can detect a pure tone or speech signal more than

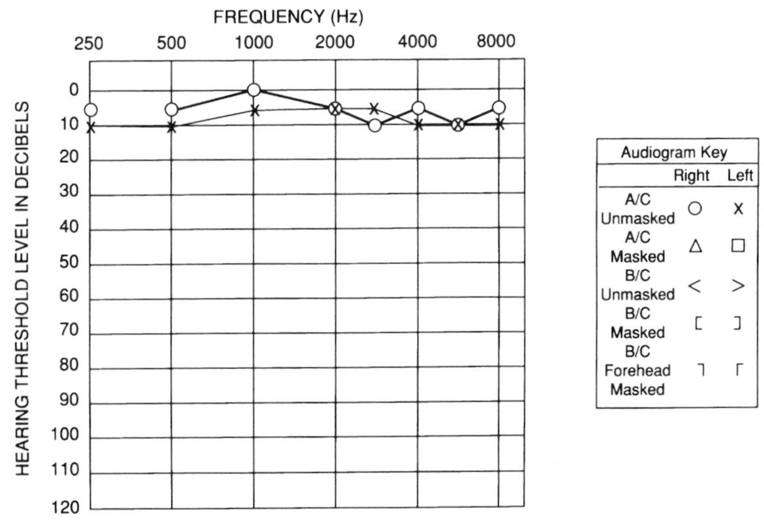

SPEECH TESTS

TESTS		R	L
Sp. Reception Threshold (SRT)		5 db	0 db
Sp. Discrim. Scores	35 db SL	98%	100%

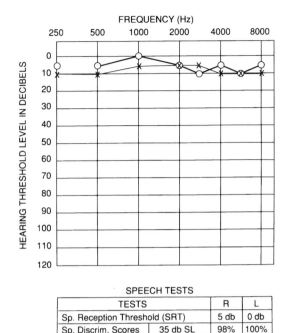

FIGURE 19.1 Normal hearing sensitivity.

50% of the time. Pure-tone air and bone thresholds are established for frequencies of 250–8,000 Hz. This frequency range is important to the detection and understanding of the speech signal. Hearing is considered normal when threshold sensitivity is 0–25 dB for frequencies of 250–8,000 Hz (Figure 19.1). Responses greater than 25 dB are classified by degree as mild, moderate, severe, moderately severe, and profound (Figure 19.2). Responses at 500 Hz, 1,000 Hz, and 2,000 Hz are averaged together to compute the *pure-tone average*.

In the measurement of bone conduction thresholds, pure-tone signals are transmitted via a bone oscillator, usually placed on the mastoid. This signal directly stimulates the cochlea, bypassing the external and middle ear. The presence of decreased air conduction threshold and normal sensitivity of bone conduction suggests abnormality in the external ear or middle ear system and is termed a *conductive hearing loss* (Figure 19.3).

The *speech reception threshold* is the lowest intensity at which an equally weighted two-syllable word is understood approximately 50% of the time. The pure-tone average and speech reception threshold should be within 7 dB of each other. Comparison of the speech reception threshold and the pure-tone average serves as a check on the validity of the pure-tone thresholds. Large discrepancies between these measures may suggest a functional or nonorganic hearing loss.

Speech discrimination is a tool used to assess an individual's ability to understand a speech signal. Most commonly, a phonetically balanced word list of 50 one-syllable words is presented to the patient at a suprathreshold level. The patient's score is represented as the number of words correct. Generally, discrimination ability decreases proportionately with an increase of hearing impairment. However, there is

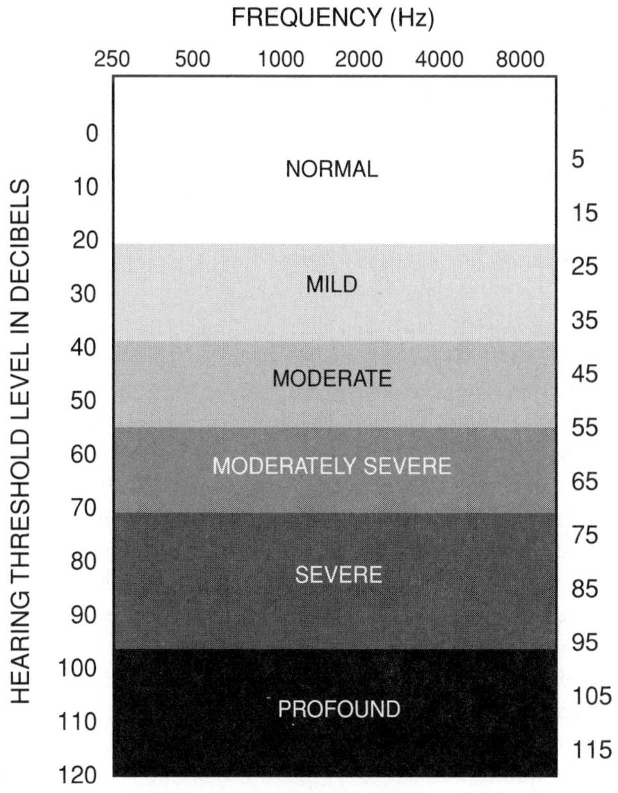

FIGURE 19.2 Classification of degree of hearing loss. (Reprinted with permission from American Speech-Language-Hearing Association. The classification of hearing disorders. Supplement No. 2. Rockville, MD: American Speech-Language-Hearing Association, 1990;25–30.)

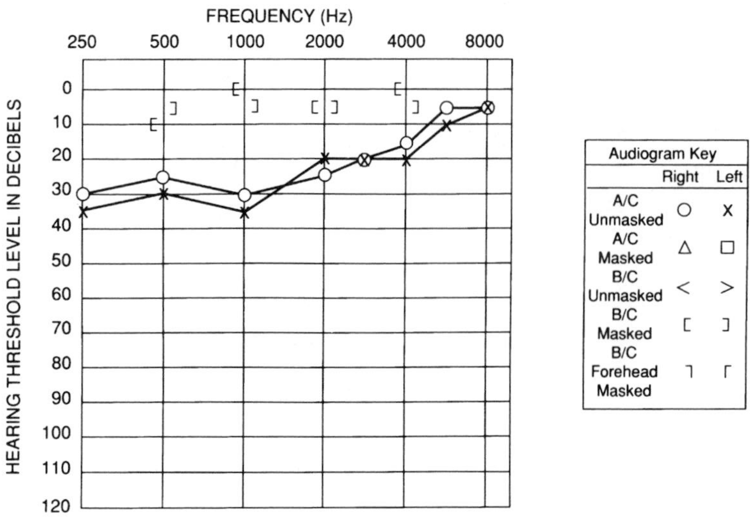

SPEECH TESTS

TESTS		R	L
Sp. Reception Threshold (SRT)		30 db	30 db
Sp. Discrim. Scores	35 db SL	98%	98%

FIGURE 19.3 Pure-tone air and bone conduction findings for a conductive hearing loss.

an exception in conductive hearing loss where discrimination ability remains relatively good because the inner ear system is normal. Poor discrimination ability in the presence of relatively good hearing sensitivity may suggest retrocochlear pathology such as acoustic neuroma and should be aggressively pursued by the clinician (Chapter 44).

Immittance Test Battery

Tympanometry, static acoustic immittance, and *acoustic reflex threshold* measures comprise the acoustic immittance test battery. Tympanometry is a measure of middle ear mobility when air pressure in the external canal is varied. Results are graphically represented with a pressure along the x axis and compliance along the y axis. Normal tympanograms have a pressure peak point of ±50 mm H_2O.

Static compliance refers to the ease of flow of acoustic energy through the middle ear. Immittance measures are obtained at +200 mm H_2O (first point of compliance, or C1) and again at the point the tympanic membrane is most compliant (second point of compliance, C2). The point at which the tympanic membrane is most compliant allows maximum transmission of energy through the middle ear cavity. Immittance of the tympanic membrane is derived by subtracting C1 from C2. Values less than 0.25 cm^3 of equivalent volume indicate a stiff or noncompliant middle ear system. Values greater than 2.0 cm^3 suggest an overly compliant system. Abnormalities associated with reduced mobility of the tympanic membrane in associated middle ear structures include otitis media, otosclerosis, and large cholesteatomas. Ossicular chain discontinuity is the most common cause of excessive tympanic membrane mobility. Examples are shown in Figure 19.4. Extremely high equivalent middle ear volume and low static compliance may suggest tympanic membrane perforation.

The acoustic reflex threshold is the lowest intensity of a pure-tone stimulus needed to elicit a contraction of the stapedius and tensor tympani muscles. The introduction of an intense sound into the ear canal results in a temporary increase in middle ear impedance. This phenomenon occurs bilaterally, but it is typically measured in one ear at a time. Contralateral reflexes are measured by stimulating one ear and measuring the reflex from the other. Ipsilateral reflexes are measured by stimulating and recording from the same ear. Reflexes occur between 70 and 100 dB sound pressure level in normal ears. Middle ear abnormalities or significant sensorineural hearing losses may elevate or obliterate the acoustic reflexes. Retrocochlear pathology and facial nerve disorders may also affect contralateral and ipsilateral acoustic reflexes.

Conductive Hearing Loss

Conductive hearing losses occur with pathology in the outer or middle ear. The bone conduction thresholds are normal, but air conduction results suggest a decrease in hearing sensitivity. The patient with a conductive hearing loss tends to have about the same loss of sensitivity for sounds of all frequencies. Sometimes hearing is better for the higher frequencies than it is for the lower ones, and occasionally the reverse may be true, but by and large the loss pattern is relatively flat across the frequencies (see Figure 19.3). Another symptom of conductive loss is that speech discrimination is relatively unimpaired. A patient with a

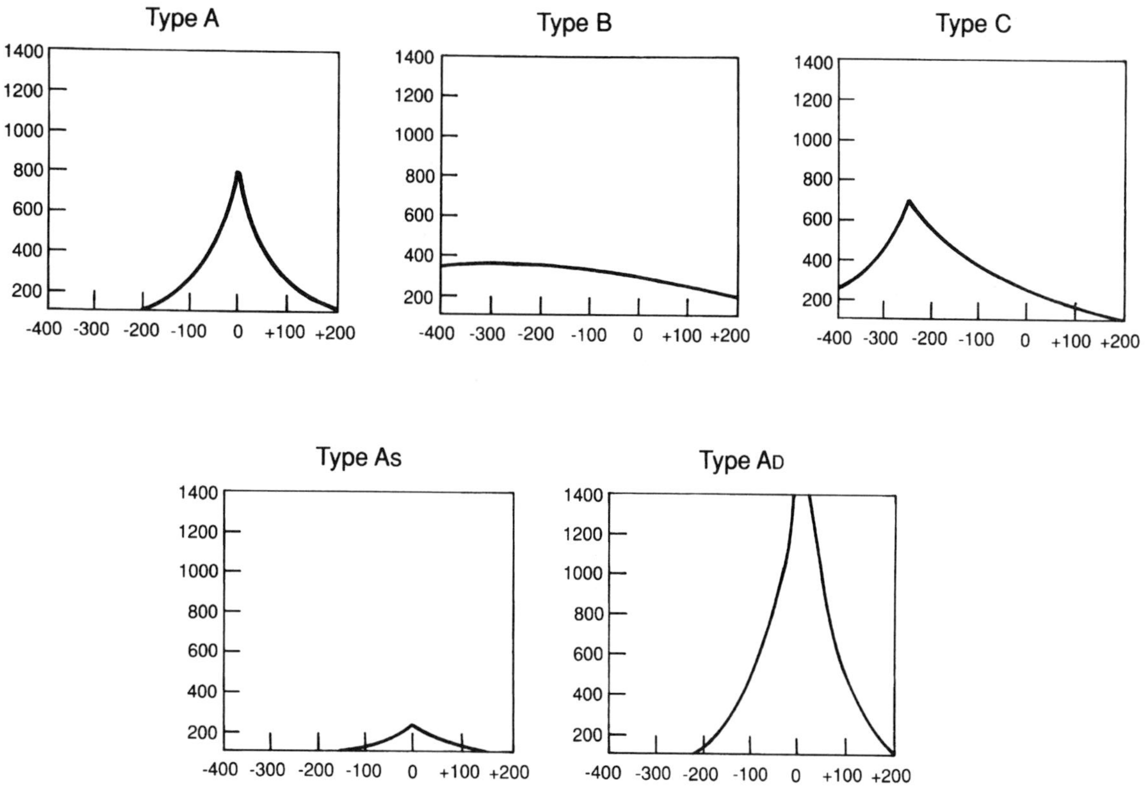

FIGURE 19.4 Representative impedance measures by tympanogram. *Type A* represents normal middle ear function. Type A curves have normal mobility and pressures and typify normal hearing and sensorineural hearing loss with normally functioning middle ear systems. *Type B* represents restricted tympanic membrane mobility. Type B curves have little or no point of maximum mobility and reduced compliance. This curve is very typical of a stiff middle ear system as is seen in otitis media. *Type C* represents significant negative pressure in the middle ear cavity. Type C curves have normal mobility and negative pressure at the point of maximum mobility (negative pressure is considered significant for treatment when more negative than –200 mm H_2O). *Type As* represents normal middle ear pressure but reduced mobility, suggesting limited mobility of the tympanic membrane and middle ear structure, commonly seen in fixation of the ossicular chain. *Type Ad* represents normal middle ear pressure but hypermobility. This pattern is indicative of a flaccid tympanic membrane due to disarticulation of the ossicular chain or partial atrophy of the eardrum.

conductive loss has good discrimination ability provided the speech is made loud enough.

Frequently, the patient with a conductive loss of hearing complains of tinnitus, which may be localized in one ear, in both ears, or unlocalized in the head. In the case of a conductive impairment, the tinnitus tends to be of relatively low pitch.

Sensorineural Loss

Sensorineural loss occurs with pathology in the inner ear or along the nerve pathway from the inner ear to the brain stem. Hearing loss from cochlear disorders alone is termed *sensory loss*. As mentioned in Chapter 44, there is some disagreement among audiologists, neurologists, and otologists over what is a *retrocochlear* and what is a *central problem*. For the purposes of this discussion, we will define *retrocochlear* as an abnormality between the cochlea and the brain stem (see below).

The term *sensorineural* includes both cochlear and retrocochlear disorders. A pure sensorineural impairment exists when the sound-conducting mechanism (outer and middle ear) is normal in every respect but a disorder is present in the cochlea or auditory nerve. Sensorineural impairment can be congenital or acquired. Congenital sensorineural hearing loss may result from hereditary factors that cause underdevelopment or early degeneration in the auditory nerve, from in utero viral infections, or from birth trauma. Acquired sensorineural hearing loss may be caused by noise exposure, acoustic tumor, head injury, infection, toxic drug effects, vascular disease, or presbycusis.

The patient with a sensorineural impairment may speak with excessive loudness of voice in situations where a loud voice is inappropriate. The configuration of the audiogram demonstrating a sensorineural hearing loss may vary sig-

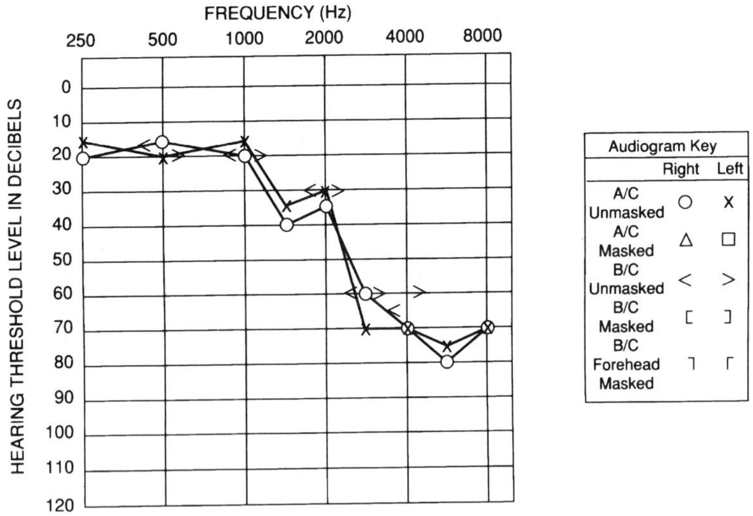

SPEECH TESTS

TESTS		R	L
Sp. Reception Threshold (SRT)		25 db	25 db
Sp. Discrim. Scores	35 db SL	72%	76%

FIGURE 19.5 Pure-tone air and bone conduction findings for a sensorineural hearing loss.

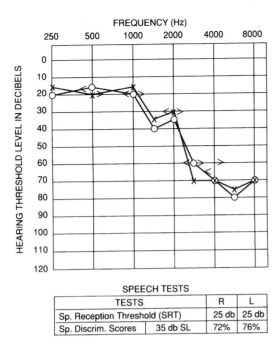

nificantly and in some instances may suggest the etiology of the loss. Many people with sensorineural losses experience a hearing loss only in the high-frequency region. These individuals have no difficulty understanding speech at normal intensities in a quiet environment since their low-frequency hearing is unimpaired. However, they do experience difficulty in understanding speech in a noisy environment. Generally, the low frequencies are defined as the range of 250–750 Hz, the middle frequencies as 1,000–2,000 Hz, and the high frequencies as 3,000–8,000 Hz on the standard audiogram.

Loudness recruitment is usually associated with sensory loss of cochlear origin, which constitutes the majority of sensorineural losses. *Recruitment* is an abnormally rapid growth of loudness with an increase in intensity (Sanders 1984). The recruiting patient with sensory loss will not hear low-intensity sounds at all and may just barely hear sounds of moderate intensity, but the recruitment of loudness may cause intense sounds to be perceived as uncomfortably loud. This disruption of normal loudness function may be painful to the individual and require the use of special circuitry should the patient pursue hearing aid use.

The patient with sensorineural hearing loss is usually subject to tinnitus of a somewhat different sort from that associated with conductive hearing loss. Generally, the patient with sensorineural loss reports a constant ringing or buzzing noise, which may be localized in either ear or may not be localized. In general, the pitch of tinnitus tends to be higher in sensorineural impairment than in conductive impairment.

In sensorineural loss, the audiometric Weber test is expected to lateralize to the better ear. Audiometrically, sensorineural loss is characterized by overlapping air and bone conduction thresholds. The tympanogram is typically normal, and acoustic reflexes may be present, elevated, or absent (Chapter 44). The audiometric findings for a typical sensorineural hearing loss are displayed in Figure 19.5.

Contrary to a commonly held misconception, sensorineural hearing loss may be helped by the use of a hearing aid. Current technology uses full dynamic range compression to significantly increase the effectiveness of amplification.

Mixed Loss

A mixed hearing loss consists of a conductive and a sensorineural component in the same ear. The patient's behavior will reflect attributes of both a conductive and a sensorineural disorder. Causes of mixed hearing loss may be any combination of the conditions described above for conductive and sensorineural hearing loss. The conductive component of the mixed hearing loss may be corrected by successful medical or surgical treatment, but the sensorineural component is not reversible. The pure-tone audiometric pattern for a mixed hearing loss is displayed in Figure 19.6. With a mixed loss, both air and bone conduction thresholds are elevated, but bone conduction thresholds are better than air conduction thresholds. The difference between the two thresholds is referred to as the *air-bone gap* and represents the amount of conductive loss present.

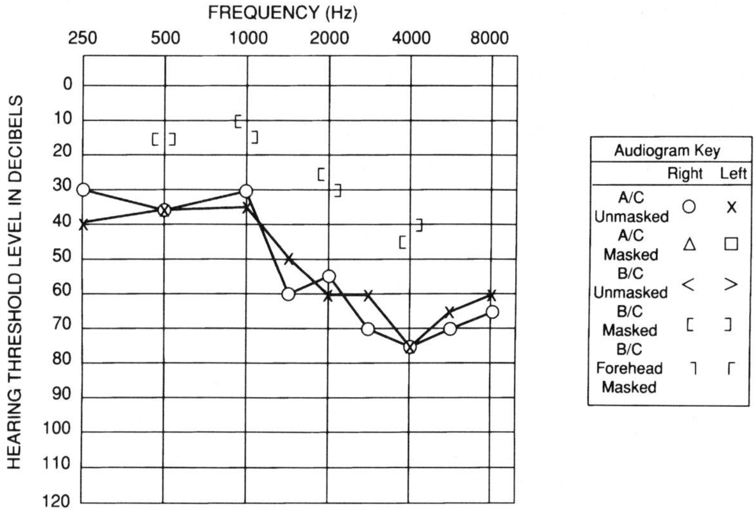

SPEECH TESTS

TESTS		R	L
Sp. Reception Threshold (SRT)		40 db	40 db
Sp. Discrim. Scores	35 db SL	84%	86%

FIGURE 19.6 Pure-tone air and bone conduction findings for a mixed hearing loss.

Sensory Versus Neural Lesions

The problems of differentiating cochlear dysfunction from eighth nerve lesions have received major emphasis during the past several years. In fact, this area has been emphasized to the extent that some audiologists have limited their concept of differential audiology primarily to those tests that assist in localizing the defect within the sensorineural mechanism. The neurologist's interest in sensorineural hearing loss is with regard to the possibility of a cerebellopontine angle tumor. Although many referrals for audiometric evaluation are made for this reason, we must emphasize that even the more sophisticated special auditory tests *cannot determine the specific pathology* underlying the disorder. Similarly, magnetic resonance imaging (MRI) may locate the presence of an abnormality, but it does not necessarily define the nature of the pathology. The audiometric tests, however, highlight patterns of auditory behavior that are generally associated with cochlear or neural involvement.

Routine pure-tone and speech testing can yield valuable information on the site of lesion during the initial phase of the differential audiological study. For example, a pure-tone configuration, which is often seen in patients with a presumptive diagnosis of Ménière's disease (a cochlear disorder), is a unilateral hearing loss most pronounced in the low frequencies. In sharp contrast, patients with eighth nerve lesions frequently present a unilateral hearing impairment most evident in the high frequencies and poor speech discrimination. Although such generalizations may describe a substantial number of cases falling into these two categories, numerous exceptions are encountered with either cochlear or neural pathology.

Central Auditory Disorders

As would be anticipated, lesions within the central auditory system are difficult to detect or localize. In fact, many central auditory dysfunctions will not be demonstrated by conventional audiological measurements. Individuals with known lesions in the central auditory tracts may not manifest any significant hearing loss when tested by conventional pure-tone audiometry (Benjamin and Troost 1988). Total removal of one hemisphere of the brain in humans has not resulted in any major change of auditory sensitivity in either ear. Measures, such as tone decay, acoustic reflex measures, acoustic reflex decay, and speech discrimination at high intensity levels, must be used to distinguish between eighth nerve, extraaxial, and intraaxial brain stem dysfunction. The auditory evoked response and MRI (see Chapter 44) are also very useful in making such a differentiation.

TINNITUS

Ear and head noises, the most common complaints presented to the audiologist or otolaryngologist, are frequently seen by the neurologist as well. As many as 32% of the adult population has tinnitus, with 20% of the population rating their condition as severe (Vernon 1984). Tinnitus may be considered a significant symptom when its intensity so overrides normal environmental sounds that it invades the consciousness. The patient experiencing tinnitus may describe the sound as ringing, roaring, hissing, whistling, chirping, rustling, clicking, or buzzing, among others. Although most patients report the presence of tinnitus to be constant, others report it to be intermittent, fluctuating, or pulsating. Tinnitus may be perceived as a high- or low-pitched tone, a band of noise, or some combination of such sounds.

The perceived loudness of tinnitus in any patient may be intense enough to be highly debilitating. Most patients with sensorineural hearing loss report tinnitus to be a high-frequency tone, but tinnitus associated with conductive hearing loss tends to be low in frequency. In sensorineural loss, the pitch of the tinnitus is usually located in the region of the maximum hearing loss. However, knowledge of the pitch of the tinnitus is of little diagnostic benefit other than allowing for the gross dichotomy of conductive versus neural pathology.

The majority of tinnitus sufferers have a concomitant loss of hearing, which may be either conductive or sensorineural. Vernon (1984) reported that no more than 8% of tinnitus patients have audiometrically normal hearing sensitivity. Tinnitus may precede or follow the onset of a loss in hearing, or the two may occur simultaneously.

Tinnitus is a symptom of an underlying disease or specific lesion when it is perceived above the intensity levels of environmental sounds. Tinnitus may be the first symptom that brings the patient to a neurologist. It may, for example, be an early symptom of a tumor in the internal auditory meatus or in the cerebellopontine angle, a glomus tumor, or a vascular abnormality in the temporal bone or skull. Because tinnitus may be a characteristic symptom of a number of disorders, a complete medical and audiological evaluation of the tinnitus sufferer is an important initial step in the management process.

Classification

Subjective tinnitus is an auditory sensation heard only by the patient. It may be present in one or both ears or localized within the head. For most patients, tinnitus is a subjective sensation. This type of tinnitus can result from a lesion involving the external ear canal, tympanic membrane, ossicles, cochlea, auditory nerve, brain stem, and cortex. The most common cause is cochlear disease. Tinnitus associated with Ménière's syndrome is often low-pitched and continuous and is described as a hollow seashell sound or very loud roaring. Tinnitus with otosclerosis is also low-pitched, is described as a buzzing or roaring sound, and may be continuous or intermittent. Continuous bilateral high-pitched tinnitus often accompanies chronic noise-induced hearing loss, presbycusis, and hearing loss due to ototoxic drugs. A number of drugs, such as aminoglycosides, quinidine, salicylates, indomethacin, carbamazepine, propranolol, levodopa, aminophylline, and caffeine, may produce tinnitus with or without associated hearing loss (Baloh 1984).

Objective tinnitus is less common than subjective tinnitus. It is perceived not only by the patient but also by the examiner. Objective tinnitus may be vascular (an arteriovenous malformation or fistula) or mechanical in origin. Objective mechanical tinnitus is due to abnormal muscular contraction of the nasopharynx or middle ear, as may occur in palatal myoclonus. Objective tinnitus of vascular origin may also be a referred bruit from stenosis in the carotid or vertebrobasilar system.

Tinnitus may be classified as mild, moderate, or severe. *Mild* tinnitus is usually noticed only in quiet environments or at bedtime. It is usually not very disturbing, and the patient can easily be distracted from the tinnitus by other stimuli. *Moderate* tinnitus is more intense and is constantly present; the patient is conscious of the tinnitus when attempting to concentrate or when trying to sleep. *Severe* tinnitus may disable individuals to the extent that they are able to concentrate on little other than the tinnitus itself.

Evaluation and Management

The complete evaluation of the tinnitus patient should be approached from a dual perspective. The patient with tinnitus, regardless of location, type, or severity, must first have a thorough otologic and audiological examination. If there are accompanying symptoms, a complete neurological examination may be appropriate. The patient with an isolated symptom of a persistent, yet unexplained, tinnitus should receive follow-up examinations at definite intervals when initial medical, otologic, and neurological studies reveal no evidence of disease. Tinnitus may be the first symptom of disorder, appearing long before any other symptom, including hearing loss. When medical and otologic examination fails to disclose a *remediable* cause for the tinnitus, or when a diagnosis is ascertained for which no known medical therapy is presently available, the tinnitus patient should undergo further evaluation to determine the most appropriate nonmedical avenue for rehabilitation.

When a specific otologic cause for the tinnitus is identified, then specific otologic management is indicated. When a specific lesion or disease process is not identifiable, however, then tinnitus management is more difficult. Given no underlying otologic disease, there is at present no effective surgery or medical therapy for the treatment of tinnitus.

Research on the effectiveness of pharmacological therapy for tinnitus, although certainly encouraging, involves medications, such as carbamazepine, lidocaine, and intravenous barbiturates, whose potentially serious side effects limit their usefulness. There is some suggestion that relatively low doses may prove effective in tinnitus management.

Masking

The use of masking as a management tool in the treatment of the tinnitus patient has met with mixed success over the years. The audiologist should remain cognizant of factors such as the patient's perception of the pitch and loudness and the overall spectral intensity of the masking signal. The referring neurologist should be aware of these issues as well.

Tinnitus maskers are designed to provide relief to the tinnitus sufferer by introducing an external masking sound into the effected ear or ears, thereby minimizing or eliminating the perception of the tinnitus. Although the use of tinnitus maskers has not proved universally successful, masking is still a feasible technique that cannot be ignored. The actual efficacy of tinnitus maskers in the average tinnitus patient is probably less than 30%. The use of a hearing aid may be beneficial by addressing the primary hearing problem.

Biofeedback

Experience with tinnitus patients has revealed that many of them have relatively high levels of anxiety, tension, or other symptoms of chronic stress. There is a significant correlation between tinnitus and tension. Biofeedback as a treatment in the management of tinnitus was first reported in the literature in the mid-1970s. These early studies reported that biofeedback was effective in the relief of tinnitus or the associated annoyance produced by it. Biofeedback is quite effective for enhancing relaxation, as are traditional relaxation procedures. When used together, muscle tension and general life stresses are reported to be reduced.

Counseling

The need for effective counseling is one important aspect of tinnitus management regardless of the management approaches taken with a given patient. Many patients are frightened by the presence of tinnitus and need a careful and clear explanation of the disorder, coupled with firm reassurance from both the neurologist and the audiologist. In light of the various effects tinnitus may have on a given patient, Tyler and Baker (1983) emphasize that counseling must be directed toward all of the patient's difficulties, not this specific problem in isolation.

REFERENCES

Baloh RW. Dizziness, Hearing Loss and Tinnitus: The Essentials of Neurotology. Philadelphia: FA Davis, 1984.

Benjamin ES, Troost BT. Central Auditory Disorders. In G English (ed), Clinical Otolaryngology. Philadelphia: Harper & Row, 1988.

Hughes GB. Textbook of Clinical Otology. New York: Thieme-Stratton, 1985.

Nadol JB Jr. Hearing loss. N Engl J Med 1993;329:1092–1102.

Sanders JW. Diagnostic Audiology. In JL Northern (ed), Hearing Disorders. Boston: Little, Brown, 1984.

Tyler RS, Baker LJ. Difficulties experienced by tinnitus sufferers. J Speech Hear Disord 1983;48:150–154.

Vernon J. Tinnitus. In JL Northern (ed), Hearing Disorders. Boston: Little, Brown, 1984.

Chapter 20
Disturbances of Taste and Smell

Pasquale F. Finelli and Robert Mair

Taste and smell rely on chemical stimuli to excite their receptors—hence the designation *chemosensory system.* The two modalities are closely related: their combination produces the sensation of flavor, and dysfunction in one is often perceived as an abnormality in the other. Disorders of the chemosensory system, though common, may be ignored by the patient as insignificant or downplayed by the physician who views testing as imprecise, time-consuming, and cumbersome. Nevertheless, accurate diagnosis is essential, as these disorders may herald a serious illness or affect the patient's life in areas of nutrition, satisfaction in eating, personal hygiene, and livelihood (as in the case of chefs, food handlers, and perfumers), while also posing the dangers inherent in the patient's failure to recognize spoiled food or the presence of natural gas and smoke.

OLFACTION

Pathophysiology

In human beings, there are two important nasal chemosensory systems: the free nerve endings of the trigeminal nerve and the sensory receptors of the olfactory system. The free nerve endings of the trigeminal system innervate the walls of the nasal passages and respond nonselectively to a large variety of volatile chemical substances. Human psychophysical studies indicate that stimulation of the trigeminal nerve contributes a sensation of general nasal irritability provoked by high concentrations of most odorants. Olfactory receptors respond to chemical stimuli at lower concentrations and with greater selectivity than do the trigeminal endings and are responsible for the discrimination of different odorous substances. In cases of total anosmia, the capacity to distinguish between odors is lost, while the response to nasal irritation is generally preserved. Thus, cases of malingering occasionally can be exposed by comparing responses to odorants that differ in their propensity to stimulate trigeminal nerve endings.

The olfactory receptor cell is a bipolar sensory neuron having a dendritic knob extending into the mucous lining of the nasal cavity and a thin unmyelinated axon that travels in bundles through the cribriform plate into the olfactory bulb (Figure 20.1). The dendritic knobs bear cilia wherein odorant transduction occurs. Receptor responses are eliminated when cilia are removed by chemical treatment but are restored as cilia subsequently grow back on surviving dendritic knobs. The receptor neurons have a limited life span, averaging 30 days, and are replaced by newly formed cells that differentiate as they migrate from the basement membrane toward the surface of the sensory epithelium. The plasticity of the receptor neuron is clinically important for two reasons: (1) treatments that affect cell division (radiation, antiproliferative agents) can disrupt olfactory receptor function by interfering with the replacement of degenerative neurons; and (2) under some circumstances, receptor function can be restored by tissue regeneration. Ciliary regrowth occurs within days, but months are required for neural regeneration.

The axons of the first cranial nerve terminate within the glomeruli of the olfactory bulb, where they form synaptic contacts with interneurons that have processes restricted to the bulb and with output neurons (mitral and internal tufted cells) that contribute axons to the lateral olfactory tract. The first cranial nerve is potentially important as a pathway for environmental toxins or viruses to enter the brain. The olfactory bulb provides a direct pathway from the periphery to important cholinergic and adrenergic systems implicated in the etiology of dementing diseases.

Axons of the olfactory tract terminate in primitive cortical areas collectively known as the *primary olfactory cortex.* In humans, this probably includes small portions of the uncus, hippocampal gyrus, amygdaloid complex, and entorhinal cortex. Olfactory auras have been ascribed to activation of the uncus or amygdala by seizures or electrical stimulation. Likewise, temporal lobectomy may impair olfactory discrimination and identification, as well as performance on the University of Pennsylvania Smell Identification Test (UPSIT), sometimes without affecting absolute olfactory sensitivity.

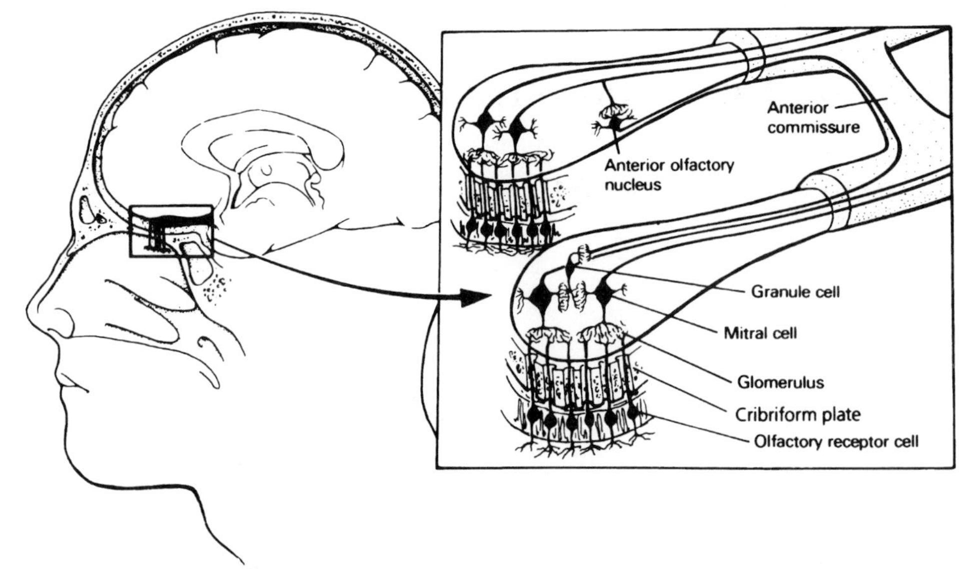

FIGURE 20.1 Olfactory nerve and bulb connections. Within the glomerulus, the olfactory receptor neuron terminals make synaptic contacts onto the dendritic branches of the mitral cells. Deep within these layers are the granule cells, whose main dendrites make synaptic contact with the secondary dendrites of the mitral cell. The mitral cells project axonal branches to the anterior olfactory nucleus, which is made up of cells in the posterior olfactory bulb. The pyramidal cells of the anterior olfactory nucleus project their main axons, after passing through the anterior commissure, to synapse with the granule cells in the contralateral olfactory bulb. The output of the bulb is carried by the axons of the mitral cells via the olfactory tract and the olfactory striae to the primary olfactory cortex. (Adapted from D Ottoson. Physiology of the Nervous System. Oxford, England: Oxford University Press, 1983.)

Clinical Evaluation of Smell

Olfactory discrimination can be disrupted by (1) nasal obstructions that prevent volatile substances from reaching the receptor epithelium (transport olfactory loss); (2) impairment of receptor or olfactory nerve function (sensory olfactory loss); and (3) pathological processes affecting central pathways from bulb to primary olfactory cortex, medial dorsal thalamic nucleus, and orbitofrontal neocortex (neural olfactory loss). The latter two processes are designated *neurogenic.*

A primary objective in assessing impaired sense of smell is to distinguish an intranasal from a neurogenic cause. Transport olfactory loss can be produced by viral upper respiratory infection, rhinitis, sinusitis, polyps, neoplasms, and abnormalities in mucus secretion. There is loss or decreased ability to detect odors (anosmia or hyposmia), distortions of normal smells (parosmia or dysosmia), increased sensitivity to some or all odorants (hyperosmia), or impaired ability to discriminate among different odors. Sensory olfactory loss produces similar symptoms and is caused by direct olfactory nerve damage (closed-head injury, viral infection, toxic substances) or impairment of normal receptor cell turnover (radiation or antiproliferative drug therapy). Neural olfactory loss can impair discrimination without producing anosmia.

Unilateral loss of smell is not recognized by the patient and, when found on examination, can be a useful sign of a neurogenic lesion. Such patients or those complaining of loss of smell should be asked about a history of head trauma, recent upper respiratory tract infection, drug use (both prescribed and abused), systemic illness, occupational exposure to toxins, dental procedures and prostheses, smoking and alcohol history, seizure disorder, radiation therapy, and pending litigation (loss of smell is a compensatable disorder). System review should include headache, visual changes, nosebleeds, nasal obstruction, menstrual history, decline in intellectual capacity, and psychiatric disturbances including mood changes such as depression. Physical examination, in addition to taste and smell testing, should carefully evaluate the ears, nose, mouth, oronasopharynx, and cranial nerves (specifically, decreased visual acuity, impaired color vision, papilledema, optic atrophy, and ocular motility abnormality). Mental status evaluation for evidence of dementia and depression is important.

In clinical practice, examination of odor discrimination or identification is sufficient to screen for deficits in transport, sensory, and neural olfactory functions. Traditionally, the sense of smell is tested by having the patient sniff a familiar odoriferous substance (small bottle of coffee, oil of cloves, oil of peppermint) held in turn beneath each nostril while the other is occluded by a finger. Suggestion is minimized by having the patient keep the eyes closed and indicating that the bottle may or may not have anything in it. If the patient detects an odor, he or she is then asked to identify the smell. Appreciation of an odor, despite the inability to name it, excludes anosmia. Hysterical patients may demonstrate unilateral anosmia on the side of an alleged neurological deficit. A

Table 20.1: Smell and taste dysfunction

- **Tumors**
  - Intracranial
    - Meningioma, olfactory groove S
    - Glioma
      - Frontal lobe S
      - Temporal lobe S
      - Cerebellum Ti
      - Pituitary S
      - Metastatic S
    - Intranasal
      - Papilloma S
      - Adenoma S
      - Squamous cell carcinoma S
      - Esthesioneuroepithelioma S
  - Systemic cancer T
  - Cholesteoatoma T
  - Jugular foramen T
- **Vascular**
  - Aneurysm, anterior cerebral S
  - Aneurysm, anterior communicating S
  - Subarachnoid hemorrhage S
  - Hemorrhage, pontine T
- **Infections, inflammation, granulomatous**
  - Encephalitis, viral S,T
  - Idiopathic midline granuloma S,T
  - Syphilis S
  - Meningitis S
  - Coryza S
  - Rhinitis, allergic-bacterial S
  - Sinusitis S
  - Bronchial asthma S
  - Ozena S,P
  - Hepatitis, acute viral S
  - Influenza S,T
  - Sjögren's syndrome S,T
  - Leprosy S
  - Sarcoid S
  - Dengue fever S
  - Gingivitis T
  - Periodontitis T
  - Sialadenitis T
  - Glossitis, bacterial-fungal T
  - Middle ear infection T
- **Systemic illness**
  - Diabetes mellitus S,T
  - Refsum's disease S
  - Paget's disease S
  - Pseudohypoparathyroidism S,T
  - Cystic fibrosis S,T
  - Adrenal insufficiency T
  - Cirrhosis S,T
  - Thermal burns T
  - Renal failure S,T
  - Familial dysautonomia T
  - Congenital adrenal hyperplasia T
  - Panhypopituitarism T
  - Hypertension T
  - Cushing's syndrome S,T
  - Hypothyroidism S,T
  - Gonadal dysgenesis (Turner's syndrome) S,T
  - Primary amenorrhea S
  - Korsakoff's psychosis Ds
  - Alcohol withdrawal OH
  - Cretinism T
  - Temporal arteritis S,T
  - Granulomatous angiitis S
- **Traumatic**
  - Olfactory nerve, olfactory bulb S,T,P
  - Chorda tympani nerve T
  - Lingual nerve T
  - Glossopharyngeal nerve T
  - Cerebral cortex S,T,Ds
- **Epileptic**
  - Uncinate seizures OH,GH
- **Psychiatric**
  - Depression P,OH,T
  - Schizophrenia GH,OH,T
  - Hysteria S
  - Malingering S
- **Drugs**
  - See Table 20.3
- **Surgical intervention or iatrogenic**
  - Thalamotomy, bilateral T
  - Rhinoplasty S
  - Laryngectomy T
  - Intracranial surgery S
  - Radiation therapy S,T
  - Middle ear surgery T
  - Orotracheal intubation T
  - Chorda tympani section T
  - Hemodialysis Ds
- **Deficiency states**
  - Niacin (B_3) T
  - Vitamin A T
  - Vitamin B_{12} S
  - Zinc S,T
- **Degenerative**
  - Parkinson's disease S,Ds
  - Alzheimer's disease S,OH
  - Multiple sclerosis S,T
  - Huntington's chorea Ds
  - Motor neuron disease S
  - Wolfram's syndrome S
- **Congenital or hereditary**
  - Kallmann's syndrome S
  - Albinism S
  - Familial S
- **Developmental**
  - Facial hypoplasia T
- **Other**
  - Idiopathic S
  - Bell's palsy T
  - Raeder's paratrigeminal neuralgia T
  - Smoking S,T
  - Dentures T
  - Pregnancy S,T
  - Inhaled toxic chemicals S
  - Hydrocephalus, obstructive S
  - Aging S,T,Ds
  - High-altitude sickness T

T = taste decreased or absent; Ti = taste increased; S = smell decreased or absent; Si = smell increased; D = discrimination decreased for taste (t) or smell (s); OH = olfactory hallucination; GH = gustatory hallucination; P = parosmia.

malingerer can be detected with ammonia, which stimulates the trigeminal nerve; if the patient denies noticing the stimulus, it is likely that the anosmia is bogus.

Doty et al. (1984) have developed the UPSIT, which uses microencapsulated odorants (the so-called "scratch and sniff" test). The test consists of 40 odorants with a forced choice of one of four alternative responses for each item. The UPSIT is practical, easily administered, reliable, and able to identify patients with a wide variety of olfactory disorders, including total and partial anosmia and malingering.

The extent of the laboratory investigation will depend on the history and physical examination. If no obvious cause can be identified, appropriate studies for an underlying systemic illness should include complete blood count, routine blood chemistries, serum vitamin B_{12}, thyroid function tests, glucose, syphilis serology, imaging examination of the skull and sinuses, and an electroencephalogram. A formal otorhinolaryngologic evaluation is essential to exclude local nasal disorders. If a cause is still not evident and the condition persists, a contrast-enhanced computed tomographic (CT) or magnetic resonance imaging (MRI) scan of the head and paranasal sinuses is needed.

Disease Entities

The causes of smell disturbances are diverse (Table 20.1), but nasal and paranasal sinus disease, disorders that fol-

Table 20.2: Causes of smell disturbance

Nasal or paranasal sinus disease	15%
Idiopathic	22%
Post–upper respiratory infection	26%
Head trauma	18%
Miscellaneous	13%
Postexposure (environmental toxins, noxious vapors, metals)	2%
Dental	2%
Medication induced	2%

low upper respiratory tract infections, head trauma, and idiopathic conditions account for more than 85% of the total (Deems et al. 1991) (Table 20.2). The high incidence of nasal and parasinus disease causing anosmia and hyposmia underscores the need for thorough otorhinolaryngological evaluation. Although intracranial causes (excluding head trauma and intracranial surgery) are rarely responsible for loss of smell, they result in the greatest morbidity if not diagnosed.

Olfactory Groove Meningioma

Anosmia may be the first symptom of an olfactory groove meningioma. In one series of 29 patients with an olfactory groove meningioma in whom smell could be tested, anosmia was bilateral in 26 and unilateral in 3. Although the majority of such patients mentioned this complaint to a physician, anosmia alone was never the cause of subsequent diagnosis in this series. The single most egregious error in dealing with a chemosensory disturbance is the failure to capitalize on the symptom of anosmia as the sole or principal feature of an olfactory groove meningioma. This diagnosable and treatable condition, if not detected, frequently enlarges and causes seizures, visual loss, and dementia. Headache is present in the majority of patients. The importance of imaging studies in this condition cannot be overemphasized. CT should be performed in all patients in whom loss of sense of smell cannot be explained by head injury, other disease, or surgical procedure of the olfactory region. Viral infection should be a diagnosis of exclusion for patients with permanent anosmia. These patients require a cerebral imaging study, preferably an MR image.

Head Trauma

Loss of smell from head trauma may result from damage to the olfactory nerve as it enters the skull at the cribriform plate of the ethmoid bone, damage to the olfactory bulb, and possibly cerebral cortical injury. Shearing forces, fracture of the anterior fossa, and direct contusion are the mechanisms most commonly responsible. Most such injuries are to the occipital or frontal areas and are associated with motor vehicle accidents. The frequency of smell dysfunction following head trauma is 10–20% and is proportional to the severity of the injury. Anosmia and hyposmia following head injury may be unilateral or bilateral, transient or permanent, and with or without fracture at the base of the skull in the anterior fossa. Recovery of smell occurs in up to 30–40% of cases following the head injury but is unlikely to occur if the loss of smell has been present for more than one year after injury (Costanzo and Becker 1986).

Aging

Olfactory changes reported with aging include reduced thresholds, intensity, identification, and discrimination. These may relate to problems at the receptor or neuronal level, to associated disease states, and to pharmacological agents, as well as to changes in hormonal and neurotransmitter levels (Schiffman 1986).

Other Causes

Impaired odor detection, discrimination, or both has been described in Parkinson's disease (Serby et al. 1985) and Alzheimer's disease (Serby et al. 1985; Koss et al. 1988). Patients with Korsakoff's psychosis retain a normal capacity to detect odors presented at threshold concentrations and yet exhibit a consistent inability to discriminate between odorants or to perform the UPSIT (Mair et al. 1986). Likewise, surgical removal of the parts of the orbitofrontal cortex receiving projections from medial dorsal thalamic nucleus produces a comparable deficit. In parkinsonian patients, no correlation has been found between degree of olfactory impairment and age, duration of disease, disease severity, cognitive impairment, and pharmacological manipulations of dopaminergic and cholinergic treatment (Doty et al. 1988, 1989). Normal olfactory function in progressive supranuclear palsy and benign essential tremor supports the distinctiveness of these disorders from Parkinson's disease (Doty et al. 1993). Significant neurofibrillary tangle formation and cell loss in the anterior olfactory nuclei, along with reduced choline acetyltransferase activity in the olfactory tubercle, have been reported in Alzheimer's disease. As with Parkinson's and Alzheimer's disease, olfactory impairment is described with other neurodegenerative conditions as motor neuron disease and Huntington's chorea (Doty 1991) as well as with granulomatous angiitis of the central nervous system (CNS), idiopathic midline granuloma, Wolfram syndrome, and hypogonadotropic hypogonadism–Kallmann's syndrome (Grange et al. 1992; Rando et al. 1992). An increased sense of smell, *hyperosmia*, is uncommon and noted in association with depression and exposure to toxic vapors (Henkin 1990).

Parosmia, the distortion of normal smell, may reflect an intracranial disease such as a temporal lobe seizure or a tumor, olfactory bulb injury from trauma, depression, or a local nasopharyngeal condition such as sinusitis. Approximately three-fourths of parosmia patients have associated hyposmia or anosmia.

Table 20.3: Drugs affecting taste and smell

Classification	*Drug*
Amebicides and antihelmintics	Metronidazole, niridazole
Anesthetics, local	Benzocaine, procaine hydrochloride (Novocain) and others, cocaine hydrochloride, tetracaine hydrochloride
Anticholesterinemic	Clofibrate
Anticoagulants	Phenindione
Antihistamines	Chlorpheniramine maleate
Antimicrobial agents	Amphotericin B, ampicillin, cefamandole, griseofulvin, ethambutol hydrochloride, lincomycin, sulfasalazine, sulfones, streptomycin, terbinafine, tetracyclines, tyrothricin
Antiproliferative, including immunosuppressive agents	Doxorubicin and methotrexate, azathioprine, carmustine, vincristine sulfate
Antirheumatic, analgesic-antipyretic, antiinflammatory agents	Allopurinol, colchicine, gold, levamisole, D-penicillamine, phenylbutazone, 5-thiopyriodoxine
Antiseptics	Hexetidine
Antithyroid agents	Carbimazole, methimazole, methylthiouracil, propylthiouracil, thiouracil
Agents for dental hygiene	Sodium lauryl sulfate (toothpaste)
Calcium channel blockers	Nifedipine, diltiazem
Diuretics and antihypertensive agents	Captopril, diazoxide, ethacrynic acid
Hypoglycemic drugs	Glipizide, phenformin and derivatives
Muscle relaxants and drugs for treatment of Parkinson's disease	Baclofen, chlormezanone, levodopa
Opiates	Codeine, hydromorphone hydrochloride, morphine
Psychopharmacological, including antiepileptic drugs	Carbamazepine, lithium carbonate, phenytoin, psilocybin, trifluoperazine
Sympathomimetic drugs	Amphetamines, phenmetrazine theoclate and fenbutrazate hydrochloride (combined)
Vasodilators	Oxyfedrine, bamifylline hydrochloride
Others	Germine monoacetate, idoxuridine, iron sorbitex, vitamin D, industrial chemicals (including insecticides), smokeless tobacco

Source: Modified from SS Schiffman. Taste and smell in disease. N Engl J Med 1983;308:1275. Reprinted by permission of the New England Journal of Medicine.

Olfactory hallucinations occur in association with Alzheimer's disease, depression, schizophrenia, alcohol withdrawal, and uncinate seizures. In seizures, the hallucinations are characteristically unpleasant or foul and rarely, if ever, appear as isolated epileptic events.

Cigarette smoking (Frye et al. 1990), a variety of drugs, both prescribed and recreational, radiation therapy, and hemodialysis (Doty et al. 1991), as well as environmental and industrial toxins, cause disturbances of smell (Table 20.3) (see Chapter 75). Abnormalities of taste and smell have been reported as an early manifestation of temporal arteritis (Schon 1988).

TASTE

In humans, the gustatory system is responsible for the perception of sweet, salty, bitter, and sour. Disturbances of taste are far less common than disturbances of smell. Although patients with chemosensory disorders frequently present with complaints that food no longer has any taste, most such patients have olfactory dysfunction with normal taste. Disorders of taste are characterized as absence of taste (ageusia), diminished sensitivity (hypogeusia), increased sensitivity to some or all taste qualities (hypergeusia), distortion of normal taste (dysgeusia or parageusia), and gustatory hallucinations.

Pathophysiology

Gustatory receptor cells are clustered in tastebuds that are located in the papillae on the surface of the tongue and, to a lesser extent, at the back of the mouth and pharynx. Taste buds are innervated by sensory fibers of the chorda tympani and greater superficial petrosal bundles of the facial nerve, the glossopharyngeal nerve, and the superior laryngeal branch of the vagus nerve. Receptor cells have a limited life span and undergo constant replacement. Unlike the olfactory system, taste receptor cells lack axons; thus, their replacement does not involve regenerative processes within the nervous system.

Taste afferent fibers from the anterior two-thirds of the tongue course through the lingual nerve, a branch of the trigeminal nerve, which they leave via the chorda tympani to join the facial nerve as the nervus intermedius portion with their cell bodies in the geniculate ganglion. The posterior one-third of the tongue, pharynx, and soft palate are subserved by taste fibers running in the glossopharyngeal nerve; the cell bodies lie in the nodose ganglion. Gustatory nerve fibers from the facial, glossopharyngeal, and vagus nerves terminate in the brain stem in the ipsilateral nucleus of the solitary tract. The central pathway from this nucleus projects via the gustatory lemniscus to the thalamus and then to the postrolandic sensory cortex. The possibilities of an alternative or accessory taste pathway through the trigeminal nerve has been considered. This is supported by a report of abnormal electrogustometric detection thresholds in patients with trigeminal neuralgia and trigeminal sensory neuropathy, with further moderate but significant threshold rise following surgical treatment (Grant et al. 1987).

Psychophysical and physiological studies have demonstrated that gustatory responses depend on the adaptive state of the tongue. For example, if the tongue is exposed (that is, adapted) to a variety of substances, then water itself becomes capable of evoking tastes (the so-called water taste). This phenomenon has important clinical implications in conditions associated with changes in the rate of flow or composition of saliva, which can be affected by food or drug consumption, diseases affecting salivary secretions such as cystic fibrosis, Sjögren's syndrome, Cushing's or Addison's disease, destruction of salivary tissue by irradiation, or periodontal conditions that add gustatory stimulants to the fluid bathing the tongue. In all cases of dysgeusia or parageusia, it is important to rule out conditions affecting salivary fluids before considering less common causes of altered taste perception.

Clinical Evaluation of Taste

Patients presenting with a disturbance of taste should be asked about any associated disorder of smell; any preexisting medical conditions and their treatment, such as ear infection, ear surgery, Bell's palsy, significant head injury, or tracheal intubation; recent upper respiratory illness; dental procedures or prostheses; and a detailed drug history.

In addition to a complete physical examination and testing of taste and smell, special attention should be paid to the oral cavity for evidence of infection, inflammation, degeneration, and masses, as well as atrophy and dryness of tongue, gums, dentition, and surrounding mucous membranes. Specific investigations are ordered to identify suspected causative considerations suggested by the clinical features. If no local cause is suggested, patients with taste abnormalities, particularly unilateral, should have audiological evaluation and imaging studies to include the area of the middle ear.

The sense of taste may be tested with natural stimuli such as aqueous solutions of sugar, sodium chloride, acetic acid, and quinine, or with electrical stimulation of the tongue (electrogustometry). A cotton applicator is used to rub the aqueous solution gently on one quadrant of the protruded tongue. The patient should not talk but rather should identify the perceived taste by pointing to cards with the words *sweet, salt, sour,* and *bitter.* The mouth is rinsed with water between tests. Electrogustometry is the evaluation of taste by applying graded electrical currents to the tongue to produce a sensation described as sour or metallic. In normal subjects, the two sides of the tongue have similar thresholds for electrical stimulation, rarely differing by more than 25%. The technique is considered to have advantages of simplicity, speed, and ease of quantification, and is capable of providing a reliable objective recording of the gustatory detection threshold.

Disease Entities

Although the cause of most cases of hypogeusia is unknown, the two most probable associated causes are nasal disorders and a prior respiratory infection. Disturbances of taste may result from local disorders involving the tongue, taste buds, or both, and damage to neural pathways in the peripheral or central nervous system.

Drugs and Physical Agents

Heavy smoking, particularly of pipe tobacco, and pharmaceutical agents, especially antirheumatic drugs, antiproliferative drugs, and drugs with sulfhydryl groups such as penicillamine and captopril, are frequent causes of taste dysfunction (see Table 20.3). Calcium channel blockers, such as nifedipine and diltiazem, antifungal agents, and smokeless tobacco have been associated with abnormalities of taste (Beutler et al. 1993; Mela 1987). Other local causes, in part related to drying of the mouth (xerostomia), including Sjögren's syndrome, radiation therapy, and pandysautonomia, illustrate the important role saliva plays in taste perception. In the elderly, the taste threshold is more than twice as high, and drugs and disease states may further decrease taste (Schiffman 1986). Loss of taste may be the initial symptom of primary amyloidosis (Ujike et al. 1987).

Bell's Palsy

Although Bell's palsy is frequently associated with ipsilateral loss of taste over the anterior two-thirds of the tongue, taste loss is usually not recognized by the patient (see Chapter 75). Loss of taste with facial palsy indicates involvement of the nervus intermedius portion of the facial nerve and localizes the lesion to the region between the pons and the point where the chorda tympani joins the facial nerve in the facial canal. Recovery of taste within the first 14 days following the onset of Bell's palsy is usually associated with complete recovery from paralysis. Impairment of taste for more than 2 weeks suggests a poor prognosis for the rapid return of facial movement. Unilateral decrease in sensitivity of taste may accompany cerebellopontine angle lesions such as an acoustic neurinoma.

Trauma

The chorda tympani is particularly vulnerable to injury in its course through the middle ear on the medial superior surface of the tympanic membrane between the malleus and the incus. Isolated involvement of the chorda tympani is rare but can occur with middle ear lesions such as cholesteatoma, otitis media, ear surgery (including tympanoplasty, stapedectomy, and mastoidectomy) (Grant et al. 1989), and head trauma. Injury to preganglionic parasympathetic fibers within the chorda tympani, with loss of salivary secretion, may contribute to long-term impairment of taste even if taste fibers regenerate.

Injury to the lingual nerve causes loss both of general somatic sensation, resulting in numbness, and of special visceral sensation, with taste loss over the anterior two-thirds of the tongue. This nerve may be injured as a result of jaw trauma and wounds, but most cases are iatrogenic due to laryngoscopy, difficult orotracheal intubation, and removal of wisdom teeth.

Head Injury

In posttraumatic head injury, taste disorders are rare and, when present, are almost always due to disturbance of smell. They may be central or peripheral in origin. The incidence of ageusia following head injury is approximately 0.5%, with about 6% of all patients with posttraumatic anosmia also having ageusia. Recovery from ageusia is much more likely than from anosmia and occurs in most over a period of a few weeks to a few months.

Areas of brain stem damage that can cause taste disturbance include the tractus solitarius and its nucleus (ipsilateral ageusia) and the pontine tegmentum involving both gustatory lemnisci (bilateral ageusia). Ipsilateral hypogeusia may follow pontine hemorrhage involving the tegmentum. Ageusia has been noted after bilateral thalamotomy, and unilateral thalamic and parietal lobe lesions have been associated with contralateral impairment of taste sensation. Gustatory hallucinations are much less frequent than olfactory ones but may occur with similar structural lesions of the temporoparietal region and with psychosis.

Dysgeusia is commonly experienced in association with dental problems, presence of dental prosthesis, poor oral hygiene, recent upper respiratory tract infection, aging, depression, and psychotic conditions. Dysgeusia with facial numbness has been noted in association with dissecting aneurysms of the carotid artery, possibly related to an alteration in blood supply to the seventh cranial nerve or branches of the chorda tympani (Francis et al. 1987) (see also Chapter 75).

Other Causes

Impaired taste may follow a focal disturbance of anatomic structures subserving taste, including jugular foramen tumors (Tan et al. 1990) and more diffuse processes such as idiopathic midline granuloma, high-altitude sickness, and diabetes mellitus (Grange et al. 1992; Doty et al. 1991). Increased sensitivity to taste, hypergeusia, is uncommon and reported in association with cerebellar glioma, the mechanism of which is unclear (Noda et al. 1989).

REFERENCES

Beutler M, Hartman K, Kuhn M, Gartmann J. Taste disorders and terbinafine. Br Med J 1993;307:26.

Costanzo RM, Becker DP. Smell and Taste Disorders in Heat Injury and Neurosurgery Patients. In HL Meiselman, RS Rivlin (eds), Clinical Measurement of Taste and Smell. New York: Macmillan 1986;565–578.

Deems DA, Doty RL, Settle G et al. Smell and taste disorders: a study of 750 patients from the University of Pennsylvania Smell and Taste Center. Arch Otolaryngol Head Neck Surg 1991;117:519–528.

Doty RL. Olfactory Dysfunction in Neurodegenerative Disorders. In TV Getchell, RL Doty, LM Bartoshuk, JB Snow (eds), Smell and Taste in Health and Disease. New York: Raven, 1991;735–751.

Doty RL, Bartoshuk LM, Snow JB. Causes of Olfactory and Gustatory Disorders. In TV Getchell, RL Doty, LM Bartoshuk, JB Snow (eds), Smell and Taste in Health and Disease. New York: Raven, 1991;449–462.

Doty RL, Deems DA, Stellar S. Olfactory dysfunction in parkinsonism: a general deficit unrelated to neurologic signs, disease stage or disease duration. Neurology 1988;38:1237–1244.

Doty RL, Golbe LI, Mkeown DA, et al. Olfactory testing differentiates between progressive supranuclear palsy and idiopathic Parkinson's disease. Neurology 1993;43:962–965.

Doty RL, Riklan M, Deems DA et al. The olfactory and cognitive deficits of Parkinson's disease: evidence for independence. Ann Neurol 1989;25:166–171.

Doty RL, Shaman P, Dann M. Development of the University of Pennsylvania Smell Identification Test: a standardized microencapsulated test of olfactory function. Physiol Behav [Monograph] 1984;32:489–502.

Francis KR, Williams DP, Troost T. Facial numbness and dysesthesia: new features of carotid artery dissection. Arch Neurol 1987;44:345–346.

Frye RE, Schwartz BS, Doty RL. Dose-related effects of cigarette smoking on olfactory function. JAMA 1990;263:1233–1236.

Grange C, Cabane J, Dubois A et al. Centrofacial malignant granulomas: clinicopath study of 40 cases and review of the literature. Medicine 1992;71:179–195.

Grant R, Ferguson MM, Strang R et al. Evoked taste thresholds in a normal population and the application of electrogustometry to trigeminal nerve disease. J Neurol Neurosurg Psychiatry 1987;50:12–21.

Grant R, Miller S, Simpson D et al. The effects of chorda tympani section of ipsilateral and contralateral salivary secretion and taste in man. J Neurol Neurosurg Psychiatry 1989;52:1058–1062.

Henkin RI. Hypersomnia and depression following exposure to toxic vapors. JAMA 1990;264:2,803.

Koss E, Weiffebach JM, Haxby JV, Friedland RP. Olfactory detection and recognition performance and disassociation in early Alzheimer's disease. Neurology 1988;38:1,228–1,232.

Mair RG, Doty RL, Kelly KM et al. Multimodal sensory discrimination deficits in Korsakoff's psychosis. Neuropsychologia 1986;24:831–839.

Mela D. Smokeless tobacco and taste sensitivity [letter]. N Engl J Med 1987;316:1165–1166.

Noda S, Hiromatsu K, Umezaki H, Yoneda S. Hypergeusia as the presenting symptom of a posterior fossa lesion. J Neurol Neurosurg Psychiatry 1989;52:804–805.

Rando TA, Horton JC, Layzer RB. Wolfram syndrome: evidence of a diffuse neurodegenerative disease by magnetic resonance imaging. Neurology 1992;42:1220–1224.

Schiffman SS. Age-Related Changes in Taste and Smell and Their Possible Causes. In HL Meiselman, RS Rivlin (eds), Clinical Measurement of Taste and Smell. New York: Macmillan, 1986;326–342.

Schon F. Involvement of smell and taste in giant cell arteritis. J Neurol Neurosurg Psychiatry 1988;51:1,594.

Serby M, Corwin J, Novatt A et al. Olfaction in dementia. J Neurol Neurosurg Psychiatry 1985;48:848–849.

Tan LC, Bordi L, Symon L, Chessman AD. Jugular foramen neuromas: a review of 14 cases. Surg Neurol 1990;34:205–211.

Ujike H, Yamamoto M, Hara I. Taste loss as an initial symptom of primary amyloidosis. J Neurol Neurosurg Psychiatry 1987; 50:111–112.

SUGGESTED READING

Doty RL. Handbook of Olfaction and Gustation. New York: Marcel Dekker, 1995.

Lie C, Yousem DM, Doty RL, Kennedy DW. Neuroimaging in patients with olfactory dysfunction. Am J Roentgenol 1994; 162:411–418.

Chapter 21
Disturbances of Lower Cranial Nerves

Maurice R. Hanson and Patrick J. Sweeney

This chapter is devoted to the clinical features of disorders of cranial nerves VII, IX, X, XI, and XII. It begins with a sufficiently detailed anatomical description of the individual cranial nerve to give the reader an understanding of how the symptoms and signs arise. This is followed by a description of the clinical findings on bedside examination. Detailed descriptions of individual functions are avoided, as they can be found in general texts, including those cited (for example, DeJong 1992). Most of the material relates to deficits of function. The exceptions are certain entities of excess of function related to the facial nerve. Comments on specific disease states are included if they are relevant to the clinical examination.

FACIAL NERVE

Anatomy

Cranial nerve VII (the facial nerve) is one of the most complex of the cranial nerves because of its multiple motor, sensory, and autonomic components and its long, tortuous intra- and extracranial course (Karnes 1992). It is concerned with the motor and sensory innervation of structures evolving from the second brachial arch.

The facial nerve is the motor nerve to the mimetic muscles of the face. It also contains secretory fibers to the salivary and lacrimal glands, as well as the mucous membranes of the oral and nasal cavities (DeJong 1992). Its exteroceptive sensory functions are modest, with some somatic pain fibers from the external auditory canal and a small strip of skin between the mastoid and the pinna. This probably accounts for the referred retroauricular pain in some patients with Bell's palsy. Finally, the facial nerve transmits taste fibers from the anterior two-thirds of the same side of the tongue.

The facial nerve has two roots—a larger motor or special visceral efferent root and a smaller sensory root, the nervus intermedius of Wrisberg. Fibers of the motor root arise from the facial motor nucleus located in the ventrolateral portion of the caudal pontine tegmentum. The motor nucleus is composed of typical motor neurons arranged somatotopically, with a dorsal group innervating the upper portion of the face and a ventral group innervating the lower portion. Intrapontine fibers run dorsomedially to sweep around the sixth nerve nucleus as the genu of the facial nerve and pass in a ventral and lateral fashion to emerge from the caudal portion of the pons. This intimate relationship of the facial nerve fibers with the sixth nerve nucleus makes it unlikely that an intramedullary lesion will produce an isolated facial palsy without abducent weakness or a gaze paresis. After leaving the pons, the motor trunk joins the nervus intermedius and eighth nerve in the cerebellopontine angle and continues through the internal auditory canal. The facial nerve and nervus intermedius enter the facial canal (fallopian aqueduct) and pass anterolaterally a short distance to the geniculate ganglion, then bend dorsolaterally and interiorly to exit through the stylomastoid foramen. Before they do so, a branch is given to the stapedius muscle and the chorda tympani. Near its exit, the facial nerve also gives off branches to the posterior belly of the digastric and stylohyoid muscles and a cutaneous posterior auricular branch. The trunk of the seventh nerve then passes through the parotid gland to terminate in branches innervating the following:

1. A superior group of muscles concerned with raising eyebrows, frowning, and moving the forehead.
2. An intermediate group involved in closing the eyelids and wrinkling the nose.
3. An inferior group of muscles involved in smiling, laughing, whistling, pouting, wrinkling the chin, and raising the upper lip.

Essentially, the facial nerve supplies all muscles of facial expression from the frontalis to the platysma, with the exception of the levator palpebrae superioris, which is innervated by the oculomotor nerve.

The facial motor nucleus is influenced by many inputs, including the corticobulbar tracts mediating voluntary facial movement. Clinical observation suggests that bilateral subcortical innervation from the deep gray nuclei is responsible for automatic and emotional movements of the face as opposed to volitional movements.

The sensory fibers of the seventh nerve travel in the intermediate nerve of Wrisberg. The perikarya reside in the geniculate ganglia. There are many preganglionic parasympathetic fibers, most of which originate in the superior salivatory nuclei, which initiate salivary, lacrimal, and mucous secretions (DeJong 1992). Preganglionic fibers involved in lacrimation course via the intermediate nerve to the geniculate ganglion and enter the greater superficial petrosal nerve to the sphenopalatine ganglion. Postganglionic fibers traverse the zygomaticotemporal nerve and the lacrimal nerve to reach the lacrimal glands. Fibers concerned with salivary gland secretion arise from the superior salivatory nucleus, traverse the seventh nerve to the chorda tympani, join the lingual branch of the fifth nerve, and synapse in the submaxillary ganglia. Postsynaptic fibers innervate the submaxillary glands, which, when stimulated, yield copious, watery mucous secretions.

Taste fibers are carried in both facial and glossopharyngeal nerves. Those from the ipsilateral anterior two-thirds of the tongue have cell bodies in the geniculate ganglion. The fibers travel through the lingual nerve and chorda tympani to the nervus intermedius and terminate in the rostral part of the nucleus solitarius.

Cutaneous nerve fibers of the facial nerve form a small component, mainly coming from the external auditory canal and the angle between the ear and the mastoid.

Symptoms and Signs

The symptoms of facial nerve disease depend on a number of factors, including the size of the lesion, the severity of the disorder, the acuteness of onset, and whether the lesion or lesions are bilateral or unilateral. A sudden, severe unilateral infranuclear paralysis, as seen in Bell's palsy, will produce, in addition to an obvious cosmetic embarrassment, significant dysarthria, pooling of saliva, and decreased tearing; it will also allow food to collect between the gum and the cheek as a result of buccinator weakness. Depending on the size of the lesion, there may also be perversion of taste and hyperacusis (Figure 21.1). On the other hand, a moderate degree of weakness of the lower face, as is seen with a unilateral corticobulbar lesion, may produce few complaints relative to the face, particularly if attention is distracted by ipsilateral limb involvement or if language dysfunction is present, as in a dominant hemisphere lesion. Bilateral corticobulbar disease, as with multiple lacunae, is much more devastating to speech and swallowing functions. Unilateral facial weakness of slow evolution, as seen with a pontine glioma, may go unnoticed by the patient although it is obvious to the examiner. This is consistent with the general clinical observation that objective neurological deficits that are more apparent to the examiner than to the patient are usually of gradual evolution.

A detailed description of the examination of the motor functions of the facial nerve can be found in standard texts of neurological diagnosis (DeJong 1992). There are, however, two observations that are helpful in examining a patient with facial paresis but that are frequently overlooked. The platysma should always be examined by having the patient retract the corners of the mouth as in a grimace; in mild degrees of facial paresis, it will often be less prominent on the involved side. It is also worth recalling that with weakness of the posterior belly of the digastric muscle innervated by the facial nerve, the jaw may deviate to the sound side when the mouth is opened wide, whereas with paralysis of the pterygoids innervated by the trigeminal nerve, the opposite is true (Karnes 1992).

A number of facial reflexes may aid in establishing or localizing lesions of the facial nerve. Some are true myotatic reflexes; others represent associated movements (DeJong 1992). A variety of stimuli, such as noise, sudden light, and pain, can elicit a blink reflex that uncovers unilateral facial weakness.

The *orbicularis oculi (blink* or *glabellar) reflex* is elicited by tapping over the supraorbital ridge or root of the nose, resulting in a bilateral blink response. It is important that this be elicited by a hand held over the top of the forehead, to avoid a visual blink response. With an early, mild, or resolving unilateral facial paresis, the glabellar reflex will be diminished. The afferent pathway is via the first division of the fifth cranial nerve, with a rapid, unilateral monosynaptic component and a delayed, bilateral polysynaptic component. A variation of this reflex is the orbicularis oculi stretch reflex elicited by grasping the lateral orbital skin between the thumb and index finger and tapping the thumb with a reflex hammer. A similar bilateral blink response is present. The afferent impulses, however, arise from stretch receptors in the muscle. A number of new neurophysiologic techniques using the brain stem reflexes including the blink reflex have been developed and validated to study these pathways and have found some diagnostic usefulness. Novel techniques using magnetic transcranial stimulation and somatosensory evoked responses are finding useful ap-

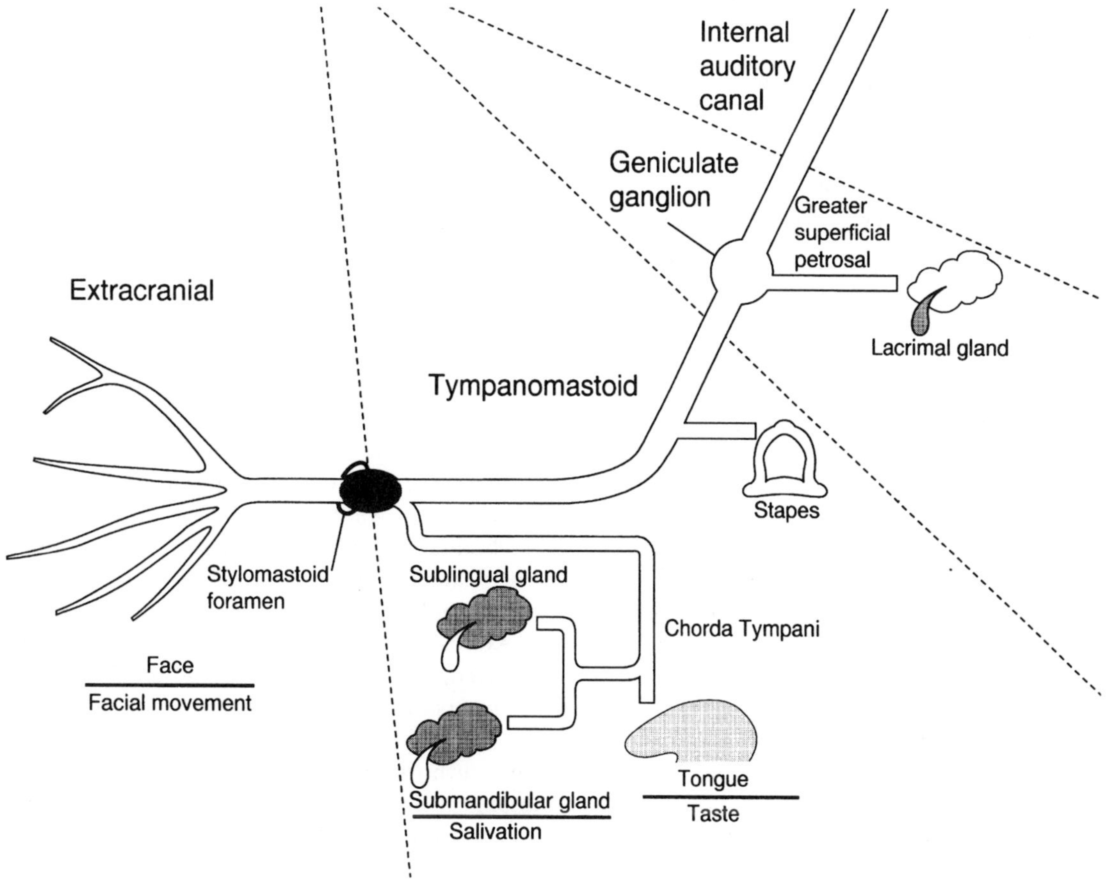

FIGURE 21.1 This schematic of the facial nerve shows the major subdivisions and illustrates the principal functions that might be impaired at the level of a lesion and distal to it. For example, a lesion at the level of the geniculate might, in addition to facial paralysis, produce impaired taste, glandular secretions, and hyperacusis.

plication to diagnosis and prognosis of facial nerve disorders (Hopf 1994).

Another stretch reflex is the *orbicularis oris reflex*, elicited by percussing the upper lip and producing elevation of the lip and angle of the mouth. Like most other myotatic responses, these reflexes are diminished or abolished by segmental dysfunction and preserved or heightened by bilateral corticobulbar lesions.

Bell's phenomenon is a true associated movement. With attempted closure of the eyes against resistance, the globes turn up and out. This normal movement can be observed with the incomplete eyelid closure in Bell's palsy.

The *stapedial reflex* is particularly helpful in diagnosis. Stapedius muscle contraction, activated by strong acoustic stimuli, pulls the stapes out of the round window, attenuating intense sound waves. Reduction or absence of this reflex results in hyperacusis or phonophobia. It can be quantified by measuring acoustic impedance but can be tested at the bedside using the stethoscope loudness imbalance test. A stethoscope is placed in the patient's ears, and a gently vibrating tuning fork is placed on the bell. With normal hearing, the perception of sound is symmetrical. With greater activation, the sound is lateralized to the side of the facial paresis (in some cases) because the attenuating effect of the stapedius muscle is reduced or absent.

The sensory functions of the seventh nerve are not easily tested. The examination of the sensory nerve at the bedside is basically limited to testing taste (DeJong 1992). Four aspects of taste are examined, including sweet, salty, sour, and bitter, using, respectively, a 4% solution of glucose, a 2.5% solution of sodium chloride, a 1% solution of citric acid, and a 0.075% solution of quinine hydrochloride. The test solution is applied to each side of the anterior portion of the tongue alternately, using a cotton-tipped applicator. The patient is instructed to keep the tongue protruded until notified otherwise. The words "sweet," "salt," "sour," and "bitter" are written on paper, and the patient points to the word describing the taste he or she perceives. After each application, the mouth is rinsed with water. Bitter is tested last because it has the strongest aftertaste.

Schirmer's test, an easily performed, semiquantitative measure of lacrimal secretion, is the only way that the secretory functions of tears and saliva can be tested accurately at the bedside without special equipment. A thin strip of filter paper, 5 × 0.5 cm, is bent at one end and inserted into each conjunctival sac. Normally, the moistened portion mi-

Table 21.1: Clinical differential features of upper motor neuron versus lower motor neuron facial weakness

Features of UMN Lesions	*Features of LMN Lesions*
Unilateral paresis of voluntary movements of lower face with sparing of the frontalis muscle	Unilateral paresis of all mimetic muscles, including the frontalis muscle
Facial muscle weakness less apparent with emotional than with voluntary action	Degree of facial weakness similar with emotional and voluntary movements
Preservation or accentuation of facial reflexes	Suppression of facial reflexes
Preserved taste, anterior two-thirds of tongue	Possible impairment of taste
Normal lacrimation	Possible abnormality of lacrimation

grates about 3 cm in 5 minutes. There will be a significant reduction on the side of a proximal facial nerve lesion above the geniculate ganglia.

Site of Lesion

With any facial paresis, it must be first determined if the lesion is affecting the upper motor or lower motor neuron. In most instances, it will be obvious. When, on occasion, it is less clear, certain critical observations can usually settle the issue (Table 21.1).

It is widely accepted that upper motor neuron disorders with unilateral facial paresis affect the voluntary movements of the lower face with relative sparing of the orbicularis oculi, frontalis, and corrugator supercilii muscles as a result of bilateral innervation of the upper face. There are certain circumstances in which this rule is violated:

1. During recovery from Bell's palsy, if the upper facial groups recover before the lower groups, and if recovery is incomplete, as may occasionally occur in incomplete acute lesions.
2. If nuclear lesions are restricted to the caudal portions of the nucleus, as seen in polio, and at some stages of motor neuron disease.
3. If an extracranial lesion involves only the lower division of the facial nerve, as seen on occasion after radical neck dissection or with parotid tumors.

In upper motor neuron lesions, there is preservation of the blink and stapedial reflexes; lacrimal and taste sensibility also remains unimpaired. This may also be true for lower motor neuron lesions. If reflex functions are involved, however, it is strong evidence that the lesion is not upper motor neuron.

In lower motor neuron lesions, the degree of weakness is the same with voluntary and emotional movements. With upper motor neuron involvement, particularly of the prefrontal cortex, the face is relatively symmetrical, with a normal emotional smile, and the movement of the involved side may actually be exaggerated, despite the unilateral weakness on voluntary contraction. This latter observation is probably the only one that consistently separates upper motor from lower motor neuron lesions.

The appearance of a severe, unilateral, infranuclear facial palsy is one of the most distinctive in clinical medicine. The most common cause of an acute, acquired, nontraumatic lesion is *Bell's palsy*, in which there is a flaccid paresis of all mimetic muscles on the involved side. The affected side is smooth and the eyebrow droops, but the palpebral fissure is widened. The angle of the mouth is depressed, and the cheek balloons on expiration. The lid remains open (*lagophthalmos*), and on attempted closure the globe turns up and out (*Bell's phenomenon*). The lower lid is everted, with excessive tearing (*epiphora*). The facial movements are paralyzed to both voluntary and involuntary contraction, and the various facial reflexes are lost. Some authors (Jepsen 1965) have proposed discrete anatomical localization along the various segments of the seventh nerve in Bell's palsy based on the test results of taste, the stapedial reflex, lacrimation, and mandibular deviation. Although there may be some validity to these observations in early lesions, in practice the localization is much less precise (see Figure 21.1). As a general rule, proximal lesions at or before the geniculate ganglion may affect taste and lacrimation as well as the stapedial reflex, whereas those distal to the geniculate ganglion produce only muscle weakness.

Mild or incomplete peripheral facial palsies can be easily overlooked. They are often suspected during the history-taking when there is a notable asymmetry of facial movement during animated conversation. The most sensitive indicators are a diminished spontaneous blink on the affected side and the presence of eyelashes that are not seen on the intact side on forceful closure of the lids.

In some cases of unilateral peripheral facial weakness, the platysma fails to contract when the angles of the mouth are pulled down voluntarily and the facial reflexes are diminished. One of the most sensitive signs of a mild, early facial paresis is the inability to wink unilaterally. However, it must be established that the patient could wink unilaterally on either side before the onset, in that a significant number of normal persons can wink only on one side (Keane 1994).

While most acute unilateral facial palsies are idiopathic (Bell's), some are due to better-defined causes including herpes zoster, Lyme disease, and sarcoid. There are usually other clues that can readily separate them. Additionally, there are less common causes of bifacial palsy, most of which have a self-limited benign course (Keane 1994).

Facial Nerve Overactivity

Heretofore, we have discussed the clinical aspects of facial nerve insufficiency. A number of interesting phenomena occur as a result of an abnormal overactivity of the facial musculature as opposed to a deficiency of movement. Several of these, including blepharospasm, facial tics, and tardive dyskinesias, are central movement disorders. Four, however, have their origin in the facial nerve: *hemifacial spasm, facial myokymia, the syndrome of aberrant reinnervation,* and *spastic paretic hemifacial contracture*. Each of these has a sufficiently characteristic clinical profile, pathophysiology, and etiologic and prognostic implication to warrant separate discussion. The use of electrodiagnosis has considerably enhanced our understanding of these entities.

Hemifacial Spasm

Hemifacial spasm (HS) was elegantly described in 1888 by Gowers, who referred to it as a *tic convulsif*. HS is characterized by rapid, irregular paroxysms of clonic twitching of one or more muscle groups innervated by the facial nerve. The twitches usually begin unilaterally about the eye and then spread to the other facial muscles, especially the perioral muscles, but never beyond the domain of the facial nerve. The contractions persist for minutes and are often precipitated by stress, fatigue, or voluntary movements of the face.

HS is one of the few movement disorders that may persist in sleep. It is not of cortical origin and is not abolished by unilateral cerebral infarction. An antecedent Bell's palsy is very rare. Facial asymmetry is not uncommon with HS and may be due to *synkinesis* (a synchronization of movement occurring with voluntary or reflex activity of different muscles that normally do not contract together; Karnes 1992), weakness, contracture, or a mild persistent spasm.

The electromyogram (EMG) picture is characteristic, with discharges of high-frequency (150–400 Hz) rhythmic bursts with synchronization (Sivak et al. 1993). If one looks closely after an attack, synkinesis may be seen. However, the use of electrophysiological recordings of the blink reflex by stimulating the superficial orbital nerve and recording from the orbicularis oculi and other facial muscles has confirmed the existence of synkinesis in virtually all patients with hemifacial spasm. The only other disorder that has this effect is aberrant reinnervation after severe facial paresis, but here the diagnosis is not in question on clinical grounds. The presence of synkinesis supports the theory that the cause of HS is ephaptic transmission.

Most of the known pathological causes of HS are extra-axial and intracranial. They include tumors, vascular malformations, and localized infectious processes. The most common appears to be vascular compression of the nerve by an aberrant arterial loop. This has recently been nicely demonstrated by magnetic resonance imaging (MRI) and magnetic tomographic angiography (Adler et al. 1992; Tash et al. 1988). Surgical decompression of the seventh nerve has led to remission in some cases, which is significant since spontaneous remission is very rare (Jannetta 1992). Botulinum toxin injection has been found to be effective.

Facial Myokymia

Facial myokymia (FM) is an uncommon condition described in 1916 by Oppenheim, who thought it was an early sign of multiple sclerosis, a prescient notion largely confirmed by time and experience. Descriptively, FM is characterized by subtle, continuous, ripplelike quivering of the facial muscles. Patients liken the sensations to a feeling of swelling and crawling of the face. FM is usually unilateral at any given time but may shift sides on occasion. Often there is a mild contracture of the facial muscles. The muscles seem to be in slight contraction so that the angle of the mouth is drawn up and the lips slightly pursed. There is a continuous flickering of the muscles that pass over the face in rapid, undulating waves. There may also be mild unilateral weakness. FM is influenced little by voluntary movement, sleep, or other exogenous or endogenous factors.

Although any intrinsic brain stem lesion may produce FM, it is most often seen in the context of multiple sclerosis and of intrinsic brain stem tumors such as pontine gliomas. In the former, the disorder is self-limited and abates after a few weeks, although it may recur. It most often develops early in the course of multiple sclerosis and rarely may be the herald symptom. By contrast, FM associated with intrinsic brain stem tumors tends to persist and progress. Other uncommon causes of FM include unilateral basilar invagination and syringomyelia and syringobulbia.

The EMG is helpful in documenting FM because there is a highly characteristic pattern on the needle examination. The motor units, which are of normal shape and duration, are grouped with a regular rhythmic discharge about every 100–200 msec but are not synchronized throughout the muscle. It is this grouped firing of more than one unit asynchronously in different parts of the muscle that causes the clinical feature of the continuous rippling of the muscle (Sivak et al. 1993).

The precise mechanism underlying FM is uncertain, but a reverberating circuit mechanism involving the facial nucleus is postulated. Once the diagnosis is established, the diagnostic procedure of choice would be MRI of the head.

Aberrant Reinnervation

Aberrant reinnervation (AR) of the facial nerve is also referred to as "facial nerve misdirection" or "facial synkinesis" (May and Galetta 1990). It differs from the two preceding disorders, however, in that there must be a history of antecedent peripheral facial paresis that was of sufficient magnitude and duration to produce axonal degeneration, since it is misdirection of regenerating fibers that underlies this syndrome (Baker et al. 1994). The most common antecedent paresis is severe Bell's palsy. AR is accompanied by contracture leading to an increased depth of the nasolabial fold and narrowing of the palpebral fissure, as well as an upward deviation of the corner of the mouth, giving the unwary examiner the impression that the palsy was on the opposite side. It is not entirely certain whether this is due to scarring of the tissues or to active contraction of muscle fibers. Supporting the latter explanation is the fact that a procaine nerve block abolishes the syndrome in some patients.

The contracture is accompanied by associated movements or synkinesis. This may take the form of a twitch of the corner of the mouth with an eyeblink or eye closure with a spontaneous smile.

The most striking outcome of AR, but a rarer one, is inappropriate unilateral lacrimation while eating, to which the term *crocodile tears* is applied (May and Galetta 1990). This is based on a misdirection of regenerating fibers originally supplying the submandibular and salivary glands rerouted to the lacrimal gland via the greater superficial petrosal nerve. The lesion must involve the nervus intermedius proximal to the origin of this nerve. As with hemifacial spasm, the EMG with blink reflexes will demonstrate the phenomenon of synkinesis.

Spastic Paretic Hemifacial Contracture

The diagnostic criteria of spastic paretic hemifacial contracture (SPFC) include progressive unilateral contracture of the facial muscles along with facial muscle weakness (May and Galetta 1990). There may be superimposed intermittent facial spasms as well as facial myokymia. In all reported cases, there have been additional signs of brain stem dysfunction, including deafness, nystagmus, ocular paresis, trigeminal sensory loss, and ataxia. All cases have been due to intrinsic brain stem lesions, usually pontine gliomas, but also including arteriovenous malformations. EMG studies show continuous high-frequency (100-Hz) discharges uninfluenced by reflex mechanisms or voluntary contraction.

SPFC is easily distinguished from the other entities previously mentioned. Aberrant regeneration always follows a severe Bell's palsy and is an isolated finding without other brain stem signs. Co-contraction of facial muscle groups, a feature of aberrant regeneration, is not part of SPFC. Facial myokymia may accompany SPFC, but it differs from that associated with multiple sclerosis in that there is little if any facial weakness associated with the latter and SPFC is progressive, whereas myokymia with multiple sclerosis remits within 3 months. SPFC may be accompanied by ipsilateral spasms and twitches. This is distinct from the more common hemifacial spasm wherein there are no accompanying brain stem signs or facial weakness.

In summary, the presence of progressive contracture in ipsilateral lower motor neuron facial weakness when accompanied by neighborhood brain stem findings is prima facie evidence of an intramedullary lesion, most often a brain stem glioma. Such a constellation merits an MRI study of the posterior fossa.

GLOSSOPHARYNGEAL AND VAGUS NERVES

Anatomy

The glossopharyngeal (ninth) and vagus (tenth) cranial nerves are usually discussed in tandem because of their intrinsic anatomical relationship, the similarity of their functions, and the difficulty in testing each separately. Of the two, the larger vagus nerve overshadows the smaller and more restricted glossopharyngeal nerve. Both contain fibers classed as special visceral efferent (SVE), general visceral efferent (GVE), visceral afferent, and general somatic afferent.

SVE fibers arise from the nucleus ambiguus, a lengthy, well-defined group of neurons situated in the lateral medullary reticular formation dorsal to the inferior olivary nucleus and ventromedial to the nucleus of the descending tract of the trigeminal nerve. A superior portion gives rise to the glossopharyngeal nerve fibers, a larger intermediate portion to vagal fibers, and a smaller caudal portion to the bulbar accessory fibers. The cells are structurally similar to typical motor neurons and innervate the striated muscles of the pharynx, larynx, and upper esophagus. The only striated muscles supplied by the glossopharyngeal nerve are the stylopharyngeus muscle and those of the anterior and posterior pillars of the fauces. GVE fibers arise from the dorsal motor (efferent) nucleus lateral to the hypoglossal nucleus below the floor of the fourth ventricle. The cells are embryologically and functionally similar to the intermediolateral gray cell column of the spinal cord.

Autonomic efferent fibers of the glossopharyngeal nerve arise from that portion of the efferent nucleus known as the "inferior salivatory nucleus." The preganglionic fibers of the glossopharyngeal nerve pass through Jacobsen's nerve, the tympanic plexus, and the lesser superficial petrosal nerve to the otic ganglion. The nerve is involved in the secretory function of the parotid gland. The visceral afferent branches of the glossopharyngeal nerve have their bipolar perikarya in the petrosal and the superior petrosal ganglia. They convey sensation from the ipsilateral posterior one-third of the tongue, fauces, tonsils, nasopharynx, inferior surface of the soft palate, uvula, eustachian tube, and tympanic cavity. The proximal branches terminate in the nucleus of the tractus solitarius.

The glossopharyngeal nerve emerges from the medulla in a groove between the inferior olive and the inferior cerebellar peduncle below the fibers for the facial cranial nerve and above those of the vagus nerve. It exits the skull through the jugular foramen with the vagus and accessory nerves. It passes between the internal jugular vein and internal carotid artery. The nerve then passes in front of the internal carotid artery and follows the inferior border of the stylopharyngeus muscle to reach the lateral wall of the pharynx.

The vagus nerve has two principal motor components. One is the visceral efferent component arising from the nucleus ambiguus and supplying all striated muscles of the soft palate save for the tensor veli palatini; all pharyngeal muscles except for the stylopharyngeus; and the cricothyroid and all intrinsic laryngeal muscles. The second motor component, the autonomic or GVE, arises from the dorsal motor nucleus and yields preganglionic parasympathetic fibers destined for the smooth muscles of the trachea, bronchi, esophagus, and gastrointestinal (GI) tract. Parasympathetic fibers are inhibitory to cardiac and upper GI muscles and secretory to the lower GI tract, liver, and pancreas. Somatic sensory fibers have cell bodies in the jugular and nodose ganglia and convey impulses via Arnold's nerve from the inferior and posterior walls of the external auditory canal. Pain fibers arise from the esophagus, trachea, and bronchi. Other fibers transmit chemoreceptor impulses from the aortic and carotid bodies terminating in the solitary nucleus.

After exiting the jugular foramen, the vagus passes interiorly within the carotid sheath between the internal jugular vein and the carotid artery, giving off some pharyngeal branches. A superior laryngeal branch gives off an external ramus to the cricothyroid muscle and an internal ramus, which gives sensory fibers to the larynx. The inferior laryngeal (recurrent) nerve turns up posteriorly under the right subclavian artery and under the aortic arch on the left. Both ascend in the tracheoesophageal sulcus to supply all of the laryngeal muscles except the cricothyroid. Further branches are autonomic to the heart, bronchi, and GI tract.

Symptoms and Signs

From a practical standpoint, the glossopharyngeal nerve is purely sensory, as the only muscle that it innervates is the stylopharyngeus, which cannot be tested separately. It should be considered the afferent arm of the palatal reflex. The sensation is tested by gently touching the palate and asking the patient to compare the two sides. Taste sensation of the posterior one-third of the tongue can be tested reliably only by galvanic current and does not lend itself to bedside analysis. Also, baroreceptive and salivary functions require elaborate testing instrumentation, which is impractical for routine analysis (Thomas and Mattias 1992).

With respect to the vagal nerve, total paralysis of one vagal nerve results in unilateral paresis of the soft palate, pharynx, and larynx, but the symptoms are quite variable as a result of bilateral representation. There is some difficulty in swallowing both liquids and solids, and the voice may have a nasal quality. Hoarseness is often present, and a vigorous cough is not possible because of failure of opposition of the vocal cords as a result of recurrent laryngeal paresis. The effects are usually transitory, and there is no respiratory difficulty.

With bilateral involvement, the nasopharynx fails to occlude, and the speech has a profound nasal quality, with regurgitation of fluids through the nose on attempted swallowing. Severe dysphagia for liquids more than solids occurs, often with aspiration. Snoring is a prominent symptom, and inspiratory stridor may supervene. If the lesions are acute, the situation is life-threatening and requires a tracheostomy. If the process develops gradually, there is adequate time for compensation and the effects are much less dramatic and more prolonged (DeJong 1992).

With a unilateral vagal lesion, the palatal arch is lowered and flattened and, on phonation, is deviated to the healthy side. During the same maneuver, the posterior pharyngeal wall is observed to contract as a result of action of the superior pharyngeal constrictor muscle. This frequently requires the examiner to depress the back of the tongue, which by itself activates the palatal reflex and causes the same movement. Unilateral paresis of the superior constrictor muscle results in a pull of the posterior pharyngeal wall toward the intact side with a motion that resembles the drawing of a curtain and is known as *Vernet's signe de rideau.*

The patient should be asked to drink from a glass of water, and observations of coordinated swallowing movements are noted. Upward movement of the larynx is normally observed, the lack of which may signify bilateral vagal paresis, as does regurgitation of fluid through the nose. Also, patients with palatal weakness will not be able to puff the cheeks out unless the nose is pinched because of posterior nasal escape of air, a symptom differentiating this condition from facial muscle weakness.

In lesions of the glossopharyngeal and vagus nerves, the palatal reflex may be lost. This takes on considerable significance if it is unilateral but is much less significant if bilateral, unless other signs are present, since there is a great variability of the gag reflex, particularly in the elderly and in smokers. Even with bilateral lesions, the response may be partially intact as a result of function of the tensor veli palatini innervated by the trigeminal nerve.

SPINAL ACCESSORY NERVE

Anatomy

The spinal accessory (eleventh) nerve has two principal components. The larger and more important is the spinal portion; the smaller branch, the accessory, is so called because of its function as accessory to the vagus. The accessory branch arises from cell bodies in the caudal prolongation of the nucleus ambiguus of the medulla oblongata. It crosses the posterior fossa in close association with fibers of the glossopharyngeal and vagus nerves, and its function cannot be distinguished from those of the vagus nerve. The cell bodies of the spinal branch are located in the posterior and lateral portion of the base of the anterior horns of cervical segments C2–C5 (Thomas and Mattias 1992). A series of rootlets emerges from the spinal cord between the dentate ligament and the posterior horns of the spinal nerves. These rootlets

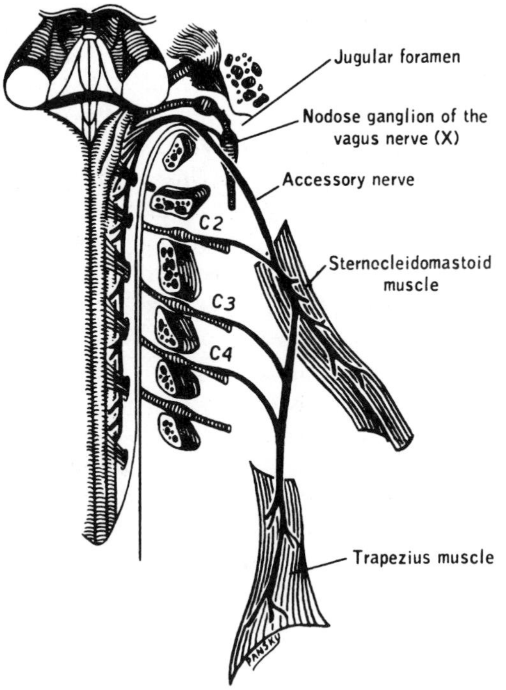

FIGURE 21.2 Course and distribution of the spinal accessory nerve. (Reprinted with permission from EL House, B Pansky. A Functional Approach to Neuroanatomy [2nd ed]. New York: McGraw-Hill, 1967.)

merge and ascend within the dura to enter the skull through the foramen magnum. The spinal and cranial branches fuse as they enter the jugular foramen and pass through this structure with the vagus and glossopharyngeal nerves. After exiting the jugular foramen, the main trunk splits into an internal ramus, which runs with the vagus nerve, and an external ramus, which continues as the spinal accessory nerve proper. In its extracranial course, the accessory nerve passes with the glossopharyngeal and vagus nerves between the internal jugular vein and internal carotid artery. It courses beneath the posterior belly of the digastric muscle, reaching the sternocleidomastoid muscle and providing a branch to this muscle. It then passes deep to the sternocleidomastoid muscle and appears at the posterior border, where it becomes quite superficial as it courses obliquely across the posterior triangle of the neck to penetrate and terminate in the upper trapezius muscle (Figure 21.2).

The accessory nerve is purely a motor nerve. The spinal portion innervates the sternocleidomastoid and trapezius muscles. The sternocleidomastoid muscle acts in concert with other cervical muscles. As it contracts, the occiput is drawn toward the side of contraction and the face is rotated to the opposite side. Contracting together, the sternocleidomastoid muscles flex the cervical spine. The trapezius retracts the head and elevates, retracts, and rotates the scapula. It also elevates the abducted arm above the horizontal. With bilateral contraction, the head is drawn back and the face up. The innervation of the trapezius is variable, but generally the upper trapezius is innervated by the accessory nerve and the lower portion by branches of the cervical plexus of segments C3 and C4. The variability of clinical findings with accessory nerve lesions probably reflects the relative contributions from these various components.

Symptoms and Signs

Despite the fact that the accessory nerve is a motor nerve, the symptoms of its dysfunction are both motor and sensory, with pain dominating the latter. Acutely, especially after inflammatory lesions, the pain is steady, severe, and well localized to the neck and top of the shoulder. This may last 1–2 weeks. The chronic pain is dull and often diffuse, involving not only the neck and shoulder but the entire arm. This aching pain is most troublesome at the end of the day and after exercise and is relieved by support of the arm at the elbow, suggesting that the pain is due to traction of fatigued muscles and ligaments. Paresthesias and numbness are common and sometimes involve the entire arm but more often affect all the fingers, in the form of coldness, pins and needles, and throbbing sensations, probably caused by traction of the heavy limb on the brachial plexus.

Weakness is the most enduring symptom with accessory nerve palsy. Patients note a reduced range of movements of the shoulder, particularly when attempting to use the arm overhead, as in reaching up to shelves, housepainting, pulling on a jacket, or combing the hair. Additional complaints relate to cosmetic effects, including drooping of the shoulder and prominence of the clavicle and scapula (Thomas and Mattias 1992).

When the sternocleidomastoid muscle is involved unilaterally, the finding is loss of bulk, best demonstrated by turning the chin against resistance (Figure 21.3). Strength is diminished only moderately as a result of participation of other cervical muscles. Bilateral sternocleidomastoid involvement is much more apparent because of the weakness of neck flexion and is most often encountered in myogenic lesions such as myotonic dystrophy. The sternocleidomastoid reflex is elicited by tapping over the clavicular origin and observing contractions of the muscle. It is lost in the unilateral lower motor neuron lesions (DeJong 1992).

The trapezius muscle, being considerably more complex, lends itself to more detailed analysis. The findings depend on the age and extent of the lesion or lesions. Let us consider a rather severe lesion more than 6 weeks old. Inspection reveals obvious drooping of the affected shoulder. With the arms hanging loosely at the sides, the fingertips touch the thigh at a lower level on the affected side. The scapula slips downward, forward, and around the axilla. This is reflected in the alignment of the clavicle, which, viewed from the front, no longer passes medial and upward laterally and back but, rather, horizontally forward and down. The clavicle becomes more prominent, especially at its medial portion.

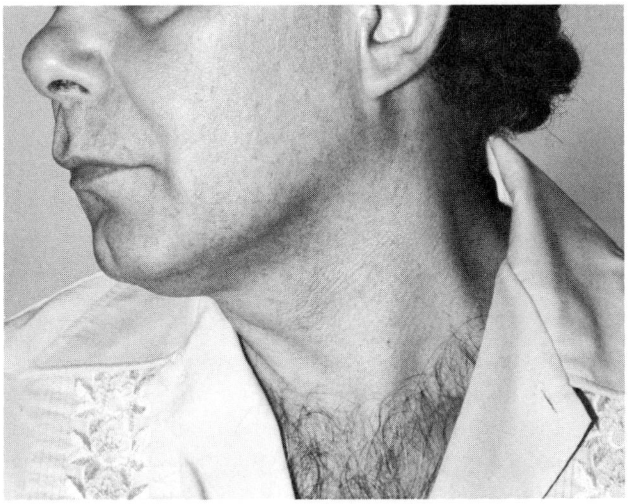

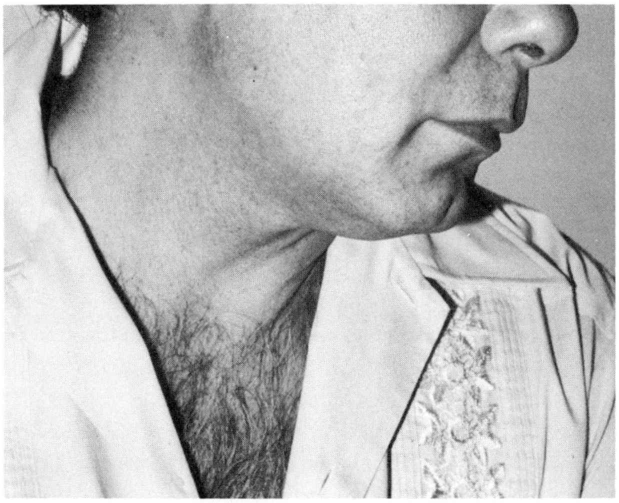

FIGURE 21.3 (Left) Normal left sternocleidomastoid muscle with forceful thrust of chin to the right. Note the prominent left sternocleidomastoid muscle. (Right) Same maneuver as the figure on the left, but to the left, showing loss of bulk of the right sternocleidomastoid muscle.

The upper one-third of the trapezius, serratus anterior, and levator scapulae muscles are necessary for scapular rotation. The upper trapezius is responsible for abduction of the arm beyond 90 degrees. This is partially compensated if the arm moves forward a little. Shoulder shrugging is a deceptive and poor test of function of the trapezius because the levator scapulae (C3, C4) does this quite well. A better test is abduction of the arm through 180 degrees. The first 90 degrees are glenohumeral (supraspinatus and deltoid), and the next 15 degrees are acromioclavicular, with the completion of the arc dependent on the trapezius. Testing must be done with the upper arm internally rotated and the hand pronated with no anterior flexion of the shoulder; otherwise, accessory muscles such as the deltoid will be activated.

Winging of the scapula is due to paresis of the middle trapezius muscle, whereas loss of abduction greater than 90 degrees is due to weakness of the upper trapezius. It is useful to contrast scapular winging of accessory nerve lesions with that due to malfunction of the long thoracic nerve (serratus anterior). With a serratus anterior palsy, there is mild deformity at rest, whereas with trapezius paresis the scapula is more prominent at rest. With serratus anterior weakness, the winging is more apparent on forward flexion of the arm, which results in movement of the inferior scapular angle away from the midline. Winging due to trapezius palsy is more prominent with abduction of the arm, as described previously, noting that the superior angle moves farther from the midline (Thomas and Mattias 1992) (Figure 21.4). In the prone position, the patient is unable to retract the shoulder or to raise it when the arm is held abducted, as lateral abduction is weakened. The palm, initially facing down, tends to twist forward and upward on attempted movement. Bilateral trapezius weakness causes the head to fall forward, as seen in motor neuron disease and myotonic dystrophy.

Evaluation

The indications for laboratory, radiological, or neurophysiological investigation depend on the initial clinical results. If the lesions involve the sternocleidomastoid and trapezius and the cause is obscure, high-resolution computed tomography through the jugular foramen may be helpful, especially if other cranial nerves, such as the glossopharyngeal, vagus, and hypoglossal nerves, are involved. This should be done with contrast because many lesions in this area are highly vascular. Alternatively, MRI may yield even better definition. Cerebrospinal fluid analysis to exclude leptomeningeal malignancy and chronic infection is indicated if there are multiple cranial nerve palsies and the imaging studies are normal.

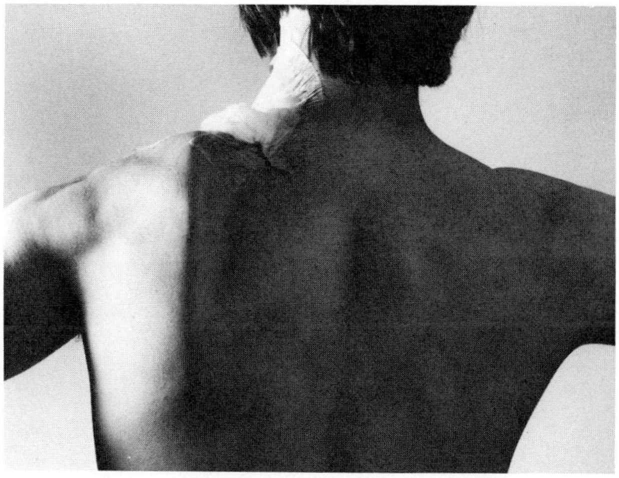

FIGURE 21.4 Spinal accessory lesion on left on attempted abduction of the left arm, demonstrating scapular winging.

EMG and conduction studies may help in some settings (Berry et al. 1991). The spinal accessory nerve is easily studied with nerve conduction by stimulating the nerve percutaneously in the posterior triangle of the neck at the midportion of the posterior border and recording from the upper trapezius. One can compare latencies and amplitudes with the sound side; a decrease in amplitude greater than 50% on the affected side indicates a substantial loss of axons.

The needle examination can confirm the degree and extent of a lower motor neuron lesion and can also be useful prognostically. If there has been prior surgery in the area of the posterior triangle, the EMG may reveal a complete or incomplete lesion. If incomplete, it is best to follow the course. If there are no units firing after several weeks, and if there are numerous fibrillations and positive waves, it may be best to explore the nerve early because surgical treatment may yield excellent results (Battista 1991).

The most common cause of accessory nerve palsies is traumatic injury at the time of lymph node biopsy or miscellaneous injuries (Berry et al. 1991). More unusual causes include bites, carotid endarterectomy, coronary artery bypass surgery, and idiopathic neuropathies.

Finally, in cases of idiopathic spinal accessory palsy, it is helpful to know if other neighboring muscles are subclinically involved. The serratus anterior, supraspinatus, infraspinatus, deltoid, and levator scapulae, as well as the rhomboids, are all easily accessible to the experienced electromyographer. Involvement of one or more along with an accessory nerve lesion is suggestive of the Parsonage-Turner syndrome (cryptogenic brachial plexopathy).

An unusual entity of isolated muscle hypertrophy has been described involving the upper trapezius after accessory lesions. Electrodiagnostic analysis suggests this is due to continuous repetitive muscular contraction similar to gastrocnemius hypertrophy after sciatic injury.

HYPOGLOSSAL NERVE

Anatomy

The hypoglossal (twelfth) nerve provides motor innervation to the extrinsic and intrinsic muscles of the tongue. It takes its origin from the hypoglossal nucleus, a somatic efferent group whose neurons are similar to the anterior horn motor neurons. The cell column consists of paired neurons beneath the floor of the fourth ventricle reaching from the most caudal part of the medulla to the striae medullaris rostrally. Axons of the hypoglossal nucleus course ventrolaterally through the reticular formation of the medulla and exit the brain stem through the ventrolateral sulcus between the pyramidal tract and the olivary eminence. About 10–15 of these rootlets coalesce to pass through the hypoglossal canal (also known as the "anterior condyloid foramen"), located less than 1 cm medial, inferior, and posterior to the jugular foramen. Outside the skull, the nerve unites as a single bundle. For several centimeters, the hypoglossal nerve courses with the glossopharyngeal, vagus, and accessory nerves between the internal jugular vein and the internal carotid artery (Hoare et al. 1993). At about the level of the mastoid, it separates and swings laterally and anterior to the internal carotid artery, looping around the occipital artery and crossing the external carotid and lingual arteries. It then passes forward above the hyoid bone and beneath the posterior digastric muscle to terminate as multiple fibers in the intrinsic and extrinsic tongue muscles (Figure 21.5). The extrinsic tongue muscles include the genioglossus, styloglossus, hypoglossus, and chondroglossus muscles. The genioglossus draws the root of the tongue forward, protruding the tip. The hypoglossi retract the tongue and depress the sides, as do the chondroglossi. The styloglossi draw the tongue upward and back. The intrinsic tongue muscles are concerned

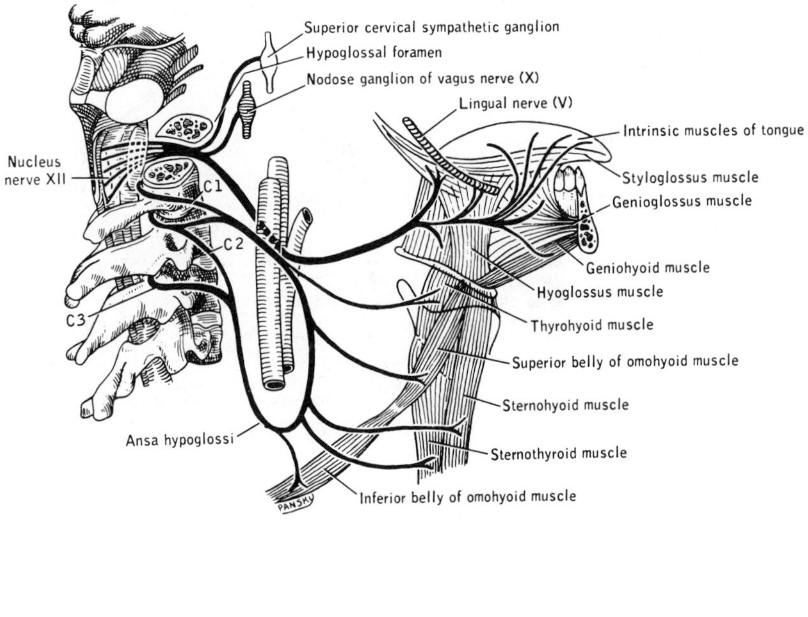

FIGURE 21.5 Origin, course, and distribution of the hypoglossal nerve. (Reprinted with permission from EL House, B Pansky. A Functional Approach to Neuroanatomy [2nd ed]. New York: McGraw-Hill, 1967.)

with altering the shape of the tongue and are important in articulation, mastication, and deglutition (DeJong 1992).

There are a number of supranuclear influences on the hypoglossal nucleus. The most important of these are the corticobulbar connections, which pass through the genu of the internal capsule and the middle of the cerebral peduncle. Probably most corticobulbar fibers are crossed. The hypoglossal nucleus contains afferent fibers, which appear to be largely spindle afferents (Thomas and Mattias 1992).

Symptoms and Signs

The symptoms of hypoglossal nerve dysfunction depend, like the other cranial nerves, on the acuteness and size of the insult and on whether the lesion or lesions are unilateral or bilateral. Unilateral lesions produce only a few symptoms, especially if the onset is gradual. Bilateral lesions, however, cause pronounced symptoms, which take the form of dysarthria, respiratory embarrassment due to prolapse of the tongue into the pharynx, and dysphagia due to inability to propel food to the back of the pharynx. Saliva tends to accumulate, and the patient stops frequently to swallow. Bilateral corticobulbar lesions are part of the *pseudobulbar syndrome*, which includes clumsy, weak tongue movements; slurred speech; an exaggerated jaw jerk; and emotional lability. This characteristic symptom complex is encountered in the lacunar states, motor neuron disease, multiple sclerosis, and high brain stem tumors.

The examination of twelfth nerve function consists largely of observation. Initially, the tongue is observed lying quiet and relaxed in the floor of the mouth. This is the optimal position for noting atrophy, fasciculations, or both (Figure 21.6). Deviations are noted with the tongue protruded, and symmetry is appreciated by observing the tongue as it moves alternately to the left and right. If the lesion or lesions are at or distal to the nucleus, the tongue will be furrowed and the median raphe will curve in a concave manner to the paralyzed side. Fasciculations are most reliably seen along the edge of the quiet tongue. Activation results in a number of movements of a vermicular type, which may be misinterpreted as fasciculations. With time, the mucosa becomes folded, dry, and thickened. Inability to protrude the tongue may be due to bilateral upper or lower motor neuron dysfunction; in addition, a short frenulum can mechanically restrict protrusion of the tongue and should be noted. If the lesion is unilateral, the tongue deviates toward the weak side because of the unopposed action of the intact contralateral genioglossus muscle. In unilateral lower motor neuron lesions, the tongue lying quietly in the mouth may deviate to the intact side because of the unopposed action of the styloglossus, which draws it up and back (Saito and Onuma 1991). The patient will be unable to push the tongue against the cheek on the sound side but will have good power toward the paretic side. With acute unilateral corticobulbar lesions, the tongue may deviate to the weak side (away from the involved hemisphere) because fibers innervating the genioglossus muscle are largely crossed. However, frequently deviation of the tongue toward the hemiparetic side is spurious and is due to the drooped paretic face. As the lesion becomes more chronic, this deviation often resolves.

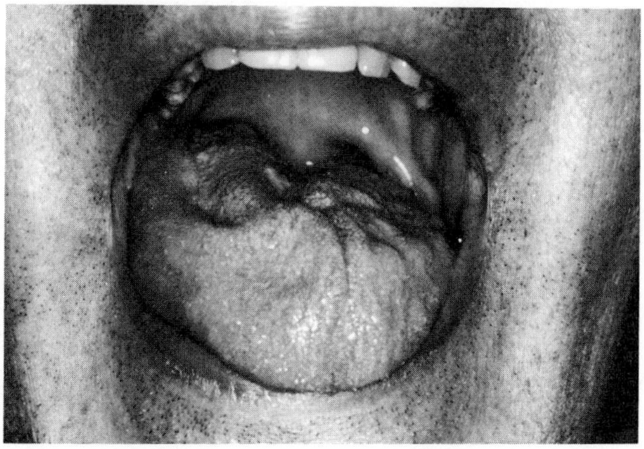

FIGURE 21.6 Bilateral hypoglossal atrophy and left vagal involvement (same patient as in Figures 21.3 and 21.4).

Evaluation

The neuroimaging evaluation of hypoglossal nerve lesions is tailored to the clinical presentation and neighborhood findings. Most destructive disorders involving this nerve are metastatic lesions invading the skull base. Plain x-rays and polytomography have been virtually replaced by high-resolution computed tomography (CT) and MRI of the skull base. These are also the procedures of choice for primary tumors of the hypoglossal nerves, most of which are extracranial neurofibromas. In rare instances, the hypoglossal nerve in the neck may be trapped by an aberrant vascular loop forcing it against the occipital artery or its branches. Hence, in undiagnosed cases of hypoglossal paralysis, angiography may be indicated.

Other unusual causes of hypoglossal dysfunction include sustained G forces, granulomas, prostatic carcinoma metastases and other tumors, Paget's disease, glomus jugulare lesions, syringobulbia, vertebral artery thrombosis, lymphoproliferative disorders, radiation, trauma, and idiopathic causes.

By far the most common cause of bilateral lower motor neuron hypoglossal nerve lesions is progressive bulbar palsy or amyotrophic lateral sclerosis. The findings are rarely restricted to the tongue but are accompanied by other motor disorders involving the trigeminal, facial, vagal, and accessory nerves; the limb and appendicular muscles; or both. In these instances, EMG may support the diagnosis by establishing denervation and motor unit abnormalities distant from the brain stem.

Table 21.2: Syndromes of the last four cranial nerves

Syndrome	*Cranial Nerve Involvement*	*Usual Lesion Location*	*Clinical Abnormality*
Vernet's	IX, X, XI	Jugular foramen	Loss of taste on posterior one-third of tongue; paralysis of vocal cord, palate, and pharynx; paralysis of trapezius plus sternocleidomastoid
Schmidt's	X, XI	Extramedullary before roots leave skull	Paralysis of soft palate, pharynx, and larynx; weakness of trapezius and sternocleidomastoid
Tapia's	X, XII	Extramedullary with involvement of hypoglossal and vagus nerves high in neck	Paralysis of pharynx and larynx; paralysis and atrophy of tongue
Jackon's	X, XI, XII	Extramedullary before roots leave skull	Paresis of palate, pharynx, and larynx; paresis of trapezius and sternocleidomastoid; paresis and atrophy of tongue
Collet-Sicard	IX, X, XI, XII	Nerves in retropharyngeal and retroparotid space	Anesthesia of palate; paresis of vocal cord and palate; weakness of trapezius and sternocleidomastoid; paresis and atrophy of tongue; hemianesthesia of pharynx and larynx
Villaret's	IX, X, XI, XII (plus cervical sympathetic)	Nerves in retropharyngeal and retroparotid space	Same as Collet-Sicard, plus Horner's syndrome

Note: Unless otherwise noted, the clinical abnormality is ipsilateral to the involved nerve or nerves.

JUGULAR FORAMEN AND ALLIED SYNDROMES

It is important to appreciate the clinical picture and diagnostic implications of multiple lower cranial nerve palsies. It is less important to recall the eponyms that are attached to the syndromes, which are summarized in Table 21.2.

Passing through the jugular foramen are the petrosal sinus; the glossopharyngeal, vagus, and spinal accessory nerves; the transverse sinus; and some meningeal branches from the occipital and ascending arteries. Hence, a skull base lesion, such as a tumor, is most likely to involve all four nerves rather than any one in isolation. Isolated involvement of two or more of the four nerves is more apt to occur outside of the skull.

The most common causes of these syndromes are tumors within the skull that extend through the foramen in a dumbbell fashion; extracranial skull base tumors, both primary and metastatic; infection of the skull base with local extension; abscess of the retropharyngeal space; and trauma and nuclear lesions such as motor neuron disease (Sawada et al. 1992).

Unusual vascular causes of these syndromes include complications of carotid artery dissection and pseudoaneurysms of the internal carotid artery. Rarely, trauma has been implicated in the Collet-Sicard syndrome.

When one establishes a combination of these palsies, the most important consideration is the presence of intrinsic brain stem findings. The presence of lower cranial nerve dysfunction in association with corticospinal signs or crossed sensory loss indicates an intramedullary tumor or vascular lesion in the brain stem or a large mass in the posterior fossa that is compressing the long tracts. The second important consideration is the presence or absence of a Horner's syndrome. The presence of a Horner's syndrome is prima facie evidence of an intramedullary lesion, particularly when accompanied by the signs noted heretofore.

Obviously, the history is crucial in a differential diagnosis. The involvement of one nerve sequentially after another suggests a neoplastic syndrome, whereas a more abrupt onset with long tract signs bespeaks a vascular lesion. Careful palpation of the neck may reveal a mass indicative of enlarged lymph nodes, a retropharyngeal tumor, or a dumbbell mass extending into the neck. One tumor that often involves the lower cranial nerves is a glomus jugulare tumor. However, it rarely does so without involving the facial and acoustic nerves, and it often erodes the tympanic cavity, presenting as a bluish mass next to the tympanic membrane.

Another entity that may produce confusion includes the postinfectious disorders referred to as a *polyneuritis cranialis*. This is a variant of the Guillain-Barré syndrome, and any combination of lesions of the lower cranial nerves may be seen.

If the signs and symptoms point to an intracranial lesion, the initial procedure of choice is an MRI of the posterior fossa. For an extracranial lesion, either a thin-section CT or MRI is acceptable. Depending on the findings, lumbar puncture to look for leptomeningeal metastasis and chronic infection is advised. If none of these are positive, the diagnosis of idiopathic polyneuropathy may be the correct one.

REFERENCES

Adler CH, Zimmerman RA, Savino PJ et al. Hemifacial spasm: Evaluation by magnetic resonance imaging and magnetic resonance tomographic angiography. Ann Neurol 1992;32:502–506.

Baker RS, Stava MW, Nelson KR et al. Aberrant reinnervation of the facial musculature in a subhuman primate: a correlative analysis of eyelid kinematics, muscle synkinesis and motoneuron localization. Neurology 1994;44:2165–2173.

Battista AF. Complications of biopsy of cervical lymph node. Surg Gynecol Obstet 1991;173:142–146.

Berry H, MacDonald EA, Mrazeh AC. Accessory nerve palsy: a review of 23 cases. Can J Neurol Sci 1991;18:337–341.

DeJong RN. The Neurological Examination (5th ed). Revised by AF Haerer. Philadelphia: Lippincott, 1992;180–200, 227–257.

Hoare TJ, Manjalay G, Proops DW. Isolated hypoglossal nerve palsy caused by carotid artery aneurysm. J Royal Soc Med 1993;86:548–549.

Hopf HC. Topodiagnostic value of brain stem reflexes. Muscle Nerve 1994;17:475–484.

Jannetta PJ. Microvascular Decompression of the Facial Nerve for Hemifacial Spasm. In CB Wilson (ed), Neurosurgical Procedures: Personal Approaches to Classic Operations. Baltimore: Williams & Wilkins 1992;154–162.

Jepsen O. Topognosis (topographic diagnosis) of facial nerve lesions. Arch Otolaryngol 1965;81:446–456.

Karnes WE. Diseases of the Seventh Cranial Nerve. In PJ Dyck, PK Thomas (eds), Peripheral Neuropathy (3rd ed). Philadelphia: Saunders, 1992;818–832.

Keane JR. Bilateral seventh nerve palsy: analysis of 43 cases and review of the literature. Neurology 1994;44:1198–1202.

May M, Galetta S. The Facial Nerve and Related Disorders of the Face. In JS Glaser (ed), Neuro-ophthalmology. Philadelphia: Lippincott, 1990;239–276.

Saito H, Onuma T. Isolated hypoglossal nerve palsy and Horner's syndrome with benign course. J Neurol Neurosurg Psychiatry 1991;54:282–283.

Sawada H, Udalia F, Kameyama M et al. Accessory nerve neuroma presenting as recurrent jugular foramen syndrome. Neuroradiology 1992;34:417–419.

Sivak M, Ochoa J, Fernandez J. Positive Manifestations of Nerve Fiber Dysfunction: Clinical Electrophysiologic and Pathologic Correlates. In WF Brown, CF Bolton (eds), Clinical Electromyography (3rd ed). Boston: Butterworth-Heinemann, 1993;128–134.

Tash RR, Kier EL, Chyatte D. Hemifacial spasm caused by a tortuous vertebral artery: MR demonstration. J Comput Assist Tomogr 1988;12:492–494.

Thomas PK, Mattias CJ. Diseases of the Ninth, Tenth, Eleventh and Twelfth Cranial Nerves. In PJ Dych, PK Thomas (eds), Peripheral Neuropathy (3rd ed). Philadelphia: Saunders, 1992;869–883.

Chapter 22
Cranial and Facial Pain

Jerry W. Swanson

Headache is a common symptom with a high prevalence in most epidemiological studies of Western populations (Rasmussen 1993). Headache is one of the ten most frequent reasons for outpatient physician visits in the United States. Patients typically present with head and facial pain because the discomfort is severe, interferes with work or other activities, or raises concerns about a serious underlying cause.

The diagnosis of a painful cephalic condition depends on three elements: the history, the neurological and general examinations, and appropriate investigations.

HISTORY

The diagnostic advice offered by the late Dr. A.L. Sahs holds well for the approach to the headache patient: "If you have 30 minutes to see a patient, spend 29 on history, one on the examination."

The method of taking a history about headache or facial pain is usually straightforward. Nevertheless, several questions are necessary, especially when dealing with a chronic condition. The scheme of questions listed in Table 22.1 can be useful for obtaining a pertinent history. This approach is fashioned, in part, after that of Blau (1986). The discussion that follows illustrates some responses and their implications.

It is usually helpful to begin by asking the patient to tell about the pain or, alternatively, simply to ask what kind of help the patient seeks. This approach allows the patient to feel at ease and to say what he or she has previously planned. Usually, the patient continues to speak for only a few minutes if not interrupted. Once the patient has had an opportunity to speak, directed but open-ended questions can be asked. The questions that follow typically contain the word *headache,* although *facial pain* could easily be substituted, if appropriate.

Types of Headaches

Many individuals, especially those with a long-standing problem, have more than one type of headache. It is valuable to establish this information at the beginning of the interview so that each type of pain can be carefully delineated. For instance, some patients have frequent or persistent headaches that are sometimes punctuated by migraine headaches. Other sufferers have clearly separated migraine and tension-type headaches (formerly called *muscle contraction* and *tension* headaches). It is also important to remember that a patient with a chronic headache disorder may develop a new headache that is a manifestation of a new disorder, such as an intracranial mass, subarachnoid hemorrhage, or intracranial infection.

Onset of Headaches

A headache disorder of many years' duration and with little change is almost always of benign origin. Migraine headaches often begin in childhood or early adulthood, and tension-type headaches are often chronic. A headache of recent onset obviously has many possible causes, including

Table 22.1: Questions for obtaining the history of headache

How many types of headache occur?
When and how did the headaches begin?
If the headaches are episodic, what is their frequency and periodicity?
How long does it take for the headaches to reach maximal intensity, and how long do they last?
When do the headaches tend to occur, and what factors precipitate a headache?
Where does the pain start, and how does it evolve?
What is the quality and the severity of the pain?
Is the pain pulsatile (throbbing)?
Are there symptoms that herald the onset or that accompany the headaches?
Does anything aggravate the pain?
What measures tend to reduce the pain?
Is there a family history of headaches?
What medications have been used to treat the headaches?
What ideas does the patient have about the headaches?
Why is the patient seeking help now?
What other medical or neurological problems does the patient have?

the new onset of either a benign condition or a more serious condition. An increasingly severe headache raises the possibility of an expanding intracranial lesion. A new headache in an elderly patient is always of concern and raises the question of an intracranial lesion or giant cell (temporal or cranial) arteritis. Headaches of instantaneous onset suggest an intracranial hemorrhage, usually in the subarachnoid space. Occasionally, mass lesions can produce intermittent acute headaches if there is interference with the cerebrospinal fluid pathways. Trauma, emotional or physical, may be an important causative factor in the pathogenesis of headache.

Frequency and Periodicity of Episodic Headaches

Migraine is episodic and does not present as a daily or constant headache for long periods. It can occur from once or twice per week to less than once per year. Cluster headaches typically occur daily for several weeks or months and are followed by a long headache-free interval, although chronic cluster headaches may occur daily for years. A related disorder, chronic paroxysmal hemicrania, occurs multiple times per day, often for years. A chronic, daily, constant headache is usually of the tension type and may be of psychogenic origin. If there is no regular periodicity, it is useful to inquire about the longest and shortest periods of freedom between headaches.

Peak and Duration of Headaches

Migraine usually peaks within 1 or 2 hours of onset and usually lasts 6–36 hours. Cluster headache is typically maximal immediately if the patient awakens with the headache in progress, or peaks within a few minutes if it begins during wakefulness. Cluster headaches characteristically last 20–60 minutes but occasionally last a few hours. "Ice-pick" head pains are momentary, lasting only seconds. Tension-type headaches commonly build up over hours and may last days to years. These headaches may merge with a headache with migraine features. This hybrid type of headache was formerly called a *mixed* or *tension-vascular* headache. A sudden severe headache that is maximal at onset and persists usually suggests an intracranial hemorrhage. Occipital neuralgia and trigeminal neuralgia are usually manifested as brief, shocklike pains, sometimes occurring in a crescendo pattern over a period of seconds to minutes. Occasionally, a duller pain in the same nerve distribution persists longer.

Time of Occurrence and Precipitating Factors

Cluster headaches often awaken patients from a sound sleep and have a tendency to occur at the same time each day in a given person. Migraine can occur at any time during the day or night but frequently begins in the morning. A headache of recent onset that disturbs sleep or is worse on waking may be due to raised intracranial pressure. Tension-type headaches are typically present during much of the day and are often more severe late in the day.

Patients with chronic recurrent headaches can often recognize factors that trigger an attack. Migraine headaches may be precipitated by bright light, menstruation, weather changes, caffeine withdrawal, sleeping longer than usual, sleeping less than usual, and ingested substances such as alcohol. Emotional factors may also precipitate migraine and tension-type headaches.

If bending, lifting, coughing, or a Valsalva maneuver produces a headache, an intracranial lesion, especially involving the posterior fossa, must be considered; however, most exertional and cough headaches are benign. Intermittent headaches that are precipitated by assuming the upright position and promptly relieved by lying down are characteristic of a cerebrospinal fluid leak. If no history of a lumbar puncture, head trauma, or a neurosurgical procedure can be identified, a spontaneous leak may be the cause.

Headache occurring during sexual activity, especially during or shortly after orgasm, may be of benign origin, especially if a headache has occurred on multiple occasions previously. A single headache in this circumstance, however, may be due to a subarachnoid hemorrhage.

Lancinating face pain triggered by facial or intraoral stimuli occurs with trigeminal neuralgia. Glossopharyngeal neuralgia is most commonly triggered by chewing, swallowing, and talking, although cutaneous trigger zones in and about the ear are occasionally present.

Location and Evolution

It is often helpful to ask the patient to delineate the location of the pain with a finger. At times, an anatomical location is indicated. For instance, the temporomandibular joint or temporalis muscle may be outlined. Trigeminal neuralgia is confined to one or more branches of the trigeminal nerve (Terrence and Fromm 1993). Often, the patient is able to localize one or more trigger points over the face or in the mouth and then outline the spread of the pain. Pain in the throat may be related to a local process or glossopharyngeal neuralgia. Pain in the lower portion of the face and neck can sometimes be produced by either a cluster or a migraine variant.

Migraine is most often unilateral, commonly in the frontotemporal region, but it may be generalized or may evolve from a unilateral location to become generalized. Cluster headaches are virtually always unilateral and are typically centered in, behind, or about the eye. A typical tension-type or muscle contraction headache is most commonly generalized or concentrated in the frontal or posterior cervico-occipital regions. Sometimes a tension-type headache begins in the nuchal muscles and spreads to the occiput; it may or may not then become generalized. When pain is localized to an eye, the intraoral region, or the ear, local processes involving these structures must be considered. Otalgia may be due to a process involving the tonsillar fossa and the posterior tongue.

Quality and Severity

Although it is often difficult for the sufferer to describe the quality of the pain, this information may be useful. It may be helpful to ask the patient to grade the severity of pain on a scale of 1–10. Headaches related to fever and hypertension often have a throbbing or pulsatile quality. Migraine often has a throbbing quality that may be superimposed on a more continuous pain. Cluster headache is characteristically severe, boring, and steady. Tension-type headaches are usually described as a feeling of fullness, tightness, or pressure, or as being like a cap, band, or vise. Headaches due to meningeal irritation, whether related to infectious meningitis or to a hemorrhage, are typically severe. Trigeminal neuralgia is severe, brief, and stabbing, occurring up to several times per minute. A milder ache may occur between paroxysms of pain. Pain due to glossopharyngeal neuralgia is similar in character to that of trigeminal neuralgia.

Premonitory Symptoms, Aura, and Accompanying Symptoms

At this juncture, leading questions may be necessary. Some patients have premonitory symptoms that precede a headache attack for hours. These can include psychological changes such as depression, euphoria, and irritability or more generalized symptoms such as constipation, diarrhea, abnormal hunger, fluid retention, or increased urination. The term *aura* refers to focal cerebral symptoms associated with a migraine attack. These symptoms most commonly last 20–30 minutes and precede the headache. At other times, the aura may continue into the headache phase or arise during the headache phase. Visual symptoms are the most frequent kind of cerebral dysfunction and may consist of either positive or negative phenomena or a mixture of both. Other hemispheric symptoms such as weakness, somatosensory disturbances (usually paresthesias), or language dysfunction may precede the headache. Aura symptoms usually have a gradual onset and spread over minutes. The slow spread is a helpful feature to differentiate these from focal neurologic symptoms due to cerebral ischemia. Symptoms of brain stem origin such as vertigo, dysarthria, ataxia, quadriparesis, and diplopia accompany basilar migraine. Migraine is occasionally accompanied by syncope. Nausea, vomiting, photophobia, phonophobia, and osmophobia characteristically accompany migraine attacks.

Ipsilateral miosis and ptosis (oculosympathetic paresis or Horner's syndrome), lacrimation, conjunctival injection, and nasal stuffiness frequently accompany cluster headache. Sweating and facial flushing on the side of the pain have been described but are uncommon. Facial swelling, usually periorbital in location, may develop with repeated attacks; infrequently, transient localized swellings of the palate are present.

Temporomandibular joint dysfunction is often characterized by jaw pain precipitated by movement of the jaw, clenching of the teeth, or both; reduction in the range of jaw movement; joint clicking; and tenderness over the joint.

Headache accompanied by fever suggests an infectious cause. Persistent or progressive diffuse or focal central nervous system symptoms suggest a structural cause for the headache. Purulent or bloody nasal discharge suggests an acute nasal or sinus cause for headaches. Likewise, a red eye raises the question of an ocular process such as infection or acute glaucoma. A history of polymyalgia rheumatica, jaw claudication, or tenderness of the scalp and superficial arteries in an elderly person raises the question of giant-cell arteritis.

A simple rule is that a headache can often be correctly diagnosed by recognizing the company it keeps.

Aggravating Factors

The worsening of headache as a result of a cough or jolt suggests an intracranial element to the pain, whereas aggravation by movement indicates a musculoskeletal component. Activity often accentuates a migraine or tension-type headache. Conversely, recumbency is usually poorly tolerated by the sufferer of a cluster headache.

Mitigating Factors

Rest, especially sleep and avoidance of light, tend to provide relief to the migraineur. Massage or heat may ameliorate the pain associated with a tension-type headache. Local application of pressure over the affected eye or ipsilateral temporal artery, local application of heat, pacing, or, rarely, short-lasting, intense physical activity may alleviate the pain of cluster headache.

Family History of Headaches

Migraine is often an inherited disorder, and a family history of migraine or sick headaches should be sought. Tension-type headaches are also frequently familial.

Prior Medications

Response to medications should be sought, including those used to treat individual headache attacks and those used prophylactically. The dose, route of delivery, dosage schedule, and duration of treatment should also be established. This information also provides an opportunity to determine whether medications such as ergot preparations and analgesics have been overused. At this point, a history of the use of caffeine-containing substances should also be elicited because they may cause or aggravate vascular headaches.

Patient Concerns

Headache pain can produce significant fear and anxiety regarding serious disease. The patient should be allowed to ventilate any concerns so that they can be appropriately addressed by the physician.

Reason for Seeking Help

The question of why the patient is seeking help may be irrelevant if the problem is of recent onset. If the problem is chronic, however, it can be useful to inquire why the patient has come for aid at this point.

Other Medical or Neurological Problems

A history of past and current medical and neurological illnesses and conditions and a history of trauma, operations, and allergies (especially to medications) should be obtained. Additionally, a history of the use of other medications unrelated to the headaches should be obtained.

EXAMINATION

In the patient with headache, the physical examination often shows no abnormalities. However, findings on examination may yield important clues as to the underlying cause. Even when the results of examination are normal, both the physician and the patient gain confidence that nothing has been overlooked. Blau's (1986) admonition that "the physician who fails to carry out a full physical examination can only give half an opinion" is an important one.

Although, strictly speaking, the history and the examination are separate parts of the evaluation, in practice the examination begins the moment the patient enters the room or the physician approaches the bedside. Careful observation helps determine whether the patient has physical or psychiatric illness or appears anxious or depressed and whether the patient's history is reliable. For instance, with respect to reliability, a patient who is unable to give a reasonably coherent history immediately is suspected of having a disordered mental state.

It is important to perform a neurological examination, including examination of the mental status, gait, cranial nerves, motor system, and sensory system, as discussed in Chapter 1. A neurovascular examination should also be performed.

The skull and cervical spine should be examined. The skull should be palpated for lumps and local tenderness. There may be tenderness over inflamed sinuses. Thickened, irregular temporal arteries with an associated reduction in pulse suggest giant cell arteritis. Occasionally, other scalp lesions may be present that point to a cause for head pain. In muscle contraction headaches, the scalp muscles may be tender.

A short neck or low hairline suggests basilar invagination or an Arnold-Chiari malformation. In an infant, separation of the sutures suggests increased intracranial pressure, most commonly due to hydrocephalus. Measuring the head circumference is always worthwhile in a child and is occasionally useful in an adult.

The cervical spine should also be tested for tenderness and mobility. Stiffness of the neck on passive flexion and Kernig's sign are evidence of meningeal irritation.

Vital signs, especially the blood pressure and pulse, should always be assessed. If there is a question of fever, the temperature should be measured. The body habitus should be noted. This observation may especially be relevant in young women with headache related to pseudotumor cerebri who tend to be obese. The general examination also includes auscultation of the heart and lungs, palpation of the abdomen, and examination of the skin.

DIFFERENTIAL DIAGNOSIS

In most cases, the history and examination are all that are needed to make a diagnosis, especially in the chronic headache sufferer. Migraine, tension-type headaches, and cluster headaches can usually be diagnosed with a high degree of certainty, especially if the headaches have been recurrent over a long period. It may then be possible to proceed directly to management.

In some situations, however, the diagnosis is uncertain. These situations specifically raise concerns of a serious organic cause for the headaches. The physician should be especially wary if the headache is of new onset, especially in middle-aged or elderly patients. Headaches that are progressive are a worrisome indication of a possible intracranial process. A new headache of abrupt onset always raises concern about an intracranial process, especially hemorrhage and sometimes a mass lesion. Headaches that interfere with sleep, though sometimes benign, must always be considered to have a potential serious cause. Headaches precipitated by exertion, change of position, cough, sneeze, or strain may be benign, although again they raise the question of intracranial lesions, especially of the posterior fossa. Systemic symptoms such as weight loss, fever, or those associated with another known systemic disease such as malignancy should be investigated with care. Headaches that are associated with neurological symptoms, except those that are typical for migraine, should raise concern.

The investigations required to evaluate a patient with headaches can include almost all of the tests used in neurology and neurosurgery, as well as various medical tests. Selection of the appropriate tests depends on the formulation after the history and physical examination. Indiscriminate use of batteries of tests is unnecessary and is poor practice.

Neuroimaging Tests

Computed Tomography Scanning

Computed tomography (CT) scanning is the single most useful test in the evaluation of headache. If a CT scan, obtained with and without intravenous contrast, is normal, then a structural intracranial lesion is extremely unlikely to be responsible for headache. Space-occupying lesions such as parenchymal tumors, intracerebral hematomas, areas of cerebral infarction, abscess formation, hydrocephalus, tumors of the pineal and pituitary regions, tumors of the cranial nerves, epidural hematomas, and acute subdural hematomas can all be detected with a high degree of reliability (see Chapter 39). Meningeal cancer can often be identified as well. With appropriate bone windows, processes affecting the skull and the base of the skull can also be detected. The posterior fossa, the cranial cavity close to the base of the skull, and the region near the foramen magnum may be difficult to visualize on a CT scan because of bony artifact.

CT scanning can also detect subarachnoid hemorrhage in most cases. If the scan is unremarkable, however, and the history is suggestive of subarachnoid hemorrhage, a cerebrospinal fluid examination should be performed.

The CT scan in migraine is typically normal, but severe migraine that is present for several days may show areas of decreased attenuation compatible with edema. This typically resolves completely unless an area of infarction has been produced. The CT scan in cluster headache, tension-type headache, and other functional headaches is normal.

The CT scan is also valuable for assessing the orbit, sinuses, facial bones, cervical spine, and soft tissues of the neck.

Skull Roentgenography

Skull films are generally unnecessary if a CT scan is obtained with the appropriate bone windows. Nevertheless, various lesions, including enlargement of the sella turcica, bony lesions of the calvarium, and congenital or developmental abnormalities of the skull are often well demonstrated.

Sinus Roentgenography

Radiological evaluation with plain films can identify opacified sinuses, which suggest the presence of sinus ostium obstruction and fluid retention in the sinus, hemorrhage, or tumor. CT and magnetic resonance imaging (MRI) scanning of the sinuses provide greater definition.

Cervical Spine Roentgenography

The role of the cervical spine in the causation of headaches escapes precise definition. However, constant or long-standing occipitonuchal pain may result from degenerative changes in the discs and facet joints of the upper cervical spine. Rheumatoid arthritis can also produce changes leading to instability and occipitonuchal pain. Tomographic films may be necessary to demonstrate the bony changes around the C1–C2 region.

Head and neck pain after hyperflexion-hyperextension whiplash injury may be accompanied by normal cervical spine films. Flexion and extension and odontoid views should be obtained. Compression of a lateral mass of a cervical vertebra can occur with a lateral flexion injury, which may require pillar views for detection. Congenital abnormalities of the cervical spine, such as the Klippel-Feil syndrome, may be associated with other disorders such as an Arnold-Chiari malformation and syringomyelia.

Other Roentgenograms

Mandibular views and tomograms or MRI scans of the temporomandibular joints may be helpful in selected patients. Degeneration of these joints may lead to the diagnosis of the temporomandibular joint diseases, but the presence of arthritic changes in this joint should not be taken as proof that the patient's headaches are related. Dental roentgenograms or roentgenograms of the face, jaw, and orbit may be useful in patients suspected of having abnormalities in these regions.

Magnetic Resonance Imaging

MRI is usually not required in the investigation of headache but is the method of choice for noninvasively examining the posterior fossa and its contents. It can, for instance, clearly demonstrate the foramen magnum region, allowing identification of lesions such as Arnold-Chiari malformation. The cervical spine and spinal cord and the soft tissues of the neck, sinuses, orbit, and temporomandibular joint can also be readily examined.

Magnetic resonance angiography (MRA) is a noninvasive method that can yield information about intracranial and extracranial vasculature. In many cases, it may demonstrate arteriovenous malformations and aneurysms. It may also demonstrate large artery dissections. MRA is quite sensitive for the delineation of intracranial venous sinus thrombosis.

Cerebral Angiography

Cerebral angiography is rarely needed in the investigation of headache in the absence of physical signs or symptoms. It may be helpful, however, in the evaluation of occlusive vascular disease, which occasionally produces headaches. It is necessary for the precise delineation of arteriovenous malformations and saccular aneurysms that give rise to subarachnoid hemorrhage. It also reliably delineates arterial dissections.

Radioisotope Studies

Radionuclide brain scanning has largely been replaced by computed tomography. Nevertheless, radioisotope scanning of the subarachnoid space is useful in one condition—namely, spontaneous cerebrospinal fluid leakage. This most frequently occurs through a tear in the arachnoid and dura in the midthoracic region after some violent physical activity. When a leak is present, it may be demonstrated as a pool of radioactivity collecting outside the confines of the neuraxis.

Cerebrospinal Fluid Tests

If the cause of headache is suspected to be intracranial infection, intracranial bleeding, or meningeal cancer, and the CT scan is negative, a lumbar puncture should be performed. Tests performed on spinal fluid are outlined in Chapters 59 and 60.

Electroencephalography

Electroencephalography (EEG) is rarely useful in the investigation of headache. No specific diagnostic EEG pattern is associated with any type of headache. EEG may occasionally be helpful in patients with focal symptoms when imaging tests are normal and in disorders associated with a change in consciousness.

General Health Tests

A few blood tests are important in the investigation of headache in the absence of systemic illness. Determining the sedimentation rate is essential in the evaluation of giant-cell arteritis. Although a normal value does not exclude the condition, it greatly reduces the likelihood (see Chapter 74). Episodic headaches associated with unusual behavior or impairment of consciousness may suggest an insulinoma, and the plasma glucose value should be determined during an attack or after a prolonged fast. Levels of carboxyhemoglobin should be measured in patients complaining of early morning headaches during the heating season, especially when several members of the same household are affected. Estimation of blood alcohol levels and drug screening may be important in certain patients. Serum total thyroxine should be measured in chronic headache sufferers because hypothyroidism may present with headaches.

Urinary concentrations of vanillylmandelic acid, metanephrines, and free catecholamines should be measured if a pheochromocytoma is suspected.

Special Examinations and Consultations

Perimetry is helpful in the delineation of visual field defects. Tonometry is necessary to document elevated intraocular pressure in glaucoma. Unless the eye is red or the cornea is cloudy, however, glaucoma is an unlikely cause of head or even eye pain. These tests are routinely done by ophthalmologists, who also have the equipment and expertise to perform slit lamp examinations and other specialized examinations.

If pain due to dental causes or temporomandibular joint dysfunction is suspected, a dentist or oral surgeon skilled in the detection and treatment of these disorders should be consulted.

Diagnosis of tumors of the sinuses, nasopharynx, and neck, as well as inflammation of the sinuses, is aided by the expertise of an otorhinolaryngologist. The cocaine test can be used to confirm a diagnosis of glossopharyngeal neuralgia. A 10% cocaine solution is applied to the tonsil and pharynx and should relieve the pain for 1–2 hours thereafter.

Temporal artery biopsy is performed to confirm giant cell arteritis (see Chapter 74).

In selected cases, psychiatric consultation may be helpful for diagnosis and management—for example, headaches presented as a chronic pain disorder with or without a history of drug abuse.

Further Observation

Sometimes a definitive diagnosis cannot be reached after history-taking, examination, and investigation. In such cases, further observation of the patient for a period of days to weeks, perhaps during a trial of therapy, will usually allow diagnosis.

REFERENCES

Blau JN. Headache: History, Examination, Differential Diagnosis and Special Investigations. In PJ Vinken, GW Bruyn, HL Klawans (eds), Handbook of Clinical Neurology. Vol. 48. New York: Elsevier, 1986;43–58.

Rasmussen BK. Epidemiology. In J Oleson, P Tfelt-Hansen, KM Welch (eds), The Headaches. New York: Raven, 1993;15–20.

Terrence CF, Fromm GH. Trigeminal Neuralgia and other Cranial Neuralgias. In J Oleson, P Tfelt-Hansen, KMA Welch (eds), The Headaches. New York: Raven, 1993;773–785.

SUGGESTED READING

Blau JN. How to take a history of head or facial pain. Br Med J 1982;285:1,249–1,251.

Davidoff, RA. Migraine: Manifestations, Pathogenesis and Management. Philadelphia: FA Davis, 1995.

Chapter 23
Brain Stem Syndromes

Michael Wall

The other chapters in this book that emphasize symptoms should be approached by beginning with the history and generating a differential diagnosis. This list of possibilities is then refined during the examination. This chapter calls for a different approach. When the neurologist evaluates a patient with a brain stem disorder, the most effective method of diagnosis often is to organize the differential diagnosis around the objective physical findings, particularly in patients with an altered mental status, such as coma. The symptoms are still integrated in the approach, but the physical findings take the center stage.

Organization around physical findings is efficient because very specific neurological localization, which limits the diagnostic alternatives, is often possible. The long tracts of the nervous system traverse the entire brain stem in the longitudinal (rostrocaudal) plane. Cranial nerve nuclei and their respective cranial nerves originate and exit at distinct levels of the brain stem. This allows for exquisite localization of function based on the findings of the neurological examination.

The chapter begins with a discussion of the brain stem ocular motor syndromes followed by miscellaneous brain stem syndromes and then brain stem stroke syndromes. The diencephalic and thalamic syndromes are also described in this chapter.

OCULAR MOTOR SYNDROMES

Combined Vertical Gaze Ophthalmoplegia

Combined vertical gaze ophthalmoplegia is defined as paresis of both upward and downward gaze. Vertical gaze ophthalmoplegia is an example of a brain stem syndrome in which the objective physical findings dictate the diagnostic approach to the problem. Symptoms of vertical gaze ophthalmoplegia, when present, are relatively nonspecific and usually occur in patients who have difficulty looking down, as in reading, eating from the table, and walking down a flight of stairs. In addition, symptoms may be unobtainable because of mental status changes due to dysfunction of the reticular formation that lies adjacent to the vertical gaze generator in the rostral midbrain (see Chapter 42).

The neurological examination will disclose the associated signs of the disorders listed in the differential diagnosis (Table 23.1). There may be coma associated with reticular system involvement. Long-tract signs and loss of pupillary reflexes are commonly associated. The syndrome of combined vertical gaze ophthalmoplegia is diagnosed when the ocular findings occur in isolation from long-tract signs.

With combined vertical gaze ophthalmoplegia, there is loss of vertical saccades and pursuit. This gaze limitation may or may not be overcome by the oculocephalic ("doll's head" or "doll's eyes") maneuver, which tests the vestibuloocular reflex (see Chapter 42). It is demonstrated by having the patient focus on an object, rotating the patient's head, and looking for a conjugate eye movement in the opposite direction. Bell's phenomenon (reflex movement of the eyes up and out in response to forced eye closure) is often absent. Skew deviation (vertical malalignment of the eyes) may occur. Absence of convergence and loss of pupillary reactions to light are common.

The location of the lesion of combined vertical gaze ophthalmoplegia is the rostral interstitial nucleus of the medial longitudinal fasciculus (riMLF) for loss of vertical pursuit and saccades (Leigh and Zee 1991).

Table 23.1: Differential diagnosis of combined vertical gaze ophthalmoplegia

Stroke
Ischemic
Hemorrhagic
Progressive supranuclear palsy
Arteriovenous malformation
Multiple sclerosis
Thalamic and mesencephalic tumors
Whipple's disease
Syphilis
Vasculitis (for example, systemic lupus erythematosus)
Metabolic disorders
Lipid storage diseases
Wilson's disease
Kernicterus
Wernicke's encephalopathy

Table 23.2: Differential diagnosis of dorsal midbrain syndrome

Pineal tumors
Stroke
Ischemic cerebrovascular disease
Thalamic hemorrhage
Trauma
Hydrocephalus
Multiple sclerosis
Transtentorial herniation
Congenital aqueductal stenosis
Metastatic tumors
Infections
Encephalitis
Cysticercosis
Midbrain arteriovenous malformation
Stereotactic midbrain surgery
Metabolic disorders
Lipid storage disease
Wilson's disease
Kernicterus
Wernicke's encephalopathy

Table 23.1 lists the disorders known to affect the rostral mesodiencephalic region (differential diagnosis) and to cause combined vertical gaze ophthalmoplegia (see Chapters 42 and 75). The most common causes of isolated combined vertical gaze ophthalmoplegia are stroke and progressive supranuclear palsy.

The diagnostic formulation varies with the age of the patient. Isolated combined vertical gaze ophthalmoplegia is usually due to infarction of the rostral dorsal midbrain (Tatemichi et al. 1992). The lesion is usually well demonstrated with computed tomography (CT) or magnetic resonance imaging (MRI). When the onset is gradual instead of abrupt, or the patient is young, the other disorders should be considered (see Table 23.1). In the elderly, progressive supranuclear palsy (PSP) (Chapter 76) is likely if the onset is gradual.

The laboratory investigations used to evaluate combined vertical gaze ophthalmoplegia include CT or, preferably, MRI. Care should be taken not to overlook lesions inferior to the floor of the third ventricle. The anatomy of this region in the transverse axial plane is complex (Wall et al. 1986). Lumbar puncture, syphilis serology, erythrocyte sedimentation rate, and an antinuclear antibody test complete the evaluation when the cause is not obvious. One should consider small-bowel biopsy if Whipple's disease remains a possible diagnosis.

Upgaze Paresis (Dorsal Midbrain or Parinaud's Syndrome)

Another brain stem syndrome that often occurs without symptoms is the dorsal midbrain syndrome. When symptoms occur, the patient has difficulty looking up and blurry distant vision, due to accommodative spasm.

On examination, there is loss of upgaze, which is usually supranuclear (that is, there is loss of pursuit and saccades with preservation of the vestibulo-ocular reflex), and normal to large pupils with light-near dissociation (that is, loss of the light reaction with preservation of pupilloconstriction in response to a near target) or pupillary areflexia. Convergence-retraction nystagmus, in which the eyes make convergent and retracting oscillations following an upward saccade, is sometimes present. Lid retraction, in addition to the previous three findings, completes the common tetrad of findings of the dorsal midbrain syndrome (Keane 1990).

Forced ductions (see Chapter 16) may be performed by grasping anesthetized sclera with forceps and moving the globe through its range of motion. The presence of restriction of movement with forced ductions implies a lesion within the orbit, such as thyroid ophthalmopathy, Brown's superior oblique tendon sheath syndrome, or congenital upgaze limitation.

The location of the lesion causing the upgaze paresis of the dorsal midbrain syndrome is the posterior commissure and its interstitial nucleus (Leigh and Zee 1991). The presence of the full syndrome implies a lesion of the dorsal midbrain (including the posterior commissure), a bilateral lesion of the pretectal region, or a large unilateral tegmental lesion.

The differential diagnosis is listed in Table 23.2. Other than the mild upgaze limitation that occurs with age, the most common cause of loss of upgaze is a tumor of the pineal region. The next most common causes are stroke and trauma. The upgaze palsy portion of the syndrome can be mimicked by (1) double elevator palsy; (2) progressive supranuclear palsy; (3) orbital causes such as thyroid ophthalmopathy and bilateral Brown's superior oblique tendon sheath syndrome; (4) pseudodorsal midbrain syndrome, secondary to myasthenia gravis, or the Guillain-Barré syndrome; and (5) congenital upgaze limitation.

The diagnostic formulation of the dorsal midbrain syndrome varies with age. In children and adolescents, pineal region tumors are usually the cause. In young and middle-aged adults, the disorder is uncommon and the cause may be trauma, multiple sclerosis, or arteriovenous malformation. In the elderly, stroke and PSP are the most common causes.

The laboratory investigation needed to evaluate the dorsal midbrain syndrome is CT or, preferably, MRI. If no tumor is present, and an infectious or inflammatory cause is suspected, a lumbar puncture should be performed.

Downgaze Paresis

Isolated downgaze paresis is uncommon. The symptoms, when they occur, are difficulty in reading, eating, and walking down stairs.

Neurological examination reveals loss of downward pursuit and saccades, although occasionally pursuit may be spared. The vertical oculocephalic maneuver may be normal or may disclose gaze limitation. Convergence may be lost, and gaze-evoked upbeating nystagmus may be present on upward gaze. In young patients one should evaluate forced ductions for evidence of congenital downgaze limitation.

The site of the lesion for isolated downgaze paresis is bilateral involvement of the lateral portions of the riMLF. The differential diagnosis is ischemic stroke, PSP, and Whipple's disease. The laboratory investigations to support the clinical diagnosis include CT or, preferably, MRI. Lesions may be detected in the rostral mesodiencephalic junction inferior to the floor of the third ventricle.

The diagnostic formulation of isolated downgaze limitation is uncomplicated: When acute in onset, it is usually due to ischemic cerebrovascular disease. PSP should be considered in an elderly patient with a progressive course.

Internuclear Ophthalmoplegia

Internuclear ophthalmoplegia (INO) is characterized by paresis of adduction of one eye, with horizontal nystagmus in the contralateral eye when it is abducted. It is due to a lesion of the MLF ipsilateral to the side of the adduction weakness.

Surprisingly, most patients with INO have no symptoms. The symptoms that may be associated with INO are diplopia, oscillopsia of one of the two images, and blurred vision. When diplopia is present, it is due to medial rectus paresis (horizontal diplopia) or skew deviation (vertical diplopia).

The MLF carries information for vertical pursuit and the vertical vestibulo-ocular reflex. Consequently, other associated findings with MLF lesions are abnormal vertical smooth pursuit and impaired reflex vertical eye movements (doll's head maneuver, Bell's phenomenon). Voluntary vertical eye movements (pursuit and saccades) are unaffected. There may also be gaze-evoked vertical nystagmus, usually on upgaze and skew deviation. Skew deviation is a pure vertical ocular deviation that is not due to a cranial nerve palsy, orbital lesion, or strabismus, but is due to disturbed supranuclear input to the third and fourth cranial nerve nuclei. The topic is discussed further in Chapter 42.

Internuclear ophthalmoplegia may occur as a false localizing sign. Cases of brain stem compression due to subdural hematoma with transtentorial herniation and cerebellar masses may cause INO. Myasthenia gravis and the Guillain-Barré syndrome may also simulate INO.

The differential diagnosis is varied. Careful examination will usually differentiate a lesion of the MLF from a partial third nerve palsy, myasthenia gravis, strabismus, or thyroid ophthalmopathy. The common causes of INO are stroke in the elderly and multiple sclerosis in the young (Leigh and Zee 1991).

The laboratory investigations to elucidate the cause include MRI. An edrophonium (Tensilon) test should be performed to rule out myasthenia gravis unless there are associated signs of obligatory brain stem dysfunction.

The diagnostic formulation for INO first necessitates accurate localization of the lesion. Limitation of adduction is initially formulated simply as an adduction deficit. It may be due to (1) a lesion of the midbrain or third cranial nerve disrupting innervation; (2) a disorder of the neuromuscular junction (myasthenia gravis); or (3) a lesion directly involving the medial rectus muscle.

Horizontal Gaze Paresis

Although there are no common symptoms of horizontal gaze paresis, this condition seldom occurs in isolation. Patients may complain of inability to see or to look to the side. Because supranuclear gaze pareses are conjugate by definition, diplopia does not occur.

On examination, with unilateral isolated involvement of the paramedian pontine reticular formation (PPRF), there is loss of ipsilateral saccades and pursuit. However, there are full horizontal eye movements with the oculocephalic maneuver.

Lesions of the sixth nerve nucleus cause horizontal gaze paresis with inability of the oculocephalic maneuver to overcome the gaze limitation, but there is always an associated ipsilateral peripheral facial palsy from involvement of the fascicle of the seventh nerve coursing over the sixth nucleus.

With bilateral lesions there is loss or limitation of horizontal saccades and (usually) pursuit in both directions. Gaze-paretic nystagmus may be present. In the acute phase, transient vertical gaze paresis and vertical nystagmus or upgaze paresis can occur. In the chronic phase, there are full vertical eye movements, although there may be nystagmus on upgaze.

The location of the lesion for horizontal gaze paresis is the frontopontine tract, mesencephalic reticular formation, PPRF, and sixth nerve nucleus. The explanation of a gaze palsy occurring with a nuclear lesion is given later in this chapter.

The differential diagnosis is varied (Leigh and Zee 1991). As with other ocular motility disorders, myasthenia gravis may cause gaze limitation that simulates a CNS lesion. The diagnostic formulation varies with age, rapidity of onset, and associated clinical findings. For patients with an acute

Table 23.3: Differential diagnosis of total ophthalmoplegia

Oculomotor apraxia
Guillain-Barré syndrome
Myasthenia gravis
Thyroid ophthalmopathy (especially in combination with myasthenia gravis)
Chronic progressive external ophthalmoplegia syndromes
Wilson's disease
Pituitary apoplexy
Botulism
Tetanus
Progressive supranuclear palsy
Anticonvulsant intoxication
Wernicke's encephalopathy
Acute bilateral pontine or mesodiencephalic lesions

onset whose age is over 50 years, cerebrovascular disease, ischemic or hemorrhagic, is a likely cause. With a subacute onset under age 50, one should consider multiple sclerosis. Congenital cases are usually due to the Möbius syndrome. Systemic lupus erythematosus, syphilis, and Wernicke's encephalopathy should be considered for any acquired cases (see Chapter 16).

The laboratory investigations for horizontal gaze paresis include MRI. Lumbar puncture may be useful for patients in whom multiple sclerosis is a diagnostic possibility.

Global Paralysis of Gaze

The common symptoms of the global paralysis of gaze are inability to look voluntarily (saccades and pursuit) in any direction (Leigh and Zee 1991). However, global paralysis of gaze rarely occurs in isolation, and signs and symptoms of involvement of other local structures are usually present.

The location of the lesion is the frontopontine tract for saccades, and the parieto-occipitopontine tract for pursuit, where they converge at the subthalamic and upper midbrain level.

The differential diagnosis for total ophthalmoplegia is given in Table 23.3. The common causes for this presentation are diseases outside the CNS such as Guillain-Barré syndrome, myasthenia gravis, and chronic progressive external ophthalmoplegia (CPEO). The differential diagnosis for intra-axial lesions is stroke, Wernicke's encephalopathy, and PSP.

The diagnostic formulation is usually concerned with extra-axial (cranial nerve, neuromuscular junction, or muscle) pathology, as isolated complete ophthalmoplegia is rarely caused by brain stem lesion. Myasthenia gravis (sometimes in combination with thyroid ophthalmopathy) and Guillain-Barré syndrome are much more likely possibilities if the onset is subacute. If the presentation is longstanding, slowly progressive, and accompanied by eyelid ptosis, the CPEO syndromes, such as Kearns-Sayre's syndrome, should be considered. In these extra-axial disorders, oculocephalics will not overcome the gaze limitations. In the elderly, PSP is a diagnostic possibility; in alcoholics and nutritionally deprived patients, Wernicke's encephalopathy should always be considered.

The laboratory investigations for patients with global paralysis of gaze should include MRI. An edrophonium test is performed when myasthenia gravis is suspected. When botulism is suspected, electromyography with repetitive stimulation and serum assay for botulinum toxin should be performed.

One-and-a-Half Syndrome

The one-and-a-half syndrome is characterized by a gaze palsy when looking toward the side of the lesion, together with internuclear ophthalmoplegia on looking away from the lesion (Leigh and Zee 1991). The common symptoms are diplopia, oscillopsia (the illusion that objects or scenes are oscillating), and blurred vision. Associated findings are skew deviation and gaze-evoked nystagmus on upgaze or lateral gaze, and less commonly on downgaze. Acutely, in the primary position there may be exotropia (one eye deviated outward). There may also be limitation of upgaze, saccadic vertical pursuit, and loss of convergence.

The location of the lesion is the paramedian pontine reticular formation or sixth nerve nucleus. The lesion extends to involve the internuclear fibers crossing from the contralateral sixth nerve nucleus, which causes the INO.

The differential diagnosis is multiple sclerosis, stroke, arteriovenous malformation, or tumor of the lower pons. A pseudo–one-and-a-half syndrome may occur with myasthenia gravis or the Guillain-Barré syndrome. The diagnostic formulation for the one-and-a-half syndrome is similar to that for INO. Prior to age 50, the cause is usually multiple sclerosis; after age 50 it is usually cerebrovascular disease.

The laboratory investigations for the one-and-a-half syndrome are MRI and, if indicated in suspected multiple sclerosis, lumbar puncture.

Syndromes Involving Ocular Motor Nuclei

Patients with lesions of the third or sixth nerve nucleus not only present with accompanying long-tract signs but also show different ocular motility disturbances than with lesions of the third or sixth cranial nerve.

Third Nerve Nucleus

The common symptoms of nuclear third nerve palsies are diplopia and eyelid ptosis.

The signs present on the side of the lesion are weakness of the inferior and medial recti and the inferior oblique muscles. Upgaze limitation is present with both eyes since the superior rectus subnucleus is contralateral and the axons cross within the nuclear complex. In addition, eyelid ptosis and dilated unreactive pupils may be present on both sides since the levator subnucleus and Edinger-Westphal nuclei are bilaterally represented.

To localize a lesion to the third nerve nucleus, both eyes must have some involvement because of the bilateral representation. The superior rectus and levator of the eyelid, however, are bilaterally represented and thus cannot demonstrate single muscle involvement. In addition, because the medial rectus subnucleus is in the most ventral portion of the nucleus and all the dorsal subnuclei send axons through it, single muscle involvement of the medial rectus may not be possible. There may be sparing of the eyelid levator subnucleus because it is located at the dorsocaudal periphery of the nuclear complex (Bryan and Hamad 1992).

The differential diagnosis is stroke (Kobayashi et al. 1986) (either ischemic or hemorrhagic), metastatic tumor, and multiple sclerosis. Of these diagnoses, only ischemic stroke is common. Disorders that simulate nuclear third nerve palsy are myasthenia gravis, CPEO, thyroid ophthalmopathy, and the Guillain-Barré syndrome.

The laboratory investigations for this syndrome are CT or, preferably, MRI, which usually demonstrate the ischemic cerebrovascular lesion.

Once the proper localization has been made, the diagnostic formulation is straightforward.

Sixth Nerve Nucleus

The sixth nerve nucleus has two populations of neurons (Leigh and Zee 1991). The abducens motor neurons terminate on the ipsilateral lateral rectus muscle. Internuclear neurons cross at the level of the sixth nerve nucleus, join the MLF, and terminate on the medial rectus subnucleus of the third cranial nerve. Therefore, a lesion of the sixth nerve nucleus causes an ipsilateral *gaze palsy*.

Patients with isolated horizontal gaze paresis are usually asymptomatic. If they do have symptoms, they complain of difficulty looking to one side.

On examination, there is conjugate horizontal gaze paresis not overcome by an oculocephalic maneuver or caloric stimulation. This occurs because the fibers mediating these responses, the vestibulo-ocular reflex, synapse in the sixth nerve nucleus. A peripheral seventh nerve palsy invariably accompanies a lesion of the sixth nerve nucleus.

The differential diagnosis is stroke, Wernicke's encephalopathy, multiple sclerosis, and a tumor of the pontomedullary junction.

The laboratory investigations for the evaluation of a lesion of the sixth nerve nucleus are CT or, preferably, MRI, lumbar puncture (when multiple sclerosis is suspected), and an edrophonium test to rule out myasthenia gravis if there are no long-tract signs obligatory for intra-axial disease.

OTHER BRAIN STEM AND ASSOCIATED SYNDROMES

Diencephalic Syndrome (Russell's Syndrome)

The common symptoms of the diencephalic syndrome are emaciation with increased appetite, euphoria, vomiting, and excessive sweating. Patients may also have an alert appearance with motor hyperactivity. Most cases occur in children under the age of 3 years.

The differential diagnosis at this stage is hyperthyroidism, diabetes mellitus, a tumor in the region of fourth ventricle, and a hypothalamic tumor. On examination there is emaciation. Most patients appear pale without anemia. Ophthalmological findings include optic atrophy and, infrequently, nystagmus.

The laboratory investigations for the diencephalic syndrome may show a serum growth hormone level that is elevated and incompletely suppressed by hyperglycemia. CT or MRI usually demonstrates a hypothalamic mass lesion. Malignant cells may be present in the cerebrospinal fluid (CSF), which is diagnostic. The CSF may also contain beta human chorionic gonadotropin in cases of germinomas. A lumbar puncture should not be performed if neuroimaging studies demonstrate a mass effect.

Thalamic Syndrome

The thalamic syndrome was first described by Dejerine and Roussy in 1906. The common symptoms of this syndrome are pain (thalamic pain), numbness, and hemisensory loss. The pain may be spontaneous or evoked by any form of stimulation. It often has a disagreeable and lasting quality. Patients may also complain of a distorted sense of taste.

On examination, there is marked hemianesthesia, which may be dissociated; that is, pain and temperature, or light touch and vibration sense, may be separately lost. However, there is usually marked proprioceptive loss, often with astereognosis. A transient hemiparesis sometimes occurs.

The location of the lesion for this type of pain is usually the ventroposterolateral nucleus of the thalamus. In addition to the thalamus, thalamic-type pain can occur with lesions of the parietal lobe (Schahmann and Leifer 1992), medial lemniscus, and dorsolateral medulla (Moffie and Hamburger 1986).

The differential diagnosis is stroke or tumor.

The diagnostic formulation depends on the rate of onset of symptoms, associated signs, and neuroimaging studies. The apoplectic onset of symptoms implicates cerebrovascular disease. Gradual onset with progressive worsening of symptoms and signs is characteristic of brain tumor. Neuroimaging studies should confirm the clinical impression.

Laboratory investigations for this disorder are CT or MRI. Somatosensory evoked responses may aid in documenting the location of the lesion.

Tectal Deafness

The symptoms associated with tectal deafness are bilateral deafness associated with other related CNS symptoms such as poor coordination, weakness, or vertigo.

The differential diagnosis of the deafness is conduction-type hearing loss, cochlear disorders, bilateral eighth nerve lesions, tectal deafness, and pure word deafness (see Chapter 19).

On examination there is deafness that usually spares pure tones. Other brain stem signs, including the dorsal midbrain syndrome, discussed earlier, are often associated.

The location of the lesion is the inferior colliculi with the most common etiologies being a tumor of the brain stem, cerebellum, or pineal region, and stroke.

The diagnostic formulation for hearing loss due to lesions rostral to the cochlear nuclei is the presence of hearing loss characterized by sparing of pure tone, with marked deterioration when background noise distortion or competing messages are added. In addition, signs of damage to adjacent nervous system structures are present. Neuroimaging studies may confirm the diagnosis.

The pertinent laboratory investigations include CT or, preferably, MRI and an audiogram. Auditory tests that reveal CNS signs of auditory loss such as distorted speech audiometry, dichotic auditory testing, and auditory brain stem evoked responses may be helpful.

Foramen Magnum Syndrome

The foramen magnum syndrome is characterized by upper motor neuron type weakness and sensory loss involving any modality below the head. This syndrome is important because it is often caused by benign tumors, such as meningiomas, which are amenable to complete removal if they are detected early in their course. Its only manifestations may be those of a high spinal cord syndrome (see Chapter 67).

The common initial symptoms are typically neck stiffness and pain, which may radiate into the shoulder. Occipital headache also may be an early symptom. Other common symptoms are weakness of the upper or lower extremities, numbness most commonly of hands or arms, and clumsiness. In addition, patients may report a gait disturbance.

The differential diagnosis at this stage is cervical spondylosis, syringomyelia, multiple sclerosis, transverse myelitis, atlantoaxial subluxation, and foramen magnum or upper cervical cord tumor.

On examination, hemiparesis or quadraparesis and sensory loss are common. The loss of sensation may involve all modalities. In some cases it may be dissociated and cape-like or occurring in a C2 distribution. In others, a hemisensory pattern below the cranium or involvement of only the lower extremities is found. Pseudoathetosis due to loss of joint position sense may be an early sign. Atrophy of muscles of the upper extremities may occur at levels well below the lesion—for instance, intrinsic muscles of the hands. Electric shock–like sensations radiating down the spine, which may be transmitted into the extremities, may occur with neck flexion (Lhermitte's symptom). This finding occurs with lesions of the posterior columns, most commonly multiple sclerosis. Lower cranial nerve palsies are infrequent. The presence of downbeating nystagmus in primary position or lateral gaze strongly suggests a lesion of the craniocervical junction. This may be missed unless the eyelids are manually elevated and the nystagmus is sought when the patient gazes laterally and slightly downward.

The differential diagnosis at this stage is a foramen magnum or upper cervical cord tumor. The tumor type is usually meningioma, neurofibroma, glioma, or metastasis. Cervical spondylosis, multiple sclerosis, syringobulbia, and the Chiari malformation are other diagnostic considerations.

The definitive laboratory investigation for evaluation of the foramen magnum syndrome is MRI.

Patients with foramen magnum tumors may have a relapsing and remitting course simulating multiple sclerosis. Since many of these tumors are meningiomas, one should be alert for patients at risk. Meningiomas occur with increased prevalence in women in their childbearing years and increase in size during pregnancy. Cervical spondylosis is usually associated with a related radiculopathy and is not accompanied by downbeating nystagmus or lower cranial nerve abnormalities. Characteristic MRI abnormalities will demonstrate a syrinx commonly accompanying a Chiari malformation.

The diagnosis requires a high index of suspicion early in the patient's course. Foramen magnum tumors are known to present difficult diagnostic problems, as signs can be minimal with a large tumor.

Syringobulbia

Syringobulbia is a disorder of the lower brain stem and spinal cord due to progressive enlargement of a fluid-filled cavity that involves the medulla and almost invariably the spinal cord (syringomyelia). The symptoms and signs are primarily those of a disorder of the region of the central spinal cord (see syringomyelia, Chapter 67).

The common symptoms of syringobulbia and syringomyelia are painless burns, hand numbness, neck and arm pain, leg stiffness, and headache together with oscillopsia, diplopia, or vertigo (Morgan and Williams 1992).

On examination there are signs of lower brain stem dysfunction. Lower motor neuron signs of the ninth through twelfth cranial nerves may be present. Nystagmus, if present, is horizontal, vertical, or rotatory. Signs of a spinal cord lesion characteristically coexist. In the upper extremities, there may be dissociated anesthesia of an upper limb or forequarter (that is, loss of pain and temperature sensation with sparing of other modalities). The sensory loss may also be in a hemisensory distribution. Absent or decreased deep tendon reflexes in the upper extremities are the rule.

Spastic paraparesis, usually asymmetrical, may occur. Loss of facial sensation can occur in an onionskin pattern emanating from the corner of the mouth. Charcot (neuropathic) joints and trophic skin disorders can appear in long-standing cases. Horner's syndrome and bowel and bladder disturbances are other occasional findings.

The location of the lesion is a rostrocaudal longitudinal cavity from the medulla (floor of the fourth ventricle) into the spinal cord. The cavity is usually located near the fourth ventricle or central canal of the spinal cord. The definitive laboratory investigation for syringobulbia is MRI, the most reliable and sensitive test to demonstrate a syrinx.

The differential diagnosis is that of an intrinsic central cord and lower brain stem lesion (syrinx, tumor, or trauma), and compressive foramen magnum syndrome caused by a tumor. Less likely causes are multiple sclerosis, spinal syphilis, and spinal arachnoiditis.

The diagnostic formulation for syringobulbia involves history, examination, and laboratory evaluation. It is usually a disease of young adults, with a peak incidence in the third and fourth decades. Painless burns and dissociated segmental anesthesia of the upper extremities are of major diagnostic significance. Multiple sclerosis requires the presence of other noncontiguous lesions. The presence of oligoclonal bands in the CSF and characteristic MRI findings permit the separation of this entity. Tumors usually produce a more rapid course.

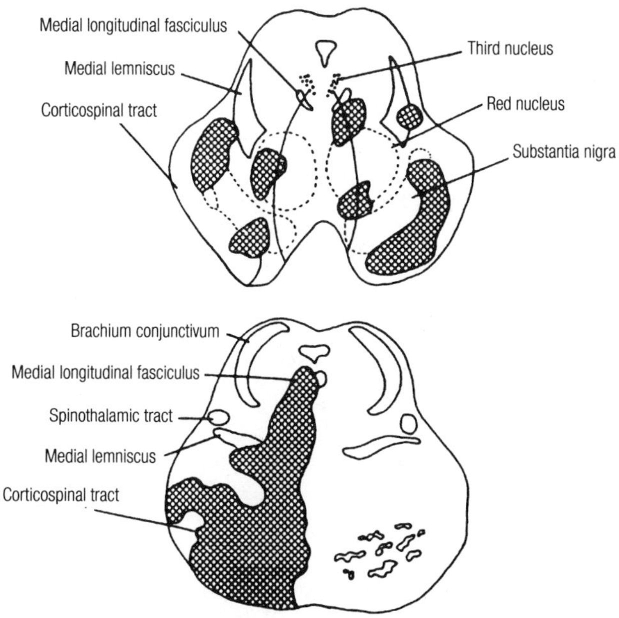

FIGURE 23.1 A postmortem examination of a patient of Kubik and Adams with embolism of the basilar artery. Note the rostrocaudal extension of the infarction along with its patchy nature. (Reprinted with permission from CS Kubik, RD Adams. Occlusion of the basilar artery: a clinical and pathological study. Brain 1946;69:73–121.)

BRAIN STEM ISCHEMIC STROKE SYNDROMES

Vertebrobasilar ischemia causes lesions with varied structural alterations (Caplan et al. 1992). These lesions often have a rostrocaudal or patchy localization (Figure 23.1) rather than the simplified transverse localization that is usually schematized. In addition, all patient's symptoms and signs may not be explainable in anatomical terms—that is, clinicopathological correlation may not be precise. The following syndromes are those classically described, but the details are variable and slightly different in each individual.

The cardinal manifestations of brain stem stroke are involvement of the long tracts of the brain stem in combination with deficits of cranial nerve nuclei. Crossed cranial nerve and motor or sensory long-tract deficits are characteristic. The cranial nerve palsy is ipsilateral to the lesion and the long-tract signs are contralateral, hence the term *crossed.* Coma, ataxia, and vertigo, which are common with vertebrobasilar stroke, are uncommon with internal carotid artery circulation stroke. INO, unreactive pupils, lower motor neuron cranial nerve impairment, and ocular skew deviation when due to stroke occur only with posterior circulation lesions. The same is usually true for nystagmus and most other ocular oscillations.

Another characteristic of vertebrobasilar ischemia is bilateral involvement of the long tracts. This can result in the *locked-in syndrome.* This syndrome, usually due to a lesion of the basis pontis, is characterized by quadriplegia with corticobulbar tract involvement and loss of the ability to produce speech. The reticular activating system is spared, and thus consciousness is preserved. Eye movements or blinking may be all that is left under voluntary control.

Another manifestation of bilateral lesions of the long tracts is *pseudobulbar palsy*. The symptoms resemble those that occur with lesions of the medulla (bulb). However, cranial nerve nuclei have been disconnected from cortical input. This causes dysarthria, dysphagia, bilateral facial weakness, extremity weakness, and emotional lability. A more descriptive term for this syndrome would be *supranuclear bulbar palsy.*

Blindness occurs with bilateral posterior cerebral artery occlusion and concomitant occipital lobe infarction.

The various ischemic stroke syndromes will be outlined in this section. These syndromes occur in isolation, as presented here and in combination. The combinations can be medial with lateral or often rostrocaudal extension.

Thalamic Stroke Syndromes

The blood supply of the thalamus is from the posterior cerebral, posterior communicating, basilar communicating (Figure 23.2), and anterior and posterior choroidal arteries. The thalamic stroke syndromes (Bogousslavsky et al. 1988; Steinke et al. 1992) are listed in Table 23.4.

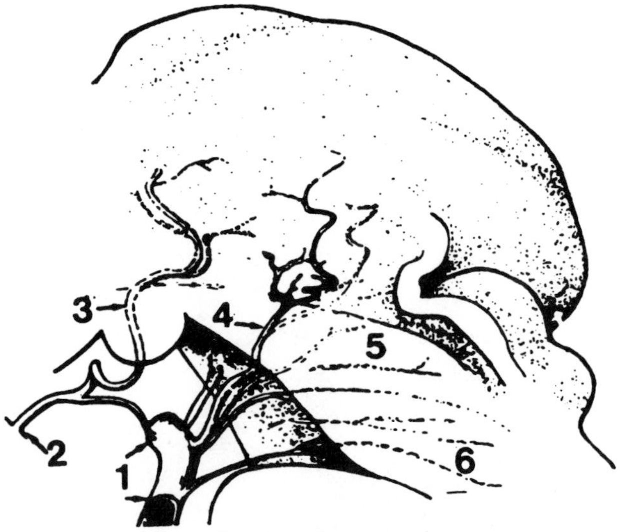

FIGURE 23.2 Diagram of branches of the basilar communicating artery as seen from a view of a sagittal section of the brain stem. (1) Thalamic polar artery, (2) posterior communicating artery, (3) posterior thalamosubthalamic paramedian artery, (4) superior, (5) inferior, and (6) mesencephalic paramedian arteries. (Reprinted with permission from G Percheron. Les artères et territoires du thalamus humain: II. Artères et territoires thalamiques paramédians de l'artère basilare communicante. Rev Neurol 1976;132:309–324.)

Midbrain Stroke Syndromes

Ischemia of the midbrain is characterized by long-tract signs in combination with deficits of the third and fourth cranial nerves. Supratentorial (anterior circulation) stroke syndromes may present with midbrain signs when rostrocaudal deterioration occurs, causing transtentorial herniation. There is much variation, and there are numerous classifications of the blood supply to the brain stem. This is nowhere more apparent than in the midbrain.

The blood supply to the upper mesencephalon is via perforating branches of the basilar communicating artery. The basilar communicating artery (P1 segment of the posterior cerebral artery, mesencephalic artery) connects the basilar artery with the posterior communicating artery. A simplified scheme used here divides the vascular territories into median and lateral transverse regions.

The medial midbrain syndromes are characterized by ipsilateral third or fourth cranial nerve palsies associated with a contralateral hemiparesis. Loss of the discriminative sensations (proprioception, vibration, and stereognosis) with involvement of the medial lemniscus may occur. The lateral syndromes are composed of contralateral loss of pain and temperature sensation and ipsilateral Horner's syndrome and loss of facial sensation. Ataxia may occur on either side. Ischemic stroke syndromes of the mesencephalon are outlined in Table 23.5.

Table 23.4: Ischemic stroke syndromes of the diencephalon

- Anterolateral
  - Common symptoms
    - Contralateral weakness, visual loss
    - Confusion
    - Disorientation
    - Language disturbance
  - Signs
    - Contralateral
      - Hemiparesis
      - Hemiataxia
      - Hemisensory loss
      - Homonymous hemianopsia
    - Right-sided lesion: visuospatial abnormalities, hemineglect, nonverbal intellect affected
    - Left-sided lesion: disorientation, aphasia
  - Arterial territory involved: thalamic polar (tuberothalamic) artery (Figure 23.3; see also Figure 23.2).
- Medial (see vertical gaze ophthalmoplegia, above)
  - Common symptoms
    - Disorientation and confusion
    - Coma with occlusion of main stem variant
    - Visual blurring
  - Signs
    - Vertical gaze ophthalmoplegia
    - Loss of pupillary reflexes
    - Loss of convergence
    - Disorientation and confusion, stupor, coma, and various neuropsychiatric disturbances
  - Arterial territory involved: posterior thalamosubthalamic paramedian artery (thalamic paramedian or deep interpeduncular profundus artery (see Figures 23.2 and 23.3)
- Lateral and posterior internal capsule
  - Common symptoms
    - Contralateral
      - Hemiparesis
      - Numbness
      - Confusion
  - Signs
    - Contralateral
      - Hemiparesis
      - Diminished pain and temperature
      - Dysarthria
      - Homonymous hemianopsia (Helgason et al. 1986); characteristically with a tongue of visual field spared along the horizontal meridian (Figure 23.4)
    - Memory impairment
    - With right-sided lesions: visuoperceptual abnormalities
  - Arterial territory involved: anterior choroidal artery (see Figure 23.3)
- Posterolateral
  - Common symptoms
    - Contralateral
      - Weakness
      - Numbness
      - Visual loss
      - Neglect
      - Confusion
  - Signs
    - Contralateral
      - Loss of touch, pain and temperature, and vibration (common)

Table 23.4: *(continued)*

Hemiparesis in some
Hemiataxia
Homonymous hemianopsia
Left hemispatial neglect
Poor attention span
Arterial territory involved: geniculothalamic artery (see Figure 23.3)

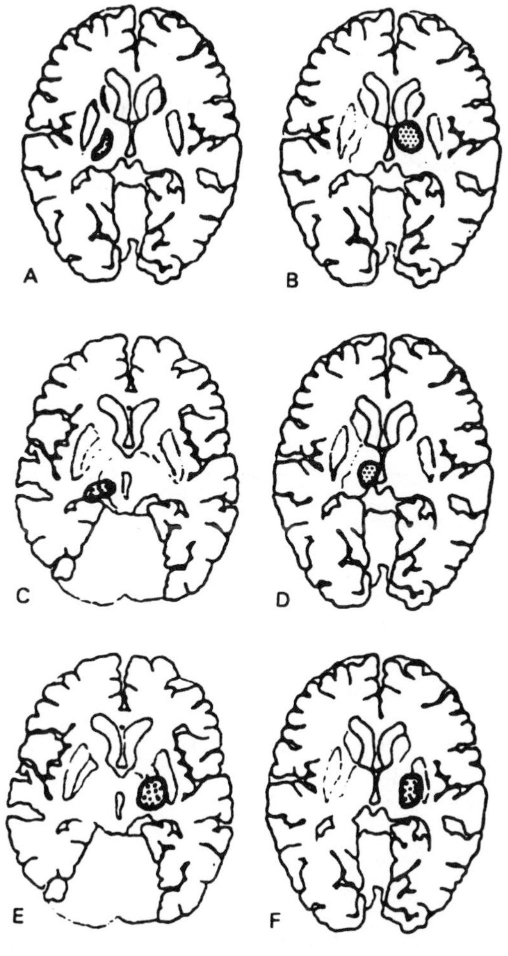

FIGURE 23.3 Schematic computed tomography sections showing the five arterial territories of the thalamus: (A) geniculothalamic (inferolateral) artery territory; (B) anterior thalamosubthalamic paramedian (tuberothalamic) territory; (C) posterior choroidal territory; (D) posterior thalamosubthalamic paramedian territory; (E, F) anterior choroidal territory. (Modified from J Bogousslavsky, F Regli, A Uske. Thalamic infarcts: clinical syndromes, etiology and prognosis. Neurology 1988;38:837–848.)

Pontine Stroke Syndromes

The pons is supplied by numerous penetrating branches of the basilar artery. These arteries have little collateral supply; consequently, lacunar syndromes commonly occur (Table 23.6). These syndromes may be clinically indistinguishable from lacunar syndromes due to lesions of the internal capsule. The medial syndromes are characterized by contralateral hemiparesis and ipsilateral ataxia, INO, and conjugate horizontal gaze paresis.

The lateral syndromes are distinguished by contralateral hemianesthesia and loss of discriminative sensation with ipsilateral Horner's syndrome, facial hemianesthesia, and ataxia. Ipsilateral lower motor neuron–type facial paresis, sixth nerve paresis, deafness, and vertigo occur with inferior pontine lesions.

Medullary Stroke Syndromes

Medial medullary ischemia can cause the crossed hypoglossal hemiparesis syndrome (Table 23.7). In addition, patients may have loss of discriminative-type sensation (position sense, graphesthesia, and stereognosis) when there is associated medial lemniscus involvement.

The lateral medullary syndrome (Wallenberg's syndrome) is one of the most dramatic clinical presentations in neurology (see Table 23.7). Long-tract signs—namely, contralateral loss of pain and temperature sensation over half of the body, ipsilateral ataxia, and Horner's syndrome—are accompanied by involvement of the nuclei and fasciculi of cranial nerves five, eight, nine, and ten. Nystagmus is often present. The critical sign that distinguishes this from a lateral pontine syndrome is involvement of the nucleus ambiguus or its fasciculus and consequent weakness of the ipsilateral palate and vocal cord. A more detailed discussion of stroke is found in Chapter 58A.

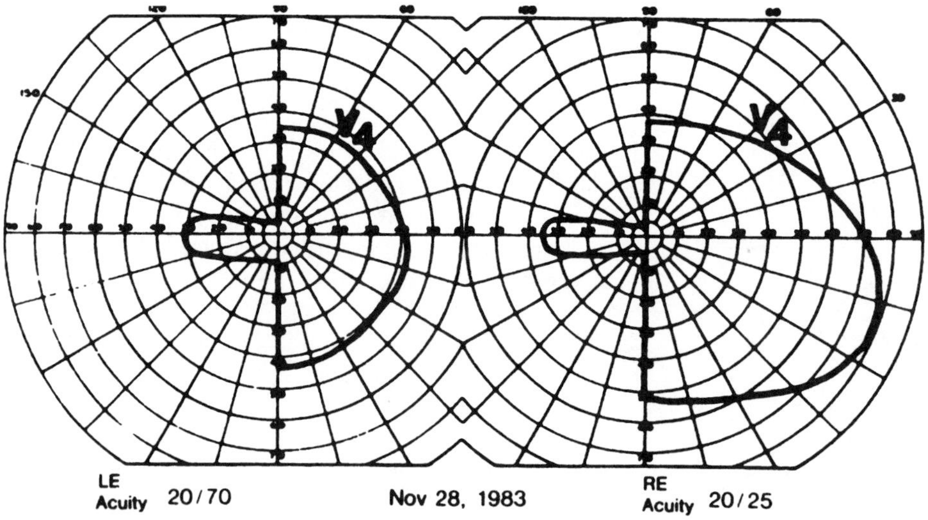

FIGURE 23.4 Typical homonymous hemianopia associated with anterior choroidal artery infarction. Notice the tongue of preserved vision along the horizontal meridian. This pattern is highly localizing to the lateral geniculate nucleus. (Reprinted with permission from C Helgason, L Caplan, J Goodwin, T Hedges III. Anterior choroidal artery—territory infarction: report of cases and review. Arch Neurol 1986;43:681–686.)

Table 23.5: Ischemic stroke syndromes of the mesencephalon

- Common symptoms:
  - Contralateral
    - Weakness
    - Ataxia
    - Numbness
  - Ipsilateral
    - Eyelid ptosis
    - Ataxia
  - Diplopia
- Signs
  - Contralateral
    - Weakness
    - Ataxia
    - Supranuclear horizontal gaze paresis
- Ipsilateral
  - Third nerve palsy
    - Nuclear
    - Fascicular
  - Internuclear ophthalmoplegia
- Arterial territory involved: median and paramedian perforating branches of the basilar or mesencephalic arteries

Middle lateral midbrain syndrome (see Figure 23.5)
- Common symptoms
  - Numbness: contralateral
  - Clumsiness: ipsilateral
- Signs
  - Contralateral
    - Hemianesthesia
    - Ataxia
  - Ipsilateral
    - Facial hemianesthesia (or contralateral)
    - Horner's syndrome
    - Ataxia (if lesion is ventral to brachium conjunctivum)
- Arterial territory involved: superior cerebellar artery

Inferior medial midbrain syndrome (Figure 23.6)
- Common symptoms
  - Diplopia
  - Contralateral weakness
  - Clumsiness
- Signs
  - Contralateral
    - Fourth nerve palsy
    - Ataxia (may be ipsilateral depending on whether the lesion is before or after the crossing of the brachium conjunctivum)
    - Hemiparesis
    - Supranuclear horizontal gaze paresis (ipsilateral if below decussation in lower midbrain)
  - Ipsilateral
    - Internuclear ophthalmoplegia
- Arterial territory involved: median branches of the basilar artery

Inferior lateral midbrain syndrome (see Figure 23.6)
- Common symptoms
  - Contralateral
    - Numbness
- Signs
  - Contralateral
    - Hemianesthesia
  - Ipsilateral
    - Hemianesthesia of face
    - Horner's syndrome

Arterial territory involved: superior cerebellar artery

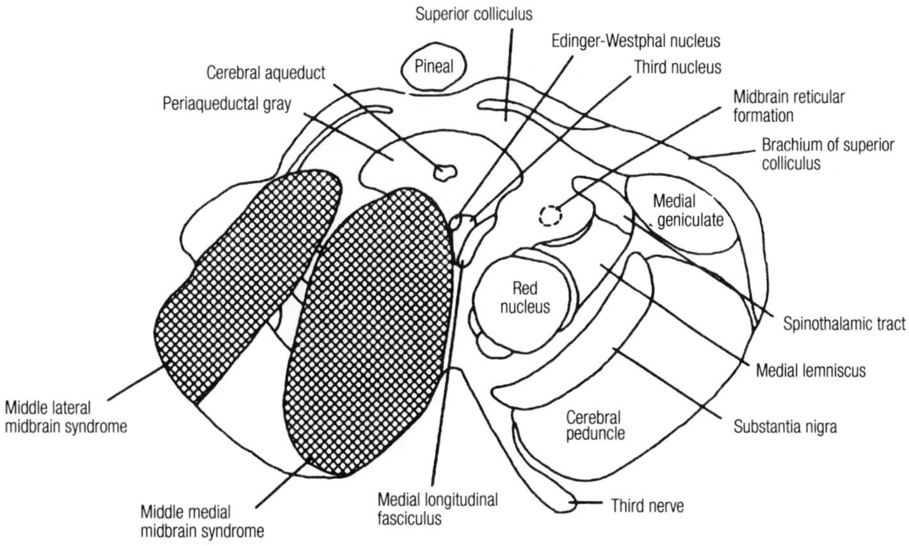

FIGURE 23.5 Midbrain at the superior colliculus level, showing the medial and lateral territories involved with occlusive stroke in this region. (Reprinted with permission from SJ DeArmond, MM Fusco, MM Dewey. Structure of the Human Brain [2nd ed]. New York: Oxford University Press, 1976.)

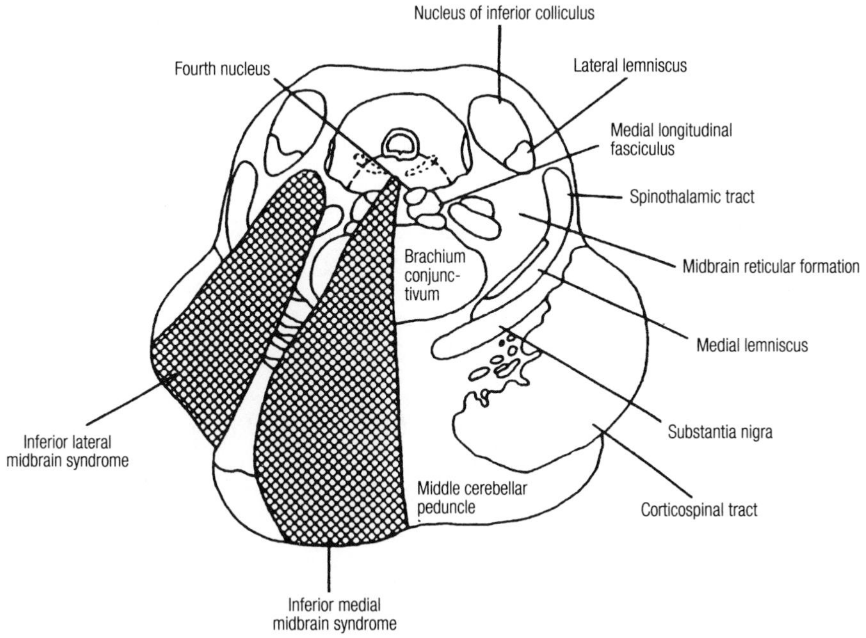

FIGURE 23.6 Midbrain at the inferior colliculus level showing the medial and lateral territories involved with ischemic stroke syndromes in this area. (Reprinted with permission from SJ DeArmond, MM Fusco, MM Dewey. Structure of the Human Brain [2nd ed]. New York: Oxford University Press, 1976.)

Table 23.6: Ischemic stroke syndromes of the pons

- Superior medial pontine syndrome (Figure 23.7)
  - Common symptoms
    - Contralateral weakness
    - Clumsiness
  - Examination
    - Signs
      - On side of lesion
        - Ataxia
        - Internuclear ophthalmoplegia
        - Myoclonus of palate, pharynx, vocal cords
      - On side opposite lesion
        - Paralysis of face, arm, and leg
  - Arterial territory involved: median branches of the basilar artery
- Superior lateral pontine syndrome (see Figure 23.7)
  - Common symptoms
    - Clumsiness: ipsilateral
    - Contralateral numbness
    - Dizziness, nausea, vomiting
  - Signs
    - On side of lesion
      - Ataxia of limbs and gait, falling to side of lesion
      - Horner's syndrome
      - Facial hemianesthesia
      - Paresis of muscles of mastication
    - On side opposite lesion
      - Hemianesthesia (trigeminothalamic tract)
      - Impaired touch, vibration, and position sense
  - Arterial territory involved: superior cerebellar artery
- Middle medial pontine syndrome (Figure 23.8)
  - Common symptoms
    - Contralateral hemiparesis
    - Ipsilateral clumsiness
  - Signs
    - On side of lesion
      - Ataxia of limbs
      - Conjugate gaze paresis toward the side of the lesion
      - Internuclear ophthalmoplegia
    - On side opposite lesion
      - Paresis of face, arm, and leg
    - With bilateral lesions, the locked-in syndrome may occur
  - Arterial territory involved: median branches of the basilar artery
- Middle lateral pontine syndrome (Figure 23.8)
  - Common symptoms
    - Numbness
    - Clumsiness
    - Chewing difficulty
  - Signs
    - Contralateral
      - Hemisensory loss
    - Ipsilateral
      - Ataxia of limbs
      - Paralysis of muscles of mastication
      - Impaired pain sensation over side of face
      - Horner's syndrome
  - Arterial territory involved: long lateral branches of basilar artery
- Inferior medial pontine syndrome (Foville's syndrome) (Figure 23.9)
  - Common symptoms
    - Contralateral weakness and numbness
    - Facial weaknesses: ipsilateral
    - Diplopia
  - Signs
    - Contralateral
      - Paralysis of arm and leg
      - Impaired tactile and proprioceptive sense over half of the body
      - Internuclear ophthalmoplegia
    - Ipsilateral
      - Paresis of conjugate gaze to side of lesion: to oculocephalic maneuver also if the sixth nerve nucleus is involved
      - One-and-a-half syndrome
      - Nystagmus
      - Diplopia on lateral gaze
      - Lower motor neuron type facial palsy
  - Arterial territory involved: median branches of the basilar artery
- Inferior lateral pontine syndrome (anterior inferior cerebellar artery syndrome) (Figure 23.9)
  - Common symptoms
    - Vertigo, nausea, vomiting
    - Oscillopsia
    - Deafness, tinnitus
    - Facial numbness
    - Dyscoordination
  - Signs
    - Contralateral
      - Impaired pain and thermal sense over half the body (may include the face)
    - Ipsilateral
      - Deafness
      - Facial paralysis
      - Ataxia
      - Impaired sensation over face
  - Arterial territory involved: anterior inferior cerebellar artery

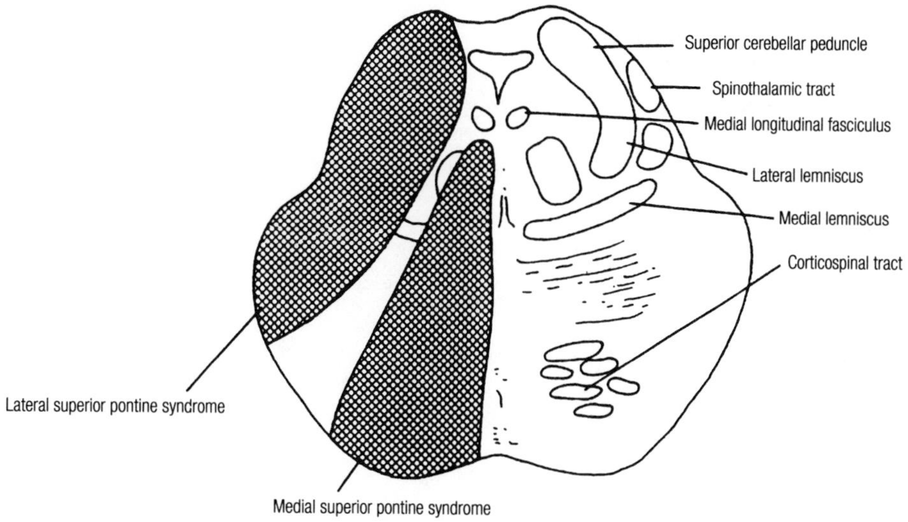

FIGURE 23.7 Superior pontine level, showing the medial and lateral territories involved with occlusive stroke in this region. (Reprinted with permission from RD Adams, M Victor. Principles of Neurology [5th ed]. New York: McGraw-Hill, 1993.)

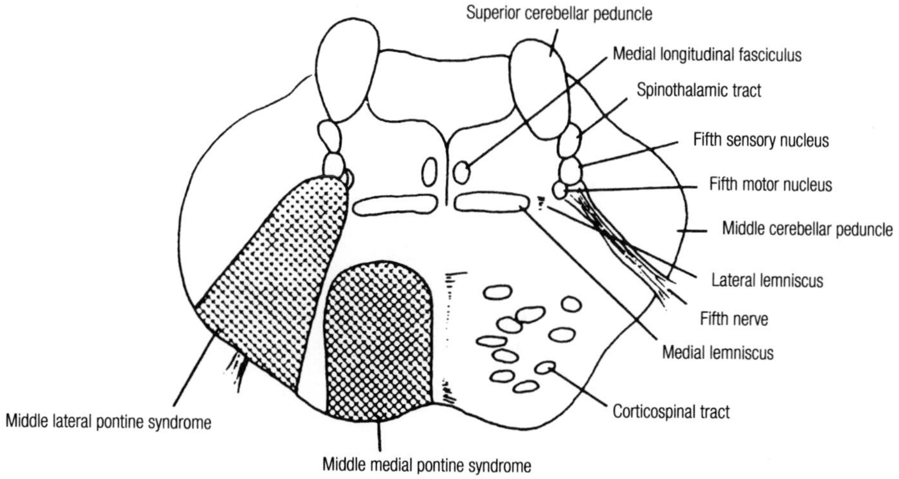

FIGURE 23.8 Middle pontine level, showing the medial and lateral territories involved with ischemic stroke syndromes in this locality. (Reprinted with permission from RD Adams, M Victor. Principles of Neurology [5th ed]. New York: McGraw-Hill, 1993.)

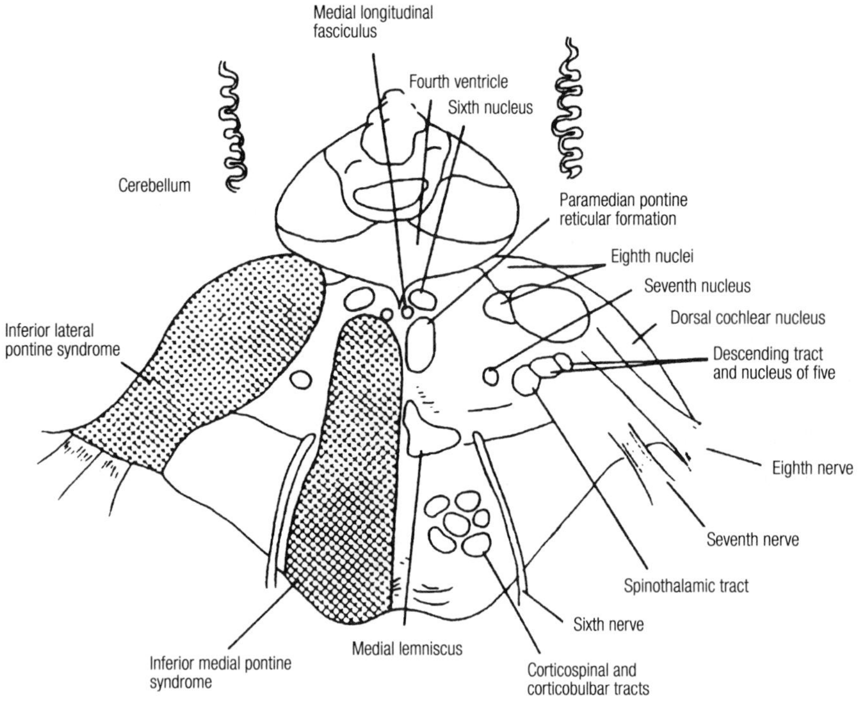

FIGURE 23.9 Inferior pons at the level of the sixth nerve nucleus, showing the medial and lateral territories involved with occlusive stroke in this area. (Reprinted with permission from RD Adams, M Victor. Principles of Neurology [5th ed]. New York: McGraw-Hill, 1993.)

Table 23.7: Ischemic stroke syndromes of the medulla

- Medial medullary syndrome (Figure 23.10)
  - Common symptoms
    - Contralateral weakness
    - Dysarthria
  - Signs
    - Contralateral
      - Paralysis of arm and leg, sparing face
      - Impaired tactile, vibratory, and proprioceptive sense over half the body
    - Ipsilateral
      - Paralysis with atrophy (late) of half the tongue
    - Primary position upbeating nystagmus
  - Arterial territory involved: occlusion of vertebral artery or branch of vertebral or lower basilar artery or anterior spinal artery
- Lateral medullary syndrome (Wallenberg's syndrome) (see Figure 23.10)
  - Common symptoms
    - Ipsilateral facial pain and numbness
    - Vertigo, nausea, and vomiting
    - Ipsilateral clumsiness
    - Diplopia, oscillopsia
    - Numbness ipsilateral or contralateral to lesion
    - Dysphagia, hoarseness
  - Signs
    - Contralateral
      - Impaired pain sensation over half the body, sometimes including the face
    - Ipsilateral
      - Impaired sensation over half the face
      - Ataxia of limbs, falling to side of lesion
      - Horner's syndrome
      - Dysphagia, hoarseness, paralysis of vocal cord
      - Diminished gag reflex
      - Loss of taste
    - Other
      - Nystagmus
        - Primary position rotatory
        - Gaze-evoked horizontal
        - Downbeating on lateral gaze
      - Ocular skew deviation
      - Hiccup
  - Arterial territory involved: occlusion of any of five vessels may be responsible: vertebral; posterior inferior cerebellar; or superior, middle, or inferior lateral medullary arteries

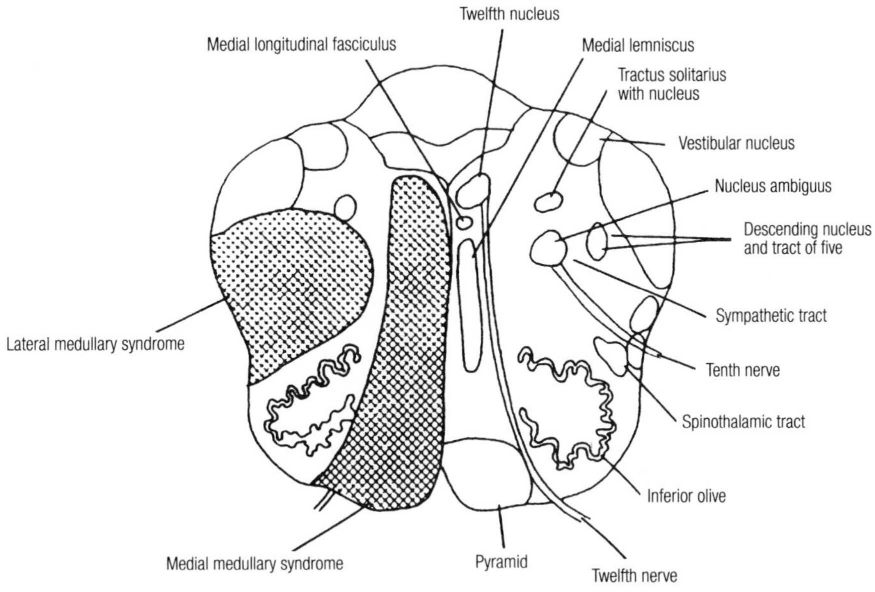

FIGURE 23.10 Cross-section of medulla at the level of the inferior olivary complex, showing the medial and the more common lateral territory involved with ischemic stroke in this brain stem site. (Reprinted with permission from RD Adams, M Victor. Principles of Neurology [5th ed]. New York: McGraw-Hill, 1993.)

REFERENCES

Bogousslavsky J, Regli F, Uske A. Thalamic infarcts: clinical syndromes, etiology and prognosis. Neurology 1988;38:837–848.

Bryan JS, Hamed LM. Levator-sparing nuclearoculomotor palsy: clinical and magnetic resonance imaging findings. J Clin Neuroophth 1992;12:26–30.

Caplan LR, Pesin MS, Mohr JP. Vertebrobasilar Occlusive Disease. In HMJ Barnett, JP Mohr, BM Stein, FM Yatsu (eds), Stroke: Pathophysiology, Diagnosis and Management. New York: Churchill Livingstone, 1992;443–516.

Helgason C, Caplan L, Goodwin J, Hedges T III. Anterior choroidal artery—territory infarction: report of cases and review. Arch Neurol 1986;43:681–686.

Keane JR. The pretectal syndrome: 206 patients. Neurology 1990;40:684–690.

Kobayashi S, Mukuno K, Tazaki Y, et al. Oculomotor nerve nuclear complex syndrome: a case with clinicopathologic correlation. Neuro-ophthalmology 1986;6:55–59.

Kubik CS, Adams RD. Occlusion of the basilar artery: a clinical and pathological study. Brain 1946;69:73–121.

Leigh RJ, Zee DS. The Neurology of Eye Movements (2nd ed). Philadelphia: FA Davis, 1991.

Moffie D, Hamburger HL. Pain and neuroma formation in Wallenberg's lateral medullary syndrome. Clin Neurol Neurosurg 1986;88:217–221.

Morgan D, Williams B. Syringobulbia: a surgical appraisal. J Neurol Neurosurg Psychiatry 1992;55;1132–1141.

Schmahmann JD, Leifer D. Parietal pseudothalamic pain syndrome. Arch Neurol 1992;49:1032–1037.

Steinke W, Sacco RK, Mohr JB et al. Thalamic stroke: presentation and prognosis of infarcts and hemorrhages. Arch Neurol 1992;49:703–710.

Tatemichi TK, Steinke W, Duncan C et al. Paramedian thalamopeduncular infarction: clinical syndromes and magnetic resonance imaging. Ann Neurol 1992;162–171.

Wall M, Slamovits TL, Weisberg LA, Trufant SA. Vertical gaze ophthalmoplegia from infarction in the area of the posterior thalamo-subthalamic paramedian artery. Stroke 1986;17: 546–555.

SUGGESTED READING

Graff-Redford NR, Damasio H, Yamada T. Nonhaemorrhagic thalamic infarction: clinical, neuropsychological and electrophysiological findings in four anatomical groups defined by computerized tomography. Brain 1985;108:485–516.

Miller NR. Walsh and Hoyt's Clinical Neuro-Ophthalmology (4th ed). Vols. 1–4. Baltimore: Williams & Wilkins, 1985–1991.

Chapter 24
Ataxic Disorders

Anita E. Harding

The term *ataxia* is derived from the Greek, literally meaning "irregularity" or "disorderliness." The symptoms and signs of ataxic disorders can nearly all be explained on the basis of irregular decomposition of the fine tuning of posture and movement normally controlled by the cerebellum and its connections. This applies not only to motor function of the limbs and trunk, but also to the eyes and bulbar musculature. Clinical assessment is complicated by the fact that few ataxic patients have pure cerebellar disease; there is often additional pathology in the brain stem, spinal cord, or elsewhere. Moreover, clinical ataxia may at times result from impaired sensory feedback or motor weakness.

SYMPTOMS OF ATAXIC DISORDERS

As in all neurological history-taking, the nature of the patient's symptoms will give the physician an indication of the anatomical diagnosis. In ataxic disorders, specific questioning about the symptoms will make this more precise and establish the most likely pathological process. This in turn is largely determined by the age of onset and the course of the illness—that is, whether symptoms have developed acutely (over minutes or hours), subacutely (over days or weeks), or chronically (over months or years), or are intermittent (Table 24.1).

Disturbances of Gait

An abnormal gait is usually the most prominent presenting feature in ataxic disorders. Patients commonly say that they walk as if they were intoxicated by alcohol. They are unable to walk in a straight line, as illustrated in observant individuals by difficulties in walking side by side with someone without bumping into him or her. Sudden changes of direction are particularly difficult. A tendency to fall or deviate consistently to one side suggests the presence of a unilateral cerebellar hemisphere lesion. Patients should be asked if they are more unsteady in the dark; ataxia largely due to sensory deafferentation or vestibular disease is much more prominent if visual cues are removed.

The duration and rate of progression of gait ataxia should be investigated in detail. Patients with slowly progressive degenerative ataxic disorders often, in retrospect, admit to poor athletic performance at school and sometimes to delayed motor milestones as well. It is also important to establish whether the gait disorder is slowly progressive, of recent onset and rapidly progressive, static after a sudden onset, or intermittent. If the last is the case, what are precipitating or relieving factors? Is there any diurnal variation? Patients who complain of morning unsteadiness that wears off later in the day, often associated with morning headache, should be strongly suspected of having raised intracranial pressure even if examination is normal.

It should be borne in mind that patients often use words rather differently from their physicians. Many refer to "giddiness" or "dizziness" when they really mean unsteadiness of gait without associated vertigo or lightheadedness.

Limb Incoordination and Tremor

Patients with cerebellar lesions tend to notice clumsiness of the arms later in the course of their illness than gait ataxia, although some are aware of difficulties in reaching for objects, opening locks, and performing tasks such as pouring

Table 24.1: Differential diagnosis of ataxic disorders based on course of illness and age at onset

Diagnosis	*Age at Onset (Years)*
Congenital nonprogressive ataxias	
Ataxic cerebral palsy	Infancy
Congenital inherited ataxias	Infancy
Acute-onset ataxias	
Cerebellar hemorrhage	Usually adult
Cerebellar infarction	Usually adult
Dominant periodic ataxias	Acute in children
Migraine	Only in children
Subacute-onset ataxias	
Viral cerebellitis	Usually before 12
Disseminated encephalomyelitis	More common in children than adults
Opsoclonus (paraneoplastic)	More common in children than adults
Paraneoplastic cerebellar syndrome	Adults
Multiple sclerosis	Mainly young adults
Hydrocephalus	Any
Foramen magnum compression	Rare in very young or old
Posterior fossa tumor	Any
Posterior fossa abscess	Any
Toxins	Any
Alcoholic cerebellar degeneration	Adults
Miller Fisher syndrome	Not infancy
Minor epileptic status	Usually children or young adults
Episodic ataxias	
Toxins, including drugs	Any
Multiple sclerosis	Usually young adults
Transient ischemic attacks	Adults
Foramen magnum compression	Rare in very young or old
Intermittent hydrocephalus (for example, cysticercosis, colloid cyst)	Adults
Dominant periodic ataxia	Before 20
Inherited metabolic ataxias	Usually infancy, <15 years
Chronic progressive ataxias	
Foramen magnum compression	Rare in very young or old
Hydrocephalus	Any
Paraneoplastic cerebellar syndrome	Adults
Infections (for example, Creutzfeldt-Jakob disease, rubella panencephalitis)	Adults and children, respectively
Alcoholic cerebellar degeneration	Adults
Vitamin E deficiency	Adults
Hypothyroidism	Young children, adults
Inherited ataxias	
Autosomal recessive	Usually before 15
Autosomal dominant	Usually over 20
Idiopathic degenerative ataxias	Usually over 30

water into a cup. Those with sensory ataxia are more likely to mention difficulties with fine motor tasks such as doing up buttons. Patients with degenerative ataxias of insidious onset are often described by relatives as being always clumsy. Tremor on action may be observed by the patient and can be a prominent symptom in diseases involving the dentatorubral pathway. This is more common in multiple sclerosis than in degenerative disease. Occasional patients are aware of head tremor (*titubation*). The combination of head tremor and action tremor in the upper limbs, with little in the way of gait disturbance, should raise the suspicion of Wilson's disease.

Many patients with cerebellar disease have difficulties in restricting movement to the required part of the body—a sort of mass action effect. This is particularly true of partly involuntary actions such as sneezing or coughing, which may lead to violent movements of the whole body, occasionally propelling the patient from his or her chair.

Dysarthria and Other Disturbances of Bulbar Function

In acute or subacute cerebellar disease, slurring of speech may be a prominent symptom, but in slowly progressive disorders neither the patient nor close relatives may be aware of quite severe dysarthria. Lack of intelligibility on the telephone is sometimes commented on early in the course of ataxic disorders. Observant musical individuals may notice difficulty in singing, particularly in sustaining notes, due to poor coordination of respiration.

Visual and Ocular Motor Symptoms

Episodic or persistent diplopia associated with ataxia should suggest a disorder in the brain stem. It is unusual in degenerative disorders, although some patients with late-onset, dominantly inherited ataxia may notice diplopia when looking into the distance. Transient blurring of vision on changing fixation may arise from overshoot ocular dysmetria. Patients with downbeat nystagmus, in whom structural foramen magnum lesions should be suspected, may complain of blurred vision on looking down and may have particular difficulties in walking down stairs. Acute or subacute oscillopsia, with chaotic involuntary eye movements observed by relatives, may be mentioned in the history of patients with viral cerebellitis, paraneoplastic cerebellar degeneration, and the dancing-eyes syndrome (opsoclonus) (see Chapter 42).

Lack of suppression of the vestibulo-ocular reflex (VOR) in cerebellar disease may give rise to oscillopsia and increased disequilibrium when moving the head rapidly, driving, attempting to follow a moving object, and reading while moving. Walking through supermarket aisles appears to be a particularly potent stimulus for symptoms caused by failure to suppress the VOR.

Some degenerative ataxias are associated with gradual visual loss, due to either optic neuropathy or retinopathy (see Chapter 77). Patients with dominantly inherited ataxia and retinal degeneration may notice visual loss before the onset of ataxia.

Other Symptoms

Headache and vomiting in association with ataxia suggest the presence of a posterior fossa mass lesion. If the history goes back over weeks or months, there should be a strong suspicion of tumor, with or without hydrocephalus. In this context, headache is usually occipital and may be worse on coughing, bending, and waking. The last also applies to nausea and vomiting; projectile vomiting may be induced by head movement in patients with posterior fossa mass lesions. Symptoms like these occurring on an intermittent basis, sometimes associated with fever and malaise, should raise the suspicion of posterior fossa cysticercosis, and a detailed travel history over the last 20 years should be sought. Presentation with catastrophic occipital headache, vertigo, vomiting, ataxia, and drowsiness suggests a diagnosis of cerebellar hemorrhage and requires urgent investigation.

Vertigo is uncommon in degenerative ataxic disorders but occurs in neoplastic, inflammatory, and vascular disease. It may be evoked by changes in position.

Symptoms of cognitive dysfunction can accompany ataxia in some of the degenerative ataxic disorders, and this combination of features with a relatively short history, often associated with urinary incontinence, suggests the presence of hydrocephalus. Urgency of micturition occurs in some degenerative ataxias and is common in multiple sclerosis. Other symptoms of dysautonomia, such as those due to postural hypotension, may be combined with ataxia and other features in multiple system atrophy. The presence of cardiac symptoms should be sought in patients with suspected Friedreich's ataxia. Skeletal deformities such as pes cavus and scoliosis occur in a number of early-onset inherited ataxias.

It is essential to take a detailed family history in patients presenting with ataxia and to ask them about consanguinity. A detailed inquiry of drug ingestion (for both medical and recreational purposes, including alcohol) and occupational exposure is also required. Systematic review should include questions relating to hypothyroidism—for example, cold intolerance, dry skin, and hair loss.

SIGNS OF CEREBELLAR DISEASE

Gait and Posture

Patients with cerebellar disease have a broad-based gait and tend to lurch from side to side. Considering their instability, they walk relatively quickly, with steps of irregular length. Their unsteadiness is more prominent on rising quickly from a chair, turning, or stopping suddenly. A tendency to fall consistently to one side suggests a unilateral cerebellar hemisphere lesion. Mild gait ataxia may be demonstrated by asking the patient to walk as if on a tightrope (heel-toe or tandem walking). More severely affected individuals have difficulties in maintaining stance; they need to have their feet placed wide apart, and they sway from side to side. This instability is not enhanced by eye closure unless there is additional proprioceptive loss or vestibular disease. Truncal ataxia may be severe enough to interfere with maintaining sitting posture.

Speech

Cerebellar speech is slow, slurred, monotonous, and irregular. Coordination of speech and respiration is abnormal, leading to excessive quietness for some words or syllables and increased volume for others (explosive speech). Slow, slurred speech with increased separation of syllables is referred to as a *scanning dysarthria*. This is specific for cerebellar disease, but many patients with ataxic disorders have only slurred speech, which can be difficult to distinguish from a spastic dysarthria. Evidence of additional corticobulbar pathology (slow tongue movements and increased facial reflexes) suggests the presence of a spastic dysarthria.

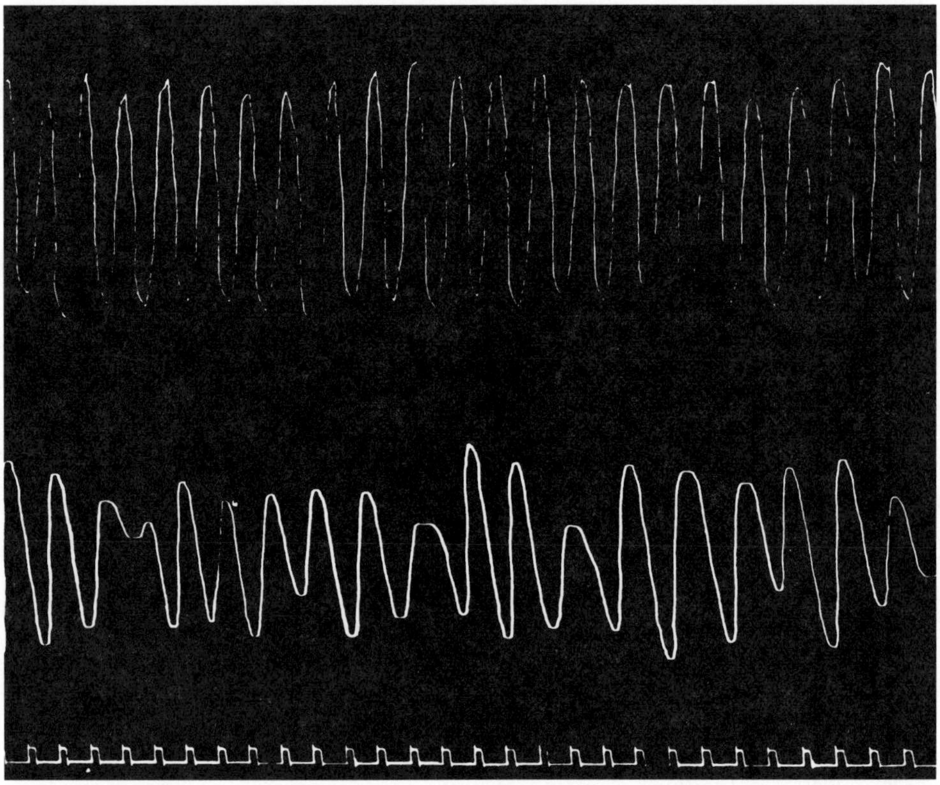

FIGURE 24.1 Tracings of alternating pronation and supination of the left (above) and right (below) arms of a patient with a right-sided cerebellar lesion. (Reprinted with permission of the publisher from G Holmes. The cerebellum of man. Brain 1939;62:1–30.)

Muscle Tone

Most neurology textbooks state firmly that cerebellar disease gives rise to hypotonia, but this is rarely detectable clinically in symmetrical slowly progressive or chronic disorders. This statement arises largely from the work of Holmes (1917) in acute unilateral cerebellar lesions, and in these circumstances there is decreased resistance to passive movement on the side of the lesion, associated with pendular knee jerks. The latter are also difficult to detect without the eye of faith in more chronic symmetrical cerebellar syndromes. The situation is complicated by the fact that many patients with ataxic disorders have disease of the spinal cord, peripheral nerves, or both, as well as the cerebellum.

The rebound phenomenon of cerebellar disease, elicited by tapping the outstretched arm or suddenly releasing the forearm flexed against resistance (which is unchecked and hits the patient's chest, known as the Stewart-Holmes sign), is often attributed to hypotonia. However, it seems more likely that this arises from incoordination between agonist and antagonist muscles.

Limb Ataxia

Limb ataxia, or *dyssynergia*, usually results from a combination of dysmetria and dysdiadochokinesis. *Dysmetria* refers to disturbance of the course or placement of the limb during movement, resulting in an erratic, jerky movement and under- or overshooting the target. The target may be reached, as in the finger-nose and heel-shin tests, by a series of oscillations (intention tremor). *Dysdiadochokinesis* means decomposition of alternating or fine repetitive movements (Figure 24.1). This can be demonstrated by asking the patient to tap one hand on the other, alternately pronating and supinating the tapping hand, rapidly opening and closing the fist, or tapping out simple rhythms on the floor with the foot. The effects of cerebellar disease on voluntary movement in humans have been reviewed by Rothwell (1987).

Abnormal performance in tests for limb ataxia is difficult to interpret if there is weakness or sensory loss. There is also a normal asymmetry in cerebellar function, with better performance, particularly for rapid alternating movements, in the dominant limb. This asymmetry is often enhanced in diffuse diseases of the cerebellum and does not necessarily imply unilateral pathology. It is interesting to note that strictly right-sided limb ataxia is more common in lesions of the right cerebellar hemisphere than is ataxia restricted to the left limbs with left-hemisphere lesions (Lechtenberg and Gilman 1978). About 40% of patients with vermis lesions do not have limb ataxia but have striking gait ataxia.

Tremor

Intention (also called *kinetic*) tremor has been mentioned previously. It is important to maximize the range of movement tested to demonstrate the presence of tremor. Gross in-

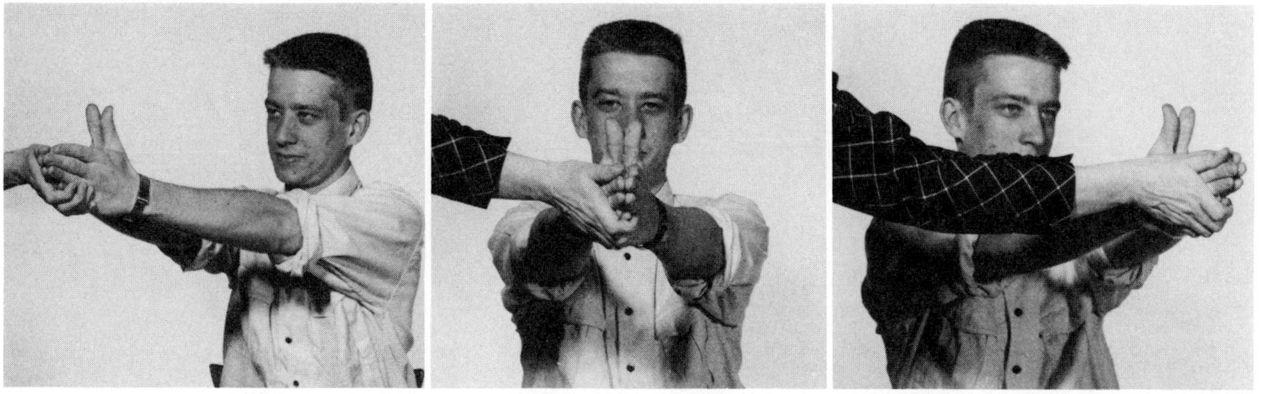

FIGURE 24.2 Test used to demonstrate failure of inhibition of the vestibulo-ocular reflex (VOR). The subject fixates on one thumbnail while rotating the upper body (position as shown) slowly from the waist. Normal individuals can maintain fixation, but those who fail to suppress the VOR cannot.

tention tremor, also present to a lesser extent on maintaining posture, is seen in some ataxic patients. This is often called *rubral* or *red nucleus tremor*, although *peduncular tremor* is probably a more accurate label. It is most commonly seen in multiple sclerosis and occasionally in late-onset degenerative ataxias. It also occurs in some patients with Wilson's disease, where it may present as a syndrome of prominent action tremor, upper limb dysdiadochokinesis, and head tremor, but with a virtually normal gait, in the absence of dystonia or parkinsonism. A nodding head tremor (titubation) with a frequency of 3–4 per second may be seen with midline cerebellar disease, and this sometimes affects the trunk as well.

Essential tremor can be distinguished from cerebellar tremor without too much difficulty (see Chapter 25), but it is not so easy to assess cerebellar function in patients with essential tremor. Normal eye movements, speech, and gait make the presence of cerebellar disease unlikely. The same difficulties apply in patients with frequent myoclonic jerks.

Eye Movements

Diseases of the cerebellum and its connections result in a host of ocular motor abnormalities, not all of which have been localized to specific parts of the cerebellum or brain stem by clinicopathological studies (see Chapters 16 and 42) (Leigh and Zee 1991). A frequent abnormality in cerebellar disease is jerkiness of smooth pursuit eye movements, particularly if there is pathology involving the vestibulocerebellum. This is often associated with inability to suppress the VOR, best demonstrated by asking the patient to fixate on an object (such as the thumbs with the arms outstretched) while the head and the object are simultaneously rotated in the horizontal plane (Figure 24.2).

Ocular dysmetria is a common abnormality seen in cerebellar disease, with relatively poor localizing value. It is analogous to limb dysmetria. The eyes overshoot when approaching a target and then undershoot on attempted correction, leading to oscillation about the target. *Square wave jerks* also occur in cerebellar disease; these are inappropriate saccades that disrupt fixation and are followed by a corrective saccade within 200 msec.

Slow saccades, often seen in both dominant and isolated cases of late-onset degenerative ataxias, are caused by pathological processes affecting the horizontal burst cells in the pons and midbrain. Such patients sometimes have difficulties in initiating saccades; they may need to blink or move the head before the eyes move. Supranuclear gaze palsy, particularly for vertical gaze, is also seen in some patients in this group, as well as in cases of hexosaminidase deficiency and Niemann-Pick disease type C (see Chapter 77). The combination of ptosis and external ophthalmoplegia in an ataxic individual suggests a diagnosis of mitochondrial myopathy, although an acute or subacute presentation, perhaps associated with vomiting, raises the possibility of Wernicke's encephalopathy.

Internuclear ophthalmoplegia in an ataxic patient usually implies a diagnosis of multiple sclerosis, particularly if it is unilateral, but bilateral internuclear ophthalmoplegia may be seen in late onset degenerative ataxias. Isolated or multiple lesions of the third, fourth, and sixth cranial nerves, in combination with ataxia, suggest intrinsic or extrinsic brain stem disease.

The eye movement disorder of ataxia telangiectasia is particularly characteristic. It has two components. There is an *ocular motor apraxia*—that is, a supranuclear gaze palsy particularly for horizontal movements, with normal saccadic velocities. Patients have difficulty in initiating voluntary eye movements and often move their heads excessively, allowing the eyes to drift back to the target using the VOR (Figure 24.3). In addition, the VOR cannot be suppressed, and there is ocular dysmetria.

Gaze-evoked nystagmus is the most common type of nystagmus associated with cerebellar disease; eccentric gaze cannot be maintained, and the slow phase of the nystagmus is toward the primary position, with rapid corrective move-

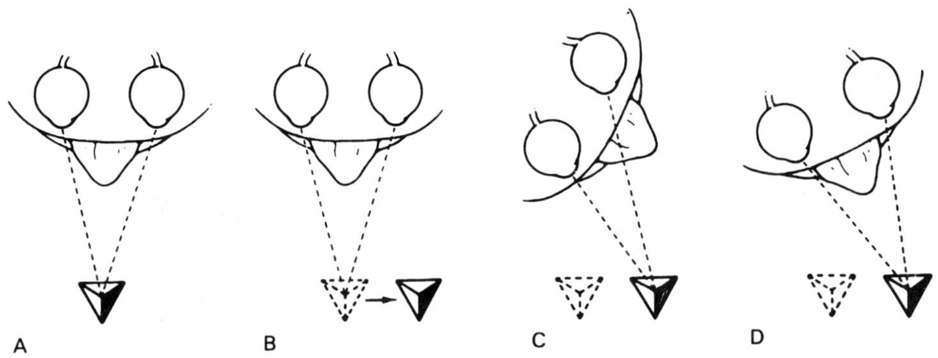

FIGURE 24.3 Gaze apraxia and head thrusting. The patient looks at the target in the primary position (A) and then cannot shift gaze to the left to follow the target (B). Fixation is changed by turning the head rapidly toward the target, and is eventually achieved by means of the oculocephalic reflex (C). Finally, the head is slowly rotated back to its original position while fixation is maintained (D). (Reprinted with permission of the authors and publisher from S Gilman, JR Blodell, R Lechtenberg. Disorders of the Cerebellum. Philadelphia: FA Davis, 1981.)

ments. It does not have much localizing value (Leigh and Zee 1991), implying midline or hemispheric cerebellar disease or brain stem disease. It may be associated with rebound nystagmus (slow- and fast-phase reversal on return to the primary position), a phenomenon that does appear to be specific for lesions of the cerebellum. Although downbeat nystagmus should raise the suspicion of a foramen magnum lesion, this is also seen in degenerative cerebellar disease.

Positional nystagmus in a patient with vertigo and unsteadiness should be attributed to benign labyrinthine disease only if it is transient, torsional, and fatigable; if it does not have these features, a posterior fossa lesion should be suspected.

Saccadic oscillations without an intersaccadic interval are called *opsoclonus* when they are vertical, horizontal, and torsional (multidirectional), and *ocular flutter* when they are restricted to the horizontal plane. Both are seen in viral cerebellitis and as a paraneoplastic phenomenon in children and adults.

Other Neurological Signs and General Examination

As the causes of ataxia are numerous, a large variety of other neurological and general physical signs may be found on examination. The range of these and their possible diagnostic significance is shown in Tables 24.2 and 24.3. Examination of the patient's relatives should be considered if there is any possibility of a genetically determined disorder.

DIFFERENTIAL DIAGNOSIS AND INVESTIGATION

Congenital, Nonprogressive Ataxia

Congenital, nonprogressive ataxias are caused by prenatal or perinatal trauma (ataxic cerebral palsy, although this diagnostic label is not excluded by a normal birth history), arrested hydrocephalus, and other nongenetic anomalies of the cerebellum (see Chapter 67), or genetically determined syndromes that are often associated with macroscopic or microscopic hypoplasia or dysplasia of posterior fossa structures (see Chapter 77). It is often difficult to determine whether an ataxic disorder is progressive in the first 2 years of life, as normal motor development requires increasing skills involving coordination. Accordingly, motor development is usually delayed in congenital ataxias, but regression does not occur. Associated mental retardation is common but unhelpful diagnostically. Computed tomography (CT) or magnetic resonance imaging (MRI) is helpful in showing developmental anomalies or evidence of trauma such as porencephalic cysts.

Ataxia of Acute or Subacute Onset

Cerebellar ataxia with extremely acute onset has two main causes: cerebellar hemorrhage (usually associated with headache, vertigo, vomiting, altered consciousness, and neck stiffness), and cerebellar infarction (in which cerebellar signs are usually combined with signs of brain stem ischemia, and the presentation may mimic that of hemorrhage). Diagnosis should be made as a matter of urgency by CT or MRI. Episodes of autosomal dominant periodic cerebellar ataxia sometimes have an acute onset in children. Acute ataxia may also be seen in children with migraine.

Subacute, reversible ataxia may occur as a result of viral infection in children 2–10 years of age. There is usually pyrexia, limb and gait ataxia, and dysarthria developing over hours or days. Recovery occurs over a period of weeks and is usually complete. In children or young adults, ataxia may also be a feature of postinfectious encephalomyelitis, particularly that related to varicella infection. A combination of ataxia, vertigo, opsoclonus, and myoclonus is sometimes seen in children (the dancing eyes syndrome) or adults

Table 24.2: Differential diagnosis of ataxic disorders: Associated neurological signs

Neurological Sign	*Found in:*
Depressed consciousness	Cerebellar hemorrhage or infarction, poisoning, minor status epilepticus
Mental retardation	Ataxic cerebral palsy, congenital ataxias, some early-onset (recessive) inherited ataxias, xeroderma pigmentosum
Dementia	Hydrocephalus, some degenerative ataxias, Gerstmann-Straüssler syndrome, Creutzfeldt-Jakob disease
Optic atrophy	Multiple sclerosis, Friedreich's ataxia (late), other inherited ataxias, alcoholism
Retinopathy	Some inherited ataxias, mitochondrial encephalomyopathies
Eye movement disorders	
Ocular motor apraxia	Ataxia telangiectasia
Supranuclear ophthalmoplegia	Dominant ataxias, idiopathic late-onset ataxias, hexosaminidase deficiency, Niemann-Pick disease type C
Internuclear ophthalmoplegia	Multiple sclerosis, rarely Wernicke's encephalopathy, degenerative ataxias
Ptosis, extraocular palsies	Mitochondrial encephalomyopathies, Wernicke's encephalopathy, Leigh's syndrome
Third, fourth, and sixth nerve palsies	Infarction, hemorrhage, multiple sclerosis, posterior fossa mass lesions
Ocular flutter, opsoclonus	Viral cerebellitis, paraneoplastic syndromes
Downbeat nystagmus	Foramen magnum lesions, degenerative ataxias
Extrapyramidal signs: dystonia, chorea, rigidity	Wilson's disease, dominant and idiopathic late-onset ataxias, ataxia telangiectasia
Myoclonus	Mitochondrial encephalomyopathy, multiple carboxylase deficiencies, ceroid lipofuscinosis, sialidosis, Ramsay Hunt syndrome, minor epileptic status, some dominant ataxias
Hyporeflexia or areflexia, often with loss of proprioception and vibration sense	Friedreich's ataxia, other inherited and degenerative ataxias, alcoholic cerebellar degeneration, vitamin E deficiency, hypothyroidism, ataxia telangiectasia, xeroderma pigmentosum, leukodystrophies, Miller Fisher syndrome
Deafness	Several inherited ataxias, mitochondrial encephalomyopathy

and is caused by viral infection or as a paraneoplastic syndrome, related to neuroblastoma in children and to carcinoma, usually of bronchial origin, in adults (see Chapter 77). Viral titers, cerebrospinal fluid (CSF) examination, urinary vanillylmandelic acid excretion, abdominal CT scan or MRI, chest x-ray, and bronchoscopy are appropriate investigations in such patients, depending on their age, after structural lesions have been excluded.

Subacute ataxia, with or without evidence of raised intracranial pressure or signs of brain stem compression, may be the presenting feature of hydrocephalus, foramen magnum compression, posterior fossa tumor (primary or secondary), abscess, or parasitic infection in any age group. These can be excluded by CT or MRI. Subacute ataxia, usually associated with vertigo and other evidence of brain stem dysfunction, is a common form of presentation or relapse in young adults with multiple sclerosis.

It is important to exclude poisoning or drug intoxication as a cause of acute or subacute onset ataxia in children and adults. Culprits include thallium, lead, barbiturates, phenytoin, piperazine, alcohol, solvents, and antineoplastic drugs (see Chapter 77).

The Miller Fisher variant of the Guillain-Barré syndrome may present with ataxia of subacute onset. There is usually areflexia, ophthalmoplegia, and facial weakness. Nerve conduction studies and CSF examination may be helpful, but the former are often normal. Another noncerebellar cause of subacute and intermittent ataxia, usually with depressed consciousness and often myoclonic jerks, is minor epileptic status, which can be diagnosed by means of the electroencephalogram.

Ataxia with an Episodic Course

In adults, drug ingestion, multiple sclerosis, transient vertebrobasilar ischemic attacks, foramen magnum compression, intermittent obstruction of the ventricular system due to a colloid cyst or cysticercosis, and dominantly inherited periodic ataxia are the main causes of episodic ataxia (probably in that order). These conditions should be distinguished largely on the basis of the history and appropriate imaging techniques. In children and young adults a metabolic disorder should be suspected, particularly defects of the urea cycle, aminoacidurias, Leigh's syndrome, and mitochondrial encephalomyopathies (Adams and Lyon 1982; see also Chapter 77). Neurological dysfunction (lethargy, ataxia, vomiting, and seizures) may be precipitated by fever, intercurrent infection, or changes in diet. There is usually residual deficit, particularly mental retardation, between attacks. Screening investigations include blood ammonia, pyruvate, lactate and amino acids, and urinary amino acids.

Table 24.3: Differential diagnosis of ataxic disorders: Associated general physical signs

System Involved	*Found in:*	*Feature*
Hair	Argininosuccinicaciduria	Brittle
	Giant axonal neuropathy	Tight curls
	Thallium poisoning, hypothyroidism, adrenoleukomyeloneuropathy	Loss
	Foramen magnum lesions	Low hairline
Skin	Ataxia telangiectasia	Telangiectases, particularly conjunctiva, nose, ears, flexures
	Xeroderma pigmentosum	Extreme light sensitivity, tumors
	Hartnup disease	Pellagra-type rash
	Cholestanolosis	Tendinous swellings
	Hypothyroidism, Refsum's disease, Cockayne syndrome	Dry skin
	Adrenoleukomyeloneuropathy	Pigmentation
Eyes	Ataxia telangiectasia	(see Skin)
	Wilson's disease	Kayser-Fleischer rings
	Cerebellar hemangioblastoma	Retinal angiomas in von Hippel-Lindau disease
	Congenital rubella, cholestanolosis, Sjögren-Larsson syndrome	Cataract
	Gillespie syndrome	Aniridia
Fever	Abscess, viral cerebellitis, cysticercosis, dominant periodic ataxia, intermittent metabolic ataxias	Fever may precipitate neurological deterioration in last two
Vomiting	Hemorrhage, infarction, demyelination, posterior fossa mass lesions, intermittent metabolic ataxias	
Hepatosplenomegaly	Niemann-Pick disease type C, some childhood metabolic ataxias, Wilson's disease, alcoholic cerebellar degeneration	
Heart disease	Friedreich's ataxia	Cardiomegaly, murmurs, arrhythmias, late heart failure, abnormal electrocardiogram
	Mitochondrial encephalomyopathy	Conduction defects
Short stature	Mitochondrial encephalomyopathy, ataxia telangiectasia, Sjögren-Larsson syndrome, Cockayne syndrome	
Hypogonadism	Recessive ataxia with hypogonadism, ataxia telangiectasia, Sjögren-Larsson syndrome, mitochondrial encephalomyopathy, adreno-leukomyeloneuropathy	
Skeletal deformity	Friedreich's ataxia, Sjögren-Larsson syndrome, many other early-onset inherited ataxias, hereditary motor and sensory neuropathy	
Immunodeficiency	Ataxia telangiectasia, multiple carboxylase deficiencies	
Malnutrition	Vitamin E deficiency, alcoholic cerebellar degeneration	

Ataxia with a Chronic Progressive Course

Most patients, children or adults, with chronic progressive ataxia have degenerative disorders that are often genetically determined (although there may not be a positive family history). Nevertheless, posterior fossa tumors, foramen magnum compression, or hydrocephalus may require exclusion by imaging studies. Infections that can cause slowly progressive ataxia include the chronic panencephalitis of congenital rubella infection in children and, in adults, Creutzfeldt-Jakob disease, particularly related to growth hormone therapy. Chronic alcoholism is one of the most common causes of cerebellar degeneration in adults. Severe vitamin E deficiency secondary to chronic liver or intestinal disease can cause a slowly progressive ataxic disorder associated with areflexia and proprioceptive loss. Multiple sclerosis only exceptionally presents as a chronic progressive cerebellar syndrome. Hypothyroidism is associated with cerebellar dysfunction in children and adults, but the clinical features of the primary diagnosis are usually obvious. Paraneoplastic cerebellar degeneration related to carcinomas of the lung or ovary or to the reticuloses usually follows a subacute course, with patients losing the ability to walk within months of onset. Although early reports suggested that the underlying neoplasm

Table 24.4: Investigation of probable degenerative ataxias

	In all cases if:		
Test or Determination	*Early Onset (1–20 Years)*		*Late Onset (Over 20 Years)*
Lipids		If hyporeflexic or areflexic	
Vitamin E		If hyporeflexic or areflexic	
Glucose	Yes		No
Electrocardiogram	Yes		If hyporeflexic or areflexic
Alpha-fetoprotein	Yes		No
Immunoglobulins	Yes		No
VLCFA, ACTH	Males		See below
Lactate	Yes		Yes
Ceruloplasmin		Yes unless NCS abnormal	
Thyroxine	Yes		Yes
Chest x-ray	Yes		Yes
NCS	Yes		Yes
CT or MRI	Yes		Yes

In selected cases with additional clinical features, think about:

1. Any age of onset, but usually <50 years:
   Muscle biopsy for mitochondrial myopathy and ceroid lipofuscinosis (fatigable weakness, dementia, strokelike episodes, myoclonus, retinopathy, short stature)
   Cholestanol (cataract, tendinous swellings)
   Gonadotrophins (hypogonadism)
   VLCFA and ACTH (spastic paraparesis, with or without axonal neuropathy, radiological evidence of white matter disease, onset earlier in males than females)
2. Particularly (but not exclusively) if early onset (2–20 years):
   Hexosaminidase (gaze palsy, neurogenic weakness, dystonia)
   Arylsulfatase A, galactocerebrosidase (dementia, psychiatric problems, optic atrophy, demyelinating neuropathy, radiological evidence of white matter disease)
   Bone marrow (gaze palsy, seizures, extrapyramidal features, dementia)
   Ammonia and amino acids (early onset, fluctuating course, mental retardation)
3. In later-onset cases (later than 20 years of age):
   Anti-Purkinje cell antibodies, pelvic imaging in females (subacute course)

VLCFA = very-long-chain fatty acids; ACTH = adrenocorticotropic hormone; NCS = nerve conduction studies; CT = computed tomography; MRI = magnetic resonance imaging.

could remain occult for several years after the onset of ataxia, this is less likely with modern investigative techniques.

Some conditions that are not generally considered primarily as ataxic disorders may present with clumsiness, tremor, or definite cerebellar signs, particularly in childhood or adolescence. These include Wilson's disease and several inherited neuropathies, such as hereditary motor and sensory neuropathy (HMSN; Charcot-Marie-Tooth disease, including the so-called Roussy-Levy syndrome). Although intention and postural tremor are quite frequent in the demyelinating type of HMSN (type I), dysarthria and pyramidal signs do not occur. These, together with marked slowing of motor nerve conduction velocity, serve to distinguish this disease from, for example, Friedreich's ataxia. Other chronic demyelinating neuropathies, such as chronic inflammatory and paraproteinemic neuropathies and Refsum's disease, may give rise to prominent tremor and ataxia; the same applies to giant axonal neuropathy. Ataxia also occurs in the mitochondrial encephalomyopathies and other metabolic disorders mentioned in Table 24.4 and in Chapter 77.

After excluding acquired causes of ataxic disorders, there remains a considerable number of patients with degenerative ataxias, not all of which are overtly genetically determined. The inherited ataxias can largely be classified according to their clinical and genetic features (see Chapter 77), and in a small proportion of cases a recognizable metabolic defect can be detected. It is important to make as accurate diagnosis as possible in these disorders for the purposes of prognosis, genetic counseling, and, occasionally, specific therapy. It is neither rational nor cost effective to investigate all possibilities in every patient, and an investigative approach to (probably) degenerative ataxias is outlined in Table 24.4. If this scheme yields negative results, then at least 90% of the residual cases can be classified on clinical and genetic grounds, as discussed in detail in Chapter 77.

REFERENCES

Adams RD, Lyon G. Neurology of Hereditary Metabolic Diseases of Childhood. New York: McGraw-Hill, 1982.

Holmes G. The symptoms of acute cerebellar injury due to gunshot injuries. Brain 1917;40:461–535.

Lechtenberg R, Gilman S. Localization of function in the cerebellum. Neurology 1978;28:376–381.
Leigh RJ, Zee DS. The Neurology of Eye Movements (2nd ed). Philadelphia: FA Davis, 1991.
Rothwell JC. Control of human voluntary movement. London, England: Croom-Helm, 1987;235–285.

SUGGESTED READING

Cole M. The foreign policy of the cerebellum. Neurology 1995 (in press).
Thompson PD, Day BL. The Anatomy and Physiology of Cerebellar Disease. In AE Harding, T Deufel (eds), Inherited Ataxias. Advances in Neurology. Vol. 61. New York: Raven 1993:15–31.

Chapter 25
Movement Disorder Symptomatology

Anthony E. Lang

The term *movement disorders* is often used synonymously with *basal ganglia* or *extrapyramidal diseases*. However, neither of the latter two terms adequately encompasses all of the disorders included under the broad umbrella of movement disorders. This field comprises the syndrome of parkinsonism and a variety of abnormal involuntary movements or dyskinesias including tremor, dystonia, athetosis, chorea, ballism, tics, myoclonus, and a few less common varieties. By convention, when considering movement disorders, most neurologists exclude the motor dysfunctions resulting from cerebellar, spinal cord, upper and lower motor neuron, peripheral nerve, and muscle disease, as well as the complex disorders of execution of movement denoted by the term *apraxia*.

Abnormal movements must be considered a clinical sign for which there are many possible causes. In the field of neurology, the standard clinical approach of deciding *where* in the nervous system the disease process is located, and then *what* that process could be, is preceded by an additional step defining the most appropriate broad class of movement disorder in which to place the problem. These curious and often bizarre spontaneous abnormal movements are sometimes difficult to categorize, and, despite attempts at uniformity in definition, errors in classification are not infrequent. Inaccuracy in diagnostic categorization occasionally has resulted in clinical, genetic, and epidemiological misinformation becoming embedded in the literature. The use of videotape documentation limits this source of confusion.

Each of the movement disorders to be described is seen in pure form with no known or established cause. These essential or idiopathic disorders must be distinguished from the symptomatic or secondary varieties. In the following sections, we will emphasize historical and clinical features that help the clinician make this distinction. Certain important historical clues are common to all movement disorder patients. For example, a careful *family history* must be obtained, including the possibility of parental consanguinity. It is crucial to recognize that symptoms distinct from those affecting the patient in question may have predominated in other family members or that the manifestations may have been limited to a forme fruste state. The additional problems that may hamper the acquisition of an adequate family history include adoption, illegitimacy, and even the deliberate withholding of important information. The onset of the disorder may not have been evident in a family member who died at an early age. In all movement disorder patients it is particularly important to exclude Wilson's disease in view of the specific therapy available and its universally fatal outcome if left untreated.

One must obtain a careful history of *birth and early developmental* abnormalities, especially emphasizing the possibility of anoxia or kernicterus. A past history of *encephalitis* must be sought. Certain *drugs* have a strong potential for causing movement disorders, particularly those that block dopamine receptors (antipsychotic drugs and the antiemetic metoclopramide) or stimulate them (such as antiparkinsonian agents and stimulants).

As well as documenting the movement disorder, *neurological examination* should search for additional findings that would help indicate the secondary nature of the problem. *General physical examination* also must be thorough. An extremely important component of this is a careful corneal evaluation, including slit-lamp examination, to exclude the presence of a Kayser-Fleischer ring, characteristic of Wilson's disease.

The nature and extent of *laboratory investigations* will depend on the clinical suspicions. Unfortunately, in the absence of clues from the history and physical examination, very few specific or special investigations assist in the diagnosis of these patients.

Movement disorders are conveniently divided into those with a loss of movement (*akinesia*), often accompanied by an increase in muscle tone (*rigidity*), and others with excessive abnormal involuntary movements (*dyskinesias*). However, these disturbances are not mutually exclusive, and numerous combinations are possible.

AKINETIC-RIGID SYNDROME (PARKINSONISM)

Many diseases of the basal ganglia present with poverty of movement (*akinesia*), often associated with an increase in muscle tone (*rigidity*). This syndrome is frequently associated with tremor as well (discussed later in this chapter). The most common cause of the syndrome is idiopathic Parkinson's disease, hence the term *parkinsonism* to describe the composite clinical picture. Patients with other, rarer conditions may display a pure parkinsonian state, but more often parkinsonism is combined with additional neurological features that provide the clue that one is not dealing with typical Parkinson's disease, but with so-called parkinsonism-plus. Table 25.1 provides a differential diagnosis of the akinetic-rigid syndrome. Throughout the following sections, we emphasize features that might aid the physician in distinguishing between Parkinson's disease and the other less common causes of parkinsonism.

Table 25.1: Etiological classification of parkinsonism (akinetic-rigid syndrome)

- Idiopathic Parkinson's disease (a single entity?)
- Secondary parkinsonism (parkinsonism-plus)
  - Due to other primary degenerative CNS diseases (many inherited)
    - Multiple-system atrophy (striatonigral degeneration, Shy-Drager syndrome, sporadic olivopontocerebellar atrophy)
    - Spinocerebellar atrophies (SCAs)*
    - Progressive supranuclear palsy
    - Parkinson-dementia-amyotrophic lateral sclerosis complex: (1) Western Pacific, (2) other
    - Alzheimer's disease
    - Pick's disease
    - Cortical-basal ganglionic (corticobasal) degeneration
    - Corticostriatospinal degeneration (spastic pseudosclerosis)
    - Machado-Joseph disease
    - Huntington's disease*
    - Familial basal ganglia calcification*
    - Pallidal degenerations*
    - Neuroacanthocytosis
    - Hallervorden-Spatz disease*
    - L-dopa-responsive dystonia-parkinsonism*
    - Others* (for example, familial depression, alveolar hypoventilation, and parkinsonism)
  - Due to other definable causes
    - Drugs* (dopamine receptor blockers, dopamine depletors, lithium, alpha-methyldopa)
    - Toxins* (manganese, MPTP, mercury, methanol, ethanol, carbon disulfide)
    - Anoxic encephalopathy* (including that due to carbon monoxide, cyanide)
    - Vascular (atherosclerotic, hypertensive, amyloid angiopathy, Binswanger's, arteriovenous malformation)
    - Postencephalitic* (encephalitis lethargica, other viral encephalitis, Creutzfeldt-Jakob disease)
    - Head injury* (including punch-drunk syndrome)
    - Brain tumor*
    - Hydrocephalus* (high pressure and normal pressure)
    - Metabolic* (Wilson's disease, acquired hepatocerebral degeneration, hypoparathyroidism, GM_1 gangliosidosis, Gaucher's disease, others)

MPTP = 1-methyl-4-phenol-1,2,3,6-tetrahydropyridine.
*Disorders that may cause juvenile parkinsonism.

Common Symptoms

Motor Abnormalities

In the strictest sense, *akinesia* refers to a lack or poverty of movement, whereas *bradykinesia* describes slowness and fatiguing of voluntary movement. Some authors have used the term *hypokinesia* to describe a reduction in amplitude of movement. Many symptoms are explained by the combination of slowness and poverty of movement and the increase in muscle tone. Early in the course of the disease, many patients are unaware of any motor deficit. Often the spouse will comment on a reduction in facial expression (frequently misinterpreted as depression), a reduction in arm swing while walking, and a slowing of many motor acts, most notably dressing, feeding, and walking. The patient may then become aware of a reduction in manual dexterity, with slowness and clumsiness interfering with activities. Parkinson's disease is often very asymmetrical, and early on only one side may be clinically affected. A painful frozen shoulder is sometimes the earliest symptom of incipient unilateral rigidity and bradykinesia. All recreational and work tasks, household chores, and self-care functions eventually become impaired. Handwriting frequently becomes slower and smaller (*micrographia*), with speed and size deteriorating as the task continues. Eventually, the writing may become illegible. Manipulation of utensils for eating becomes difficult, chewing is laborious, and choking while swallowing may occur. If the latter is an early and prominent complaint, one must consider bulbar involvement in one of the parkinsonism-plus syndromes. Dressing tasks, such as doing small buttons or getting arms into sleeves, are frequently difficult. Maintenance of hygiene becomes impaired. As with most other tasks, disability is greater if the dominant arm is most affected. For example, shaving and particularly brushing teeth become difficult. Climbing in and out of the bathtub causes problems, and patients frequently may be showering only. Many patients interpret these difficulties as due to "weakness." Generalized loss of energy and easy fatiguability are also common complaints.

Speech loses its volume (*hypophonia*), and patients are often asked to repeat themselves. A large number of additional speech disturbances may occur, including stuttering and *palilalia* (repetition of a phrase involuntarily with increasing rapidity). Early pronounced voice changes could indicate a diagnosis other than idiopathic Parkinson's disease. Another problem related to impairment of bulbar function is excessive salivation and drooling. Initially this may occur only at night, but later it can be present throughout the day, at times requiring the constant use of a tissue or handkerchief.

Rising from a deep chair may require a push off with the arms or more than one attempt. Walking becomes slowed. When involvement is asymmetrical, one leg may drag behind the other. Stride then becomes shortened and turns require multiple steps. Later, patients may note a tendency to advance rapidly with short steps (*festination*), at times seemingly propelled forward with a secondary inadequate attempt to maintain the center of gravity over the legs. When this occurs, a nearby wall or an unobstructed fall may be the only method of stopping. Alternatively, the feet may seem to become glued to the floor, the so-called freezing phenomenon. Early on, this is appreciated when attempting to initiate walking (*start hesitation*), when turning (especially in an enclosed space), or when attempting to walk through an enclosed area such as a doorway (an elevator door is a common precipitant). When combined with poor postural stability, prominent freezing results in the tendency to fall forward or to the side while turning. Later, impaired postural reflexes may cause falls without a propulsion or freezing precipitant. Importantly, the early occurrence of falls suggests a diagnosis other than true Parkinson's disease.

Turning over in bed and adjusting the bedclothes often become difficult. Patients may have to sit up first and then turn, and later the spouse may have to help roll the person over or adjust his or her position for comfort.

Cognitive, Autonomic, and Sensory Abnormalities

The complaints of patients suffering from akinetic-rigid syndromes are not limited to the motor system. Dementia may be seen in a variety of akinetic-rigid syndromes, as outlined in Table 25.2. Depression also is a common problem, and in addition, patients often lose their assertiveness and become more passive and less interested in daily activities. The term *bradyphrenia* has been used to describe the slowness of thought processes and inattentiveness that are often seen.

Complaints related to autonomic dysfunction are also common. In all parkinsonian syndromes, constipation is a frequent complaint and may reach severe proportions. However, incontinence of stool is not seen in Parkinson's disease unless the motor disability is such that the patient cannot maneuver to the bathroom or dementia is superimposed. Bladder complaints such as frequency, nocturia, and the sensation of incomplete bladder emptying may occur. A mild to moderate degree of *orthostatic hypotension* is common in akinetic-rigid syndromes, and the problem is often further aggravated by antiparkinsonian drugs (see Chapter 76). If these features are early, prominent, and otherwise inexplicable, however, one must consider the possibility of the Shy-Drager syndrome. In addition to presyncope and fainting, patients with severe orthostatic hypotension experience a variety of confusing complaints such as posturally induced fatigue and weakness, alteration in vision with dimming or blurring, a disconnected feeling, neck and shoulder pain, vertigo, and even true drop attacks without loss of consciousness. The Shy-Drager syndrome also causes early impotence in males, often years before the onset of other problems. As motor disability progresses, it is common for all akinetic-rigid syndrome patients to note sexual dysfunction, caused at least in part by the motor disability. A helpful historical differentiating point here is the loss of nocturnal or morning erections in patients with autonomic degenerations.

Visual complaints are usually not a prominent feature, with the following specific exceptions. In Parkinson's disease, diplopia on reading secondary to impaired convergence is not uncommon. Other akinetic-rigid syndromes, particularly progressive supranuclear palsy and the olivopontocerebellar atrophies, sometimes have visual complaints (see Chapter 76). *Oculogyric crises* in the absence of neuroleptic drug exposure are virtually pathognomonic of parkinsonism following encephalitis lethargica. Sensory loss usually indicates a parkinsonism-plus syndrome. However, patients

Table 25.2: Diseases causing dementia and parkinsonism

Idiopathic Parkinson's disease with
Concomitant Alzheimer's disease
Cortical Lewy body disease
No good explanation for dementia
Alzheimer's disease
Progressive supranuclear palsy
Multiple-system atrophy
Huntington's disease
Cortical-basal ganglionic degeneration
Pick's disease
Parkinson-dementia-amyotrophic lateral sclerosis complex
Creutzfeldt-Jakob disease
Multi-infarct state (atherosclerotic parkinsonism)
Normal-pressure hydrocephalus
Cerebral anoxia (including carbon monoxide poisoning)
Dementia pugilistica
Wilson's disease
Hallervorden-Spatz's disease
Calcification of basal ganglia (primary or secondary)
Others (for example, manganese poisoning, neurosyphilis, Lafora body disease, ceroid lipofuscinosis)

Source: Reprinted with permission of the authors and publisher from WJ Weiner, AE Lang. Movement Disorders: A Comprehensive Survey. Mount Kisco, NY: Futura, 1989.

with akinetic-rigid syndromes, including Parkinson's disease, may have poorly explained positive sensory complaints such as numbness and tingling, aching, and painful sensations, which are sometimes quite disabling.

Onset and Course

As in other movement disorders, the age of onset of a parkinsonian syndrome is clearly important in considering a differential diagnosis. Although the majority of patients are adults, parkinsonism can be seen in childhood (see Table 25.1). The natural history of the disorder is also helpful. Idiopathic Parkinson's disease usually has a slow onset and very gradual progression. Other disorders (such as those due to toxins, cerebral anoxia, or infarction) may present abruptly or progress more rapidly (resulting in so-called malignant parkinsonism) and may even improve spontaneously (as in those due to drugs, multiple infarcts, and certain forms of encephalitis).

The Examination

Clinical Signs

The diagnosis of parkinsonism is often immediately apparent on first contact with the patient. The facial expression, voice characteristics, tremor, poverty of movement, and flexed posture give an immediate and irrevocable first impression. However, the physician must remember the need for detailed assessment in attempting to distinguish between the various causes of this picture.

Loss of *facial expression* is often an early sign. Occasional patients demonstrate a wide-eyed, anxious expression. Frequency of blinking is usually reduced, although *blepharoclonus* (repetitive spasms of the lids on gentle eye closure) and *reflex blepharospasm* (for example, precipitated by shining a light into the eyes or manipulation of the lids) also may be seen. Spontaneous blepharospasm and apraxia of lid opening occur less often. In addition to the facial characteristics, parkinsonian patients develop excessive greasiness of the skin and seborrheic dermatitis, characteristically seen over the forehead, eyebrows, and malar area.

The *voice* of parkinsonism is hypophonic, monotonous, often hesitant, stuttering, and more rapid than normal. One must attempt to discern the presence of additional pseudobulbar or cerebellar features that suggest alternative diagnoses. Palilalia and *echolalia* (involuntary repetition of words and phrases spoken by others) occur in several akinetic-rigid disorders. Careful observation of facial and voice characteristics may be immediately rewarding. For example, the combination of poor eye contact due to the disturbance of refixation eye movements, furrowing of the brow, and deepening of the nasolabial folds secondary to facial spasticity, and a harsher, higher-pitched nasal quality of the voice, which is quite distinctive from the hypophonic monotone of Parkinson's disease, can all suggest the diagnosis of progressive supranuclear palsy (PSP) within a few minutes of a patient's entering the room.

Various types of *tremor,* most notably resting and postural varieties (see the next section for definitions), often accompany akinetic-rigid syndromes. A true intention tremor, suggesting involvement of cerebellar connections, is much less common but is more helpful in limiting the diagnostic possibilities.

Rigidity is an increase in muscle tone, usually equal in flexors and extensors and best appreciated using slow, passive movements. This contrasts with the distribution and velocity-dependent nature of spasticity. *Paratonia* (or *gegenhalten*), on the other hand, seems to increase further with attempts to get the patient to relax. It may be difficult to distinguish between milder forms of paratonia and rigidity, especially in the legs. Characteristically, rigidity is brought out or aggravated by the performance of movements in the opposite limb (such as opening and closing the fist, or abduction-adduction of the shoulder), a phenomenon known as *activated rigidity* (Froment's sign). Superimposed on the rigidity one may appreciate a tremor or cogwheeling phenomenon. This, like the milder forms of rigidity, is better appreciated by placing one hand over the muscles being tested (for example, the left thumb over the biceps and the remaining fingers over the triceps while flexing and extending the elbow with the right hand). The distribution of the rigidity is sometimes helpful in differential diagnosis. For example, pronounced nuchal rigidity with much less hypertonicity in the limbs suggests the possibility of PSP, whereas an extreme degree of unilateral arm rigidity might suggest cortical-basal ganglionic degeneration.

Akinesia and *bradykinesia* may be appreciated on examination in a variety of ways. Movements normally expressed in conversation, such as the use of the hands while speaking, crossing and uncrossing the legs, and repositioning the body in the chair, are reduced or absent. Rapid, repetitive, and alternating movements such as finger tapping, opening and closing of the fist, pronation-supination of the forearm, and foot tapping, are performed slowly, with a gradual reduction in amplitude and degree of completion. In addition to fatiguing, there may be hesitation in initiating movement and arrests in ongoing movement. The severely afflicted patient may be barely able to perform the task. There is a tendency for rapid, repetitive movements to take on the frequency of an accompanying tremor. In such cases the patient should be instructed to slow the movement and attempt to complete it voluntarily.

Watching the patient write is an important part of the examination. Observation may reveal great slowness and effort even in someone with minimal change in the size of the script. In addition to micrographia, writing and drawing show a tendency to fatigue with a further reduction in size as the task proceeds, as well as a concomitant action tremor.

Postural disturbances are common in akinetic-rigid syndromes. The head usually tilts forward and the body becomes stooped, often with pronounced kyphosis and varying degrees of scoliosis. The arms become flexed at the elbows and wrists, with varying postural deformities in the hands, the most common being flexion at the metacarpophalangeal joints and extension at the interphalangeal joints with adduction of all the fingers and opposition of the thumb to the index finger. Flexion also occurs in the joints of the legs. Again, variable foot deformities occur, the most common being hammertoe-like disturbances in most of the toes, occasionally with extension of the great toe (the so-called striatal foot), which may be misinterpreted as an extensor plantar response. Initially, abnormal foot posturing may be action-induced, occurring only while walking or bearing weight. The flexed or simian posture is sometimes extreme, with severe flexion at the waist and maintenance of the hands above the belt line because of flexion of the elbows. Occasional patients remain upright or even demonstrate a hyperextended posture. Hyperextension of the neck is particularly suggestive of PSP.

Postural instability is characteristic of akinetic-rigid syndromes. In rising from a sitting position, poor postural stability, slowness, and failure to reposition the feet beneath them often combine to cause patients to fall back into the chair "in a lump." Rising may require several attempts, a push off the arms of the chair, or a pull from an assistant. Gait disturbances in typical parkinsonism include lack of arm swing, shortened and later shuffling stride, freezing in the course of walking (especially at a door frame), and in more severe cases propulsion and spontaneous falls. In addition, a resting tremor is frequently brought out by walking. To assess postural instability, the physician performs the pull test. Standing behind the patient, the examiner pulls the patient backward by the shoulders (or by a hand on the sternum), carefully remaining close behind to prevent a possible fall. Once postural reflexes are impaired, there may be *retropulsion* or multiple backward steps in response to the postural perturbation. Later, there is a tendency to fall en bloc without retropulsion or even normal attempts to recover or to cushion the fall.

The base of the gait is usually narrow, and tandem gait is performed relatively well. When the gait is wide-based, a superimposed ataxia must be considered, as is seen in the olivopontocerebellar atrophies (OPCAs). Toe walking (cock-walk) is seen in some parkinsonian disorders, and a peculiar loping gait may indicate the rare patient with akinesia in the absence of rigidity. The so-called magnetic foot or *marche à petits pas* of senility (also seen in multiple infarctions, Binswanger's disease, and normal pressure hydrocephalus) more commonly results in a lower half parkinsonism; the striking discrepancy of involvement between the lower body and the upper limbs (with relatively normal or even excessive arm swing) provides an important clue (see Chapter 26).

Differential Diagnosis

The four major characteristics of parkinsonism—tremor, rigidity, akinesia, and postural disturbances (making up the acronym TRAP)—account for most of the clinical abnormalities described here. Although dementia does occur in a proportion of patients with Parkinson's disease, this feature must alert the physician to consider other possible diagnoses (see Table 25.2), including the coincidental association of unrelated causes of cognitive decline. Eye movements must be examined carefully. Prominent disturbances are especially helpful in distinguishing the olivopontocerebellar atrophies, postencephalitic parkinsonism, and PSP. It is important to assess optokinetic nystagmus, where, for example, the dominant abnormality in PSP is a loss of vertical fast components. The oculocephalic ("doll's head") maneuver must be performed where ocular excursions are limited, seeking supportive evidence for a supranuclear gaze palsy. Although obvious pyramidal tract dysfunction usually suggests another diagnosis or additional pathology, mild rigidity can accentuate the reflexes. When the parkinsonism is asymmetrical, this may cause confusing reflex changes. Primitive reflexes, including the inability to inhibit blinking in response to tapping over the glabella (*Myerson's sign*), are nonspecific and commonly present in many akinetic-rigid disorders. A pathologically brisk jaw jerk, however, suggests additional corticobulbar tract pathology. A grasp response indicates disturbance of the frontal lobes and the possibility of a concomitant dementing process. Occasionally, a pronounced flexed posture in the hand may be confused with a grasp reflex, and the examiner must be convinced that there is active contraction in response to stroking the palm. The abnormalities of rapid, repetitive, and alternating movements described earlier must not be confused with the disruption of rate, rhythm, and force typical of the dysdiadochokinesia of cerebellar disease. A helpful maneuver in testing for the presence of associated cerebellar dysfunction is to have the patient tap with the index finger on a hard surface. Watching and, in particular, listening to the tapping often allow a distinction between the slowness and fatiguing of pure bradykinesia and the irregular rate and force of cerebellar ataxia.

Testing for apraxia should also be performed. However, in the later stages of many parkinsonian disorders, the degree of bradykinesia for other extrapyramidal motor disturbances may make it difficult to interpret the dysfunction seen on these tests.

The presence of other abnormal movements in an untreated patient may indicate a diagnosis other than Parkinson's disease. Stimulus-sensitive myoclonus (discussed below) should be sought by using light touch or pinprick in the digits and the proximal palm or the sole of the foot. Easily elicitable and nonfatiguing myoclonic jerks in response to these stimuli may be seen in cortical-based ganglionic degeneration and multiple-system atrophy.

Despite a variety of sensory complaints, patients with true idiopathic Parkinson's disease do not show prominent abnormalities on the sensory examination, aside from the normal increase in vibration threshold that occurs with age. Wasting and muscle weakness are also not characteristic of Parkinson's disease, although later in the course severely disabled individuals demonstrate disuse atrophy and severe problems in initiating and maintaining muscle activation, which are often difficult to separate from true weakness. Combinations of upper and lower motor neuron weakness may be seen in several other akinetic-rigid syndromes listed in Table 25.1.

Autonomic function must be assessed carefully. At the bedside, this includes an evaluation of orthostatic changes in blood pressure and pulse and, in appropriate circumstances, the response to the Valsalva maneuver, mental arithmetic, and the cold pressor test, among others.

Finally, it is important to emphasize the need for sequential examinations over time, carefully searching for the development of additional findings that may provide a clue to the diagnosis. Several of the akinetic-rigid syndromes present as pure parkinsonism; only later, as the disease progresses, do other signs develop.

TREMOR

Tremor can be defined as a rhythmic oscillation of a body part, produced by either alternating or synchronous contractions of reciprocally innervated antagonistic muscles. Tremors usually have a relatively fixed periodicity, although the rate may appear irregular clinically. The waveform and amplitude of the stereotypic rhythmic movements can vary considerably, depending on both physiological and psychological factors. Tremor is usually further categorized on the basis of the position, posture, or motor performance necessary to elicit it. A *resting tremor* is seen with the body part in complete repose. Maintenance of a posture such as extending the arms parallel to the floor reveals a *postural tremor;* moving the body part to and from a target brings out an *intention* tremor. The use of other descriptive categories in the literature has caused some confusion in tremor terminology. *Static tremor* has been used to describe both resting and postural tremors. *Action tremor* has been used for both postural and intention tremors. One source of confusion here is the fact that many postural tremors appear on approaching a target. The term *terminal tremor* probably avoids this confusion most successfully. In contrast, an intention tremor is present throughout goal-directed movement but is also exaggerated as the target is neared. The term *kinetic tremor* may be more accurate but is unlikely to replace the longer-standing *intention tremor. Ataxic tremor* has been used to refer to a combination of this type of tremor plus limb ataxia. Table 25.3 provides a list of differential diagnoses for the three major categories of tremor, as well as other rhythmic movements that occasionally might be confused with tremor.

Common Symptoms

Symptoms are described under the various different categories of tremor. All people have a normal or physiological tremor that can be demonstrated with sensitive recording devices. Two common pathological tremor disorders that are often confused are parkinsonian resting tremor and essential tremor. Although both conditions are discussed in detail in Chapter 76, helpful distinguishing points are discussed next in view of the frequency of misdiagnosis.

Resting Tremor

A classical *resting tremor* occurs with the body part in complete repose and often dampens or subsides entirely with action. For this reason, patients with pure resting tremor experience greater social embarrassment than functional disability. Indeed, in some cases, it is a family member or friend who first observes the tremor, which is noticeable to the patient only later. Alternatively, some patients complain of the sensation of trembling inside long before a resting tremor becomes overt. Early on, resting tremor may be intermittent and is often precipitated only by anxiety or stress. Most types of tremor are experienced first in the arms, often beginning quite asymmetrically. In the face, resting tremor usually affects the lips and jaw, and the patient may note a rhythmic clicking of the teeth. In the limbs, the tremor is usually most pronounced distally in the fingers ("pill rolling"), wrist, forearm, and ankle. In severe forms, however, it may be conducted more proximally, causing the entire body to shake. The complaint of prominent head tremor (*titubation*) is rarely due to Parkinson's disease unless there is concomitant severe limb tremor with conduction to the trunk and head. Tremor in the legs, and especially in the feet while sitting, is usually due to a parkinsonian resting tremor. A history of progression from unilateral arm tremor to involvement of the arm and the ipsilateral leg suggests parkinsonism rather than essential tremor. Once the tremor has become noticeable to the patient, a variety of methods are used to conceal the movement—for example, holding one hand with the other, sitting on the affected hand, or crossing the legs to dampen a tremulous lower limb. Many patients find that they can abort the tremor transiently at will.

Postural Tremor

In contrast to a pure resting tremor, *postural tremors,* especially with pronounced terminal accentuation, can result in significant disability. Many such patients are mistakenly thought to have "bad nerves." Individuals who perform delicate work with their hands (e.g., jewelers and surgeons) will become aware of this form of tremor earlier than most. The average person usually first appreciates tremor in the acts of feeding and writing. Carrying a cup of liquid, pouring, or eating with a spoon often brings out the tremor. Writing is tremulous and sloppy, and the patient's signature on a check may be questioned. Again, anxiety and stress worsen the tremor, and patients frequently notice that their symptoms are especially bad in public.

Patients often adopt compensatory mechanisms to lessen the disability caused by tremor. Many give up certain tasks, such as serving drinks and eating specific foods (e.g., soup), especially in public. When the tremor is very asymmetrical, patients often switch to using the less affected hand for many tasks, including writing. Two hands may be used to

Table 25.3: Classification and differential diagnosis of tremor

- Resting tremors
  - Parkinson's disease
  - Other parkinsonian syndromes (less common)
  - Midbrain (rubral) tremor: Rest < postural < intention
  - Wilson's disease (also acquired hepatocerebral degeneration)
  - Essential tremor—only if severe: Rest < < postural and action
    - Postural and action (terminal) tremors
  - Physiological tremor
  - Exaggerated physiological tremor; these factors can also aggravate other forms of tremor
    - Stress, fatigue, anxiety, emotion
    - Endocrine—hypoglycemia, thyrotoxicosis, pheochromocytoma, Cushing's disease
    - Drugs and toxins—adrenocorticosteroids, beta agonists, dopamine agonists, amphetamines, lithium, tricyclic antidepressants, neuroleptics, theophylline, caffeine, valproic acid, alcohol withdrawal, mercury ("hatter's shakes"), lead, arsenic, others
  - Essential tremor (familial or sporadic)
    - ?Subtypes
  - Primary writing tremor and other task-specific tremors
  - Orthostatic tremor
  - With other CNS disorders
    - Parkinson's disease
    - Other akinetic-rigid syndromes
    - Idiopathic dystonia, including focal dystonias
  - With peripheral neuropathy
    - Charcot-Marie-Tooth disease (termed the Roussy-Levy syndrome)
    - Other peripheral neuropathies
  - Cerebellar tremor
- Intention tremors
  - Disease of cerebellar outflow (dentate nuclei, interpositus nuclei, or both, and superior cerebellar peduncle): multiple sclerosis, trauma, tumor, vascular, Wilson's disease, acquired hepatocerebral degeneration, drugs, toxins (such as mercury), others
- Miscellaneous rhythmic movement disorders
  - Psychogenic tremor
  - Rhythmic movements in dystonia (dystonic tremor, myorrhythmia)
  - Rhythmic myoclonus (segmental myoclonus—for example, palatal or branchial myoclonus, spinal myoclonus)
  - Oscillatory myoclonus
  - Asterixis
  - Clonus
  - Epilepsia partialis continua
  - Hereditary chin quivering
  - Spasmus nutans
  - Head bobbing with third ventricular cysts
  - Nystagmus

Source: Reprinted with permission of the authors and publisher from WJ Weiner, AE Lang. Movement Disorders: A Comprehensive Survey. Mount Kisco, NY: Futura, 1989.

bring a cup to the mouth; later, a straw may be required. Writing may require the other hand to steady the paper or the writing hand itself. Patients frequently switch to printing, and heavier or thicker writing instruments sometimes make the script more legible.

Other Types of Tremor

Various types of *writing disturbances* may be combined with tremor. *Primary writing tremor* is one form of *task-specific tremor* that affects the writing act in isolation, with little or no associated postural or terminal tremor interfering with other acts. *Dystonic writer's cramp* (discussed later in this chapter) can involve additional tremulousness on writing. This must be distinguished from the voluntary excessive squeezing on the pen or pressing onto the page often seen in patients with postural tremor (or primary writing tremor) attributable to their attempts to lessen the effect of tremor on writing. In addition, patients with postural tremor may consciously slow their writing down to improve accuracy, but this is a voluntary compensatory mechanism unassociated with the micrographia and fatigue that accompany parkinsonism.

Tremor in the head and neck, or titubation, can occur in isolation or can be combined with a postural tremor elsewhere, especially in the arms. As discussed later, this and other postural tremors are often associated with symptoms indicative of additional dystonia. Head tremor is rarely a source of physical disability but may create considerable social embarrassment. Patients occasionally complain of a similar tremor of the voice. This is particularly noticeable to others who are listening to the patient on the telephone, and many patients are asked whether they are sad or have been crying.

Less often, patients with postural tremors note a similar tremor in the legs and trunk. The awareness of this form of tremor clearly depends on the activity being performed. One unusual form of postural tremor has been termed *orthostatic tremor*. Here, patients note the tremor in the legs only after standing for variable periods of time. Characteristically, the tremor subsides if the individual can walk about, lean against something, or sit down.

Other Clues in the History

Although patients with a variety of different types of tremor may relate that alcohol transiently reduces their shaking, especially if they are intoxicated, a striking response to small amounts of alcohol is particularly characteristic of essential tremor. Clues to the possible presence of factors aggravating the normal physiological tremor (see Table 25.3) must also be sought by further inquiry.

The Examination

With the patient in a seated or standing position, head tremor may be evident as a vertical nodding (*tremblement affirmatif*) or a side-to-side horizontal shake (*tremblement negatif*). There may be combinations of the two, with rotatory movements. Head tremors usually range from 1.5–5.0 Hz and are most commonly associated with essential tremor or cervical dystonia, as well as diseases of the cerebellum and its outflow pathways. A parkinsonian resting tremor may involve the jaw and lips. A similar tremor of the perioral and nasal muscles, the so-called *rabbit syndrome,* has been associated with antipsychotic drug therapy but also occurs in Parkinson's disease. In many disorders, voluntary contraction of the facial muscles induces an action tremor. In addition, a postural tremor of the tongue is often present on tongue protrusion. In the case of tremors of head and neck structures, it is important to observe the palate at rest for the slower rhythmic movements of palatal myoclonus. Occasionally, the palate is spared, with similar movements affecting other branchial structures. A voice tremor is best demonstrated by asking the patient to hold a note as long as possible. Superimposed on the vocal tremulousness may be a harsh, strained quality or abrupt cessations of air flow during the course of maintaining the note, suggesting a superimposed dystonia of the larynx (spasmodic dysphonia).

A parkinsonian resting tremor is characteristically in the 4- to 6-Hz range. The frequency of postural arm tremors varies depending on cause and severity. Essential tremor is usually in the range of 5–10 Hz, with the greater-amplitude tremors tending to be slower. Exaggerated physiological tremor has a frequency of 8–12 Hz. Many patients with parkinsonism demonstrate a combination of slower resting and faster postural tremors. Some patients with slower, larger-amplitude forms of essential tremor have a definite resting component.

A resting tremor in the limbs is seen with the muscles in complete repose. Even a small amount of muscle activity, as may occur if the patient is somewhat anxious or the limb is not completely at rest, may bring out a faster-frequency postural tremor. It is sometimes impossible to abate this postural tremor during a stressful office interview. An occult resting tremor also may be brought out by stress or concentration, such as the performance of serial 7s. Although a resting tremor characteristically subsides on maintaining a posture, such as holding the arms outstretched parallel to the floor, after a few seconds it may recur. Carrying out goal-directed movements, such as finger-to-nose testing, usually causes the tremor to dampen further or subside completely. On the other hand, a typical postural tremor usually is seen without significant latency after the initiation of a posture and may worsen further at the end points of goal-directed movement (terminal tremor). The slower intention tremor of cerebellar disease is seen throughout the movement but also worsens as the target is reached. Occasionally, pronounced bursts of muscle activity in a patient with terminal tremor cause individual separate jerks, which give the impression of superimposed myoclonus (to be discussed).

Having the patient point the index fingers at each other under the nose (without touching the fingers together or touching the face) with the arms abducted at the sides and the elbows flexed will demonstrate both a distal tremor in the hands and proximal tremors, such as the slower wing-beating tremor of cerebellar outflow pathway disease, as may be seen in Wilson's disease. Tremor during the course of slowly pronating and supinating the forearms with the arms outstretched or with forceful abduction of the fingers may be seen in patients with primary writing tremor. Holding a full cup of water with the arm outstretched will often amplify a postural tremor, and picking up the full cup, bringing it to the mouth, and tipping it to drink will enhance the terminal tremor, often causing spillage. In addition to writing, one should have the patient draw with both hands separately. Useful drawing tasks include an Archimedes spiral, a wavy line from one side of the page to the other, and an attempt to draw carefully a line or spiral between two well-defined, closely opposed borders.

In the legs, in addition to the standard heel-to-shin testing, which will bring out terminal and intention tremors, it may be possible to demonstrate a postural tremor by having the patient hold the leg off the bed and attempt to touch the examiner's finger with the great toe. With the legs flexed at the knees and abducted at the hips, the feet held flat on the bed, synchronous rhythmic 3-per-second abductions of the thighs may be seen in patients with atrophy of the anterior vermis, as seen in alcoholic cerebellar degeneration.

On standing with the feet together, patients with orthostatic tremor develop rapid rhythmic contractions of leg muscles, causing the kneecaps to bob up and down. This dampens or subsides on walking. In contrast, cerebellar disease results in a slower titubation of axial structures and head seen in the upright position. Observing the gait often helps differentiate between upper-limb resting tremor and postural tremor that persists at rest as a result of stress. The former is usually clearly evident during walking, whereas the latter typically subsides. Obviously, observing additional features of the gait is helpful in making these distinctions as well.

Certain tremors persist in all positions. Disease in the midbrain involving the superior cerebellar peduncle near the red nucleus (possibly also involving the nigrostriatal fibers) results in the so-called *midbrain* or *rubral tremor.* Characteristically, this form of tremor combines features of the three different tremor classes. It is often present at rest, increases with postural maintenance, and increases still further—sometimes to extreme degrees—with goal-directed movement.

Tremor also may be a feature of psychiatric disease, representing a conversion reaction or even malingering. Usually certain features are atypical or incongruous. This type of tremor differs from most organic tremors in that the frequency is often quite variable, and concentration and distraction often abate the tremor instead of increasing it.

CHOREA

The term *chorea* is derived from the Greek *choreia,* meaning "a dance." This condition consists of irregular, unpredictable, brief, jerky movements that flit from one part of the body to another in a random sequence. The movements are brisk and abrupt in some conditions—for instance, Sydenham's chorea—whereas in others they are somewhat slower and more flowing, as in Huntington's disease. The term *choreo-athetosis* has been used in this latter situation, where chorea may be combined with features of dystonia and athetosis (to be discussed). The numerous possible causes of chorea are listed in Table 25.4.

Common Symptoms

Initially, patients often are unaware of the presence of involuntary movements, and the family may simply interpret the chorea as normal fidgetiness. The earliest patient complaints are usually those of clumsiness and incoordination—for example, dropping or bumping into things. The limbs occasionally strike closely placed objects. In more moderate to severe cases, patients may complain of the abnormal involuntary jumping or jerking of the limbs and trunk. They rarely complain of the presence of abnormal movements of the face. This discrepancy is particularly striking in the case of tardive dyskinesia, where the patient often appears completely unaware of or indifferent to constant and severe choreic movements of the mouth and tongue. Alternatively, it may be impossible to maintain dentures in place, teeth may be ground or cracked, and there may be constant biting of the tongue or inner cheek. Speech may be slurred and periodically interrupted, especially in Huntington's disease, in which speech disturbances are severe and often fail to correlate with the severity of chorea. Here, in addition to dysarthria, there is usually a considerable reduction in the spontaneity and quantity of speech output. Problems with feeding are due to a combination of limb chorea, which causes sloppiness, and swallowing difficulties, which can result in choking and aspiration. Eating is particularly difficult for patients with neuroacanthocytosis (choreoacanthocytosis), where severe orolingual dystonia can cause the tongue to push the food out of the mouth almost as quickly as the patient puts it in. Here, patients often place food at the back of the tongue and throw the head back to initiate swallowing.

Disturbances of stance and gait can be early complaints. The patient may note a tendency to sway and jerk while standing, as well as an unsteady, uneven gait often likened to a drunken stagger. Later still, added postural instability in Huntington's disease can result in falls. Respiratory dyskinesias may cause the patient to feel short of breath or unable to obtain enough air. Patients with involvement of the pelvic region may complain bitterly of thrusting and rocking movements in the lower trunk and pelvis. Respiratory and pelvic involvement are sources of complaint more often in tardive dyskinesia than in other choreic movement disorders.

Table 25.4: Etiological classification of chorea

Developmental and aging choreas
Physiological chorea of infancy
Cerebral palsy—anoxic, kernicterus
Minimal cerebral dysfunction
Buccal-oral-lingual dyskinesia and edentulous orodyskinesia
In elderly, senile chorea (probably several causes)
Hereditary choreas
Huntington's disease
Benign hereditary chorea
Neuroacanthocytosis
Other CNS degenerations: olivopontocerebellar atrophy, Machado-Joseph's disease, ataxia telangiectasia, tuberous sclerosis, Hallervorden-Spatz's disease, familial calcification of basal ganglia, others
Neurometabolic disorders: Wilson's disease, Lesch-Nyhan's syndrome, lysosomal storage disorders, amino acid disorders, Leigh's disease, porphyria
Drug-induced—neuroleptics (tardive dyskinesia), antiparkinsonian drugs, amphetamines, tricyclics, oral contraceptives
Toxins—alcohol intoxication and withdrawal, anoxia, carbon monoxide, manganese, mercury, thallium, toluene
Metabolic
Hyperthyroidism
Hypoparathyroidism (various types)
Pregnancy (chorea gravidarum)
Hyper- and hyponatremia, hypomagnesemia, hypocalcemia
Hypo- and hyperglycemia (the latter may cause hemichorea, hemiballism)
Acquired hepatocerebral degeneration
Nutritional—for example, beriberi, pellagra, vitamin B_{12} deficiency in infants
Infectious
Sydenham's chorea
Encephalitis lethargica
Various other infectious and postinfectious encephalitides, including Creutzfeldt-Jakob disease
Immunological
Systemic lupus erythematosus (including antinuclear antibody-negative cases with lupus anticoagulant)
Henoch-Schönlein purpura
Others rarely—sarcoidosis, multiple sclerosis, Behçet's disease, polyarteritis nodosa
Vascular (often hemichorea)
Infarction
Hemorrhage
Arteriovenous malformation
Polycythemia rubra vera
Migraine
Tumors
Trauma, including subdural and epidural hematoma
Miscellaneous, including paroxysmal choreoathetosis

Source: Adapted from I Shoulson. On chorea. Clin Neuropharmacol 1986;9:585.

Other Clues on History

It is obvious from a review of Table 25.4 that it is impractical to discuss additional historical clues for every cause of chorea. I will limit discussion here to a few practical and important points.

Age of onset and manner of progression will vary depending on the cause. A helpful distinction can be made here between benign hereditary chorea and Huntington's disease. In the former, chorea typically begins in childhood with a slow progression and little cognitive change, whereas Huntington's disease presenting in childhood is more often of the akinetic-rigid variety, with severe mental changes and rapid progression.

In most cases the onset of chorea is slow and insidious. An abrupt or subacute onset is more typical of many of the symptomatic causes of chorea, such as neuroleptic drug withdrawal (withdrawal emergent syndrome), hyperthyroidism, systemic lupus erythematosus (SLE), or multiple infarcts, as opposed to Huntington's disease and other neurodegenerative disorders. A pattern of remissions and exacerbations suggests the possibility of drugs, SLE, and rheumatic fever, whereas brief (minutes to hours) bouts of involuntary movement indicate a paroxysmal dyskinesia (see below).

A recent history of streptococcal throat infection, and of musculoskeletal or cardiovascular complaints in a child, suggests a diagnosis of Sydenham's chorea. One may obtain a previous history of rheumatic fever, particularly in women developing chorea during pregnancy or while taking the birth control pill. In women, chorea during pregnancy or a history of previous fetal loss suggests the possibility of SLE, even in the absence of other features of collagen vascular disease. Symptoms isolated to one side of the body suggest a structural lesion in the contralateral basal ganglia. Many patients who complain of unilateral involvement, however, will have abnormalities of both sides on examination.

A careful family history is crucial. The most common cause of inherited chorea is Huntington's disease, which has fully penetrant autosomal-dominant transmission. It is important to remember that the family history can be misleading and that the manifestations of the disease in other family members may have been quite dissimilar from those of the patient. A wide range of behavioral and psychiatric disturbances may be most prominent and the chorea hardly noticed.

The Examination

A wide range of flowing, brief, jerky movements can involve almost any somatic muscle. Although the movements usually appear random, prolonged observation often reveals a pattern that recurs in a somewhat stereotypical manner—for instance, lip pursing with downward movement of the chin. In tardive dyskinesia, however, the movements are often much more stereotypical and repetitive. Therefore, orofacial dyskinesia is discussed separately at the end of this section.

The range of choreiform movements is quite broad—for example, eyebrow lifting or depression, lid winking, lip pouting or pursing, cheek puffing, lateral or forward jaw movements, tongue rolling or protruding, head jerking in any plane (a common pattern is a sudden backward jerk followed by a rotatory sweep forward), shoulder shrugging, trunk jerking or arching, pelvic rocking, and flitting movements of the fingers, wrists, toes, and ankles. Patients can be seen to incorporate choreic jerks into voluntary movement, perhaps in part to mask the presence of the dyskinesia (so-called *parakinesis*).

Performance of various tasks, such as finger-to-nose testing and rapid alternating movements, is frequently altered by the chorea, which can cause a jerky, interrupted performance. Standing and walking frequently aggravate the chorea. Particularly in Huntington's disease, the gait has additional bizarre characteristics that are not simply explained by increased chorea. The gait is usually wide-based despite the absence of typical ataxia. Patients may deviate from side to side in a zigzag fashion, with lateral swaying and additional spontaneous flexion. In addition, the stride is usually shortened and the speed slowed, with some features similar to a parkinsonian gait, such as loss of arm swing, festination, propulsion, and retropulsion.

Respiratory irregularities are common, especially in tardive dyskinesia, and periodic grunting, respiratory gulps, and sniffing are frequently seen.

Other movement disorders are often combined with chorea. Dystonic features are probably the most common and are seen in many different conditions. Less frequent but well recognized are parkinsonism (e.g., with Huntington's, neuroacanthocytosis, and Wilson's), tics (e.g., in neuroacanthocytosis), myoclonus (e.g., in Huntington's and others), and tremor (e.g., in Wilson's and Huntington's). Tone is usually normal to reduced. Muscle bulk is typically preserved, although weight loss and generalized wasting are commonly seen in Huntington's disease. When distal weakness and amyotrophy are present, one must consider accompanying anterior horn cell or peripheral nerve disease as in neuroacanthocytosis, ataxia telangiectasia, *Machado-Joseph's disease*, and olivopontocerebellar atrophies. Here the reflexes may be reduced. On the other hand, chorea often results in a so-called hung-up reflex, probably due to the occurrence of a choreic jerk following the usual reflex muscle contraction.

Depending on the cause (see Table 25.4), a variety of other neurological disturbances may be associated with chorea. In Huntington's disease, for example, cognitive changes, motor impersistence (such as difficulty maintaining eyelid closure, tongue protrusion (*trombone tongue*), or constant hand grip), apraxias (especially orolingual), and oculomotor dysfunction are all quite common (see Chapter 76).

Tardive Dyskinesia

It is worth separating the usual movements seen in tardive dyskinesia from those of classical chorea because there are distinguishing factors that help in the differential diagnosis (Table 25.5). In contrast to the random and unpredictable flowing nature of chorea, tardive dyskinesia usually demonstrates repetitive stereotypic movements, which are most pronounced in the orolingual region—for example, chewing and smacking

Table 25.5: Features distinguishing between oromandibular dystonia (OMD), tardive dyskinesia (TD), and Huntington's disease (HD)

	OMD	*TD*	*HD*
Nature of the movements			
Repetitive stereotypic chorealike movements	–	++	–
Flowing choreic movements	–	±	++
Prolonged dystonic movements	++	±	±
Rhythmic tremulous movements	+	–	–
Akathitic movements	–	+	–
Sites of involvement			
Forehead involvement	+	–	+
Blepharospasm	+	±	±
Oral-buccal-lingual dyskinesia (including masticatory muscles)	++	++	±
Platysma	++	±	±
Nuchal muscles	+	±	+
Respiratory dyskinesia	–	+	±
Trunk, legs	–	+	++
Additional features and other movement disturbances			
Ocular motor disturbances and head thrusts	–	–	++
Impersistence of tongue protrusion	±	–	++
Improvement of facial movements on tongue protrusion	–	++	–
Facial dyspraxia	–	–	++
Dysarthria	++	–	++
Milkmaid grip	–	–	++
Body rocking movements	–	+	±
Marching in place	–	+	–
Stuttering, bizarre ataxic gait	–	–	++
Postural instability	–	–	++
Dementia	–	±	++
Progressive course	+	–	++

++ = extremely common; + = commonly present; ± = occasionally present; – = usually absent.
Source: Adapted from S Fahn, personal communication, 1992.

of the mouth and lips, rolling of the tongue in the mouth or pushing against the inside of the cheek ("bon-bon sign"), and periodic protrusion or fly-catcher movements of the tongue. The speed and amplitude of these movements can increase markedly when concentrating on performing rapid alternating movements in the hands. Patients often have a striking degree of voluntary control over the movements and may be able to suppress them for a prolonged period when asked to do so. On distraction, however, the movements return immediately. Despite severe facial movements, voluntary protrusion of the tongue is rarely limited, and this act often dampens or completely inhibits the ongoing facial movements. This contrasts with the pronounced impersistence of tongue protrusion seen in Huntington's disease, which is far out of proportion to the degree of choreic involvement of the tongue.

Several other clinical factors help distinguish between Huntington's disease and tardive dyskinesia. One feature is the occurrence of stereotypic movements in other body locations such as the hands, pelvis, and feet. Despite the rocking movements of the pelvis, tapping of the feet, and shifting of the weight from side to side while standing (some of which may be due to akathisia, to be discussed), the gait is practically normal in most patients, in contrast to the strikingly abnormal gait in many other choreatic disorders, especially in Huntington's disease.

Tardive dyskinesia due to chronic neuroleptic drugs is not the only cause for these stereotypic bucco-linguo-masticatory movements. Other drugs, particularly dopamine agonists in Parkinson's disease, anticholinergics, and antihistamines, cause a similar form of dyskinesia. Multiple infarctions in the basal ganglia and possibly lesions in the cerebellar vermis result in similar movements. Elderly individuals, especially the edentulous, often have a milder form of orofacial movement, usually with minimal lingual involvement. Here, as in tardive dyskinesia, inserting dentures in the mouth may dampen the movements considerably, and placing a finger to the lips can also suppress them. Another important diagnostic consideration and source of clinical confusion is idiopathic oromandibular dystonia (see later). Table 25.5 also lists features that help distinguish tardive dyskinesia from this disorder.

BALLISM

Ballism or *ballismus* is probably the least common of the well-defined dyskinesias. Derived from the Greek word meaning "to throw," these movements are wide in amplitude, violent, and flinging or flailing in nature. As in chorea, they are rapid and poorly patterned. The prominent involvement of more

Table 25.6: Causes of ballism

Infarction or ischemia, including transient ischemic attacks
Usually lacunar disease, hypertensive, diabetic, atherosclerosis, vasculitis, polycythemia, thrombocytosis, other causes
Hemorrhage
Tumor
Metastatic
Primary
Other focal lesions—for example, abscess, arteriovenous malformation, tuberculoma, multiple sclerosis plaque, encephalitis, subdural hematoma
Hyperglycemia (nonketotic hyperosmolar state)
Drugs (phenytoin, dopamine agonists in Parkinson's disease)

proximal muscles of the limbs usually accounts for the throwing or flinging nature. Smaller-amplitude distal movements also may be seen, and occasionally there is even intermittent prolonged dystonic posturing (see below). Some authors have emphasized the greater proximal involvement and the persistent or ceaseless nature of ballism in contrast to chorea. It is more likely, however, that ballism and chorea represent a continuum rather than distinct entities. The coexistence of distal choreic movements, the discontinuous nature in less severe cases, and the common evolution of ballism to typical chorea during the natural course of the disorder or with treatment all support this concept. Ballism is most often confined to one side of the body, when it is referred to as *hemiballismus*. Occasionally only one limb is involved (*monoballism*), and rarely both sides may be affected (*biballism*) or both legs (*paraballism*).

Table 25.6 lists the various causes of hemiballism. These flinging movements are often extremely disabling to patients, who frequently drop things from the hands or damage closely placed objects. Self-injury is common, and examination often reveals multiple bruises and abrasions. Additional signs and symptoms depend on the cause, location, and extent of the lesion, which is usually placed in the contralateral subthalamic nucleus or striatum (see Chapter 76).

DYSTONIA

Dystonia can be defined as a disorder dominated by sustained muscle contractions, which frequently cause twisting and repetitive movements or abnormal postures. The term *dystonia* has been used in three major contexts. It may be used to describe the specific form of involuntary movements described above—that is, a *physical sign*. It also may be used to refer to a *syndrome* caused by a large number of different disease states (Table 25.7). The concept of dystonia as a syndrome is akin to the use of the term *parkinsonism* to describe an akinetic-rigid syndrome. Finally, the term has been used synonymously with the idiopathic form of dystonia (that is, to refer to a *disease*), also known as *idiopathic torsion dystonia* or dystonia musculorum deformans.

Dystonic movements may be slow and twisting. When these are located distally, they are referred to as *athetosis*.

Table 25.7: Etiological classification of dystonia

Primary dystonia
Generalized dystonia (dystonia musculorum deformans, idiopathic torsion dystonia)
Hereditary (primarily autosomal dominant)
Sporadic
Focal, segmental, multifocal
Cranial dystonia (Meige's syndrome, blepharospasm, oromandibular dystonia)
Spasmodic torticollis
Writer's cramp and other occupational dystonias
Spasmodic dysphonia
Others
Idiopathic paroxysmal dystonias
Kinesigenic
Nonkinesigenic
Secondary dystonia
Diseases with known metabolic defect: Wilson's disease, GM_1 gangliosidosis, GM_2 gangliosidosis, metachromatic leukodystrophy, Lesch-Nyhan's syndrome, glutaric acidemia, methylmalonic acidemia, homocystinuria, dystonic lipidosis (Niemann-Pick's disease), Hartnup's disease, others
Diseases with presumed (but undefined) metabolic defect: Hallervorden-Spatz's disease, calcification of basal ganglia, Leigh's disease, bilateral necrosis of basal ganglia (with or without Leber's optic neuropathy), ataxia telangiectasia, neuroacanthocytosis, ceroid lipofuscinosis
Degenerative CNS diseases: X-linked dystonia-parkinsonism (Philippines), L-dopa–responsive dystonia, Parkinson's disease, progressive supranuclear palsy, Huntington's disease, pallidal degenerations, olivopontocerebellar atrophy, Machado-Joseph's disease
Nondegenerative CNS disorders
Perinatal anoxia/kernicterus (may be delayed)
Head trauma (often delayed)
Cerebral infarction/hemorrhage (often delayed)
Arteriovenous malformation
Tumor
Encephalitis (various types)
Toxins (especially manganese)
Postoperative (after thalamotomy)
Multiple sclerosis (often paroxysmal)
Drugs (especially neuroleptics, dopamine agonists)
Psychogenic dystonia
Disorders simulating dystonia
Orthopedic disorders: rotational atlantoaxial subluxation
Neurological: seizures, posterior fossa tumor causing torticollis, hemianopia, strabismus
Miscellaneous: hiatal hernia in childhood (Sandifer's syndrome), congenital neck muscle lesions, abnormal posture in utero, others

Prolonged dystonic spasms result in the characteristic posturing, to be described later. In addition, however, dystonic movements may be quite rapid, resembling the shocklike jerks of myoclonus (discussed later). There may be additional rhythmic movements, especially when the patient attempts to resist the involuntary movement actively. Here, if the patient is asked to relax and allow the limb to move as it pleases, the abnormal dystonic posturing usually becomes evident, and the rhythmic *dystonic tremor* lessens. A faster distal postural tremor also may occur. It is the varied nature of these movements that often results in the misdiagnosis of dystonia as some other type of movement disorder.

Another common error in diagnosis is the mislabeling of dystonia as hysteria. The movements are typically aggravated by stress and anxiety and are improved by rest and even hypnosis. A variety of peculiar tricks can be used to lessen or even completely abate the dystonic movements and postures (discussed later in this chapter and in Chapter 76). The abnormal movements and postures may occur only during the performance of certain acts and not others that use the same muscles. Examples of this *action dystonia* are involvement of the hand only on writing but not with other manual tasks such as using utensils (writer's cramp or graphospasm), dystonia of the oromandibular region only on speaking or eating, and dystonia in a leg only on walking forward but not on walking backward, climbing stairs, or running. A final source of confusion with hysteria is the occurrence of spontaneous remissions in idiopathic dystonias, particularly in patients with involvement of neck muscles (cervical dystonia/spasmodic torticollis).

Common Symptoms

Dystonia can affect almost all the striated muscle groups. Common symptoms include forced eyelid closure (*blepharospasm*); jaw clenching, forced jaw opening, or involuntary tongue protrusion (*oromandibular* or *lingual dystonia*); a harsh, strained, or sometimes breathy voice (laryngeal dystonia or *spasmodic dysphonia*); involuntary deviation of the neck in any plane or combination of planes (*cervical dystonia/spasmodic torticollis*); spasms of the trunk in any direction that variably interfere with lying, sitting, standing, or walking (*axial dystonia*); interference with manual tasks (often only specific tasks in isolation: the occupational palsies, such as *writer's cramp*); and finally involvement of the leg, usually with inversion and plantar flexion of the foot causing the patient to walk on the toes. All of these disorders may slowly progress to the point of complete loss of voluntary function of the affected part. On the other hand, only certain actions may be impaired, and the disorder may remain quite focal in distribution. Chapter 76 deals with each of these forms of dystonia in more detail.

The age of onset and distribution of dystonia are often helpful in determining the possible cause. There are a large number of causes of secondary dystonia (see Table 25.7). Although many of these have additional historical and clinical features, some can present initially with a pure dystonic syndrome. Generalized involvement may occur irrespective of the cause (idiopathic or symptomatic) when dystonia begins at an early age. On the other hand, dystonia beginning in adult life is usually limited to one or a small number of contiguous regions (focal or segmental dystonia; see Table 25.7). Generalized involvement or onset in the legs in an adult always suggests the possibility of a secondary cause. Involvement of one side of the body (*hemidystonia*) is strong evidence for a lesion in the contralateral basal ganglia.

Most patients complain of the dystonia brought out by specific actions but initially show little abnormality at rest. Certain disorders cause paroxysmal episodes of dystonia (see later). The complaint of early constant abnormal posturing of the body part (dystonia at rest) also suggests the possibility of a secondary cause. A fixed posture maintained during sleep implies superimposed contractures or a musculoskeletal disturbance mimicking the postures of dystonia. Although many patients find that dystonia is lessened by rest and sleep, some note a striking diurnal variation, with little or no dystonia on rising in the morning, followed by the progressive development of problems as the day goes on, sometimes to the point of becoming unable to walk late in the day. This diurnal variability strongly suggests a possible diagnosis of L-dopa–responsive dystonia. The nature of the onset of the symptoms (sudden versus slow) and their course, whether rapid progression, slow changes, or episodes of spontaneous remission, all provide important clues to the possible cause.

The family history must be reviewed in considerable detail, with the awareness that affected relatives may have limited or distinctly different involvement from that of the patient. A careful birth and developmental history must be obtained in view of the frequency of dystonia after birth trauma, birth anoxia, and kernicterus. As with the other dyskinesias, a history of such features as previous encephalitis, drug use, and head trauma must be sought. There is also increasing support for the ability of peripheral trauma to precipitate various forms of dystonia, and occasionally this is combined with the syndrome of reflex sympathetic dystrophy.

The Examination

Action dystonia is commonly the earliest manifestation of idiopathic dystonia. It is clearly important to observe patients performing the acts that they complain are most affected. Later, other tasks precipitate similar problems, the use of other parts of the body causes the dystonia to become evident in the originally affected site, and the dystonia may overflow to other sites. Still later, dystonia is evident periodically at rest, and even later the posturing may be persistent and difficult to correct passively, especially when secondary joint contractures develop. A significant deviation from this progression, particularly with the appearance early on of dystonia at rest, should encourage the physician to search carefully for a secondary cause (see Table 25.7).

It is important to recognize the natural variability of dystonia and particularly the effects of stress and anxiety, which may be somewhat paradoxical. This is especially the case with blepharospasm, in which the increased concentration or anxiety associated with a visit to the doctor frequently reduces the severity of the problem. If reliance is placed only on the degree of disability seen in the office, the physician may underestimate the severity of the blepharospasm, and may misdiagnose the problem as hysterical.

Depending on the cause of the dystonia, a variety of neurological abnormalities may accompany the movement disorder. The diverse nature of dystonic movements has been outlined earlier. When present concomitantly with dystonia, the two movement disorders that clearly indicate a need to consider a secondary cause are chorea and an akinetic-rigid syndrome. Obviously, Wilson's disease is the most important, though not the exclusive, consideration in this case. Many of the disorders listed in Table 25.7 will result in additional psychiatric or cognitive disturbances, seizures, or pyramidal tract or cerebellar dysfunction. Oculomotor abnormalities may suggest a diagnosis of Leigh's disease, dystonic lipidosis, ataxia telangiectasia, Machado-Joseph's disease, Huntington's disease, or OPCA. Optic nerve or retinal disease raises the possibility of Leigh's disease, dystonia with striatal lucencies, Hallervorden-Spatz's disease, GM_2 gangliosidosis, and ceroid lipofuscinosis. Lower motor neuron and peripheral nerve dysfunction may be seen with neuroacanthocytosis, ataxia telangiectasia, metachromatic leukodystrophy, Machado-Joseph's disease, and other multisystem degenerations. It must be remembered that the dystonia itself may cause additional neurological problems such as spinal cord or cervical root compression from long-standing torticollis, and peripheral nerve entrapment from limb dystonia. Also independent of the cause, long-standing dystonic muscle spasms often result in hypertrophy of affected muscles (for instance, the sternocleidomastoid in cervical dystonia).

Although the general medical examination must be thorough, it is usually unrevealing. As always, the systemic signs of Wilson's disease must be carefully sought. Abdominal organomegaly also may indicate a storage disease. Severe self-mutilation is typical of Lesch-Nyhan's syndrome. Minor tongue and lip mutilation is seen in neuroacanthocytosis, where orolingual action dystonia may be prominent. Oculocutaneous telangiectasia and evidence of recurrent sinopulmonary infections suggest ataxia telangiectasia. Musculoskeletal abnormalities may stimulate dystonia and, rarely, dysmorphic features of a mucopolysaccharidosis may be present.

TICS

Tics are the most varied of all movement disorders. Patients demonstrate motor or vocal tics as well as a wide variety of associated symptoms. *Motor* and *vocal tics* can be further subdivided as *simple* or *complex*. Tics are usually abrupt, transient, stereotypical, coordinated movements, which vary in intensity and are repeated at irregular intervals. The movements are most often brief and jerky (*clonic*); however, slower, more prolonged movements (*tonic* or dystonic tics) also occur. Several other characteristic features are helpful in distinguishing this movement disorder from other dyskinesias. Patients usually experience an inner urge to make the movement, which is temporarily relieved by its performance. Tics are voluntarily suppressible for variable periods of time, but this occurs at the expense of mounting inner tension and the need to allow the tic to occur. Indeed, a large proportion of these patients, when questioned carefully, admit that the movements or sounds that make up their tics are produced intentionally (in contrast to most other dyskinesias) in response to the uncontrollable inner urge to perform them.

Table 25.8: Classification of tics

Simple motor tics: eye blinking, eyebrow raising, nose flaring, grimacing, mouth opening, tongue protrusion, platysma contractions, head jerking, shoulder shrugging or abduction, neck stretching, arm jerks, fist clenching, abdominal tensing, pelvic thrusting, buttock or sphincter tightening, hip flexion or abduction, kicking, knee extension, foot dorsiflexion, toe curling
Simple phonic tics: sniffing, grunting, throat clearing, shrieking, yelping, barking, growling, squealing, snorting, coughing, clicking, hissing, humming, moaning
Complex motor tics: head shaking, teeth gnashing, wrist shaking, finger cracking, touching, hitting, jumping, skipping, stamping, squatting, kicking, smelling hands or objects, rubbing, finger twiddling, echopraxia, copropraxia, spitting, exaggerated startle
Complex vocal tics: coprolalia (wide variety, including shortened words), unintelligible words, whistling, "Bronx cheer" or "raspberry," panting, belching, hiccough, stuttering, stammering, echolalia, palilalia (also mental coprolalia and palilalia)

Source: Reprinted with permission of the authors and publisher from WJ Weiner, AE Lang. Movement Disorders: A Comprehensive Survey. Mount Kisco, NY: Futura, 1989.

Table 25.8 provides examples of the various types of tics. Simple motor tics are random, brief, irregular muscle twitches of isolated body segments, particularly the eyelids and other facial muscles, the neck, and the shoulders. In contrast, complex motor tics are coordinated patterned movements involving a number of muscles in their normal synergistic relationships. A wide variety of other motor disturbances may be associated with tic disorders, and it is sometimes difficult to separate complex tics from some of these—for example, obsessive-compulsive behavior, copropraxia (obscene gestures), echopraxia (mimicked gestures), hyperactivity with attentional deficits and impulsive behavior, and externally directed and self-destructive behavior, including self-mutilation.

Simple and complex phonic tics comprise a wide variety of sounds, noises, or formed words (see Table 25.8). Possibly the best known (although not the commonest) example of the complex vocal tics is *coprolalia,* the pronunciation of obscene words. Obscenities are frequently slurred or shortened or may intrude into the patient's thoughts but not become verbalized (so-called mental coprolalia).

Like most dyskinesias, tics usually increase with stress. In contrast to other dyskinesias, however, relaxation—for instance, watching television at home—also frequently re-

Table 25.9: Etiological classification of tics

Idiopathic
Acute simple transient tic (<1 year)
Persistent simple or multiple tic of childhood (remits before adulthood)
Chronic simple or multiple motor tics (persist throughout life)
Adult-onset or senile tic
Gilles de la Tourette's syndrome
Secondary tics
Postencephalitic (especially encephalitis lethargica: klazomania)
Postrheumatic chorea
Head injury
Carbon monoxide poisoning
Poststroke
Neuroacanthocytosis
Drugs: stimulants, levodopa, neuroleptics (tardive Tourette's), carbamazepine, phenytoin, phenobarbital
Mental retardation syndromes, including chromosomal abnormalities
Others
Related disorders
Mannerisms
Stereotypies
Habitual manipulations of the body
Hyperactivity syndrome
Compulsions
Excessive startle
Jumping Frenchmen of Maine, Latah, Myriachit

Source: Reprinted with permission of the authors and publisher from WJ Weiner, AE Lang. Movement Disorders: A Comprehensive Survey. Mount Kisco, NY: Futura, 1989.

sults in an increase in the tics, probably because the patient does not feel the need to suppress them voluntarily. Distraction or concentration usually diminishes tics, which also differs from most other types of dyskinesia. Many patients with idiopathic tics note spontaneous waxing and waning in their nature and severity over weeks to months, and periods of complete remission are possible. A large proportion of individuals with tics are only mildly affected, and many are even unaware that they demonstrate clinical features. This must be kept in mind when reviewing the family history. Finally, tics are one of the few movement disorders that can persist during all stages of sleep.

Common Symptoms

The causes of tic disorders are listed in Table 25.9. Most are primary or idiopathic, and within this group the majority of cases present in childhood. Males are affected more often than females. Idiopathic tics occur on a spectrum from a mild, transient, single, simple motor tic to chronic multiple simple and complex motor and phonic tics (Gilles de la Tourette's syndrome).

Patients and their families complain of a wide variety of symptoms (see Table 25.8). They may have seen numerous other subspecialists—for example, allergists for repetitive sniffing, otolaryngologists for throat clearing, ophthalmologists for excessive eye blinking or eye rolling, and psychologists and psychiatrists for the neurobehavioral abnormalities. The true diagnosis often is first questioned after someone close to the patient has learned about it in the media. Children may verbalize few complaints or feel reluctant to speak of the problem, especially if they have been the object of ridicule by others. Even young children, when questioned carefully, can provide the history of sensation of urge to perform the movement that gradually culminates in the release of a tic, as well as the ability to control the tic voluntarily at the expense of mounting inner tension. Children may be able to control the tics for prolonged periods of time but often complain of difficulty concentrating on other tasks while doing so. Some give the history of requesting to leave the school room and then releasing the tics in private, for instance, in the washroom. Peers and siblings often chastise or ridicule the patient, and parents or teachers, failing to appreciate the nature of the disorder, may scold or punish the child for what are thought to be voluntary bad habits (indeed, an older term for tics is *habit spasms*).

The past history may include an exposure to stimulants for hyperactivity. The family history must be reviewed for the wide range of potential manifestations (especially obsessive-compulsive behavior). Additional neurological complaints, including other dyskinesias, suggest the possibility of a secondary cause for the tics.

The Examination

In most patients with tics, the neurological examination is entirely normal. In patients with primary tic disorders, the presence of other neurological, cognitive, behavioral, and neuropsychological disturbances may simply relate to extension of the underlying cerebral dysfunction beyond the core that accounts for pure tic phenomena. Patients with both primary and secondary forms of tics may demonstrate other involuntary movements, such as mild chorea or dystonia. Careful interview stressing the subjective features that accompany tics usually allows the distinction between true dystonia and dystonic tics. Many of the secondary tic disorders show additional neurological or systemic features, which vary depending on the cause (see Table 25.9).

Despite bitter complaints by the family, it is common for patients to show no evidence of a movement disorder during an office appointment. Aware of this, the physician must attempt to observe the patient at a time when he or she is less likely to be exerting voluntary control—for example, in the waiting room. If no movements have been witnessed during the interview, the physician should seemingly direct attention elsewhere—for instance, to the parents—while observing the patient out of the corner of the eye. The patient often releases the tics while changing in the examining room, particularly if they have been held back during the interview. The physician should attempt to view the patient at this time, or at least listen for the occurrence of vocal tics. Despite these maneuvers, one may have to resort to having the patient voluntarily mimic the movements. This, in combination with associated symptoms such as urge, voluntary release and control, and the often varied and complex nature of the movements, is usually enough to provide the diagnosis, even without witnessing the spontaneous dyskinesia in the office.

MYOCLONUS

Myoclonus can be defined as sudden, brief, shocklike involuntary movements that may be caused by both active muscle contraction (*positive myoclonus*) or inhibition of ongoing muscle activity (*negative myoclonus*). The differential diagnosis of myoclonus is broader than that of any other movement disorder (Table 25.10). To exclude muscle twitches such as fasciculations due to lower motor neuron lesions, some authors have insisted that an origin in the central nervous system (CNS) be a component of the definition. Although the vast majority of causes of myoclonus originate in the CNS, occasional cases of brief shocklike movements, clinically indistinguishable from CNS myoclonus, occur with peripheral nerve disease.

There is a wide range of clinical patterns of myoclonus. The frequency varies from single, rare jerks to constant repetitive contractions. The amplitude may range from a small contraction that fails to move a joint to a very large jerk that moves the entire body. The distribution ranges from focal involvement of one body part, to segmental (involving two or more contiguous regions), to multifocal, to generalized. When the jerks occur bilaterally, they may be symmetrical or asymmetrical. When they occur in more than one region, they may be synchronous in two body parts (within milliseconds) or asynchronous. Myoclonus is usually arrhythmic and irregular, but in some patients it is very regular (rhythmic), and in others there may be jerky oscillations that last for a few seconds and then fade away (oscillatory). Myoclonic jerks may occur spontaneously without a clear precipitant or in response to a wide variety of stimuli. This stimulus sensitivity may occur in response to sudden noise, light, visual threat, pinprick or touch, or muscle stretch. Attempted movement (or even the intention to move) may initiate the muscle jerks (action or intention myoclonus).

Common Symptoms

As may be seen from the foregoing description and the long list of possible causes for myoclonus, the symptoms in these patients are quite varied. For simplification, we briefly review the possible symptomatology with respect to the four major etiological subcategories in Table 25.10.

Table 25.10: Etiological classification of myoclonus

Physiological myoclonus (normal subjects)
- Sleep jerks (hypnic jerks)
- Anxiety-induced
- Exercise-induced
- Hiccough (singultus)
- Benign infantile myoclonus with feeding

Essential myoclonus (no known cause and no other gross neurological deficit)
- Hereditary
- Sporadic

Epileptic myoclonus (seizures dominate and no encephalopathy, at least initially)
- Fragments of epilepsy
  - Isolated epileptic myoclonic jerks
  - Epilepsia partialis continua
  - Idiopathic stimulus-sensitive myoclonus
  - Photosensitive myoclonus
  - Myoclonic absences in petit mal
- Childhood myoclonic epilepsies
  - Infantile spasms
  - Myoclonic astatic epilepsy (Lennox-Gastaut's)
  - Cryptogenic myoclonus epilepsy (Aicardi's)
  - Awakening myoclonus epilepsy of Janz
- Benign familial myoclonic epilepsy (Rabot's)
- Progressive myoclonus epilepsy: Baltic myoclonus (Unverricht-Lundborg's)

Symptomatic myoclonus (progressive or static encephalopathy dominates)
- Storage disease
  - Lafora body disease
  - Lipidoses, such as GM_2 gangliosidosis, Tay-Sachs, Krabbe's
  - Ceroid-lipofuscinosis (Batten's, Kuff's)
  - Sialidosis (cherry-red spot)
- Spinocerebellar degeneration
  - Ramsay Hunt syndrome (many causes)
  - Friedreich's ataxia
  - Ataxia telangiectasia
- Basal ganglia degenerations
  - Wilson's disease
  - Torsion dystonia
  - Hallervorden-Spatz's disease
  - Progressive supranuclear palsy
  - Huntington's disease
- Parkinson's disease
- Cortical-basal ganglionic degeneration
- Pallidal degenerations (usually with involvement of the dentate nucleus among other locations)
- Multiple system atrophy

Mitochondrial encephalopathies, including MERRF

Dementias
- Creutzfeldt-Jakob disease
- Alzheimer's disease

Viral encephalopathies
- Subacute sclerosing panencephalitis
- Encephalitis lethargica
- Arbovirus encephalitis
- Herpes simplex encephalitis
- Postinfectious encephalitis

Metabolic
- Hepatic failure
- Renal failure
- Dialysis syndrome

Table 25.10: *(continued)*

Hyponatremia
Hypoglycemia
Infantile myoclonic encephalopathy (polymyoclonus) (with or without neuroblastoma)
Nonketotic hyperglycemia
Multiple carboxylase deficiency
Toxic encephalopathies
Bismuth
Heavy metal poisons
Methyl bromide, DDT
Drugs, including levodopa, tricyclics
Physical encephalopathies
Posthypoxia (Lance-Adams's)
Posttraumatic
Heat stroke
Electric shock
Decompression injury
Focal CNS damage
Poststroke
Postthalamotomy
Tumor
Trauma
Olivodentate lesions (palatal myoclonus)
Spinal cord lesions (segmental or spinal myoclonus)

MERRF = myoclonic epilepsy and ragged-red fibers.
Source: Adapted from S Fahn, CD Marsden, MH van Woert. Definition and classification of myoclonus. Adv Neurol 1986;43:1.

Physiological forms of myoclonus occurring in normal subjects vary depending on the precipitant. Probably the most common form is the jerking that most of us have experienced on falling asleep. This very familiar phenomenon is rarely a source of concern. Occasionally patients do become concerned by anxiety or exercise-induced myoclonus. The history is usually clear and there is little to find (including abnormal movements) when the patient is seen.

In the *essential myoclonus* group, patients usually complain of isolated muscle jerking in the absence of other neurological deficits (with the possible exception of tremor and dystonia). The movements may begin any time from early childhood to late adult life and may remain static or progress slowly over many years. The family history may be positive, and some patients note a striking beneficial effect of alcohol. Associated dystonia, present in some patients, also may respond to ethanol.

Myoclonus occurring as one component of a wide range of seizure types is called *epileptic myoclonus.* Most of these patients give a clear history of seizures as the dominant feature. Myoclonic jerks may be infrequent and barely noticeable to the patient or may occur frequently and cause pronounced disability. Myoclonus on waking in the morning or an increasing frequency of the myoclonic jerks may forewarn of a seizure soon to come. The clinical pattern of myoclonus in this instance also varies considerably. Sensitivity to photic stimuli as well as other sensory input may be prominent. Occasional patients demonstrate isolated myoclonic jerks in the absence of additional seizure activity. In these cases, the family history may be positive for seizures, and the electroencephalogram (EEG) often demonstrates a typical centrencephalic seizure pattern that is otherwise asymptomatic (such as a 3-per-second spike and wave pattern). In others, myoclonus and seizures are equally prominent (the myoclonic epilepsies). These may or may not be associated with an apparent progressive encephalopathy (most often with cognitive dysfunction and ataxia) in the absence of a definable underlying symptomatic cause.

In the disorders classified as causing *symptomatic myoclonus,* seizures may occur, but the encephalopathy (either static or progressive) is the feature that predominates. All manner of myoclonic patterns are seen in this broad category. As can be appreciated from review of Table 25.10, a plethora of other neurological and systemic symptoms may accompany the encephalopathy. Two clinical subcategories of this larger grouping have been distinguished to assist in differential diagnosis. In *progressive myoclonic epilepsy,* myoclonus, seizures, and encephalopathy predominate, while in *progressive myoclonic ataxia* (often termed *Ramsay Hunt syndrome*), myoclonus and ataxia dominate the clinical picture with less frequent or severe seizures, mental changes, and so forth.

The Examination

Considering the varied causes, a wide range of neurological findings are possible. Alternatively, despite the complaint of abnormal movements, some patients with myoclonus (like those with tics and certain paroxysmal dyskinesias) have little to reveal on examination. This is particularly the case for the physiological forms of myoclonus, as well as those associated with epilepsy and some symptomatic causes. When myoclonus is clearly present on examination, the physician should try to characterize the movement as outlined in the introduction to this section. When the jerks are single or repetitive but arrhythmic, one must differentiate these movements from tics. Myoclonus is usually briefer and less coordinated or patterned. At times, it is difficult to distinguish the two clinically, and it is important to rely on the associated subjective symptoms (and additional history) that occur with tics. Rhythmic forms of myoclonus may be confused with tremors. Here, the pattern of movement is more one of repetitive, abrupt-onset "square wave" movements, in contrast to the smoother sinusoidal activity of tremor. Rhythmic myoclonus is usually in the 1- to 4-Hz range, in contrast to the faster frequencies seen in most types of tremor. The oscillations of so-called oscillatory myoclonus may be faster. These are distinguished by their bursting or shuddering nature, usually precipitated by sudden stimulus or movement, lasting for a few seconds and then fading away.

The distribution of the myoclonus is helpful. Focal myoclonus may be more common in disturbances of an isolated region of the cerebral cortex. Segmental involvement, particularly when rhythmic, may occur with brain stem lesions (such as branchial or palatal myoclonus) or spinal lesions (spinal myoclonus). Multifocal or generalized myoclonus suggests a more diffuse disorder, particularly involving the reticular substance of the brain stem. When multiple regions of the body are involved, it is helpful to attempt to estimate whether they are occurring in synchrony. It is sometimes difficult to do this clinically, and multichannel electromyographic (EMG) monitoring may be required (see below).

Through the course of the examination, it is important to define whether the movements occur spontaneously, with various precipitants, or both. A number of special sense and somesthetic sensory inputs should be tested. In addition, it is important to evaluate the effects of passive and active movement. In the case of action or intention myoclonus, jerking occurs during voluntary motor activity, especially when the patient attempts to perform a fine motor task such as reaching for a target. This disturbance is often confused with severe ataxia. Action myoclonus may be evident in such activities as voluntary eyelid closure, pursing of lips or speaking, holding the arms out, finger-to-nose testing, writing, bringing a cup to the mouth, holding the legs out against gravity, heel-to-shin testing, and walking. In addition to the positive myoclonus that results from a brief active muscle contraction, negative myoclonus also may occur. Although clinically these, too, appear as brief jerks, they are due to periodic inhibition of ongoing muscle activity and sudden loss of muscle tone. The most common example of negative myoclonus is *asterixis,* which may be seen in liver failure and, to a lesser extent, in other metabolic encephalopathies, and occasionally with focal brain lesions. The best recognized location of asterixis is the forearm muscles, where it causes a flapping, irregular tremorlike movement when the wrists are held extended. When mild and of low amplitude, this may be confused with 5- to 6-Hz postural tremor. A similar form of negative myoclonus accounts for the periodic loss of postural tone in axial and leg muscles in some patients with action myoclonus syndromes, such as postanoxic action myoclonus. This results in a bobbing movement of the trunk while standing and may culminate in falls.

MISCELLANEOUS MOVEMENT DISORDERS

Hemifacial spasm is a common disorder in which irregular tonic and clonic movements involve the muscles innervated by one seventh cranial nerve. Eyelid twitching usually is the first symptom, followed at variable intervals by lower facial muscle involvement. Rarely, both sides of the face are affected, in which case the spasms are asynchronous on the two sides, in contrast to other pure facial dyskinesias such as cranial dystonia.

The term *akathisia* refers to a sense of restlessness and the feeling of a need to move. This was first used to describe what was thought to be a hysterical condition, and later the term was applied to the restlessness and motor impatience seen in patients with idiopathic and postencephalitic parkinsonism. The syndrome is now most commonly seen as a side effect of major tranquilizing drugs or neuroleptics. Akathitic movements occur in response to the subjective inner feeling of restlessness and need to move, although some authors believe that the subjective component is not mandatory. The movements of akathisia are quite varied and complex—for example, repetitive rubbing, crossing and uncrossing the arms, stroking the head and face with the hands, repeatedly picking at clothing; abducting and adducting, crossing and uncrossing, swinging, or up and down pumping of the legs; and shifting weight, rocking, marching in place, or pacing while sitting and standing. Occasionally, patients demonstrate a variety of vocalizations such as moans, grunts, and shouts. Akathisia can be an acute or delayed complication of antipsychotic drug therapy (acute akathisia and tardive akathisia, respectively). It also occurs in Parkinson's disease and in certain confusional states or dementing processes.

Another disorder in which movements occur secondary to the subjective need to move is the *restless legs syndrome.* Here, unlike in akathisia, the patient typically complains of a variety of sensory disturbances in the legs, including pins and needles, creeping or crawling, aching, itching, stabbing, heaviness, tension, burning, or coldness. Occasionally, similar symptoms are appreciated in the upper limbs. These complaints are usually experienced during recumbency in the evening and are often associated with insomnia. This condition is commonly associated with another movement disorder, *periodic movements of sleep* (sometimes inappropriately termed "nocturnal myoclonus"). These periodic, slow, sustained (1- to 2-second) movements range from synchronous or asynchronous dorsiflexion of the big toes and feet to triple flexion of one or both legs. More rapid myoclonic movements or slower prolonged dystonic-like movements of the feet and legs also may be present in these patients while awake. Table 25.11 lists the movement disorders that usually persist or occur primarily during sleep.

Another uncommon but well-defined movement disorder of the lower limbs has been termed *painful legs and moving toes.* Here, the patient typically complains of a deep pulling or searing pain in the lower limb and foot associated with continuous wriggling or writhing of the toes, occasionally the ankle, and less commonly more proximal muscles of the leg. Rarely, a similar problem is seen in the upper limb as well. In some cases, there is a history of nerve injury, and the examination may demonstrate evidence of peripheral nerve dysfunction.

Some dyskinesias occur intermittently rather than in a persistent fashion. This is typical of tics and certain forms of myoclonus. Dystonia often occurs only with specific actions, but this is usually a consistent response to the action rather than periodic and unpredictable. A small group of patients with chorea, dystonia, or both have bouts of sudden-onset, short-lived involuntary movements known as

Table 25.11: Abnormal involuntary movements occurring in sleep*

Hypnic jerks
Nocturnal myoclonus
Periodic leg movements in sleep
Seizures, including epilepsia partialis continua
Segmental myoclonus
Tics
Paroxysmal hypnogenic dystonia
Dystonic postures when contractures supervene or disorders that simulate dystonia (for example, orthopedic)
Hemifacial spasm
Painful legs and moving toes (movements may or may not be present in sleep)

*Other dyskinesias (such as tremor and chorea) may persist in the earlier sleep stages and subside in deeper stages of sleep.

Table 25.12: Differential diagnosis of paroxysmal dyskinesias

Idiopathic (familial or sporadic)
Paroxysmal kinesigenic choreoathetosis
Paroxysmal nonkinesigenic (dystonic) choreoathetosis
Intermediate form (occurring after prolonged exercise)
Paroxysmal hypnogenic dystonia*
Symptomatic
Seizures (especially involving the supplementary motor area)
Multiple sclerosis
Transient ischemic attacks
Drugs
Head trauma
Cerebral palsy
Metabolic disturbances, such as hypoparathyroidism, hyperthyroidism, Hartnup's disease, pyruvate decarboxylase deficiency, D-glyceric acidemia
Degenerative disorders (rarely)
Psychogenic

*Most if not all cases of "paroxysmal hypnogenic dystonia" are probably examples of frontal seizures.
Source: Adapted from DE Riley, AE Lang. Dystonia. In C Kennard (ed), Recent Advances in Clinical Neurology. Edinburgh, Scotland: Churchill Livingstone, 1987:175.

paroxysmal choreoathetosis (Table 25.12). Certain features characterize these disorders and sometimes help to separate them into diagnostic categories (such as precipitants, duration, frequency, age of onset, family history) (see Chapter 76). The dyskinesia is most often dystonic, although chorea or a combination of both also occurs. In many cases the movements are so infrequent that they are never witnessed by the physician, and so a careful history is required to determine the nature of the disorder.

Finally, there are a number of disorders in which an abnormal or excessive response to *startle* occurs (Table 25.13). In some patients, one simply finds an exaggerated startle response, which habituates poorly after repeated stimuli. In others, there is an abnormal response to the stimuli that normally evoke startle. *Hyperekplexia* (Chapter 76), also known as *startle disease,* may be more akin to certain forms of myoclonus than to a normal startle response.

Table 25.13: Startle and related syndromes

Startle reflex
Normal
Exaggerated
Hyperekplexia
Reticular reflex myoclonus
Startle epilepsy
Startle reflex plus Moro reflex
Exaggerated startle in Tourette's syndrome
Jumping Frenchmen of Maine, Latah, Myriachit

Source: Adapted from DE Wilkins, M Hallett, MM Weiss. Audiogenic startle reflex of man and its relationship to startle syndromes. Brain 1986;109:561.

A variety of other unusual disorders, first described in the nineteenth century together with Tourette's syndrome, manifest excessive startle. The jumping Frenchmen of Maine, Latah, and Myriachit also involve sudden striking out, echo phenomena, automatic obedience, and several other less common features. It is now believed that these disorders are quite distinct from Tourette's syndrome and possibly represent culturally related operant-conditioned behavior rather than true neurological disease, although this point remains somewhat controversial.

INVESTIGATION OF MOVEMENT DISORDERS

As mentioned in the introduction to this chapter, the nature and extent of the investigation of a patient presenting with a movement disorder vary depending on the clinical circumstances. When the historical and clinical features are typical of certain conditions, further investigations may be unnecessary. Examples of these include normal physiological tremor and myoclonus, essential tremor (especially if familial), adult-onset focal dystonias, and childhood tic disorders. However, one must always be mindful of the possibility of additional occult aggravating factors (as listed in the tables) superimposed on a known preexisting movement disorder. The reverse is also possible, where the presumed cause is actually an aggravating factor or simply a coincidental association, particularly in the case of patients thought to have drug-induced disturbances. For example, chorea apparently due to the birth control pill (or chorea gravidarum) may be a manifestation of underlying SLE. When dealing with presumed neuroleptic-induced movement disorders, it is important to consider the possibility that the antipsychotic drug was given for initial psychiatric manifestations of a disease that is now causing the movement disorder in question. Huntington's disease and Wilson's disease are two examples in which this may occur.

The importance of *excluding Wilson's disease* cannot be overemphasized in view of its treatability and universally fatal outcome if left undiagnosed. Among other things, this will include slit-lamp examination, measurement of serum ceruloplasmin and copper, liver function tests, and, if nec-

Table 25.14: Investigation of movement disorders

	Movement Disorder					
Investigation	*A*	*C*	*B*	*D*	*T*	*M*
Routine hematology (including sedimentation rate)	+	+	+	+	−	+
Routine biochemistry (including Ca^{++}, uric acid, liver function tests)	+	+	+	+	±	+
Serum Cu, ceruloplasmin (with or without 24-hour urine Cu, liver biopsy, radiolabeled Cu studies)	++	++	−	++	±	+
Slit-lamp examination	++	++	−	++	±	+
Thyroid function	±	++	−	++	±	+
Antistreptolysin O test, antihyaluronidase	−	+	−	±	±	−
Antinuclear factor, LE cells, other immunological studies (also anticardiolipin antibody, VDRL)	±	++	+	+	±	+
Blood acanthocytes	+	+	−	+	+	±
Lysosomal enzymes	+	+	−	+	±	+
Urine organic and amino acids	±	+	−	+	−	+
Urine oligosaccharides and mucopolysaccharides	±	+	−	+	−	+
Serum lactate and pyruvate	±	+	−	+	−	+
Bone marrow for storage cells (including electron microscopy)	±	+	−	+	−	+
Electron microscopy of leukocytes; biopsy of liver, skin, conjunctiva	±	+	−	+	−	+
Nerve, muscle biopsy	±	+	−	+	−	+
Oligoclonal bands	±	+	+	+	−	±
CT scan*	±	±	−	±	−	−
MRI scan*	++	++	++	++	±	++
Electroencephalography	+	+	−	+	+	++
Electromyography and nerve conduction studies	+	+	−	+	+	+
Evoked potentials	+	+	−	+	−	++
Electroretinogram	±	+	−	+	−	+

Note: The extent of investigation will depend on factors such as age of onset, nature of progression, and presence of historical or clinical atypical features suggesting a secondary cause of the movement disorder in question.
A = akinetic-rigid syndrome; C = chorea; B = hemiballism; D = dystonia; T = tics; M = myoclonus; LE = lupus erythematosis.
++ = very important or frequently useful; + = sometimes helpful; ± = questionably helpful; − = rarely if ever helpful.
*CT scan ratings apply where MRI is also available (e.g., evaluates calcification of the basal ganglia not seen on MRI). If MRI is unavailable, the value of the usefulness of CT scan recorded in the columns increases toward but does not reach those listed for MRI scan.

essary, measurement of 24-hour urinary copper excretion and liver biopsy. Children and adolescents presenting with parkinsonism, chorea, or a dystonic or myoclonic syndrome require additional careful hematological and biochemical assessment, as indicated in Table 25.14.

These investigations are less rewarding in adults; however, certain more common associations must be considered. Very few *biochemical tests* are helpful in patients with parkinsonism. Rarely, neuroacanthocytosis (blood acanthocytes, elevated serum creatine kinase, altered nerve conduction studies) presents in this fashion, as well as causing chorea, dystonia, and tics. Occasionally, acanthocytosis is not present in the patient but is found in other members (often asymptomatic) of the family. Biochemical screening may reveal evidence for hypoparathyroidism, which can cause calcification of the basal ganglia, resulting in several different movement disorders. Hyperthyroidism, polycythemia rubra vera, and SLE are common enough causes of undiagnosed chorea in an adult to require exclusion in all cases. In the last situation, chorea may be the first manifestation of the disorder. Early clues are a history of recurrent fetal loss, an elevated partial thromboplastin time, a falsely positive VDRL, and thrombocytopenia indicating the presence of antiphospholipid immunoglobulins such as the lupus anticoagulant and anticardiolipin antibodies. Although Sydenham's chorea is now uncommon, antistreptolysin O titer, antihyaluronidase, and electrocardiogram should still be performed in a child presenting with chorea of unknown origin. In a patient with hemiballism, one should search for potential risk factors for vascular disease by measuring levels of blood sugar, hemoglobin, platelets, erythrocyte sedimentation rate, cholesterol, and triglycerides. Adults with generalized dystonia or dystonia beginning in the legs must be suspected of having a symptomatic cause and investigated accordingly. Myoclonus may be caused by a wide variety of systemic or primary neurological disorders, and the extent of the investigation clearly depends on clinical suspicions. If such a patient is approached with the four major etiological categories in mind (see Table 25.10), the direction and extent of further investigation is greatly simplified.

Imaging studies such as computed tomography (CT) and magnetic resonance imaging (MRI) are particularly useful in certain disorders. In the large majority of patients with hemidystonia, there is a definable lesion in the contralateral basal ganglia (most often the putamen). Hemiballism or hemichorea is usually caused by a structural lesion in the contralateral subthalamic nucleus or striatum. The cause is commonly a small lacunar infarction, and so MRI may be more successful than CT in localizing the lesion. In patients with parkinsonism, imaging must assess the possibility of hydrocephalus (either obstructive or communicating), midbrain atrophy (as in PSP), and cerebellar and brain stem atrophy (as in OPCA). MRI is clearly much more effective in demonstrating these posterior fossa abnormalities than is CT scanning. Atrophy of the head of the caudate nucleus is found in Huntington's disease, but it is not specific for this disorder and does not correlate with the presence or severity of chorea. Multiple infarctions, intracerebral calcification (better seen on CT), mass lesions (such as tumors and arteriovenous malformations), and basal ganglia lucencies (as seen in a variety of disorders) may be found in patients with several different movement disorders such as parkinsonism, chorea, and dystonia. Further developments in MRI promise to improve our ability to differentiate among various degenerative disorders, especially if they are associated with characteristic pathological features such as deposition of pigments or heavy metals. An excellent example of this is the pronounced low-intensity signal, possibly representing iron deposition, seen in the posterior putamen on heavily T2-weighted images in many patients with striatonigral degeneration. Positron emission tomography using fluorodeoxyglucose, fluorodopa, and other radiolabeled compounds has shown reproducible changes in such disorders as Huntington's disease and parkinsonian disorders. The patterns of abnormalities seen may be predictive of the underlying pathological changes and thus may be useful in differential diagnosis.

Routine *electrophysiological testing,* including EEG, somatosensory evoked potentials, EMG, and nerve conduction studies, may provide supportive evidence of disease involving structures outside the basal ganglia. EMG analysis of the activity in various muscle groups has been used extensively in the study of most movement disorders, and tremor can be further documented by accelerometric recordings. Although these and other electrophysiological procedures have contributed to the understanding of the pathophysiology of movement disorders, they have been most crucial to the study of myoclonus. Here, a variety of different disturbances may be found on routine EEG, such as spikes, spike and wave, and periodic discharges. Occasionally, spikes are seen to precede EMG myoclonic discharges, particularly if the myoclonus is associated with epilepsy. In the majority of cases, however, it is impossible to determine a correlation between spike discharges and myoclonic jerks by simple visual inspection. Special electrophysiological techniques averaging cortical activity that occurs preceding a myoclonic jerk (so-called triggered back-averaging) may show focal contralateral central negativity lasting 15–40 msec preceding the muscle jerk by 10–25 msec in the upper limbs or 30–35 msec in the legs. This is evidence for so-called cortical myoclonus, indicating that the cortical activity results in the muscle jerks.

In other forms of myoclonus that originate in subcortical areas, cortical discharges may be seen but are not time-locked in the same fashion to the jerks. In these cases, there may be generalized 25- to 40-msec negativity preceding, simultaneous with, or following the muscle jerking. The muscle bursts as seen on EMG are typically synchronous in antagonistic muscles and are usually less than 50 msec in duration. In one form of essential myoclonus, so-called ballistic reflex myoclonus, the EMG bursts show alternating activity in antagonists, which lasts 50–150 msec. With multichannel EMG recording, it may be possible to demonstrate the activation order of muscles. In cortical myoclonus, muscles are activated in a rostrocaudal direction, with cranial nerve muscles firing in descending order before the limbs. In myoclonus originating from subcortical or reticular sources, it may be possible to show that the myoclonus propagates in both directions from a point source, up the brain stem, usually starting in muscles innervated by the eleventh cranial nerve, and down the spinal cord.

Somatosensory evoked potentials and late EMG responses (C reflexes) are often enhanced in patients with myoclonus. Giant sensory evoked potentials can be seen in the hemisphere contralateral to the jerking limb in patients with cortical myoclonus. This is particularly the case in patients with focal myoclonus sensitive to a variety of sensory stimuli applied to the affected part (cortical reflex myoclonus). The cortical components of the sensory evoked potentials are usually not enhanced in subcortical or spinal myoclonus, but the latencies may be prolonged, depending on the location of the disease process.

Progress in the field of molecular biology promises to have an increasing impact on the diagnosis, understanding, and management of genetically determined neurological diseases. In the area of movement disorders this has been exemplified by the characterization of the genetic abnormality in Huntington's disease. Now it is not only possible to confirm the diagnosis in a clinically affected patient and provide accurate predictive testing in at-risk individuals, but it is also possible to provide a rough idea of the expected age of onset in an affected fetus at the time of prenatal screening. This field is advancing extremely rapidly. Similar testing is also becoming available for other genetically determined diseases manifesting as movement disorders, such as a number of the autosomal dominant cerebellar ataxias (ADCAs). The obvious hope and expectation is that these developments will be translated into effective therapy.

Finally, it is worth reiterating that in caring for a patient with a movement disorder the clinician must always keep an open mind to the possibility of finding a secondary cause. This should be the case even where the onset, progression, and clinical features of the movement disorder in question are typical of an idiopathic condition, and the preliminary laboratory testing has failed to reveal another cause. Thorough neurological examination should be repeated periodically in a search for clues that might indicate the need to pursue the investigation further.

REFERENCES

Fahn S, Marsden CD, Van Woert MH. Definition and classification of myoclonus. Adv Neurol 1986;43:15.

Riley DE, Lang AE. Dystonia. In C Kennard (ed), Recent Advances in Clinical Neurology. Edinburgh: Churchill Livingstone, 1987;175–200.

Shoulson I. On chorea. Clin Neuropharmacol 1986;9:S85–S99.

Weiner WJ, Lang AE. Movement disorders: a comprehensive survey. Mount Kisco, NY: Futura, 1989.

Wilkins DE, Hallett M, Weiss MM. Audiogenic startle reflex of man and its relationship to startle syndromes. Brain 1986; 109:56–73.

Chapter 26
Walking Disorders

Philip D. Thompson and C. David Marsden

GAIT

The maintenance of an upright posture and the act of walking are among the first and ultimately the most complex motor skills humans acquire. From an early age, these skills are modified and refined. In later years the interplay between voluntary and automatic control of posture and walking provides such a rich and complex repertoire of movement that individuals can be recognized by their distinctive pattern of walking. In the same way that walking may be viewed as an individual's "motor fingerprint," many diseases of the motor system produce characteristic disturbances of gait and posture that permit identification of an underlying disease by the way gait is altered.

Physiological and Biomechanical Aspects of Gait

Humans assume a stable upright posture before beginning to walk. Mechanical stability when standing is based on musculoskeletal linkages. Dynamic equilibrium in the upright posture is maintained by a hierarchy of postural reflexes. These postural responses are generated by the integration of visual, vestibular, and proprioceptive inputs in the context of voluntary intent and ongoing changes in the environment in which the subject is moving. Postural responses consist of coordinated synergistic axial and lower limb muscle contraction, correcting for and controlling body sway and maintaining a vertical posture of the trunk. These reflexes range from automatic *righting reflexes* keeping the head upright on the trunk, *supporting reactions* controlling antigravity muscle tone, *anticipatory postural reflexes* before limb movement (feed forward) or in response to perturbation during movement (feedback), and *reactive postural responses* counteracting body perturbations, to those modified by voluntary control in accordance with the circumstances, *rescue reactions* (a step or windmill arm movements), and *protective reactions* to prevent injury or break a fall.

Once the trunk is upright and stable, locomotion may begin. The initiation of gait is heralded by a complex shift in the center of pressure beneath each foot, first posteriorly, then laterally toward the stepping foot, and finally away toward the stance foot to allow the stepping foot to swing forward (Elble et al. 1994). This sequence is then followed by the stereotyped stance, swing, and step phases of the gait cycle.

Anatomical Aspects of Gait

The neuroanatomical structures responsible for these components of normal walking are poorly understood in humans. Studies in lower species suggest two basic anatomical components. Supraspinal centers signal when to start walking, when to stop, the speed of locomotion, and the size and direction of stepping. These signals descend to the spinal level where spinal locomotor centers elaborate walking patterns of muscle activity.

In quadripedal animals, *spinal locomotor centers* are capable of maintaining and coordinating rhythmic stepping movements after spinal transection. This *spinal stepping* is generated by assemblies of interneurons, referred to as *central pattern generators*, which activate limb muscles in a locomotor synergy. They exist for the hindlimb, forelimb, and trunk and are interlinked by propriospinal networks to facilitate interlimb coordination (Armstrong 1988). In monkeys, spinal stepping requires preservation of the ventrolateral tracts of the spinal cord containing descending reticulospinal and vestibulospinal pathways. The isolated spinal cord in humans can produce spontaneous movements but cannot generate rhythmic stepping or maintain truncal balance. Higher brain stem and cortical connections are therefore necessary for bipedal walking. Brain stem structures are important in maintaining *postural righting reflexes* that control axial extensor tone. Lesions of the medial brain stem interrupt descending reticulo-, vestibulo-, and tectospinal systems that innervate proximal and axial muscles, resulting in dysequilibrium. Brain stem locomotor centers are present in lower species and also probably exist in humans. High-frequency trains of stimuli in the region of the *mesencephalic locomotor region* in the posterior midbrain elicit locomotor activity in the thalamic monkey (Eidelberg et al. 1981). This region overlaps with the pedunculopontine nucleus, which is thought to be important in rhythm generation.

Walking is also influenced by other areas of the central nervous system. *Basal ganglia* lesions interfere with postural control, the initiation of walking, and the quality of stepping. The connections of the basal ganglia mediating these effects may involve the brain stem structures described above. The *cerebellum* is important in modulating the rate, rhythm, amplitude, and force of voluntary movement and accordingly regulates these aspects of stepping. Midline cerebellar structures also are important in postural reflex control and maintaining balance. The *cerebral cortex* is required for precision movements of the legs when walking. Corticospinal activation modifies spinal locomotor activity (consistent with the voluntary control of when to start and stop walking) and sensory feedback during the walking cycle in turn modifies motor cortical activity. In primates, the frontal cortex also appears to be important in postural control (unlike quadripeds).

HISTORY AND COMMON SYMPTOMS

A detailed account of the walking difficulty and its evolution provides important clues to the underlying diagnosis. Patients with walking difficulties describe only a limited number of complaints. Each may be produced by disorders at many levels of the peripheral and central nervous systems. For example, tripping and stumbling with falls may be due to upper motor neuron, extrapyramidal, or cerebellar syndromes, or to a proprioceptive sensory loss, peripheral neuropathy, or lower motor neuron problem. Accordingly, when evaluating the history it is helpful to note the particular circumstances in which the walking difficulty occurs, the leg movements most affected, and any associated symptoms. This approach will provide the first clues to whether the problem is primarily motor, due to muscle weakness or a more global defect of motor control, or imbalance.

Uneven ground will exacerbate most walking difficulties and will therefore often provide an additional complaint. A ligamentous ankle strain or even a bony fracture may result from tripping and falling in this situation and may be the presenting symptom of a gait disorder. Indeed, a fear of falling may lead to a variety of voluntary protective measures to minimize the risk of injury. In some patients this element may come to dominate the clinical picture and may be a presenting feature.

Weakness

Weakness of the legs may be described in various ways. Complaints of stiffness, heaviness, or "legs that do not do what they are told" may be the presenting symptoms of a spastic paraparesis or hemiparesis. Patients with spastic paraparesis may report that they drag their legs along to walk or their legs may suddenly give way, causing them to stumble and fall. Weakness of certain muscle groups also may be described in terms of difficulties in performing particular movements. A tendency to trip due to catching or scraping the toe on the ground may be the presenting symptom of hemiplegia (due to the spastic equinovarus foot posture) or a foot drop due to weakness of ankle dorsiflexion. In the former, the whole leg is described as abnormal, whereas only the distal leg is affected in the latter. Associated symptoms such as back pain or radicular sensory change in the leg provide further clues to a peripheral origin. If the symptoms are bilateral and have a distal emphasis, a peripheral neuropathy should be considered. Similarly, weakness of certain movements may first become apparent in particular situations; for example, difficulty in climbing stairs or rising from a seated position suggests proximal muscle weakness and is most commonly due to a myopathy. Rarely, these complaints may be the presenting symptoms of an acute inflammatory polyneuropathy (Guillain-Barré syndrome). Weakness of knee extension (due to a femoral neuropathy) may impose difficulty walking down stairs.

Slowness

Slowness of walking and limb stiffness are common symptoms in extrapyramidal disease. These symptoms are produced by difficulty in engaging the limbs in brisk motion and increased muscle tone (rigidity). This slowness of movement may be accompanied by shuffling with small steps. Such patients often report difficulty initiating the first few steps as they start walking, with pronounced shuffling for a few steps and freezing at the slightest obstacle or distraction. Conversely, some patients overcome the shuffling and facilitate walking by carefully watching and treading over lines or objects. These symptoms are most commonly observed in Parkinson's disease.

Difficulty rising from a chair may be an associated symptom. It can be due to a loss of truncal mobility and axial rigidity, in addition to muscle weakness. Similarly, muscle fatigue while walking may be described but does not usually imply a defect of neuromuscular transmission.

Other extrapyramidal diseases, such as multiple-system atrophy and progressive supranuclear palsy (Steele-Richardson-Olszewski syndrome), diffuse cerebrovascular disease, and hydrocephalus also may present with similar slowness of walking and shuffling steps. Patients with these conditions frequently complain of falls (either backward or forward) when walking. The history of falls in the early stages of an akinetic-rigid syndrome strongly suggests the possibility of one of the aforementioned conditions, rather than Parkinson's disease.

The circumstances in which leg stiffness occurs when walking may be revealing. For example, the presenting symptom of idiopathic torsion dystonia in childhood may be stiffness of one leg, a tendency to walk on the toes, and inversion and plantar flexion of the foot due to an action dystonia of the leg or foot, evident only when walking or running. Patients with dopa-responsive dystonia and prominent diurnal fluctuation develop their symptoms only in the afternoon.

Loss of Balance

Symptoms of poor balance, unsteadiness, and a tendency to fall are cardinal features of the ataxic syndromes caused by midline (vermis) cerebellar disease, or proprioceptive sensory loss. The patient with a cerebellar gait ataxia complains of an inability to walk in a straight line or difficulty turning suddenly without veering to one side or staggering. Observers may remark that the patient staggers as if intoxicated. A sensory ataxia may first give rise to symptoms of unsteadiness on walking in the dark, when visual compensation for proprioceptive loss is not possible. Patients with impaired proprioceptive sensation and sensory ataxia complain of being uncertain of the exact position of their feet when walking and of an inability to appreciate the texture of the ground. Abnormal sensations in the feet may create the impression of walking on a spongy surface or cotton wool. Falls commonly accompany the symptoms of unsteadiness in all ataxic syndromes.

Sensory Symptoms and Pain

The distribution of any accompanying sensory complaints provides further information as to the site of the lesion producing walking difficulties. A common example is found in patients with cervical spondylosis and myelopathy who present with cervical radicular pain, paresthesias, or both and a spastic paraparesis. Paresthesias and tight bands around the trunk, or a combination of trunk and limb sensory symptoms and a spastic paraparesis, suggest a myelopathy. Distal, symmetrical paresthesias affecting the limbs point toward a peripheral neuropathy.

It is important to determine whether complaints of leg pain and weakness in patients with difficulty walking share a common cause or whether the pain is of musculoskeletal origin and is exacerbated by walking. An example of the former is exercise-induced pain and weakness of the legs due to neurogenic intermittent claudication of the cauda equina. These symptoms are frequently accompanied by transient paresthesias or radicular sensory loss, relieved by sitting and leaning forward. This should be distinguished from vascular intermittent claudication of calf muscles where ischemic muscle pain interrupts walking. Skeletal pain due to degenerative joint disease, which is common in elderly patients, is often present at rest and aggravated by leg movement. The normal pattern of walking is often modified in these situations. The patient may voluntarily use various strategies to minimize pain by avoiding bearing the full weight on the affected limb and by limiting its range of movement (*antalgic gait*).

Incontinence

Spinal cord lesions interfere with the voluntary control of sphincter function and sexual potency in the male. Loss of sphincter control should also remind the physician to consider parasagittal cerebral lesions as a possible cause of a spastic paraparesis. Such lesions include frontal lobe tumors, such as parasagittal meningioma, frontal lobe infarction due to anterior cerebral artery disease, and hydrocephalus. Higher mental function may also be impaired.

EXAMINATION OF POSTURE AND WALKING

The examination of posture and walking is summarized in Table 26.1. A convenient starting point is to observe the overall pattern of whole body movement as the patient walks. Normal walking progresses in a smooth and effortless manner, with an upright posture of the trunk, free swinging motion of the legs, regular and appropriately sized strides, and flowing associated synergistic head, trunk, and upper limb movement. Careful observation of the overall pattern of body movement during walking often enables the experienced clinical observer to decide whether the gait problem is due to a focal leg abnormality, muscle weakness, or a more generalized disorder of movement, and whether it is unilateral or bilateral.

Table 26.1: Checklist for the clinical examination of posture and gait

- Posture
  - Trunk posture (upright or stooped)
  - Stance (narrow- or wide-based)
  - Postural reflexes
- Walking
  - Initiation (start hesitation, shuffling, magnetic feet)
  - Stepping
    - Rhythm (regular, irregular)
    - Length (normal, short)
    - Trajectory (shallow, high-stepping)
  - Speed
  - Festination
  - Freezing
  - Associated trunk movement and arm swing
- Special maneuvers
  - Heel-toe walking
  - Romberg's test
  - Walking backward or running
- Formal motor and sensory examination (supine)
  - Leg size and length
  - Range of joint movement
  - Muscle bulk
  - Muscle tone
  - Muscle strength
  - Voluntary movement
    - Arm and hand dexterity
    - Trunk (rolling over)
    - Leg movement when not standing
  - Tendon reflexes
  - Sensation: proprioception
  - Heel-shin test

Posture

Trunk Posture

The trunk is normally upright during standing and walking. Flexion of the trunk is a prominent feature of extrapyramidal diseases but may also be seen in cautious gait syndromes where the center of gravity is lowered to minimize body sway and the risk of falling. Characteristic changes in axial posture include neck extension in progressive supranuclear palsy and an exaggerated lumbar lordosis due to hip girdle weakness in proximal myopathies. Paraspinal muscle spasm and rigidity also produce an exaggerated lumbar lordosis. This is a striking feature of the "stiff man syndrome." A variety of axial muscle spasms are seen in torsion dystonia, the most common being exaggerated flexion of the trunk and hip when walking. Abnormal thoracolumbar postures also may result from spinal ankylosis and spondylitis. The finding of a restricted range of spinal movement and persistence of the abnormal posture when supine or during sleep is a useful pointer toward a bony spinal deformity as the cause of an abnormal trunk posture. Truncal, particularly lumbar, posture also may be altered to compensate for a shortening of one lower limb, disease of the hip, knee, or ankle, or leg pain.

Stance

Stance base and the distance between the feet during quiet standing and walking give some indication of balance. Classically, wide-based gaits are seen in patients with cerebellar or sensory ataxia but also may be seen in patients with diffuse cerebral vascular disease and frontal lobe lesions (Table 26.2). It is important to remember that people whose balance is insecure for any reason tend to adopt a wider stance and a posture of mild generalized flexion and take shorter steps. Widening the stance base is an efficient method of reducing body sway in the lateral and anteroposterior planes (Day et al. 1993). Those who have attempted to walk on ice or other slippery surfaces will recognize this phenomenon.

Postural Reflexes

Postural reflexes are examined while standing by gently pushing the patient backward or forward. The examiner should stand in front of or behind the patient and be prepared to catch or support the patient to prevent him or her from falling. An impairment of postural righting reactions will be evident after each displacement by a few short shuffling steps backward (*retropulsion*) or forward (*propulsion*). Severe loss of postural reflexes may render the patient susceptible to falls after only minor perturbations, without any reflex stepping or compensatory arm movements to adjust posture and restore balance or the rescue reaction of an outstretched arm to break a fall. The presence of injuries to the knees, shins, face, or back of the head sustained during falls provides a clue to the loss of these postural reactions.

Walking

Initiation of Gait

Difficulty initiating the first step (*start hesitation*) and episodes of *freezing* are features of Parkinson's disease and frontal lobe disease and occasionally are seen in relative isolation in the syndrome of *gait ignition failure* (Atchison et al. 1993). Start hesitation ranges in severity from a few shuffling steps to small shallow steps on the spot without forward progress ("slipping clutch"), to complete immobility with the feet seemingly glued to the floor ("magnetic feet"). Patients may move their upper bodies in an effort to engage their legs in motion. Once underway, freezing may interrupt walking with further shuffling and start hesitation.

Stepping

Once walking is underway, the *rhythm* of stepping and the *length* and *trajectory* of each step should be noted. The short, regular, and shallow steps of shuffling are characteristic of the akinetic-rigid syndromes. Shuffling may be most evident when starting to walk, stopping, or turning corners.

Table 26.2: Summary of the major clinical features distinguishing different types of gait ataxia

Feature	*Cerebellar Ataxia*	*Sensory Ataxia*	*Frontal Lobe Ataxia*
Trunk posture	Stooped: leans forward	Stooped: upright	Upright
Stance	Wide-based	Wide-based	Wide-based
Postural reflexes	±	Intact	Impaired or absent
Initiation of gait	Normal	Normal	Start hesitation
Steps	Staggering, lurching	High-stepping	Short, shuffling
Speed	Normal, slow	Normal, slow	Very slow
Heel-toe	Unable	±	Unable
Turning corners	Veers away	Minimal effect	Freezing, shuffling
Romberg's test	±	Increased unsteadiness	±
Heel-shin test	Usually abnormal	±	Normal
Falls	Uncommon	Yes	Very common

± = variable.

Repeatedly observing these maneuvers may highlight a subtle tendency to shuffle. Jerky steps of irregular rhythm and variable length and trajectory suggest an ataxic syndrome. Abnormal leg and foot trajectories occur in sensory ataxia, foot drop, spasticity, and dystonia. Each is associated with a distinctive leg posture during stepping.

The *speed* of walking is revealing. Slowness is characteristic of the akinetic-rigid syndromes but is also seen in ataxic and spastic syndromes. *Festination* (increasingly rapid, small steps) is common in Parkinson's disease but rare in other akinetic-rigid syndromes, which frequently are associated with poor balance and falls rather than festination. A reduction in *associated trunk movement* and *arm swing* is most evident in unilateral upper motor neuron, extrapyramidal, and acute ataxic syndromes. Bilateral loss of synergistic arm movement when walking is a valuable sign of Parkinson's disease in the early stages when most symptoms are unilateral.

Special Maneuvers

Subtle degrees of cerebellar ataxia may be unmasked by asking the patient to walk in a straight line heel-to-toe (tandem gait), to stand on one leg, or to walk and turn quickly. If vision is important in helping maintain balance, as in sensory ataxia due to proprioceptive loss, the removal of vision will greatly exaggerate the ataxia. This is the basis of Romberg's test in which eye closure leads to a dramatic increase in unsteadiness and even falls in the patient with sensory ataxia. In contrast, this effect is not apparent in cerebellar ataxia provided the patient is standing comfortably and securely before the test is performed. When performing Romberg's test, it is important that the patient be standing comfortably before eye closure. Remember that normal subjects and patients with cerebellar ataxia will also show a modest increase in body sway with eye closure.

It may be necessary to examine the patient running to identify an action dystonia of the legs in the early stages of idiopathic torsion dystonia. Similarly, difficulty walking forward may not be evident when walking backward.

Formal Motor and Sensory Examination

Having observed the patient walking, examine motor and sensory function in the limbs with the patient supine in the conventional examination position. The size and length of the limbs should be measured in any child presenting with a limp. An asymmetry in leg size suggests a congenital malformation of the spinal cord or brain or (rarely) local overgrowth of tissue. The spinal column should be inspected for scoliosis and the lumbar region for skin defects or hairy patches indicative of spinal dysraphism.

Changes in muscle tone such as spasticity, rigidity, or *gegenhalten* (an increase in muscle tone or inability to relax during passive manipulation of the limb) point toward diseases of the upper motor neuron, basal ganglia, and frontal lobes, respectively. In the patient who complains of symptoms in only one leg, a detailed examination of the other leg is important. If signs of an upper motor neuron syndrome are present in both legs, then a disorder of the spinal cord is likely.

Muscle bulk and strength are examined and evidence of muscle wasting and the presence and distribution of muscle weakness documented. Examination will reveal whether the abnormal posture of the leg in a patient with a foot drop (Table 26.3) is due to spasticity or weakness of ankle dorsiflexors, which in turn may be due to motor neuron disease, a peripheral neuropathy, a peroneal compression neuropathy, or an L5 root lesion. Subtle degrees of ankle dorsiflexion weakness may be detected by observing the patient walking on his or her heels. The sense of joint position should be carefully examined for defects of proprioception in the ataxic patient.

Several conditions are notable for producing minimal, abnormal signs on physical examination of the recumbent patient, in striking contrast with the observed difficulty walking. Patients with a cerebellar gait ataxia due to a pure vermis lesion may perform the heel-shin test normally when supine but be quite unable to walk heel-to-toe. The finding of normal muscle strength, muscle tone, and tendon reflexes is common in dystonic syndromes where an action

Table 26.3: Causes of foot drop or equinovarus foot posture when walking

Peripheral nerve
L5 radiculopathy
Lumbar plexopathy
Sciatic nerve palsy
Peroneal neuropathy (compression)
Peripheral neuropathy (bilateral)
Motor neuropathy (motor neuron disease)
Myopathy
Scapuloperoneal syndromes
Spasticity
Dystonia
Sensory ataxia

dystonia causes abnormal posturing of the feet only when walking. Similarly, paratonia or *gegenhalten* (with or without brisk tendon reflexes) may be the only abnormal signs in the legs of the recumbent patient with a frontal lobe lesion, hydrocephalus, or diffuse cerebrovascular disease who is totally unable to walk. Moreover, such patients may be able to perform the heel-shin test and make bicycling movements of their legs when lying on a bed. A similar discrepancy can be seen in patients with spastic paraplegia due to hereditary spastic paraplegia, cerebral palsy (Little's disease), or cervical spondylotic myelopathy, who may exhibit only minor changes in muscle tone, strength, and tendon reflexes when examined supine but have profound leg spasticity when walking.

Elderly patients with walking difficulties and falls often have signs of multiple deficits. The most common are cervical spondylotic myelopathy with a mild spastic paraparesis and a degree of proprioceptive loss and a peripheral neuropathy with loss of ankle reflexes and proprioceptive loss. Visual and hearing loss also may be evident, giving rise to multiple sensory deficits. In this group of patients musculoskeletal factors also may interfere with mobility, as may hypotension, particularly postural hypotension. Finally, due account must be taken of the fear of falling that frequently accompanies gait difficulties. It may lead to a marked loss of confidence and a cautious or protected gait. Such patients may be unable to walk without support yet improve dramatically when support is provided and fall when it is removed.

PHYSICAL SIGNS AND INVESTIGATION

Spastic Gait

Spasticity of the arm and leg on one side produces the characteristic clinical picture of a *spastic hemiparesis*. The arm is held abducted and is internally rotated at the shoulder and flexed at the elbow, with pronation of the forearm and flexion of the wrist and fingers. The leg is slightly flexed at the hip and extended at the knee, with plantar flexion and inversion of the foot. The swing phase of each step is accomplished by slight lateral flexion of the trunk toward the unaffected side, hyperextension of the hip on that side to allow the slow circumduction of the stiffly extended paretic leg, as it is swung forward from the hip, dragging the toe or catching it on the ground beneath. There is a minimum of associated arm swing on the affected side. The stance may be slightly wide-based, and the speed of walking is slow. Balance may be poor because the hemiparesis interferes with corrective postural adjustments on the affected side. Muscle tone in the affected limbs is increased, there may be clonus, and the tendon reflexes are abnormally brisk with an extensor plantar response. Examination of the sole of the shoe may reveal wear of the toe and outer borders of the shoe, suggesting that the spastic gait is of long standing.

After identifying a spastic hemiparesis, the next step is to determine the level of the lesion responsible. Attention should be paid to the face, for an upper motor neuron facial weakness on the same side indicates that the level lies above the pons. The most common cause of this is cerebral infarction, which will be suggested by a history of acute onset. Alternatively, a slower evolution may indicate a space-occupying lesion and is most conveniently investigated by computed tomography (CT) or magnetic resonance imaging (MRI) of the brain. A lower facial weakness on the side opposite the hemiparesis (crossed hemiparesis) suggests a pontomedullary lesion. When the face is not involved, clues to the site of the lesion must be sought by examining the motor function of the lower cranial nerves. Weakness of shoulder shrugging on the same side points to a lesion above the foramen magnum. A cervical spinal cord lesion will involve the arm and leg only, whereas a lesion of the thoracic cord will affect only the leg. Where lesions of the spinal cord are suspected, myelography or MRI of the cord is indicated.

Spasticity of both legs gives rise to a *spastic paraparesis*. The legs are stiffly extended at the knees, plantar flexed at the ankles, and slightly flexed at the hips; the gait is slow, and patients appear to walk by dragging themselves forward one step after the other. Both legs circumduct, and there is often a tendency to pronounced adduction of the legs, particularly when the disorder begins in childhood. This appearance gave rise to the term *scissor gait*. These postures are determined by the distribution of increased muscle tone. The causes of a spastic paraparesis include *hereditary* spastic paraplegia, where the arms and sphincters are unaffected and there may be little or no leg weakness; *compressive* spinal lesions (including neoplastic infiltration or deposits, epidural abscess, or cervical spondylosis); *vascular* myelopathies (such as anterior spinal artery thrombosis); or *demyelinating* disorders of the spinal cord (such as multiple sclerosis). An indication of the extent and level of the spinal cord lesion will be obtained by noting the presence or absence of weakness or sensory loss in the arm, a spinothalamic sensory level or posterior column sensory loss, and alterations in sphincter function. The majority of patients with paraparesis of recent onset should be investigated with MRI of the spinal cord to exclude potentially treatable causes such as spinal cord compression.

Occasionally, bilateral leg dystonia (dystonic paraparesis) may mimic a spastic paraparesis. It typically occurs in dopa-responsive dystonia in childhood, which may be misdiagnosed as hereditary spastic paraplegia or cerebral diplegia (Little's disease). Separation of these conditions can be difficult. Brisk tendon reflexes may occur in both, and spontaneous extension of a great toe in patients with striatal disorders may be interpreted as a Babinski's response. Fanning of the toes and knee flexion suggest the latter. Other distinguishing features include changes in muscle tone, spasticity in hereditary spastic paraparesis, and rigidity in dystonic paraparesis. In young children the distinction is an important one, as a proportion of such patients will be successfully treated with levodopa (see Chapter 76).

Cerebellar Ataxia

The gait disorder that accompanies disease of the cerebellar vermis and anterior lobe consists of a decomposition of normal leg movement and a loss of normal truncal balance and equilibrium. The patient adopts a wide-based stance and may flex the hips slightly to crouch forward and minimize body sway. He or she steps with care, tending to stagger in an irregular and lurching fashion from side to side or backward and forward. There may be rhythmic swaying of the trunk, head, or both (*titubation*) in addition to truncal instability. Movements of the legs are irregular and variable in timing (*dyssynergia*) and the steps are erratic (*dysmetria*). These defects are made worse when the patient attempts to walk heel-to-toe in a straight line or to turn a corner rapidly around a chair. With lesions confined to one cerebellar hemisphere, these abnormalities will be limited to the affected (ipsilateral) limb and will affect coordination of limb movement more than balance, if the vermis is not involved. Conversely, pure truncal ataxia may be the sole feature of a midline (anterior lobe vermis) cerebellar syndrome and may escape notice if the patient is not examined when walking. Leg coordination as judged by the heel-shin test may be relatively normal when the patient with a vermis lesion is examined while supine.

Cerebellar ataxia may be dramatically improved by minor support, such as holding the patient's hand during walking. In contrast, the ataxia is greatly exacerbated by the rapid postural adjustments needed when turning corners, avoiding obstacles, and stopping or starting to walk. Vision influences the disturbances of gait and equilibrium in cerebellar lesions by helping compensate and plot a secure path ahead; eye closure may increase the patient's anxiety about falling.

One of the most common causes of cerebellar gait ataxia is malnutrition in alcoholism, where relatively selective damage appears to affect the cerebellar vermis and anterior lobes (see Chapter 64). It affects almost exclusively the legs and gait, while sparing the ocular movements, speech, and upper limbs. A similar gait disorder may also be a feature of midline cerebellar masses and of paraneoplastic cerebellar degeneration.

Spastic Ataxia

A combination of spasticity and ataxia produces a characteristic springing or bouncing gait. Such gaits may be seen in multiple sclerosis, the Arnold-Chiari malformation, and hydrocephalus in young people. The gait is wide-based, and clonus is readily elicited by stretching the leg muscles when examining muscle tone or tapping the tendon reflexes. Even voluntary leg movements may precipitate clonus, which will throw the ataxic patient off balance. Compensatory reflex and voluntary movements, made in an effort to regain balance, set up a vicious cycle of ataxic movements, clonus, and increasing unsteadiness, so that such patients may be totally unable to stand and walk. Bouncing gaits must be distinguished from action myoclonus of the legs and from leg and trunk tremors seen in cerebellar disease (see below).

Sensory Ataxia

The loss of proprioceptive input from the legs deprives the patient of knowledge of the position in space, the progress of any ongoing movement, the state of muscle contraction, and finer details of the texture of the surface of the ground. Patients without such information tend to adopt a wide base and to take slow steps, advancing cautiously with the aid of visual guidance. The feet are thrust out in front of the patient with each step, and the sole of the foot strikes the floor forcibly, giving rise to a slapping noise (*slapping gait*). Patients with sensory ataxia find it very difficult to walk on uneven surfaces or at night. Lesions at any point in the sensory pathways that interrupt large-diameter proprioceptive afferent fibers may produce this clinical picture. Peripheral neuropathies, posterior root and ganglion lesions such as tabes dorsalis, posterior column lesions such as multiple sclerosis, or a combination of these such as produced by vitamin B_{12} deficiency are examples of such lesions.

Akinetic-Rigid Gait

The classic and most common akinetic-rigid gait disturbance is that seen in Parkinson's disease. The patient is usually elderly and adopts a stooped posture with flexion of the shoulders, neck, and trunk. Tremor of the upper limbs may be evident when walking, but parkinsonian tremor affects the legs less commonly. The gait is typically slow and shuffling, with small, shallow paces on a narrow base. This disability may be dramatically reversed by levodopa treatment. There is little associated body movement; arm swing is reduced or absent. The arms are held immobile at the

Table 26.4: Differential diagnosis in the patient presenting with an akinetic-rigid syndrome and a gait disturbance

Parkinson's disease
Drug-induced parkinsonism
Multiple-system atrophy
Striatonigral degeneration
Shy-Drager's syndrome (idiopathic orthostatic hypotension)
Olivopontocerebellar atrophy
Progressive supranuclear palsy (Steele-Richardson-Olszewski's syndrome)
Pick's disease
Corticobasal degeneration
Creutzfeldt-Jakob disease
Cerebrovascular disease
Hydrocephalus
Frontal lobe tumor
Senile gait disorder of the elderly
Juvenile Huntington's disease
Wilson's disease
Cerebral anoxia
Neurosyphilis

sides or slightly forward of the trunk. A characteristic feature is the tendency to begin walking with a few rapid, very short, shuffling steps (start hesitation) before breaking into a more normal walking rhythm. Walking, once underway, may be interrupted by further shuffling or even complete cessation of movement (freezing) if a doorway or other obstacle is encountered. The posture of generalized flexion of the patient with Parkinson's disease exaggerates the normal tendency to lean forward when walking and renders patients susceptible to falling forward. To maintain balance when walking and avoid falling, the patient may advance forward with a series of rapid small steps (*festination*). Retropulsion and propulsion are similar manifestations of a flurry of small-sized parkinsonian steps made in an effort to preserve equilibrium in response to external perturbations. Instead of a single large step, a series of small steps are taken to restore balance. If these compensatory festinating steps are too small to maintain or restore balance, the patient may fall forward. Other causes of falls in Parkinson's disease include tripping or stumbling over rough surfaces because each step is too small or shallow to clear obstacles, and profound start hesitation or freezing. In each of these examples, falling stems from the lack of normal-sized, rapid, compensatory voluntary movements. This phenomenon is a manifestation of the defect in voluntary movement in Parkinson's disease. Late in the illness falls may occur either spontaneously or after minor perturbations for which the foregoing reasons cannot account. These are due to loss of postural and righting reflexes. Impaired postural reflexes late in the disease do not respond to levodopa medication, unlike the hyopkinetic steps and flexed truncal posture early in the disease.

A similar slowness of leg movement and shuffling when walking may occur in a variety of other akinetic-rigid syndromes (Table 26.4). These include multiple-system atrophy, cerebrovascular disease, and progressive supranuclear palsy. Subtle clinical signs help distinguish these conditions (Table 26.5). In progressive supranuclear palsy, the typical neck posture is one of extension rather than flexion as in Parkinson's disease. A stooped posture with exaggerated neck flexion is sometimes a feature of multiple-system atrophy. Patients with cerebrovascular disease and hydrocephalus may exhibit an upright posture with an exaggerated arm swing giving their gait a military appearance. A striking and distinguishing feature of degenerative diseases such as progressive supranuclear palsy or multiple-system atrophy is their tendency to produce an early loss of postural and righting reflexes in comparison to their relative preservation in Parkinson's disease until the late stages of the illness. There also may be an element of ataxia in these akinetic-rigid syndromes, which is not evident in Parkinson's disease. Accordingly, the patient who presents with falls and an akinetic-rigid syndrome is more likely to have symptomatic parkinsonism due to one of the foregoing conditions than Parkinson's disease itself. Finally, a dramatic response to levodopa is typical of idiopathic Parkinson's disease, though some cases of multiple-system atrophy will respond partially for a short period of time.

Dystonic Gait

Of all gait disturbances, dystonic syndromes may produce the most bizarre and often the most difficult diagnostic problems. The classic presentation of childhood-onset idiopathic torsion dystonia (dystonia musculorum deformans) is an action dystonia of a leg with a sustained abnormal posture of the foot (typically, plantar flexion and inversion) on attempting to run. In contrast, walking forward or backward or even running backward may be entirely normal at an early stage. An easily overlooked sign in the early stages is tonic extension of the great toe (*the striatal toe*) when walking. This may be a subtle finding but occasionally is so pronounced that a hole is worn in the toe of the shoe. With the passage of time the disorder may progress to involve the whole leg and then become generalized.

More difficult to identify are those dystonic syndromes that present with bizarre, seemingly inexplicable postures of the legs and trunk when walking. A characteristic feature common to all these dystonic postures is excessive flexion of the hip when walking. These patients may hop or walk sideways in a crablike fashion, with hyperflexion of the hips producing an attitude of general body flexion in a simian posture, or with a birdlike (peacock) gait with excessive flexion of the hip and knee and plantar flexion of the foot during the swing phase of each step. Many of these unfortunate patients have been thought to be hysterical because of the bizarre nature of their gait disturbance and because formal neurological examination is often normal if the patient is examined when lying supine. This observa-

Table 26.5: Summary of the clinical features that help differentiate between Parkinson's disease and symptomatic or secondary parkinsonism in patients with an akinetic-rigid gait syndrome

Feature	*Parkinson's Disease*	*Symptomatic Parkinsonism*
Posture	Stooped (trunk flexion)	Stooped or upright (trunk flexion or extension)
Stance	Narrow	Often wide-based
Initiation of walking	Start hesitation	Start hesitation: magnetic feet
Stride length: steps	Small, shuffling	Small, shuffling
Freezing	Common	Common
Leg movement	Stiff, rigid	Stiff, rigid
Speed	Slow	Slow
Festination	Common	Rare
Arm swing	Minimal or absent	Reduced or excessive
Heel-toe walking	Normal	Poor (truncal ataxia)
Postural reflexes	Preserved in early stages	Absent at early stage
Falls	Late (forward: tripping)	Early and severe (backward: tripping or without apparent reason)

tion reinforces the action-specific or action-related nature of dystonic syndromes. Furthermore, each of these patterns of gait disturbance has been described in association with identifiable secondary dystonic syndromes, including postencephalitic illness, manganese poisoning, and Wilson's disease. Finally, tardive dystonia following the ingestion of neuroleptic drugs may also produce similar bizarre abnormalities of gait.

It is always important to look for asymmetry in the assessment of childhood-onset dystonia, as a hemidystonic syndrome should be investigated to exclude symptomatic causes. Similarly, an isolated dystonic leg should also point toward symptomatic causes in an adult, though not in childhood. Should there be an early loss of postural responses and righting reflexes in association with a dystonic gait disturbance, attention should also be directed toward excluding underlying secondary causes.

Dystonia with diurnal fluctuation (dopa-responsive dystonia) characteristically presents with walking difficulties in childhood. Typically, the child is normal in the early morning but as the day progresses develops increasing rigidity and dystonic posturing of the legs with difficulty walking. These dystonic leg postures frequently become evident or worsen after exercise. Examination reveals a dystonic foot posture of plantar flexion and inversion, with the additional feature of brisk tendon reflexes. Some of these patients respond dramatically to levodopa-containing preparations, and early recognition is important. Indeed, all children presenting with a dystonic foot or leg should have a therapeutic trial of levodopa before other therapies such as anticholinergic drugs are commenced.

Paroxysmal dyskinesias also may present with difficulty walking. Paroxysmal kinesigenic choreoathetosis may present with the sudden onset of difficulty walking as a result of dystonic postures and involuntary movements of the legs, which often appear after standing from a seated position. Similarly, dystonia of the legs, either paroxysmal or exercise-induced, may interfere with walking.

Choreic Gait

The random and chaotic movements of chorea may be superimposed on or even interrupt all voluntary movements, including those of walking. This combination often provides a spectacular series of movements as the patient incorporates the choreic movements into his or her voluntary movements and compensates for them. The patient may describe an irregular path. The violent movements of Sydenham's chorea or chorea gravidarum may be sufficient to cause patients to be thrown off their feet and unable to walk at all. In contrast, chorea of this severity is uncommon in Huntington's disease, in which the involuntary movements may only cause the patient to lurch and take a step backward or occasionally stumble. Slowness of walking is characteristic of Huntington's disease. The stance is wide-based, the patients sway excessively, and the steps are variable in length and timing. Spontaneous knee flexion and leg raising are also common. Dopamine antagonists reduce the chorea but do not improve the gait. Balance and equilibrium are usually maintained until the terminal stages of Huntington's disease, when an akinetic-rigid syndrome may supervene.

Mixed Movement Disorders and Gait

Many conditions—for example, athetoid cerebral palsy—may produce a range of motor signs that reflect abnormalities at many levels of the nervous system. All interfere with and disrupt normal patterns of walking. These include spasticity of the legs, truncal and gait ataxia, and dystonic spasms and postures affecting the trunk and limbs. Difficulties may arise in distinguishing such patients from those with idiopathic torsion dystonia, which may begin at a similar age in childhood. The patient with cerebral palsy usually has a history of hypotonia and delayed achievement of developmental milestones. Often there is a history of perinatal injury or birth asphyxia, but in a substantial proportion of patients such an event cannot be identified. A major distinguishing feature is poor balance at an early age, which may be a contributing factor to the delay in sitting and later walking. As the child begins to walk, the first signs of dystonia and athetosis appear. The presence of spasticity and ataxia also help the physician distinguish this condition from idiopathic or primary dystonia.

Childhood neurodegenerative diseases also may first manifest themselves as a disorder of walking with a combination of motor syndromes. A progressive course should raise the possibility that the syndrome is symptomatic and secondary to an underlying cause.

Action Myoclonus and Tremor of the Legs

Some causes of involuntary movements of the legs when standing or walking are listed in Table 26.6.

Action myoclonus and reflex myoclonus affecting the legs are rare but striking disorders. The former, frequently seen in patients with postanoxic myoclonus, often is severe. Attempts to use the legs to stand or walk produce repetitive myoclonic jerks, which interrupt normal muscle activity to throw the patient off balance. The lapses of muscle activity between the jerks (negative myoclonus) cause patients to sag toward the ground. This sequence of events gives rise to an exaggerated bouncing appearance, which the patient is able to sustain for only a few seconds before falling or sitting down. Indeed, difficulty in walking is one of the major residual disabilities of this condition, and many patients remain wheelchair-bound. The stance is wide-based, and there is often an element of cerebellar ataxia, although this may be difficult to distinguish from the severe action myoclonus. Stimulus-sensitive reflex myoclonus also may produce a striking disorder of stance and gait, with reflex myoclonic jerks of leg muscles, particularly the quadriceps. The clinical appearance is similar to that just described. Investigation of these syndromes is directed toward the causes of myoclonus.

An action tremor of the legs may produce a similar but less severe disturbance of standing and walking. Significant leg tremor is present in up to 25% of patients with benign essential tremor. Another form of leg tremor is orthostatic tremor. In both conditions the symptoms are maximal when the patient is standing still and are minimized by walking or sitting down. The differentiation among leg tremors is best made by analysis of the electromyographic activity of leg muscles during these involuntary movements and their frequency. Benign essential tremor of the legs has a frequency on the order of 6 Hz, whereas orthostatic tremor is much faster at 16 Hz (Thompson et al. 1986). Muscle contractions at this high frequency of tremor are visible only as a rippling of the quadriceps muscles. Clonazepam has been reported to be of value in the latter condition, whereas a beta-blocker, such as propranolol, is the treatment of choice in essential tremor.

Table 26.6: Differential diagnosis of involuntary movements of the legs when standing

Action myoclonus of legs (as in postanoxic myoclonus)
Benign essential tremor
Orthostatic tremor
Clonus in spasticity
Spastic ataxia

Gait in the Elderly

Healthy, neurologically normal, elderly people tend to walk at slower speeds than their younger counterparts. The slower speed of walking is related to shorter and shallower steps with reduced excursion at lower limb joints. In addition, stance width may be slightly wider than normal, and synergistic arm and trunk movements are less vigorous. The rhythmicity of stepping is preserved. Such changes give the normal elderly gait a cautious or guarded appearance. Factors contributing to this general decline in mobility of the elderly include degenerative joint disease, reduced range of limb movement, and decreased cardiovascular fitness, limiting exercise capacity. The reduced speed of walking and associated changes in gait pattern in the elderly also may represent one method of providing a more secure base to compensate for a subtle age-related deterioration in balance. These elements of a *cautious gait* may be superimposed on any decline in walking ability and balance and may dominate the clinical picture.

In unselected elderly populations there is a more pronounced deterioration in gait. Steps are shorter, stride length is reduced, and the stance phase of walking is increased, leading to a dramatic reduction in walking speed, particularly in those who fall. Neurological causes of walking difficulty in the elderly, such as myelopathy, parkinsonism, cerebellar disease, and imbalance due to sensory loss, accounted for approximately half of the cases in one survey (Sudarsky and Ronthal 1983). In a further 20%, a frontal gait disorder or gait apraxia was identified, and in 14% a cause was not found. The latter remain the subject of much contention and debate. The following discussion summarizes the broad groups of walking difficulty encountered in the elderly that cannot be explained adequately by upper motor neuron lesions, weakness, sensory loss, parkinsonism, and cerebellar disease (Table 26.7) and is based on the classification of Nutt et al. (1993).

Imbalance may have several causes in the elderly. In many elderly patients, multiple sensory deficits affecting vision and vestibular and proprioceptive function cause imbalance, resulting in an insecure gait and loss of confidence when walking. The cumulative effects of lesions at many sites can interfere with walking without any one lesion being severe enough to explain the observed difficulty. Multiple mild sensory deficits of peripheral nerve or posterior column origin, combined with modest leg weakness of peripheral nerve or corticospinal tract origin—for example, in cervical and lum-

Table 26.7: Comparison of terms used to describe the clinical patterns of gait in the elderly with those from previous publications

Proposed Terminology	*Previous Terms*	*Lesions*
Cautious	Elderly gait Senile gait	Musculoskeletal Peripheral nervous system lesions Central nervous system lesions
Gait ignition failure	Gait apraxia Magnetic apraxia Slipping clutch phenomenon Lower-half parkinsonism Arteriosclerotic parkinsonism Trepidant abasia (Petren's gait)	Frontal lobe connections with brain stem (?)
Frontal gait disorder	*Marche à petits pas* Magnetic gait apraxia Arteriosclerotic parkinsonism Parkinsonian ataxia Lower-half parkinsonism Lower-body parkinsonism	Frontal lobe and connections
Frontal dysequilibrium	Gait apraxia Frontal ataxia Astasia, abasia	Frontal lobe and connections
Subcortical dysequilibrium	Tottering Astasia, abasia Thalamic astasia	Brain stem (upper) Basal ganglia Thalamus

Source: Modified from JG Nutt, CD Marsden, PD Thompson. Human walking and higher-level gait disorders, particularly in the elderly. Neurology 1993;43:268–279.

bar spondylosis—is a common example of this clinical picture. *Subcortical dysequilibrium* refers to the inability to stand because of inadequate postural reflexes and a tendency to fall backward or forward, often with injury. There are no frontal lobe release signs, incontinence, or cerebellar ataxia of the limbs. There may be postural abnormalities of the trunk, rigidity, bradykinesia, dysarthria, and ocular motor signs. Acute vascular lesions of the thalamus (Masdeu and Gorelick 1988), basal ganglia (Labadie et al. 1989), or midbrain produce this clinical picture. Similar postural and balance difficulties are found in progressive supranuclear palsy syndrome and multiple-system atrophy. Impaired central vestibular function may account for isolated dysequilibrium in some elderly patients and correlate with an increase in body sway (Fife and Baloh 1993). Dysequilibrium also may be prominent in frontal lobe disease (see below).

The disturbances of gait that accompany lesions of the frontal lobes have long been the subject of interest, and the mechanisms responsible are poorly understood (see Table 26.7). Frontal lobe tumors (glioma or meningioma), anterior cerebral artery infarction, obstructive or communicating hydrocephalus (especially normal pressure hydrocephalus), and diffuse cerebrovascular disease (multiple lacunar infarcts and Binswanger's disease) all produce a similar disturbance of gait. The clinical appearance of the gait of patients with such lesions varies from a predominantly wide-based ataxic gait to an akinetic-rigid gait with slow, short steps and a tendency to shuffle. A common presentation of patients with the foregoing conditions is a combination of these features. In the early stages, the gait is wide-based, with an upright posture of the trunk, and short, shuffling steps (*frontal gait disorder*). This may be most noticeable on starting to walk or turning corners. There may be episodes of freezing. Arm swing is often normal or even exaggerated when walking, but the normal fluidity of trunk and limb motion is lost, giving the appearance of a "military two-step" gait. Formal examination often reveals normal voluntary upper limb and hand movements and a lively facial expression (Thompson and Marsden 1987).

This lower-half parkinsonism is commonly seen in diffuse cerebrovascular disease. The *marche à petits pas* of Dejerine and *atherosclerotic parkinsonism* of Critchley refer to a similar clinical picture. Patients with this clinical syndrome are commonly misdiagnosed as having Parkinson's disease. The normal arm function, upright truncal posture, upper motor neuron signs including a pseudobulbar palsy, and the absence of a resting tremor distinguish this syndrome from Parkinson's disease. In addition, the lower-half parkinsonism of diffuse cerebrovascular disease does not respond to levodopa treatment, further distinguishing it from Parkinson's disease (see Table 26.4). Similarly, the slowness of movement and the relative lack of heel-shin ataxia when the patient is examined supine distinguish the syndrome from cerebellar gait and leg ataxia due to an anterior lobe-vermis lesion.

As the underlying condition progresses, the elements of ataxia and parkinsonism become more pronounced. There may be great difficulty in initiating a step, the feet being apparently glued to the floor (the magnetic foot response). Attempts to take a step require assistance, with the patient clutching at nearby objects or persons for support. There may be excessive upper body movement as the patient tries to free the feet to initiate walking, and when underway shuffling becomes even more pronounced. Such patients rarely exhibit the festination of Parkinson's disease, but a few steps of propulsion or retropulsion may be taken. Postural and righting reactions are impaired and eventually lost, and falls are common at the slightest perturbation. In contrast with this difficulty in walking, these patients often can move their legs with greater facility when seated or lying supine. They may be able to make stepping, walking, or bicycling leg movements when lying but be quite unable to do so when standing.

At an advanced stage, such patients may develop profound truncal ataxia with a loss of truncal mobility, so that they are unable to stand or sit, or even turn over when lying in bed (*frontal dysequilibrium*). Walking then becomes impossible, and even simple leg movements are slow and clumsy when lying down. Paratonic rigidity of the arms and legs (gegenhalten) is common, the tendon reflexes may be brisk, and the plantar responses are extensor. Grasp reflexes in the hands and feet may be elicited. Urinary incontinence and dementia frequently occur in the evolution of this syndrome. Investigation by MRI or CT of the brain will reveal the majority of conditions causing this syndrome.

In some patients fragments of this clinical picture are observed. Those with *gait ignition failure* exhibit profound start hesitation without disturbance of stepping once walking is underway, or of balance while standing or walking. Initiation of the first step is hampered by shuffling, and walking may be interrupted by freezing (Atchison et al. 1993). Sensory cues may facilitate stepping. These findings are similar to walking in Parkinson's disease but speech and upper-limb function are normal and there is no response to levodopa. Imaging of the brain is normal. The cause of this syndrome is not known, but the slowly progressive evolution of symptoms suggests a degenerative condition. Occasionally, patients exhibit *isolated festination*, again without any other signs of parkinsonism, or a response to levodopa. The cause of this syndrome is not known.

There remain elderly patients in whom walking difficulties resemble those described in frontal lobe disease but in whom there is no evidence of structural disease and no underlying cause can be found. In the *essential senile gait disorder of the elderly* or *senile paraplegia*, parkinsonism and ataxia similar to those in frontal gait disorders are seen. The history is one of gradual onset, without stroke-like episodes or identifiable structural lesions of the frontal lobes or cerebral white matter. MRI and CT of the brain are normal. The cause of this disorder remains unknown. It does not fulfill the criteria for normal-pressure hydrocephalus, and there is no evidence of more generalized cerebral dysfunction such as occurs in Alzheimer's disease. Indeed, it is rare for patients with Alzheimer's disease to develop difficulty in walking until the later stages of the disease.

Early descriptions of these frontal gait syndromes emphasized the ataxic components, and the term *frontal ataxia* was used to reflect the perceived involvement of the frontopontocerebellar pathways as the most likely mechanism. Indeed, the gait ataxia of many midline cerebellar lesions associated with obstructive hydrocephalus can be out of proportion to the degree of lower limb ataxia (heel-shin ataxia) and may be largely relieved by the insertion of a ventricular drain or shunt. This confirms the importance of hydrocephalus in the gait ataxia associated with these lesions. Others were impressed by the slowness of movement and a discrepancy between the pronounced disability when attempting to walk and the preservation of leg movements when lying or sitting. This combination of signs was considered a form of limb-kinetic apraxia and referred to as *frontal apraxia* and later *gait apraxia* (Meyer and Barron 1960). *Gait apraxia* is defined as "the loss of ability to properly use the lower limbs in the act of walking which cannot be accounted for by demonstrable sensory impairment or motor weakness." Gait apraxia comprises ataxia plus hypokinesia, rigidity (gegenhalten), and brisk reflexes, the latter signs distinguishing it from cerebellar ataxia. The combination of bradykinesia and ataxia in frontal lobe or diffuse cerebral white matter disease can be explained by interruption of the connections between motor, premotor, and supplementary motor cortex and other subcortical motor areas such as the cerebellum and basal ganglia. However, the use of the term *apraxia* in this context remains controversial and probably encompasses a spectrum of higher gait syndromes (see Table 26.7) (Nutt et al. 1993).

Myopathic Weakness and Gait

Weakness of proximal leg and hip girdle muscles interferes with the stabilization of the pelvis and legs on the trunk during all phases of the gait cycle. Failure to stabilize the pelvis produces exaggerated rotation of the pelvis with each step (*waddling* or *Trendelenburg gait*), the hips are slightly flexed as a result of weakness of hip extension, and there is an exaggerated lumbar lordosis. Weakness of hip extension interferes with the ability to stand from a squatting or lying position (*Gowers's sign*) and makes running impossible. The classic descriptions of this gait were of patients with Duchenne's muscular dystrophy, but any myopathy that affects these muscles will result in such a picture. Similarly, neurogenic weakness of proximal muscles—for example, spinal muscular atrophy and occasionally the Guillain-Barré syndrome—may mimic this waddling gait.

Neurogenic Weakness and Gait

Muscle weakness of peripheral nerve origin, as in a peripheral neuropathy, typically affects distal muscles of the legs and results in a *steppage gait*. This refers to a weakness or paralysis of ankle dorsiflexion that makes the patient lift the leg and foot high above the ground. When this clinical picture is confined to only one leg (unilateral foot drop), a common peroneal or sciatic nerve palsy or an L5 radiculopathy is the usual cause. Rarely, myopathic weakness of the peroneal muscles (scapuloperoneal syndromes) may produce foot drop.

A femoral neuropathy—for instance, due to diabetes mellitus—is another example of a strategic mononeuropathy that may disable walking. Weakness of knee extension allows the knee to buckle when walking or standing and causes the patient to collapse on the floor. This may first be evident when walking down stairs. Such focal weakness also may be the presenting feature of the progressive muscular atrophy in motor neuron disease.

Psychogenic Gait Disorders

The wide range of abnormalities of gait that can be seen in lesions of different parts of the nervous system make psychogenic gaits among the most difficult to diagnose. Occasionally patients will have complete inability to use a leg when walking but will display normal power of synergistic movements of the leg when they are examined lying down or observed when changing position. This discrepancy is illustrated by *Hoover's sign*. The patient with an apparently paralyzed leg or legs is examined when lying down. The patient is asked to lift up one leg, and the examiner then places his or her hand under the other leg to feel for the presence of synergistic hip extension in the apparently paralyzed leg. The apparent severe weakness often presents little disability or inconvenience to such patients. In contrast, other patients with hysterical paraplegia may be totally confined to bed and may even develop contractures from lack of leg movements. A variety of patterns, including transient fluctuations in posture while walking, knee buckling without falls, gross slowness, a crouched or stooped (or other abnormal) posture of the trunk with hip, knee and ankle flexion, exaggerated body sway, and trembling "weak" legs, have been described (Keene 1989; Lempert et al. 1991). Suggestibility and improvement with distraction are common features. Other hysterical symptoms may be present in up to 75% of cases.

The more acrobatic hysterical disorders of gait indicate the extent to which the nervous system is functioning normally. These patients are able to take advantage of high-level motor skills and coordination to perform their various maneuvers. This is an important observation in the assessment of suspected hysterical gait disorders, as is a rapid, dramatic, and complete recovery. One must be cautious in accepting a diagnosis of hysteria, however, as a bizarre gait may be a presenting feature of idiopathic torsion dystonia.

MISCELLANEOUS

Agoraphobia and Gait

Marks (1981) described a syndrome of space phobia in which middle-aged people developed an inability to walk in open spaces. These patients sought the support of nearby fences and walls. Many had fallen in the course of their illness. Other neurological symptoms and general medical abnormalities were common. It was proposed that the disorder was distinct from agoraphobia and might represent a disturbance of central vestibulo-ocular mechanisms.

Painful Gaits

Most people at one time or another will suffer from a limp due to a painful or injured leg. Limps and gait difficulties that are caused by joint disease or by local bony or soft-tissue injury are not usually accompanied by muscle weakness or by reflex or sensory change. Limitation of the range of movement at the hip, knee, or ankle joints may lead to short steps with a fixed leg posture.

Pain in the leg caused by intermittent claudication of the cauda equina is most commonly due to lumbar spondylosis and rarely to a spinal tumor. Diagnosis is confirmed by MRI. Occasionally it may be difficult to distinguish this syndrome from claudication of the calf muscles due to peripheral vascular disease. Examination of the patient after inducing the symptoms by exercise may resolve the issue by revealing a depressed ankle jerk or radicular sensory loss, with preservation of arterial pulses in the leg.

Skeletal Deformity and Joint Disease

Degenerative osteoarthritis of the hip may produce leg shortening, in addition to mechanical limitation of leg movement at the hip, giving rise to a waddling gait or a limp.

Leg shortening with limping in childhood may be the presenting feature of hemiatrophy due to a cerebral or spinal lesion. Such walking difficulties between the ages of 1 and 5 years are the most common mode of presentation of spinal dysraphism. On examination, a variety of additional abnormalities may be detected, including lower motor neuron signs in the legs and sensory loss with trophic ulcers of the feet. Occasionally, upper motor neuron signs, such as a brisk knee reflex, will be present in the same limb. Lumbosacral vertebral abnormalities (spina bifida), bony foot deformities, and a cutaneous hairy patch over the lumbosacral region are clues to the diagnosis. In adult life, spinal dysraphism (diastematomyelia with a tethered cord) may first become symptomatic after a back injury, with the development of walking difficulties, leg and lower back pain, neurogenic bladder disturbances, and sensory loss in a leg. MRI or CT myelography will reveal the abnormality.

Epileptic Falls in Childhood

Seizure disorders of the myoclonic or akinetic-atonic type typically produce falls but may present as an unsteady or uncoordinated gait in childhood. Tonic seizures or flexor spasms also may produce this clinical picture (Ikeno et al. 1985). Simultaneous video, electroencephalographic, and electromyographic recordings are helpful in diagnosing and identifying these various seizure patterns.

REFERENCES

Armstrong DM. The supraspinal control of mammalian locomotion. J Physiol (Lond) 1988;405:1–37.

Atchison PR, Thompson PD, Frackowiak RSJ et al. The syndrome of isolated gait ignition failure: a report of six cases. Move Disord 1993;8:285–292.

Day BL, Steiger MJ, Thompson PD et al. Influence of vision and stance width on human body movements when standing: implications for afferent control of lateral sway. J Physiol 1993;469:479–499.

Eidelberg E, Walden JG, Nguyen LH. Locomotor control in macaque monkeys. Brain 1981;104:647–663.

Elble RJ, Moody C, Leffler K et al. The initiation of normal walking. Move Disord 1994;9:139–146.

Fife TD, Baloh RW. Dysequilibrium of unknown cause in older people. Ann Neurol 1993;34:694–702.

Ikeno T, Shigematsu H, Miyakoshi M et al. An analytic study of epileptic falls. Epilepsia 1985;26:612–621.

Keene JR. Hysterical gait disorders: 60 cases. Neurology 1989;39:586–589.

Labadie EL, Awerbach GI, Hamilton RH et al. Falling and postural deficits due to acute basal ganglia lesions. Arch Neurol 1989;45:492–496.

Lempert T, Brandt T, Dietrich M, Huppert D. How to identify psychogenic disorders of stance and gait. J Neurol 1991; 238:140–146.

Marks I. Space "phobia": a pseudo-agoraphobic syndrome. J Neurol Neurosurg Psychiatry 1981;44:387–391.

Masdeu JC, Gorelick PB. Thalamic astasia: inability to stand after unilateral thalamic lesions. Ann Neurol 1988;23:596–603.

Meyer JS, Barron D. Apraxia of gait: a clinico-pathological study. Brain 1960;83:61–84.

Nutt JG, Marsden CD, Thompson PD. Human walking and higher level gait disorders, particularly in the elderly. Neurology 1993;43:268–279.

Sudarsky L, Ronthal M. Gait disorders among elderly patients: a survey of 50 patients. Arch Neurol 1983;40:740–743.

Thompson PD, Marsden CD. Gait disorder of subcortical arteriosclerotic encephalopathy: Binswanger's disease. Move Disord 1987;2:1–8.

Thompson PD, Rothwell JC, Day BL et al. The physiology of orthostatic tremor. Arch Neurol 1986;43:584–587.

Chapter 27
Hemiplegia and Monoplegia

Frank R. Freemon

As long as there has been an art of medicine, weakness in one or two limbs has challenged the diagnostic acumen of the clinician. Healers in the ancient world knew that lesions of the nervous system could produce focal weakness. The Alexandrian Greeks observed paralysis in a limb after the nerve to that limb was cut. The leading physician of the ancient world, Galen, cut the spinal cord at various levels and noted paralysis below the level of the lesion. Aretaeus of Cappadocia observed that a lesion in one cerebral hemisphere produced paralysis on the opposite side of the body; he related this crossed paralysis to the visible decussation of fibers at the base of the brain.

Definitions can be difficult, especially when one confuses the original languages with modern meaning. *Monoplegia* is paralysis of one arm or one leg. *Hemiplegia* is the paralysis of the arm and leg on the same side of the body. If a person is hemiplegic (half-paralyzed) on one side of the body and develops a hemiplegia involving the other side, this unfortunate victim is said to be tetraplegic or quadriplegic (paralyzed in all four limbs). Direct translation from the Latin and Greek into English produces confusion to the point of humor: In the English translation, one-half plus one-half equals four! These terms do not make arithmetic sense, but neurological principles explain these syndromes with good biological sense.

CLINICAL EVALUATION

The characteristics of hemiplegia or monoplegia depend on the location and duration of the underlying causative lesion. From the characteristics of the weakness, and from associated findings, the clinician should be able to determine what portion of the nervous system has suffered damage: cortex, deep white matter, internal capsule, brain stem, spinal cord, or peripheral nervous system. The time course of the symptoms gives information about the type of the lesion. The lesion that is maximal in severity from its onset is generally caused by an acute brain infarction. Alternately, a lesion that slowly infiltrates around nerve cells rather than destroying them can reach a huge size and cause significant mental aberration without greatly affecting motor function.

The first step in the examination evaluates the general appearance of the patient. The arm of the hemiplegic patient may lie limply at the side or may be drawn across the chest. The clinician should observe the outward rotation of the hemiplegic foot; this is an ancient observation, as shown in Figure 27.1. If the hemiplegia results from a lesion of the cerebral hemisphere, one may note associated psychological dysfunction involving language or attention. The patient with a nondominant hemisphere lesion often exhibits poor posture; he or she is slumped in a wheelchair or crumpled up in one portion of the bed.

The clinician should attempt to judge the severity of the weakness. One must separate true weakness, as determined by formal muscle testing, from a disorder of movement due to awkwardness or pain. A person with an arm that is essentially useless due to ataxia or apraxia may have normal strength. As summarized in Table 27.1, a number of scales have been developed to record the degree of weakness. I have observed that the numerical scale gradations mean different things to different physicians and often complicate rather than improve communication among doctors. These numerical systems are not linear since the patient with a gradation of 4 is not twice as strong as a patient with a gradation of 2. The Medical Research Council scale has an advantage in being absolute and is reproducible from observer to observer provided it is conducted accurately. This is the most widely used clinical system. However, I recommend the descriptive scale in Table 27.1. One should note that

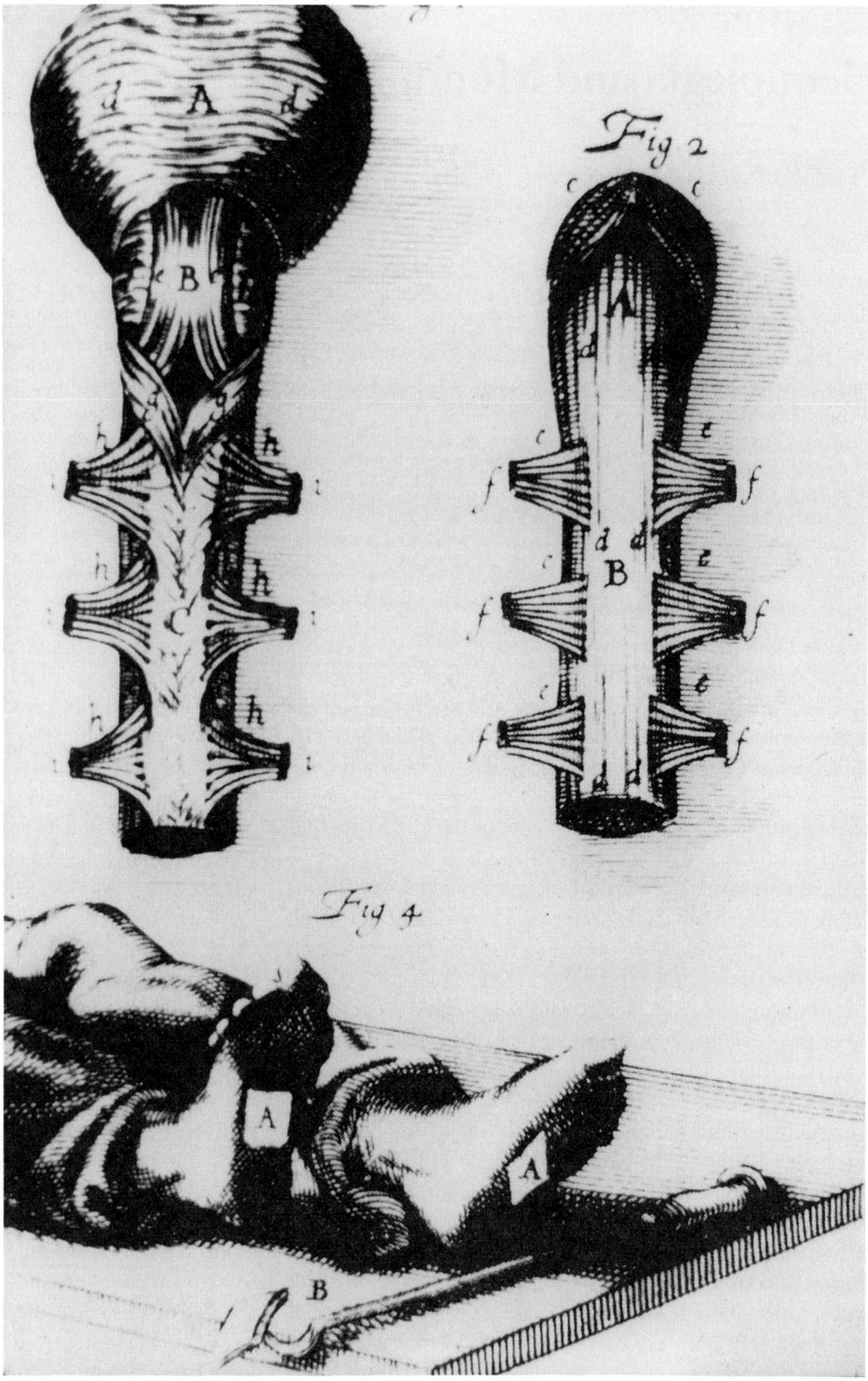

FIGURE 27.1 The outward rotation of the hemiplegic foot was first illustrated by Domenico Mistichelli in 1709. Mistichelli was the first physician after Aretaeus to correlate a lesion in one hemisphere with contralateral hemiplegia. He related this association to the visible decussation of fibers in the caudal medulla as shown in his dissections.

the term *hemiplegia* should be restricted to *total paralysis*; partial weakness should be termed *hemiparesis*. If the speaker wishes to ensure that it is recognized that the patient has total paralysis on one side of the body, the term *dense hemiplegia* can be used, though this is a tautology.

When judging the degree of weakness, it is important to eliminate the effect of pain. If the patient gives way with a groan when strength is tested, weakness may not be present at all. Sometimes the examiner is able to judge strength for just the instant before the onset of pain; sometimes the clinician must admit that the degree of weakness cannot be evaluated.

The clinician can detect patients with very slight hemiparesis. The patient is asked to extend both arms; the arm that is slightly weak may drift downward. In the most slightly affected patient, the arm will not drift but the little finger will move outward and upward; this is the *digiti quinti* sign. Some clinicians have found that arm drift is best seen when patients are asked to turn their hands with palms

Table 27.1: Grading weakness

I. The five-point system of the Medical Research Council
5: Normal strength
4: Weak movement against resistance
3: Can move limb against gravity but not against resistance
2: Can move limb with gravity eliminated (i.e., horizontally) but not against gravity
1: Muscle contraction without movement of a joint
0: No muscle contraction at all
II. The four-point Mayo Clinic system
0: Normal strength
–1: Mild weakness (25% loss)
–2: Moderate weakness (50% loss)
–3: Severe weakness (75% loss)
–4: No contraction
III. Descriptive system (recommended)
Normal strength
Slight but definite weakness
Moderate weakness
Movement across the bed but cannot lift against gravity
Muscle contraction without limb movement
Total paralysis
Unclassifiable due to give-way or pain

upward, as though they were holding two pies in front of them. If one hand assumes a twisted posture but there is no drift, the clinician should suspect very mild dysfunction within the contralateral hemisphere. Drift can also be tested in the legs with the patient lying in bed.

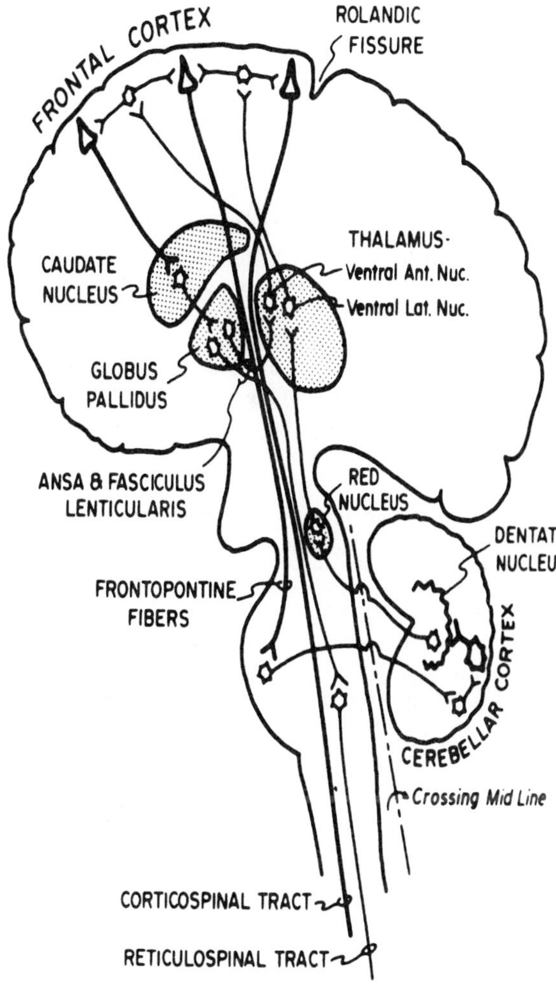

FIGURE 27.2 While the corticospinal tract is important in understanding the neuroanatomical basis of hemiplegia, the cerebral cortex, basal ganglia, cerebellum, and reticular formation interact in the control of movement.

ANATOMICAL DIAGNOSIS

Hemiplegia results from lesions in several locations within the central nervous system. The term *pyramidal tract* has two meanings: (1) the fibers running through the medullary pyramids, and (2) the long axons of the pyramid-shaped cells, including the Betz cells, located in the motor gyrus. The pyramidal tract, defined in either way, has important functions in the control of movement (Davidoff 1990). Hemiplegia is not produced solely by transection of this pathway but is due to the destruction of several interacting neural systems. Figure 27.2 illustrates the neuroanatomy of the motor system. Hemiparesis can result when damage occurs in the cerebral cortex, in the deep white matter or internal capsule, in the brain stem, or in the spinal cord. Monoparesis can occur from a lesion in any of these locations or from damage of the peripheral nerve fibers from their origin in the anterior horn of the spinal cord to their termination in the muscles.

As summarized in Table 27.2, a lesion of the convexity of the cerebral hemisphere affects arm strength more than leg; weakness of the lower face is obvious, and the tongue deviates toward the weak side. Lesions of the paramedian region of the central hemisphere produce weakness of one or both legs. Table 27.3 summarizes the signs and symptoms that occur if the corticospinal fibers are damaged in the internal capsule; this lesion also damages the outflow of the globus pallidus. The arm and the leg are often equally weak; the lower face may be weak but may be spared if the lesion only involves the most posterior portion of the posterior limb of the internal capsule.

Lesions of the brain stem produce a hemiparesis with nearly equal weakness of arm and leg. The face may or may not be involved depending on whether the lesion is above or below the point at which the corticobulbar fibers cross the midline to terminate in the facial nucleus. These findings are summarized in Table 27.4. Brain stem lesions that cause hemiplegia usually also produce other neurological dysfunction. The cranial nerve abnormalities associated with contralateral hemiplegia are associated with the names of the physicians who first described this association, as summarized in Table 27.5.

Patients demonstrate abnormal psychological function depending on the side of lesion. Damage to the hemisphere that is

Table 27.2: Characteristics of the hemiplegia resulting from a lesion of the cerebral cortex

1. The arm is weaker than the leg; the face is involved, the tongue deviates toward the weak side.
2. Usually there is an associated somatosensory loss, vague in description, but the examination shows poor graphesthesia.
3. Some patients have a homonymous visual field defect on the side of the weakness.
4. Patients demonstrate abnormal psychological function depending on which cerebral hemisphere is damaged:
   a. The side dominant for speech, usually the left: aphasia, emotional depression, motor apraxia (even in the left arm).
   b. The side not dominant for speech, usually the right: spatial dysfunction, constructional apraxia, denial of the weakness (or even of the existence) of the hemiplegic left limbs, emotional flatness, apparently uncomfortable postures.

Table 27.3: Characteristics of the hemiplegia with a lesion in the region of the internal capsule

1. The arm and leg are equally weak. The face may be weak but may be spared if the lesion only involves the posterior portion of the posterior limb of the internal capsule.
2. There is usually no sensory loss, but hemihypesthesia may be marked due to involvement of the adjacent thalamus.

Table 27.4: Characteristics of the hemiplegia with a lesion in the brain stem

1. The arm and leg are equally weak.
2. The face is completely normal in lesions of the lower brain stem, but may be quite weak in more rostral lesions.
3. Somatosensory examination of the body is normal.
4. Cranial nerve abnormalities are often present.
5. Other common findings are internuclear ophthalmoplegia and Horner's syndrome.

Table 27.5: Eponyms associated with hemiplegia

Eponym	
Brain stem lesion:	Contralateral hemiplegia plus ipsilateral
Weber	Third nerve palsy
Raymond	Sixth nerve palsy
Foville	Gaze palsy (often with seventh nerve palsy)
Millard-Gubler	Seventh nerve palsy
Jackson	Ninth, tenth, eleventh, and twelfth nerve palsies
Spinal cord lesion:	Ipsilateral hemiplegia plus contralateral
Brown-Séquard	Loss of pinprick and fine touch sensations

dominant for speech, usually the left, produces aphasia, emotional depression, and apraxia. Lesions of the cerebral hemisphere that is not dominant for speech produce an emotional flatness and a loss of abilities requiring knowledge of spatial relationships. The patient is unable to copy simple designs such as a cube, may leave food on the left half of the plate, and may improperly clothe the left half of the body. In the most severely damaged individual, there may be denial of the paralysis of the left arm (*anosognosia*) or even of the existence of the left arm.

Sensory signs and symptoms help the clinician localize the lesion. Abnormalities on pinprick and fine-touch sensation examinations generally parallel motor dysfunction. If the lesion is subcortical, a decrease of these sensations will occur on one-half the body and face; this hemihypesthesia is on the same side as the hemiplegia. The person with pinprick and fine-touch sensory loss on one side of the body and hemiplegia on the other has suffered a hemisection of the high cervical spinal cord. The patient with damage involving the cerebral cortex may complain of abnormal sensation over one-half of the body; this loss can be vague in description, but the examination shows an inability to identify numbers written on the palm (*agraphesthesia*) or small objects placed within the hand (*astereognosis*). A diminution of vibration sense indicates a subcortical site of damage.

Damage to the corticospinal tract produces a loss of superficial skin reflexes (*superficial abdominal* and *cremasteric reflexes*) and a *Babinski's sign* (Table 27.6). A lesion of the frontal lobe can produce a contralateral *palmomental reflex*. A lesion in the posterior portion of the hemisphere can produce contralateral homonymous *visual field loss*. This chapter devotes special attention to these associated findings: deviation of the head and eyes, decreased corneal reflex, and the special characteristics of facial and tongue weakness.

Deviation of the Head and Eyes

An inherent balance exists between two centers for gaze in the two frontal lobes. When one center is destroyed, the other is unopposed. Therefore the patient who has just suffered an acute brain infarction in one cerebral hemisphere may turn his or her head and eyes away from the side of the paralysis. After a variable period, the undamaged center adapts to the disappearance of the balancing action in the opposite frontal lobe. A person with severe damage to the right hemisphere may disregard the left portion of his or her personal space for several weeks or even months. Relatives who wish to communicate with the stroke victim should sit on the right side. (When President Woodrow Wilson suffered a severe right hemisphere stroke in 1919, his wife, as advised by the consulting neurologist Francis X. Dercum, arranged for visiting politicians to address the stricken president from his right side.)

Facial Weakness

Most patients with hemiplegia experience weakness of the face as well as of the arm and leg. Many patients with arm weakness alone, without leg weakness, demonstrate an associated facial weakness. If only slightly affected, the patient may show only a loss of the nasolabial fold that is overcome by voluntary movement of the face. In general, only the lower half of the face is affected. The patient may have severe drooping of

Table 27.6: Upper versus lower motor neuron dysfunction

	Upper	Lower
Atrophy	Mild	Severe (if chronic)
Tone	Increased	Decreased
Tendon reflexes	Increased	Decreased or absent
Abdominal reflexes	Absent	Present (except lower thoracic lesions)
Babinski's sign	Present	Not present

the muscles around the mouth but can corrugate the forehead quite normally and hold the eyes closed against pressure.

An upper motor lesion causes weakness only of the lower portion of the face. This is an old neurological saying that is usually, but not always, correct. The rostral half of the facial nerve nucleus in the floor of the fourth ventricle sends fibers to the muscles of the upper face; the caudal portion of the nucleus sends fibers to the lower face. At one time it was thought that the rostral half of the nucleus received direct input from both hemispheres; therefore, a lesion restricted to one hemisphere would not produce weakness of the upper face. Subsequent research has shown that, in most people, the central portion of the precentral gyrus sends corticobulbar fibers mainly to the caudal portion of the contralateral facial nucleus (Jenny and Saper 1987), while the rostral portion of the facial nucleus receives direct input from the surrounding reticular formation. However, the details of innervation of the facial nucleus vary from person to person, so that it is not unusual to encounter a patient with severe weakness of the lower face and significant weakness of the upper face due to a lesion in the cerebral hemisphere.

Upper motor neuron facial weakness can be overcome by emotion and by involuntary movements such as a yawn. Both sides of the face move normally in spontaneous laughter, but a smile given voluntarily is only half of a smile. Apparently, the limbic system has significant input to the facial nucleus via the pontine reticular formation (Hopf et al. 1992).

Tongue Weakness

Upper motor neuron tongue weakness is similar in nature to facial weakness, though less marked. The corticobulbar fibers cross the midline to innervate the contralateral hypoglossal nucleus. When a patient with damage to this pathway voluntarily protrudes the tongue, the contralateral hypoglossal nucleus is inadequately stimulated and the tongue may protrude toward the side of the dysfunctioning nucleus, or away from the side of the cerebral lesion. As with facial innervation, the tongue is only weak when voluntary movements are undertaken. The patient will lick his or her lips normally when this action is undertaken spontaneously.

Corneal Reflex

A decreased contralateral corneal reflex will be present for several days in the patient who has experienced sudden damage to one cerebral hemisphere. The corneal reflex is monosynaptic: touching the cornea stimulates the fifth nerve, the fibers of which synapse in the brain stem on the seventh nerve nucleus, causing the orbicularis oculi muscle to be activated and the eye to close. The entire reflex pathway is some distance from the site of the lesion, yet the corneal response is temporarily depressed or even absent. One surmises that the monosynaptic reflex is facilitated by corticobulbar fibers that are interrupted by a hemispheric lesion. This may be an example of the neurological mechanism known as "diaschisis."

ETIOLOGICAL DIAGNOSIS

The clinician tries to answer two questions: *Where is the lesion (anatomy)?* and *What is the lesion (pathology)?* The careful examination almost always answers the first question, while the clinical history is most valuable to answer the second.

The discussion to this point has emphasized the effect of the exact site of the lesion on the clinical characteristics of the resulting weakness. Another important variable is time. A small lesion that occurs suddenly may produce a devastating disability; a huge lesion that develops slowly may produce very little motor dysfunction. If the lesion damages brain tissue suddenly, as with an acute brain infarction, several signs and symptoms occur that one can expect will be transient. Transient findings after an acute brain lesion include forced deviation of the eyes and head, the depressed corneal reflex, and denial of hemiplegia.

Common causes of hemiplegia and monoplegia are presented in Table 27.7. The clinician must emphasize the discovery of an underlying cause that may respond to specific therapy. Less common but potentially reversible causes receive greatest emphasis; dissection of the carotid artery is an example. Compassionate care of the patient with hemiplegia due to a malignant tumor is also important. The diagnostic evaluation of the patient is discussed in subsequent chapters of this work.

MONOPLEGIA

Upper Versus Lower Motor Neuron Lesion

Monoplegia can result from central nervous system lesions. Unlike hemiparesis, however, weakness of one limb can fol-

Table 27.7: Causes of hemiparesis

I.	Potentially reversible causes
	Hypoglycemic hemiplegia
	Hemiplegic migraine
	Subdural hematoma
	Postictal paresis
	Meningioma or other benign brain tumor
	Arteritis
	Thrombosis in evolution
	Arteriovenous malformation
	Aortic or cerebral arterial dissection
	Contusion of brain or spinal cord
	Brain abscess
	Multiple sclerosis
II.	Treatable causes, without expectation of complete recovery
	Acute brain infarction, completed
	Intracerebral hematoma
	Cerebral or pontine glioma
	Sickle cell crisis
	Cerebral lymphoma
	Special forms of encephalitis or encephalomalacia
	Moyamoya disease
	Brain metastases of systemic cancer

low damage to peripheral nerve fibers. Therefore, the initial diagnostic decision made by the clinician faced with a patient with monoparesis involves deciding whether it is an upper motor neuron or a lower motor neuron lesion. Does the weakness result from a lesion between the cortex and the anterior horn cell, or between the anterior horn cell and the muscle?

The upper motor lesion usually produces increased tone in the weak muscles. This lesion is generally associated with hyperactive tendon reflexes, pathological reflexes such as Babinski's sign, and the disappearance of superficial reflexes such as the abdominal and cremasteric. The lower motor neuron lesion produces flaccid muscles; tendon reflexes are usually absent because of damage to the afferent limb of the reflex arc. If the disease is chronic, damage to the lower motor neuron produces severe muscle atrophy. Most chronic upper motor neuron diseases produce only mild atrophy.

The patient with monoplegia can be a challenging diagnostic problem. If the face is weak as well as the arm, then an upper motor lesion is certain, or the patient has two problems. If the weak limb shows increased tone to passive stretch, an upper motor lesion is present. Similarly, if the tendon reflexes in the weak limb are definitely increased, as compared to the normal limb, the clinician strongly suspects disease of the brain or high spinal cord. On the other hand, if the weakness is in a specific nerve distribution, or if the accompanying sensory loss is in a clear dermatomal distribution, the clinician can be reasonably certain that the disorder involves the peripheral nervous system. The electromyogram can help differentiate these two classes of disorders, but sometimes there can be both an upper and a lower motor neuron lesion.

Pathological reflexes are a great help since they are present only in upper motor neuron lesions. In monoparesis of the lower limb, the clinician should devote a major effort to elicit Babinski's sign or similar associated signs. The inexperienced clinician may mistake the *triple response of Babinski* (flexion at hip and knee as well as extension of the large toe) for a *withdrawal reflex*. The examiner should attempt to elicit an upgoing toe with other stimuli such as downward stroking the ridge of the tibia (*Oppenheim's reflex*), squeezing the calf muscles (*Gordon's reflex*), scratching the dorsolateral surface of the foot (*Chaddock's reflex*), touching the dorsal surface of the large toe with a sharp stick (*Bing's reflex*), and twisting the small toe (*Rossolimo's reflex*). To elicit the reflex properly, the clinician may need to induce discomfort.

For the upper limb, the *Hoffmann's reflex* (flexion of the thumb or rapid flicking of the partly flexed middle finger) indicates an upper motor neuron lesion. Pathological reflexes more homologous to Babinski's sign are the *grasp reflex* and the *Wartenberg thumb sign*. The latter reflex, sometimes called the *Klippel-Feil sign*, is elicited when the clinician tests the resistance of the tips of the four fingers to extension. If the sign is present, the thumb contracts at the distal interphalangeal joint and may move across the palm to nearly touch the base of the little finger. If the fingers are paralyzed, the sign cannot be elicited. These pathological reflexes, if present, indicate an upper motor neuron lesion of the brain or spinal cord.

Upper Limb Monoparesis

A common cause of monoparesis of the arm is a small infarction involving the central portion of the precentral gyrus (Boiten and Lodder 1991). A small mass lesion in this area can also produce upper limb monoparesis.

Benign focal amyotrophy or monomelic amyotrophy is a poorly understood disorder of progressive wasting of the upper limb, usually beginning in the hand. Electromyography suggests that this disorder is due to degeneration of the anterior horn cells of the cervical spinal cord. This disorder usually stabilizes, although it may come to involve both arms. Motor neuron disease (amyotrophic lateral sclerosis [ALS]) can begin in one arm and progress to involve all four extremities.

Lesions of the brachial plexus can produce severe paralysis. Obvious causes include gunshot wounds, lacerations, trauma involving stretch of the arm over the head, and surgical procedures. Complications of delivery include traction on the upper (*Erb's palsy*) and lower (*Klumpke's palsy*) portions of the brachial plexus. Infiltrative tumors are perhaps the most common cause of brachial plexus lesions. The mysterious entity of idiopathic brachial plexus neuropathy (or brachial plexitis) can produce a flaccid arm. A proximal lesion produces winging of the scapula and loss of pinprick sensation over the back. A high cervical proximal lesion produces paralysis of the diaphragm while involvement of the C8 or T1 nerves may cause Horner's syndrome. Mononeuropathies and monoradiculopathies of the upper limb are easily diagnosed by the pattern of sensory loss and by the involvement of muscles innervated by a specific nerve or root.

Illustrative Case History of Upper Limb Monoplegia

A 61-year-old man with severe vasculopathy due to diabetes mellitus underwent amputation of a gangrenous foot. Two days after the surgery, the patient awoke with a profound weakness of his right hand. When he held his arms to the front, the right hand dangled helplessly at the wrist. His surgeon thought this was radial nerve palsy. The neurological consultant found that all of the intrinsic muscles of the hand were paralyzed and the patient could move the hand at the wrist only with the greatest difficulty. The biceps and triceps muscles were slightly weak; all the shoulder muscles were strong. The sensory examination and the entire remainder of the neurological examination were normal. Deep tendon reflexes including finger flexion reflexes were normal throughout. The patient was too weak to allow testing of the Wartenberg thumb sign. The weak hand seemed flaccid except for a hint of increased muscle tone in the fingers. Since the weakness involved muscles innervated by all the major nerves of the forearm, the neurologist diagnosed a small acute brain infarction in the central portion of the motor gyrus. The electromyogram and cranial computed tomographic (CT) scan were normal. Two months later the patient thought that his strength had returned to normal but his hand was awkward in movements. Examination showed only the slightest weakness of the intrinsic muscles of the right hand; a Wartenberg's thumb sign was now present. The CT scan remained normal.

Lower Limb Monoparesis

The patient with a weak leg, but with normal strength in arm and face, may have suffered a lesion in the medial (parasagittal) portion of the cerebral hemisphere. The most common cause of lower limb monoparesis is an infarction in the distribution of the anterior cerebral artery territory (Bogousslavsky and Regli 1990). Occlusion of small penetrating branches of the basilar artery can also produce weakness in one leg; bilateral Babinski's signs are often present. Ischemia of the area between the middle and anterior cerebral arteries, the so-called watershed infarct, can produce weakness of the opposite leg. Rolandic vein thrombosis may produce intermittent leg weakness and cortical sensory loss: Sometimes the leg, hip, and shoulder are profoundly weak while the face and arm are spared. Spinal hemisection below the cervical enlargement produces weakness of the ipsilateral and sensory loss in the contralateral leg (Brown-Séquard's syndrome). This lesion can follow trauma or be due to tumor or multiple sclerosis. Painless and progressive footdrop, even unilateral, raises the suspicion of ALS. More proximal weakness is usually also present and careful examination may reveal fasciculations. Lower motor neuron lesions that produce leg weakness include lumbar radiculopathy, lumbosacral plexopathy, and mononeuropathies of the sciatic or peroneal nerves. Electromyography discloses signs of denervation in these conditions.

Figure 27.3 presents a patient with a monoparesis of the leg. This 49-year-old man with cutaneous evidence of neurofibromatosis developed progressive weakness of the right leg. Atrophy of the right leg was visible. Knee and ankle tendon reflexes were increased on the right and a Babinski's sign was present. The magnetic resonance image of the brain showed a lesion, probably an arteriovenous malformation, involving the medial portion of the precentral gyrus.

PARTICULAR TYPES OF HEMIPLEGIA

Hemiplegia in Children and Infants

In his remarkable monograph *Hemiplegia in Children*, Sigmund Freud noted that hemiplegia not infrequently afflicts infants and children. Acute cerebral hemispheric infarction in an infant produces weakness of the contralateral arm and leg but never involves the face, because the corticobulbar fibers from the precentral gyrus to the facial nucleus in the pons have not yet developed. This phenomenon can produce unusual findings when the patient becomes an adult.

Illustrative Case History

At the age of 1 year, a male infant experienced the sudden onset of left arm and leg weakness, but his face was spared. No cause was determined, but a marked improvement in the weakness gradually occurred. The patient developed normally and completed 2 years of college. At the age of 32, the patient was suddenly afflicted by paralysis of the mouth and tongue. He was unable to talk but could communicate fully by writing. He weakly wrinkled his forehead and could barely open his eyes against resistance. His mouth drooped and he drooled continuously. Although he was unable to move the corners of his mouth on command, the patient responded to a humorous joke with a vigorous smile. The tongue lay in the midline of the mouth and could not be voluntarily moved. The patient had normal strength of his arms and legs. Deep tendon reflexes were brisk but symmetrical. A Babinski's sign was present on the left. Imaging studies showed an abscess located in the central region of the precentral gyrus on the right. This was treated medically with intravenous antibiotics. The patient recovered completely and the abscess disappeared on subsequent imaging studies.

In this patient, because of an infantile right cerebral infarct, the central portion of the left motor cortex provided the corticobulbar tract to both facial nuclei. Therefore, when this area was involved by a focal lesion (a cerebral abscess), both facial nuclei lost their voluntary input and the patient was unable to initiate voluntary movements of the bulbar musculature. Limbic input was not involved so

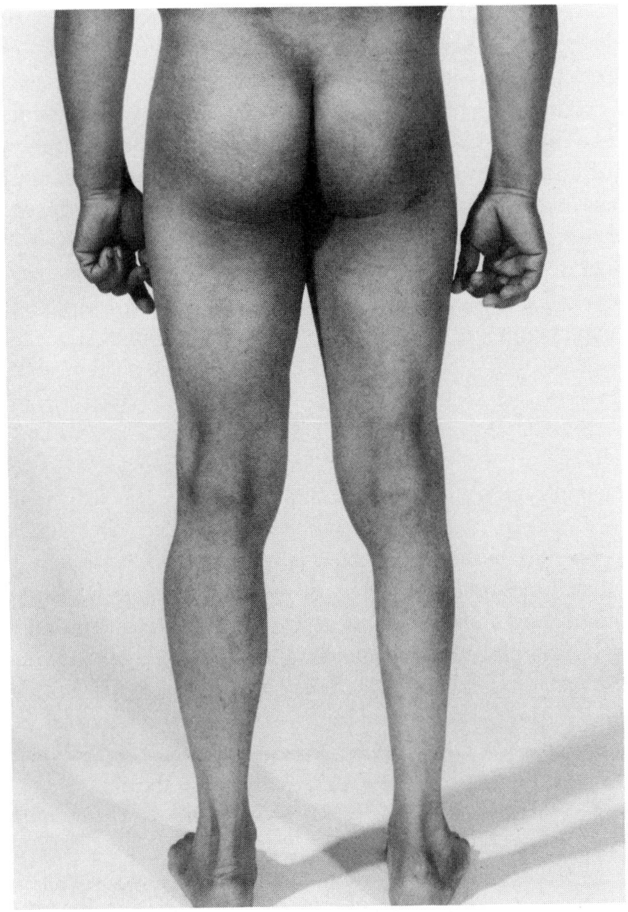

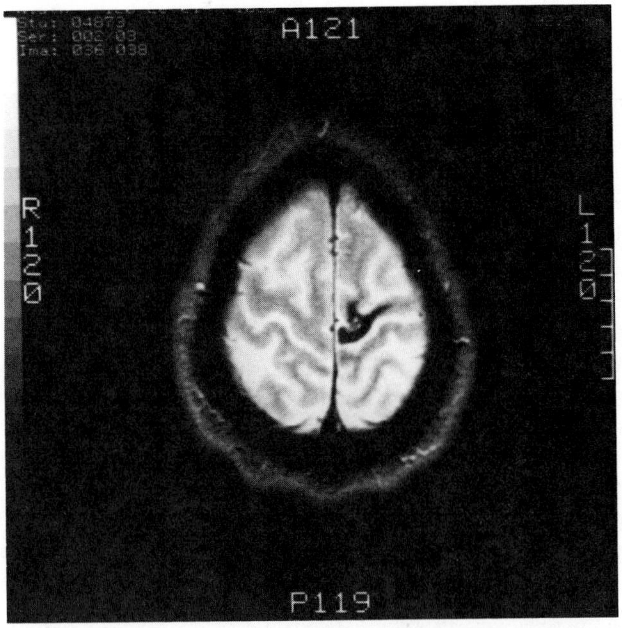

FIGURE 27.3 A patient with atrophy and weakness of the right leg. The magnetic resonance imaging study shows a small lesion, presumably an arteriovenous malformation, involving the medial portion of the precentral gyrus. (Patient of Dr. David Goldblatt.)

that involuntary or emotional facial movements were retained. The usual innervation from the right hemisphere had never developed because of the stroke in infancy.

Hypoglycemic Hemiplegia

Occasionally, a patient is encountered who develops hemiplegia, always on the same side, whenever the blood sugar falls to a low level. Such patients always have preexisting brain damage in a focal distribution, usually in one hemisphere. When the blood sugar falls, all brain cells become slightly dysfunctional, but those areas of the brain that have been previously damaged become symptomatic; the degree of hypoglycemia that brings out focal symptomatology depends on the degree of underlying damage.

Illustrative Case History

A 55-year-old diabetic man was hospitalized for adjustment of his insulin dosage. He had suffered an acute brain infarction in the right hemisphere the previous year but was thought to have recovered completely. On the morning after admission, the patient awoke with a dense left hemiplegia, involving the face, arm, and leg, but without any other signs. His blood glucose level was measured and the patient was given glucose intravenously in a bolus injection. The hemiplegia disappeared completely within 30 seconds. His examination was then normal. The blood glucose level at the time of the recurrent hemiplegia was 30 mg/100 ml, revealing a serious hypoglycemia. The insulin dosage was reduced, but two further similar events occurred until the correct dosage was achieved.

Ataxic Hemiparesis

Very frequently, a patient with a mild or moderate hemiparesis has an associated awkwardness. In some cases this apparent ataxia is actually due to weakness. In others, the damage that produced the hemiplegia also causes dysfunction of the cerebellocerebral system as shown graphically in Figure 27.2. Output from the cerebellum courses through the superior cerebellar peduncle, across the midline, through the red nucleus, to the ventral anterior thalamus, then to the frontal granular cortex. The circuit is then completed by frontopontine fibers passing from the cortex, through the anterior limb of the internal capsule to the nuclei of the basis pontis, then across the midline, entering the cerebellum through the middle cerebellar peduncle. Landau (1988) has carefully analyzed the anatomical and physiological basis of hemiparesis with and without awkwardness and has concluded that the concept of ataxic hemiparesis has no special localizing or clinical value.

Pure Motor Hemiplegia

The concept of pure motor hemiplegia refers to paralysis without any associated signs or symptoms—that is, without sensory loss, without visual field abnormality, and without psychological or speech dysfunction. Facial paralysis may or may not be present with the hemiplegia. Descending motor pathways can be damaged in many regions of the brain and spinal cord to produce pure motor findings, but the most common sites are the posterior limb of the internal capsule and the paramedian pons (Nighoghossian et al. 1993). The underlying lesion in the patient with pure motor hemiplegia is usually a small infarct.

Some people speak of a lacunar hemiparesis; however, it is not good to mix pathological and clinical terms. A small vascular lesion can cause hemiplegia, particularly pure motor hemiplegia. One should note that the radiological or pathological picture of a lacuna takes weeks to months to develop. Therefore, if a patient has the sudden onset of a pure motor hemiplegia, and if the imaging study shows one or more lacunae, one can tentatively conclude that the hemiplegia is due to a new vascular lesion of a lacunar nature, not yet visualized.

Hysterical or Functional Hemiplegia

Hysteria is a term with a specific psychiatric definition. Hysterical hemiparesis is a weakness of the arm and leg that is not due to any organic disease. In the absence of the specific features of hysteria, the term *functional hemiplegia* is preferred since it does not presume whether the defect is voluntary or involuntary. The diagnosis is made on the basis of important items from the history and from the examination. Several specific findings have been recommended as valuable in the diagnosis of functional hemiplegia; I think they are often more confusing than helpful.

Some observers think that the hemihypesthesia that often accompanies functional hemiplegia is characteristic in that the change from the hypesthetic to normal sensation occurs exactly at the midline. In "real" hemihypesthesia, the change occurs 1–2 cm before the midline on the abnormal side because of the crossover of superficial nerves. However, many patients with hemihypesthesia due to damage to the spinothalamic tract report the change from decreased to normal pinprick sensation exactly at the midline of body and face. I have found valuable a "surprise" hemihypesthesia; the patient with the hysterical hemiplegia reports no abnormal sensory feelings but when formally tested a hemihypesthesia appears. The patient who suffers a true decrease of pinprick sensation over one-half of the body and face usually knows about this before formal testing.

A physical finding that is sometimes erroneously advanced as an aid in the diagnosis of functional hemiplegia is weakness of head turning. If a patient with right hemiparesis has weakness turning the head to the right, the young clinician may claim that the hemiplegia is not due to organic illness, since the left sternocleidomastoid muscle is contracted when the head turns to the right. However, weakness of the right side of the body does not cause a weakness of turning the head to the left. The clinician must remember the dictum of Hughlings Jackson that the higher motor centers are organized in terms of movements, not in terms of muscles. Cortical damage produces weakness of head turning away from the side of the lesion (weakness of the ipsilateral sternocleidomastoid muscle). This is not a sign of hysterical hemiplegia.

One special motor examination that helps in the diagnosis of functional hemiplegia is the Hoover sign. With the patient supine, the examiner places one hand below the heel and then instructs the patient to raise the other leg against the examiner's pressure. The patient who is truly hemiplegic will have difficulty with this maneuver bilaterally because it requires the contraction of muscles of both legs; one leg pushes down while the other is raised. The patient with a functional hemiplegia will be unable to raise the paretic leg, but the examiner will feel no downward pressure from the normal leg. When the strength of the normal leg is tested, the downward pressure from the paretic leg will be quite strong.

Needless to say, functional hemiplegia is not associated with any of the objective findings that usually accompany brain lesions: facial weakness, unilateral hyperreflexia, absence of abdominal and cremasteric reflexes, Babinski's sign, and decreased corneal reflex. Inconsistency of the weakness can usually be detected by methodical examination. For example, the patient may be able to walk on the toes, yet during formal testing the examiner overcomes flexion at the ankle with the slightest pressure. A careful examination that gauges strength in different situations is more important in differentiating organic from functional hemiparesis than any special examination tricks.

Illustrative Case History

A 40-year-old deputy sheriff presented to the emergency room because of the inability to use his right arm. His arm was flexed on his chest and he walked with a right-sided limp. When formally tested, all muscles of the right arm and right leg were totally without power. The patient related that 2 days prior to the onset of the hemiplegia, he had shot and killed a burglar. The psychiatric consultant hypothesized that the sheriff was unable to deal with two conflicting emotions: joy that he had terminated a criminal and guilt that he had killed a fellow human being. His shooting hand and arm had become paralyzed so that he would never again be faced with the decision to shoot someone. The patient changed his job, underwent psychotherapy, and the hemiplegia disappeared.

Todd's Paralysis

Pronounced hemiparesis occasionally follows focal seizure activity involving the same side of the body. This postictal or *Todd's paralysis* is often associated with numbness of the limbs, and if the seizure discharge involves the dominant hemisphere, with aphasia. This transient neurological dysfunction is probably due to exhaustion of all energy stores within that portion of the brain that has been involved in the repetitive depolarization and repolarization associated with continuous seizure activity. Poor blood flow to the region of seizure discharge exacerbates energy depletion. Strength usually returns to normal in a very short time.

A rare patient may experience episodes of hemiplegia associated with the simultaneous electroencephalographic recording of epileptiform activity over the central portion of the opposite hemisphere. This may represent some form of inhibitory seizure discharge.

An especially difficult clinical problem is the patient who presents to the emergency room with a new hemiplegia and who has a known cerebral lesion that produces seizures. Is the hemiplegia due to postictal exhaustion (Todd's paralysis), to ongoing inhibitory seizure discharges, or to an enlargement or worsening of the underlying lesion? A very careful history relating seizure activity to the onset of the hemiparesis may help evaluate Todd's paralysis; an electroencephalogram recorded during the hemiparesis may rule out inhibitory seizure discharge; an imaging study of the brain can be compared with a previous study to evaluate worsening of the underlying lesion. This situation, like so many instances of hemiparesis and monoparesis, requires careful evaluation and mature clinical judgment.

REFERENCES

Bogousslavsky J, Regli F. Anterior cerebral artery territory infarction in the Lausanne stroke registry: clinical and etiologic patterns. Arch Neurol 1990;47:144–150.

Boiten J, Lodder J. Isolated monoparesis is usually caused by superficial infarction. Cerebrovasc Dis 1991;1:337–340.

Davidoff RA. The pyramidal tract. Neurology 1990;40:332–339.

Hopf HC, Muller-Forell W, Hopf NJ. Localization of emotional and volitional facial paresis. Neurology 1992;42:1918–1923.

Jenny AB, Saper CB. Organization of the facial nucleus and corticofacial projection in the monkey: a reconsideration of the upper motor neuron facial palsy. Neurology 1987;37:930–939.

Landau WM. Ataxic hemiparesis: special deluxe stroke or standard brand? Neurology 1988;38:1799–1801.

Nighoghossian N, Ryvlin P, Trouillas P et al. Pontine versus capsular pure motor hemiparesis. Neurology 1993;43:2197–2201.

Chapter 28
Paraplegia and Spinal Cord Syndromes

Thomas N. Byrne and Stephen G. Waxman

The clinical presentations of spinal cord disease are diverse. Patients may present with vague numbness or weakness. Alternatively, their first complaint can be pain without neurological signs, which may be incorrectly attributed to musculoskeletal disease or visceral pathology. The protean manifestations may mislead even the most astute clinician. Since it is essential to evaluate and treat patients with spinal cord disease expeditiously, a thorough understanding of its clinical manifestations, as well as those of the non-neurological diseases that may mimic spinal disease, is necessary. The purpose of this chapter is to provide an understanding of the clinical pathophysiology of the spinal cord and to demonstrate methods of history-taking and physical examination helpful in assessing the patient suspected of harboring spinal disease.

The localization of spinal cord pathology is described by the following anatomical coordinates: (1) the "level" in the rostrocaudal axis, and (2) the extent, in the transverse plane, of spinal cord involvement. These coordinates are determined by clinically assessing neurological functions served by both nerve roots and tracts. The time course of evolution of spinal cord dysfunction is the third coordinate and is often important in predicting the etiology and the physiological response of the cord to injury and determining prognosis (Byrne and Waxman 1990).

SEGMENTAL INNERVATION

Ventral Root Dysfunction

Ventral root dysfunction is usually manifested by characteristic motor disturbances that are quite distinct from those arising from corticospinal tract disease or from plexus or peripheral nerve disease. Important aspects of the physical examination are the assessment of muscle strength, tone, and bulk. The pattern of weakness is often the most important physical finding that distinguishes root disease from peripheral nerve disease.

Muscle strength or power may be determined by individual muscle testing or by functional assessment. Since each muscle is usually innervated by multiple roots, lower motor neuron paralysis of a muscle or muscle group typically signifies plexus or peripheral nerve disease rather than a monoradiculopathy. Despite this fact, with a monoradiculopathy a single muscle often suffers greater dysfunction than others. Such muscles have been termed "segment-pointer" muscles. Table 28.1 lists a group of muscles that may "point" the examiner to a specific nerve root (Schliack 1969). This listing, however, should not be considered infallible, since some individuals have prefixed or postfixed plexuses.

Some common causes of muscular atrophy are disuse, endocrinological disturbance, malnutrition, and denervation (*neurogenic atrophy*). Neurogenic atrophy develops in cases of radiculopathy. With a monoradiculopathy, however, the atrophy is not as prominent as that occurring with peripheral nerve injury since most muscles receive innervation from multiple nerve roots. In cases of chronic radiculopathy, such as that due to cervical spondylosis, atrophy may precede weakness. Alternatively, in cases of acute radiculopathy, due, for instance, to acute disc herniation, weakness may precede atrophy. Neurogenic atrophy may be associated with *fasciculations*, which represent spontaneous contraction of a group of muscle fibers innervated by a single motor neuron (a motor unit). They are usually seen as a rippling movement just beneath the skin. Fatigue, cold, medications, and metabolic derangements often cause similar movements. Fasciculations are commonly seen in motor neuron disease. In cases of compressive root lesions, fasciculations may be restricted to the myotomal distribution of the compressed root. These fasciculations are different than those seen in anterior horn cell disease in that they occur repetitively in the same fasciculus during minimal contraction and are absent during complete rest. *Benign fasciculations* typically occur only after contraction of the muscle and are not associated with weakness or atrophy.

Muscle tone is often a very valuable sign in distinguishing the site of a lesion causing weakness. When measuring muscle tone it is important that the muscles be relaxed, and it is often helpful to distract the patient's attention. In cases of radiculopathy, muscle tone is either not affected or tone is decreased unless there is muscle spasm, as often occurs with pain. Alternatively, *spasticity* and *rigidity* refer to common forms of increased muscle tone due to central nervous system disease. In spasticity, the increased tone is due to an exaggeration of the stretch reflex. Consequently, if the muscle is slowly stretched, tone may be normal; however, if the muscle is stretched more rapidly, increasing amounts of resistance are found. Spasticity has been referred to as rate-sensitive for this reason. Spasticity (and the weakness associated with it) preferentially involves the flexors in the upper extremities and extensors in the lower extremities, whether due to cortical or corticospinal tract disease. Spasticity usually results from dysfunction of the descending tracts, including the corticospinal tract (Ditunno and Formal 1994).

Rigidity, commonly due to extrapyramidal disease or a side effect of antidopaminergic drugs, refers to increased muscle tone, which does not depend on the rate of movement. Unlike spasticity it is found equally in both extensors and flexors.

Table 28.1: Segment-pointer muscles

Root	*Muscle*	*Primary Function*
C3	Diaphragm	Respiration
C4	Diaphragm	Respiration
C5	Deltoid	Arm abduction
C5	Biceps	Forearm flexion
C6	Brachioradialis	Forearm flexion
C7	Triceps	Forearm extension
L3	Quadriceps femoris	Knee extension
L4	Quadriceps femoris	Knee extension
L4	Tibialis anterior	Foot dorsiflexion
L5	Extensor hallucis longus	Great toe dorsiflexion
S1	Gastrocnemius	Plantar flexion

Source: Adapted from H Schliack. Segmental Innervation and the Clinical Aspects of Spinal Nerve Root Syndromes. In PJ Vinken, GW Bruyn (eds), Handbook of Clinical Neurology. Vol. 2. Amsterdam: North-Holland Publishing, 1969:157–177.

Dorsal Root Dysfunction

Disturbance of dorsal root function most commonly produces pain and, to a lesser extent, sensory impairment. The pain may be local or projected elsewhere in a radicular or nonradicular distribution.

Pain

Local Pain. Local or regional back or neck pain is usually secondary to irritation or damage of innervated structures of the spine. The periosteum, ligaments, dura, and apophyseal joints are innervated structures. The clinical characteristics of local pain are that it is appreciated in the region of the spine and that it is deep, aching, and exacerbated by activity that places an increased load on the diseased structures. Patients suffering from pain due to epidural tumor often report that their pain is made worse by the supine position, whereas those suffering from spondylosis and musculoligamentous strain generally favor bed rest (Byrne 1992).

Palpation or percussion of the involved structures may exacerbate the local pain regardless of the cause. In addition to irritation of local innervated structures, muscle spasm often causes local pain. Such pain is usually diffuse and aching, and spasm may be palpable.

Projected Pain. *Projected pain* is pain that arises from one anatomical site but is projected to a site some distance from the location of the pathology. When the spine is the source of projected pain, it may be either radicular or nonradicular in nature. Projected pain that arises from irritation of posterior nerve roots is of a radicular type, whereas that due to irritation of other spinal structures is usually of a nonradicular type, herein termed *referred pain.* Although these forms of pain are not always easy to differentiate, it is important to distinguish between them since radicular pain has strong localizing value whereas nonradicular pain does not.

Referred Pain. McCall and associates (1979) studied the pattern of pain referral in normal volunteers after injection of 6% saline into the apophyseal joints of L1–2 and L4–5. The pain was cramping and aching in quality. As shown in Figure 28.1, there was overlap in the regions of pain referral from upper and lower lumbar injections with most of the pain being referred to the flanks, buttocks, groins, and thighs. It is of clinical interest that referred pain did not project below the knee despite the fact that the L4–5 level was stimulated. These investigators concluded that unlike radicular pain, referred pain does not follow segmental dermatomes and is not helpful in localization.

Although there may be paresthesias in the cutaneous area of pain referral, as well as tenderness to deep palpation of the muscles, there are no neurological abnormalities found in cases of referred pain of nonradicular origin. This situation is in contrast to cases of radicular pain, where disturbance of the nerve root may often be present in the form of sensory loss, hyporeflexia, ventral root dysfunction, or a combination of these. Referred pain is generally aggravated and relieved by the same maneuvers that alter local pain.

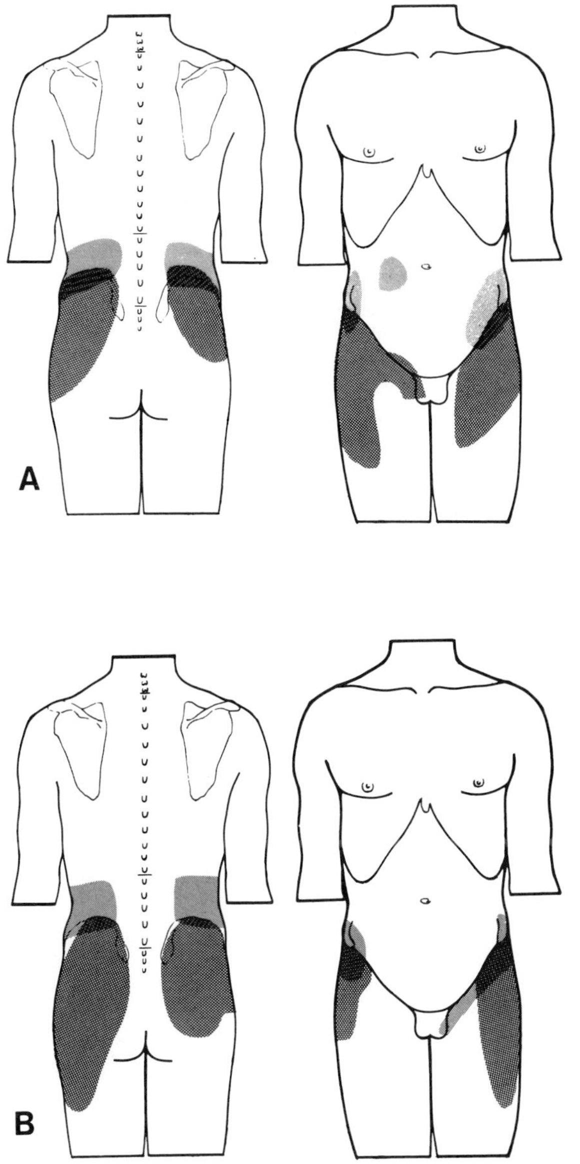

FIGURE 28.1 Patterns of referred pain. The distributions of pain referral from L1–2 (diagonal lines) and L4–5 (crosshatching) are superimposed following intracapsular (A) and pericapsular (B) injections of 6% saline into the apophysial joints. Overlap of the patterns is shown in the region of the iliac crest and the groin. (Reprinted with permission from IW McCall, WM Park, JP O'Brien. Induced pain referral from posterior lumbar elements in normal subjects. Spine 1979;4:441–446.)

Radicular Pain. Radicular pain, which has great localizing value, arises from irritation of dorsal roots, with pain being projected to the dermatome of the nerve root. Tables 28.2 and 28.3 list the differential diagnosis of lesions of the cervical and lumbrosacral nerve roots and the common sites to which pain of radicular origin is projected.

Radicular pain often has a sharp stabbing quality. Maneuvers that stretch or further compress the nerve root, such as Valsalva maneuver, coughing, straight leg raising, and neck flexion, generally aggravate the pain. The patient may avoid certain activities and postures that place further stretch on the nerve. For example, in the case of sciatica (pain in the distribution of the sciatic nerve) due to a compressive L5 radiculopathy, the patient may maintain the leg in a flexed posture at the hip and knee and plantar flex the foot. Such a posture may result in a rather characteristic gait. Cutaneous paresthesias and tenderness of tissues in the region of pain projection are common. However, in radicular pain, unlike referred pain, there may be sensory disturbances and, at times, reflex and motor abnormalities corresponding to the injured nerve root.

Sensory Disturbances: Dermatomes

A knowledge of the dermatomal map is very valuable in recognizing and localizing radicular syndromes. Figure 28.2 illustrates a currently recognized dermatomal map that has considerable clinical value. A few points deserve emphasis:

1. On the trunk the C4 and T2 dermatomes are contiguous.
2. The thumb, middle finger, and fifth digits are innervated by C6, C7, and C8, respectively.
3. The nipple is at the level of T4.
4. The umbilicus is at the T10 level.
5. In the posterior axial line of the leg (medial thigh) the lumbar and sacral dermatomes are contiguous.

Finally, it should be recognized that there are variations in dermatomal maps between individuals that may make problematic clinical conclusions based on sensory testing alone.

Deep Tendon Reflexes

In addition to motor and sensory disturbances, deep tendon reflex abnormalities can be of precise localizing value. When deep tendon reflexes are segmentally hypoactive, they can be very sensitive indicators of specific root disturbance. When they are hyperactive below a specific spinal level, they may indicate a myelopathy at or above that level.

The combination of hypoactive reflexes at a segmental level with hyperactive reflexes caudal to that level is commonly found with cervical spine disease. For example, cervical spondylosis may cause hyporeflexia of the biceps, brachioradialis, or triceps due to impingement on C5, C6, or C7 roots, respectively, and hyperreflexia below this level secondary to an associated myelopathy. At times, attempts to elicit the brachioradialis reflex produce no direct response but paradoxically cause contraction of the finger flexors rather than flexion and supination of the hand. Such a response is called *inversion of the radial reflex*.

Nerve Root Versus Peripheral Nerve Lesion

Monoradiculopathies rarely cause paralysis of a single muscle or muscle group. Alternatively, with peripheral nerve dis-

Table 28.2: Differential diagnosis of lesions of the cervical nerve roots

Roots	*C5*	*C6*	*C7*	*C8*	*T1*
Sensory supply	Lateral border upper arm	Lateral forearm including thumb	Over triceps, midforearm, and middle finger	Medial forearm to include little finger	Axilla down to the olecranon
Sensory loss	As above	As above	Middle fingers	As above	As above
Area of pain	As above, and thumb and index finger	As above, especially thumb and index finger	As above, and medial scapula border	As above	Deep aching in shoulder and axilla to olecranon
Reflex arc	Biceps jerk	Supinator jerk	Triceps jerk	Finger jerk	None
Motor deficit	Deltoid Supraspinatus Infraspinatus Rhomboids	Biceps Brachioradialis Brachialis (pronators and supinators of forearm)	Latissimus dorsi Pectoralis major Triceps Wrist extensors Wrist flexors	Finger flexors Finger extensors Flexor carpi ulinaris (thenar muscles in some patients)	*All* small hand muscles (in some thenar muscles via C8)
Some causative lesions	Brachial neuritis Cervical spondylosis Upper plexus avulsion	Cervical spondylosis Acute disc lesions	Acute disc lesions Cervical spondylosis	Rare in disc lesions or spondylosis	Cervical rib Thoracic outlet syndromes Pancoast tumor Metastatic carcinoma in deep cervical nodes

Source: Adapted from J Patten. Neurological Differential Diagnosis. New York: Springer-Verlag, 1977.

Table 28.3: Differential diagnosis of lesions of the lumbosacral nerve roots

Roots	*L2*	*L3*	*L4*	*L5*	*S1*
Sensory supply	Across upper thigh	Across lower thigh	Across knee to medial malleolus	Side of leg to dorsum and sole of foot	Behind lateral malleolus to lateral foot
Sensory loss	Often none	Often none	Medial leg	Dorsum of foot	Behind lateral malleolus
Area of pain	Across thigh	Across thigh	Down to medial malleolus	Back of thigh, lateral calf, dorsum of foot	Back of thigh, back of calf, lateral foot
Reflex arc	None	Adductor reflex	Knee jerk	None	Ankle jerk
Motor deficit	Hip flexion	Knee extension	Inversion of the foot	Dorsiflexion of toes and foot (latter L4 also)	Plantar flexion and eversion of foot
Some causative lesions	Neurofibroma Meningioma Metastasis Intervertebral disk prolapse Lumbar canal stenosis Ependymoma Lesions associated with spinal dysraphism				

Source: Adapted from J Patten. Neurological Differential Diagnosis. New York: Springer-Verlag, 1977.

ease, it is common for paralysis of such muscle groups to occur. A knowledge of innervation of muscle groups is important in making the distinction. The sensory examination may be very helpful in distinguishing peripheral nerve lesions from radiculopathies. Finally, autonomic disturbances may be valuable in distinguishing peripheral nerve lesions from root disturbances. Ordinarily, monoradiculopathies are not associated with autonomic disturbances such as sweat loss, whereas peripheral nerve injuries frequently are associated with autonomic complaints. Tables 28.2 through 28.5 review the locations of sensory loss, projected pain, reflex loss, motor deficit, and some causative lesions of the more common radiculopathies and peripheral neuropathies.

LOCALIZATION OF LESIONS IN THE TRANSVERSE PLANE

Motor Disorders

As mentioned above, the findings of lower motor neuron dysfunction are weakness associated with atrophy, hypoto-

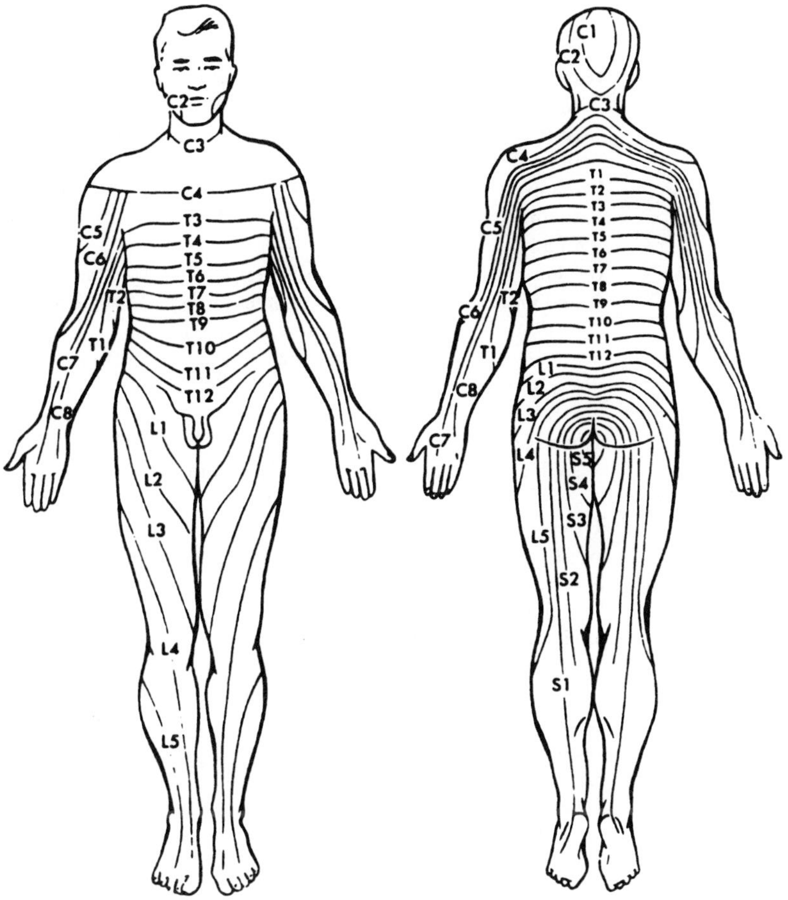

FIGURE 28.2 A dermatomal map. (Reprinted with permission from W Haymaker. Bing's Local Diagnosis in Neurological Disease [15th ed]. St. Louis: Mosby, 1969:57–59.)

nia, fasciculations, and depressed reflexes. In contrast, corticospinal tract disease often manifests with spasticity, hyperreflexia, and Babinski's sign (note the exception of spinal shock), as well as weakness that usually involves more than a single extremity. In cervical spine disease, one may find a combination of lower motor neuron disturbance involving the upper extremity and upper motor neuron findings in one or both lower extremities.

Perhaps the most important clue suggesting a spinal origin to weakness is the pattern of weakness. Hemiparesis involving the face, arm, and leg usually localizes the problem to the brain. Proximal muscle weakness of the arms and legs with intact sensation and normal deep tendon reflexes direct the examiner to myopathic disorders. When the pattern is distal and associated with stocking-glove sensory loss and decreased deep tendon reflexes, peripheral neuropathies are considered. In patients with paraparesis or quadriparesis, the examiner is usually directed to the spinal cord. Monoparesis creates the greatest diagnostic confusion. Early in the development of spinal cord disease, the patient may present with unilateral leg weakness, and examination may not reveal findings in the contralateral leg or the arms.

Lesions of the craniocervical junction and cervical spine often present with a pattern of unilateral arm weakness before progressing to ipsilateral leg weakness, and then contralateral involvement (Byrne and Waxman 1990). However, although weakness involving an ipsilateral arm and leg with sparing of the face suggests a high cervical lesion, it should be recognized that cerebral disturbances or medullary pyramidal infarction may account for this localization (Ropper and Poskanzer 1978).

The Babinski response, or upgoing toe, is a sign of corticospinal tract disease. Plantar stimulation is therefore tested in patients with leg weakness in an attempt to differentiate upper motor neuron causes from other etiologies.

Sensory Disturbances

Subjective sensory complaints generally precede objective sensory signs and therefore sensory complaints without abnormal sensory signs may be the first sign of serious underlying neurologic disease. One corollary is that in the absence of sensory complaints, the sensory examination is usually normal.

Dysfunction of the dorsal (or posterior) columns and of the lateral spinothalamic pathways usually causes different characteristic symptoms. Tingling paresthesias, which may be vibratory in nature, are sometimes reported below the level of a dorsal column lesion. Subjective reports of the skin

Table 28.4: Differential diagnosis of lesions of upper-limb peripheral nerves

Nerves	*Axillary*	*Musculocutaneous*	*Radial*	*Median*	*Ulnar*
Sensory supply	Over deltoid	Lateral forearm to wrist	Lateral dorsal forearm and back of thumb and index finger	Lateral palm and lateral fingers	Medial palm and 5th and medial half ring finger
Sensory loss	Small area over deltoid	Lateral forearm	Dorsum of thumb and index (if any)	As above	As above but often none at all
Area of pain	Across shoulder tip	Lateral forearm	Dorsum of thumb and index	Thumb, index, and middle finger Often spreads up forearm	Ulnar-supplied fingers and palm distal to wrist Pain occasionally along course of nerve
Reflex arc	Nil	Biceps jerk	Triceps jerk and supinator jerk	Finger jerks (flexor digitorum sublimis)	Nil
Motor deficit	Deltoid (teres minor cannot be evaluated)	Biceps Brachialis (coracobrachialis weakness not detectable)	Triceps Wrist extensors Finger extensors Brachioradialis Supinator of forearm	Wrist flexors Long finger flexors (thumb, index, and middle finger) Pronators of forearm Abductor pollicis brevis	All small hand muscles excluding abductor pollicis brevis Flexor carpi ulnaris Long flexors of ring and little finger
Some causative lesions	Fractured neck of humerus Dislocated shoulder Deep IM injections	Very rarely damaged	Crutch palsy Saturday night palsy Fractured humerus In supinator muscle	Carpal tunnel syndrome Direct trauma to wrist	Elbow: trauma, bed rest, fractured olecranon Wrist: local trauma, ganglion of wrist joint

Source: Reprinted with permission from J Patten. Neurological Differential Diagnosis. New York: Springer-Verlag, 1977.

being "too tight" or an extremity or trunk being "wrapped in bandages" may also be due to dorsal column disturbances. Spinothalamic tract disturbance is often first manifest by poorly characterized and localized pain. It should be recognized that many of the complaints of patients with intramedullary lesions are not associated with any abnormal signs early in their course, so that the complaints may be inappropriately dismissed after a negative sensory examination.

Pain sensation, usually measured by pinprick, and temperature sensation are conveyed via the lateral spinothalamic tract. These pathways are somatotopically organized so that the sacral fibers are most peripheral and the cervical fibers are most central. Since a laterally placed extramedullary lesion will compress the peripheral fibers before the more centrally located fibers, a compressive lesion in the rostral spine may give rise to an apparently ascending loss of pain and temperature sensation. These findings underscore the importance of recognizing that *a rostral lesion may give rise to a sensory level far below the site of the compression.* In practical terms, therefore, when spinal cord compression is suspected one may need to image the entire spine rostral to the sensory level to exclude a lesion above the sensory level.

Position and vibration sensation are transmitted through the posterior columns and are generally very easily evaluated. Ataxia due to spinal lesions is not as readily recognized. Disturbances of posterior columns or possibly the spinocerebellar tracts may result in an ataxic gait. This may be particularly evident in vitamin B_{12} deficiency. Light touch is conveyed by both lateral and posterior columns and is usually not impaired as early in spinal cord disease as the more specific modalities described above.

Several incomplete lesions of the spinal cord result in characteristic sensory signs. A hemisection of the spinal cord results in the *Brown-Séquard syndrome*, in which there is loss of appreciation of pain and temperature contralateral to the lesion and loss of sensation for position and vibration and upper motor neuron paralysis ipsilateral to the lesion (Figure 28.3).

An early intramedullary lesion such as a syrinx, intramedullary tumor, or contusion may give rise to a *dissociated sensory loss* in which the decussating fibers at the level, mediating sensation of pain and temperature, are lost or decreased, whereas the position and vibratory sensibilities remain unimpaired. Central cord lesions may also result in a *suspended sensory level* (see Figure 28.3). In such cases, sacral sensation is preserved until late in the course since these fibers are most peripheral in the lateral spinothalamic tracts and they tend to be involved later.

Table 28.5: Differential diagnosis of lesions of lower-limb peripheral nerves

Nerves	Obturator	Femoral	Sciatic Nerve: Peroneal Division	Sciatic Nerve: Tibial Division
Sensory supply	Medial surface of thigh	Anteromedial surface of thigh and leg to medial malleolus	Anterior leg, dorsum of ankle and foot	Posterior leg, sole, and lateral border of foot
Sensory loss	Often none	Usually anatomical	Often just dorsum of foot	Sole of foot
Area of pain	Medial thigh	Anterior thigh and medial leg	Often painless	Often painless
Reflex arc	Adductor reflex	Knee jerk	None	Ankle jerk
Motor deficit	Adduction of thigh	Extension of knee	Dorsiflexion, inversion and eversion of the foot (+lateral hamstrings)	Plantar flexion and inversion of foot (+medial hamstrings)
Some causative lesions	Pelvic neoplasm Pregnancy	Diabetes Femoral hernia Femoral artery aneurysm Posterior abdominal neoplasm Psoas abscess	Pressure palsy at fibula neck Hip fracture or dislocation Penetrating trauma to buttock Misplaced injection	Very rarely injured even in buttock Peroneal division more sensitive to damage

Source: Reprinted with permission from J Patten. Neurological Differential Diagnosis. New York: Springer-Verlag, 1977.

Autonomic and Respiratory Disturbances

Dysfunction of the spinal cord and cauda equina are often manifested as symptoms and signs of bladder, bowel, and sexual dysfunction. A high cervical cord lesion may cause respiratory compromise.

Although the diaphragm, intercostal muscles, and abdominal muscles are used for normal respiration, individuals may ventilate adequately with only the diaphragm intact (see Table 28.1). In cases of complete cord transection above C3, respiration cannot be maintained. Trauma, foramen magnum tumors, atlantoaxial dislocation, and congenital disturbances of the craniocervical junction are frequent causes of upper cervical spine injury.

The urinary bladder is innervated by (1) sympathetic nerves beginning in the intermediolateral cell column at the lumbar level (primarily L1 and L2); (2) parasympathetic nerves exiting at S2–S4; and (3) somatic efferent nerves to the skeletal muscles of the external urethral sphincter exiting at S2–S4 to form the pudendal nerves. In complete transverse lesions of the cord, the bladder immediately becomes flaccid. In unilateral lesions, as demonstrated by ventrolateral cordotomy, voluntary control of micturition is not lost. This corresponds to the clinical observation in spinal cord compression in which it is unusual to have sphincter function disturbed early when there is only unilateral or equivocal bilateral lower-extremity weakness or sensory disturbance. The most common exception is when the conus medullaris or sacral nerve roots are compressed.

Immediately following many cases of acute spinal cord injury there is an initial period of *spinal shock*, which is often accompanied by urinary retention and overflow incontinence; later, a *reflex (neurogenic* or *spastic) bladder* typically develops. If the disturbance of upper motor neuron function evolves slowly, then the reflex bladder may develop without a preceding period of spinal shock and flaccid bladder.

The reflex bladder is characterized by overactivity of both the detrusor muscle and the external sphincter. This causes incontinence of urine. In addition, the bladder capacity is diminished due to the detrusor contraction. The sensation of bladder distention may be lost if ascending tracts are involved. The anal reflex is often intact in cases of reflex bladder. On cystometry the detrusor muscle demonstrates excessive contraction to small increments of fluid volume.

In contrast to the reflex bladder, when the damage occurs in the region of the conus medullaris or the cauda equina, a *decentralized* or *autonomous flaccid bladder* develops. Voluntary control over bladder function is impaired or abolished entirely. In such cases detrusor tone is lost and the bladder distends to the point that overflow incontinence occurs. Bladder sensation is impaired. Control over the anal sphincter and the anal reflex is usually lost. A region of saddle anesthesia may be present (see Figure 28.3). Unlike the situation in the reflex bladder, the cystometrogram usually demonstrates diminished or absent contractions of the detrusor muscle.

The anatomical pathways subserving bowel function are similar to those controlling the urinary bladder. Spinal shock is generally associated with ileus, and a neurogenic megacolon may develop. The anal reflex is usually lost in cases of spinal shock. In lesions above the sacral level that evolve slowly, voluntary control of the sphincter ani may be lost, but in such cases the anal reflex remains intact unless complete cord transection occurs, in which case it may be absent. In disturbances of the conus medullaris and cauda equina (nerve roots S3–5), fecal incontinence and a flaccid anal sphincter with loss of the anal reflex may be a

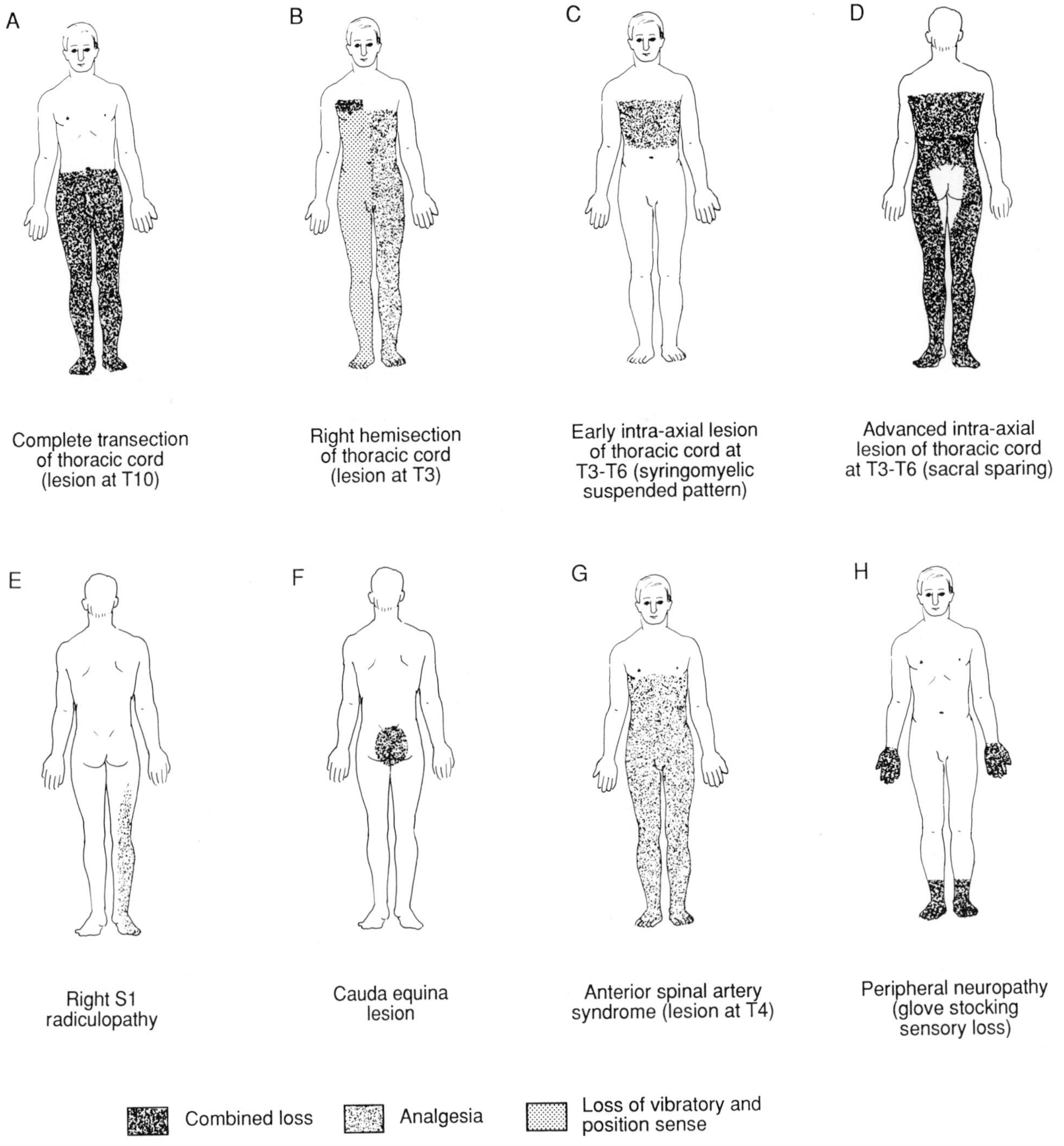

FIGURE 28.3 Characteristic sensory disturbances found in various spinal cord lesions in comparison to peripheral neuropathy. (Reprinted with permission from TN Byrne, SG Waxman. Spinal Cord Compression: Diagnosis and Principles of Treatment. Contemporary Neurology Series. Philadelphia: FA Davis, 1990.)

presenting manifestation of neurological disease. Saddle anesthesia is often seen in such cases. Partial impairment may be present in any of these syndromes before frank paralysis and a flaccid sphincter ensues.

Disturbances of sexual function are common in spinal cord disease, especially in males. The descending pathways from the neocortex, limbic system, and hypothalamus course adjacent to the corticospinal tracts in the lateral funiculi. Penile erection occurs via the sacral parasympathetics (S3 and S4) and the pudendal nerves and nervi erigentes, and via inhibition of the sympathetic vasoconstrictor center located in the intermediolateral cell column at L1–2 and then through the superior hypogastric plexus. Ejaculation is performed via the reflex arc beginning with the afferent limb arising in the genital epithelium and passing centrally via the dorsal nerve of the penis and pudendal nerve to the S3 and S4 dorsal roots. The perineal branch of the pudendal nerve is an important peripheral efferent pathway (Haymaker 1969).

COMMON SPINAL CORD SYNDROMES

Spinal Shock

A complete transverse lesion of the spinal cord results in total loss of motor and sensory functions below the level of the lesion. If the lesion is slow in development, such as may occur with a benign tumor or cervical spondylosis, or if it is incomplete, then spinal reflexes such as hyperactive deep tendon reflexes and Babinski's signs are generally present. Alternatively, if the lesion is acute in development, a condition known as "spinal shock" ensues, in which there is loss of all spinal reflex activity below the level of the lesion along with motor paralysis and sensory loss.

The condition of spinal shock is characterized by flaccid, areflexic paralysis of skeletal and smooth muscles. There is a complete loss of autonomic functions below the level of the lesion, which results in a loss of urinary bladder tone and paralytic ileus. Sweating and piloerection are also diminished or absent below the lesion. Since vasomotor tone is lost, dependent lower extremities may become edematous and temperature regulation may be a major problem. Genital reflexes such as penile erection, the cremasteric reflex, and bulbocavernosus reflexes are lost. Sensation below the level of the lesion is completely absent.

Incomplete Lesions of the Spinal Cord

Unilateral Transverse Lesion

A unilateral lesion or hemisection of the spinal cord produces a Brown-Séquard syndrome. In reality such pure unilateral lesions are rare and therefore most clinical cases are described as a "modified Brown-Séquard" syndrome.

The clinical presentation of a pure Brown-Séquard syndrome is that of ipsilateral weakness and loss of position and vibration below the lesion as well as contralateral loss of pain and temperature caudal to the lesion. The loss of pain and temperature is usually manifest a few segments below the level of the lesion due to the fact that the decussating fibers enter the spinothalamic tract a few segments rostral to the level of entry of the nerve root. At the level of the insult there may be a small ipsilateral area of anesthesia, analgesia, and lower motor neuron weakness since the segmental afferent and efferent pathways are disrupted (see Figure 28.3).

Trauma is probably the most common cause of the Brown-Séquard syndrome (Haymaker 1969). Spinal metastases rarely present with a Brown-Séquard syndrome. In the large series of spinal metastases published by Stark et al. (1982), of 106 patients with signs of myelopathy, only two had a pure Brown-Séquard syndrome. An additional eight patients had greater weakness ipsilateral to the lesion and more marked pain and temperature loss contralateral to the lesion, but there were no dorsal column signs in these patients. The latter group would be considered to have "modified Brown-Séquard syndromes." Radiation necrosis has also been reported to present with a Brown-Séquard syndrome (Gutin et al. 1991).

Central Cord Syndrome

The central cord syndrome is due to an intra-axial lesion disturbing the normal structures of the central or paracentral region of the spinal cord. Such disturbances are usually either acute, in which case they are usually due to hemorrhage or contusion following trauma, or chronic, in which case they may be due to tumor or syringomyelia. Although a demyelinating process may occasionally cause a similar syndrome, it is usually not confused with the other more typical causes. While clinically distinct, the presentations of these disorders share some common features. Contusions following trauma and syringomyelia frequently occur in the cervical spine and cervicothoracic junction. Spontaneous hematomyelia generally presents with the acute onset of severe back or neck pain followed by paralysis.

When the cervical spine or cervicothoracic junction is the site of a central cord syndrome, the upper extremities show weakness of a lower motor neuron type. Characteristically, there is loss of sensation in the upper extremities of a dissociated type, with loss of pain and temperature sensation and preservation of position and vibration sensation. This is due to the decussating fibers destined for the spinothalamic tracts being interrupted, while those projecting within the dorsal columns are spared (see Figure 28.3). As a result of the laminated structure of the spinothalamic tract, sensation from the more caudal regions is preserved, with *sacral sparing* of pain and temperature sensation being the rule.

Anterior Spinal Artery Syndrome

Spinal cord infarction has been recognized much more frequently in recent years, in part due to an increased number of invasive procedures such as vascular and thoracoabdominal surgery and improved survival after cardiac arrest and hypotension (Aminoff 1992).

As demonstrated in Figure 28.4, the anterior horns and anterolateral tracts are involved in this syndrome. Initially spinal shock is expected. Subsequently, corticospinal deficits develop below the level of the infarction; dysfunction of autonomic pathways occurs, causing loss of bowel, bladder, and sexual functions, and a sensory disturbance develops in which posterior column function remains intact whereas the spinothalamic tracts are disrupted.

Anterior spinal artery syndrome is differentiated from acute central cord syndrome, as occurs in traumatic contusions and hematomyelia, by the sacral sensory sparing that tends to occur in the latter. Moreover, the anterior spinal artery syndrome may be differentiated from that of acute complete transverse myelopathy due to the loss of posterior column function in the latter (Ropper and Poskanzer 1978).

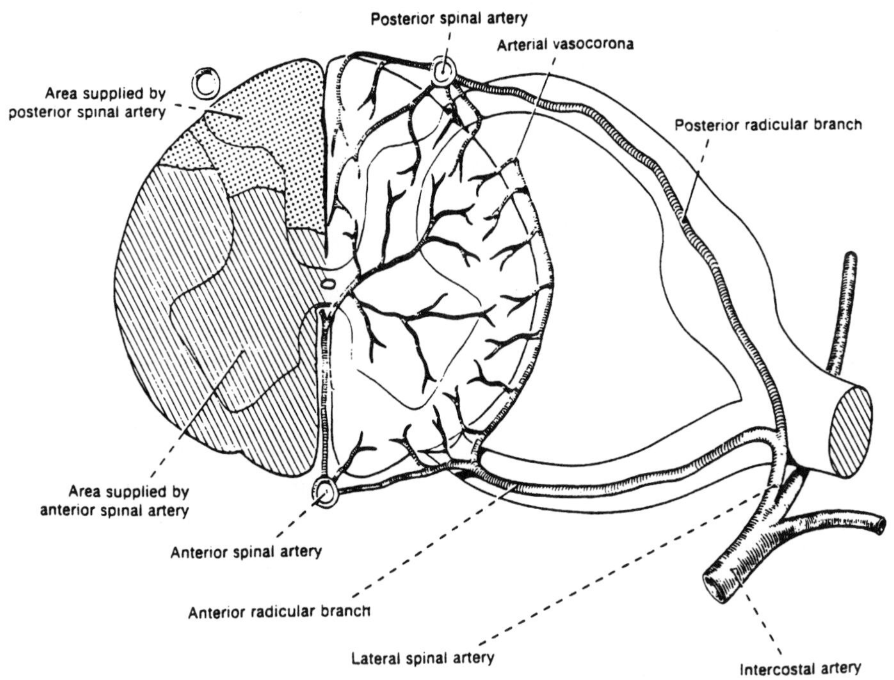

FIGURE 28.4 The arterial supply of the spinal cord. (Reprinted with permission from RN DeJong. The Neurologic Examination [4th ed]. Hagerstown, MD: Harper & Row, 1979.)

Anterior Horn and Pyramidal Tract Syndrome

Disturbances of the anterior horns and pyramidal tracts alone with sparing of the sensory functions and autonomic nervous system are seen in motor neuron disease. Clinically, one typically finds a combination of both lower motor neuron weakness with its attendant atrophy and fasciculations (and fibrillations on electromyography) and upper motor weakness with spasticity, hyperreflexia, and Babinski's signs. Virtually diagnostic is the presence of lower and upper motor neuron signs in the same muscle group. Alternatively, either the lower motor neuron or upper motor neuron disturbance may predominate for months or years. Ultimately, as the lower motor neuron disease progresses, there is increasingly severe atrophy and evolution from hyperreflexia to hyporeflexia.

Combined Posterior and Lateral Column Disease

The clinical presentation of loss of posterior column and lateral column (pyramidal) function is that of spastic ataxic gait. The ataxia is of a sensory type and may be bizarre in its appearance. Although Friedreich's ataxia may cause such a syndrome, the classic cause for this is subacute combined degeneration associated with vitamin B_{12} deficiency.

CHARACTERISTIC CLINICAL FEATURES OF LESIONS AT DIFFERENT LEVELS

Spinal lesions at different levels often present with characteristic symptoms and signs referable to the segmental levels involved. In cases of extramedullary compression, disturbances at the segmental level usually herald the presentation. Conversely, intramedullary diseases frequently do not present with segmental disturbances but rather with tract dysfunction.

Foramen Magnum

Lesions of the foramen magnum, which include trauma, tumors, syringomyelia, multiple sclerosis, Arnold-Chiari malformation, atlantoaxial dislocation, and other bony abnormalities of the craniocervical junction, present a most challenging diagnostic problem for the clinician because symptoms are often vague or may be distant from the foramen magnum.

Occipital or neck pain, often increased by neck movement, is a common initial manifestation. The pain may also radiate into the shoulders or the ipsilateral arm. In the latter situation the pain may be similar to that of cervical spondylosis (Byrne and Waxman 1990; Saunders and Bernini 1992).

The neurological signs associated with foramen magnum tumors may also be perplexing. Cranial nerve symptoms and signs are inconstant; nystagmus, often downbeating, impaired sensation over the face (due to involvement of the descending tract of cranial nerve V), and dysarthria, dysphonia, and dysphagia are present in some patients.

Motor system involvement characteristically presents as spastic weakness. The corticospinal tracts compression causes weakness that typically begins in the ipsilateral arm and is followed by weakness of the ipsilateral leg and then the contralateral leg and then arm.

Alternatively, it has been long recognized that foramen magnum tumors may cause signs of lower motor neuron weakness, atrophy, and depressed reflexes in the arms and hands. The mechanism of this lower motor neuron disturbance well below the level of the tumor has never been fully elucidated but is thought to be possibly secondary to circulatory disturbances affecting the distribution of the anterior spinal artery.

Sensory disturbances consisting of pain and numbness are early manifestations of foramen magnum tumors. In the series of Symonds, pain and paresthesias affecting the same upper extremity first involved by spastic weakness was an early finding. The sensory disturbances found in these patients are often of the dissociated type so that patients suffer from loss of pain and temperature sensation but have preserved tactile sensation. In addition, a suspended sensory loss has also been reported in some cases. This pattern of sensory loss may be due to a secondary syrinx, which may direct attention away from the causative lesion at the cervicomedullary junction. Magnetic resonance imaging (MRI) has become the test of choice for imaging the craniocervical junction.

Upper Cervical Spine

Compressive lesions of the upper cervical spine have similar clinical characteristics to those arising at the foramen magnum. Pain in the neck, occipital region, or shoulder is a very common presenting complaint. The second cervical root innervates the posterior aspect of the scalp, which explains the pattern of radicular pain. If the compression is at the third or fourth cervical level, radicular pain may be projected to the neck or top of the shoulder. When pain does occur, it is usually provoked by neck movements, resulting in marked limitation of head turning and nodding.

With progressive compression, upper-extremity weakness usually becomes apparent on the side of pain. The weakness may be of an upper or lower motor neuron type. Some patients may therefore have spasticity and hyperreflexia and others may have atrophy and hyporeflexia of a portion or of the entire upper extremity including the hand. When upper motor neuron findings develop in the ipsilateral leg, a spinal hemiplegia is present. Weakness may then progress to the contralateral lower extremity and then the contralateral upper extremity.

Lower Cervical and Upper Thoracic Spine

Spinal cord and root compression at the levels of C5–T1 most frequently betray their presence by radicular symptoms at the affected level in the shoulder or upper extremity in the form of pain and later reflex, motor, and sensory disturbances. With lesions at the C4–C6 level, pain and sensory disturbances are frequently reported along the radial aspect of the arm, forearm, and thumb (see Figure 28.2 and Table 28.2). With intramedullary neoplasms, pain is also frequent at these levels, but the localization is usually more diffuse and less typically radicular in nature.

At the C7–T1 levels, pain and sensory symptoms frequently are localized to the ulnar aspect of the arm, forearm, and hand. Tumors at the T1 and T2 levels often cause pain to radiate into the elbow and hand, together with sensory complaints along the ulnar border of the hand. As at other locations, intramedullary neoplasms usually give rise to more diffuse symptoms, which are often bilateral. Conversely, extramedullary compression frequently presents with exquisite localizing symptoms.

Weakness usually follows pain, particularly at the affected segmental level. As might be expected based on the myotomal map of the upper extremity, intramedullary and extramedullary lesions at C4–C6 show a predilection to involve the muscles in the shoulder and upper arm (see Table 28.2). Atrophy and weakness of the hand can rarely occur with lesions at C4–C6. This may be due to vascular factors affecting the lower cervical segments. Such a pattern of weakness and atrophy is usually due to a lesion at the C7–T2 level.

The pattern of extremity weakness may be a guide in distinguishing intramedullary from extramedullary disorders. Although exceptions will be encountered, extramedullary lesions tend to affect the ipsilateral upper and lower extremity before involving the contralateral side. In contrast, intramedullary lesions may involve both upper extremities before the lower extremities are affected or show bilateral arm and leg involvement from the onset.

The deep tendon reflexes are very helpful in localizing the segmental level of involvement in the cervical spine. Disease at the C5–C6 levels is often associated with depressed biceps (C5), brachioradialis reflex (C6), or both (see Table 28.2). Alternatively, one may encounter depressed biceps and brachioradialis reflexes associated with a hyperactive triceps reflex if there is a compressive myelopathy at the C5–C6 levels. Although not specific for cervical spondylosis, a depressed brachioradialis (C6) reflex with hyperactive finger flexors (C8–T1) is often seen in individuals who have a C6 radiculopathy with myelopathy; neoplasms or other diseases at the C6 level may cause a similar clinical presentation. When the lesion is at the C7 level, the triceps reflex may be depressed.

With lesions at C8 and T1, the finger flexor response may be impaired. Hoffman's sign is performed by dorsiflexing the patient's wrist and then flicking the distal phalanx of the middle finger with the examiner's thumb (DeJong 1979). The patient's middle finger is thus flexed and suddenly extended. When Hoffman's sign is present, this maneuver is followed by reflex flexion of the patient's thumb and other fingers. When present bilaterally, the Hoffman's sign is usually an indication of hyperactive deep tendon reflexes. Although disease of the pyramidal pathways may be responsible, healthy individuals with hyperactive reflexes may have bilateral Hoffman's signs such as in the case of anxiety, hyperthyroidism, and stimulatory drugs. When Hoffman's sign is present unilaterally, it usually signifies disease of the nervous system. In such cases, the examiner must distinguish between disease of the pyramidal tract causing a pathological Hoffman's sign and disease of the peripheral nervous system, such as the

Table 28.6: Differentiation of conus lesions from cauda equina lesions

	Conus Medullaris	*Cauda Equina*
Spontaneous pain	Unusual and not severe; bilateral and symmetrical in perineum or thighs	Often very prominent and severe, asymmetrical, radicular
Motor findings	Not severe, symmetrical Fibrillary twitches are rare	May be severe, asymmetrical, fibrillary twitches of paralyzed muscles are common
Sensory findings	Saddle distribution, bilateral, symmetrical, dissociated sensory loss (impaired pain and temperature sensibility with sparing of tactile sensibility)	Saddle distribution, may be asymmetrical, no dissociation of sensory loss
Reflex changes	Epiconus: only Achilles reflex absent Conus: Achilles and patellar present	Patellar and Achilles reflexes may be absent
Sphincter disturbance	Early and marked (both urinary and fecal incontinence)	Late and less severe
Male sexual function	Impaired early	Impairment less severe
Onset	Sudden and bilateral	Gradual and unilateral

Source: Adapted from RN DeJong. The Neurologic Examination (4th ed). Hagerstown, MD: Harper & Row, 1979; W Haymaker. Bing's Local Diagnosis in Neurological Disease (15th ed). St. Louis: Mosby, 1969;57–59.

C8–T1 nerve roots or the lower brachial plexus (such as a Pancoast tumor), resulting in a unilateral loss of a Hoffman's reflex in an individual with diffuse hyperreflexia.

Thoracic Levels

The thoracic dermatomal landmarks that guide the examiner to the level of involvement are the nipple (T4), the umbilicus (T10), and the inguinal ligament (L1). Pain or sensory alterations in a radicular distribution are localized to a specific dermatome using these levels as points of reference.

The relatively small vertebral canal and the vascular watershed area of the spinal cord in the thoracic region make the thoracic spinal cord extremely vulnerable to injury from compression. Consequently, the temporal course of symptoms of cord compression is often shorter in this region than elsewhere in the spine (Schliack and Stille 1975). Thus, pain often evolves rapidly into weakness, sensory loss, and reflex abnormalities caudal to the lesion. Sphincter disturbances ultimately develop.

Conus Medullaris and Cauda Equina

Lesions of the cauda equina and conus medullaris (Table 28.6) cause similar symptoms and signs including local, referred, and radicular pain, sphincter disturbances, loss of buttock and leg sensation, and leg weakness. While it may be relatively easy to establish the level of a single radiculopathy based on sensory, motor, and reflex changes, it is much more difficult to assign the cause and localization when there are several lumbosacral levels involved. In such situations one must consider the possibility of a lower spinal cord lesion or a cauda equina syndrome. Although there has been a long effort to differentiate conus medullaris lesions from those of the cauda equina, it is not always possible to accurately discriminate between lesions injuring the lower spinal cord and those arising from the cauda equina.

Although rare in its pure form, the conus medullaris syndrome presents with sphincter disturbances, saddle anesthesia (S3–5), impotence, and absence of lower-extremity abnormalities. If the cauda equina is involved, patients may experience difficulty with external rotation and extension of the thigh at the hip, flexion of the knee, and weakness of all muscles below the knee.

DISTINGUISHING INTRAMEDULLARY FROM EXTRAMEDULLARY LESIONS

The earlier sections of this chapter describe several features that help distinguish between intramedullary lesions and extramedullary compressive lesions of the spinal cord. However, as stressed, this may be a vexing clinical problem that ultimately requires radiographic elucidation. The explanation for this clinical experience has been provided by a clinicopathological study by McAlhany and Netsky (1955) of extramedullary spinal neoplasms. These authors demonstrated that extramedullary compression can cause ischemia and demyelination in the posterior and lateral column with relative sparing of the anterior columns regardless of the location of the extramedullary tumor. Both "coup" and "contre-coup" injuries occurred in the spinal cord. The areas of infarction and demyelination were often deep and did not follow a specific pattern. In some instances the pathological findings were more marked ipsilateral to the tumor and in other cases they were primarily contralateral to the mass. It would follow, therefore, that stereotypical clinical patterns of evolution would not be expected.

Table 28.7: Differential diagnosis of diseases affecting the spinal cord

- **Compressive lesions**
  - Non-neoplastic
    - Trauma
    - Spondylosis
    - Intervertebral disc herniation
    - Spinal stenosis
    - Infectious disorders (e.g., abscess, tuberculosis)
    - Inflammatory (e.g., rheumatoid arthritis, ankylosing spondylitis, sarcoid)
    - Spinal hemorrhage
    - Syringomyelia
    - Congenital disorders
    - Arachnoid cysts
    - Paget's disease
    - Osteoporosis
  - Neoplastic
    - Epidural
    - Intradural-extramedullary (e.g., meningioma, neurofibroma, and leptomeningeal metastasis)
    - Intramedullary
- **Noncompressive myelopathies**
  - Demyelinating (e.g., multiple sclerosis, acute disseminated encephalomyelitis)
  - Viral myelitis (e.g., zoster, AIDS-related myelopathy, HTLV-1)
  - Vitamin B_{12} deficiency and other nutritional deficiencies
  - Infarction
  - Spirochetal diseases (syphilis and Lyme disease)
  - Toxic myelopathies (e.g., radiation-induced)
  - Autoimmune diseases (e.g., lupus, Sjögren's)
  - Paraneoplastic
  - Neuronal degenerations
  - Acute and subacute transverse myelitis of unknown cause

CLASSIFICATION OF DISEASES AFFECTING THE SPINAL CORD

This chapter has emphasized the clinical pathophysiology of spinal cord disorders. Although thorough discussions of specific diseases affecting the spinal cord can be found elsewhere in this book, Table 28.7 lists a classification of disorders that may help the clinician approach the individual patient. Diseases are classified according to their etiology and location. With the availability of MRI, this classification permits the clinician to consider the differential diagnosis both before and after the imaging has been obtained. Furthermore, since compressive lesions may be surgical emergencies, this classification considers the therapeutic nature of many of the diseases that need to be considered.

Metastatic Epidural Spinal Cord Compression

Metastatic epidural spinal cord compression (MESCC) deserves special comment since it affects approximately 20,000 cancer patients in the United States annually (Byrne 1992). Figure 28.5 demonstrates the location of tumors of the spine, distinguishing among intramedullary, extramedullary-intradural, and extradural tumors.

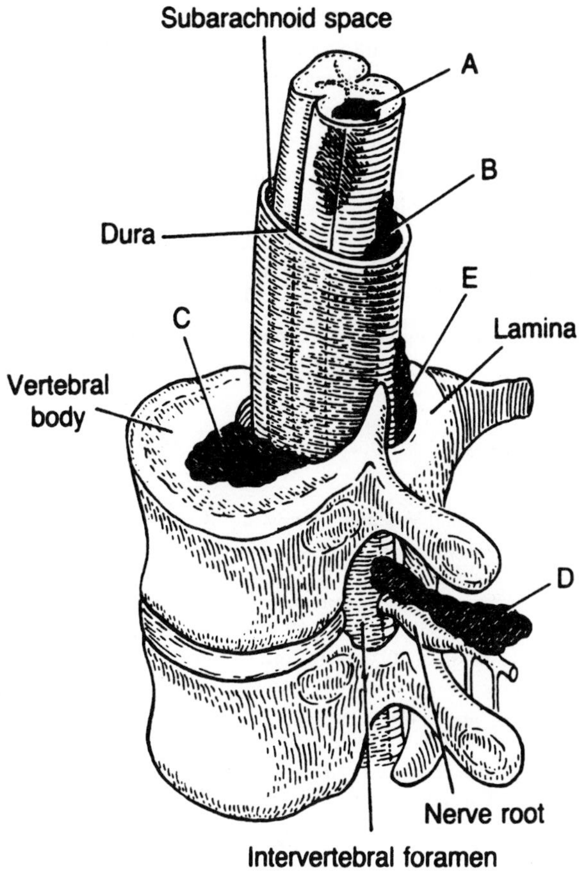

FIGURE 28.5 Anatomical locations of spine metastases. Intramedullary metastasis is located within the spinal cord (A). Leptomeningeal metastasis is in the subarachnoid space and is extramedullary and intradural (B). Epidural metastases arise from the extension of metastases located in one of the adjacent structures: vertebral column (C); the paravertebral spaces via the intervertebral foraminae (D), or, rarely, the epidural space itself (E). As these epidural metastases grow, they compress adjacent blood vessels, nerve roots, and spinal cord resulting in local and referred pain, radiculopathy, and myelopathy. (Reprinted with permission from TN Byrne, SG Waxman. Spinal Cord Compression: Diagnosis and Principles of Treatment. Contemporary Neurology Series, Philadelphia: FA Davis, 1990.)

As with other causes of spinal cord compression, the major presenting clinical signs and symptoms of MESCC are pain, weakness, sensory loss, and autonomic disturbance. In approximately 95% of adults and 80% of children, progressive axial, referred, and/or radicular pain is the most common initial complaint of both vertebral metastasis and MESCC (Gilbert et al. 1978; Lewis et al. 1986). Since the neurologic prognosis depends directly on the level of neurologic function at the time of initiation of therapy, there is a great incentive to make an early diagnosis while the patient is still ambulatory.

The diagnostic imaging test of choice in evaluating patients for MESCC is MRI when available in a timely fashion (Byrne 1992). Alternatively, myelography should be performed when management is delayed by inability to schedule MRI in a timely fashion, in patients unable to undergo MRI (for instance, those with pacemakers and pain precluding recumbency), or when a technically adequate MRI cannot be obtained. The mainstays of treatment include corticosteroids, radiotherapy, and, in selected patients, surgical decompression of the cord. Approximately 80% of patients who are ambulatory at the initiation of radiotherapy remain so at the end of treatment, whereas fewer than 10% who are paraplegic at the beginning of radiotherapy recover ambulation (Byrne 1992).

REFERENCES

Aminoff M. Spinal Vascular Disease. In E Critchley, A Eisen (eds), Diseases of the Spinal Cord. London: Springer-Verlag, 1992; 281–299.

Byrne TN. Spinal cord compression from epidural metastases. N Engl J Med 1992;327:614–619.

Byrne TN, Waxman SG. Spinal Cord Compression: Diagnosis and Principles of Treatment. Contemporary Neurology Series. Philadelphia: FA Davis, 1990.

DeJong RN. The Neurologic Examination (4th ed). Hagerstown, MD: Harper & Row, 1979.

Ditunno J, Formal C. Chronic spinal cord injury. N Engl J Med 1994;330:550–556.

Gilbert RW, Kim JH, Posner JB. Epidural spinal cord compression from metastatic tumor: diagnosis and treatment. Ann Neurol 1978;3:40–51.

Gutin P, Leibel S, Sheline G. Radiation Injury to the Nervous System. New York: Raven, 1991.

Haymaker W. Bing's Local Diagnosis in Neurological Disease (15th ed). St. Louis: Mosby, 1969;57–59.

Lewis DW, Packer RJ, Raney B et al. Incidence, presentation, and outcome of spinal cord disease in children with systemic cancer. Pediatrics 1986;78:438–442.

McAlhany HJ, Netsky MG. Compression of the spinal cord by extramedullary neoplasms: a clinical and pathological study. J Neuropath Exp Neurol 1955;14:276–287.

McCall IW, Park WM, O'Brien JP. Induced pain referral from posterior lumbar elements in normal subjects. Spine 1979;4:441–446.

Patten J. Neurological Differential Diagnosis. New York: Springer-Verlag, 1977.

Ropper AH, Poskanzer DC. The prognosis of acute and subacute transverse myelopathy based on early signs and symptoms. Ann Neurol 1978;4:51–59.

Saunders R, Bernini P (eds). Cervical Spondylitic Myelopathy. Boston: Blackwell, 1992.

Schliack H. Segmental Innervation and the Clinical Aspects of Spinal Nerve Root Syndromes. In PJ Vinken, GW Bruyn (eds), Handbook of Clinical Neurology. Vol. 2. Amsterdam: North-Holland Publishing, 1969;157–177.

Schliack H, Stille D. Clinical Symptomatology of Intraspinal Tumors. In PJ Vinken, GW Bruyn (eds), Handbook of Clinical Neurology. Vol. 19. Amsterdam: North-Holland Publishing, 1975:23–49.

Stark RJ, Henson RA, Evans SJW. Spinal metastases: a retrospective survey from a general hospital. Brain 1982;105:189–213.

Chapter 29
Proximal, Distal, and Generalized Weakness

Valerie A. Cwik and Michael H. Brooke

Weakness is decreased muscle strength as measured by the force of a maximal contraction. Fatigue is a failure to maintain the expected contraction. Weak muscles are always more easily fatigued than normal muscles, but fatigue may occur in the absence of weakness. Both weakness and fatigue may be features of dysfunction at any level of the neuraxis or may accompany systemic disease. Weakness caused by disorders of the neuraxis can be localized to the upper motor neuron or to the *motor unit* by the clinical features. The motor unit consists of an anterior horn cell, its motor axon and branches, the neuromuscular junctions, and all the skeletal muscle fibers it innervates.

In general, neuropathic disorders cause distal limb weakness, and disorders of the neuromuscular junction or muscle cause proximal weakness. However, these broad generalizations are of little help when attempting to narrow down the differential diagnosis in a patient with weakness, and exceptions to the rules are expected. Fortunately, neuromuscular diseases are relatively few in number. More important, the initial clinical features are often sufficiently distinctive to suggest the correct diagnosis or a limited differential list. Patients with weakness have nonspecific and specific clinical features; the nonspecific characteristics confirm that a patient is truly weak, while the specific features help establish the diagnosis.

SYMPTOMS OF WEAKNESS

The symptoms that people experience when their muscles begin to fail depend more on which muscles are involved than on the cause of involvement. A complicating factor is the layperson's *interpretation* of the word *weak*. Although the physician may unequivocally use the word to denote a loss of muscle power, the patient may use the word more loosely. In addition to weak muscles, one may have weak eyesight, weak willpower, weak excuses, and weak tea; in all, the word has a slightly different meaning. Thus, the complaint of weakness should not be taken at face value but should be probed until it is clearly shown to mean a loss of muscle strength. Less predictably, patients with early symptoms of weakness may not recognize it as such and may describe their problems as clumsiness, numbness, stiffness, or fatigue.

Symptoms of weakness, as they affect various body parts, are fairly stereotyped, but nonspecific as to cause. They may be broadly divided into symptoms of ocular weakness, facial and neck weakness, shoulder and arm weakness, and hip and leg weakness.

Ocular Muscles

Symptoms of ocular muscle weakness are usually easy to recognize. Drooping of the eyelids may be noticed by the patient when looking in the mirror or it may be pointed out by friends. Mild diplopia may be noticed as blurring of vision, leading to the conclusion that the patient's eyeglasses need adjusting. It may occur only in particular situations—for example, when faced with the oncoming headlights of approaching cars at night or when trying to read. Occasionally, the complaint relates not to the eyes at all but to the position of the head. Lateral tilt with fourth nerve palsies and backward tilt compensating for bilateral ptosis are well-known examples. It is worth asking the patient if closing one eye corrects the diplopia, because neuromuscular weakness is not among the many causes of monocular diplopia.

Face and Neck

Facial weakness is usually experienced by the patient as a feeling of stiffness or sometimes numbness. Drinking through a straw and blowing up balloons are particularly difficult tasks and may be sensitive tests for facial weakness. Acquaintances may notice that the patient's expression is somehow changed; a common observation is a tendency for the patient to sleep with the eyes open. A pleasant smile may turn into a snarl because of weakness of the perioral muscles. The development of pharyngeal, palatal, and tongue weakness disturbs speech and swallowing. A flaccid palate is associated with nasal regurgitation, choking spells, and aspiration of liquids. In bilateral upper motor neuron lesions affecting swallowing, nasal regurgitation is less frequently seen. In this instance, the more common complaint is of choking sensations and aspiration, as the stiff and uncoordinated muscles fail to propel the food bolus along in an orderly fashion (see Chapter 79).

Neck muscle weakness is first noticed in situations in which they are called on to stabilize the head. Riding as a passenger in a car when the brake or the accelerator is used, particularly in an emergency situation, may be very disconcerting for the patient with neck weakness. Similarly, when the patient is stooping or bending forward, weakness of the posterior muscles may cause the chin to fall on the chest. A patient with neck flexion weakness often notices difficulty lifting the head off the pillow in the morning.

Shoulders and Arms

Weakness of the shoulders is often expressed by the patient as a feeling of tiredness. Fatigue is a normal phenomenon in everyone; for example, anyone would feel fatigue after trying to carry a 100-pound weight for a long distance. In a patient with shoulder weakness, the weight of the arms is sufficient to bring on such fatigue. Thus, early in the history, the patient will experience fatigue on performing sustained tasks with the hands held over the head, which may include painting the ceiling, combing the hair, or simply trying to lift an object off a high shelf. Hand and forearm weakness is similarly noticed for the first time when the patient needs to exert full power. Such efforts as opening a tightly closed screw-capped jar, trying to turn on a faucet, using a key, or opening a car door may all present problems depending on the severity of the weakness.

Hips and Legs

The importance of the muscles of the hip and leg is reflected by the fact that they are often responsible for the earliest symptoms experienced by patients who develop weakness. Patients notice that they have difficulty arising from the floor or from a deep chair and have to use the support of the hands or knees. This is often interpreted by older patients as arthritis or some similar minor problem, rather than what it really represents. Walking becomes clumsy, and patients stumble. In descending stairs, the patient with quadriceps weakness tends to keep the knee locked and stiff. If the knee bends slightly as the weight of the body is transferred to the lower stair, the knee may collapse; hence, the patient feels insecure. Patients who have more symptoms coming down stairs than going up usually have quadriceps weakness; the reverse is true of those who have hip extensor weakness. Weakness of the anterior tibial and ankle evertor group may again be perceived incorrectly by the patient, who may simply complain of spraining the ankle repeatedly. If the weakness becomes severe, a foot drop is noted, and the gait assumes a slapping quality. Weakness of both anterior and posterior muscles of the lower leg frequently gives an instability to the stance, which causes the patient to complain of poor balance.

EXAMINATION OF THE WEAK PATIENT

The four parts to the examination of patients with muscle weakness are inspection, palpation, muscle strength evaluation, and examination of tendon reflexes.

Inspection

Inspection is probably the most important part of the examination. Although it is possible to detect weakness by examining the strength of individual muscles, it is often more useful to observe how the patient functions and what posture is adopted at rest. Head and neck, shoulders, arms, torso, and legs are evaluated separately.

Ptosis may be obvious in the head and neck inspection; the more severe the ptosis, the more the tendency to throw the head backward. The patient usually elevates the eyebrows and wrinkles the forehead in an attempt to raise the upper lids. This is sometimes so successful that the ptosis is only apparent when the examiner smooths out the wrinkled forehead and allows the eyebrows to assume a more normal position. Hysterical ptosis is easy to detect because, in addition to the lowered upper lid, there is also a contraction of the lower lid (blepharospasm).

Weakness of the face that has been present since childhood may give a smooth, unlined appearance to the adult face. In addition, facial expression is diminished or altered. A smile may become a grimace or snarl, with eversion of the upper lip. The normal blink may be altered by incomplete closure of the eyelid, and the sclera may be visible the entire time. On opening the mouth, the normal preservation of the arch of the upper lip may be lost, and the mouth may assume a tented or straight-line configuration. Actual wasting of the facial muscles is difficult to see, but temporal and masseter atrophy produces a characteristic scalloped

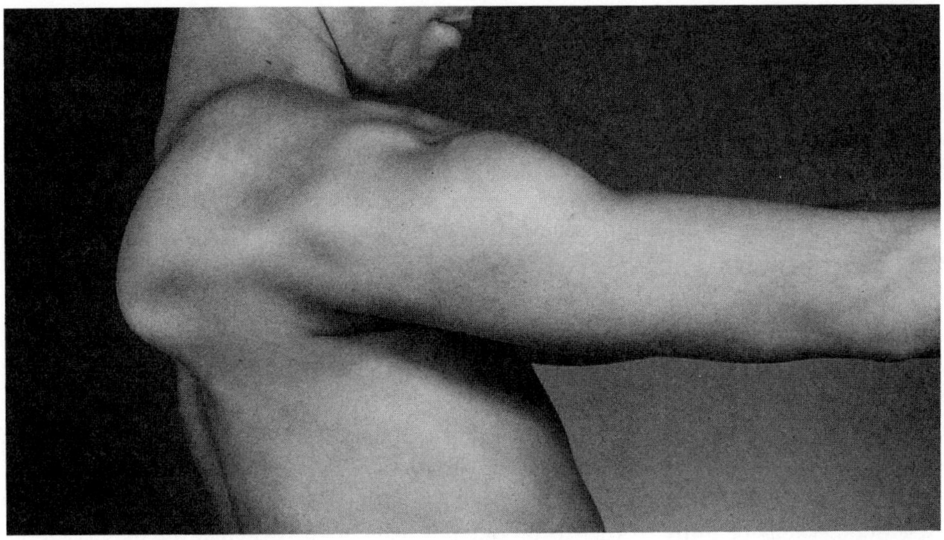

FIGURE 29.1 The scapular winging of facioscapulohumeral muscular dystrophy is distinguished by the prominent protrusion of the inferior medial border of the scapula. When viewed from the front, the elevation of the scapula under the trapezius muscle produces the "trapezius hump."

appearance above and below the cheekbone. Since patients often rearrange their hairstyles to cover this wasting, the examiner should make a conscious effort to check for it. Facial weakness, particularly when associated with palatal weakness, causes drooling, and the patient may sit with a tissue in readiness. The tongue should be inspected for atrophy and fasciculations, which should not be confused with the normal quivering movements of the tongue.

Speech is affected by facial weakness, and the normal labials (*p* and *b*) are softened. Speech is also altered in other ways, which can be detected by the examiner with a practiced ear. Lower motor neuron involvement of the palate and tongue gives the speech a hollow, echoing timbre, whereas upper motor neuron dysfunction causes the speech to be monotonous, forced, and strained. Laryngeal weakness may also be noticed in speech when the voice becomes harsh or brassy, often associated with the loss of the glottal stop (the small sound made by the larynx closing, as at the start of a cough).

Weakness of the shoulder muscles causes a characteristic change in posture. Normally the shoulders are braced back by the tone of the muscles, so that when the arms are held by the side, the thumbs tend to face forward. As the shoulder muscles lose their tone, the point of the shoulder rotates forward, rather like the curling of the corner of a piece of paper. This forward rotation of the shoulder is associated with a rotation of the arm, so that the backs of the hands now face forward. Additionally, the loss of tone is associated with rather loose swinging movements of the arm in normal walking. When shoulder weakness is severe, the patient may fling the arm by using a movement of the trunk, rather than lifting the arm in its normal fashion. In the most extreme example, the only way the patient can get the hand above the head is to use a truncal movement to throw the whole arm upward and forward so that the hand rests on the wall, and then to creep the hand upward by using finger movements.

Another effect of shoulder weakness that may be seen, particularly in the presence of atrophy of the pectoral muscles, is an upward sloping crease of the anterior axillary fold, which takes on the appearance of a folded corner of a piece of paper.

Winging of the scapula is a characteristic finding in weakness of the serratus anterior muscles and trapezii that normally fix the scapula to the thorax. As these muscles become weak, any attempted movement of the arm will cause the scapula to rise off the back of the rib cage and protrude like small wings. The arm and shoulder may be thought of as a crane; the boom of the crane is the arm and the base is the scapula. Obviously, if the base is not fixed, any attempt to use the crane will result in the whole structure falling over. So it is with attempting to elevate the arm; the scapula simply pops off the back of the chest wall in a characteristic fashion. In the most usual type of winging, the entire medial border of the scapula protrudes backward. In some diseases, particularly facioscapulohumeral muscular dystrophy, the inferomedial border angle juts out first, and the entire scapula rotates and rides up over the back. Viewed from the front, this is often associated with a trapezius hump, in which the middle part of the trapezius muscle, in the web of the neck, is mounded over the upper border of the scapula (Figure 29.1). A word of caution pertains to the examination of the slender person, particularly a child. In such an individual there may be a prominent shoulder blade. The shoulder configuration returns to normal, however, when the individual attempts to use the arm forcibly, as in a pushup.

Weakness and wasting of the intrinsic muscles of the hand produces the characteristic claw hand, in which the thumb rotates outward so that it lies in the same plane as the fingers; the interphalangeal joints are slightly flexed and the metacarpophalangeal joints are slightly extended. Wasting of the small muscles leaves the bones easily visible through the skin, resulting in the characteristic guttered appearance of the back of the hand.

Muscle mass is so variable among people that it is sometimes difficult to decide whether the muscles of the leg are wasted. Any marked asymmetry indicates an abnormality, but it is often difficult to decide whether a particular individual has a slender thigh or quadriceps muscle atrophy. One way to try to distinguish this is to ask the patient to tighten the knee as firmly as possible. The firm medial and lateral bellies of the normal quadriceps that bunch up in the distal part of the thigh just above the knee fail to appear in the wasted muscle. The same technique may be used to evaluate anterior tibial wasting. In a severely wasted muscle, a groove on the lateral side of the tibia (which should be filled by the anterior tibial muscles) is apparent. A moderate degree of wasting is hard to distinguish from a thin leg, but if the patient is asked to dorsiflex the foot, the wasted muscle fails to develop the prominent belly seen in a normal muscle.

Finally, all the limbs should be examined to determine the presence or absence of *fasciculations*. These brief, shocklike twitches of isolated muscle bundles may be difficult to differentiate from *myokymia*, which is a more rhythmic writhing and slower contraction of the motor unit. Fasciculations may be difficult or impossible to see in infants or obese individuals. They can be present in normal people, however, so fasciculations in the absence of wasting or weakness are probably of no significance. Nevertheless, fasciculations that are widespread and seen on every examination may indicate denervating disease, particularly anterior horn cell disease. Fasciculations are exacerbated by mental or physical fatigue, caffeine, cigarette smoking, or drugs such as amphetamines. Patients whose fasciculations appear benign should be reevaluated after avoiding exposure to exacerbating factors.

Palpation of Muscle and Testing for Range of Motion

Palpation and percussion of muscle provide additional information. Fibrotic muscle may feel rubbery and hard, whereas denervated muscle may sometimes separate into separate strands that can be rolled under the fingers. Muscle in inflammatory myopathies or rheumatological conditions may be tender to palpation, but severe muscle pain on palpation is unusual and is much more characteristic of hysteria than neuromuscular disease. An exception to this is the patient experiencing an acute phase of viral myositis or rhabdomyolysis, whose muscles may be very sensitive to either movement or touch.

In addition to its diagnostic value, the presence or absence of *muscle contracture* across a joint may cause disability, even in the absence of weakness. Thus an evaluation of range of motion at major joints is an important part of the clinical examination. In a standard examination, contractures are evaluated at the elbows, wrists, hips, knees, and ankles. It is important to realize that wrist flexor contractures can only be evaluated with the fingers extended; otherwise the dorsiflexion of the wrist is compensated for by flexion of the fingers. At the hips, both flexion and iliotibial band contractures should be evaluated. Percussion of muscle may produce the phenomenon of *myotonia*, in which a localized contraction of the muscle persists for some seconds after percussion. This phenomenon, which is characteristic of myotonic dystrophy and myotonia congenita, is to be distinguished from *myoedema*, which is occasionally found in patients with thyroid disorders and other metabolic problems. In myoedema, the percussion is followed by the development of a dimple in the muscle, which then mounds to form a small hillock.

Table 29.1: The Medical Research Council scale for grading muscle strength

0	No contraction
1	Flicker or trace of contraction
2	Active movement, with gravity eliminated
3	Active movement against gravity
4	Active movement against gravity and resistance
5	Normal power

Evaluation of Muscle Strength

Evaluation of individual muscle strength is an important part of the clinical examination. Many methods are available, but most clinicians rely on manual muscle testing. Such a method has to be reproducible and consistent (see also Chapter 27). The method discussed here is based on the Medical Research Council grading system (Table 29.1). This is adequate for use in an office situation, particularly if it is supplemented by the functional testing described later in this section. A scale of 0–5 is used. Grade 5 is normal strength. A 5– grade is only used if the examiner is uncertain that a muscle is weak and should not be used for muscles that are slightly weak. Muscles that can move the joint against resistance may vary quite widely in strength; grades of 4+, 4, and 4– are often used to indicate differences, particularly between one side of the body and the other. The fact that grade 4 represents a wide range of strength, from slight weakness to moderate weakness, is a disadvantage. For this reason, the scale has been more useful in following the average strength of many muscles during the course of a disease, rather than the course of a single muscle. Averaging the scores of many muscles smooths out the stepwise progression noted in a single muscle and may demonstrate a steadily progressive decline in an illness. Grade 3+ is used when the muscle can move the joint against gravity and can exert a tiny amount of resistance but then collapses under the pressure of the examiner's hand. It is not used to denote the hysterical phenomenon of sudden give. Grade 3 indicates that the muscle can move the joint throughout its full range against gravity, but not against any added resistance. Sometimes, particularly in muscles acting across large joints, the muscle is capable of moving the limb partway against gravity, but not through the full range of movement. A muscle that cannot extend the knee horizontally when in a sitting position but can extend the knee within to 30–40 degrees of horizontal is graded 3–. Grades 2, 1, and 0 are as defined in Table 29.1.

Although it is commendable and sometimes essential to examine each skeletal muscle separately, most of us test groups of muscles rather than individual muscles. In our clinic, we test neck flexion, neck extension, shoulder abduction, internal rotation, external rotation, elbow flexion and extension, wrist flexion and extension, finger abduction and adduction, thumb abduction, hip flexion and extension, knee flexion and extension, ankle dorsiflexion and plantar flexion, and dorsiflexion of the great toe.

Much information about muscle strength can be gained by observing the patient perform certain tasks. The three most useful tasks are walking, arising from the floor, and stepping onto an 8-inch–high stool.

Walking

Gait is altered by weakness of muscles of the hip and back, the leg, and the shoulder. In normal walking, when the heel hits the ground, the shock is taken up by the action of the hip abductors, which stabilize the pelvis. In a sense, the hip abductors act as shock absorbers; their weakness disturbs the normal fluid movement of the pelvis during walking, so that when the heel hits the ground the pelvis dips to the other side; when the weakness is bilateral, this results in a waddle. Additionally, weakness of the hip extensors and back extensors makes it difficult for the patient to maintain a normal posture. Ordinarily the body is carried so that the center of gravity is slightly forward of the hip joint. To maintain an erect posture, the hip and back extensors are in continual activity. If these muscles become weak, the patient often throws the shoulders back so that the weight of the body falls behind the hip joints. This accentuates the lumbar lordosis. Alternatively, if there is much weakness of the quadriceps muscles, the patient stabilizes the knee by throwing it backward. When the knee is hyperextended, it is locked; it derives its stability from the anatomy of the joint, not from the support of the muscles. Finally, weakness of the muscles of the lower part of the leg may result in a steppage gait, in which dorsiflexion of the foot is effected by a short throw at the ankle midswing. The foot is then brought rapidly to the ground before the toes fall back into plantar flexion.

Shoulder weakness may be noted as the patient walks; the arms hang loosely by the sides and tend to swing in a pendular fashion, rather than with a normal controlled swing.

Arising from the Floor

The normal method for arising from the floor depends, to a certain extent, on the age of the patient. The young child can spring rapidly to his or her feet without the average observer being able to dissect the movements. The elderly patient may turn to one side, place a hand on the floor, and rise to a standing position with a deliberate slowness, not to mention a certain amount of creaking of the joints. In spite of this variability, abnormalities caused by muscle weakness are easily detected. The patient with hip weakness will turn to one side or the other to put the hand on the floor for support. The degree of turning is proportional to the severity of the weakness. Some patients have to turn all the way around until they are in a prone position before they draw their feet under them to begin the standing process. Most people will arise to a standing position from a squatting position, but the patient with hip extensor weakness finds it easier to keep the hands on the floor and raise the hips high in the air. This has been termed the *butt-first maneuver*; the patient forms a triangle, with the hips at the apex and the base of support provided by both hands and feet on the floor, and then laboriously rises from this position, usually by pushing on the thighs with both hands to brace the body upward. The progress of recovery or progression of weakness can be documented by noting whether the initial turn is greater than 90 degrees, whether unilateral or bilateral hand support is used on the floor and thighs, whether this support is sustained or transient, and whether there is a butt-first maneuver. The entire process is known as *Gower's maneuver*, but it is useful to break it up into its component parts (Figure 29.2).

Stepping onto a Stool

For a patient with hip and leg weakness, stepping onto an 8-inch–high foot stool is equivalent in difficulty to a normal person's stepping onto a table. This analogy is apt because similar maneuvers are performed in both cases. Whereas the patient with normal strength will readily approach a footstool and easily step onto it, the patient with weakness will often hesitate in front of the stool while contemplating the task. When the weight is transferred from the foot on the ground to the foot placed on the stool, the pelvis will dip toward the floor as the leading leg takes up the strain. Finally, if the weakness is severe, patients may either use hand support on the thighs or gather themselves in and throw their bodies onto the footstool. Analysis of the various components—the hesitation, the hip dip, and the throw—together with the presence or absence of hand support may provide a sensitive measure of changes in an illness.

INVESTIGATING THE WEAK PATIENT

Before embarking on exhaustive investigations that carry some risk and expense, it is important to be certain that a patient is truly weak. If the patient has no objective weakness at the time of the examination, the clinician must rely on the history. Patients with weak muscles have a fairly stereotypical set of symptoms, including difficulty getting out of deep chairs or bathtubs, climbing stairs (during which they have to help themselves up with the railing or by pushing on the knee), lifting heavy objects from shelves, opening

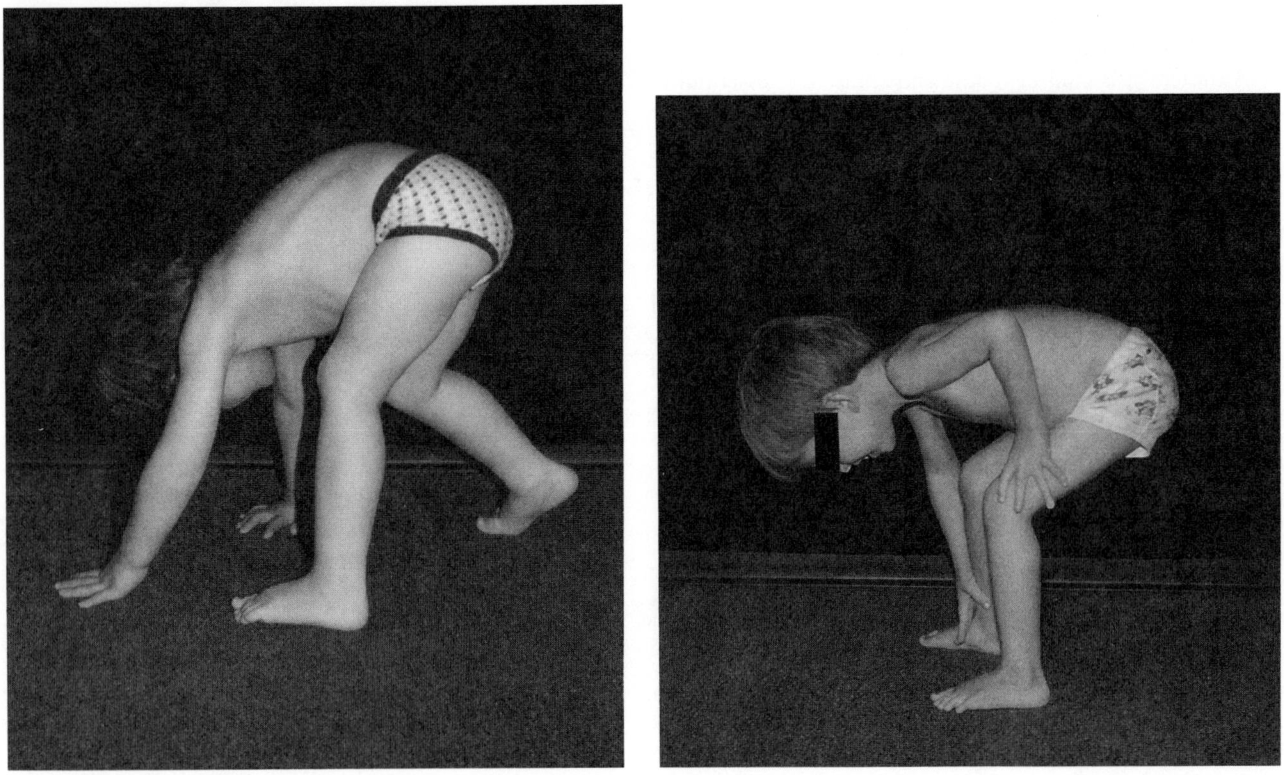

A B

FIGURE 29.2 The Gowers' maneuver. A. "Butt-first" maneuver as the hips are hoisted in the air. B. Hand support on the thighs.

door handles, and so on. The patient whose weakness is caused by a disturbed mental state (such as depression or malingering) has much vaguer symptoms, and if leading questions are avoided, the stereotypical symptoms of weakness are seldom volunteered. Instead, patients make statements such as "I have no strength to do the housework," "I just can't do the task," "I can't climb the stairs because I get so tired and have to rest," and the like. If the patient is pressed on these symptoms, it soon becomes apparent that specific details are lacking. Patients who cannot get out of a deep chair because of weakness will explain exactly how they have to maneuver themselves into an upright position—pushing on the chair arms, leaning forward in the seat, and bracing their hands against the furniture. Patients whose history is vague may be asked what they would do to escape if there were a fire in the room. Patients with real weakness often say that they might have to slide out of the chair and crawl out of the room. Patients whose weakness is less substantive often say that they are so tired that they do not think they could get out of the room. At the risk of belaboring the point, it is important that the examiner not provide patients with the details for which they are searching. Asking patients whether they have to push on the arms of the chair to stand up provides patients with information that will be used later in response to your baffled successors.

It is also possible to differentiate real weakness from *hysterical weakness* on examination. The primary characteristic of hysterical weakness is that it is unpredictable and fluctuating. Muscle strength may suddenly give when being evaluated. The patient has a difficult time knowing exactly how much strength is expected and therefore cannot adequately counter the examiner's resistance. This gives rise to a wavering, collapsing force. Tricks may be used to bring out the discrepancy in muscle performance when the patient is being tested and not aware of being observed. For example, if the thigh cannot be lifted off the chair in a seated position because of weakness, then the legs should not be able to swing up onto the mattress when the patient is asked to sit on the examining table. If I suspect that weakness of shoulder abduction is feigned, I will often put the patient's arm in abduction, put my hand on the elbow, and instruct the patient to push toward the ceiling. At first the downward pressure is kept very light and the patient is unable to move the examining hand toward the ceiling. However, the arm does not fall down either, and as the downward pressure is gradually increased by the examiner, continued exhortation to push the examiner's hand upward results in increasing resistance to the downward pressure. The examiner ends up putting maximum weight on the outstretched arm, which remains in abduction. The examiner concludes that the strength is normal. Patients do not realize this since, as far as they are concerned, they did not move the examiner's hand upward and therefore must be weak.

For patients whose weakness is real and whose diagnosis is not evident on clinical grounds, laboratory investigations may help with defining the disease. In the investigation of diseases of the motor unit, the most helpful tests are measurement of the serum concentration of creatine kinase, electrodiagnosis, and muscle biopsy, which are available to virtually all physicians. In addition, if facilities are available, exercise testing can provide useful information. Genetic testing is also being used increasingly for definitive diagnosis.

Serum Creatine Kinase

The usefulness of measuring the serum creatine kinase (CK) concentration in the diagnosis of neuromuscular diseases is to differentiate between neurogenic disease, in which there may be mild to moderate elevations of CK, and myopathies in which the CK may be markedly increased. Serial CKs are also used to follow the progress of the disease. Neither of these uses is devoid of problems. Foremost is the determination of the "normal" level. A survey of 250 hospitals in Ontario showed a surprising ignorance of the basic mechanisms involved in the test as well as the way in which normal values were derived. Some hospitals were ignorant that race, gender, age, and activity level must be taken into account in determining normal values. When blood samples are obtained from truly normal controls and not a population of inactive hospital patients who happen not to have overt muscle disease, the normal serum concentration of CK is higher than anticipated. Furthermore, all studies on CK show that the values are not normally distributed. A log transformation does much to convert this to a normal distribution curve, but even then the results are not perfect. In a survey of 1,500 hospital employees, using carefully standardized methods, it was possible to detect three "populations," each with characteristic CK values. The upper limits of normal (97.5th percentile) are as follows:

Black men only: 520 U/liter
Black women, nonblack men: 345 U/liter
Nonblack women: 145 U/liter.

The "nonblack" population included Hispanics, Asians, and whites. Because the upper limit is expressed as a percentile, it must be understood that by definition 2.5% of the normal population will be above that. Although this does not seem to be a large number, in a town of 100,000 it means that 2,500 are candidates for the muscle clinic if they have their serum CK analyzed. The point is that the upper limit of normal CK is not rigid and should be interpreted intelligently.

The serum CK concentration can be useful in determining the course of an illness, although, again, judgment should be used since changes in CK values do not always mirror the clinical condition. In treating inflammatory myopathies with immunosuppressive drugs or corticosteroids, a steadily declining CK level is a reassurance, whereas levels that are creeping back up again when the patient is in remission are not.

Serum CK concentrations can also be used to determine if an illness is monophasic. A bout of myoglobinuria may be associated with very high concentrations of CK. When this is followed over the next week or so, the concentration declines steadily by about 50% every 2 days. This indicates that a single episode of muscle damage has occurred. Patients with CK concentrations that do not decline in this fashion or that vary from high to low on random days have an ongoing illness that should be treated as such. It must be remembered that CK concentrations elevated as high as 10 times normal may also be seen with denervating disorders such as amyotrophic lateral sclerosis (ALS) and spinal muscular atrophy (see Chapter 79). Finally, exercise may cause a marked elevation in CK, which usually peaks 12–18 hours after the activity, but may be days later. CK concentrations are more likely to rise in people who are sedentary and then undertake unaccustomed exercise than in a trained individual.

Electromyography

As with all laboratory tests, an experienced electromyographer is essential to interpret electromyography (EMG) correctly. The principles of EMG are discussed in Chapter 37. The EMG may give much useful information. An initial step in the assessment of the weak patient is determination of whether the disease is due to denervation or myopathy. Nerve conduction studies and needle electrode examination are particularly sensitive for identifying neuropathic disorders and localizing the abnormality to anterior horn cells, or nerve root or peripheral nerve territories (see Chapters 80 and 81). Repetitive nerve stimulation and single-fiber EMG can aid in elucidating disorders of the neuromuscular junction. Needle electrode examination may help establish the presence of a myotonic disorder or an inflammatory myopathy.

Muscle Biopsy

The use of muscle histochemistry evaluation as well as electron microscopy may provide a specific diagnosis. Histochemical evaluation is now within reach of most hospitals; an elaborate setup is not necessary. The details of muscle biopsy are reviewed in Chapter 84, but a word about the selection of the muscle to be biopsied is appropriate here. In all biopsies there is a risk of sampling error. Not all muscles are equally involved in any given disease, and it is important to select a muscle that is likely to give the most useful information. The gastrocnemius muscle is often chosen for muscle biopsy but has the disadvantage of demonstrating type 1 fiber predominance in the normal individual. Also, it seems to show more than its fair share of random pathological changes, such as fiber necrosis and small inflammatory infiltrates, even when there is no clinical suspicion of a muscle disease. For this reason, it might be preferable to select either the quadriceps femoris or the biceps brachii if either of these muscle is weak. Never biopsy a muscle that is the site of a recent EMG or intramuscular injection. If such a muscle has to be biopsied, allow at least 2–3 months before performing the biopsy.

In the patient with a relatively acute (duration of weeks) disease, it is wise to select a muscle that is obviously clinically weak. In patients with long-standing disease, it may be better to select a muscle that is clinically fairly normal to avoid an end-stage muscle. Sometimes an apparently normal muscle is selected for biopsy. For example, in a patient who is suspected of having motor neuron disease and who has wasting and weakness of the arms, with EMG changes of denervation in the arms but no apparent denervation of the legs, biopsy of the biceps muscle would show the expected denervation and would not add any useful information. If a biopsy of a quadriceps muscle showed denervation, this would provide support for widespread denervation, supporting the diagnosis of motor neuron disease. Similarly, if the biopsy from the quadriceps muscle was normal, this would make the diagnosis of ALS less likely, since even strong muscles in patients with ALS usually show some denervation.

Genetic Testing

The details of genetic testing and counseling are covered in Chapter 47. Genetic analysis has now become a routine part of the clinical investigation of neuromuscular disease and, in certain situations, may supplant muscle biopsy and other diagnostic tests. This is a distinct advantage to the patient for whom a blood test may be substituted for a muscle biopsy. The use of genetic testing as a diagnostic test in an isolated individual implies that the gene is well characterized and that intragenic probes are available that allow the determination of whether or not the gene in question is abnormal. Examples are the deletion in the dystrophin gene seen in many cases of Duchenne's dystrophy and the expansion of the myotonic dystrophy gene. For the more traditional purpose of identifying those who are at risk for the disease or those who may be carriers, linkage studies using probes that are close to the gene may suffice.

Linkage studies are possible when the location of the gene is known. The success of such studies depends on having probes that are close to the gene even though the gene is not completely characterized. By using these closely situated probes it can often be demonstrated that the individual is or is not carrying the part of the chromosome on which a "bad" gene must have occurred in another family member. For linkage studies to be successful there must be a sufficient number of family members available for testing, both with and without the illness, to allow an identification of the segment of the chromosome at fault. This type of study is hampered by the tendency of bits of the chromosome to become detached during meiosis and to be exchanged with parts of another chromosome, a phenomenon known as "recombination." The closer the probe is to the actual gene, the less likely recombination is to separate them. Genetic counseling based on linkage studies is less likely to be successful when only one or two patients with the illness and few family members are available.

Exercise Testing

Exercise testing is an important part of the investigation of muscle disease, particularly metabolic disorders. The two primary types of exercise tests that are used are forearm exercise and bicycle exercise. Forearm (grip) exercise has been designed to provide a test of glycolytic pathways, particularly those involved in power exercise. Incremental bicycle ergometry gives additional information in regard to the relative use of carbohydrates, fats, and oxygen.

Forearm exercise is performed according to several schedules. The traditional method was to ask the patient to grip a dynamometer repetitively, with a cuff occluding the circulation. If the work performed by the patient is sufficiently strenuous, the cuff is unnecessary, since the muscle is working at a level that surpasses the ability of blood-borne substances to sustain it. An adequate level of forceful exercise is maintained for 1 minute, and then venous blood is drawn at intervals following the exercise to monitor changes in metabolites. In the normal individual the energy for such work is derived from intramuscular glycogen. Lactate is formed when exercise is relatively anaerobic, as it is when the exercise is strenuous. Additionally, serum concentrations of hypoxanthine and ammonia are elevated. Patients with defects in the glycolytic pathways produce normal to excessive amounts of ammonia and hypoxanthine, but no lactate. Patients with adenylate deaminase deficiency show the reverse situation; no ammonia or hypoxanthine appear, but lactate production is normal. In patients who cannot cooperate with the testing and whose effort is poor, neither lactate nor ammonia concentrations are very high. This test is also useful for defining the mechanical fatigue that occurs in some illnesses such as myasthenia gravis or the metabolic myopathies. In mitochondrial disorders and other instances of metabolic stress, the production of both lactate and hypoxanthine is excessive.

Incremental bicycle ergometry allows one to measure the oxygen consumption and carbon dioxide production associated with varying workloads. The patient pedals a bicycle at a steady rate. The workload is increased every minute or two. Excessive oxygen consumption for a given work level suggests an abnormality in the energy pathway in muscle. In addition, the *respiratory exchange ratio* (RER)—the ratio of carbon dioxide produced to oxygen consumed—is characteristic for various fuel sources. Carbohydrate metabolism results in an RER of 1. Fat, on the other hand, has an RER of 0.7. The resting RER in normal individuals is around 0.8. For technical reasons, at the end of an incremental exercise test, the RER is often as high as 1.2 in the normal individual. Patients with disorders of lipid metabolism often have an unusually high RER because they preferentially metabo-

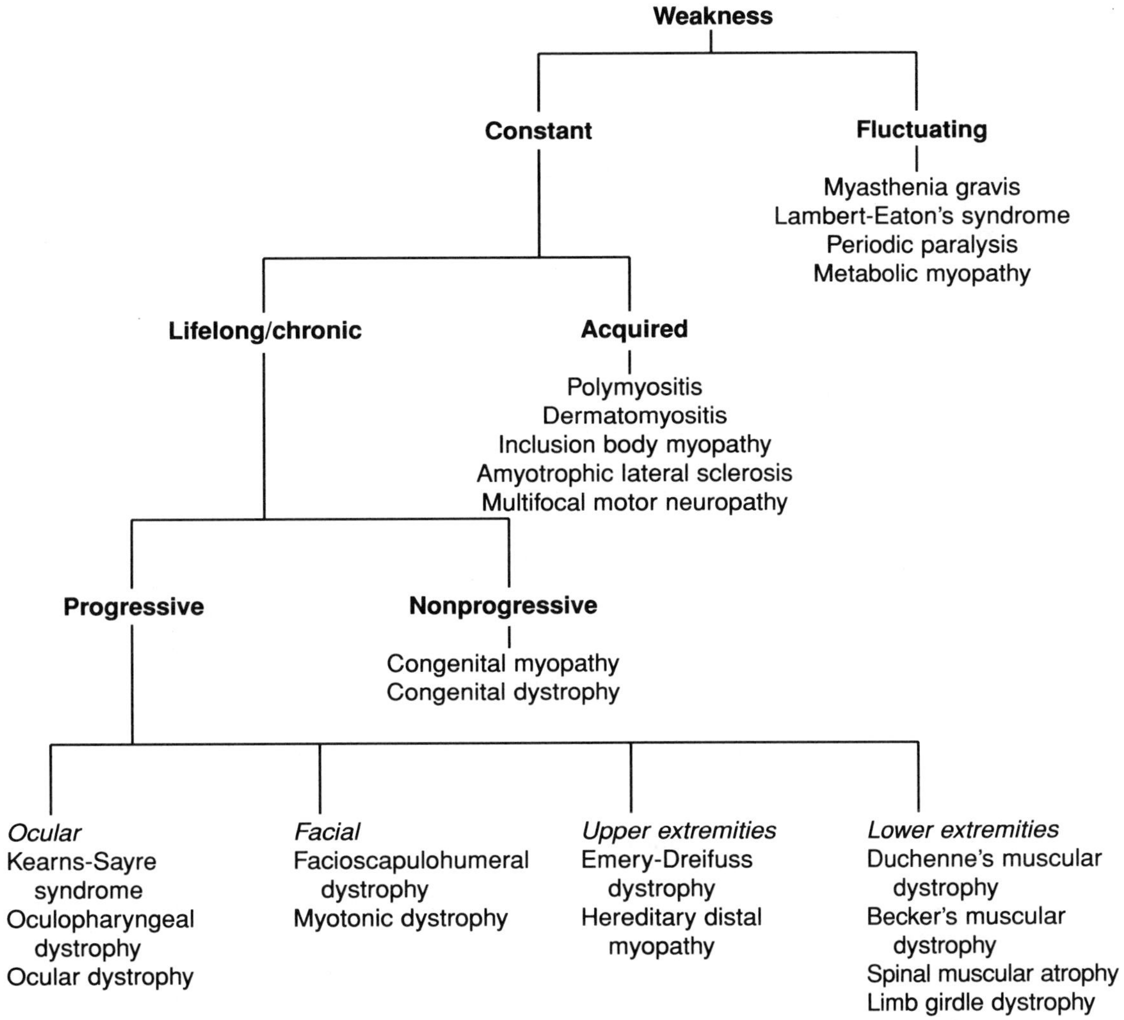

FIGURE 29.3 An algorithm for the approach to the patient with weakness.

lize carbohydrates, whereas patients with disorders of carbohydrate metabolism may never increase RER to greater than 1 because they preferentially metabolize lipids.

PATIENTS WITH DEFINITE WEAKNESS

Once it is established that a patient has weakness, either by history or examination, the clinical features may be so characteristic that the diagnosis is obvious. At other times the clinician may be uncertain. Figure 29.3 displays an outline of diagnostic considerations based on the characteristics of the weakness, such as whether it is fluctuating or constant. The following sections amplify this approach.

Fluctuating Weakness

The first step is to determine if the weakness is constant or fluctuating. Even constant weakness may vary according to how the patient feels; this is expected. We are all capable of better physical performance on the days when we feel energetic and cheerful and do less well on days when we are depressed or sick. Such factors also affect the patient with neuromuscular weakness. Specific inquiries should be made to determine how much variability exists. Is the fluctuation related to exercise or time of day? Symptoms and signs that are provoked by exercise imply disorder in the physiological or biochemical mechanisms governing muscle contraction. Pain, contractures, and weakness following exercise are often characteristic of abnormalities in the biochemistry of muscle contraction. Pathological fatigue is the hallmark of neuromuscular junction abnormalities.

Factors other than exercise may result in a worsening or improvement of the disease. Some patients notice that fasting, carbohydrate loading, or other dietary manipulations make a difference in their symptoms. Such details may provide a clue to underlying metabolic problems. Patients with a defect in lipid-based energy metabolism will be weaker in the fasting state and may carry a candy bar or sugar with them. The patient with hypokalemic periodic paralysis may have noticed that attacks are precipitated by a heavy carbohydrate meal.

Disorders of the Neuromuscular Junction

Weakness that fluctuates markedly on a day-to-day basis or within a space of several hours is more often caused by a defect in neuromuscular transmission or a metabolic abnormality such as periodic paralysis than by one of the muscular dystrophies. Most neurologists recognize that the cardinal features of myasthenia gravis are ptosis, ophthalmoparesis, dysarthria, dysphagia, and axial weakness (see Chapter 83). On clinical examination the hallmark of myasthenia gravis is pathological fatigue. Normal muscles fatigue if exercised sufficiently, but in myasthenia gravis fatigue occurs with little effort. Failure of neuromuscular transmission may prevent maintenance of the arms in an outstretched position for more than a few seconds or maintenance of sustained upgaze. One of the problems with the diagnosis of myasthenia is that the patient may be relatively normal when examined in the office; the history and ancillary studies (acetylcholine receptor antibodies and EMG with repetitive stimulation or single fiber EMG) must be relied on to establish the diagnosis.

In the Lambert-Eaton's syndrome, fluctuating weakness of the shoulder and hip girdles predominates, but bulbar, ocular, and respiratory muscles are spared. Reflexes are typically reduced. Exercise may improve the weakness and enhance the reflexes. The electrophysiological correlate of this phenomenon is the demonstration of an incremental response to rapid repetitive nerve stimulation.

Fluctuating Weakness Exacerbated by Exercise

Fatigue and muscle pain provoked by exercise, the most common complaints in the muscle clinic, are often unexplained, and diagnoses such as fibromyalgia and the aches, cramps, and pain syndrome are used to cloak our ignorance (see Chapter 30). Biochemical defects are being found in an increasing number of patients with exercise-induced fatigue and myalgia. The metabolic abnormalities that impede exercise are disorders of carbohydrate metabolism, lipid metabolism, and mitochondrial function. The patient's history may give some clue to the type of defect.

Fatty acids provide the main source of energy metabolism for resting muscle. The initiation of vigorous exercise requires the use of intracellular stores of energy, since blood-borne metabolites are initially inadequate. It takes some time for the cardiac output to rise, for capillaries to dilate, and for the blood supply to muscle to be increased, and an even longer time for fat stores in the body to be mobilized so that the level of fatty acid rises in the blood. Muscle must use its glycogen stores in the initial phase of heavy exercise. Thus, defects of glycogen metabolism cause fatigue and muscle pain in the first few minutes of exercise. As exercise continues in the normal individual, the blood supply increases, resulting in an increased supply of oxygen, glucose, and fatty acids. After 10–15 minutes, the muscle begins to use a mixture of fat and carbohydrate. The use of carbohydrate cannot be tolerated for long periods, since it would deplete the body's glycogen stores and might result in hypoglycemia. After 30–40 minutes of continued endurance exercise, the muscle is chiefly using fatty acids as an energy source. Patients with a defect of fatty acid metabolism can exercise in the initial phase very easily but may become incapacitated with endurance exercise lasting 30–60 minutes. Similarly, in the fasting state, the body is more dependent on fatty acids, which it uses to conserve glucose. The patient with a disorder of fatty acid metabolism may complain of increased symptoms when exercising in the fasting state. Ingestion of a candy bar may give some relief, as this boosts the blood sugar. Patients with fatty acid metabolism defects often have well-developed muscles, because their favorite exercise is relatively intense, brief power exercise, such as weight lifting.

Disorders of mitochondrial metabolism are of three types. In one there are recurrent encephalopathic episodes, often noted in early childhood and resembling Reye's disease (see Chapter 69). The second type is associated with particular weakness of the extraocular and often other skeletal muscles. In another type, usually affecting young adults, the symptoms are predominantly of exercise intolerance. Defects occur in the electron transport system or cytochrome chain that uncouple oxygen consumption from the useful production of adenosine triphosphate. This causes metabolic pathways to run at their limit, even to keep up with the demands of a light exercise load. Resting tachycardia, high lactic acid levels in the blood, excessive sweating, and other indications of hypermetabolism are noted. This may lead to an erroneous diagnosis of hyperthyroidism. It is always worth measuring the serum lactic acid concentration if a mitochondrial myopathy is suspected. In addition to lactate, ammonia and hypoxanthine concentrations may also be elevated. Patients with suspected metabolic defects require forearm exercise and bicycle exercise tests. Myoglobinuria may occur during an exercise test, so the patient should be cautioned about the possibility.

Several disorders characterized by episodic weakness are associated with specific abnormalities of the sodium channel (see Chapter 84), including hyperkalemic periodic paralysis and paramyotonia congenita. Hypokalemic periodic paralysis shares some clinical features, but the basic abnormality is in a calcium channel.

In these disorders bouts of weakness of varying severity occur, sometimes making it impossible for the patient to get out of bed. Nevertheless, respiratory function is not compromised. Within a day or so the patient's strength usually returns to normal even without treatment. These features separate this group from other fluctuating diseases.

In hypokalemic paralysis, attacks that may last from a few hours to a day are associated with low serum potassium. Rest after exercise, high carbohydrate meals, and emotional stress may precipitate an attack. In the hyperkalemic group, the attack lasts minutes to hours and the potassium levels are normal or high. The patient may notice that consumption of orange juice or other potassium-containing foods may bring on an attack. Rest after activity also may precede an attack of hyperkalemic paralysis. In paramyotonia congenita, cooling of the muscle is associated with flaccid weakness.

Constant Weakness

All weakness shows some fluctuation; people have good and bad days. With "constant" weakness the course is one of stability or steady deterioration. Without treatment, the periods of sustained, objective improvement or major differences in strength on a day-to-day basis are lacking. The division of this group into acquired and chronic also needs clarification. "Acquired" means that weakness appeared over weeks to months in a previously healthy person. In contrast, "chronic" weakness implies a much less definite onset. While the patient may say that the weakness came on suddenly, a careful history elicits symptoms that go back many years. This division is not absolute. Patients with polymyositis, an acquired disease, may have a slow, ingravescent course mimicking a dystrophy. Patients with dystrophy may have a slow increase in weakness and suddenly lose a specific function, such as standing from a chair or climbing stairs, and believe their disorder to be acute.

Acquired Disorders Causing Weakness

Acquired disorders producing weakness are usually either motor neuron diseases, inflammatory diseases of muscle, or peripheral neuropathies, which are considered in Chapter 81. The first task is to determine whether the weakness is due to denervation or myopathy. If strength and tendon reflexes have declined out of proportion to the muscle bulk, one may suspect a myopathy. Muscle biopsy, EMG, and determination of serum CK are helpful.

ALS is a common illness with a relatively rapid course often presaged by the occurrence of night cramps in the calf muscles. Examination shows wasting and often widely distributed fasciculations. If pseudobulbar palsy, with difficulty swallowing and speaking, is also present the diagnosis is relatively simple. Hyperreflexia is often seen because of the associated involvement of the upper motor neuron. A weak, wasted muscle, associated with an abnormally brisk reflex, is almost pathognomonic of ALS. The diagnosis is confirmed by the finding of denervation in at least one arm and leg—some say three limbs—together with upper motor neuron signs. It is important to rule out a local spinal cord lesion or a multifocal motor neuropathy if the illness is limited to the arms or legs. Multifocal motor neuropathy mimics ALS, but there are no bulbar features or hyperreflexia, and the EMG findings are characteristic. Sporadic forms of juvenile spinal muscular atrophy or adult-onset spinal muscular atrophy occur in which the progression of weakness is slower, fasciculations are less prominent, and upper motor neuron and bulbar involvement are lacking.

If the changes on EMG are myopathic, one must consider a muscular dystrophy, inflammatory myopathies, or inclusion body myopathy (see Chapter 84). Inflammatory myopathies, as exemplified by polymyositis, often run a steadily progressive downhill course, although some fluctuation may be noted, particularly in children. If an associated skin rash is present, there is little doubt about the diagnosis of dermatomyositis. In its absence, polymyositis may be difficult to differentiate from any of the other causes of proximal weakness. Sometimes the illness occurs as part of an overlap syndrome, in which fragments of other autoimmune diseases, such as scleroderma, lupus, or arthritis, are involved. Polymyositis is sometimes difficult to differentiate from limb girdle muscular dystrophy, even after a muscle biopsy; some inflammatory changes may be seen in the latter, and the characteristic perifascicular atrophy is not always noted in the former. Other signs of systemic involvement, such as malaise, transient aching pains, mood changes, and loss of appetite, are more common in polymyositis than in limb girdle dystrophy.

Inclusion body myopathy may also mimic polymyositis clinically. Clues to the diagnosis are male gender and age over 40 years. Usually there is slowly progressive weakness of the limb girdle musculature associated, in a significant number of patients, with distal weakness, especially of the hands. Inclusion body myopathy, unlike polymyositis, is unresponsive to immunosuppressive therapy and has rimmed vacuoles and intracytoplasmic and intranuclear filamentous inclusions in muscle fibers.

Lifelong Disorders

Most patients seen in the neuromuscular clinic have lifelong, presumably inherited disorders of progressive weakness. In some the responsible genetic abnormality has been identified. An important point in the differential diagnosis of muscle disease is to determine if weakness is truly progressive. Surprisingly, hospital charts often fail to document progression. The examiner should ask questions until the progressive or nonprogressive nature of the disease is certain. The severity of the disease is often taken as proof of progression. It is hard to imagine that a 16-year-old girl, confined to her wheelchair with spinal muscular atrophy and scoliosis and having difficulty breathing, has a relatively nonprogressive disorder, but careful questioning may show that there has been no loss of function for the last 8–9 years. Neither is it sufficient to ask the patient in vague and general terms whether the illness is progressive. Questioning should be specific, such as: "Are there tasks that you cannot perform this year [or month or week] that you could perform last year [or month or week]?" One must also be alert for denial, which is common in young patients with increasing weakness. The 18-year-old boy with limb girdle dystrophy may claim to be the same now as in years gone by, but questioning may reveal that he was able to climb stairs well when he was in high school, whereas he now needs assistance in college.

Lifelong, Nonprogressive Disorders. Some patients complain of lifelong weakness that has been relatively unchanged over many years. Almost by definition such disorders have to start in early childhood. Nonprogression of weakness does not preclude severe weakness. Later-life progression of such weakness may occur as the normal aging process further weakens muscles that have very little functional reserve. One major group of such illnesses is the congenital nonprogressive myopathies, including central core disease, nemaline myopathy, and congenital fiber-type disproportion. The typical clinical picture in these diseases is that of a slender dysmorphic individual with diffuse weakness (Figure 29.4A). There may be associated skeletal abnormalities, such as high-arched palate, pes cavus, and scoliosis. Deep tendon reflexes are depressed or absent. Although it is unusual, severe respiratory involvement has occasionally been noted in all of these diseases. The less severe (non–X-linked) form of myotubular (centronuclear) myopathy may be suspected because of the occurrence of ptosis, ocular weakness, and facial diplegia. Muscle biopsy can usually be relied on to provide the diagnosis in the congenital myopathies.

Several varieties of congenital muscular dystrophy are recognized. The weakness in congenital muscular dystrophy is usually severe, contractures are prominent, and there may be associated findings. For example, in Fukuyama's dystrophy, there are associated mental retardation and seizures. Other signs of damage to the central nervous system may be present, such as increased tendon reflexes and extensor plantar responses. Most patients with Fukuyama's dystrophy are severely disabled, both physically and intellectually. The serum CK concentration may be markedly elevated. The muscle biopsy is very different from that in the congenital nonprogressive myopathies and shows fiber necrosis with fibrosis and phagocytosis.

There are also patients whose biopsies show dystrophic changes but whose illnesses are much milder. One such illness has been termed "stick man dystrophy" because of the almost skeletal appearance of the limbs, with severely atrophic muscles (see Figure 29.4B). Although there is diffuse weakness, the atrophic muscles generate more force than one would expect on the basis of their bulk. Patients also have severe heel cord contractures and often have contractures of the posterior cervical muscles.

Lifelong Disorders Characterized by Progressive Weakness. Most diseases in this category are inherited, progressive disorders of anterior horn cells or of muscle. Mild day-to-day fluctuations in strength may occur, but the overall progression is steady. That is, if a disorder is slowly progressive from the start it will remain that way; it will not suddenly change course and become rapidly progressive. As mentioned earlier, patients may experience long periods of stability when their disease is seemingly nonprogressive.

Attempts to categorize disorders of weakness by particular body regions are artificial at best, as most inherited progressive disorders have widespread or diffuse weakness or affect multiple regions. However, characteristic patterns of weakness sometimes suggest specific diagnoses. For example, facioscapulohumeral dystrophy and oculopharyngeal dystrophy are so named because of their selective involvement of muscles.

Disorders with Prominent Ocular Weakness. In oculopharyngeal muscular dystrophy, a steadily progressive weakness of the eye muscles, causing ptosis and external ophthalmoplegia, is associated with difficulty in swallowing. This disorder is an autosomal-dominant trait and does not seem to shorten life. A number of patients also have facial weakness and hip and shoulder weakness. Swallowing difficulty may become severe enough to necessitate gastrostomy tube placement.

The Kearns-Sayre syndrome is a distinctive collection of physical findings, including ptosis, extraocular palsies, pigmentary degeneration of the retina, cerebellar ataxia, pyramidal tract signs, short stature, mental retardation, and cardiac conduction defects, that accompany an abnormality of the mitochondria in muscle and other tissues. It may be slowly progressive or nonprogressive.

Disorders with Distinctive Facial Weakness. Facioscapulohumeral muscular dystrophy is often noted early in adult life. Weakness of the face may lead to difficulty with whistling or blowing up balloons and may be severe enough to give the face a smooth, unlined appearance with an abnormal pout to the lips (Figure 29.5A). Weakness of the muscles around the shoulders is always seen, although the deltoid muscle is surprisingly well preserved. When the patient attempts to hold the arms extended in front, there is winging of the scapula that is quite characteristic. The whole scapula may slide upward on the back of the thorax. The inferomedial border always juts backward, producing the appearance of a triangle at right angles to the back, with the base of the triangle still attached to the thorax. In addition, a discrepancy in power is often seen between the wrist flexors, which are strong, and the wrist extensors, which are weak. Similarly the plantar flexors may be strong, while the dorsiflexors of the ankles are weak. It is common for the weakness to be asymmetrical, with one side much less involved than the other. The disorder is inherited as an autosomal dominant trait, although mild forms of the illness may be missed in the parents.

Related to facioscapulohumeral dystrophy is scapuloperoneal dystrophy, which has similar features but lacks the facial weakness. The two are differentiated because the scapuloperoneal distribution of weakness may be seen in some other congenital nonprogressive myopathies, which may lead to some confusion in the diagnosis.

Myotonic dystrophy is a common illness with distinctive features, including distal predominance of weakness. It is inherited as an autosomal dominant trait, but often no family history is reported because the patients may be unaware that other family members have the illness. The diagnosis may be suspected in any patient with muscular dystrophy

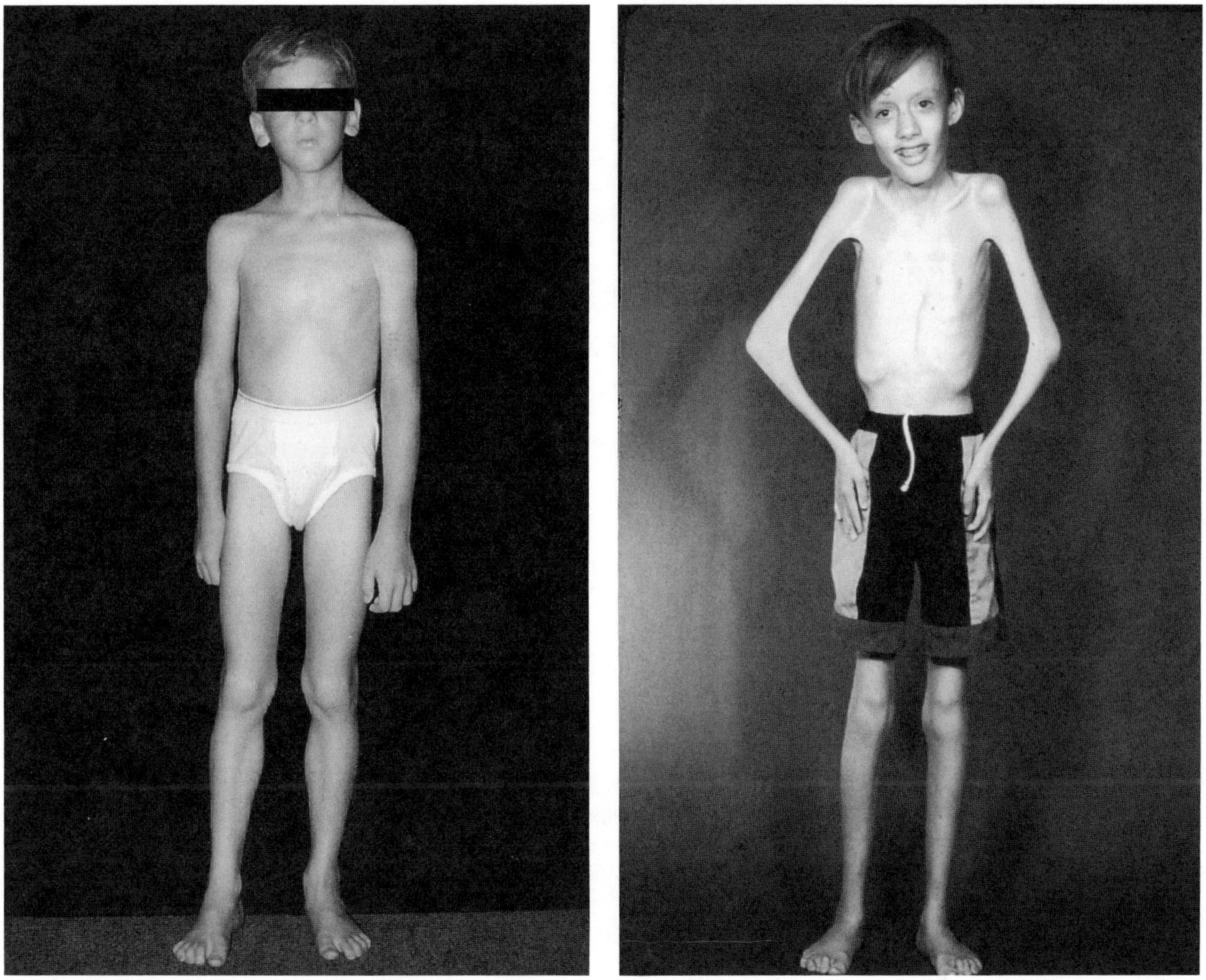

A B

FIGURE 29.4 A. The patient with a congenital dystrophy is slender, without focal atrophy. Shoulder girdle weakness is apparent from the horizontal set of the clavicles. B. The patient with congenital muscular dystrophy of the "stick man" type is distinguished by his skeletal appearance and the presence of prominent contractures.

and predominantly distal weakness. The neck flexors and temporal and masseter muscles are often wasted. More characteristic than the distribution of the weakness is the long, thin face with hollowed temples and hooded eyes (ptosis) and frontal balding (see Figure 29.5B). Percussion myotonia and grip myotonia are seen in most patients after age 13 years. An EMG can be diagnostic. Muscle biopsy may also show characteristic changes, and genetic testing shows the characteristic chromosome 19 gene expansion.

Disorders with Distinctive Shoulder Girdle or Arm Weakness. In Emery-Dreifuss's disease, an abnormal gene on the X chromosome produces wasting and weakness of muscles around the shoulders, the upper arms, and the lower part of the leg, with contractures of the elbow, the posterior part of the neck, and the Achilles tendon. Cardiac conduction abnormalities are common, and death may occur as a result of acute heart block.

Although prominent distal weakness is generally associated with denervating disorders, two muscular dystrophies are predominantly distal: myotonic dystrophy, which has already been discussed, and hereditary distal myopathy. In hereditary distal myopathy the weakness usually starts in the muscles of the forearms and hands, which become clumsy. The onset of weakness is often after age 35 and may slowly spread to involve the lower part of the leg, particularly the anterior tibial compartment. The finger extensors are often involved unequally so that when the patient is asked to extend the hand, individual fingers assume different postures. Weakness sometimes begins in the distal part of the legs rather than in the arms.

Disorders with Prominent Hip Girdle or Leg Weakness. While patients with these disorders often have more diffuse weakness, including arm and shoulder girdle weakness, it is the hip and leg weakness that brings them to medical attention.

Acute infantile spinal muscular atrophy (Werdnig-Hoffmann's disease) is a severe and usually fatal illness with marked weakness of the limbs and respiratory muscles. Children with the intermediate form of spinal muscular atrophy

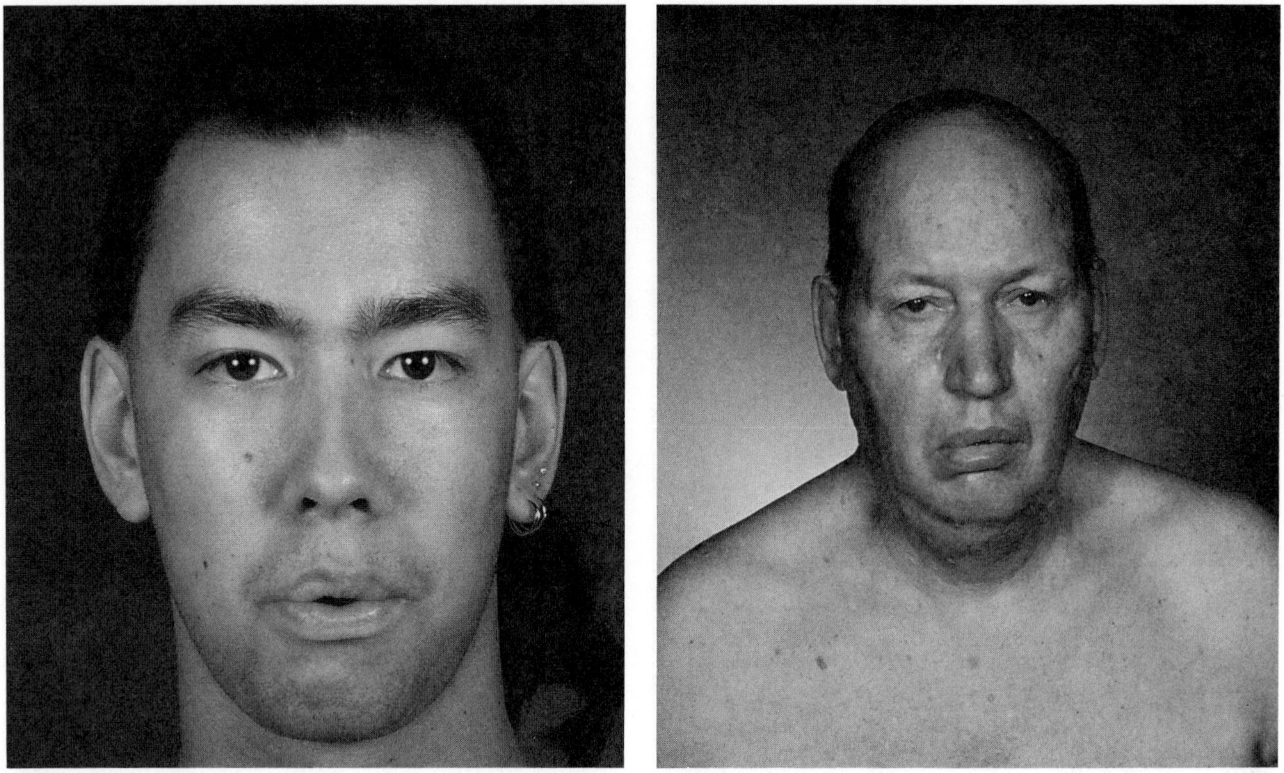

A B

FIGURE 29.5 Facial weakness is a prominent feature of both facioscapulohumeral dystrophy (FSH) and myotonic dystrophy. However, the characteristic features are so distinctive that they are readily recognizable and not easily confused. A. The patient with FSH dystrophy is unable to purse his or her lips when attempting to whistle. B. The typical appearance of a patient with myotonic dystrophy includes frontal balding, temporalis muscle wasting, ptosis, and facial weakness.

(chronic Werdnig-Hoffmann's disease, or spinal muscular atrophy type 2) are also severely affected, rarely maintaining the ability to walk for more than a few years, so that they are confined to a wheelchair in adult life. The progression of the illness is not steady; plateaus last for some years, interspersed with more rapid deterioration. Scoliosis is very common. In the intermediate form of spinal muscular atrophy, a fine tremor of the outstretched hands is characteristic.

Although it is a disorder of anterior horn cells, in juvenile spinal muscular atrophy the weakness is more severe proximally. The illness begins sometime during the first decade, and patients walk well into the second decade or even into early adult life. Scoliosis is less common than in the infantile form.

The inherited muscular dystrophies also cause progressive, nonfluctuating weakness. Duchenne's muscular dystrophy is an X-chromosome–linked recessive disorder associated with an absence of dystrophin. Clinically, the combination of greater proximal than distal weakness with hypertrophic muscles and contractures gives the clue to the diagnosis. The serum CK concentration is markedly elevated and the muscle biopsy is diagnostic (see Chapter 84). The clinical features of Becker's muscular dystrophy are identical except for later onset and slower progression.

Severe childhood autosomal recessive muscular dystrophy (SCARMD) is caused by deficiency in muscle of a dystrophin-associated glycoprotein and has been linked to chromosomes 13 and 17. SCARMD is phenotypically similar to Duchenne's muscular dystrophy, including the calf hypertrophy, but affects both males and females.

The limb girdle dystrophies are a well-accepted diagnostic classification, despite their clinical heterogeneity. Weakness begins in the hips, shoulders, or both and spreads gradually to involve the rest of the limbs and the trunk. The diagnosis is often established by exclusion of everything else. The most helpful test is the muscle biopsy, which shows dystrophic changes, separating limb girdle dystrophy from other (inflammatory) myopathies and from denervating diseases.

OTHER

No scheme of analysis is perfect in clinical medicine, and many exceptions exist to the guidelines provided above. Most notable are disorders that are restricted to various parts of the body. The etiology and the reasons for such localized illness are not clear, but examples include branchial myopathy and quadriceps myopathy, as well as the focal form of motor neuron disease, which often remains in one segment of the body for years to decades. These diseases are often "benign" in that they do not shorten life. The weakness may cause disability although it is usually mild.

SUGGESTED READING

Astrand PO, Rodahl K. Textbook of Work Physiology. New York: Mc-Graw-Hill, 1986.

Brooke MH. A Clinician's View of Neuromuscular Disease. Baltimore: Williams & Wilkins, 1986.

Guarantors of Brain. Aids to the Examination of the Peripheral Nervous System (2nd ed). London: Balliere-Tindall, 1986.

Harris EK, Wong ET, Shaw ST. Statistical criteria for separate reference intervals: race and gender groups in creatine kinase. Clin Chem 1991;37:1580–1582.

Henderson AT, McQueen MJ, Patten RL et al. Testing for creatine kinase-2 in Ontario: reference ranges and assay types. Clin Chem 1991;38:1365–1370.

McArdle WD, Katch FI, Katch VL. Exercise Physiology: Energy, Nutrition, and Human Performance. Philadelphia: Lea & Febiger, 1986.

Chapter 30
Muscle Pains and Cramps

Robert B. Layzer

Muscle pain and spasm are among the most common of all medical complaints. Generally the symptoms are transitory, and even when they persist long enough to cause a patient to seek medical advice, they seldom have any serious significance. This chapter presents a diagnostic approach that will help physicians recognize and identify the serious or disabling causes of muscle pains and cramps.

Muscle pain is a sensation; a *cramp* or *spasm* (the terms are interchangeable) is an involuntary contraction of muscle. In taking a medical history, it is important to distinguish between these two symptoms from the outset, or the diagnostic process may go completely awry. Muscle cramps are often painful, but most painful conditions of muscle do not involve cramp or spasm. However, many patients use the word *cramp* to signify a tight, pulling pain that *feels* the way a cramp (or its after-effect) feels. If the patient complains of cramps, one should ask whether the affected muscles appear to contract, whether the muscles become palpably hard and knotted or resist stretching, and whether the cramp causes involuntary movement such as flexion of the toes or ankle.

MUSCLE PAIN

Pain Mechanisms

Animal experiments have shown that muscle pain receptors are sensitive to a variety of stimuli. Some nerves are most readily excited by mechanical stimuli such as pressure, pinching, cutting, or stretching. Others are excited by chemical substances that accumulate in inflamed tissues: bradykinin, prostaglandins, serotonin, and histamine. Other chemical mediators of muscle pain may exist that have not been identified.

For clinical purposes, muscle pain syndromes can be divided into five categories, based on their physiological mechanism.

1. *Mechanical pain.* Excessive muscle tension accounts for the immediate pain caused by a muscle cramp, the lingering pain of reflex muscle spasm or extrapyramidal rigidity, and the pain produced by a muscle mass such as a hematoma. However, a forceful cramp can injure the muscle, and the longer-lasting pain that results is related to inflammation.
2. *Inflammatory pain.* Extensive muscle necrosis, as well as mechanical disruption of muscle fibers, can produce an inflammatory reaction that is accompanied by long-lasting pain, tenderness, and swelling. The serum enzyme concentration is elevated. Polymyositis, rhabdomyolysis, and delayed muscle soreness after exercise are examples of this mechanism. Other inflammatory disorders cause myalgia without muscle weakness, tenderness, or swelling; there is no muscle fiber damage, and the serum enzyme concentrations are normal. The myalgia associated with fever, infection, and systemic diseases like giant cell arteritis is of this type.
3. *Ischemic pain.* In normal persons, ischemic exercise eventually causes a deep, aching, squeezing muscle pain that subsides quickly when the circulation is restored. The pain is not associated with muscle cramp or spasm. This is the pain of intermittent claudication, and the same mechanism probably contributes to the exertional pain experienced by patients with certain disorders of muscle energy metabolism. However, patients with McArdle's disease and related disorders of carbohydrate metabolism also suffer exertional muscle cramps, which cause mechanical pain, and they often sustain exertional muscle damage, which causes long-lasting inflammatory pain.
4. *Referred pain.* The pain of nerve root irritation is often felt as a deep, aching discomfort in the muscles supplied by that root. Muscles affected by referred pain may even be tender. A similar pain occurs in some peripheral nerve diseases, especially ischemic focal neuropathies.
5. *Mysterious pain.* Many pain syndromes that affect the muscles or limbs are poorly understood, partly because there are no abnormal clinical or laboratory findings. This category includes the "growing pains" of childhood, the restless legs syndrome, and generalized fibromyalgia (fibrositis).

Table 30.1: Causes of focal muscle pain

With swelling, tenderness, or induration
Acute alcoholic myopathy
Coma from drug overdose
Exertional muscle injury
Gas gangrene
Hematoma
Influenza myopathy in children
Ischemic necrosis
Neoplasm
Parasitic infection
Pyomyositis
Ruptured synovial cyst
Ruptured tendon
Thrombophlebitis
Without swelling, tenderness, or induration
Growing pains
Lumbar canal stenosis
Painful legs and moving toes syndrome
Painful neuropathies
Parkinsonism
Restless legs syndrome (Ekbom's syndrome)

Table 30.2 Causes of nonfocal muscle pain

Exertional muscle pain
Carnitine palmityltransferase deficiency
Hypothyroidism
Ischemia
Lumbar canal stenosis
McArdle's disease and related muscle glycogenoses
Mitochondrial myopathies
Myoadenylate deaminase deficiency
Generalized muscle pain without weakness
Collagen-vascular disease
Corticosteroid withdrawal
Fever or infection
Fibromyalgia (fibrositis)
Hypothyroidism
Muscle pain-fasciculation syndrome
Parkinsonism
Polymyalgia rheumatica
Muscle pain, weakness, and elevated serum creatine kinase concentration
Acid maltase deficiency
Alcoholic myopathy
Drugs: clofibrate, emetine, beta blockers, aminocaproic acid, gemfibrozil, lovastatin
Hypothyroidism
Muscular dystrophies
Myoglobinuria
Polymyositis, dermatomyositis
Toxoplasmosis
Trichinosis
Weakness and bone pain with normal serum creatine kinase
Aluminum osteodystrophy
Chronic hypophosphatemia
Chronic renal failure
Hyperparathyroidism
Vitamin D deficiency (including chronic phenytoin therapy)
Vitamin D resistance

Diagnostic Approach

In taking a medical history, it is useful to inquire whether the pain occurs at rest or only during exercise. If it occurs at rest, is it constant or does it occur at a specific time of day? Is the pain focal, multifocal, or generalized? In the physical examination the physician should look for abnormalities of the skin over affected muscles (such as the livid discoloration of rhabdomyolysis); swelling, mass, or induration of muscle; muscle tenderness, spasm, or resistance to stretch; and muscle weakness.

The single most useful laboratory test is the serum creatine kinase (CK) concentration. An elevated value indicates the presence of muscle damage, and levels over 10,000 IU are often accompanied by myoglobinuria. In contrast, a normal serum CK concentration excludes a necrotizing myopathy. Soft-tissue imaging by ultrasound and especially by computed tomography or magnetic resonance imaging is very useful for defining the location and nature of a muscle hematoma, tumor, or abscess. Radionuclide scanning with gallium can detect muscle abscesses in patients with pyomyositis, and technetium scans may show focal uptake of isotope in regions of muscle necrosis. Electromyography (EMG) helps confirm a clinical diagnosis of myopathic or neuropathic muscle weakness but rarely provides more specific information. Muscle biopsy is essential for the diagnosis of a few diseases, such as polymyositis, focal myositis, trichinosis, and genetic myopathies; in most cases of muscle pain, however, muscle biopsy adds no specific diagnostic information.

After an initial clinical and laboratory evaluation, the diagnostic approach can be simplified by classifying the pain problem into one of several syndromes. In patients with focal pain, muscle enlargement, tenderness, or induration may be present or absent (Table 30.1). Pain may occur only in muscles that are being exercised (Table 30.2); in such cases there is usually no pain at rest except for lingering discomfort in muscles recently injured by exercise.

Generalized pain at rest, without muscle weakness, is characteristic of various nonmyopathic disorders (see Table 30.2); the serum CK concentration is normal except in hypothyroidism, where it is usually elevated even in patients without myopathy. The two most important diseases in this category are polymyalgia rheumatica and primary fibromyalgia (fibrositis). *Polymyalgia rheumatica*, a symptom of giant cell arteritis, occurs after age 50 and is characterized by muscle pain and stiffness mainly located in the proximal limbs and trunk, often accompanied by weight loss and low-grade fever. As in other rheumatic disorders, the pain occurs during movement, especially after a period of inactivity, and when severe can confine the patient to bed. The muscles are not tender, and passive movement of the limbs and joints is not painful. The erythrocyte sedimentation rate (ESR) is almost always elevated. *Primary fibromyalgia* is a common diagnosis by rheumatologists to describe ill-defined muscle pain. The syndrome is characterized by generalized myalgia with tender spots in muscles; there are no objective clinical or laboratory abnormalities, and psychiatric symptoms are commonly associated (Bohr 1995). Sleep deprivation of any cause can produce a similar syndrome.

Necrotizing myopathies are characterized by generalized muscle pain, weakness, and elevated serum CK concentrations (see Table 30.2). An atrophic myopathy associated with metabolic bone disease should be suspected in patients with pain and myopathic weakness but a normal serum CK concentration. The pain originates in the bones, which hurt during movement and are tender to pressure or percussion.

Even after extensive laboratory investigations, a definite disease diagnosis cannot be determined in many patients with generalized muscle pain. This is particularly true when pain occurs at rest and the neuromuscular and neurological examinations are normal. In such cases, a reasonable laboratory screening panel consists of an ESR, serum CK, thyroid function tests, and an antinuclear antibody test. If these tests are normal, more elaborate tests, such as EMG and muscle biopsy, are very unlikely to be diagnostically rewarding.

MUSCLE CRAMPS AND STIFFNESS

Diagnostic Approach

Muscle rigidity and spasms are recognized features of dystonia and other extrapyramidal disorders (see Chapter 76), but this discussion is limited to the motor unit hyperactivity states (Layzer 1993). These states produce twitching, myokymia, stiffness or rigidity, slow relaxation, and cramps or spasms. An accurate history and physical examination usually point toward the correct diagnosis, based on the presence of one or more of the following clinical features: muscle stiffness at rest, slow relaxation, spontaneous spasms, exertional spasms, and muscle irritability to percussion (Table 30.3).

When the diagnosis is uncertain, EMG is an extremely useful way to analyze the abnormal muscle activity (see Chapter 37). The standard EMG can distinguish between the electrically silent contracture of McArdle's disease, the muscle fiber irritability of myotonia, the peripheral nerve discharges of neuromyotonia or tetany, and the spinal cord discharges of tetanus or the "stiff man syndrome." In unusual cases, EMG analysis can be supplemented by anesthetic block at the level of the spinal roots, peripheral nerves, or neuromuscular junctions. Muscle activity that persists after anesthetic block at a given location must arise distal to the block. Unfortunately, the reverse is not necessarily true; for example, if a nerve block abolishes motor hyperactivity, this effect could have been achieved by block of afferent or gamma efferent motor nerve fibers rather than of alpha efferent motor fibers. The excitability of spinal motor neurons can be assessed by recording the amplitude of F-wave responses and by examining muscle responses to cutaneous nerve stimulation. Inhibitory reflexes can be assessed by recording the silent period during the muscle stretch reflex.

The effect of various drugs on abnormal motor activity is of limited diagnostic value because most drugs act at many levels in the nervous system. Diazepam and baclofen act at the level of the spinal cord or higher; phenytoin and carbamazepine act at a cerebral level but also reduce the irritability of spinal cord axons, peripheral nerves, and muscle; and dantrolene reduces the contractility of muscle by interfering with excitation-contraction coupling.

Table 30.3: Causes of muscle stiffness

Stiffness at rest
Malignant hyperthermia (only during anesthesia)
Myopathy with complex repetitive discharges
Neuromyotonia
Progressive encephalomyelitis with rigidity
Schwartz-Jampel syndrome
Stiff man syndrome
Tetanus, strychnine poisoning
Slow muscle relaxation
Lambert-Brody syndrome
Myotonic disorders[a]
Myxedema[a]
Neuromyotonia
Pseudomyotonia in cervical radiculopathy
Spontaneous muscle spasms
Ordinary cramps
Progressive encephalomyelitis with rigidity
Stiff man syndrome
Tetanus, strychnine poisoning
Tetany
Exertional muscle spasms
Lambert-Brody syndrome
McArdle's disease[b]
Myotonia with painful spasms[b]
Myxedema[b]
Neuromyotonia
Ordinary cramps[b]
Other myotonic disorders
Pseudomyotonia in cervical radiculopathy
Progressive encephalomyelitis with rigidity[b]
Stiff man syndrome[b]
Tetanus, strychnine poisoning[b]

[a]Muscle irritable to percussion. In myxedema, only local mounding occurs (myoedema); in myotonia, the entire muscle contracts and relaxes slowly.
[b]Painful spasms.

Clinical Syndromes

Although Table 30.3 provides a useful scheme for analyzing the leading symptoms of patients with muscle hyperactivity, a *logical* classification requires an understanding of the pathophysiology of these disorders. The simplest such classification is based on the anatomical origin of the abnormal motor unit activity.

Muscle Contracture

In physiological terms, a contracture is an active muscle contraction that is not dependent on excitation of the outer muscle membrane; the EMG is electrically silent. Contracture can result from inappropriate release of calcium from intracellular stores in the sarcoplasm reticulum (as in malignant hyperthermia), or from abnormally slow reuptake of calcium by the sarcoplasmic reticulum during relaxation (as in the Lambert-Brody syndrome). Other mechanisms may exist but have not been identified. The term *contracture* is also used clinically to describe fibrosis and contraction of muscle and tendons such as in muscular dystrophy.

The cramps of *McArdle's disease* (muscle phosphorylase deficiency) are electrically silent contractures, and the same symptom occurs in other enzymatic defects of glycogen or glucose breakdown (see Chapter 84). The biochemical mechanism of contracture in defects of carbohydrate metabolism is not well understood (Layzer 1994). The cramps never occur spontaneously; they are brought on by forceful exertion and can always be provoked by ischemic exercise, usually within 30 seconds. Because exercise tends to injure muscle, patients with these disorders have elevated concentrations of serum CK much of the time.

The *Lambert-Brody syndrome* is a congenital disorder characterized by myotonia-like slowness of muscle relaxation, with increasing muscle stiffness during exercise. It is caused by a hereditary deficiency of the calcium-dependent ATPase of the sarcoplasmic reticulum, which is greatly reduced in its ability to take up calcium. Slow reuptake of calcium also accounts for some of the painful muscle stiffness associated with myxedema.

Malignant hyperthermia is a rare anesthetic reaction consisting of widespread muscle contractures, provoked in susceptible persons by exposure to succinylcholine or various volatile anesthetic agents, which trigger the intracellular release of calcium. The sustained contractures cause hyperthermia and metabolic acidosis, which can be rapidly fatal. Patients who survive the acute episode may have severe rhabdomyolysis, which in turn causes acute renal failure and hyperkalemia. Pretreatment with dantrolene helps prevent this series of events. Dantrolene and rapid cooling are the essential emergency treatments of the developing syndrome. Malignant hyperthermia is genetically heterogeneous; about 50% of cases are caused by mutations of the gene for the calcium release channel of the sarcoplasmic reticulum (Ball and Johnson 1993).

Myotonia

Myotonia is a hyperexcitable state of the muscle membrane, characterized by slow relaxation of voluntary contraction, and an excessive, prolonged contractile response to muscle percussion. The inappropriate muscle contraction is caused by discharges of muscle action potentials without accompanying nerve activity. Active myotonia is usually observed as delayed relaxation of the hand grip after forceful flexion of the fingers. Percussion myotonia is most easily shown by striking the extensor muscles of the forearm while the hand hangs free in flexion; the wrist or fingers extend briskly upward and then descend slowly and haltingly. Myotonia does not cause spontaneous muscle spasms, and there is no muscle stiffness at rest except in the rare Schwartz-Jampel syndrome, which combines myotonia with continuous, spontaneous muscle fiber discharges.

Myotonia is always accompanied by EMG abnormalities consisting of high-frequency bursts of muscle fiber action potentials, often provoked by electrode movement. The frequency waxes and wanes during the discharge, giving rise to the well-known "dive bomber" sound. Abnormal mechanical irritability persists after block of neuromuscular transmission, because myotonia is a disorder of the electrically excitable muscle membrane itself. The symptom of myotonia may respond to treatment with membrane-stabilizing drugs such as quinine, procainamide, phenytoin, carbamazepine, or mexiletine (Kwiecinski et al. 1992).

Myotonia is not usually painful, but rare patients with true myotonia have prolonged, painful spasms during exercise that are probably contractures, because they are electrically silent. Patients with *paramyotonia congenita* also experience a combination of contracture and true myotonia on exposure to cold.

The term *pseudomyotonia* has been applied to patients with cervical osteoarthritis who have difficulty opening one hand. Muscle relaxation is actually normal, but attempts at active extension of the fingers produce paradoxical flexion of the fingers as a result of misdirected regeneration of the C7 nerve root fibers.

Tetany

Carpopedal spasms in patients with hypocalcemia or alkalosis are caused by spontaneous, repetitive discharges arising in peripheral nerves. Similar discharges in the sensory nerves cause the pins-and-needles paresthesias that always precede and accompany the spasm. The characteristic hand posture—extension and adduction of the fingers, flexion of the metacarpal-phalangeal joints—reflects early activation of the longest nerves supplying the most distal muscles.

Ischemia induces hand spasm in patients with latent tetany (the *Trousseau test*). EMG of the hand muscles during this test at first shows regular, repetitive firing of single or grouped motor unit potentials at a rate of 5–15 Hz; as the spasm intensifies, the discharges resemble a maximal interference pattern.

Neuromyotonia

The complete expression of neuromyotonia (Isaac's syndrome) consists of myokymia, muscle stiffness at rest and increasing with activity, and delayed relaxation after voluntary contraction; myokymia is not a constant feature. Distal limb muscles are usually affected more severely than proximal muscles, but the face, throat, and tongue can be involved. Muscles respond normally to percussion despite the resemblance to myotonia.

The abnormal activity arises primarily in the distal axons and nerve terminals of motor nerves. EMG of stiff muscles shows spontaneous activity consisting of prolonged, irregular discharges of action potentials, some of which resemble muscle fiber discharges, while others resemble motor unit potentials. Voluntary or electrical activation of nerves elicits a prolonged after-discharge of similar activity. The spontaneous activity is diminished but not abolished by peripheral nerve block and is completely abolished by neuromuscular blockade. All symptoms respond to treatment with either phenytoin or carbamazepine. An autoimmune etiology is postulated, and a few cases have had a paraneoplastic origin (Sinha et al. 1991).

Tetanus

Tetanus toxin causes a hyperexcitable state of motor neurons by blocking spinal and brain stem inhibitory pathways. The clinical syndrome consists of rapidly worsening rigidity and painful muscle spasms provoked by movement or sensory stimulation. Spasm of jaw closure (trismus) is an early and characteristic feature. EMG of the contracting muscles shows a continuous or intermittent discharge of motor unit potentials, resembling voluntary activity. The silent period of the stretch reflex is typically abolished in affected muscles, indicating loss of reflex central inhibition, while the amplitude of the F waves is increased as a result of hyperexcitability of the motor neuron pool. Strychnine poisoning, which blocks glycine-mediated postsynaptic inhibition, produces a similar picture, except that spasms are more prominent than rigidity.

Stiff Man Syndrome

Stiff man syndrome shares many clinical features with tetanus but progresses slowly over months and years and does not cause trismus. The EMG findings are also similar, except that the silent period of the stretch reflex is preserved, showing that the inhibitory influence of Renshaw's cells on motor neurons is not impaired. The origin of motor neuron hyperexcitability in stiff man syndrome is uncertain but is believed to involve descending influences from the brain stem. Elevated concentrations of immunoglobulin G and the presence of oligoclonal bands in the cerebrospinal fluid (CSF) suggest an autoimmune pathogenesis. Serum antibodies to glutamic acid decarboxylase have been detected in many cases (Solimena et al. 1988).

The stiffness and spasms may respond partially to diazepam, clonazepam, baclofen, or centrally acting noradrenergic blocking agents. Immunosuppressive therapy has caused remission in some cases.

Rigidity and spasms also occur in a rare type of progressive encephalomyelitis. Patients with this syndrome, unlike those with ordinary stiff man syndrome, have neurological deficits and an increased protein concentration and pleocytosis in the CSF, but glutamic acid decarboxylase antibodies have been shown in several such cases, suggesting a common pathogenesis with stiff man syndrome (Mitsumoto et al. 1991).

Ordinary Muscle Cramps

Muscle cramps are familiar to nearly everyone as an occasional normal occurrence. They are explosive in onset and variable in rate of resolution. A painful and palpable contraction in one muscle is seen. Cramps are stimulated by a trivial movement or a forced contraction and are usually terminated by passive stretching of the muscle.

Frequent muscle cramps are associated with lower motor neuron disorders such as motor neuron disease, radiculopathies, and peripheral neuropathies; dehydration caused by diuretic therapy, diarrhea, vomiting, or renal dialysis; pregnancy; myxedema; and uremia. Contrary to common belief, hypokalemia does not cause muscle cramps, and most people with frequent cramps are normal.

EMG during a cramp shows a high-frequency discharge of motor unit potentials that resemble a voluntary contraction. Fasciculations are often seen at the beginning and end of the spasm. The site of origin of muscle cramps is unknown. A spinal cord origin is often assumed, but the available evidence favors an origin in the motor nerves or nerve terminals (Layzer 1994). Cramps can be induced by repetitive motor nerve stimulation distal to a nerve block, and such cramps are terminated by muscle stretching (Bertolasi et al. 1993). Cramps can usually be prevented by prophylactic treatment with membrane-stabilizing drugs. Carbamazepine is the most effective.

REFERENCES

Ball SP, Johnson KJ. The genetics of malignant hyperthermia. J Med Genet 1993;30:89–93.

Bertolasi L, DeGrandis D, Bongiovanni LG, et al. The influence of muscular lengthening on cramps. Ann Neurol 1993;33: 176–180.

Bohr TW. Fibromyalgia syndrome and myofascial pain syndrome. Do they exist? Neurol Clin 1995;13:365–384.

Kwiecinzki H, Ryniewicz B, Ostrzycki A. Treatment of myotonia with antiarrhythmic drugs. Acta Neurol Scand 1992;86: 371–375.

Layzer RB. Classification of Motor Unit Hyperactivity States. In RB Layzer, G Sandrini, G Piccolo et al (eds), Motor Unit Hyperactivity States. New York: Raven, 1993;1–21.

Layzer RB. Muscle Pain, Cramps, and Fatigue. In AG Engel, C Franzini-Armstrong (eds), Myology (2nd ed). New York: McGraw-Hill, 1994;3462–3497.

Mitsumoto H, Schwartzman MJ, Estes ML et al. Sudden death and paroxysmal autonomic dysfunction in stiff-man syndrome. J Neurol 1991;238:91–96.

Sinha S, Newsom-Davis J, Mills K et al. Autoimmune etiology for acquired neuromyotonia (Isaac's syndrome). Lancet 1991; 338:75–77.

Solimena M, Folli F, Denis-Donini S, et al. Autoantibodies to glutamic acid decarboxylase in a patient with stiff-man syndrome, epilepsy, and type I diabetes mellitus. N Engl J Med 1988; 318:1012–1020.

Chapter 31
The Hypotonic Infant

Gerald M. Fenichel

DEFINITIONS

Hypotonia is one of the more common presentations of neurological dysfunction in newborns (birth–30 days) and infants (1 month–1 year). Hypotonia is caused by abnormalities at several sites in the central or peripheral nervous systems. The first decision point in evaluating a "floppy" infant is to determine whether the site of abnormality is in the central nervous system, in the peripheral nervous system, or in both places. That determination requires an understanding of the mechanisms of normal and abnormal tone and the means by which it is assessed in newborns and infants.

Tone can be defined operationally as the resistance of muscle to stretch. Two kinds of tone are measured clinically: phasic and postural. *Phasic tone* is a brief contraction to a high-intensity rapid stretch. The tendon reflexes are the best test of phasic tone. When a hammer strikes the patellar tendon, the quadriceps muscle is stretched and the spindle apparatus, sensing the stretch, sends an impulse through the afferent nerve to the spinal cord. This information is transmitted to the alpha motor neuron and the quadriceps muscle contracts (monosynaptic reflex). The phasic mechanism of tone does not normally respond to the low-intensity stretch of gravity. However, this happens when inhibitory suprasegmental influences on the monosynaptic reflex are impaired.

Postural tone is a prolonged contraction to a low-intensity stretch. Gravity is the stimulus that provokes a steady, low-amplitude stretch on antigravity muscles, which respond with prolonged contraction. When postural tone is depressed, the infant is less able to maintain the body and limbs against gravity and looks floppy. Therefore, the hypotonic infant is one whose postural tone is unable to resist the stretch caused by gravitational forces. An infant with poor postural tone can also be spastic; consider a child with cerebral palsy who is floppy when lying or sitting but whose limbs extend because of increased adductor and extensor tone (spasticity) when lifted vertically against gravity (see Chapter 67). Both the decreased postural tone and the increased phasic tone are caused by abnormal suprasegmental influences on the segmental mechanism of tone

The maintenance of normal tone requires that the central and peripheral nervous systems are intact and that skeletal muscle is healthy. Therefore, it is not surprising that hypotonia is encountered in diseases of the brain, spinal cord, nerves, and muscles (Table 31.1). One anterior horn cell and all the muscle fibers that it innervates make up a *motor unit.* A primary disorder of the anterior horn cell body is a *neuronopathy* (see Chapter 79), of the axon or its myelin covering is a *neuropathy* (see Chapters 80 and 81), and of the muscle fiber is a *myopathy* (see Chapter 84). During infancy and childhood, diseases of the brain are far more common than diseases of the motor unit. The term *cerebral hypotonia* is used to encompass all causes of postural hypotonia due to cerebral disease or defect.

APPEARANCE OF HYPOTONIA

Inspection

An infant's resting posture is an important clue to neurological status. All normal newborns (32–40 weeks' gesta-

Table 31.1: Differential diagnosis of infantile hypotonia (gene location)

Cerebral hypotonia
Chromosome disorders
Prader-Willi syndrome (15q11–13)
Trisomy
Chronic nonprogressive encephalopathy
Cerebral malformation
Perinatal distress
Postnatal disorders
Peroxisomal disorders
Cerebrohepatorenal syndrome (Zellweger's)
Neonatal adrenoleukodystrophy
Other genetic defects
Familial dysautonomia
Oculocerebrorenal syndrome (Lowe's)
Other metabolic defects
Acid maltase deficiency
Infantile GM_1 gangliosidosis
Spinal cord disorders
Hypoxic-ischemia myelopathy
Injuries
Spinal muscular atrophies
Acute infantile (5q11–q13)
Chronic infantile (5q11–q13)
Congenital cervical (restricted) spinal muscular atrophy
Infantile neuronal degeneration
Neurogenic arthrogryposis
Vaccine-induced poliomyelitis
Polyneuropathies
Congenital hypomyelinating neuropathy
Giant axonal neuropathy
Hereditary motor-sensory neuropathies
Disorders of neuromuscular transmission
Genetic myasthenic syndromes
Infantile botulism
Transitory myasthenia gravis
Fiber-type disproportion myopathies
Central core disease (19q13)
Congenital fiber type disproportion myopathy
Myotubular (centronuclear) myopathy
Acute (Xq28)
Chronic
Nemaline (rod) myopathy (1q21–q23)
Infantile myositis
Metabolic myopathies
Acid maltase deficiency (17q23)
Cytochrome-*c*-oxidase deficiency
Carnitine deficiency
Phosphofructokinase deficiency (1cenq32)
Phosphorylase deficiency (11q13)
Muscular dystrophies
Congenital muscular dystrophy
Cerebroocular dystrophy
Fukuyama type
Leukodystrophy
Congenital myotonic dystrophy (19q13)
"Benign" congenital hypotonia

tion) and infants lie with some degree of abduction at the thighs and flexion at the elbows, hips, and ankles (Figure 31.1). Newborns delivered from breech positions are sometimes an exception and keep their legs extended. At 25–30 weeks' gestation, the arms are flexed but the legs may be either flexed or extended. Abduction tone in the thighs is present even at 25 weeks gestation.

Table 31.2: Differential diagnosis of arthrogryposis

Nonneurologic causes
Oligohydramnios: malformations of fetal mouth and esophagus
Oligohydramnios: malformations of fetal urinary tract
Twinning
Uterine abnormalities
Cerebral disorders
Cerebrohepatorenal syndrome
Cerebral malformations
Chromosomal disorders
Motor unit disorders
Congenital cervical (restricted) spinal muscular atrophy
Congenital fiber type disproportion myopathy
Congenital hypomyelinating neuropathy
Congenital muscular dystrophy
Genetic myasthenic syndromes
Infantile neuronal degeneration
Myotonic dystrophy
Neurogenic arthrogryposis (spinal muscular atrophy)
Phosphofructokinase deficiency
Transitory neonatal myasthenia

When lying in the supine position all hypotonic newborns and infants look very much the same without regard to underlying cause or site of abnormality within the nervous system. Spontaneous limb movement is decreased, the legs are fully abducted with the lateral surface of the thighs against the examining table, and the arms lie either extended at the sides of the body or flexed at the elbow with the hands beside the head. Pectus excavatum is present when there is long-standing weakness in the muscles of the chest wall. Infants who lie motionless eventually develop flattening of the occiput and loss of hair on the portion of the scalp in constant contact with the crib sheet. When placed in a sitting posture, the head falls forward, the shoulders droop, and the limbs hang limply.

Newborns who are hypotonic in utero may be born with either dislocation of the hips, *arthrogryposis*, or both. Dislocation of the hip is a common feature of intrauterine hypotonia because the formation of a normal hip joint requires the forceful contraction of muscles to pull the head of the femur into the acetabulum. Arthrogryposis is joint fixation at birth. It varies in severity from clubfoot, the most common manifestation, to symmetrical flexion deformities of all limb joints. Joint contractures are believed to be a nonspecific consequence of intrauterine immobilization. However, among the several disorders that equally decrease fetal movement, some regularly produce arthrogryposis and others never do. The differential diagnosis of arthrogryposis is summarized in Table 31.2. Nonfetal causes are usually due to abnormalities of the uterus or abnormal fetal positioning, as caused by twinning. Fetal causes not due to nervous system disease include primary bone

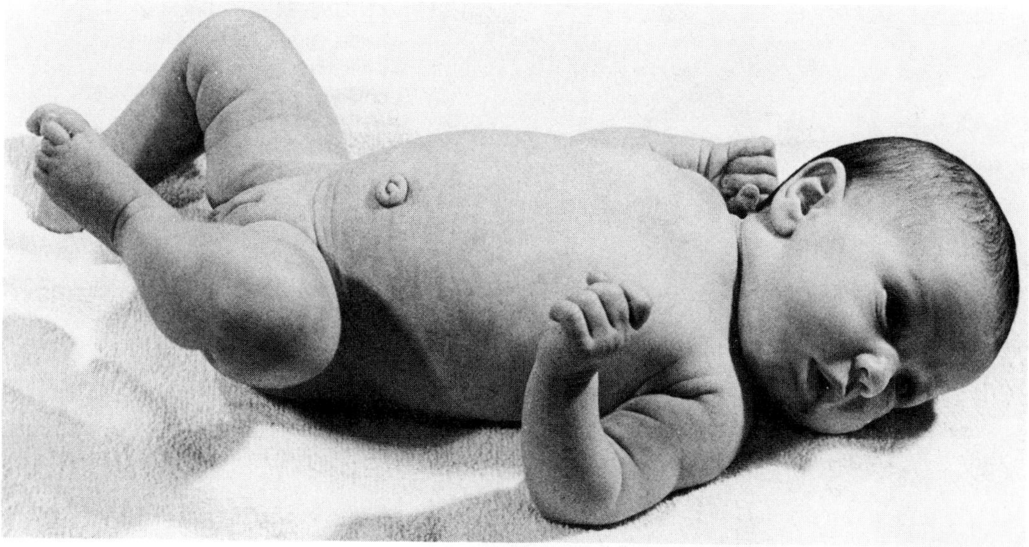

FIGURE 31.1 Normal resting tone. There is always some abduction of the thighs and flexion at the elbows, hips, and ankles.

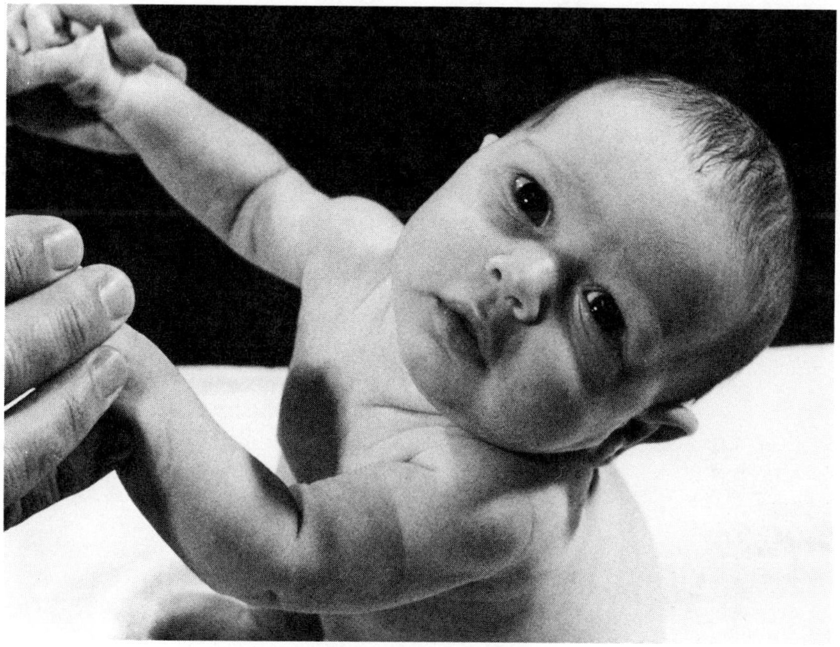

FIGURE 31.2 The traction response. When the child is pulled to sitting, the head lifts from the surface with the body and is held in the midline when the sitting position is attained.

and joint disturbances and failure to produce amniotic fluid due to urinary tract malformations. Those conditions due to abnormality in the fetal brain or motor unit are also part of the differential diagnosis of infantile hypotonia.

After inspection is completed, tone is further evaluated by lifting the child against gravity. Three tests should be done in sequence: the traction response, vertical suspension, and horizontal suspension.

Traction Response

Traction response is the most sensitive measure of postural tone. The response is initiated by grasping the hands and pulling the child to a sitting position. Normal full-term newborns lift the head immediately with the body. When the sitting position is attained, the head is held erect in the midline. During traction, the examiner should feel the child pulling back against traction, and there is flexion at the elbows, knees, and ankles. A traction response is not present in premature infants of less than 33 weeks' gestation. After 33 weeks, there is considerable head lag, but the neck flexors consistently respond to traction by lifting the head. At term, only minimal head lag is present, but when the sitting posture is attained, the head may continue to lag or may become erect momentarily and then fall forward (Figure 31.2).

The presence of more than minimal head lag and failure to counter traction by flexion of the limbs is abnormal and indicates hypotonia in full-term newborns and infants (Figure 31.3).

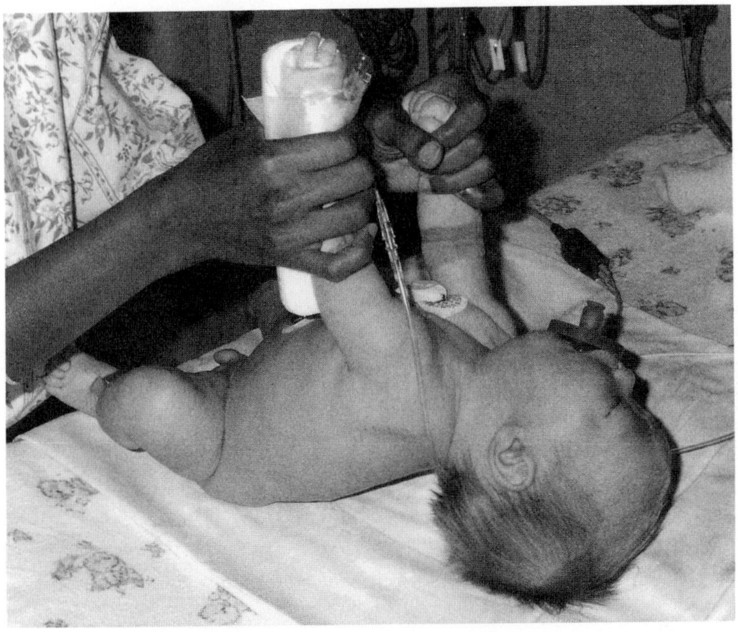

FIGURE 31.3 Abnormal traction response. As the child is pulled to sitting, the head falls backward and no effort is made to flex the arms at the elbow.

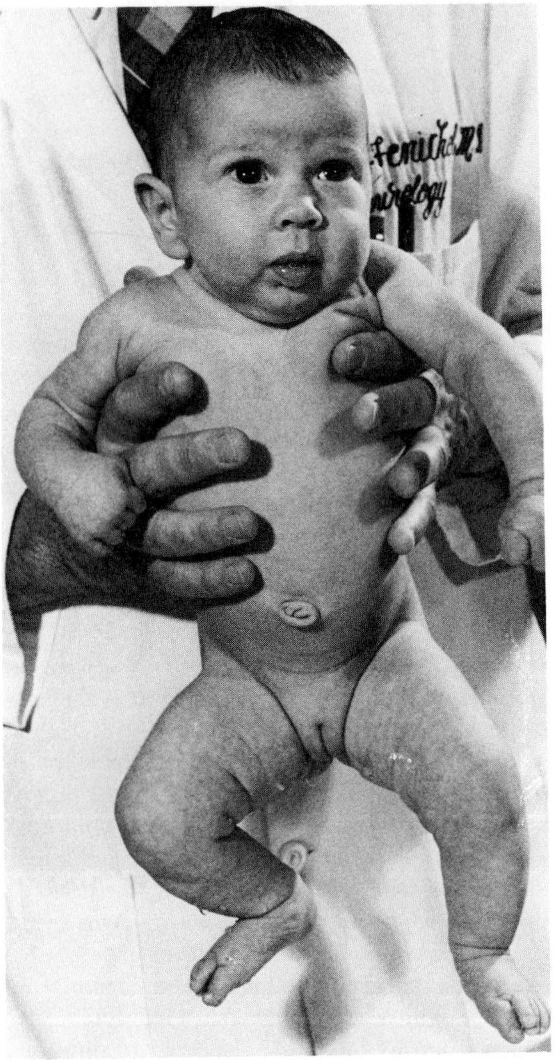

FIGURE 31.4 Vertical suspension. The head is held erect and the legs flex against gravity.

Vertical Suspension

The examiner places both hands in the child's axillae and without grasping the thorax lifts straight up. In the normal full-term newborn and infant, the muscles of the shoulders should be strong enough to press down against the examiner's hands and allow the child to suspend vertically without falling through (Figure 31.4). While the child is in vertical suspension, the head is held erect in the midline and the legs are kept flexed at the knee, hip, and ankle. When the hypotonic infant is suspended vertically, the head falls forward, the legs dangle, and there is a tendency to slip through the examiner's hands because of weakness in the muscles of the shoulder.

Horizontal Suspension

A normal infant suspended horizontally in prone position keeps the head erect, maintains the back straight, and demonstrates flexion at the elbow, hip, knee, and ankle (Figure 31.5). A healthy term newborn makes intermittent efforts to maintain the head erect, the back straight, and the limbs flexed against gravity. Hypotonic newborns and infants drape over the examiner's hands with the head and legs hanging limply.

Tendon Reflexes

Tendon reflexes in newborns and infants cannot be tested with an adult-sized percussion hammer. The pediatric-sized "Queen's Square" hammer with a flexible plastic handle is the best instrument. The patella reflex is the only tendon reflex consistently present at birth, but it may be difficult to elicit on the first day postpartum and its absence is not

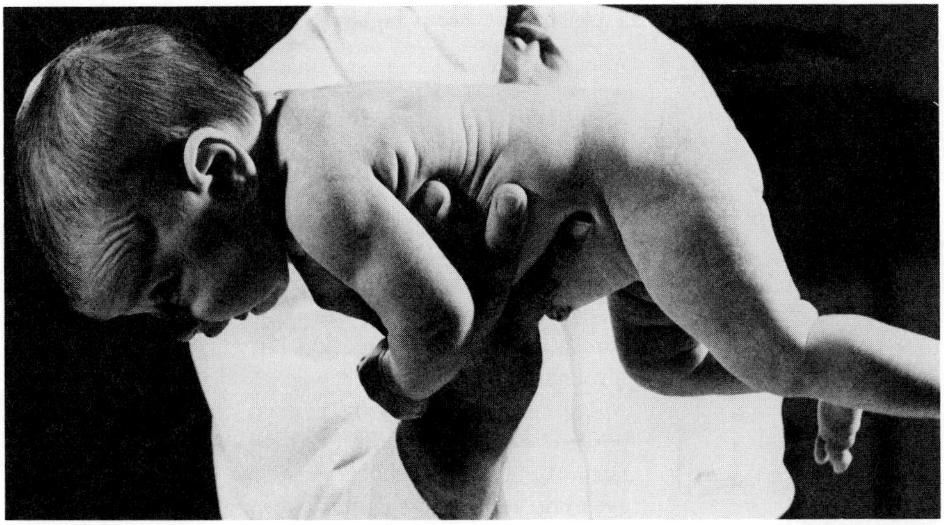

FIGURE 31.5 Horizontal suspension. The head is held erect and the legs flex against gravity.

Table 31.3: Clues to cerebral hypotonia

Abnormalities of other brain function
Dysmorphic features
Fisting of the hands
Malformations of other organs
Movement through postural reflexes
Normal or brisk tendon reflexes
Scissoring on vertical suspension

abnormal. When testing the patella tendon reflex in children from birth to 3 months, the head must be placed with the face in the midline or asymmetries will be imposed by the tonic-neck reflex (see discussion below); the knee jerk is exaggerated on the side to which the head is turned and depressed on the opposite side.

The biceps and Achilles tendon reflexes are inconstant at birth but become increasingly easy to elicit with each succeeding month. A few beats of ankle clonus may be present in normal newborns, but sustained clonus is abnormal. The activation of clonus requires a constant state of stretch in the muscle. It is difficult to accomplish by forceful dorsiflexion of the foot and is better elicited by stretching the tendon to a variety of lengths to find the point of excitation for clonus. Ankle clonus can be present during an acute encephalopathy when the patella tendon reflex cannot be elicited and can serve to indicate that the motor unit is intact.

The absence of tendon reflexes usually suggests dysfunction in the motor unit but does not exclude cerebral disorders. Newborns with an acute encephalopathy are frequently areflexic for several days postpartum. Eventually the reflexes return and may become exaggerated.

The plantar response, so dear to adult neurologists, is not worth annoying an infant to elicit. It is normally extensor throughout much of the first year and sometimes into the second year. There is such variability in the time of transition from extensor to flexor as to render the response useless for diagnosis.

APPROACHES TO DIAGNOSIS

The first step in diagnosis is to determine if the site of pathology is cerebral, spinal, or motor unit.

Cerebral Hypotonia

Hypotonia is a common feature of cerebral disorders in newborns and infants. In contrast, hypertonia is very unusual in the newborn. Spasticity develops during the first year and dystonia during the second.

There are several clues to the diagnosis of cerebral hypotonia in newborns and infants (Table 31.3). Most important is the presence of other abnormal brain functions, such as states of decreased consciousness and seizures in newborns (see Chapter 85) and global developmental delay in infants (see Chapter 67). Tendon reflexes are generally normal or brisk, and clonus may be present as well. Cerebral malformation is the probable explanation for hypotonia in an infant with dysmorphic features or malformations in other organs.

A tightly fisted hand in which the thumb is constantly enclosed by the other fingers and does not open spontaneously (*fisting*) and adduction of the thigh so that the legs are crossed when the infant is suspended vertically (*scissoring*) are considered precursors of spasticity and indicate cerebral dysfunction.

Postural reflexes, such as the Moro reflex and the tonic-neck reflex, may be elicited in newborns and infants with cerebral hypotonia even when there is a paucity of spontaneous movement (Fenichel 1993). Their presence shows that the motor unit is intact.

The *Moro reflex* is a startle reaction, normally present from birth to 3–6 months, that allows observation of coordinated extension and flexion movements. The best stimulus for startle in the newborn is the sensation of falling. With the child held in supine position, the head is allowed

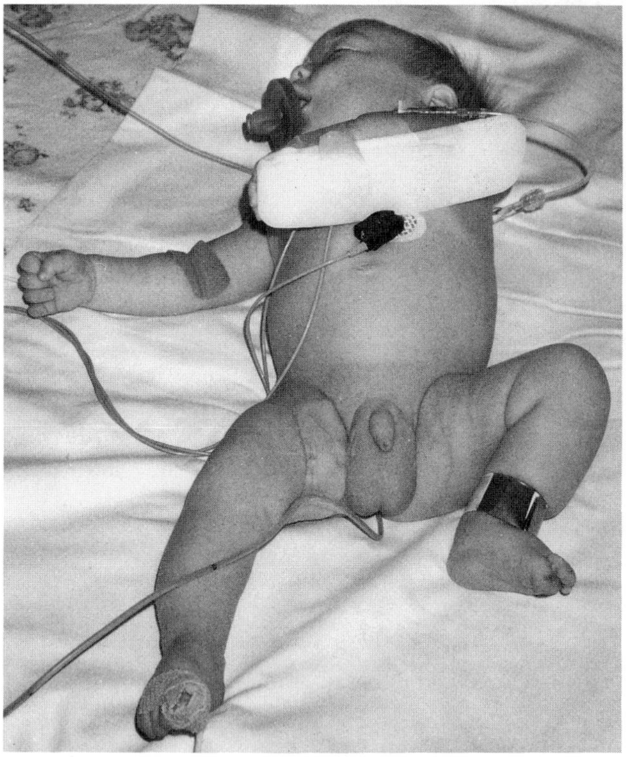

FIGURE 31.6 Obligatory tonic-neck reflex. The child remains with the right limbs extended and the left limbs flexed as long as the head is turned.

to fall a few centimeters, rapidly but gently, in the examiner's hands. The first response is a spreading movement; the arms abduct and extend and the hands open. This is followed by a clutching movement in which the arms adduct and flex over the body and the fists close. The spreading movement, but not the clutching, is seen routinely at 28 weeks' gestation.

Complete absence of the spreading movement is abnormal and is most often observed in newborns with severe cerebral depression or disorders of the motor unit. Asymmetrical movements of the arms may indicate a brachial plexus palsy. An exaggerated Moro reflex, either because of a low threshold or excessive clutching, is often seen in newborns with mild hypoxic-ischemic encephalopathy (see Chapter 85) and in some metabolic disorders (see Chapter 69).

The *tonic-neck reflex* is a primitive vestibular reflex, present from birth to 3 months, that must be suppressed before the child can turn over. With the head held in the midline, the limbs are in their resting flexion attitude. As the head is slowly turned to the right, extension tone increases in the right limbs and flexion tone increases in the left limbs. The only consistent visible evidence of these postural changes is extension of the arm. Extension of the leg is variable, and increased flexion in the contralateral limbs is rarely seen. After observing the response to turning the head to the right, the head is rotated to the left to reverse the posture.

Table 31.4: Clues to motor unit disorders

Absent or depressed tendon reflexes
Failure of movement on postural reflexes
Fasciculations
Muscle atrophy
No abnormalities of other organs

The tonic neck reflex is abnormal if the responses are excessive and obligatory (Figure 31.6). In newborns with severe hemispheric dysfunction but an intact brain stem, turning of the head produces full extension of both ipsilateral limbs and tight flexion on the contralateral side. These postures are maintained for as long as the head is kept rotated. A unilateral obligatory response indicates brain damage in the hemisphere opposite the extended limbs.

Spinal Cord Injury

Only in the newborn is spinal cord injury part of the differential diagnosis of hypotonia. Injuries to the cervical spinal cord occur almost exclusively during vaginal delivery; approximately 75% are associated with breech presentation and 25% with cephalic presentation. Because the injuries always occur on a background of a difficult and prolonged delivery, states of decreased consciousness are common and hypotonia may be falsely attributed to asphyxia or cerebral trauma. However, the presence of impaired sphincter function and loss of sensation below the midchest should suggest myelopathy.

Motor Unit Disorders

Disorders of the motor unit are not associated with malformations of other organs except for joint deformities and the secondary maldevelopment of bony structures. The face sometimes looks dysmorphic when facial muscles are weak or the jaw is underdeveloped (Table 31.4).

Tendon reflexes are absent or depressed. The complete absence of tendon reflexes in muscles with residual movement is more likely to be caused by neuropathy than myopathy, while diminished reflexes consistent with the degree of weakness are more often encountered in myopathy than neuropathy. Muscle atrophy suggests motor unit disease but does not exclude cerebral hypotonia. Failure of muscle growth and even atrophy can be considerable in brain-damaged infants. The combination of atrophy and fasciculations is strong evidence for denervation. The observation of fasciculations in newborns and infants, however, is often restricted to the tongue, and it is difficult, if not impossible, to distinguish fasciculations from normal random movements of the tongue unless atrophy is present.

Postural reflexes such as the tonic-neck and positive supporting reaction cannot be elicited from weak muscles. The

Table 31.5: Combined cerebral and motor unit hypotonia

Acid maltase deficiency
Familial dysautonomia
Giant axonal neuropathy
Hypoxic-ischemic encephalomyopathy
Infantile neuronal degeneration
Lipid storage diseases
Mitochondrial (respiratory chain) disorders
Neonatal myotonic dystrophy
Perinatal asphyxia secondary to motor unit disease

motor unit is the final common pathway of tone; limbs that will not move voluntarily cannot be moved reflexively.

Combined Cerebral and Motor Unit Disorders

Newborns and infants with combined cerebral and motor unit disorders have clinical features of both and can be challenging diagnostic problems (Table 31.5). The brain and the peripheral nerves are concomitantly involved in some lipid storage diseases, mitochondrial disorders with a deficiency of respiratory chain enzymes (see Chapter 69), and familial dysautonomia. Both brain and skeletal muscles are abnormal in acid maltase deficiency and neonatal myotonic dystrophy. Several motor unit disorders produce sufficient hypotonia at birth to impair respiration and produce brain damage by the mechanism of perinatal asphyxia. Finally, newborns with spinal cord injuries have frequently been born during long, difficult deliveries in which brachial plexus injuries and depressed cerebral function from asphyxia are present as well.

DIFFERENTIAL DIAGNOSIS

Cerebral Hypotonia

This section discusses cerebral disorders with hypotonia as a prominent and presenting feature. Hypotonia is also a feature of many progressive degenerative disorders of infancy (i.e., lipid storage diseases, neuroaxonal dystrophy), but these are not considered here because the presenting feature is developmental delay or regression (see Chapter 8).

Chromosome Disorders

Despite considerable syndrome diversity, common characteristics of autosomal chromosome aberrations in the newborn are dysmorphic features of the hands and face and profound hypotonia (Table 31.6) (de Grouchy and Turleau 1990). For this reason, chromosome studies are indicated in any hypotonic newborn with dysmorphic features of the hands and face, with or without other organ malformation (see Chapter 67).

Table 31.6: Hypotonia and dysmorphic features

Cerebral dysgenesis
Cerebrohepatorenal syndrome
Chromosomal aberrations
Fiber-type disproportion myopathies
Neonatal adrenoleukodystrophy
Neonatal myotonic dystrophy
Prader-Willi syndrome

Chronic Nonprogressive Encephalopathy

Cerebral dysgenesis may be due to known or unknown noxious environmental agents, chromosomal disorders, or genetic defects (see Chapter 67). In the absence of an acute encephalopathy, hypotonia may be the only symptom at birth or during early infancy. Hypotonia is usually worse at birth and tends to lessen with time. Cerebral dysgenesis should be suspected when hypotonia is coupled with malformations in other organs or abnormalities in head size and shape (see Chapter 67). Unenhanced magnetic resonance imaging (MRI) of the head is advisable when cerebral malformation is suspected. The identification of a major cerebral malformation provides useful information not only for prognosis but also for assessing the costs and benefits of aggressive therapy to correct malformations in other organs.

Brain injuries occur in the perinatal period and less commonly during infancy secondary to anoxia, intracranial hemorrhage, infection, and trauma. The sudden onset of hypotonia in a previously well newborn or infant, with or without signs of encephalopathy, should always suggest a cerebral cause. Infantile spinal muscular atrophy and botulism are the important exceptions. The premature newborn who demonstrates a decline in spontaneous movement and tone may have an intraventricular hemorrhage (see Chapter 85). Hypotonia is an early feature of meningitis in both full-term and premature newborns. During the acute phase, tendon reflexes may be diminished or absent.

Chronic Progressive Encephalopathy

Children with inborn errors of metabolism are often hypotonic. Because several organ systems may be affected in infants with inborn errors of metabolism, hypotonia may be overlooked or blamed on systemic disease (see Chapter 69). Hypotonia is especially prominent in peroxisomal disorders and may be an initial feature.

Motor Unit Disorders

Spinal Muscular Atrophies

Spinal muscular atrophies are a heterogenous group of genetic disorders characterized by the degeneration of anterior horn cells in the spinal cord and motor nuclei of the

Table 31.7: Polyneuropathies with possible onset in infancy

Demyelinating
Congenital hypomyelinating neuropathy
Chronic inflammatory demyelinating polyneuropathy
Globoid cell leukodystrophy
Hereditary motor-sensory neuropathy I
Hereditary motor-sensory neuropathy III
Metachromatic leukodystrophy
Postinfectious polyradiculoneuropathy
Axonal
Familial dysautonomia
Hereditary motor-sensory neuropathy II
Idiopathic with encephalopathy
Infantile neuronal degeneration
Subacute necrotizing encephalopathy

Table 31.8: Difficulty of feeding in the alert newborn

Familial dysautonomia
Genetic myasthenic syndromes
Hypoplasia of bulbar motor nuclei
Infantile neuronal degeneration
Myophosphorylase deficiency
Myotonic dystrophy
Neurogenic arthrogryposis
Prader-Willi syndrome
Transitory neonatal myasthenia

brain stem (neuronopathy). They are believed to represent a disorder of apoptosis, or programmed cell death. The onset of symptoms is at any age from the newborn to adult life. Some spinal muscular atrophies have a generalized distribution of weakness and others affect specific muscle groups. Those with onset in infancy have generalized weakness and present as infantile hypotonia. Infantile spinal muscular atrophy is one of the more common disorders of the motor unit causing infantile hypotonia.

Two clinical syndromes of infantile spinal muscular atrophy, both transmitted by autosomal inheritance, can be distinguished. One is an acute fulminating form with onset before birth or within 6 months of age, and the other is a chronic slowly progressive form with onset after 3 months of age. The value of this classification is questionable because both forms are caused by defects at the same site on chromosome 5 (Munsat et al. 1990) and the overlap in clinical features is considerable (Russman et al. 1992).

Vaccine-induced poliomyelitis must be considered in infants who develop acute denervation generalized or limited to one or more limbs. The interval between vaccine administration and onset of illness ranges from 11 to 58 days (Strebel et al. 1992).

Polyneuropathies

Polyneuropathies are uncommon in childhood and even more uncommon during infancy. Table 31.7 lists the polyneuropathies that have their onset during infancy. They are divided into those that primarily affect the myelin (demyelinative) and those that primarily affect the axon (axonal). In the newborn and infant, the term *demyelinative* also includes disorders in which myelin has failed to form (hypomyelination). Only congenital hypomyelinating neuropathy regularly presents as a hypotonic infant. Some cases, especially those with a family history of the disease, may represent an infantile form of hereditary motor and sensory neuropathy type III (Balestrini et al. 1991).

Acute inflammatory demyelinating polyneuropathy (the Guillain-Barré syndrome) is rare and perhaps nonexistent during infancy. Reports are mainly in older literature, and, in retrospect, it seems that most were probably cases of infantile botulism (Ouvrier et al. 1990). Chronic inflammatory demyelinating polyneuropathy sometimes has a neonatal onset. The distinction is important since the latter is corticosteroid-responsive. The initial symptom in the other conditions is more likely to be a progressive gait disturbance or developmental retardation.

Disorders of Neuromuscular Transmission

Botulism and myasthenia gravis cause hypotonia in newborns and infants. Botulism produces the more profound limb hypotonia of the two (Glauser et al. 1990), and the weakness of myasthenia gravis may be restricted to the cranial nerves.

Transitory neonatal myasthenia, a form that occurs only in newborns of myasthenic mothers, and familial infantile myasthenia are the myasthenic conditions most likely to produce infantile hypotonia (see Chapter 83). Feeding difficulty is a common feature in myasthenic newborns (Table 31.8).

Congenital Myopathies and Dystrophies

The common muscle disorders that cause infantile hypotonia are congenital myopathies and congenital dystrophies (see Chapter 84). Congenital myopathies are diagnosed only by muscle biopsy. The common feature is that type I fibers are greater in number, but smaller in size, than type II fibers. This fiber type predominance, in the absence of fiber degeneration, is referred to as *congenital fiber type disproportion myopathy*. Fiber type disproportion myopathies are probably not primary diseases of muscle but rather are developmental abnormalities of innervation. Indeed, most infants with hypotonia and type I fiber predominance are later shown to have a cerebral abnormality (Kyriakides et al. 1993).

Some congenital myopathies have a unique histologic feature in addition to type I predominance: *myotubular (centronuclear) myopathy*, *nemaline (rodbody) myopathy*, and *central core disease*. They are difficult to distinguish from each other by clinical features alone. Some useful guidelines are (1) hypotonia is most severe in myotubular myopathy and respiratory distress is common (Table 31.9), (2) axial and facial weakness are most prominent in nemaline my-

Table 31.9: Motor unit disorders with perinatal respiratory distress

Acute infantile spinal muscular atrophy
Congenital hypomyelinating neuropathy
Familial infantile myasthenia
Myotonic dystrophy
Neurogenic (spinal muscular atrophy) arthrogryposis
X-linked myotubular myopathy

Table 31.10: Evaluation of motor unit disorders

Serum creatine kinase
Electrodiagnosis
Electromyography
Nerve conduction studies
Repetitive stimulation
Muscle biopsy
Nerve biopsy
Tensilon test

opathy, and (3) extraocular and facial muscles are affected in myotubular neuropathy and always spared in central core disease.

Congenital muscular dystrophy is not a nosological entity but rather a collection of conditions in which muscular dystrophy is present at birth. Most cases are sporadic, but in others, siblings are involved or parental consanguinity has occurred, suggesting autosomal recessive inheritance. Four forms are recognized: (1) with normal intelligence, (2) with cerebral dysplasia, (3) with leukodystrophy, and (4) with ocular abnormalities (Fenichel 1992).

A neonatal form of myotonic dystrophy sometimes occurs in the offspring of affected mothers. The disease is caused by an unstable DNA region on chromosome 19 that expands in successive generations, causing more severe disease (Harley et al. 1992). The prominent clinical features are facial diplegia in which the mouth is oddly shaped so that the upper lip forms an inverted V, generalized muscular hypotonia, joint deformities ranging from bilateral clubfoot to arthrogryposis, and gastrointestinal dysfunction.

Metabolic Myopathies

Infants with inborn error of metabolism usually have disorders of many organ systems and do not present with hypotonia alone (see Chapter 69). Of the conditions listed in Table 31.1, acid maltase deficiency is the one most likely to pose a problem in the differential diagnosis of infantile hypotonia. The major clinical features suggesting the diagnosis are cardiomegaly and symptoms of cardiac failure.

Infantile Myositis

There have been only 11 case reports of infantile myositis; three were newborns. It is unlikely that these represent a single nosologic entity. The diagnosis is important, because the condition responds to corticosteroids.

Benign Congenital Hypotonia

Benign congenital hypotonia is a retrospective term referring to infants who are hypotonic at birth or shortly thereafter but later develop normal tone. It encompasses many different pathological processes affecting the brain, the motor unit, or both. A large subset of such children probably have cerebral hypotonia. Despite the recovery of normal muscle tone, an increased incidence of mental retardation, learning disabilities, and other sequelae of cerebral abnormality are evident in those children later in life.

LABORATORY DIAGNOSIS

Cerebral Hypotonia

In most newborns and infants with cerebral hypotonia, the diagnosis is based on the clinical features. When laboratory diagnosis is needed, the choice of tests should be planned as indicated by the differential diagnosis and were therefore discussed in the previous section.

Motor Unit Disorders

A limited number of tests readily define the anatomy and often the etiology of disorders affecting the motor unit (Table 31.10). The sequence in which they are done is important.

Serum Creatine Kinase

Increased serum concentrations of creatine kinase (CK) are a reflection of skeletal or cardiac muscle necrosis. The serum CK concentration should be studied prior to the performance of electromyography (EMG) or muscle biopsy, because either procedure will cause elevation. The total concentration of CK and its isoenzymes increases significantly with acidosis. Levels as high as 1,000 IU/liter may be recorded in severely asphyxiated newborns, but even normal newborns have a higher than normal concentration during the first 24 hours postpartum. Newborns born in prolonged and traumatic deliveries may have elevated concentrations of serum CK for a week.

Normal CK in a hypotonic infant is strong evidence against a rapidly progressive myopathy but does not exclude congenital myopathies and some metabolic myopathies. Conversely, a mild elevation in the concentration of CK is sometimes encountered in rapidly progressive neuronopathies (spinal muscular atrophy).

Electrodiagnosis

Electrophysiological studies are extremely useful in the diagnosis of infantile hypotonia when the study is performed by an experienced physician (see Chapter 37B). EMG is able to predict the final diagnosis in 82% of infants less than 3 months of age with hypotonia of motor unit origin. Fewer than 5% of hypotonic infants with a normal EMG have abnormal results on muscle biopsy.

Studies of nerve conduction velocity are useful to distinguish axonal from demyelinating neuropathies; demyelinating neuropathies cause greater slowing of conduction velocity. Repetitive nerve stimulation studies demonstrate disturbances in neuromuscular transmission.

Muscle Biopsy

Muscle biopsy should not be undertaken unless the tissue can be processed by histochemical techniques. Electron microscopy is helpful in selected cases but is rarely essential for diagnosis. The muscle selected for biopsy should be mild to moderately weak but still able to move. When there is symmetrical weakness, the muscles of one limb should be studied by EMG and the muscles of the other limb reserved for biopsy. Adequate tissue can be obtained either by needle or by open biopsy depending on the physician's preference. Histochemistry is essential to demonstrate fiber types and storage materials (see Chapter 84).

Nerve Biopsy

Sural nerve biopsy is indicated only in patients with electrodiagnostic evidence of sural neuropathy. Nerve biopsy is useful in differentiating axonal from demyelinating neuropathies and can be diagnostic in demonstrating storage material by use of histochemical techniques or electron microscopy.

Tensilon Test

Edrophonium chloride (Tensilon) is a rapidly acting anticholinesterase that produces a temporary reversal of weakness in patients with myasthenia. Reversal of ptosis is the most reliable measure of efficacy. Rare patients are supersensitive to edrophonium and may stop breathing due to depolarization of endplates or an abnormal vagal response. Equipment for mechanical ventilation should always be available when the test is performed. In newborns and infants the total dose is 0.15–0.20 mg/kg given intravenously at one quarter increments each minute until a response is seen. Subcutaneous injection can be used when venous access is difficult. The total dose of 0.15 mg/kg is given as a single injection and there is a 10-minute delay to response.

REFERENCES

Balestrini MR, Cavaletti G, D'Angelo A et al. Infantile hereditary neuropathy with hypomyelination: report of two siblings with different expressivity. Neuropediatrics 1991;22:65–70.

de Grouchy J, Turleau C. Autosomal Disorders. In AEH Emery, DL Rimoin (eds), Principle and Practice of Medical Genetics (2nd ed). Edinburgh: Churchill Livingstone, 1990;247–271.

Fenichel GM. Congenital Myopathies. In G Miller, JC Ramer (eds), Static Encephalopathies of Infancy and Childhood. New York: Raven, 1992;343–350.

Fenichel GM. The neurological examination of the newborn. Child Brain 1993;15:403–410.

Glauser TA, Maguire HC, Sladky JT. Relapse of infant botulism. Ann Neurol 1990;28:187–189.

Harley HG, Brook JD, Rundle SA et al. Expansion of an unstable DNA region and phenotypic variation in myotonic dystrophy. Nature 1992;355:545–546.

Kyriakides T, Silberstein JM, Jongpiputvanich S et al. The clinical significance of type 1 fiber predominance. Muscle Nerve 1993;16:418–423.

Munsat TL, Skerry L, Korf B et al. Phenotypic heterogeneity of spinal muscular atrophy mapping to chromosome 5q11.213.3 (SMA 5q). Neurology 1990;40:1831–1836.

Ouvrier R, McLeod JG, Pollard J. Peripheral Neuropathy in Children. New York: Raven, 1990;39–40.

Russman BS, Iannacone ST, Bucher CR et al. Spinal muscular atrophy: New thoughts on the pathogenesis and classification schema. J Child Neurol 1992;7:347–353.

Strebel PM, Sutter RW, Cochi SL et al. Epidemiology of poliomyelitis in the United States one decade after the last reported case of indigenous wild virus-associated disease. Clin Infect Dis 1992;14:568–579.

Chapter 32
Sensory Abnormalities of the Limbs and Trunk

Thomas R. Gordon, Jonathan M. Goldstein, and Stephen G. Waxman

This chapter outlines an approach to the diagnosis of sensory disorders excluding those of the head and neck. Pertinent anatomy is presented in context. Discussions of specific diseases are included elsewhere in this book, although some clinical details must be included here, especially for certain unusual disorders with unique patterns of sensory loss. In taking this approach, the chapter outlines those principles of sensory function that are relevant to the clinical neurosciences. The specific modalities of sensation under consideration consist of those transduced by receptors in the skin—namely, superficial pain, temperature (warm and cold), and light touch—and those transduced by deep receptors—namely, deep pain, pressure, and joint position sense. Pacinian corpuscles, both superficial and deep, provide vibratory sensation.

Human experience is mediated through the senses and therefore the content of consciousness is, at least in part, a manifestation of the senses. This statement is more obviously true for the special senses transmitted by cranial nerves, but it also applies to sensation in the limbs and trunk. In addition, sensation, conscious or unconscious, is necessary for proper motor function. For example, a patient with impaired joint position sensation may have incapacitating sensory ataxia that superficially resembles cerebellar ataxia, or may have gross random finger movements, termed *pseudoathetosis* or *pseudochoreoathetosis*, despite normal strength. It is apparent, then, that the clinical approach to sensory disorders must take other systems into account, including motor systems.

The diagnosis of sensory abnormalities relies on a careful history and examination and confirmatory laboratory tests. A patient may complain of sensory loss or of unpleasant or unusual sensations. With disorders devoid of positive symptoms, the patient may be unaware of a deficit, and an abnormality will be found only on examination. Patients may express symptoms inaccurately. A patient may complain of "weakness" but have a profound sensory loss with little loss in strength, or complain of "numbness" with normal sensation but with marked weakness when tested. As all clinicians know, the sensory examination can be an exercise in frustration. A successful sensory examination requires a cooperative, attentive, relaxed subject who can report sensation without being too meticulous about equivocal differences. The subjective nature of the examination is obvious. Limb withdrawal to noxious stimuli in a comatose patient is perhaps the most objective finding one can elicit, but most sensory disorders must be found with a wisp of cotton, a pin, tuning forks, vials of warm and cold water, and passive joint movement. In the demented patient, a wince to pinprick may be more helpful than a verbal response. Higher discriminatory sensory function is tested by having the patient identify familiar objects by the sense of touch *(stereognosis)*, identify numbers traced on the skin *(graphesthesia)*, and test the ability to discriminate between one and two pins placed on the skin *(two-point discrimination)*. A sensation that reaches consciousness when presented alone may be extinguished when presented in the context of a similar competing stimulus applied to the same location on the opposite side in double simultaneous stimulation *(extinction)*.

Perhaps most important is the clinician's ability to discern how detailed an examination to conduct without losing the attention of the patient. This is qualitatively different from most other forms of clinical examination, in which, for example, the clinician may have difficulty resolving various faint heart sounds but at least the heart will be indifferent to the stethoscope. Methods for quantification of the sensory examination are available but are not yet routinely used at the bedside; the interested reader should see Munsat (1989) for details. Aspects of the sensory examination pertinent to lesions at different levels of the nervous system are discussed in the appropriate sections of this chapter. Many

Table 32.1: Causes of mononeuropathy and monoradiculopathy

Compression	
	Trauma
	Intervertebral disc (monoradiculopathy)
	Entrapment syndromes (for example, carpal tunnel)
	Tumor mass
	Inherited tendency to develop pressure palsies
Vasculopathy	
	Vasculitis
	Diabetes mellitus
	Embolic or thrombotic arterial occlusion
Infiltration by non–nervous system tumor	
Primary nervous system tumor	
Freezing injury	
Ionizing radiation	
Leprosy	
Herpes zoster	
Herpes simplex (dysesthesias)	
Malaria (rare complication)	
Lyme disease (uncommon complication)	

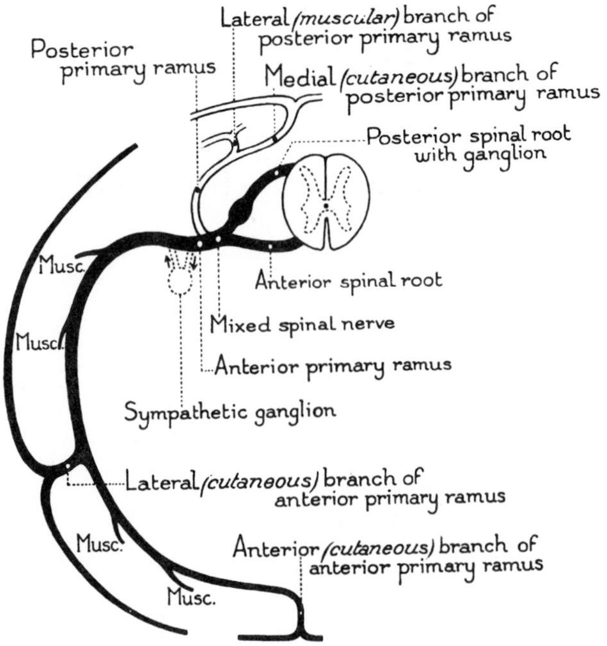

FIGURE 32.1 The components of a segmental nerve. (Musc. = the muscular branches of the anterior primary ramus.) (Reprinted with permission from W Haymaker, B Woodall. Peripheral Nerve Injuries: Principles of Diagnosis. Philadelphia: Saunders, 1945.)

specifics of the examination can be found in textbooks of neurological physical diagnosis, such as Haerer (1992).

CLINICAL PATTERNS OF SENSORY LOSS AND THEIR PATHOLOGICAL SIGNIFICANCE

Mononeuropathies and Monoradiculopathies

This section reviews pertinent anatomy of the spinal roots and peripheral nerves and discusses sensory disturbances that accompany lesions thereof. Details of the clinical presentation of specific neuroradiculopathies and of motor and autonomic deficits are discussed in Chapters 80 and 81 and in specialized texts such as Stewart (1987). Table 32.1 lists common and uncommon causes of this problem. The diagnosis of sensory disturbances secondary to radiculopathy or mononeuropathy depends primarily on anatomical knowledge of the sensory distribution of the involved root or nerve. Motor involvement will often clarify the localization of a lesion. The clinical history and signs and symptoms often lead to a diagnosis that can be confirmed with neuroimaging, neurophysiological tests, and other laboratory tests.

The 31 pairs of spinal nerves consist of eight cervical, 12 thoracic, five lumbar, five sacral, and one coccygeal. Each spinal nerve is formed by the joining of a ventral root and a dorsal root (Figure 32.1). Although the ventral root is generally considered to carry only motor fibers, up to 25% of the fibers are unmyelinated; while some of these loop back and enter the spinal cord via the dorsal roots, others may convey small-fiber sensation to the cord via the ventral roots. This fact may be, in part, the reason that dorsal root surgical section for the control of pain is not always successful. The spinal nerves, which contain both motor and sensory fibers, exit through the intervertebral foramina beneath the vertebral bodies at the appropriate level (Figure 32.2) and subsequently divide into anterior and posterior primary rami. The posterior rami innervate the muscle and skin of the back and neck, with the exception of the first cervical root, which is only motor. The posterior rami provide sensory innervation to the skin in a segmental fashion, with the adjacent segments overlapping. The anterior rami provide sensory and motor innervation to the limbs and to the ventral and ventrolateral trunk of the body. The anterior rami supply sensory fibers to the trunk in a segmental fashion; the sensory field of an anterior ramus overlies the muscles innervated by that segment. The anterior rami supplying the head and the limbs unite in the cervical, brachial, lumbar, and lumbosacral plexuses, which branch and form peripheral nerves comprising fibers from several segments.

The sensory distribution of individual nerve roots *(dermatomes)* has been determined in several different ways, including mapping the sensory deficits of patients with discrete root compression secondary to vertebral disc herniation and by sectioning nerve roots for several segments above and below the level of interest, to demonstrate the entire sensory distribution of a root in isolation. Because of the overlap in the distribution of sensory nerves from different adjacent roots, transection of a single root may cause little or no sensory loss.

Studies of subhuman primates suggest that there may be even greater variability in dermatomal maps than previously thought (Dykes and Terzis 1981). Nevertheless, the currently recognized dermatomal maps (see Figure 28.2) have considerable value. In the clinical assessment of sensory status, a few points should be stressed. Since in many patients there is no C1 dorsal root, there is no C1 dermatome (when a C1 dermatome does exist, as an anatomic variant, it covers a small area in the central part of the scalp). The C4 and T2 dermatomes border each other over the anterior trunk. The C6, C7, and C8 dermatomes include the thumb, middle finger, and fifth digit, respectively. The nipple is at the level of T4. The umbilicus is at the level of T10.

With complete transection of a nerve *(neurotmesis)*, all function of that nerve will be abruptly halted. In a mixed nerve, sensory, motor, and autonomic functions will cease. Complete loss of sensation *(anesthesia)* will occur in the region of skin that is supplied by that nerve alone. The area of skin that is also innervated by adjacent nerves will show decreased sensation, with light touch sensation deficient in a larger area than that of pinprick. The complete transection of a nerve will usually involve a history of trauma. Figures 32.3 and 32.4 show the cutaneous distribution of a number of peripheral nerves.

Partial nerve injury severe enough to sever the axon but leave the epineurium and perineurium intact is termed *axonotmesis*. A discrete traumatic injury, or any other local pressure phenomenon such as that due to a mass, can cause this kind of lesion. The immediate clinical manifestation will be similar to that of a severed nerve—that is, complete dysfunction in the distribution that is unique to that nerve—with partial loss in surrounding regions that have overlapping innervation. With a crush injury leading to axonotmesis, the epineurium and perineurium provide a milieu for outgrowth of axons from the proximal segment of the injured axon. The severed distal axon segment degenerates and is resorbed. Consequently, there can be almost complete symptomatic recovery after such an injury. Over the course of axonal regeneration, which occurs at a rate of 1.0–1.5 mm per day, an area of anesthesia will have gradual recovery of sensation. During this period, the skin may be excruciatingly sensitive to touch *(hyperpathia)*, and sensory stimuli may lead to a burning sensation or a sensation of pins and needles. These unpleasant sensations may occur spontaneously *(paresthesias)*. In 1864 Weir Mitchell described a particularly severe form of posttraumatic pain termed *causalgia*. This painful syndrome generally affects the hand or foot and can occur after a gunshot wound or other high-velocity penetrating injury of a peripheral nerve or nerves, including the brachial or lumbosacral plexus. Trophic changes of the involved extremity, including shiny, taut skin, osteoporosis, and loss of motion of the joints, occur subsequent to the onset of the pain. The trophic changes are thought by some authors to be secondary to immobility. The immobility is due to the nature of the severe, burning pain, which can interfere with sleep and dominate the patient, who will go to great ends to protect the involved extremity. Although sympathectomy can relieve causalgia, the pathophysiology of this disorder is not known.

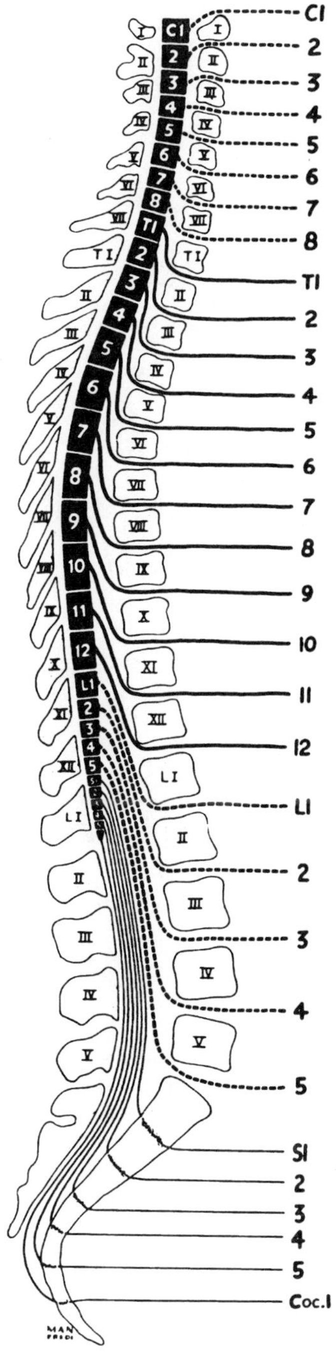

FIGURE 32.2 The relationship between spinal nerves and vertebrae. Cervical nerves exit through intervertebral foramina above their respective vertebral bodies; other nerves exit below these bodies. (Reprinted with permission from W Haymaker, B Woodall. Peripheral Nerve Injuries: Principles of Diagnosis. Philadelphia: Saunders, 1945.)

In addition to *causalgia*, other "neuropathic pain" syndromes such as *reflex sympathetic dystrophy* (RSD) and *sympathetically maintained pain* are the subject of scientific controversy. An attempt at developing criteria for the dif-

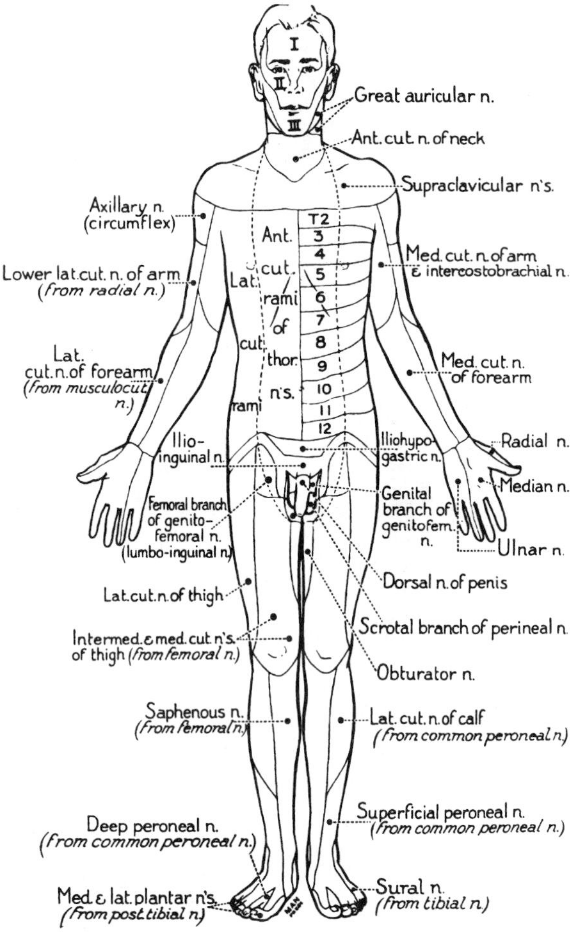

FIGURE 32.3 The cutaneous fields of peripheral nerves from the anterior aspect. The numbers on the left side of the trunk refer to the intercostal nerves. On the right side are shown the cutaneous fields of the lateral and medial branches of the anterior primary rami. The area beneath the scrotum is in the field of the posterior cutaneous nerve of the thigh. (Reprinted with permission from W Haymaker, B Woodall. Peripheral Nerve Injuries: Principles of Diagnosis. Philadelphia: Saunders, 1945.

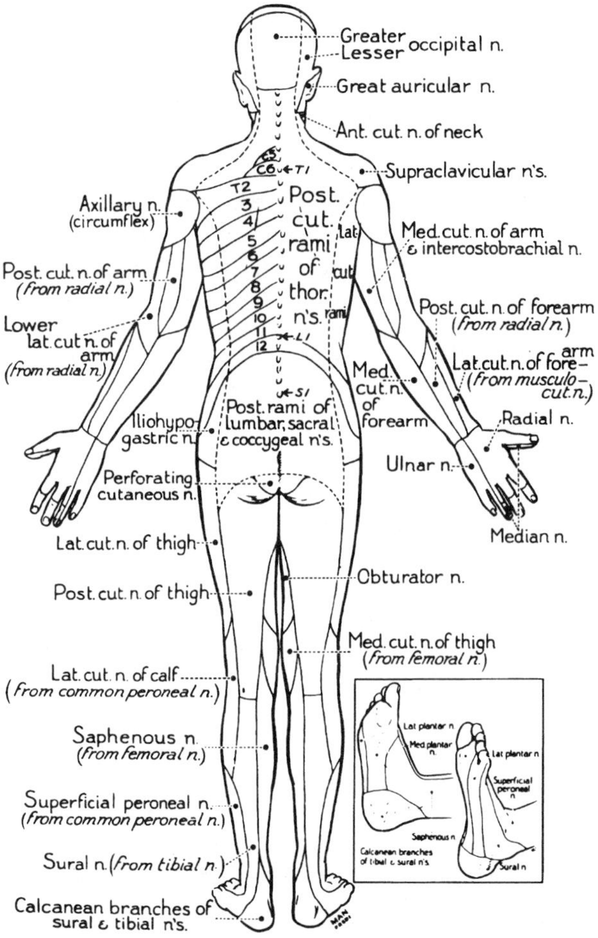

FIGURE 32.4 The cutaneous fields of peripheral nerves from the posterior aspect. The boundaries of cutaneous supply of the posterior primary rami are indicated by broken lines. The distributions of branches of the posterior and anterior primary rami are indicated; the spinous processes of T1, L1, and S1 are also indicated. (Reprinted with permission from W Haymaker, B Woodall. Peripheral Nerve Injuries: Principles of Diagnosis. Philadelphia: Saunders, 1945.)

ferent pain syndromes has not completely resolved the problem. As a result, there is disagreement on the pathophysiology of neuropathic pain.

In the International Association for the Study of Pain classification, the key difference between RSD and causalgia is the lack of direct damage to a peripheral nerve and the associated sympathetic hyperactivity in RSD (Dotson 1993). Possible etiologies for the pain include tonic activity in mechanoreceptor afferents with tonic firing in multireceptive neurons, which are part of the central nociceptive pathway. It is interesting, in this respect, that cutaneous and muscular afferent axons possess different types of sodium channels, which may underlie different firing patterns after injury (Honmou et al. 1994). Other theories have suggested a peripheral nervous system location for these pain syndromes (Campbell et al. 1992).

In contrast to the above physiological theories for neuropathic pain, theories promoted by other investigators have stressed the importance of a psychogenic etiology in some cases (Ochoa 1993; Verdugo and Ochoa 1993). These investigators raise the important point that physiological and pathological involvement of specific peripheral and central pain pathways have not been conclusively demonstrated. In fact, placebo effect may account for a significant number of patients with neuropathic pain who "respond" to therapeutic maneuvers such as sympathetic block.

The treatment of neuropathic pain remains as controversial as the definition of the disease. Sympathetic blockade, morphine injection, and systemic corticosteroids have all been reported helpful. Double-blind controlled studies of placebo and sympathetic blocking drugs have failed to confirm an etiological role for the sympathetic nervous system

(Verdugo and Ochoa 1994; Verdugo et al. 1994). Only through careful scientific investigation using appropriate placebo controls will a clearer understanding of the mechanism and treatment of neuropathic pain develop.

Other forms of sensory disturbance that occur after nerve injury include deep aches or darting and lancinating pains. All these forms of sensation, including paresthesias and numbness, can be manifest in the *phantom limb syndrome* after amputation. The tangle of nerve fibers *(neuroma)* that forms at the amputation site of a severed nerve can be the source of paresthesias, particularly with tactile stimuli. When such neuromas are resected, however, phantom limb sensation can persist although painful sensations are decreased.

A common form of sensory disturbance is that due to pressure-induced transient ischemia. Ischemia can lead to conduction block and loss of sensation, the familiar sensation of a limb "going to sleep" (Bostock et al. 1991). Subsequent restoration of blood flow leads to paresthesias, which are generated in the nerve at the site of pressure rather than in the sensory end organ (Burke and Applegate 1989; Strupp et al. 1990). A more persistent pressure can result in focal demyelination and more persistent conduction block without disruption of the axon. This occurs in immobile and comatose patients and is the source of so-called Saturday night palsy in alcoholics. Paresthesias in the distribution of the involved nerve can accompany recovery that is complete from a clinical standpoint. The accumulation of extraneous sodium channels in neuromas may lead to inappropriate bursting, resulting in persistent paresthesis (Devor et al. 1981). However, there is experimental evidence that there are persistent anatomical changes after functional recovery from a focal crush injury, including shortened internodes and persistent myelin remodeling.

Symmetrical Distal Sensory Syndrome

The symmetrical distal sensory syndrome, a common problem in clinical practice, is a manifestation of a wide variety of systemic illnesses and chronic intoxications. In its mild form, some or all sensory modalities may be slightly compromised. Symptoms include dysesthesias in the form of pins and needles, and burning and aching pain, usually presenting in the feet but occasionally in both upper and lower extremities. These dysesthesias can cause an abnormal gait, as if the patient were walking on a bed of hot coals, and can interfere with sleep when the patient dwells on the discomfort. More severe forms may cause a sensory ataxia because the patient is unable to locate the position of the limbs in space; Romberg's sign indicates this loss of position sensation in the legs. The distribution of sensory loss is often referred to as *stocking and glove*, with the distal region of abnormality gradually blending into more proximal normal regions. *Abruptly demarcated anesthesia* in a stocking or glove distribution is more likely to be feigned or psychogenic. Some patients will manifest a greater sensory loss of one modality than another; for instance, pain and temperature loss may be worse than vibratory, joint position, and discriminatory sense loss. If the discrepancy is great, then a modality-specific or nerve fiber diameter–specific disorder is present.

An example of a *modality-specific disorder* is familial amyloid polyneuropathy, which initially presents as a loss of pain and temperature sensation in the feet or as severe shooting pain. Electrophysiological recordings and biopsies of sural nerves from patients with this disorder show absent C fiber potentials and reduced A delta potentials (small diameter); these are the fibers that carry pain and temperature information, respectively (Lambert and Dyck 1984). In Friedreich's ataxia, joint position and discriminatory sensory loss are selectively impaired due to the loss of the large, heavily myelinated A alpha fibers carrying joint position and discriminatory sensory information. This correlates with decreased compound action potential amplitudes of A alpha fibers, with sparing of A delta and C fiber potentials.

This is not to say that different peripheral fiber types are affected whenever there is a discrepancy between the sensory losses of different modalities. Focal pathology involving particular spinal cord tracks can result in modality-specific sensory deficits. For example, in some cases of multiple sclerosis (MS), posterior column function is impaired, with consequent vibratory, position, and discriminatory sense loss, but peripheral nerves are intact.

Symmetrical distal sensory loss is often a manifestation of what is termed *polyneuropathy* or, more loosely, *peripheral neuropathy*, and may be associated with motor and autonomic deficits as well (see Chapter 81). The term *polyneuroradiculopathy* is probably more accurate in some disorders, such as diabetes, where the nerve roots are also involved (see Chapter 80). The onset is often gradual and can be asymptomatic until brought to the patient's attention. However, some disorders cause a subacute or acute sensory loss, which may be associated with a previously diagnosed disease or can be the new presentation of a systemic disease. Common causes include diabetes mellitus and alcoholism (Figures 32.5 and 32.6). See Chapter 81 for other causes of the syndrome of symmetrical distal sensory loss. Not all of the disorders included in the differential diagnosis of this syndrome are polyneuropathies. For example, *mononeuritis multiplex*, a syndrome of multiple mononeuropathies, can mimic symmetrical polyneuropathy if enough individual nerves are involved. When it is due to infarction of multiple nerves, deterioration occurs in a discrete, stepwise fashion. *Tabes dorsalis*, which is secondary to disease of the dorsal root entry zones, can be associated with symmetrical sensory disturbances in the extremities (see Chapter 80).

One pathological distinction that has been made is that of *dying-back change*, a term first used to describe spin-

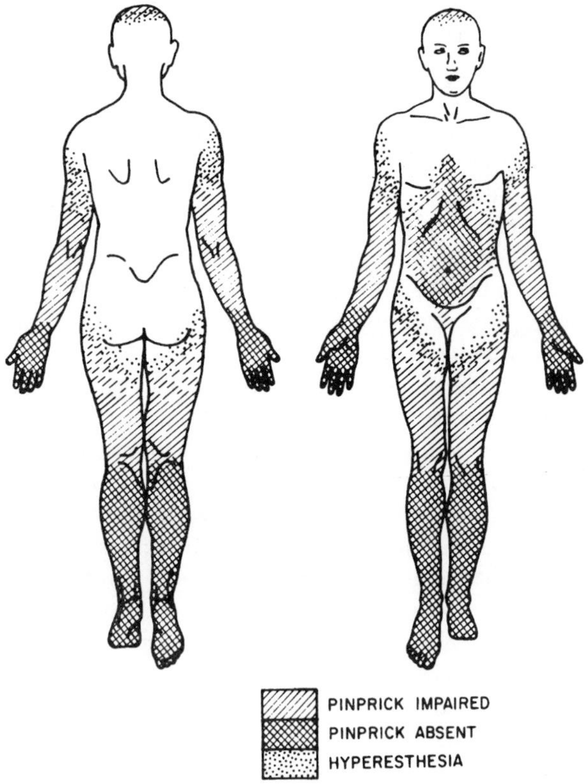

FIGURE 32.5 Sensory loss in a patient with diabetes. Note the involvement of the top of the head and the sparing of the posterior trunk. (Reprinted with permission from W Haymaker, B Woodall. Peripheral Nerve Injuries: Principles of Diagnosis. Philadelphia: Saunders, 1945.)

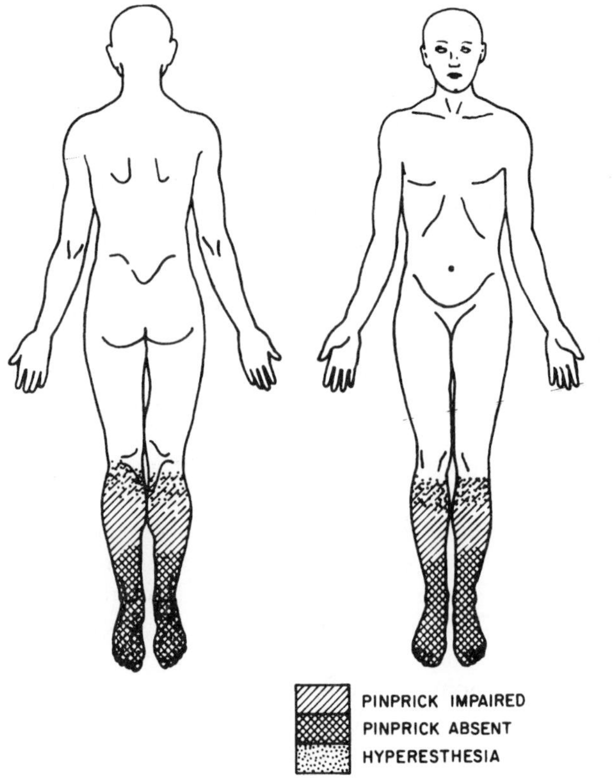

FIGURE 32.6 Sensory loss in a patient with alcoholism. (Reprinted with permission from TD Sabin, N Geschwind, SG Waxman. Patterns of Clinical Deficits in Peripheral Nerve Disease. In SG Waxman [ed], Physiology and Pathobiology of Axons. New York: Raven, 1978.)

ocerebellar degenerations as opposed to multifocal polyneuropathies. As the name implies, the primary feature of dying-back neuropathies is an axonal degeneration of the most distal nerve segments, with subsequent distal clinical deficit worse than proximal clinical deficit. These disorders can be produced by toxic exposure to a variety of agents such as acrylamide, isoniazid (in large doses), organophosphates, and hexacarbons.

Spencer and Schaumburg (1984) prefer the term *central and peripheral distal axonopathy* to *dying-back*, to emphasize that the largest axons in the spinal cord are also degenerating. Pathological changes occur initially in the distal segments of the longest heavily myelinated axons and may be multifocal and limited to distal, preterminal regions (Spencer and Schaumburg 1984). Evidence favors the view that the primary insult in dying-back neuropathy is peripheral, rather than reflecting primary pathology at the cell body. In these axonopathies, the presumably healthy cell body is unable to meet the metabolic needs of the damaged distal axon.

Another pathological pattern associated with distal symmetrical sensory loss is that of *multifocal proximal and distal lesions*. Examples in which this pattern can be seen include lead-induced neuropathy manifested as multifocal demyelination, alcoholic neuropathy, and diabetic symmetrical sensory neuropathy. In these disorders, multifocal lesions located along the nerve, both proximally and distally, are associated with a symmetrical distal sensory syndrome indistinguishable at the bedside from those disorders secondary to a dying-back pathology of axons. This pattern of sensory loss is thought to occur because longer distal nerve fibers will inevitably have more lesions than shorter ones and are therefore more likely to have lesions that cause conduction block. Furthermore, multiple sites of segmental demyelination may lead to temporal dispersion of the nerve action potentials, with subsequent degradation of distal sensory information. Computer simulations of nerves with multifocal areas of conduction block are in accord with these mechanisms of sensory loss.

Evidence indicates that in the symmetrical peripheral neuropathy associated with diabetes mellitus, the primary insult is probably ischemia leading to multifocal axonal degeneration and demyelination. When the disease is moderately advanced, the summation of multifocal lesions results in sensory loss in the distal limbs but also in territories innervated by distal segments of the truncal nerves. Thus, initially the anterior trunk and the top of the head are affected; subsequently, the neck, back, and chest may become involved (see Figure 32.5). If only the anterior trunk is tested, these neuropathies can be confused with myelopathies. Consequently, when there appears to be a midthoracic spinal cord sensory level, both anterior and posterior sensory testing must be done to rule out this possibility.

A wide variety of diseases can present as symmetrical distal sensory loss (see Chapter 81). Moreover, diagnosis is often not made on the basis of history and sensory examination. Because some of the causes are treatable, it is important to undertake thorough laboratory investigation of such patients.

Sensory Loss in Leprosy

Although leprosy is rare in the United States, it is a common treatable cause of neuropathy in underdeveloped countries and is not uncommon in Japan, Korea, Portugal, Spain, and Mexico (Said 1990; see Chapter 81). There are areas of Florida, Louisiana, and Texas in which leprosy is endemic, and, with the influx of Southeast Asians into the United States in the 1970s and 1980s, it is a diagnosis that must be considered in an appropriate clinical setting. The disorder represents the rare situation where nerves are directly invaded by microorganisms (the acid-fast bacillus *Mycobacterium leprae*). The interaction of bacillary growth requirements and host immune response leads to several unique and characteristic patterns of sensory loss.

Indeterminate leprosy, which is most common in children, presents as a single hypopigmented macule, which may have some degree of sensory loss, particularly to pinprick. It may resolve spontaneously or, less commonly, progress to one of the forms outlined below.

Tuberculoid leprosy occurs in patients with a normal cell-mediated immune response. It is characterized by one or several hypopigmented, asymmetrically distributed, macular, dry, scaly skin lesions with distinct raised red borders. The dramatic granulomatous cellular immune response both confines the lesion and causes tissue damage. Cutaneous nerve endings are destroyed, leading to a patch of sensory deficit coinciding with the skin lesion (Figure 32.7). Furthermore, the inflammatory response can affect the underlying nerve trunk and cause a mononeuropathy in the distribution of that nerve. Thus, the deficit is initially sensory and subsequently involves both sensory and motor function. The predominant sensory loss, particularly for pain, can lead to painless trauma, with subsequent deformity and autoamputation of digits and, over years, an entire distal extremity *(acrodystrophy)*. Sharp-dull differentiation may be intact, but the pinprick is not painful. In tuberculoid leprosy, treatment may be curative but may be associated with new lesions and worsening mononeuropathy as a result of increased cell-mediated immunity. This *reversal reaction* may be countered with appropriate anti-inflammatory treatment.

Lepromatous leprosy is characterized by symmetrical bacillary infiltration of the skin, with a propensity for cooler regions such as the pinna of the ear, the dorsum of the hands and feet, the dorsomedial forearm, the dorsolateral legs, the tip of the nose, and the malar region of the face. Sensation in warmer areas, such as under the hairline and in the inguinal crease, popliteal fossa, axilla, and nasolabial fold, is relatively preserved and is lost only when the disease is far advanced. The skin will have multiple nodules, papules, macules, and ulcerations, or there may be diffuse cutaneous involvement with a waxy or somewhat red appearance. Focal weakness can occur as a result of involvement of nerves containing motor fibers at sites where they run close to the body surface. Ulnar weakness is particularly common. Interestingly, deep tendon reflexes are usually preserved in lepromatous leprosy. Mononeuropathy occurs later in lepromatous than in tuberculoid leprosy because the immune response, which mediates this complication, is depressed in lepromatous leprosy. Figure 32.8 shows an example of the sensory loss in lepromatous leprosy.

Borderline leprosy is characterized by more symmetrical involvement than tuberculoid because there is hematogenous spread. Multiple patches of involvement without central healing are typical. The cutaneous sensory loss is less well localized to the patches, and because the host immune system is more intact than in lepromatous disease, there may be multiple superficial nerve trunks involved by inflammation leading to mononeuritis multiplex. This form of leprosy is unstable. It may undergo a reversal reaction with subsequent healing or a downgrading reaction with greater bacillary proliferation, spread, and subsequent lepromatous disease.

Sensory Loss in Porphyria

The hereditary hepatic porphyrias include acute intermittent porphyria, variegate porphyria, and hereditary coproporphyria. Approximately half of the cases are associated with sensory disturbance. Cardiac arrest and respiratory failure from motor involvement represent life-threatening manifestations of these disorders (see Chapter 81).

Porphyric neuropathy generally begins with pain in the back and extremities preceding or coincident with weakness in those regions. Weakness may be either symmetrical or asymmetrical and may present proximally or distally. Occasionally sensory symptoms occur first, with motor symptoms soon to follow. Dysesthesias in the extremities, face, trunk, or buttocks may occur in a patchy or contiguous fashion. Sensory abnormalities at the onset of an attack are most apt to be paresthesias or numbness in the feet or buttocks. Loss of vibratory sense is less common. Cranial nerves are often involved. Deep tendon reflexes may or may not be depressed. Psychiatric disturbance, urinary retention, fecal incontinence, and seizures may accompany an attack. Tachycardia is almost always present, worsens with the onset of neuropathy, and improves with its resolution. Ab-

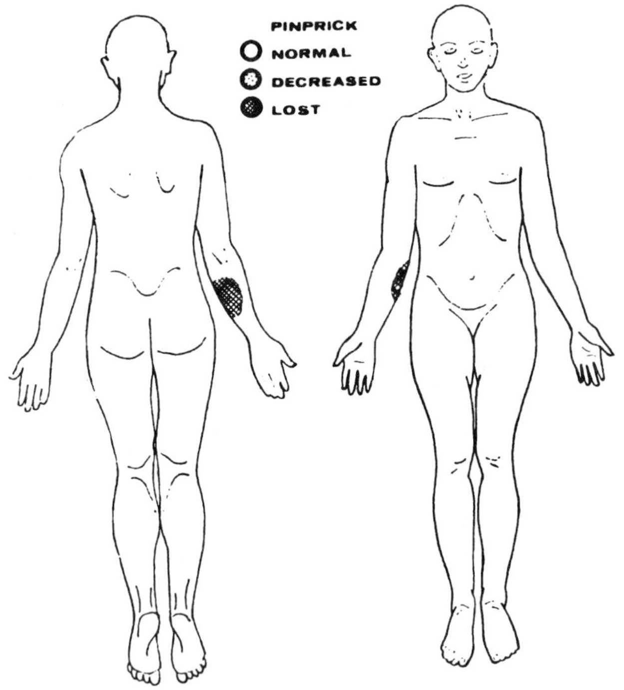

FIGURE 32.7 Sensory loss in a patient with tuberculoid leprosy. (Reprinted with permission from TD Sabin, N Geschwind, SG Waxman. Patterns of Clinical Deficits in Peripheral Nerve Disease. In SG Waxman [ed], Physiology and Pathobiology of Axons. New York: Raven, 1978.)

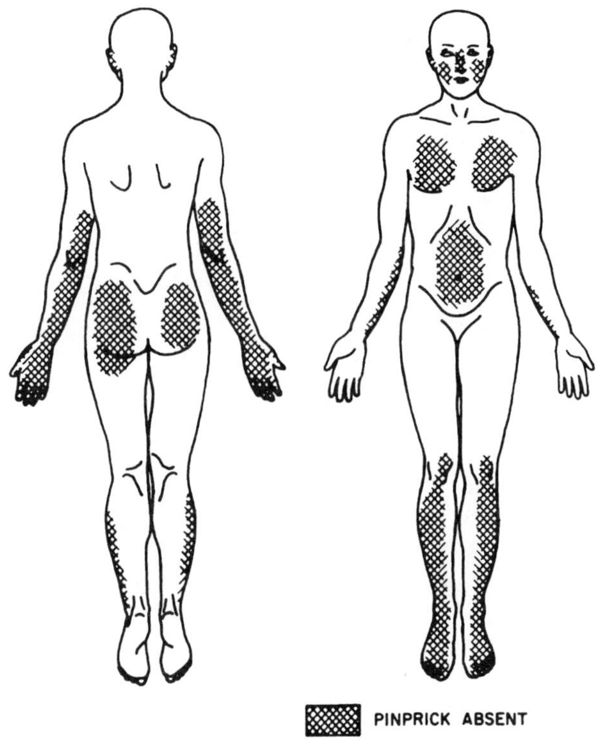

FIGURE 32.8 Sensory loss in a patient with lepromatous leprosy. Note the distribution to cooler areas. (Reprinted with permission from TD Sabin, TR Swift. Leprosy. In PJ Dyck, PK Thomas, EH Lambert et al [eds], Peripheral Neuropathy [2nd ed]. Philadelphia: Saunders, 1984;1955–1987.

dominal pain, which may appear to be psychogenic, is common in acute intermittent porphyria.

There is a pattern of sensory loss that, though not pathognomonic, is quite striking in porphyria. It is characterized by *proximal sensory loss* and occurs approximately 2 weeks after the onset of the attack, at which time motor symptoms are generally prominent. This pattern is that of proximal involvement with distal sparing. Consequently, the area of involvement may resemble long underwear in severe disease, or swimming trunks or a wide band of loss around the proximal arms or thighs in milder disease. The reason for the frequent proximal involvement in porphyria, implicating short rather than long nerves, has not yet been explained. Sabin (1986) has discussed pathophysiological mechanisms that may underlie this unusual pattern of sensory loss.

The distribution of sensory loss may be similar to that seen in distal symmetrical sensory loss, although the concomitant clinical picture and family history in porphyria aid in differentiation. The main disorders in the differential diagnosis are the Guillain-Barré syndrome and the toxic neuropathies, including diphtheritic neuropathy. In the Guillain-Barré syndrome, the spinal fluid has a high protein content, as opposed to the normal or only moderately elevated (rarely greater than 100 mg/dl) level in porphyria; tachycardia, if present in the Guillain-Barré syndrome, is less pronounced. Urine and stool porphyrin analysis (see Chapter 81) will aid greatly in diagnosis. Lead intoxication can resemble acute intermittent porphyria, but the differentiation can be made by history and appropriate laboratory tests.

Attacks of porphyria can be precipitated by a wide variety of drugs, including sulfonamides and barbiturates; if the diagnosis is considered, the clinician must exercise great caution in prescribing drugs.

Spinal Cord Levels

Because of the closely organized structure of the spinal cord, it is unusual to find a purely sensory disorder related to compressive lesions, except early in the course of disease. However, sensory signs are important for localization of the rostrocaudal level of a lesion. The structures involved in sensory abnormalities of the cord (Figures 32.9 and 32.10) include the posterior, lateral, and anterior white matter columns, posterior gray matter, and anterior white commissure. The ascending fibers of the posterior columns are large myelinated fibers arising from ipsilateral dorsal root ganglion cells. The fibers enter medial to the posterior horn;

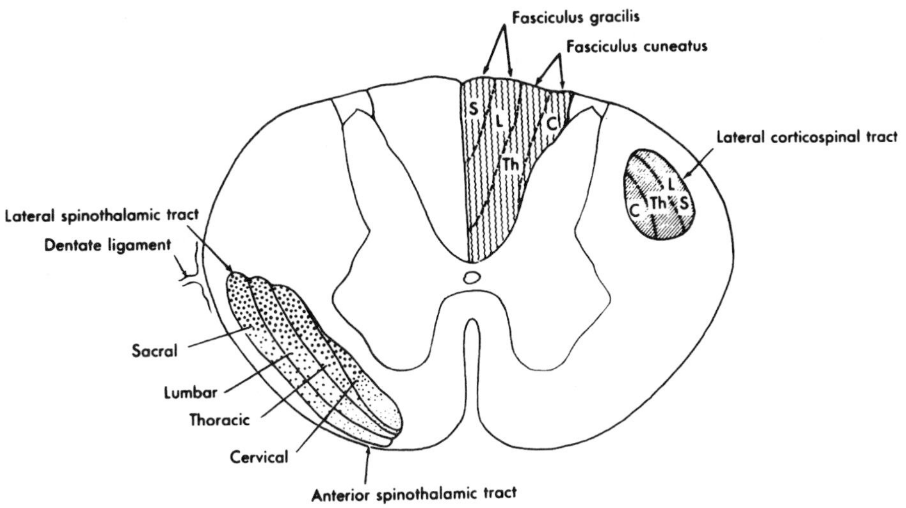

FIGURE 32.9 Lamination of the posterior column, lateral and anterior spinothalamic tracts, and corticospinal tract. (C = cervical, Th = thoracic, L = lumbar, S = sacral.) (Adapted from O Foerster. The dermatomes in man. Brain 1933;56:1–39.)

sacral and lumbar fibers are displaced posteromedially by fibers entering from higher levels. The greatest number of fibers enter at the lumbar and cervical levels, reflecting the great amount of sensory information received from the limbs. The medial aspect of the posterior column, the fasciculus gracilis, carries sensory information from the legs and lower trunk, and its fibers synapse in the nucleus gracilis in the medulla. The fasciculus cuneatus, in the lateral posterior column, carries fibers from the ipsilateral upper extremity to the nucleus cuneatus at the cervicomedullary junction. The fibers in the fasciculi gracilis and cuneatus cross the midline in the medulla, enter the medial lemniscus, and ascend to the ventral posterolateral (VPL) nucleus of the thalamus. Joint position sense, discriminatory touch, and vibratory and deep pressure sense are sensory modalities carried in the posterior columns. Several disorders that can involve the posterior columns are MS and vitamin B_{12} deficiency. Fibers conveying the sensory modalities of pain, temperature, and nondiscriminatory light touch are found in the anterior and lateral spinothalamic tracts (see Figure 32.9). Sensory fibers enter the cord through posterior roots and synapse with neurons mainly in Rexed's laminae I, IV, and V. The fibers from these neurons cross the midline in the anterior white commissure within several spinal segments and ascend to the VPL nucleus of the thalamus (see Figure 32.10). The anterior spinothalamic tract has somatotopic organization, with fibers of most caudal origin placed laterally. This tract carries light touch sensation. The lateral spinothalamic fibers carry pain and temperature information, also arranged somatotopically; fibers of caudal origin are dorsolateral to those of more rostral origin.

This somatotopic arrangement is of clinical importance. An extramedullary laterally placed compressive lesion, such as a metastatic tumor deposit, can cause contralateral cutaneous pain and temperature sensory loss caudal to the level of the lesion. Quite often the sensory level will ascend with the progression of a lesion that is fixed at a more rostral level. Thus, the sensory level cannot be used as a precise indicator of the level of the lesion until late in the clinical course. Conversely, sacral sensation will often be spared when the pathological process affects intramedullary regions of the cord, sparing laterally located fibers. This pattern of sacral sparing is useful, but not obligatory, in the diagnosis of the central cord syndrome. It may be seen in disorders such as intrinsic cord tumors, intramedullary hemorrhage secondary to contusion or to rupture of a vascular malformation, and syringomyelia.

With *complete transection* of the cord, all sensory modalities are affected, although the response to pinprick is the most useful in determining the level of the lesion. Because the cord is shorter than the spine, the cord level will be lower than the vertebral body level. Both ventral and posterior trunk sensation should be tested as severe polyneuropathies can affect sensation over the ventral trunk causing confusion with a myelopathy.

The simplified anatomy presented herein has proved clinically useful but remains incomplete. For example, surgical lesions of the dorsal columns do not permanently affect the gross qualities of joint position sense, and surgical section of the spinothalamic tracts for pain control does not always provide persistent relief. This may be due to multisynaptic pathways within the cord, which can bypass the surgical lesions. Alternatively, previously silent pathways may be activated following injury to the usual route of sensory transmission (Wall 1988). Additionally, there are a small number of fibers that ascend to the medulla ipsilaterally, chiefly in the anterior spinothalamic tract, with sacral segments having the greatest bilateral representation.

The *Brown–Séquard syndrome*, resulting from hemisection of the spinal cord, consists of ipsilateral weakness below the lesion due to interruption of upper motor neuron fibers, and loss of joint position, vibratory, and discriminatory sensation on the side of the lesion below the hemisec-

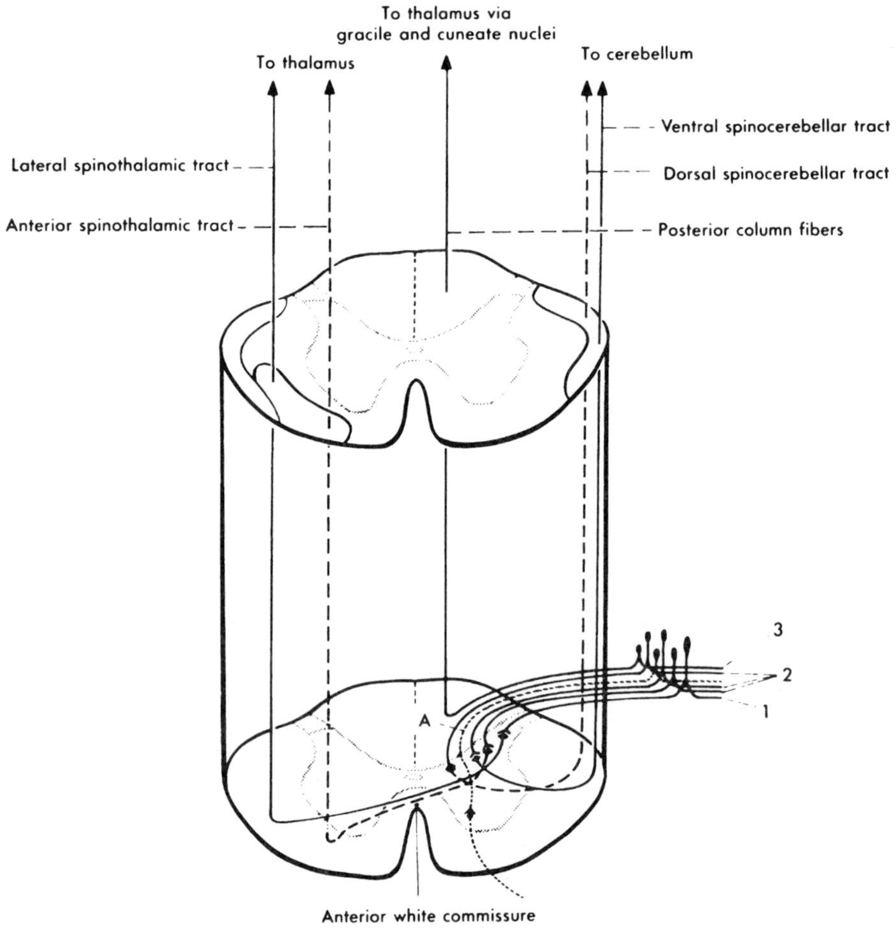

FIGURE 32.10 Ascending tracts of the spinal cord. Some fibers from the posterior root ganglia synapse upon entering the cord (1) or shortly thereafter (2), whereas those that form the dorsal columns synapse in the medulla. (Reprinted with permission from W Haymaker. Bing's Local Diagnosis in Neurological Disease [15th ed]. St. Louis: Mosby, 1969.)

tion due to section of the dorsal column. Contralaterally, there is loss of pain and temperature sense below the level of the lesion due to transection of the spinothalamic fibers carrying impulses from the opposite side of the body. In practice, the syndrome is often incomplete.

Multiple sclerosis can present with minor sensory symptoms due to focal spinal cord demyelination. For example, paresthesias may occur in a small area of an extremity, more commonly in a lower than in an upper extremity, and sometimes bilaterally. A small cutaneous region of a finger or several fingers may be the only areas affected; these often evanescent symptoms may be dismissed initially as insignificant. With progression of the demyelinating process, localization to the appropriate level of the cord becomes simpler, particularly if there is involvement of motor tracts. With clinical evidence of other lesions isolated spatially and in time, such as optic neuritis and internuclear ophthalmoplegia, the diagnosis will be more obvious. Although *Lhermitte's sign,* which is due to abnormal mechanosensitivity of damaged axons, commonly occurs in patients with MS, it is also present in other spinal cord disorders and is therefore not pathognomonic (Vollmer et al. 1991; see Table 32.2).

Sensory Loss in Syringomyelia

Syringomyelia is a cavitary disorder of the spinal cord gray matter (see Chapter 67). The syrinx is located most commonly over several segments in low cervical and high thoracic regions, although it can present in the lower brain stem, where it is known as *syringobulbia* (see below), or in the lumbosacral cord. Rarely, it may extend almost the entire length of the cord.

A common presentation is with loss of pain and temperature sense in the ulnar aspects of the hands and forearms or in a capelike distribution over the shoulders, arms, and upper back. Depending on the exact placement of the lesion in the cord, there may be asymmetrical involvement. With a lumbosacral lesion there will be loss of sensation for pain and temperature in the lumbosacral levels. Because of the location of the lesion, the sensory loss is dissociated in that posterior column function is spared initially, while early in the course of the disease crossing pain and temperature sensation fibers in the midline of the cord are damaged. A more anterior location of the lesion, or its expansion, will lead to loss of anterior horn cells and consequent denervation, reflex loss, and weakness of muscles

Table 32.2: Disorders associated with Lhermitte's sign

Multiple sclerosis
Nitrous oxide myeloneuropathy
Vitamin B_{12} deficiency
Cisplatin myeloneuropathy
Cervical spondylotic myelopathy
Radiation myelitis
Prolapsed cervical disc
Atlantoaxial subluxation
Lateral cervical puncture
Fractured odontoid process
Traumatic central cord syndrome
Syringomyelia
Spinal cord tumors (extrinsic and intrinsic)
Behçet's disease
Tonsillar (cerebellar) ectopia
Herpes zoster (shingles)

Source: TL Vollmer, LM Brass, SG Watman. Lhermitte's sign in a patient with herpes zoster. J Neurol Sci 1991;106:153–158.

with atrophy, most commonly of the intrinsic muscles of the hands. Posterior column function may be affected with further enlargement of the syrinx. A lesion that is located in a posterior horn may cause a sensory deficit resembling that of radiculopathy, but the loss will be dissociated, with sparing of posterior column function. Spasticity and paresis of an upper motor neuron type may occur below the level of the lesion if corticospinal tract fibers are damaged by an enlarging syrinx. If this occurs, it is usually late in the course of the disease.

Syringomyelia can be associated with mutilating deformities of the hands, due to painless trauma, which are similar to those of leprosy, but other clinical features should differentiate the two disorders. Other intramedullary lesions, as noted previously, may present similarly to syringomyelia. Magnetic resonance imaging (MRI) has made the diagnosis simpler than in the past because the lesion may be directly imaged without the need for radiopaque contrast agents, which may fail to demonstrate the lesion even with computed tomography (CT) scanning.

Foramen Magnum Tumors

Extramedullary tumors in the region of the foramen magnum are associated with a variety of sensory disturbances. Nuchal and suboccipital pain, particularly with motion, often leads to head tilt or torticollis. This pain is frequently accompanied by loss of tactile sensation over the back of the head in the distribution of the upper cervical roots that are compressed. Pain referred to the C2 distribution, followed by numbness, is particularly characteristic. Loss of pain and temperature sensation or loss of proprioception, worse in the upper than in the lower extremities, may accompany motor loss. The motor loss often begins in a single upper extremity, progresses to the ipsilateral lower and thence to the contralateral lower extremity, and leads finally to quadriparesis. Thus, the progression of symptoms is "around the clock." The sensory abnormalities may reflect this progression or may be in a Brown-Séquard pattern, or can simulate syringomyelia.

Occasionally there may be patches of truncal sensory loss or stimulus-induced dysesthesias in an apparent segmental distribution at several different levels, suggesting lesions at multiple spinal cord levels. Patients with anteriorly placed lesions may complain of a pronounced sensation of cold, sometimes associated with piloerection. Sudden "electrical" pains occurring with neck flexion down the spine and into the upper extremities (Lhermitte's sign) are often reported. Loss of vibratory sense over the clavicles and acromion processes has also been reported.

Sensory complaints with foramen magnum tumors, particularly patchy loss over the trunk, might initially be dismissed as psychogenic or might lead to false localization. The fact that this is a treatable condition emphasizes the need to keep this diagnosis in mind.

Sensory Abnormalities Associated with Lesions of the Brain Stem

Lesions above the level of the foramen magnum may make themselves known by sensory disturbances. Because the tracts and nuclei in the brain stem are so closely packed, a lesion there will usually involve cranial nerves and other descending motor tracts. The consequent signs and symptoms will usually fit into a recognized brain stem syndrome (see Chapter 23). For example, with occlusion of a vertebral artery or a posterior inferior cerebellar artery, ischemia of the lateral medulla may occur. The resulting disorder, often referred to as *Wallenberg's syndrome*, includes pain and temperature sensory loss of the ipsilateral face and contralateral limbs and trunk. Damage to the lateral aspect of the cuneate nucleus may lead to impaired light touch and joint position sensation in the ipsilateral upper extremity. In addition to these sensory abnormalities, ipsilateral Horner's syndrome, hoarseness, dysphagia, vertigo, nausea, nystagmus, and ipsilateral ataxia of a cerebellar type are present in Wallenberg's syndrome as a result of damage to cranial nerve nuclei and associated white matter.

A different pattern of sensory loss, bifacial sensory loss and nystagmus, is seen with intrinsic tumor in the midline of the medulla or with syringobulbia. Since virtually all cases of syringobulbia are associated with extension of a cervical syrinx, signs of syringomyelia will usually be present with this lesion.

Ischemia of the inferolateral pons due to occlusion of the anterior inferior cerebellar artery can disrupt the spinothalamic tract and lead to contralateral loss of pain and temperature sensation of the limbs, the trunk, and occasionally the face. If the lateral medial lemniscus is also damaged, then vibratory, position, and discriminatory sensation will be impaired contralaterally. In addition, vertigo, nausea, nystagmus, ipsilateral deafness and facial sensory loss, and paresis of conjugate gaze to the side of the lesion are present with this disorder.

Signs of cranial nerve dysfunction can serve to localize sensory abnormalities of the limbs and trunk to the brain stem, as demonstrated earlier. Rarely, a laterally placed lesion in the superior medulla may cause a contralateral hemianesthetic syndrome, which may spare the face. The presentation of hemisensory loss without other abnormalities, however, suggests a supratentorial process, namely a thalamic lesion. See Chapter 23 for further examples and discussion of brain stem syndromes.

Hemianesthetic Syndrome and Other Sensory Abnormalities Associated with Supratentorial Lesions

Thalamic lesions may cause a pure contralateral hemisensory deficit, often sparing the face. Although tumors can occur in the thalamus, usually the onset of thalamic sensory loss is acute or subacute and is due to a lacunar infarct. With thalamic lesions, discriminatory sensation is often affected more than pain and temperature sensation. Sometimes direct testing will not demonstrate sensory loss, but subjectively sensation is impaired. Excruciating pain, described in graphic detail, may accompany the sensory loss or may exist independently. This thalamic pain syndrome may occur with small lesions and may be paroxysmal and severely incapacitating. Tactile stimuli may precipitate painful dysesthesias. A lesion of the thalamus, with its characteristic contralateral hemisensory loss, may be associated with mild hemiparesis due to damage to the internal capsule, usually secondary to compression from swelling in the thalamus. Furthermore, there are cases of dominant-hemisphere thalamic lesions associated with aphasia. However, the sensory problem will usually be most prominent with thalamic lesions. CT and MRI are particularly valuable for localization of the lesion in equivocal cases.

Lesions of the *sensory cortex* may cause sensory loss corresponding to the affected region of the sensory homunculus (Figure 32.11). A pure sensory loss will not be extensive because a lesion affecting the sensory cortex that is large enough to affect more than a small area of the body will also affect other cortical functions, for example, of speech or movement. The presence of neglect, or a hemi-inattention syndrome, in the context of a left-sided sensory abnormality, suggests a nondominant cortical lesion, especially affecting the parietal region, although neglect can occasionally occur with thalamic lesions.

In some cases of right-hemispheric disorders, the patient may be unaware of (or unconcerned about) a dense left-sided sensory abnormality because of the associated inattention syndrome *(anosagnosia)*. This is often associated with visual and auditory hemi-inattention. Usually there will be evidence of upper motor neuron damage, often with initial flaccid paresis and subsequent spasticity contralateral to the side of the lesion. Babinski's sign will be present in most cases.

With the initial presentation of a stroke in evolution or with a transient ischemic attack affecting sensory cortex, there may be no evidence of the aforementioned signs of cortical dysfunction so that there is pure sensory loss; but with progression, the diagnosis is usually clarified by the appearance of these signs of cortical damage.

Sensory abnormalities may be associated with an epileptic focus. Sensations of movement can occur with a focus in the postcentral cortex. Pins and needles, numbness, tingling, throbbing, pain, and sensations of buzzing, quivering, crawling, electricity, or water running down an arm suggest a lesion in the precentral and postcentral cortex. Various thermal sensations, including hot, cold, or burning, suggest a lesion in the temporoparietal cortex. The abnormal sensations may progress, or march, to anatomically adjacent regions in the same fashion as focal motor seizures or may remain contained. Because of their disproportionately large cortical representations, hand or perioral regions are commonly involved. Reflecting the organization of the cortical homunculus, sensory abnormalities can march from hand to face or vice versa. The episode may suggest a transient ischemic attack. Careful history, neuroimaging studies, and electroencephalography can help clarify the problem.

LOCALIZATION OF SENSORY ABNORMALITIES

The foregoing discussion has presented an approach to the diagnosis of sensory abnormalities based on pathophysiology, neuroanatomy, and clinical signs and symptoms. Because sensorimotor abnormalities of the limbs and trunk can be due to lesions in both the peripheral and the central nervous system, quite remote from the sites of impaired sensation, the intellectual step of localization ("Where is the lesion?") must consciously be made by the clinician to initiate appropriate diagnostic studies and rational therapy. We now briefly review some of the steps involved in localization, beginning with the differentiation of cortical from subcortical lesions on the basis of the neurological examination.

Tactile identification of different shapes (stereognosis), recognition of numbers traced on the skin (graphesthesia), localization of stimuli on the skin, and two-point discrimination are all considered to be cortical sensory functions. With cortical lesions, these higher sensory modalities may be impaired in the context of preservation of the elementary sensory modalities, such as pinprick and vibration. This pattern of sensory loss usually signals contralateral cortical disease. As noted earlier, however, thalamic and other deep hemispheric disorders occasionally interfere with higher discriminatory functions.

An abnormality anywhere between the peripheral sensory receptors and the cortex might compromise the transmission of the basic sensory information. Thus, loss of

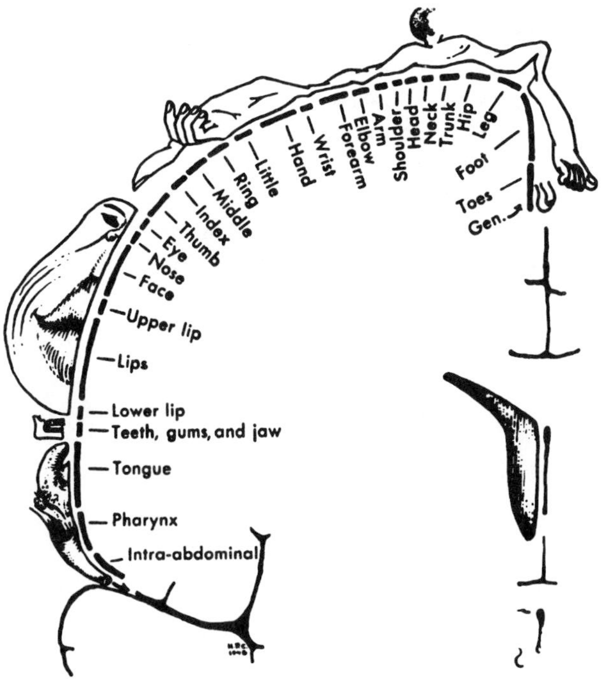

FIGURE 32.11 The sensory homunculus. The extent of sensory cortex represented by a given part of the body is indicated by the drawing and, more accurately, by the length of the underlying line. (From Penfield and Rasmussen 1950. Copyright © 1950 by Macmillan Publishing Co, renewed 1978 by T. Rasmussen. Reprinted by permission of author and publisher.)

cortical modes of sensation, in the context of severe impairment of elementary modes of sensation, has little localizing value. One must look at the constellation of signs and symptoms to arrive at the most likely diagnosis. Some examples will clarify this.

The presence of dysphasia with dominant hemispheric lesions, hemi-inattention with nondominant lesions, and hemiparesis in the pattern associated with upper motor neuron lesions and concomitant ipsilateral sensory loss implies a cortical abnormality, as does the presence of focal seizures of any kind. Although thalamic lesions may be associated with motor and language deficits, this is atypical; motor deficits, if present, are usually not prominent. Predominantly hemisensory loss is typical of a thalamic lacunar infarct.

Brain stem lesions cause a variety of syndromes, usually with motor and sensory dysfunction as well as involvement of cranial nerve nuclei. In exceptional cases a pure hemisensory deficit may be secondary to a laterally placed lesion in the superior medulla, but abnormalities of the brain stem typically are associated with signs of cranial nerve dysfunction. Abnormalities of eye movements, sensory abnormalities that are crossed with respect to the face and the rest of the body, vestibular dysfunction with concomitant vertigo and nausea, hearing deficit, and dysphagia all suggest a brain stem lesion. The pattern of abnormality will point to the appropriate level of the neuraxis and to the lateralization of the lesion within the brain stem. Evidence of nystagmus or cranial nerve dysfunction must place a lesion above the level of the foramen magnum, or there must be multiple sites of disease, as occur with MS and metastatic tumor.

A number of findings can point to a disease process involving the spinal cord. The presence of spasticity always indicates a disorder in the central nervous system. Thus, a minor sensory abnormality in an extremity, associated with spasticity, or the presence of Babinski's sign implies disease in the spinal cord or higher. The absence of other signs of cortical or brain stem disorder, noted previously, leaves the spinal cord as the probable site. The presence of bilateral hyperreflexia with a sensory or sweating level of the extremities, or both, without other findings, also suggests spinal cord disease. An exception to this is the rare case of a parasagittal meningioma located over primary sensory cortex, which may lead to bilateral proximal lower extremity sensory loss without other findings.

The loss of deep tendon reflexes implies a peripheral nerve or root disorder, or damage to anterior horn cells. A process that damages anterior horn cells at the level of the lesion, associated with sensory loss, will usually also damage corticospinal tracts, leading to hyperreflexia below the level of the lesion. An exception to this is in syringomyelia that has progressed to involve anterior horn cells but not lateral white matter. Sacral sparing is a useful, but not necessary, finding in the central cord syndrome. Symmetrical distal sensory loss with loss of reflexes almost defines peripheral neuropathy. Severe polyneuropathy can mask signs of cord compression. The presence of Babinski's sign and brisk reflexes points to the diagnosis of a central problem, but these signs can be attenuated by a superimposed peripheral neuropathy. The presence of a level circumferentially on the trunk, below which there is absence or impairment of pinprick sensation, demarcated at the superior edge by the inferior margin of a dermatome, and associated with spasticity below the sensory level, is diagnostic of cord compression.

Mononeuropathies lead to loss of sensation in the distribution of the sensory branches of the involved nerves. Radiculopathies typically cause lancinating, shooting pain. A monoradiculopathy is unlikely to cause an appreciable sensory deficit but may be the source of painful sensory symptoms. Sensory neuroradiculopathy may be seen in disorders such as diabetes mellitus. The findings with this disorder may be clinically indistinguishable from those of symmetrical polyneuropathy due to some other cause, but electromyography will often show the presence of spinal root involvement, inferred from the presence of denervation potentials in paraspinous and other proximal muscles.

When there are features that are atypical for a common clinical syndrome, a consideration of the differential diagnosis is essential. For example, although numbness and muscle atrophy in the hands may be due to bilateral carpal tunnel syndrome, the presence of medial hand involvement should raise the possibility of syringomyelia, even in cases where nerve conduction studies show a decrease in median nerve conduction across the wrists. As previously noted, ataxia is not solely a sign of cerebellar dysfunction but may be due to interruption of impulses carried in the posterior columns. The presence of a sign referable to a certain level of the nervous system implies the presence of a lesion at that level or *higher*. An example is a laterally placed compressive lesion of the cervical spinal cord. The resultant damage to spinothalamic tract fibers may lead to a sensory deficit confined to the contralateral lower extremity.

Another important step in the process of localization is the decision about whether to attribute abnormal physical findings to a lesion at a single site or multiple sites. For example, sensory loss in the distribution of the lateral cutaneous nerve of the thigh associated with ischemic optic neuropathy indicates a lesion at two sites, even though a single pathological process, such as diabetes mellitus, might underlie both abnormalities. Neuroanatomical knowledge allows the determination of what is clinically possible with a single lesion.

These points are of more than academic importance. The clinician is responsible for helping the radiologist direct imaging studies toward the correct sites. Despite MRI and CT, localization of neurological abnormalities by reference to the clinical history and physical examination remains the most important tool of the practicing physician for the diagnosis of neurological illness.

FACTITIOUS SENSORY DISORDERS

Part of the clinical presentation of certain organic disorders includes sensory abnormalities that are difficult to explain on purely anatomical grounds. Some of these conditions may have a prominent affective and psychiatric component. Causalgia, acute intermittent porphyria, foramen magnum tumors with patchy truncal sensory deficits, the thalamic pain syndrome, minor sensory complaints in MS, and perhaps focal sensory epileptic seizures present complex pictures of sensory dysfunction, which can be confused with those associated with functional illness. Some patients will have sensory abnormalities associated with psychogenic illness (conversion reactions), Munchausen's syndrome, or malingering. The diagnosis of such a cause, which may present along with organically based neurological illness, rests in part on the demonstration of inconsistency in the results of different tests of the same function or in demonstration of anatomical inconsistency.

For example, a hemisensory deficit in response to pinprick that splits perfectly at the midline is inconsistent with the fact that cutaneous nerves innervate somewhat across the midline. Loss of vibratory sensation over a midline bone when the tuning fork is moved over a short distance from one side of the midline to the other is not anatomically valid. Some patients will have a hemisensory deficit that includes loss of hearing and vision on the same side of the body. Others will respond "no" to a pinprick each time they "do not feel it." Such inconsistencies are not compatible with anatomical pathways. Nevertheless, because some patients embroider an organic illness with a psychological overlay, a thorough evaluation must be done to rule out the possibility of organic illness coexisting with an overlay of psychogenic illness.

REFERENCES

Bostock H, Baker M, Grafe P et al. Changes in excitability and accommodation of human motor axons following brief periods of ischemia. J Physiol (Lond) 1991;441:513–535.

Burke D, Applegate C. Paraesthesia and hypasthesia following prolonged stimulation of cutaneous afferents. Brain 1989;112:913–929.

Campbell JN, Meyer RA, Raja SN. Is nociceptor activation by alpha 1 adrenoreceptors the culprit in sympathetically mediated pain? Am Pain Soc 1992;1:3–11.

Devor M, Keller CH, Deerinck TJ et al. Na channel accumulation on axolemna of afferent endings in neuromas in Apteronotus. Neurosci Lett 1989;102:149–154.

Dotson RM. Causalgia-reflex sympathetic dystrophy. Sympathetically maintained pain: Myth and reality. Muscle Nerve 1993;16:1049–1055.

Dykes RW, Terzis JK. Spinal nerve distribution in the upper limb: organization of the dermatome and afferent myotome. Phil Trans Royal Soc 1981;293:509–594.

Foerster O. The dermatomes in man. Brain 1933;56:1–39.

Haerer AF (ed). DeJong's The Neurologic Examination (5th ed). Lippincott, 1992:42–83.

Haymaker W. Bing's Local Diagnosis in Neurological Disease (15th ed). St. Louis: Mosby, 1969.

Haymaker W, Woodall B. Peripheral Nerve Injuries: Principles of Diagnosis. Philadelphia: Saunders, 1945.

Honmou O, Utzschneider DA, Rizzo MA et al. Delayed depolarization and slow sodium currents in cutaneous afferents. J Neurophysiol 1994;71:1627–1638.

Lambert EH, Dyck PJ. Compound Action Potentials of Sural Nerve In Vitro in Peripheral Neuropathy. In PJ Dyck, PK Thomas, EH Lambert, R Bunge (eds), Peripheral Neuropathy (2nd ed). Philadelphia: Saunders, 1984:1030–1034.

Munsat T (ed). Quantitation of Neurologic Deficit. London: Butterworth, 1989.

Ochoa JL. Guest editorial: Essence, investigation, and management of "neuropathic" pains: hopes from acknowledgment of chaos. Muscle Nerve 1993;16:997–1008.

Sabin TD. Classification of peripheral neuropathy: the long and short of it. Muscle Nerve 1986;9:711–719.

Sabin TD, Geschwind N, Waxman SG. Patterns of Clinical Deficits in Peripheral Nerve Disease. In SG Waxman (ed), Physiology and Pathobiology of Axons. New York: Raven, 1978.

Sabin TD, Swift TR. Leprosy. In PJ Dyck, PK Thomas, EH Lambert et al. (eds), Peripheral Neuropathy (2nd ed). Philadelphia: Saunders, 1984;1955–1987.

Said G. Studies on the Mechanism of Nerve Lesions in Leprous Neuropathies. In G McKhann (ed), Childhood Neuropathy. New Issues in Neuroscience, Vol. 2. New York: Wiley, 1990;85–94.

Spencer PS, Schaumberg HH. Experimental Models of Primary Axonal Disease Induced by Toxic Chemicals. In PJ Dyck, PK Thomas, EH Lambert et al. (eds), Peripheral Neuropathy (2nd ed). Philadelphia: Saunders, 1984;636–649.

Stewart JD. Focal Peripheral Neuropathies. New York: Elsevier, 1987.

Strupp M, Bostock H, Weigl P et al. Is resistance to ischemia in motor axons in diabetes subjects due to depolarization? J Neurol Sci 1990;99:271–280.

Verdugo RJ, Campero M, Ochoa JL. Phentolamine sympathetic block in painful polyneuropathies. II. Further questioning of the concept of "sympathetically maintained pain." Neurology 1994;44:1010–1014.

Verdugo RJ, Ochoa JL. Use and misuse of conventional electrodiagnosis, quantitative sensory testing, thermography, and nerve blocks in the evaluation of painful neuropathic syndromes. Muscle Nerve 1993;16:1056–1062.

Verdugo RJ, Ochoa JL. "Sympathetically maintained pain." I. Phentolamine block questions the concept. Neurology 1994;44:1003–1010.

Vollmer TL, Brass LM, Waxman SG. Lhermitte's sign in a patient with herpes zoster. J Neurol Sci 1991;106:153–158.

Wall PD. Recruitment of Ineffective Synapses After Injury. In SG Waxman (ed), Functional Recovery in Neurological Disease. New York: Raven, 1988;387–400.

Chapter 33
Sexual and Sphincter Dysfunction

David N. Rushton

Neurological lesions at different sites may result in characteristic patterns of sexual and sphincter dysfunction, but distinguishing those patterns reliably often requires investigational as well as clinical data. This chapter describes some of these patterns of dysfunction and the physiological bases on which they arise. It does not attempt to give an account of specific diseases or investigations. It is intended to serve as the background for considering the specifics of neurourological investigations, findings, and diagnoses, which are discussed in Chapter 45.

The available physiological and clinical knowledge may also throw some light on a group of functional or "psychological" disorders (for example, adult enuresis, detrusor instability, urethral sphincter spasm, and primary anorgasmia), where it might be concluded that an occult neurological disorder (that is, a disorder for which there is no other clinical evidence) may be present.

Patients with complaints relating to sexual and sphincter dysfunction may seek a wide range of medical specialists, including neurologists, urologists, gynecologists, and psychiatrists. These specialists need to take an interest in the exact disturbances and the available choice of investigation and treatment methods, because effective medical and surgical treatments are now available for many of these disorders. Special neurourological investigations are often essential, principally cystometry, urodynamics, videocystourethrography, urethral pressure profile recording, ultrasonography, sphincter and pelvic floor electromyography, and electrophysiological testing of pelvic and pudendal nerve conduction and reflexes. These techniques often allow precise diagnosis of incontinence and voiding difficulties of every sort and are detailed in Chapter 45.

It is in recognition of the development of this new field of investigation that the term *neurourology* has come into common use. Because neurourology is oriented in two directions, two systems of classification are needed: a urological classification and a neurological classification. The patient has urological symptoms that may require treatment, and these symptoms may help localize the neurological lesion. One urologically based symptomatic classification is the International Continence Society's system, describing detrusor, urethral, and sensory functions in a three-by-three structure (Table 33.1). One obvious limitation of this structure is that it takes no account of variations with time. One neurological classification recognizes five major central pathways that may be disrupted (Table 33.2) and nine major peripheral pathways (Table 33.3).

This chapter attempts to use these classification structures to consider, in terms of the diagnostic significance of the history and examination and the planning of investigation and treatment, approaches to some specific urogenital symptom complexes that may have neurological causes. Non-neurological causes, such as prostatic hypertrophy or urethral stricture, will be considered only as differential diagnoses and not discussed in detail. Disorders of erection, ejaculation, and orgasm are often treatable. If the neurological diagnosis is known or if the clinical diagnosis belongs to the functional group of disorders, trials of probable forms of treatment can often be instituted without invasive investigation.

Table 33.1: Urological classification of urinary faults

Detrusor Vesicae Function	*Urethral Sphincter Function*	*Bladder and Urethral Sensation*
Normal	Normal	Normal
Overactive	Overactive	Hypersensitive
Underactive	Incompetent	Hyposensitive

Table 33.2: Central sensorimotor pathways concerned with micturition and sphincter control

Pathway	*Origin or Destination*	*Function*
Higher CNS loop	Brain stem Frontal lobe Basal ganglia	Initiates and inhibits switching between filling and voiding states
Lower CNS loop	Brain stem Conus medullaris	Coordinates and sustains detrusor and sphincter contraction and relaxation
Detrusor reflex loop	Detrusor afferents Pudendal motoneurons	Promotes sphincter relaxation when detrusor is active
Urethral reflex loop	Urethral afferents Pudendal motoneurons	Maintains sphincter tone when detrusor is inactive
Corticospinal pathway	Motor cortex Pudendal motoneurons	Voluntary control of sphincters and pelvic floor

ANATOMY AND PHYSIOLOGY OF BLADDER AND SPHINCTER CONTROL

Pathways

Uniquely among smooth muscles, the detrusor vesicae is subject to voluntary activation and inhibition. There is a cortical level of control, allowing determination of the social and behavioral circumstances under which micturition occurs. There are suprasegmental (pontine) and segmental (conus) centers responsible for the organization of voiding reflexes (Figure 33.1). It is believed that the functional control and reflex pathways include the following:

1. Afferents from the bladder wall excite the detrusor nucleus and inhibit Onuf's sphincteromotor nucleus. This segmental reflex helps initiate the voiding state.
2. Afferents from the urethra excite sphincter contraction and inhibit the detrusor, except in the voiding state, when their action is switched to maintain voiding. During voiding the stimulus provided by the flow of urine serves to maintain detrusor contraction and inhibit the sphincters. Efficient switching of this reflex requires supraspinal control, and failure of such switching results in uninhibited detrusor contraction, detrusor-sphincter cocontraction (*dyssynergia*), or both.
3. Sensations of bladder fullness can facilitate triggering of the pontine micturition center; triggering activates the detrusor reflex and inhibits the sphincters.
4. The pontine micturition center can normally be both activated and inhibited from the frontal cortex, so that rather than functioning automatically, the bladder is under conscious control. Lesions of the superomedial frontal cortex or of the linking pathways usually result in automatic voiding when the bladder is full, with loss of the ability to initiate or inhibit voiding consciously.

Table 33.3: Nerve roots supplying peripheral sensorimotor pathways concerned in micturition, sphincter control, erection, and ejaculation

Functional Pathway	*Nerve Roots**
Parasympathetic innervation of detrusor	S2, **S3**, S4
Somatic innervation of urethral sphincter	**S3**, S4
Somatic innervation of anal sphincter	S3, **S4**
Detrusor afferents	S2, S3, S4
Urethral afferents	?S2, S3, S4
Genital afferents	S2, S3
Sympathetic innervation of bladder neck and urethra	T11, **T12**, L1
Sympathetic erectile and antierectile pathways	T11, **T12**, L1
Parasympathetic erectile pathway	**S2**, S3
Sympathetic ejaculatory pathway	T11, **T12**, L1

*Dominant root supply in bold.

5. The functions of the anatomically well-demarcated pathways between the pontine micturition center and the cerebellar vermis and basal ganglia are unknown. Uninhibited detrusor contraction (Berger et al. 1987) and perhaps sphincter bradykinesia can occur in Parkinson's disease. However, it is not clear whether there is any characteristic urodynamic pattern in Parkinson's disease apart from such changes as might be seen in other elderly subjects (Malone-Lee 1994). Uninhibited detrusor contractions are described in patients with apparently pure cerebellar disorders.

Cerebral Cortex

Lesions of the superomedial frontal cortex, particularly if bilateral, result in uninhibited voidings occurring in response to bladder filling; occasionally there may be inability to void.

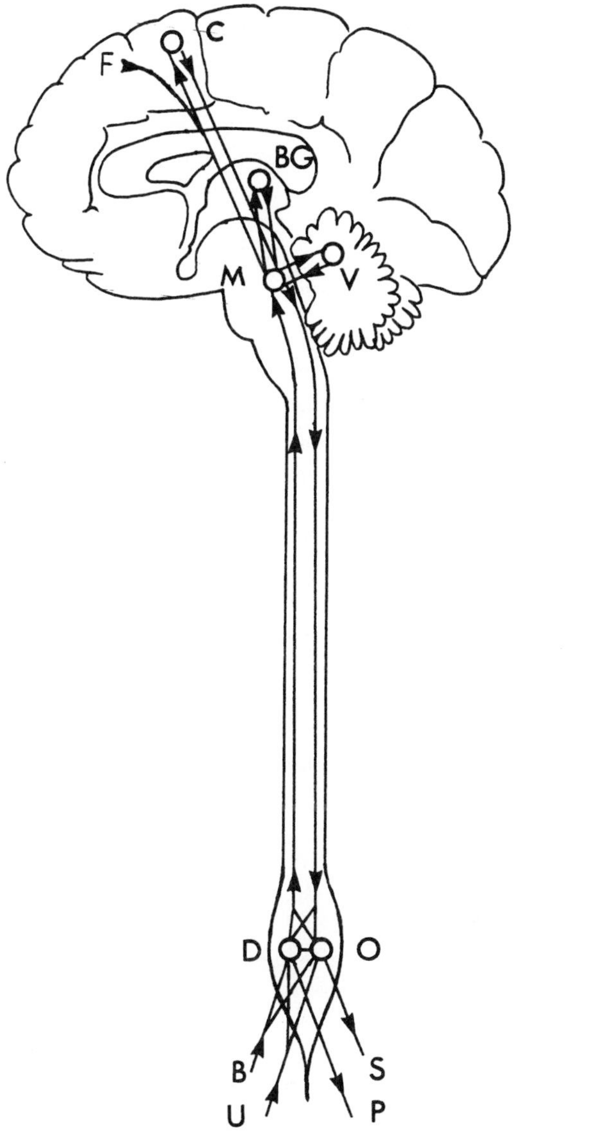

FIGURE 33.1 Principal spinal and supraspinal pathways involved in the control of micturition. Afferent pathways are shown on the left, efferent pathways on the right. (D = detrusor motor nucleus; O = Onuf's sphincteromotor nucleus; B = afferent pathways from bladder wall; U = afferent pathways from urethra; S = somatic sacral outflow to sphincters and pelvic floor; P = parasympathetic sacral outflow; M = pontine micturition center; V = cerebellar vermis; BG = basal ganglia connections; C = sensorimotor cortical pathway to and from sphincters; F = frontal micturition regulating area.)

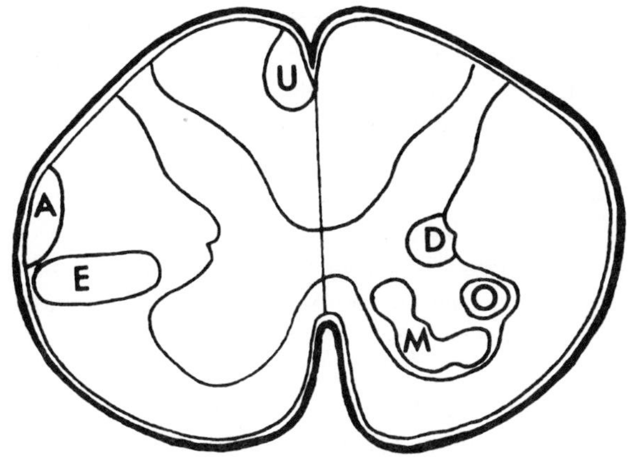

FIGURE 33.2 Spinal tracts and nuclei concerned in the control of micturition. Long tracts are shown in the left half, and motor nuclei in the right half. In reality both are bilateral, and unilateral lesions often cause little lasting disability. The evidence about long tract location is derived partly by studying the patterns of deficit in patients with bilateral cordotomies (usually for cancer pain), with postmortem study of degeneration patterns in the cord. (Left: A = approximate location of bladder wall afferents; E = approximate location of motor tracts to detrusor and sphincters; U = approximate location of urethral afferents. Right: D = location of detrusomotor neuron colonies in the sacral intermediolateral horns, at S2–S4 segmental level; O = Onuf's sphincteromotor nucleus, innervating urethral and anal sphincters; M = motoneuron colonies to extrinsic muscles of the pelvic floor.)

Patients with this sort of reflex incontinence may be embarrassed or not, depending on the site and extent of the cerebral lesion. The cerebral influence is normally dominant, in that fullness alone (within normal capacity) does not initiate detrusor contractions. Even during voiding, the active detrusor can be switched off. This is achieved by sphincter closure, following which the detrusor contraction dies away, and urine is "milked back" into the bladder by the closure of the striated sphincter, proximal urethra, and bladder neck. The initial sphincter closure removes the reflex stimulus to continued voiding that arises from urethral flow. The voluntary sphincter closure is cortical in origin; a fast corticospinal pathway to the sphincters has been demonstrated.

Pontine Micturition Center

The basic reflex organization of the filling and voiding states, and the reciprocal inhibition of the detrusor and sphincter mechanisms, is at the pontine level. There, nuclei in the locus coeruleus, the pontomesencephalic gray matter, and the nucleus tegmentolateralis dorsalis are believed, on the basis of animal experimental evidence, to receive both pudendal and detrusor afferents, and to project densely to neurons in the intermediolateral cell column at conus level.

Spinal Long Tracts

In the spinal cord, impulses for the modalities of bladder and rectal sensation and for urethral pain and temperature travel in the lateral columns superficially in the equatorial region (Figure 33.2, left). At conus level, the pudendal afferents appear anatomically to bear more segmental collaterals than detrusor afferents. Pudendal afferents for urethral touch, pressure, and tension probably travel in the posterior column. Impulses for the initiation and organization of voiding contractions travel in the lateral columns near the intermediolateral horn bilaterally, while impulses controlling the sphincters and pelvic floor travel a little more laterally. These impulses enable conscious control of both voiding and defecation, and the latter impulses enable control of the pelvic and perineal muscles. Unilateral lesions often have no lasting effect on these functions, and even bilateral sensory lesions do not always abolish all sense of bladder and bowel fullness. However, the vague sensations that remain after a transverse cord lesion do not allow distinction between feces and flatus, control of loose stool, or accurate assessment of bladder fullness.

Conus Medullaris and Peripheral Innervation

At conus level, somatic motor fibers originating in Onuf's sphincteromotor nucleus (see Figure 33.2, right) traverse S2–S4 (mainly S3) anterior roots to the intrinsic urethral striated sphincter mechanism, probably via supralevator branches of the pelvic nerves. Periurethral striated muscle and anal sphincter innervation is via S3–S4 and the pudendal nerves. Parasympathetic neurons in the intermediolateral sacral cell column innervate the detrusor via S2–S4 (mainly S3) and the pelvic ganglia and nerves.

A sparse sympathetic motor innervation of the dome and a dense innervation of the neck of the bladder are derived from motor neurons of the intermediolateral cell column, most commonly between T10 and L1, through the corresponding roots and the pelvic ganglia and nerves.

The structure and functions of the pelvic ganglia in humans are poorly understood, though there is a good deal of animal evidence that sympathetic and parasympathetic pathways interact there. There is evidence of a wide range of neurotransmitter substances in the pelvic ganglia (Hoyle et al. 1994). In addition to acetylcholine there is evidence that enkephalin, neuropeptide Y, noradrenaline, somatostatin, VIP, dopamine, and ATP occur there either as transmitters or cotransmitters.

In the detrusor most sympathetic endings are beta-adrenergic and may modulate transmission in parasympathetic ganglia, inhibiting it during the filling phase. Parasympathetic postganglionic fibers either run in bundles containing synaptic vesicles located on axon varicosities, or innervate detrusor smooth muscle fibers by close contact. In humans the postganglionic parasympathetic transmission is mainly cholinergic muscarinic, whereas in species that use urine for territorial marking, ATP is prominent. There is evidence that nitric oxide (NO) is an inhibitory neurotransmitter in the urethra (Andersson et al. 1992). Adjacent smooth muscle cells may communicate via low-impedance gap junctions. In the male there is a dense sympathetic innervation of the preprostatic genital sphincter (see section below on ejaculatory failure), and in both sexes there is alpha- and beta-adrenergic innervation of the bladder neck.

The detrusor muscle fibers are arranged in well-defined bundles in a collagen framework. In the trigone, the fiber bundles are smaller and mainly alpha-adrenergic. In the urethra, smooth muscle is in a matrix of collagen and elastin, lined by transitional epithelium more proximally and by squamous epithelium distally; the latter contains pudendally innervated sensory receptors.

DISORDERS OF BLADDER FUNCTION

Urgency of Micturition and Urgency Incontinence

Urinary urgency is a common symptom, which can result from a wide range of causes. The causes can be grouped under sensory, motor, obstructive, and idiopathic headings.

Sensory Urgency

The functional capacity is reduced because abnormal patterns of sensory impulses occur, signaling that the bladder is full before the normal capacity is reached. The voiding reflex itself is intact, but, depending on the site and pathology of the lesion, the act of voiding itself may well be painful. Mechanical urethritis or bacterial cystitis are common causes of sensory urgency, but any other source of inflammation of the epithelium of the lower urinary tract will cause similar symptoms. Some of these causes of inflammation are listed in Table 33.4, together with their characteristics, where applicable. Most of these causes of urgency can be diagnosed with the help of urine culture, intravenous pyelography, ultrasound, blood chemistry, and, if necessary, cystoscopy and biopsy. These causes are not primarily neurological, although secondary sensory urgency may occur as a result of urinary infection, which is common in patients with neurological problems who void poorly.

Motor Urgency

The reduced functional bladder capacity of patients with motor urgency is caused by abnormal excitability or failure of inhibition of the voiding reflex, and it is therefore the type of urgency incontinence most usually associated with neurological disease (Table 33.5). Motor urgency symptoms are etiologically nonspecific, but the pattern of urgency incontinence has some anatomical localizing value, as between cerebral and spinal lesions. As noted above, diffuse or appropriately located cerebral lesions may result in loss of control of the pontine micturition center, so that voiding occurs prematurely and involuntarily. There may also be loss of ability to initiate voiding voluntarily. The reflex voiding act itself remains intact, with a normal flow pattern and voiding to completion. Loss of detrusor inhibition also means that interrupting voiding is difficult or impossible; if achieved at all, it is done by voluntary striated sphincter closure against a continuing detrusor contraction.

Table 33.4: Differential diagnosis of sensory urgency of micturition

Group Causes of Sensory Urgency	*Underlying or Predisposing Causes*
Bacterial cystitis	Anatomical anomaly
	Indwelling catheter
	Retention of urine
	Diabetes mellitus
Mechanical urethritis	Catheter
	Sexual intercourse
	Urethral foreign body
Viral infection	Hemorrhagic adenovirus (in children)
	Herpes zoster (with mucosal vesicles)
	Herpes simplex type II
	Condylomata acuminata
Other cystitis	Interstitial cystitis
	Eosinophilic cystitis (bilharzia, toxocara, or nonparasitic)
	Allergic cystitis (many foods, molds, pollen, and dusts)
	Radiation cystitis
	Chemical cystitis (e.g., cyclophosphamide, turpentine, or thiotepa instillation)
Tumors	Carcinoma
	Myoblastoma
	Leiomyosarcoma
	Rhabdomyosarcoma
	Pheochromocytoma (hypertensive crisis on voiding)
	Pelvic lipomatosis
	Desmoid tumor
Metaplasia	Nephrogenic metaplasia
	Intestinal-type metaplasia
	Endometriosis (cyclical hematuria)
Others	Actinomycosis (forms fistula)
	Amyloidosis
	Cholesteatoma

Incomplete spinal cord lesions often result in urgency incontinence, but here the voiding pattern itself is usually abnormal. *Detrusor-sphincter dyssynergia* is often present, and the detrusor contractions may be poorly sustained, so that voiding is irregular and incomplete, resulting in hesitant and interrupted micturition and an increased residual volume (Torrens and Morrison 1987).

Obstructive Urgency

Detrusor instability can also occur as a result of outflow obstruction. Whether the obstruction is structural or neurological, there may be urgency and frequency, because the functional capacity of the bladder is reduced by the large residual volume. Urgency then coexists with hesitancy and difficulty of voiding and poor or intermittent flow. The common causes of infravesical obstruction include prostatic hypertrophy or malignancy, and urethral stone, cyst, or stricture (Table 33.6). Most of the causes can be differentiated by clinical examination, urodynamic testing, and micturating cystogram, but some will require sphincter electromyography (EMG). Neurological functional obstruction can occur at the bladder neck or at the striated sphincter level. The causes and characteristics of such obstruction are discussed in the section on disorders of urethral function.

Table 33.5: Differential diagnosis of motor urgency of micturition

Group Causes of Motor Urgency	*Common Conditions*
"Idiopathic"	?Subclinical spinal cord or cerebral disease
	?Developmental anomaly
	?Maturational failure
	?Aging, without other evidence of disease
System disorders	Progressive autonomic failure
	Multiple-system atrophy
	Parkinson's disease
	Familial dysautonomias
Local brain diseases	Inferomedial frontal lesions
	Hydrocephalus
	Parasagittal meningioma
	Callosal glioma
Diffuse brain diseases	Alzheimer's disease
	Pick's disease
	Huntington's disease
	Parenchymatous syphilis
	AIDS encephalopathy
Spinal cord diseases	Cord injury, tumor, or compression
	Multiple sclerosis
	Spondylotic myelopathy
	Transverse myelitis
	Late syringomyelia

Idiopathic Urgency Incontinence

Detrusor instability is usually present in patients with urgency incontinence, and there may be no associated abnormalities to find on investigation. Detrusor instability is defined as the occurrence of uninhibited systolic detrusor contractions greater than 15 cm H_2O on bladder filling, occurring during cystometry at a volume of less than 300 ml. There may be a long or lifelong history of urgency, and sometimes delayed resolution of childhood enuresis. There is by definition no evidence of causative structural urological abnormality or neurological disease. It is often thought of as a failure of maturation of bladder control and is sometimes associated with adult nocturnal enuresis.

Difficulty and Hesitancy of Micturition

Neurological Causes

Neurological causes of difficulty and hesitancy of micturition include lesions causing detrusor areflexia, such as acute

Table 33.6: Differential diagnosis of infravesical obstruction causing acute or chronic urinary retention

Type	*Diagnostic Tests and Features*
Bladder neck dyssynergia	Micturating cystourethrogram (MCUG), urodynamics, response to adrenergic blockers
Detrusor-sphincter dyssynergia	MCUG, urethral pressure profile (UPP)
Striated sphincter spasm	Sphincter electromyography, UPP
In young men	
In young women	
In women with sphincter reinnervation	
In women with Kline-Levin syndrome	
In association with urethritis	
Psychogenic (pseudodyssynergia)	
Structural in male	Cystoscopy, MCUG
Prostatic hypertrophy, trapping, inflammation, or carcinoma	
Urethral valves or stricture	
Meatal stricture or phimosis	
Male cystocoele	Follows abdominoperineal resection
Structural in female	Cystoscopy, MCUG, gynecological examination
Trigonocele or posterior descensus	
Urethral valves	
Urethral caruncle	
Urethral fibrosis or stricture	If atrophic, may respond to estrogens

spinal cord lesions (spinal shock phase), lesions of the conus or cauda equina, and spinal cord lesions that result in infravesical obstruction (bladder neck dyssynergia, sphincter spasticity or spasm, or detrusor-sphincter dyssynergia). Examples of these main nonobstructive classes of retention are listed in Table 33.7. Some of the obstructive causes of retention and poor stream are listed in Table 33.6, as obstruction is part of the differential diagnosis of poor voiding.

Any cause of an *acute* cord lesion, complete or incomplete, can engender spinal shock. Hesitancy or voiding difficulty in *chronic* cord lesions, however, is likely to have some other cause, particularly one of the causes of functional infravesical obstruction listed under Group 4 in Table 33.7. Non-neurological causes of acute retention may act directly (infravesical obstruction), reflexively (pelvic or urethral pain), or in an uncertain, perhaps partly mechanical, way (postoperative, constipation).

Detrusor Failure

Detrusor decompensation can occur following chronic retention, with fibrosis and loss of detrusor shortening ability. The sensation of bladder filling and reflex detrusor contractions may also be reduced. Even if an obstruction is removed, the residual volume may be only incompletely relieved, and voiding may be aided by straining. A similar situation may occur temporarily following severe acute retention, when voiding may subsequently be impaired for a time by what is believed to be a traction neuropathy of the terminal parasympathetic nerve fibers. In acute or chronic detrusor decompensation, the bladder atony may cause confusion, with the atony resulting from a preganglionic parasympathetic lesion, caused for example by cauda equina compression from a central lumbar disc prolapse.

Table 33.7: Differential diagnosis of neurological urinary retention

Group	*Pathology*
1. Spinal areflexia	Spinal shock
	Conus infarction or destruction
	Transverse myelitis
2. Sensorimotor neuropathy	Central disc prolapse
	Trauma involving cauda equina
	Lumbar canal stenosis
	Guillain-Barré polyneuropathy
	Herpes zoster of sacral nerves
	Cauda equina tumors
	Diabetes mellitus
	Tabes dorsalis
3. Autonomic neuropathy	Diabetes mellitus
	Multiple-system atrophy
	Shy-Drager syndrome
	Radical pelvic surgery
4. Infravesical obstruction	Structural obstructions (see Table 33.6)
	Detrusor-sphincter dyssynergia
	Bladder neck dyssynergia
	Sphincter spasm (pseudodyssynergia)
5. Unknown mechanism (possibly reflex)	Constipation
	Alcohol intoxication
	Postoperative

DISORDERS OF URETHRAL FUNCTION

Stress Incontinence

Stress incontinence as a symptom means the immediate involuntary loss of a significant amount of urine when abdominal pressure is raised, for example by coughing, laughing, or lifting. However, only some patients with such symptoms have the condition termed *genuine stress incontinence* (GSI). The reason is that to diagnose GSI, it must be shown that incontinence occurs when intravesical pressure exceeds the maximum urethral closure pressure and that the resulting incontinence occurs without any accompanying detrusor contraction (Cardozo 1994). GSI can thus only be diagnosed on the basis of both clinical and urodynamic evidence. GSI is common and may coexist with a neurological lesion causing urgency incontinence. Cure of the urgency incontinence may then reveal the stress incontinence, which may need to be treated in its own right. The forms of stress incontinence caused by pelvic floor incompetence and by denervation of the Onuf's nucleus are both accompanied by prominent anorectal incontinence, so they are dealt with under the disorders of anal function.

Stress Incontinence in Women

GSI occurs most commonly in postpartum women, in association with anterior or posterior suspension defects and descent of the bladder neck, or incompetence of the pelvic floor. The normal bladder neck and proximal urethra, like the bladder itself, are within the abdominal pressure zone, so that a rise in intra-abdominal pressure does not force urine into the urethra, but abnormal descent of the bladder neck takes it out of the abdominal pressure zone, so that additional hydrostatic pressure in the bladder can overcome the urethral closing pressure, and stress incontinence may result, even if the sphincter closing pressure is normal.

In addition, any disease causing incompetence of the bladder neck closure mechanism can also be a cause of stress incontinence, particularly in women. Examples include pelvic surgery, suspension defects, irradiation, degenerative or inflammatory changes, or hormone withdrawal. However, an open bladder neck seen on videocystourethroscopic screening in women does not necessarily imply that stress incontinence will be present (Versi 1991). Urinary incontinence due to bladder neck descent, unlike that due to pelvic floor incompetence, is not usually associated with anorectal incontinence.

Detailed consideration of the treatment of prolapse and stress incontinence is discussed by Cardozo (1994). Treatment methods available include pelvic floor exercises, alpha-adrenergic drugs, surgical elevation of the bladder neck, or surgical implantation of an artificial urethral sphincter.

Stress Incontinence in Men

In men, stress incontinence usually occurs only where both proximal and distal sphincter mechanisms are impaired. Causes include combined bladder neck resection and external sphincterotomy, with resection below the verumontanum, or infiltration of proximal and distal sphincter mechanisms by prostatic cancer.

Treatment may be by alpha-adrenergic drugs, artificial sphincter, or external drainage device. Surgical methods have been reviewed by Kirby and Christmas (1994).

Stress Incontinence in Paraplegia

A combined sphincterotomy and bladder neck resection has been popular in paraplegic men in the past, having the aim of promoting urinary drainage; it intentionally causes severe stress incontinence, which is then managed using a urine-collecting device. This combined procedure has never been indicated for paraplegic women, because of the lack of a satisfactory urine-collecting system for women. Incontinent paraplegics with poor or dyssynergic reflex voiding can usually be provided with good voiding and continence by intermittent self-catheterization (with anticholinergic drugs if necessary). Increasingly, these patients are being managed using the sacral anterior root stimulator implant (SARSI) (Brindley and Rushton 1990). The stimulator is used in combination with a sacral deafferentation, which cures reflex incontinence and sphincter dyssynergia and restores bladder compliance. The restoration of a controlled voiding pressure obviates the need for sphincter surgery.

Pseudo–Stress Incontinence

Stress incontinence can be mimicked by reflex incontinence, when exertion causing raised abdominal pressure triggers a detrusor contraction. When there is no sensation of detrusor contraction, as is sometimes the case, then there need be no sense of urgency before incontinence occurs. Such reflex incontinence is therefore urgency incontinence in disguise, and the causes are the same as those of urgency incontinence. "Giggle incontinence" is one form of reflex incontinence that is often idiopathic and is usually seen in young women. One might surmise that the rapid fluctuations in abdominal pressure that occur in laughter are a potent stimulus to detrusor contraction in some people.

Uninhibited Urethral Relaxation

Urethral relaxation normally precedes detrusor contraction in voluntary voiding. Correspondingly, when uninhibited detrusor contractions occur, they are often preceded by an uninhibited urethral relaxation. Therefore, uninhibited urethral relaxation is often associated with urge incontinence, whether due to cerebral or spinal cord lesions. This sort of uninhibited urethral relaxation can also occur in the absence of a subsequent detrusor contraction, so that episodes of dribbling incontinence occur.

Bladder Neck Dyssynergia

Bladder neck dyssynergia (BND) is characterized by failure of the bladder neck to open or to remain open during attempted voiding. It may be idiopathic and can be clearly distinguished from striated sphincter dyssynergia by videocystourethrography. Idiopathic BND is believed to be caused either by an abnormal arrangement of smooth muscle at the bladder neck, so that it narrows instead of funnelling during voiding, or by alpha-adrenergic overactivity in the bladder neck and preprostatic sphincter. BND also occurs in a small proportion of patients with spinal cord lesions. The mechanism is unknown but may be related to adrenergic supersensitivity in association with anterolateral cell column loss at T12–L2. It may be associated with autonomic dysreflexia. The idiopathic form of BND is a cause of recurrent episodes of retention in young men (the so-called nervous bladder of young men). Most forms of BND can be successfully treated with $alpha_1$-adrenergic blockers such as prazosin, alfuzosin, or indoramin.

Detrusor-Striated Sphincter Dyssynergia

Functional obstruction is commonly seen at the striated sphincter level and is particularly associated with cord lesions where the conus medullaris is intact. *Detrusor-sphincter dyssynergia* (DSD) implies the loss of reciprocal inhibition between the rhabdosphincter and detrusor, so that the sphincter fails to relax when a detrusor contraction occurs, or relaxes only incompletely, or intermittently, or after a delay. Consequently, there can be a high-pressure, low-flow, delayed, or intermittent pattern of voiding, with an increased residual volume.

Pseudo–Detrusor-Striated Sphincter Dyssynergia

In neurologically intact subjects, the symptoms of DSD may be mimicked by painful conditions of the urethra, resulting in sphincter contraction when urine enters the urethra. Pseudo–DSD can also occur in voiding difficulty due to psychological disturbance. Pseudo–DSD can often be distinguished from genuine DSD by its shorter length of urethral closure seen on micturating cystogram (McGuire 1984).

Sphincter Spasm in Young Women

Apart from pseudo–DSD, recurrent acute retention in neurologically normal young women may be associated with a form of sphincter spasm that has a characteristic EMG picture (and sound), with motor unit bursts of descending frequency. On single-fiber EMG there is a complex repetitive discharge of low jitter, and evidence of ephaptic transmission between sphincter muscle fibers. It may be associated with evidence of sphincter denervation and reinnervation and with polycystic ovaries (Fowler et al. 1985).

Failure of Bladder Neck Closure

Failure of bladder neck closure sometimes causes stress incontinence, particularly in women with bladder neck descent or pelvic floor incompetence. As noted above, the common incidental finding of an open bladder neck on videocystourethrography does not necessarily imply that stress incontinence will be present (Versi 1991). It does, however, suggest that the strength of the rhabdosphincter will be critical.

Failure of bladder neck closure also follows bladder neck resection and occurs in patients taking alpha-adrenergic blockers. Other specific causes include a central or peripheral sympathetic lesion—for example, resulting from a long spinal cord lesion extending from T10 to L2—or acute or chronic autonomic neuropathy, or pelvic injury or surgery.

Abnormal Urethral Responses to Bladder Filling

Urethral pressure normally rises slightly during bladder filling. This response may be lost if there is a lesion of urethral afferents or of the smooth muscle at the bladder neck. Urethral pressure normally falls just before the onset of a detrusor contraction. This response is lost in prostatic obstruction and where the pressure rise is caused by a noncompliant bladder. It is often lost in voiding contractions initiated in the spinal bladder. Uninhibited urethral relaxation responses (often seen in association with uninhibited detrusor contractions) may occur spontaneously on bladder filling in the presence of lesions of the spinal cord or brain.

DISORDERS OF ANAL SPHINCTER FUNCTION

Normal Mechanisms

Fecal continence is maintained by the combined actions of the puborectalis muscle sling, which forms and maintains the anorectal angle and flap-valve mechanism, and the anal sphincters (external striated sphincter and internal smooth muscle sphincter), which form the necessary length of high-pressure zone distal to the anorectal angle. The striated sphincter is conventionally described as comprising subcutaneous, superficial, and deep components. The puborectalis part of the system is thought to be more concerned with major continence of solid feces, and the sphincters with the prevention of fecal soiling and the control of loose stool and flatus. Voluntary contraction of the striated sphincter inhibits rectal contractions; conversely, rectal contractions cause reflex relaxation of the internal and external anal sphincters, via the intrinsic innervation networks rather than a spinal pathway.

Anal Sphincter Failure

Denervation or surgical division of the sphincters causes loss of control of flatus and loose stool, while denervation or loss of the puborectalis muscle causes solid fecal incontinence. On the sensory side, loss of anal canal sensation in pudendal neuropathy or cauda equina lesions may also be associated with fecal incontinence. Anorectal incontinence may therefore occur in disorders of the sensory roots, conus, motor roots (S3, S4), or peripheral nerves (pelvic or pudendal neuropathy). Pelvic floor neuropathy and system degenerations affecting the sphincters are of particular interest and are discussed below.

Stress and Fecal Incontinence Due to Pelvic Floor Incompetence

The problem of pelvic floor incompetence has been reviewed by Swash (1993). It is often accompanied by electrophysiological evidence of injury to the terminal pudendal nerve branches innervating the sphincters and pelvic floor. Anorectal incontinence (ARI) is common and is often accompanied by stress incontinence of urine. There is clinical and EMG evidence of pelvic floor and sphincter denervation, and abnormal descent of the pelvic floor can be observed during straining. In addition, partial or complete rupture of the anal sphincter mechanism can often be demonstrated ultrasonographically (Deen et al. 1993) and is believed to be a major factor causing ARI. A lesser degree of pudendal nerve damage is very common following childbirth and may also occur in chronic constipation. Regeneration and recovery may occur but are not always complete. This condition may be distinguished from stress incontinence caused by prolapse through pelvic examination with straining and through pelvic electromyography. Treatment is surgical, by sphincter repair or post–anal repair as appropriate. If these conventional procedures fail, an artificial anal sphincter can be fashioned using a conditioned and activated gracilis sling (Abercrombie and Williams 1995).

Stress and Fecal Incontinence Due to Onuf Denervation

In autonomic failure due to multiple-system atrophy (MSA) or Shy-Drager syndrome, there is selective degeneration of Onuf's nucleus (see Figure 33.2) and consequently selective denervation of Onuf-innervated muscles, with incontinence as a result. Conversely, in motor neuron disease there is relative preservation of Onuf-innervated muscles, even when there is extensive denervation of the pelvicaudal muscles of the pelvic floor; hence, in motor neuron disease continence is typically preserved. The status of the puborectalis muscle is uncertain in motor neuron disease, as embryologically and by innervation it seems to be pelvicaudal and not Onuf-innervated, and it is believed to be important for fecal continence.

Anal Sphincter Spasm

It has long been suspected that anal sphincter spasm might be a cause of proctalgia fugax, a sharp, short-lasting but recurrent, usually nocturnal anal pain syndrome that is very common. Alternatively, given that anal manometry and proctoscopy are usually found to be normal, it has often been held to be of psychological origin. The difficulties with this conclusion are (1) that it is hard to arrange to do manometry when the pain is present and (2) that there are often no associated features of psychological disturbance.

A hereditary myopathy localized to the internal anal sphincter has been described in a family in whom the affected members complained of constipation and severe proctalgia fugax (Kamm et al. 1991). The internal sphincter was greatly thickened, with PAS–positive polyglycosan bodies in the fibers and endomysial fibrosis. In this group at least, anal canal pressure was often sustained at abnormally high levels. This familial myopathic form of proctalgia should probably be thought of as separate from the common idiopathic form, whose cause is still unknown.

DISORDERS OF SEXUAL FUNCTION

Sexual disorders of mainly psychological origin have been well described (Masters and Johnson 1970), are very common, and are outside the scope of this chapter. The normal sexual response in both males and females is conventionally divided into four phases: excitement, plateau, orgasm, and resolution. Nevertheless, the neurological disorders of sexual function tend to be gender-specific and are discussed as such.

Sensory Mechanisms

Receptor density in the glans penis or clitoris, comprising 90% free and 10% encapsulated endings, is higher than in any other body tissue. Both rapid-adapting (RA) and slow-adapting (SA) free endings are represented, with encapsulated SA endings (Ruffini type) located distally and RA endings (lamellated type) located proximally, on the glans penis of the dog. Receptor sensitivity increases with erection and with temperature rise. The primary afferents synapse segmentally, onto reflex erectomotor and long-tract secondary sensory pathways in the spinothalamic tract.

Neural Control of Secretions

In the first two phases of the sexual response cycle, lubricating mucus is secreted by the bulbourethral and Littre's glands in the male, and Bartholin's glands in the female, which may be parasympathetically controlled. Increased vaginal blood flow, thought to be sympathetic and mediated by vasoactive intestinal peptide (VIP), also leads to secretion by way of an increased formation of plasma transudate (there are no glands in the vaginal wall). Secretory function in the seminal vesicles may involve noradrenaline (NA), acetylcholine (ACh), and 5-hydroxytryptamine in a poorly understood combination. Prostatic contraction is noradrenergic, while secretion there is probably cholinergic.

Erection

Normal Peripheral Mechanisms of Erection

During erection of the corpora cavernosa penis, arterial resistance falls by a large factor (so that inflow rate and then cavernosal pressure rises), and resistance to venous drainage rises. The rise in venous resistance is not merely a passive consequence of engorgement because at the onset of penile detumescence, venous outflow resistance falls greatly. The venous obstruction of the erect cavernosa enables the erect penis to withstand squeezing to above systolic pressure without subsidence. Such squeezing can be exerted, to provide extra stiffness, by the bulbocavernosus and bulbospongiosus muscles. Erection of spongy tissue, as in the glans and corpus spongiosum penis, and of the clitoris and labia minora, on the other hand, is not associated with venous obstruction, and the blood can be easily squeezed out. The neural control of the arterial and venous resistance in the penis is complicated, with several mechanisms present. Some of the evidence in animals and humans as to the nature of these mechanisms is as follows:

1. Alpha-adrenergic blockers (such as phenoxybenzamine or phentolamine) and depleters of adrenergic nerve terminals (guanethidine), like directly acting smooth-muscle relaxant drugs (papaverine, thymoxamine), will all induce intracavernosal arterial opening and venous closure, and hence full cavernosal erection, when injected intracavernosally (Virag 1982; Brindley 1983). Intracavernosal metaraminol (Brindley 1984) will quickly abolish such erections, whereas atropine has little effect on erections in humans (Stief et al. 1989), although there is evidence that VIP and ACh may be cotransmitters in erectile function in the cat and dog.
2. Strong stimulation of S2 or (occasionally) S3 ventral roots causes erection in many but not all paraplegic men and vaginal lubrication in many women. These effects are not reflex, as they occur in patients who have undergone sacral deafferentation. Electrical stimulation must be stronger than that required for a maximal contraction of skeletal muscles. This suggests that these functions are served by way of fine myelinated fibers in the parasympathetic outflow.
3. There is evidence that NO serves a role as a neurotransmitter mediating erection, among other functions, in several species (de Groat and Booth 1993).
4. Strong electrical stimulation of the hypogastric plexus in men and in experimental animals induces erection, or penile shrinkage followed by erection, as well as seminal emission. This probably indicates a sympathetic erectile pathway, although the possibility of a reflex mechanism has not been eliminated. The roots involved are T11–L2, and the shrinkage is probably due to activation of the sympathetic antierectile pathway noted in (1) above. Lesions of the superior hypogastric plexus may occur in men—for example, following para-aortic lymph node dissection. Such lesions, if complete, cause failure of seminal emission (though not loss of orgasmic sensation), but only in a minority of men do they also cause erectile failure.
5. The sympathetic and parasympathetic erectile pathways probably link in the inferior hypogastric plexus and may share some of the same postganglionic axons.
6. The dense alpha-adrenergic cavernosal innervation, which is believed to be tonically active in the detumescent penis, co-localizes there with other neurotransmitters such as VIP, neuropeptide Y, and adenosine triphosphate (ATP).
7. There is some evidence that VIP may be released from cavernosal endothelium, not neurally but in direct response to increased cavernosal blood flow (Ralevic et al. 1992).

Normal Central Mechanisms of Erection

These have been reviewed by de Groat and Booth (1993). In intact men, erection usually has both psychogenic and reflex components, which are hard to study separately in a satisfactory way, because it is difficult to avoid synergy between them. Vibration of the glans is a strong reflex stimulus to erection (and ejaculation) in both normal and spinal men. However, in normal men the response can often be prevented by painful stimuli applied elsewhere, or by mental arithmetic; so the reflex can be inhibited and may require facilitation. It is not known whether psychogenic impulses selectively facilitate the lumbar sympathetic erectile pathway, the sacral parasympathetic, or both. In the rat there is evidence for an erection-inhibitory descending pathway originating in the nucleus paragigantocellularis. The D-1 dopaminergic neurons in the medial preoptic area seem to be important in erectile facilitation in several species. Lasting loss of libido and impotence have been reported following a fairly localized lesion of the ansa lenticularis. Nocturnal erections occurring during rapid eye movement sleep are evidently brain-initiated and may use different descending pathways from waking psychogenic erection, because nocturnal erections often occur in patients with "primary constitutional impotence" (Brindley 1994). One can conclude (Figure 33.3, left) that there is a reflex center for erection in the conus medullaris, with a parasympathetic erectile outflow at the S2,3 level. There are sympathetic erectile and antierectile outflows at about the T12 level. There are descending erectile and probably antierectile pathways in the lateral columns.

Individual Variations

It is not known why there is more than one pathway for erection, but as noted below there is evidence in humans of individual variation in the relative importance of the sympathetic and parasympathetic erectile pathways. Since in normal men cavernosal alpha-blockade nearly always causes some (though not always full) erection, it may be concluded that the adrenergic antierectile pathway is constantly present and tonically active.

Erectile Disorders

Disorders of penile erection have been traditionally divided into vascular, psychological, and neurological groups (Table 33.8). Vascular disorders are outside the scope of this chapter. Brindley (1994) argued for a four-group classification, recognizing constitutional, vascular, psychological, and overtly neurological causes, based on clinical criteria. The "constitutional" group could represent an occult neurological disorder, possibly of the nitrergic system. Differentiating this group from the psychological group is discussed later. Erectile failure is not necessarily accompanied by anorgasmia or ejaculatory failure.

Erectile Function in Paraplegia

In paraplegic men with a cord level above T12 and evidence of an intact conus, there is a great variation in reflex erections. In some, they can be elicited by handling the penis, or catheterization, or spontaneously; in others they are unobtainable. Obviously, the psychogenic pathway in these patients has been interrupted, and the sympathetic erectomotor pathway may or may not (depending on the extent of the cord lesion) be damaged or disconnected from the sacral sensory signals.

Similarly, the majority of men with a SARSI show an erectile response to appropriate electrical stimulation, usually strong stimulation of the S2 roots at about 10 Hz. This is not reflex, because it works as well in patients who have been deafferented from S2 to S4 as in those who have not. However, about 30% of men with otherwise normal sacral root responses (that is, with no sign of motor root damage) have little or no erectile response (Brindley and Rushton 1990). This suggests that the sacral parasympathetic erectomotor pathway is subject to individual variation. It is not known whether this minority of men who show no response to sacral stimulation corresponds to the minority of individuals who develop impotence following a hypogastric nerve lesion. If so, it would suggest that some individuals rely on their sympathetic erectile pathway and some on the parasympathetic. Whether the sympathetic erectomotor pathway in man is constantly present is not known. In many but not all men with a complete cord or cauda equina lesion with its upper level below T12, psychogenic erections may occur, no doubt via the sympathetic outflow, reflex erections being absent.

Other Spinal Cord Lesions

Incomplete spinal cord lesions add information to the above only where the anatomy of the lesion is clear. Patients

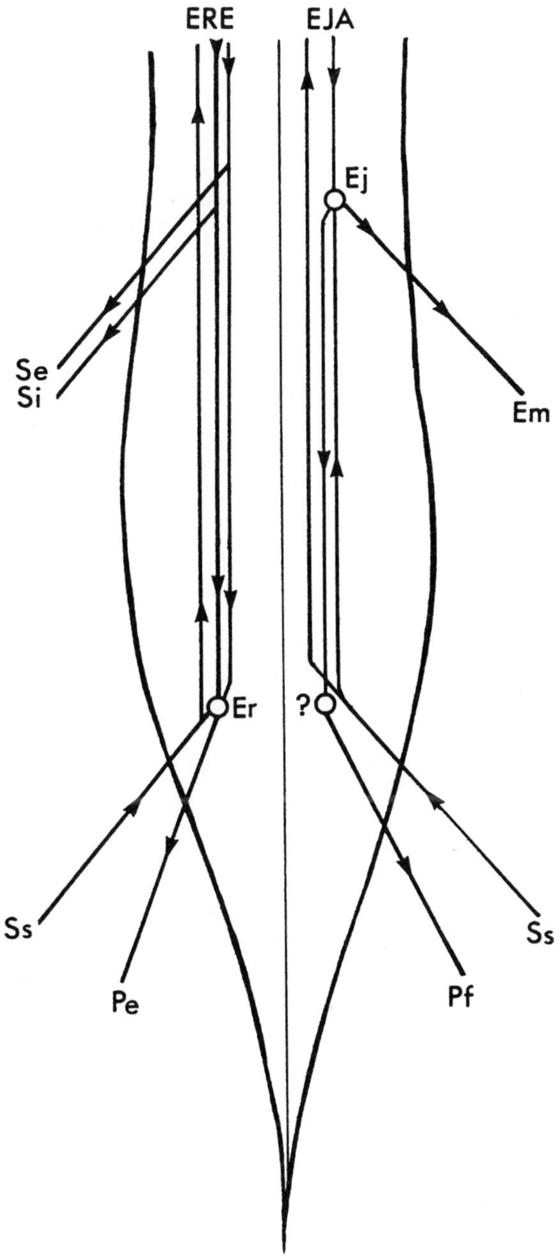

FIGURE 33.3 Probable pathways and nuclei involved in penile erection and ejaculation. Erectile pathways (ERE) are shown on the left, ejaculatory (EJA) on the right. Both are in reality bilateral. Some of the evidence for the existence and function of these pathways is noted in the text. (Left: Ss = sacral sensory pathway serving reflex erection and erotic sensation (S2–S3); Pe = parasympathetic erectile motor pathway; Se = sympathetic erectile motor pathway; Si = sympathetic erectile inhibitory pathway; Er = conus-located synapse for reflex erection. Right: Em = sympathetic nerves causing seminal emission; Ej = postulated ejaculatory center at about L1 cord level; ? = postulated generator of rhythmic pelvic floor contractions, site unknown; Ss = sacral sensory pathway whose impulses are integrated in Ej to an orgasm level.) Collaterals pass to the brain, probably in the spinothalamic tract. (Pf = pudendal nerves carrying impulses for rhythmic contractions of ejaculation.)

Table 33.8: Differential diagnosis of erectile impotence

Group Cause	*Mechanisms*
Idiopathic	Primary
	Secondary (age-related)
Psychological disturbance	Secondary
Neuropathic	Diabetes mellitus
	Alcoholism
	Amyloid neuropathy
	Vitamin B_{12} deficiency
	Tabes dorsalis
Cord lesion	Trauma, tumor, compression
	Occlusion of artery of Adamkiewicz
	Infarct, hemorrhage, angioma
	Multiple sclerosis, other myelitis
	Spina bifida
Penile arterial insufficiency	Aortic coarctation, aneurysm, dissecting aneurysm
	Aortic or internal iliac atheroma
	Pudendal artery occlusion
Cavernous fistula	Primary
	Acquired
Cavernous thrombosis	Postpriapism
	Sickle cell disease
Hormonal insufficiency	Pituitary disease
	Testicular disease
	Androgen suppression

with thoracic cordotomies aimed at bilateral section of the spinothalamic tracts may report loss of erection and ejaculation, or loss only of erotic and orgasmic sensations, with preserved ejaculation. Patients with pure posterior column lesions rarely report such changes, although the posterior columns are believed to carry impulses signaling urethral touch, stretch, and pressure.

Peripheral Nervous System Disorders and System Degenerations

Autonomic neuropathy is a common cause of erectile failure, and psychogenic and reflex erections are usually equally affected, the lesion being peripheral. Some neuropathic causes are noted in Table 33.8. Diabetes mellitus is the most common cause of symptomatic autonomic neuropathy, including neuropathic impotence. In diabetes mellitus, it has been found that there is a good correlation between a sensory neuropathy affecting unmyelinated fibers (loss of sensitivity to warmth) and erectile failure (Fowler et al. 1988). Similarly, there is a good correlation between erectile failure and other symptoms of autonomic neuropathy. Erectile failure is present in at least 50% of men with diabetes mellitus requiring oral hypoglycemic drugs or insulin treatment for 5 years or more, and it usually begins years before there is any other symptom of autonomic failure. Erectile failure may be correlated with a loss of cavernosal VIP, acetylcholinesterase, and NO formation. Similarly, erectile failure may be an early symptom of progressive autonomic system failure, whether isolated or combined with MSA.

Occult, Idiopathic, and Psychological Disorders

Secondary erectile failure in young men with no demonstrable autonomic or vascular disease, diabetes, or neurological disorder is common and has been considered to be usually psychogenic. However, this may not always be the case. Brindley (1994) has proposed criteria for diagnosing a psychological cause: for example, impotence with one partner but potency with another, or permanent cure of the impotence following psychotherapy, psychotropic drug treatment, or intracavernosal self-injection of a vasoactive drug. At the other extreme, there is a group in whom there is an identifiable organic lesion, either vascular or neurological. They can be recognized because they have no nocturnal or early-morning erections. But there is a group in between, who have nocturnal erections, but who are impotent under all other circumstances and show no evidence of a psychological cause (though they may be depressed as a result of their impotence). It may conceivably be that the central pathway for sleep erections is intact in a group of men who have a constitutional disorder of the mechanisms of sexually evoked erection and its maintenance.

Ejaculation

Normal seminal ejaculation occurs in two phases, one being a sympathetic reflex mechanism and the other a somatic reflex mechanism. Sustained contraction of the adrenergic smooth muscle of the bladder neck, prostate, seminal vesicles, and vasa deferentia propel semen into the urethra and prevent its reflux into the bladder. In some species at least, ATP, ACh, and VIP are cotransmitters with NA in these motor functions (reviewed by Hoyle et al. 1994). Involuntary (reflex) rhythmic contractions of the intrinsic striated sphincter, bulbospongiosus, pelvic floor, and ischiocavernosus muscles propel the semen to the exterior. Normally these two phases are coordinated, but either may fail in disease. The functions call for intersegmental coordination between the T12 and S3 cord segments (see Figure 33.3, right).

Ejaculation and Spinal Cord Lesions

Many men with complete or incomplete spinal cord lesions above T10 have reflex erections but fail to ejaculate during intercourse or masturbation. Probably this is because of loss of a descending facilitation. However, strong vibration of the glans often induces ejaculation in these men. The extent to which the coordinated pelvic floor contractions are preserved in paraplegia is variable. Usually they are abnormal in distribution and rhythm.

The ejaculatory reflex mechanism in the lumbosacral cord may also be facilitated by subcutaneous physostigmine (Chapelle et al. 1983). Ejaculation may then be achievable during intercourse or masturbation. Intrathecal prostigmine (a technique no longer used because it can cause dangerous hypertension) will cause a series of spontaneous seminal emissions. These observations suggest that the summating point in the ejaculatory reflex mechanism in the spinal cord involves cholinergic mechanisms. Facilitated reflex ejaculation is not obtainable if the cord lesion involves destruction of segments T12–L2, suggesting that the reflex center is at T12–L2 (Chapelle et al. 1988). If reflex ejaculation cannot be achieved (at least part of the sympathetic outflow at T12–L2 being preserved), then seminal emission can be evoked by transrectal electrical stimulation of the preganglionic sympathetic fibers in the hypogastric plexus, or by an implanted hypogastric plexus stimulator (Brindley and Hendry 1992).

In patients with spinal cord lesions below L2, reflex ejaculation is absent but emission in response to strong psychological sexual stimulation may occur. This suggests the possibility of neuronal plasticity, supersensitivity, or upregulation, because ejaculation in response to psychological stimuli alone is said to be very rare in normal men.

Retrograde Ejaculation

External ejaculatory failure may be due to complete ejaculatory failure or retrograde ejaculation. Complete failure is associated with severe sympathetic lesions, such as occur in autonomic system degenerations or pelvic surgery. Retrograde ejaculation is present if urine passed after ejaculatory failure contains semen. It is often associated with an early autonomic lesion, because of preprostatic sphincter weakness, and it may be painful. It may be an early symptom of diabetic autonomic neuropathy and may sometimes be reversed by augmenting peripheral phasic adrenergic function with an adrenergic reuptake blocker such as desipramine. Retrograde ejaculation also commonly follows bladder neck surgery or prostatectomy, when it is not amenable to drug treatment.

Anorgasmia

Anorgasmia, or delayed or altered orgasm, may be associated with spinal cord lesions, particularly affecting the equatorial regions, with sensory neuropathy, with autonomic failure, and with advanced age. The cause of these sorts of secondary anorgasmia is usually evident. Age-related changes in the duration and intensity of orgasm and the length of the refractory period have been well described. However, primary anorgasmia, defined as inability ever to achieve an orgasm in the waking state, is often found not to be associated with any other evidence of overt neurological disease.

Anorgasmia in Women

Primary anorgasmia is much more common among women than men. In women, it is believed to be due in many cases to ignorance of methods of masturbation and failure of a partner to stimulate her adequately. Most women who present with a complaint of primary anorgasmia will reach orgasm when stimulated adequately; use of a vibrator is conventional. Once the woman is familiar with the cycle of sexual excitation, the problem may be solved. However, some women do not respond to the vibrator. It is uncertain whether this is due to a powerful psychological inhibition or an occult neurological constitutional disorder; a constitutional disorder seems possible, because failure to respond orgasmically to clitoral vibration is correlated with absence of the tonic glandipudendal reflex and of vaginal vascular responses to stimulation.

The tonic glandipudendal reflex is a sustained reflex contraction of the pudendally innervated muscles, in response to vibratory or other sexual stimulation. It is lateralized to the side of the stimulus and normally occurs in both sexes. It is at least partly segmental, because it is often preserved in patients with complete suprasacral spinal cord lesions.

Anorgasmia in Men

In men, primary anorgasmia is much less common than in women, perhaps because in the past male masturbation has been more socially acceptable, and the method is more obvious. However, male primary anorgasmia in coitus may be more common in religious groups that strictly forbid male masturbation (Brindley 1994).

Anorgasmia may, however, be more of a disability in men than women, because it is a cause of infertility as well as frustration. Male primary anorgasmia may be associated with endocrine or neurological disease, but when it is not, it may often be cured using the vibrator, as in women. Failure of the vibrator is again associated with absence of the glandipudendal reflex, and a hypothetical occult neurological defect may be invoked. Men with primary anorgasmia do not necessarily have erectile impotence (Lemaire 1984).

REFERENCES

Abercrombie JF, Williams NS. Implants for Ano-Rectal Function. In GS Brindley, DN Rushton (eds), Baillières Clinical Neurology 3.3: Neuroprostheses. London: Baillière Tindall, 1995;21–34.

Andersson KE, Garcia PA, Persson K et al. Electrically-induced nerve-mediated relaxation of rabbit urethra involves nitric oxide. J Urol 1992;147:253–259.

Berger Y, Blaivas JG, DeLaRocha ER et al. Urodynamic findings in Parkinson's disease. J Urol 1987;138:836–838.

Brindley GS. Cavernosal alpha-blockade: A new technique for investigating and treating erectile impotence. Br J Psychiatry 1983;143:332–337.

Brindley GS. New treatment for priapism. Lancet 1984;2: 220–221.

Brindley GS. Impotence and Ejaculatory Failure. In DN Rushton (ed), Handbook of Neuro-Urology. New York: Marcel Dekker, 1994;329–348.

Brindley GS, Hendry WF. Hypogastric plexus stimulators. Urodinamica 1992;1:47–48.

Brindley GS, Rushton DN. Long-term follow-up of patients with sacral anterior root stimulator implants. Paraplegia 1990; 28:469–475.

Chapelle PA, Blancart F, Puech AJ, Held JP. Treatment of anejaculation in the total paraplegic by subcutaneous injection of physostigmine. Paraplegia 1983;21:30–36.

Chapelle PA, Roby-Brami A, Yakorleff A, Bussel B. Neurological correlations of ejaculation and testicular size in men with a complete spinal cord section. J Neurol Neurosurg Psychiatry 1988;51:197–202.

Deen KI, Kumar D, Williams JG et al. The prevalence of anal sphincter defects in fecal incontinence: A prospective endosonic study. Gut 1993;34:685–688.

De Groat WC, Booth AM. Neural Control of Penile Erection. In CA Maggi (ed), The Autonomic System. Vol 3. Nervous Control of the Urogenital System. London: Harwood Academic Publishers, 1993;465–522.

Fowler CJ, Ali Z, Kirby RS et al. The value of testing for unmyelinated fibre sensory neuropathy in diabetic impotence. Br J Urol 1988;61:63–67.

Fowler CJ, Kirby RS, Harrison MJG. Decelerating bursts and complex repetitive discharges in the striated muscle of the urethral sphincter associated with urinary retention in women. J Neurol Neurosurg Psychiatry 1985;48:1004–1009.

Hoyle CHV, Lincoln J, Burnstock G. Neural Control of Pelvic Organs. In DN Rushton (ed), Handbook of Neuro-Urology. New York: Marcel Dekker, 1994;1–54.

Kamm MA, Hoyle CHV, Burleigh DE et al. Hereditary internal anal sphincter myopathy causing proctalgia fugax and constipation. Gastroenterology 1991;100:805–810.

Kirby RS, Christmas TJ. Surgical Management of the Neurogenic Bladder. In DN Rushton (ed), Handbook of Neuro-Urology. New York: Marcel Dekker, 1994;369–383.

Lemaire A, Burat-Herbault M, Fourlinnie JC et al. Resultats des Investigations et du Traitement dans Bocas d'Anejaculation sans Orgasme. In J Buvel, P Jouannet (eds), L'ejaculation et Ses Perturbations Simep. Lyon: 1984;71–87.

Malone-Lee J. Lower Urinary Tract Function in Late Life. In DN Rushton (ed), Handbook of Neuro-Urology. New York: Marcel Dekker, 1994;349–368.

Masters W, Johnson VE. Human Sexual Inadequacy. London: Churchill, 1970.

McGuire FJ. The Neuropathic Urethra. In AR Munday, TP Stephenson, AJ Wein (eds), Urodynamics: Principles, Practice and Application. London: Churchill Livingstone, 1984.

Ralevic V, Lincoln J, Burnstock G. Release of Vasoactive Substances from Endothelial Cells. In US Ryan, GM Rubyani (eds), Endothelial Regulation of Vascular Tone. New York: Marcel Dekker, 1992:297–328.

Stief C, Benard F, Bosch R et al. Acetylcholine as a possible neurotransmitter in penile erection. J Urol 1989;141:1444–1448.

Swash M. Faecal Incontinence. Br Med J 1993;307:636–637.

Versi E. The significance of an open bladder neck in women. Br J Urol 1991;68:42–43.

Virag R. Intracavernous injection of papaverine for erectile failure. Lancet 1982;2:938.

SUGGESTED READING

Abrams PH, Farra DJ, Turner-Warwick R et al. The results of prostatectomy: A symptomatic and urodynamic appraisal of 152 patients. J Urol 1979;121:640–642.

Cardozo L (ed). Urogynaecology. London: Churchill Livingstone, (in press).

Cardozo L. Sex and the bladder. Br Med J 1988;296:587–588.

Galloway NT. Urethral sphincter abnormalities in Parkinsonism. Br J Urol 1983;55:691–693.

Gelber DA, Good DC, Laven LJ et al. Causes of urinary incontinence after acute hemispheric stroke. Stroke 1993;24:378–382.

Hodgkinson CP, Ayers MA, Drukker BH. Dyssynergic detrusor dysfunction in the apparently normal female. Am J Obstet Gynecol 1963;87:717–730.

Krane RJ, Siroky MB (eds). Clinical Neuro-Urology (2nd ed). Boston: Little, Brown, 1991.

Levine SB. Sexual Life: A Clinician's Guide. New York: Plenum, 1992.

Morrell MJ, Sperling MR, Stecker M et al. Sexual dysfunction in partial epilepsy: a deficit in physiologic sexual arousal. Neurology 1994;44:243–247.

Parks AG. Anorectal incontinence. Proc Royal Soc Med 1975;68:681–690.

Rushton DN (ed). Handbook of Neuro-Urology. New York: Marcel Dekker, 1994.

Torrens MJ, Morrison JFB. The Physiology of the Lower Urinary Tract. Berlin: Springer-Verlag, 1987.

Chapter 34
Arm and Neck Pain

Thomas R. Swift and Kapil D. Sethi

Pain in the arm and neck frequently brings the patient to consult with the neurologist. The varied causes necessitate a careful history, physical examination, and appropriate investigations to arrive at a correct diagnosis. In this discussion, diseases causing arm and neck pain are considered as either neurological or non-neurological.

NEUROLOGICAL CAUSES OF ARM AND NECK PAIN

This discussion of neurological conditions considers the causes from central to peripheral.

Spinal Cord Lesions

Lesions of the spinal cord usually cause what is best described as *deep segmental pain.* It differs from radicular pain in that it is not as sharp and not as well localized. It is usually not influenced by coughing, sneezing, or straining. The examination may reveal segmental atrophy in the upper limbs and tendon reflex changes appropriate to the level of the lesion. Some patients with anterior spinal artery syndrome may develop severe burning, stinging, or aching pain that is diffuse and involves all four extremities and the trunk (Beric 1993).

The lesions responsible for causing segmental pain are intramedullary tumors, arteriovenous malformations, and occasionally extramedullary tumors. Syringomyelia, though characteristically associated with segmental and dissociated anesthesia, may at times produce deep, boring, and continuous pain affecting the arm and neck. An additional type of pain in syringomyelia may be due to neuropathic arthropathy of the shoulder and sometimes of other joints (Figure 34.1). Occasionally, acute transverse myelitis may involve the cervical cord, with neck pain and subsequent rapid development of neurological deficits.

Myelography, computed tomographic (CT) scanning, and magnetic resonance imaging (MRI) usually help in identifying the nature of the intraspinal lesion responsible for causing pain (Figure 34.2).

Diseases of Cervical Nerve Roots

Herniation of Intervertebral Discs

Herniation of intervertebral discs is the most common cause of combined arm and neck pain. Anatomically, the nerve root is compressed by the prolapsed disc and further distorted by secondary changes in the cervical vertebrae and the joints. To understand the symptoms and signs, it is best to consider some anatomical facts about cervical nerve roots. The nerve roots at the cervical level exit through the intervertebral foramen above the corresponding vertebrae. The cervical and lumbar vertebrae are the most mobile parts of the vertebral column. The intervertebral discs are composed of nucleus pulposus and surrounding annulus fibrosus. The jellylike nucleus pulposus has a high water content at birth, which gradually diminishes with age. In the normal infant the water content is 90%, diminishing in old age to less than 70%. This makes the nucleus less resilient. There is also concomitant loss of cushioning and narrowing of the space between the vertebrae. The annulus fibrosus may develop clefts through which the nucleus pulposus may bulge, anteriorly, laterally, and posterolaterally. The anterior and lateral herniations are of little clinical consequence. It is the posterior and posterolateral herniations that usually cause neurological problems because of their proximity to intervertebral foramina and nerve roots. Reactive changes occur in the surrounding tissues with the formation of osteophytes. In addition, the facet joints of Luschka, which are formed between the two adjacent vertebrae, are a frequent site of degeneration and osteophyte formation. These osteophytes are immediately posterior to the cervical nerve roots and may compress them.

A carefully obtained history often reveals preceding mild trauma or prolonged abnormal posture of the head, such as painting the ceiling or twisting the neck, or a recent episode of painful locking (a "crick" in the neck). We believe the crick in the neck represents involvement of cervical nerve roots by a herniated disc, although the classical radicular symptoms are not present in the majority of patients. Herniated cervical discs are more common in men than women. Pain in the neck and shoulder occurs in a significant number of patients with cervical disc herniation at various levels and is thus of little localizing value. Pain tends to be poorly localized in this region of the body and does not clearly follow a dermatomal pattern. Pain in the arm occurs with C5, C6, or C7 disc herniations and is thus also of poor localizing value. Pain in the forearm is frequent and may be accompanied by paresthesias. Pain in the lateral forearm and hand occurs more often in C6 or C7 root lesions, while in C5 root involvement the pain does not involve the forearm. Elbow pain is more often due to C8 involvement but can occasionally be due to C7 involvement as well, whereas the pain on the dorsal aspect of the forearm is most often due to C7 involvement.

In contrast to the poor localizing value of arm and shoulder pain, paresthesias of the hands are of great localizing significance. Thumb paresthesias are most often seen with C6 root involvement. In lesions of the C7 root, the paresthesias involve the index, the middle, and rarely the ring finger. With a C8 radiculopathy, the paresthesias usually involve the third, fourth, and fifth fingers. In general, paresthesias are of more value in localization than is the pain itself.

Sensory loss is found in only about one-fourth of patients and usually conforms to the distribution of paresthesias. Muscle weakness is common. Nerve roots supplying different muscles are shown in Table 34.1. Subjective weakness is found in about one-third of patients, and objective weakness may be demonstrated in three-fourths. Examination of the tendon reflexes often reveals a diminished triceps reflex with either C7 or C8 root lesions, whereas the biceps reflex is diminished in C5 or C6 root lesions (Haerer 1992) (Table 34.2). Electromyography (EMG) and nerve conduction studies usually reveal evidence of denervation in the muscles supplied by the appropriate root when weakness, wasting, and fasciculations are present. EMG abnormalities may not be found in about one-third of the patients with clinically unequivocal radiculopathy. Abnormalities in somatosensory evoked responses may be seen more often, but they are more difficult to interpret (Leblhuber et al. 1988). Denervation potentials take 10–14 days to develop and may not be of much help in the acute phase of the illness unless disc herniation with nerve root involvement had been present in previous episodes.

X-rays may reveal straightening of the cervical spine, with loss of normal lordosis due to paraspinal muscle contraction. Oblique views of the cervical spine must be obtained. Positioning for cervical spine films must be done carefully; both the head and the body must be oblique so that the intervertebral foramina are seen. In an acute disc prolapse there may be no chronic radiological changes of spondylosis. However, both acute and chronic changes may

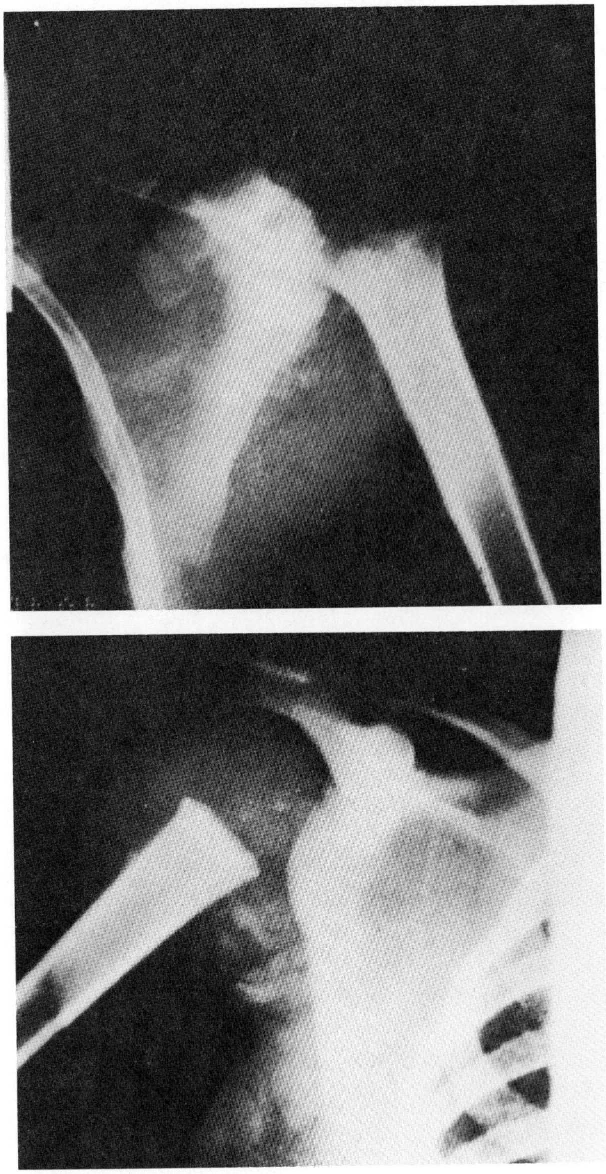

FIGURE 34.1 Shoulder x-rays. Destruction of the humeral head and irregularities of glenoid fossa in patients with syringomyelia. (Reprinted with permission from JC Sackellares, TR Swift. Shoulder enlargement as the presenting sign in syringomyelia: report of two cases and review of the literature. JAMA 1976;236: 2878–2879.)

coexist. Previously, CT scan and myelography were needed to establish the diagnosis. At present, MRI is the imaging modality of choice in the diagnosis of herniated intervertebral discs (Figure 34.3) (see Chapter 39).

In addition to compression of nerve roots by herniated intervertebral discs, cervical roots may be involved by other pathological processes. Extradural lesions, such as abscess or metastasis, may cause pain that is bilaterally symmetrical,

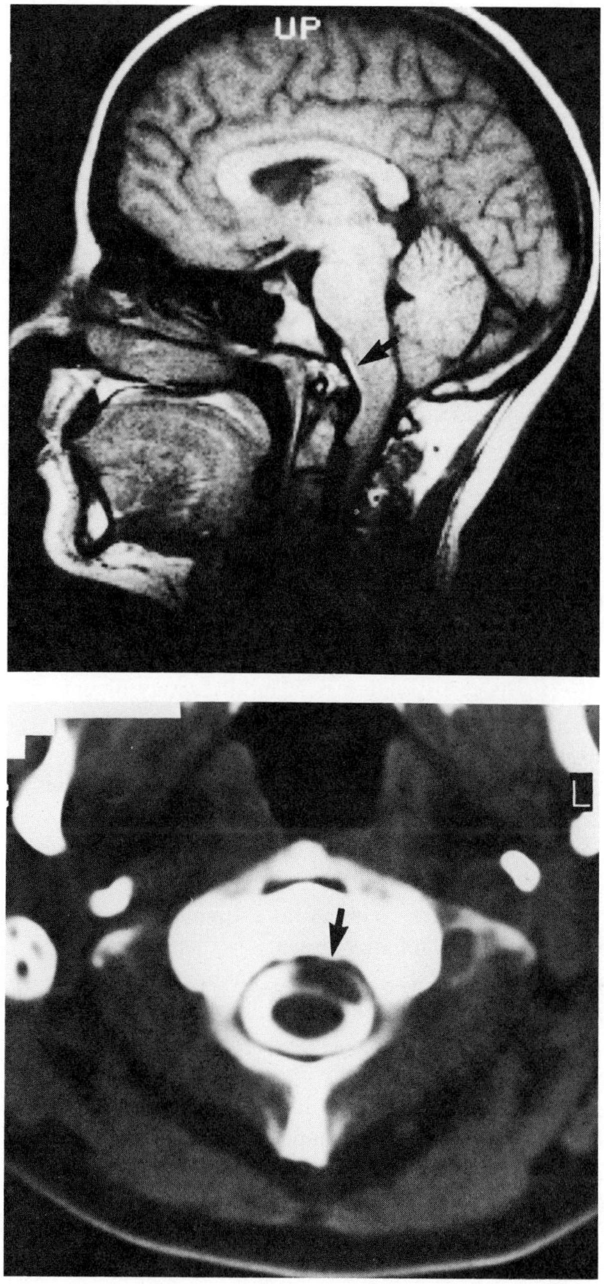

FIGURE 34.2 Magnetic resonance imaging. Extramedullary tumor, possibly epidermoid, anterior to the medullospinal junction in a patient with neck and interscapular pain.

Table 34.1: Spinal roots innervating upper-extremity muscles

Root	*Muscles Supplied*
C4	Levator scapulae
	Rhomboids
C5	Serratus anterior
	Supraspinatus
	Infraspinatus
	Deltoid
	Biceps
	Subscapularis
	Brachialis
	Brachioradialis
C6	Pectoralis major (clavicular portion)
	Deltoid
	Subscapularis
	Biceps
	Brachialis
	Brachioradialis
C7	Pectoralis major (sternal portion)
	Triceps
	Extensor carpi radialis longus
	Extensor carpi radialis brevis
	Extensor carpi ulnaris
	Extensor digitorum communis
	Abductus pollicis longus
	Extensor pollicis brevis
	Extensor pollicis longus
C8	Extensor carpi ulnaris
	Adductor pollicis longus
	Extensor pollicis brevis
	Extensor pollicis longus
	Palmaris longus
	Flexor digitorum sublimis
	Flexor digitorum profundus
	Flexor carpi ulnaris
	Flexor pollicis longus
	Abductor pollicis brevis
	Opponens pollicis
	Flexor pollicis brevis
	Interossei
T1	Flexor pollicis longus
	Abductor pollicis brevis
	Opponens pollicis
	Flexor pollicis brevis
	Hypothenar muscles
	Interossei
	Abductor pollicis

Source: Mayo Clinic. Clinical Examinations in Neurology (6th ed). St Louis: Mosby, 1991;193–220.

and these lesions may be accompanied by local tenderness to percussion and deformity of the spine. Extramedullary intradural tumors, usually schwannomas (neurofibromas), can cause root pain on one side before involving the spinal cord and causing myelopathy. A useful radiological sign of schwannoma is enlargement of the corresponding intervertebral foramen seen on oblique views. More rarely, meningiomas may cause root pain. Cervical arachnoiditis may involve nerve roots and cause intractable pain.

Nerve Root Trauma

Trauma may involve the cervical roots by stretching from subluxation of joints, by compression from protrusion of intervertebral discs, or by actual avulsion of roots from the spinal cord. A root avulsion typically occurs in injuries where shoulder and neck are separated forcibly, as frequently occurs in motorcycle accidents. In addition to the severe muscle wasting and anesthesia of the arm with a flail

Table 34.2: Distribution of signs and symptoms in nerve root lesions

Root Involved	*Distribution of Pain*	*Distribution of Paresthesias*	*Weak Muscles*	*Reflex Change*
C5	Neck, shoulder, or lateral aspect of arm	Not usual	Deltoid, supraspinatus, infraspinatus	Diminished biceps and brachioradialis
C6	Shoulder, neck, lateral aspect of forearm	Thumb, occasionally index fingers	Biceps, brachioradialis, wrist extensors	Diminished biceps and brachioradialis
C7	Back of arm, interscapular area, back of forearm	Middle finger, occasionally index and ring fingers	Triceps, wrist extensors	Diminished biceps
C8	Ulnar side of hand and distal forearm	Little and ring fingers	Intrinsic muscles of hand, long flexor of thumb, extensor of index finger	Diminished triceps
T1	Ulnar forearm	Ulnar forearm	Intrinsic muscles of hand, long flexor of thumb, extensor of index finger	No reflex change

upper limb, the root avulsion may cause chronic incapacitating pain as well; even amputation of the limb may fail to cure this pain. Nerve conduction studies may be helpful; in avulsion of a root, the dorsal root ganglia typically remain connected to their peripheral processes, and the finding of a normal digital sensory nerve action potential in a totally numb extremity is strongly suggestive of root avulsion as the cause.

Herpes Zoster

Herpes zoster is a viral infection that usually involves one cervical root, but two or more are occasionally affected. In C2 herpes zoster the pain may precede the appearance of vesicles by days, and the vesicles, when they do appear, may be few and hidden by the patient's hair or ear, necessitating careful examination.. The eruption of herpes zoster in some cases may be followed by severe pain that can be lancinating or burning (postherpetic neuralgia). This pain may last weeks to months and can be very difficult to treat.

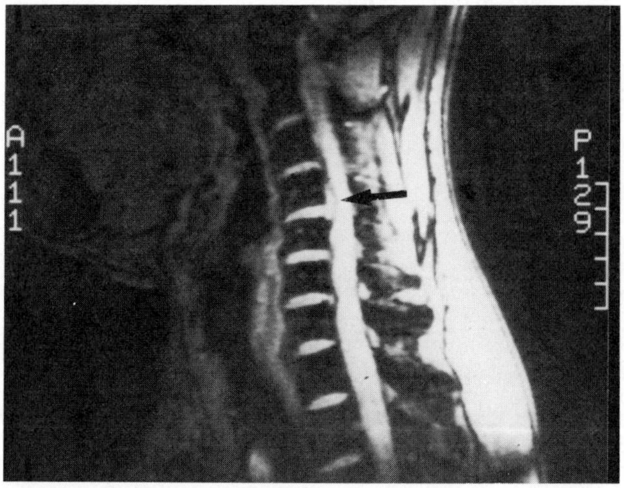

FIGURE 34.3 Magnetic resonance imaging. Intervertebral disc prolapse at C4–C5 level (arrow).

Cervical Spondylosis

Disc degeneration with secondary reactive changes in vertebral bones, formation of osteophytes, loss of disc substance, and straightening of the cervical lordosis contribute to the changes of spondylosis. The discs may or may not protrude. About 75% of people above age 65 show the typical radiological changes of cervical spondylosis. In healthy people the roots are free of adhesions, but in spondylosis the sleeves become thickened and adhesions form between the filaments. There is fibrosis of the arachnoid membrane as well. The neurological picture may consist of radicular arm and neck pain, a combination of pain and myelopathy, or progressive myelopathy alone. C7–T1 disc herniation is very rare, so that wasting of the intrinsic muscles of the hand is extremely unusual in cervical spondylosis. Examination of a patient with cervical spondylosis may reveal weakness and wasting of the upper limbs and spasticity of the lower limbs. The reflexes may be brisk in all four limbs, or one or more of the upper limb reflexes may be absent. A helpful sign pointing to the high cervical spine as the site of the lesion is the finding of a normal jaw jerk with hyperreflexia of all four limbs. Radiological examination reveals osteophyte formation with abnormalities of the articular surfaces of joints of Luschka and with projection of the osteophytes into the intervertebral foramen or the spinal canal (Figure 34.4). Myelography reveals indentation of the subarachnoid space by the protruded disc anteriorly, or by transverse osteophytic bars anteriorly and by redundant and hypertrophied ligamenta flava posteriorly.

Diseases of the Brachial Plexus

Brachial plexus lesions causing arm and neck pain can affect either the upper or lower parts of the brachial plexus or the entire plexus. The pain of a brachial plexus lesion usually involves the shoulder but may radiate down the lateral side of the arm and forearm and extend upward into the neck as well. The pain may be increased by movement but,

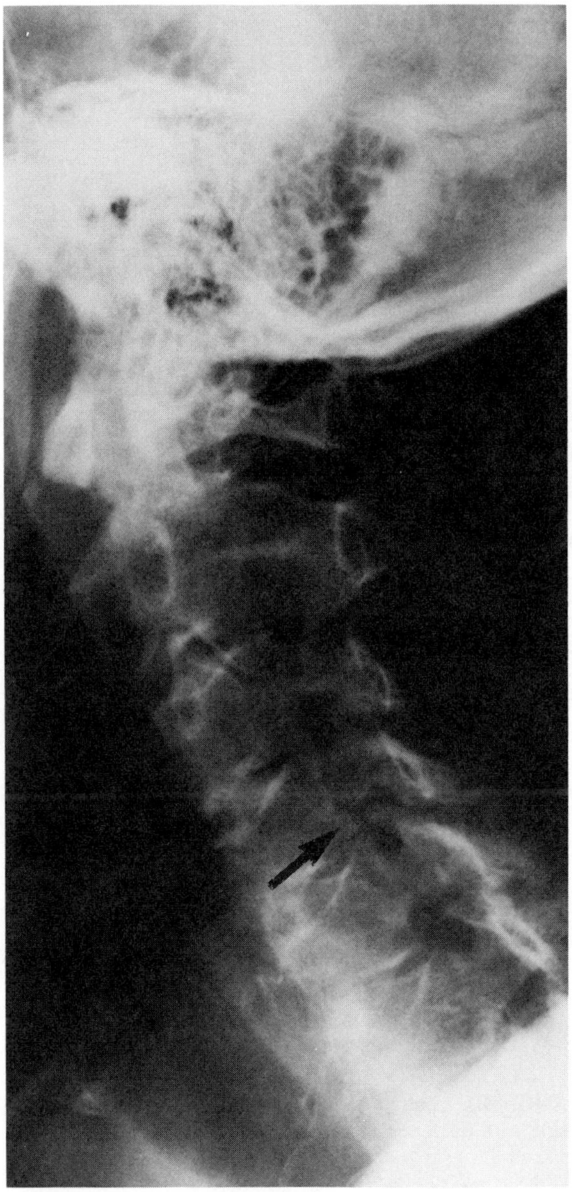

FIGURE 34.4 Oblique view of the cervical spine. Osteophytes projecting into the intervertebral foramen (arrow).

unlike root pain, is not markedly aggravated by sneezing or coughing. The distribution of muscle wasting and weakness helps to localize the lesion in the brachial plexus. Examination of the neck may reveal a mass, x-irradiation changes, or a palpable cervical rib. There are many diseases affecting the brachial plexus.

Trauma

Trauma takes many forms. Penetrating injuries may directly lacerate the plexus. Fractures, dislocations, and subluxation may cause stretch injuries to the plexus. Gunshot and missile wounds may cause widespread dysfunction, with transient block of conduction in addition to the anatomic injury. Open injuries usually involve the upper, more exposed portions of the plexus; the lower, more protected parts of the plexus are less likely to be traumatized. The most common injury, however, is due to traction, the prototype of which occurs in motorcycle accidents.

Radiation-Induced Plexopathy and Malignant Infiltration

The development of a brachial plexus lesion in a patient with a previous breast cancer and radiotherapy may suggest either malignant infiltration or radiation plexopathy. In general, the malignant infiltration is painful and involves the lower part of the plexus. Examination may reveal a mass in the neck. A malignant tumor of the apex of the lung (Pancoast's tumor) may involve the lower plexus, causing arm pain and Horner's syndrome. Radiation plexopathy can follow radiation to the plexus after a few months to several years. This may involve the entire plexus or the upper plexus alone. It is typically painless. CT or MRI of the neck and shoulder may be helpful in differentiating radiation plexopathy and malignant infiltration; electromyographically recorded myokymic discharges suggest radiation plexopathy (Harper et al. 1989). In some cases, however, surgical exploration may be required to establish the diagnosis.

Idiopathic Brachial Plexus Neuropathy (Brachial Neuritis)

Idiopathic brachial plexus neuropathy, also called brachial neuritis, neuralgic amyotrophy, and the Parsonage-Turner syndrome, has a rather abrupt onset in a previously healthy individual, although sometimes there is a history of antecedent infection, vaccination, or surgery. Men are more often affected than women; the usual age of onset is in the third to seventh decade, although no age is exempt. Pain may awaken the patient at night and can be severe. In as many as one-third of cases, the pain may be bilateral, with both sides becoming involved simultaneously or sequentially. The pain lasts anywhere from hours to several weeks and is followed by severe muscle weakness with subsequent muscle wasting, usually involving the shoulder girdle. Rarely, the wasting may be more distal. Sensory changes are less impressive. Most patients improve within months, and 80–90% recover within 2–3 years. EMG and nerve conduction studies help differentiate the plexus lesion from root lesion due to disc herniation and spondylosis (see Chapter 37B). Other differential diagnoses of brachial plexopathy include radiation-induced plexopathy and serum sickness plexitis.

Familial Brachial Plexopathy

Occasional families have been described in which there are repeated episodes of painful brachial plexopathy. Sometimes other limb nerves may be involved. Sural nerve biopsy may reveal sausagelike areas of myelin thickening (tomaculous neuropathy) (see Chapter 81).

Thoracic Outlet Syndrome

Thoracic outlet syndrome is an unfortunate term applied to a variety of conditions that are poorly understood by physicians, in part because of the hopeless confusion that exists in the literature. There are three general categories under this heading: cervical rib and band syndrome; droopy shoulder syndrome; and a variety of other structural lesions, which may be conveniently grouped together. Because of the confusion that exists, it is appropriate to discuss these entities in more detail.

Symptoms in cervical rib and band syndrome are produced by a developmental anomaly consisting of either a rib or an elongation of the transverse process of the seventh cervical vertebra. The rib curves down to articulate with the superior surface of the first true thoracic rib or, more commonly, is replaced in its distal portion by a band connected to the first thoracic rib (Figure 34.5). Most commonly this rib and band compress the lower portion of the brachial plexus. Rarely, the rib and band may compress the middle or upper portion of the plexus. Symptoms of pain, paresthesias, and numbness in the hand are usually referable to compression of the lower trunk or medial cord of the plexus, which results in wasting of intrinsic muscles of the hand and sensory loss over the last three digits. Because of the syndrome's developmental nature, the entire arm and hand frequently are smaller on the affected side (Figure 34.6). Vascular insufficiency, though frequently mentioned in the literature, is rarely apparent clinically, although angiography may show severe angulation, poststenotic dilation, or actual obstruction of the subclavian artery. Vascular symptoms in the arm rarely occur because of the rich collateral circulation. However, vertebral artery emboli have been reported in some cases.

The condition rarely is bilateral. It is important to stress that the mere presence of cervical ribs, particularly if they are small, does not imply causation of the patient's arm and neck pain since they may be a normal finding, and other causes should be sought. Various diagnostic maneuvers to demonstrate obliteration of the arterial pulse at the wrist with head turning, deep breathing and shoulder movement are of no value, being positive in up to 80% of normal subjects. Likewise, the scalenus anticus syndrome does not exist, and scalenotomy, formerly in fashion, is of no value in treatment. Somatosensory potentials and F latencies may be prolonged in the affected arm (see Chapter 37A and B). The treatment of the cervical rib and band syndrome is operative removal of the offending rib and band from above the clavicle; in no instance should the first thoracic rib be removed.

The droopy shoulder syndrome accounts for the largest group of patients with the so-called thoracic outlet syndrome. Pain occurs in the shoulder, arm, and hand, and less frequently in the neck and head. Symptoms are produced by

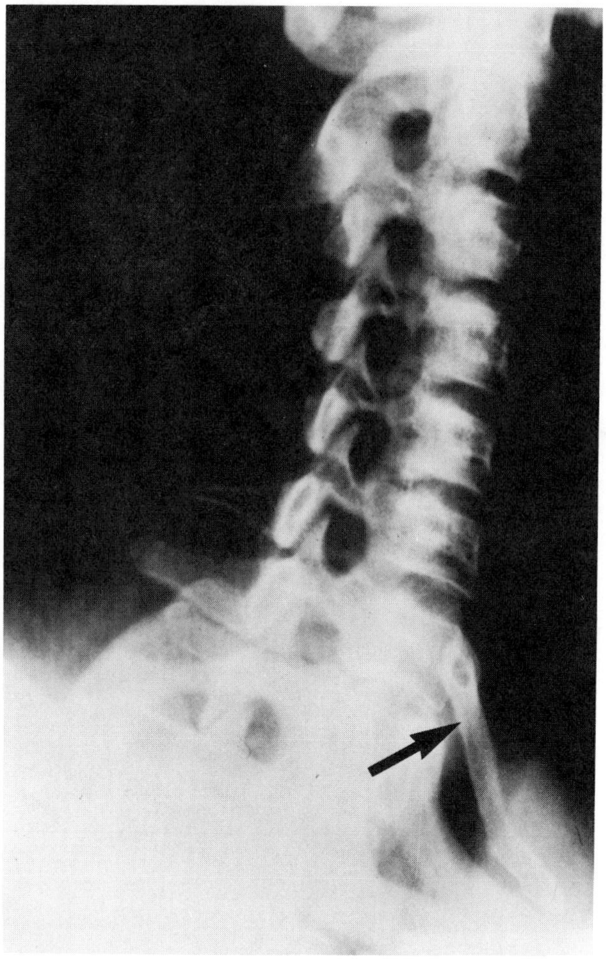

FIGURE 34.5 Lateral radiograph of the neck. Cervical rib articulating with the first true thoracic rib (arrow).

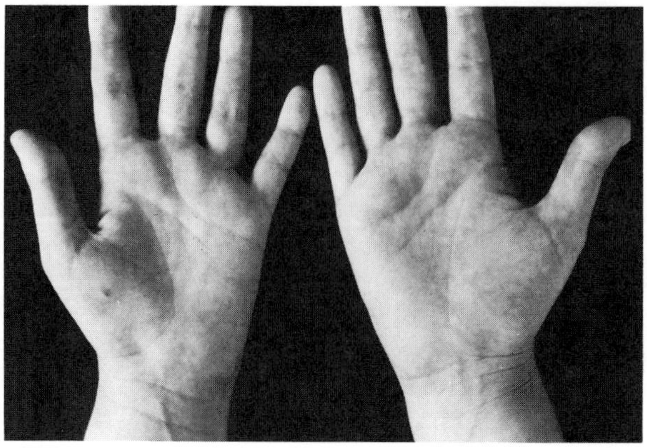

FIGURE 34.6 Wasting of the left thenar eminence muscles in a patient with a left cervical rib. Note the smaller left hand.

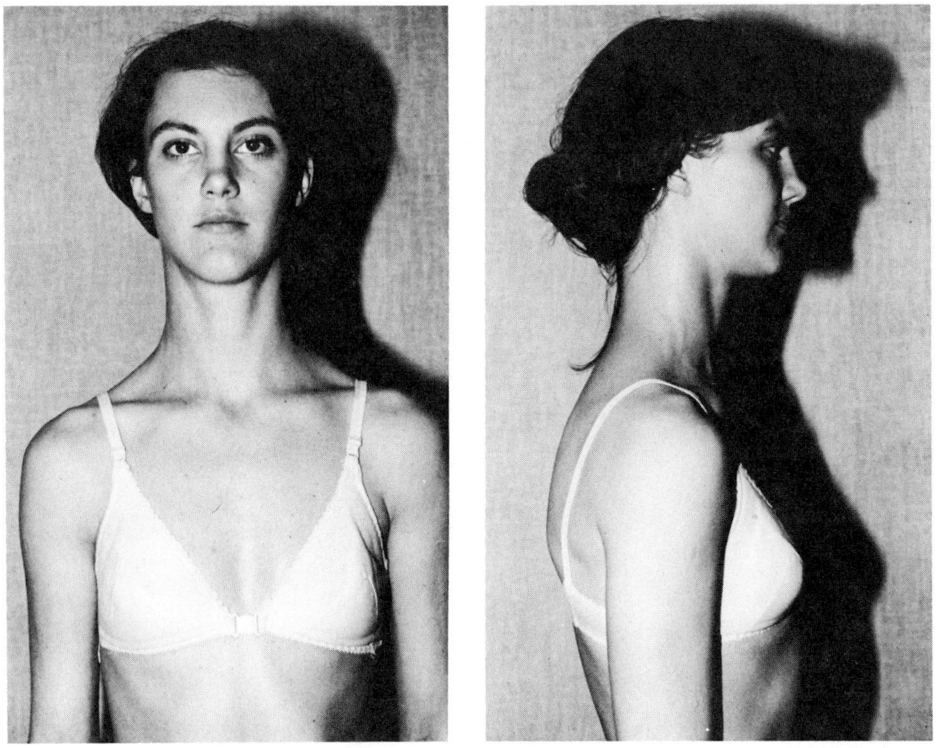

FIGURE 34.7 A patient with the droopy shoulder syndrome. Note the long neck and horizontal clavicles. The right shoulder is lower than the left.

chronic stretch of the brachial plexus occasioned by the low-hanging shoulders. Almost all of these patients are women between ages 20 and 40 who have low-hanging shoulders and long necks. Tapping over the plexus will cause paresthesias in the arm and hand and is quite uncomfortable. If the arms are forcibly pulled down, the symptoms are immediately worsened. Conversely, if the arms are pushed up, symptoms rapidly disappear. Neurological examination is normal despite the sensory symptoms, and vascular problems do not occur. Symptoms of pain and paresthesias are usually worse in the dominant arm, which is lower, even in normal subjects. On looking at the patient, one is struck by the long neck, low shoulders, and horizontal or down-sloping clavicles (Figure 34.7). Lateral cervical spine films are important because the upper two to four thoracic vertebrae can be seen, with the low shoulders out of the plane of projection. Nerve conduction studies are normal. The syndrome is treated with physical therapy to strengthen the shoulder suspension muscles. Unfortunately, many patients are subjected to removal of the first thoracic rib through a transaxillary approach. There are no controlled data to show that this operation is beneficial, and many patients are in worse condition after surgery, possibly because the shoulder hangs even lower when the first rib is removed.

A variety of other structural lesions occur about the brachial plexus and can cause symptoms referred to as the thoracic outlet syndrome. Many of these are congenital anomalies occurring in the fascia, muscles, bone, and other structures in the area, and usually are associated with abnormal physical findings about the shoulder. Muscles may appear to have anomalous insertions, a mass may be palpated above the clavicle, the shoulder on the affected side may be higher, and the arm and hand may be smaller. A common anomaly is the development of a ring of tight connective tissue about the brachial plexus, encircling the divisions or cords. Patients complain of numbness, pain, and paresthesias in hand or arm, and less commonly in the shoulder. Muscle wasting and weakness may occur. Electrophysiological studies may reveal evidence of denervation, absent sensory potentials, or delayed or absent somatosensory responses. Treatment of this diverse group of conditions must be individualized; the removal of constricting fibrous bands is often followed by disappearance of the symptoms.

Diseases of the Peripheral Nerves

Suprascapular Nerve Entrapment

Suprascapular nerve entrapment is a rare entrapment syndrome that occurs as the nerve passes through the suprascapular notch. It may be due to trauma or may be spontaneous. The primary symptom is deep, throbbing pain located at the upper border of the scapula. Flexing the shoulder increases the pain. Examination reveals wasting and weakness of the infraspinatus and, less commonly, the supraspinatus muscle. External rotation of the arm is weak. Tenderness over the scapular notch is another helpful sign.

Carpal Tunnel Syndrome

Carpal tunnel syndrome is the most common of all entrapment neuropathies. The carpal tunnel is bounded dorsally and to the sides by bones and on the flexor aspect by the thick transverse carpal ligament. Tendons, median nerve, and vessels pass through this crowded space. Any disease in this area may compress the median nerve.

Carpal tunnel syndrome is three times more common in women than in men. The usual age of onset is 40–60 years. Classically, the presenting complaint is numbness of the thumb, index, and middle fingers, and of the radial half of the ring fingers. Many patients cannot describe this well, however, and may report that all digits are involved.

Pain can extend from the hand to the forearm, the elbow, and even the shoulder. Hence, the carpal tunnel syndrome must be considered in the differential diagnosis of arm pain. The pain or paresthesias may appear after prolonged use of the hand, or the patient may be awakened from sleep during the night, as a result of sleeping with the wrists flexed or extended. Usually, rubbing or shaking the hand will relieve the pain. Early in the process there may be no neurological deficit on physical examination, but later there may be hypesthesia in the distribution of the digital branches of the median nerve. It is important to note that the palmar branch of the median nerve leaves the main trunk 3 cm proximal to the transverse carpal ligament and hence is uninvolved in the carpal tunnel syndrome. This palmar branch supplies sensation to the thenar eminence. Therefore, lack of sensory symptoms and signs on the palm help differentiate the carpal tunnel syndrome from high lesions of the median nerve. Tinel's sign is produced by gently tapping over the flexor wrist skin crease. A positive response is tingling or electric shock–like sensations extending into the median-innervated digits. It is less sensitive, but more specific, than Phalen's test, which is carried out by placing the wrist in an unforced but complete flexion. Reproduction or exacerbation of symptoms of the carpal tunnel syndrome constitutes a positive response. In normal subjects, paresthesias arise in the ring and middle digits after 30 seconds. In patients with the carpal tunnel syndrome, symptoms arise in less than 20 seconds. Less commonly, in addition to the sensory abnormalities, wasting and weakness of the thenar eminence muscles may occur. Electrophysiological testing reveals decreased amplitude and increased median sensory latencies (Chapter 37B). Comparison of median sensory conductions in both hands and comparison with ulnar sensory responses will enhance the sensitivity of electrophysiological testing for median nerve entrapment at the carpal tunnel. The motor conduction across the carpal tunnel is slowed less often, and in advanced cases electromyographic examination may reveal denervation abnormalities in the median-innervated muscles (Dawson et al. 1990).

The diseases causing the carpal tunnel syndrome include rheumatoid arthritis and other granulomatous arthritides, gouty arthritis, amyloidosis, sarcoidosis, fractures, acromegaly, hypothyroidism, mucopolysaccharidoses, and other conditions. Some cases are occupationally induced or occur during pregnancy, but most cases occur in otherwise healthy people.

Median Nerve Entrapment in the Region of the Elbow

Pronator Teres Syndrome. The median nerve below the elbow passes beneath the thick fascial band between the biceps and the forearm fascia, and then between the heads of the pronator teres muscle. It can be compressed at either of these two sites. The symptoms usually begin insidiously or after prolonged use of the arm. The pain may radiate into the hand or shoulder. Numbness is ill defined and is not changed by wrist position. Tenderness may be found in the proximal arm. There may be weakness of flexor pollicis longus and abductor pollicis brevis muscles. Sensory findings are usually poorly defined but include the palm. Nerve conduction and EMG studies help localize the point of compression.

Anterior Interosseous Nerve Syndrome. Anterior interosseous nerve syndrome involves the last major branch of the median nerve in the forearm. The compression causes pain in the elbow and proximal forearm. Examination is striking, particularly because of absence of flexion of the distal interphalangeal joint of the thumb and index fingers, due to the weakness of the flexor pollicis longus and flexor digitorum profundus muscles, respectively. The patient is therefore unable to form the letter O with the thumb and index fingers. There may be paralysis of the pronator quadratus muscle, which may be tested after completely flexing the elbow; this helps diminish the contribution of the pronator teres muscle to pronation. EMG is very helpful in confirming this condition.

Ulnar Nerve Entrapment at the Elbow. Ulnar nerve entrapment at the elbow is the second most common upper-extremity compression neuropathy. Most patients initially have intermittent numbness in the ulnar nerve distribution that is aggravated by elbow movement. The ulnar nerve may be involved just proximal to the epicondylar notch at the elbow or just distal (cubital tunnel syndrome). Light tapping of the skin over the nerve usually reveals the location of the lesion. Pain around the elbow or in the ulnar nerve distribution may occur. Examination may reveal hypesthesia of the palmar aspect of the fifth and ulnar half of the fourth digits. There may be diminution of sensation on the dorsum of the hand and the fourth and fifth digits due to involvement in the distribution of the dorsal branch of the ulnar nerve. There may be wasting and weakness of the adductor pollicis, interosseous, and hypothenar muscles. Clawing of the fourth and fifth digits may be found as a result of weakness of the third and fourth lumbricals. Nerve conduction studies may show conduction delay at the elbow, and EMG examination will show denervation changes in the forearm and hand muscles supplied by the ulnar nerve. At times only the hand muscles will show changes.

Ulnar Nerve Entrapment at the Wrist. The most common wrist lesion of the ulnar nerve is compression of the deep palmar branch. It is usually painless and does not cause sensory loss. Occasionally, wrist pain with radiation into the digits may be a complaint. Electrophysiological testing helps in the localization of the lesion. The flexor carpi ulnaris muscle is spared with compression at the wrist, and the dorsal digital sensation is normal as the dorsal sensory branch leaves the ulnar nerve before it reaches the wrist. Other intrinsic hand muscles supplied by the ulnar nerve are affected. If the lesion is distal to branches to the hypothenar muscles, these will be spared. Motor latency from the wrist to the first dorsal interosseous muscle is prolonged in the affected hand.

Radial Nerve Entrapment. In high axillary lesions of the radial nerve, the triceps and brachioradialis muscles may be involved. Pain may occur in the area, and tenderness and Tinel's sign may be elicited in the area of nerve damage. The muscles involved are usually the extensors of the forearm, with a prominent wrist drop. In addition, however, the patient may have difficulty making a strong grip, which is due to difficulty in fixing the position of the wrist.

Posterior Interosseous Nerve Compression. Two types of compression syndromes can occur as the nerve passes under the arcade of Frohse in the supinator muscle. The motor syndrome consists of weakness and wasting of the extensor muscles of the forearm. The other syndrome is the resistant tennis elbow. Signs and symptoms are similar to those of lateral epicondylitis. The primary symptom is lateral arm pain. The pain is generally a dull ache, located deep in the extensor muscle area, which may radiate proximally and distally. Nighttime pain may occur. Tenderness may be elicited over the posterior interosseous nerve; this tenderness is maximal distal to the radial head. Pain is increased on resisted active supination of the forearm. The extension of the elbow, wrist, and middle fingers under resistance increases the lateral elbow pain. This painful syndrome can occur after manual labor and also may be seen in typists.

Painful Polyneuropathies. Some neuropathies can be very painful, and the pain may affect the rest of the body, especially the lower extremities. These include alcoholic neuropathy, some other toxic neuropathies, and erythema nodosum leprosum reaction and nerve abscess in leprous neuritis.

Causalgia, Reflex Sympathetic Dystrophy, and Sympathetically Mediated Pain. Causalgia, reflex sympathetic dystrophy, and sympathetically mediated pain are a complex group of disorders that cause spontaneous and stimulus-induced pain and vasomotor, sudomotor, or skeletomotor dysfunction (Dotson 1993). They may follow partial injury to peripheral nerve trunks. In the upper extremity it is usually found in the distribution of the median nerve and is associated with hyperalgesia and hyperesthesia. In advanced cases there may be trophic changes in skin and subcutaneous tissues. The usual causes are trauma, surgery, occlusive vascular disease, and other vascular disorders.

NON-NEUROLOGICAL CAUSES OF ARM AND NECK PAIN

Neck Pain

Diseases of the Cervical Spine

Rheumatoid Arthritis. Rheumatoid arthritis usually involves the atlantoaxial articulation. Disease at this joint can cause pain and stiffness and, with them, destruction of the ligament restraining the odontoid. Craniocervical dislocations may occur, which can compress the spinal cord in the high cervical region and cause quadriparesis. Evidence of rheumatoid arthritis in the joints of the extremities and a positive rheumatoid factor will help in the diagnosis of this illness. Spine films should be obtained with careful flexion and extension views to look for excessive separation of the odontoid from the atlas.

Ankylosing Spondylitis. Ankylosing spondylitis rarely involves the cervical spine but usually involves the lumbar and lower thoracic region. Plain films may show ankylosis of the spine. The presence of HLA B–27 will help support the diagnosis.

Osteomyelitis. Osteomyelitis of the cervical vertebrae can cause severe local pain and tenderness. The pain may radiate to the shoulder area as well. The presence of fever, leukocytosis, and positive gallium bone scan and the use of cervical spine x-rays, CT, and MRI will help make the diagnosis.

Diseases of the Muscles and Soft Tissues

Whiplash Injury. Whiplash injury is a common problem faced by clinicians. It typically occurs in rear-end automobile collisions in which the victim is seated in a stationary vehicle that is struck from the rear by another vehicle. The patient complains of pain and stiffness in the neck and tenderness of the neck and shoulder girdle muscles. The pain may radiate into the upper anterior chest or the upper limbs. Neurological abnormalities are rare. Cervical spine x-rays may be normal except for a straightening of the spine from muscle contraction, or may show preexisting spondylosis. The mechanism of injury seems to be the stretching and tears of muscles and ligaments, and intertissue hemorrhages, with resulting secondary inflammation. The integrity of uncovertebral joints may be violated, and secondary degenerative changes may appear. There are often strong psychological concomitants, and litigation frequently is involved. EMG studies are normal, but preexisting spondylosis may complicate the situation.

Meningeal Irritation. All types of meningitis and subarachnoid hemorrhage may cause pain and stiffness of the muscles in the neck. The pain is worsened by flexion of the neck, and rotation may be painless. The presence of fever, headache, and other signs of meningeal irritation, such as the Kernig's and Brudzinski's signs, are helpful in establishing the diagnosis.

Miscellaneous Conditions

Carotid Artery Dissection. Spontaneous or trauma-induced dissection can occur in children, adolescents, and adults. Typically, the pain of carotid artery dissection involves the neck, the ipsilateral head, and the periorbital area. Arteriography and associated neurological deficits may be helpful in diagnosing this entity. MRI is very useful in defining the extent of the dissecting aneurysm.

Carotidynia. Carotidynia is not one entity but may be produced by a variety of pathological processes. Patients may have pain in the neck, face, ear, jaw, or teeth. There is tenderness over the common carotid artery at its bifurcation, with some swelling of the overlying tissues. Rarely, carotidynia may occur in giant cell arteritis or cluster headache. Displacement of the carotid artery by a tumor may produce the same syndrome.

Glomus Jugulare Tumor. Glomus jugulare tumor occurs in the region of the jugular foramen and may extend into the neck. In addition to the neck pain, there may be evidence of ninth, tenth, and eleventh cranial nerve palsies.

Retropharyngeal Space Infections. Retropharyngeal space infections occur predominantly in children and occasionally in adults. The inflammation in adults may not be as acute. There is a low-grade fever and pain in the neck aggravated by movement. Lateral spine x-rays with careful measuring of soft-tissue shadows behind the pharynx and subsequent investigations such as CT and needle aspiration will help in the diagnosis.

Tension Headache. Usually the tension headache patient complains of pain in the back of the neck that radiates into the vertex and as far forward as the forehead. The pain is usually a dull ache, which may occasionally be severe. Tension headache tends to last longer than the classical vascular headaches and is usually relieved by analgesics. It does not interfere with the patient's sleep or wake the patient from sleep during the middle of the night.

Arm Pain

Skin and Subcutaneous Tissue Diseases

In skin and subcutaneous tissue diseases, pain is usually superficial but may occasionally extend into the adjacent skin or joint. It is well localized and is associated with tenderness and usually with visible changes in the skin.

Cellulitis, erythema nodosum associated with sarcoid, tuberculosis, and rheumatoid arthritis may cause pain and visible skin changes. Thrombophlebitis will cause arm pain and tenderness, with visible inflammation of the superficial veins.

Musculoskeletal Diseases

The various synovial bursae may be inflamed as a result of trauma, rheumatoid arthritis, gout, or bacterial infection. The inflammation of the subdeltoid and subacromial bursae may cause severe local pain and tenderness, with marked decrease in the activity and mobility of the involved joints. In longstanding cases the pain may diminish and fibrotic changes may occur. In addition, even passive movements may be diminished. Subdeltoid bursitis involves the supraspinatus tendon as well. Pain may be felt in the shoulder and is sometimes more intense in the arms. Abduction and internal rotation aggravate the pain. Night pain may occur. The mobility of the shoulder joint is limited initially by pain and subsequently by lesions of the capsule, leading to decreased passive range of motion. This is a common cause of frozen shoulder. Occasionally, it can occur after hemiplegia with immobility. Immobility due to other causes of shoulder pain, such as disc disease, will cause problems in making the differential diagnosis between this disease and frozen shoulder.

Painful Diseases of the Muscles

Localized tenderness and swelling may follow local trauma or severe unaccustomed exercise. Polymyalgia rheumatica, which occurs in elderly people, presents with malaise and aching pain in the proximal muscles of the lower extremity and the shoulders. There is usually a marked elevation of sedimentation rate.

Pyomyositis is a rare condition characterized by the sudden appearance of single or multiple muscle abscesses caused by *Staphylococcus* in otherwise healthy individuals in the tropics or in AIDS patients. Polymyositis may cause proximal limb pain and mild tenderness.

Painful arthritis of the arm and hand can be due to infectious, degenerative, posttraumatic, metabolic (for instance, gout), or autoimmune (such as rheumatoid arthritis) causes. Acute swelling, redness, pain, and tenderness usually suggest infectious or inflammatory causes. Appropriate radiological investigations and joint aspiration will help establish the diagnosis.

Hypertrophic osteoarthropathy and clubbing occur predominantly with a malignancy in the thorax but can occur as a result of chronic pulmonary infections as well. The characteristic changes in the terminal fingers and a positive chest x-ray will help in the diagnosis.

Osteomyelitis can cause acute arm pain associated with fever and leukocytosis. This may follow surgery, discograms, or systemic bacteremia. Bone scan and x-rays may be helpful in establishing the diagnosis.

Fibromyalgia

A condition referred to as fibromyalgia (also called fibrositis, myofacial pain syndrome) consists of widespread pain, tender points, morning stiffness, sleep disturbance, and other symptoms (see Chapter 78). Criteria have been developed for diagnosis, but the authors themselves admit to an absence of "hard" findings, and often concomitant painful diseases such as arthritis are present (Wolfe et al. 1990). Arm and neck pain could conceivably be part of the syndrome. Axial pain and tender points are invariably present. It is unlikely that fibromyalgia exists as a discrete disease entity.

Diseases of the Blood Vessels

Acute Arterial Occlusion. Arteriosclerosis rarely extends beyond the subclavian arteries in the upper extremity. However, acute arterial occlusion may result from cardiogenic emboli, resulting in severe acute pain and ischemic changes. Chronic arterial occlusions may occur in thromboangiitis obliterans. Rarely, the subclavian steal syndrome, which is due to stenosis of the subclavian artery proximal to the origin of the vertebral artery, may cause arm pain on exercise accompanied by symptoms of vertebrobasilar insufficiency, such as dizziness, visual disturbances, and loss of balance.

Painful Vasospastic Conditions. Raynaud's disease is a benign symmetrical disease of unknown cause. It usually affects women in their early teens or twenties. Cold and emotional strain may precipitate the attacks. The fingers of both hands may blanch on exposure to cold, followed by cyanosis. During recovery, hyperemia occurs. Paresthesias may occur during the white and blue stages, and throbbing pain may accompany the phase of reactive hyperemia.

Raynaud's phenomenon is usually secondary to underlying disease. Onset may occur at any age, and female predominance is not seen. The condition may be symmetrical and associated with excessive use of the hands, as in pneumatic drill users. It also may be secondary to a collagen-vascular disease, rheumatoid arthritis, paraproteinemia, and occasionally trauma.

Miscellaneous Causes of Arm Pain

Glomus Tumor. Glomus tumor is a highly vascular lesion usually found under the nail and can cause severe pain.

Ischemic Heart Disease. Angina pectoris may present with crushing substernal pain radiating to the left and, rarely, to the right arm and neck. The pain is usually precipitated by exercise and emotional excitement. In myocardial infarction, similar pain may be longer lasting and may be accompanied by sweating and vomiting. Electrocardiogram, serum enzyme changes, and exercise stress testing where indicated are helpful in diagnosing arm pain due to ischemic heart disease.

Dressler's Syndrome. Dressler's syndrome follows myocardial infarction and is characterized by fever and pleural chest pain. It is thought to be due to an autoimmune pericarditis, pleuritis, and pneumonitis. The pain is usually substernal but may radiate into the neck and the shoulder region as well. It is relieved by leaning forward and by deep breathing. It responds to corticosteroids and indomethacin.

Shoulder-Hand Syndrome. In the shoulder-hand syndrome, pain and stiffness of the left arm and shoulder may occur. In contrast to Dressler's syndrome this is possibly related to immobility.

Metastasis. Metastasis to the upper-extremity bones may occur from primary malignancies of the breast, lung, thyroid, kidney, or gastrointestinal tract. It may be multiple in Hodgkin's disease. Bone scan and plain x-rays will help establish the diagnosis.

Lateral Epicondylitis (Tennis Elbow). The extensor tendons of the forearm take a common origin from the back of the lateral epicondyle of the humerus. Excessive use of the arm in sports and manual labor can cause lateral epicondylitis. Although it has been called tennis elbow, its victims are not limited to tennis players. The pain is located in the lateral part of the elbow and radiates into the forearm. Extension of the wrist aggravates the pain, and tenderness is found behind the lateral epicondyle. Elbow x-rays are usually normal.

De Quervain's Disease. De Quervain's disease is due to tenosynovitis of the abductor pollicis brevis and extensor pollicis brevis muscles. Typically, ulnar deviation of the hand with the thumb flexed into the palm reproduces the pain (Finkelstein's test).

REFERENCES

Beric A. Central pain: "new" syndromes and their evaluation. Muscle Nerve 1993;16:1017–1024.

Dawson DM, Hallet M, Millenda LH. Entrapment Neuropathies (2nd ed). Boston: Little, Brown, 1990;25–92.

Dotson RM. Causalgia-reflex sympathetic dystrophy-sympathetically maintained pain. Myth and reality. Muscle Nerve 1993;16:1049–1055.

Haerer AF. The Neurologic Examination (5th ed). Philadelphia: Lippincott, 1992;343.

Harper CM, Thomas JE, Cascino TL et al. Distinction between neoplastic and radiation-induced plexopathy with emphasis on the role of EMG. Neurology 1989;39:502–506.

Leblhuber F, Reisecker F, Boehm-Jurkovic H et al. Diagnostic value of different electrophysiologic tests in cervical disk prolapse. Neurology 1988;38:1879–1881.

Mayo Clinic. Clinical Examinations in Neurology (6th ed). St. Louis: Mosby, 1991;193–220.

Sackellares JC, Swift TR. Shoulder enlargement as the presenting sign in syringomyelia: report of two cases and review of the literature. JAMA 1976;236:2878–2879.

Wolfe F, Smyth HA, Yunns MB et al. The American College of Rheumatology 1990. Criteria for the classification of fibromyalgia. Report of the Multicenter Criteria Committee. Arthritis Rheum 1990;33:160–172.

Chapter 35
Low Back and Lower-Limb Pain

Walter G. Bradley

Low back pain is the most common specific complaint leading to consultation with primary-care physicians. About 70% of all adults have an episode of low back pain at some time during their life, and 40% have an episode of sciatica (pain radiating from the back or buttocks into the lower limb) (Frymoyer 1988; Hardy 1993). Five percent of the population suffers an acute attack of low back pain in any one year. In the United States about 200 million person-days of work are lost and 200,000 surgical procedures are performed each year for this syndrome. It ranks sixth in the diagnoses responsible for the greatest use of hospital bed-days annually. At any one time, about 5 million Americans are completely disabled by low back pain and another 11 million are partially disabled. The social, economic, and medical costs of low back pain in the United States may be as much as $30 billion per year.

The most frequently diagnosed causes of low back and lower-limb pain are musculoskeletal conditions, although the differential diagnosis is extensive (Table 35.1). Despite full investigations, it is frequently difficult to arrive at a firm diagnosis, and many patients are left with a diagnosis of "idiopathic low back pain." Investigations used to help achieve a diagnosis, such as magnetic resonance imaging (MRI) are costly. It is thus important in planning investigations to consider cost-effectiveness and risk-benefit factors. There are many clues in the history that can point to the possible diagnosis. Grasping the significance of these clues allows the neurologist to search during the examination for evidence to confirm or refute a given hypothesis for the cause of the symptoms. Evidence of psychogenic or compensation features, or both, may call into question the organic nature of the disorder. After completion of a careful interactive history and examination, the neurologist should be able to plan a logical series of investigations based on the differential diagnosis. These may demonstrate the cause of the condition, or may all be normal. After coming to a diagnosis, the neurologist should be able to discuss this diagnosis and its prognosis with the patient and plan the treatment.

Most of the conditions mentioned in this chapter are fully described in the chapters dealing with diseases of the spine (Chapter 78), peripheral nerves, nerve roots, and plexuses (Chapters 80 and 81).

ANATOMICAL CONSIDERATIONS

A knowledge of the nerve roots innervating individual muscles (Figure 35.1), those subserving the tendon reflexes (Table 35.2), and those innervating individual dermatomes (see Figure 28.2), and of the anatomy of the lumbosacral plexus (Figure 35.2) is essential to interpret the abnormalities found in the neurological examination.

The low back region comprises the whole of the lumbar, sacral, and coccygeal segments of the spine. Pain from this region can arise from the vertebral bodies, intervertebral synovial joints, discs, ligaments, and joint capsules. The cauda equina comprises all of the lumbar, sacral, and coccygeal nerve roots, which lie within the subarachnoid space, where they can be exposed to any infectious, inflammatory, neoplastic, or compressive process. Each nerve root exits through its intervertebral foramen, where it lies adjacent to the intervertebral disc, the synovial joints, and the ligaments. Any process that narrows the spinal canal, such as congenital or acquired spinal stenosis or an intraspinal space-occupying lesion, may cause low back and lower-limb pain and nerve root damage. The conus medullaris ends at the lower border of the first lumbar vertebra, and therefore a lesion of the spine at or above the L1 can cause upper motor neuron dysfunction in the sacral levels. This may produce an extensor plantar response and a spastic bladder, combined with lower motor neuron signs in the lumbar myotomes, such as wasting

Table 35.1: Causes of low back and lower-limb pain, arranged by anatomical origin

- Spine
  - Intervertebral disc disease
    - Herniated disc
    - Discitis
  - Bone disease
    - Paget's disease
    - Neoplasm
    - Infections (such as osteomyelitis)
    - Fracture
  - Joint disease
    - Osteoarthritis
    - Rheumatoid or ankylosing spondylitis
    - Spondylolisthesis
    - Spondylolysis
    - Spinal stenosis
      - Congenital
      - Acquired
- Epidural space
  - Abscess
  - Hematoma
  - Metastasis
- Nerve roots and cauda equina
  - Tumor
  - Perineurial cyst
  - Inflammation
  - Diabetes mellitus
  - Chronic meningitis or arachnoiditis
- Lumbosacral plexus
  - Compression (hematoma, neoplasm, enlarged uterus, aneurysm)
  - Diabetes mellitus
  - Lumbosacral inflammatory plexopathy
- Nerve
  - Entrapment
  - Mononeuropathy
  - Polyneuropathy e.g., Guillain-Barré syndrome
  - Reflex sympathetic dystrophy or causalgia
- Muscle or connective tissue
  - Fibromyalgia (fibrositis)
  - Myositis
- Referred pain
  - Pelvic organs
- Leg
  - Bone disease
    - Infection
    - Tumor
    - Fracture
  - Joint disease
    - Osteoarthritis
    - Trauma
  - Venous disease
    - Arterial insufficiency
- Psychogenic
- Malingering

and paralysis of the quadriceps and anterior tibialis muscles, as well as loss of reflexes at the knee and ankle.

After exiting from the intervertebral foramina, the spinal nerves interconnect to form the lumbosacral plexus. For simplicity, the lumbosacral plexus can be divided into two parts: the upper lumbar plexus, which gives rise to the femoral, iliohypogastric, ilioinguinal, lateral femoral cutaneous, genitofemoral, and obturator nerves, all of which exit anterolaterally from the pelvis; and the lower lumbosacral plexus, which gives rise to the sciatic, gluteal, pudendal, and posterior cutaneous nerves of the thigh, all of which exit posteriorly from the pelvis. This division is clinically important because conditions that damage the upper lumbar plexus and upper lumbar roots tend to cause anterior thigh and leg pain, whereas those of the lower lumbosacral plexus and lower lumbar and sacral roots cause buttock, posterior thigh, and leg pain. In addition, the differential diagnostic possibilities for lumbar and lumbosacral plexus lesions are somewhat different (Chad and Bradley 1987; see Chapter 80).

Table 35.2: Nerve roots involved in reflexes of the lower limbs

Cremasteric reflex	T12
Knee jerk	L2, L3, L4
Adductor reflex	L3, L4
Medial hamstring reflex	L4, L5
Ankle reflex	L5, S1

The femoral, sciatic, and obturator nerves innervate the muscles and convey superficial sensation in the lower limbs, while the pudendal nerves innervate the anal and urethral sphincters that are responsible for continence. Compromise of any of these nerves may cause pain and a characteristic sensorimotor deficit. Many of the nerves exiting from the pelvis do so through anatomically tight canals, where nerve entrapment can lead to pain (Stewart 1987; see Chapter 81). However, pain in the back and lower limbs can also arise from diseases of many other structures in the back and legs, such as the bones, joints, muscles, and connective tissue, as well as the arteries and veins. All have characteristic features in the history and physical examination that help in achieving a diagnosis.

HISTORY

It is important to allow patients to use their own words in presenting their history, but this process should be interactive. Ideally, in the end the physician should have as clear a picture of the development and character of the symptoms as if the physician had experienced them personally. This can be illustrated in terms of the pain (Table 35.3).

EXAMINATION

After completing the history, the physician should have a clear idea of the likely origin of the pain and its anatomical distribution. The examination is aimed at investigating the parts of the low back and the lower limbs for the origin of the pain, with particular reference to such regions as indicated by the

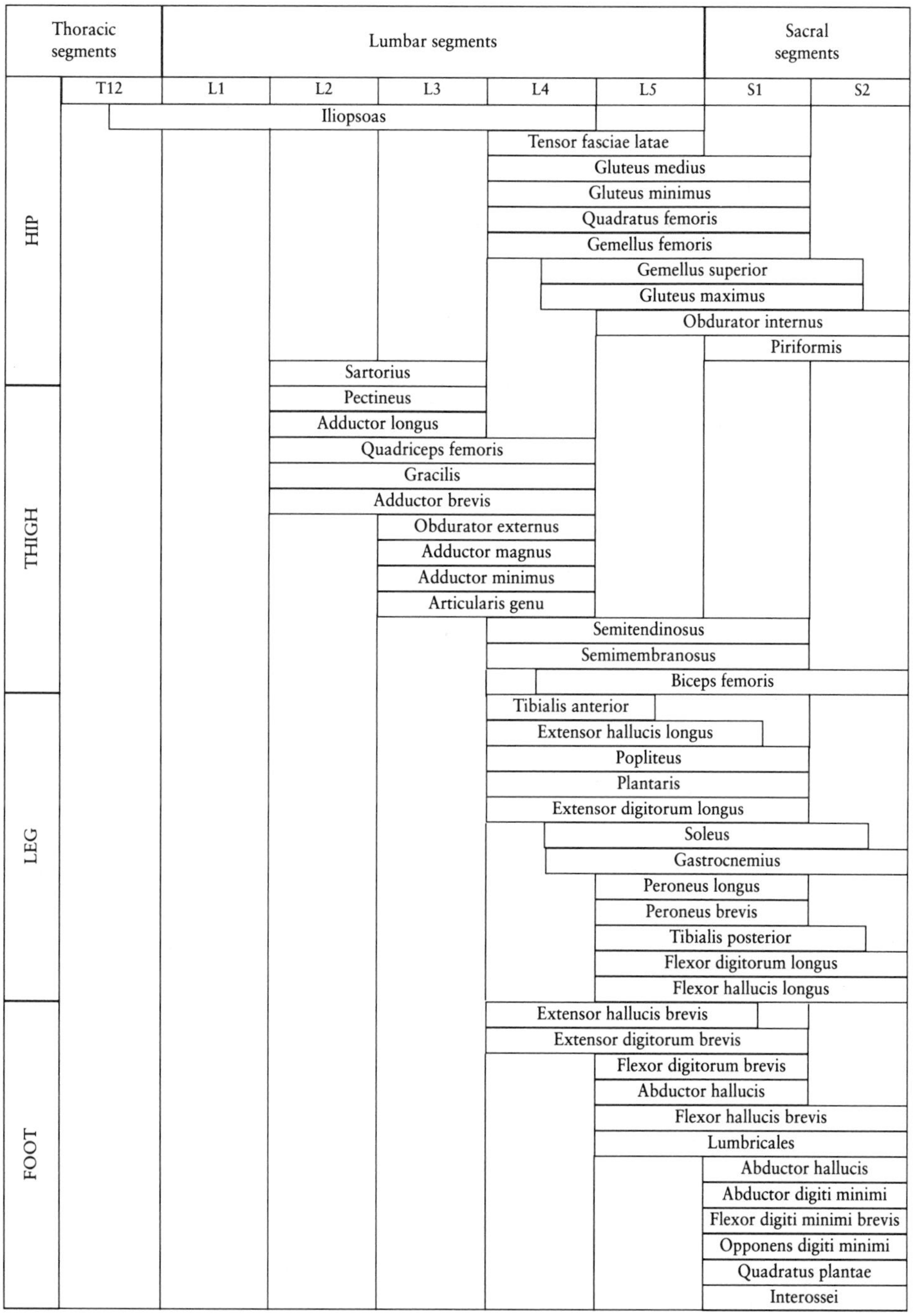

FIGURE 35.1 Segmental innervation of the muscles of the lower extremity. (Reprinted with permission from WR Brain, JN Walton. Diseases of the Nervous System. London: Oxford University Press, 1969;34–36.)

history. For instance, if the history suggests a lumbar disc syndrome with pain radiating down the back of the leg to the ankle, then it is important that straight leg raising, the ankle jerk, the power of dorsiflexion of the hallux, and sensation on the foot be carefully examined. If the history suggests a spinal metastasis, then search for spinal tenderness to percussion and the primary source of the tumor are required.

It is important that the examination be complete and that it look for abnormalities of all the relevant systems (Table 35.4). The examination should concentrate on the parts of the body that the history indicates might be abnormal.

The patient should be examined while standing, walking, and lying on the couch. Abnormalities of gait include a limp, foot drop, and difficulty in rising on the toes or in walking on the heels. Alterations of the normal lumbar lordosis and the presence of scoliosis should be sought. Paravertebral muscle spasm is common wherever there is back pain, irrespective of the cause.

The posture of the pelvis when standing and walking may indicate joint or muscle problems. A patient with degenerative arthritis of one hip will tend to dip the pelvis on that side while standing and walking, as a result of pain

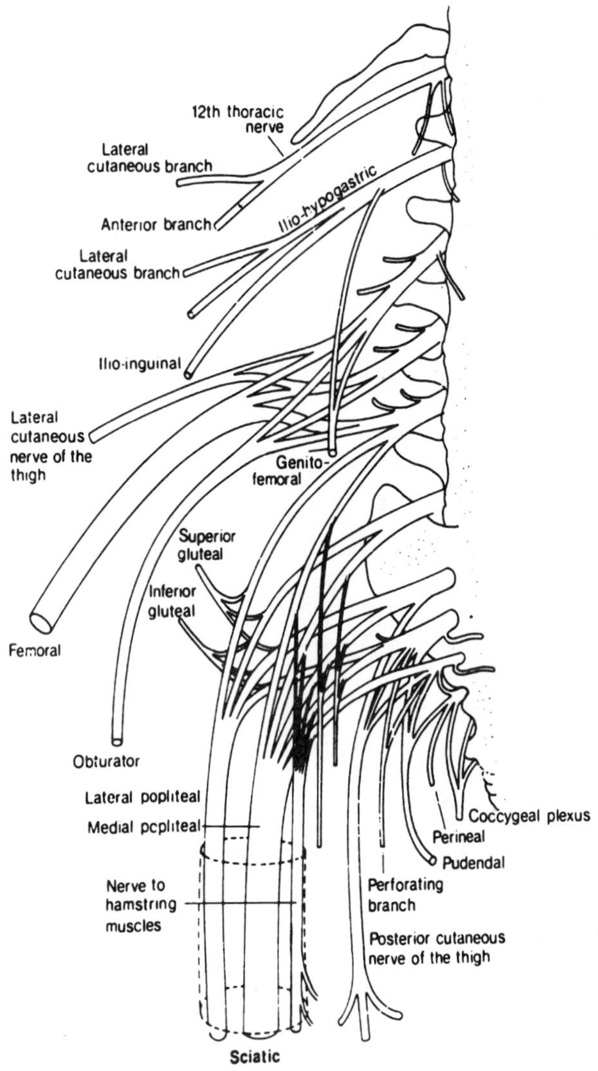

FIGURE 35.2 Anatomy of the lumbosacral plexus. (Reprinted with permission from WG Bradley. Disorders of Peripheral Nerves. Oxford, England: Blackwell, 1974:29.)

and limitation of hip joint mobility. A patient with weak ileopsoas and gluteus maximus muscles will have an increased lumbar lordosis and protuberant abdomen (the aldermanic posture) due to downward rotation of the anterior pelvis. A patient with weak hip abductors will have a positive Trendelenburg test. In this test, when a normal subject lifts one leg, the opposite gluteus medius muscle contracts to stabilize the pelvis on the weight-bearing leg and to lift the pelvis on the side of the elevated leg. Weakness of the gluteus medius muscle prevents this stabilization, and the pelvis dips downward on the side of the elevated leg (a positive Trendelenburg test). When a patient with weak gluteus medius muscles walks, the gait is waddling (a Trendelenburg gait). These abnormalities are often seen as the result of a proximal myopathy or muscular dystrophy, and the consequent strain on the ligaments and joints frequently produces back and leg pain.

Table 35.3: Important features of pain

Character: What is the quality of the pain? Is it sharp, dull, lancinating, burning, tingling, or throbbing?

Anatomical distribution: Where is the pain maximal, and to where does it radiate? Is the distribution anatomically explicable or not? In this context, it must be remembered that pain is a primitive sensation, which is often poorly localized, and patients may have difficulty in providing such details.

Temporal sequence: When did the pain begin, and have there been periods of relief, remissions, or relapses? Did it appear acutely when lifting and lock the patient in the flexed position?

Severity pattern: What is the pattern of severity? For instance, was the pain most severe at onset, waning thereafter, or did it begin gradually and progressively increase?

Precipitating and alleviating features: Does bending, straining, sneezing, exercise, rest, or the menstrual periods have any effect? Does it make the pain worse or better? Does the pain wake the patient from sleep?

Associated features: Is there numbness, tingling, weakness, wasting, sphincter disturbance, or alteration in gait? Is there associated fever, malaise, or weight loss? Are the joints red or swollen? Are there distal trophic changes such as ulcers or black toes?

Other relevant illnesses: Is there any past or present illness that might be the cause of the low back and leg pain? Is there diabetes mellitus, vascular disease, tuberculosis, arthritis, or carcinoma? Are any current medications of potential relevance, such as corticosteroids or anticoagulants? Is the patient a smoker?

Work and compensation relationships: Did the symptoms begin at work, and were they related to an injury? Is the patient receiving insurance compensation? Is there a lawsuit or compensation claim as a result of the injury?

The response of the patient to elicited pain can be instructive. Histrionic responses may point to a psychogenic cause or malingering, although it must be remembered that response to pain varies greatly from patient to patient. The range of motion of the major joints of the back and legs should be examined. Is the patient able to touch the toes without bending the knees, run the thumb down the outer aspect of the leg to at least the level of the knee on lateral flexion, extend the spine by 30 degrees, and rotate the spine by 130 degrees in both directions? If not, is the restriction greater in one direction of movement than in the others? Movements of flexion, extension, and internal and external rotation of the hip joints should be examined, because referred pain from hip disease is frequently diagnostically confusing. Pain on moving the sacroiliac joint by crossed flexion of the thigh on the trunk may indicate inflammation of that joint. Deep percussion of the lumbosacral spine may reveal exquisite focal tenderness suggesting a fracture, osteomyelitis, abscess, or metastasis. Auscultation of the spine may reveal the bruit of an arteriovenous malformation.

The straight leg–raising test will be limited in all conditions in which the lower lumbosacral nerve roots are irritated or compressed, be it by an intervertebral disc prolapse, an intraspinal tumor, or an inflammatory radicu-

Table 35.4: Major areas to be examined in patients with low back and lower-limb pain

Location	*Feature*
Spine	Posture, deformity, tenderness, range of motion
Joints	Sacroiliac, hip, knee, ankle
	Range of motion; capsule, ligaments, soft tissues
Nerve root irritation	Straight-leg–raising, femoral stretch test
Muscle	Bulk and strength of major muscle groups
Reflexes	Abdominal, knee, ankle, anal, plantar
Sensation	Pinprick, light touch in each of the dermatomes and major sensory nerve territories; vibration at bony prominences, joint position sense at the hallux, ankle, knee, and hip
	Trophic changes
Autonomic nervous system	Sphincter tone, sweating, color, temperature
Blood vessels	
Arteries	Bruits, pulses in feet, abdominal aneurysm
Veins	Varicosities, Homan's sign
Abdomen	Masses, bruits
Soft tissues	Masses

lopathy. The radicular origin of the pain can be confirmed by dorsiflexing the foot at the extreme of pain-free elevation of the straight leg, at which time there would be a marked exacerbation of the pain in the low lumbar region radiating down to the back of the calf. The normal young individual should be able to sustain an 80–90-degree flexion of the straight leg on the trunk. The femoral nerve stretch test is the reverse of the straight leg–raising test, with the patient lying prone or on the other side. Extension of the hip with the knee flexed should be possible to about 15 degrees beyond the straight line. Restriction of the femoral stretch test and pain suggest a high lumbar disc prolapse or compression of the lumbar plexus.

The neurological examination is designed to demonstrate impairment of the roots, nerves, plexuses, or muscles. Is there any atrophy of the muscles, and if so, is it asymmetrical? Is there a difference in circumference of the limbs? Is the power of all the muscles normal, or is there weakness? If so, this should be graded on the Medical Research Council scale (Table 35.5). Can the amount of weakness be explained by the pain that is present, or does it indicate a motor nerve deficit? Are the deep tendon reflexes normal or diminished (Table 35.6)? Loss of reflexes indicates impairment of the reflex arc, which consists of the muscle, the nerve and nerve roots, and the synapses within the spinal cord. For instance, the loss of the ankle jerk points to damage to the S1 nerve root, perhaps due to prolapse of the L5–S1 intervertebral disc. The function of the lower sacral nerve roots can be examined by testing for anal sphincter tone and the anal reflex. Weakness of the extensor hallucis longus muscle may be the only abnormal sign of an L5 radiculopathy.

The examination of sensation is the most difficult part of the neurological examination because of its subjectivity. The patient should first be asked to outline with one finger any area of impaired or altered sensation. Usually the examiner should look specifically for focal abnormalities in the dermatomes suggested to be involved from the history, and can examine the remainder of the sensory system in the back and legs in less detail. Thus, a diminution of pinprick sensation on the outer aspect of the left ankle in a patient with recurrent episodes of low back and left lower-limb pain may indicate damage of the S1 root. This diminution of pinprick is most easily determined by comparing the sensation on the inner and outer aspects of the ankle.

Examination of the abdomen and vascular systems in the legs is a necessary part of the examination. The presence of an abdominal mass or an abdominal aortic aneurysm may explain the low back and lower-limb pain. Enlarged lymph

Table 35.5: The Medical Research Council scale of muscle strength

Grade	*Muscle Strength*
Grade 5	Normal power
Grade 4	Active movement against gravity and resistance (grades 4–, 4, and 4+ may be used to indicate movement against slight, moderate, and strong resistance, respectively)
Grade 3	Active movement against gravity
Grade 2	Active movement, with gravity eliminated
Grade 1	Flicker or trace of contraction
Grade 0	No contraction

Source: Aids to the Examination of the Peripheral Nervous System. Medical Research Council Memorandum No. 45. London: Her Majesty's Stationery Office, 1976.

Table 35.6: Recommended grading scale for tendon reflexes

Grade	*Reflexes*
0	Absent
±	Present only with reinforcement
1	Present but depressed
2	Normal
3	Increased
4	Sustained clonus

nodes in the groin may indicate the presence of a neoplasm causing back and lower-limb pain. The absence of pulses in the feet indicates that the patient has peripheral arterial disease, which may be unilateral or bilateral and may be responsible for exercise-induced pain in the legs.

Venous insufficiency can cause leg pain. Varicose veins due to proximal obstruction to venous return or valvular incompetence can cause chronic back pressure in the veins of the lower limbs, with consequent pain in the legs on standing. A second type of venous insufficiency occurs in deep vein thrombosis, with acute swelling and tenderness of the calf, fever, an increased temperature of the leg, and a positive Homan's sign—that is, pain on dorsiflexion of the foot with the leg extended.

PATIENT WITH LOW BACK AND LOWER-LIMB PAIN

The pattern of presentation of patients with low back and leg pain may be described in a number of ways (Table 35.7). The reason for making such distinctions is that they permit a separation of conditions that have potentially different causes.

The patient may have a high lumbar or lumbosacral lesion, involving either the nerve roots or the plexuses. Pain from high lumbar lesions affects the midback and anterior thigh, whereas pain from low lumbar and sacral lesions affects the low back and posterior and lateral leg region. Though it is often thought that lumbar disc prolapse is the most common cause of either syndrome, most patients have no definable cause. There is a higher likelihood of a diabetic ischemic neuropathy or carcinomatous infiltration in patients with the high lumbar syndrome.

Another way of describing patients with low back pain, leg pain, or both is according to the rapidity of development of the symptoms. Were they acute, subacute, chronic progressive, or acute recurrent? The acute syndrome is more likely to be due to an acute disc prolapse or nerve ischemia, whereas chronic progressive syndromes are more probably due to nerve root compression or infiltration by slowly expanding tumors. Chronic recurrent syndromes are more typical of recurrent disc prolapses or mechanical musculoskeletal syndromes, such as the facet syndrome due to osteoarthritis affecting the zygoapophysial joints of the vertebrae.

Determination of anatomical distribution is very important, both to allow localization of the site of the lesion and to indicate different causes. This is especially true in the case of patients with pain restricted to the low back, those with pain restricted to the leg, and those in whom pain involves both the leg and back. The last of these possibilities is especially likely to indicate intraspinal damage of both the vertebra and the cauda equina.

The final way of separating patients with low back and leg pain depends on the presence or absence of neurological signs. The presence of neurological signs indicates nerve or nerve root damage. Because there is generally little recovery of severe proximal damage, there is a need for urgent surgery to decompress the nerve roots if there is neurological damage or loss of sphincter control. Thus, a patient with an acute central lumbar disc prolapse frequently develops bilateral sciatica and cauda equina compression with loss of bowel and bladder sphincter function, leading to urinary retention or urinary and fecal incontinence. Urgent removal of the herniated disc is required, because this may lead to recovery in many patients. A delay in diagnosis and treatment, however, may result in permanent incontinence and lower limb paralysis.

Table 35.7: Patterns of presentation of low back and leg pain

Acute, subacute, chronic progressive, acute recurrent
Upper lumbar or lower lumbosacral disorders
Low back alone, lower limb alone, both low back and lower limb
With or without signs of neurological involvement

It must be remembered that the absence of signs of neurological damage, such as absent ankle jerk or loss of pinprick sensation on the outer border of the ankle, does not rule out mild nerve root damage. Specialized electrophysiological investigations may be needed to reveal motor nerve damage (Chapter 37B). The absence of sensory abnormality can be explained by the overlap of nerve root territories even though there may be significant sensory root damage.

SPECIFIC SYNDROMES OF LOW BACK AND LOWER-LIMB PAIN

Low Back Pain Alone

The *acute or subacute* presentation of low back pain alone may be due to a vertebral fracture or collapse, to intervertebral disc prolapse, or to one of several soft-tissue injuries (see Chapter 78). The presence of fever and malaise may indicate an osteomyelitis or epidural abscess. Previous corticosteroid therapy or advanced age may indicate compression fracture from osteoporosis. Preceding weight loss and malaise may indicate the presence of vertebral metastases. A recurrent acute syndrome is likely to be due to a disc prolapse or other mechanical musculoskeletal disorder.

Chronic or recurrent back pain, sometimes with minor radiation into the buttock and upper thigh, is frequently due to disorders of the soft tissues, facet joints, ligaments, intervertebral discs, or sacroiliac joints.

Chronic progressive pain, slowly extending over months, suggests a slowly growing intraspinal tumor, such as a cauda equina ependymoma, neurofibroma, chordoma, or chondroma (see Chapter 59).

If bending, lifting, straining, coughing, and sneezing make the pain worse, particularly with radiation of the pain down the legs (see below), it is likely that there is an intraspinal lesion compressing nerve roots. These maneuvers increase the pressure in the venous epidural plexuses and the cerebrospinal fluid, compressing an already painful nerve root.

If the symptoms are worsened by extension and eased by moderate flexion of the lumbar spine, then either lumbar canal stenosis or spondylolisthesis is the likely diagnosis (see Chapter 78). Flexion tends to increase the spinal canal diameter, giving the nerve roots more room and thereby easing the pressure on the nerve roots. As a result, patients who cannot walk 100 yards without developing severe neurogenic claudication may be able to ride an exercise bicycle for 30 minutes in the slightly flexed position.

Focal exquisite tenderness of the lumbar spine on deep percussion suggests the presence of an intervertebral disc prolapse, metastasis, osteomyelitis, or epidural abscess. Symptoms that are much worse on waking in the morning, with generalized stiffness, particularly if there is a low-grade fever, weight loss, and chronic progression, suggest the presence of ankylosing spondylitis or some other rheumatological disorder.

A diffuse cervical, thoracic, and lumbosacral back pain, often with discrete "trigger points" to deep pressure over the muscles of the back, suggests the ill-defined myofascial syndrome (fibromyalgia, fibrositis).

Lower-Limb Pain without Neurological Involvement

Patients with pure leg pain may have one of several conditions that are not neurological but which must be considered in the differential diagnosis of back and leg pain. Rarely a lumbar disc prolapse causes pure leg or foot pain without back pain.

Pain in the calves on exertion that is eased by rest is generally due to arteriosclerotic arterial insufficiency (intermittent claudication). It may be unilateral or bilateral. Rarely, it is due to other vascular diseases such as a vasculitis. The characteristic pain develops at a reproducible distance, such as one-half mile or 100 yards of walking, and the distance diminishes as the arterial insufficiency worsens. The pain is a deep aching in the muscle that causes limping. The patient is unable to walk through the pain. Rest produces relief within seconds. After a few minutes of rest the patient is able to walk the same distance before the pain returns. The explanation for this phenomenon is that during walking, the metabolic demand of the muscle increases twenty- to fifty-fold over the resting level. The pain results from inability of the restricted blood flow to provide sufficient oxygen and glucose and to remove metabolites such as lactic acid and carbon dioxide. The resting blood flow is generally only slightly diminished in such patients. Hence, when the exercise stops, the resting blood flow is able to remove metabolites quickly, with rapid relief of pain.

Exertional pain can result from neurological causes (see below), where the characteristic feature is that pain remains for 5–20 minutes after rest (neurogenic claudication).

Pain from arthritis is generally easy to diagnose. The history may point to one or more joints (see Chapter 78), and the examination shows the arthropathy with limitation of range of movement of the joint, crepitus, and pain on active and passive movement. Sacroiliitis is less easy to diagnose. Pain on cross-flexion of the thigh on the abdomen, x-rays of the joints, and abnormalities on rheumatological blood studies may all be required to make the diagnosis. It is important to remember that referred pain can cause confusion. For instance, pain in the knee can originate in arthritis of the hip. A hot joint may be infected. Recurrent episodes of joint pain are likely to be due to gout. Multiple joint involvement suggests rheumatoid arthritis, particularly if the maximal involvement is distal. Other features in the history may point to the diagnosis; for instance, the presence of hemophilia suggests a hemarthrosis, and intravenous drug abuse suggests a septic arthritis.

The presence of a painful mass lesion can be due to a sarcoma, inflammatory focal myositis, a Baker's cyst in the popliteal fossa, or a metastasis. Several of these may present as painless masses. Osteomyelitis is relatively rare now but should always be considered in a patient with a painful leg in whom the pain is poorly localized or maximal at the end of a long bone.

Lower-Limb Pain with Neurological Involvement

The presence of neurological damage is of great help in achieving a diagnosis, but the neurological damage may be clinically silent, requiring electrophysiological studies for demonstration.

The pain may be in the distribution of one nerve, often with neurological deficits in the same distribution. For instance, there may be pain radiating from the buttock down the back of the thigh to the calf and foot, with weakness of dorsiflexion and plantar flexion of the ankle and impairment of sensation below the knee. If there is no back pain, then an intrapelvic compressive lesion such as a carcinoma or lymphoma, a lesion of the pelvic bones such as an osteogenic sarcoma or metastasis, or sciatic nerve entrapment at the sciatic notch must be considered. An occupational sciatic neuropathy occurs in tilers, who sit on their heels for many hours. An intraneural neurofibroma and diabetic ischemic neuropathy are other possible causes of a painful sciatic nerve lesion. A disc prolapse at the L5–S1 level may occasionally cause a similar syndrome, but usually there is accompanying low back pain (see below).

Meralgia paresthetica is the syndrome of pain, tingling, and numbness in the anterolateral aspect of the thigh, which may be unilateral or bilateral, and is due to entrapment of the lateral cutaneous nerve of the thigh as the nerve exits through the inguinal ligament or fascia lata (see Chapters 80 and 81). It typically occurs in obese or pregnant individuals or where the bulk of the quadriceps muscle is increasing or decreasing rapidly.

A painful femoral neuropathy is frequently due to the proximal ischemic neuropathy of diabetes mellitus. Less commonly it can be due to vasculitis or nerve compression from a hematoma deep to the iliacus fascia in patients with hemophilia or who are receiving anticoagulants or who have suffered abdominal trauma. Carcinomatous compression or infiltration of the lumbar plexus can also be responsible. In about one-third of the cases of lumbosacral plexopathy, no cause can be found. These cases are probably due to an autoimmune inflammatory plexopathy, which usually shows a slow spontaneous resolution (see Chapter 80). Occasionally, a high lumbar disc lesion must be considered in the diagnosis of thigh pain, but usually this is associated with back pain (see below).

There are a number of specific nerve entrapments that cause distal nerve pain, including Morton's metatarsalgia and the tarsal tunnel syndrome (see Chapter 81). The anterior tibial compartment syndrome (split shins) is another cause of pain in the leg. In such compartment syndromes, unusual exercise causes muscle swelling in a tight anatomical compartment leading to ischemic necrosis of muscle.

If the neurological lesion is in the distribution of a nerve root, then generally an intervertebral disc prolapse is responsible and there is coexisting back pain (see below). Occasionally a slow-growing cauda equina tumor, such as a schwannoma, may cause lower-limb pain and nerve root damage without back pain.

If the neurological deficit involves one or both lower limbs with a patchy distribution, with no clear anatomical localization, a lumbosacral plexopathy is likely to be present (see Chapter 80). In some patients, the cause may be obvious, as in late pregnancy when pressure of the fetal head may compress the lumbosacral plexus against the pelvic brim. In most cases, however, further investigation will be required to identify such causes as a vasculitis, diabetic ischemic proximal plexopathy, carcinomatous infiltration, or compression. Radiation plexopathy, such as that due to external irradiation of retroperitoneal malignant nodes, usually causes a painless progressive motor deficit (see Chapter 79).

Intraspinal inflammatory pathology, such as the late effects of a bacterial meningitis, sarcoidosis, or other uveomeningitic syndromes, and idiopathic chronic arachnoiditis can cause leg pain and patchy neurological deficits (see Chapter 78). In all of these conditions there is usually spinal cord involvement, with upper motor neuron signs and sphincter impairment.

If the distribution of the neurological deficit indicates a distal symmetrical polyneuropathy, there can be many causes (see Chapter 81). A burning, painful polyneuropathy is likely to be due to a metabolic cause such as diabetes mellitus or malabsorption. A small-fiber neuropathy affecting pain and temperature sensation and autonomic function may be due to primary amyloidosis. Tingling and numbness are usually due to large-fiber involvement, for which there are many causes; toxins, vitamin deficiencies, and paraneoplastic causes are among the most common.

Three further syndromes of leg pain must be mentioned: phantom limb pain, causalgia, and reflex sympathetic dystrophy. Phantom limb pain is described as pain perceived in a part of a limb that has been amputated. Occasionally this can be due to a painful neuroma in the limb stump, but usually no cause can be found. Causalgia, a syndrome of a burning pain, made worse by contact, loud noise, or anxiety, with shiny red skin in the affected part, follows a partial injury to a large nerve such as the sciatic nerve (see Chapter 81) Reflex sympathetic dystrophy has some of the features of causalgia, with particular signs of sympathetic dysfunction in the affected part, such as vasoconstriction or dilation, and loss of or excessive sweating. Osteoporosis of the adjacent bones is frequently found. There is considerable controversy concerning the nature and diagnoses of causalgia and reflex sympathetic dystrophy.

Low Back and Lower-Limb Pain

The combination of low back and leg pain clearly indicates a spinal origin for the pain, with nerve root involvement causing referred pain to the legs. The only other explanation is multifocal lesions. If the location of the lesion is intraspinal, it will generally worsen with movements of the lumbar spine and with maneuvers that increase the intraspinal pressure, such as coughing, straining, or sneezing.

Anatomical features are important, not only in localizing the lesion but in determining its cause. Pain in the high lumbar region, focal tenderness over the second lumbar vertebra, pain radiating down to the anterior aspect of the thigh, and an absent knee jerk indicate an L2–L3 nerve root lesion, possibly an intervertebral disc herniation or an extradural metastasis. The former causes a rapid onset of pain, while the latter is slower. Ischemic diabetic plexopathy rarely causes back pain. Pain in the low lumbar region radiating into the buttock and down the back of the leg may be due to an L5–S1 herniated intervertebral disc. If no disc lesion is identified, the diagnosis is an idiopathic mechanical musculoskeletal syndrome.

Other features may aid in the diagnosis. The acute onset of severe pain while lifting a heavy weight, causing locking of the lumbar spine with inability to straighten, is likely to be due to an acute intervertebral disc prolapse. A past history of similar episodes supports this diagnosis or that of some other mechanical musculoskeletal syndrome. If a neurological deficit is also present, such as the absence of an ankle jerk and diminished sensation on the outer aspect of the foot, then nerve root compression by an intervertebral disc prolapse is likely. The sudden onset of low back and leg pain with a neurological deficit, but with an associated severe headache and meningism, is likely to be due to a subarachnoid hemorrhage from a spinal arteriovenous malformation. A slowly progressive picture over months or years, with a bilateral and sometimes asymmetrical neurological deficit, indicates an expanding intraspinal tumor, which is likely to be an ependymoma, schwannoma, chondroma, or chordoma (see Chapter 59).

A fever with marked diffuse spinal tenderness to percussion is likely to be due to an epidural abscess. A similar syndrome with a marked focal spinal tenderness is likely to be due to discitis, particularly if there has recently been spinal surgery (see Chapter 78). In a patient with a known carcinoma or inexplicable weight loss and malaise, the subacute progression of backache and nerve root pain, with or without neurological involvement, is likely to indicate a metastasis to the vertebral body or epidural space.

Referred Pain from the Pelvic Organs

Diagnosis of referred (or projected) pain from disease of the pelvic organs is often difficult, usually requiring the exclusion of other causes for back and leg pain, and the demonstration of an intrapelvic disorder. There is generally low back and proximal leg pain. Confirmation may come from relief of pain by treatment of the pelvic disorder. Causes include pelvic inflammatory disease, endometriosis, intrauterine disorders, and an abdominal aortic aneurysm. The latter can erode the anterior bodies of the lumbosacral spine, causing pain, although this only rarely causes lower-limb pain.

Psychogenic Syndromes

Three psychogenic syndromes must be considered in patients with low back and leg pain, namely malingering, conversion-somatization, and secondary psychological overlay of a primary organic disorder. The correlation between back pain and the degree of disability is poor. Patients with sports-related injuries are much less likely to suffer chronic disability than those with work-related back pain.

All patients with severe chronic pain have secondary psychological side effects. In some patients, anxiety about what the diagnosis may be and the severity of the pain produce a subconscious or conscious amplification of the signs. This may be the patient's way of seeking recognition by the physician that he or she has a severe disease. Thus, a histrionic reaction to mild pain or apparently feigned weakness, indicated by a variable effort and contraction of the antagonist muscles, should not be immediately construed as indicating that the whole syndrome is due to malingering. Nevertheless, signs of a functional type and symptoms in a nonanatomical distribution raise the possibility of a subconscious or conscious psychogenic cause of the pain.

It is important in such cases to search for the underlying basis, such as a lawsuit, insurance compensation, or secondary gain from the attention of others. The way in which the neurologist seeks evidence about the secondary gain may determine the success of that search. If a patient is asked flatly whether there is a compensation claim in progress, or what advantage the patient might get from disability, then it is unlikely that a meaningful answer will be elicited. On the other hand, if the approach is sympathetic and includes comments that the injury must have been very painful and the financial loss severe, and that there must have been considerable strain on the family, then the question whether compensation has been offered will usually lead to a revelation of this side of the picture. The patient should be asked whether a report of this consultation should be sent to a lawyer.

If the search reveals underlying secondary gain, then some attempt should be made to determine whether the patient is unaware of the effect of this or whether there is conscious malingering. It is impossible to make this separation with certainty, but most experienced neurologists develop an intuition for the diagnosis based on the patient's demeanor and other signs. For instance, a patient who says that the pain has been so bad that he has been virtually bedbound for the last 2 months is unlikely still to have grimy, calloused hands and dirty fingernails. Occasionally it is worth having the patient surreptitiously observed while leaving the hospital and in home circumstances. A malingerer may lose his limp and run for a bus after a neurological examination that has indicated marked leg weakness and pain.

Exertional Syndromes

Pain in the legs on exertion (intermittent claudication) is a typical result of severe arterial insufficiency, with the characteristics that have been described earlier. The most important feature is the rapid relief of pain within a few minutes of resting. Several other exertional pain syndromes can also be recognized.

Neurological (or neurogenic) claudication is generally caused by a structural lesion compressing the nerve roots of the cauda equina, often due to spinal stenosis. It may be due to congenital spinal stenosis with a constitutionally narrow spinal canal or acquired spinal stenosis from a combination of hypertrophic osteoarthropathy of the facet joints, a bulging of the intervertebral discs, and posterior osteophyte formation from the vertebral bodies. Spondylolisthesis, whether congenital or acquired through degenerative osteoarthropathy of the spine, may also cause the syndrome of neurogenic claudication.

There are two typical features of neurogenic claudication. The first is that in addition to the pain there are neurological symptoms, such as paresthesias and numbness, or weakness in excess of that expected from the pain. The second is that the pain and the neurological symptoms may remain for 5–20 minutes after stopping exercise, compared to relief within 1–2 minutes in the case of vascular claudication. Some patients are aware that exercise in a flexed position, such as an exercise bicycle, will produce less pain.

Neurogenic claudication has been suggested to arise from chronic compromise of the vascular supply of the nerve roots.

Table 35.8: Logical sequence of investigations of low back and lower-limb pain

Stage I	Plain lumbrosacral spine x-rays including lateral flexion and extension views, blood studies
Stage II	Electrophysiological studies, CT or MRI of the lumbosacral spine
Stage III	Myelogram (with or without follow-up CT)*
Stage IV	Arteriography, discography, facet block, surgical biopsy, or exploration (depending on individual features)*

*Now rarely required if MRI is available.

The firing of action potentials increases the metabolic rate of nerve tissue by 50–100% over the resting state, compared to the ten-fold to fifty-fold rise in muscles. Hence, exercise of partially ischemic nerve or muscle will cause pain from the accumulation of metabolites such as lactic acid. The metabolic demand of the exercised nerve roots falls only slowly after rest, and hence the pain and neurological symptoms resolve only slowly after the cessation of exercise. Typical neurogenic claudication occasionally occurs in the absence of cauda equina compression, perhaps due to aortoiliac vascular insufficiency.

Not all exercise-induced neurological syndromes are due to ischemia of the cauda equina. Common leg cramps ("charley horse") are of unknown origin but arise from reflex overactivity of the muscles of the calf and foot, with consequent pain. Muscle cramps and pain on exertion can be due to several disorders of muscle metabolism. These include deficiencies of the enzymes myophosphorylase, phosphofructokinase, and carnitine palmityl transferase.

An occasional patient has exertional increase in neurological symptoms in the legs due to spinal cord disease. On examination, such patients have upper motor neuron and long-tract sensory abnormalities at rest, with increase of these abnormal signs on exercise. Most of these patients have multiple sclerosis, although occasionally patients with cervical spondylotic myelopathy complain of exertional increase in symptoms. The basis seems likely to be similar to that described earlier for peripheral nerve claudication, although here the origin lies in the damaged spinal cord.

Atypical Syndromes

Patients do not always follow textbook descriptions. Thus the neurologist must be willing to make a diagnosis even though some of the "essential" features are missing. Rarely, for example, an acute intervertebral disc prolapse may cause painless nerve root damage. The neurologist needs a great deal of experience to know how likely this is and should make the diagnosis with caution while considering all other possibilities.

INVESTIGATIONS

At the end of taking the history and performing the examination, the neurologist should have a clear idea about the differential diagnosis of the problem. Investigations should be carefully planned to help confirm or reject each of the conditions on the differential diagnostic list. A neurologist who does not know what he or she is looking for when ordering an investigation will probably miss the true diagnosis and find some abnormality that is not the cause of the patient's complaints.

The investigations can be grouped into a series of increasingly invasive or expensive procedures (Table 35.8) and should be performed in a logical sequence. How far along this sequence the neurologist chooses to go, and the urgency of investigation, must be tailored to the individual patient. A patient with excruciating leg pain and a severe sensorimotor deficit in one or both legs and urinary retention demands complete and urgent investigation. A patient with a mild recurrent back pain for many years and rare twinges of pain in one hip, in whom the neurological and general examinations are normal, often requires no laboratory or radiological investigation.

The remainder of this section reviews the types of investigations that may be needed in appropriate patients, and the information that can be gleaned from them.

Blood studies are directed at finding evidence of an underlying disease responsible for the patient's complaints. A high sedimentation rate, antinuclear antibody level, and rheumatoid factor titers may point to a chronic rheumatological condition. A high sedimentation rate and polymorphonuclear leukocytosis may indicate the presence of an infection such as an epidural abscess. A paraproteinemia may indicate the presence of a plasma cell dyscrasia. High blood sugar and increased glycohemoglobin concentration indicate the presence of diabetes mellitus.

Electrophysiological studies (see Chapter 37B) are directed to find abnormalities of the peripheral nerves and muscles and to define their anatomical origin. The electromyographer needs to be given a brief summary of the patient's history and findings on examination, as well as the question being asked by the referring neurologist. Verbal contact with the referring physician is often helpful. In the context of pain in the low back and lower limb, damage to specific nerves and nerve roots should be sought. Denervation changes in the paraspinal muscles may confirm the presence of nerve root damage. If the damage is of less than 3 weeks' duration, there may be no changes in the electromyogram at rest, since muscle fibrillation potentials only appear after about 3 weeks of denervation. The knowledgeable electromyographer searches for the distribution of the muscles sharing these changes, since this points toward the anatomical localization of the lesion. A detailed knowledge of neuroanatomy is essential here. Nerve conduction studies may indicate slowing of conduction through areas of nerve entrapment. Compression of nerve roots can be demonstrated by slowing of the late waves (H-reflex and F-wave, see Chapter 37B), or by somatosensory evoked potential studies from the lower limb nerves (see Chapter 37A). Nerve root stimulation may be helpful in investigating proximal motor nerve involvement.

Imaging techniques (Chapter 39) are often required to come to an anatomical diagnosis in patients with low back and lower-limb pain. Plain x-rays of the lumbosacral spine and pelvis should be obtained in all patients with significant chronic pain. Radiographs in the extreme range of motion can demonstrate instability of the vertebrae. The presence of bony erosion suggests a metastasis or slowly growing tumor. Changes in the disc space and osteophyte formation may indicate an intervertebral disc prolapse. Alterations of the bones or their alignment, as occurs in the presence of spondylolisthesis, may be important. A radionuclide bone scan may help reveal the presence of a metastasis or infection of the bone. There is controversy concerning the role, if any, of thermography in the diagnosis of back and leg pain.

Computed tomography (CT) of the lumbosacral spine is frequently needed to investigate the bones and intervertebral discs. Unfortunately, a large number of cuts are required to study the whole of the lumbosacral spine, and thus this investigation should be accurately directed at the clinically relevant anatomical level. MRI, which is now the investigation of choice for patients with low back pain, is more helpful in the examination of the nerve roots and soft tissues but generally reveals little about the nature of the bones. Myelography with a water-soluble radiopaque dye may be required to study the intrathecal contents and is frequently combined with CT. These imaging techniques can help demonstrate if there is a lesion compressing the nerves or distorting the bones, which is responsible for the pain.

Vascular studies, including arteriography, may be required in appropriate patients. Abdominal ultrasound is of help for the localization and determination of the likely nature of an intra-abdominal mass. Finally, at times it may be necessary to carry out surgical procedures such as biopsy of a nerve, muscle, or bone to reveal the exact cause of the condition.

It is important to realize that imaging studies are not required for the majority of patients with low back and leg pain. In those in the 20- to 60-year age group with the common presentation of an acute, subacute, or recurrent backache that remits within 6 weeks and in which there are no significant neurological abnormalities, special investigations are not required. The MRI in particular is so sensitive that many normal individuals are found to have some degree of lumbar disc bulging that can easily be misinterpreted as the cause of low back pain.

DIAGNOSTIC SYNTHESIS

The object of the investigations is to rule out the presence of most diseases on the differential diagnostic list and to confirm the presence of one. At times there is no absolute confirmatory test for a disease, and the diagnosis must be one of exclusion. At other times, an abnormality in an investigation is so frequent in control individuals of the same age that the possibility that the abnormality caused the symptoms must be viewed with skepticism.

After full investigations, up to half of the patients with low back and lower-limb pain fail to have any demonstrated abnormality. This is particularly the case in younger individuals. The cause of the pain syndrome in such patients is still controversial; suggestions range from inflammation of nerves, fascia, connective tissue, ligaments, and joints to mechanical derangements of the complex interaction of the intervertebral joints and discs. The natural history of most of these conditions is benign, although often it can be recurrent. Time will usually reveal the benign prognosis, as will the response to anti-inflammatory analgesics and a program of back muscle strengthening exercises (see Chapter 78).

Low back and lower-limb pain, with or without neurological involvement, presents a diagnostic challenge even to the experienced neurologist. There are many clues in the history and examination, and many laboratory investigations to aid the neurologist. The art is to make use of these clues and investigations in a well-planned, efficient manner.

REFERENCES

Bradley WG. Disorders of Peripheral Nerves. Oxford, England: Blackwell, 1974;29.

Brain WR, Walton JN. Diseases of the Nervous System. London: Oxford University Press, 1969;34–36.

Chad DA, Bradley WG. Lumbosacral plexopathy. Semin Neurol 1987;7:97–107.

Frymoyer JW. Back pain and sciatica. N Engl J Med 1988; 318:291–300.

Hardy RW Jr. (ed). Lumbar Disc Disease (2nd ed). New York: Raven, 1993.

Stewart JD. Focal Peripheral Neuropathies. New York: Elsevier, 1987.

Part II

Neurological Investigations and Related Clinical Neurosciences

Chapter 36
The Place of Laboratory Investigations in Diagnosis and Management of Neurological Disease

Walter G. Bradley, Robert B. Daroff, Gerald M. Fenichel, and C. David Marsden

In Chapter 1 in Part I, we emphasized the primacy of the history and neurological examination in the diagnosis of patients with neurological disease. However, laboratory investigations embodied in a number of clinical neuroscience disciplines have come to play an increasingly important role in neurological diagnosis. An understanding of these disciplines is essential for the application of the information in Part III: The Neurological Diseases.

Laboratory investigations define and quantify the extent to which a body system functions normally or abnormally. The results of tests are often diagnostic and determine the response to treatment. Neurologists can only use laboratory tests judiciously if they first understand their yield, interpretation, risks, and costs. Part II, Neurological Investigations and Related Clinical Neurosciences, covers the neurodiagnostic investigations that constitute clinical neurophysiology, neuropsychology, neuroimaging, neuro-ophthalmology, neuro-otology, and neurourology. Part II also discusses related disciplines that play an essential role in understanding neurological disease. For example, neurogenetics provides the DNA studies needed for genetic counseling; neuroendocrinology deals with the interactions of the neurons and endocrine systems and with the neuropeptides, which are becoming increasingly important in clinical neurology; neuroepidemiology plays a key role in understanding neurological disease and is vital to determining the cause of an outbreak of a new disease, such as the toxic cerebellar syndrome due to organic mercury poisoning around the Bay of Minamata in Japan (see Chapter 65). Neuroimmunology and neurovirology offer investigations that help diagnose many inflammatory and infectious diseases of the nervous system, such as multiple sclerosis and encephalitis. Neurosurgical exploration and biopsy may be needed to diagnose a tumor, abscess, or vasculitis of the nervous system.

Neuropathology is the keystone of the clinical neurosciences. We do not believe it can be covered in a single chapter and have asked authors to address the pathology of individual diseases in Part III. The coverage there, however, is no substitute for a comprehensive study of neuropathology.

GENERAL PRINCIPLES FOR THE USE OF LABORATORY TESTS

The laboratory investigations used in the diagnosis of neurological disease continue to change rapidly. Computed tomography (CT), the standard for neuroimaging when the first edition of this book was published, is rapidly being replaced by magnetic resonance imaging (MRI) for most conditions, and we anticipate that magnetic resonance arteriography (MRA) may soon replace conventional arteriography.

The neurologist must be sufficiently knowledgeable about each laboratory test to be able to request it appropriately and to interpret the results intelligently. Two particular practices in the use of laboratory tests should be avoided. The first is to substitute studies for competent history and physical examination, and the other is ordering tests that do not substantially affect management. The neurologist who orders tests before developing a differential diagnosis is unlikely to make the right choices or to use the information wisely. Test results only have meaning in the context of the clinical features; we treat patients, not test results.

Diagnostic tests comprise a large part of health care expense. They should be purchased only if the result influences a diagnostic or therapeutic decision. Plain skull roentgenograms, once considered mandatory to an adequate standard of care in head-injured patients, have been shown not to improve diagnosis and rarely to alter management in patients with mild head injury (Masters et al. 1987). Further, it increases the cost of health care to order a head CT because it is more readily available than MRI, when MRI is the definitive test that must be done no matter what the CT shows. Finally, tests are intended to manage patients and not to protect neurologists from litigation. When used judiciously they serve both purposes; when ordered indiscriminately, they serve neither.

Diagnostic Yield

The plethora of available laboratory tests tempts the inexperienced neurologist to put the patient through a general screening of all of the functions of the nervous system. However, such screening subjects patients to unnecessary investigations, which increase the risk and cost and often mislead by detecting irrelevant abnormalities. When choosing tests, neurologists should decide what information will discriminate between the diseases on the differential diagnostic list. A test is justified if the result will confirm or rule out a certain disease or alter patient management, and if the risk is not excessive.

Most of the specialized laboratory tests require the neurologist to interact with a laboratory specialist. The neurologist should provide full clinical information to the colleague performing an investigation and should highlight the important questions.

Interpretation of Results

Normal variation and statistics must be taken into account when evaluating the results of a test. Every biological function has a range of normal values that can be described in mathematical terms. The "normal range" for a laboratory test may be set at plus or minus two standard deviations from the mean value, which encompasses 96% of the population, or at plus or minus three standard deviations, which encompasses 99%. Even when the ninety-ninth percentile is used, one normal person in 100 is expected to have a value outside the normal range. Therefore, an "abnormal" result may not indicate disease.

It is important to know the parameters of the "normal" population used to standardize a laboratory test. Ranges that were normalized using adults are often incorrect for children and almost never correct for newborns and infants. Ranges that were normalized using a hospitalized population may not be accurate for people who are ambulatory; an example is serum creatine kinase (CK).

Abnormal test results are sometimes caused by disorders or situations that are concurrent to the major illness being considered. For example, an elevated serum CK concentration can result from recent electromyography or intramuscular injections, pregnancy, liver disease, or myocardial infarction in addition to a primary muscle disease. A common problem for pediatric neurologists is the electroencephalographic (EEG) report of centrotemporal spikes in a child with headache or learning disability who has never had a seizure. The EEG should not have been ordered in the first place, and to act on it with anticonvulsant drugs would convert poor judgment in diagnosis to worse judgment in management.

A laboratory report is only as good as its interpreter, who, even if well informed, may not fully understand the clinical problem. Hence, the neurologist must look carefully at the results, particularly with neuroimaging studies. For example, the CT scan of a patient with clinical features of a brain stem lesion may show an appearance that is of diagnostic significance though the neuroradiologist is unwilling to call it abnormal because artifacts are so frequent in that region. Similarly, a pathologist may correctly report that the muscle biopsy from a patient with clinical findings suggestive of polymyositis is nondiagnostic, yet the neurologist will use the presence of a few necrotic fibers and interstitial lymphocytes as the basis for starting treatment with immunosuppressant drugs.

Proper use of a test requires considerable understanding of its strengths and limitations. A clinician who orders an EEG, for instance, should recognize the significance of various features that may be disclosed, such as periodic lateralized epileptiform discharges or isolated spikes and slow waves, and interpret them in the context of the patient's disease (see Chapter 37). Similarly, clinicians should not order an MRI without knowing the possible associations of areas of increased T2-weighted signal in the deep white matter of the brain (see Chapter 39). The chapters in Part II give this information.

RISK AND COST

Some investigations are more uncomfortable, risky, or expensive than others. If different tests provide equivalent information, the physician should choose the one that causes the least pain and risk. Cost needs to be considered in every country in the world. The diagnostic capability of various tests may not be identical, and the least expensive test may not be the best. The cost of tests should be considered as part of the total cost of illness. An expensive test that shortens a hospital stay may be cost-effective. The selection of laboratory tests and the sequence in which they are performed is an important component of good medical practice.

Risk-Benefit Analysis

The practicing neurologist makes risk-benefit judgments every day; the sequence presented in Figure 36.1 is illustrative. Although rarely written out, a written procedure helps clarify why some diagnostic tests are ordered and others are not. Some examples will help clarify these principles.

Lumbar Puncture

The risks and benefits of a lumbar puncture (LP) must be carefully weighed. The diagnostic benefits can be important, and LP may yield a specific diagnosis, such as subarachnoid hemorrhage or bacterial meningitis. More often, the information is less specific but still helpful. A fourfold increase in the cerebrospinal fluid (CSF) protein concentration suggests one of the following diagnoses: an acute or chronic inflammatory demyelinative polyradiculoneuropathy, schwannoma or meningioma within the CSF pathways, or spinal compression that obstructs the flow of CSF (Froin's syndrome). Increased numbers of lymphocytes, an increased gamma-globulin concentration, and oligoclonal bands in the CSF point to an immunological process in the central nervous system, such as multiple sclerosis. LP may help confirm the diagnosis (such as by showing raised intracranial pressure in benign intracranial hypertension). It may be required for intrathecal administration of drugs such as methotrexate to treat fungal or carcinomatous meningitis.

LP unfortunately carries significant risks, the most disastrous being cerebral or cerebellar herniation. The sudden

FIGURE 36.1 Flowchart of the decisional process involved in choosing investigations to elucidate the diagnosis in an 80-year-old man with a 3-month history of a progressive dementia. The differential diagnosis includes Alzheimer's disease, Creutzfeldt-Jakob disease, cerebral vasculitis, and cryptococcal meningitis. A brain biopsy was not performed, and an electroencephalogram did not show typical changes of Creutzfeldt-Jakob disease. The analysis suggests that an arteriogram will be justified to look for a vasculitis, but the lumbar puncture revealed cryptococcal meningitis before the angiogram was performed.

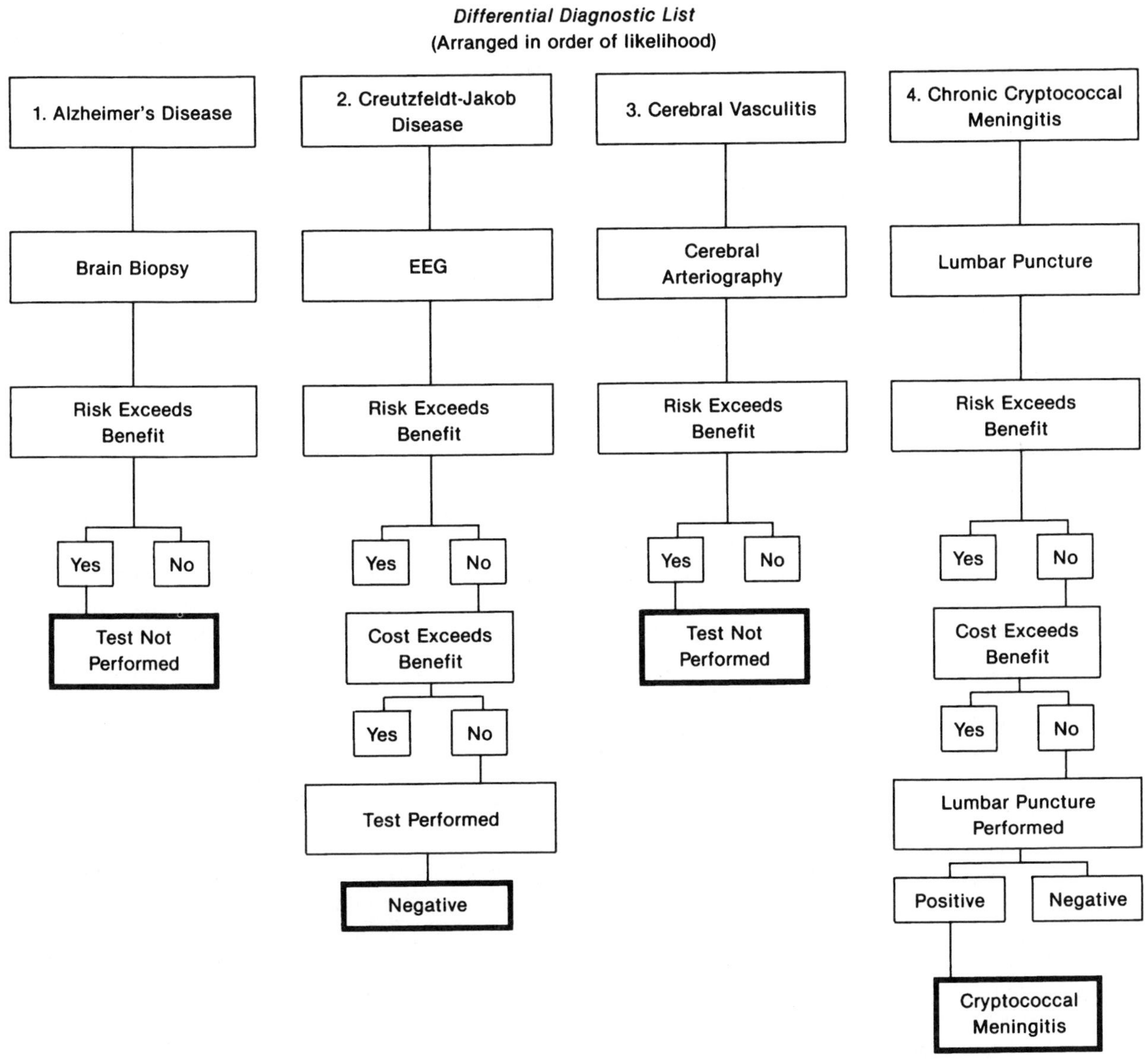

release of elevated CSF pressure may allow an expanding supratentorial lesion to force the medial temporal lobe through the tentorium cerebelli to compress the brain stem; an expanding infratentorial lesion may push the cerebellar tonsils through the foramen magnum and compress the medulla and spinal cord (see Chapters 57 and 59). These herniations can be fatal, and an LP should never be performed without carefully considering the risk-benefit analysis when an intracranial space–occupying lesion or raised intracranial pressure of any cause is suspected. In patients with critical spinal cord compression, LP may produce rapid deterioration by a similar mechanism. Whenever such risks are present, a neurosurgical consultation should be obtained *before* performing the procedure. Other risks of LP include the introduction of an infection into the CSF, the production of a postlumbar puncture (low-pressure) headache, or the later development of an implantation dermoid (if the needle is inserted without the trochar).

LP is justified in some situations despite increased intracranial pressure. The prime example is acute meningitis; examination of the CSF is essential to establish the diagnosis and identify the organism.

Cerebral Arteriography

The question of whether to request cerebral arteriography (see Chapter 39) requires analysis of the risks and benefits to each patient. In a stroke patient, the study can show thrombotic or embolic occlusion of arteries and abnormalities of the arterial wall, including arteriosclerotic plaques, fibromuscular hyperplasia, medial dissection, and arteritis. It can also demonstrate an intracranial aneurysm or arteriovenous malformation. Any of these findings can help clarify the diagnosis, treatment, and prognosis.

The arteriogram has risks, however. In a study of 5,000 catheter arteriograms, the total complication rate was 1.4%, of which 10% were major (Mani et al. 1978). Serious cerebral complications occurred in 40 patients, 20 of whom were left with permanent hemiparesis. Ten patients died. Local complications at the catheter site that necessitated embolectomy or thrombectomy occurred in five cases.

The likelihood that a patient being considered for cerebral arteriography will experience a particular complication is influenced by age and the presence of arteriosclerosis or other disease. Therefore, the probability of the complication in the general population must be weighted by a factor based on features specific to the patient. These patient-specific probabilities must be balanced, in turn, against the benefits that arteriographic information may produce. Finally, the probability of benefit from discovering a treatable disease must be weighted by a factor based on the probability of demonstrating the disease. The process sounds complicated but is simple in practice. Thus, arteriography is definitely indicated in a previously well 35-year-old woman with an acute transient right hemiplegia and aphasia and a left carotid artery bruit, especially where carotid ultrasound studies suggest an internal carotid artery stenosis. Invasive angiography is clearly not indicated in a 75-year-old woman with congestive cardiac failure and advanced carcinoma of the breast who suffers a similar transient ischemic attack.

Two noninvasive techniques may prove to be sufficiently accurate in many instances to replace cerebral angiography. Carotid Doppler ultrasound and transcranial Doppler studies in well-experienced hands can be as reliable as angiography for demonstrating intra- and extracranial occlusive disease.

MRA is a technique that visualizes main intracranial vessels noninvasively. It may obviate the need for invasive angiography in patients with such conditions as intracranial occlusive disease, arteriovenous malformations, or a family history of intracranial aneurysms.

Craniotomy and Brain Biopsy

Another procedure that requires careful risk-benefit analysis is brain biopsy in a patient who has CT evidence of an intraparenchymal brain tumor. The risk-benefit analysis of tumor biopsy is influenced by the availability of computer-assisted stereotactic technology. When such technology is available, tumor biopsy is almost always recommended. It provides tissue diagnosis that confirms the suspicion of tumor and allows the development of a treatment plan using radiation and chemotherapy.

Open biopsy of an intraparenchymal brain tumor is quite another matter. Age, other diseases, tumor location, and the patient's wishes must all be taken into account. Biopsy carries relatively little risk of producing a permanent neurological deficit if the lesion is in a "silent" area of the brain, such as the nondominant frontal lobe. It has a high risk of worsening the neurological deficit (unless that deficit is already total) if the tumor is located in the sensorimotor cortex, Broca's speech area, or the internal capsule. Treatability of the tumor must be added into the equation. Almost invariably, a meningioma is benign and removal is curative. Thus, if meningioma is the likely diagnosis, risk-benefit analysis argues for removing at least part of the lesion. A primary lymphoma of the brain will respond to radiotherapy; thus confirmatory biopsy to separate a lymphoma from a glioma should be attempted. Because histological diagnosis is so important to the treatment and prognosis of a patient with a brain tumor, biopsy is generally recommended unless there is a strong contraindication.

Cost-Benefit Analysis

Cost-benefit analysis must be approached carefully because it may place society's interests in conflict with the patient's. MRI and MRA are safer procedures than arteriography for diagnosing an arteriovenous malformation, but may be more costly. The rapid expansion of expensive technologies puts a strain on health resources in rich countries as well as developing nations. Where limited funding is available for health care, consideration must be given to purchasing the best care for the most people. Whatever the circumstances, physicians should acquaint themselves with the cost of every test.

Order of Testing

Tests are generally undertaken in order of their diagnostic specificity, invasiveness, and benignity. Thus, blood studies precede neuroimaging and lumbar puncture. Sometimes a therapeutic trial is used as an investigation. For instance, in a patient with possible herpes simplex encephalitis, the neurologist uses risk-benefit analysis to assess the benefits of performing an EEG, which may show typical changes of the disorder, followed by an MRI scan, which may show abnormality in the inferior frontal and temporal areas. A therapeutic trial of acyclovir may then be reasonable without a potentially risky brain biopsy. If there is no improvement, diagnosis may require arteriography and eventually a brain biopsy. Time may also be used as an investigation. For instance, occasionally a stroke can be difficult to differentiate from a tumor on neuroimaging studies. A reasonable plan is to follow the patient and repeat the scan in 2–4 weeks rather than immediately schedule a brain biopsy.

QUANTITATIVE DIAGNOSTIC METHODS AND DECISION ANALYSIS

The development of a new laboratory test requires an analysis of its *sensitivity*, the frequency with which the test is abnormal in patients with a confirmed diagnosis, and its *specificity*, the frequency with which the test is negative in a normal population. The false-positive rate for the test is 1 minus the specificity. These two variables can be used in Bayesian analysis to quantitate the extent to which a test result makes a diagnosis of a certain disease more or less likely. Plante (1991) reviewed the Bayesian methodology and decision analysis in the first edition of this textbook. Decision analysis forces the clinician to derive quantitative estimates of each of the many parameters entering into a decision and to calculate the risk-benefit ratio of each management decision. The old-fashioned diagnostic tool, namely the global experience of the clinician, uses a similar though usually not so explicit process to arrive at these decisions. Decision analysis is an excellent teaching tool, though often crucial quantitative data are not available. The analysis then prompts a search for such data, either from the literature or through new research. Decision analysis can also help recognize the basic weakness of diagnostic and management methods that are based on too little information and biased by insufficient experience. The outcome effects of important parameters in decision analysis can be computer-modelled and may play an increasing role in defining management and research protocols (Sox et al. 1988).

RESEARCH INVESTIGATIONS

Since many readers may be neurologists-in-training, we briefly mention the use of investigations in teaching and research centers. Clinical research is well regulated in most parts of the world, and researchers cannot perform an investigation until a protocol is approved by an institutional review board (IRB) or an ethics-in-research committee. The peer review process is interactive and is designed to ensure that the risks of the investigation are justified, taking into account the patient's particular disease and the likely benefits of the research. If the plan is approved, the IRB ensures that the patient receives full information contained in an informed consent form and understands the risks of the test and what is likely to be learned from the research. No patient should be coerced, knowingly or unknowingly, into participating in a research procedure. Once the IRB gives permission for a research project, it continues to monitor the research to ensure that it conforms to approved standards.

In a teaching hospital, the attending neurologist is ethically and legally responsible for the care of a patient with neurological disease. The attending neurologist must ensure that every investigation is justified for diagnostic and management purposes. We are ethically bound to ensure that the patient understands and approves the reason for each investigation and gives informed consent. The neurologist-in-training must learn to use tests judiciously and not to perform them simply to gain information. The two-way discussion with the senior neurologist about the rationale and risk-benefit analysis of each investigation is an important learning process for the neurologist-in-training.

THE PLACE OF LABORATORY INVESTIGATIONS IN THE MANAGEMENT OF NEUROLOGICAL DISEASE

The standard neurological examination is directed more at detecting abnormal function for diagnostic purposes than at quantifying the neurological abnormality. Laboratory investigations are helpful in both diagnosis and management of disease. Generally, abnormal values return toward normal as a disease improves and become increasingly abnormal as it worsens; visual acuity in a patient with optic neuritis or vital capacity in a patient with the Guillain-Barré syndrome are two examples where the change in laboratory values parallels the severity of disease. This is not always true. In Duchenne's muscular dystrophy, the serum CK concentration falls as the disease progresses because fewer muscle fibers remain to release enzyme into the serum. Thus, monitoring laboratory values cannot always be used as an index of disease state or response to treatment.

Other limitations on the use of laboratory tests to monitor disease progression are sampling errors, test sensitivity limitations, and test specificity. The best example of a sampling problem is muscle or brain biopsy where only a very small piece of a large organ is inspected. "Test sensitivity limitations" refers to studies that tend to be either normal or abnormal and do not correlate well with organ function; an example is the visual evoked response in patients with optic neuritis. Test specificity asks, "What is being tested?" An abnormal EEG in patients with an acute encephalitis may be caused by cerebral inflammation. When the inflammation subsides, the EEG may return to normal despite considerable residual cerebral abnormality. Therefore, the EEG is a useful measure of acute inflammation but not of cerebral function.

Quantitative tools provide important information for measuring a patient's status objectively during the course of a disease. Quantitative tools can be as simple as visual acuity measurement, how many serial numbers from 1 to 100 a patient can count on a single breath, or the frequency and severity of headaches each month. They can be sophisticated measurements such as the force of maximum voluntary muscle contraction or the temperature perception threshold for an area of skin. They can be summated scores of qualitative assessments such as the Kurtzke scale, devised to follow patients with multiple sclerosis, the Norris score for amyotrophic lateral sclerosis, or the Z scores of muscle strength (Munsat 1989). When used routinely, quantitative measures of neurological function may allow better patient management than do the routine neurological interview and examination, particularly during treatment of the disease.

CONCLUSIONS

Laboratory investigations and quantification of neurological function play an increasingly important role in neurological practice. The discipline of *decision analysis* provides the neurologist with a better understanding of diagnosis and management and the application of quantitative methods to this clinical field. However, the patient and society may be badly served unless the neurologist understands the nature and basis of the investigations. We therefore urge the reader to remember the general principles outlined in this chapter when reading the chapters in Part II.

REFERENCES

Mani RL, Eisenberg RL, McDonald EJ et al. Complications of catheter cerebral angiography: analysis of 5,000 procedures. Am J Radiol 1978;131:861–865.

Masters JS, McClean PM, Arcarese JS et al. Skull x-ray examinations after head trauma. N Engl J Med 1987;316:84–91.

Munsat TL. Quantification of neurologic deficit. Boston: Butterworth, 1989.

Plante D. Quantitative Diagnostic Methods and Decision Analysis. In WG Bradley, RB Daroff, GM Fenichel et al. (eds), Neurology in Clinical Practice. Stoneham, MA: Butterworth, 1991; 423–428.

Sox HC, Blatt MA, Higgins MC et al. Medical Decision Making. Stoneham, MA: Butterworth, 1988.

Chapter 37
Clinical Neurophysiology

A. ELECTROENCEPHALOGRAPHY AND EVOKED POTENTIALS

Timothy A. Pedley and Ronald G. Emerson

The techniques of applied electrophysiology are of practical importance in the diagnosis and management of certain categories of neurological disease. Modern instrumentation permits the clinician to investigate selectively various functional aspects of the central and peripheral nervous systems. The *electroencephalogram* (EEG) and *evoked potentials* (EPs) are measures of electrical activity generated by the central nervous system. With the exception of positron emission tomography (PET) and magnetoencephalography (MEG), research techniques not yet in widespread use, EEG and EPs are currently the only available laboratory tests of brain physiology. As such, they are generally complementary to anatomic imaging techniques such as computed tomography (CT) or magnetic resonance imaging, especially when it is desirable to document abnormalities that are not associated with detectable structural alterations in brain tissue. Furthermore, EEG provides the only continuous measure of cerebral function over time.

This chapter is not intended as a comprehensive account of all aspects of EEG and EPs. Rather, it is designed to provide clinicians with an appreciation of their scope and limitations as currently used.

ELECTROENCEPHALOGRAPHY

Physiological Principles of the Electroencephalogram

EEG signals are generated by the cerebral cortex. Spontaneous EEG activity reflects currents flowing in the extracellular space generated by the summation of excitatory and inhibitory synaptic potentials occurring on thousands, or even millions, of cortical neurons. Individual action potentials do not contribute directly to EEG activity. Conventional EEG is a continuous graph over time of the spatial distribution of changing voltage fields at the scalp surface that result from ongoing synaptic activity in the underlying cortex.

In addition to reflecting the spontaneous intrinsic activities of cortical neurons, the EEG depends very much on important afferent inputs from subcortical structures, including the thalamus and brain stem reticular formation. Thalamic afferents, for example, are probably responsible for entraining cortical neurons to produce the rhythmic oscillations that characterize such normal patterns as the alpha rhythm and sleep spindles. Similarly, an EEG abnormality may occur directly from disruption of cortical neural networks or indirectly from modification of subcortical inputs onto cortical neurons.

The EEG is not the same as the *electrocorticogram*, and not all potentials recorded at the cortical surface are detectable at the scalp. In the case of epileptiform activity, it has been estimated that 20–70% of *cortical spikes* will not appear in the EEG, depending on the region of cortex involved. This is largely because of the pronounced voltage attenuation that occurs from overlying cerebrospinal fluid and dura. Thus, relatively large areas of cortex need to be involved in similar activity for a discharge to appear in the EEG. Furthermore, potentials involving surfaces of gyri are more readily recorded than are potentials arising in the walls and depths of sulci. Activity generated over the lateral convexities of the hemispheres is more accurately recorded than is activity coming from interhemispheric, mesial, or basal areas.

These considerations limit the usefulness of EEG. First, surface recordings cannot be used to determine unambigu-

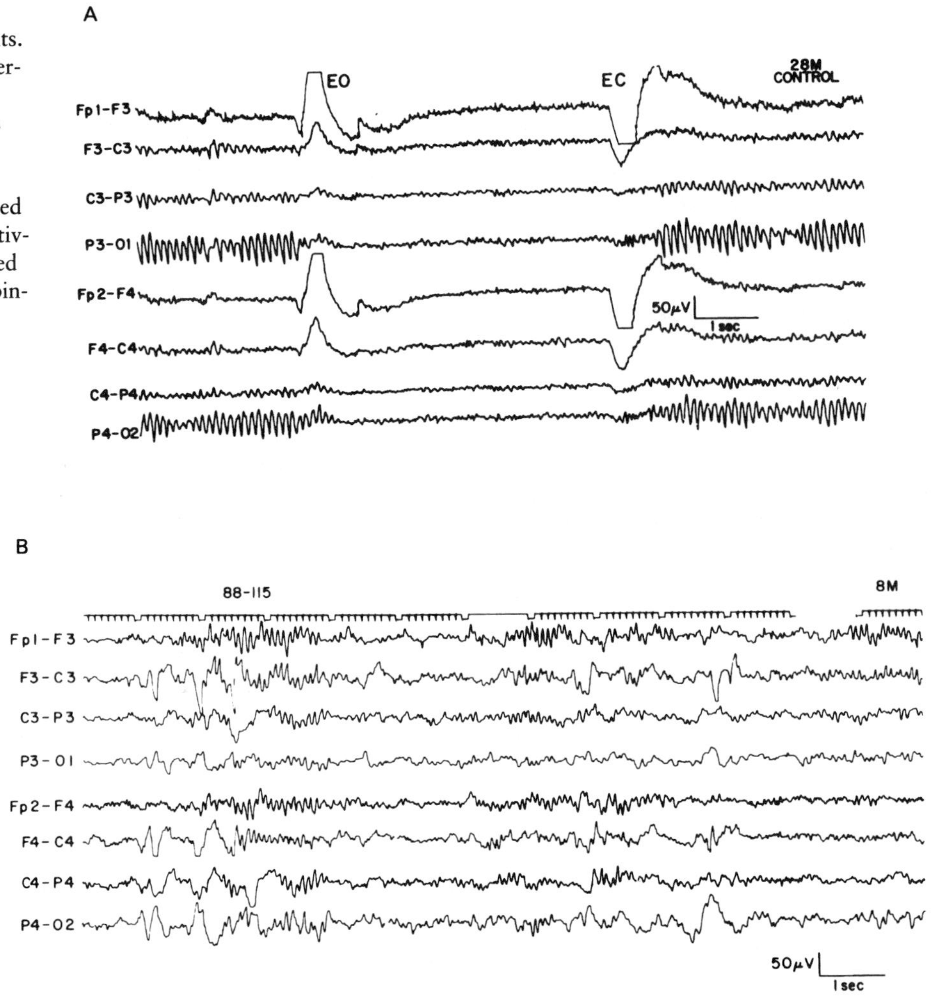

FIGURE 37A.1 Samples of normal EEG from two patients. A. Waking activity is characterized by a 9-Hz alpha rhythm that attenuates when the eyes are opened (EO) and returns when eyes are closed (EC). B. Stage 2 sleep is characterized by 2- to 5-Hz background activity, on which are superimposed vertex (V) waves and sleep spindles.

ously the nature of synaptic events contributing to a particular EEG wave. Second, the EEG is rarely specific as to cause, because different diseases and conditions produce similar EEG changes. In this regard, the EEG is analogous to findings on the neurological examination; hemiplegia caused by a stroke cannot be distinguished by physical findings alone from one caused by a brain tumor. Third, many potentials occurring at the brain surface involve such a small area or are of such low voltage that they cannot be detected at the scalp. The EEG may then be normal despite clear indications from other data of focal brain dysfunction. Finally, abnormalities in brain areas inaccessible to EEG recording electrodes (some cortical areas and virtually all subcortical and brain stem regions) do not affect EEG directly but may exert remote effects on patterns of cortical activity.

Normal Electroencephalogram Activities

Spontaneous fluctuations of voltage potential at the cortical surface are in the 100- to 1,000-mV range but at the scalp are only 10–100 μV. Different parts of the cortex generate relatively distinct potential fluctuations, which also differ in the waking and sleep states.

In most normal adults, the waking pattern of EEG activity consists mainly of sinusoidal oscillations occurring at 8–12 Hz, which are most prominent over the occipital area (*alpha rhythm*) (Figure 37A.1A). The alpha rhythm is attenuated (or blocked) by eye opening, mental activity, and drowsiness. Activity faster than 12 Hz (*beta activity*) is normally present over the frontal areas and may be especially prominent in patients receiving barbiturate or benzodiazepine drugs. Activity slower than 8 Hz is subdivided into *delta activity* (1–3 Hz) and *theta activity* (4–7 Hz). Adults may normally show a very small amount of theta activity over the temporal regions; the percentage of intermixed theta frequencies increases after the age of 60. Delta activity is not normally present in adults when they are awake but appears when they fall asleep (Figure 37A.1B). The amount and amplitude of slow activity (theta and delta) correlate closely with the depth of sleep. Slow frequencies are abundant in the EEG of newborns and young children, but these disappear progressively with maturation.

Common Types of EEG Abnormalities

Focal Arrhythmic (Polymorphic) Slow Activity. *Polymorphic slow activity* is irregular or amorphous activity in the delta (1–4 Hz) or theta (4–7 Hz) range, which, when continuous, has a high correlation with a localized cerebral lesion such as infarction, hemorrhage, tumor, or abscess. Intermittent focal slow activity may also indicate localized parenchymal dysfunction but is less predictive.

Intermittent Rhythmic Slow Waves. *Paroxysmal bursts* of generalized, bisynchronous rhythmic theta or delta waves usually indicate thalamocortical dysfunction and may be seen with metabolic or toxic disorders, obstructive hydrocephalus, deep midline or posterior fossa lesions, and also as a nonspecific functional disturbance in patients with generalized epilepsy. Focal bursts of rhythmic waves lateralized to one hemisphere usually indicate deep (typically thalamic or periventricular) abnormalities, often of a structural nature.

Generalized Arrhythmic (Polymorphic) Slow Activity. Diffuse disturbances in background rhythms marked by excessive slow activity and disorganization of waking EEG patterns are seen in encephalopathies of metabolic, toxic, or infectious origin, and in persons with brain damage due to a static encephalopathy.

Voltage Attenuation. Voltage attenuation is caused by cortical disease. Generalized voltage attenuation is usually associated with diffuse depression of function such as occurs following anoxia or with certain degenerative diseases (for instance, Huntington's disease). The most severe form of generalized voltage attenuation is *electrocerebral inactivity*, which is corroborative evidence of brain death in the appropriate clinical setting. Focal voltage attenuation reliably indicates localized cortical disease such as porencephaly, atrophy, or contusion, or an extra-axial lesion, such as a meningioma or subdural hematoma.

Epileptiform Discharges. Epileptiform discharges are spikes or sharp waves that occur interictally in patients with epilepsy and sometimes in individuals who themselves do not have seizures but have a genetic predisposition to epilepsy. Epileptiform discharges may be focal or generalized depending on seizure type.

Recording Techniques

The following outline summarizes the recording methods in common use. Details are provided in the American EEG Society's *Guidelines* (1994).

1. A series of small gold, silver, or silver-silver chloride discs are symmetrically positioned over the scalp on both sides of the head in standard locations (the International Ten-Twenty System).
2. These recording electrodes are then interconnected in chains, and the potential difference between pairs of electrodes is recorded. In practice, 16–20 or more channels (one pair of electrodes equals one amplifier channel) of EEG activity are recorded simultaneously. Electrode pairs are interconnected in different arrangements called "montages" to permit a comprehensive survey of the brain's electrical activity. Typically, montages are designed to compare symmetrical areas of the two hemispheres, as well as anterior versus posterior regions, or parasagittal versus temporal areas in the same hemisphere.
3. Spontaneous brain wave activity is recorded for 30–45 minutes. In addition, most patients are routinely subjected to two types of activating procedures: *hyperventilation* and *photic stimulation.* In some patients, these techniques provoke abnormal focal or generalized alterations in activity that are of diagnostic importance and would otherwise go undetected (Figure 37A.2).
4. Sleep, sleep deprivation, and placement of additional electrodes at other recording sites are useful in detecting specific kinds of epileptiform potentials.
5. Other maneuvers are carried out depending on the clinical question posed. For example, epileptiform activity may occasionally be activated only by movement or specific sensory stimuli. Vasovagal stimulation may be important in some types of syncope.

Digital Electroencephalography

Computer-based EEG machines are increasingly finding a place in routine EEG laboratories. Borrowing on technology developed mainly for epilepsy monitoring units, *digital EEG machines* have several advantages over conventional analog instruments. The term *digital* refers to the fact that for EEG information to be stored and processed by a computer, the analog EEG signal (which is a graph of voltage plotted against time) must be transformed into a series of numbers that specify the original signal sequentially at short time intervals. This process is termed *analog-to-digital conversion.* Digitized EEG data can be manipulated advantageously in several ways. First, data can be transmitted by network or removable media (e.g., floppy disk) to remote review stations for either off-line or on-line analysis. Second, portions or all of the EEG can be reformatted retrospectively using different time scales, filters, or montages for optimal display of abnormalities. Third, because the EEG is stored in computer memory and displayed on a high-resolution video monitor, the recording process is essentially paperless. Fourth, innovative display methods can be used to present EEG results to nonelectroencephalographers. And finally, archiving is simpler, less expensive, and more compact because digitized EEG can be stored on com-

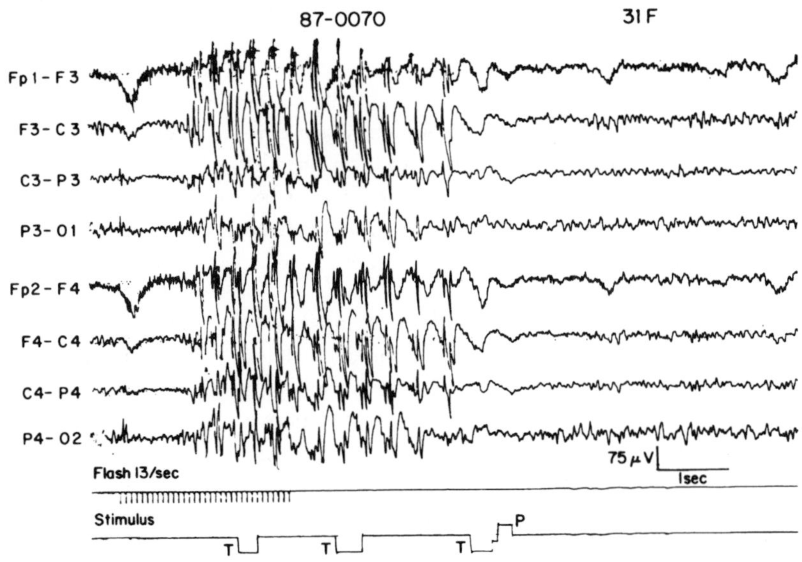

FIGURE 37A.2 Intermittent stroboscopic light stimulation at 13 per second elicited generalized bursts of 4- to 5-Hz spike-wave activity, termed a photoparoxysmal (photoconvulsive) response. The spike-wave paroxysm was associated with a brief absence, as documented by the patient's (P) inability to respond to a tone given by the technologist (T). Normal responsiveness returned immediately on cessation of the spike-wave activity. The remainder of the EEG was normal.

puter hard disks, tape drives, or optical disks rather than as complete paper records, selected paper samples, or microfilm rolls. When necessary, a hard copy of any EEG segment can be made using a printing device. As computers continue to evolve at an extraordinarily rapid pace, it is likely that digital EEG machines will incorporate additional desirable features allowing, for example, improved network and communication functions, a wide range of signal-processing options, and versatility for interfacing with other physiological and computer equipment.

Clinical Uses of the Electroencephalogram

The EEG assesses physiological alterations in brain activity. Many changes are nonspecific but some are highly suggestive of specific entities (epilepsy, herpes encephalitis, metabolic encephalopathy). The EEG is also useful in following the course of patients with altered states of consciousness and may, in certain circumstances, provide prognostic information. It is especially important in the determination of brain death.

EEG is not a screening test but is ordered to answer a particular problem posed by the patient. Sufficient clinical information must be provided so that an appropriate test can be designed that allows a meaningful electrographic clinical correlation. The question to be addressed by the EEG should be specifically stated on the request.

EEG interpretation should be rational and based on a systematic analysis that uses consistent parameters that permit comparisons to be made with findings expected from the patient's age and circumstances of recording. Accurate interpretation requires high-quality recording. This depends on trained technologists who understand the importance of meticulous electrode application, proper use of instrument controls, recognition and, where possible, elimination of artifacts, and appropriate selection of recording montages to allow optimal display of cerebral electrical activity.

Epilepsy

EEG is usually the most helpful laboratory test when a diagnosis of epilepsy is considered. Because the onset of seizures is unpredictable and their occurrence is relatively infrequent in most patients, EEG is usually obtained when the patient is asymptomatic. Fortunately, electrical abnormalities in the EEG occur in most patients with epilepsy even between attacks. Interictal findings, however, must always be interpreted with caution. Although certain patterns of abnormality may support a diagnosis of epilepsy, most *epileptiform discharges* correlate poorly with the frequency and likelihood of recurrence of epileptic seizures. In certain cases, they may not even help in distinguishing epilepsy from other paroxysmal but nonepileptic conditions. Furthermore, a substantial number of patients with unquestionable epilepsy have normal EEGs on any given occasion. The most convincing proof that a patient's episodic symptoms are epileptic is obtained by recording an *electrographic seizure discharge* during a typical behavioral attack. Although ictal EEG tracings greatly increase EEG sensitivity in assessing the pathophysiology of specific behavioral episodes, the clinician must still be aware of limitations inherent in such recordings (discussed later).

The only EEG finding that has a high correlation with epilepsy is epileptiform activity, a term used to describe *spikes* and *sharp waves* that are clearly distinct from ongoing background activity. Both clinical and experimental evidence supports a specific association between epileptiform discharges and seizure susceptibility. Only about 2% of

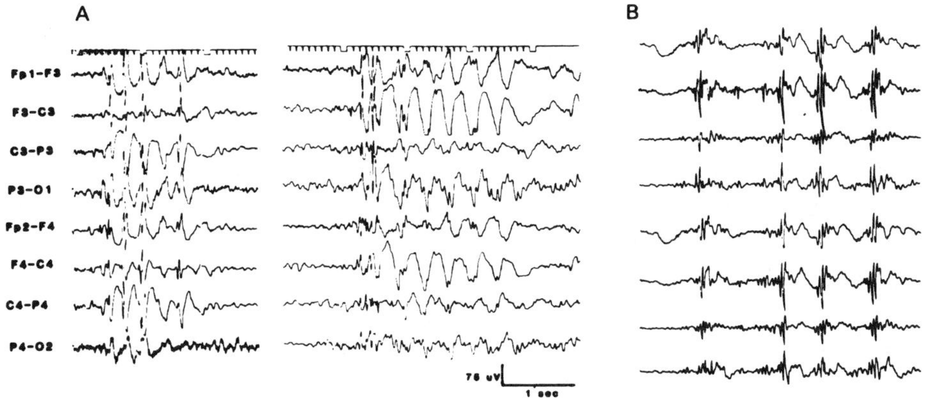

FIGURE 37A.3 Examples of generalized spike-wave patterns from different patients with primary generalized (idiopathic) epilepsy. The patient in A had mainly tonic-clonic seizures, with occasional absence attacks. The patient in B had juvenile myoclonic epilepsy.

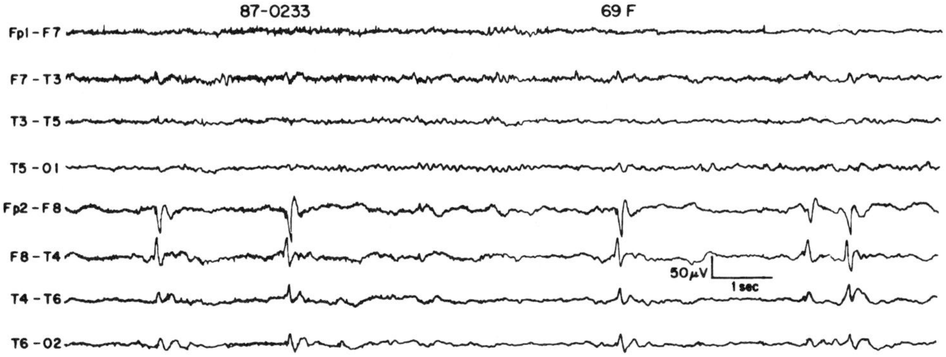

FIGURE 37A.4 Focal right anterior temporal spikes occurring in a 69-year-old woman with complex partial seizures following a stroke involving branches of the right middle cerebral artery.

nonepileptic patients have epileptiform EEGs, while as many as 90% of patients with epilepsy show epileptiform activity, depending on the circumstances of recording and the number of studies obtained.

In addition to epileptiform patterns, EEGs in patients with epilepsy often show excessive focal or generalized slow wave activity. Less often there may be asymmetries of frequency or voltage. These findings are not unique to epilepsy and may be seen in other conditions such as static encephalopathies, brain tumors, migraine, and trauma. In patients with unusual spells, nonspecific changes on EEG should be weighed cautiously and not considered direct evidence for a diagnosis of epilepsy. On the other hand, when clinical data are unequivocal, or when epileptiform discharges occur as well, the degree and extent of background EEG changes may provide information important for judging the likelihood of an underlying focal cerebral lesion, a more diffuse encephalopathy, or a progressive neurological syndrome. Additionally, EEG findings may help determine prognosis and aid in the decision to discontinue antiepileptic medication (Callaghan et al. 1988).

The type of epileptiform activity on EEG is helpful in classifying a patient's seizure type correctly and sometimes in identifying a specific epileptic syndrome. Clinically, generalized tonic-clonic seizures may be generalized from the outset or secondary to spread from a focus. Lapses of awareness with automatisms may be a manifestation either of a generalized nonconvulsive form of epilepsy (*absence seizures*) or of focal epileptogenic dysfunction (*temporal lobe epilepsy*). The initial clinical features of a seizure may be uncertain because of postictal amnesia or nocturnal occurrence. In these and similar situations, the EEG can provide information crucial to correct diagnosis and appropriate therapy.

In generalized seizures of nonfocal origin, the EEG typically shows bilaterally synchronous diffuse bursts of spikes and spike-wave discharges (Figure 37A.3). All generalized EEG epileptiform patterns share certain common features, although the exact expression of the spike-wave activity varies depending on whether the patient has pure absence, tonic-clonic, myoclonic, or atonic-astatic seizures. The EEG may also distinguish between primary and secondary generalized epilepsy. In the former instance there is no demonstrable cerebral disease, whereas in the latter, evidence can be found for diffuse brain damage. Typically, primary (idiopathic) generalized epilepsy is associated with normal or near-normal EEG background rhythms, whereas secondary (symptomatic) epilepsy is associated with some degree of generalized slow wave activity.

Consistently focal epileptiform activity is the signature of partial (focal) epilepsy (Figure 37A.4). With the exception of the *benign focal epilepsies of childhood* (Lerman 1992),

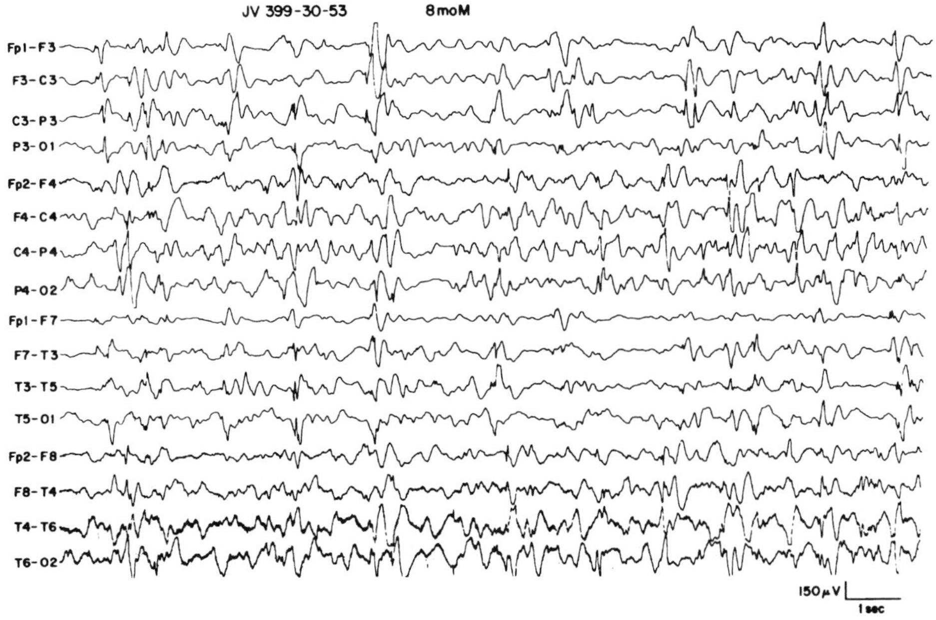

FIGURE 37A.5 EEG pattern termed hypsarrhythmia from an 8-month-old boy with infantile spasms. Background activity is high voltage and unorganized with abundant multifocal spikes.

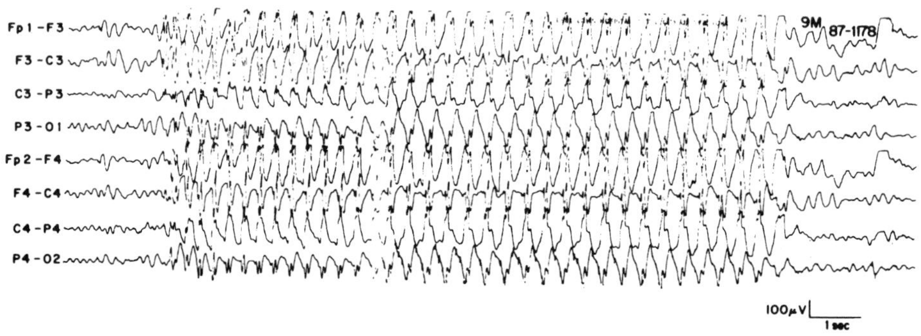

FIGURE 37A.6 A 3-Hz spike-and-wave paroxysm from a 9-year-old boy with absence seizures (petit mal epilepsy). During this 12-second discharge, the child was unresponsive and had rhythmic eye blinking.

focal epileptiform activity is caused by neuronal dysfunction associated with demonstrable brain disease. The waveform of focal epileptiform discharges is largely independent of localization, but there is a reasonable correlation between spike location and the type of ictal behavior. *Anterior temporal spikes* are almost always associated with complex partial seizures, *rolandic spikes* with simple motor or sensory seizures, and *occipital spikes* with primitive visual hallucinations or diminished visual function as an initial feature.

In addition to distinguishing epileptiform from nonepileptiform abnormalities, EEG analysis sometimes identifies specific electroclinical syndromes such as *hypsarrhythmia* with infantile spasms (West's syndrome) (Figure 37A.5); *3-Hz spike-and-wave activity* associated with typical absence attacks (petit mal epilepsy) (Figure 37A.6); *generalized multiple spikes and waves* (polyspike-wave) with myoclonic epilepsy, including so-called juvenile myoclonic epilepsy of Janz (see Figure 37A.3B); *generalized sharp and slow waves* (slow spike and wave) with Lennox-Gastaut syndrome (Figure 37A.7); *central-midtemporal spikes* with benign rolandic epilepsy (Figure 37A.8); and *periodic lateralized epileptiform discharges* with acute destructive cerebral lesions including hemorrhagic cerebral infarction, a rapidly growing malignancy, or herpes simplex encephalitis (Figure 37A.9).

The increased availability of special monitoring facilities for simultaneous closed-circuit television, EEG recording, and ambulatory EEG cassette recorders has improved diagnostic accuracy and the reliability of seizure classification. Prolonged, continuous recordings through one or more complete sleep-wake cycles are the best way to document ictal episodes and should be considered in patients whose interictal EEGs are normal or nondiagnostic, and in clinical dilemmas that can only be resolved by recording actual behavioral events. Although EEG documentation of an ictal discharge establishes the epileptic nature of a corresponding behavioral change, the converse is not necessarily true. Sometimes the EEG recording is so obscured by muscle or movement artifacts that it is impossible to know if any EEG change has occurred. In these circumstances, postictal slowing is usually indicative of an epileptic event if similar slow waves are not present elsewhere in the recording, and if the EEG subsequently returns to its baseline condition. In addition, focal seizures that are not accompanied by alteration in consciousness occasionally have no detectable scalp correlate. On the other hand, per-

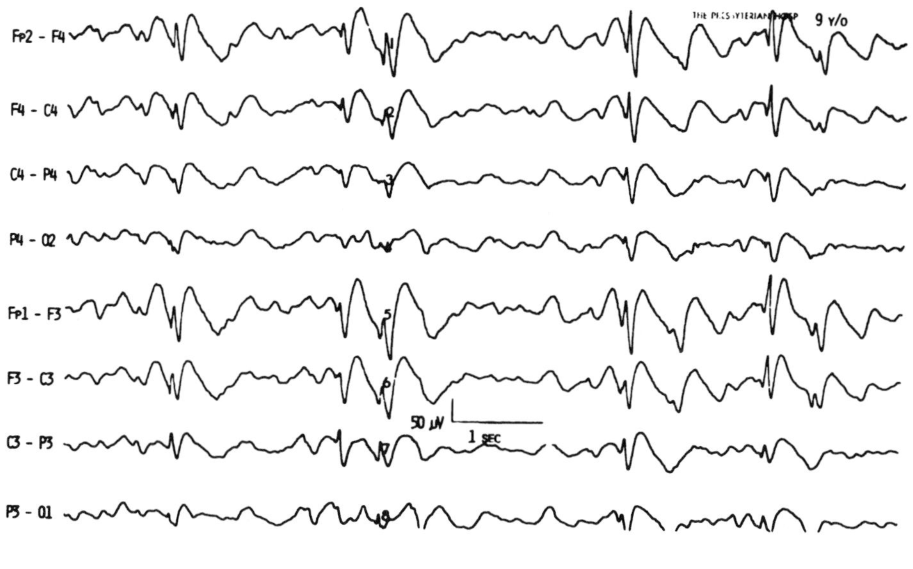

FIGURE 37A.7 Generalized sharp and slow wave discharges in a 9-year-old child with mental retardation and uncontrolled atypical absence, tonic and atonic generalized seizures. This constellation of clinical and EEG features constitutes the Lennox-Gastaut syndrome.

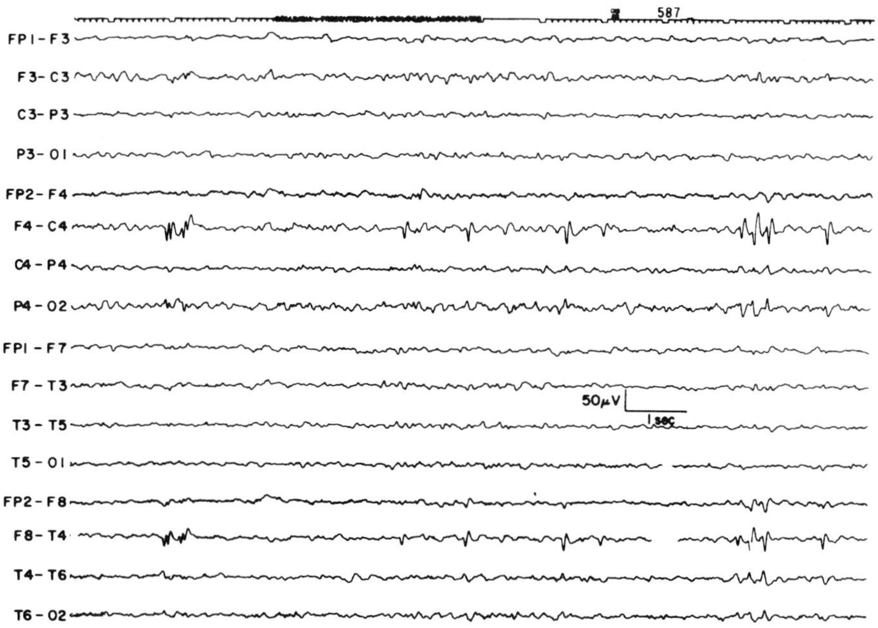

FIGURE 37A.8 EEG obtained during drowsiness in a 10-year-old boy with benign rolandic epilepsy. Stereotyped di- or triphasic sharp waves occur in the right central-parietal and midtemporal regions.

sistence of alpha activity and absence of slowing during and after an apparent convulsive episode are inconsistent with an epileptic generalized tonic-clonic seizure.

Focal Cerebral Lesions

The use of the EEG to detect focal cerebral disturbances has declined in the last 15 years because of the development and widespread availability of computerized anatomical imaging techniques. Nonetheless, the EEG has a role in documenting focal physiological dysfunction in the absence of discernible structural pathology, and in evaluating the functional disturbance produced by known lesions.

Focal delta activity is the usual EEG sign of a local disturbance. A structural lesion is likely if the delta activity is continuously present; shows variability in waveform, amplitude, duration, and morphology (so-called arrhythmic or polymorphic activity); and persists during changes in wake-sleep states (Figure 37A.10). The localizing value of focal delta is increased when it is topographically discrete or associated with depression or loss of superimposed faster background frequencies. Superficial lesions tend to produce restricted EEG changes, while deep cerebral lesions produce hemispheric, or even bilateral, delta activity.

Bilateral paroxysmal bursts of rhythmic delta waves (Figure 37A.11) with frontal predominance were once attributed to subfrontal, deep midline, or posterior fossa lesions, but they are nonspecific and seen more often with diffuse encephalopathies. *Focal or lateralized intermittent bursts of rhythmic delta waves* as the prominent EEG ab-

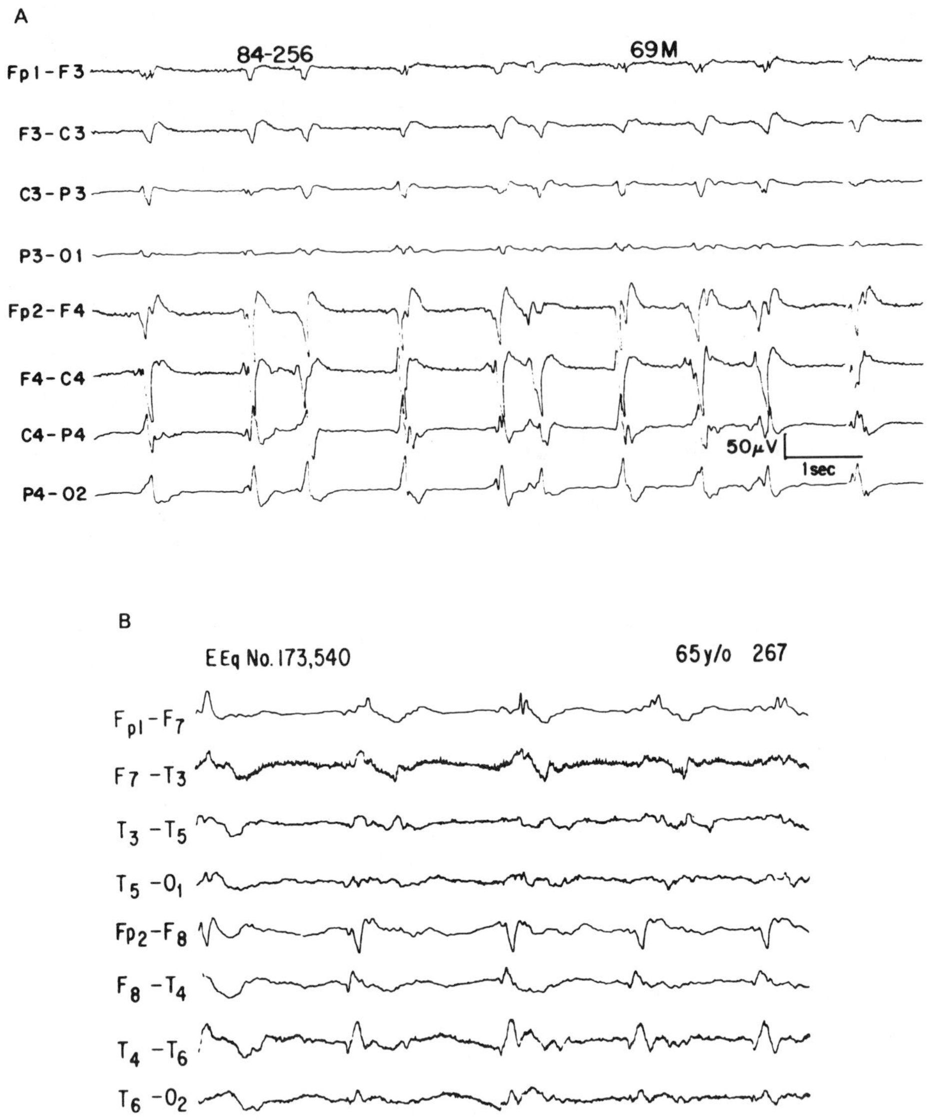

FIGURE 37A.9 Two examples of periodic lateralized epileptiform discharges (PLEDs). A. Right parasagittal PLEDs in a 69-year-old man with severe brain damage due to meningitis with multiple cerebral infarctions. B. A 65-year-old woman with herpes simplex encephalitis. PLEDs are bilateral, but with a right-sided predominance.

normality suggest a deep supratentorial (periventricular or diencephalic) lesion.

The character and distribution of the EEG changes caused by a focal lesion depend on its size, its distance from the cortical surface, the specific structures involved, and its acuity. A small stroke critically located in the thalamus may produce widespread hemispheric slowing and alteration in sleep spindles and alpha rhythm regulation. The same-sized lesion located at the cortical surface produces few, if any, EEG findings.

Single lacunae usually produce little or no change in the EEG. Similarly, transient ischemic attacks not associated with chronic cerebral hypoperfusion or imminent occlusion of a major vessel do not significantly affect the EEG outside the symptomatic period. Superficial cortical or large, deep hemispheric infarctions are usually associated with localized EEG abnormalities. If the infarction is nonhemorrhagic, the CT scan may be normal at the same time that the EEG clearly documents a functional disturbance. In addition to showing the functional effects of acute infarction, EEG occasionally shows bilateral focal abnormalities in a patient with stroke, suggesting more extensive disease or emboli. Cortical laminar necrosis rarely produces CT abnormalities but often causes focal or widespread EEG changes. Marginal regional perfusion and impending infarction may be suggested by EEG and confirmed by regional cerebral blood flow studies in the absence of CT change. Consensus has not been reached on the use of EEG in prognosis following stroke.

Focal EEG changes (and other nonepileptiform abnormalities) are common in migraine. The likelihood of an abnormal EEG, and the severity of the abnormality, are related to the timing and character of the migraine attack. EEGs are more likely to be focally abnormal with complicated rather than with common migraine, and during rather than between headaches.

FIGURE 37A.10 A. A 46-year-old man with a glioblastoma involving the right temporal and parietal lobes. B. The EEG shown demonstrates continuous arrhythmic slowing over the right temporal and parieto-occipital areas. In addition, there is loss of the alpha rhythm and overriding faster frequencies seen in corresponding areas of the left cerebral hemisphere.

A

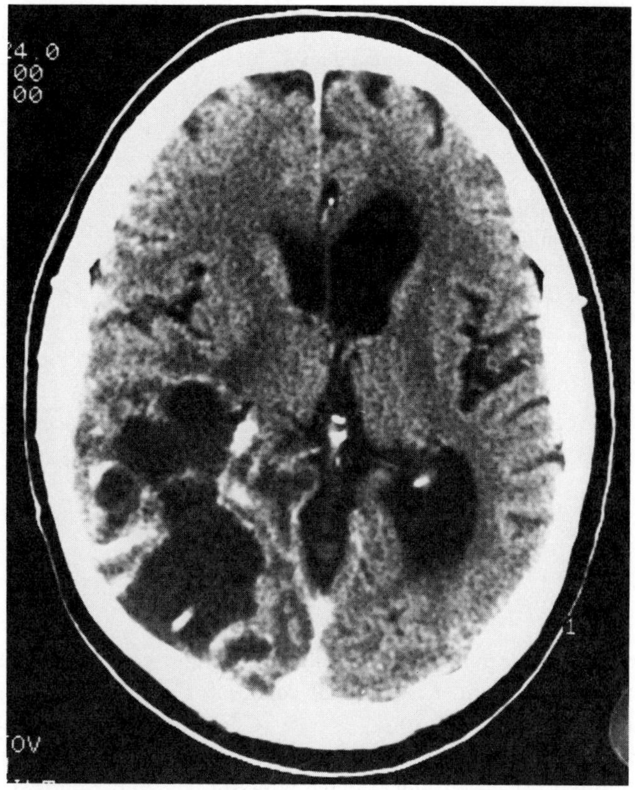

B

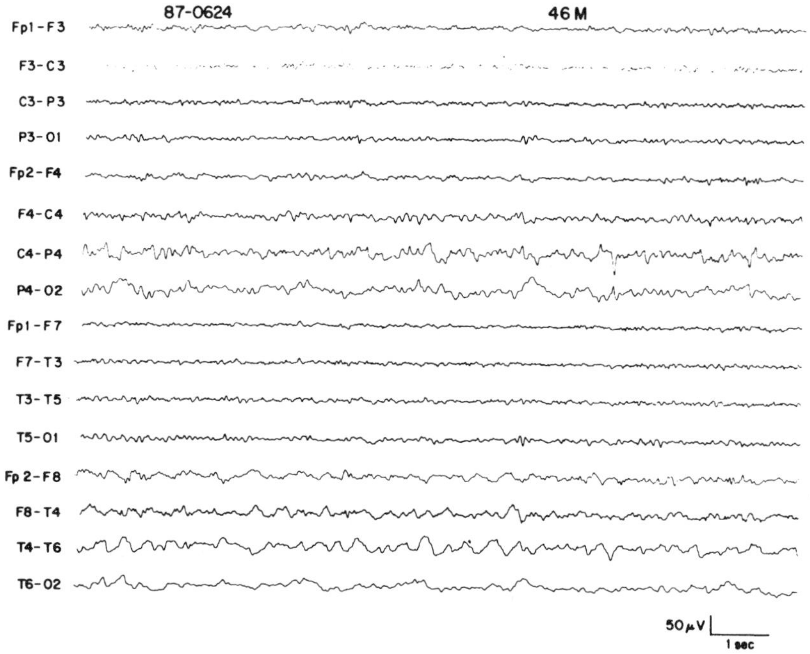

EEG changes seen with brain tumors are caused by disturbances in bordering brain parenchyma; tumor tissue is electrically silent. Focal EEG changes are caused by interference with patterns of normal neuronal synaptic activity; by destruction or alteration of the cortical neurons; and by metabolic effects caused by changes in blood flow, cellular metabolism, or the neuronal microenvironment. More diffuse EEG changes are the consequence of increased intracranial pressure, shift of midline structures, or hydrocephalus. EEG is especially helpful in following the extent of cerebral dysfunction over time, in distinguishing between direct effects of the neoplasm and superimposed

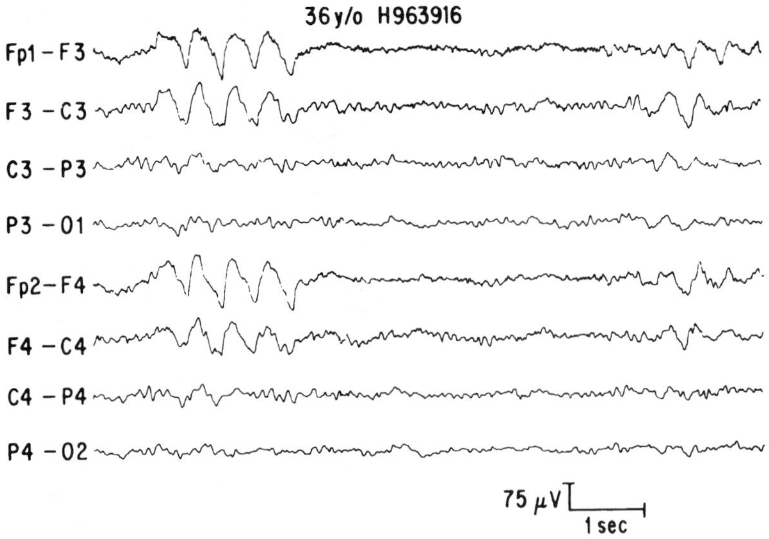

FIGURE 37A.11 Bursts of intermittent rhythmic delta waves in a 36-year-old man with primary generalized epilepsy and tonic-clonic seizures. Generalized spike-wave activity occurred elsewhere in the EEG. The intermittent rhythmic delta waves are a nonspecific manifestation of his generalized epileptic disorder. (Courtesy of Dr. Bruce J. Fisch.)

metabolic or toxic encephalopathies, and in differentiating among epileptic, ischemic, and noncerebral causes for episodic symptoms.

The role of EEG in the management of patients with head injuries is limited. Transient generalized slowing is common after concussion. A persistent area of continuous localized slow wave activity suggests cerebral contusion even in the absence of a focal clinical or CT abnormality, and unilateral voltage depression suggests subdural hematoma. EEG in the first 3 months after injury does not predict posttraumatic epilepsy.

Altered States of Consciousness

The EEG retains a major role in the evaluation of patients with altered levels of consciousness. It complements the clinical examination when consciousness is significantly depressed, because EEG permits a reasonably critical assessment of supratentorial brain function. Abnormalities are typically nonspecific with regard to etiology. There is, however, a generally good correlation with the clinical state. Some findings are more suggestive of particular causes than of others and are occasionally prognostically useful as well. Specific questions that the EEG may help answer, depending on the clinical presentation, are the following:

1. Are psychogenic factors playing a major role?
2. Is the process diffuse, focal, or multifocal?
3. Is unrecognized epileptic activity depressing consciousness (*nonconvulsive status epilepticus*)?
4. Is there evidence of improvement despite relatively little change in the clinical picture?
5. Are there findings that assist in assessing prognosis?

Metabolic Encephalopathies. Metabolic derangements affecting the brain diffusely are one of the most common causes of altered mental function in a general hospital. Generalized slow wave activity is the main indication of decreased consciousness. The degree of EEG slowing parallels closely the patient's mental status and ranges from only minor slowing of alpha rhythm frequency (slight inattentiveness and decreased alertness) to continuous delta activity (coma). Slow wave activity sometimes becomes bisynchronous and assumes a high-voltage and sharply contoured triphasic morphology, especially over the frontal head regions (Figure 37A.12). These *triphasic waves* were originally considered diagnostic of hepatic failure but are now known to occur with equal frequency in other metabolic disorders, such as uremia, hyponatremia, hyperthyroidism, anoxia, and hyperosmolarity (Fisch and Klass 1988). The value of triphasic waves is that they suggest a metabolic cause in an unresponsive patient.

Some EEG features increase the likelihood of a specific metabolic disorder. Prominent, generalized rhythmic beta activity raises the suspicion of drug intoxication in a comatose patient. Severe generalized voltage depression indicates impaired energy metabolism and suggests hypothyroidism if anoxia and hypothermia can be excluded. A photoconvulsive response is seen more often with uremia than with other causes of metabolic encephalopathy. Focal seizure activity is common in patients with hyperosmolar coma.

Hypoxia. Hypoxia, with or without circulatory arrest, produces a wide range of EEG abnormalities depending on the severity and reversibility of the brain damage. EEGs obtained 6 hours or more following the hypoxic insult may show patterns that have prognostic value. The validity of such findings is strengthened if sequential EEGs are obtained. EEG abnormalities associated with poor neurological outcome are *alpha coma*, *burst suppression*, and *periodic patterns*.

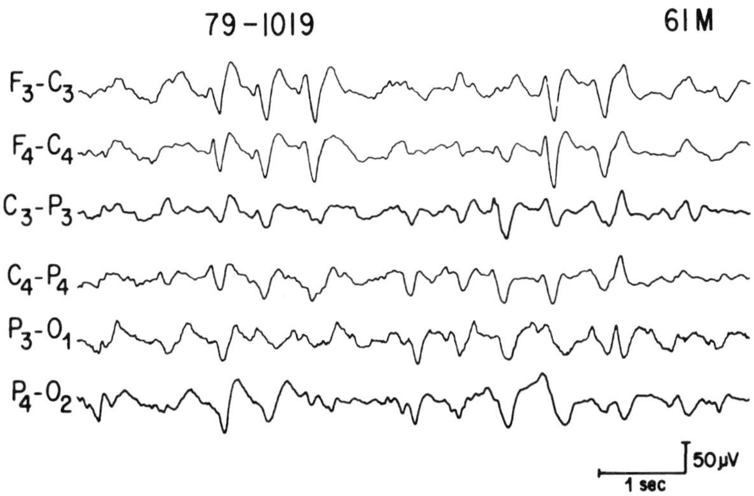

FIGURE 37A.12 Triphasic waves in a 61-year-old man with hepatic failure. (Courtesy of Dr. Bruce J. Fisch.)

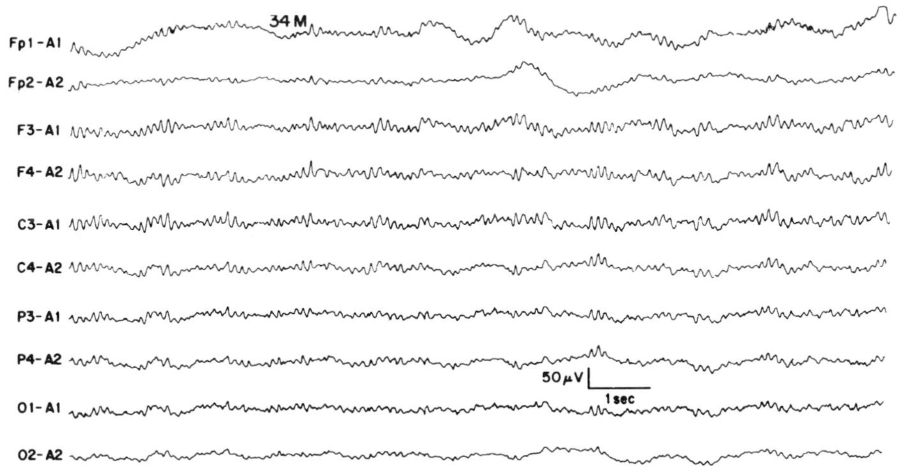

FIGURE 37A.13 Alpha coma in a 34-year-old man with severe hypoxic-ischemic brain damage following subarachnoid hemorrhage with diffuse prolonged cerebral vasospasm. Unlike the normal alpha rhythm, the alpha range activity in this comatose patient is widespread but maximal frontally, unreactive, and superimposed on low-voltage arrhythmic delta frequencies.

The term *alpha coma* refers to the apparent paradoxical appearance of monorhythmic alpha frequency activity in the EEG of a comatose patient; the EEG may appear normal to the inexperienced observer (Figure 37A.13). In contrast to normal alpha activity, that seen with alpha coma is generalized, often maximal frontally, and unreactive to external stimuli.

The burst suppression pattern consists of occasional generalized bursts of medium- to high-voltage mixed-frequency slow wave activity, sometimes with intermixed spikes, with intervening periods of severe voltage depression or cerebral inactivity (Figure 37A.14). The bursts may be accompanied by massive myoclonic body jerks.

The periodic pattern consists of generalized spikes or sharp waves that recur with a relatively fixed interval, typically 1–2 per second (Figure 37A.15). Sometimes the periodic sharp waves occur independently over each hemisphere. A postanoxic periodic pattern is usually accompanied by myoclonic jerks of the limbs or whole body.

The prognostic value of these patterns is related exclusively to cause. Similar findings are seen with potentially reversible causes of coma including deep anesthesia, drug overdose, and severe liver or kidney failure.

Infectious Diseases. Of all infectious diseases affecting the brain, EEG is most useful in the initial assessment of patients with possible herpes simplex encephalitis. Early and accurate diagnosis is important because the response to acyclovir is best when treatment is started early. Although a definitive diagnosis is made only by brain biopsy, characteristic EEG changes in the clinical setting of encephalitis help select patients for early treatment and biopsy. The EEG is usually abnormal and suggestive of herpes infection before CT lesions are recognized.

Viral encephalitis is expected to cause diffuse polymorphic slow wave activity and a normal EEG raises doubt about the diagnosis. With herpes simplex encephalitis, the majority of patients show focal temporal or frontal-temporal slowing that may be unilateral or, if bilateral, asymmet-

FIGURE 37A.14 Suppression burst pattern in a 53-year-old woman with anoxic encephalopathy following cardiorespiratory arrest. The patient died several days later. (Courtesy of Dr. Barbara S. Koppel.)

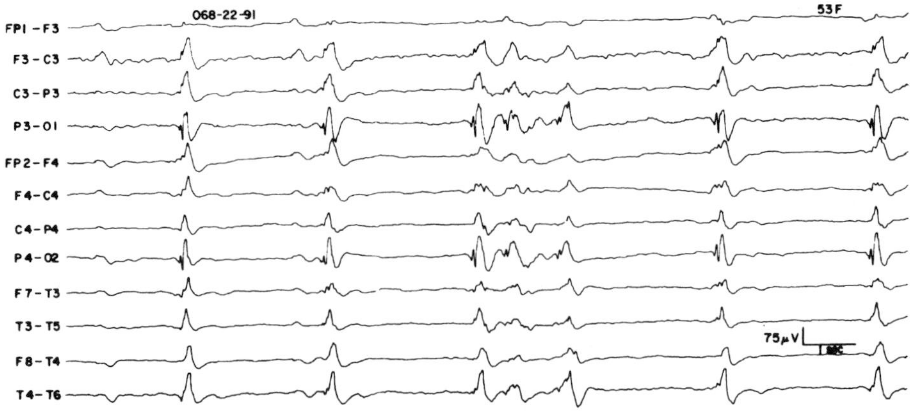

rical. Periodic sharp wave complexes over one or both frontotemporal regions (occasionally in other locations and sometimes generalized) add additional specificity to the EEG findings (see Figure 37A.9B). These diagnostic features usually appear between the second and fifteenth day of illness and are sometimes detected only with serial tracings.

Bacterial meningitis causes severe and widespread EEG abnormalities, typically profound slowing and voltage depression, but viral meningitis produces little in the way of significant changes. Although CT has replaced EEG in the evaluation of patients with suspected brain abscess, focal EEG changes may be seen in the early stage of cerebritis, before an encapsulated lesion is demonstrable on CT.

EEG abnormalities usually diminish as the patient recovers, but the rate of resolution of clinical deficits and the electrographic findings may be different. It is not possible to predict either residual neurological morbidity or postencephalitic seizures by EEG criteria. An early return of normal EEG activity does not exclude the possibility of persistent neurological impairment.

Brain Death. The diagnosis of brain death rests on strict clinical criteria that, when satisfied unambiguously, permit a conclusive determination of irreversible loss of brain function. In the United States, *brain death* is defined as "irreversible cessation of all functions of the entire brain,

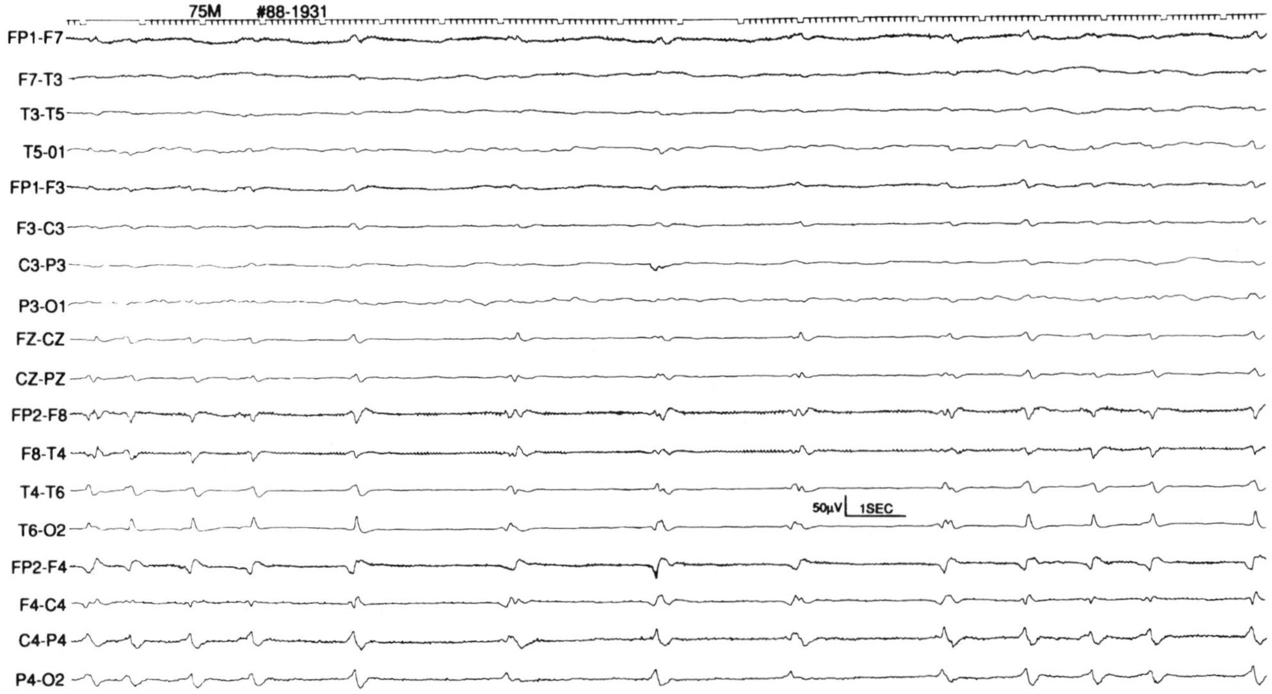

FIGURE 37A.15 Periodic pattern in a patient with anoxic encephalopathy following cardiorespiratory arrest. The patient was paralyzed with pancuronium because of bilateral myoclonus.

including the brain stem" (President's Commission 1981). Because the EEG is a measure of cerebral, especially cortical, function, it has been widely used to provide objective evidence that brain function is lost. Several studies have demonstrated that enduring loss of cerebral electrical activity (termed *electrocerebral inactivity* or *electrocerebral silence*) accompanies clinical brain death and is never associated with recovery of neurological function. Determination of electrocerebral inactivity is technically demanding and requires a special recording protocol. Reference should be made to criteria established by the American EEG Society (1986).

Temporary and reversible loss of cerebral electrical activity can be seen immediately following cardiorespiratory resuscitation, drug overdose from central nervous system depressants, and severe hypothermia. Therefore, accurate interpretation of an EEG demonstrating electrocerebral inactivity must take into account these exceptional circumstances.

Occasional patients who satisfy clinical criteria for brain death have residual evidence of minimal EEG activity. If clinical criteria have been rigorously met, there is no evidence that this residual electrical activity indicates survival (Grigg et al. 1987). On the other hand, rare patients in a chronic vegetative state with evidence of brain stem function have isoelectric EEGs, probably reflecting total neocortical death. As a result, determination of death on neurological grounds in the United Kingdom, unlike the United States, places sole emphasis on demonstration of (1) irreversible structural brain damage, (2) apneic coma, and (3) loss of brain stem reflexes.

Although some hospital protocols in the United States require EEG proof of cerebral inactivity as part of the brain death determination, we agree with the medical consultants to the President's Commission (1981) that the EEG is best viewed as a confirmatory test. In this context, the EEG may be helpful in ensuring diagnostic accuracy and in providing objective documentation in support of clinical findings.

Aging and Dementia

Because the EEG is a measure of cortical function, it should theoretically be useful in the diagnosis and classification of dementia. However, the utility of single EEG examinations in the evaluation of patients with known or suspected dementing illnesses is often disappointing. Two important reasons for this are (1) problems encountered in distinguishing the effects on cerebral electrical activity of normal aging from those caused by disease processes, and (2) absence of generally accepted quantifiable methods of analysis and statistically valid comparison measures.

With increasing age over 65, there is normally a slight reduction in alpha rhythm frequency and in the total amount of alpha activity. Normal elderly persons also show slightly increased amounts of theta and delta activity, especially over the temporal and frontotemporal regions, as well as changes in sleep patterns. Early in the course of some dementing illnesses, there may be no apparent EEG abnormality (this is the rule with Alzheimer's disease, for example), or the normal, age-related changes may become exaggerated, differing more in degree than in kind.

In practice, the EEG can assist in the evaluation of suspected dementia by confirming abnormal cerebral function where there is the possibility of a psychogenic disorder, and by delineating whether the process is focal or diffuse. Sequential EEGs are usually more helpful than a single tracing, and an early test in the course of the illness may provide more specific information than a later one. Overall, the degree of EEG abnormality shows a good correlation with the degree of dementia.

EEG findings in Alzheimer's disease are highly dependent on timing. The EEG is initially normal or shows an alpha rhythm at or just below the lower limits of normal. Generalized slowing appears as the disease progresses. In patients with focal cognitive deficits, there may be accentuation of slow frequency activity over the corresponding brain area. Continuous focal slowing is sufficiently unusual as to raise the possibility of another diagnosis. Prominent focal or bilateral independent slow wave activity, especially if seen in company with a normal alpha rhythm, favors multifocal disease—for example, multiple cerebral infarcts. Sometimes a specific cause may be suggested. For example, an EEG showing generalized typical *periodic sharp wave complexes* in a patient with dementia is virtually diagnostic of Creutzfeldt-Jakob disease (Figure 37A.16).

Event-related evoked potentials have been applied to the study of dementia (Goodin and Aminoff 1992). These are long-latency events (that is, potentials occurring more than 150 msec following the stimulus) that are heavily dependent on psychic and cognitive factors. Ideally, they measure the brain's intrinsic mechanisms for processing certain types of information and are potentially valuable in the electrophysiological assessment of dementia. The best known of the event-related potentials is the *P300,* or *P3, wave.* The place of these long-latency evoked potentials in the evaluation of dementia is still under investigation, but it may be possible to help distinguish among types of dementia by the pattern of electrophysiological abnormality.

Computerized Electroencephalography and Topographic Brain Mapping

Topographic mapping of computerized EEG activity is achieving a certain popularity, and numerous mapping systems are now commercially available. Topographic mapping refers to the display of EEG data using procedures that emphasize the spatial relationships of selected EEG characteristics (Plate 37A.I) (Nuwer 1990). Like conventional EEG, topographic maps of brain electrical activity rely on visual inspection for analysis. In addition, topographic maps offer the potential advantage of displaying statistical values derived from quantitative comparisons.

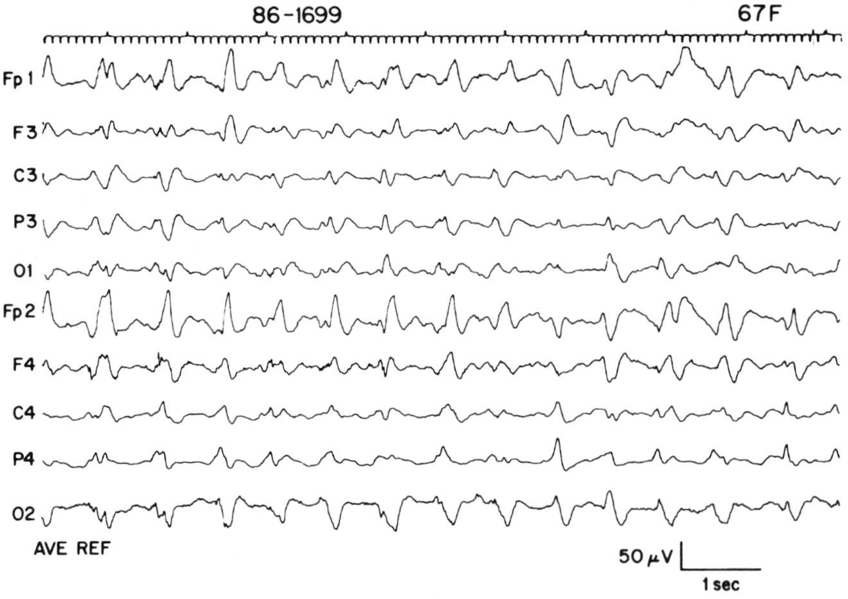

FIGURE 37A.16 Periodic sharp-wave pattern in a 67-year-old woman with Creutzfeldt-Jakob disease. There are generalized, bisynchronous diphasic sharp waves occurring about 1.5–2.0 per second.

Currently, topographic maps are used to display (1) EEG voltage distributions at a particular point in time (time domain mapping), (2) features derived from frequency analysis of EEG background (frequency domain mapping), and (3) statistical comparisons (statistical mapping). Examples of voltage maps include averaged epileptiform spikes and evoked potentials. Spike averaging may reveal the presence of widespread or unexpected field distributions that cannot otherwise be appreciated. Frequency domain topographic mapping of background activity is usually accomplished by plotting some aspect of the frequency spectrum derived from a fast Fourier transform. The major practical limitation of frequency domain topographic maps has been the lack of any general consensus regarding normal limits for any particular spectral feature.

Until statistically reliable normal limits for mapped values are determined and agreed on, clinical use of topographic mapping should serve mainly to inform the electroencephalographer of possible additional information that may be obtained from reinspection of the conventional EEG or evoked potential record. At this time, we do not believe that findings from topographic mapping of cerebral electrical activity should be used as clinical evidence for brain dysfunction in the absence of significant changes by routine testing methods (Fisch and Pedley 1989; Lopes da Silva 1990).

Magnetoencephalography

MEG is a measure of brain function equivalent to EEG (Sato et al. 1991). The same neuronal sources that generate electrical activity also give rise to magnetic fields. Because of the shielding requirements and the complex and costly instrumentation necessary to measure neuromagnetic fields, MEG has been, and is likely to remain, limited to research applications. To date, MEG has been used mainly to localize sources of evoked potentials and focal epileptiform activity (Rose et al. 1987; Sutherling et al. 1988). It has also been applied, in a more limited way, to investigations of patients with psychiatric disorders, stroke, and migraine.

MEG differs from EEG in several ways that are theoretically useful. For example, EEG potentials are volume conducted and are thus easily attentuated by the overlying cerebrospinal fluid, dura, and skull. Magnetic fields are less affected by these structures. In addition, EEG measures cortical current sources oriented in all directions but emphasizes radially oriented dipoles. MEG more accurately measures tangential dipoles that are parallel to the cortical surface. Finally, MEG has a higher degree of spatial resolution for some current sources than does scalp EEG. There may be fewer differences, however, between MEG and EEG if MEG is compared not to conventional scalp EEG but to EEG recordings obtained using voltage topography and source localization techniques. A note of caution is warranted, however. Dipole models, whether used in EEG or MEG, employ a number of assumptions that, if applied without recognition of their limitations, can result in anatomically and physiologically erroneous conclusions.

EVOKED POTENTIALS

Evoked potentials are electrical signals generated by the nervous system in response to sensory stimuli. The timing and location of these signals are determined by the sensory system involved and the sequence in which different neural structures are activated. The stimulus paradigms used in clinical practice are chosen so that the responses they evoke are sufficiently stereotyped to allow the limits of normal to be clearly defined. Violation of these limits indicates dysfunction of the sensory pathways being studied. An overview of recording methodology, criteria for abnormality, and limitations of use is provided by the American EEG Society's "Recommended Standards for the Clinical Practice of Evoked Potentials" (1994).

Because of their low voltage, evoked potentials are generally not discernible without computer averaging to resolve them from ongoing EEG activity and other sources of electrical noise. Exceptions are the visual responses evoked by transient flash stimuli, which can be seen in the routine EEG as photic driving. Typically, however, it is necessary to present the stimulus repeatedly, averaging the time-locked brain or spinal cord responses to a series of identical stimuli, while allowing unrelated noise to average out.

In the clinical setting, evoked potential studies are properly viewed as an extension of the neurological examination. Like any neurological sign, they help reveal the existence and often suggest the location of neurological lesions. Evoked potentials, therefore, are most useful when they detect clinically silent abnormalities that might otherwise go unrecognized, or when they assist in resolving vague or equivocal symptoms and findings. Like EEG, evoked potentials are tests of function; they are not usually etiologically specific.

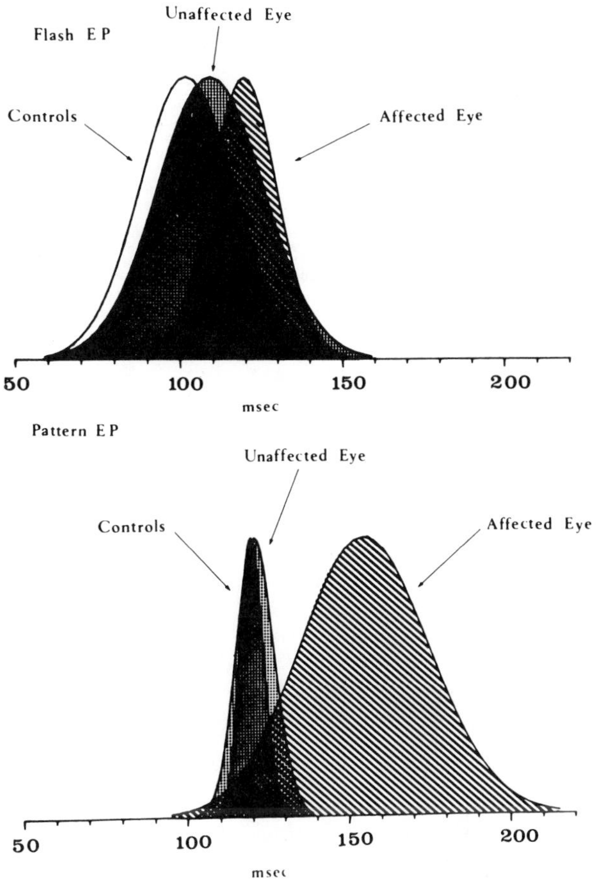

FIGURE 37A.17 Distributions of latencies of the major occipital positivity to flash (upper panel) and pattern-shift (lower panel) stimulation in healthy controls, and in the affected and unaffected eyes of patients with optic neuritis. The superior sensitivity of pattern-shift VEP to demyelinating lesions is clearly demonstrated. (Reprinted with permission from AM Halliday. The Visual Evoked Potential in the Investigation of Diseases of the Optic Nerve. In AM Halliday [ed], Evoked Potentials in Clinical Testing. New York: Churchill Livingstone, 1982.)

Visual Evoked Potentials

Cerebral visual evoked potentials (VEPs) are responses of the visual cortex to appropriate stimuli. The composite retinal response to visual stimuli, the *electroretinogram*, may be recorded separately, and the procedure may be indicated in certain clinical situations (for review, see Celesia 1993). The cerebral VEP is obtained by averaging the responses from occipital scalp electrodes generated by 100 or more sequential stimuli. Stimulus characteristics are critically important in determining what portion of the visual system will be tested by the VEP and what the sensitivity of the test will be to the presence of lesions. Initial clinical applications of VEPs employed a stroboscopic flash stimulus, but the utility of the *flash evoked VEP* is severely limited by the great variability of responses among normal individuals and its relative insensitivity to clinical lesions (Figure 37A.17). Occasionally, flash VEPs may provide limited information about the integrity of visual pathways when the preferred *pattern reversal stimulus* cannot be used, as in infants or other patients unable to cooperate for more sensitive testing methods.

Normal Visual Evoked Potential

More sensitive and reliable responses are obtained using a pattern reversal stimulus. The subject focuses on a high-contrast checkerboard of black and white squares displayed on a video or optical projection screen. The stimulus is the change of black squares to white and white squares to black (pattern reversal). When appropriate check sizes are used (15–40 minutes of arc at the subject's eye), the VEP is generated primarily by foveal and parafoveal elements. Monocular full-field stimulation is almost always employed so that the test is most sensitive to lesions of the optic nerve anterior to the chiasm. It is possible, however, to modify the stimulus presentation so that only selected portions of the visual field are stimulated, thus permitting detection of postchiasmatic abnormalities as well. VEPs elicited by pattern reversal stimuli show less intersubject variability than do flash VEPs and are much more sensitive to lesions affecting the visual pathways.

A few investigators have further refined the pattern-shift stimulus by using a black and white sinusoidal grating rather than a checkerboard pattern. This appears to enhance test sensitivity by permitting selective stimulation of retinal elements responsive to specific spatial frequencies,

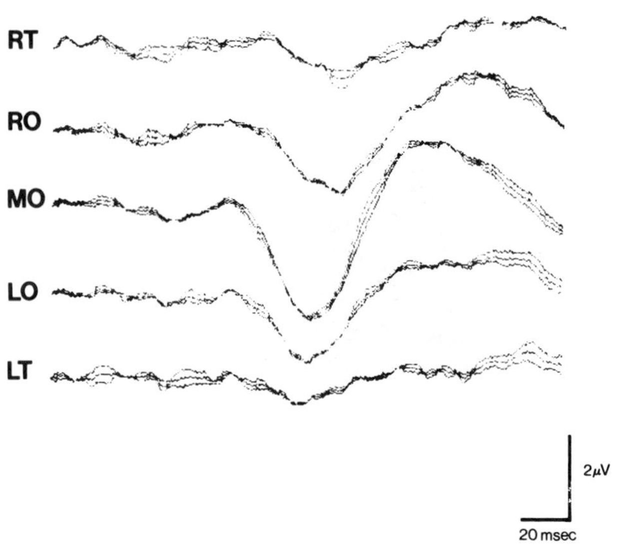

FIGURE 37A.18 Normal pattern reversal VEP to full-field monocular stimulation. The MO electrode is in the posterior midline over the occiput. RO and RT are 5 and 10 cm, respectively, to the right of MO, and LO and LT are 5 and 10 cm, respectively, to the left of MO. All electrodes are referred to Fpz. The response is largest at MO and symmetrically distributed left and right of midline.

and of cortical elements sensitive to both spatial frequency and orientation.

A normal pattern reversal VEP to full-field monocular stimulation is illustrated in Figure 37A.18. The VEP waveform is deceptively simple. It is the sum of many waveforms generated simultaneously by various areas of the retinotopically organized occipital cortex. By selectively stimulating portions of the visual field, it is possible to dissect the full-field VEP into its component waveforms. For example, Figure 37A.19, recorded from the same individual as Figure 37A.18, illustrates VEPs to right and left hemifield stimulation. It is apparent that the full-field VEP is the sum of the two hemifield responses. In principle, it is possible to divide the visual fields into progressively smaller and smaller components, and to record the VEP to each independently.

Clinical interpretation of the pattern reversal VEP is based primarily on measurement of the *latency of the P100 component* (the major positive wave having a nominal latency of about 100 msec in normal subjects) following stimulation of each eye separately. Less emphasis is placed on measurement of P100 amplitude, although intereye differences of more than 50–60% may be significant. The absolute P100 latency is measured for each eye, and then the intereye P100 latency difference is determined. These values are compared to the laboratory's normative data and a conclusion reached regarding whether the responses are normal or abnormal. Finally, the clinical significance of the findings should be interpreted, whenever possible, in light of other relevant clinical data.

Because optic nerve fibers from the temporal retina decussate at the chiasm, unilateral prolongation of P100 latency following full-field monocular stimulation implies an abnormality anterior to the optic chiasm on that side. Bilateral delay of the P100, demonstrated by separate stimulation of each eye, can be caused by bilateral lesions either anterior or posterior to the optic chiasm, or by a chiasmal lesion. Unilateral hemispherical lesions do not alter the latency of the full-field P100 (because of the contribution from the intact hemifield), but do alter the scalp topography of the response.

FIGURE 37A.19 Normal pattern-shift VEP to right and left hemifield stimulation of one eye. Same subject as Figure 37A.18. Partial field responses are asymmetrical about the midline, with the largest positivities ipsilateral to the stimulated field.

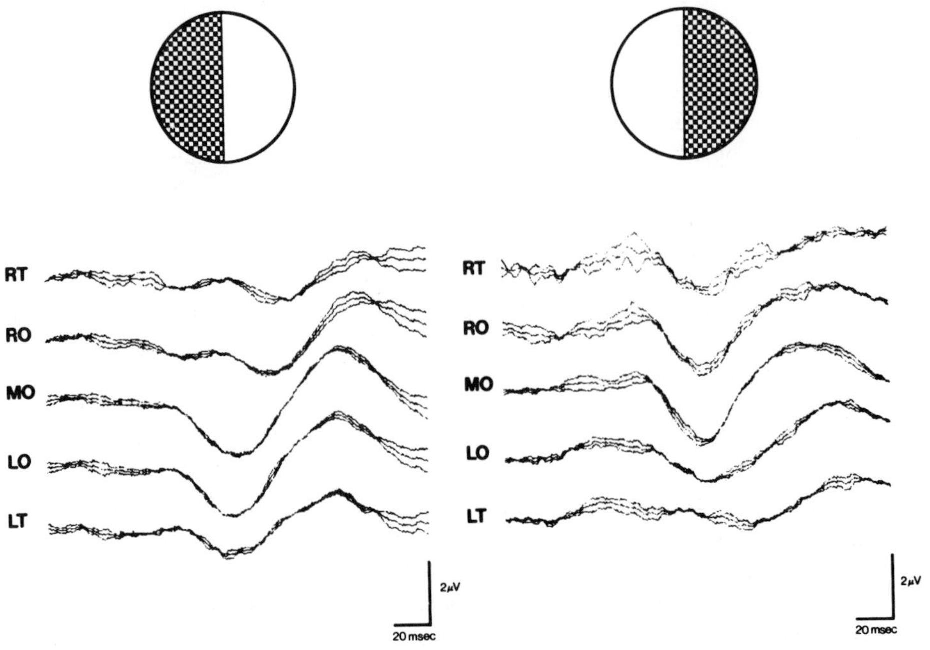

Visual Evoked Potentials in Neurological Disease

Acute optic neuritis is accompanied by marked attenuation or loss of P100 amplitude following pattern reversal stimulation of the affected eye. Following the acute attack, the VEP shows some recovery, but P100 latency almost always remains prolonged, even if functionally normal vision is restored. In patients with a history of optic neuritis, P100 latency is typically prolonged, but waveform amplitude and morphology are often relatively well preserved (Figure 37A.20). Factors contributing to changes in P100 probably include the combined effects of patchy conduction block, areas of variably slowed conduction, temporal dispersion of the afferent volley in the optic nerve, loss of some components of the normal VEP, and the appearance of previously masked components.

Pattern-shift VEPs are abnormal in nearly 100% of patients with a definite history of optic neuritis. More important, the pattern-shift VEP is a sufficiently sensitive indicator of optic nerve demyelination that it can reveal asymptomatic and clinically undetectable lesions. Thus, 70–80% of patients with definite multiple sclerosis but no history of optic neuritis or visual symptoms have abnormal VEPs. Many patients with abnormal VEPs have normal neuro-ophthalmological examinations.

Pattern reversal VEPs are highly sensitive to demyelinating lesions but are not specific for multiple sclerosis. A partial list of other causes of abnormal VEPs is given in Table 37A.1.

VEPs may be helpful in distinguishing hysteria or malingering from blindness. A normal pattern reversal VEP is strong evidence in favor of psychogenic illness. Rare cases have been reported, however, in which essentially normal VEPs were present in cortical blindness due to bilateral destruction of area 17, with preservation of areas 18 and 19, or bilateral occipital infarcts with preservation of area 17 (Celesia 1993).

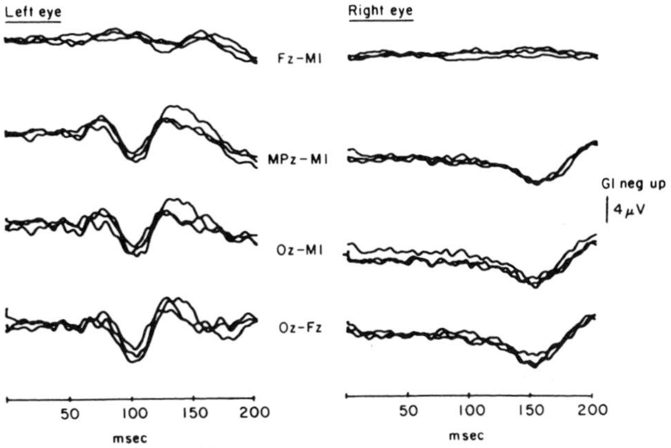

FIGURE 37A.20 Pattern-shift VEPs in a patient with right optic neuritis illustrating marked delay of the P100 component from the right eye. As is typical of demyelinating optic neuropathies, waveform is relatively preserved.

Brain Stem Auditory Evoked Potentials

Brain stem auditory evoked potentials (BAEPs) are signals generated in the auditory nerve and brain stem following an acoustic stimulus. A brief stimulus, usually a sharp click, is given to one ear through an earphone, while the opposite ear is masked with white noise to prevent its stimulation by transcranially conducted sound. The normal BAEP consists of a series of waves that occur within the first 10 msec after the stimulus. The BAEP is extremely low voltage (only about 0.5 μV), and typically about 1,000–2,000 recordings need to be averaged to resolve the BAEP waveform.

Normal Brain Stem Auditory Evoked Potential

Unlike VEPs, which are cortical responses, BAEPs are generated entirely from subcortical sites. They are characteristically much more resilient than cortical ones. This means that the subject's cooperation is not essential for their recording; in the absence of anatomical lesions, BAEPs persist essentially unchanged into deep coma or in the presence of general anesthesia.

A normal BAEP is illustrated in Figure 37A.21. The components designated by roman numerals are produced by summated neuronal activity in anatomical structures that are activated sequentially by the afferent sensory volley. Uncertainty exists regarding the relative contributions to the scalp-recorded BAEP of synaptic potentials occurring in nuclear structures and compound action potentials in fiber tracts. Although the following electroanatomical relationships may be somewhat oversimplified, they are useful for purposes of clinical localization. *Wave I*, corresponding to N1 of the electrocochleogram, represents the auditory nerve compound action potential and arises in the distalmost por-

Table 37A.1: Some causes of abnormal visual evoked potentials

Ocular disease
Major refractive error
Lens and media opacities
Glaucoma
Retinopathies
Compressive lesions
Extrinsic tumors
Optic nerve tumors
Noncompressive lesions
Demyelinating disease
Ischemic optic neuritis
Nutritional and toxic amblyopias (including pernicious anemia)
Leber's hereditary optic atrophy
Diffuse CNS disease
Adrenoleukodystrophy
Spinocerebellar degenerations
Parkinson's disease

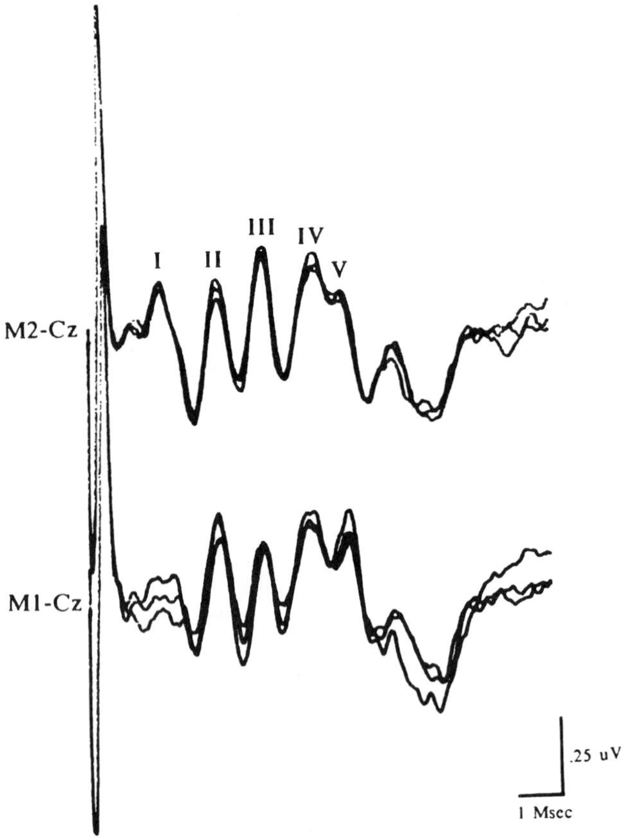

FIGURE 37A.21 Normal BAEP. Major components are labeled with roman numerals and discussed more fully in the text. M2 is an electrode over the mastoid process ipsilateral to the stimulated ear, in this case the right. Left and right mastoid electrodes are connected to an electrode at the vertex (Cz).

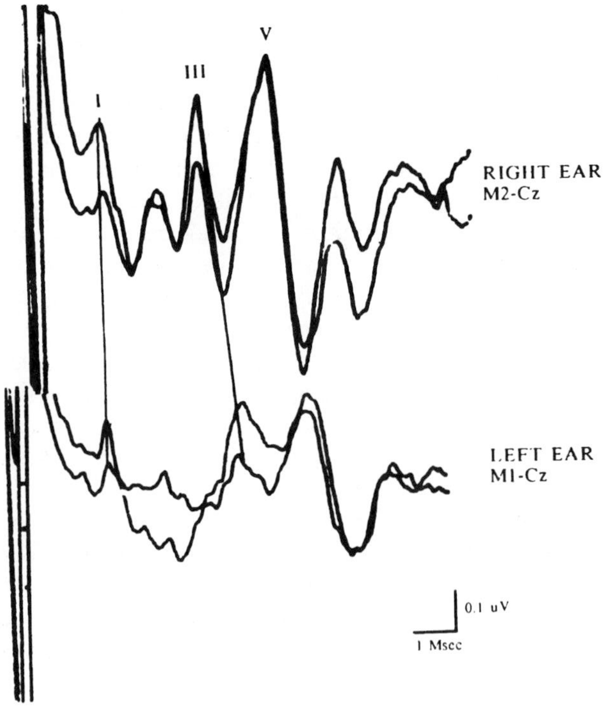

FIGURE 37A.22 BAEPs in a patient with a left acoustic neurinoma. There is prolongation of the I–III interval on that side, and the overall response is not as well formed as that from the normal ear.

tion of the nerve. *Wave II* is generated mainly in the proximal eighth nerve but probably also includes a contribution from the intra-axial portion of the nerve and perhaps the cochlear nucleus as well. *Wave III* is generated in the lower pons, in the region of the superior olive and trapezoid body. The generators of *waves IV and V* lie in the upper pons and the midbrain, as high as the inferior colliculus. Waves II and IV are inconsistently identified in some normal individuals, and therefore clinical interpretation of BAEPs is based primarily on latency measurements of waves I, III, and V. Despite decussation of brain stem auditory pathways at multiple levels, clinical experience indicates that unilateral BAEP abnormalities usually reflect lesions ipsilateral to the stimulated ear.

Brain Stem Auditory Evoked Potentials in Neurological Disease

Auditory nerve pathology has several effects on the BAEP, in part related to the nature and size of the lesion. Findings range from prolongation of the I–III interpeak interval, to preservation of wave I with distortion or loss of later components, to loss of all BAEP components. Any of these abnormalities can be seen with acoustic neurinomas and other cerebellopontine angle tumors (Figure 37A.22). In fact, the BAEP is perhaps the most sensitive screening test for acoustic neurinoma, detecting abnormalities in more than 90% of patients (Hart et al. 1983). The sensitivity of the test can be further extended by changing stimulus intensity over a range of values and evaluating the effect on components of the BAEP (*the "latency intensity" function*). With very small intracanalicular tumors, an abnormal latency intensity function may be the only clue to the lesion (Legatt et al. 1988) (Figure 37A.23).

In patients with focal brain stem lesions that impinge on the auditory pathways, the BAEP is abnormal and the type of abnormality reflects the lesion's location and extent. For example, Figure 37A.24 illustrates a BAEP obtained from a patient with a brain stem hemorrhage that involved the rostral two-thirds of the pons but spared the caudal third. Waves IV and V are absent but waves I, II, and III are relatively normal. BAEPs are normal when brain stem lesions do not involve auditory pathways, as is often the case in the locked-in syndrome produced by ventral pontine infarction, or with Wallenberg's lateral medullary syndrome. In contrast, pontine gliomas nearly always produce abnormal BAEPs.

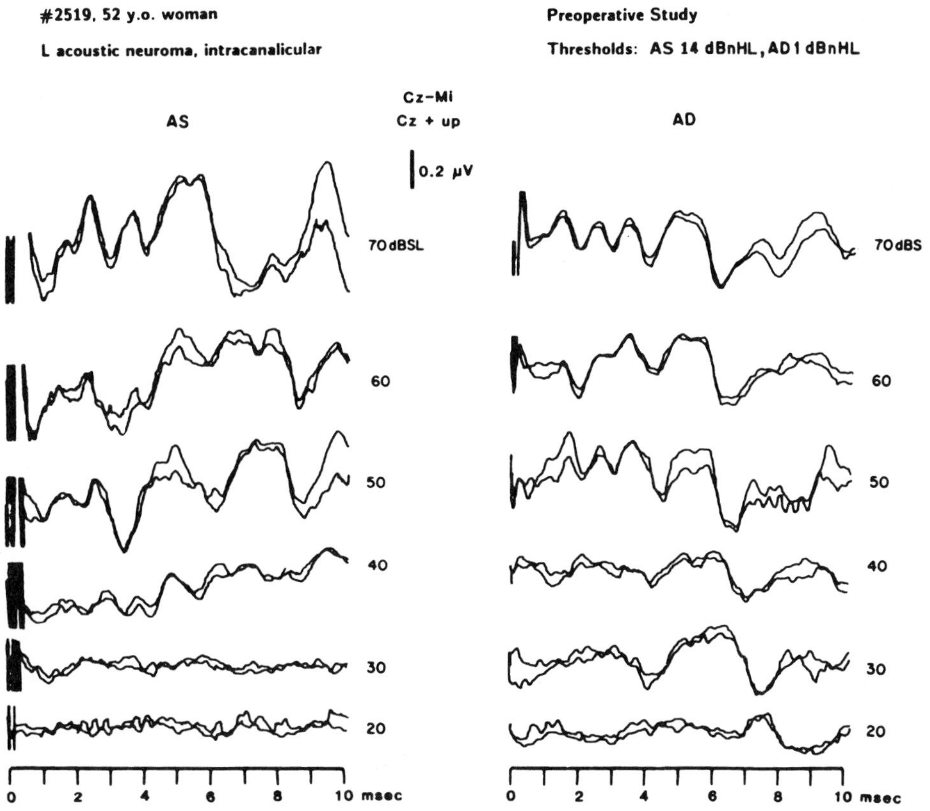

FIGURE 37A.23 BAEP wave V latency plots as a function of increasing stimulus intensity from 20 to 70 dBSL in a woman with a left intracanalicular acoustic neurinoma. BAEPs at 70 dBSL are normal bilaterally, but responses at lower intensities are quite asymmetrical, and the response threshold is elevated on the left.

Nearly 50% of patients with definite multiple sclerosis have abnormal BAEPs. Of greater clinical importance, about 20% of patients with possible or probable multiple sclerosis have an abnormal BAEP, even in the absence of clinical signs or symptoms referable to the brain stem. In such cases, abnormalities usually consist of absence or decreased amplitude of BAEP component waves, most often of waves IV and V, or increased III–V interpeak latency. Occasionally there will be prolongation of the I–III interpeak interval, probably reflecting involvement of the central myelin, which covers the proximal and immediately intra-axial portion of the auditory nerve.

BAEPs may document brain stem involvement in patients with nonfocal neurological disease, especially those affecting myelin such as metachromatic leukodystrophy and adrenoleukodystrophy. In such diseases, the BAEP may also show electrophysiological abnormalities in clinically asymptomatic heterozygotes.

BAEPs are used to assess hearing in young children and in patients otherwise unable to cooperate for standard audiological testing. A latency intensity study, discussed above, permits characterization of the response threshold for wave V as well as the relationship between wave V latency and stimulus intensity (Stapellus 1989). Such testing allows estimation of hearing threshold and may distinguish between conductive and sensorineural types of hearing impairment). However, brain stem audiometry is not really a hearing test per se but, rather, a measure of the brain stem's sensitivity to auditory input. The BAEP is normal in the rare patient with deafness resulting from bilateral cortical lesions. On the other hand, patients with multiple sclerosis or a pontine glioma often have abnormal BAEPs but normal hearing (although their ability to localize sound accurately in space may be diminished). One limitation to using BAEPs to test hearing is that the brain stem must be intact, so that BAEP alterations reflect dysfunction in the peripheral hearing apparatus.

Somatosensory Evoked Potentials

Following electrical stimulation of a peripheral nerve, recordings from electrodes placed over the spine and scalp reveal a series of waves that reflect sequential activation of neural structures along the afferent somatosensory pathways. The dorsal column–lemniscal system is the major substrate of the somatosensory evoked potential (SEP), although other non-lemniscal systems, such as the dorsal spinocerebellar tract, have been shown to contribute to SEP generation. In clinical practice, SEPs are usually elicited by stimulation of the median nerve at the wrist, the common peroneal nerve at the knee, or the posterior tibial nerve at the ankle.

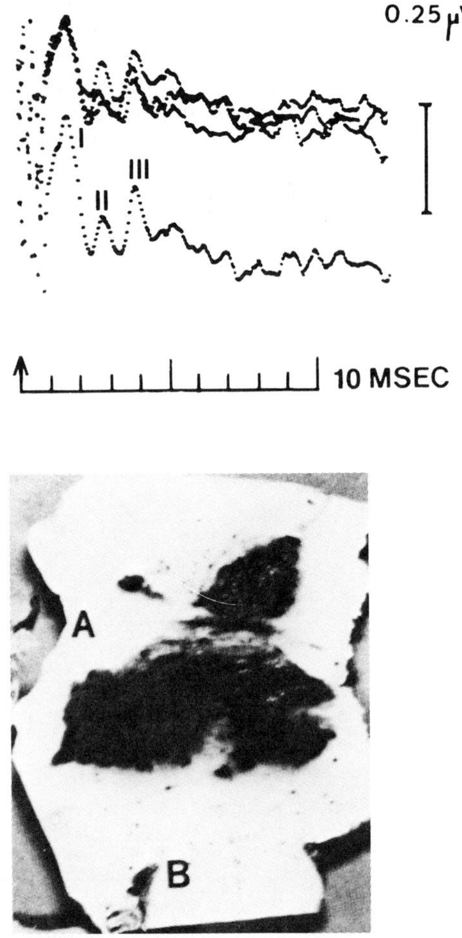

FIGURE 37A.24 BAEP recorded from a patient with a brain stem hemorrhage sparing the lower third of the pons. Waves I, II, and III are preserved but later components are lost. The figure shows a coronal section through the pons. A is at the pontomesencephalic border. B is at the pontomedullary border. (Reprinted with permission from KH Chiappa. Evoked Potentials in Clinical Medicine. In AB Baker, LH Baker [eds], Clinical Neurology. New York: Harper & Row, 1985.)

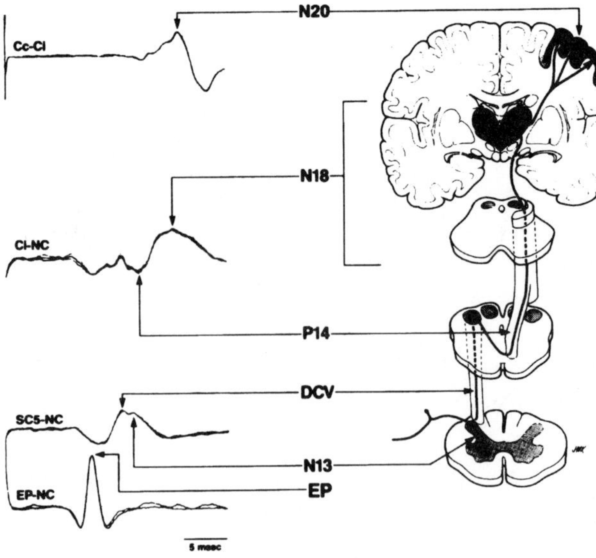

FIGURE 37A.25 Presumed generator sources of median nerve somatosensory evoked potential. Cc and Ci are central-parietal scalp locations contralateral (Cc) and ipsilateral (Ci) to the stimulated nerve. They are 2 cm posterior to the C3 and C4 placements of the International Ten-Twenty System. EP and SC5 are electrodes located over Erb's point and the spinous process of the fifth cervical vertebra, respectively. NC is a noncephalic (such as elbow) reference.

Normal Median Nerve Somatosensory Evoked Potential

Figure 37A.25 shows a normal SEP elicited by median nerve stimulation. The accompanying diagram indicates presumed generator sources for the various components of the SEP (Emerson and Pedley 1990). An electrode at Erb's point ipsilateral to the stimulated arm registers the afferent volley as it passes through the brachial plexus. The Erb's point potential serves as a reference point against which the latencies of subsequent components are measured. Electrodes over the midcervical dorsal spine record two independent but partially overlapping waveforms that reflect local activity in the spinal cord. The first of these, designated *DCV* (for *dorsal column volley*), is the afferent volley in the cuneate tract. The second, *N13*, represents postsynaptic activity in the central gray matter of the cervical cord generated by input from axon collaterals off the primary large fiber afferents. N13 is accompanied by a simultaneous potential of opposite polarity (*P13*) over the anterior neck. Lesions such as syringomyelia, which disrupt the central gray matter, may selectively affect the N13/P13.

SEP components generated in the brain stem are best recorded by an electrode placed on the scalp away from the primary sensory area. This electrode "sees" subcortical activity that is volume-conducted to the scalp surface. The *P14 wave* is generated in the cervicomedullary region, probably by the caudal medial lemniscus. This is followed by a long-duration negative wave, *N18*, whose origin is uncertain but probably includes postsynaptic and tract activity from multiple generators in the rostral brain stem. Activity in thalamic sensory nuclei may also contribute to N18. Figure 37A.26 illustrates preservation of the P14 but loss of the N18 and all later waves in a patient with an arteriovenous malformation of the right pons. This is probably the electrophysiological equivalent of functional transection of the medial lemniscus at a pontine level.

The initial cortical response to the afferent sensory volley is designated *N20* and is best recorded by a scalp electrode placed directly over the primary sensory cortex contralateral to the stimulated side. The N20 is also a composite waveform made up of signals from multiple generators within or close to the primary cortical receiving area. This can be demonstrated by selective stimulation of cutaneous and muscle spindle afferent fibers in the median nerve, which are known to project to adjacent but distinct cortical regions, or by observation of state-dependent changes in the

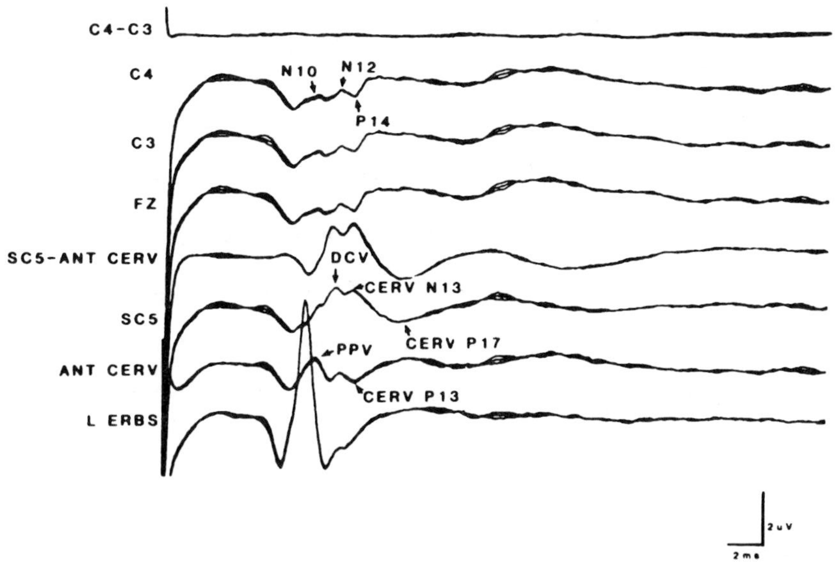

FIGURE 37A.26 Left median nerve SEP in a patient with a right pontine arteriovenous malformation. All components after P14 (cervicomedullary potential) are absent. Unless otherwise labeled, a right elbow reference was used.

N20 (Figure 37A.27). Sleep, for example, attenuates small inflections that are often present on the waking N20, a phenomenon probably due to downward modulation of some generators contributing to N20 and to alterations in thalamic input to cortex during sleep.

Normal Posterior Tibial Nerve Somatosensory Evoked Potential

SEPs to posterior tibial nerve stimulation are, in many ways, analogous to median nerve SEPs. When the posterior tibial nerve is stimulated, recordings from electrodes over the lumbar spine show two distinct potentials (Figure 37A.28). One (*PV*) is produced by the afferent volley in the lumbar nerve roots and gracile tract, and the other (*N22*) is a summated synaptic potential generated in the gray matter of the lumbar cord. Because of its stability, fixed latency, and relatively high voltage, the N22 lumbar potential is used clinically as a reference point against which latencies of subsequent components are measured. Additionally, determination of the spinal level where N22 voltage is maximal provides an approximate indication of the position of

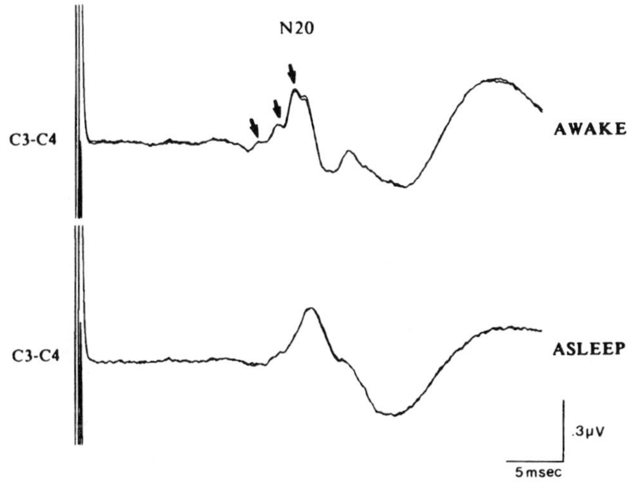

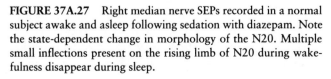

FIGURE 37A.27 Right median nerve SEPs recorded in a normal subject awake and asleep following sedation with diazepam. Note the state-dependent change in morphology of the N20. Multiple small inflections present on the rising limb of N20 during wakefulness disappear during sleep.

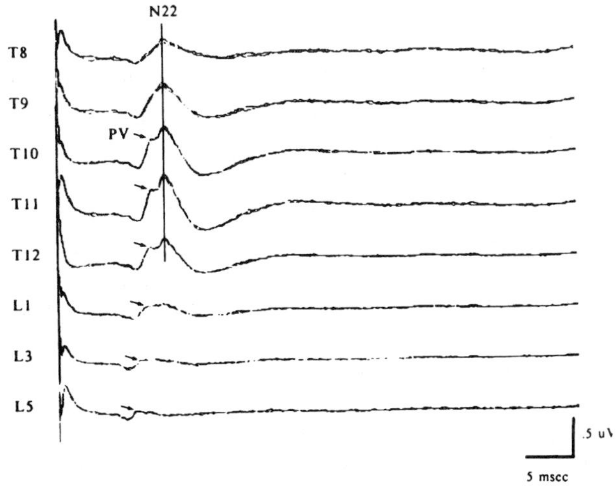

FIGURE 37A.28 Recordings over the lumbar and lower thoracic spine following posterior tibial nerve stimulation. Recording electrodes are referenced to the iliac crest. Note the increasing latency of the propagated volley (PV) and the appearance at T12 of a second, stationary potential (N22). See text for further details.

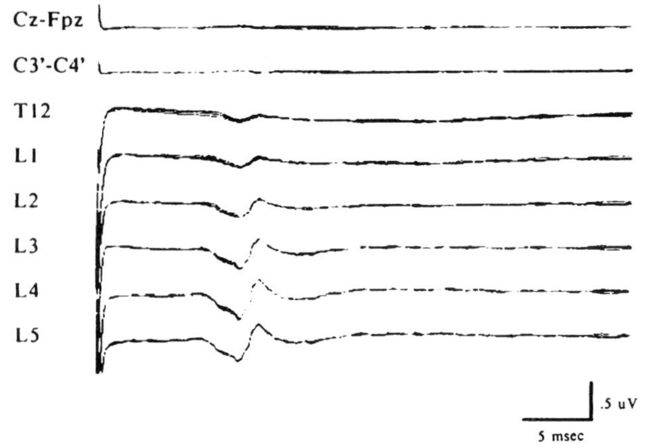

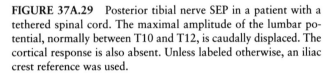

FIGURE 37A.29 Posterior tibial nerve SEP in a patient with a tethered spinal cord. The maximal amplitude of the lumbar potential, normally between T10 and T12, is caudally displaced. The cortical response is also absent. Unless labeled otherwise, an iliac crest reference was used.

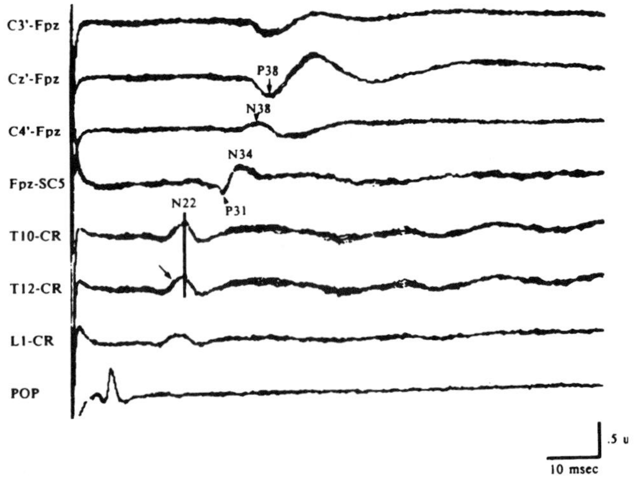

FIGURE 37A.30 Normal posterior tibial SEP. The lower channel is a bipolar recording between two electrodes over the popliteal fossa.

the lumbar cord enlargement. This is sometimes clinically useful if there is a question of spinal cord tethering (Emerson 1988) (Figure 37A.29).

Subcortical activity from posterior tibial nerve stimulation consists of a positive wave, *P31*, followed by a long-duration negative wave, *N34* (Figure 37A.30). These components are analogous to the P14 and N18 following median nerve stimulation, and are probably generated by the afferent volley in the caudal medial lemniscus and by postsynaptic activity in the rostral brain stem, respectively.

The initial cortical response to posterior tibial nerve stimulation is a prominent positivity (*P38*) that is recorded from scalp electrodes placed at the vertex and central parasagittal regions, close to the cortical areas representing the leg (see Figure 37A.30). This positive potential is usually maximal just lateral to the vertex, ipsilateral to the stimulated nerve. This apparently paradoxical localization of the P38 reflects the mesial location of the primary sensory area for the leg and foot within the interhemispheric fissure (Emerson and Pedley 1990).

Somatosensory Evoked Potentials in Neurological Disease

SEP abnormalities are produced by a wide variety of conditions that disturb conduction within the somatosensory system. These include focal lesions (tumors, strokes, cervical spondylosis) and diseases that affect the nervous system more diffusely (hereditary ataxias, subacute combined degeneration, vitamin E deficiency). Ninety percent of patients with definite multiple sclerosis have either upper- or lower-limb SEP abnormalities. Furthermore, an abnormal SEP is found in 50–60% of multiple sclerosis patients even in the absence of symptoms or signs referable to the large-fiber sensory system. Other diseases that affect myelin, such as Pelizeus-Merzbacher's disease, metachromatic leukodystrophy, adrenoleukodystrophy, and adrenomyeloneuropathy, also produce SEP abnormalities. In cases of adrenoleukodystrophy and adrenomyeloneuropathy, SEP abnormalities can be demonstrated in heterozygotes.

Many lesions alter the SEP by producing a conduction delay or block. This results in prolonged interpeak latencies or in attenuation or even loss of one or more SEP components. Abnormally large SEPs, involving exaggeration of cortical components occurring after N20 (median nerve), are characteristic of patients with progressive myoclonus epilepsy, some patients with photosensitive epilepsy, and children with late infantile ceroid lipofuscinosis (Figure 37A.31).

Motor Evoked Potentials and Magnetic Coil Stimulation

It is possible to assess the functional integrity of the descending motor pathways using *motor evoked potentials* (MEPs) (Eisen and Shtybel 1990). MEP studies generally entail stimulating the motor cortex and recording the evoked potential compound action potential over appropriate target muscles. Although the clinical utility of MEPs is not fully defined, they provide information about motor pathways that complements data about sensory pathways obtained from SEPs. MEPs also offer insights into the pathophysiology and evolution of disorders affecting the motor system. Finally, transcranial magnetic coil stimulation has been used to study transcallosal signal transmission, language, and visual perception (Cracco et al. 1990).

MEPs are elicited by stimulating the motor cortex either by directly passing a brief, high-voltage electrical pulse

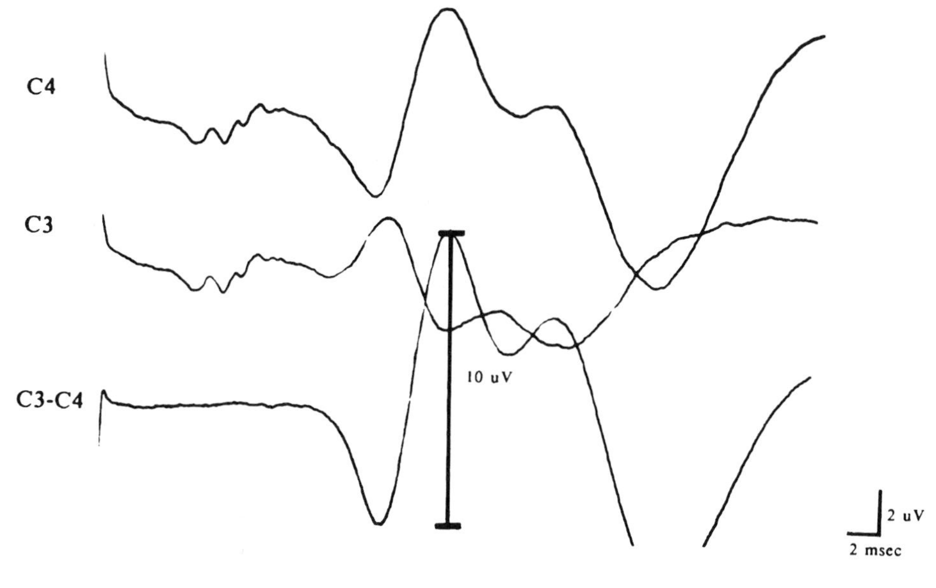

FIGURE 37A.31 Recording from central-parietal scalp electrodes following median nerve stimulation in a patient with cortical myoclonus. There is marked exaggeration of later cortical components. A noncephalic reference was used in the upper two tracings.

through the scalp or by using a time-varying magnetic field to induce an electrical current within the brain. MEPs evoked by transcranial magnetic stimulation are more labile and occur at slightly greater latency than those evoked by electrical stimulation. These differences arise because transcranial electrical stimulation seems to activate corticospinal neurons directly, whereas magnetic coil stimulation acts presynaptically. In awake patients, transcranial electrical stimulation is painful, whereas magnetic coil stimulation is not.

MEPs are often delayed in patients with multiple sclerosis and may be more sensitive to demyelinating lesions than SEPs (Eisen and Shtybel 1990). Patients with cerebral palsy may have enhanced MEPs in some muscle groups because of aberrant corticospinal projections. MEP latencies are normal in Parkinson's disease, but the amplitude of responses may be increased because of spinal disinhibition or corticomotoneuronal hyperexcitability (Kandler et al. 1990). In motor neuron disease, pyramidal tract conduction delays can be demonstrated in patients without upper motor neuron signs (Small et al. 1993). In patients with chronic spinal cord injury, MEPs may assist in predicting recovery (Levy et al. 1987).

Intraoperative Monitoring

Electrophysiological monitoring to assess the functional integrity of the brain and spinal cord during neurosurgical and orthopedic procedures has become routine at many centers. Such monitoring reduces neurologic morbidity by detecting adverse effects at a time when prompt correction of the cause can avoid permanent neurologic injury. In addition, monitoring may provide information about the mechanisms of postoperative neurologic abnormalities and occasionally lead to changes in surgical approach or technique.

Monitoring can be done using EEG, sensory evoked potentials (usually BAEPs or SEPs), and MEPs. Which monitoring modality or combination of modalities is used depends on the type of surgery, the neural structures judged to be most at risk, and previous experience with complications of the particular surgical procedure. Because neurological injury can occur suddenly and may be irreversible, the ideal monitoring method is one that detects impending, not permanent, damage. A certain percentage of false-positive results is therefore highly desirable. Experienced monitoring teams learn that small changes in recorded signals are common during surgery due to clinical and technical factors that have negligible effects on outcome. Other variables that affect electrical signals are the type of anesthesia, temperature, blood pressure, and neuromuscular blockade. Determining what constitutes a significant and reproducible change that warrants alerting the surgeon or anesthesiologist is a critical aspect of monitoring.

Patients occasionally experience a new postoperative neurological abnormality despite uneventful monitoring. It is rare, if it occurs at all, for a major neurological complication to occur in a part of the nervous system that was monitored directly and accurately judged to be normal throughout the operation. More often, complications arise from involvement of structures not monitored directly (e.g., infarction of the ventral spinal cord when only dorsal column function was monitored using SEPs), or when a significant pre-existing abnormality masks even moderate changes from baseline. Minor and usually transient neurological symptoms and signs (e.g., sensory dysesthesias, mild weakness, temporary neurogenic bladder) occur occasionally in the face of stable intraoperative electrophysiologic measures.

EEG monitoring has been used extensively in patients undergoing carotid endarterectomy, during embolization of arteriovenous malformations, and for clipping or removal of some aneurysms. Computer-assisted methods are commonly used to process primary EEG data to compress what is otherwise an unmanageable amount of information and to present the data in a more easily interpretable manner. Monitoring is especially helpful in selecting patients for shunting during occlusion of the carotid artery. With monitoring, overall intraoperative major morbidity for endarterectomy should be reducible to 1%.

Monitoring auditory nerve function using BAEPs, with or without electrocochleography, is useful in any neurosurgical or neuro-otological procedure that risks injury to the eighth cranial nerve. Risk of hearing loss is minimized in patients with small, especially intracanalicular, acoustic neurinomas and other cerebellopontine angle tumors, as well as in patients undergoing microvascular decompression for hemifacial spasm or trigeminal neuralgia. Monitoring facial nerve function by recording compound nerve or muscle action potentials following direct stimulation of the intracranial portion of the seventh nerve has greatly reduced the incidence of permanent facial palsy following cerebellopontine angle surgery.

SEPs are used routinely to monitor baseline and spinal cord function during neurosurgical and orthopedic procedures. They provide useful and sensitive feedback information about the integrity of the dorsal column somatosensory system. MEPs are particularly sensitive to the effects of spinal cord ischemia, compression, distraction, and blunt trauma. A clinical application of MEPs is to monitor spinal cord function during surgical procedures (Adams et al. 1993). They complement SEPs, because SEPs may not detect surgical injuries that are limited to the lateral and anterior spinal cord.

REFERENCES

Adams DC, Emerson RG, Heyer EJ et al. Monitoring of intraoperative motor-evoked potentials under conditions of controlled neuromuscular blockade. Anesth Analg 1993;77:913–918.

American EEG Society. Guidelines in EEG and evoked potentials. J Clin Neurophysiol 1994;11:1–143.

Callaghan N, Garrett A, Goggin T. Withdrawal of anticonvulsant drugs in patients free of seizures for two years: a prospective study. N Engl J Med 1988;318:942–946.

Celesia GG. Visual Evoked Potentials and Electroretinograms. In E Niedermeyer, F Lopes da Silva (eds), Electroencephalography: Basic Principles, Clinical Applications, and Related Fields. Baltimore: Williams & Wilkins, 1993:911–936.

Chiappa KH. Evoked Potentials in Clinical Medicine. In AB Baker, LH Baker (eds), Clinical Neurology. New York: Harper & Row, 1985.

Cracco JB, Amassian VE, Cracco RQ et al. Brain stimulation revisited. J Clin Neurophysiol 1990;7:3–15.

Eisen AA, Shtybel W. AAEM minimonograph #35: clinical experience with transcranial magnetic stimulation. Muscle Nerve 1990;13:995–1011.

Emerson RG. The anatomic and physiologic basis of posterior tibial nerve somatosensory evoked potentials. Neurol Clin 1988;6:735–750.

Emerson RG, Pedley TA. Somatosensory Evoked Potentials. In DD Daly, TA Pedley (eds), Current Practice of Clinical Electroencephalography (2nd ed). New York: Raven, 1990;679–705.

Fisch BJ, Klass DW. The diagnostic specificity of triphasic wave patterns. Electroencephalogr Clin Neurophysiol 1988;70:1–8.

Fisch BJ, Pedley TA. The role of quantitative topographic mapping or "neurometrics" in the diagnosis of psychiatric and neurological disorders: The cons. Electroencephalogr Clin Neurophysiol 1989;73:5–9.

Goodin DS, Aminoff MJ. Evaluation of dementia by event-related potentials. J Clin Neurophysiol 1992;9:521–525.

Grigg MM, Kelly MA, Celesia GG et al. Electroencephalographic activity after brain death. Arch Neurol 1987;44:948–954.

Halliday, AM. The Visual Evoked Potential in the Investigation of Diseases of the Optic Nerve. In AM Halliday (ed), Evoked Potentials in Clinical Testing. New York: Churchill Livingstone, 1982.

Hart RG, Gardner DP, Howieson J. Acoustic tumors: Atypical features and recent diagnostic tests. Neurology 1983;33:211–221.

Kandler RH, Jarratt JA, Sagar HJ et al. Abnormalities of central motor conduction in Parkinson's disease. J Neurol Sci 1990;100:94–97.

Legatt AD, Pedley TA, Emerson RG et al. Normal brain stem auditory evoked potentials (BAEPs) with abnormal latency-intensity studies in patients with acoustic neuromas. Arch Neurol 1988;45:1326–1330.

Lerman P. Benign Partial Epilepsy with Centro-Temporal Spikes. In J Roger, M Bureau, C Dravet et al. (eds), Epilepsy Syndromes in Infancy, Childhood, and Adolescence (2nd ed). London: John Libbey & Co. 1992;189–200.

Levy WJ, McCafferty M, Hagichi S. Motor evoked potential as a predictor of recovery in chronic spinal injury. Neurosurgery 1987;20:138–142.

Lopes da Silva FH. A critical review of clinical applications of topographic mapping of brain potentials. J Clin Neurophysiol 1990;7:535–551.

Nuwer MR. The development of EEG brain mapping. J Clin Neurophysiol 1990;7:459–471.

President's Commission for the Study of Ethical Problems in Medicine and Biomedical and Behavioral Research. Guidelines for the determination of death. JAMA 1981;246:2184–2186.

Rose DF, Sato S, Smith PD et al. Localization of magnetic interictal discharges in temporal lobe epilepsy. Ann Neurol 1987; 22:348–354.

Sato S, Balish M, Muratore R. Principles of magnetoencephalography. J Clin Neurophysiol 1991;8:144–156.

Small GA, Pullman S, Emerson R et al. Central motor delay in the motor neuron diseases [abstract]. Electroenceph Clin Neurophysiol 1993;87:S71.

Stapells DR. Auditory brain stem response assessment of infants and children. Semin Hearing 1989;10:229–251.

Sutherling WW, Crandell PH, Cahan LD et al. The magnetic field of epileptic spikes agrees with intracranial localizations in complex partial epilepsy. Neurology 1988;38:778–786.

B. ELECTRODIAGNOSIS OF NEUROMUSCULAR DISORDERS

Jun Kimura

NERVE CONDUCTION STUDIES

Principles

Electrical stimulation of a nerve initiates an impulse that travels along motor, sensory, or mixed nerves. Conduction characteristics of motor fibers are assessed by studying compound evoked potentials recorded from the muscle; sensory fibers are assessed by compound evoked potentials recorded from the nerve. The use of standard methods allows precise lesion localization and accurate characterization of peripheral nerve function (Campbell and Robinson 1993). Nerve conduction studies primarily measure the latency of the fastest conducting fibers from the time of stimulation to the onset of the evoked potential.

The routine conduction studies are those for the motor and sensory fibers of the median, ulnar, and radial nerves; the motor fibers of the peroneal and tibial nerves; the sensory fibers of the sural and superficial peroneal nerves; and the motor fibers of the facial and accessory nerves. The basic principles of testing are the same for all nerves, but the approach may vary because of the anatomic peculiarities of the individual nerve being tested. Studies of the blink reflex, the F wave, and the H reflex supplement routine conduction studies to assess the central or most proximal segment of the nerve. This section reviews the fundamental concepts of nerve stimulation techniques and discusses their proper clinical application.

Techniques

Stimulation and Recording Stimulators

Two different kinds of electric stimulators are used in nerve conduction studies. Constant voltage stimulators regulate voltage output so that current varies inversely with the impedance of the system including the skin and subcutaneous tissues. Constant current stimulators change voltage according to impedance, so that the amount of current that reaches the nerve is specified within the limits of skin resistance. In either type, the range of stimulus output must be adequate to elicit maximal muscle and nerve action potentials in all patients. As the current flows between the cathode (negative pole) and anode (positive pole), negative charges accumulate under the cathode, depolarizing the nerve, and positive charges under the anode hyperpolarize the nerve. In bipolar stimulation, both electrodes are placed over the nerve trunk, with the cathode closer to the recording site to avoid anodal conduction block of the propagated impulse. Some electromyographers prefer to use monopolar stimulation by inserting a needle electrode subcutaneously close to the nerve because less current is needed to elicit the same response (Pease et al. 1989). The anode may be a surface electrode located on the skin nearby or a second needle electrode inserted in the vicinity of the cathode.

Surface and Needle Electrodes. Surface recording allows measurement of the *onset latency* (conduction time of the fastest fibers) and the *amplitude* (approximate number of available axons) of the *compound muscle action potential* (CMAP) (Figure 37B.1). Surface electrodes are also used for recording sensory and mixed nerve action potentials. Ring electrodes are convenient to record the antidromic sensory potentials from digital nerves over the proximal and distal interphalangeal joints.

Needle electrodes register only a small portion of the muscle or nerve action potential, but with less interference from neighboring discharges. They improve the recording from small atrophic muscles, or a proximal muscle not excitable in isolation. Needle electrodes placed perpendicular to the nerve improve the signal-to-noise ratio by about five times and, when averaging, considerably reduce the time required to reach the same resolution.

Optimal Recording. A prepulse preceding the stimulus triggers the sweep, which is adjusted based on the response latency. The amplifier sensitivity determines the amplitude of the potential. Overamplification truncates the response and underamplification prevents accurate measurements of the takeoff from baseline. Digital averaging is a major improvement over isolated recording of individual responses (Normand and Daube 1992). Signals time-locked to the stimulus summate at a constant latency and appear as an evoked potential, distinct from the background noise. The signal-to-noise ratio increases in proportion to the square

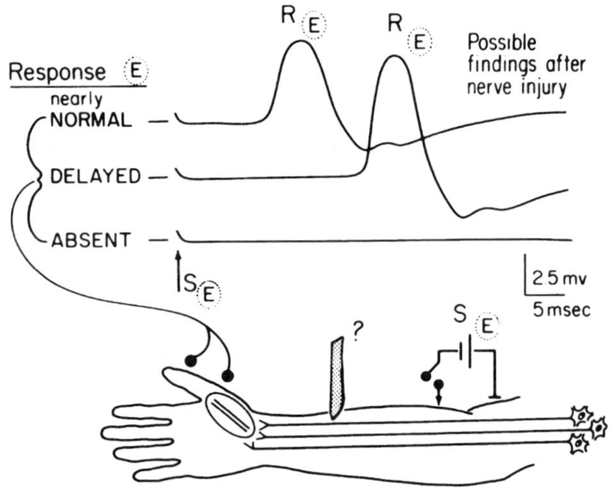

FIGURE 37B.1 Three basic types of alteration in the compound muscle action potential occur after a presumed nerve injury distal to the site of stimulation. The response may be mildly reduced in amplitude but nearly normal in latency (top). It may be essentially normal in amplitude but substantially increased in latency (middle). Or it may be absent or markedly reduced in amplitude even with a stimulus of supramaximal intensity (bottom). (Reprinted with permission of the author and publisher from J Kimura. Electrodiagnosis in Diseases of Nerve and Muscle: Principles and Practices [2nd ed]. Philadelphia: FA Davis, 1989.)

root of the trial number. For example, four trials give twice as big a response as a single stimulus, whereas nine trials give three times the amplitude. Modern instruments digitally indicate the latency and amplitude when the desired spot on the waveform is marked. The comparison of successively elicited potentials is facilitated by displaying a series of responses with a stepwise vertical shift of the baseline on a storage oscilloscope.

Motor Nerve Conduction

Stimulation and Recording. The nerve is stimulated at two or more points along its course with pulses of moderate intensity. Stimulation with maximal intensity excites all nerve fibers and provides the full size of the CMAP. It is customary to stimulate at 20–30% supramaximal, which guarantees the activation of all nerve axons.

A pair of recording electrodes consists of an active lead (G1) placed on the belly of the muscle and an indifferent lead (G2) on the tendon (belly-tendon recording). The propagating muscle action potential, originating under G1 located near the motor point, gives rise to a simple biphasic waveform with initial negativity (Kincaid et al. 1993). Initial positivity suggests incorrect positioning of the active electrode or a volume-conducted potential from distant muscles, activated by anomalous innervation or by accidental spread of stimulation to other nerves.

Amplitude, Duration, Latency, and Conduction Velocity. The usual measurements are *amplitude* from baseline to the negative peak, *duration* from onset to the positive peak or to final return to baseline, and *latency* from stimulus artifact to onset of the negative response. Electronic integration provides the area under the waveform, which shows linear correlation with the product of the amplitude and duration measured by conventional means.

Onset latency is the sum of nerve conduction time, neuromuscular transmission time, and propagation time along the muscle membrane. Because neuromuscular transmission time and propagation time are common to any stimulus site, the latency difference between two points is the time for the nerve impulse to travel from one stimulus point to the other.

The *conduction velocity* is derived by dividing the nerve length between the two stimulation points by the corresponding latency difference. The length of the nerve segment is estimated by measuring the surface distance along the course of the nerve.

$$\text{Conduction velocity} = \frac{D}{Lp - Ld} \text{ m/s}$$

where D is the distance between the two stimulus points in millimeters, and Lp and Ld, the proximal and distal latencies in milliseconds.

A 10-cm separation of the two stimulation points improves the accuracy of surface measurement and consequently the determination of conduction velocity. In the evaluation of a focal lesion such as compressive neuropathy, inclusion of the unaffected segments in calculation dilutes the effect of slowing at the injured site and decreases the sensitivity of the test. Therefore, incremental stimulation across the shorter segment helps localize an abnormality that might otherwise escape detection.

Residual Latency. For the evaluation of the most distal segment, the *terminal latency* from the most distal stimulus point to the muscle is compared to the normal range using either premeasured distance or anatomic landmarks for electrode placement. The actual conduction time in the terminal segment (Ld) slightly exceeds the value calculated for the same distance based on the conduction velocity of more proximal segments (Ld'). The difference (Ld' – Ld), known as the *residual latency*, provides a measure of the conduction delay at the nerve terminal and at the neuromuscular junction.

Sensory Nerve Conduction

Stimulation and Recording. Sensory conduction in the arms is studied either by stimulation of digital nerves to elicit an *orthodromic sensory potential* at a proximal site, or by stimulation of the nerve trunk to elicit an *antidromic digital potential* (Winkler et al. 1991). Stimulation of the ulnar or median nerves at the wrist elicits a mixed nerve potential along the nerve trunk at the elbow. Because the thresholds of some motor axons are similar to those of large myelinated sensory axons, superimposition of action potentials from distal muscles may obscure antidromically recorded sensory potentials. Fortunately, onset latency can still be measured accurately because the large-diameter sensory fibers conduct 5–10% faster than motor fibers. This relationship may change in disease states that selectively affect different fibers.

Although surface electrodes provide adequate and reproducible results, the improved signal-to-noise ratio of needle electrodes may be needed to define small late components that result from demyelinated, remyelinated, or regenerated fibers.

Amplitude, Duration, and Waveform. The waveform of a *sensory nerve action potential* (SNAP) is influenced by the position of the recording electrodes. The orthodromic SNAP is triphasic with an initial positive deflection when recorded with the active (G1) electrodes on the nerve and reference (G2) electrode at a remote site. Placing G2 near the nerve at a distance more than 3 cm from G1 makes the SNAP tetraphasic, by adding a final negative deflection. The antidromic digital SNAP does not have an initial positive deflection when recorded with a pair of ring electrodes. Its amplitude is greater than the orthodromic response recorded from the nerve trunk, because the digital nerves lie closer to the surface.

SNAP amplitude is measured either from the baseline to the negative peak or between the negative and positive peaks. This value varies substantially among individuals, and to a lesser extent between the two sides in the same subject when recording with surface or needle electrodes. *SNAP duration* is measured from the initial deflection to the intersection between the descending phase and the baseline, or to the negative or positive peak.

Latency and Conduction Velocity. The calculation of *sensory conduction velocity* requires stimulation at a single site, because the latency consists only of the nerve conduction time from the stimulus point to the recording electrode. Distal latency of the median and ulnar nerves may be shorter using orthodromic than antidromic stimulation, but either method is satisfactory for clinical practice.

The latency of the orthodromic SNAP is measured to the initial positive peak or to the subsequent negative peak. The waveforms of SNAPs elicited by stimulation at different sites along the nerve vary because of temporal dispersion between fast and slow fibers; the interval between the positive and negative peaks increases in proportion to the distance. Therefore, the conduction velocity calculated by using the latency to the negative peak does not necessarily correspond to the fastest-conducting sensory fibers.

The high resolution of most modern amplifiers allows measurement of sensory latency to the initial positive peak. If latency is measured to the negative peak instead of the preceding smaller positive peak, the conduction distance is then determined to the midpoint of G1 and G2 to compensate for the discrepancy between the arrival of the impulse and the appearance of the negative peak.

The onset latency of the biphasic digital potential recorded antidromically is measured to the initial takeoff of the negative peak. This corresponds to the conduction time of the fastest fibers from the cathode to G1. The use of the peak latency is not justified for antidromically recorded digital potentials, which are considerably larger in amplitude than orthodromic potentials.

Segmental Stimulation in Short Increments

Routine conduction studies are sufficient to approximate the site of involvement in entrapment neuropathies (Kimura 1989). More precise localization requires inching the stimulus in short increments along the course of the nerve. The study of short segments provides better resolution of restricted lesions. Assume a nerve impulse conducting at a rate of 1.0 cm/0.2 msec (50 m/second) except for a 1-cm segment where demyelination has doubled the conduction time to 0.4 msec/cm. In a 10-cm segment, normally covered in 2.0 msec, a 0.2-msec increase would constitute a 10% change, or approximately one standard deviation, well within the normal range of variability. The same 0.2-msec increase, however, would represent a 100% change in latency if measured over a 1-cm segment. The large per-step increase in latency more than compensates for the inherent measurement error associated with stimulating multiple times in short increments.

This technique is particularly useful in assessing sensory conduction in patients with carpal tunnel syndrome. With stimulation of a normal median nerve in 1-cm increments across the wrist, the latency changes approximately 0.16–0.21 msec/cm from midpalm to distal forearm (Figure 37B.2). A sharply localized latency increase across a 1-cm segment indicates a focal abnormality of the median nerve (Figure 37B.3). An abrupt change in waveform usually accompanies the latency increase across the site of compression.

Late Responses

Routine nerve conduction studies mainly apply to the distal segments of the peripheral nerves. The F wave and H reflex supplement routine studies to assess central conduction (Fraser and Olney 1992).

A supramaximal stimulus applied at any point along the course of a motor nerve elicits a small late response (*F wave*) following the CMAP (*M response*). This long latency response F wave results from backfiring of antidromically activated motor neurons (Figure 37B.4). The *F-wave latencies* (Table 37B.1) measured from the stimulus artifact to the beginning of the evoked potential vary by a few milliseconds from one stimulus to the next (Dengler et al. 1992). Therefore, an adequate study requires that more than 10 F waves be clearly identified; 15–20 trials are often required. The most sensitive criterion of abnormality in a unilateral disorder affecting a single nerve is a latency difference between the two sides, or between two nerves in the same limb. Absolute latencies are only useful for sequential

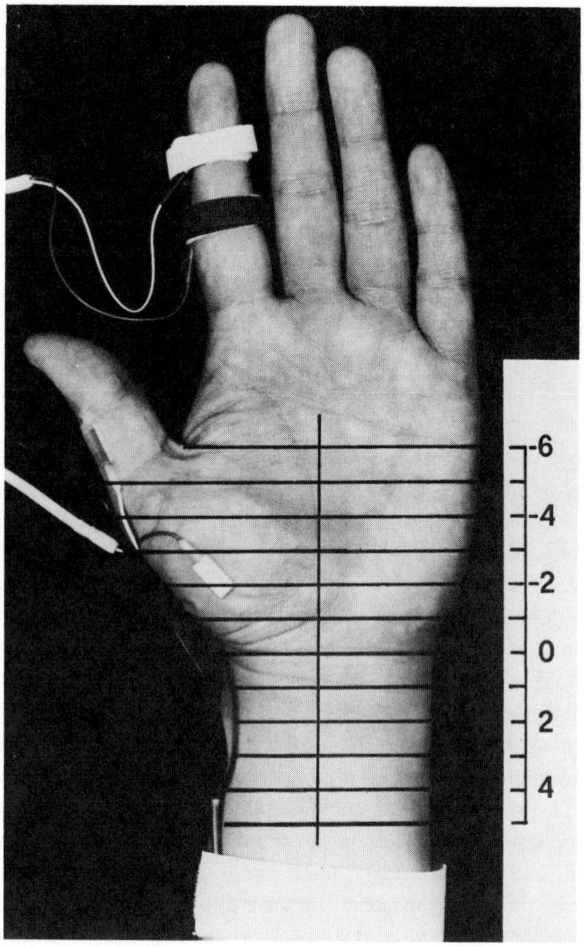

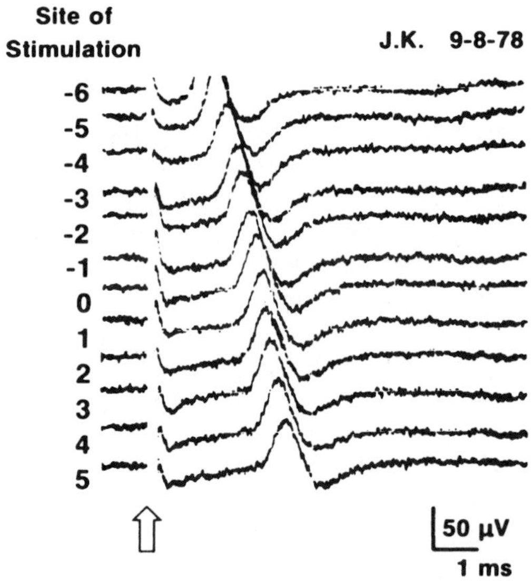

FIGURE 37B.2 (Left) Twelve sites of stimulation in 1-cm increments along the length of the median nerve. The 0 level is at the distal crease of the wrist, corresponding to the origin of the transverse carpal ligament. Sensory nerve and muscle action potentials are recorded from the second digit and abductor pollicis brevis, respectively. (Right) Sensory nerve potentials in a normal subject recorded after stimulation of the median nerve at multiple points across the wrist. The site of each stimulus is indicated on the left. The latency increased linearly as the stimulus site was moved proximally in 1-cm increments. (Reprinted with permission of the author and publisher from J Kimura. The carpal tunnel syndrome: Localization of conduction abnormalities within the distal segment of the median nerve. Brain 1979;102:619–635.)

reassessment of the same nerve. The *F wave conduction velocity* provides a better comparison between proximal and distal segments. The degree of scatter among consecutive F waves, as determined by the difference between the minimal and maximal F wave latencies, indicates the range of motor conduction velocities in the nerve.

The *H reflex*, named after Hoffmann for his original description, is an electrical counterpart of the stretch reflex elicited by a mechanical tap to the tendon. The group 1A sensory fibers and alpha motor neurons form the afferent and efferent arcs of this predominantly monosynaptic reflex (Figure 37B.5). In contrast, the F wave can be elicited from any distal limb muscle. The H reflex and F wave can be distinguished by increasing stimulus intensity. The H reflex is best elicited by a long-duration stimulus, *sub*maximal to produce an M response (Panizza et al. 1989), whereas the F wave requires *supra*maximal stimulus intensity. The H reflex of the triceps surae is the one most commonly used in clinical practice. It is recorded from the soleus after stimulation of the tibial nerve at the knee. The reflex latency, determined by the sensory and motor conduction of the nerve, is better than routine nerve conduction studies in the detection of early neuropathy. The H reflex is also a sensitive indicator for mild neuropathies, maturational changes in the proximal versus distal segment of the tibial nerve, and S_1 radiculopathy (White 1991).

Magnetic Stimulation

The magnetic stimulator is capable of depolarizing any nerve. It was originally designed to stimulate the peripheral nervous system. Unlike electrical stimulation, it allows the painless stimulation of otherwise inaccessible deep nerves. Nonetheless, experience indicates no particular advantage of magnetic stimulation over conventional bipolar electrical stimulation in routine nerve conduction studies (Evans 1991; Olney et al. 1990).

Magnetic stimulation fails to achieve the accuracy of electrical stimulation because of marked intertrial variability of latencies, uncertainty about the point of stimulation, and instability in evoked waveform by minor shifts in stimulator position. The exact site of impulse generation in the

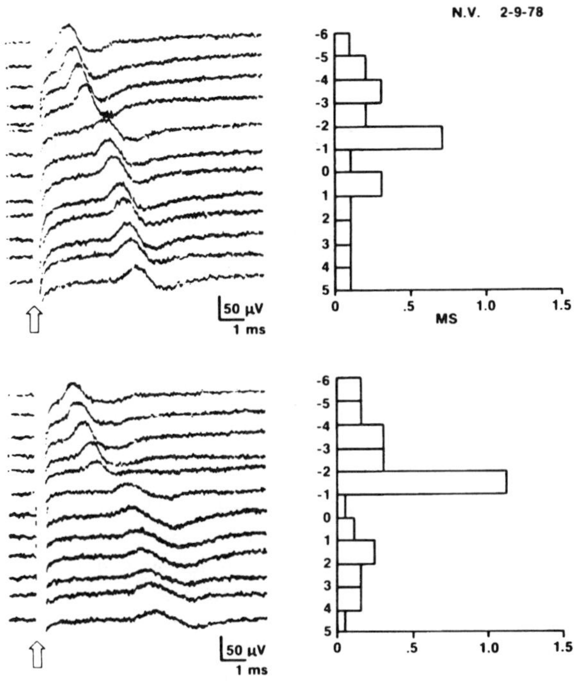

FIGURE 37B.3 Sensory nerve potentials in a patient with the carpal tunnel syndrome. A sharply localized showing was found from –2 to –1 in both hands, representing a segmental conduction velocity of 14 m/second on the left (top) and 9 m/second on the right (bottom). Note a distinct change in waveform of the sensory potential at the point of localized conduction delay. Double-humped appearance at –2 on the left suggests sparing of some sensory axons at this level. (Reprinted with permission of the author and publisher from J Kimura. The carpal tunnel syndrome: Localization of conduction abnormalities within the distal segment of the median nerve. Brain 1979;102:619–635.)

distal peripheral nerve is difficult to determine, and supramaximal responses are hard to elicit (Olney et al. 1990).

In contrast, magnetic stimulation of proximal segments is reliable to measure peripheral conduction time when estimating central conduction time. Paravertebral magnetic stimulation at the neck activates the nerve roots at their exit from the spine (Bischoff et al. 1993). The configuration of M responses elicited by proximal magnetic stimuli varies from one trial to the next, because an F wave, intermittently generated, overlaps the M response. This variability therefore reveals proximally activated F waves, which can be recorded by consecutive subtraction of sequentially elicited M responses. This circumvents the use of collision as the method of separating the F wave from the overlying M response when evaluating the radicular segment. Measurement of the onset latencies of the proximally evoked F waves, using the collision method or subtraction technique, allows assessment of radiculopathies and proximal neuropathies such as the Guillain-Barré syndrome.

Normal and Abnormal Results

Motor Conduction

Nerve Versus Individual Fibers. Three types of abnormalities occur when a motor nerve is stimulated proximal to a presumed lesion (see Figure 37B.1): (1) reduced amplitude with normal or slightly increased latency, (2) increased latency with relatively normal amplitude, and (3) absent response. The abnormal features associated with lesions of the nerve as a whole compared to individual fibers are more complicated because different types of abnormalities tend to coexist. Further, small reductions in the amplitude of the recorded response may escape detection because amplitudes vary among normal individuals.

Demyelination. In *demyelination* it is characteristic that stimulation distal to the lesion elicits a normal CMAP, while proximal stimulation elicits a response with reduced amplitude. This finding, elicited during the first few days after nerve injury, is consistent with either a partial nerve lesion causing *neurapraxia* or early *axonotmesis* before the onset of distal degeneration. To distinguish between these two possibilities, the nerve is stimulated below the lesion several days later, when degenerating axons would have lost their excitability. If the distally evoked CMAP still has higher amplitude than the proximally elicited response, this indicates partial neurapraxia with demyelination. In contrast, a reduced amplitude from stimulation above or below the lesion indicates axonotmesis.

In general, demyelination prolongs conduction time. In the absence of neurapraxia, stimulation proximal to the lesion produces a slowed conduction time and a relatively normal amplitude. These changes imply primary segmental demyelination affecting most nerve fibers. Incomplete proximal compressive lesions may also slow conduction along the distal nerve segment as the result of distal paranodal demyelination.

With neurapraxia, the CMAP elicited by stimulation above the lesion is smaller than the response elicited by stimulation below the lesion. Reduced size may also result from *phase cancellation* between peaks of opposite polarity because of abnormally increased temporal dispersion. Such *excessive desynchronization* often develops in acquired demyelinative neuropathies. If the distal and proximal responses have dissimilar waveforms, the discrepancy in amplitude or area between the two may in part represent a phase cancellation rather then true conduction block.

Axonal Degeneration. Selective loss of many fast-conducting fibers associated with more than a 50% reduction in mean amplitude can slow conduction velocity to 70–80% of normal because the value now represents the remaining physiologically slow-conducting fibers. If CMAP amplitudes are less than half the control value, a reduction to 80–90% of normal conduction velocity is attributable to axonal degeneration of fast-conducting fibers. Greater slowing of con-

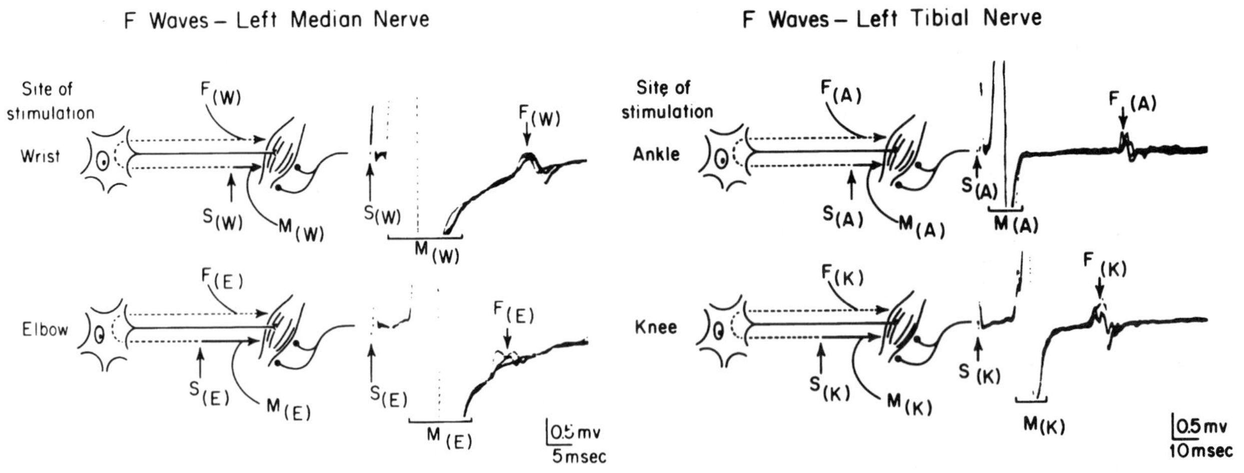

FIGURE 37B.4 (Left) Normal M response (horizontal brackets) and F wave (small arrows) recorded from the thenar muscles through surface electrodes. Sites of supramaximal stimulus to the median nerve are shown, with these consecutive traces superimposed for each. As the stimulus was moved from the wrist to the elbow, the latency of the M response increased, whereas that of the F wave decreased. The figures on the left are schematic illustrations showing the centrifugal (solid arrows) and centripetal (dotted arrows) impulses carrying the M response and F wave, respectively. (Modified from J Kimura. F-wave velocity in the central segment of the median and ulnar nerves: A study in normal subjects and in patients with Charcot-Marie-Tooth disease. Neurology [Minneapolis] 1974;24:539–546.) (Right) Normal M response (horizontal brackets) and F wave (small arrows) recorded from the abductor hallucis through surface electrodes. Supramaximal stimulus was delivered to the tibial nerve at the ankle (top tracing) and knee (bottom tracing). Three consecutive traces are superimposed for each. As the stimulus was moved from ankle to knee, the latency of the M response increased, whereas that of the F wave decreased. (Reprinted with permission from J Kimura, P Bosch, GM Lindsay. F-wave conduction velocity in the central segment of the peroneal and tibial nerves. Arch Phys Med Rehabil 1975; 56:492–497.)

duction velocity suggests the presence of a demyelinating process. The loss of large anterior horn cells in motor neuron degenerations and myelopathies can lead to the motor conduction velocity being slowed to 70% of the mean normal value with reduction of amplitude to less than 10% of normal. A conduction velocity to less than 60% of the mean normal value suggests a peripheral neuropathy with demyelination rather than anterior cell damage.

Sensory Conduction

The types of abnormalities described for motor conduction apply in principle to sensory conduction (Bromberg and Albers 1993). Demyelination slows conduction velocity substantially, whereas axonotmesis reduces the amplitude of response from distal stimulation. Sensory fibers degenerate only when the lesion is distal to the sensory ganglion; the presence of distal sensory potentials in anesthetic digits in a patient with upper limb trauma suggests preganglionic root avulsion rather than plexopathy. Selective impairment of the SNAPs of the first and second digits indicates C6 involvement, of the third digit indicates C7 involvement, of the fourth and fifth digits indicates C6 involvement, of the third digit indicates C7 involvement, and of the fourth and fifth digits indicates C8 involvement. In contrast, plexopathy tends to affect multiple digits. This type of assessment must take into account the relative amplitudes of the SNAP for each digit.

Interpretations

Clinical Values

Optimal application of nerve conduction studies requires an understanding of the principles and pitfalls of the technique. These techniques, when used appropriately, offer important diagnostic information (Bleasel and Tuck 1991; Robinson et al. 1992). Nerve conduction studies precisely delineate the extent and distribution of nerve lesions, and distinguish between axonal and demyelinating involvement. In vitro recordings from the sural nerve biopsy clearly delineate a close relationship between histological and physiological findings in axonopathies, though correlations are poorer in demyelinating neuropathies.

Hereditary and demyelinating neuropathies can be distinguished by the overall pattern of nerve conduction abnormalities. Diffuse slowing with little difference from one nerve to another characterizes hereditary demyelinating neuropathies. The findings may be similar in several members of the same family. Because different nerve fibers are similarly involved, temporal dispersion is limited despite considerable increases in latency. In contrast, acquired demyelinating neuropathies tend to affect certain segments of the nerve disproportionately. Therefore, the abnormalities are less symmetrical and temporal dispersion is substantially increased.

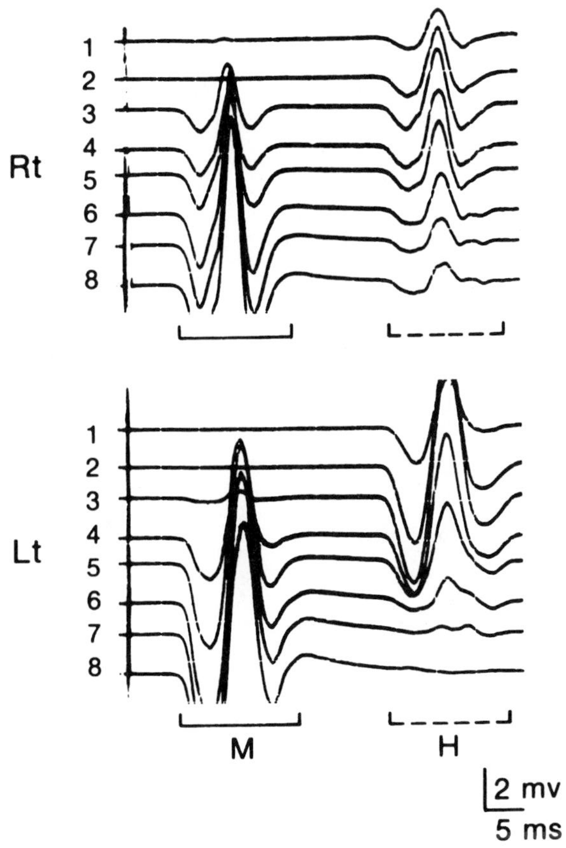

FIGURE 37B.5 H reflex recorded from the soleus after stimulation of the tibial nerve at the knee. Shock intensity was gradually increased from subthreshold level (1) to supramaximal stimulation (8). Note initial increase and subsequent decrease in amplitude of the reflex potential with successive stimuli of progressively higher intensity. The H reflex normally disappears with shocks of supramaximal intensity that elicit a maximal M response.

Common Sources of Error

The major pitfalls in nerve conduction studies usually result from technical errors in the stimulating or recording systems (Kimura 1989). The most common problems are easily corrected. They are (1) spread of the stimulating current to a nerve not under study, eliciting an unwanted potential from distant muscles; (2) anatomical variability, such as the presence of an anastomosis between the median and ulnar nerves in the forearm, and anomalous innervation of the extensor digitorum brevis (EBB) by the accessory deep peroneal nerve; (3) the effect of temporal dispersion; and (4) errors in the measurement of nerve length and conduction time.

Stimulation Current

A low-stimulus intensity may not activate the fastest-conducting, largest-diameter fibers. Failure to propagate impulses in some fibers distorts the waveform in a way that mimics a conduction block. An excessive stimulus intensity can cause an erroneously short latency because spread of stimulus current depolarizes the nerve a few millimeters away from the cathode, and the surface length between the two cathodal points no longer corresponds to the conduction distance of the nerve segment under study.

When recorded with a high sensitivity, a small negative peak, probably originating from small nerve fibers near the motor point, may precede the main negative component of the muscle action potential. This may lead to miscalculation of nerve conduction, especially if it is seen with stimulation at one point and not at a second point. If the evoked potentials obtained by stimulation at different sites are of dissimilar shapes, this precludes accurate calculation of conduction velocity, because the two onset latencies may represent motor fibers of different conduction characteristics.

Inappropriately high stimulus intensity may cause current spread to nerves or muscles not being tested. Visual inspection of the contracting muscle helps confirm selective activation of the intended nerve. Needle electrodes allow recording from a limited area when studying the innervation of individual motor branches or patterns of abnormality, although they do not reliably record the size of compound muscle action potentials.

Assessment of the median or ulnar nerve is difficult if both nerves are activated simultaneously at the axilla because of their proximity. To overcome this difficulty, we use a physiological nerve block applied distally to the nerve not under study (Figure 37B.6). The antidromic impulse from the wrist collides with the orthodromically directed impulse from the axilla in the ulnar nerve, allowing only the median impulse to reach the muscle. The ulnar response induced by the distal stimulus occurs much earlier and does not obscure the median CMAP. Similarly, distal stimulus to induce a physiological block of the median nerve enables selective recording from ulnar-innervated muscles when both nerves are coactivated at the axilla (see Figure 37B.6).

Anomalies

In the *Martin-Gruber anastomosis*, anomalous fibers cross from the median to the ulnar nerve in the forearm. The communicating branch usually consists of motor axons that supply the ulnar-innervated intrinsic hand muscles, with an inconsistent contribution from sensory axons. The anomaly represents a small bundle of ulnar fibers that descend with the median nerve as far as the elbow before branching off to join the ulnar nerve in the forearm.

Electrophysiological assessment establishes the presence of the anomaly, which occurs in 15–20% of people. Stimulation of the median nerve at the elbow activates both the median nerve and the anomalous ulnar fibers, but stimulation at the wrist evokes a smaller thenar potential without the ulnar component. Stimulation of the ulnar nerve causes the reverse; the evoked hypothenar potential is smaller from stimulation at the elbow than the wrist, because the distal stimulation activates the additional anomalous fibers. A

Table 37B.1: F waves in normal subjects[a]

Number of Nerves Tested	*Site of Stimulation*	*F-Wave Latency to Recording Site (m/sec)*	*Difference Between Right and Left (m/sec)*	*Central Latency[b] to and from the Spinal Cord (m/sec)*	*Difference Between Right and Left (m/sec)*	*Conduction Velocity[c] to and from the Spinal Cord (m/sec)*	*F Ratio[d] Between Proximal and Distal Segments*
122 median nerves from 61 subjects	Wrist	26.6 ±2.2 (31)[f]	0.95 ±0.67 (2.3)[f]	23.0 ±2.1 (27)[f]	0.93 ±0.62 (2.2)[f]	65.3 ±4.7 (56)[g]	—
	Elbow	22.8 ±1.9 (27)	0.76 ±0.56 (1.9)	15.4 ±1.4 (18)	0.71 ±0.52 (1.8)	67.8 ±5.8 (56)	0.98 ±0.08 (0.82–1.14)[f,g]
	Axilla[e]	20.4 ±1.9 (24)	0.85 ±0.61 (2.1)	10.6 ±1.5 (14)	0.85 ±0.58 (2.0)	—	—
130 ulnar nerves from 65 subjects	Wrist	27.6 ±2.2 (32)	1.0 ±0.83 (2.7)	25.0 ±2.1 (29)	0.84 ±0.59 (2.0)	65.3 ±4.8 (55)	—
	Above elbow	23.1 ±1.7 (27)	0.68 ±0.48 (1.6)	16.0 ±1.2 (18)	0.73 ±0.52 (1.8)	65.7 ±5.3 (55)	1.05 ±0.09 (0.87–1.23)
	Axilla[e]	20.3 ±1.6 (24)	0.73 ±0.54 (1.8)	10.4 ±1.1 (13)	0.76 ±0.52 (1.8)	—	—
120 peroneal nerves from 60 subjects	Ankle	48.4 ±4.0 (56)	1.42 ±1.03 (3.5)	44.7 ±3.8 (52)	1.28 ±0.90 (3.1)	49.8 ±3.6 (43)	—
	Above knee	39.9 ±3.2 (46)	1.28 ±0.91 (3.1)	27.3 ±2.4 (32)	1.18 ±0.89 (3.0)	55.1 ±4.6 (46)	1.05 ±0.09 (0.87–1.23)
118 tibial nerves from 59 subjects	Ankle	47.7 ±5.0 (58)	1.40 ±1.04 (3.5)	43.8 ±4.5 (53)	1.52 ±1.02 (3.6)	52.6 ±4.3 (44)	—
	Knee	39.6 ±4.4 (48)	1.25 ±0.92 (3.1)	27.6 ±3.2 (34)	1.23 ±0.88 (3.0)	53.7 ±4.8 (44)	1.11 ±0.11 (0.89–1.33)

[a]Mean ± standard deviation (SD).
[b]Central latency = F – M, where F and M are latencies of the F wave and M response, respectively.
[c]Conduction velocity = 2D/(F – M – 1), where D is the distance from the stimulus point to C7 or T12 spinous process.
[d]F ratio = (F – M – 1)/2M with stimulation with the cathode on the volar crease at the elbow (median). 3 cm above the medial epicondyle (ulnar), just above the head of fibula (peroneal) and in the popliteal fossa (tibial).
[e]F(A) = F(E) + M(E) – M(A), where F(A) and F(E) are latencies of the F wave with simulation at the axilla and elbow, respectively, and M(A) and M(E) are latencies of the corresponding M response.
[f]Upper limits of normal calculated as mean +2 SD.
[g]Lower limits of normal calculated as mean –2 SD.
Source: J Kimura. Electrodiagnosis in Diseases of Nerve and Muscle: Principles and Practices (2nd ed). Philadelphia: FA Davis, 1989.

collision technique selectively blocks unwanted impulses transmitted via the anomalous fibers (Figure 37B.7). Without using collision, an accurate conduction velocity cannot be calculated.

The EDB muscle is normally innervated by the deep peroneal nerve, a major branch of the common peroneal nerve. In 20–30% of individuals, the EDB is also innervated by the accessory deep peroneal nerve, an anomalous branch of the superficial peroneal nerve. Stimulation of the deep peroneal nerve at the ankle elicits a smaller CMAP than stimulation of the common peroneal nerve at the knee. Stimulation of the accessory deep peroneal nerve behind the lateral malleolus activates the anomalously innervated lateral portion of the muscle. The presence of this anomaly causes lesions of the deep peroneal nerve to spare the lateral portion of the EDB, leading to incorrect localization.

Temporal Dispersion

Onset latency allows calculation of the maximal motor or sensory velocities, and waveform analysis helps estimate the size and distribution of the functional units. They are equally important in the assessment of peripheral neuropathies and other conduction abnormalities.

Although the size of the recorded response approximates the number of excitable fibers, an amplitude discrepancy between the proximal and the distal sites of stimulation does not necessarily indicate a conduction block. The velocity of impulses in slow-conducting fibers lags increasingly behind those of fast-conducting fibers as conduction distance increases. Such temporal dispersion may result in a physiological reduction both in amplitude and area under the waveform. Nevertheless, regarding the motor fibers, stimuli of supramaximal intensity elicit nearly identical

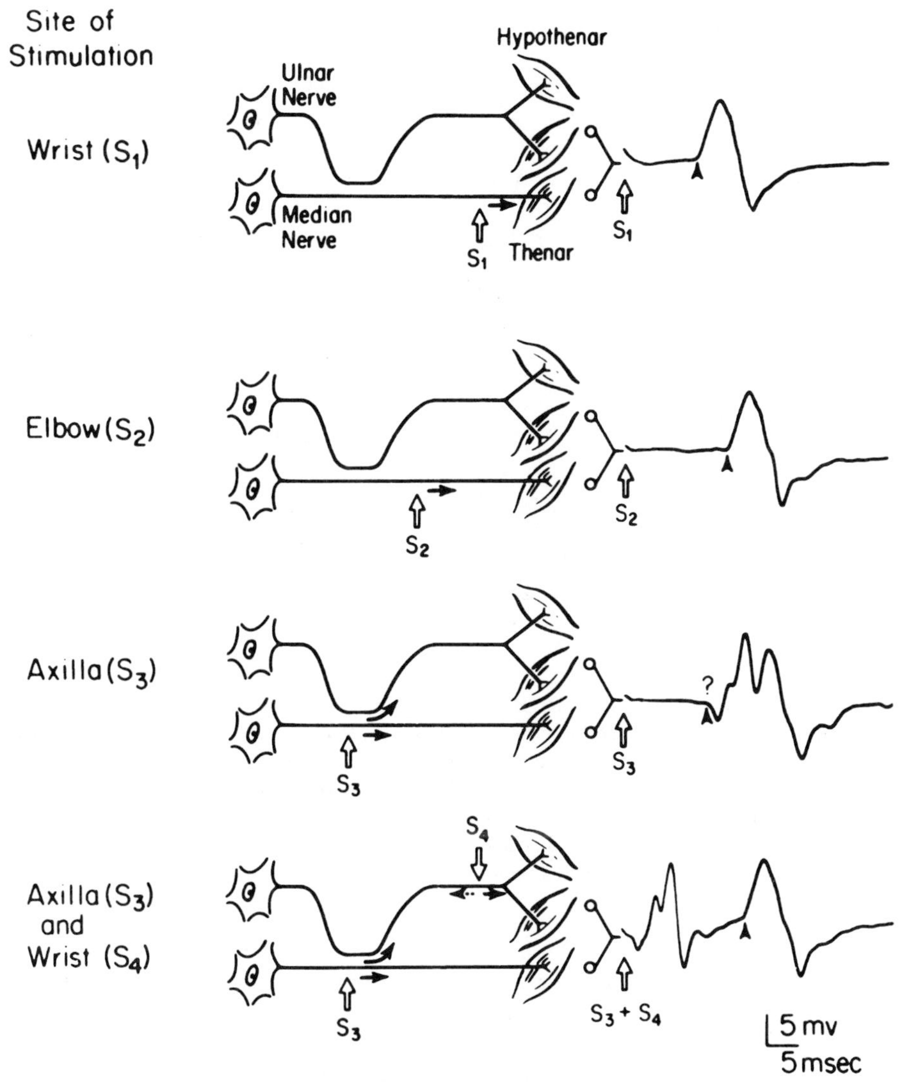

FIGURE 37B.6 A 39-year-old man with carpal tunnel syndrome. The stimulation of the median nerve at the wrist (S1) or elbow (S2) elicited a muscle action potential with increased latency in the thenar eminence. Spread of axillary stimulation (S3) to the ulnar nerve (third tracing from top) activated ulnar-innervated thenar muscles with shorter latency. Another stimulus (S4) applied to the ulnar nerve at the wrist (bottom tracing) blocked the proximal impulses by collision. The muscle action potential elicited by S4 occurred much earlier. The diagnosis on the left shows collision between the orthodromic (solid arrows) and antidromic (open arrows) impulses. (Reprinted with permission from J Kimura. Collision technique. Physiologic block of nerve impulses in studies of motor nerve conduction velocity. Neurology [Minneapolis] 1976;26:680–682.)

CMAPs regardless of the sites of stimulation. Thus, physiological temporal dispersion does not drastically alter the waveform of the CMAP.

In contrast, SNAPs become substantially smaller in amplitude and longer in duration with increasing distance between stimulating and pickup electrodes. Further, contrary to common belief, the area under the waveform also diminishes. For the same number of conducting fibers activated by the stimulus, the size of SNAPs changes almost linearly with the length of the nerve segment. Indeed, stimulation at Erb's point or the axilla often fails to elicit identifiable digital potentials without the use of an averaging technique.

Physiological temporal dispersion may affect SNAPs more than CMAPs because of the difference in duration of individual unit discharges between nerve and muscle (Figure 37B.8). With short-duration diphasic sensory spikes, a slight latency difference could line up the positive peaks of the fast fibers with the negative peaks of the slow fibers and cancel both (Figure 37B.9). In longer-duration motor unit potentials, the same latency shift would only partially superimpose peaks of opposite polarity, and cancellation would be less of a factor (Figure 37B.10).

Physiologic Variability

Effect of Temperature. Nerve impulses propagate faster by 2.4 m/second or approximately 5% per degree centigrade from 29° to 38°C of body temperature. Conversely, distal latencies increase when the hand is cooled. Cooling increases the amplitude of nerve and muscle potential in the squid axon, and in human nerves, probably because slowed Na^+ channel inactivation.

To reduce this type of variability, skin temperature is measured with a plate thermistor that correlates linearly with the subcutaneous and intramuscular temperatures. If the skin temperature falls below 34°C, indicating a muscle temperature of less then 37°C, it is necessary to warm the limbs with an infrared heat lamp or by immersion in warm water. Adding 5% of the calculated conduction velocity for each degree below

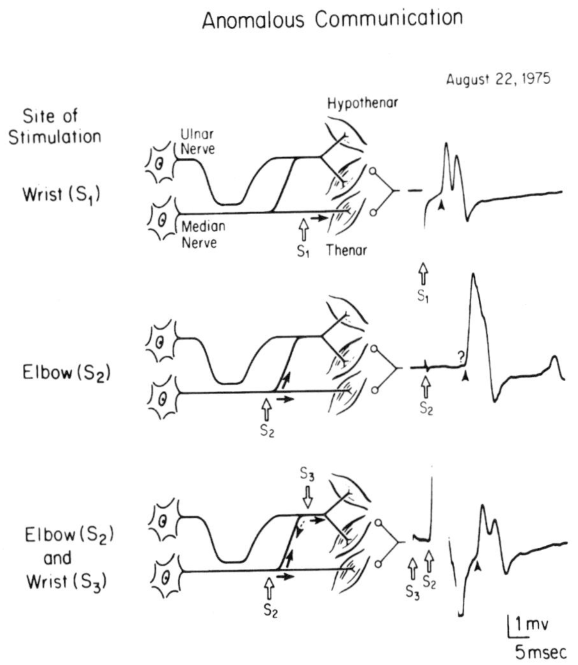

FIGURE 37B.7 A 55-year-old man with the carpal tunnel syndrome in the presence of an anomalous communication from the median to the ulnar nerve. The median nerve was stimulated at the wrist (S1) or elbow (S2), and the muscle potential was recorded by surface electrodes from the thenar eminence. Spread of the elbow stimulation (S2) to the ulnar nerve through the anomalous communication (middle tracing) activated ulnar-innervated thenar muscles, obscuring the onset (arrowhead) of the muscle response under study. Another stimulus (S3) applied to the ulnar nerve at the wrist (bottom tracing) blocked the impulses transmitted through the communicating fibers. The stimulus at the wrist (S3) was delivered 4 msec before the stimulation at the elbow (S2) to avoid an overlap of the muscle responses elicited by these two stimuli. (Reprinted with permission of the author and publisher from J Kimura. Collision technique. Physiologic block of nerve impulses in studies of motor nerve conduction velocity. Neurology [Minneapolis] 1976;26:680–682.)

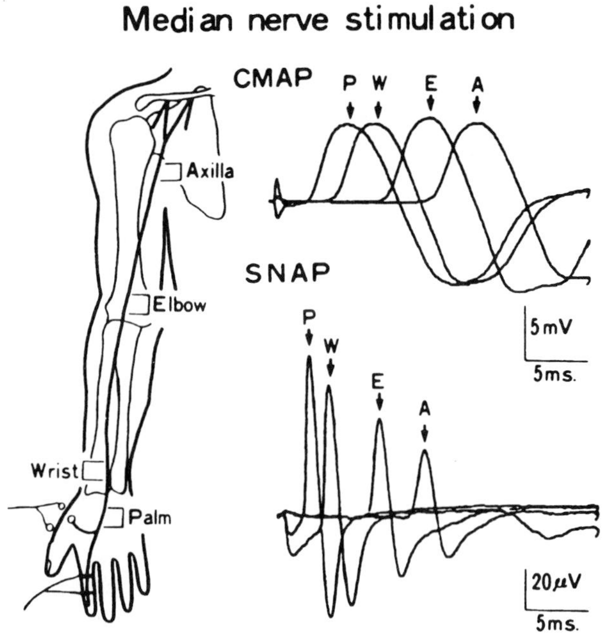

FIGURE 37B.8 Simultaneous recordings of compound muscle action potentials (CMAPs) from the thenar eminence and sensory nerve action potentials (SNAPs) from index and middle fingers after stimulation of the median nerve at palm, wrist, elbow, and axilla. With progressively more proximal stimulation, CMAPs remained nearly the same; for SNAPs, however, both amplitude and the area under the waveform became considerably smaller.

34°C theoretically normalizes the result. However, such conversion factors are based on experience with healthy individuals and may not apply to those with peripheral neuropathy.

Nerves and Nerve Segments. The conduction velocities of the peroneal and tibial nerves are 7–10 m/second slower than the median and ulnar nerves. This cannot be explained by the small reduction in temperature of the leg as compared to the arms. An inverse relationship between height and nerve conduction velocity suggests that longer nerves generally conduct slower than shorter nerves. Possible factors to account for the length-related slowing include abrupt distal axonal tapering, progressive reduction in axonal diameter, shorter internodal distances, or lower distal temperatures. Nerve impulses propagate faster in the proximal than the distal nerve segments for the same reason. This type of velocity gradient is documented by conventional nerve conduction studies and measurements of the F-wave latency, although such analyses show no significant difference between cord-to-axilla and axilla-to-elbow segments.

Effects of Age. Nerve conduction velocity increases with myelination from roughly half the adult value in full-term newborns to adult values at 3–5 years (Figure 37B.11). Conduction velocity in premature newborns ranges from 17 to 25 m/second in the ulnar nerve and from 14 to 28 m/second in the peroneal nerve. The conduction velocities of 23- to 24-week fetuses is roughly one-third of term newborns. Table 37B.2 summarizes the conduction velocity data in children compiled by Gamstorp in 1963.

Both motor and sensory conduction velocities tend to increase in the arms and decrease in the legs during childhood up to 19 years as a function of age and growth in length (Stetson et al. 1992). Conduction velocities slowly decline after 30–40 years of age. The mean conduction rate is reduced about 10% at 60 years of age. Aging also causes a diminution in amplitude and changes in the shape of the evoked potential, especially at the common sites of compression. The latencies of the F wave and somatosensory evoked potentials also gradually increase with advancing age.

Other Factors. Pneumatic tourniquet-induced ischemia causes a substantial change in nerve excitability, resulting in progressive slowing in conduction velocity, decrease in

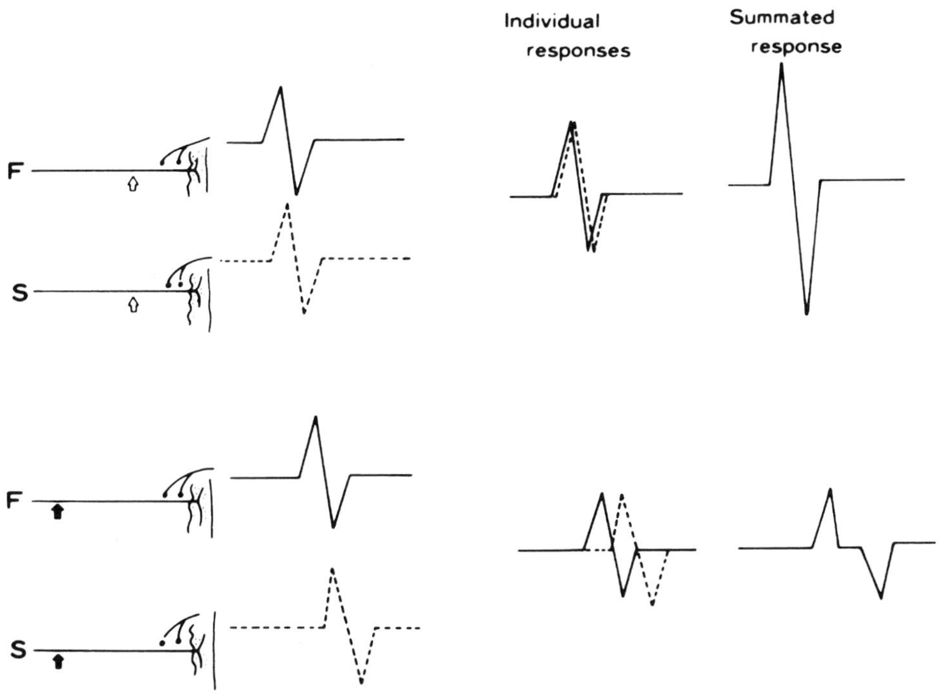

FIGURE 37B.9 Sensory action potentials. A model for phase cancellation between fast-conducting (F) and slow-conducting (S) sensory fibers. With distal stimulation, two unit discharges sum in phase to produce a sensory action potential twice as large. With proximal stimulation, a delay of the slow fiber causes phase cancellation between the negative peak of the fast fiber and positive peak of the slow fiber, resulting in a 50% reduction in size of the summated response. (Reprinted with permission from J Kimura, M Machida, T Ishida et al. Relation between size of compound sensory or muscle action potentials and length of nerve segment. Neurology 1986;36:647–652.)

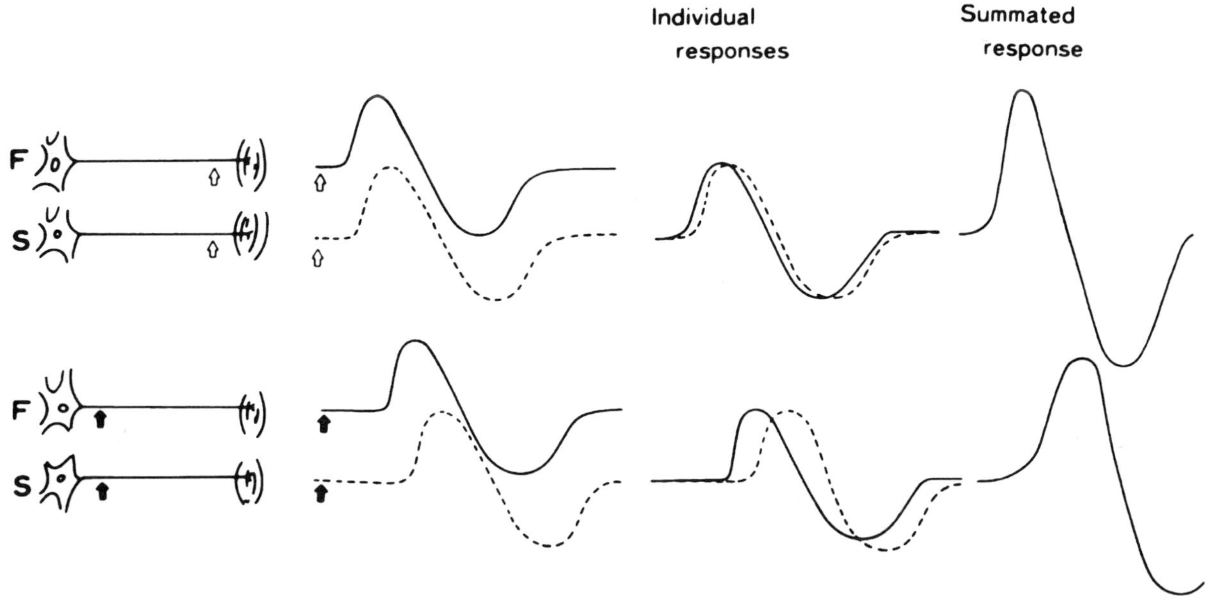

FIGURE 37B.10 Compound muscle action potentials. Same arrangements as in Figure 37B.9 to show the relationship between fast-conducting (F) and slow-conducting (S) motor fibers. With distal stimulation, two-unit discharges representing motor unit potentials sum to produce a muscle action potential twice as large. With proximal stimulation, motor unit potentials of long duration still superimpose nearly in phase despite the same latency shift of the slow motor fiber as the sensory fiber shown in Figure 37B.10. Thus, a physiologic temporal dispersion alters the size of the muscle action potential only minimally, if at all.

Phase cancellation increases substantially when the latency difference between fast- and slow-conducting fibers is increased by a demyelinating neuropathy. This gives the false impression of motor conduction block.

amplitude, and increase in duration of the action potential (Parry and Kohzu 1990). The effect is greater in patients with carpal tunnel syndrome than in normal controls when testing the median nerve. Conversely, ischemia alters peripheral nerve function less in elderly patients and in those with diabetes or uremia.

ELECTROMYOGRAPHY

Principles

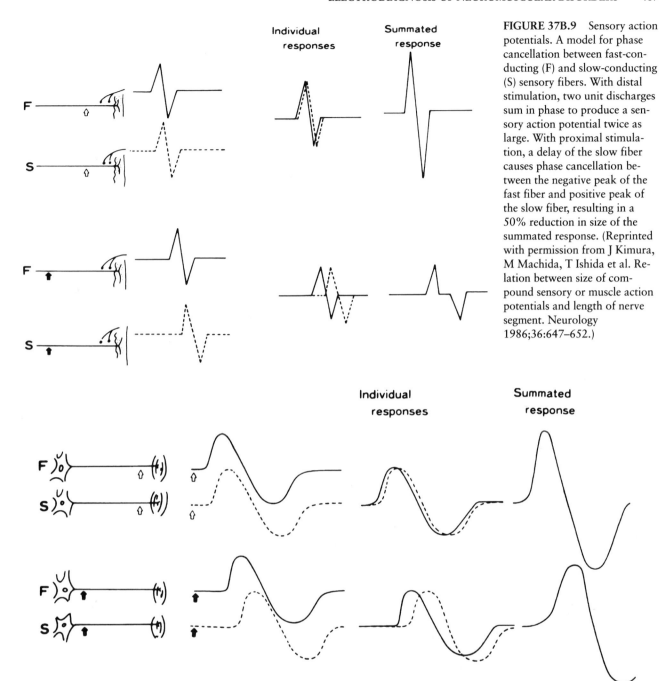

The *motor unit* consists of a single motor neuron and all the muscle fibers it innervates. It is the smallest unit capable

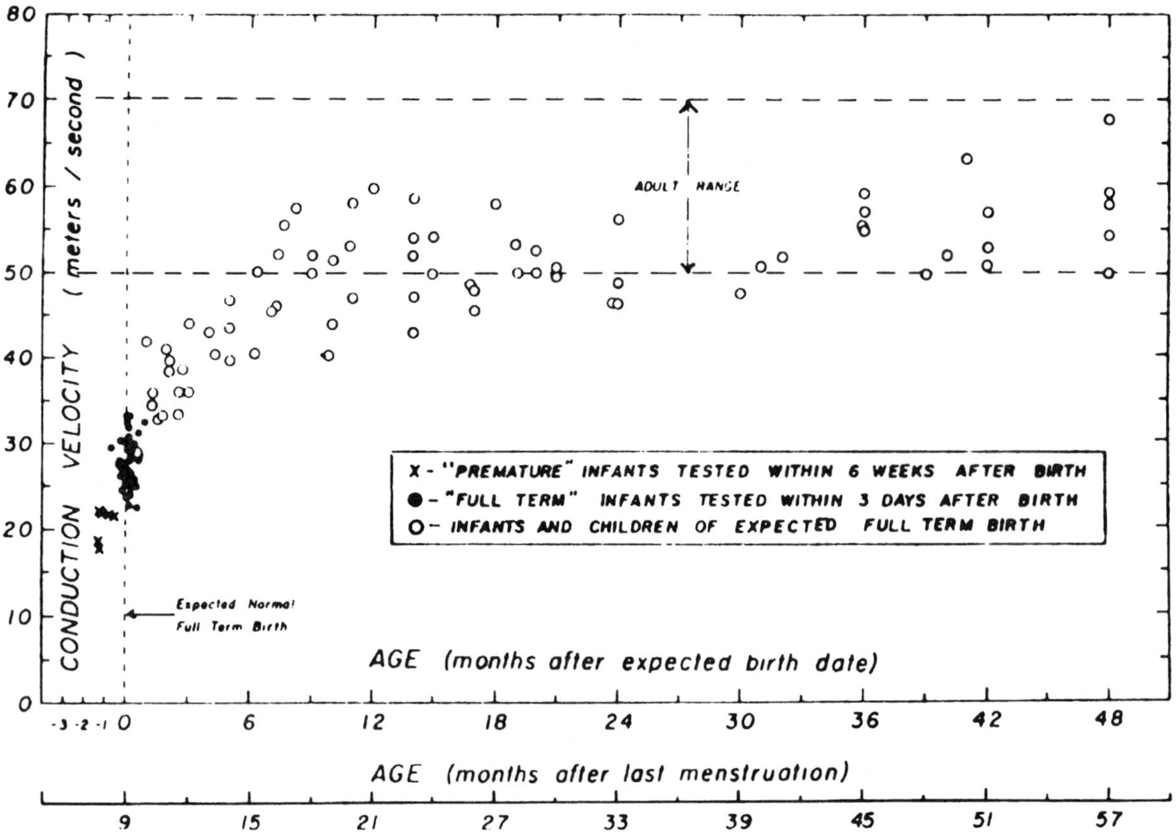

FIGURE 37B.11 Relation of age to conduction velocity of motor fibers in the ulnar nerve between the elbow and wrist. Velocities in normal young adults range from 47 to 73 m/second, with the majority of values between 50 and 70 m/second. Ages plotted indicate the month after the expected birth date based on calculation from the first day of last menstruation. (Reprinted with permission from JE Thomas, EH Lambert. Ulnar nerve conduction velocity and H reflex in infants and children. J Applied Physiol 1960;15:1–9.)

of individual excitation and thus the unit of all voluntary and reflex muscle contraction. All muscle fibers in one motor unit discharge simultaneously when stimulated by synaptic input to the motor neuron or by electrical stimulation of the axon. The ratio of muscle fibers per motor neuron (*motor unit ratio*) ranges from three to one for extrinsic eye muscles to between many hundreds to one for limb muscles. The smaller ratio generally occurs in muscles that perform fine gradations of movement. The distribution of muscle fibers in a fascicle is such that there is considerable overlap among different motor units. A single motor unit consists of either type I or type II muscle fibers, but never both (see Chapter 84).

Each muscle fiber has a motor endplate, which is the site of the neuromuscular junction. A needle electrode in proximity to the endplate records potentials that result from summation of miniature endplate potentials at the nerve terminal. The muscle fiber has a resting potential of 90 mV, with negativity inside the cell. The generation of an action potential reverses the transmembrane potential, which then becomes positive inside the cell. An extracellular electrode, as used in electromyography (EMG), records the activity resulting from this switch of polarity as a negative potential. As a rule, electrical potentials recorded in a volume conductor give rise to triphasic, positive-negative-positive waveforms. However, when recording near a damaged region, action potentials consist of a large positivity followed by a small negativity.

Techniques

Single-Fiber Electromyography

Single-fiber needles allow the recording of single-muscle fiber action potentials (Gilchrist 1992). Single-fiber electromyography (SFEMG) is most useful in clinical practice to determine *fiber density* (the number of single fibers firing within the recorded radius) and *jitter* (the variability of the interpotential interval between two or more single fibers belonging to the same motor unit) (Trontelj and Stålberg 1991).

A small side port on the canula of the needle serves as the pickup area. It records from a circle of 300-mm radius, as compared to the l-mm radius of a conventional EMG needle. The amplifier must have an impedance of 100 megaohms or greater to counter the high electrical

Table 37B.2: Normal sensory and motor nerve conduction velocities (m/sec) in different age groups[a]

	Age Group					
	10–35 Years (30 cases)		*36–50 Years (16 cases)*		*51–80 Years (18 cases)*	
Nerve	*Sensory*	*Motor*	*Sensory*	*Motor*	*Sensory*	*Motor*
Median nerve						
Digit-wrist	67.5 ±4.7	—	65.8 ±5.7	—	5.4 ±4.9	—
Wrist-muscle	—	3.2 ±0.3	—	3.7 ±0.3	—	3.5 ±0.2
Wrist-elbow	67.7 ±4.4	59.3 ±3.5	65.8 ±3.1	55.9 ±2.6	62.8 ±5.4	54.5 ±4.0
Elbow-axilla	70.4 ±4.8	65.9 ±5.0	70.4 ±3.4	65.1 ±4.2	66.2 ±3.6	63.6 ±4.4
Ulnar nerve						
Digit-wrist	64.7 ±3.9	—	66.5 ±3.4	—	57.5 ±6.6	—
Wrist-muscle	—	2.7 ±0.3[b]	—	2.7 ±0.3	—	3.0 ±0.35
Wrist-elbow	64.8 ±3.8	58.9 ±2.2	67.1 ±4.7	57.8 ±2.1	56.7 ±3.7	53.3 ±3.2
Elbow-axilla	69.1 ±4.3	64.4 ±2.6	70.6 ±2.4	63.3 ±2.0	64.4 ±3.0	59.9 ±0.7
Common peroneal nerve						
Ankle-muscle	—	4.3 ±0.9	—	4.8 ±0.5	—	4.6 ±0.6
Ankle-knee	53.0 ±5.0	49.5 ±5.6	50.4 ±1.0	43.6 ±5.1	46.1 ±4.0	43.9 ±4.3
Posterior tibial nerve						
Ankle-muscle	—	5.9 ±1.3	—	7.3 ±1.7	—	6.0 ±1.2
Ankle-knee	56.9 ±4.4	45.5 ±3.8	49.0 ±3.8	42.9 ±4.9	48.9 ±2.6	41.8 ±5.1
H reflex,	—	71.0 ±4.0	—	64.0 ±2.1	—	60.4 ±5.0
popliteal fossa	—	27.9 ±2.2	—	28.2 ±1.5	—	32.0 ±2.1

[a]Values are means ±1 standard deviation.
[b]Latency in milliseconds.
Source: J Kimura. Electrodiagnosis in Diseases of Nerve and Muscle: Principles and Practices (2nd ed). Philadelphia: FA Davis, 1989.

impedance of the small lead-off surface. The gain is set higher for SFEMG recordings than for conventional EMG, the sweep speed is faster, and the filter allows much higher frequencies.

A mild voluntary contraction produces a biphasic potential with a duration of about 1 msec and an amplitude that varies with the recording site. Single-fiber potentials suitable for study must have a peak-to-peak amplitude greater than 200 μV, rise time less than 300 μs, and a constant waveform. The needle is rotated, advanced, and retracted until a potential meets these criteria. A delay line allows the entire waveform to be viewed even though the single-fiber potential triggers the sweep.

Fiber density is determined by the number of single-fiber potentials firing almost synchronously with the initially identified single-fiber potential. Increased muscle fiber clustering indicates collateral sprouting (see Chapter 84). Simultaneously firing single-fiber potentials within 5 msec after the triggering single-fiber unit are counted at 20–30 sites. In the extensor digitorum communis muscle, single fibers fire without nearby discharges in 65–70% of random insertions; with only two fibers discharging in 30–35%; and with three fibers discharging in 5% or fewer.

If the variability in interpotential intervals between repetitively firing paired single-fiber potentials (jitter) exceeds a certain value, the second potential fails to appear. This phenomenon, called *blocking*, results primarily from motor endplate instability and is used as a sensitive test for disorders of the neuromuscular junction. Other neuromuscular disorders can also increase jitter. Age and other factors can affect the jitter value, but blocking in more than one fiber or jitter greater than 55 msec is definitely abnormal.

Jitter measurements require identifying 10 paired single-fiber potentials and determining the latency difference between takeoff of the earliest and latest second potentials. The average latency difference for five sampling sites is multiplied by 0.37 to give the *mean value of consecutive difference*. Jitter can be determined manually or by using a commercially available computer software program.

SFEMG may be abnormal in 1 of 20 recorded potentials in healthy subjects, so that increased jitter or blocking must appear in 2 or more of 20 pairs of potentials to indicate defective neuromuscular transmission. The degree of jitter varies from muscle to muscle in myasthenic patients; ocular myasthenics may have increased jitter only in the facial muscles. In the Lambert-Eaton myasthenic syndrome, higher jitter value up to 500 msec may occur (see Chapter 83). Jitter and blocking decrease with higher stimulus rate and increase with rest.

Conventional Electromyography Needle Examination

EMG evaluation is performed in four steps (Daube 1991):

1. Inserting or slightly moving the needle causes *insertional activity* that results from injury of muscle fibers by the needle.
2. *Spontaneous activity* is assessed in relaxed muscle by moving the needle a small distance and pausing a few

seconds. The needle is relocated in four quadrants of the muscle from a single insertion to make these evaluations.

3. A minimal contraction is obtained to assess several different *motor unit potentials* (MUPs), which are measured on the oscilloscope or hard copy.
4. The intensity of muscle contraction is increased to assess the *recruitment* of previously inactive MUPs. Maximal contraction normally fills the screen, producing the *interference pattern.*

Oscilloscope sweep speeds of 5–10 mV/cm best define spontaneous and voluntary activity; slower sweeps are used to study recruitment pattern. Most laboratories use an amplification of 50–100 μV/cm for spontaneous activity and 200 μV/cm to 1 mV/cm for voluntary activity. Our laboratory uses a low filter 10–20 Hz and high filter of 10 KHz.

Quantitative Measurements

EMG abnormalities can be assessed with reasonable certainty based on the visual display of waveforms and their audio characteristics. Such assessment may fail to delineate subtle abnormalities or mixed patterns that require *quantitative MUP measurement* (Engstrom and Olney 1992). A standardized objective method also allows meaningful comparison of test results obtained sequentially or in different laboratories. Findings often vary among different muscles in the same patient or even from one site to another in a given muscle. An adequate study requires exploration in different parts of the limb and sampling each muscle in several areas. Muscles with minimal dysfunction may be normal, and very severely diseased muscles may show only nonspecific end-stage change. Therefore, an optimal examination should include muscles that are moderately affected but not totally destroyed.

It is also possible to automatically analyze MUP using analog or digital techniques. The MUP is converted into a digital equivalent for analysis of duration, amplitude, polarity, number of phases, and integrated area under the waveform. MUPs are selected by visual inspection using a monitor scope; only MUPs whose peak-to-peak amplitude exceeds a predetermined value are accepted. Computer analysis, which can be conducted quickly and automatically, can discriminate typical neuropathic and myopathic changes, showing no major discrepancy compared to the results of manual quantification. Automated techniques do not always resolve borderline cases in which conventional methods provide equivocal information.

Normal and Abnormal Results

Insertional Activity

Origin and Characteristics. Brief bursts of electrical discharges accompany insertion of a needle electrode into the muscle and each repositioning, slightly outlasting the movement of the needle. On average, insertional activity lasts for a few hundred milliseconds. It appears as a cluster of positive or negative repetitive high-frequency spikes, which make a crisp static sound over the loudspeaker. The term *injury potential* implies that insertional activity originates from muscle fibers injured or mechanically stimulated by the penetrating needle.

Decreased Versus Prolonged Activity. A marked reduction or absence of insertional activity suggests either fibrotic or severely atrophied muscles or functionally inexcitable muscles such as occur during attacks of familial periodic paralysis. In contrast, an abnormally prolonged insertional activity indicates instability of the muscle membrane, often seen in conjunction with denervation, myotonic disorders, or certain myopathies such as myositis.

Insertional Positive Waves. Needle insertion often provokes sustained *positive sharp waves* and, less frequently, *fibrillation potentials* in denervated muscles. These discharges fire 3–30 impulses per second and last several seconds to minutes after needle movement ceases. They are initiated by needle movement but are otherwise identical to the spontaneous discharges recorded from denervated muscle at rest. This activity signals early denervation (10 days to 2 weeks after nerve injury), chronic denervation, or rapidly progressive degeneration of muscle fibers.

Myotonic Discharge

Myotonic discharges are a special type of insertional activity. They appear either as a sustained run of sharp positive waves, each followed by a slow negative component of longer duration, or as a sustained run of negative spikes with a small initial positivity. Myotonic discharges are recurring single-fiber potentials, showing, like those of denervation, two types of waveforms depending on the spatial relationship between the recording surface of the needle electrode and the discharging muscle fibers.

Of the two types, the positive sharp waves are usually initiated by needle insertion injuring muscle membrane, whereas the negative spikes, resembling fibrillation potentials, tend to occur at the beginning of slight volitional contraction. Both positive sharp waves and negative spikes typically wax and wane in amplitude over the range of 10 μV to 1 mV, varying inversely to the rate of firing. Their frequency range, 50–100 impulses per second, gives rise to a characteristic noise over the loudspeaker, simulating an accelerating or decelerating motorcycle or chain saw.

Endplate Activity

Endplate Noise. The tip of the needle approaching the endplate region frequently registers recurring irregular negative potentials, 10–50 μV in amplitude and 1–2 msec in duration (Figure 37B.12). The extracellularly recorded

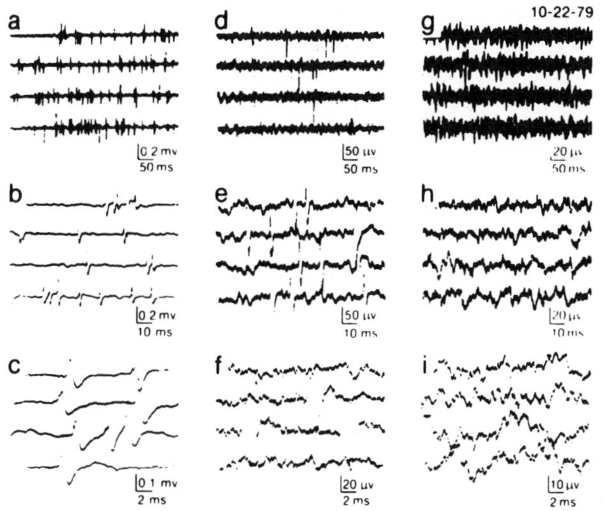

FIGURE 37B.12 Normal endplate activity. Endplate spikes (a, b, c) are of much greater amplitude than endplate noise (g, h, i). Usually these are seen together (d, e, f). (Reprinted with permission of the author and publisher from J Kimura. Electrodiagnosis in Diseases of Nerve and Muscle: Principles and Practices [2nd ed]. Philadelphia: FA Davis, 1989.)

miniature endplate potentials are nonpropagating depolarizations caused by spontaneous release of acetylcholine (ACh) quanta. They produce a characteristic sound much like a seashell held to the ear.

Endplate Spike. Endplate noise is intermixed with intermittent spikes, 100–200 μV in amplitude, and 3–4 msec in duration, firing irregularly at 5–50 impulses per second (see Figure 37B.12). The endplate spikes are discharges of single muscle fibers excited by activation of intramuscular nerve terminals irritated by the needle. The similarity of the firing pattern of endplate spikes to discharges of muscle spindle afferents suggests that they may originate in the intrafusal muscle fibers.

The waveform of endplate spikes is indistinguishable from initially negative fibrillation potentials recorded with the tip of the recording electrode at the endplate region. However, their irregular pattern of high-frequency discharge is not seen in fibrillation potentials. Slight relocation of the needle tip near the source of discharge may reverse the polarity of the initially negative endplate spikes, and endplate spikes can appear as positive sharp waves without negative spikes if the recording needle injures the cell membrane at the endplate region.

Spontaneous Activity

Types of Discharges. Spontaneous activity includes *fibrillation potentials, positive sharp waves, fasciculation potentials, myokymic discharges,* and *complex repetitive discharges.* Fasciculation potentials and complex repetitive discharges may cause detectable movement over a localized area, but neither fibrillation potentials nor positive sharp waves can be seen at the skin surface. Myokymic discharges often give rise to sustained contractions, which have an undulating appearance beneath the skin ("bag of worms").

Both fibrillation potentials and positive sharp waves are generated by spontaneous discharge of single muscle fibers (Daube 1991). The waveform of the potential is dictated by the physical relationship between the firing unit and the recording electrode. If the tip of the needle damages the membrane, the sustained standing depolarization prevents the appearance of a negative spike. Propagating action potentials approach the site of injury as a sharp positive discharge, followed by low-amplitude negative deflection.

Fasciculation potentials are isolated spontaneous discharges of a motor unit, and myokymic discharges are grouped fasciculations caused by repetitive firing. Complex repetitive discharges result from rapid firing of many muscle fibers in sequence, driven ephaptically at a point of lateral contact. A spontaneously activated single fiber serves as a pacemaker that regulates the frequency and pattern of discharge by two different and usually independent, mechanisms: rate of rhythmic depolarization of the denervated muscle fiber and circus movements of currents among muscle fibers.

A numerical grading is used to semiquantitate fibrillation potentials and positive sharp waves. +1 represents transient runs of positive discharges after moving the needle electrode (i.e., insertional positive waves). +2 represents occasional spontaneous potentials at rest in more than two different sites. +3 represents spontaneous activities present at rest, regardless of the position of the needle electrode. +4 represents abundant spontaneous potentials nearly filling the screen of the oscilloscope.

Fibrillation Potentials. Fibrillation potentials are diphasic or triphasic with initial positivity (Figure 37B.13). They range 15 msec in duration and 20–200 μV in amplitude when recorded with a concentric needle electrode. If the needle electrode is placed near the endplate zone, they resemble physiological endplate spikes with an initial negativity.

Fibrillation potentials are triggered by spontaneous oscillations in the membrane potential. They typically fire in a regular pattern at a rate of 1–30 impulses per second with an average frequency of 13 impulses per second. A very irregular firing pattern usually indicates that more than one fiber is firing but may also originate from the same muscle fiber.

The sound produced by fibrillation potentials is crisp and clicking, reminiscent of the sound caused by wrinkling tissue paper or frying fat in a pan. Discharge frequency increases by warming the muscle or after administration of cholinesterase inhibitors, and decreases with moderate cooling of the muscle or hypoxia.

Although fibrillation potentials may occasionally occur in otherwise healthy muscles, the presence of reproducible discharges in at least two different areas of the muscle usually suggests lower motor neuron disorders. Because of the 2- to 3-week latent period before fibrillations appear after nerve in-

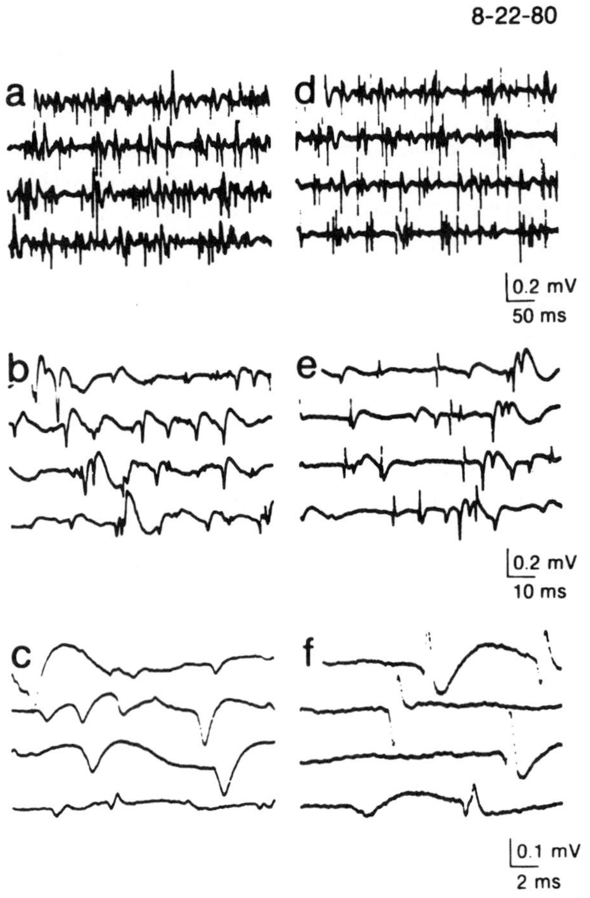

FIGURE 37B.13 Spontaneous activity recorded from the paraspinal muscle in a patient with radiculopathy, showing positive sharp waves (a, b, c) and fibrillation potentials (d, e, f). (Reprinted with permission of the author and publisher from J Kimura. Electrodiagnosis in Diseases of Nerve and Muscle: Principles and Practices [2nd ed]. Philadelphia: FA Davis, 1989.)

jury, their absence does not preclude recent denervation. The distribution of spontaneous potentials is useful to localize lesions in the spinal cord, root, plexus, or peripheral nerve.

Fibrillation potentials are recorded in some myopathic processes, especially the muscular dystrophies and inflammatory myopathies (see Chapter 84). Spontaneous activity may also result from increased membrane irritability or inflammation of intramuscular nerve fibers.

Positive Sharp Waves. These discharges often follow insertion of the needle but also occur spontaneously, at regular intervals. The initial positivity and the subsequent slow negativity, much lower in amplitude but longer in duration, gives a characteristic sawtooth appearance. Recording near the damaged part of the muscle fiber incapable of generating an action potential accounts for the absence of negative spike. Although usually seen together, positive sharp waves tend to precede fibrillation potentials after nerve section, possibly because they can be triggered by the insertion of a needle in already irritable muscle membrane.

Like fibrillation potentials, positive sharp waves are seen not only in denervated muscles but also in several myopathic conditions, especially muscular dystrophies and inflammatory myopathies. Positive sharp waves may also form part of myotonic discharges, triggered by insertion of the needle or mild voluntary contraction. Despite similarities in waveform, positive sharp waves associated with denervation do not have the characteristic waxing and waning appearance seen in myotonia.

Fasciculation Potentials. Fasciculation potentials originate in the axon or anywhere along the length of the peripheral nerve and may also originate in the spinal cord. Voluntary motor unit potentials mimic fasciculation potentials, but fasciculation potentials undergo slight changes in amplitude and waveform from time to time, have a much slower firing rate, and are unaffected by slight voluntary contraction of agonist or antagonist muscles.

Fasciculation potentials are most commonly seen in diseases of anterior horn cells, but the differential diagnosis includes radiculopathy, entrapment neuropathy, the cramps-fasciculation syndrome, and cervical spondylotic myelopathy. Fasciculation potentials appear in the legs with cervical compression and abate following decompression. They are also seen in tetany, thyrotoxicosis, and overdose of anticholinesterase medication (Daube 1991). Grouped fasciculation potentials from multiple units suggest amyotrophic lateral sclerosis, progressive spinal muscular atrophy, or other degenerative diseases of the anterior horn cells, such as poliomyelitis and syringomyelia.

Myokymic Discharges. Myokymia results from complex bursts of repetitive discharges in which the same motor units fire repetitively, usually with 2–10 spikes discharging at 30–40 impulses per second. Each burst recurs at regular intervals of 0.1–10.0 seconds (Figure 37B.14). Myokymic bursts probably originate ectopically in demyelinated motor nerve fibers and accordingly are amplified by increased axonal excitability, such as after hyperventilation-induced hypocapnea. Myokymic discharges in the facial muscles suggest a brain stem glioma or multiple sclerosis, and myokymic discharges in limb muscles suggest chronic neuropathies such as the Guillain-Barré syndrome and radiation plexopathies.

Normal muscle sometimes shows single or grouped spontaneous discharges that may cause cramps. Waveform analysis of action potentials cannot reliably distinguish this form of fasciculation potential from those associated with motor neuron disease. The frequency of discharge may separate the two; those seen in motor neuron disease discharge irregularly at an average interval of 3.5 seconds as compared with 0.8 second in *benign fasciculation syndrome*. The association of fasciculation potentials with either fibrillation potentials or positive sharp waves suggests a disease of the lower motor neuron at any level from the anterior horn cells to axon terminals.

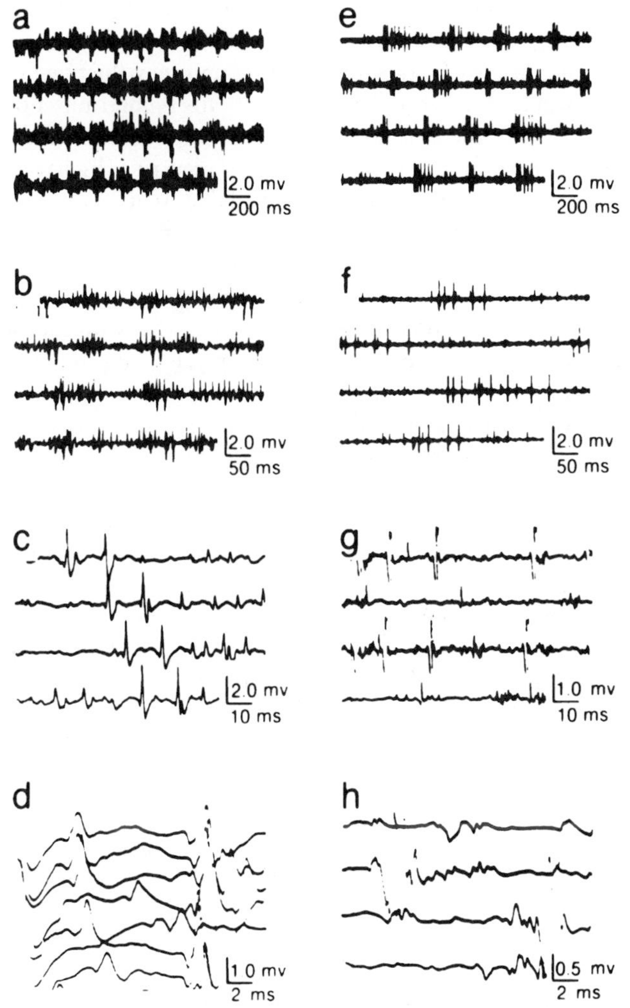

FIGURE 37B.14 Myokymic discharges from the orbicularis oris (a, b, c, d) and orbicularis oculi (e, f, g, h) muscles of a patient with multiple sclerosis. The repetitive pattern of the waveform is shown in d, in which a recurring potential triggered the sweep. (Reprinted with permission of the author and publisher from J Kimura. Electrodiagnosis in Diseases of Nerve and Muscle: Principles and Practices [2nd ed]. Philadelphia: FA Davis, 1989.)

Complex Repetitive Discharges. Complex repetitive discharges result from the near-synchronous firing of a group of muscle fibers. The discharges range from 50 μV to 1 mV in amplitude and up to 50–100 msec in duration. Each burst contains 10 or more distinct MUPs separated by intervals that range from less than 0.5 msec to as much as 100–200 msec. One fiber in the complex serves as a pacemaker, driving one or several other fibers ephaptically so that the individual spikes within the complex fire in the same order as the discharge recurs.

One of the late-activated fibers reexcites the principal pacemaker to repeat the cycle. The entire sequence recurs at slow or fast rates, usually in the range of 5–100 impulses per second. The polyphasic and complex waveform remains uniform from one discharge to another, although the shape may change suddenly. These discharges typically begin abruptly, maintain a constant rate of firing for a short period, and cease as abruptly as they started when the chain reaction eventually blocks. They produce a noise that mimics the sound of a machine gun. The spike components of complex repetitive discharges often have higher amplitude than fibrillation potentials. This is probably why the electrical field associated with this repetitive pattern effectively induces ephaptic activation of neighboring muscle fibers.

This discharge occurs most commonly in Duchenne's muscular dystrophy, spinal muscular atrophy, and Charcot-Marie-Tooth's disease, but is also seen in other chronic myopathies and neuropathies. Complex repetitive discharges are also found in the striated muscle of the urethral sphincter of women with urinary retention, and in deep muscles such as the iliopsoas of apparently healthy individuals, probably implying a clinically silent irritative process.

Continuous Muscle Fiber Activity. Continuous muscle fiber activity occurs in neuromyotonia (see Chapter 30). Muscle fibers fire repetitively at 100–300 Hz, either continuously or in recurring bursts, producing a "pinging" sound. The discharge continues during sleep and, unlike myokymia, also persists after procaine block of the nerve. Other conditions associated with continuous muscle fiber activity include anticholinesterase poisoning, tetany, and chronic spinal muscular atrophies.

Cramp Discharges. Cramps are sustained, usually painful, involuntary muscle contractions (see Chapter 30). An EMG cramp discharge consists of motor unit potentials usually firing at a rate of 40–60 per second, with abrupt onset and cessation. Cramps most often occur in healthy individuals, but are exaggerated by hyponatremia, hypocalcemia, myxedema, pregnancy, postdialysis states, and early stages of motor neuron disease.

Motor Unit Potentials

Motor Unit Profile. The amplitude, rise time, duration, and number of phases together characterize an MUP (Daube 1991). The waveform is dictated by the inherent properties of the MUP and the spatial relationships between the needle and individual muscle fibers. Slight repositioning of the electrode causes major changes in the electrical profile of the same motor unit. Therefore, one motor unit can give rise to many MUPs of different amplitude at different recording sites.

Amplitude. MUP amplitudes range from several hundred microvolts to a few millivolts with a concentric needle, and substantially greater with a monopolar needle. The amplitude of MUP falls to less than 50% at a distance of 200–300 mm from the source and to less than 1% a few millimeters away. Therefore, of all the individual muscle fibers in a motor unit discharging in near-synchrony, only the small number located near the tip of the recording electrode determine the amplitude of an MUP; probably less than 20 muscle fibers lying within a 1-mm radius of the electrode tip. In general, amplitude indicates muscle fiber density and not the motor unit territory.

Rise Time. Rise time is the time lag from the initial positive peak to the subsequent negative peak. Closeness between the recording tip of the electrode and the discharging motor unit shortens the rise time and produces a crisp sound, which is an important clue of proximity of the unit to the electrode. Distant units have a greater rise time because the resistance and capacitance of the intervening tissue act as a high-frequency filter. A distant discharge has a dull sound, indicating the need to reposition the electrode closer to the source. Rise time confirms the suitability of the recorded potential for quantitative assessment of amplitude. A unit accepted for quantitative measurement should have a rise time less than 500 msec, and preferably 100–200 msec.

Duration. MUP duration reflects the activity from most muscle fibers belonging to a motor unit because potentials generated more than 1 mm away from the electrode contribute to the initial and terminal low-amplitude portions of the potential. The duration, measured from the initial takeoff to the return to the baseline, indicates the degree of synchrony among many individual muscle fibers with variable length, conduction velocity, and membrane excitability. A slight shift in needle position influences duration much less than the amplitude. The duration normally varies from 5 to 15 msec, depending on the age of the subject. The duration of the MUP is a good index of the motor unit territory. For meaningful assessment, one must compare the measured value to the normal range established in the same muscle for the same age group by the same technique.

Phases. A phase constitutes the portion of a waveform that departs from and returns to the baseline. The number of phases equals the number of negative and positive peaks extending to and from the baseline, or the number of baseline crossings plus one. Most normal MUP have four phases or less; 5–15% have five phases or more. An increased number of *polyphasic MUPs* suggests desynchronized discharge or loss of individual fibers within a motor unit. Some action potentials have a serrated pattern with several "turns" or directional changes without crossing the baseline; this also indicates desynchronization among discharging muscle fibers. The number of polyphasic units is increased in myopathy, neuropathy, and neuronopathy. Polyphasia indicates temporal dispersion of muscle fiber potentials within a motor unit. Excessive temporal dispersion, in turn, results from differences in conduction time along the terminal branch of the nerve or over the muscle fiber membrane.

Stability. Waveform variability of a repetitively firing MUP indicates deficient neuromuscular transmission. Motor units normally discharge semirhythmically, with successive potentials showing nearly identical configuration. The amplitude of a repetitively firing unit may fluctuate or diminish steadily if individual muscle fibers intermittently block within the unit. Such is the case in patients with defective neuromuscular transmission, as recurring discharges deplete the store of immediately available ACh.

This observation is especially useful in muscles not accessible by conventional nerve stimulation techniques. MUP instability is consistent with not only myasthenia gravis, the myasthenic syndrome, and botulism, but also with motor neuron disease, poliomyelitis, syringomyelia, and the early stages of reinnervation. In myotonia congenita, a characteristic decline in amplitude of the successive discharges typically recovers during continued contraction.

Discharge Pattern. A motor unit may fire twice (doublet) or thrice (triplet) at very short intervals. Doublet discharges suggest two action potentials maintaining the same relationship to one another at intervals of 2–20 msec, whereas *paired discharges* are a set of spikes with longer intervals, ranging from 20 to 80 msec. The intervals also range from 2 to 20 msec for triplets, although the middle spike discharges closer to the first than to the third. Multiple discharges occur in latent tetanus, hyperventilation, myotonic dystrophy, and other hyperexcitable states of the motor neuron pool. They are also seen in poliomyelitis, motor neuron disease, the Guillain-Barré syndrome, radiculopathy, and at the beginning and termination of voluntary contraction in normal muscles.

Lower Motor Neuron Versus Myopathic Disorders. The amplitude and duration of the MUP are altered in different ways in myopathies as compared to neuropathies. Amplitude and duration increase in lower motor neuron diseases and decrease in myopathies (see Chapters 79 and 84). Electromyography and histochemical findings from muscle biopsies have an overall concordance of 90% or greater, except in some very chronic degenerative neuromuscular disorders.

The increased size of the MUP in neuropathic disorders could be caused by simultaneous discharge of two or more motor units because of abnormal synchronization at the spinal cord level or ephaptic activation near the terminal axons, but the usual explanation is anatomic reorganization of the motor unit by axon sprouting from healthy neurons. The incorporation of denervated fibers within the territory of the surviving axon increases muscle fiber density, which in turn increases MUP amplitude. Increased MUP duration is probably caused by the variability in length and conduction time of regenerating axon terminals rather than the enlarged territory.

Destructive myopathic disorders may lead to the random loss of parts or all of functional muscle fibers from each motor unit. If only a single muscle fiber is left in a motor unit, its MUP is equivalent to a fibrillation potential. In such cases, the voluntary activation of short 1- to 2-msec–duration spikes of the MUPs produces a high-frequency sound over the loudspeaker that sounds like spontaneously discharging fibrillation potentials. On the other hand, mild metabolic and endocrine myopathies usually cause little or no alteration in the duration or amplitude of the MUP.

The dichotomy between myopathic and neuropathic changes in the MUP is to some extent an oversimplification and does not always correlate with the clinical diagnosis. "Sick" axon terminals in a distal neuropathy may result in random loss of muscle fibers within a motor unit and an appearance on EMG suggesting myopathy. During early reinnervation, immature motor units consist of only a few muscle fibers. In both examples, the MUP may be polyphasic, low in amplitude, and short in duration, which changes typify myopathy. Conversely, long-duration MUPs may occur in myopathies with regenerating muscle fibers, erroneously suggesting a neuropathic process. These long-duration potentials are usually distinct from the main unit and were called "satellite" or "parasite" potentials but are now called *late components*. Further, if fiber density increases during regeneration, the amplitude of the MUP may be greater than expected in myopathy.

Recruitment

Recruitment Pattern. During constant contraction, a healthy individual initially excites only 1–2 motor units semirhythmically with slowly increasing, then decreasing interspike intervals. The motor units activated early are primarily those with small, type I muscle fibers. Large, type II units participate later during strong voluntary contraction. Greater muscle force brings about not only recruitment of previously inactive units but also more rapid firing of already active units, both mechanisms operating simultaneously (Petajan 1991).

Recruitment frequency is a measure of motor unit discharge, defined as the firing frequency at the time an additional unit is recruited. In normal muscles, mild contraction induces isolated discharges at a rate of 5–10 impulses per second, depending on the types of motor units studied. The reported ranges for healthy individuals and those with neuromuscular disorders overlap considerably. The normal recruitment ratio, defined as the average firing rate divided by the number of active units, should not exceed five with, for example, three units each firing less than 15 impulses per second (Daube 1991). A ratio of 10, with two units firing at 20 impulses per second each, indicates a loss of motor units.

With greater contraction, many motor units begin to fire rapidly, making recognition of individual unit potentials difficult—hence the name *interference pattern*. A number of factors influence the spike density and the average amplitude of the summated response. These include descending input from the cortex, number of motor neurons capable of discharging, firing frequency of each motor unit, waveform of individual potentials, and phase cancellation. Because of such complexity, analysis of the summated response provides only a semiquantitative means to evaluate the number of firing units during maximal muscle contraction.

Lower and Upper Motor Neuron Disorders. Recruitment is limited in disorders with a reduced number of excitable motor neurons. During increasing effort, surviving motor neurons must fire at an inappropriately rapid rate to compensate for the loss in number. In the extreme, a single MUP discharges at a high rate, producing the discrete "picket fence" or *single-unit interference pattern* at maximal effort (Figure 37B.15).

Failure of descending impulses also limits recruitment, although here the excited motor units discharge more slowly than expected for normal maximal contraction. Thus, a slow rate of discharge in an upper motor neuron or hysterical paralysis stands in sharp contrast to a fast rate of discharge of a lower motor neuron weakness, even though both have a reduced interference pattern. Irregular tremulous firing of motor units, not seen in genuine paresis, suggests hysterical weakness or poor cooperation.

Myopathy

Low-amplitude, short-duration MUPs produce a smaller force per unit than normal MUPs. The efficiency of motor unit discharge is inversely related to the number of units required to maintain a given force. Many units must be recruited instantaneously to support a slight voluntary effort in patients with advanced myopathy or disorders of neuromuscular transmission. When motor units recruit early, a full interference pattern is attained at less than maximal contraction, but its amplitude is low because fiber density is decreased in individual motor units. In advanced myopathic disorders, loss of muscle fibers is so extensive that whole motor units disappear, resulting in limited recruitment and an incomplete interference pattern, mimicking a neuropathic change.

Interpretation

The results of the needle EMG study supplement but do not replace the clinical evaluation (Figure 37B.16). The electromyographer must first take a history and examine the patient to design the best EMG study. The content of the study depends on the clinical situation and the EMG findings in muscles already tested. The testing physician must know the normal values in different muscles, how EMG findings differ in different diseases, and how to recognize some EMG findings as nonspecific.

Upper Motor Neuron Lesions

Patients with upper motor neuron lesions have normal insertional activity, spontaneous activity is not present at rest, and the MUPs are normal in size and morphology. The only abnormality is a reduced interference pattern and a slow

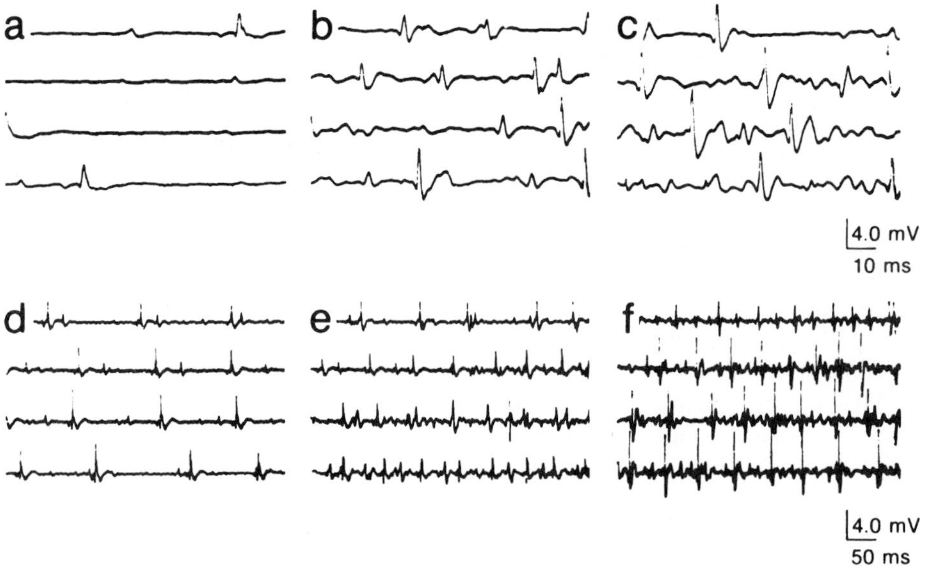

FIGURE 37B.15 Abnormal recruitment in the tibialis anterior muscle of a patient with motor neuron disease, with rapid discharge of a single motor unit during strong contraction. (Reprinted with permission of the author and publisher from J Kimura. Electrodiagnosis in Diseases of Nerve and Muscle: Principles and Practices [2nd ed]. Philadelphia: FA Davis, 1989.)

rate of motor unit discharge (Shahani et al. 1991). Hysterical weakness produces a similar firing pattern, except that motor unit firing is irregular. Recruitment, measured by either recruitment frequency or ratio of firing rate to number of firing units, is normal in patients with upper motor neuron lesions or hysteria.

Lower Motor Neuron Lesions

Insertional activity is usually increased and outlasts movement of the needle. Insertional positive waves may appear within 2 weeks after denervation injury. Late in the course, muscles that are fibrotic or severely atrophied show no insertional activity. Spontaneous activity, appearing 2–3 weeks after nerve injury, consists of fibrillation potentials and positive sharp waves. Complex repetitive discharges occur mainly in chronic lower motor neuron disorders such as spinal muscular atrophy and Charcot-Marie-Tooth's disease but also in certain myopathic disorders such as muscular dystrophy and polymyositis. Fasciculation potentials accompany electrical denervation changes in diseases of the anterior horn cells, roots, and peripheral nerves, but do not have pathological significance when they appear alone. Myokymic discharges in the facial muscles are usually associated with multiple sclerosis and brain stem gliomas, but also occur with polyradiculopathies and Bell's palsy. Myokymia in the limbs is associated with radiation plexopathy.

Reinnervation causes first an increased number of phases and then an increased amplitude and duration of the MUP (Lester et al. 1993). Amplitude generally reflects fiber density and duration reflects motor unit territory. The expected MUP from lower motor neuron lesions is a long-duration, high-amplitude polyphasic unit. The exceptions are distal axonopathy and early reinnervation in which loss of muscle fibers in the motor units results in brief, small polyphasic motor units.

Recruitment frequency and ratio increase because fewer motor units fire for a given strength of contraction (Daube 1991). In the extreme case, only a single motor unit fires rapidly, producing a picket fence pattern.

The distribution of denervation potentials in different muscles can be used to localize lesions at the root, plexus, peripheral nerve, and anterior horn cell. For example, paraspinal muscle abnormalities suggest a radiculopathy because the lesion must be proximal to the division of the spinal nerve into anterior and posterior rami. Paraspinal findings may also be part of a diffuse neuropathic process, and multiple levels must be assessed for precise localization. EMG also provides a means to estimate prognosis in disorders such as the Guillain-Barré syndrome and idiopathic facial palsy (Albers 1993). In these conditions, the presence of spontaneous activity indicates axonal damage, and recovery requires reinnervation, which is a much longer process than remyelination.

Myopathic Disorders

Insertional activity is usually normal except in the late stage of the disease when it is reduced by atrophy and fibrosis. Spontaneous activity is absent except in some cases of Duchenne's muscular dystrophy, fascioscapulohumeral dystrophy, limb girdle dystrophy, oculopharyngeal dystrophy, myotubular myopathy, and trichinosis.

The amplitude and duration of the MUP are reduced because of random loss of fibers from the motor unit (Wilbourn 1993). Regeneration of muscle fibers sometimes gives rise to long-duration spikes, as well as satellite potentials. Findings vary from muscle to muscle and even within the same muscle; the most diagnostic results are obtained from moderately affected muscles. The MUP is often normal in mild metabolic or endocrine myopathies.

Early recruitment is the rule because more motor units are needed to maintain a given force in compensation for

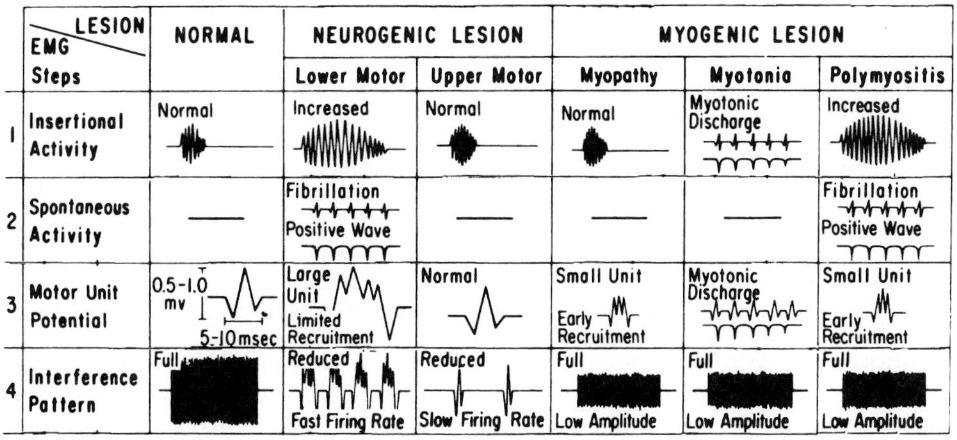

LESION
EMG Steps
NORMAL
NEUROGENIC LESION
Lower Motor
Upper Motor
MYOGENIC LESION
Myopathy
Myotonia
Polymyositis
1 Insertional Activity
Normal
Increased
Normal
Normal
Myotonic Discharge
Increased
2 Spontaneous Activity
Fibrillation
Positive Wave
Fibrillation
Positive Wave
3 Motor Unit Potential
0.5-1.0 mv
5-10 msec
Large Unit
Limited Recruitment
Normal
Small Unit
Early Recruitment
Myotonic Discharge
Small Unit
Early Recruitment
4 Interference Pattern
Full
Reduced
Fast Firing Rate
Reduced
Slow Firing Rate
Full
Low Amplitude
Full
Low Amplitude
Full
Low Amplitude

FIGURE 37B.16 A summary of characteristic electromyography findings in normal persons, patients with neurogenic lesions, and those with myogenic lesions. Insertional activity is increased in lower motor neuron lesions and polymyositis and consists of myotonic discharges in myotonia. Spontaneous activity generally occurs in lower motor neuron disorders and in inflammatory myopathy. Motor unit potentials are usually large and polyphasic, with reduced recruitment in lower motor neuron conditions; in myopathies and polymyositis motor units are small with early recruitment. Interference pattern is reduced in both upper and lower motor neuron lesions, as well as in hysterical weakness; however, firing rate is rapid in lower motor neuron lesions and normal in upper motor neuron lesions, and also hysteria (in which the rate may also be irregular). Interference pattern is full but of low amplitude in myopathic lesions. (Reprinted with permission of the author and publisher from J Kimura. Electrodiagnosis in Diseases of Nerve and Muscle: Principles and Practices [2nd ed]. Philadelphia: FA Davis, 1989.)

the small size of individual units. The interference pattern develops before contraction is maximal. Minimal effort causes several units to fire concomitantly; the patient cannot recruit only one or two single motor units.

Myotonia occurs in myotonic dystrophy, myotonia congenita, paramyotonia congenita, hyperkalemic periodic paralysis, and chondrodystrophic myotonia. Myotonic discharges are initiated by needle movements or voluntary muscle contractions. Early recruitment causes a reduced-amplitude full-interference pattern. Myotonic discharges may at times occur in polymyositis, type II glycogen storage (acid maltase deficiency) disease, and, rarely, chronic denervation.

Inflammatory myopathies typically show increased insertional activity, fibrillation potentials, and positive waves. These findings may occur only in paraspinous muscles. As in other myopathies, MUPs are often brief, low-amplitude, and polyphasic, with early recruitment. Spontaneous activity in polymyositis stops a few weeks after successful corticosteroid therapy and can be used to assess treatment efficacy. The presence of spontaneous discharges is also helpful in differentiating exacerbation of myositis from a corticosteroid-induced myopathy.

REFERENCES

Albers JW. Clinical neurophysiology of generalized polyneuropathy. J Clin Neurophysiol 1993;10:149–166.

Bischoff C, Meyer B-U, Machetanz J et al. The value of magnetic stimulation in the diagnosis of radiculopathies. Muscle Nerve 1993;16:154–161.

Bleasel AF, Tuck RR. Variability of repeated nerve conduction studies. Electroencephalogr Clin Neurophysiol 1991;81: 417–420.

Bromberg MB, Albers JW. Patterns of sensory nerve conduction abnormalities in demyelinating and axonal peripheral nerve disorders. Muscle Nerve 1993;16:262–266.

Campbell WW, Robinson LR. Deriving reference values in electrodiagnostic medicine. Muscle Nerve 1993;16:424–428.

Daube JR. AAEM Minimonograph #11: needle examination in clinical electromyography. Muscle Nerve 1991;14:685–700.

Dengler R, Kossev A, Wohlfart K et al. F waves and motor unit size. Muscle Nerve 1992;15:1138–1142.

Engstrom JW, Olney RK. Quantitative motor unit analysis: the effect of sample size. Muscle Nerve 1992;15:277–281.

Evans BA. Magnetic stimulation of the peripheral nervous system. J Clin Neurophysiol 1991;8:77–84.

Fraser JL, Olney RK. The relative diagnostic sensitivity of different F-wave parameters in various polyneuropathies. Muscle Nerve 1992;15:912–918.

Gilchrist JM. Single fiber EMG reference values: a collaborative effort. Ad hoc committee of the AAEM special interest group on single fiber EMG. Muscle Nerve 1992;15:151–161.

Kimura J. F-wave velocity in the central segment of the median and ulnar nerves: A study in normal subjects and in patients with Charcot-Marie-Tooth disease. Neurology (Minneapolis) 1974;24:539–546.

Kimura J. Collision technique. Physiologic block of nerve impulses in studies of motor nerve conduction velocity. Neurology (Minneapolis) 1976;26:680–682.

Kimura J. The carpal tunnel syndrome: localization of conduction abnormalities within the distal segment of the median nerve. Brain 1979;102:619–635.

Kimura J. Electrodiagnosis in Diseases of Nerve and Muscle: Principles and Practices (2nd ed). Philadelphia: FA Davis, 1989.

Kimura J, Bosch P, Lindsay GM. F-wave conduction velocity in the central segment of the peroneal and tibial nerves. Arch Phys Med Rehabil 1975;56:492–497.

Kimura J, Machida M, Ishida T et al. Relation between size of compound sensory or muscle action potentials and length of nerve segment. Neurology 1986;36:647–652.

Kincaid JC, Brashear A, Markand ON. The influence of the reference electrode on CMAP configuration. Muscle Nerve 1993;16:392–396.

Lester JM, Soule NW, Bradley WG et al. An augmented computer model of motor unit reorganization in neurogenic diseases of skeletal muscle. Muscle Nerve 1993;16:43–56.

Normand MM, Daube JR. Interaction of random electromyographic activity with averaged sensory evoked potentials. Neurology 1992;42:1605–1608.

Olney RK, So YT, Goodin DS et al. A comparison of magnetic and electrical stimulation of peripheral nerves. Muscle Nerve 1990;13:957–963.

Panizza M, Nilsson J, Hallett M. Optimal stimulus duration for the H reflex. Muscle Nerve 1989;12:576–579.

Parry GJ, Kohzu H. Acute changes in blood glucose affect resistance to ischemic nerve conduction failure. Neurology 1990; 40:107–110.

Pease WS, Fatehi MT, Johnson EW. Monopolar needle stimulation: Safety considerations. Arch Phys Med Rehabil 1989; 70:412–414.

Petajan JH. AAEM Minimonograph #3: motor unit recruitment. Muscle Nerve 1991;489–502.

Robinson LR, Rubner DE, Wahl PW, et al. Factor analysis. A methodology for data reduction in nerve conduction studies. Am J Phys Med Rehabil 1992;71:22–27.

Shahani BT, Wierzbicka MM, Parker SW. Abnormal single motor unit behavior in the upper motor neuron syndrome. Muscle Nerve 1991;14:64–69.

Stetson DS, Albers JW, Silverstein BA et al. Effects of age, sex, and anthropometric factors on nerve conduction measures. Muscle Nerve 1992;15:1095–1104.

Thomas JE, Lambert EH. Ulnar nerve conduction velocity and H reflex in infants and children. J Applied Physiol 1960;15:1–9.

Trontelj JV, Stålberg EV. Single motor endplates in myasthenia gravis and LEMS at different firing rates. Muscle Nerve 1991;14:226–232.

White JC. The ubiquity of contraction enhanced H reflexes: Normative data and use in the diagnosis of radiculopathies. Electroencephalogr Clin Neurophysiol 1991;81:433–442.

Wilbourn AJ. The electrodiagnostic examination with myopathies. J Clin Neurophysiol 1993;10:132–148.

Winkler T, Stålberg EV, Haas LF. Uni- and bipolar surface recording of human nerve responses. Muscle Nerve 1991;133–141.

SUGGESTED READING

Aminoff MJ. Electrodiagnosis in Clinical Neurology (3rd ed). New York: Churchill Livingstone, 1992.

Brown WF, Bolton CF. Clinical Electromyography (2nd ed). Boston: Butterworth-Heinemann, 1993.

Delagi EF, Perotto A, Iazzetti J, Morrison D. Anatomic Guide for the Electromyographer (2nd ed). Springfield, IL: Charles C Thomas, 1980.

Johnson EW. Practical Electromyography (2nd ed). Baltimore: Williams & Wilkins, 1988.

Stålberg E, Trontelj JV. Single Fibre Electromyography. Surrey, England: Mirvalle Press, 1979.

Chapter 38
Noninvasive Craniovascular Studies

Roger E. Kelley

NONINVASIVE ASSESSMENT OF THE EXTRACRANIAL AND INTRACRANIAL CIRCULATION

Direct tests of the vascular integrity include the following:

1. Palpation
2. Bruit auscultation
3. Bruit analysis
4. Ultrasound imaging (B-mode and Doppler)

The carotid bifurcation is the most accessible and important area for ultrasound visualization. The common carotid artery (CCA) typically bifurcates into the internal carotid artery (ICA) and external carotid artery (ECA) at the fourth cervical vertebral level (Figure 38.1). The ICA can usually be visualized for several centimeters distal to its origin. This is the most clinically relevant area of interest because of the predilection of obstructive atheromatous plaque to occur at the ICA origin. It is also possible to directly visualize a section of the vertebral arteries as they course through the posterior neck.

The effect of occlusive disease on the more distal (retinal or intracranial) circulation can be assessed by so-called indirect tests (Ackerman and Cardia 1994). These tests typically demonstrate alteration of the more distal circulation when there is hemodynamically significant proximal arterial stenosis. The most commonly used tests of the distal carotid circulation include the following:

1. Periorbital Doppler ultrasound
2. Oculoplethysmography (OPG)
3. Oculopneumoplethysmography (OPPG)
4. Transcranial Doppler ultrasonography (TCD), which provides indirect information about the extracranial circulation and direct information about the intracranial circulation.

From a practical standpoint, a noninvasive laboratory should help guide the clinician in optimal management of patients with carotid artery disease. The basic questions to be answered by the carotid scan are whether there is occlusive disease of the vessel and, if present, how severe is the stenosis. Reports that are difficult to interpret generally raise questions about the reliability of the laboratory. If the report suggests that further tests may be warranted, then one can assume that the visualization or the interpretation was suboptimal. This is a major reason for the performance of indirect tests.

Despite modern duplex scanners, which combine the anatomical information of B-mode imaging with the physiological information provided by Doppler ultrasonography, certain patients have a carotid bifurcation that is difficult to insonate. These are especially patients with short, thick necks as well as patients with a high carotid bifurcation, diffuse vessel wall calcification, or anatomical variations. In such instances, an indirect test, which reliably determines if there is a hemodynamically significant proximal lesion, can be invaluable.

The vertebral duplex scan can provide useful information in selected circumstances. The vessels can be imaged to only a limited extent because of the anatomy and the insonation window available. The flow pattern can be altered by nonspecific kinking of the vessel or by tortuosity. The diagnostic yield of noninvasive imaging of the vertebral arteries is greatest when the information provided by duplex scan is combined with that provided by TCD. From a practical standpoint, one needs to know whether there is patency of the vessel, whether the flow is anterograde or not, and whether there is evidence of flow disturbance.

Ultrasonography

B-Mode Scan

The characteristics of the B-mode scanner are summarized in Table 38.1. This scanner provides a real-time image,

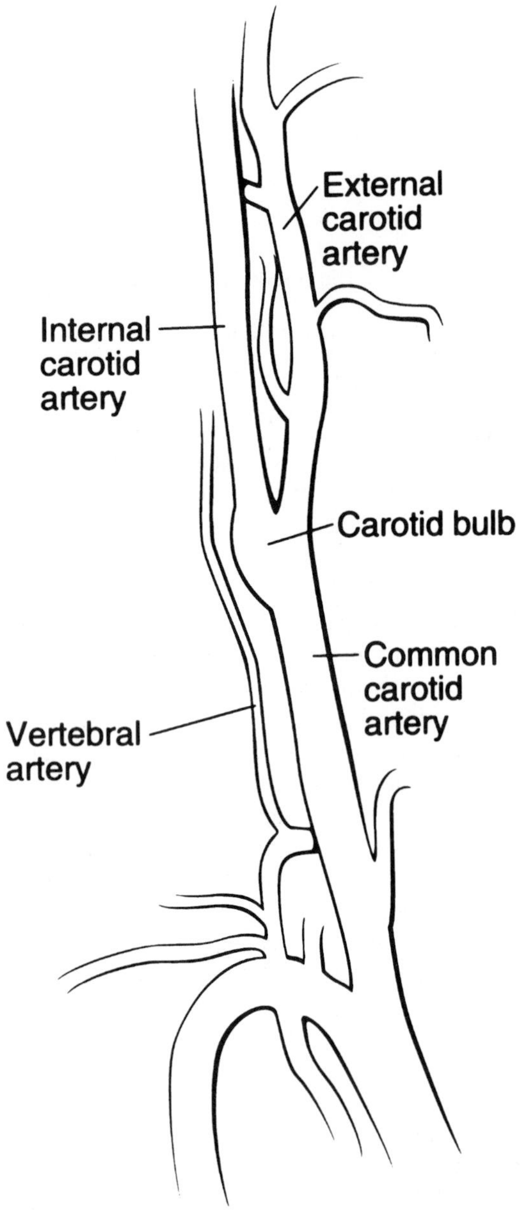

FIGURE 38.1 Right extracranial arterial distribution.

which results from generation of ultrasound pulses into the vessel wall via a properly placed transducer. The returning echoes are simultaneously received and displayed on an oscilloscope, the brightness being a function of the intensity of the signal. The brightness reflects the variation in the acoustical impedance of the particular tissue, which is why the brightness-modulated image is termed *B-mode scan.* The image is generated in two dimensions, along either the longitudinal plane or transverse plane (Figure 38.2).

The image generated represents the anatomy of the vessel wall. The real-time nature of this type of scanning is reflected by the actual pulsation of the vessel seen on the display screen. Typically, the lumen of the vessel is sonolucent (dark) while calcific plaque is sonodense (white). A calcific plaque within the origin of the ICA is shown in Figure 38.3.

Table 38.1: Characteristics of B-mode scanners

1. High-frequency (5–10 MHz) real-time transducer
2. Can image in longitudinal and transverse planes
3. Echogenicity is reflective of the acoustical impedance of the tissues being insonated
4. Primarily provides anatomical information about the vessel wall

Doppler Ultrasound

Doppler ultrasound is based on the change in Doppler frequency as the signal is reflected off the moving column of blood. There are two types of Doppler imaging: continuous-wave (CW) and pulsed-wave (PW) (Table 38.2). Both types of Doppler can detect the direction of change of the Doppler signal. This direction of change is proportional to the direction of flow. When flow is directed toward the probe (anterograde), the reflected signal is higher than that transmitted. When flow is directed away from the probe (retrograde), the reflected signal is less than that transmitted.

CW Doppler is obtained by two transducers, one emitting and the other receiving the ultrasound continuously. An image of the vessel as a function of the blood flowing through its lumen is produced. The major advantage of CW Doppler is that it can detect a broad spectrum of flow velocity changes, including the fast velocities associated with high-grade stenosis.

PW Doppler is obtained with one transducer. It allows specific localization of the reflected signal within the moving column of blood. This is particularly pertinent in that PW Doppler is coupled with the B-mode image to produce the duplex scan. Furthermore, only by having localization of the Doppler signal reflection can one effectively identify the artery of interest with TCD. Thus, this advantage of being able to select the depth of insonation, by gating of the Doppler signal, is only feasible with PW Doppler.

Doppler Velocity Analysis

The Doppler waveform envelope can be analyzed to detect alterations in the velocity pattern reflective of stenosis. The shift in the Doppler signal represents a spectrum of frequencies. The amplitude of each frequency, in turn, is proportional to the number of red blood cells producing a particular Doppler shift for a particular sample volume. Multiple spectral lines are generated, and each spectral line contains the entire frequency content of the particular sample volume for that instant in time.

Qualitative assessment of the Doppler velocity spectrum includes determination of the maximum frequency envelope and the degree of diastolic flow, audible interpretation of the degree of turbulence of the flow through a stenotic vessel, and evaluation of the amount of spectral broadening (Figure 38.4), which is the expansion of the area beneath the systolic velocity envelope. By audible analysis, a high-

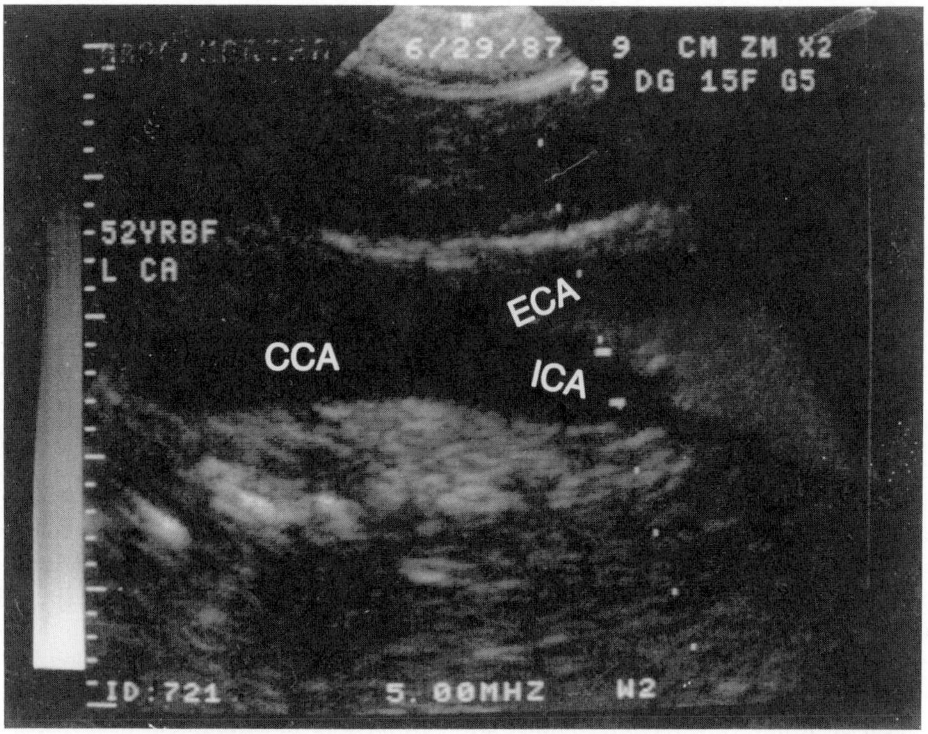

FIGURE 38.2 Normal B-mode scan of the carotid bifurcation, which demonstrates common carotid artery (CCA), internal carotid artery (ICA), and external carotid artery (ECA).

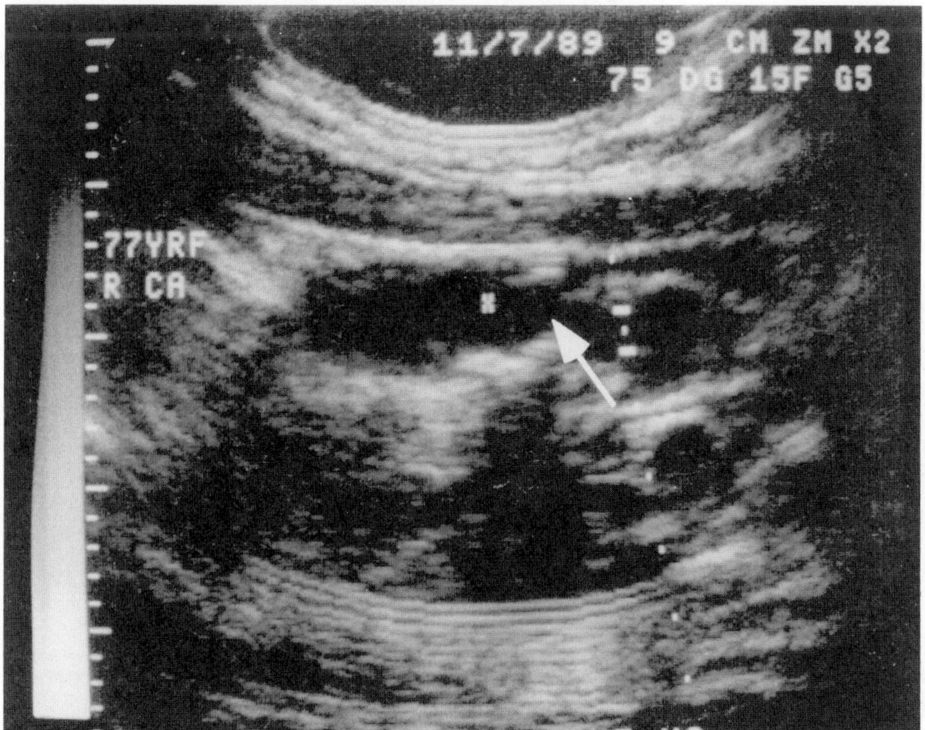

FIGURE 38.3 Carotid B-mode scan that demonstrates calcific plaque (arrow) at the origin of the internal carotid artery. Note that the plaque is present along the posterior wall, where it is most prominent, as well as the anterior wall of the vessel—that is, it is circumferential.

frequency harsh Doppler signal is the most reliable indication of high-grade stenosis. As a general rule, the broadening of the Doppler envelope is proportional to the turbulence of the flow.

Quantitative analysis of Doppler spectral waveforms can be accomplished by spectrum analysis of either CW Doppler signals or PW Doppler signals with use of a real-time analyzer. This allows actual measurement of the peak systolic Doppler frequency shift, which is the most important factor in determining the degree of stenosis. The peak systolic velocity (PSV) is derived from the peak systolic Doppler shift under the assumption that the angle of in-

Table 38.2: Features of continuous-wave versus pulsed-wave Doppler ultrasonography

Continuous-Wave Doppler	*Pulsed-Wave Doppler*
Consists of two transducers with one emitting and the other receiving the ultrasound continuously	Obtained with one transducer
Generates an image that reflects the moving column of blood	Doppler signal can be positioned so that discrete volumes of blood can be sampled along the vessel lumen
Has greater capacity for the detection of fast-flow velocities seen with high-grade stenosis	Can allow better characterization of the flow pattern proximal to, within, and distal to the region of stenosis

sonation can be accurately measured from the B-mode scan while the Doppler shift is provided by the Doppler spectrum analyzer.

A major point of confusion that continues to this day is the designation of hemodynamically significant ICA stenosis based on imaging criteria. It is generally felt that a 50% diameter stenosis corresponds to a 75% area reduction, and it is at this point that one begins to see reduction of more distal ICA flow. The results of the North American Symptomatic Carotid Endarterectomy Trial (NASCET) (1991) and the European Carotid Surgery Trial (ECST) (1991) indicated that endarterectomy was beneficial for stroke prevention in symptomatic carotid linear stenosis of greater than 70%. The formula to calculate the percentage reduction of diameter stenosis is:

$$1 - (d/n) \times 100$$

where d = maximal diameter reduction at the site of stenosis and n = an estimate of normal vessel diameter. These values must be derived from estimates of normal vessel diameter and the region of greatest stenosis on biplanar B-mode scan or biplanar angiography. The derivation options are illustrated in Figure 38.5. As can be seen from the figure, the B-mode scan cannot adequately determine the widest diameter beyond the proximal stenosis because of insonation limitations.

The Doppler signal alteration takes on added significance because of this limitation. The major Doppler determinants of hemodynamically significant stenosis include a peak frequency shift of 4–8 KHz, or a correlative PSV of 120–150 cm/sec or greater, an end-diastolic frequency of greater than 4.5 KHz, marked spectral broadening, and pronounced turbulence of the Doppler signal by analysis of the audio signal.

Another criterion for determination of critical stenosis has been the determination of the systolic to diastolic Doppler shift (or velocity) in the CCA or comparison of the CCA value to the corresponding value in the carotid bulb. The ratio of the PSV (A) to the end diastolic velocity (D) of the CCA, calculated as R = (A – D)/A, should be below 0.75 in the normal flow state. The ratio of the peak systolic ICA velocity to the peak systolic CCA velocity is below 0.8 in normal vessels, greater than 1.5 in stenoses of 60% or

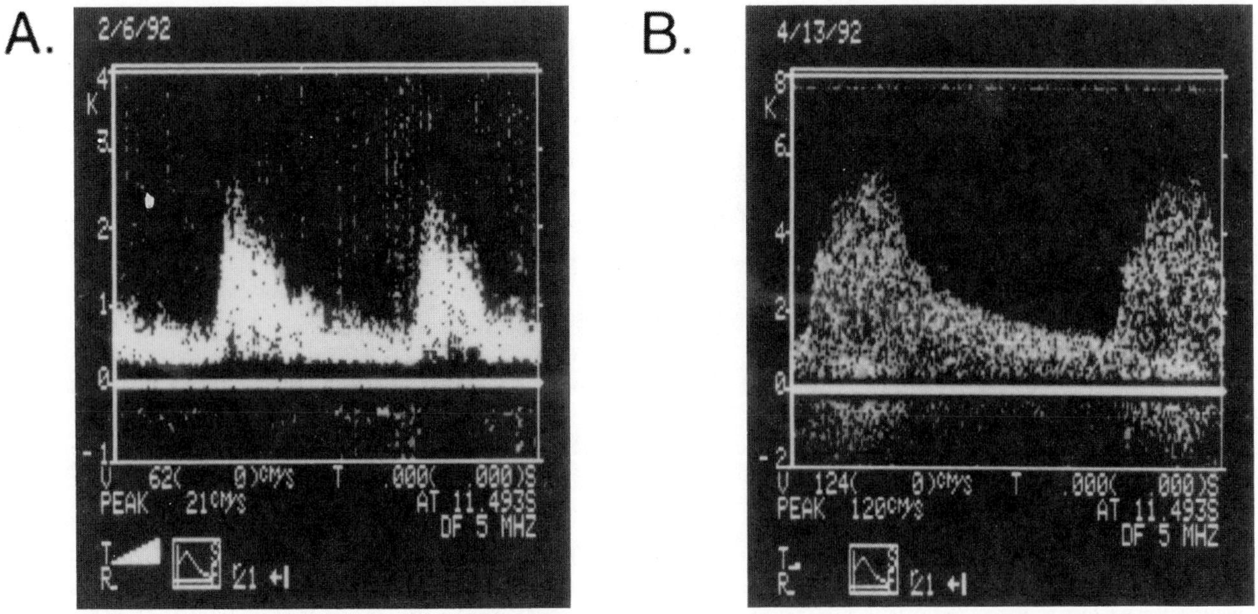

FIGURE 38.4 A. Normal Doppler spectral pattern within the internal carotid origin associated with a Doppler shift of 2.5 KHz. B. Increased Doppler shift of 6 KHz at the origin of an internal carotid artery where there is 60–70% stenosis. Note the associated spectral broadening compared to the waveform in A.

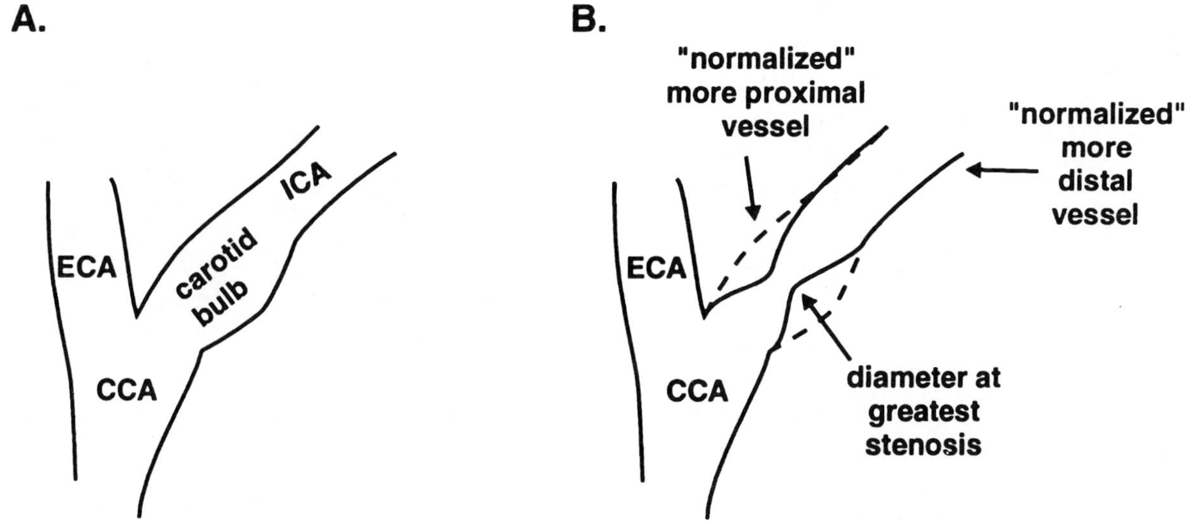

FIGURE 38.5 A. Schematic diagram of a normal carotid bifurcation. B. Illustration of how the degree of carotid bulb narrowing can be calculated from the "normal" linear diameter estimated in reference to the area of stenosis campared to a maximal "normal" diameter more distal to the region of stenosis.

greater, and between 0.8 and 1.5 in about two-thirds of vessels with mild diameter reduction.

In a study of the association between ICA residual lumen diameter and maximal velocity of the ICA, as measured by spectral analysis of PW Doppler, a maximal velocity of more than 80 cm/sec was associated with more than 50% diameter reduction at a sensitivity of 87% and a specificity of 93% (Nordal et al. 1993). The criteria for detection of clinically relevant stenosis—that is, 50%—are listed in Table 38.3.

Detection of vertebral or basilar artery stenosis by Doppler velocity analysis may be much less reliable than carotid evaluation. This is related to the narrower vertebral artery lumen, the limited insonation window, and the susceptibility of these posterior circulation vessels to kinking, tortuosity, and ectasia. Adequate insonation of the vertebral arteries is not possible in roughly one-third of patients. Generally, the origin and proximal vertebral artery can be insonated along with intertransverse segments from C3 to C6 (Figure 38.6). The normal mean systolic velocity ranges from 20 to 40 cm/sec, but elevation of the peak systolic frequency and spectral broadening are less reliably associated with flow-limiting stenosis. Directional CW Doppler of the distal vertebral arteries can allow detection of basilar artery occlusive disease in subjects with 60% or greater luminal diameter reduction, however.

Table 38.3: Criteria for detection of 50% or greater internal carotid artery stenosis by Doppler

1. Peak systolic frequency shift greater than 4 KHz or peak systolic velocity of 120–150 cm/sec or greater
2. Maximal velocity of greater than 80 cm/sec
3. Ratio of internal carotid artery to common carotid artery peak velocity or Doppler shift of more than 1.5
4. End-diastolic frequency greater than 4.5 KHz
5. Prominent turbulence of the Doppler signal with poststenotic spectral broadening

Color Doppler Imaging

Color Doppler imaging (CDI) is the latest advance in ultrasonographic vascular imaging. It represents a combination of duplex scanning with two-dimensional, color-coded, real-time flow imaging. The shift in the pulsed Doppler signal is quantitated as to magnitude and variance, as well as to whether the flow is toward or away from the probe. The flow is coded by either red or blue with the flow velocity proportional to the degree of color saturation. A reduction in color saturation is recorded as the flow velocity increases.

There is disruption of the normal flow pattern with stenosis. The normal pattern of flow is characterized by cylindrical laminae coursing through the vessel as a function of their distance from the vessel wall, with the slowest flow nearest the vessel wall. This produces an elliptical moving column of blood, which is termed *laminar flow*. The normal CDI scan of laminar flow is replaced by turbulence with distortion of the color-coding. With prominent stenosis, a jet flow pattern evolves consisting of a mixture of white, blue, and red colors. This allows easier detection of a stenotic lesion as long as one recognizes the limitations of CDI (Erickson et al. 1989).

CDI allows easier vessel identification and, generally, more readily distinguishes a normal from an abnormal flow pattern. It can allow more efficient screening of the vessel surface, and one can complement the information with that

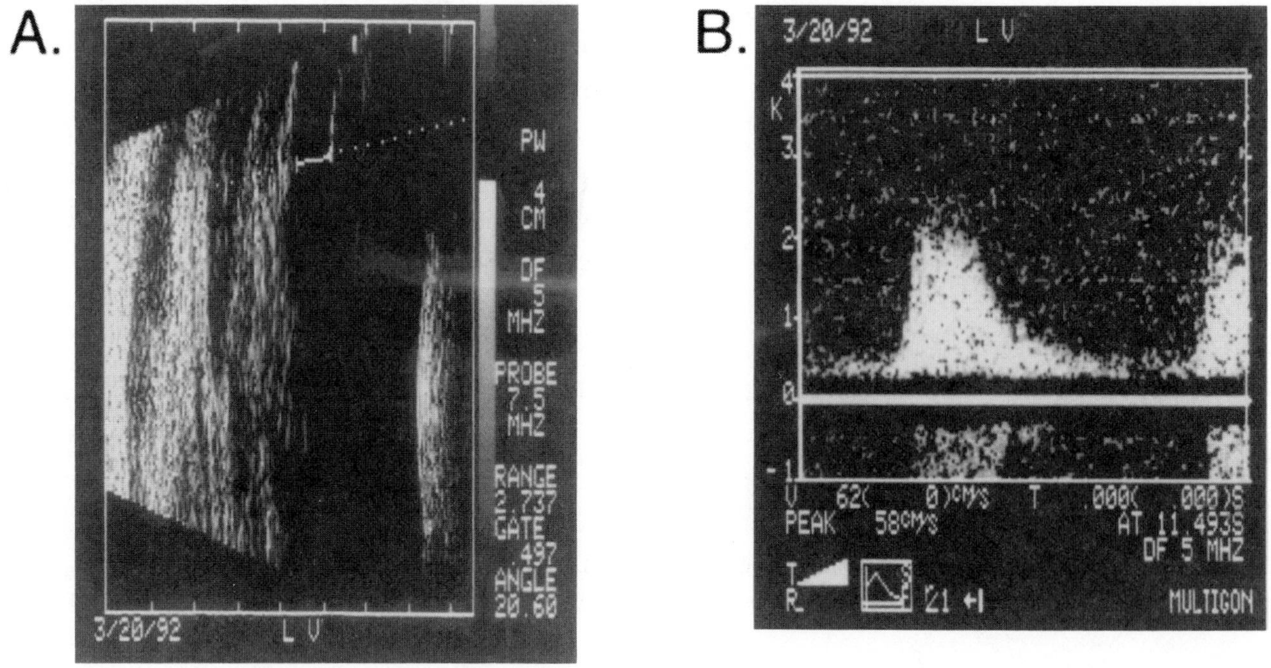

FIGURE 38.6 A. B-mode scan of the left vertebral artery (arrow) that reveals a patent vessel in the region insonated. B. The correlative pulsed-wave Doppler waveform. This is a normal-appearing waveform with a Doppler shift of 2 KHz.

provided by the routine PW Doppler of the duplex system once an area of abnormality has been identified. In addition, CDI appears to be superior to other modalities for imaging the vertebral arteries and for evaluating other structural abnormalities of the carotid bifurcation, such as carotid body tumors.

Periorbital Doppler Ultrasound

Directional Doppler ultrasound of the supraorbital and supratrochlear arteries can provide important information about the collateral circulation in hemodynamically significant carotid stenosis. The flow of the periorbital arteries is anterograde in the normal state—that is, the flow is from the orbit toward the face. If the degree of carotid stenosis is such that the ECA branches provide collateral flow to the intracranial circulation via the periorbital arteries, then one will see retrograde flow of the supraorbital or supratrochlear artery, or both.

Generally, the supratrochlear artery flow direction is more specific but less sensitive than the supraorbital artery flow direction. A particularly specific finding is the return of the flow direction from retrograde to anterograde with compression of the ipsilateral superficial temporal artery. This compression reduces the pressure head of the extracranial conduit such that there can be temporary reconstitution of normal flow direction through the periorbital arteries.

Periorbital Doppler ultrasound is of limited value in the carotid noninvasive battery because of its limited sensitivity and specificity. The flow dynamics required to produce a positive test are often not seen unless there is 90% or greater ipsilateral ICA stenosis. It can help to identify a particularly high-grade stenosis, however, and this is its primary value.

Other Noninvasive Techniques

Bruit Analysis with Carotid Phonoangiography

Bruit analysis requires the presence of a clinically recognizable bruit. Typically, a carotid bruit is heard when the residual lumen diameter is 2.5–3.0 mm or less. It is important to note that the bruit usually disappears as the residual lumen diameter falls to 0.5–0.8 mm or less. The most cost-effective, but least accurate, method of bruit analysis is by auscultation with a stethoscope. A high-pitched or harsh bruit that is prolonged, especially if it extends into diastole, and that is heard best at the angle of the jaw, is most likely to be associated with greater than 50% ICA stenosis.

Direct bruit analysis involves placing a microphone over multiple carotid locations to assess the relationship of the amplitude of the bruit to time in the cardiac cycle. The primary use of this technique is to distinguish a bruit from a radiated murmur and to determine if the bruit extends into diastole. The limited practical utility of this technique and its low specificity render it primarily of historical interest.

Quantitative carotid phonoangiography accomplished via spectral bruit analysis allows fairly accurate determination of the residual lumen diameter of a stenotic lesion

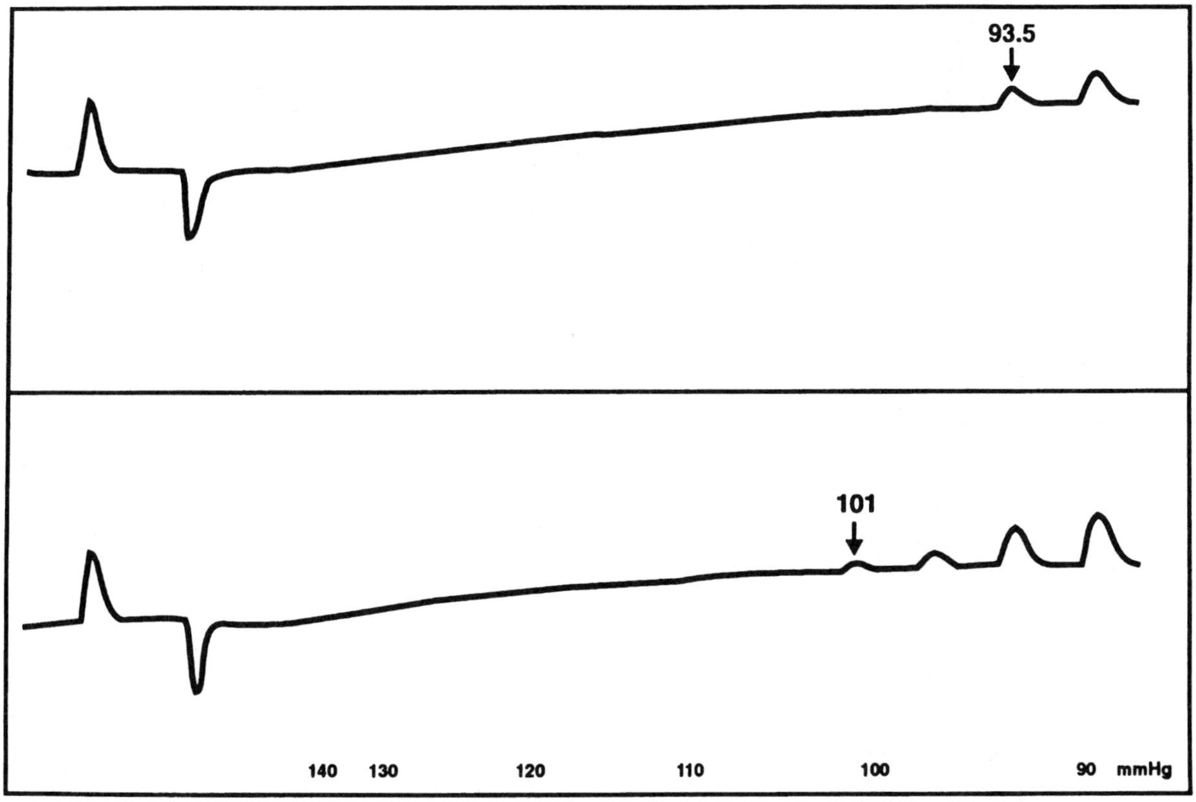

FIGURE 38.7 Illustration of abnormal oculopneumoplethysmography. Ophthalmic artery pulsations appear at a systolic pressure of 93.5 mm Hg on the top and 101 mm Hg on the bottom. A difference of 5 mm Hg or more between the two sides usually reflects hemodynamically significant stenosis on the lower side.

when a bruit is present. Unfortunately, it has been estimated that up to one-third of high-grade carotid stenoses are not associated with a bruit and, thus, this technique is of limited clinical value.

Oculoplethysmography and Oculopneumoplethysmography

OPG and OPPG require eyecups over the globe to assess ocular hemodynamics as a reflection of ipsilateral carotid occlusive disease. OPG monitors the ocular pulse wave to assess for a difference between the two eyes. A delayed pulse wave is presumably reflective of an ipsilateral hemodynamically significant ICA stenosis. This technique is limited by suboptimal sensitivity, especially when there are bilateral carotid occlusive disease and patient intolerance of the eyecups.

OPPG has been found to be a sensitive indicator of hemodynamically significant carotid stenosis, and a correction can be made for bilateral high-grade ICA stenosis. This method involves external pressure on the globe to the point that intraocular pressure is raised above systolic pressure in the ophthalmic artery. At this point, ophthalmic artery perfusion falls such that the patient experiences transient blindness. As the intraocular pressure falls, with release of pressure, ocular pulsations reappear on the ocular pressure tracing (Figure 38.7). One can correct for the possible presence of bilateral stenosis with reference to a regression line of the ipsilateral brachial blood pressure. In experienced hands, OPPG has a reported overall accuracy of 92.5%. The limitations of OPG should not be confused with those of OPPG as the latter technique clearly has value in detecting hemodynamically significant ICA stenosis. This is important in identifying stroke-prone patients, including those most likely to benefit from carotid endarterectomy (North American Symptomatic Carotid Endarterectomy Trial Collaborators 1991).

Assessment of Plaque Morphology

Anatomical Imaging with B-Mode Scan

B-mode scanning has been touted as a technique that can readily detect plaque, can accurately determine residual lumen diameter, and can assess for ulceration of the plaque and for intraplaque hemorrhage. There is no doubt that B-mode scanning can provide a superb image of the carotid bifurcation in the majority of patients. However, the claim that B-mode scanning, even when coupled to PW Doppler in the duplex scan, can provide accurate assessment in 95% or more of subjects is questionable.

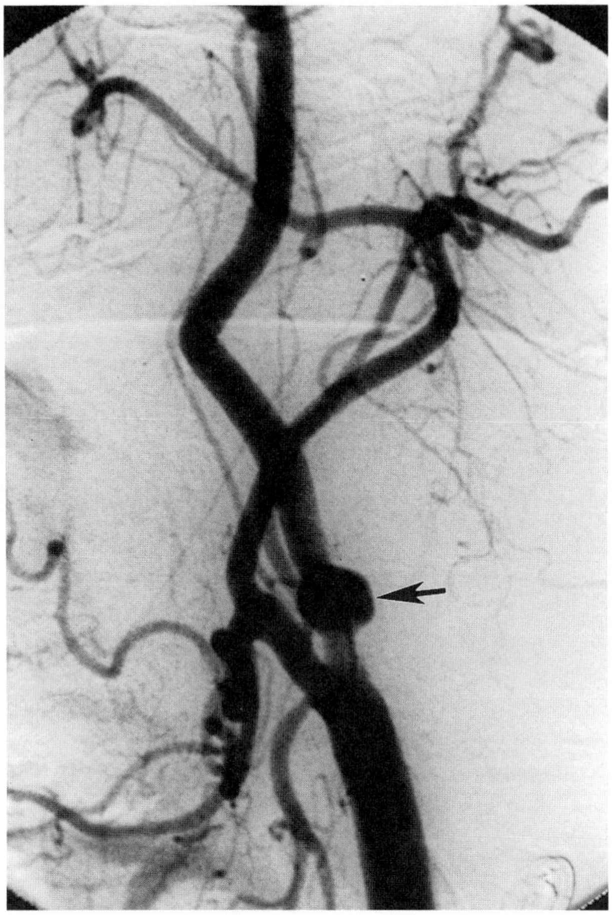

FIGURE 38.8 Cerebral arteriogram that demonstrates a large bulbous enlargement of the right internal carotid artery just distal to the origin (arrow). Plaque formation was noted within the right internal carotid artery by B-mode scan associated with moderate turbulence by Doppler. At surgery, this was found to be a large, complicated fibrofatty plaque.

Experienced ultrasonographers recognize the potential shortcomings of duplex scanning. The duplex scan may correlate with cerebral angiography in only 60–70% of cases, according to some studies, but the potential for much greater accuracy is realized in superior noninvasive laboratories. It is very important to recognize that the results are subject to interpretation, and that 5–10% of scans are uninterpretable.

Ulcerated Plaque

The detection of excavation within the plaque, *ulceration,* is felt to be clinically relevant by some authors. However, both carotid ultrasonography and routine angiography can be limited in this regard. In Figure 38.8, we see what was called a *pseudoaneurysm* by angiography, although the carotid duplex scan demonstrated circumferential plaque formation at the origin. At surgery, the ballooning of the proximal ICA was found to be the result of a very complicated calcific plaque with two distinct areas of focal narrowing.

Intraplaque Hemorrhage and Sonolucent Plaque

Intraplaque hemorrhage and sonolucent plaque may be more dangerous from the standpoint of stroke risk. Soft plaque is primarily detected by sonolucency on B-mode with turbulence by Doppler. Such a plaque might represent recent hemorrhage or echolucent fibrofatty tissue. Intraplaque hemorrhage is detected on B-mode scan by a central area of sonolucency within an echodense outer layer (Figure 38.9) due to calcium. In a radio frequency–based ultrasonic assessment of atherosclerotic plaque (Urbani et al. 1993), the authors reported that determination of the echogenic characteristics could be enhanced by direct assessment of the radio frequency signal. Their system allowed measurement of a two-dimensional integrated backscatter index. This index allowed delineation of the very low backscatter values of intraplaque hemorrhage, the intermediate values of fibrofatty plaque, and the relatively high values of calcific plaque.

Color Doppler Imaging

CDI study of symptomatic versus asymptomatic high-grade stenoses may show distinct morphological features in the two groups. For example, calcific plaques are more common in asymptomatic subjects, echolucent plaques, presumably representing mural wall thrombi, are more frequent in symptomatic subjects, while there appears to be no difference in the frequency of homogeneous and heterogeneous plaques in the two groups. Notably, the hemodynamic pattern, such as jet flow, poststenotic turbulence or reversed flow, is not different in the two groups. Overall, comparisons of plaque surface analysis by CDI agree with angiographic findings in 70% of subjects.

Determination of Stenosis

Implications for Carotid Endarterectomy

A symptomatic linear ICA stenosis of 70% or greater is optimally treated by surgery *if* the patient is a good surgical candidate and a technically excellent surgeon is available (NASCET 1991). The three studies of carotid endarterectomy were based on carotid duplex scanning as a screening procedure. The accuracy of the duplex scan in such an endeavor has been questioned (Barnett and Warlow 1993), but this can be ascribed to the interpretative nature of B-mode scanning and also applies, to a lesser degree, to angiographic interpretation.

Accuracy of Noninvasive Tests in Carotid Stenosis

There is no doubt that noninvasive tests can achieve an accuracy of 90% or greater in detecting carotid artery plaque formation and stenosis. In one study (Sitzer et al. 1993), the positive predictive value for color duplex was 0.84 and

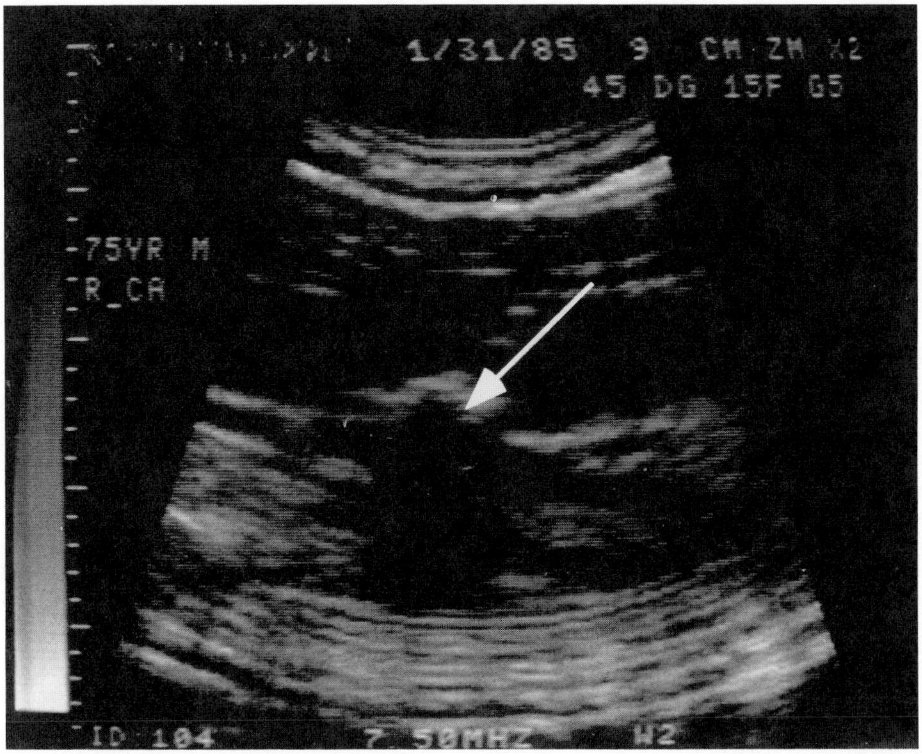

FIGURE 38.9 Calcific plaque along the posterior wall of the internal carotid artery at the origin. There is a sonolucent central area (arrow) compatible with intraplaque hemorrhage.

the negative predictive value was 0.98 in detecting 70–99% ICA stenosis. The duplex scan may actually be more accurate than angiography in determining "true" anatomic stenosis, since angiography tends to underestimate the degree of stenosis.

Accuracy of Noninvasive Tests in Vertebral Artery Stenosis

Studies that have correlated duplex scanning and CDI with angiography in vertebral occlusive disease have been limited. In one study, adequate visualization with duplex scan was achieved in only 86 of 117 patients. In healthy subjects, however, the visualization is more readily obtained. CDI certainly appears to be a promising technique for evaluating the vertebral arteries, but the visualization is limited in roughly two-thirds of subjects. It can be concluded that both duplex scanning and CDI are limited in the assessment of proximal vertebral artery occlusive disease. The information can be combined with TCD and magnetic resonance angiography, however, to enhance the reliability.

Vascular Dissection

CW Doppler can provide a rather characteristic pattern in extracranial carotid artery dissection. Typically, there is a high-resistance Doppler flow pattern. The spectral pattern often has a high-amplitude Doppler signal, pronounced reduction of the systolic Doppler frequencies, and an alternating flow direction. Duplex ultrasound may show (1) tapering of the ICA lumen distal to the bulb, (2) the presence of double lumen with the false lumen having no flow, (3) an irregular membrane that crosses the lumen of vessel, or (4) absence of Doppler signal if there is total occlusion. It is possible to noninvasively monitor the resolution of the dissection, once the diagnosis has been established by routine angiography, with duplex scanning or CDI.

Transcranial Doppler Ultrasonography

Basic Principles

With a low-frequency (2-MHz) high-energy pulsed Doppler probe, one can insonate the basal cerebral arteries including the middle cerebral arteries (MCAs), anterior cerebral arteries (ACAs), posterior cerebral arteries (PCAs), the ophthalmic arteries, the carotid siphons, the basilar artery, and the distal vertebral arteries (Figure 38.10).

The basic principle behind TCD is that there is an inverse relationship between vessel diameter and flow velocity. Thus, disease processes that narrow the vessel lumen, including intracranial arterial stenosis and post–subarachnoid hemorrhage vasospasm, produce an increase in the flow velocity. In addition, a more proximal occlusive process, such as carotid stenosis in the region of the carotid bifurcation, produces distal reduction of the flow velocity and flow acceleration.

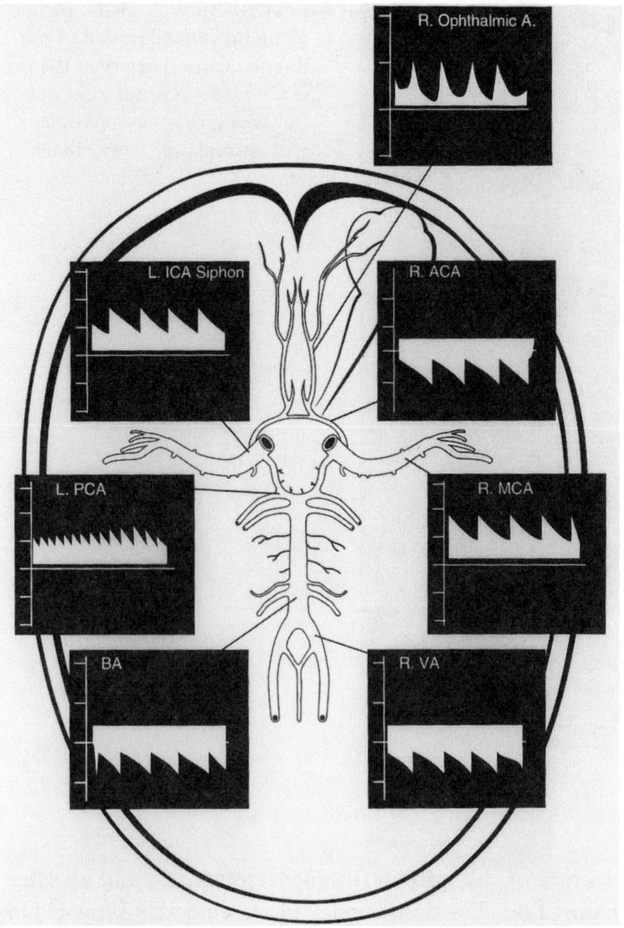

FIGURE 38.10 Schematic diagram of the transcranial Doppler directional findings within the circle of Willis in a normal individual. The Doppler waveform above the 0 horizontal line is flow that is anterograde (toward the probe) while a waveform directed below the 0 horizontal line is retrograde flow (away from the probe).

Clinical Uses of Transcranial Doppler

Intracranial Stenosis

The MCA is the most readily insonated of the intracranial vessels, is the most clinically relevant in terms of vascular involvement, and provides the most reliable TCD information. Stenosis of the MCA results in an increased flow velocity within the stenotic segment while the flow velocity is reduced beyond the area of stenosis. Reversed flow through the A1 segment of the ipsilateral ACA is seen when there is hemodynamically significant MCA stenosis or total occlusion. Following total occlusion, one can sometimes see reestablishment of the MCA flow pattern over time, with a diminishing flow velocity as the vessel is recanalized. Reversed flow through both the ACA and ipsilateral ophthalmic artery, with dampened or absent flow through the ipsilateral MCA, is highly suggestive of ICA occlusion on that side.

Ley-Pozo and Ringelstein (1990) reported on the sensitivity, specificity, and overall accuracy of TCD in detecting MCA and carotid siphon occlusive disease. For MCA stenosis, they reported a sensitivity of 85.7%, a specificity of 98.7%, and an accuracy of 97.6%. For MCA occlusion, they reported a sensitivity of 90.9%, a specificity of 99.4%, and an accuracy of 98.8%. The corresponding values for any MCA lesion were 92%, 98.6%, and 97.6%. For carotid siphon stenosis, the sensitivity was 94.1%, the specificity 96.7%, and the accuracy 96.4%. For carotid siphon occlusion, the sensitivity was 85.7%, the specificity 100%, and the accuracy 99.3%. The corresponding values for any carotid siphon lesion were 91.7%, 96.5%, and 95.7%.

TCD can assess the flow characteristics of the distal vertebral arteries and proximal basilar artery. It is primarily useful for determining whether the flow signal is normal and whether it is in the normal direction. Information provided by TCD can be useful in the clinical realm. It may help to explain the mechanism of the stroke in a noninvasive fashion. It can allow serial noninvasive monitoring that might influence patient management. In addition, TCD can provide prognostic information, since markedly attenuated or absent flow signal within the MCA, as determined by TCD, carries a less favorable prognosis in acute hemispheric brain infarction.

Evaluation of Extracranial Carotid Stenosis

A carotid bifurcation stenosis or occlusion often reduces the flow velocity of the intracranial basal arteries supplied by the ipsilateral ICA. However, the absolute flow velocity values can be unreliable as the velocity values depend on age, pCO_2, hemorrheologic factors, metabolic factors, wakefulness, and the presence of coexistent intracranial occlusive disease. On the other hand, the flow acceleration, which represents the time that the upstroke of the Doppler waveform envelope reaches peak velocity (Figure 38.11), is the most useful TCD measurement for detecting extracranial ICA stenosis (Kelley et al. 1993b). For ICA stenosis of 70–100%, the sensitivity is 82%, the specificity 73%, and the accuracy is 78%.

Intracranial Vascular Dissection

TCD can detect flow velocity alteration secondary to carotid or vertebral dissection. Using a criterion of abnormal flow velocity defined as a value two standard deviations higher or lower than normal values, Mullges et al. (1992) reported on the potential value of TCD in ICA dissections. When combined with extracranial sonography and MRI, TCD was able to detect flow velocity disturbance in 12 of 13 consecutive patients whose dissection was confirmed by angiography.

Vasospasm Secondary to Subarachnoid Hemorrhage

One of the most clinically relevant uses for TCD is to detect preclinical vasospasm. A baseline TCD study of ACAs, MCAs,

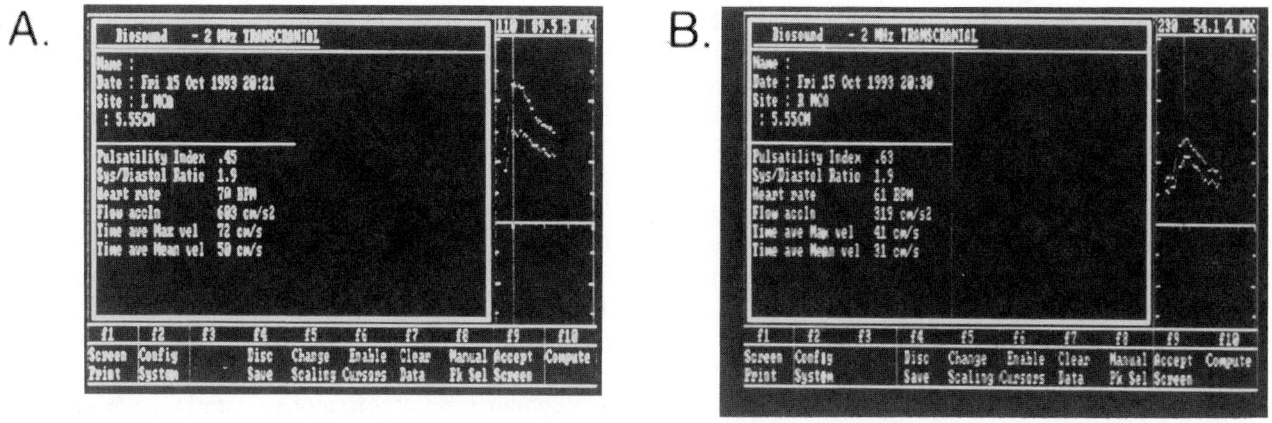

FIGURE 38.11 Comparison of a middle cerebral artery transcranial Doppler waveform ipsilateral to an unobstructed left ICA (A) compared to a middle cerebral artery Doppler waveform ipsilateral to a high-grade stenotic right ICA (B). The flow acceleration and flow velocities are both lower on the right than the left.

and PCAs should be obtained at the time of presentation. The study is repeated at least once daily to assess for an increasing flow velocity reflective of vessel narrowing. The criteria for clinically relevant vasospastic changes vary, but an elevation of the flow velocity to two standard deviations above baseline, or what is considered to be normal for a particular patient, is a useful cutoff. In addition, a relatively rapid increase in the flow velocity—that is, 50 cm/sec/24 hours—may also identify subjects at risk for symptomatic vasospasm. In one study, mean velocities up to 120 cm/sec correlated with less than 25% vessel narrowing by angiography, mean velocities of 120–200 cm/sec correlated with 25–50% narrowing, and values greater than 200 cm/sec correlated with 50% or greater narrowing.

Sloan et al. (1989) looked at sensitivity and specificity of TCD in detecting vasospasm, using a mean velocity of 120 cm/sec as an indicator of vasospasm. For their 34 consecutive subjects, who all had an angiogram within 24 hours of the TCD study, the sensitivity was 58.6% and the specificity was 100%. Table 38.4 summarizes some of the more commonly used criteria for detecting of vasospasm. TCD findings in the preoperative period may help screen patients who are more likely to have vasospastic complications of early aneurysm surgery.

Subclavian Steal

TCD can assess flow direction in the vertebral arteries and basilar artery via the foramen magnum. Typically, the flow is retrograde (away from the probe) within the distal vertebrals and at the area of insonation of the basilar artery. Reversal of the normal flow direction secondary to "steal" into the subclavian circulation can be detected by TCD.

Table 38.4: Criteria used to detect vasospasm following subarachnoid hemorrhage

1. Elevation of the flow velocity by two standard deviations or more above the baseline value
2. Mean velocities of 120–200 cm/sec or greater
3. A relatively rapid increase in the flow velocities—i.e., 50 cm/sec/24 hr or greater, during serial monitoring

Cerebrovascular Reactivity

The concept of cerebrovascular reserve capacity (CVRC) is that compensatory vasodilatation of cortical arterioles can effectively counteract a drop in perfusion pressure. This maintenance of cerebral perfusion in the face of an occlusive or hemodynamic process has a particular threshold, beyond which cerebral ischemia results. If the resistance arteries are maximally dilated, an additional vasodilatory stimulus, such as hypercapnia, will not increase cerebral blood flow. TCD flow velocity measurements of the basal cerebral arteries correlate with cerebral blood flow *if* it can be assumed that the caliber of the insonated vessels remains constant. Theoretically, if this assumption holds, TCD can be used to noninvasively assess the effect of CO_2 arterial concentration on the CVRC. This CO_2 reactivity can be accomplished by having the subject breathe various concentrations of CO_2 or by the intravenous administration of acetazolamide, which is a carbonic anhydrase inhibitor.

Maeda et al. (1993) assessed CO_2 cerebrovascular reactivity with TCD in three types of ischemic cerebrovascular disease: (1) unilateral carotid artery stenosis, (2) lacunar infarction, and (3) cortical infarction. The authors reported a diminished CO_2 reactivity ipsilateral to carotid occlusive disease or cortical infarction compared to the uninvolved side, while lacunar infarction was associated with bilateral reduction when compared to normal controls. It has been hypothesized that impaired CVRC can allow identification of patients at high risk for ischemic infarction, but this capability has not been verified to date.

Cerebral Activation

It is possible to assess the circulatory correlates of mental activity with TCD. Visual stimulation, for example, is associated with an elevation of the flow velocity within the PCAs. A selective increase within both MCAs and the left PCA can be observed during the playing of a commercial video game and a selective increase within the right MCA is seen during performance of a spatial task (Kelley et al. 1993a). Although primarily of research interest, such a noninvasive objective monitoring of cognitive activity may have practical applications in evaluating vascular-mediated disease states and possibly in assessing drugs given in an effort to improve mental function.

Sickle Cell Disease

Adams et al. (1992) studied 190 patients with sickle cell disease over an average follow-up of 29 months. Six of the seven strokes that developed occurred among the 23 subjects with a TCD flow velocity of 170 cm/sec or more. The authors concluded that TCD is capable of identifying subjects with sickle cell disease who are at greatest risk for cerebral infarction.

Intracranial Circulatory Arrest and Brain Death

Absent or reversed diastolic flow, or small early systolic spikes, in at least two basal cerebral arteries have been reported with brain death. Three successive stages of circulatory arrest have been described: (1) oscillating flow, (2) systolic spike flow, and (3) zero flow. Increasing intracranial pressure, which precedes intracranial circulatory arrest, results in three successive high-resistance profiles: (1) low diastolic flow velocity, (2) absent flow pattern, and (3) reversed diastolic flow velocity.

Monitoring of Therapy

A valuable potential use of TCD would be to noninvasively assess response to medical or surgical therapy. Assessment of the efficacy of thrombolytic therapy for acute MCA occlusion and monitoring during carotid endarterectomy are two examples. Some studies suggest that TCD may be more sensitive than electroencephalography in detecting hemodynamic changes.

Embolization Detection

TCD can detect embolic material traveling through the intracranial circulation. The Doppler signal associated with cerebral embolus is characterized by (1) brief duration of 0.01–0.10 second, (2) random occurrence, and (3) amplitude of 10 db when compared to the background Doppler signal. These high-intensity transient signals have been termed "HITS." Audible characteristics include a harmonic tone with a whistling or chirping quality (Spencer et al. 1990).

Cerebral emboli can be detected during carotid endarterectomy and from cardiogenic sources (Klotzsch et al. 1994; Siebler et al. 1994). In vitro, different types of embolic material can be distinguished (thrombus, platelet, atheroma, fat) based on the TCD signal characteristics. It is possible that TCD monitoring for cerebral emboli during cardiac or vascular procedures may influence how the procedure is performed in an effort to prevent perioperative stroke.

Newer Developments in Neurovascular Ultrasound Imaging

Three-Dimensional Transcranial Doppler Blood Flow Mapping

The combination of a headpiece with Doppler probes interfaced with a computer, which allows three-dimensional reconstruction of the flow-generated image, results in a blood flow map of the arteries associated with the circle of Willis. This procedure provides a more complete view of the intracranial circulation. It has been reported to be useful in detecting intracranial stenoses with greater than 50% diameter reduction, in assessing the collateral circulation when there is extracranial occlusive disease, and in detecting intracranial vascular anomalies.

The detection of intracranial flow disturbances may be enhanced with the use of a color Doppler system, although there continue to be problems with calculation of absolute velocity values unless the incident angle is precisely known. Furthermore, in approximately 10–20% of subjects, there are marked limitations in insonating through the skull. For subjects who can be adequately studied, however, there has been reported to be a 90% correlation between three-dimensional color flow mapping results and angiography.

Transcranial Color Duplex Sonography

The addition of B-mode imaging to TCD allows more precise determination of the angle of the artery's course to the Doppler beam. With use of a computer-based dual-frequency (2.0/2.5 MHz) sector scan transducer, a color display Doppler flow map can be superimposed on the B-mode image. Traditionally, one has to calculate the flow velocity based on an estimate of the insonation angle. This carries with it a potential error of 15% for insonation of one vessel and the potential error could, theoretically, approach 30% when comparing homologous vessels. Although in its infancy in terms of clinical use, a TCCD system can provide more accurate flow velocity determinations in both the anterior and posterior cerebral circulation.

Contrast-Enhanced Transcranial Color Sonography

In an effort to improve resolution, agents are being developed that can enhance reflection of the ultrasound beam. As an example, microparticle-based agents, such as galactose, can be given by intravenous injection during TCCD to enhance the echodensity of blood. This transpulmonary ultrasound contrast agent allows delineation of peripheral branches of the MCAs, ACAs, and PCAs, as well as the posterior communicating arteries, cerebellar arteries, and deep cerebral veins.

CARDIAC ASSESSMENT WITH ULTRASOUND IN CEREBROVASCULAR DISEASE

Transthoracic Echocardiography Principles

All echocardiographic methods are characterized by transmission of sound energy to and through the heart. The sound energy is reflected back to the transducer as a function of each acoustic interface encountered. The time from transmission of the sound to the reception of the reflected echo, for a particular cardiac structure, is displayed in a pattern of distance to reflector over time. As a number of depth samples are insonated in sequence, a two-dimensional echocardiogram is generated. Repeated sampling of the structure of interest over one cardiac cycle results in a motion (M-mode) scan.

Contrast Imaging

Contrast imaging is achieved with intravenous administration of suspended particles or microbubbles. The contrast agent produces an acoustical interface to enhance the reflection of registered sound on the two-dimensional echocardiogram. In addition, the flow of contrast can be monitored, which enhances the detection of septal defects.

Doppler Echocardiography

Doppler echocardiography, in a fashion analogous to carotid Doppler, allows determination of the direction and velocity of blood. The Doppler signal can either be pulsed-wave or continuous-wave. The latter method is superior for recording the movement of blood at high speed, which is particularly useful in assessing the flow characteristics of stenotic valves. Both methods produce a spectral display of frequency (or velocity) over time that corresponds to a gray scale of frequency (or velocity) shifts. In color-flow Doppler mapping, a color map, which corresponds to the pulsed-wave Doppler frequency shifts, is superimposed over the two-dimensional image.

Transesophageal Echocardiography

Transesophageal echocardiography (TEE) uses the same methodology as described for transthoracic echocardiography. To optimize insonation of the atria, cardiac valves, and aorta, however, the transducer is attached to a flexible endoscope so that it can be positioned within the esophagus. This is generally a well-tolerated procedure.

Table 38.5: Structural cardiac abnormalities that can result in cerebral embolus

1. Hypokinetic left ventricle with or without demonstrated mural wall thrombus, aneurysm, or both
2. Valvular stenosis or regurgitation
3. Left atrial enlargement with or without demonstrated thrombus
4. Valvular vegetations, which can be infectious, marantic, or related to systemic lupus erythematosus (Libman-Sacks)
5. Septal defect including patent foramen ovale with or without septal aneurysm
6. Mitral valve prolapse with or without myxomatous degeneration
7. Atrial myxoma

Clinical Value of Echocardiography in Ischemic Stroke

There are a number of potential structural cardiac sources of cerebral embolus, as outlined in Table 38.5. In addition, aortic atherosclerotic plaque formation and dissection can be detected especially well with TEE. It is estimated that a potential cardiac source of embolus can be found in approximately 30% of patients with cerebral ischemia, but in roughly 10% there is coexistent cerebrovascular occlusive disease, which could explain the symptoms.

Global Left Ventricular Hypokinesis

A markedly reduced ejection fraction associated with global hypokinesis of the left ventricle is a common setting for thromboembolic disease. The risk is enhanced when there is coexistent ventricular aneurysm formation, mural wall thrombus formation, or both. Mural wall thrombi form in 20–60% of patients who die from myocardial infarction, although systemic embolism complicates transmural myocardial infarction in only 3–10% of subjects.

The echocardiographic appearance of the thrombus can have value in the determination of risk for embolization. Thrombi are mobile through the cardiac cycle and those that protrude into the left ventricular cavity are the most dangerous (Figure 38.12). The risk of thrombus formation in dilated cardiomyopathy tends to parallel the degree of global hypokinesis. Most subjects with left ventricular thrombus formation in association with dilated cardiomyopathy have evidence of congestive heart failure. It is important to point out that systemic embolism can complicate dilated cardiomyopathy without echocardiographic evidence of thrombus.

Valvular Cardiac Disease

Echocardiography is of value in the assessment of both prosthetic heart valves and rheumatic valvular disease. It can be used to assess for stenosis, regurgitation, and dehiscence of the valve and to detect the presence of vegetations. CW Doppler ultrasonography can be used to measure the

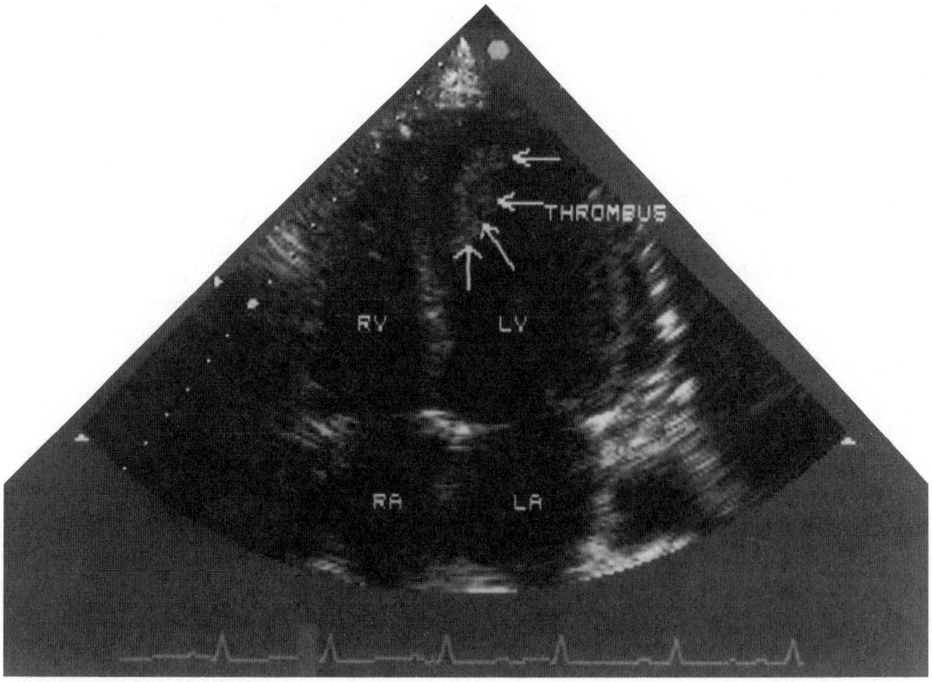

FIGURE 38.12 Echocardiogram that reveals a thrombus (arrows) within the left ventricle (LV).

gradient across a diseased valve, and the information correlates well with that provided by cardiac catheterization.

Mitral valve prolapse continues to be of questionable importance in terms of stroke risk. Associated factors such as redundant and thickened leaflets, mitral insufficiency, tricuspid valve prolapse, myxomatous change, and mitral annulus abnormalities are more readily detected by TEE.

Atrial Septal Aneurysm and Patent Foramen Ovale

Atrial septal aneurysm represents a ballooning of the atrial septum through the fossa ovalis with protrusion into the right or left atrium, or both. It is often seen in association with a patent foramen ovale (PFO), which is the most common type of atrial septal defect, and is associated with a fourfold increased risk of stroke. This has led to a much more aggressive pursuit of the presence of PFO with the combination of TEE and contrast. Contrast TEE, in the evaluation of right-to-left atrial shunt, has a markedly enhanced sensitivity to PFO compared to either contrast transthoracic echocardiography or TCD (Figure 38.13). It must be realized, however, that approximately 10% of controls have a PFO.

Cabanes et al. (1993) looked at 100 consecutive patients with cryptogenic ischemic stroke who were less than 55 years of age and who underwent TEE. They found that both atrial septal aneurysm, especially with more than 10 mm excursion, and PFO were significantly associated with cryptogenic stroke, while mitral valve prolapse was not. Studies suggest, however, that paradoxical cerebral embolism, resulting from PFO, is not the major mechanism of stroke in most instances, despite the presence of a PFO.

Transthoracic Versus Transesophageal Echocardiography in the Assessment of Cerebral Ischemia

TEE is more expensive and more invasive than transthoracic echocardiography, but it also has a higher yield in the detection of a potential cardiogenic source of embolus. Studies that have supported the diagnostic utility of TEE in stroke, however, have demonstrated that many of these potential cardiac sources of embolus include anomalies that are of questionable clinical significance, such as mitral valve prolapse, PFO, and mitral annulus calcification. TEE is clearly superior for detecting left atrial appendage thrombus, valvular abnormalities, and stasis of blood within the left atrium, all of which are associated with increased stroke risk. Thus, if it is felt that detecting a potential cardiogenic source of cerebral embolism will affect clinical management, TEE is the procedure of choice.

REFERENCES

Ackerman RH, Cardia MR. Identifying clinically relevant carotid disease [editorial]. Stroke 1994;25:1–3.

Adams R, McKie V, Nichols F et al. The use of transcranial ultrasonography to predict stroke in sickle cell disease. N Engl J Med 1992;326:605–610.

Barnett HJM, Warlow CP. Carotid endarterectomy and the measurement of stenosis [editorial]. Stroke 1993;24:1281–1284.

Cabanes L, Mas JL, Cohen A et al. Atrial septal aneurysm and patent foramen ovale as risk factors for cryptogenic stroke in patients less than 55 years of age. A study using transesophageal echocardiography. Stroke 1993;24:1865–1873.

Erickson JJ, Mewissen MW, Foley WD et al. Stenosis of the internal carotid artery: assessment using color Doppler imaging

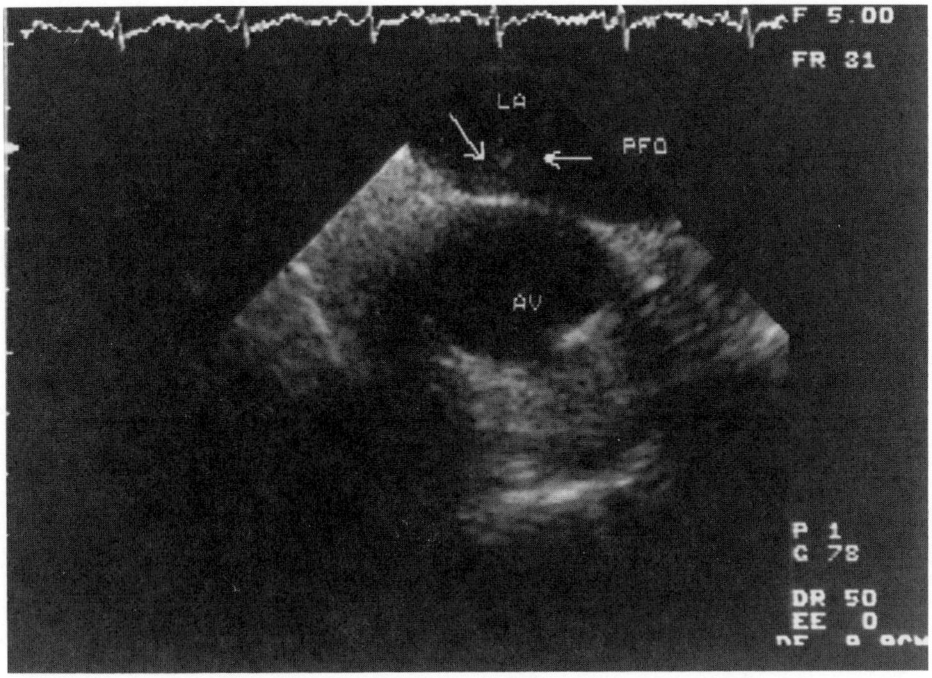

FIGURE 38.13 Echocardiogram that demonstrates contrast that is spontaneously entering the left atrium (LA) from the right atrium representing a patent foramen ovale (PFO). In the foreground is the aortic valve (AV).

compared with angiography. Am J Roentgenol 1989;152: 1299–1304.

European Carotid Surgery Trialists' Collaborative Group. MRC European Carotid Surgery Trial: interim results for symptomatic patients with severe (70–99%) or with mild (0–29%) carotid stenosis. Lancet 1991;337:1235–1243.

Kelley RE, Chang JY, Suzuki S et al. Selective increase in the right hemisphere transcranial Doppler velocity during a spatial task. Cortex 1993a;29:45–52.

Kelley RE, Namon RA, Mantelle LL et al. Sensitivity and specificity of transcranial Doppler ultrasonography in the detection of high-grade carotid stenosis. Neurology 1993b;43:1187–1191.

Klötzsch C, Janßen G, Berlit P. Transesophageal echocardiography and contrast-TCD in the detection of a patent foramen ovale: experiences with 111 patients. Neurology 1994;44:1603–1606.

Ley-Pozo J, Ringelstein EB. Noninvasive detection of occlusive disease of the carotid siphon and middle cerebral artery. Ann Neurol 1990;28:640–647.

Maeda H, Matsumoto M, Hand A et al. Reactivity of cerebral blood flow to carbon dioxide in various types of ischemic cerebrovascular disease: evaluation by the transcranial Doppler method. Stroke 1993;24:670–675.

Mullges W, Ringelstein EB, Leibold M. Non-invasive diagnosis of internal carotid artery dissections. J Neurol Neurosurg Psychiatry 1992;55:98–104.

Nordal HJ, Dullerud R, Amthor K-F. Grading stenoses of the internal carotid artery by estimation of blood velocity with pulsed Doppler ultrasound. Eur Neurol 1993;33:38–43.

North American Symptomatic Carotid Endarterectomy Trial Collaborators. Beneficial effect of carotid endarterectomy in symptomatic patients with high-grade carotid stenosis. N Engl J Med 1991;325:445–453.

Siebler M, Kleinschmidt A, Sitzer M et al. Cerebral microembolism in symptomatic and asymptomatic high-grade internal carotid artery stenosis. Neurology 1994;44:615–618.

Sitzer M, Fürst G, Fischer H et al. Between-method correlation in quantifying internal carotid stenosis. Stroke 1993;24:1513–1518.

Sloan MA, Haley Jr EC, Kassell NF et al. Sensitivity and specificity of transcranial Doppler ultrasonography in the diagnosis of vasospasm following subarachnoid hemorrhage. Neurology 1989;39:1514–1518.

Spencer MP, Thomas GI, Nicholls SC et al. Detection of middle cerebral artery emboli during carotid endarterectomy using transcranial Doppler ultrasonography. Stroke 1990;21:415–423.

Urbani MP, Picano E, Parenti G et al. In vivo radio frequency-based ultrasonic tissue characterization of the atherosclerotic plaque. Stroke 1993;24:1507–1512.

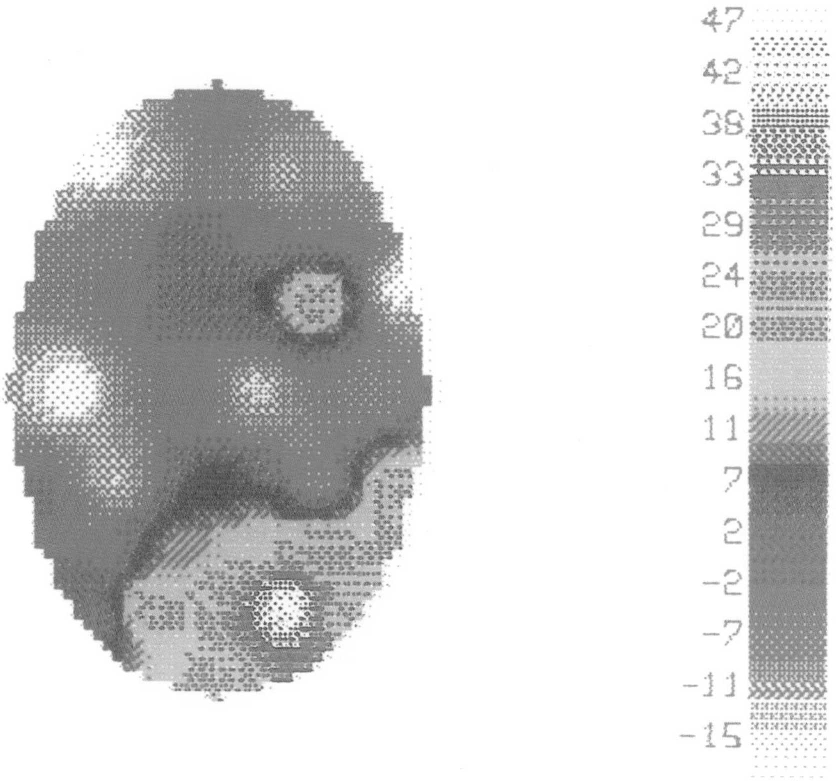

PLATE 37A.1 Frequency domain topographic brain map obtained from a 32-channel bipolar EEG recording. The patient was a 53-year-old man with hemodynamically significant left carotid stenosis. This map demonstrates an asymmetry over the occipital regions during eye opening, reflecting relative failure of left-hemisphere alpha activity to attenuate normally. The color scale at the right reflects percentage change in EEG activity going from the eyes-closed to eyes-open state. (Courtesy of Dr. Bruce Fisch.)

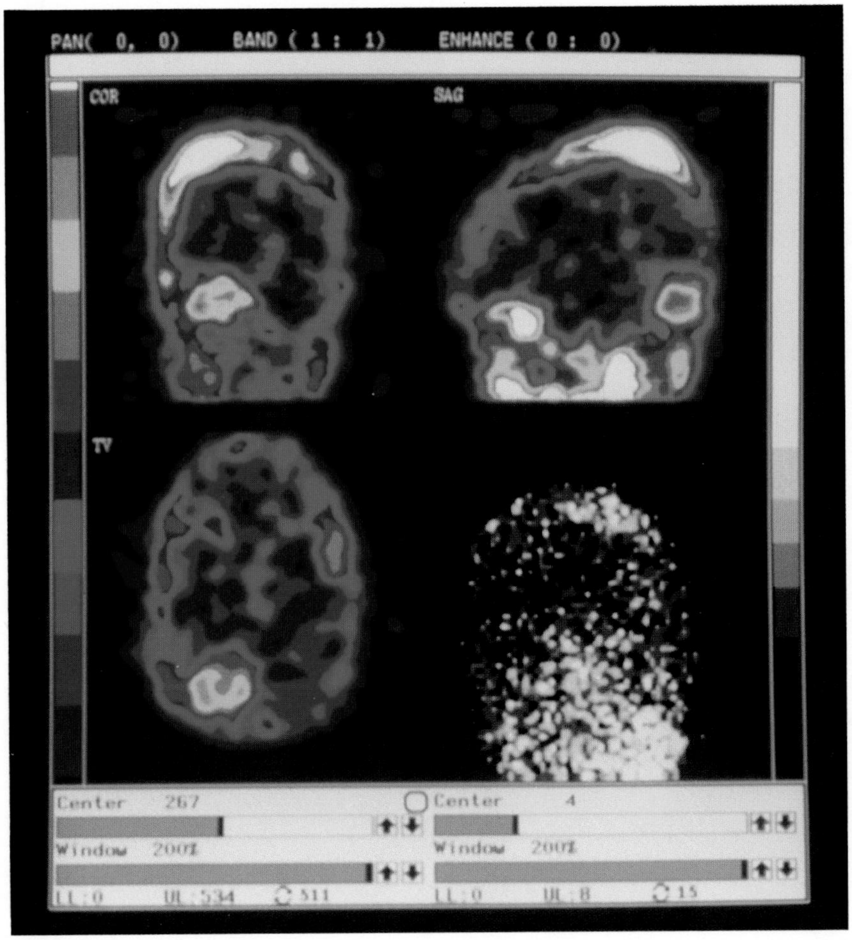

PLATE 39.1 Brain SPECT images with thallium-201 demonstrate a focal region of increased uptake corresponding to the same location as the lesion seen on CT (see Figure 39.36). This is a biopsy-proven lymphoma. (Reprinted with permission from A Ruiz, WL Ganz, MJD Post et al. Use of thallium-201 brain SPECT to differentiate cerebral lymphoma from toxoplasma encephalitis in AIDS patients. Am J Neuroradiol 1994;15:1885–1894.)

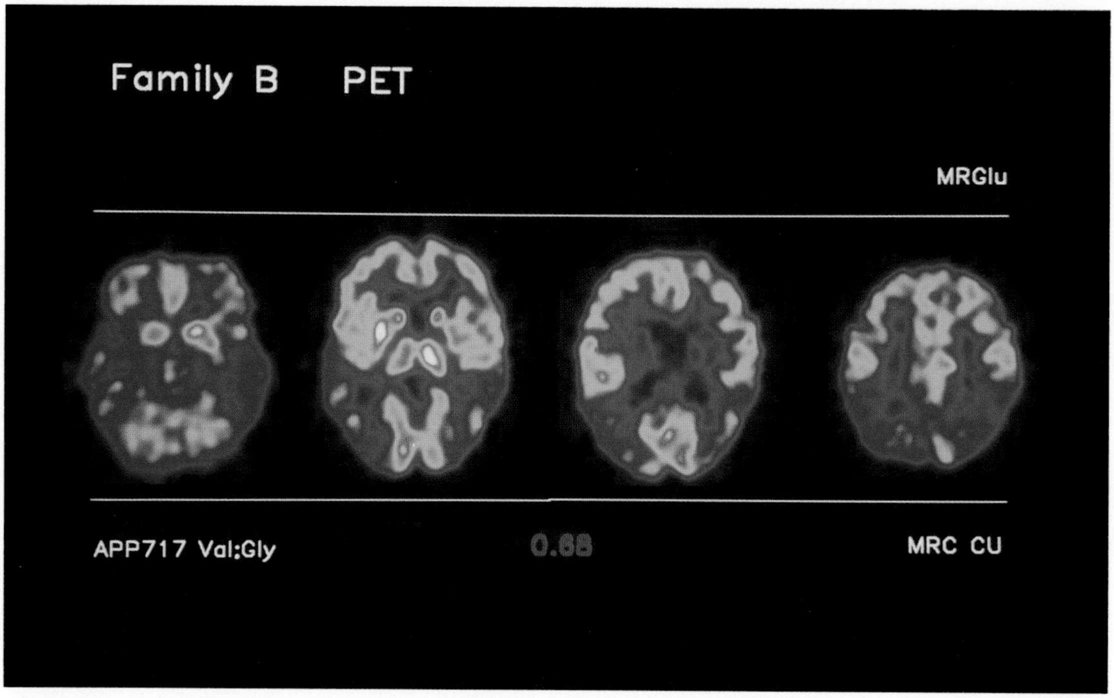

PLATE 40.I PET scans of the posterior parietal and temporal abnormalities of metabolism obtained with 18FDG-PET in Alzheimer's disease. This is the characteristic pattern seen in early disease.

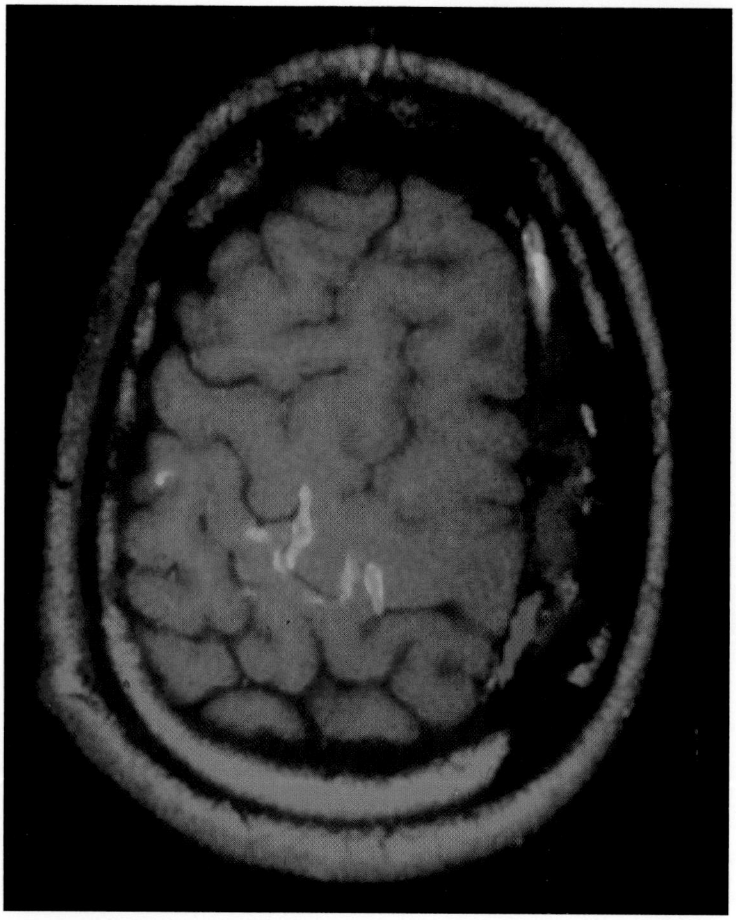

PLATE 40.II Functional MRI studies: The corresponding activation image (see Figures 40.2A and 40.2B) superimposed on the anatomical MRI. Cortical activity can clearly be seen running along the central sulcus, the maximal signal increase being about 4%.

Chapter 39
Neuroimaging

Evelyn M.L. Sklar and Robert M. Quencer

Major technological developments in neuroradiology have resulted in the detection and characterization of neurological diseases that heretofore were not demonstrated by earlier imaging methods. Magnetic resonance imaging (MRI) in particular has had the greatest impact on the practice of neurology since the arrival of computed tomography (CT) two decades ago.

The purpose of this chapter is to review the basic principles involved in the major imaging techniques, particularly CT and MRI, and to illustrate and describe the findings in a wide range of neurological diseases.

BASIC PRINCIPLES OF NEUROIMAGING PROCEDURES

Computed Tomography

CT provides a cross-sectional image of the body. The images produced are based on the principle of tissue absorption of x-rays. A beam of x-rays is transmitted through the body and the x-ray attenuation of a volume of tissue (*voxel*) is recorded. Shades of gray are then applied to the voxels depending on the amount of x-ray absorption. A scan is thus produced as shades of black and white. Differences in the shades of gray directly reflect the differences in x-ray attenuation of different tissues. Tissues have different attenuation properties depending on the atomic number of their constituent atoms and physical density. The attenuation of a material can be described as an attenuation coefficient, which is then translated to a CT number on an arbitrary scale (*Hounsfield units*). The images are acquired in an axial or coronal plane and then may be reformatted in any desirable plane.

Contrast agents have increased the sensitivity and specificity of CT in comparison to noncontrast studies. The mechanism of enhancement is based on disruption of the blood-brain barrier. This barrier restricts the movement of many substances from the bloodstream to the brain. On CT (and, as shall be seen in the next section, on MRI), only those areas where the blood-brain barrier is damaged enhance, such as tumors and inflammatory processes.

Magnetic Resonance Imaging

In MRI, the images result from the varying intensities of radio wave signals emanating from the tissue where hydrogen nuclei have been excited by a radio frequency (RF) pulse. Contrast in the MR image is the result of these differences in signal intensities. The initial level of intensity and its rate of decay depend on different physical properties of tissues, and therefore different tissues show different intensity signals depending on the time between radio frequency excitation and the sampling time chosen. Hydrogen is the most frequently used nucleus for MR imaging because of its abundance in biological tissues.

When placed in a magnetic field the majority of the hydrogen atoms align in the direction of the field. A 90-degree pulse produced by an RF transmitter causes the net magnetization vector to rotate away from its primary alignment to produce net magnetization in a different plane. It is the resulting transverse component of the field that is responsible for the production of the MR signal.

The loss of magnetization from the transverse plane occurs by two distinct relaxation processes: *spin lattice* and *spin-spin relaxation*. Spin-lattice relaxation is the return of magnetization to equilibrium with the applied magnetic field (z-direction). This process is represented by the *time constant T1*. One T1 period is the amount of time in which 63% of the longitudinal magnetization has been regained. Spin-spin relaxation is the loss of nuclear spin phase coherence. The protons dephase, resulting in a decrease in the transverse magnetization, causing a decrease in signal. Dephasing due to molecular interaction alone is termed *T2*. Dephasing produced by molecular interactions and spatial variation of the external magnetic field is termed *T2**. Signal is measured at a time interval, *echo time* (TE), following the RF excitations. The time between excitations is called *repetition time* or TR.

For the different pulse sequences used in MRI, the reader is referred to more extensive texts for a thorough description involved in MRI (Stark and Bradley 1992).

The four major types of magnets are permanent, hybrid, resistive, and superconducting. The field strength achievable with a resistive magnet is limited, whereas it is possible to achieve magnetic fields of much greater strength with superconductive magnets. A set of coils called "shim coils" are used to adjust the static field to establish a high degree of homogeneity within the magnetic field.

Contrast agents in MRI have been widely used. As in CT the mechanism of enhancement of central nervous system (CNS) pathology is based on disruption of the blood-brain barrier. Unlike conventional contrast agents used in CT that are directly visualized, those used in MRI (termed *paramagnetic contrast agents*) produce local alterations in the magnetic environment that influence the MR signal intensity. It is the effect on proton relaxation that appears on the MR images, not the contrast material itself.

Angiography

There are many indications for cerebral angiography, including subarachnoid hemorrhage and intracerebral hemorrhage in which the cause has not been determined clinically or with CT or MRI. Angiography is also used in the evaluation of patients with thromboembolic stroke, especially for evaluation of the carotid vessels in the neck and the intracranial vasculature. In patients with arterial dissections, vasculitis, or tumors at the base of the skull, angiography is also indicated.

Currently, angiography is performed by puncture of the femoral artery and threading a catheter up the iliac artery and into the aortic arch with subsequent selective catheterization of the carotid or vertebral arteries. After entering the desired vessel, an iodine-containing contrast agent is injected and serial films of the vasculature are obtained for approximately 10 seconds to demonstrate arterial, capillary, and venous phases of the cerebral circulation. More recently *digital subtraction angiography* has been substituted for cut film angiography in which a computer subtracts the background image and transmits it to a television monitor.

In addition, newer advances in angiographic techniques have allowed for expansion in the field of interventional neuroradiology. These procedures include embolization of vascular malformation and tumors, occlusion of cavernous carotid fistulas by detachable balloons, and angioplasty. The advent of the tracker catheter system and its variants has greatly promoted this field, and the reader is referred to other sources for further reading in these areas (Halbach et al. 1989).

Myelography

Myelography is still carried out in certain cases in which MRI cannot be performed, such as in postoperative patients in whom multiple clips or metallic hardware may produce too many artifacts. CT myelography may also define nerve root avulsions or dural tears better than MRI.

This procedure is performed by the injection of an iodinated water-soluble agent into the subarachnoid space and subsequently obtaining x-ray images of the spine. Tilting of the myelogram table allows the contrast to be moved throughout the spine. The contrast agents can be introduced by a lumbar, a C1–C2, or a cisternal puncture.

Intraoperative Neurosonography

The development of a high-resolution, portable, real-time sonographic scanner that can be used in the operating room allows the visualization of intraspinal or intracranial abnormalities and permits the surgeon and radiologist to assess the progress and final result of surgery before the operation is completed.

The images are obtained using a 7.5-MHz or a 5.0-MHz in-line transducer, with the optimal focus varying depending on the transducer's RF. The transducer is most commonly placed in a water bath at the laminectomy site in the case of intraoperative spinal sonography, or at the craniotomy or burr hole site in the case of intraoperative cranial sonography.

Intraoperative neurosonography (IONS) is performed in multiple planes. Images are obtained in each plane by gradually moving the transducer across the operative field. Filmed images are obtained throughout the study.

Magnetic Resonance Angiography

Magnetic resonance angiography (MRA) is a very sensitive method for detecting and characterizing flow. It produces a blood flow map where the vessel visualization is based on the physical differences between moving and stationary protons. Image intensity reflects velocity and flow patterns.

There are two major types of MRA techniques: time of flight angiography and phase contrast angiography. The differentiation between moving and stationary protons depends on the degree of longitudinal or transverse magnetization. Time of flight angiography deals with longitudinal magnetization and is amplitude-sensitive, while phase contrast angiography deals with transverse magnetization and is phase-sensitive.

Time of flight angiography relies on inflow of unsaturated protons into an imaging plane. A volume is repeatedly pulsed, and since stationary nuclei are unable to remagnetize fully when the repetition period is smaller than the relaxation time T1, their signal is smaller than that of the fully magnetized nuclei flowing into the excited volume. Inflowing blood therefore has a higher signal than stationary tissue, and it is the differentiation between the signals of stationary and flowing protons that produces a time of flight MRA.

Phase contrast MRA relies on velocity-induced phase shifts of moving protons. A bipolar gradient is applied, and if the proton is stationary, there is no phase shift. If, however, the proton is moving, there will be a phase shift. The faster the proton moves, the greater the phase shift. Velocity-induced changes in the transverse magnetization will distinguish moving from stationary protons.

MRA can be performed with either a two- or three-dimensional Fourier transformation (2DFT or 3DFT) gradient echo technique. In 2DFT techniques, each slice is individually acquired and even relatively slow flow will be identified. In 3DFT or volume acquisition, data are acquired from an entire volume simultaneously. Very thin sections can be obtained with 3DFT and therefore high resolution can be attained.

The maximum-intensity projection is a ray-tracing technique performed at a specific angle. It processes a series of acquired slices by projecting a straight line through these slices. It selects only those pixels along the ray with the highest signal intensity, and therefore only vascular structures are represented in the final image. The procedure is repeated using parallel rays until a full two-dimensional projection is generated. The use of MRA with arteriovenous malformations is illustrated in the section on vascular malformations below.

The source images are the individually reconstructed 2DFT or 3DFT partitions, while the collapsed view refers to the maximum-intensity projection that pancakes all the images into one.

INTRACRANIAL LESIONS

Intra-Axial Brain Tumors (see Chapter 59)

Supratentorial Gliomas

Primary cerebral gliomas comprise 40–45% of all intracranial tumors; their incidence peaks in the second decade of life. In adults, most of these are supratentorial, whereas in children, they are mostly located in the posterior fossa. The degree of malignancy is variable, ranging from low-grade pilocytic astrocytomas to glioblastomas.

MR is more sensitive than CT for tumor detection and delineation, even after contrast administration.

Oligodendrogliomas. Oligodendrogliomas are usually heterogeneous in signal on MRI with small cystic regions and areas of hemorrhage. Edema is usually not significant. Calcification on CT has been reported in 50–90% of these tumors. One-half of the cases demonstrate contrast enhancement (Figure 39.1).

Low-Grade Astrocytoma. Low-grade astrocytoma (grades I and II) is an irregular nonhomogeneous lesion with calcifications present in approximately 15% of cases. Usually, there is little edema around the lesion, and in general, it is nonencapsulated and poorly demarcated from the surrounding parenchyma. With contrast, grade I astrocytomas may show minimal or no enhancement, and grade II astrocytomas enhance in approximately 89% of cases (see Figure 39.1).

Ganglioglioma. Ganglioglioma mostly affects children and young adults and is composed of both neural and glial elements. Most gangliogliomas are supratentorial, the temporal lobe being the predominant site. In imaging studies, they are well circumscribed and typically cystic and often have calcification.

Glioblastoma Multiforme. Glioblastomas represent the most malignant end of the spectrum of glial tumors. They represent 15–20% of all intracranial tumors, are the most common supratentorial neoplasm in an adult, and show a male predominance. Peak incidence is between 45 and 55 years of age. They are located most commonly in the frontal lobe, followed by the temporal lobe. A "butterfly" pattern is the characteristic distribution in those glioblastomas with bihemispheric involvement and intervening corpus callosum infiltration. There is a tendency for glioblastomas to invade the leptomeninges and dura.

MRI usually shows marked tumoral heterogeneity (Figure 39.2), with necrosis and cystic changes. These tumors have a tendency to bleed, but calcification is rare. The majority of these lesions enhance with contrast, and the enhancement pattern is heterogeneous. One can see ringlike enhancement with thick irregular nodular areas surrounding necrotic regions (see Figure 39.2). Regions that enhance correlate with areas of tumor tissue at pathology; hence, enhancement is helpful in guiding surgical biopsy. It should be emphasized that one cannot distinguish the exact margins of the tumor from edema. As with all infiltrative gliomas, there is no clear margin microscopically where tumor cells stop and reactive gliosis, edema, or normal brain begins (Atlas 1991).

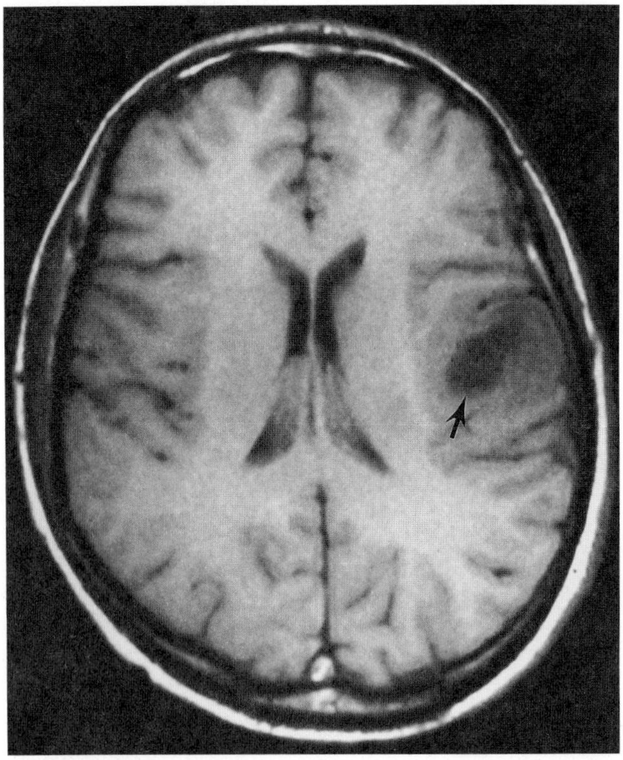

A

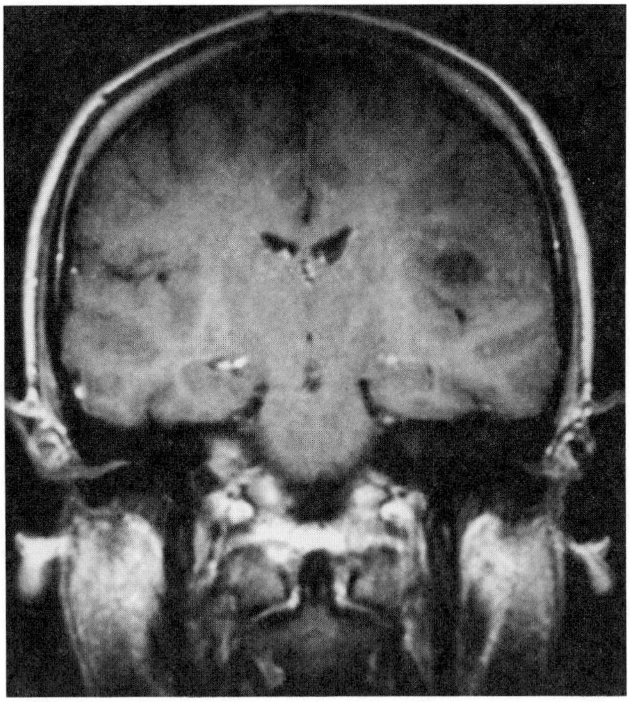

C

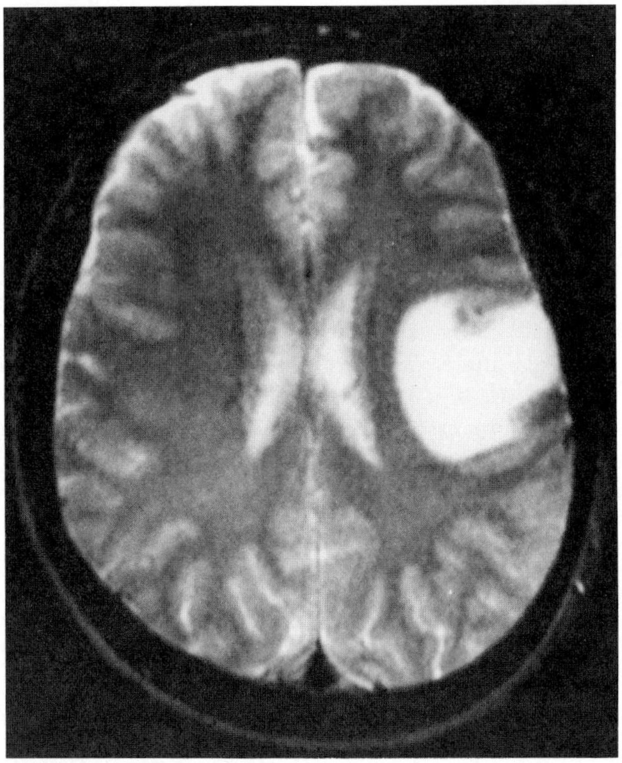

B

FIGURE 39.1 Oligodendroglioma. A. Axial T1-weighted MRI shows a predominantly hypointense left temporal-parietal mass, which exhibits no mass effect other than compression and narrowing of surrounding sulci and subarachnoid space. The central well-defined hypointense region (arrow) represents a cystic component of the tumor, whereas the smaller punctate areas of hypointensity were small areas of calcifications. B. Axial T2-weighted MR demonstrates the well-defined hyperintense mass with no surrounding edema or mass effect. C. Postcontrast (Gd-DTPA) coronal T1-weighted images show no enhancement of the mass. This combination of findings is typical for a low-grade astrocytoma or oligodendroglioma.

Subependymal Giant Cell Astrocytoma. The classic setting of a subependymal giant cell astrocytoma is a mass in the region of the foramen of Monro in a young adult with tuberous sclerosis. The mass is an astrocytic neoplasm projecting into the ventricle from a subependymal location. It is found in up to 10% of patients with tuberous sclerosis, and it is very rare outside the clinical setting of this disease. MRI and CT findings in subependymal giant cell astrocytoma include the typical location, a heterogeneous hyperintense mass with evidence of contrast enhancement, and hydrocephalus (Figure 39.3). Central regions of hypointensity on MRI may be due to calcifications.

Posterior Fossa Tumors

The posterior fossa is the most common site of primary intracerebral tumors in the child. The most common tumors of the posterior fossa seen in children are, in order of decreasing frequency, cerebellar astrocytomas, primitive neuroectodermal tumors (PNETs), ependymomas, and brain stem gliomas. In the adult, infratentorial tumors make up

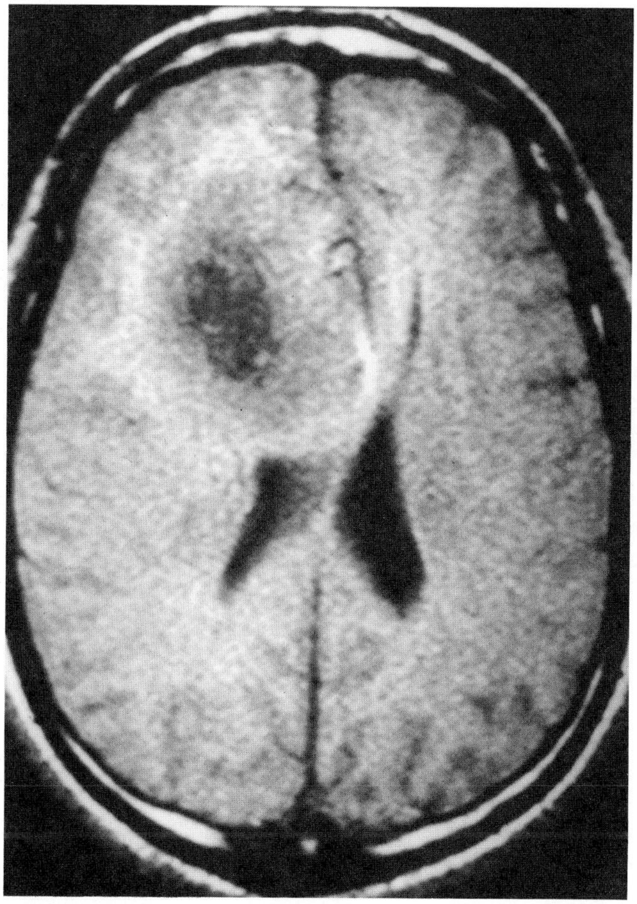

A

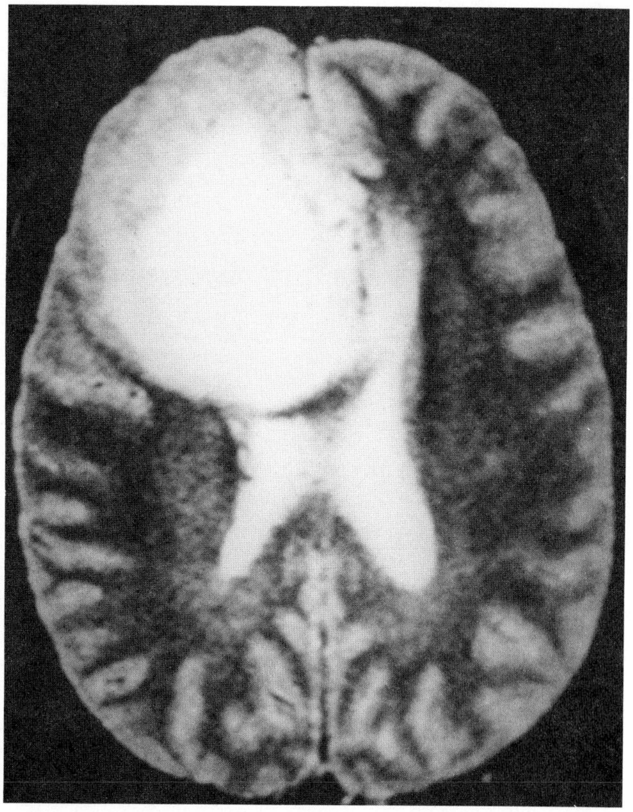

B

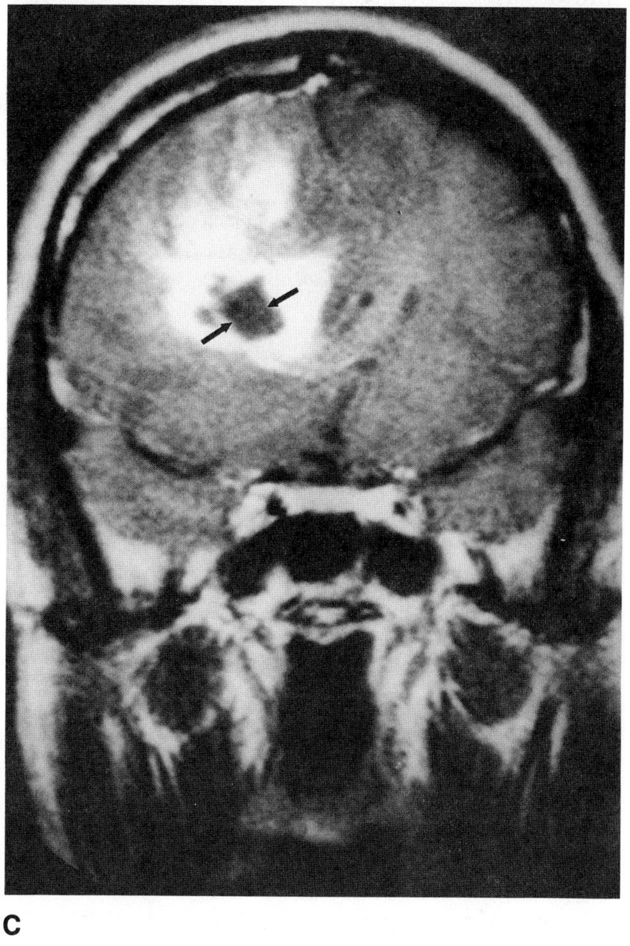

C

FIGURE 39.2 Glioblastoma multiforme. Axial T1-weighted image (A) and T2-weighted image (B) reveal a mass lesion compressing the frontal horn and producing shift of the midline. This lesion is iso- to hypointense on T1 weighting and becomes hyperintense on T2 weighting. C. Postcontrast T1 coronal image shows irregular enhancement of this lesion with a central area of hypointensity representing a tumor cyst or necrotic tissue (arrows).

only 15–20% of all intra-axial brain tumors, the most common being hemangioblastoma and metastasis.

Cerebellar Astrocytoma. The cerebellar astrocytoma is the most common posterior fossa neoplasm in the child. The typical findings of a juvenile pilocytic astrocytoma on MRI include a mass made up of a single large cyst with a solid nodular portion in the wall of the cyst. The solid portion of the tumor enhances with contrast, while the cyst wall may or may not enhance. The solid portion is hyperintense to normal brain on T2-weighted sequences, whereas the cystic portion is isointense to cerebrospinal fluid (CSF). Cerebellar astrocytomas may not be cystic, and if solid they are usually homogeneous in signal intensity. Twenty percent calcify.

Primitive Neuroectodermal Tumors. PNETs are a group of CNS tumors thought to originate from primitive or un-

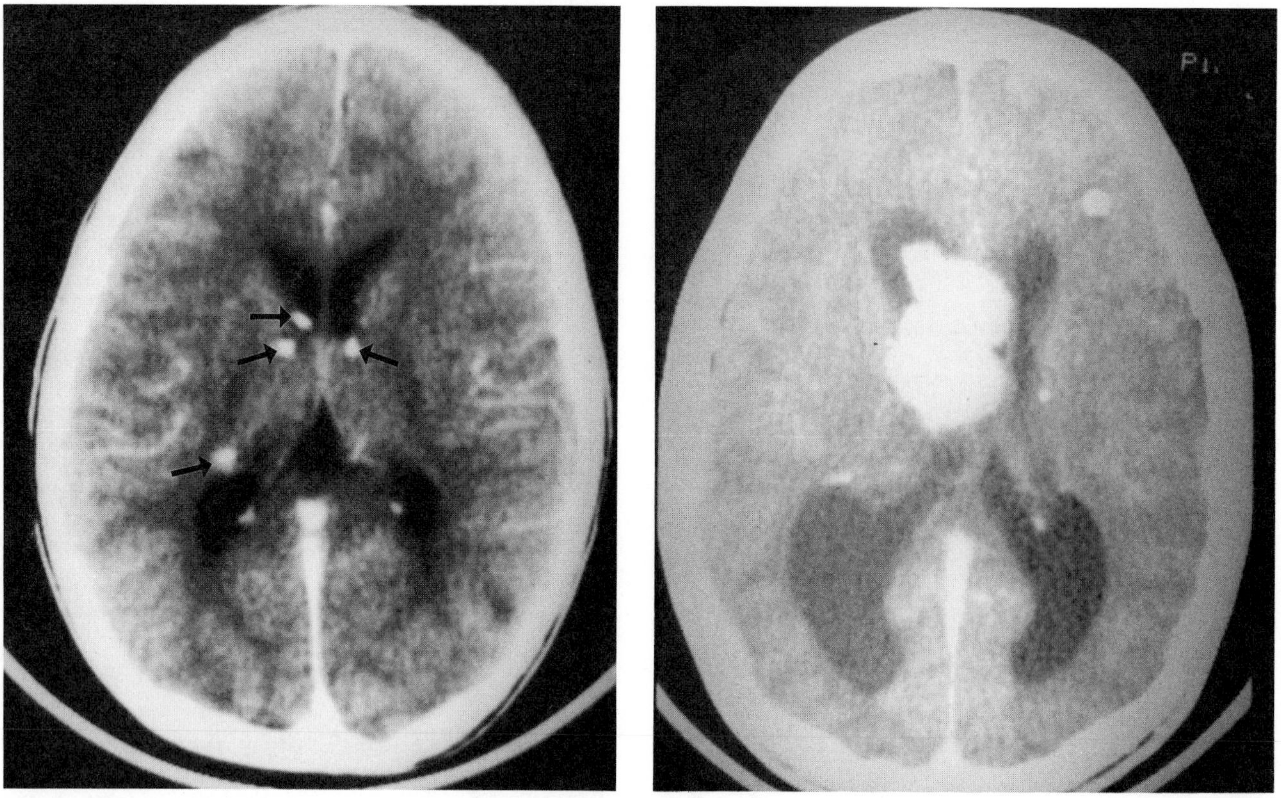

A B

FIGURE 39.3 Tuberous sclerosis. A. Multiple calcified periventricular lesions (arrows) are seen on this CT axial scan. B. In another patient an enhancing mass lesion is noted in the region of the foramen of Monro with associated hydrocephalus. The diagnosis was subependymal giant cell astrocytoma.

differentiated neuroepithelial cells. The prototype of these tumors is the medulloblastoma. Other tumors included in this category are ependymoblastoma, cerebral neuroblastoma, pinealoblastoma, medulloepithelioma, and pigmented medulloblastoma.

The cerebellar PNET, the medulloblastoma, makes up 25% of all intracerebral tumors in children, second only to cerebellar astrocytoma. They originate most frequently in the midline filling the fourth ventricle. These malignant tumors tend to invade the leptomeninges and seed the CSF.

On CT, these tumors are high-density lesions that enhance and produce hydrocephalus. On MRI, they have homogeneous to mixed signal intensity (Figure 39.4). On T2-weighted images, the lesions are nearly isointense to brain parenchyma. These tumors enhance intensely after contrast administration (see Figure 39.4).

Ependymoma. Ependymomas are common tumors in children (10% of pediatric CNS neoplasms), and two-thirds are located in the posterior fossa. They are usually intimately associated with the fourth ventricle or its outlet foramina, and tend to arise from the floor and track along its lateral recesses into the cerebellopontine angle. The next most common location is the body of the lateral ventricle, although they may also be found in the brain parenchyma, outside the ventricular system.

Ependymoma most frequently presents as a partially cystic, calcified, and sometimes hemorrhagic mass. They can extend through the foramen magnum and compress the dorsal aspect of the spinal cord (plastic ependymoma). Virtually all of them enhance with contrast. Seeding of the CSF occurs less frequently than with the PNET lesions.

Brain Stem Astrocytoma. Brain stem astrocytoma comprises 10% of all childhood brain tumors. It is characteristically located in the pons. The great majority are of the diffuse (infiltrative) fibrillary type, and a small minority constitute the more benign juvenile pilocytic astrocytoma. The MRI appearance of brain stem astrocytoma is variable with regard to signal intensity and enhancement. MRI demonstrates these lesions as poorly defined areas of high intensity on long TR-long TE images (Figures 39.5 and 39.6). The MRI is much better for demonstrating this lesion than the CT. When gross enlargement of the brain stem occurs, the size of the cisternal spaces decreases, and when the growth becomes exophytic there may be encase-

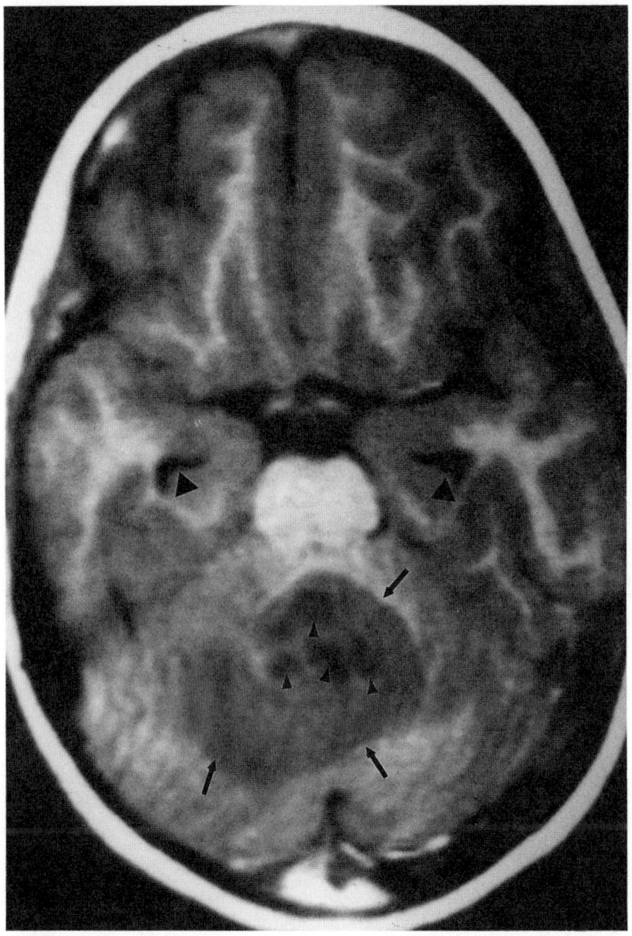

A

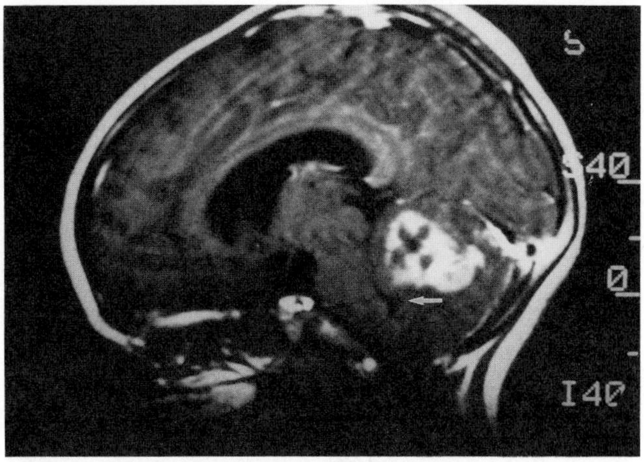

B

FIGURE 39.4 Medulloblastoma. A. Axial T1-weighted MRI shows a mixed intensity (isointense to hypointense to gray matter) midline posterior fossa mass (arrows). The hypointense areas (arrowheads) represent cysts within the mass. B. The postcontrast sagittal T1-weighted image shows dense enhancement throughout the mass, except for the areas of cyst formation. The mass extends from the cerebellar vermis into the right cerebellar hemisphere. Compression of the fourth ventricle (arrow in B) and early hydrocephalus (see dilatation of the temporal horns—large arrowheads in A).

ment of the basilar artery. Contrast enhancement occurs in approximately half the cases and is often irregular (see Figure 39.6).

Hemangioblastoma

Hemangioblastoma is the most common primary posterior fossa intra-axial neoplasm of the adult (Atlas 1991). This lesion has a high association with Von Hippel-Lindau syndrome in which there are retinal angiomas, cysts and angiomas of the liver and kidney, renal cell carcinoma, and pheochromocytoma (Atlas 1991). Although the cerebellum is the most frequent site of involvement, supratentorial hemangioblastoma may occasionally be seen.

Pathologically and in imaging studies, hemangioblastomas are commonly well-demarcated cystic masses with highly vascularized nodules within the wall of the cyst. Importantly, the cyst wall is not tumorous. The vascular nidus always abuts pia mater, giving rise to the alternate theory of origin that this is primarily a meningeal-based tumor (Figure 39.7). Entirely solid hemangioblastomas occur in 30–40% of cases, especially in the supratentorial compartment.

On MRI, the majority of these lesions are cystic and have a peripheral pial-based mural nodule of solid tissue that enhances markedly, and there may be large vessels within or at the periphery of the mass. The cysts can be isointense to CSF on all sequences or slightly hyperintense to CSF on T1-weighted images, a fact that relates to their high protein content. The mural nodule is slightly hyperintense to gray matter on long TR images.

Pineal Tumors

Pineal tumors are uncommon, representing 1% of all intracranial tumors. MR is excellent at distinguishing true pineal masses from parapineal masses, a differentiation that has clear surgical relevance. Two major groups of pineal tumors are recognized: germ cell tumors and tumors derived from pineal parenchymal cells.

Germ Cell Tumors. The majority of pineal tumors are of germ cell origin. These include the germinoma, teratoma, embryonal carcinoma, choriocarcinoma, and mixed types. Of these, germinomas are the most common.

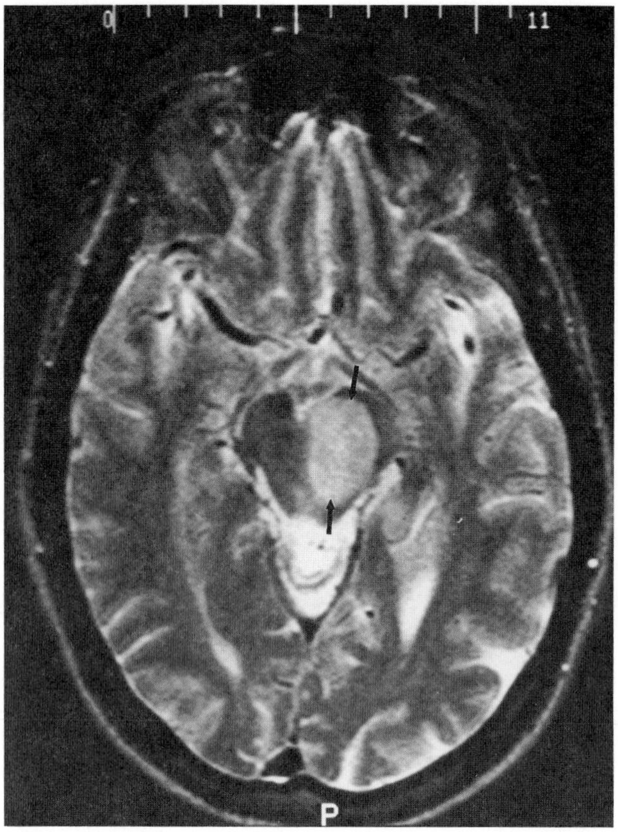

A

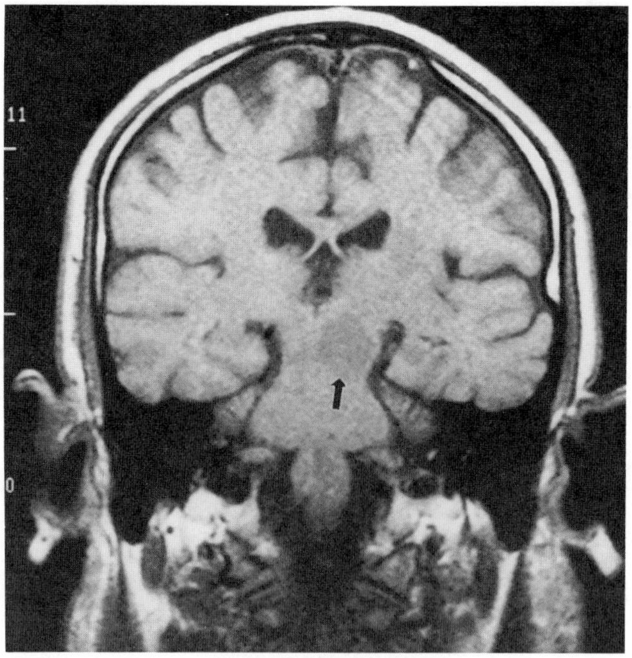

B

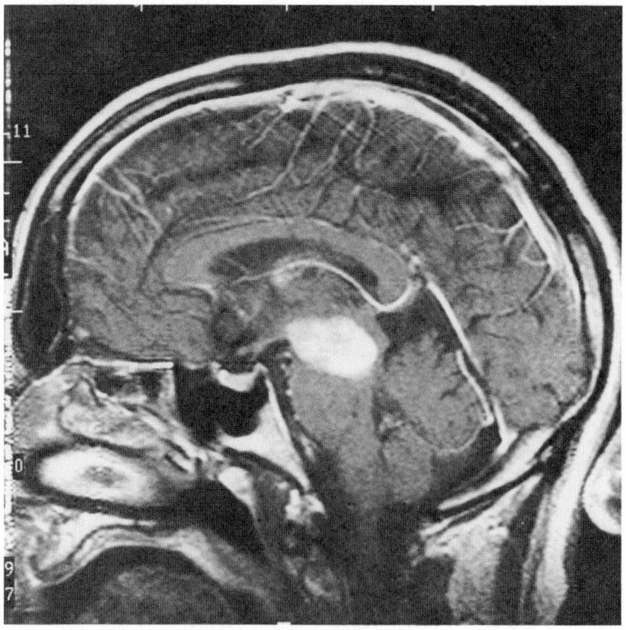

C

FIGURE 39.5 Brain stem astrocytoma. A. T2-weighted axial image shows a hyperintense lesion (arrows) located in the midbrain. This lesion is obliterating the cisterns ventrally. B. Coronal T1-weighted image shows a midbrain lesion that is hypointense in signal intensity (arrow). C. Postgadolinium T1-weighted sagittal image shows an enhancing lesion in the midbrain with little involvement of the quadrigeminal plate.

They frequently seed the subarachnoid space and invade adjacent brain parenchyma. The second most common pineal germ cell tumor is the teratoma, occurring in an earlier age group than germinomas. These can contain hair, teeth, bone, and fat.

Pineal germinomas are well-circumscribed, relatively homogeneous lesions. Nonhemorrhagic germinomas can be of low signal intensity on T2-weighted image, and they enhance markedly with intravenous contrast. Teratomas, on the other hand, are very heterogeneous, and their enhancement is variable.

Pineal Cell Tumors. *Pinealoblastoma* (a PNET) is a highly cellular tumor that tends to disseminate early through the subarachnoid pathways with leptomeningeal and subependymal seeding (Figure 39.8). Pinealoblastoma tends to be isointense to gray matter on T1-weighted images (similar to other PNET tumors) and to enhance densely with contrast.

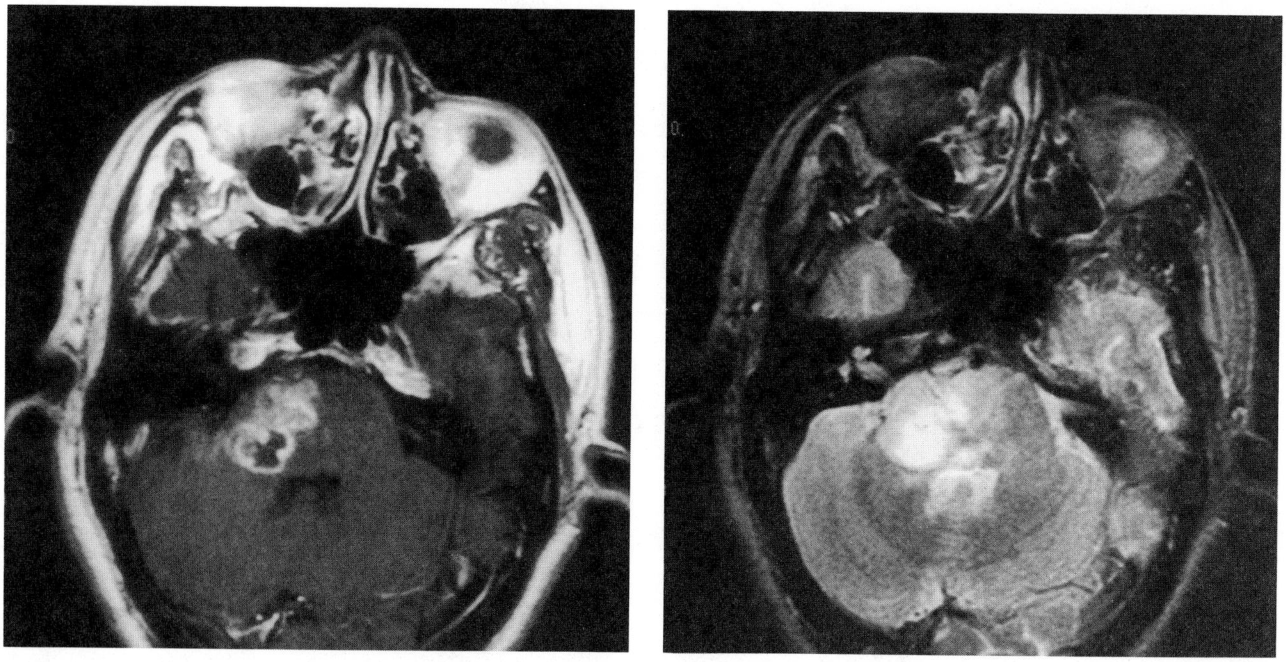

A B

FIGURE 39.6 Pontine astrocytoma. A. Axial MRI scan after gadolinium administration demonstrates a lesion on the right side of the pons, with irregular borders and nonhomogeneous enhancement, which is producing enlargement of the pons. B. The T2-weighted image shows a high-intensity lesion with heterogeneous signal.

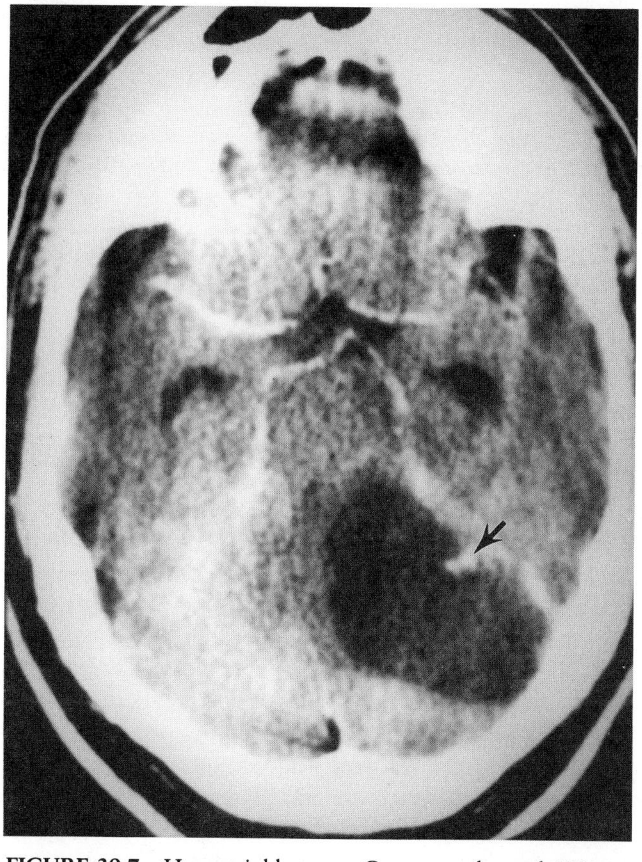

FIGURE 39.7 Hemangioblastoma. Contrast-enhanced CT scan demonstrates a cystic lesion with an enhancing mural nodule (arrow), which is peripheral and pial-based.

Pinealocytoma is a tumor of adults that is more benign than pinealoblastoma. It is a well-differentiated densely enhancing mass, which has a high signal on T2-weighted sequences. Calcifications are seen more frequently with pinealocytomas.

Colloid Cysts

Colloid cysts are benign lesions derived from infolding of the neuroepithelium, which is probably developing choroid plexus. The majority of these lesions are located in the anterosuperior aspect of the third ventricle. They represent the most common form of neuroepithelial cysts and contain dense mucoid material and various ions, some of which are paramagnetic.

On MRI, colloid cysts are varied in their signal, ranging from hypointense to markedly hyperintense on both T1- and T2-weighted images. Peripheral contrast enhancement may occur (Figure 39.9).

Lymphoma

Primary CNS lymphoma represents approximately 1% of all primary brain tumors, although this incidence has been steadily increasing in the past decade due to its frequent occurrence in patients with acquired immune deficiency syndrome (AIDS). Focal intracerebral masses are the most common initial presentation of primary CNS lymphoma, and multiplicity is common. To be contrasted are intracra-

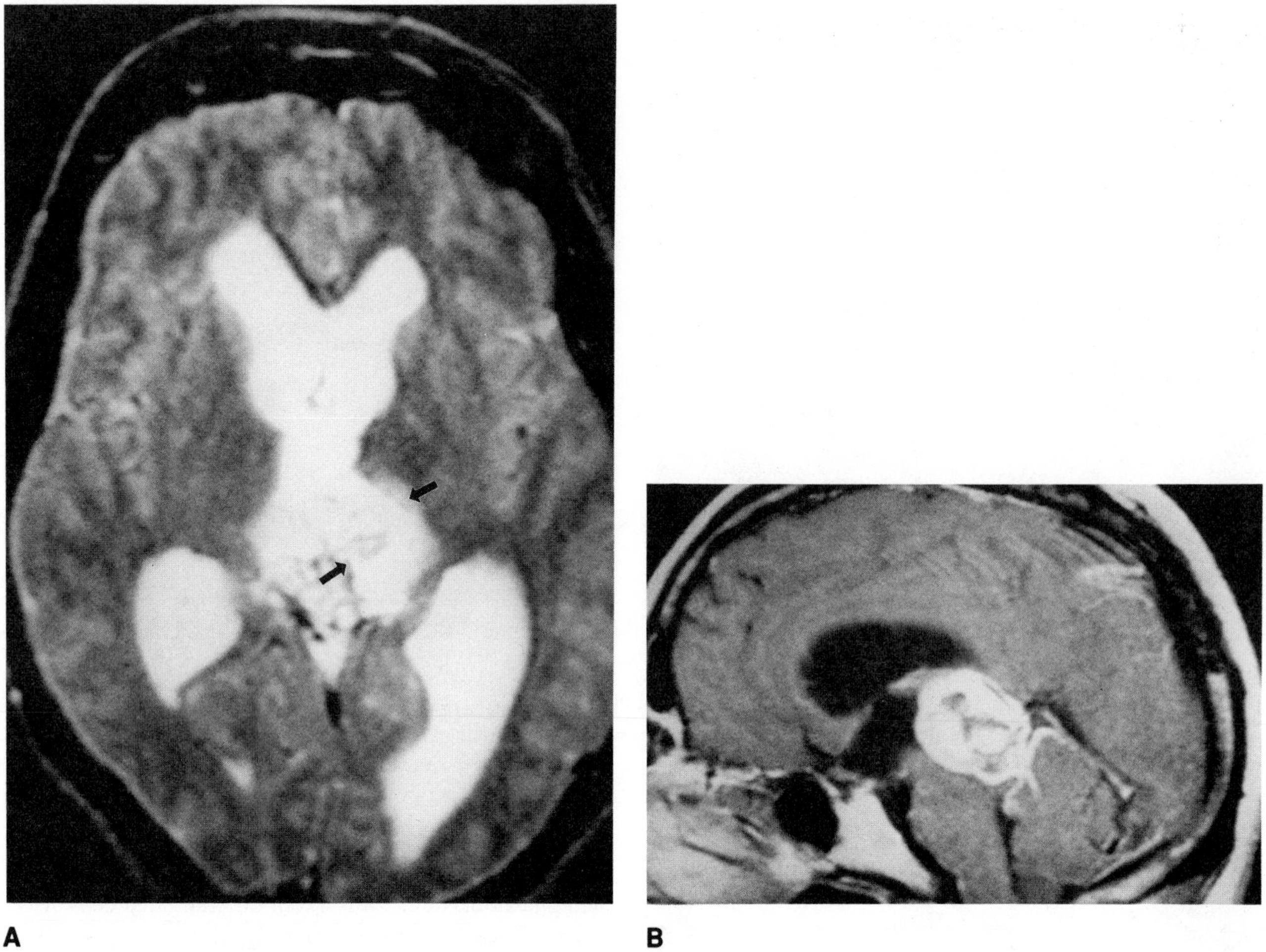

FIGURE 39.8 Pinealoblastoma. A. Axial T2-weighted image shows a mass (arrows), which is hyperintense and produces mass effect on the posterior portion of the third ventricle. B. Postcontrast-enhanced MR sagittal image demonstrates the mass and its effect on the colliculi and on the aqueduct of Sylvius with resultant hydrocephalus.

nial metastases from systemic lymphoma that tend to spread via the leptomeninges (with or without parenchymal involvement).

The appearances of parenchymal lymphoma on neuroimaging studies include masses that involve the deep gray matter structures, periventricular regions, and corpus callosum. The amount of edema seen on MRI is proportionately less than that seen with primary gliomas or metastases. Signal intensity is variable, but when these lesions are deep they are often isointense to gray matter on T2-weighted images. In the majority of lymphomas, enhancement is dense and homogeneous (Figures 39.10, 39.11). Secondary brain involvement is indistinguishable from primary CNS lymphoma, but parenchymal as opposed to meningeal involvement is more common with primary lymphoma. Postcontrast MRI is more sensitive than CT for detecting leptomeningeal seeding. Lymphoma in AIDS patients tends to have more necrosis than in non-AIDS patients and therefore appears as lesions with ring enhancement and more prominent edema than in non-AIDS patients.

Metastatic Disease

Cerebral metastases comprise 26% of all clinically detected brain tumors (Atlas 1991) and 80–85% of them are supratentorial in location. The optimal screening examination for the detection of intracerebral metastases is the postcontrast MRI. Intraparenchymal metastases are most common, with the tumors of the lung and breast being the most common primary sites. Most intracerebral metastases are multiple, but solitary metastases are not infrequent (30–50% of cases of metastases). They are found at the gray-white junction, are usually well circumscribed and round, and are frequently surrounded by considerable edema (Figure 39.12). The extent of edema bears no relationship to the size of the metastasis or the clinical status of the patient.

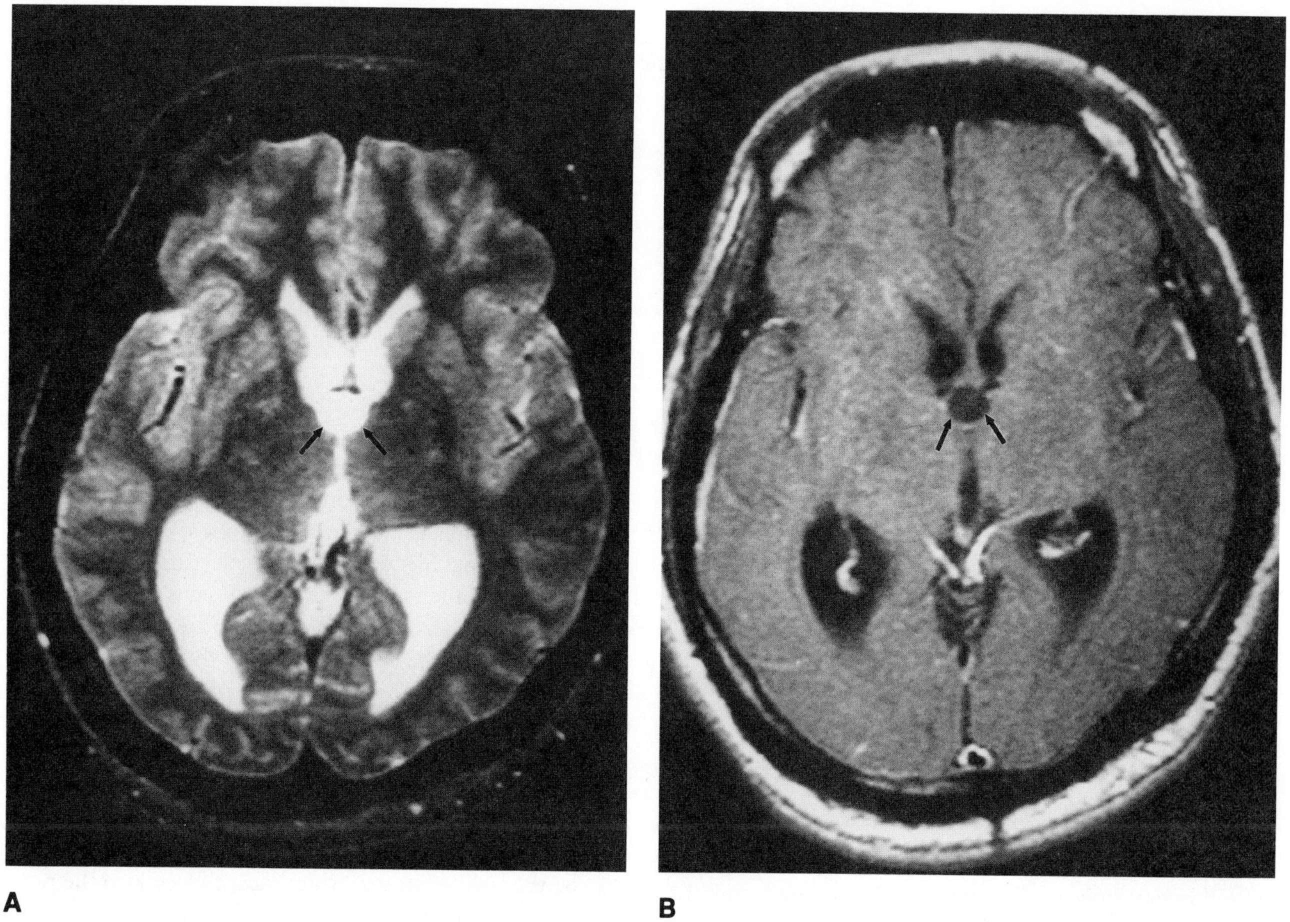

FIGURE 39.9 Colloid cyst. A. There is a rounded lesion in the region of the foramen of Monro, which is hyperintense on T2-weighted image (arrows). There is associated hydrocephalus. B. Post–contrast T1-weighted image shows a hypointense lesion with slight peripheral enhancement (arrows).

On MRI, metastases can be distinguished from edema on T2-weighted images as the metastasis is of variable intensity within an area of high-intensity edema. Peritumoral edema is usually prominent and is identified as fingerlike projections following white matter boundaries. Intratumoral hemorrhage occurs in 20% of metastases.

Contrast increases the ability to detect metastases. CT is highly sensitive to intraparenchymal metastatic disease, but contrast-enhanced MRI detects many lesions that are not detected on CT. In one study, Yuh et al. (1992) found that high-dose (triple-dose) gadolinium-enhanced MRI examinations have advantages over the standard 0.1 mmol/kg examinations in detecting small metastases. In addition, magnetization transfer (a new technique that uses special saturation pulses to produce greater than normal enhancement of cortical and subependymal veins and other gadolinium-containing structures) with single-dose gadolinium-enhanced MRI improves sensitivity to metastases and doubles the relative contrast of enhancing brain lesions. In general, metastases have more edema and mass effect than inflammatory processes and primary gliomas, a sign that can be helpful in differential diagnostic considerations.

Extra-Axial Brain Tumors

Several criteria help establish the location of a lesion as extra-axial. A broad dural-based margin is strongly suggestive of an extra-axial lesion. Other characteristics of extra-axial tumors include bony hyperostosis, invasion of the bone, displaced gray matter, buckled white matter, inwardly displaced pial vascular structures, and CSF clefts (Atlas 1991).

Meningiomas

Meningiomas, the most common primary nonglial intracranial tumors, have a peak incidence in the middle and later decades of life (Atlas 1991). Meningiomas have a predilection for certain locations: parasagittal, convexity, sphenoid

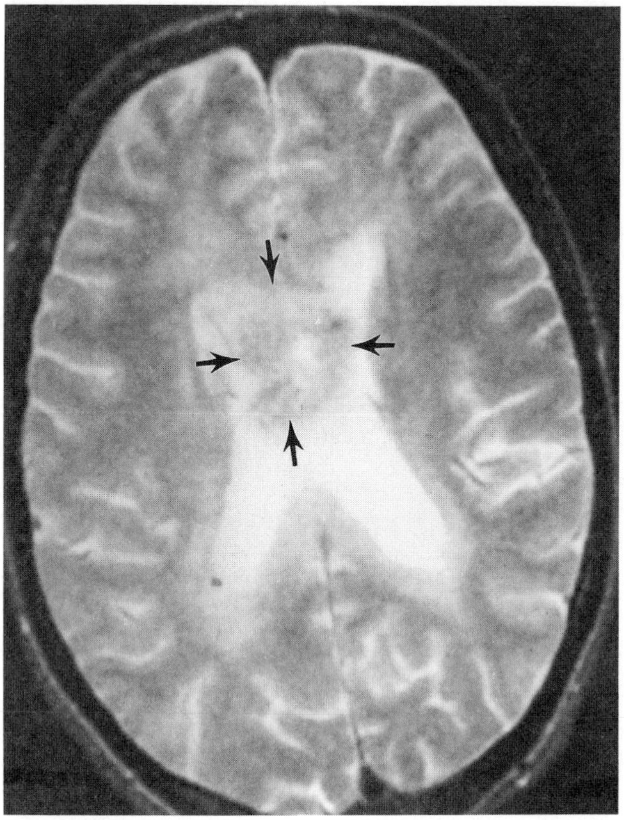

FIGURE 39.10 Lymphoma. Mass involving the body of the corpus callosum (arrows) is isointense to gray matter on this T2-weighted axial image.

wings, tuberculum sellae, parasellar, olfactory groove, cerebellopontine angle, clivus, and tentorium. They are usually broad-based and are attached to the adjacent dura.

If high field strength magnets are used, the detection rate on noncontrast MRI for the meningiomas is comparable to that of contrast CT. MRI is superior to CT in determining dural sinus invasion with occluded venous flow and in defining tumor vascularity and arterial encasement. On T1-weighted images, meningiomas are iso- to hypointense to gray matter, and on T2-weighted images approximately half are isointense and half hyperintense to gray matter (Figure 39.13). There is a good correlation between tumor histology and tumor intensity on T2-weighted images, though exact histological typing by MRI is not possible. Almost all the meningiomas that are hyperintense to gray matter on T2-weighted images are of either the synctial or angioblastic type, whereas fibroblastic and transitional cell type are hyperintense to gray matter on T2-weighted images. The majority of meningiomas demonstrate a heterogeneous intensity pattern. Tumor vascularity has been identified in approximately one-third of the cases, seen as punctate and curvilinear hypointensities. Calcification, seen in 20% of meningiomas, appears as coarse, irregular regions of hypointensity on both T1- and T2-weighted sequences. Routine MR imaging may not distinguish complete from near-total venous sinus obstruction, and MRA or routine angiography may be needed in these cases for proper surgical planning.

Brain edema is seen in approximately 50% of meningiomas (Atlas 1991), with the most significant edema associated with meningiomas of the synctial or angioblastic cell types. Angioblastic meningiomas are considered histologically identical to hemangioblastomas and show tumor neovascularity. A less common variety of meningioma that is clinically more aggressive is histologically similar to the extracranial hemangiopericytoma.

Sellar and Parasellar Tumors

Pituitary Adenoma. Pituitary adenomas of less that 10 mm are termed microadenomas, and those greater than 10 mm are called macroadenomas. The most common of the actively secreting adenomas is the prolactinoma. Nonfunctional pituitary adenomas present with signs and symptoms due to compression or invasion of structures adjacent to the adenoma, such as the optic chiasm and the cavernous sinus.

Most commonly, the MRI image of the pituitary adenoma shows low signal intensity on T1-weighted images and high signal on T2-weighted images when compared to normal pituitary tissue. Hyperintensity on T1-weighted images most often represents subacute collections of blood (Figure 39.14). This hemorrhage is usually subclinical but may be the indication that a significant bleed into the pituitary tumor occurred (Atlas 1991). Gadolinium-DTPA enhancement can detect adenomas that otherwise would be occult by differentially enhancing the normal gland tissue and the nonenhancing microadenoma (Figure 39.15). Enhanced MRI is the best way to detect small adenomas found in Cushing's disease. Delayed images can sometimes demonstrate a reversal of the image contrast due to accumulation of gadolinium-DTPA in the adenoma and washout from the rest of the normal gland (Atlas 1991).

A macroadenoma characteristically is seen as a hypointense mass on T1-weighted images. The visualization of the cavernous carotid arteries and the middle and anterior cerebral arteries obviates the need for preoperative angiography. Lateral extension of the tumor into the cavernous sinus is common and may be associated with extremely high prolactin levels. It is frequently impossible to determine if the cavernous sinus is invaded or compressed by the adenoma since the medial wall of the cavernous sinus is very thin. However, the placement of abnormal tissue between the lateral wall of the cavernous sinus and the cavernous carotid is a reliable indicator of cavernous sinus invasion (Atlas 1991). Marked constriction or occlusion of the cavernous carotid artery by a pituitary adenoma is rare.

Craniopharyngioma. Craniopharyngiomas commonly present in the suprasellar cistern. However, intrasellar craniopharyngiomas are occasionally found. Craniopharyn-

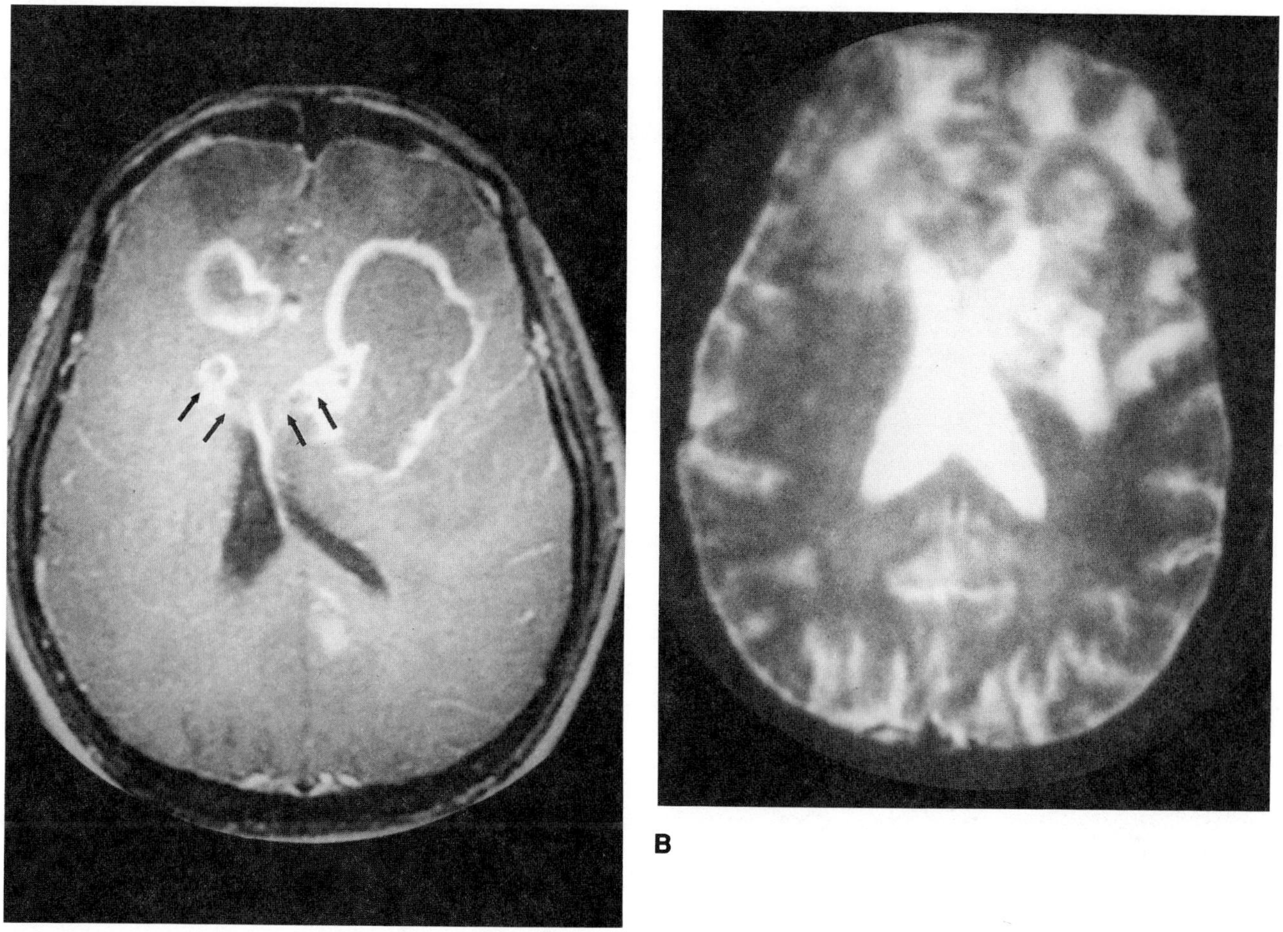

A

B

FIGURE 39.11 Lymphoma. A. Postgadolinium T1-weighted image in a patient with lymphoma shows multiple ring-enhancing lesions in the frontal lobes and one lesion in the left occipital parasagittal location. Arrows indicate subependymal enhancement B. Axial T2-weighted image demonstrates iso- to hyperintense lesions in the frontal lobes bilaterally corresponding to the ring-enhancing lesions.

giomas may have both solid and cystic components, and calcification is seen in most tumors but is less common in adults (Atlas 1991).

On MRI craniopharyngiomas are heterogeneous suprasellar masses, with components that may be hyperintense on both T1- and T2-weighted images. If contrast is given the solid portions usually enhance moderately (Figure 39.16). The extension of these masses can be quite remarkable, growing beneath the frontal and temporal lobes and extending inferiorly along the clivus.

Meningioma. Ten percent of meningiomas occur in the parasellar region. On MRI, they are frequently isointense relative to gray matter on T1-weighted images; 50% are isointense on T2-weighted images and 40% are hyperintense. Vascular encasement is a frequent finding with a meningioma in the cavernous sinus. Meningiomas enhance intensely with gadolinium-DTPA, and therefore those arising from the walls of the cavernous sinus can be difficult to separate from the enhancing venous blood in the cavernous sinus.

Chiasmatic and Hypothalmic Glioma. The distinction between gliomas that arise in either the optic chiasm or hypothalamus is arbitrary since the lesion frequently involves both areas. These gliomas are seen mostly in children (Atlas 1991), particularly in those with neurofibromatosis (Figure 39.17). Tumors of the chiasm are more aggressive than those arising from the optic nerves.

On T1-weighted images, the gliomas are usually isointense and on T2-weighted images they are moderately hyperintense. Because they can extend posteriorly along the optic radiations, T2-weighted images of the entire brain are necessary. If intraorbital extension is possible, then fat-suppressed MR images are helpful.

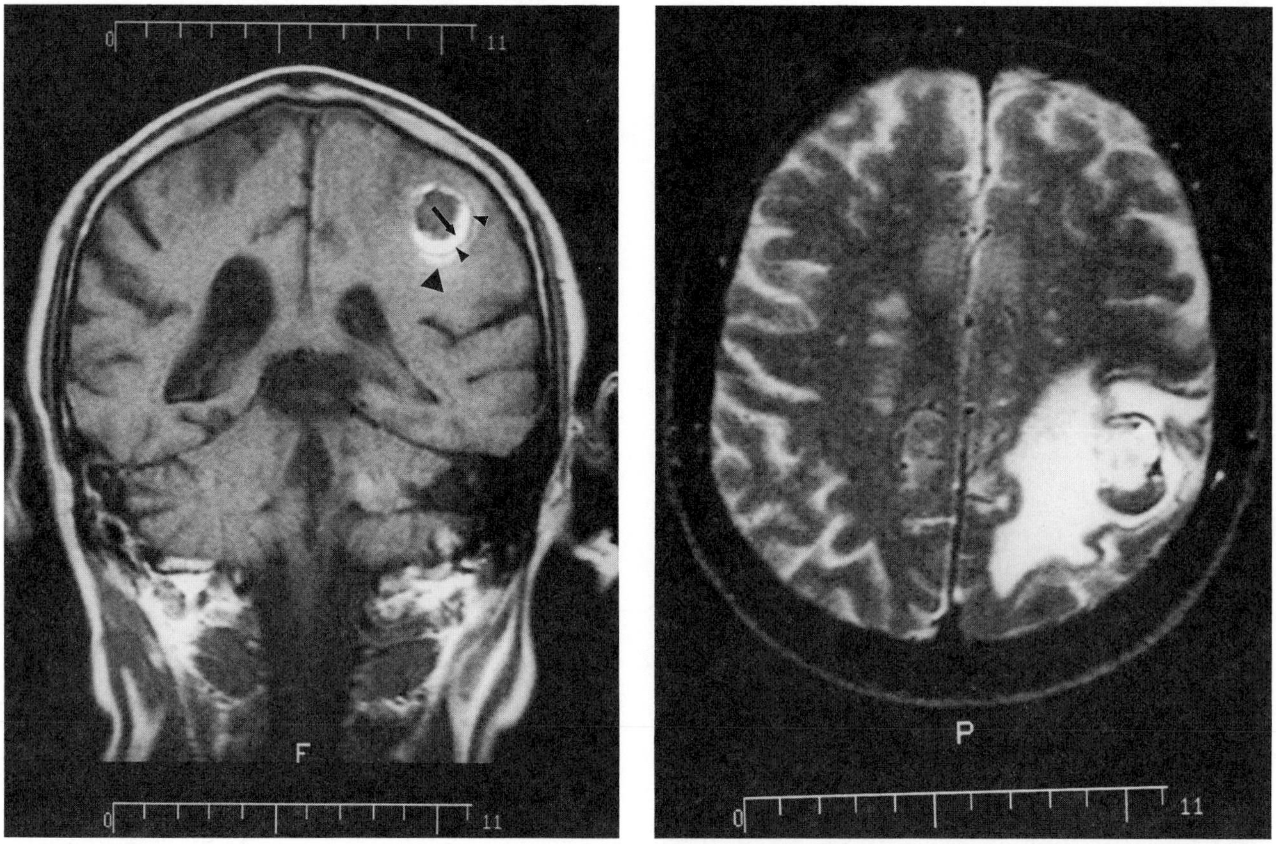

A

B

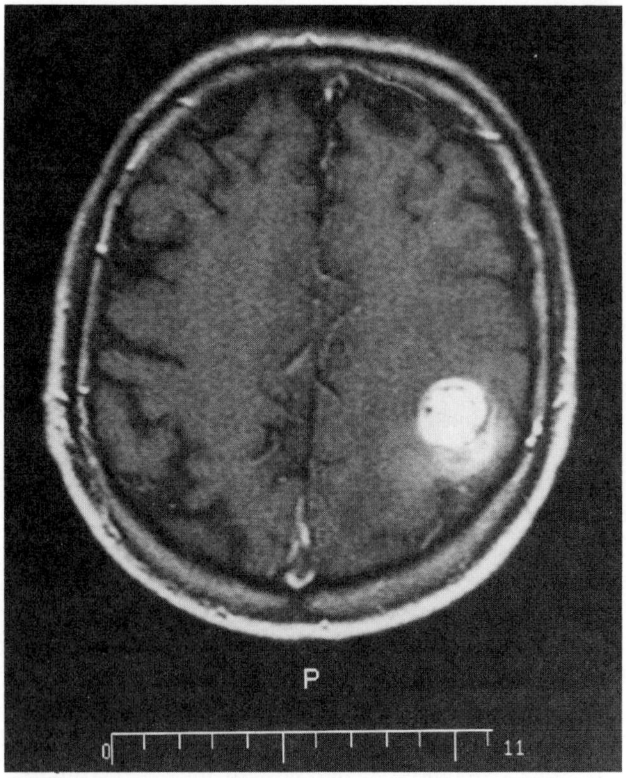

C

FIGURE 39.12 Hemorrhagic metastasis. A. Precontrast coronal T1-weighted MR shows a well-defined left parietal mass with a hypointense center and irregular thick hyperintense periphery (arrow) consistent with subacute hemorrhage, a thin hypointense rim (small arrowheads) likely secondary to hemosiderin deposits, and less well-defined hyperintense area (large arrowhead), which represents either blood or a free radical reaction, shortening T1 relaxation. Hemispheric mass effect is evident with compression of the atrium of the left lateral ventricle. B. Fingerlike projections of edema in the white matter, associated with the mixed hypo- and hyperintense signals of the metastatic lesion itself and blood, are seen on the T2-weighted axial image. C. Dense contrast enhancement is identified on the postcontrast T1 image. The finding of abundant edema in the face of relatively small parenchymal mass, the location of the mass at the cortical-medullary junction, and hemorrhage all favor metastasis, despite the presence of just one lesion.

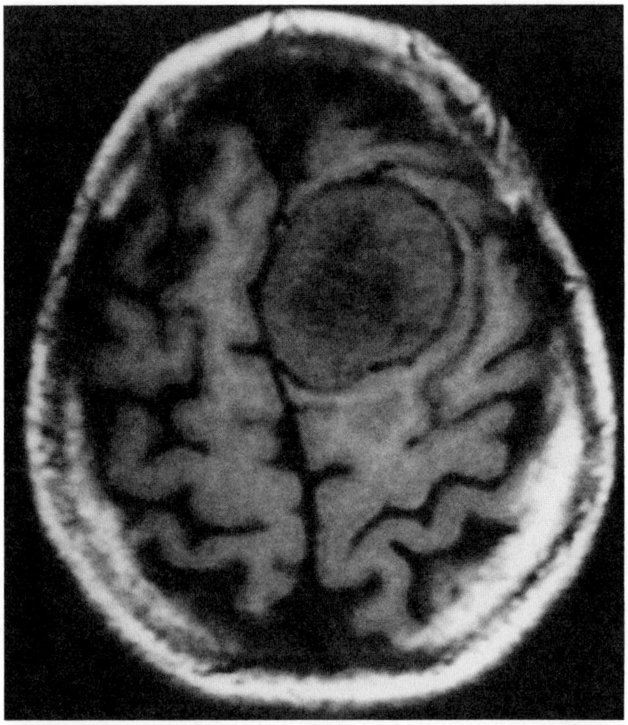

A

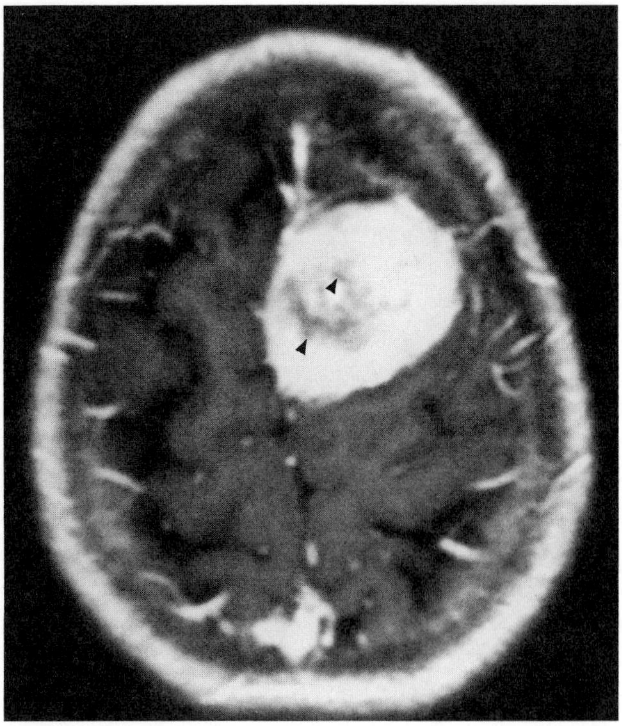

C

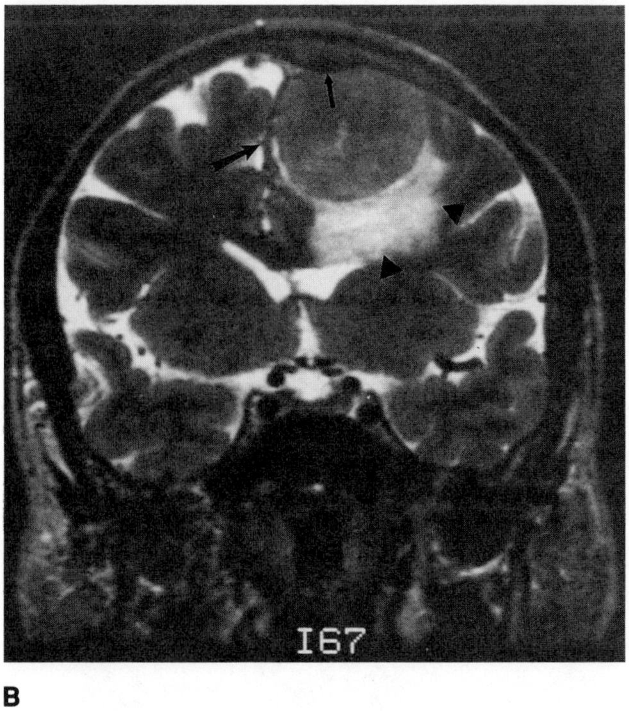

B

FIGURE 39.13 Meningioma. A. Axial T1-weighted MR shows a well-defined predominantly isointense (to gray matter) mass in the left parasagittal region. Scattered low signal within the mass was areas of calcification. B. The coronal T2-weighted image shows a dural-based isointense parasagittal mass, thickening of the adjacent inner table (small arrow), shift of the falx (large arrow) to the right, peritumoral edema (arrowheads), and ventricular compression. C. Axial postcontrast T1-weighted image shows dense enhancement of the mass. The few areas within the mass that do not enhance (small arrowheads in C) represent calcifications.

Acoustic Neurinoma

Acoustic neurinomas (or schwannomas) arise from the vestibular portion of the eighth cranial nerve and are seen frequently with type 2 neurofibromatosis (Figure 39.18).

On MRI, most tumors are visualized on thin-section T1-weighted images, where these tumors are well demarcated from CSF. On T2-weighted images the tumors are hyperintense. The pattern of signal is frequently heterogeneous due to their internal composition, which is quite varied and includes different cells, mucinous and microcystic changes, regions of focal calcification, and blood vessels. Significant

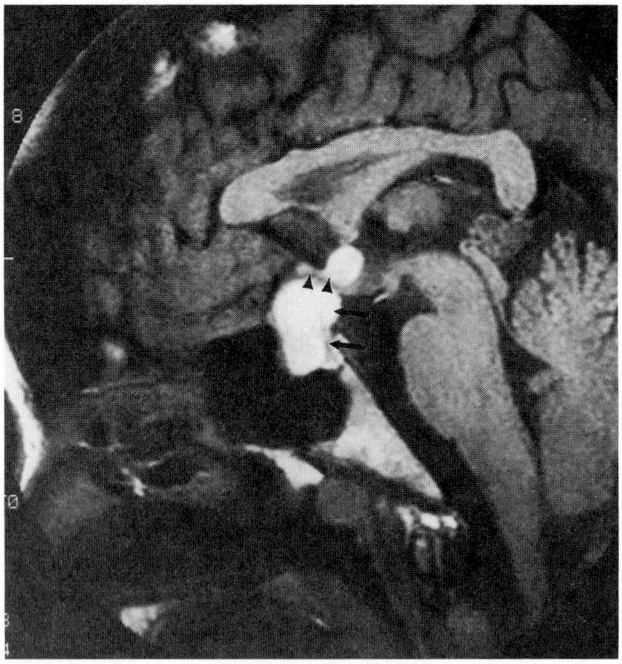

A

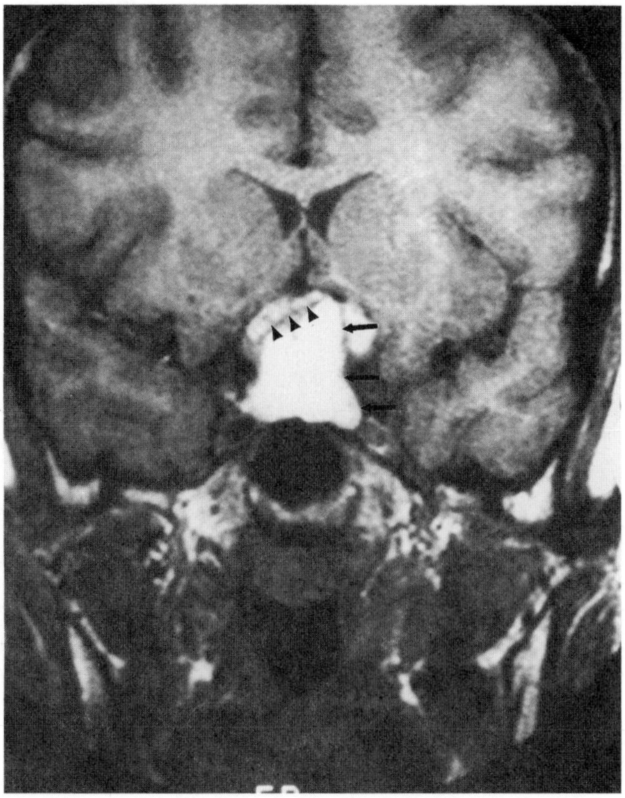

B

FIGURE 39.14 Hemorrhagic pituitary macroadenoma. Sagittal (A) and coronal (B) noncontrast T1-weighted images show a hyperintense signal (subacute blood) in a sellar and suprasellar mass (arrows). This patient presented with pituitary apoplexy and sudden visual loss, which is explained by the compression of the optic chiasm and hemorrhage into the chiasm (arrowheads in A and B). Incidentally noted is the multicystic pineal gland in A (pineal cyst).

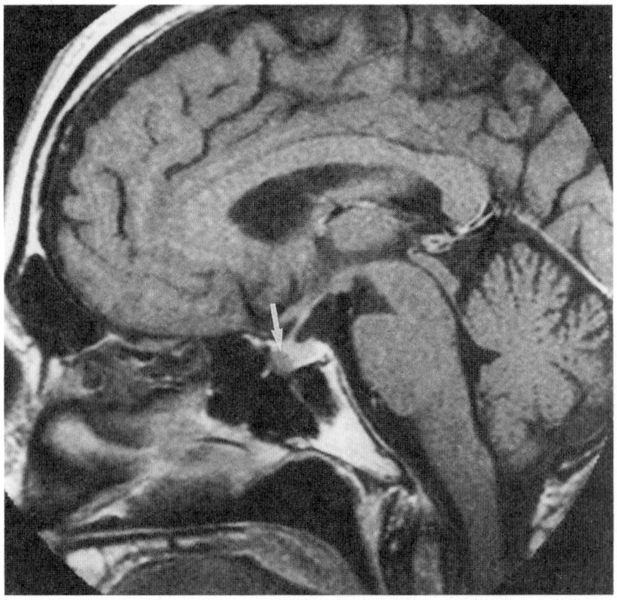

A

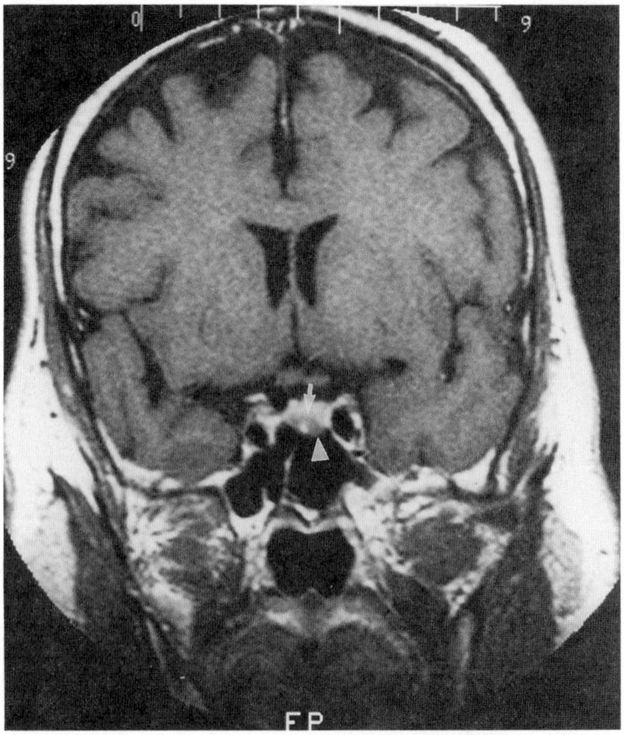

B

FIGURE 39.15 Pituitary microadenoma. Post–contrast T1-weighted images in sagittal (A) and coronal (B) planes show a nonenhancing lesion in the anterior inferior aspect of the gland (white arrow). Note the sloping of the floor of the sella (arrowhead).

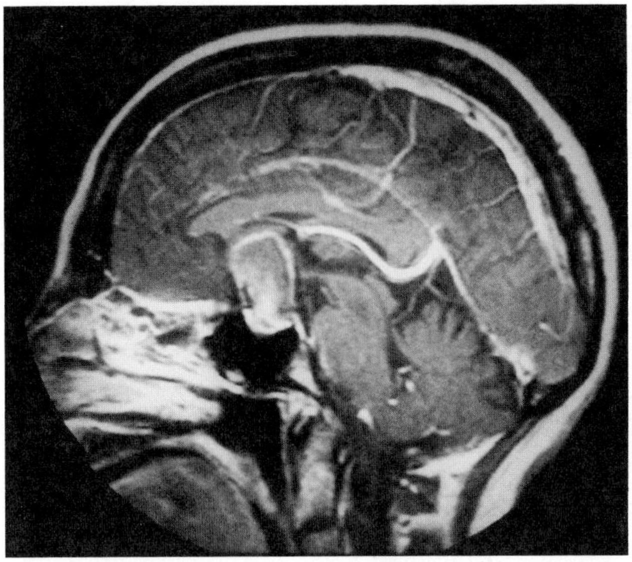

A

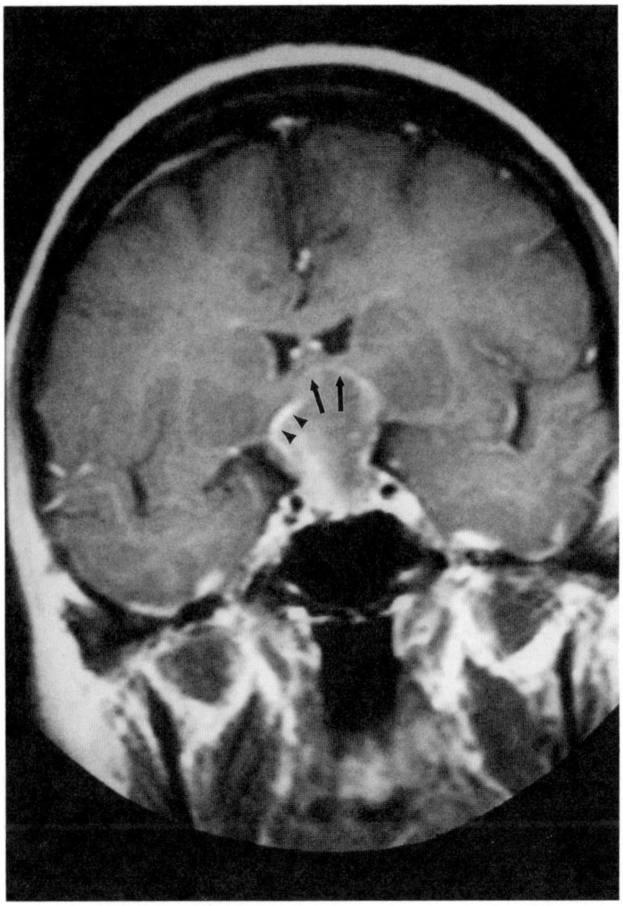

B

FIGURE 39.16 Craniopharyngioma. A large suprasellar mass with nonuniform enhancement is seen on these post–contrast T1 sagittal (A) and coronal (B) images. There is intense enhancement around the periphery of the mass, a portion of which may represent slowed flow in the A1 segment of the right anterior cerebral artery (arrowheads in B) and a portion of which represents rim enhancement (capsule) (arrows in B). The cavernous carotid arteries are clearly separated from the mass. The major differential lies between a pituitary adenoma with suprasellar extension and craniopharyngioma. Note in A and B that the sella turcica is not enlarged, a point distinctly against this being a pituitary adenoma.

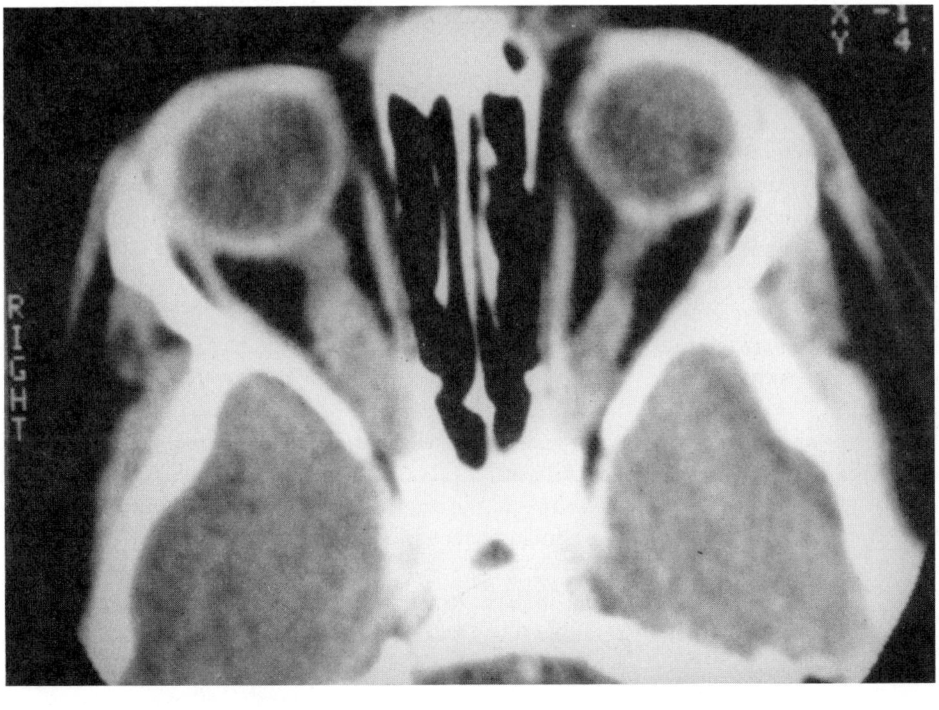

FIGURE 39.17 Neurofibromatosis. Bilaterally enlarged optic nerves in a patient with NF1. Patient also was noted to have an optic chiasm glioma.

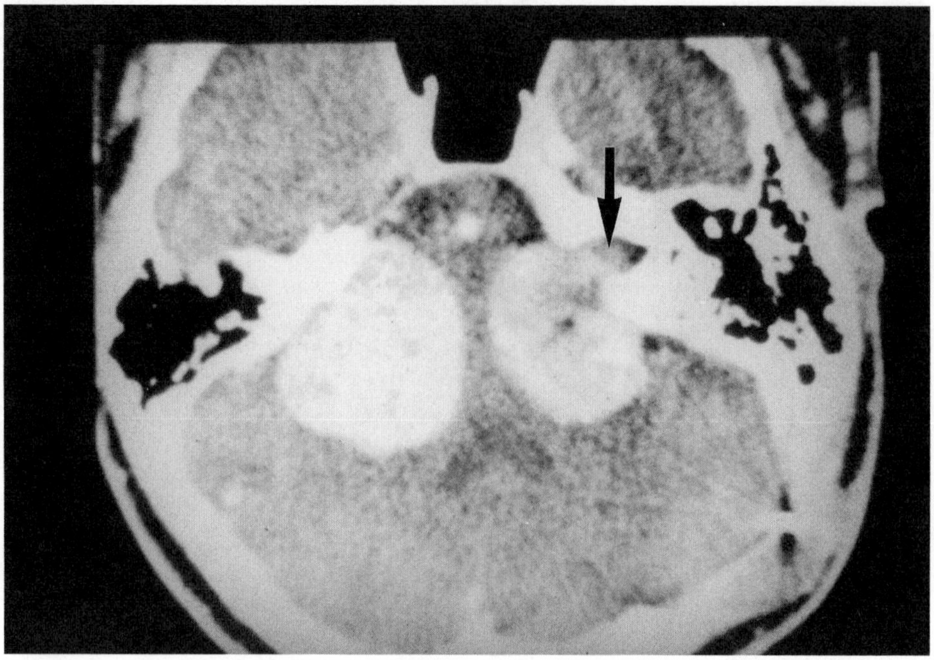

FIGURE 39.18 Acoustic neurinomas. Bilateral acoustic neurinomas in a patient with NF2. CT axial scan after contrast administration demonstrates bilateral rounded cerebellopontine angle masses. Note the extension of the left cerebellopontine angle mass into a widened internal auditory canal (arrow).

heterogeneity on MRI is more typical of acoustic neurinomas than meningiomas, which is the other lesion frequently found in the cerebellopontine angle (Figure 39.19). Acoustic neurinomas can be demonstrated on noncontrast MRI when they are 5 mm or greater. Usually there is an intracanalicular portion of the tumor associated with a cisternal mass. Approximately 20% of acoustic neurinomas have no intracanalicular component, and in those cases the differential diagnosis from meningiomas is difficult. Small intracanalicular tumors can be demonstrated with contrast enhancement.

Epidermoid Cysts

Epidermoid cysts are congenital lesions of ectodermal origin and usually do not present until the third or fourth decade of life. They are frequently located in the cerebellopontine angle, suprasellar and parasellar regions, and middle cranial fossa.

On CT they are hypodense, do not enhance with contrast, and may be difficult to differentiate from arachnoid cysts. Their external surface, however, is lobulated, unlike the smooth surface of arachnoid cysts. On T1-weighted images epidermoid tumors are hypointense, but internal structure can be seen, and on T2-weighted images the tumors are markedly hyperintense (Figure 39.20).

Neurodegenerative Disorders

Atrophy

With normal aging, there is mild to moderate progressive enlargement of the ventricles, sulci, and cisternal spaces. In neurodegenerative disorders, atrophy is excessive and premature.

Periventricular white matter hyperintense lesions range from normal capping of the frontal horns to confluent abnormal high-signal regions extending into the deep white matter. The amount of periventricular hyperintensity increases with age and is increased in patients with vascular disease. Subcortical lesions, ischemic in nature, are located outside the periventricular region in the cerebral white matter, deep gray matter (basal ganglia), or pons. The extent of these lesions also increases with age and in patients with pathology such as multi-infarct dementia (MID).

Hypointensity compared to gray matter on T2-weighted images is normally seen in the globus pallidus, red nucleus, substantia nigra, and dentate nuclei due to iron deposition. With aging, there is a progressive decrease in signal in the putamen and caudate. Many neurodegenerative disorders are associated with excessive signal loss in the extrapyramidal nuclei and thalami.

Dementia

Alzheimer's Disease. In Alzheimer's disease (AD), generalized atrophy is seen on MRI as well as symmetric or asymmetric enlargement of the temporal horns, sylvian fissures, and suprasellar cistern. The degree of atrophy is in general greater than in normal aging. Medial temporal lobe atrophy and the number and size of white-matter hyperintense foci are generally greater than in normal aging.

Multi-Infarct Dementia. MID may result from cortical or multiple subcortical infarcts, or both, and is associated with hypertension. Extensive periventricular hyperintensity, corti-

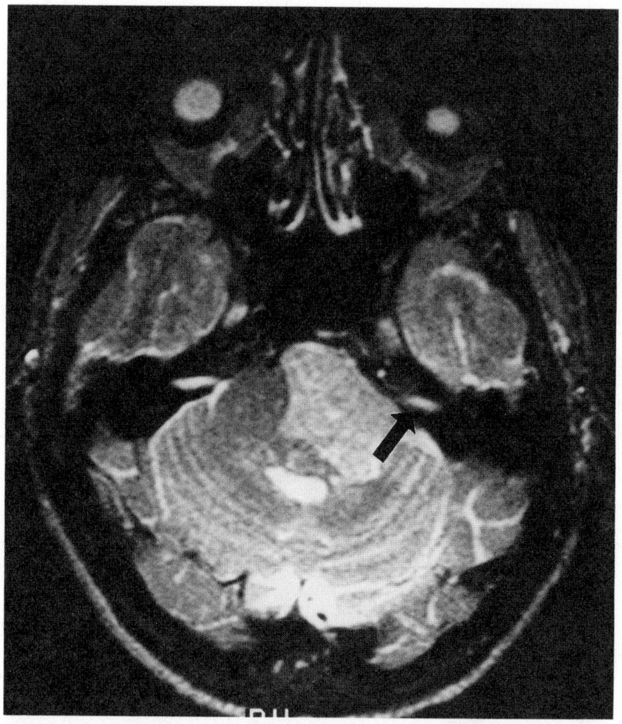

A

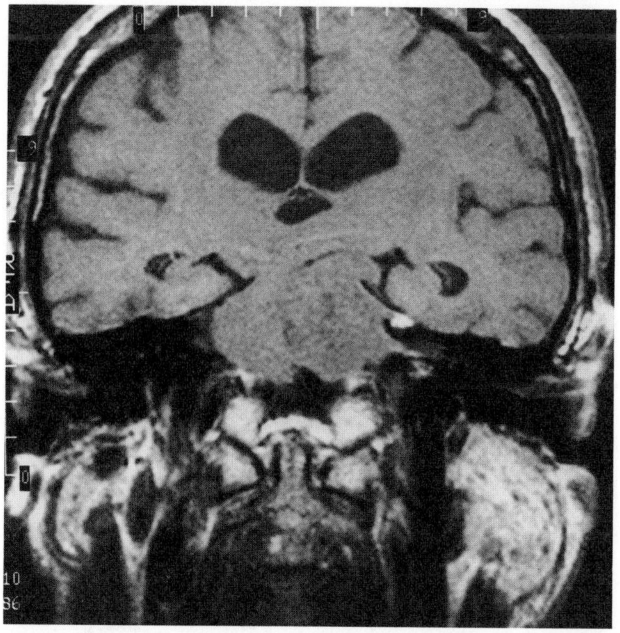

B

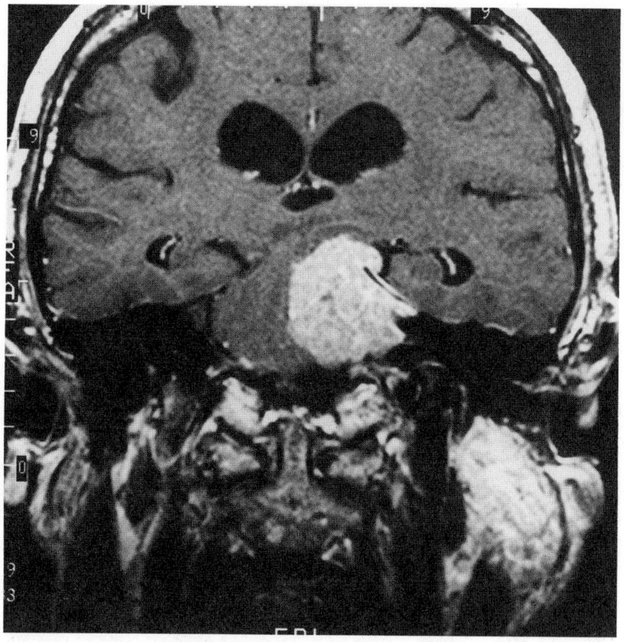

C

FIGURE 39.19 Meningioma. A. T2-weighted axial image demonstrates a broad-based hyperintense mass located in the left cerebellopontine angle. The internal auditory canal (arrow) is not involved by the lesion. Coronal T1-weighted images before (B) and after (C) gadolinium administration demonstrate the lesion, which is displacing the brain stem to the right. Note the lack of extension into the left internal auditory canal.

cal infarcts, and basal ganglia lacunar infarcts in a patient with dementia favor a clinical diagnosis of MID or mixed MID and AD. If one suspects AD instead of MID, an MR scan demonstrating prominent white-matter signal changes, particularly subcortical lesions, favors MID over AD (Figure 39.21). Lacunar infarcts may be found in all forms of MID.

Pick's Disease

Grossly, Pick's disease is characterized by lobar atrophy that may be asymmetric, with the frontal and temporal lobes most commonly affected. This atrophy is well demonstrated on CT and MR images.

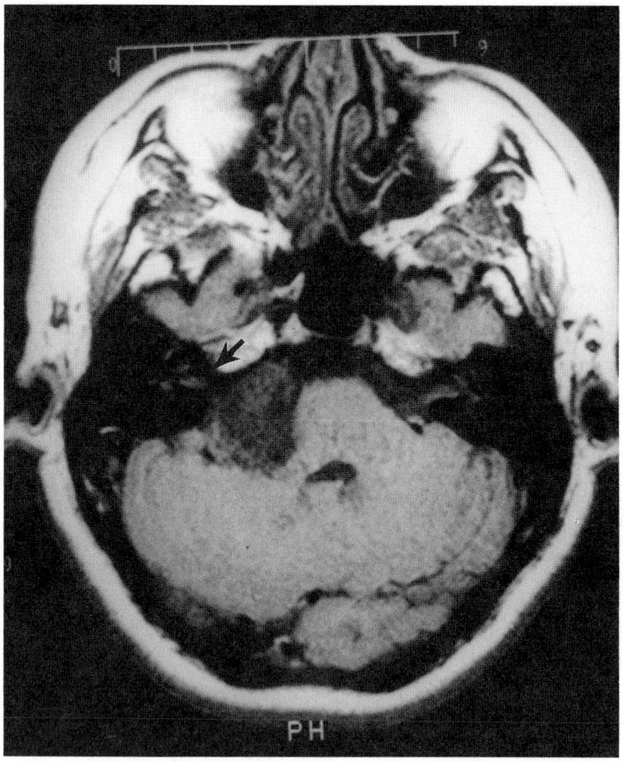

A

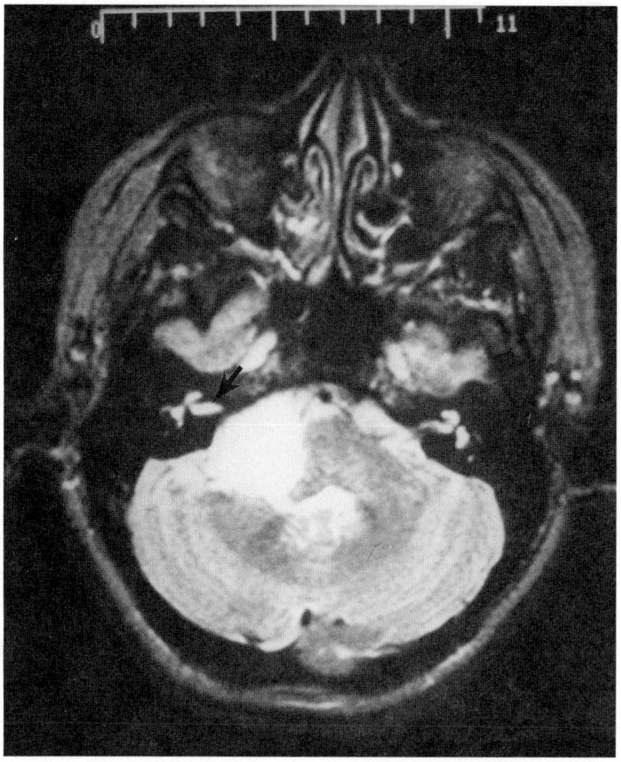

B

FIGURE 39.20 Epidermoid cyst. There is a lesion located in the right cerebellopontine angle, which is hypointense (slightly higher than CSF) on T1-weighted image (A) and hyperintense on T2-weighted image (B). The right internal auditory canal is normal (arrows).

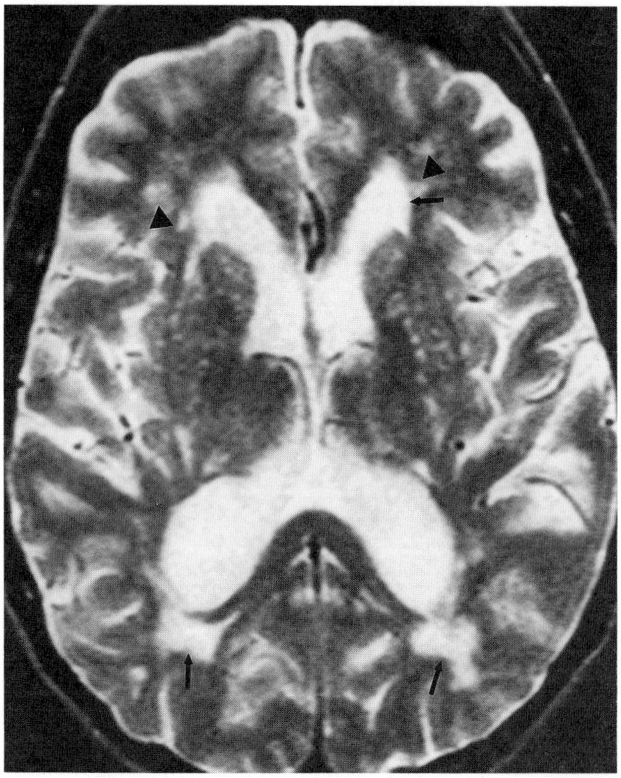

A

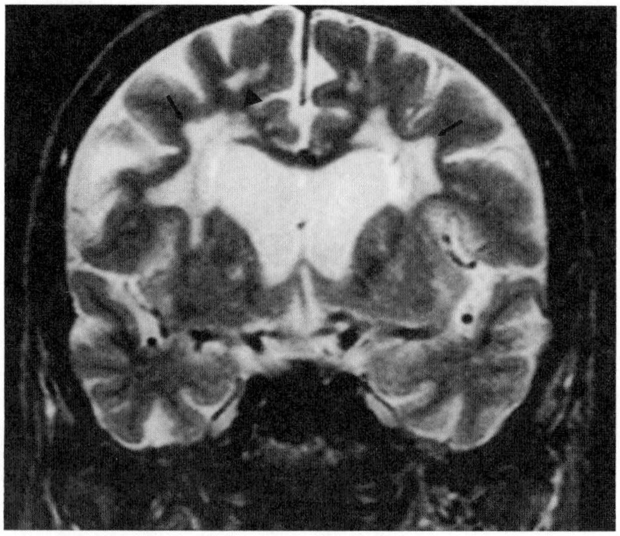

B

FIGURE 39.21 Multi-infarct dementia. T2-weighted axial (A) and coronal (B) images demonstrate periventricular hyperintensity (arrows) as well as multiple subcortical lesions (arrowheads). Prominent perivascular spaces are seen in the basal ganglionic region.

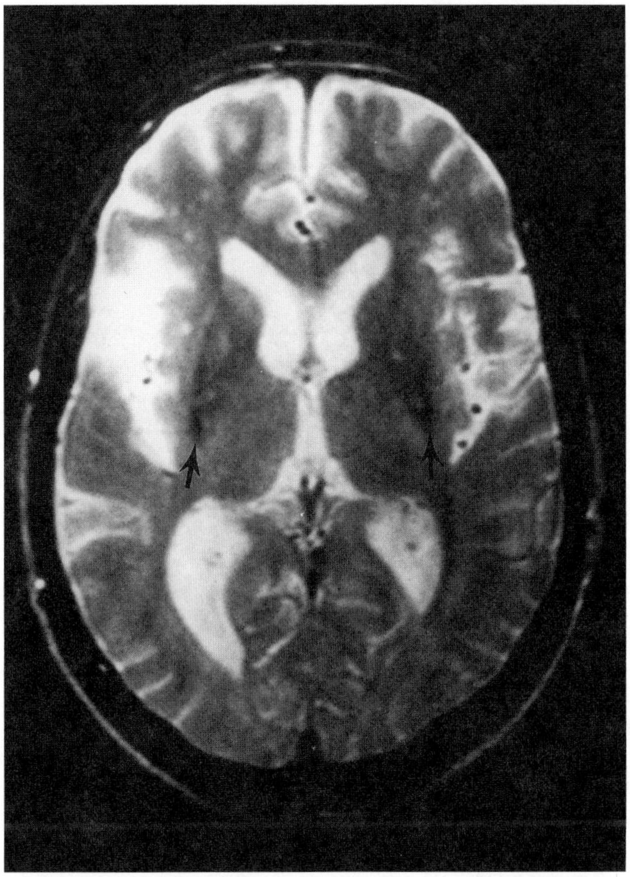

FIGURE 39.22 Shy-Drager syndrome. This T2-weighted axial image shows hypointensity in the region of the putamen (arrows). Right temporal lobe atrophy (widened sylvian fissure) and ventriculomegaly are present.

Creutzfeldt-Jacob Disease. CT scanning is used to exclude focal lesions as a cause for the patient's symptoms, but CT scanning uncommonly shows any focal parenchymal abnormalities. Most frequently CT scans are normal, but in approximately 20% of cases atrophy is present. Approximately half of the cases demonstrate atrophy only on MR scanning, whereas in the remaining cases, abnormal high signal intensity is noted on T2-weighted images in the caudate nuclei, striatum, thalamus, cortex, basal ganglia, and periventricular white matter. Cortical gray matter involvement without diffuse cerebral atrophy may represent an early phase of the disease.

Movement Disorders (see Chapter 76)

Parkinsonism. Parkisonism includes several conditions, such as Parkinson's disease (PD), the Shy-Drager syndrome, olivopontocerebellar atrophy (OPCA), progressive supranuclear palsy, striatonigral degeneration, and corticobasal ganglionic degeneration.

Parkinson's Disease. The imaging findings in Parkinson's disease are frequently indistinguishable from normal aging. There may be decreased width of the pars compacta, decreased signal in the putamen, or both. The latter finding is more likely to be observed in patients with Parkinson's-plus syndromes. Patients with Shy-Drager syndrome associated with striatonigral degeneration (SND) have MRI findings of striatonigral degeneration (Figure 39.22) (Atlas 1991), while those with pure autonomic failure have normal MRIs. Neuroimaging and pathological examination in SND show atrophy of the striatum with signal changes in the putamen. Specifically, at 1.5 T the signal of the putamen is as hypointense as the globus pallidus, and the width of the pars compacta is diminished. The MR in OPCA shows atrophy and abnormal signal in the pons and cerebellum (Figure 39.23). There is atrophy of the pons, middle cerebellar peduncles, cerebellum, and inferior olives. On long TR images, slight hyperintensity is seen involving the pontocerebellar pathways and olives.

Mitochondrial Encephalopathies

Four syndromes of mitochondrial dysfunction are described: myoclonus epilepsy with ragged-red fibers (MERRF); mitochondrial encephalopathy, lactic acidosis and strokelike episodes (MELAS); Kearns-Sayre syndrome; and subacute necrotizing encephalomyelopathy, Leigh's disease, which is a severe and often fatal mitochondrial disease. In Leigh's disease, necrosis and capillary proliferation occur in the basal ganglia, spinal cord, and brain stem. CT scans usually show low-density areas in the putamen and caudate nuclei that do not enhance following the administration of contrast. T2-weighted MRIs show striking symmetric hyperintense foci in the globus pallidus, putamen, and caudate. The imaging changes most commonly seen in the brain in MELAS are those of cerebral infarcts. Both large and multifocal infarcts occur, and the occipital lobes are the most common sites of involvement. Imaging findings in MERRF syndrome may be similar to MELAS syndrome or may show atrophic changes in the cerebral cortex, brain stem, and cerebellum.

White-Matter Disease

Demyelinating Diseases

Demyelinating diseases cause normal myelin to be destroyed; multiple sclerosis (MS) is the most common of the demyelinating diseases.

Multiple Sclerosis (see Chapter 61). On MRI, MS plaques appear as rounded areas of increased signal on T2-weighted images (Figure 39.24). Gadolinium enhancement and possibly mass effect may be seen during the acute

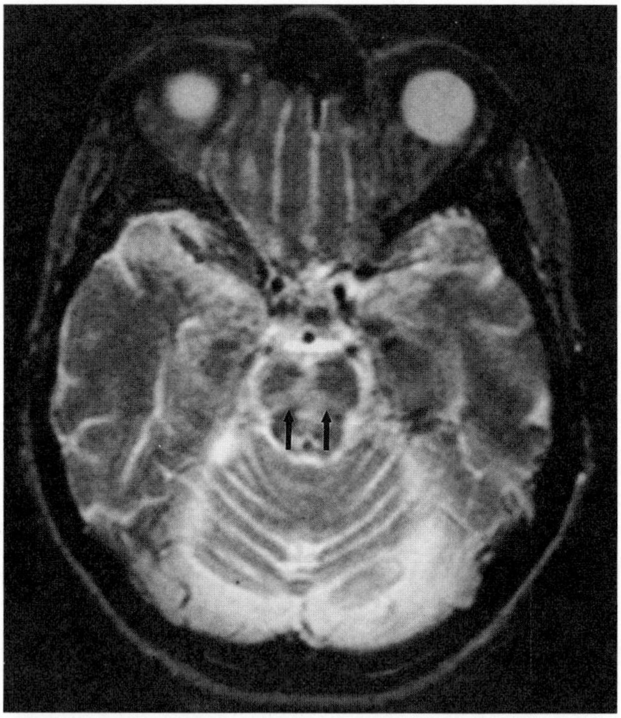

A

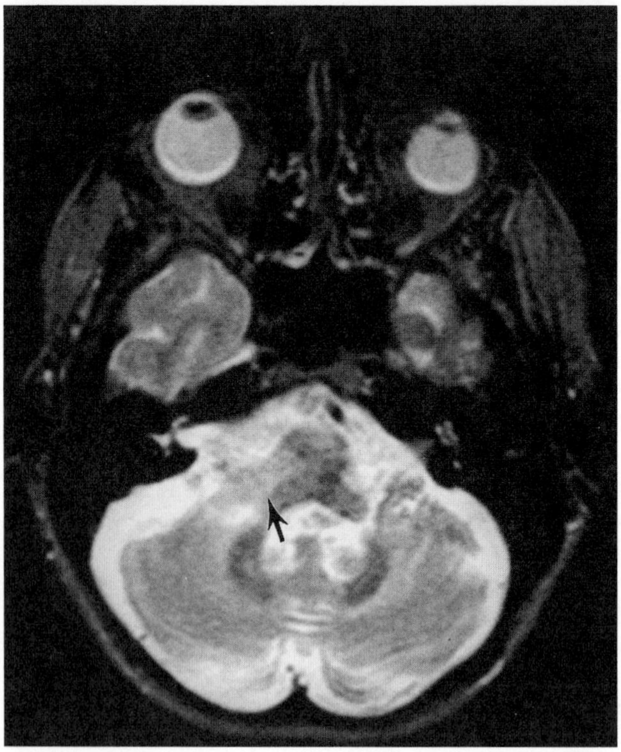

B

FIGURE 39.23 Olivopontocerebellar atrophy. A. Axial T2-weighted image through the pons shows abnormal hyperintense signal of transverse pontine fibers (between the tegmentum and the base of the pons) (arrows). Cerebellar atrophy is present. B. A more inferior section shows abnormal hyperintense signal of the right middle cerebellar peduncle (arrow). Also note atrophy of the brain stem with enlargement of the cisterns and the fourth ventricle.

phase. In time, the area of inflammation decreases in size and leaves a plaque of high intensity on T2-weighted images. Plaques are common in the periventricular regions, internal capsule, corpus callosum, pons, and brachium pontis. Plaques located in the periventricular region may not be well seen on long TR, long TE images, where CSF within the ventricles is bright and may obscure the plaques. Proton-density images (long TR, short TE) will better define the MS lesions.

Acute Disseminated Encephalomyelitis (see Chapter 61). In acute disseminated encephalomyelitis (ADEM) the MR shows bright lesions on T2-weighted images, most being located in the subcortical white matter with relative symmetric involvement of both hemispheres (Atlas 1991). Enhancement can be seen with ADEM, and lesions usually regress in response to corticosteroid treatment.

Central Pontine Myelinolysis. On MRI, in T2-weighted images, high-intensity lesions may be seen throughout the brain, but these are most prominent in the pons. The pontine lesion is typically central with sparing of the periphery of the pons.

Leukodystrophies (see Chapter 81)

The MRI picture is that of progressive white-matter lesions and diffuse cerebral atrophy. There are some distinguishing features between the leukodystrophies early in the course of the disease.

Krabbe's Disease. On CT, there is increased density in the thalami, caudate, and corona radiata. On MRI, lesions involve the basal ganglia and white matter in a symmetrical fashion.

Metachromatic Leukodystrophy. CT and MRI reveal diffuse white-matter lesions (Figure 39.25).

Adrenoleukodystrophy. On CT and MRI there are symmetric areas of white-matter abnormality that surround the atria of the lateral ventricles and span the splenium of the corpus callosum. At the lateral margin of the zones of demyelination, contrast enhancement may occur. Demyelination along certain tracts, such as the lateral lemniscus, is occasionally identified.

Miscellaneous Lesions of White Matter

Radiation and Chemotherapy. Arteritis and secondary ischemic lesions of brain may result from chemotherapy and radiation treatment. Deciding whether a patient's symptoms are due to an exacerbation of the neoplasm or to the effects of treatment (i.e., radiation necrosis) can be difficult. Most recurrent or residual tumors appear as focal areas of enhancement with surrounding edema. The

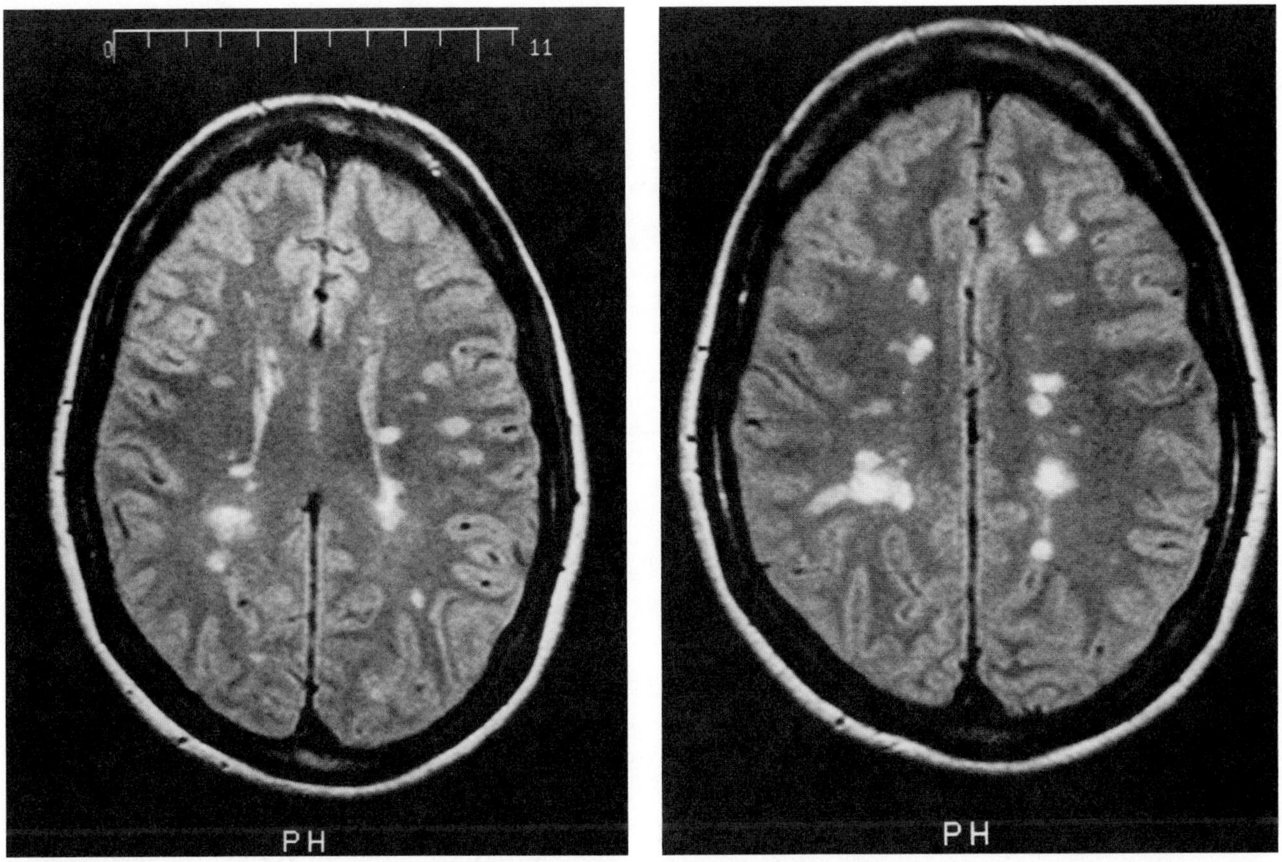

A B

FIGURE 39.24 Multiple sclerosis. Proton-weighted axial images demonstrate hypertense lesions in the periventricular region (A) and in the centrum semiovale (B) in a patient with multiple sclerosis.

white-matter lesions caused by radiation endarteritis may be transient or permanent.

Areas of radiation necrosis can be focal or disseminated within the white matter. Radiation necrosis is seen on T2-weighted images as an area of high-intensity signal with variable gadolinium enhancement on T1-weighted images. Mass effect and edema are common early in radiation necrosis, though later, atrophy predominates.

Head Trauma

CT is the study to be obtained in the initial evaluation of the acutely unstable patient who has a head injury to determine if there is a surgical lesion, such as a subdural or epidural hematoma. However, many lesions are identified by MR imaging, such as cortical contusions, small subdural hematomas, and diffuse axonal injury that may not be seen on CT examination. In addition, MRA can play an important role in evaluating the trauma patient, identifying vascular abnormalities such as arterial occlusion and dissection, arteriovenous fistula, and venous sinus occlusion.

Diffuse Axonal Injury

Diffuse axonal injury (DAI) occurs when the brain has been subjected to an angular acceleration force, causing one hemisphere to move in relation to the other, thus tearing the connecting white-matter fibers (axons). DAI or shear injury is a common posttraumatic lesion and is well seen on MR images. Lesions are commonly less than 1 cm in diameter and are seen in the lobar white matter, the corpus callosum, the dorsolateral aspect of the rostral brain stem, and at the corticomedullary junction (Figure 39.26). Patients with such injuries present with loss of consciousness and significant neurological impairment.

The majority of shear injuries are nonhemorrhagic and MRI, especially the T2-weighted sequence, is more sensitive than CT in detecting them.

Cortical Contusion

Cortical contusions, another common type of traumatic lesion, involve the superficial cortex, tend to be multi-

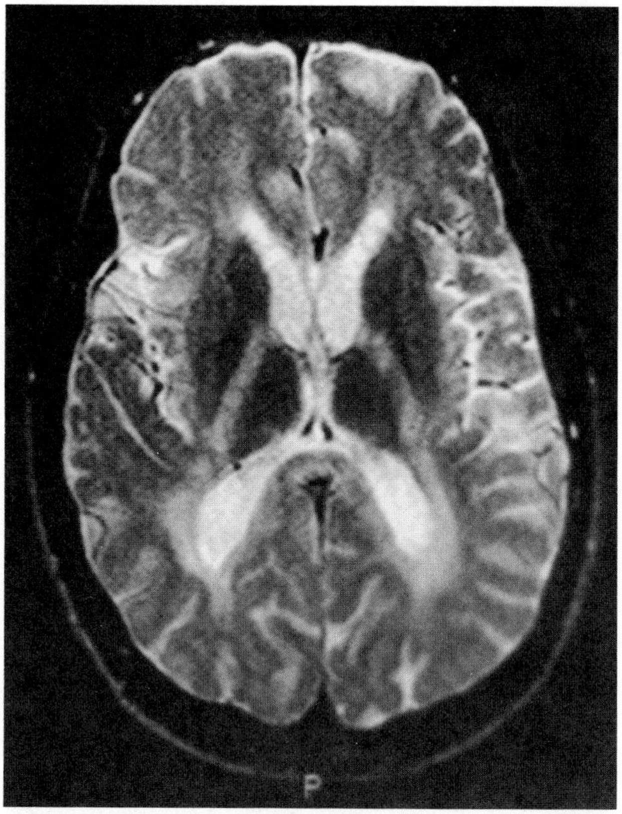

FIGURE 39.25 Metachromatic leukodystrophy. A 26-year-old patient with progressive neurological deterioration. Diffuse high-intensity signal is noted in the periventricular white matter and internal capsules bilaterally in this T2-weighted axial scan. The absolute symmetry of the abnormal high signals is a clue that a white-matter disease other than multiple sclerosis or vascular disease is responsible.

ple, are usually larger (2–4 cm) than diffuse axonal injuries, are less likely to be associated with severe impairment of consciousness, and most commonly occur in the temporal and frontal lobes. A higher percentage of cortical contusions are hemorrhagic than are those of DAI. MRI and CT are sensitive in detecting hemorrhagic cortical contusions, but MRI, particularly the T2-weighted sequence, is more sensitive in detecting nonhemorrhagic contusions (Figure 39.27).

Subdural Hematoma

Subdural hematomas (SDHs) evolve in a pattern similar to parenchymal hematomas in the acute and subacute phase but differ from parenchymal hematomas in the chronic phase, as explained later. The time categories used in this discussion are: *Acute* means less than 1 week old; *early subacute* indicates more than 1 week and less than 2 weeks; *late subacute* means more than 2 weeks and less than 1 month; and *chronic* indicates a duration of more than 1 month. The acute SDHs are characterized by hypointensity on T2-weighted images, reflecting the presence of deoxyhemoglobin. A late SDH shows high signal on all pulse sequences due to the presence of extracellular methemoglobin (Figure 39.28). SDHs in a chronic phase are hypointense on short TR and TE images. This loss of T1 shortening results from a decrease in the concentration of methemoglobin due to dilution, absorption, and/or degradation. Enhancement of the periphery of the SDH is expected in the chronic phase because of the presence of a vascular capsule.

Epidural Hematoma

Epidural (or extradural) hematomas may arise from arterial or venous bleeding. When arterial, they usually are due to a laceration of a meningeal artery and are associated with skull fractures (Figure 39.29). On MRI the dura can often be seen displaced away from the inner table of the skull, as a thin low-signal line between the brain and the hematoma.

Subarachnoid Hemorrhage

On CT, subarachnoid hemorrhage is seen as high density in the basal cisterns, sylvian fissures, interhemispheric fissure, sulci, or some combination of these. The majority of the increased density rarely lasts more than a few days because the blood becomes diluted in the subarachnoid space and is resorbed over the cerebral convexities. MRI is less successful in depicting acute subarachnoid hemorrhage, so CT is still the preferred study in suspected subarachnoid hemorrhage.

This relative insensitivity of MRI to blood in the subarachnoid space is related to the high pO_2 in the CSF. Conversion of oxyhemoglobin to deoxyhemoglobin and subsequently to methemoglobin requires a narrow range of oxygen tension. In the CSF, significant quantities of methemoglobin are not formed until several days after the hemorrhage, and if the subarachnoid hemorrhage is mild the red blood cells may be resorbed before significant amounts of methemoglobin are formed. For these reasons, CT is advocated for the early diagnosis of acute subarachnoid hemorrhage. However, for subacute and chronic subarachnoid hemorrhage, MRI may be superior to CT.

Intracerebral Hematoma

Traumatic intracerebral hematomas may range from a few millimeters to several centimeters in size. The differentiation of hematomas from hemorrhagic contusions and shear injuries is difficult but important. Unlike intracerebral hematomas, the hemorrhage in the latter two types of injuries is interspersed between areas of edematous brain. Although most of these lesions develop immediately after trauma, some may develop during the first 48 hours after injury. This may be either because the swelling of the brain decreases, thus allowing more cap-

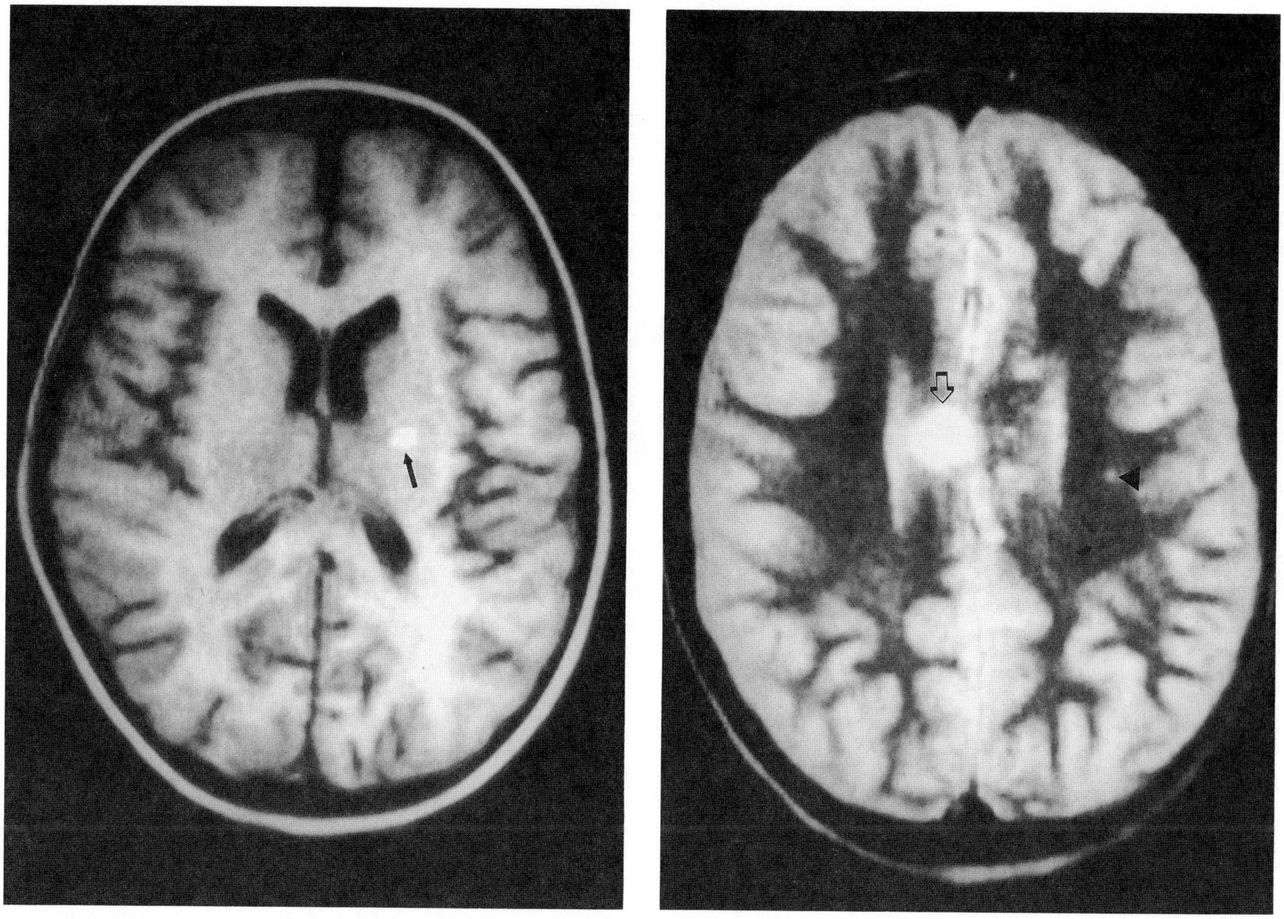

A B

FIGURE 39.26 Diffuse axonal injury. A. Axial short TR-TE MR scan of a patient with hemorrhagic and nonhemorrhagic diffuse axonal injury. A hemorrhage is seen in the posterior limb of the left internal capsule (arrow). B. Axial long TR-TE image at a higher level demonstrates a lesion in the corpus callosum (open arrow) as well as a smaller lesion in the left centrum semiovale (arrowhead). (Reprinted with permission from EML Sklar, RM Quencer, BC Bowen et al. Magnetic resonance application in cerebral injury. Radiol Clin North Am 1992;30:353–366.)

illary bleeding, or because the change in oxygen tension alters the brain perfusion, thus increasing the chances of delayed hemorrhage.

Vascular Injuries: Role of Magnetic Resonance Angiography

Vascular injuries can be either arterial or venous. The most common abnormality of the major arteries after trauma is arterial occlusion (Sklar et al. 1992), which is attributed to severe spasm and emboli from mural thrombi in areas of intimal disruption. Arterial dissections frequently occur near the junction of the cervical and petrous segments of the internal carotid artery where it enters the carotid canal. The etiology is frequently idiopathic, but trauma can be the cause.

Routine spin-echo MRI is useful in imaging carotid-cavernous fistulas. The MRA findings are characteristic even though the exact site and dynamic character of the fistula are not as well shown as on conventional angiography (Figure 39.30). A sign of a carotid-cavernous fistula on routine MR is significant enlargement of a draining vein, such as the superior ophthalmic vein.

Cerebral Infections

MR is the imaging procedure of choice for CNS infection and inflammation. With intravenous contrast administration, areas of enhancement on MR scans indicate sites of blood-brain barrier disruption and meningeal inflammation.

Viral Infections

Herpes Simplex Encephalitis. On MRI, hyperintensity involving the cortex and white matter in the temporal and inferior frontal lobes is noted in T2-weighted images. The areas of involvement then enlarge and coalesce. MR often demonstrates bitemporal involvement, and hemor-

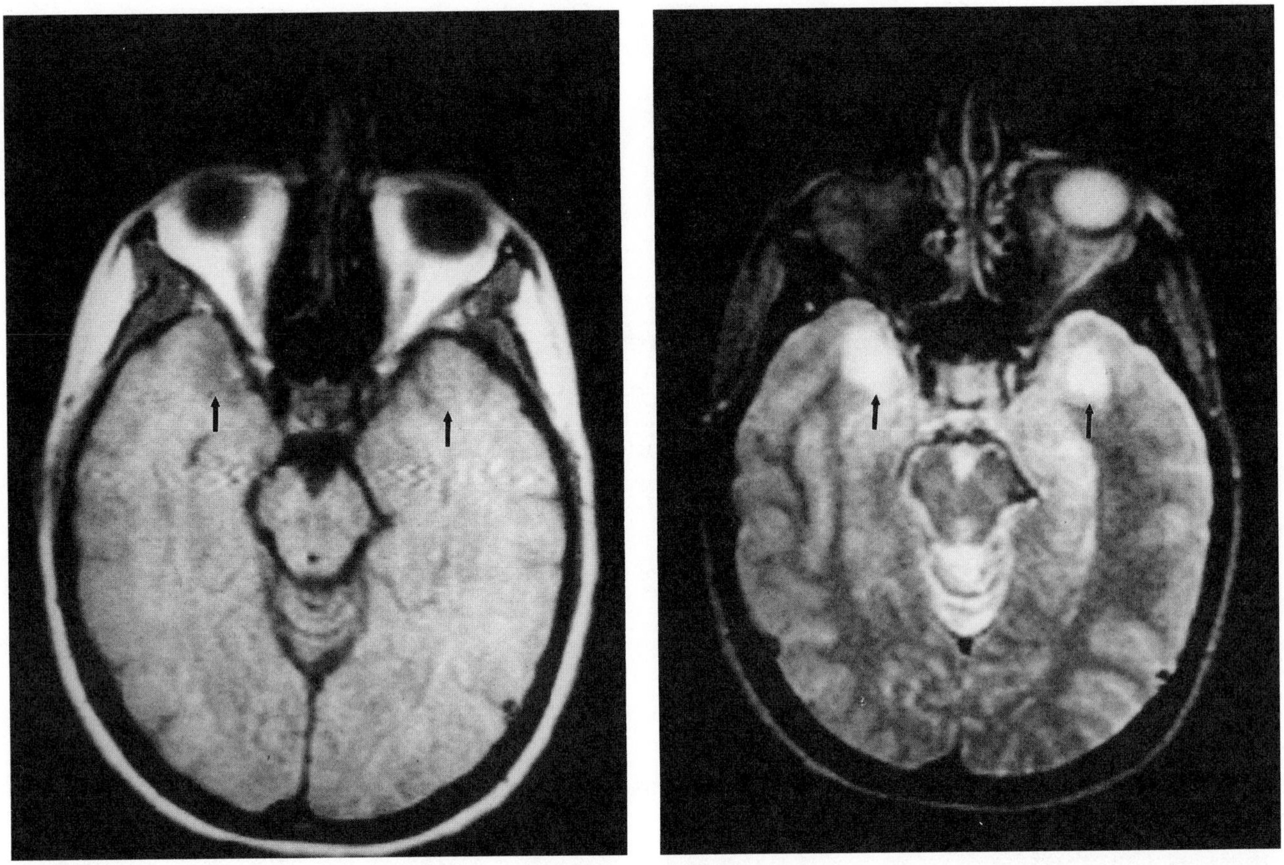

A B

FIGURE 39.27 Contusion. Nonhemorrhagic cortical contusions in the temporal lobes (arrows). Areas are much more clearly seen on T2-weighted (B) than on T1-weighted (A) images. (Reprinted with permission from EML Sklar, RM Quencer, BC Bowen et al. Magnetic resonance application in cerebral injury. Radiol Clin North Am 1992;30:353–366.)

rhage may be detected (Figure 39.31). Atrophy is seen late in the course of the disease.

Bacterial Infection (see Chapter 60A)

Cerebritis-Abscess. Cerebritis is a poorly demarcated localized area of parenchymal softening with necrosis, edema, vascular congestion, and perivascular inflammation. A focus of cerebritis may progress to abscess formation, in which a central zone of necrosis liquefies and becomes better defined and eventually encircled by a vascularized fibrotic capsule surrounded by a zone of gliosis. Most abscesses form because of hematogenous spread of organisms at the gray matter–white matter junction, most commonly in the frontal and parietal lobes.

On MRI, an abscess on T1-weighted images has a central cavity, which is hypointense to brain parenchyma; on T2-weighted images it is hyperintense. The rim, which is iso- to hypointense on T1-weighted images and is hypointense on T2-weighted images is not identical to the ring of enhancement seen with gadolinium. The ring of enhancement is usually smooth and relatively thin walled when compared to the peripheral enhancement seen with malignant tumors; however, occasionally, the wall may be thick and simulate a necrotic neoplasm (Figure 39.32). Edema in the white matter around an abscess is usually greater in volume than the abscess itself. Abscesses tend to "point" toward the ventricle and may rupture into the ventricle.

Meningitis. Unenhanced MRI scans usually show no abnormality. Gadolinium-enhanced MRI scans may show prominent leptomeningeal enhancement with a gyral pattern in severe cases. Complications of meningitis include cerebral infarction, cerebritis-abscess, subdural empyema, hydrocephalus, and ventriculitis. These complications are best detected by MRI.

Mycobacterium Tuberculosis. Infection by *Mycobacterium tuberculosis* (TB) or certain fungi causes a granulomatous inflammatory reaction, which may involve the meninges or brain parenchyma. Characteristically, a thick gelatinous exudate is found in the basal cisterns. The capsule of the granuloma is often thicker than that of a pyogenic abscess. TB may produce a vasculitis that can result in an infarction. Basal cisternal and diffuse meningeal enhancement is a predominant feature of tuberculous meningitis (Figure 39.33).

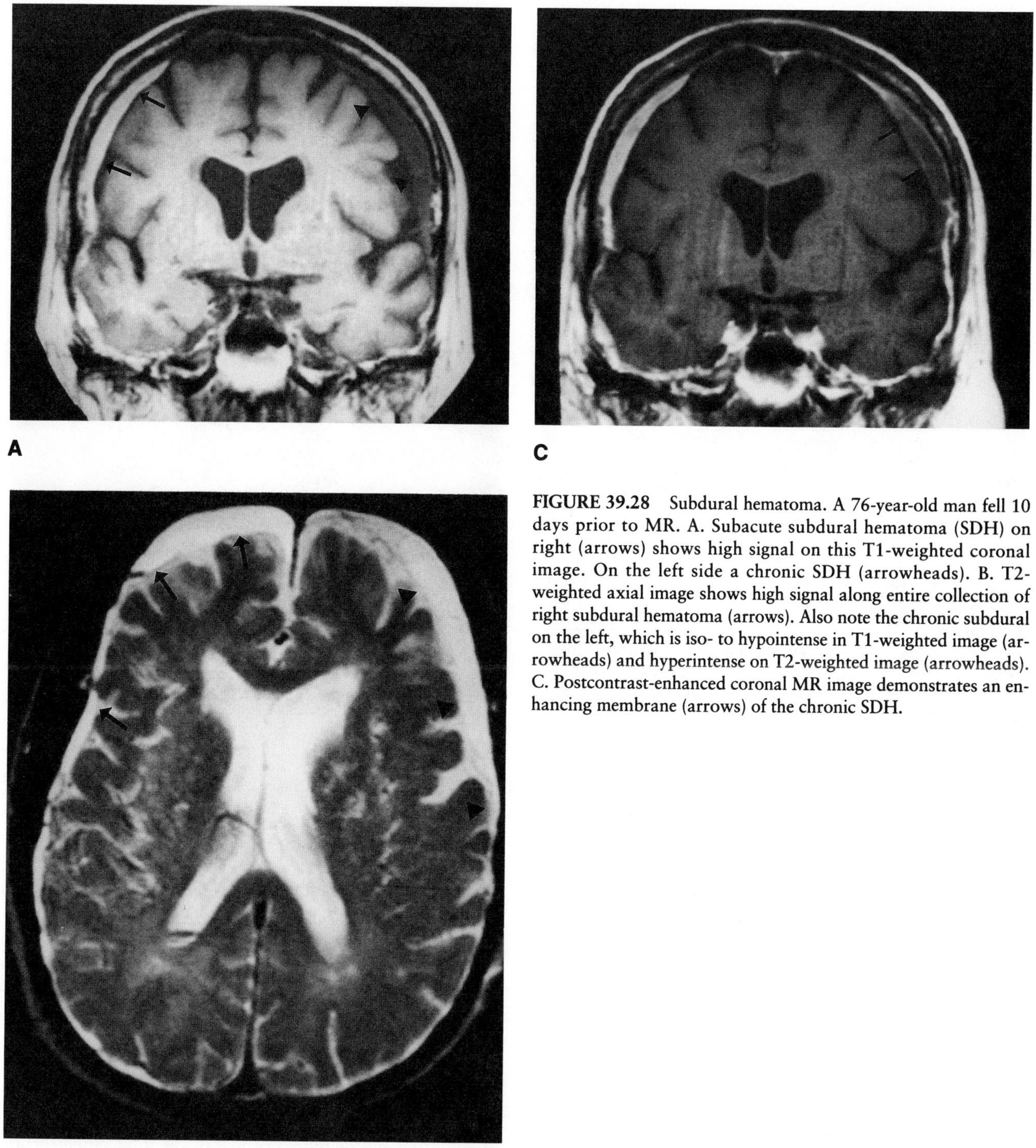

FIGURE 39.28 Subdural hematoma. A 76-year-old man fell 10 days prior to MR. A. Subacute subdural hematoma (SDH) on right (arrows) shows high signal on this T1-weighted coronal image. On the left side a chronic SDH (arrowheads). B. T2-weighted axial image shows high signal along entire collection of right subdural hematoma (arrows). Also note the chronic subdural on the left, which is iso- to hypointense in T1-weighted image (arrowheads) and hyperintense on T2-weighted image (arrowheads). C. Postcontrast-enhanced coronal MR image demonstrates an enhancing membrane (arrows) of the chronic SDH.

Tuberculomas can be located anywhere in the cerebrum or cerebellum, as well as in subarachnoid, subdural, and epidural spaces. Intraparenchymal granulomas are found at the corticomedullary junction and in the periventricular regions. In general, there is less edema in the brain surrounding a tuberculoma than that surrounding a pyogenic abscess. With intravenous contrast administration, tuberculomas enhance intensely in a nodular or ringlike fashion.

Cysticercosis

Cysticercosis is the most common parasitic infection of the human CNS worldwide. The causative agent is the pork tapeworm, *Taenia solium*. There are four types of neurocysticercosis: parenchymal, subarachnoid, intraventricular, and mixed. Following initial infection, the cysticercus develops into a cyst within which is the scolex (Figure 39.34).

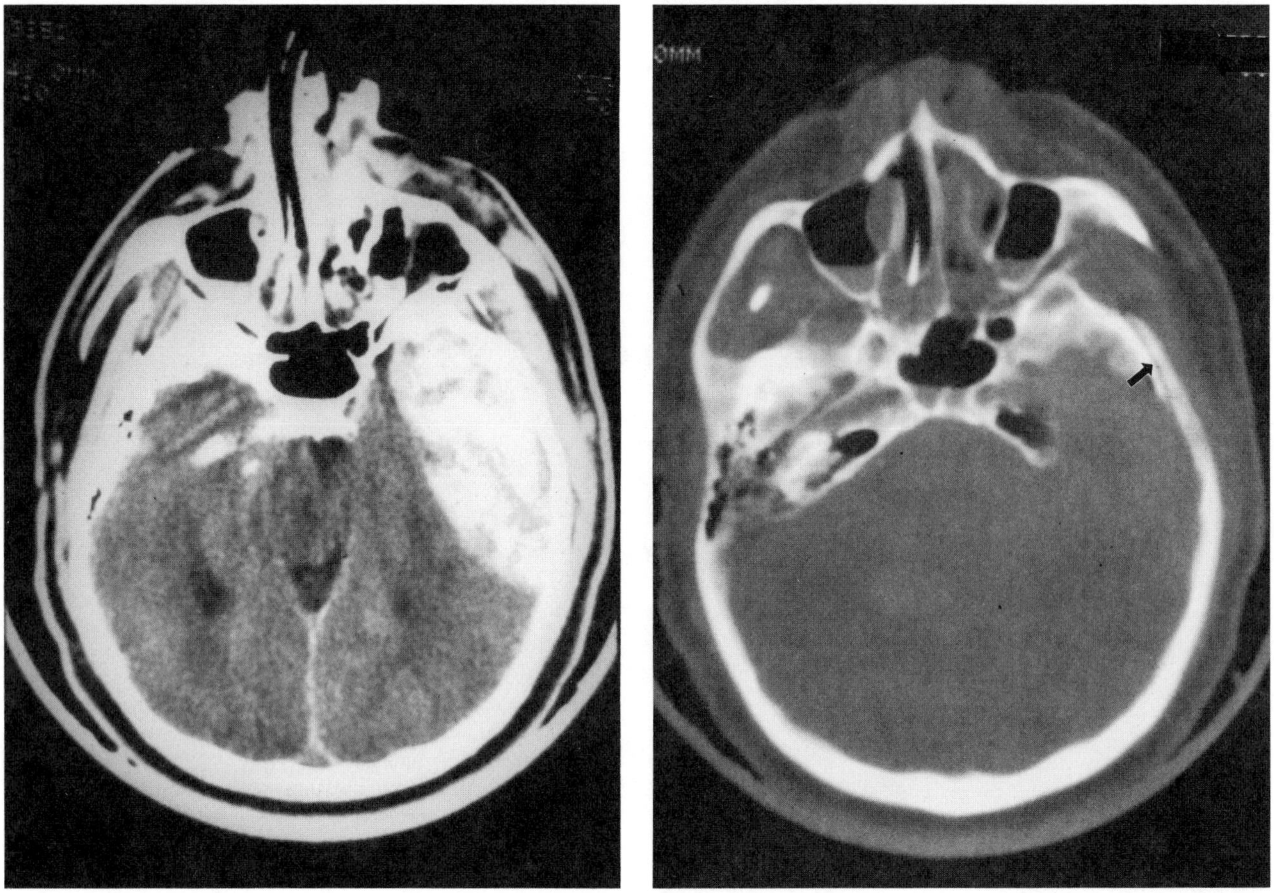

A B

FIGURE 39.29 Epidural hematoma. A. CT axial section shows a biconvex peripheral high-density lesion consistent with an epidural hematoma. B. A fracture (arrow) is seen on the bone windows of the same section.

As the organism dies, metabolic products leak from the wall of the cyst and incite an inflammatory reaction. Edema may then develop and the cyst becomes turbid. The cyst then collapses and calcifies (see Figure 39.34). If the cyst becomes multiloculated, it resembles a cluster of grapes, known as the "racemose form," which typically occurs in the basilar cisterns.

Intraventricular and subarachnoid cysts can be difficult to visualize on CT and are better seen on MR. The fourth ventricle is the most common site of intraventricular cysticercosis (see Figure 39.34B).

Autoimmune Deficiency Syndrome (see Chapter 60D)

Neuroimaging plays a crucial role in the investigation of AIDS patients with CNS disease. CT and MR are the most commonly used modalities in evaluating AIDS patients with CNS pathology; however, in recent years nuclear medicine has become very important in defining mass lesions. Specifically, thallium-201 brain single-photon emission computed tomography (SPECT) can be used to differentiate inflammatory from neoplastic lesions, thus helping to distinguish toxoplasma encephalitis from CNS lymphoma, the two primary pathologic lesions in this population (Ruiz et al. 1994).

MR is more sensitive than CT in detecting diffuse white-matter disease, which commonly is seen in AIDS. T2-weighted images are required in the evaluation of neurologically symptomatic AIDS patients.

Toxoplasma Encephalitis

Toxoplasma encephalitis is caused by the intracellular protozoan *Toxoplasma gondii*, the most common infectious agent in the brain in AIDS. In noncontrast CT, toxoplasma encephalitis is seen as multiple areas of iso- or hypodensity with a predilection for the corticomedullary junction and basal ganglia. The lesions may vary in size from less than 1 cm to over 3 cm, and hemorrhage, although unusual, has been reported in both the treated and the untreated patient. There is surrounding edema and mass effect and postcontrast CT demonstrates ring, solid, or nodular enhancement (Figure 39.35), although ring enhancement is most common. Double-dose delayed CT is more effective in detecting these lesions.

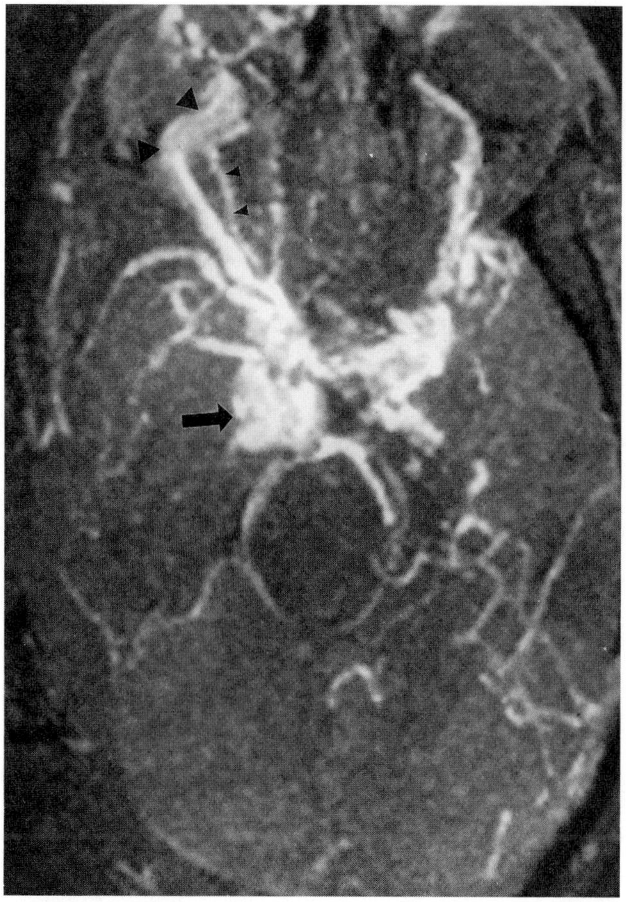

A

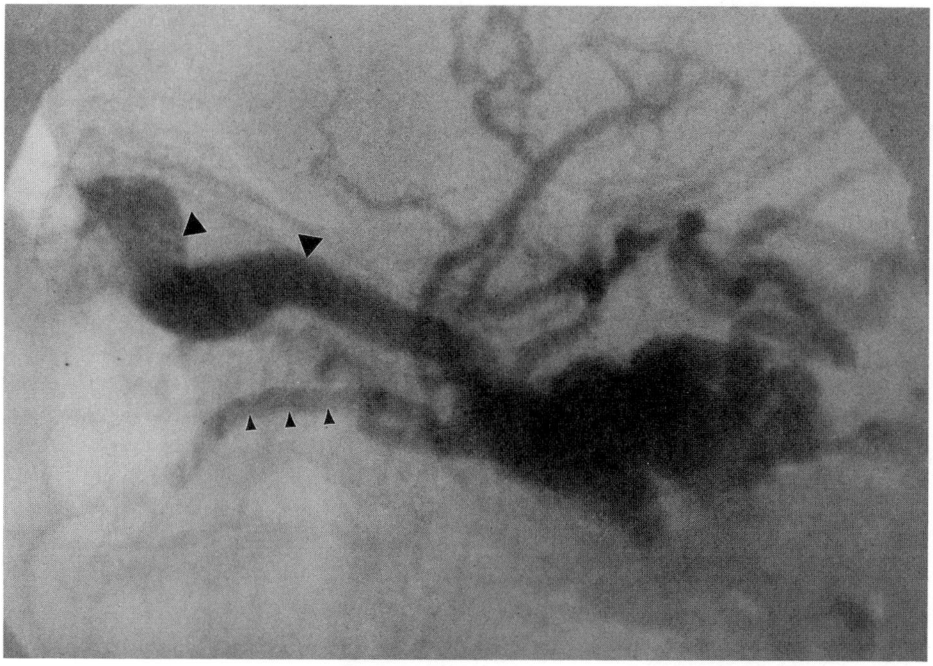

B

FIGURE 39.30 Bilateral carotid-cavernous fistulas. A 34-year-old woman with extensive facial injuries and proptosis of the right eye following a motor vehicle accident reported double vision and hearing a pulsating noise in the right side of her head. A. Three-dimensional time of flight MRA acquired as a transaxially oriented slab and displayed as a semiaxial maximum-intensity projection oriented 20 degrees to the horizontal plane. There is abnormal time of flight enhancement and enlargement of the right cavernous sinus, superior ophthalmic vein (large arrowheads), and inferior ophthalmic vein (small arrowheads). A large "venous pouch" projects posteriorly from the right cavernous sinus (long thick arrow). Abnormal time of flight enhancement is also present in the left cavernous sinus and superior ophthalmic vein. B. Conventional right internal carotid angiogram, midarterial phase, lateral projection. The superior (large arrowheads) and inferior (small arrowheads) ophthalmic veins are identified, as is the venous pouch. (Reprinted with permission from EML Sklar, RM Quencer, BC Bowen et al. Magnetic resonance application in cerebral injury. Radiol Clin North Am 1992;30:353–366.)

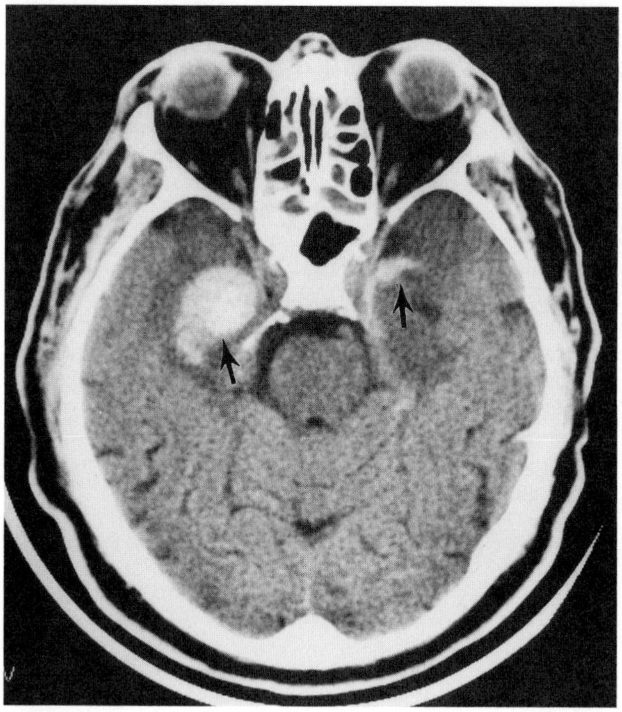

FIGURE 39.31 Herpes encephalitis. Noncontrast axial CT shows bilateral hemorrhagic lesions (arrows). These medial and inferiorly located temporal lobe lesions of blood, edema, and inflammatory tissue are characteristics of herpes encephalitis.

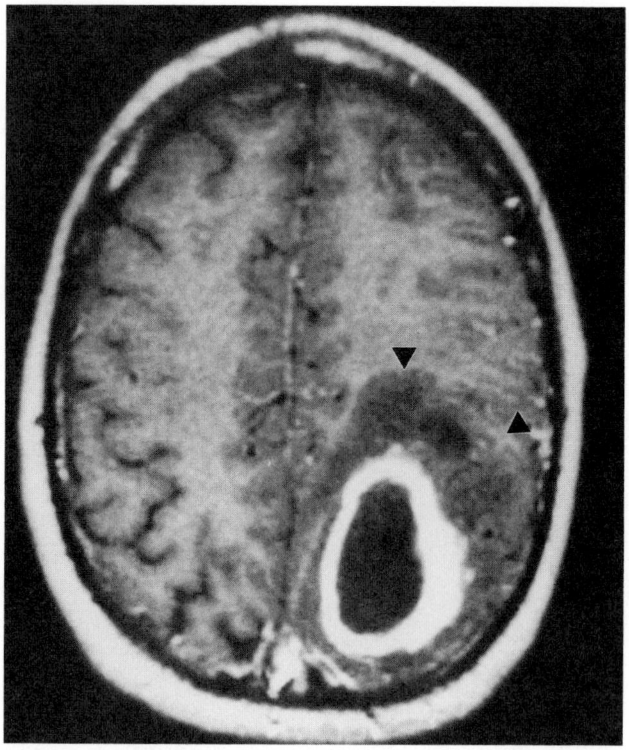

FIGURE 39.32 Intracerebral abscess. Contrast-enhanced axial T1-weighted MRI shows a ring of enhancement surrounded by edema (arrowheads) and considerable hemispheric mass effect producing obliteration of sulci and crowding of the gyri. Because of the thick rim of enhancement and necrotic center, one would commonly consider a malignancy the primary diagnosis, but this was a surgically proved *Streptococcus viridans* abscess.

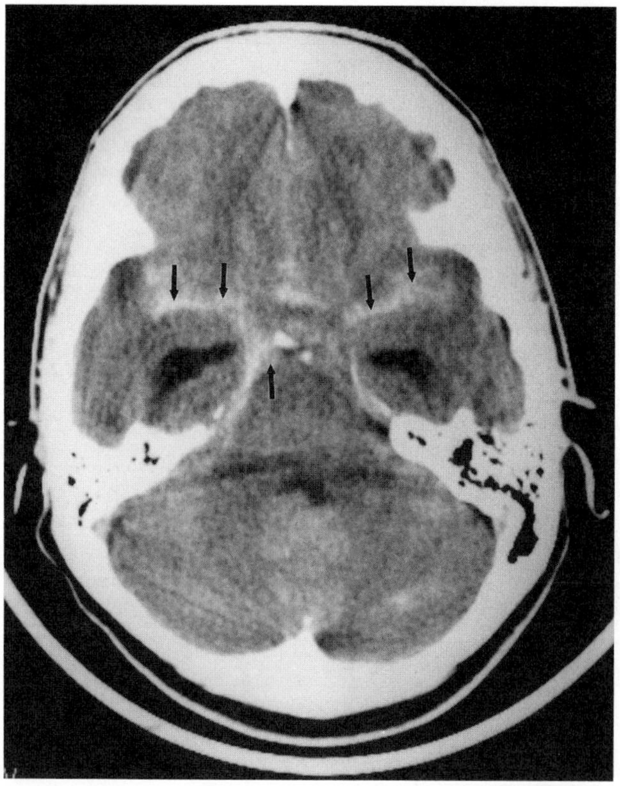

FIGURE 39.33 Tuberculous meningitis. Postcontrast CT scan reveals diffuse cisternal enhancement (arrows) compatible with diffuse meningitis.

After the patient is on treatment, scans should show a decrease in the number and size of the lesions and a reduction in edema and mass effect within 2–4 weeks after initiating treatment. Treated lesions have a variable appearance on CT. The areas of prior involvement may appear normal, may show encephalomalacia, may calcify, or, rarely, may show areas of petechial hemorrhage. Reduction or resolution of the lesions on serial scans is presumptive evidence that toxoplasma was the causative agent for the lesions. Toxoplasma encephalitis will recur if treatment is discontinued and therefore lifelong therapy is required. If the lesions do not improve with specific antitoxoplasma therapy, alternative diagnoses must be considered.

MRI without and with gadolinium is more sensitive to lesions of toxoplasma encephalitis than postcontrast CT. On T1-weighted images, the lesions are iso- to hypointense to brain parenchyma. On T2-weighted images, active lesions are of variable intensity. The lesions may be hyperintense to brain parenchyma or may be isointense to hypointense to brain centrally and surrounded by high-signal edema referred to as the "target sign." The enhancement pattern is similar to that on CT. Only 14% of patients with toxoplasmosis demonstrate a solitary lesion; therefore, lack of multiplicity should raise the possibility of a different diagnosis.

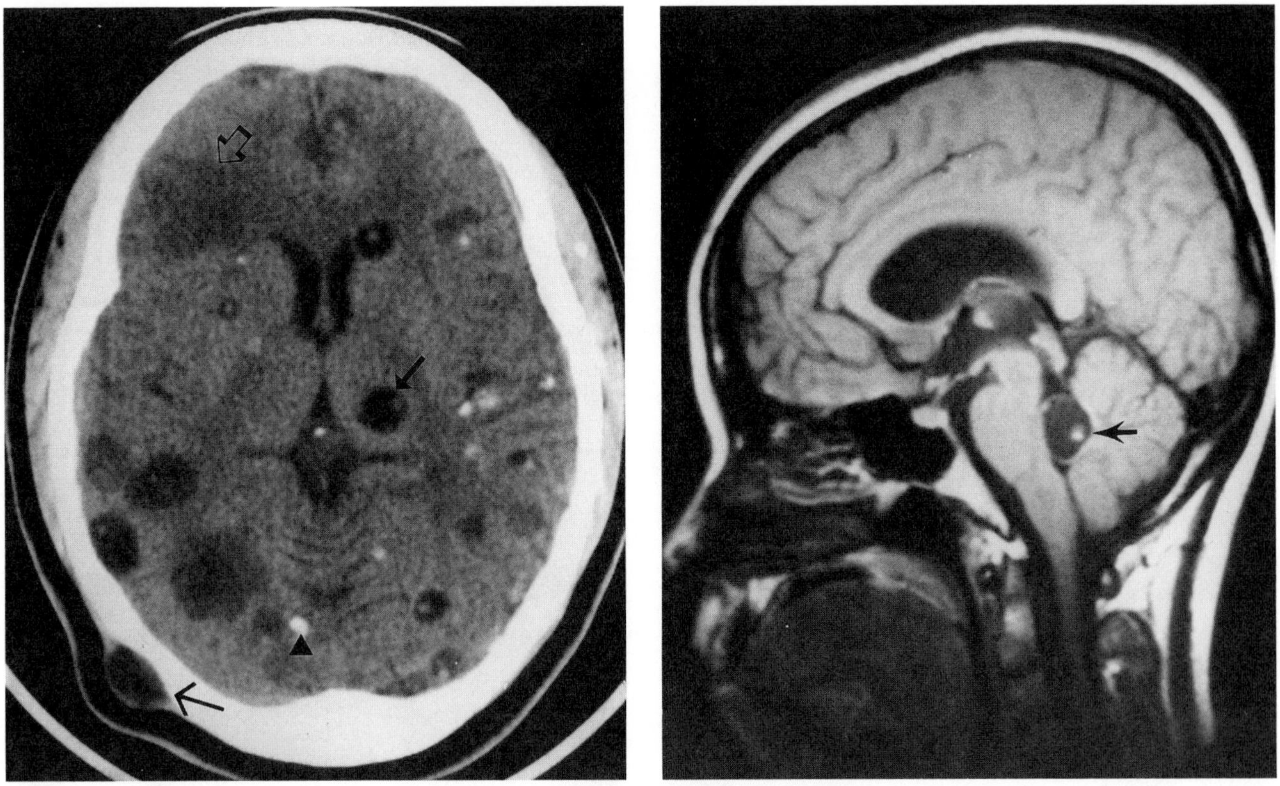

A B

FIGURE 39.34 Cysticercosis. A. Noncontrast axial CT demonstrates multiple lesions of cysticercosis in various stages of evolution. Note the multiple cysts with scolices (arrows) as well as the calcified lesion (arrowhead). There is also a hypodense lesion in the right frontal lobe representing a degenerating cysticercus with edema (open arrow). Note scalp lesion (long arrow). B. Sagittal T1-weighted MRI of another patient shows a cysticercosis cyst in the fourth ventricle (arrow).

Primary CNS lymphoma and toxoplasma encephalitis may be very difficult to distinguish from each other, and since treatment is very different, it is important to distinguish these two lesions. Thallium-201 brain SPECT has become valuable in making this distinction, since tumors have increased uptake (Figure 39.36, Plate 39.I) while infectious lesions do not (Ruiz et al. 1994).

Human Immunodeficiency Virus Encephalitis

MRI is more sensitive than CT in demonstrating the effects of human immunodeficiency virus (HIV) infection. Hyperintense lesions are seen on T2-weighted images in the periventricular white matter and centrum semiovale and correspond to foci of demyelination and vacuolation. MRI may demonstrate atrophy and signal changes in the white matter but does not demonstrate the microglial nodules and multinucleated giant cells seen on histologic sections. MRI is abnormal in approximately 70% of patients with AIDS, regardless of the presence of neurologic symptoms.

Proton MR spectroscopy has also been used to detect abnormalities in the brains of HIV-infected patients. One study found abnormal spectra in ten patients with AIDS, while routine MR images of these same patients revealed no significant abnormalities. Proton spectroscopy may therefore hold promise of early diagnosis of biochemical alterations in HIV-infected patients.

Progressive Multifocal Leukoencephalopathy

On CT, progressive multifocal leukoencephalopathy (PML) appears as a focal area of hypodensity in the white matter without mass effect and usually without enhancement. MRI has greater sensitivity than CT in imaging PML. On T2-weighted images, PML has increased signal in the periventricular or subcortical white matter, or both (Figure 39.37), sometimes with a bilateral multifocal distribution. Any lobe may be affected, but the frontal and parieto-occipital locations are most common. PML may be difficult to distinguish from HIV-related demyelination, but the latter is more often diffuse, symmetric, and periventricular in location, while PML is more multifocal and asymmetric and has a predilection for the subcortical white matter.

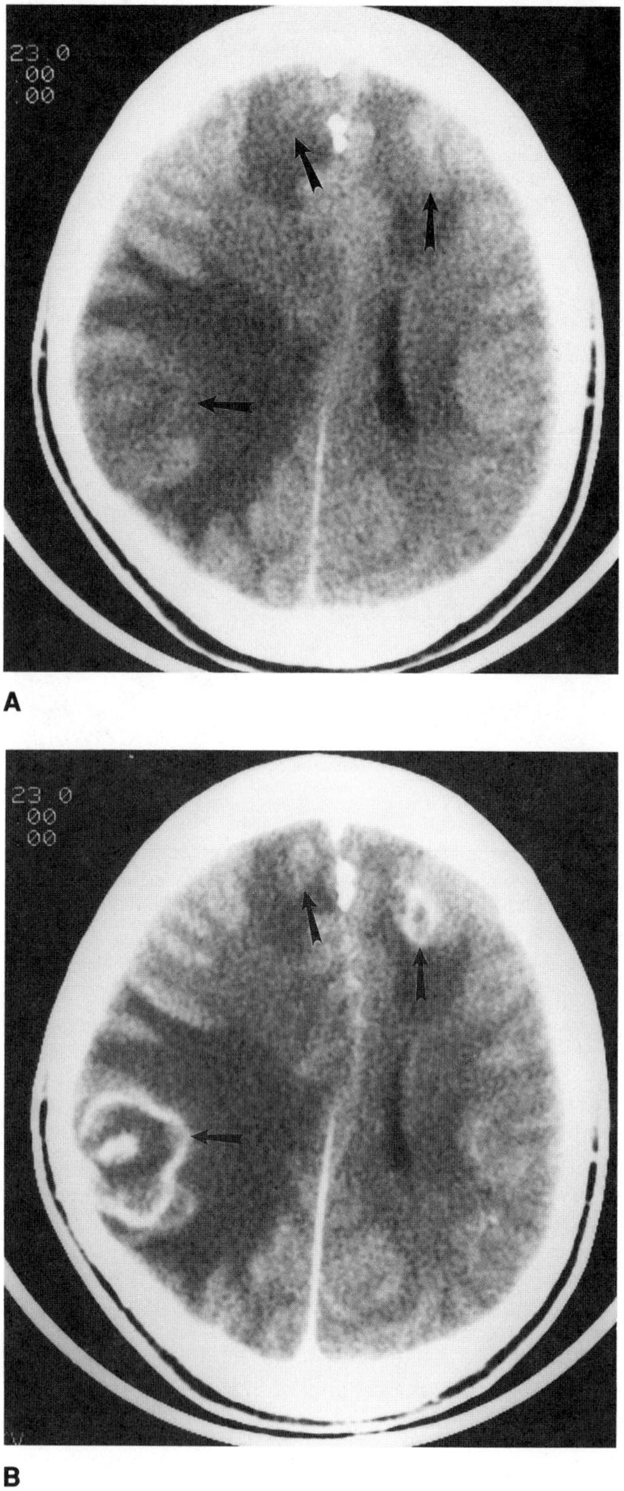

A

B

FIGURE 39.35 Toxoplasma encephalitis. A. Noncontrast CT scan of an HIV-seropositive patient shows lesions that are iso- to hypodense with extensive mass effect and edema (arrows). B. Postcontrast CT scan (double-dose delayed technique) reveals multiple enhancing lesions (arrows).

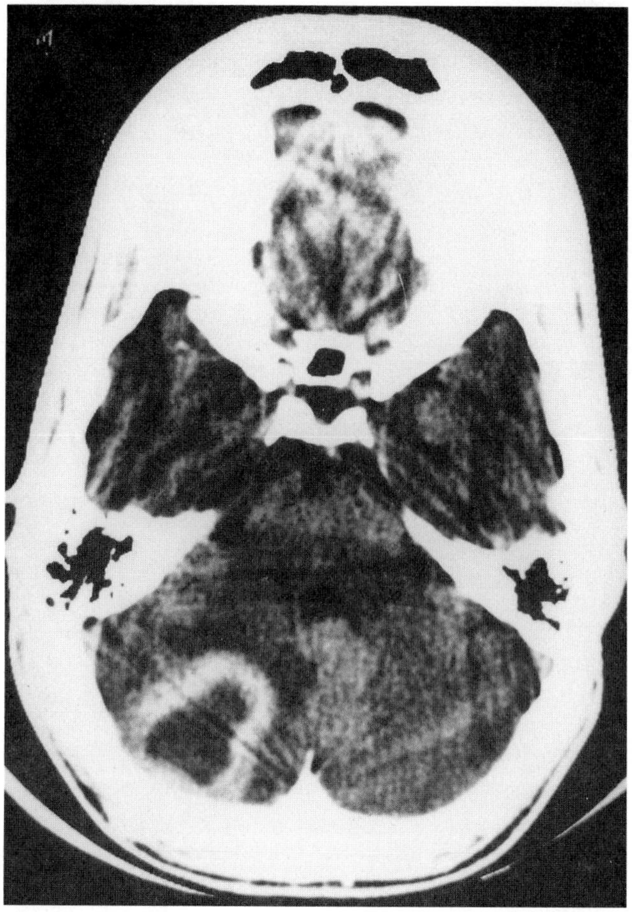

FIGURE 39.36 Lymphoma. Postcontrast CT scan demonstrates a ring-enhancing lesion with a necrotic center in the right cerebellar hemisphere. See Plate 39.I for brain SPECT images. (Reprinted with permission from A Ruiz, WL Ganz, MJD Post et al. Use of Thallium-201 brain SPECT to differentiate cerebral lymphoma from toxoplasma encephalitis in AIDS patients. Am J Neuroradiol 1994;15:1885–1894.)

Cytomegalovirus

Cytomegalovirus (CMV) is a frequent pathogen in patients with AIDS. On CT, atrophy is the most frequent finding, and hypodensity of the white matter may be seen. Periventricular and subependymal enhancement may be present, however. CT may grossly underestimate the degree of involvement (Post et al. 1988). MRI has greater sensitivity than CT in detecting CNS CMV and its extent. MRI may demonstrate increased signal in the periventricular white matter on T2-weighted images and subependymal enhancement after contrast administration.

Cryptococcosis

Cryptococcus neoformans is the most common fungus to involve the CNS in AIDS patients. Imaging findings in cryptococcal meningitis are often negative, but gadolinium studies

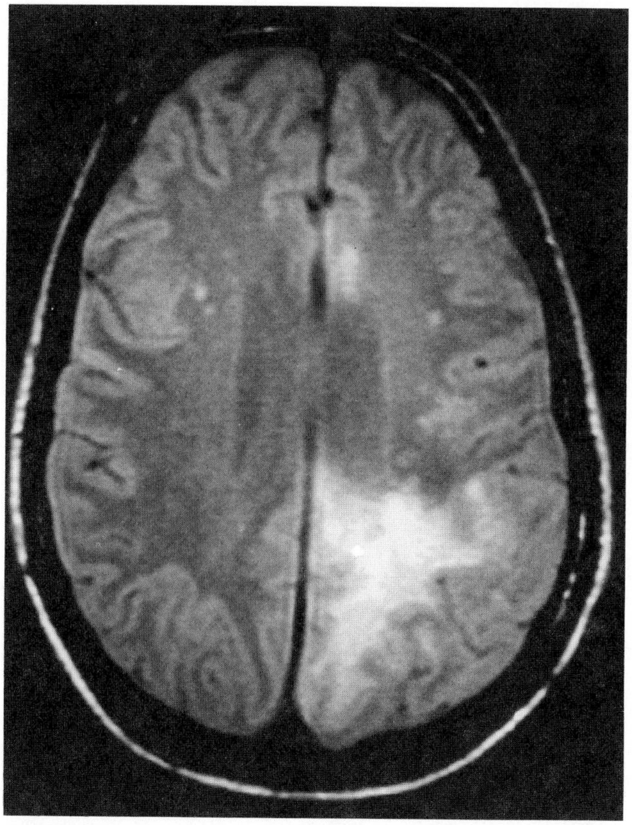

FIGURE 39.37 Progressive multifocal leukoencephalopathy (PML). Proton-density–weighted image shows a high-intensity lesion located in the white matter in the left posterior parietal lobe consistent with PML.

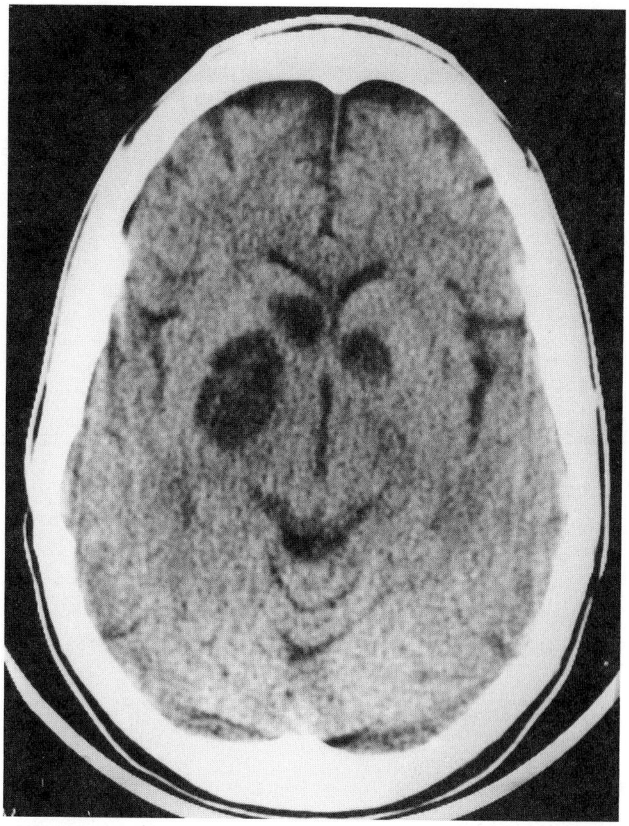

FIGURE 39.38 Cryptococcal pseudogelatinous cysts. Noncontrast CT scan shows gelatinous pseudocysts in the basal ganglia in a patient with AIDS.

may show meningeal enhancement. Parenchymal disease may include mass lesions, dilated Virchow-Robin's spaces, and leptomeningeal nodules. The mass lesions may be subdivided into gelatinous pseudocysts, fibrogranulomatous masses, or abscesses. CT may demonstrate hypodense lesions with solid or ring enhancement, particularly in the basal ganglia. The parenchymal disease is less widely distributed and incites less edema than toxoplasma encephalitis. Septated gelatinous pseudocysts do not enhance with contrast and are frequently seen in the basal ganglia (Figure 39.38); in T2-weighted images, these are seen as hyperintense foci.

Lymphoma

Primary CNS lymphoma is the most frequent CNS neoplasm seen in HIV-infected patients. AIDS-related CNS lymphomas are more frequently peripheral in location and tend to demonstrate necrosis more often compared to non–AIDS-related lymphomas. Up to 25% of CNS lymphomas occur infratentorially. Non-AIDS lymphomas appear as hyperdense masses on noncontrast CT exams, whereas AIDS-related CNS lymphoma lesions may be hypodense, probably related to a greater degree of necrosis. On MR, the dense cellularity of lymphoma renders these lesions iso- to hypointense on all sequences. Enhancement in non-AIDS lymphoma may be homogeneous, whereas in AIDS-related lymphoma enhancement may be heterogeneous or ringlike, which again may be related to the greater degree of necrosis (see Figure 39.36).

Congenital Lesions (see Chapter 67)

Two major types of congenital disorders of the CNS can be described. *Disorders of organogenesis* are those in which an alteration of CNS development occurs. *Disorders of histogenesis* are those with normal development but with abnormal cell differentiation. The disorders of organogenesis include abnormalities of diverticulation, closure migration, and CSF flow (Chapter 67). The disorders of histogenesis include the phakomatoses (Chapter 70).

Disorders of Diverticulation

Disorders of diverticulation are due to failure of the primitive prosencephalon to develop into cerebral hemispheres, and various degrees of separation of the brain and ventricles may occur.

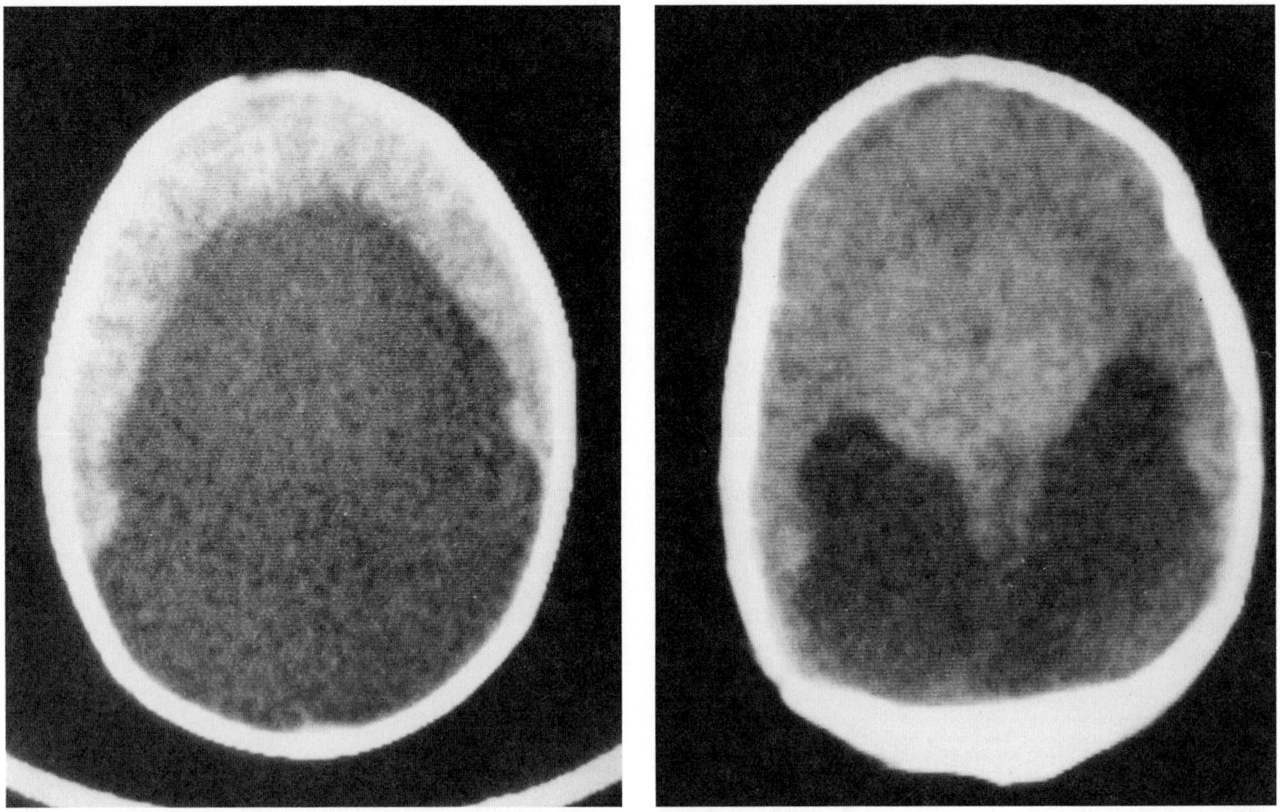

FIGURE 39.39 Alobar holoprosencephaly. A. Axial CT scan demonstrates a large central monoventricular cavity with a peripheral rim of cortical tissue. B. The thalami are fused and the third ventricle cannot be identified.

Holoprosencephaly. Holoprosencephaly represents absence of cleavage of the forebrain (prosencephalon). Three types are seen, depending on the severity of the lesion (from most severe to least severe): alobar, semilobar, and lobar. Alobar is the extreme form of holoprosencephaly resulting in a single monoventricular cavity with thin cortical tissue (Figure 39.39).

Septo-Optic Dysplasia. Septo-optic dysplasia involves the anterior midline structures of the brain. It consists of an absent septum pellucidum and hypoplasia of optic nerves, chiasm, and infundibulum. On CT and MR, there is absence of the septum pellucidum, atrophic optic nerves, and large ventricles.

Disorders of Closure

Agenesis of Corpus Callosum. In agenesis of the corpus callosum, a large bundle of fibers (bundles of Probst) persists passing anteroposteriorly on the medial aspect of the ventricles. On CT or MR there is wide separation of the lateral ventricles, occipital horns may show relative dilatation, and there may be interposition of the third ventricle between the bodies of the lateral ventricles (Figure 39.40). On sagittal MR images, there is absence of the corpus callosum. In addition, the sulcal markings and gyri in the parasagittal area have a more vertical course.

Disorders of Cerebrospinal Fluid Flow

Chiari Malformations. In the Chiari type I malformation the cerebellar tonsils are positioned below the foramen magnum, but the cerebellum is normal otherwise and the fourth ventricle is in normal position. Syringohydromyelia is a frequent concurrent lesion with an incidence of 20–25% in Chiari I malformation (Figure 39.41).

The Chiari II malformation is a dysgenesis of the hindbrain, which results in a caudally displaced fourth ventricle and medulla (Naidich et al. 1983). The essential feature is the pathological downward displacement of the fourth ventricle extending into the cervical canal so that nonvisualization of the fourth ventricle is common. Anomalies associated with Chiari II are the following: lukenschadel skull (pitting of the skull), clivus and petrous scalloping, enlarged foramen magnum, myelomeningocele, dural anomalies (widened tentorial incisura), hindbrain and midbrain anomalies (beaking of the tectum) (Figure 39.42), and forebrain anomalies.

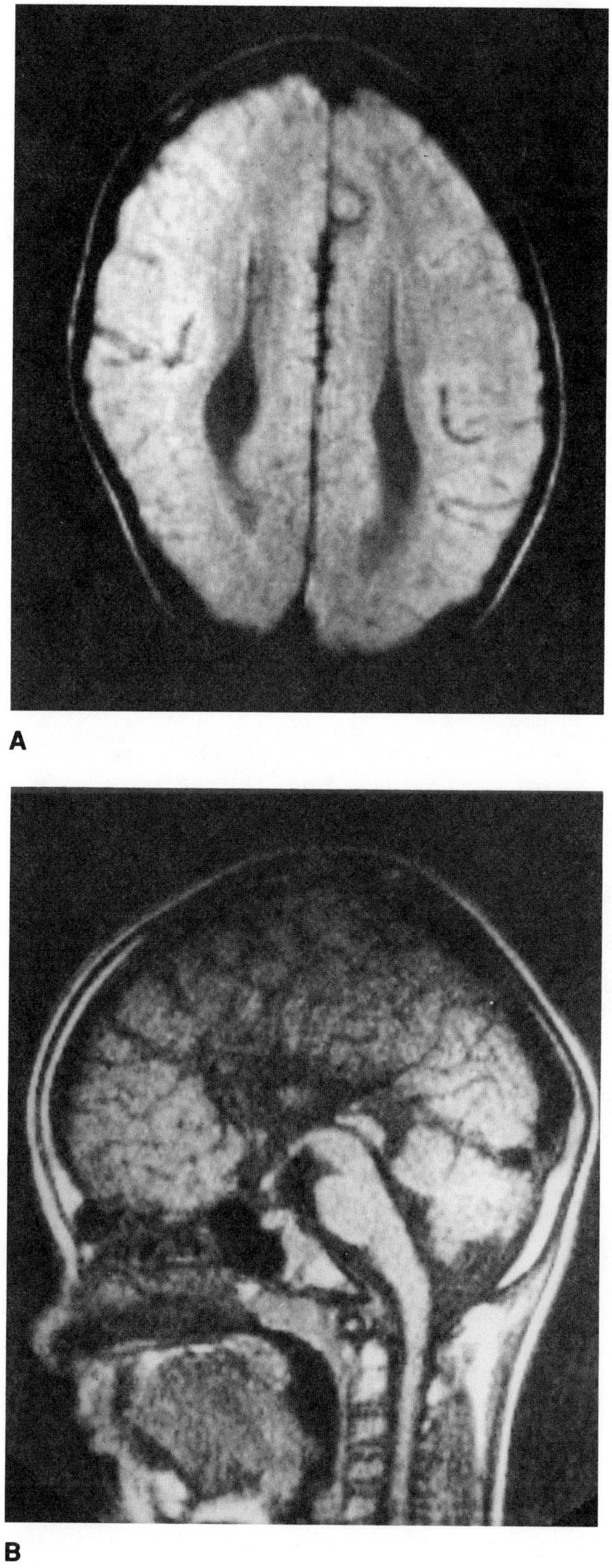

FIGURE 39.40 Agenesis of corpus callosum. A. T1-weighted axial image shows separated and parallel lateral ventricles. B. Sagittal T1-weighted image shows absence of a midline corpus callosum.

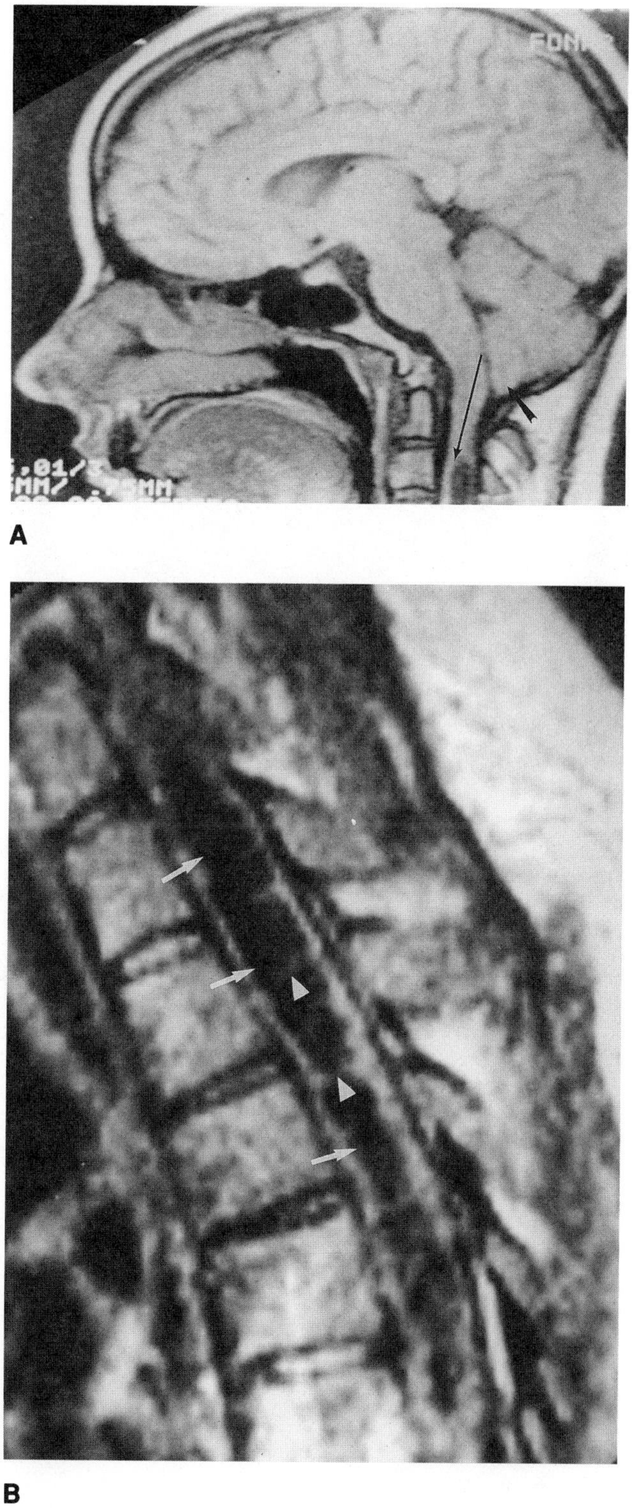

FIGURE 39.41 Chiari I malformation with syringohydromyelia. A. Sagittal T1-weighted image shows the tonsils extending below the foramen magnum (arrow). The very superior aspect of an intramedullary cyst is seen (long black arrow). B. The sagittal T1-weighted image of the cervical spine in the same patient demonstrates a syringohydromyelia of the cervical spine (white arrows). There are multiple septations (white arrowheads) within the syrinx and the cord is widened.

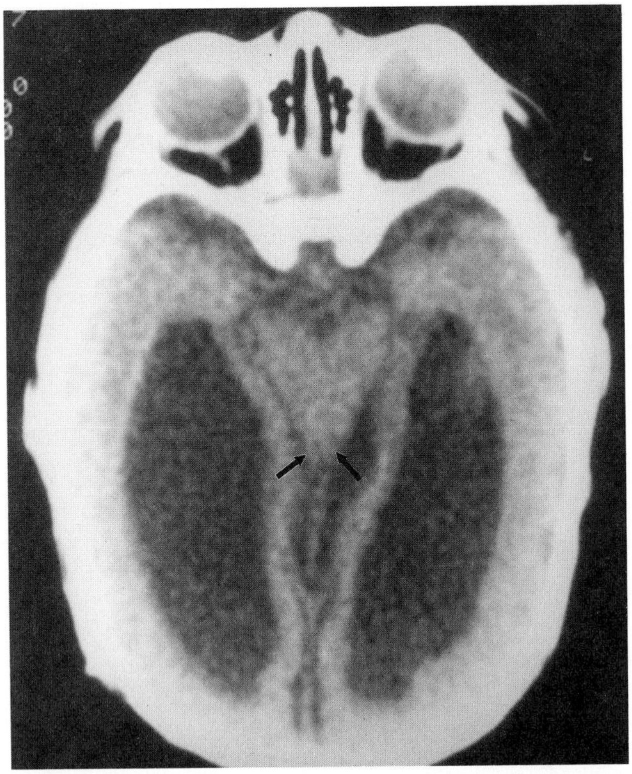

A

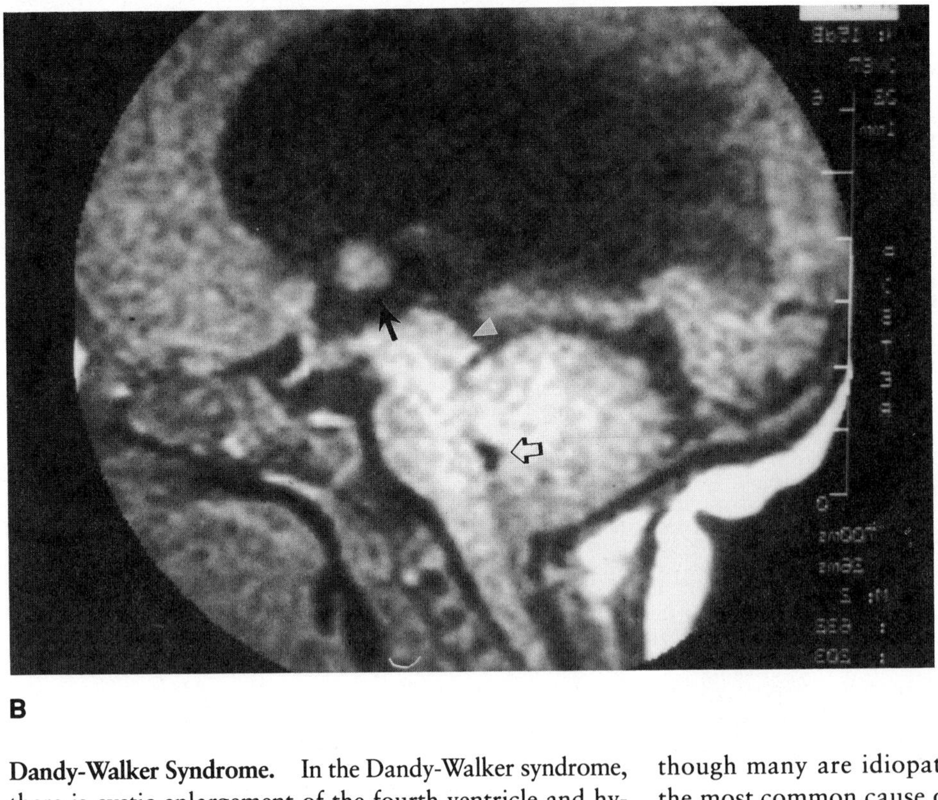

B

FIGURE 39.42 Chiari II malformation. A. Beaking of the tectum (arrows) is demonstrated in the axial CT scan of a patient with Chiari II malformation. B. T1-weighted sagittal image in another patient shows marked hydrocephalus, an enlarged massa intermedia (arrow), and beaking of the tectum (white arrowhead). The fourth ventricle (open arrow) is not caudally displaced in this patient.

Dandy-Walker Syndrome. In the Dandy-Walker syndrome, there is cystic enlargement of the fourth ventricle and hypoplasia of the vermis (Figure 39.43). The tentorium, torcula, straight sinus, and vein of Galen are displaced superiorly.

Aqueductal Stenosis. The causes of aqueductal stenosis include infection, Chiari II malformation, and neoplasm, though many are idiopathic. Chiari II malformation is the most common cause of hydrocephalus and aqueductal stenosis in early childhood. The lateral and third ventricles are moderately to severely enlarged (Figure 39.44). If Chiari II malformation is not present, the fourth ventricle is usually normal in size (see Figure 39.44).

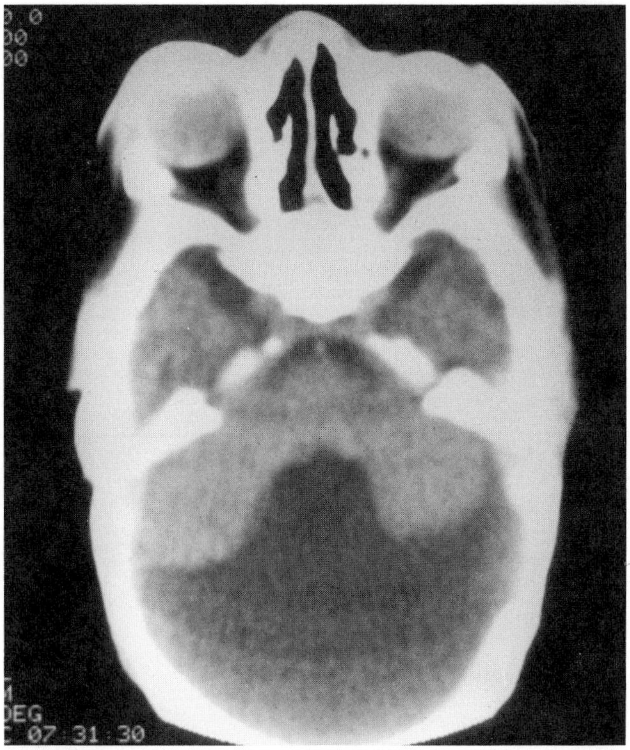

FIGURE 39.43 The Dandy-Walker syndrome. The fourth ventricle is replaced by an enlarged midline cyst in the axial CT scan of a patient with the Dandy-Walker syndrome. Note the hypoplasia of the vermis.

Disorders of Sulcation and Migration

Heterotopias. Heterotopias have classically been separated into three forms:

1. The *nodular form* consists of subependymal nodules of gray matter that are usually bilateral.
2. The *bulk form* consists of islands of gray matter that are usually isolated in the hemispheric white matter (Figure 39.45).
3. In band heterotopia, alternating layers of gray-white-gray-white matter are symmetric throughout both hemispheres.

Schizencephaly. Schizencephaly is a disorder in which there are clefts spanning the cerebral hemispheres. Pathologically, these clefts are characterized by an infolding of the gray matter along the cleft from the cortex into the ventricles. There are two groups: (1) those in which the walls of the cleft are fused (*closed lip schizencephaly*) (Figure 39.46), and (2) those in which the walls of the cleft are separated (*open lip schizencephaly*).

Destructive Lesion

Hydranencephaly. In hydranencephaly, there is virtual absence of the cerebral hemispheres except for the basal ganglia. The infratentorial structures are intact (Figure 39.47). A severe and early intrauterine vascular accident is the presumed cause.

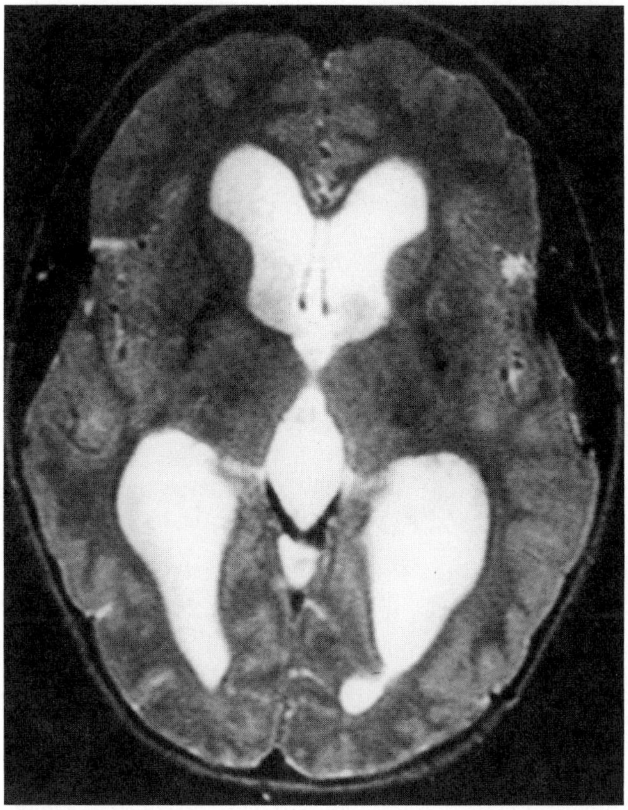

A

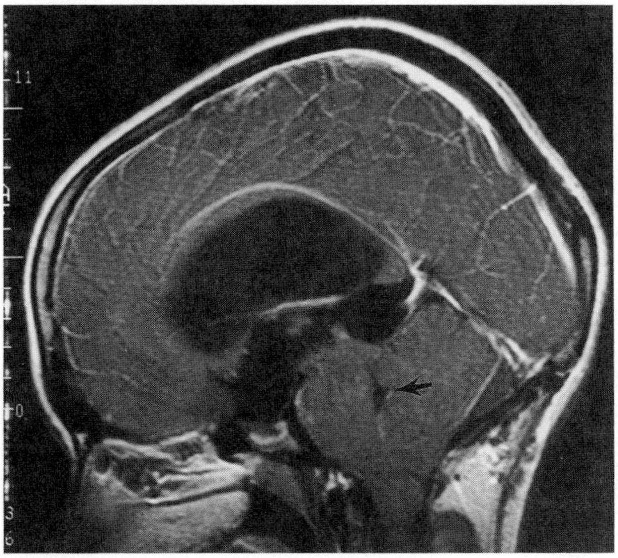

B

FIGURE 39.44 Aqueductal stenosis. A. T2-weighted axial MRI demonstrates markedly dilated lateral and third ventricles. B. The sagittal T1-weighted image (postcontrast) shows the marked dilatation of the lateral and third ventricles, but a small fourth ventricle (arrow). The posterior fossa is small and the aqueduct is not well seen.

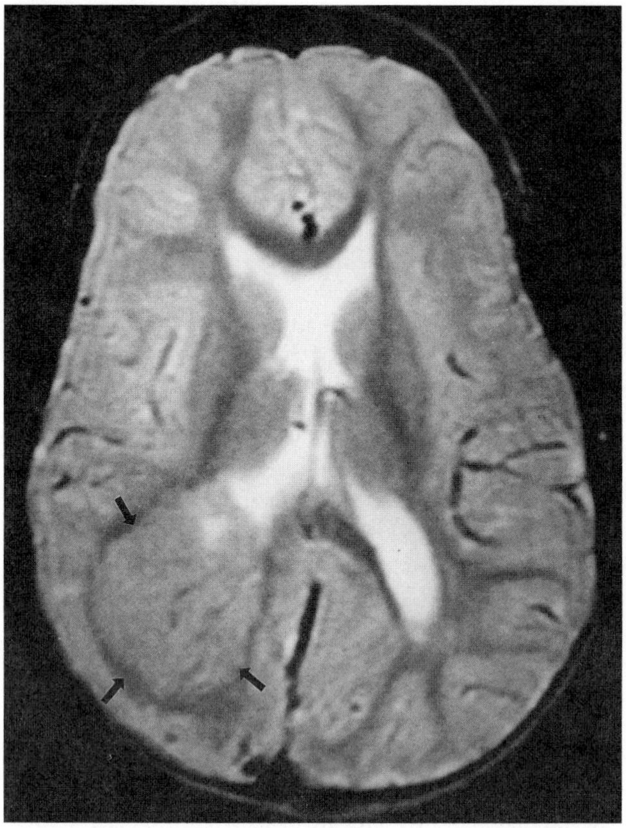

FIGURE 39.45 Heterotopia. Bulk form of heterotopia is seen as an island of gray matter that is isolated in the hemispheric white matter. This island of tissue (arrows) has the signal characteristics of gray matter on this T2-weighted image.

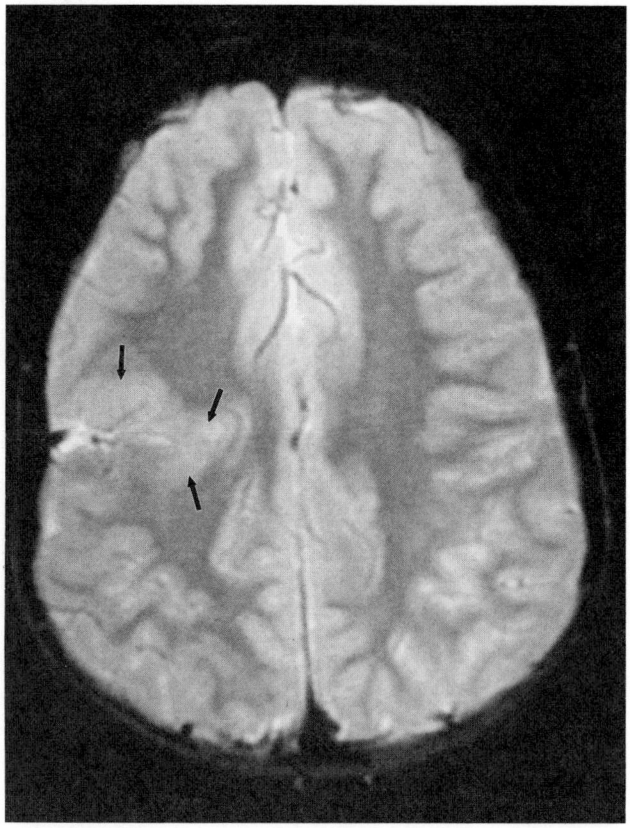

FIGURE 39.46 Schizencephaly. Closed lip schizencephaly appears as a cleft lined by gray matter extending through the full thickness of the cerebral mantle. The island of tissue has the signal characteristics of gray matter on this T2-weighted image (arrows).

Disorders of Histogenesis (see Chapter 70)

Tuberous Sclerosis. Hamartomas, the most frequent lesion seen on MR in patients with tuberous sclerosis, are isointense on T1 and hyperintense on T2-weighted images. Subependymal nodules are usually multiple and bilateral, they frequently calcify, and are usually iso- to hyperintense on T1-weighted images and are hyperintense on T2-weighted images. These subependymal hamartomas may degenerate into a giant cell astrocytoma (see Figure 39.3), which is most frequently found at the foramen of Monro.

Neurofibromatosis. Neurofibromatosis (NF) is the most common of the neurocutaneous syndromes. It has been classified into two main types, NF1 and NF2.

Neurofibromatosis 1. NF1 is inherited as an autosomal dominant disease and is referred to as *peripheral NF* or *von Recklinghausen's disease*. The CNS and calvarial manifestations are diverse and include gliomas of the optic nerves and chiasm (see Figure 39.17); gliomas in other areas of the brain; neuromas and neurofibromas of the cranial, spinal, and peripheral nerves; dysplasia of the sphenoid bone and orbit; plexiform neurofibromas of the scalp and elsewhere; and hyperintense brain lesions demonstrated on MR with T2-weighted images (Atlas 1991).

Neurofibromatosis 2. NF2, also called *central neurofibromatosis*, is inherited in a dominant fashion. The diagnostic criteria for NF2 include bilateral eighth nerve schwannomas (see Figure 39.18) or a unilateral eighth nerve schwannoma with two of the following: neurofibroma or schwannoma in a different location, meningioma, glioma, or a relative with NF2. This is a genetically different entity from NF1, and hence optic nerve gliomas, skeletal dysplasias, and cutaneous neurofibromas are rare.

Vascular Disorders

Vascular Malformations (see Chapter 58)

Vascular malformations have been divided into four major pathological types: (1) arteriovenous malformation, (2) cavernous angiomas, (3) capillary telangiectasia, and (4) venous angioma.

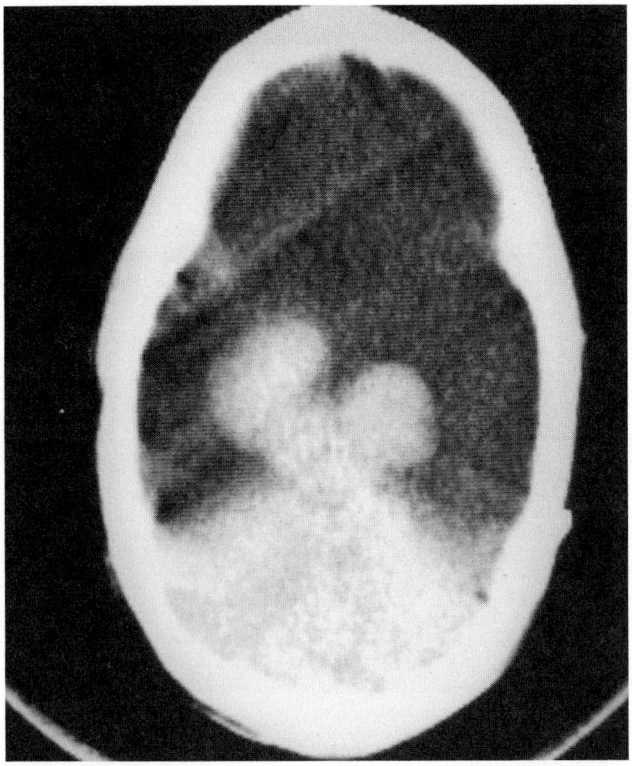

FIGURE 39.47 Hydranencephaly. Absence of the cerebral hemispheres, with intact basal ganglia and infratentorial structures.

Arteriovenous Malformation. Cerebral angiography is the definitive method of accurately delineating the vascular supply and venous drainage of intracranial arteriovenous malformations (AVMs). Morphologically, AVMs appear as wedge-shaped clusters of vessels with the apex directed toward the ventricular surface. The typical AVM appears on spin-echo MRI as a cluster of focal round lesions or serpentine areas of signal void (Figure 39.48). At this time, conventional angiography is superior to MRA in depicting the arterial supply and venous drainage of the AVM.

Cavernous Angiomas. Cavernous angiomas are discrete multilobulated berrylike lesions that contain hemorrhage in various stages of evolution. They may be found in any part of the brain; most are supratentorial and are found mostly in the frontal and temporal lobes. In the posterior fossa, the pons and cerebellar hemispheres are the most common sites.

Most are angiographically occult, but occasionally a faint blush can be seen in the late capillary or venous phase. On CT, these lesions may be isodense to hyperdense in noncontrast scans and calcification is common. MR scans may show a popcorn-like lesion of mixed signal consistent with hemorrhage in different stages.

Venous Angioma. Venous angiomas are clinically silent malformations of venous drainage without an arterial component. Imaging studies delineate typical curvilinear vascular channels receiving drainage from a "spoke wheel–appearing" collection of small tapering veins arranged in a radial pattern (Figure 39.49). The larger draining veins empty into a large cortical vein, a dural sinus, or a subependymal ventricular vein.

Spinal Arteriovenous Malformations

Most spinal vascular malformations are AVMs or arteriovenous fistulas (AVFs). AVMs have a nidus of vessels and are fed by enlarged feeding arteries and drain via large veins. AVFs drain directly into enlarged venous outflow tracts.

Spinal vascular malformations have been subdivided into four groups. Type I is a dural AVF, which is mostly found in the dorsal aspect of the lower thoracic spine. Type II are intramedullary AVMs that drain into a venous plexus that surrounds the cord and are usually located in the cervicomedullary junction. Type III are larger vascular masses that involve the cord and often have extramedullary extension. Type IV are intradural extramedullary AVFs. Most are anterior to the spinal cord and occur near the conus medullaris.

MRI may show foci of flow void within enlarged vessels. The cord may be atrophic and often has high signal intensity on T2-weighted images. MRA is a very good modality for evaluation of these lesions, although spinal angiography has been the definitive diagnostic procedure for the evaluation of spinal AVMs. Myelography may show filling defects caused by the enlarged vessels, but since the advent of MR, the flow voids, the enhancement of flow in enhanced veins, and flow-related enhancement on MRA make myelography unnecessary in the vast majority of cases.

Aneurysms (see Chapter 58C)

Conventional angiography remains the modality of choice for the diagnosis of an aneurysm (Figure 39.50) (Atlas 1991). MRI cannot be used definitively to exclude the presence of an aneurysm, though it can diagnose aneurysms based on the identification of regions of flow void. In the face of a subarachnoid hemorrhage with a completely negative cerebral angiogram, repeat angiography is recommended in an effort to discover an aneurysm that for various reasons may not have been seen on the first study.

Patients with perimesencephalic subarachnoid hemorrhage have a better prognosis and have negative cerebral angiograms. In these patients the subarachnoid hemorrhage is found in the interpeduncular and prepontine cisterns. The hemorrhage may be related to the clival venous plexus.

Cerebral Infarction

In the first 24 hours after an arterial occlusion with infarction, 80% of MR scans are positive, compared to 50% of CT scans. These infarcts are seen as regions of increased signal on T2-weighted images. At this stage the abnormalities are mostly in the gray matter. In infarcts 2 days to 3 weeks old,

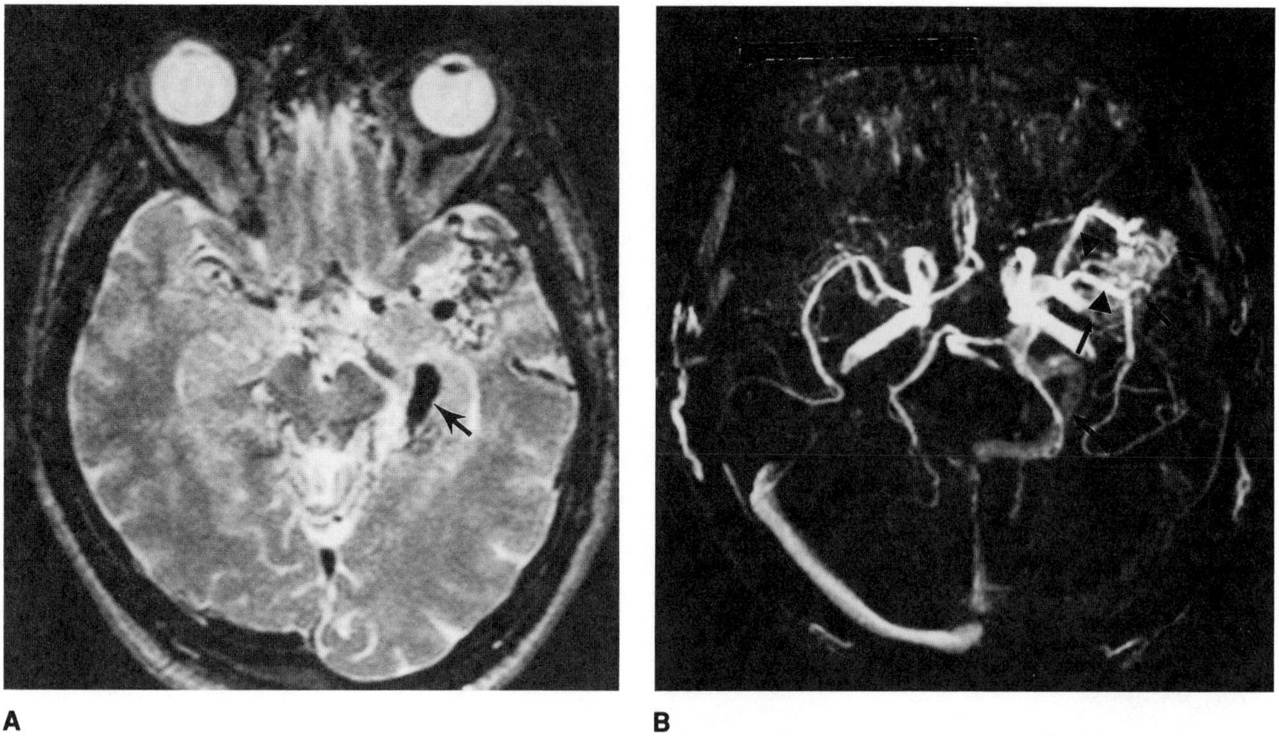

FIGURE 39.48 Arteriovenous malformation (AVM). A. Long TR-TE spin-echo MR shows a wedge-shaped cluster of vessels in the left temporal lobe seen as linear and round areas of signal void. Note enlarged draining vein (arrow). B. MRA formed by a three-dimensional time of flight volume slab through the base of the skull and circle of Willis shows an AVM (outlined by arrows) in the left temporal lobe. Feeding vessels (arrowheads) arise from the left middle cerebral artery. There is a large medially draining vein (probably a perimesencephalic vein—large arrow).

the subtle signal intensity changes seen initially become more obvious with increasing signal intensity on long TR images. White- and gray-matter abnormalities are then seen. In 20% of cases there will be a hemorrhagic component with increased signal seen on T1-weighted images if the stroke is greater than approximately 48 hours old. More acute hemorrhagic strokes reveal hypointense to isointense areas on MRI, with factors such as field strength and pulse sequence playing an important role in the appearance. MRI is the most sensitive, accurate, and practical means of imaging acute strokes.

The MRI of an infarct 3–6 weeks old is characterized by a smaller and better-defined zone of signal changes. The signal intensity on T2-weighted images is greater due to cystic cavitation. Focal atrophy is also present due to a loss of tissue volume.

A crucial factor in the management of strokes is the determination of a hemorrhagic component in the infarct (Figure 39.51). Acute hemorrhage may not be as obvious on MR, especially if gradient echo scans have not been done (Atlas 1991). Hyperacute hemorrhagic lesions may not have adequate time for the accumulation of deoxyhemoglobin, so it may therefore be appropriate to continue to perform CT scans in the early stroke.

The pattern of cerebral infarction resulting from blood vessel occlusion depends on vascular anatomy, and the signal changes closely follow the anatomic distribution of the arteries (Figure 39.52). In the case of proximal disease and

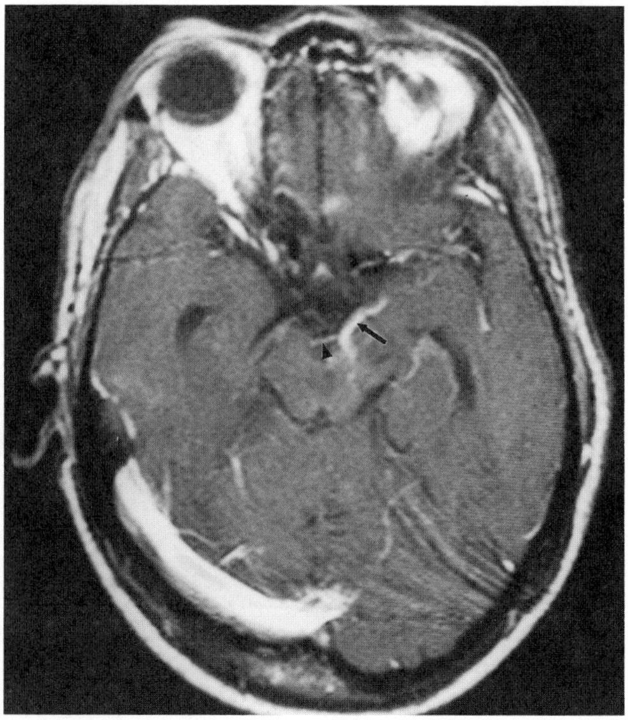

FIGURE 39.49 Venous angioma. Postcontrast axial T1-weighted image shows a prominent vein coursing within the left crural cistern (arrow). It is receiving multiple small feeding veins (arrowhead) from within the substance of the midbrain. These findings are typical of a venous angioma.

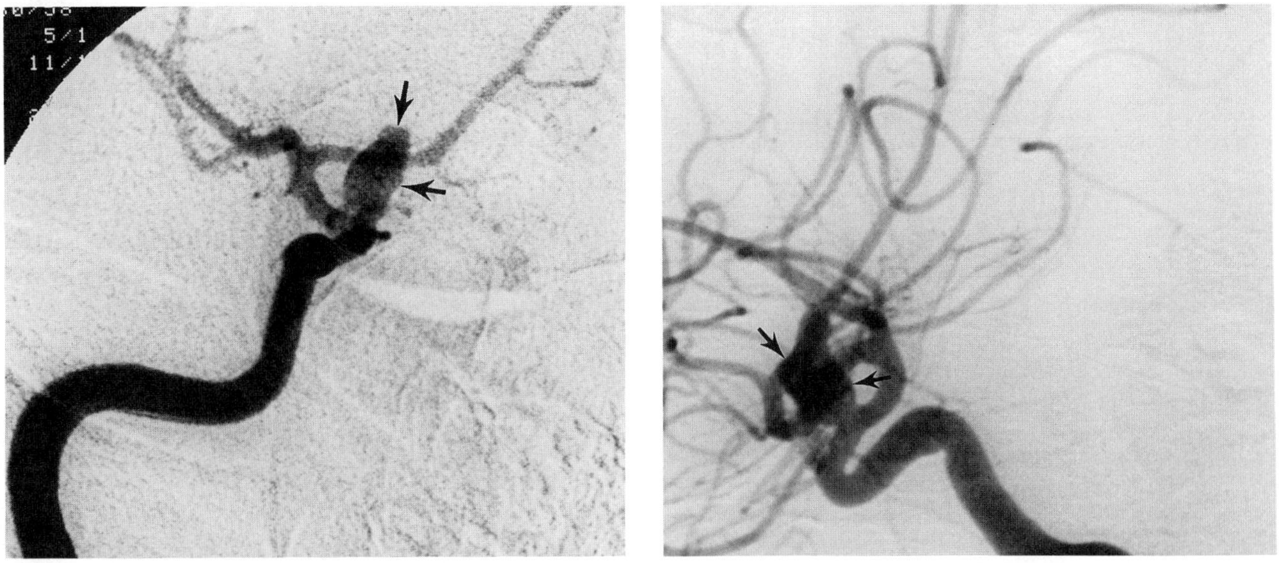

A B

FIGURE 39.50 Cerebral arterial aneurysm. An ophthalmic artery aneurysm (arrows) is shown in these oblique (A) and lateral (B) views of a right internal carotid artery angiogram.

Table 39.1: Blood breakdown products

		Signal Intensity	
Time		*T1WI*	*T2WI*
0–24 hrs	Oxyhemoglobin	↓/=	↑
First 24 hrs to 3–5 days	Deoxyhemoglobin	↓/=	↓↓
3–7 days	Intracellular methemoglobin	↑	↓↓
1 wk to months	Extracellular methemoglobin	↑	↑
1–2 wks to yrs	Hemosiderin	=/↓	↓↓

↓ = decreased; ↓↓ = marked decreased; ↑ = increased; = = unchanged.

infarcts due to systemic hypotension the anastomotic border zones (*watershed zones*) between major vascular territories are most severely involved.

MRI is superior to CT in the evaluation of infarcts in posterior fossa structures because CT resolution is limited by skull-base artifacts. Infarcts in the brain stem are small in relation to the extent of clinical damage. The small size of these lesions, in addition to the fact that these patients may be neurologically devastated and therefore poor candidates for MRI, make these lesions sometimes difficult to evaluate.

The vessel most frequently involved in embolic disease is the middle cerebral artery. Smaller, more peripheral infarcts are often seen with embolic disease. If emboli are multiple, more than one vascular territory may be involved.

The etiology for small, deep infarcts in the capsular and ganglionic regions is unclear. During the chronic stage, these small infarcts resolve to become very small cystic lesions—the typical *lacunae.*

Hemorrhage and Magnetic Resonance Imaging

Acute hemorrhage consists of intact red blood cells (RBCs) and plasma. Intracellular oxyhemoglobin is converted to deoxyhemoglobin (Figure 39.53), which is then oxidized to methemoglobin (from the periphery to the center). Subsequently, as a result of RBC lysis, intracellular methemoglobin becomes free methemoglobin and concomitantly hemosiderin appears in the periphery. Eventually methemoglobin is resorbed and only a hemosiderin cleft remains (Gomori et al. 1985). As the hemorrhage evolves, each of the stages has unique T1 and T2 relaxation times on MRIs. This allows us to determine the age of these hematomas (Table 39.1).

Hydrocephalus

Hydrocephalus is considered to be present when there are enlarged ventricles in the absence of atrophy or dysgenic

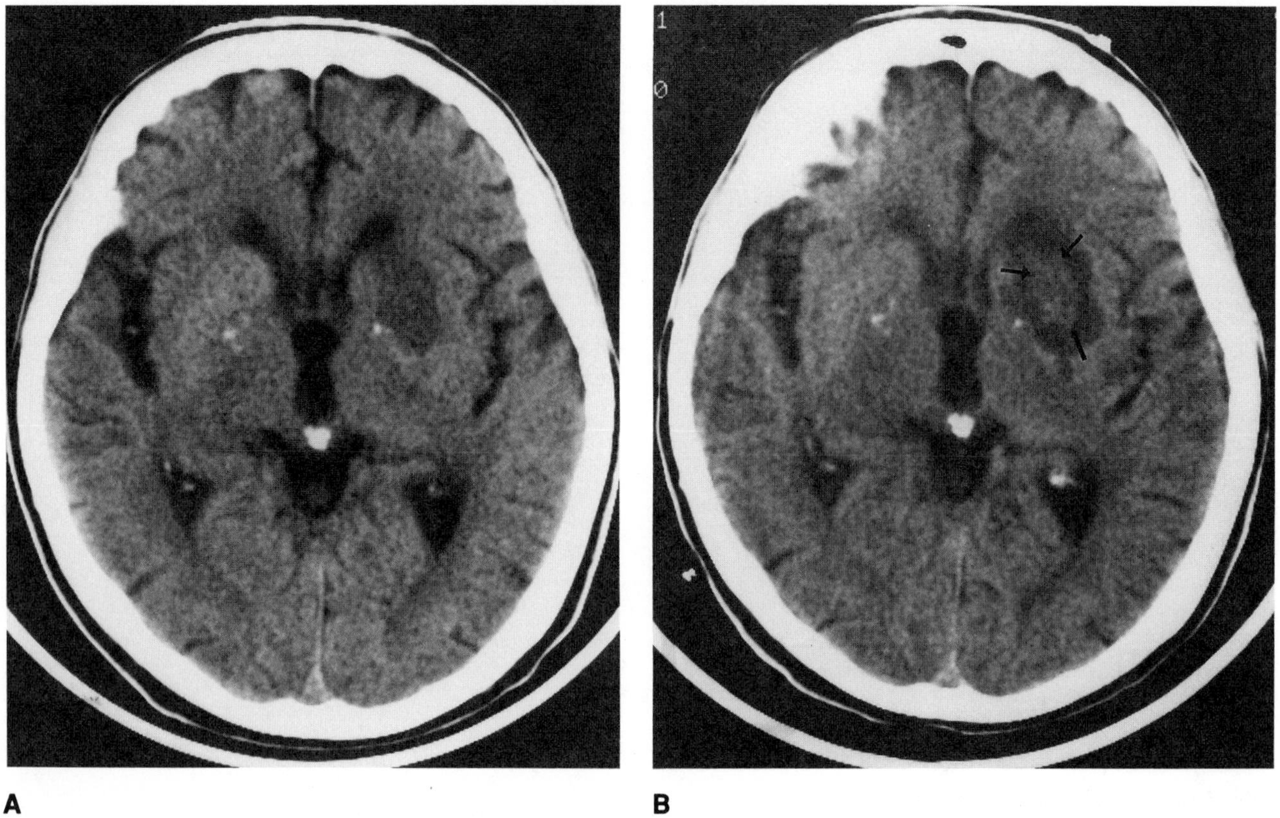

FIGURE 39.51 Cerebral infarct. A. Noncontrast CT scan shows infarct involving left basal ganglia. Incidental basal ganglionic calcifications are seen. B. Three days later the CT scan shows hemorrhage (arrows) in the area of infarction.

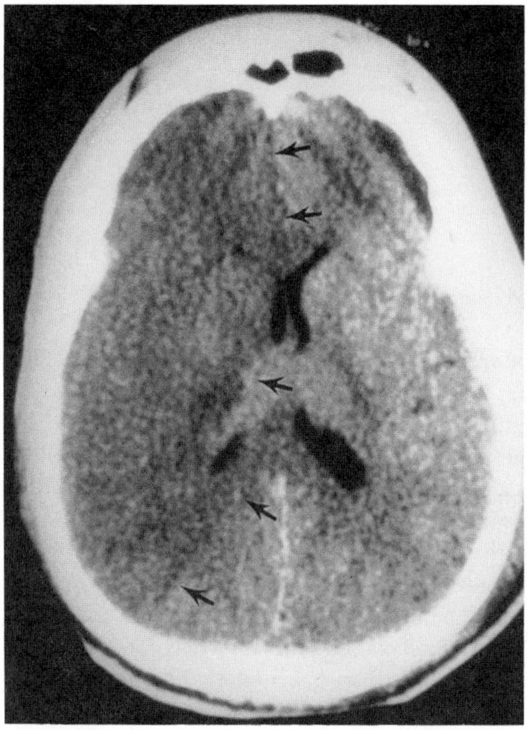

FIGURE 39.52 Right hemisphere infarct. Noncontrast CT scan demonstrates a low-density lesion involving the right frontal, temporal, and parietal lobes (arrows) in a patient who sustained a bullet injury to the skull base with injury to the right internal carotid artery.

brain (see Chapter 66). Therefore, a clear difference exists between hydrocephalus and ventriculomegaly, since the latter indicates large ventricles regardless of the cause. CT and MR can characterize the different patterns of ventricular enlargement to determine the etiology.

Obstructive Hydrocephalus or Noncommunicating Hydrocephalus

The hallmark of obstructive noncommunicating hydrocephalus is ventriculomegaly proximal to the site of obstruction with the frequently associated finding of periventricular edema secondary to transependymal flow of CSF. The site of obstruction is determined by the characteristic ventricular dilatation. Aqueductal obstruction will produce dilatation of the third and lateral ventricles, while the fourth ventricle remains normal (see Figure 39.44). A colloid cyst of the third ventricle produces only dilatation of both lateral ventricles. Cerebellar tumors may compress the fourth ventricle and cause obstructive hydrocephalus.

Communicating Hydrocephalus

In communicating hydrocephalus, the normal flow of CSF over the cerebral convexities and its resorption are altered. The most common causes are subarachnoid hemorrhage and meningitis. However, seeding of meninges by metastatic

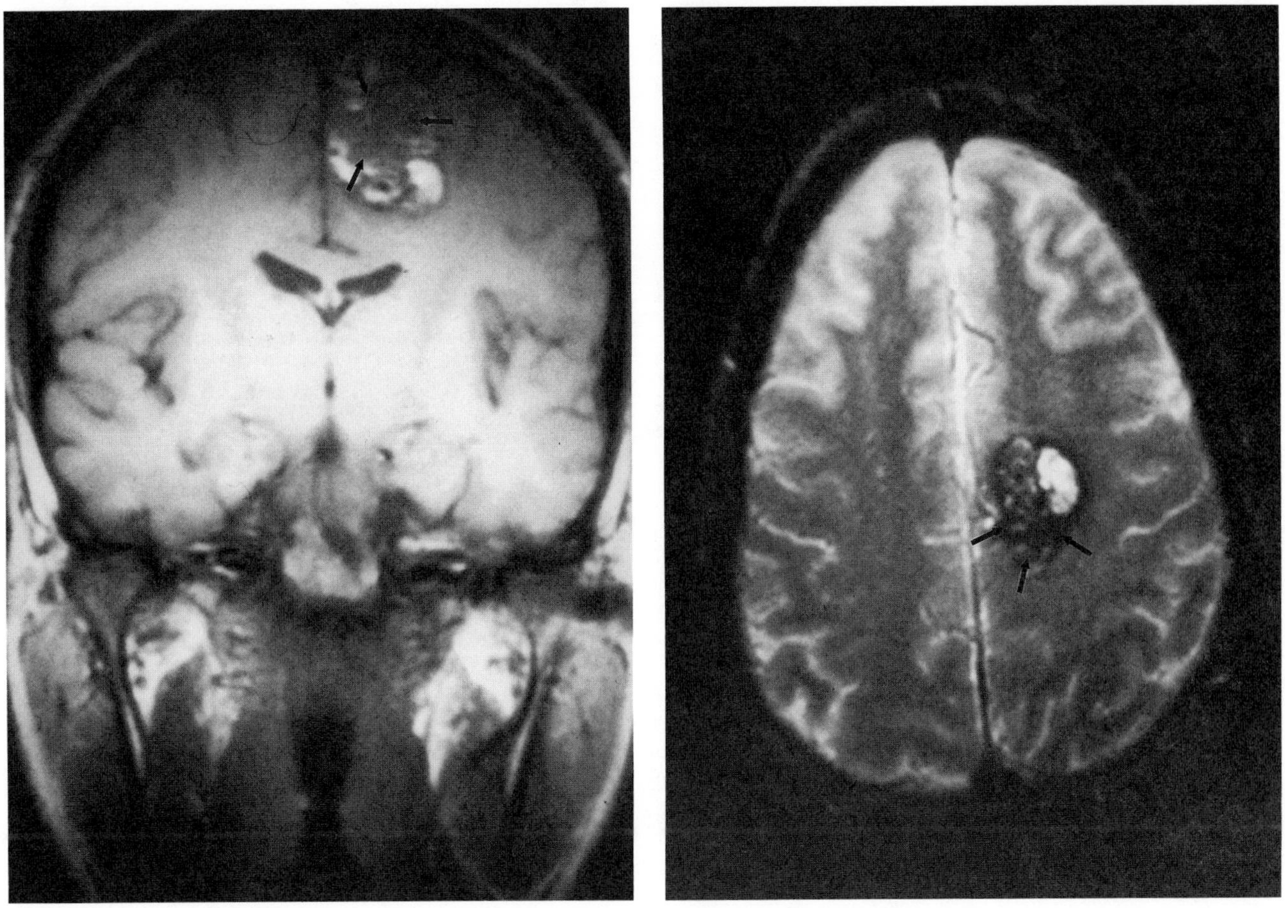

A B

FIGURE 39.53 Acute hematoma. There is a central area that is isointense to brain (arrows) on T1-weighted image (A) and hypointense (arrows) on T2-weighted image (B), consistent with intracellular deoxyhemoglobin, and a peripheral area that is hyperintense on both T1 and T2 images consistent with extracellular methemoglobin.

diseases and chronic meningoencephalitic diseases like sarcoidosis may also result in hydrocephalus. On imaging, all the ventricles are dilatated and the sulci are effaced.

Normal-Pressure Hydrocephalus

The classic clinical triad of normal-pressure hydrocephalus (NPH) is dementia, gait apraxia, and urinary incontinence (see Chapter 66). Positive isotope cisternography of NPH shows reflux of the isotope into the ventricles after injection of the isotope into the lumbar thecal sac but no passage of isotope over the cerebral convexities. Degenerative disorders, however, may also show abnormal CSF flow, so this study is not entirely conclusive. The distinction on MRI or CT of atrophy versus NPH is difficult. NPH usually causes uniform thinning and elevation of the corpus callosum and distention of the third ventricle causing dilatation of the optic and infundibular recesses. The normal CSF flow void in the aqueduct may be accentuated in NPH. There may or may not be periventricular transudation of fluid into the parenchyma in NPH.

Skull Base Lesions

MR has become an essential part of the evaluation of skull base lesions; it can show the margin of the tumor relative to vital structures such as the cavernous sinus and the relationship to the carotid artery. Often, it can differentiate tumor from an obstructed paranasal sinus. Considerable fat is found between the various muscle groups beneath the skull base. As the tumor invades this fat, the normal high signal on T1-weighted images is obliterated by the intermediate signal of the tumor. This is especially important in detecting tumor extension through the various neural foramina. For definition of fine cortical bony erosion at the base of the skull, CT is needed.

Nasopharyngeal Carcinoma

Squamous cell carcinoma, the most malignant tumor seen in the nasopharynx, tends to be locally invasive and erode through the skull base into the intracranial cavity (Figure 39.54). Tumor may extend through the petroclival suture

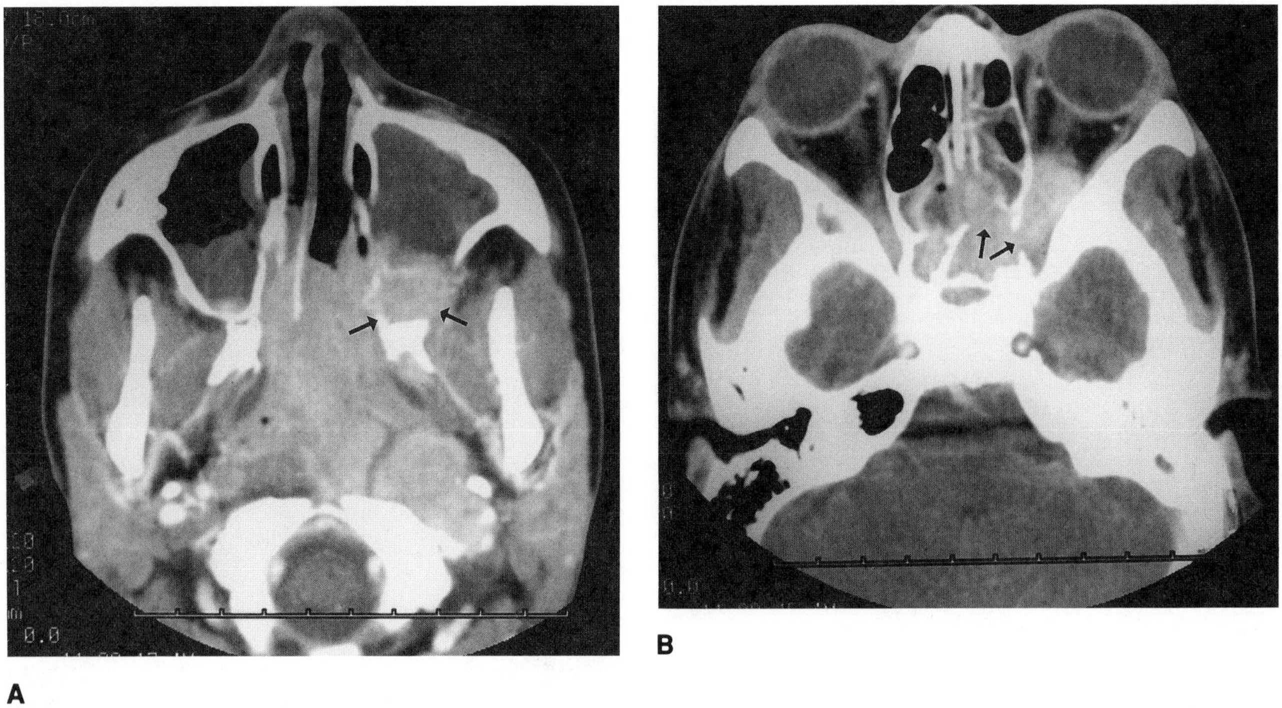

FIGURE 39.54 Nasopharyngeal carcinoma. A. Axial CT scan after contrast administration demonstrates a mass in the nasopharynx, which extends anteriorly to involve the nasal cavity and left maxillary sinus. The lesion is invading the left pterygopalatine fossa (arrows). There is bony destruction of the posterior walls of the left maxillary sinus and lateral wall of the nasal cavity. The mass extends posteriorly to the prevertebral space and laterally involves the left carotid space. B. The mass extends superiorly to involve the ethmoids and left orbit (arrows).

and foramen lacerum into the posterior fossa and into the inferior aspect of the cavernous sinus.

Petrous Apex Lesions

The two major lesions occurring in the petrous apex are the *primary cholesteoma* or *epidermoid tumor*, and the *granulomatous cholesterol cyst*. The latter results from air cells that have been partially obstructed by chronic otitis media and filled with liquid cellular debris and hemorrhage. An epidermoid ("pearly tumor") tends to be low signal on T1-weighted images and bright on T2-weighted images. The granulomatous cholesterol cyst is bright on both sequences due to the recurrent hemorrhage.

Glomus Jugulare Tumor

Glomus jugulare tumor (paraganglioma) arises in the lateral portion of the jugular foramen. There can be significant extension inferiorly beneath the temporal bone and intracranially. On T1-weighted images these lesions are usually of intermediate signal intensity and on T2-weighted images they are hyperintense (Figure 39.55). Signal voids representing blood flow scattered throughout the lesion are very characteristic.

Chordoma

Chordoma is a tumor of notochordal origin that is mainly seen in the sacrum and the clivus. Those originating at the clivus level usually grow and spread through the dura into the middle or posterior cranial fossa and compress the brain stem. They may extend anteriorly into the nasopharynx and frequently develop calcification. In T1-weighted MR images, a chordoma is seen as a moderately hypointense lesion that replace the hyperintense clival fat (Figure 39.56). On T2-weighted images chordomas are usually hyperintense, and calcifications that may be present are seen as hypointensities within the mass (Figure 39.57). CT will show the bony erosion and calcification to best advantage.

ORBITAL LESIONS

Orbital Tumors

Hemangiomas

Hemangiomas are the most common primary tumor of the orbit. Capillary hemangiomas are seen in childhood and cavernous hemangiomas in adults. Capillary hemangiomas

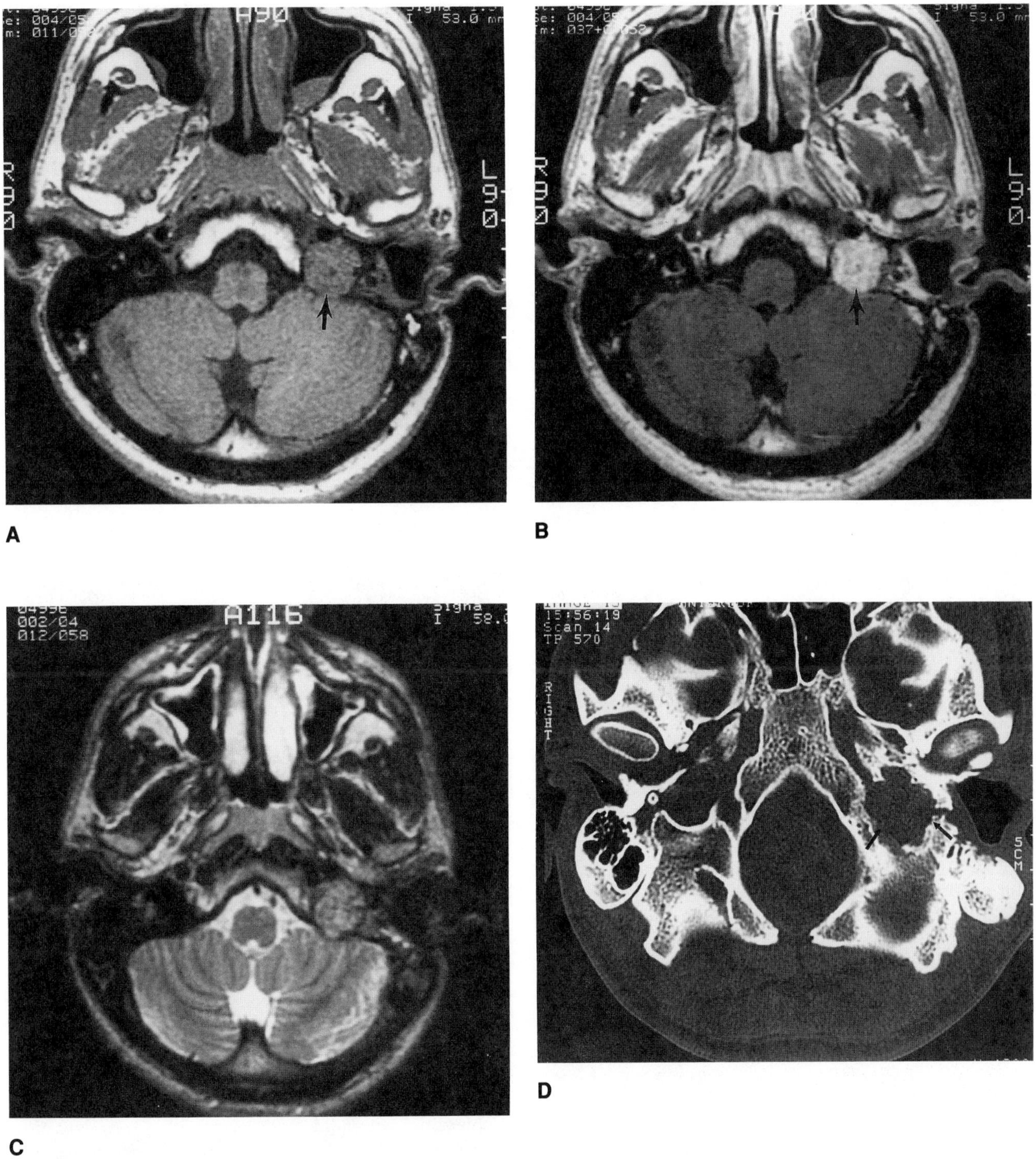

FIGURE 39.55 Glomus jugulare tumor. Axial T1-weighted images before (A) and after (B) intravenous administration of gadolinium show a lesion in the region of the jugular foramen, which enhances densely (arrows). C. Axial T2-weighted image demonstrates an iso- to hyperintense lesion, which has a few signal voids. D. CT scan using bone technique through the skull base shows erosion of the jugular foramen (arrows).

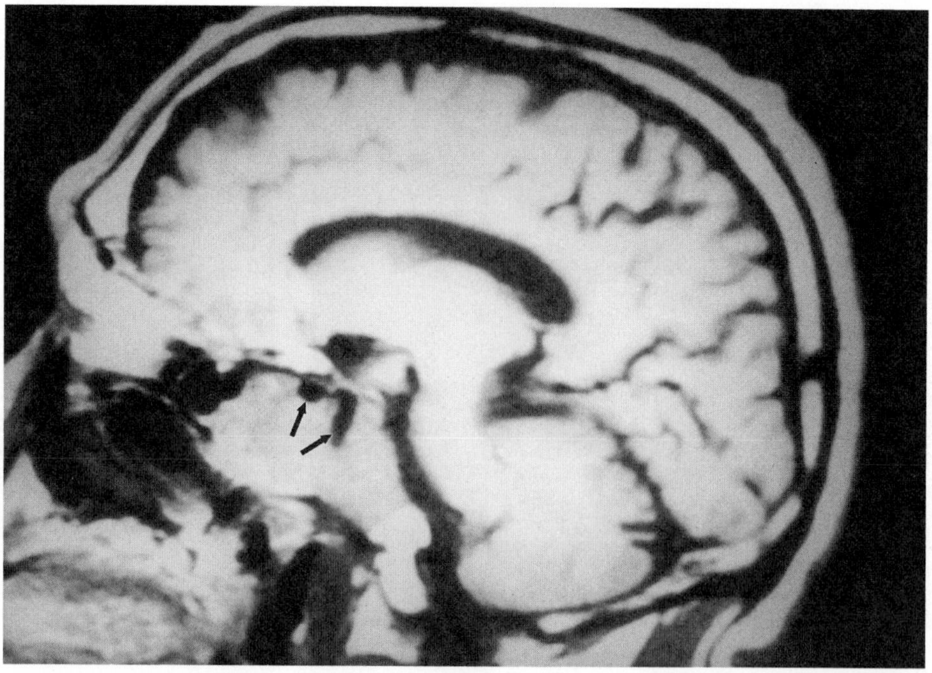

FIGURE 39.56 Clival chordoma. Sagittal T1-weighted image demonstrates lesion involving the clivus with destruction of the clivus and extension to the prepontine cistern and apparent encasement of the carotid artery (arrows).

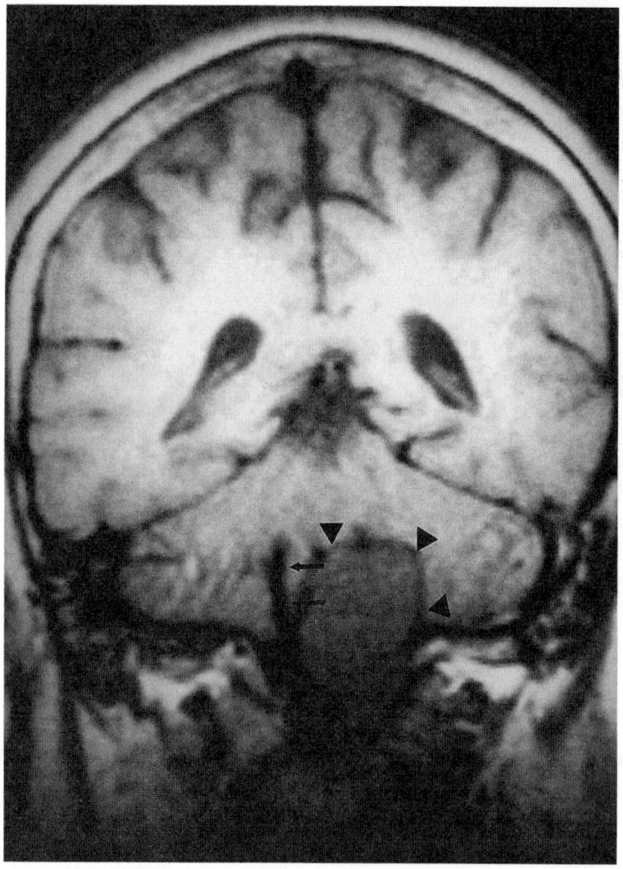

A

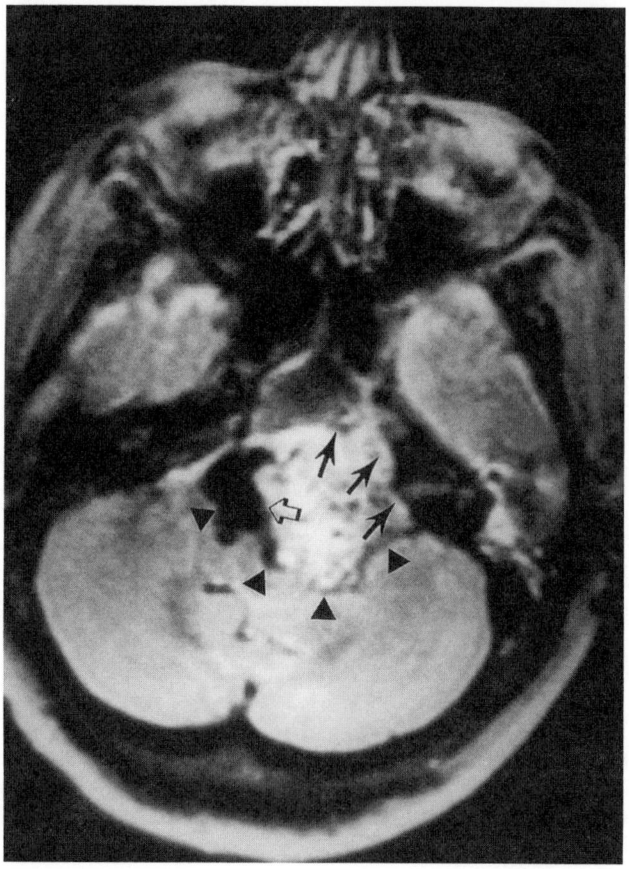

B

FIGURE 39.57 Chordoma. Coronal T1-weighted (A) and T2-weighted axial (B) images show a well-defined mass (arrowheads) present in the prepontine cistern. Its extra-axial nature is suspected because of the presence of erosion of the clivus and petrous apex (arrows in B). The small punctate areas that do not enhance are flecks of calcification within the tumor. The displaced basilar artery is outlined with arrows in A. The findings here are typical for a primary clival chordoma. A meningioma is the major differential possibility for an extra-axial mass in this location, but the presence of bone erosion (B) would be atypical. The large area of marked signal loss to the right of the lesion (open arrow) represents a combination flow void in the basilar artery and probable tumoral calcification.

appear during the neonatal period and not later than the first two-and-one-half years of life. They show an infiltrating growth (Figure 39.58) but may regress spontaneously. Cavernous hemangiomas have an insidious onset and never disappear on their own. They are well circumscribed and have an encapsulated pattern (Sklar et al. 1986). On imaging, the cavernous hemangioma demonstrates a well-circumscribed intraconal orbital lesion (Figure 39.59). On MRI these lesions are of low intensity on T1-weighted images, are markedly hyperintense on T2-weighted images, and enhance with contrast. With MRI one can determine the precise delineation of the mass and its relation to the optic nerve and muscle cone, which is important in the surgical planning.

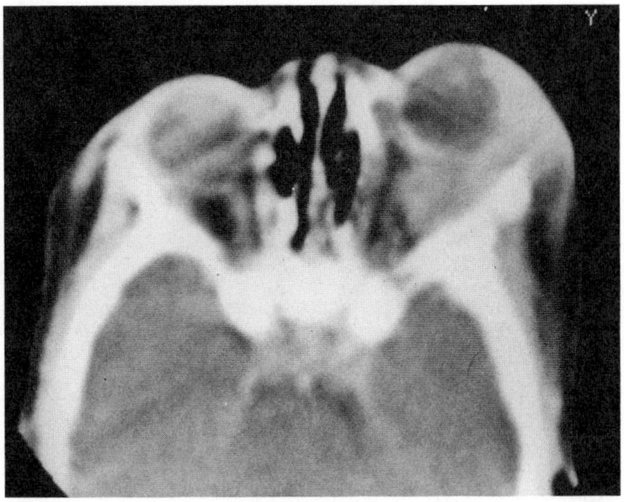

FIGURE 39.58 Capillary hemangioma. Orbital CT of a capillary hemangioma after administration of contrast material. A large mass is noted, primarily temporally within the left orbit. (Reprinted with permission from EML Sklar, RM Quencer, SF Byrne et al. Correlative study of the computed tomographic, ultrasonographic and pathologic characteristics of cavernous versus capillary hemangiomas of the orbit. J Clin Neuro-ophthalmol 1986;6:14–21.)

Lymphangioma

Lymphangioma is a vascular lesion that is less frequent than the hemangioma. Most of these lesions present at a young age. They show slow progressive growth without regression, and because they are likely to hemorrhage, sudden symptoms such as proptosis are possible. On MRI these lesions are heterogeneous with areas of hemorrhage of varying ages and with regions of cystic change.

Dermoid Lesions

Dermoid lesions are derived from congenital epithelial cell rests. They contain sebaceous glands and other skin appendages. In their growth, they may expand the inner and outer tables of the skull and produce sharply demarcated bone defects with well-defined borders and slightly sclerotic margins. The usual site is in the orbital roof, near the orbital zygomatic suture, and the growth extends to involve the frontal bone. Less often they arise in the lateral wall and rarely in the inferior wall. Focal areas of fat are easily identified on MR. These lesions do not usually enhance.

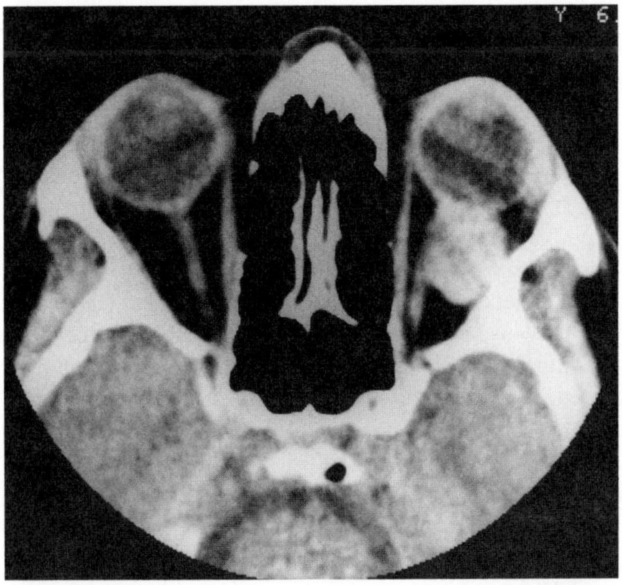

FIGURE 39.59 Cavernous hemangioma. Orbital CT shows a well-circumscribed intraconal mass located in the temporal portion of the left muscle cone. (Reprinted with permission from EML Sklar, RM Quencer, SF Byrne et al. Correlative study of the computed tomographic, ultrasonographic and pathologic characteristics of cavernous versus capillary hemangiomas of the orbit. J Clin Neuro-ophthalmol 1986;6:14–21.)

Orbital Pseudotumor

An inflammatory lesion with acute onset usually occurring in middle age, orbital pseudotumor is difficult to differentiate clinically from a true orbital tumor. Some show spontaneous recovery, while others require aggressive therapy, including systemic or local corticosteroid therapy or orbital decompression.

Pseudotumor causes diffuse inflammation and resultant edema. Thickening of the sclera may be seen (uveal-scleral pseudotumor), whereas in other cases there is a mass, extraocular muscle thickening, or diffuse orbital infiltration. Fluid surrounding the optic nerve may be seen as a thickened optic nerve. Obliteration of retrobulbar fat planes may be seen, as well as an isolated lacrimal or retrobulbar mass. If the insertion of an extraocular muscle into the globe is involved, pseudotumor is a more likely diagnosis than thyroid eye disease.

On MRI, these lesions are isointense to muscle on T1-weighted images, but on T2-weighted images they are hyperintense, making a distinction between pseudotumor and lymphoma possible, since orbital lymphoma is most commonly hypointense on T2-weighted images.

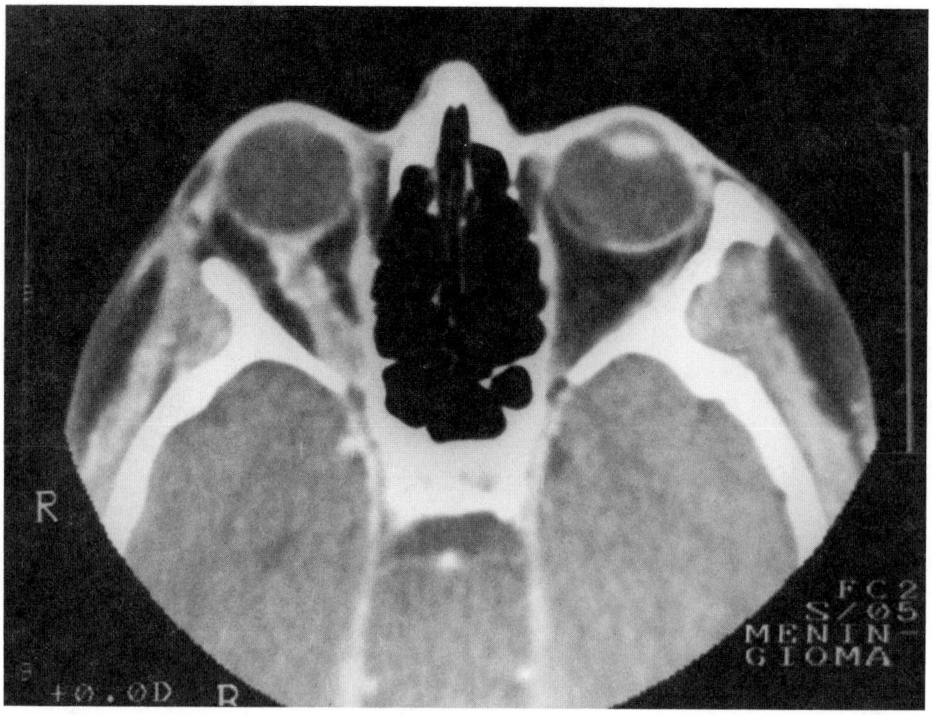

FIGURE 39.60 Optic nerve meningioma. Contrast-enhanced CT shows the typical thickening and peripheral enhancement of the right optic nerve characteristic of a perioptic meningioma. Extension from the intrascleral portion of the optic nerve posteriorly to the orbital apex is noted.

Optic Nerve Glioma

Optic gliomas are low-grade pilocytic astrocytomas, which may be isolated abnormalities or may be associated with neurofibromatosis, especially if bilateral. Three-fourths present by age 10 years. Some gliomas have extensive thickening of the perioptic meninges (peritumoral arachnoidal hyperplasia), which may be characteristic of patients with neurofibromatosis (Atlas 1991).

Optic nerve gliomas are isointense to normal white matter on T1-weighted images, and enhancement with contrast is common. In evaluating a patient with an optic glioma, the entire visual pathway needs to be studied, since a large number of these tumors involve the chiasm (see Figure 39.17) and retrochiasmal pathways extending to the level of the lateral geniculate bodies (Atlas 1991). A significant proportion of visual pathway gliomas are restricted to the chiasm and retrochiasmal tracts, sparing the intraorbital optic nerve. The signal intensity varies with the site of involvement of the visual pathway (Atlas 1991). Specifically, intraorbital optic nerve masses are of relatively low intensity on T2-weighted images, which may correlate with arachnoid hyperplasia. The chiasmal and retrochiasmal lesions tend to be hyperintense on T2-weighted images.

Optic Nerve Meningioma

Perioptic meningiomas account for one-third of primary tumors of the optic nerve or sheath. Bilateral perioptic meningiomas may be associated with neurofibromatosis. In general, perioptic meningiomas are most common in adults and optic nerve gliomas occur in children.

These lesions frequently calcify and enhance markedly on CT (Figure 39.60). MRI has a major advantage in evaluating optic nerve lesions; MRI allows visualization of the optic nerve directly and separates it from surrounding subarachnoid space and therefore distinguishes optic nerve lesions from sheath lesions. MRI can also evaluate the intracanalicular portion of the optic nerve (Atlas 1991). MRI signal intensity patterns are variable depending on the site of the lesions (i.e., perioptic versus extraconal intraorbital location). The majority of perioptic meningiomas enhance with contrast, and fat-suppression techniques with contrast are very helpful in delineating regions of gadolinium enhancement.

Ocular Lesions

Melanoma

Malignant melanoma is the most common intraocular malignancy in adults and is usually unilateral. MRI aids in the differential diagnosis of these lesions, since there are other entities (such as choroidal metastases, choroidal nevi, choroidal hemangiomas, sarcoidosis, granulomas, and choroidal detachment) that can simulate a melanoma. Also, MRI helps delineate extraocular extension, which occurs in 13% of cases.

On MRI, melanomas are focal masses that extend into the vitreous (Atlas 1991) and enhance after contrast, a characteristic common to most ocular neoplasms (Figure 39.61). In one series, the majority of melanomas were hyperintense on T1-weighted images and on T2-weighted images were hypointense due to their content of melanin, which has the paramagnetic characteristic of shortening of T1 and T2 re-

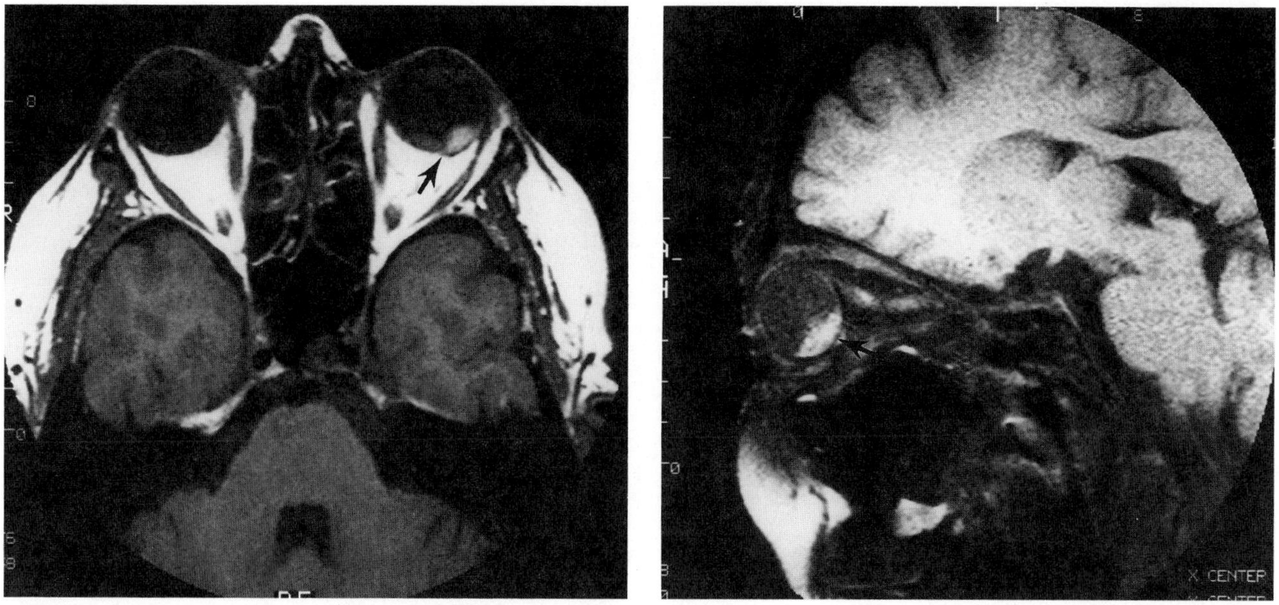

A B

FIGURE 39.61 Choroidal melanoma. A. Axial T1-weighted image demonstrates a lesion in the posterior aspect of the globe, which is partially hyperintense (arrows). This is consistent with a melanotic melanoma. B. Sagittal fat-suppressed image shows the hyperintense lesion located in the inferior aspect of the globe (arrow). No retrobulbar extension is seen.

laxation times. Melanomas, however, may vary in their degree of pigmentation, and lesions may be amelanotic and then indistinguishable from other ocular lesions.

These lesions can be confusing because they can exhibit varying paramagnetic behavior when they are melanotic or hemorrhagic and they are frequently associated with hemorrhagic retinal detachments. In general, MRI can distinguish a melanotic melanoma from an associated hemorrhagic (or nonhemorrhagic) subretinal fluid collection and from an amelanotic neoplasm on the basis of their intensity signals.

Retinoblastoma

Retinoblastoma is the most common intraocular malignancy of childhood. The average age at diagnosis is 18 months. The roles for imaging include (1) to limit the diagnostic possibilities since the differential of leukokoria (reflection from a white mass within the eye giving the appearance of a white pupil) is extensive; (2) to define the extension of the lesion since retinoblastoma can spread in a variety of ways, including to the retrobulbar orbit and to the CSF spaces, seeding the CNS; and (3) to determine if the contralateral orbit is affected since bilateral lesions are common (up to one-third of patients). Also, the "trilateral" retinoblastoma (bilateral retinoblastoma associated with a pineal tumor) can be detected by MRI.

On MRI, retinoblastoma has variable signal intensity. Histopathologically, retinoblastoma is very similar to other PNET tumors of the CNS and therefore has signal intensity patterns similar to them. These tumors also demonstrate hemorrhage and necrosis. The classic CT finding of retinoblastoma is retinal calcification. Because of the insensitivity of MRI for calcification, CT remains the initial diagnostic imaging study of choice when a retinoblastoma is suspected (Atlas 1991).

SPINAL LESIONS

Spinal Tumors

Extramedullary Intradural Tumors

The two most common extramedullary intradural tumors are the neurinoma (or neurilemmoma) and meningioma. As with any other extramedullary intradural mass lesion, these tumors cause displacement of the cord and widening of the ipsilateral subarachnoid space.

Nerve Sheath Tumors. Nerve sheath tumors are the most common intraspinal neoplasm. Neurinomas can occur at any spinal level, are equally common in both sexes, and often present in the fourth decade of life. Although these tumors are most commonly extramedullary intradural in location, they can also be purely extradural or dumbbell-shaped, with both an extradural and an intradural component.

On MRI these tumors tend to have slightly increased intensity compared with muscle in T1- and T2-weighted images. These lesions enhance intensely and homogeneously (Figure 39.62), except when there is an intratumoral cyst.

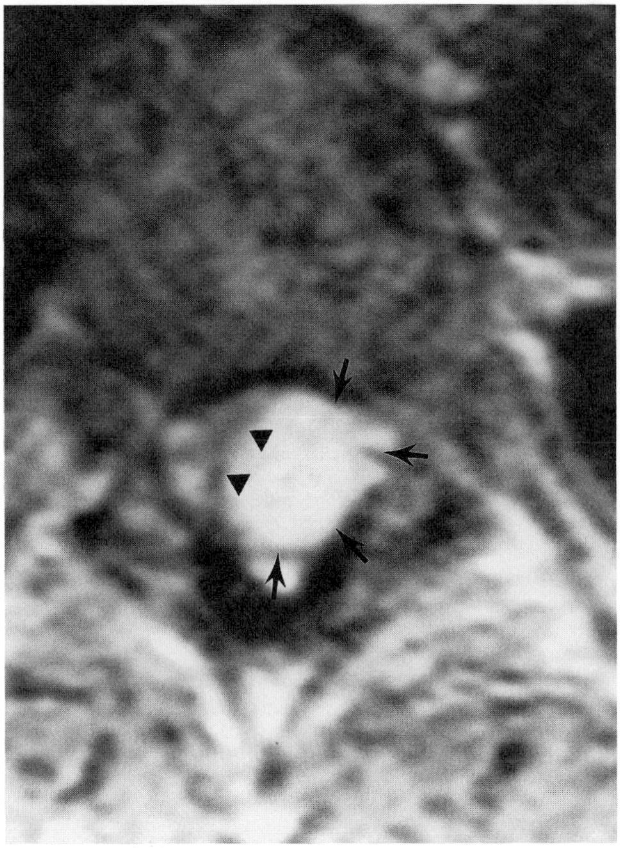

A

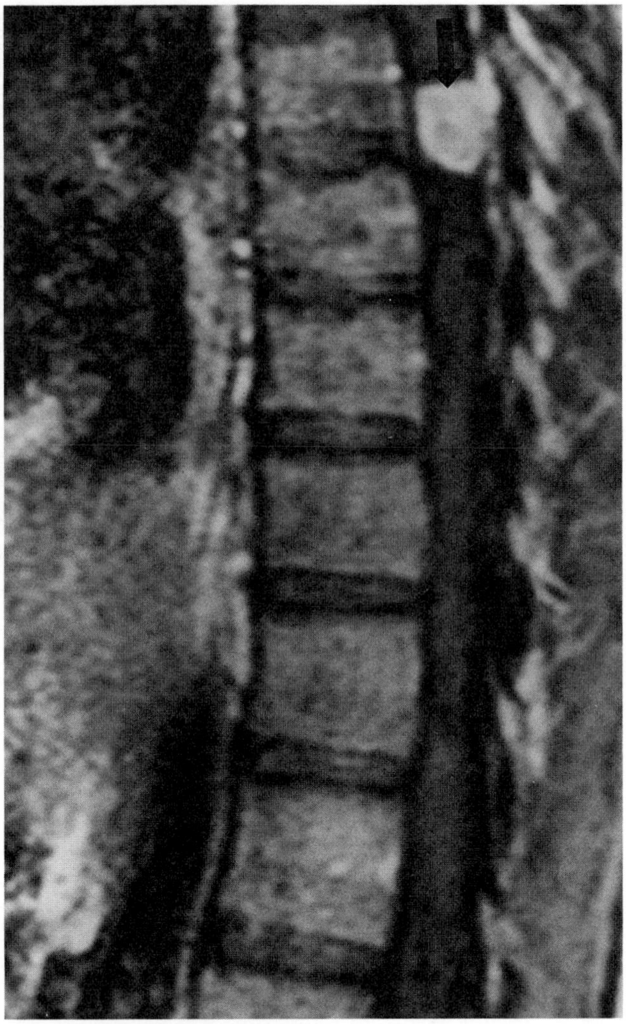

B

FIGURE 39.62 Neurofibroma. Postgadolinium T1-weighted axial (A) and (B) sagittal images demonstrate an enhancing intradural extramedullary mass (arrows) on the left, displacing the cord (arrowheads) to the right. C. On intraoperative spinal sonography in a sagittal plane, the mass is noted displacing the cord anteriorly (arrows).

C

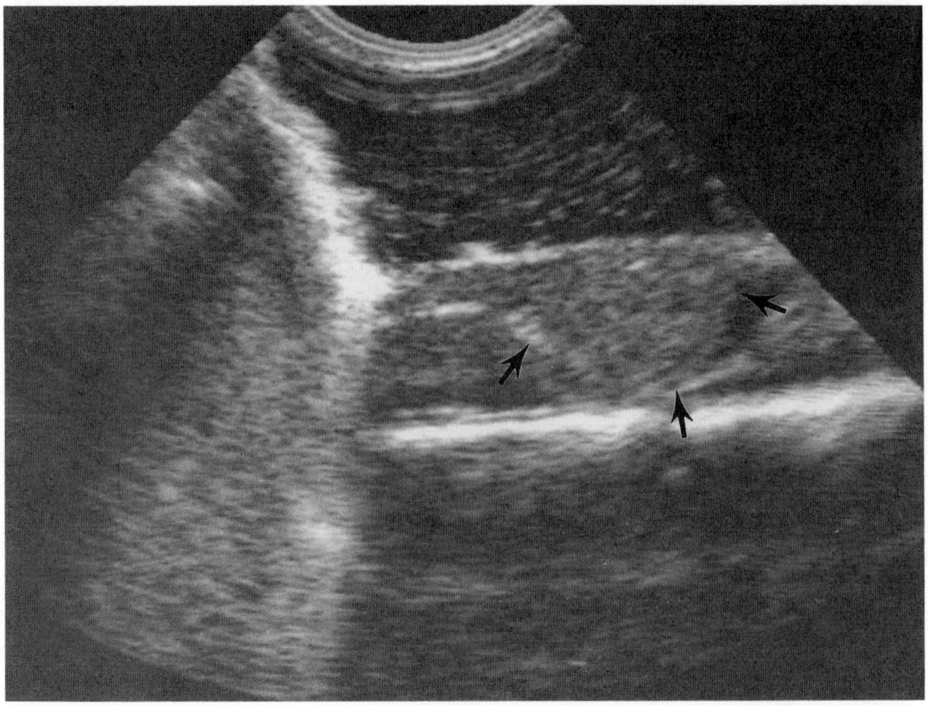

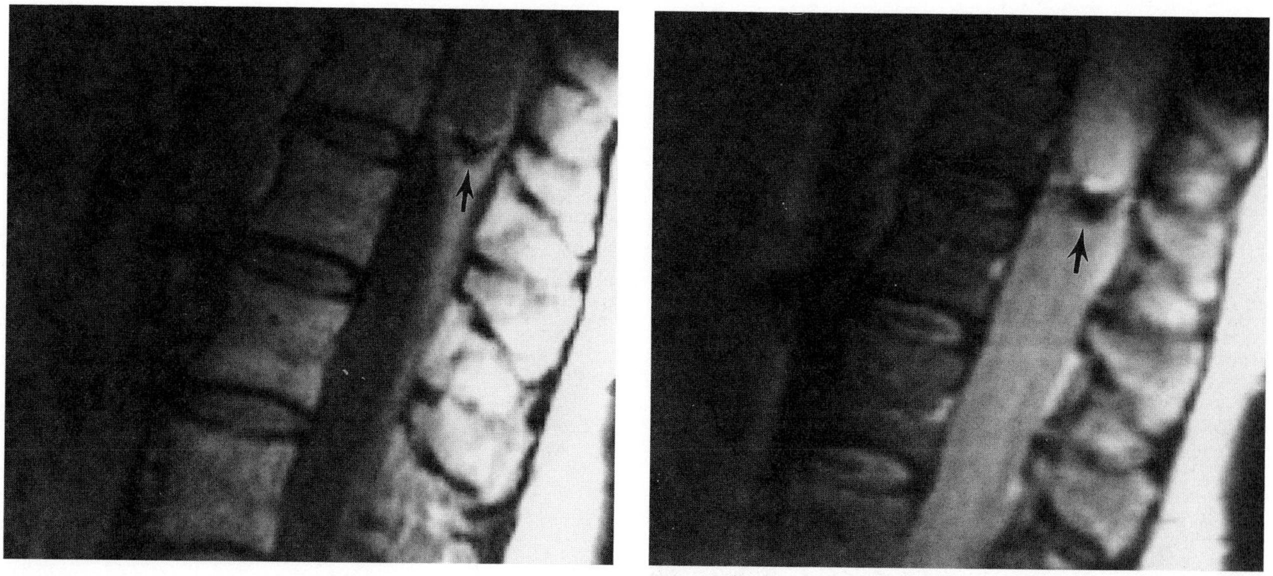

A B

FIGURE 39.63 Ependymoma. T1 (A) and T2 (B) sagittal images demonstrate spinal cord widening at the conus. The lesion is hypointense on short TR images and hyperintense on long TR images. Hemosiderin deposition is noted at the inferior borders of the tumor (arrows).

Meningiomas. Meningiomas are typically found in adults. They usually occur in the thoracic spine or at the foramen magnum and are seen more frequently in females than males. They are primarily extramedullary and intradural in location, but they can also be both intradural and extradural or purely extradural.

On MRI, with short TR images these lesions are hypo- to isointense to spinal cord, and T2-weighted images show meningiomas to be slightly hyperintense to the spinal cord. These lesions enhance relatively homogeneously and intensely after gadolinium administration.

Intramedullary Tumors

In the extradural and in the extramedullary intradural space, MRI has proved to be as effective as CT myelography (CTM) while being noninvasive (Atlas 1991). However, for lesions within the cord, MRI is superior to CTM. Although noncontrast MRI scans generally detect lesions, gadolinium can help in further delineating them.

Astrocytomas. The peak incidence of spinal astrocytomas is in the third and fourth decades of life, but they are not uncommon in children. They are most often located in the thoracic cord, but in children holocord involvement can be found.

On MRI with T1-weighted images astrocytomas are hypointense to normal cord, while on T2-weighted images they are hyperintense. The margins of the lesions are poorly defined. After intravenous contrast administration, these lesions almost always enhance, either with a homogeneous or inhomogeneous pattern. MRI is also helpful in distinguishing tumor cysts from benign cysts associated with tumor; tumor cysts are surrounded by enhancement while the walls of benign cysts lack enhancement.

Ependymomas. Ependymoma usually presents in patients in the fourth and fifth decades of life, in men more commonly than women. It is the most common primary cord tumor of the lower spinal cord, conus medullaris, and filum terminale.

Noncontrast MRI demonstrates cord widening (Figures 39.63 and 39.64). The lesion is hypointense or hyperintense on T2-weighted images. Areas of hemorrhage may appear and intratumoral cysts are common. Hemosiderin deposition is frequently encountered at the superior and inferior borders (see Figures 39.63 and 39.64). After intravenous contrast, ependymomas tend to enhance intensely and homogeneously.

Extradural Tumors

Metastases are the most common of the extradural tumors. They can cause destruction of the vertebral bodies and can extend into the spinal canal, causing displacement of the subarachnoid space and spinal cord. The tumor and adjacent bony changes, as well as the extent of the epidural and paraspinal involvement, are well demonstrated on MR (Figure 39.65).

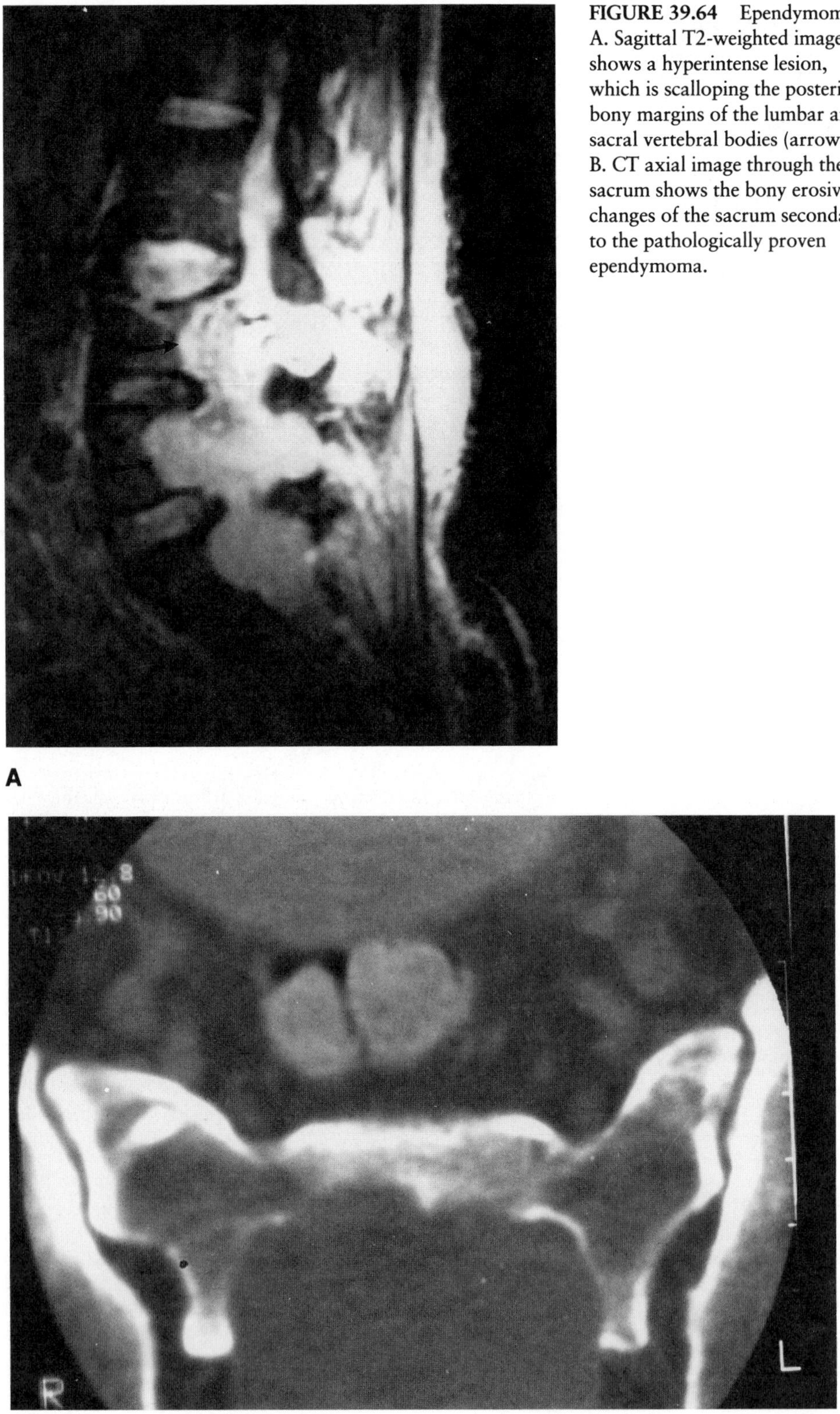

A

B

FIGURE 39.64 Ependymoma. A. Sagittal T2-weighted image shows a hyperintense lesion, which is scalloping the posterior bony margins of the lumbar and sacral vertebral bodies (arrows). B. CT axial image through the sacrum shows the bony erosive changes of the sacrum secondary to the pathologically proven ependymoma.

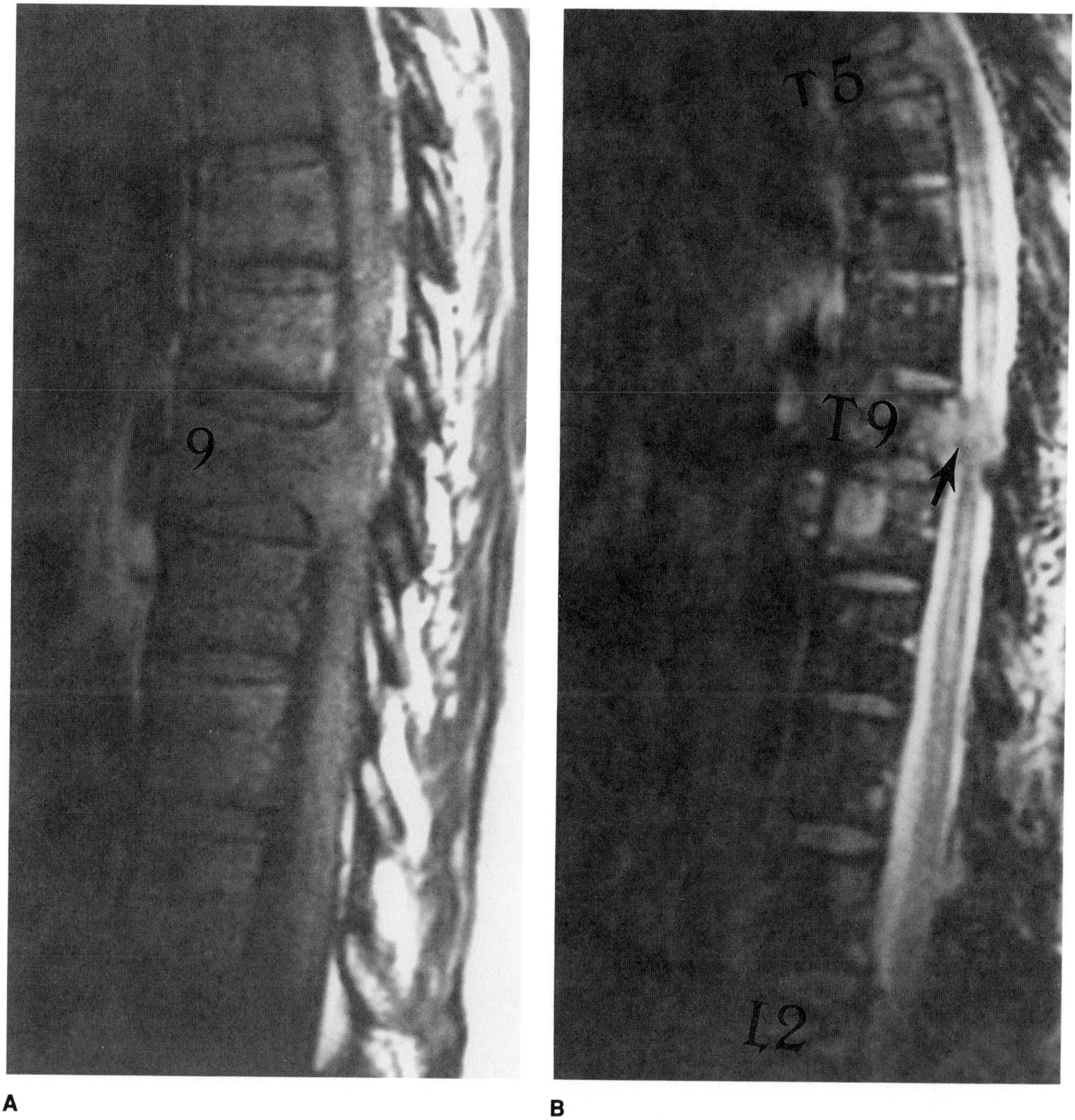

FIGURE 39.65 Spinal metastases. A. Sagittal T1-weighted image demonstrates a metastatic lesion involving the T9 body with epidural extension of soft-tissue tumor into the ventral aspect of the canal. B. On T2-weighted image (with a larger field of view) multiple levels are involved with high signal lesions. Also, there is compression of T5, T9, and L2. Epidural extension of tumor is noted at T9 with compression of the cord (arrows).

Degenerative Disease of the Spine

Degenerative Disc Disease (see Chapter 78)

As an intervertebral disc degenerates, it loses water, and fibrous tissue replaces nuclear material as the disc collapses. Annular fibers weaken, resulting in disc bulging, and annular tears predispose to disc herniation.

Disc Herniation. A *bulging disc* is one that extends diffusely beyond the adjacent vertebral body margins, though the concentric annular fibers are intact. An *extruded disc* is one that extends through all the layers of the annulus and appears as a focal soft-tissue mass (Figure 39.66). These disc herniations may be subligamentous (anterior to the posterior longitudinal ligament) or may rupture through and be posterior to the posterior longi-

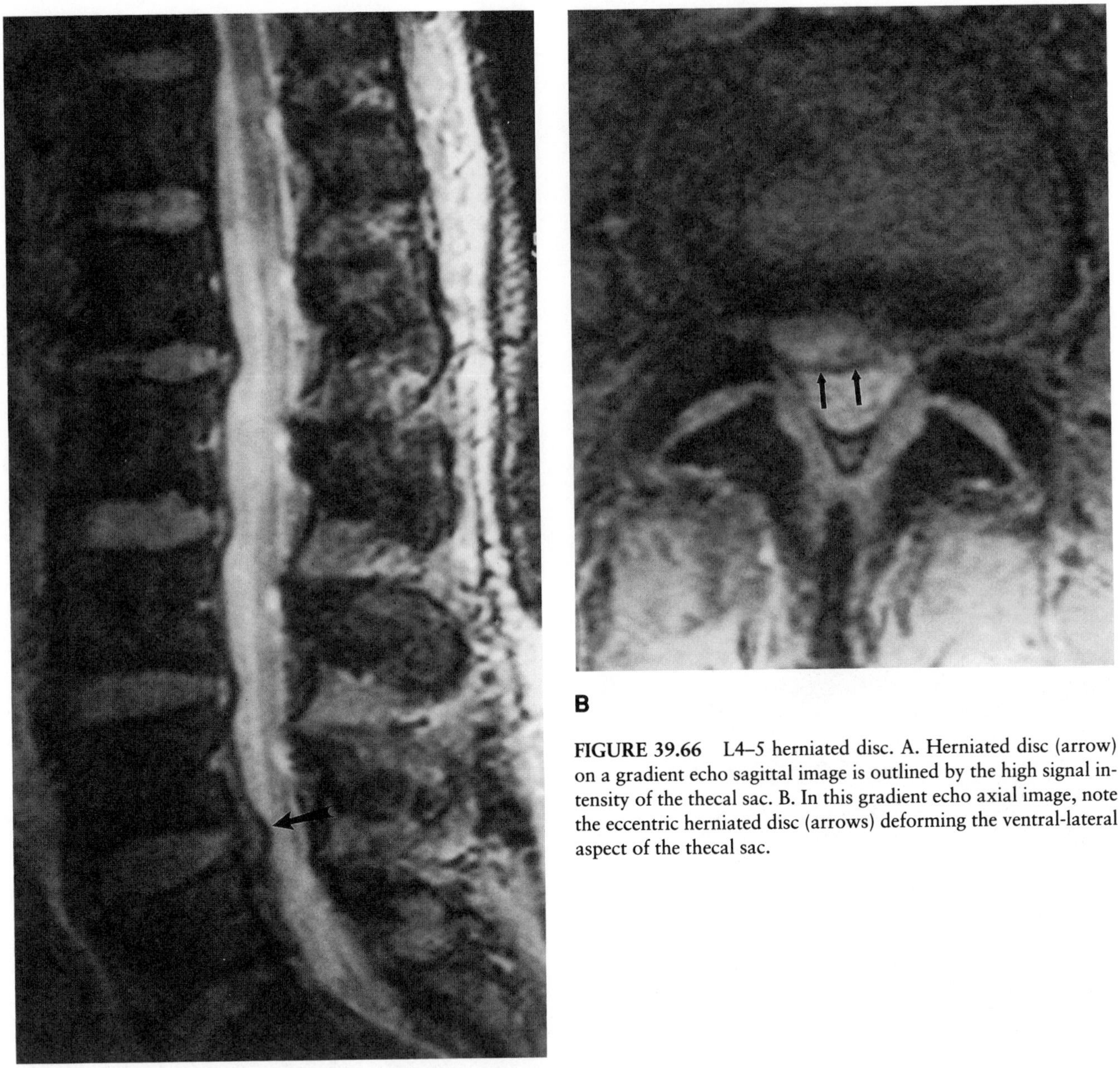

A

B

FIGURE 39.66 L4–5 herniated disc. A. Herniated disc (arrow) on a gradient echo sagittal image is outlined by the high signal intensity of the thecal sac. B. In this gradient echo axial image, note the eccentric herniated disc (arrows) deforming the ventral-lateral aspect of the thecal sac.

tudinal ligament. A free disc fragment is herniated disc material that has separated from the parent disc and may migrate to a position quite removed from the original disc space. Approximately 90% of lumbar herniated discs occur at L4–5 or L5–S1, 7% at the L3–4 level, and 3% at L1–2 or L2–3.

On MRI, most bulging discs extend beyond the vertebral body margin in a diffuse manner and have decreased signal intensity on T2-weighted images because of disc degeneration and loss of water, whereas a herniated disc is seen as a focal soft-tissue mass displacing the epidural fat or thecal sac (see Figure 39.66) and can show enhancement along the periphery of the disc because of the presence of reactive vascular connective tissue.

Spinal Stenosis and Spondylosis

The most common degenerative process of the spine is *spondylosis deformans* (*osteophytosis*). Osteophytes occur because of underlying disc disease (Atlas 1991). Osteoarthritis refers to degenerative arthritis involving the synovial joints such as the facet joints. These terms are often used synonymously because the conditions often coexist. Both lead to narrowing of the spinal canal or neural foramina and as a result can cause cord compression, root entrapment, or both.

Lumbar Spinal Stenosis. The term *lumbar spinal stenosis* includes stenosis of the spinal canal, the lateral recess, and

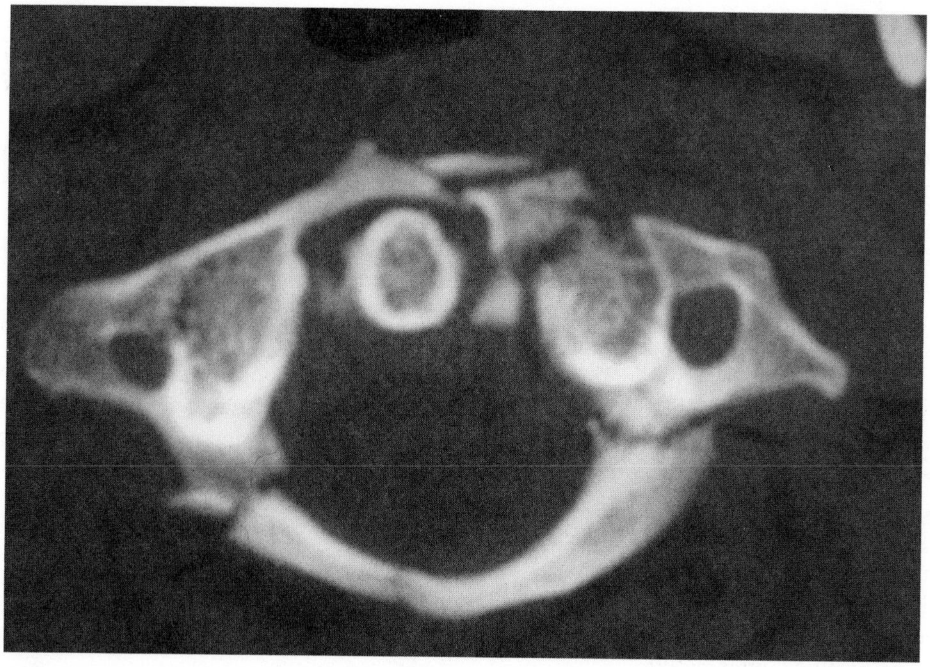

A

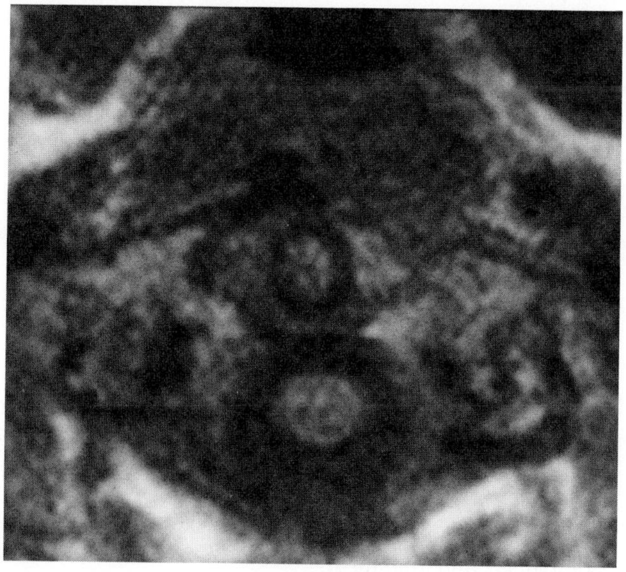

B

FIGURE 39.67 Jefferson fracture. A. Axial CT shows multiple fracture through C1. B. MRI at the same level is shown to demonstrate the difficulty frequently encountered in diagnosing fractures with MR. The spinal cord and the surrounding subarachnoid space at the level are normal.

the foramina. Canal stenosis is most common at L2–3 to L4–5 and causes radiculopathy. Stenosis may be due to a combination of diffuse disc bulging, facet hypertrophy, and ligamentous thickening.

Cervical Spinal Stenosis. Cervical canal stenosis is most often due to spondylosis deformans and ligamentous thickening (Atlas 1991). Foraminal stenosis is due to hypertrophy of the uncinate process and superior articular facet. Patients are at particular risk for myelopathy or radiculopathy if the anteroposterior diameter of the cervical canal is less than 11 mm.

T2*-weighted gradient echo images are most effective for evaluating cervical spondylosis because spurs can be distinguished from discs and the anteroposterior diameter of the canal can be measured. CT scans have been considered the procedure of choice for the diagnosis of neural foraminal stenosis. However, with three-dimensional gradient-echo techniques, thin sections may be obtained to evaluate the neural foramina, and the accuracy of these approaches that of high-resolution CT myelography.

Spinal Trauma

Imaging plays a key role in evaluating spinal trauma because the information obtained facilitates the surgical and clinical management of acute and chronic spinal injuries. In choosing a particular imaging protocol, numerous factors should be taken into account. These include the neurologic status of the patient, the level of injury, the age of the lesion, and the potential benefit that might be derived from each of the different imaging modalities.

Plain radiography remains indispensable in evaluating bony injury and is the foundation on which the initial clinical treatment of spinal injuries is based. CT has replaced conventional tomography in the evaluation of bony injuries to the spine (Figure 39.67), and advances in CT technology with spiral CT allow extremely rapid acquisition of CT data. The ability of helical CT to reformat slices in a multiplanar format allows total bony assessment. These examinations should be tailored using plain x-ray films to localize the area of concern. Advantages of CT include the ability to assess the spinal canal and impingement by bony fragments and to evaluate the paravertebral soft tissues.

MRI in patients with acute or chronic spinal cord injuries allows visualization of soft-tissue (particularly spinal cord) abnormalities such as edema, hemorrhage, cysts, and subarachnoid cysts. CTM with nonionic contrast agents is used when MR is not available or cannot be performed. CTM may be indicated in the evaluation of nerve root avulsions and dural tears. Intraoperative sonography plays an important role in monitoring the surgical procedures used to treat patients with both acute and chronic spinal trauma (Quencer 1988).

Spinal Injury and Associated Osseous Abnormalities

A three-column approach to spinal trauma was described by Denis in 1983 with reference to spinal stability and neurologic sequelae. The *anterior column* includes the anterior longitudinal ligament, anterior annulus fibrosus, and anterior vertebral body. The *middle column* includes the posterior longitudinal ligament, posterior annulus fibrosus, and posterior vertebral body. The *posterior column* consists of all structures posterior to the posterior longitudinal ligament. Stability is present when the middle column is intact.

Classically, certain forces and mechanisms have been described as responsible for particular injuries. These include flexion, extension, rotation, axial compression, distraction, shearing, and often a combination of these. Various forces and injury classification schemes are based on these mechanisms.

Hyperflexion Injuries. Flexion injuries comprise the majority of fractures of the thoracolumbar region. Flexion results in compression of the anterior column. On sagittal views, loss of height of the vertebral bodies may be appreciated. The "seat belt" injury (*Chance fracture*) is one type of flexion distraction injury. The majority of these occur from L1 to L3. A seat belt injury produces a horizontal fracture of the vertebral body, pedicles, laminae, and spinous processes, as well as disruption of the ligaments and distraction of the intervertebral disc and facet joint. These injuries are unstable because the middle column is affected.

Axial Compression Fracture. In axial compression fractures, vertical compression forces cause the intervertebral disc to herniate through the endplate and result in "bursting" of the vertebra from within. There is disruption of the anterior and middle columns. These injuries usually occur from T4 to L5 and are most common at L1. Radiographs show widened interpediculate distance, vertical vertebral fracture, anterior wedging, and retropulsed bony fragments. CT and MRI show equally well the compromise of the spinal canal caused by displaced fracture fragments, but the cord is better shown by MRI.

Spinal Injury and Soft-Tissue Abnormalities

Cord Injuries. MRI is best able to detect traumatic cord injury. With MRI, T1- and T2-weighted images are acquired both in the sagittal and axial planes. These images show intracanalicular bone fragments, herniated discs, and extradural hematomas and their effect on the cord. They also depict hemorrhage and edema in the cord.

Edema and hemorrhage in the cord cause swelling within hours of an acute spinal cord injury. Edema is shown as high signal zones on T2-weighted images and usually less well as low signal on T1-weighted images (Figure 39.68). Hemorrhagic cord injuries (Figure 39.69) are best demonstrated on gradient echo T2* images, because of the sensitivity of that pulse sequence to acute blood (Quencer 1988). The prognosis for neurological improvement is extremely poor if blood rather than edema is seen in an injured spinal cord. If only edema and not hemorrhage is identified in the cord, some neurologic improvement may be seen, and if improvement does not occur there may be a previously undetected abnormality such as a herniated disc, extradural hematoma, or bone fragment compressing the cord.

Extradural Lesions

Traumatic disc herniations are usually single but may be multiple. In one series, the cervical spine was the most frequent site of involvement (Figure 39.70). In patients with fracture dislocations who are to undergo stabilization, the discovery of an associated herniated disc may indicate the need for a prompt surgical intervention, specifically a decompressive anterior discectomy and fusion. Spinal epidural hematomas are focal collections of blood located outside the dura, which must be decompressed immediately if rapid progression of neurological dysfunction occurs. These lesions are well demonstrated with MRI.

Sonography

Intraoperative sonography has been recommended for cases in which stabilization procedures for acute spine injuries are performed. Real-time sector scanning helps define the relationship of bone fragments and disc material to the spinal cord and subarachnoid sac and helps identify edema, hemorrhage, and alignment.

Chronic Sequelae of Spinal Cord Trauma

Posttraumatic spinal cord cysts (Figure 39.71) are cavitations within the spinal cord that develop after severe trauma to the spinal cord. They may occur at all levels of the spinal cord and may progress from one level to another either in a cephalad or caudal direction from the prior site of trauma (Quencer et al. 1986). Even though previously quiescent, they can cause new or progressive neurologic deficits that develop months to years after the original injury. A multilevel examination may be required as they may be quite large and extend well beyond the site of the original injury. Sagittal and axial T1-weighted sequences and a sagittal T2-weighted scan are recommended in the evaluation.

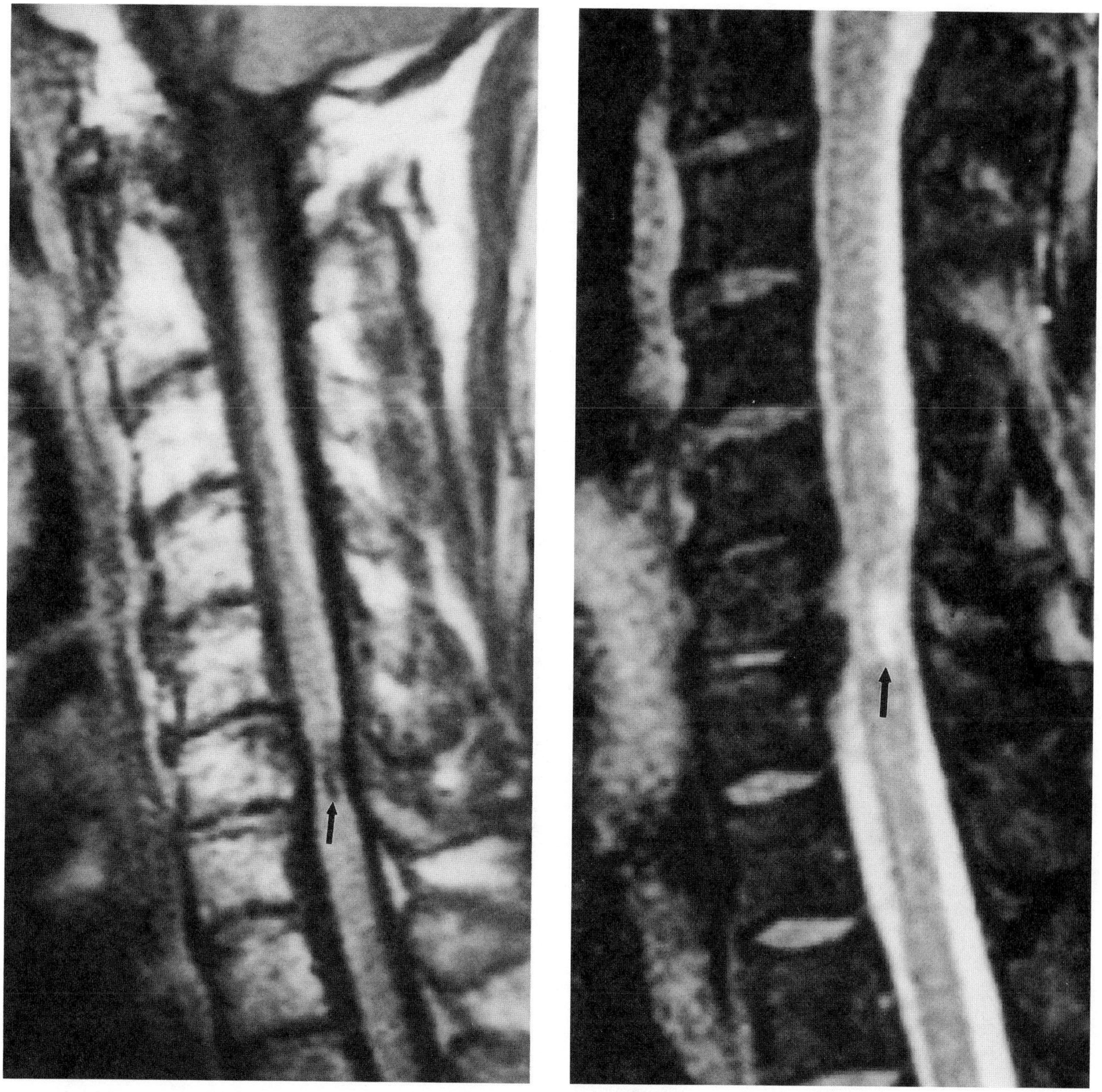

A B

FIGURE 39.68 Cord edema. A. Focal lesion in the cord, which is hypointense on T1-weighted image (A) and hyperintense on T2-weighted image (B), consistent with an area of edema (arrows) in patient with acute spine injury. On the T2-weighted image, the markedly hypointense areas at C5–6 and C6–7 disc spaces represent calcified osteophytes.

One needs to distinguish myelomalacia from cyst, as the latter requires a different clinical approach (Figure 39.72). Although this distinction may be difficult, certain features may be helpful. A spinal cord cyst usually has a sharp interface on T1-weighted images between the hypointense area within the cord and surrounding normal cord. There is usually no internal signal within the cord cyst, which usually extends through several levels. If the lesion is small, the distinction between a nonpulsatile cyst and myelomalacia is clinically less important because cysts of that size are usually not shunted.

Subarachnoid cysts (SACs) may occur as a sequela of trauma. MRI is the most efficient preoperative study in diagnosing and characterizing acquired SACs and associated abnormalities. An SAC is seen as a low-intensity signal collection on T1-weighted images that are high intensity on T2-weighted images, paralleling CSF intensity. These collections usually produce mass effect with indentation of the cord. In some instances, the SAC may be loculated and not in direct communication with the subarachnoid space. In other cases, the cyst freely communicates with the subarachnoid space.

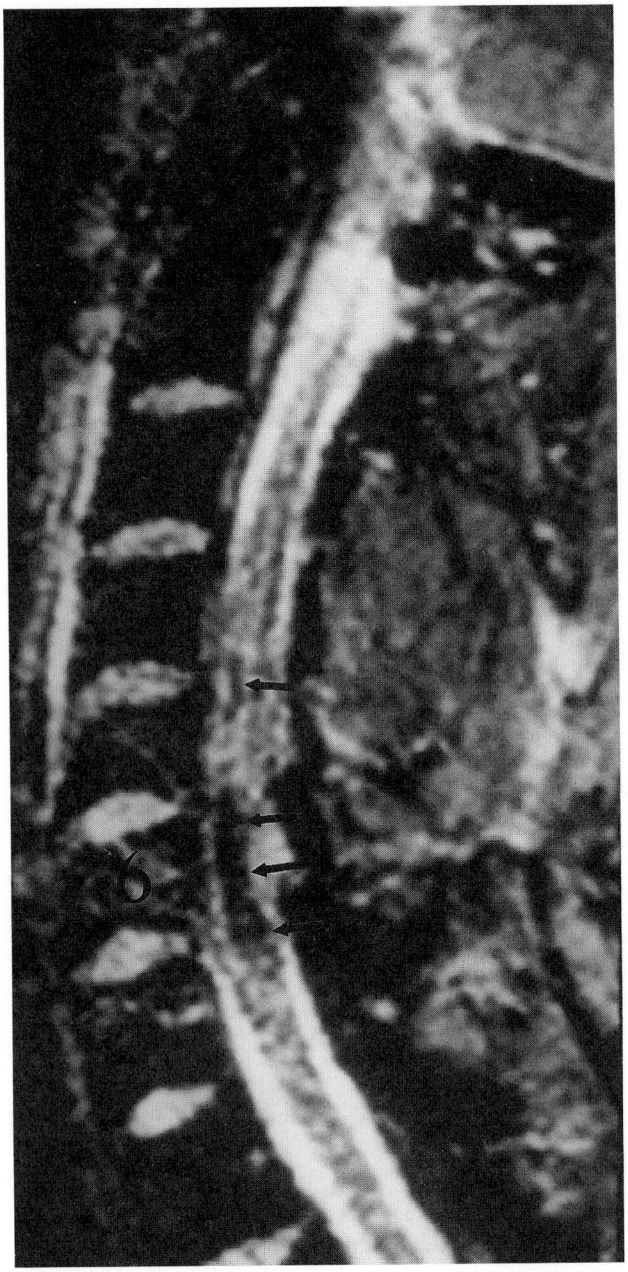

FIGURE 39.69 Cord hematoma. T2* gradient echo sagittal image shows hypointensity within the cord from C4 to C7 (arrows) consistent with acute hemorrhage (deoxyhemoglobin) in the cord.

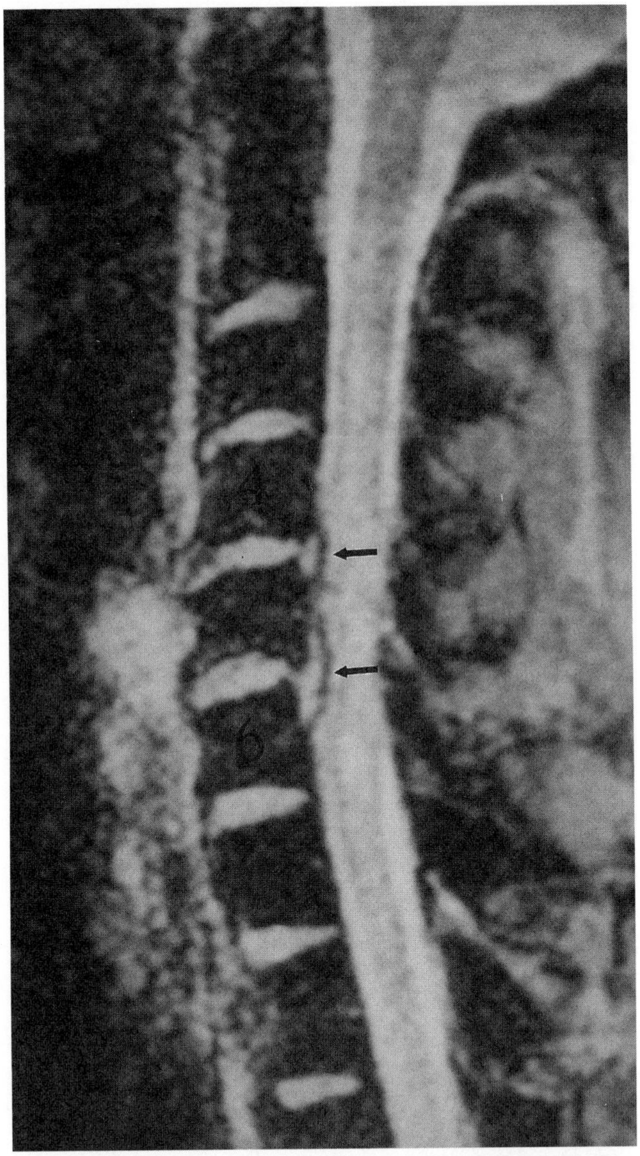

FIGURE 39.70 Posttraumatic cervical herniated disc. Gradient echo sagittal image demonstrates cervical herniated discs at the C4–5 and C5–6 levels (arrows).

Infection of the Spine (see Chapter 78)

Infections of the spine often involve the vertebral body or disc space. The organism most often implicated is *Staphylococcus aureus* (60% of infections), even in AIDS patients (Post et al. 1988). Although CT is useful in detecting bone destruction associated with vertebral osteomyelitis, its depiction of the intraspinal soft tissue structures is limited. Because MRI is able to detect bony changes earlier and is able to show associated soft-tissue abnormalities, it is the imaging study of choice for the evaluation of inflammatory disease of the spine.

Discitis and Vertebral Osteomyelitis

Pyogenic Infections. Pyogenic infections have a peak incidence in the sixth to seventh decades. Infectious spondylitis involves both the vertebral body and adjacent disc space. The most common site of pyogenic infection is the cancellous bone adjacent to the endplate, due to its rich vascularity. The infection then spreads into the disc space. Two-thirds of patients have infection limited to the disc space and the adjacent vertebral bodies, and one-fourth have involvement at more than one level.

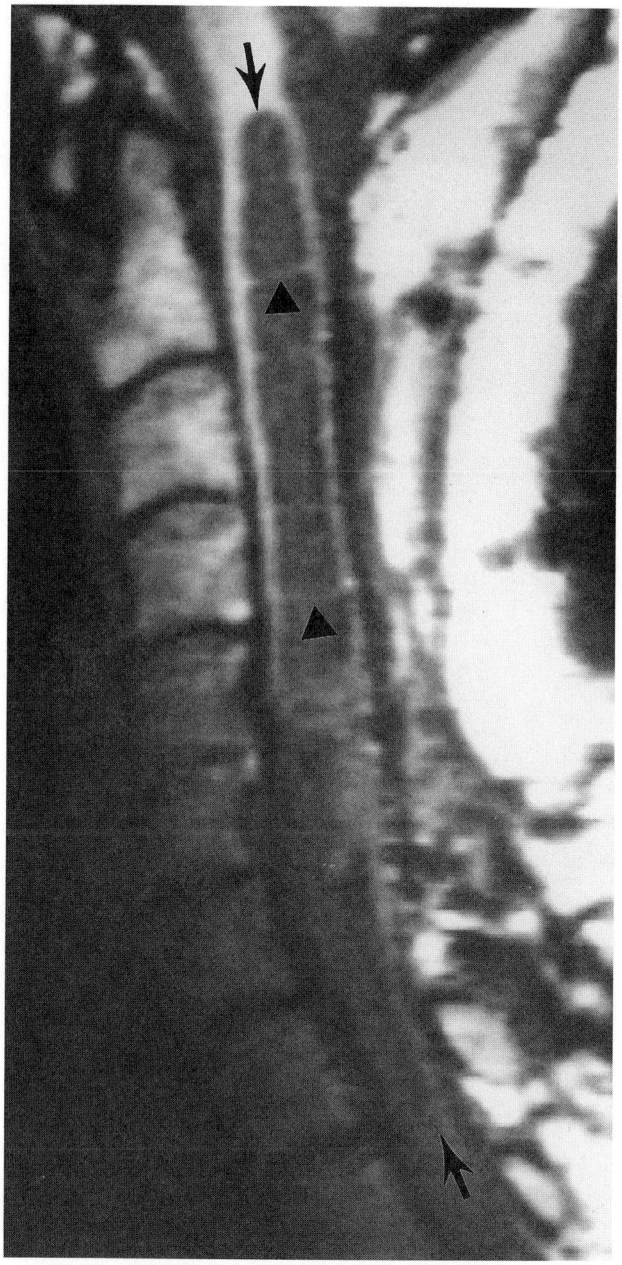

FIGURE 39.71▲ Posttraumatic intramedullary cyst. A large, multisegmented intramedullary cyst is present from C1 to T1 (between arrows). This patient was worsening neurologically after a fracture-subluxation in the distant past and had a prior wide posterior laminectomy. Note within the cyst linear bands (arrowheads), which represent fibroglial scars traversing the cyst.

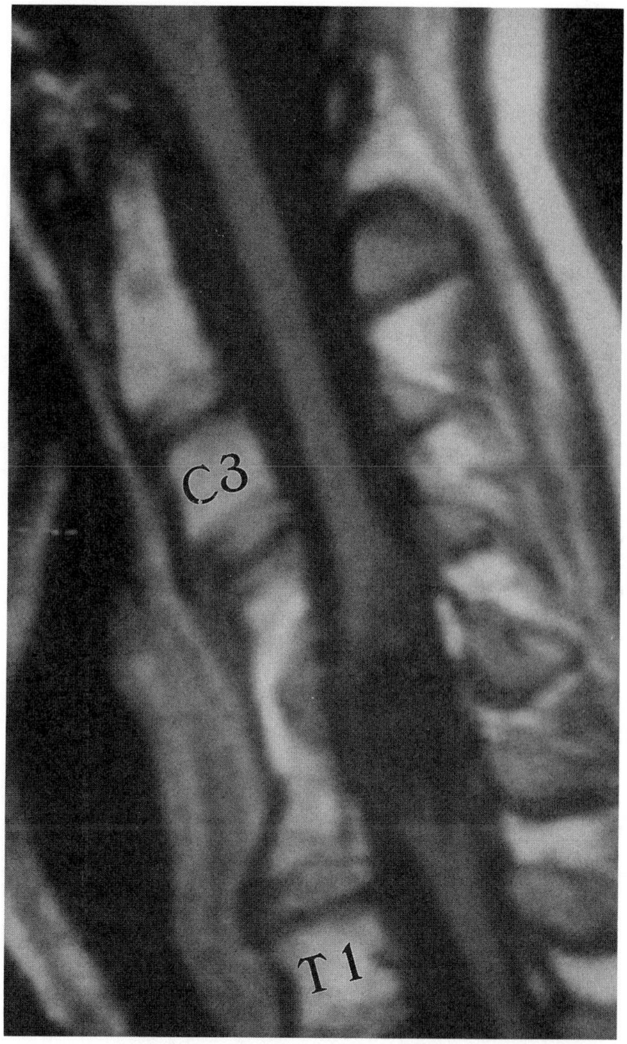

A

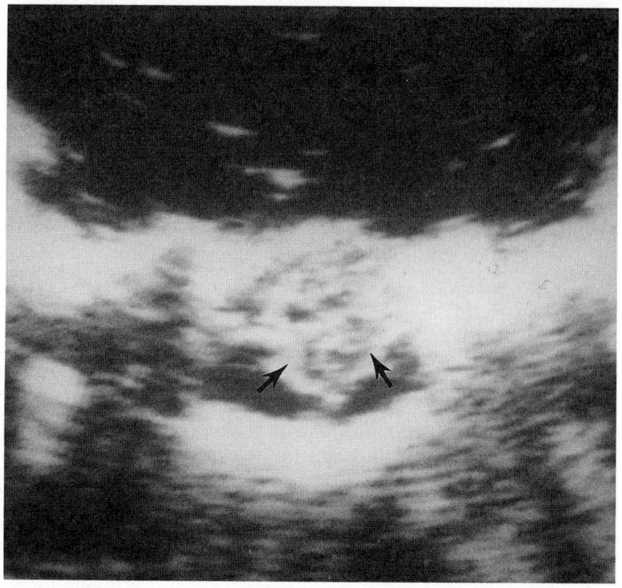

B

FIGURE 39.72 ▶ Posttraumatic myelomalacia. Sagittal T1-weighted MR from C5 to C7 shows postsurgical anterior cervical decompression and fusion from C4 through C6. The cord at C5 appears expanded with an ill-defined hypointensity. The differential diagnosis was between a posttraumatic syrinx and a microcystic myelomalacia with tethering of the cord anteriorly and posteriorly to the surrounding dura. A laminectomy was performed at C5, and transverse intraoperative sonography (B) shows no evidence of a cyst but rather a cord of mixed echogenicity (arrows surrounding cord), a finding compatible with myelomalacia.

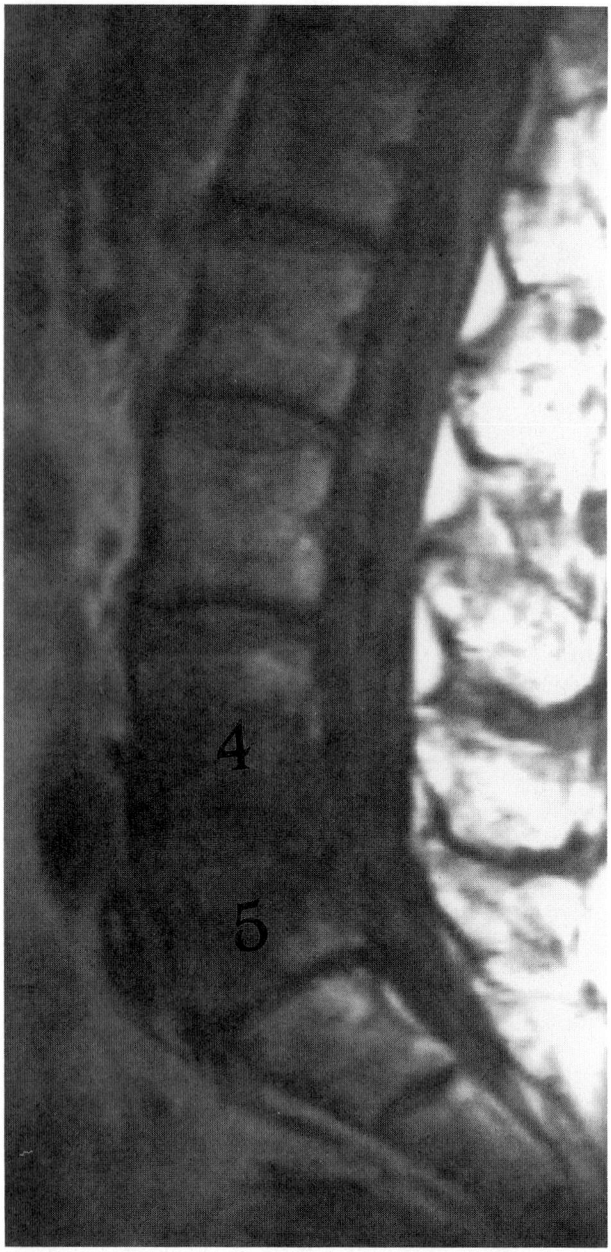

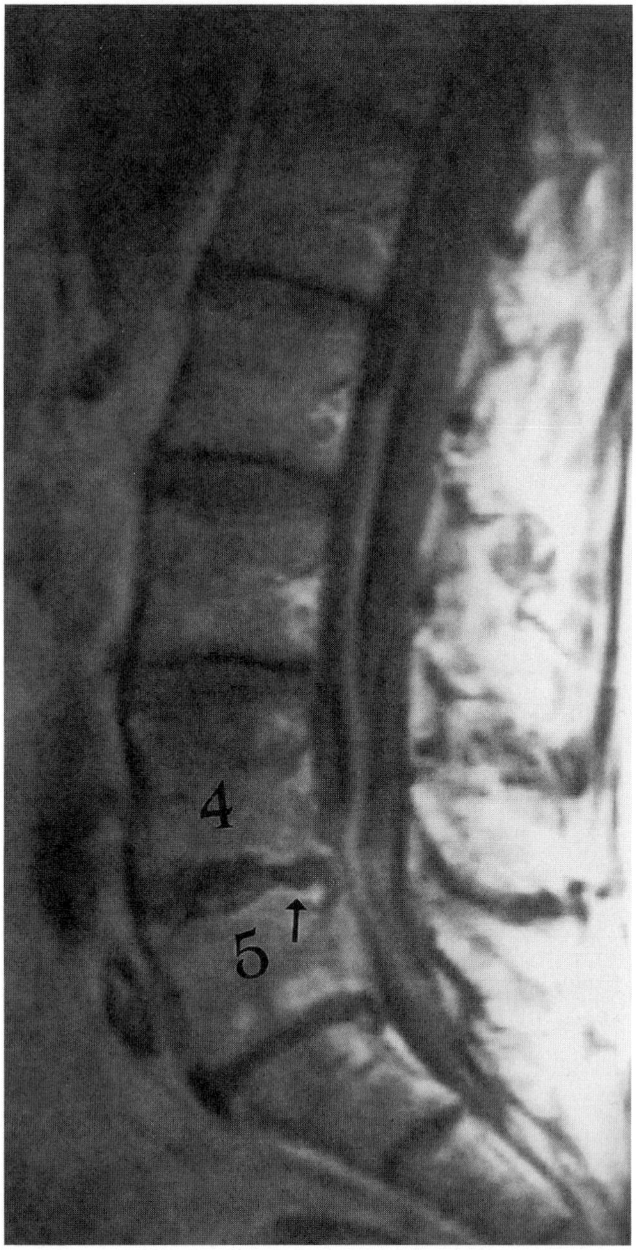

FIGURE 39.73 Disc space infection. L4–5 disc space infection in a 65-year-old intravenous drug abuser with blood cultures positive for *Staphylococcus aureus*. MR scans reveal changes consistent with disc space infection and osteomyelitis at L4–5. A. T1-weighted image shows abnormally low signal in the L4 and L5 bodies. B. Postcontrast-enhanced T1-weighted image demonstrates linear enhancement of the L4–5 disc (arrow) and some epidural enhancement.

MRI is able to detect infection earlier than other imaging modalities. The replacement of marrow by inflammatory tissue is seen as abnormally low signal intensity within the vertebral body on T1-weighted images (Figure 39.73). Disc space involvement is seen usually as narrowing of the disc space and a slight loss of signal of the nucleus pulposus on T1-weighted images and high–intensity signal in the disc on T2-weighted images. In many patients these changes in the bone and disc are associated with adjacent inflammatory tissue anteriorly or posteriorly in the epidural space in the spinal canal. Following contrast administration, enhancement is seen in the infected disc space and vertebral bodies.

Tuberculous Infections. The most common site of infection of tuberculous spondylitis is at L1, the frequency being much less in the cervical and sacral regions. Classically, spinal tuberculosis is thought to begin in the anterior-inferior portion of the vertebral body. The infection can spread

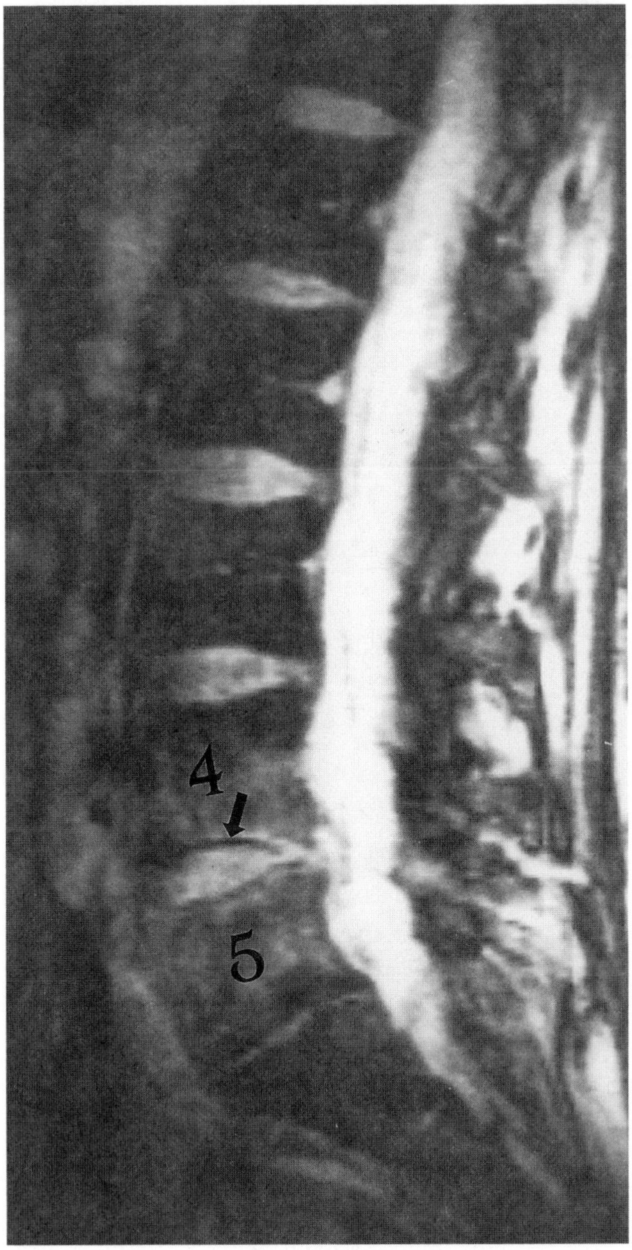

C

FIGURE 39.73 *(continued)* C. The T2-weighted image shows a uniform hyperintense signal in the disc (arrow) with absence of the normal low signal intranuclear cleft (compare with the other disc spaces).

beneath the anterior longitudinal ligament involving adjacent vertebral bodies. Bone destruction is typically more extensive than in pyogenic infections. Contiguous vertebral body involvement with destruction of the disc occurs in half the cases, and spread of infection beneath the anterior longitudinal ligament may cause involvement of noncontiguous vertebral bodies. This multiplicity of vertebral body involvement makes differentiation from metastatic disease sometimes difficult.

Paraspinal infection and gibbus deformity are common in tuberculous spondylitis. The size of the paraspinal lesion has been noted to be generally larger in tuberculosis than in pyogenic infections. These paravertebral abscesses may calcify and thus may be better identified on CT.

Epidural Abscess

An epidural abscess, although an uncommon entity when not associated with osteomyelitis or discitis, is important to recognize because early diagnosis greatly improves patient outcome. MRI generally facilitates the diagnosis and may be positive earlier than a radionuclide scan. Timely diagnosis is important because timely decompression can save neurologic function.

Although MRI has been described to be as sensitive (91%) as CT myelography (92%) in detecting epidural abscesses, it offers the advantage of distinguishing epidural abscesses from other entities, such as herniated discs, spinal tumor, or spinal hematoma (Sklar et al. 1993). Another advantage of MRI over CT myelography is its noninvasive nature, avoiding the potential of spreading the infection to produce meningitis via the spinal puncture required for myelography.

On plain MRI, an epidural abscess appears as a mass that is isointense to spinal cord on T1-weighted images and frequently has high-intensity signal on T2-weighted images (Figure 39.74). The epidural abscess may go unrecognized if its signal is similar to that of adjacent CSF. With contrast enhancement, however, an epidural abscess can be clearly delineated on MR imaging. Most epidural abscesses enhance in a homogeneous fashion, occur adjacent to an infected disc space level, and involve two to four spinal segments. The organism most commonly responsible for epidural abscesses is *S. aureus*, as in vertebral osteomyelitis.

REFERENCES

Atlas SW (ed). Magnetic Resonance Imaging of the Brain and Spine. New York: Raven, 1991.

Gomori JM, Grossman RI, Goldbert HI et al. Intracranial hematomas: imaging by high-field MR. Radiology 1985;157:87–93.

Halbach VV, Higashida RT, Hirshima GP. Interventional neuroradiology. Am J Roentgenol 1989;153:467–476.

Naidich TP, McLore DC, Fulling KH. The Chiari II malformation: Part IV. The hindbrain deformity. Neuroradiology 1983; 25:179–197.

Post MJD, Berger JR, Hensley GT. The Radiology of Central Nervous System Disease in Acquired Immunodeficiency Syndrome. In JM Taveras, JT Ferruci (eds), Radiology: Diagnosis-Imaging-Intervention. Vol. 3. Philadelphia: Lippincott, 1988;1–26.

Quencer RM. The injured spinal cord, evaluation with magnetic resonance and intraoperative sonography. Radiol Clin North Am 1988;26:1025–1045.

Quencer RM, Sheldon JJ, Post MJD et al. Magnetic resonance imaging of the chronically injured cervical spinal cord. Am J Neuroradiol 1986;7:457–464.

Ruiz A, Ganz WL, Post MJD et al. Use of thallium-201 brain SPECT to differentiate cerebral lymphoma from toxoplasma en-

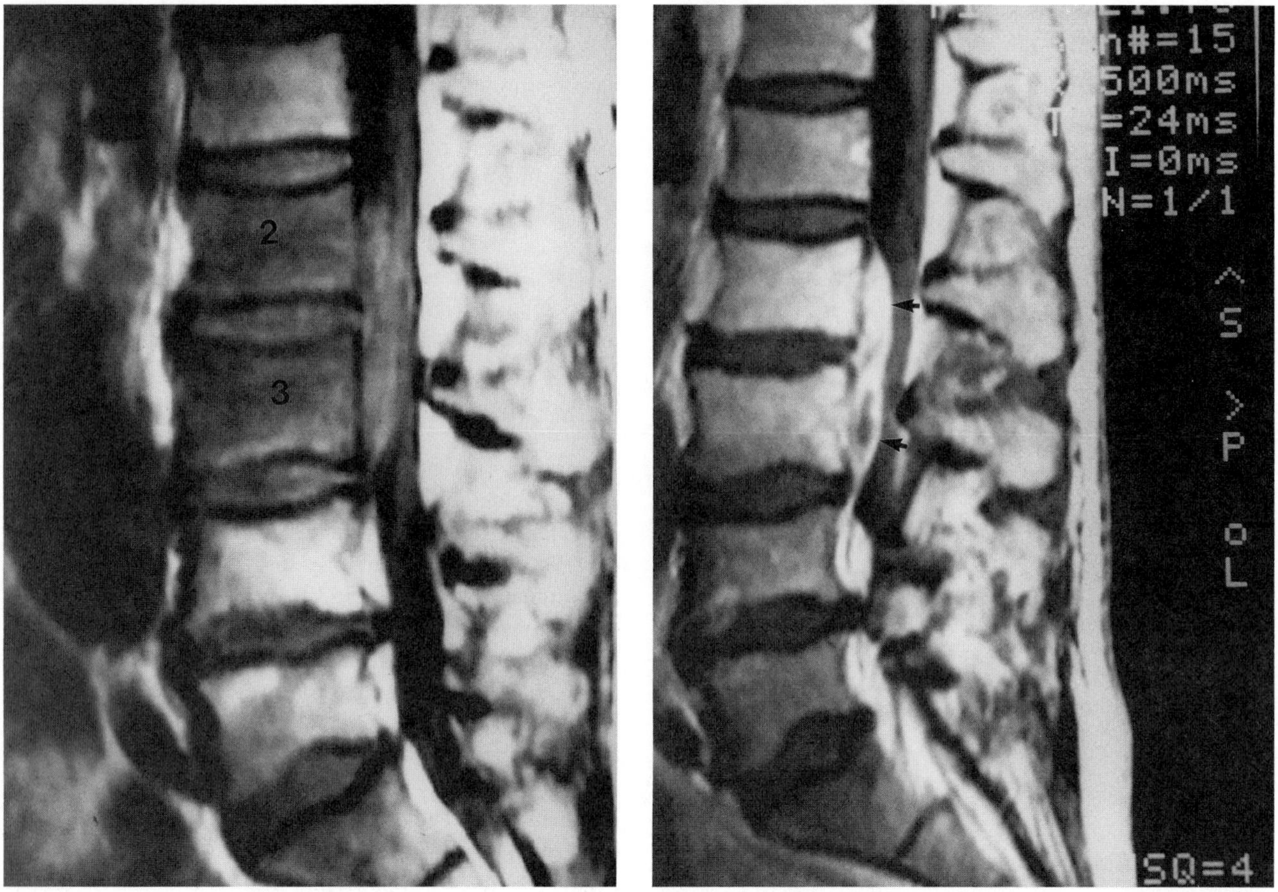

A B

FIGURE 39.74 L2 and L3 osteomyelitis and epidural abscess. Sagittal T1-weighted image demonstrates abnormally low signal in the bodies of L2 and L3 (A), which enhances on the gadolinium-enhanced MR images (B). An epidural soft-tissue mass extends from L2 to the lower margin of L3, which enhances diffusely and intensely with gadolinium administration (arrows). (Reprinted with permission from EML Sklar, MJD Post, NH Lebwohl. Imaging of infection of the lumbosacral spine. Neuroimaging Clin North Am 1993;3:577–590.)

cephalitis in AIDS patients. Am J Neuroradiol 1994;15: 1885–1894.

Sklar EML, Post MJD, Lebwohl NH. Imaging of infection of the lumbosacral spine. Neuroimaging Clin North Am 1993; 3:577–590.

Sklar EML, Quencer RM, Bowen BC et al. Magnetic resonance application in cerebral injury. Radiol Clin North Am 1992;30:353–366.

Sklar EML, Quencer RM, Byrne SF et al. Correlative study of the computed tomographic, ultrasonographic and pathologic characteristics of cavernous versus capillary hemangiomas of the orbit. J Clin Neuro-ophthalmol 1986;6:14–21.

Stark DD, Bradley WG (eds). Magnetic Resonance Imaging (2nd ed). St. Louis: Mosby, 1992.

Yuh WTC, Engelke JD, Muhonen MC et al. Experience with high-dose gadolinium MR imaging in the evaluation of brain metastases. Am J Neuroradiol 1992;13:335–345.

SUGGESTED READING

Braffman BH, Bilanium LT, Zimmerman RA. The central nervous system manifestations of the phakomatoses on MR. Radiol Clin North Am 1988;26:773–800.

Brant-Zawadski M, Norman D (eds). Magnetic Resonance Imaging of the Central Nervous System. New York: Raven, 1987.

Harwood-Nash DC, Fitz CR. Neuroradiology in Infants and Children. St. Louis: Mosby, 1976;1167–1226.

Savoiardo M, Girotti F, Strada L et al. Magnetic Resonance Imaging in Progressive Supranuclear Palsy and Other Parkinsonian Disorders. In E Tolosa, R Duvoisin, FF Cruz-Sánchez (eds), Progressive Supranuclear Palsy: Diagnosis, Pathology and Therapy. New York: Springer-Verlag, 1994;93–110.

Schoene WC. Degenerative Diseases of the Central Nervous System. In RL Davis, DM Robertson (eds), Textbook of Neuropathology. Baltimore: Williams & Wilkins, 1985;788–823.

Chapter 40
Functional Neuroimaging

Richard S. J. Frackowiak and David G. Gadian

Functional neuroimaging methods fall broadly into two classes: methods that provide information about synaptic activity, often called *functional mapping* or *activation studies*, and those that provide information of a *chemical* or *neurochemical nature*. The former methods usually depend on some form of perfusion mapping because of the tight coupling between glucose metabolism and blood flow locally in the brain at rest and at times of altered synaptic activity. The latter methods depend on identifying a chemical species of interest, either by using an appropriate radioligand or by using the intrinsic magnetic properties of a compound.

FUNCTIONAL MAPPING

Functional mapping is concerned with describing neural activity in the brain that is associated with some physiological, cognitive, or pathological state of interest (Frackowiak 1989). Modern, noninvasive methods of recording the distribution of brain activity are based on radiotracers or on magnetic resonance techniques. The radiotracer methods include positron emission tomography (PET) and single-photon emission computed tomography (SPECT). Magnetic resonance methods include imaging (MRI) and spectroscopy (MRS).

Positron Emission Tomography and Single-Photon Emission Computed Tomography

The essential difference between PET and SPECT is one of sensitivity. PET can measure distributions of radioactivity in the brain in absolute units; in other words, the signals can be calibrated. Calibration in absolute units of activity is possible because the sensitivity for the detection of radiation by PET is uniform throughout the scanned head; an accurate correction for the attenuation of signal caused by the brain, skull, and skin can be measured; and the field of view can be precisely and electronically delineated. These features result in better image quality for very substantially less radiation exposure than is possible with SPECT. PET is more expensive than SPECT, and this is the main advantage of the latter technique, in which attenuation correction is approximate, sensitivity decreases as the square of the distance from the detector surface, and the field of view must be constrained by heavy collimation that results in a substantial loss of counts and hence sensitivity. However, there are operational advantages to SPECT that mean it can be useful in evaluating certain clinical situations that will be described below.

MAGNETIC RESONANCE

MRI data are often recorded completely noninvasively—that is, without the need for the injection of radioisotopes, although contrast agents can be useful adjuncts for functional imaging. Another major advantage is the versatility of measurements that can be recorded with magnetic resonance techniques. With the radio tracer–based techniques, versatility is provided by the range of different chemical species that can be labeled as informative biological tracers. However, on the down side, magnetic resonance methods are also intrinsically less sensitive than PET scanning. The signals that are recorded and used to image brain anatomy depend on the magnetic properties of protons in, among other species, fat and water. These properties can be exploited to generate images of functional significance in a number of ways, and these are discussed below.

MRS uses the principles of spectroscopy, developed initially for the analysis of pure chemical samples, to generate information about chemicals in the body. The concentrations of many of the chemicals of biological interest in vivo are small, especially in comparison to the amounts of fat and water in the brain. The ability to register signals from chemical species of biological interest in small areas of the brain is therefore quite limited. To study tissue metabolism by detecting signals from ATP, phosphocreatine, and inorganic phosphate, ^{31}P-MRS has been used. It is also possible to measure the intracellular pH from the chemical shift of the inorganic phosphate signal peak. To measure lactate and *N*-acetyl aspartate, a proposed neuronal marker, ^{1}H-MRS, has been used with considerable success. Other chemical species of neurochemical interest, present in sufficient concentrations, can also be detected. Clinical applications of these techniques have emerged, notably in the study of the physiology of exercise and of muscle disease.

PERFUSION MAPPING

Interesting new data are available from functional mapping based on scanning perfusion changes in the brain that accompany brain activity. For example, functionally specialized cortical areas associated with different aspects of vision have been localized in human brain (Watson et al. 1993). Such basic studies of the functional organization of the normal brain constitute an active area of ongoing investigation with PET and more recently with functional MRI (fMRI).

fMRI is one of the more remarkable of developments in the use of magnetic resonance, for it now provides a means of visualizing brain function completely noninvasively. It is likely that this new MRI approach, together with other neuroimaging methods, will lead to major advances in our understanding of normal and abnormal brain function. However, the impact of functional imaging on diagnosis and management is still comparatively restricted, especially if one compares it with the major impact that conventional MRI, and for that matter x-ray computed tomography (CT), have had on individual patient management in the last two decades.

OTHER METHODS

There are a number of other functional imaging techniques under development, including magnetoencephalography, electroencephalographic (EEG) mapping, and event-related potential mapping. They provide the best information available on the temporal aspects of neural activity and hence are of particular interest to epileptologists. Electron spin resonance–based methods are low in sensitivity but promise a way of noninvasively monitoring free-radical formation in tissue and are experimental at present.

FUNCTIONAL NEUROIMAGING IN DISEASE

Dementia and Other Neurodegenerative Disorders

The neurodegenerative disorders have been studied extensively with functional techniques because many such diseases manifest at the end stage of a chronic process when there is already a considerable degree of neuronal attrition. The possibility of diagnosing such diseases before they manifest clinically is a goal that has many therapeutic and prognostic implications.

Alzheimer's Disease

In Alzheimer's disease ^{15}O and ^{18}FDG-PET studies consistently indicate an impairment of oxygen and glucose metabolism (Kennedy and Frackowiak 1994). These abnormalities are mirrored by an equivalent decrease of blood flow and are centered on the parietal and posterior temporal regions of the brain. There is a tendency for such focal scanning abnormalities to start asymmetrically in some Alzheimer's patients. The abnormalities can be detected early, in some cases even before dementia is established, or when minor impairment of memory is the only clinical finding or complaint (Plate 40.I).

Patients with early familial Alzheimer's disease show the same pattern. Also, at-risk individuals from such families have been described with similar scanning abnormalities at a stage when signs and symptoms were minimal or absent. Invariably such individuals soon manifest features of the disease. The disease is also predicted by the typical parietotemporal scanning abnormalities in patients with mild cognitive abnormalities that are insufficient to satisfy formal criteria for the diagnosis of sporadic Alzheimer's disease.

Functional scanning cannot differentiate familial from sporadic Alzheimer's dementia because the pattern of dysmetabolism in the two is very similar, if not identical. A similar parietotemporal pattern of dysmetabolism has been described in patients receiving radiotherapy to ports centered on the parietotemporal regions, in patients with combined Parkinson's disease and dementia, and rarely in patients with biparietal strokes.

Late Alzheimer's disease is characterized by focal abnormalities of metabolism in frontal regions additional to those in the parietotemporal region. These frontal changes are superimposed on markedly impaired metabolism throughout the brain. The distribution of scanning abnormalities in severe cases encompasses all the association cortices, but the visual and motor cortices and the cerebellum remain relatively spared.

There is little impairment of ^{18}F-DOPA uptake in the basal ganglia of patients with Alzheimer's disease. The uptake of ^{18}F-DOPA, which is an indicator of presynaptic nigrostriatal function, is markedly impaired in Parkinson's disease (see below). There is no abnormality of ^{18}F-DOPA uptake into the basal ganglia of patients with dementia in whom rigidity is a prominent associated, but secondary, feature. Such rigidity is often clinically of a nonparkinsonian type and is almost invariably associated with apraxia (Tyrrell et al. 1990).

Pick's Disease

The characteristic pattern of functional scanning findings in Pick's disease is that of an inferior frontal impairment that is often also seen in the inferomedial temporal lobes and basal ganglia (Kamo et al. 1987). This pattern has also been reported with SPECT perfusion scanning in patients with frontal lobe dementia associated with amyotrophy.

Creutzfeldt-Jacob Disease

Very few patients with Creutzfeldt-Jacob dementia have undergone functional imaging. A generalized decline in cerebral metabolism without focal emphasis is the most consistently encountered pattern (Goto et al. 1993).

Dementia Associated with Human Immunodeficiency Virus

Little has been established in functional scanning terms for dementia associated with human immunodeficiency virus (HIV). Abnormalities of interregional correlations of cerebral metabolism have been described, but the body of knowledge remains small. Increases in basal ganglion metabolism as well as generalized cortical metabolic abnormalities have been described. However, functional imaging serves no diagnostic purpose in this disorder at present. The differentiation of central nervous system (CNS) lymphomas, which show high glucose uptake with ^{18}FDG-PET, from other intracranial lesions may also become useful in AIDS patients (Hoffman et al. 1993).

Vascular Dementia

The distribution of functional scanning abnormalities is random in vascular dementia. Abnormalities are most often found in middle cerebral arterial territory. Hypometabolism is matched by equivalent decreases in blood flow. Occasional discrepancies between MRI or CT scan findings and PET have been demonstrated, but in general, MRI is the most sensitive indicator of ischemic tissue damage.

Small vessel disease, or Binswanger's syndrome, is associated with abnormalities of metabolism in the white matter and in the overlying cortex (Yao et al. 1990). The appearances differ little from the changes seen in dementia associated with larger vessel disease, though there is a less focal emphasis to the abnormalities.

The focal metabolic and blood flow abnormalities seen in the different types of dementia, and particularly in the most common diagnostic groups, lend themselves to imaging with SPECT because there is preserved coupling between flow and metabolism. Hence measurement of the distribution of one variable reflects that of the other. The relative distribution of perfusion is readily imaged using tracers such as ^{99m}technetium (Tc)-labeled hexa-methyl propylene amine oxine (HMPAO) which distinguishes between the typical patterns observed in Alzheimer's disease and those seen with vascular dementia.

Lewy Body Disease

The patterns of dysfunction associated with Lewy body dementia are not well characterized. This disorder is thought by some to account for approximately 10–20% of dementia in the elderly, but the differential diagnosis remains difficult and is not presently aided by functional imaging.

Dementia Associated with Depression

The dementias associated with depression ("pseudodementias") are characterized, with SPECT, by a uniform distribution of blood flow. However, PET scans indicate, in group studies, that there are resting abnormalities of flow and metabolism in medial and left lateral frontal regions. The contrast between parietotemporal changes in Alzheimer's disease and a uniform distribution of perfusion in depression-associated dementia has discriminant value (Bench et al. 1992).

MOVEMENT DISORDERS

Parkinsonism

A number of degenerative disorders manifest clinically with a parkinsonian syndrome. They are often difficult to distinguish on structural scanning grounds, especially early in the disease. Clinical features are often the best guide, though up to 20% of clinical diagnoses of idiopathic Parkinson's disease (PD) may be erroneous on postmortem criteria. Functional imaging with tracers of the dopaminergic system has been found useful in establishing suspected clinical diagnoses in these disorders.

Parkinson's Disease

PD is associated with a decrease in the uptake and retention of ^{18}F-DOPA in the basal ganglia (Brooks 1993). Good scanners can monitor the progression of impairment with advancing disease from the ventrolateral aspects of the putamen to the more anterior and dorsal parts. Relative sparing of the caudate nucleus is characteristic of idiopathic PD. Clinical parkinsonism manifests when there is degeneration of over 50% of the pigmented nigral cells that project to the striatum. There is, therefore, at least theoretically, scope for the detection of preclinical disease (Sawle 1993). Scan abnormalities have been found in at-risk subjects from families with hereditary parkinsonism. Scan abnormalities of nigrostriatal function have also been shown in a subgroup of patients with drug-induced rigidity that fail to recover on drug withdrawal, and in certain patients with drug-induced tremors that do not resolve with the cessation of treatment.

The ^{18}F-DOPA technique is sensitive and can be used to monitor the progression of nigrostriatal dysfunction in patients scanned sequentially. The scanning abnormalities are frequently asymmetrical in early disease, mirroring the typical asymmetrical clinical presentation, with the abnormal putamen found contralateral to the clinically affected limbs. Abnormalities become symmetrical as the disorder progresses. The technique is the only one available, at present, that permits direct monitoring of the viability of transplanted fetal mesencephalic graft tissue in patients so treated (Lindvall et al. 1992)

Other tracers of presynaptic dopaminergic function have been used—for example, ^{11}C-nomifensine, a dopamine reuptake site inhibitor—but the greatest image contrast is still obtained with ^{18}F-DOPA. Novel SPECT tracers of dopamine reuptake sites, such as ^{99m}Tc-labeled CIT, seem very promising but require further evaluation.

Patients with PD can develop cognitive impairment or even frank dementia. A typical Alzheimer's-like scanning pattern has been shown in a PD patient with clinical dementia. However, in a pathologically verified case with such scanning abnormalities, there were no changes of Alzheimer's disease associated with the typical striatonigral degeneration. It is difficult to be sure how typical these single observations are, or indeed whether, as seems likely, they form a spectrum of overlapping phenotypes. The differential diagnosis of cortical Lewy body disease with dementia, PD with dementia, or PD with coincidental Alzheimer's disease cannot be helped by functional scanning at present. This is largely because there is insufficient information about the correlation of scan appearances with pathologically verified diagnoses.

Multiple-System Atrophy

Multiple-system atrophy (MSA) encompasses a clinical spectrum ranging from striatonigral degeneration (SND) through olivopontocerebellar atrophy (OPCA) to pure autonomic failure (PAF). The pattern of ^{18}F-DOPA uptake is abnormal and severe as in idiopathic PD. However, the caudate nucleus is not relatively spared as it is in PD. In addition, PAF is not normally associated with a decline in striatal ^{18}F-DOPA uptake, though a patient with an abnormal scan has been described who subsequently developed more extensive signs and symptoms of MSA. Scans of the striatum with D_2 receptor ligands, such as ^{11}C-raclopride, have shown diagnostically insignificant changes in PD. Though there are small decreases in putaminal D_2 ligand binding in MSA patients, they are also insufficient to be of diagnostic use (Brooks et al. 1992).

Metabolic scans have shown significant abnormalities in some MSA patients. This finding contrasts with the usual absence of metabolic changes in PD patients. There are decreases in frontal cortical metabolism that can also affect the cerebellum in MSA. For distinguishing MSA syndromes from PD, ^{18}FDG is a more promising tracer than ^{18}F-DOPA (Eidelberg et al. 1993). In SND there is a profound decline in striatal metabolism, often associated with frontal and cerebellar hypometabolism. In OPCA striatal metabolism is normal but frontal and cerebellar metabolism are abnormal. In PAF there are few metabolic changes. However, it should be recognized that these patterns are not inevitably found in the different disorders; for example, SND without ataxia is associated with normal cerebellar metabolism. Normal ^{18}F-DOPA and ^{18}FDG uptake occur in PAF, but such a pattern can also be associated with OPCA.

Progressive Supranuclear Palsy

Progressive supranuclear plasy is an akinetic-rigid syndrome associated with pronounced cognitive impairment, often of a frontal lobe type. In both caudate and putamen, ^{18}F-DOPA scans show uniform impairment of uptake, distinguishing this disease from idiopathic PD (Burn et al. 1994). This is a reliable differential diagnostic feature enabling correct assignation in approximately 90% of cases. Scanning of D_2 receptors indicates a possible small decrease of the binding potential (a composite index of receptor density and affinity) in this disorder, which also contrasts with findings in PD, but that is insufficient to be useful for differentiating the diseases in individual cases.

Metabolic scans consistently show a relative impairment of frontal activity, though in early cases this may not be severe. This feature does not always distinguish supranuclear palsy from PD. The relatively focal frontal abnormality is often present against a background of mild diffuse impairment of cortical function. There is also striatal hypometabolism, which is a feature that distinguishes progressive supranuclear palsy from PD.

Friedreich's Ataxia and Cerebellar Degenerative Syndromes

In patients with Friedreich's ataxia who are ambulant, there is a characteristic widespread increase of resting glucose metabolism throughout the cortex, basal ganglia, and cerebellum. When the disease progresses to a stage that patients become chairbound, the metabolic rate declines to normal values in all areas except in the caudate and lenticular nuclei (Gilman et al. 1990). Studies of the distribution of benzodiazepine receptors in cerebellar degenerative syndromes have failed to show any consistent abnormalities.

In alcoholic cerebellar degeneration ^{18}FDG scanning shows hypometabolism in the superior cerebellar vermis and in the medial frontal cortex. Such changes are not seen in alcohol-dependent patients who do not manifest cerebellar dysfunction clinically.

Idiopathic Torsion Dystonia

In idiopathic torsion dystonia there are no differences in the distribution of perfusion at rest between patients and normal subjects. Activation scans show overactivity of the supplementary motor area, lateral premotor area, lateral prefrontal regions, parietal association cortices, and contralateral cerebellum during arm movement (Ceballos-Baumann et al. 1994). There is no consensus among reported studies about changes of metabolism in the basal ganglia, though there is a suggestion that increases also occur in the putamen. A modest decrease of ^{18}F-DOPA uptake into the putamen has been seen in groups of patients. However, this is not great enough to qualify as a diagnostic feature in individuals, some of whom show uptake values that fall into the normal range.

In sporadic generalized dystonia the uptake of ^{18}F-DOPA into the striatum is similar to that found in idiopathic torsion dystonia. Resting perfusion scans are normal.

DOPA-Responsive Dystonia

DOPA-responsive dystonia usually presents in early life. However, rarely the disease can present in adult life as a DOPA-responsive parkinsonian syndrome that is distinguishable with difficulty from idiopathic PD. In DOPA-responsive dystonia, unlike idiopathic PD, ^{18}F-DOPA uptake into the striatum is normal or only slightly reduced (Sawle et al. 1991a). Interestingly, the akinetic-rigid syndrome associated with manganese intoxication is also associated with normal striatal ^{18}F-DOPA uptake, implying structural integrity of the nigrostriatal neurons but a deficit in the functional pathway of which these neurons are a component.

Corticobasal Degeneration

Hypometabolism that is often asymmetrical is found in the posterior frontal, inferior parietal, and superior temporal areas in corticobasal degeneration (neuronal achromasia), which is a pattern opposite to that found in Pick's disease. The thalami and hippocampus also variably show hypometabolism. There is a profound associated impairment of ^{18}F-DOPA uptake that is equal in caudate and putamen but asymmetrical, being most marked on the side opposite the more affected limbs (Sawle et al. 1991b). There is evidence to suggest that mesial frontal ^{18}F-DOPA uptake is also impaired, which is not the case in PD patients.

Wilson's Disease

In Wilson's disease there are abnormalities of glucose metabolism and ^{18}F-DOPA uptake. Impaired metabolism is found in the striatum, with both the caudate and putamen affected. Cerebellar metabolism is also markedly impaired, and there are less-prominent metabolic abnormalities in the thalami and cerebral cortex (Kuwert et al. 1992). Striatal hypometabolism is most marked in patients who have recently begun treatment, and there is evidence that improvement of putaminal and cortical metabolism is associated with clinical improvement resulting from long-term chelation therapy. Uptake of ^{18}F-DOPA is impaired in the striatum of symptomatic patients but not in those who are asymptomatic. However, once the striatum shows abnormalities of ^{18}F-DOPA uptake, it does not revert to normal even after prolonged penicillamine treatment, indicating that some permanent damage has occurred in the nigrostriatal pathways.

Huntington's Disease

Caudate glucose metabolism is impaired in Huntington's disease, a dominantly inherited disorder. The impairment may precede clinical features, and hypometabolism in the caudate can be used as a marker of the asymptomatic carrier state in at-risk asymptomatic relatives of patients with the disorder (Baxter et al. 1992). As a marker of the carrier state, functional imaging is more sensitive than the presence of chorea, subtle clinical abnormalities of motor control, or caudate atrophy on structural imaging. Hypometabolism in the carrier state has also been described in the putamen and globus pallidus, and hypermetabolism has been found in the precentral gyrus. There is some controversy about whether hypometabolism is present when there is a complete absence of motor signs or symptoms. However, with identification of the Huntington's gene and a description of the genetic mechanism for the production of disease, this matter is now largely academic.

Neuroacanthocytosis and Other Choreas

Neuroacanthocytosis comprises a mixture of akinetic-rigid features and chorea in addition to seizures, axonal neuropathy, and orolingual self-mutilation. Uptake of ^{18}F-DOPA is decreased in a manner identical to early idiopathic PD, with the posterior putamen being most affected (Brooks et al. 1991). In addition, there is loss of ^{11}C-raclopride binding in the caudate and putamen as judged by the ratio of the uptake of this D_2 receptor ligand to uptake in the cerebellum. There is, therefore, evidence of both nigrostriatal and intrinsic striatal damage in this disorder. Additionally, striatal and frontal cortical glucose metabolism are impaired.

Chorea, from whatever cause, is generally associated with striatal hypometabolism (Otsuka et al. 1993). Such a pattern has been described in Wilson's disease, Huntington's disease, sporadic chorea with dementia, and the pseudo-Huntington's variant of dentatorubropallidoluysian atrophy. Only benign hereditary chorea is not associated with a similar striatal metabolic change.

EPILEPSY

Hemispheric Dominance

Localization of hemispheric dominance for language is traditionally carried out using the invasive Wada test. In this test a short-acting barbiturate is injected into each internal carotid artery in turn during the performance of language and memory tasks. The pattern of induced behavioral change, especially in terms of language dysfunction, is observed and conclusions are drawn about dominance. Activation mapping can be used very effectively to determine language dominance by scanning during the performance of single-word generation and verbal fluency tasks and comparing patterns of activity with those recorded at rest (Pardo and Fox 1994). Preliminary experience with fMRI suggests that this modality will give equally informative results.

Localizing Epileptic Foci

There is marked, focal, interictal hypometabolism in the temporal lobes in patients with partial seizures of temporal lobe origin (Engel 1991). Ictally, the changes are in the opposite direction, with marked increases in local blood flow and glucose metabolism, but oxygen metabolism is not augmented to the same extent, which leads to an uncoupling between glucose and oxygen consumption. Interictally, the extent of hypometabolism is often much larger than any underlying structural abnormality. It is thought that this, in part, reflects decreased activity in local neuronal circuits in the region of the epileptic focus. Over 70% of patients with partial epilepsy show interictal regions of hypometabolism. These are most commonly found in temporal lobe patients, but extratemporal foci are less easily identified. The dissociation between blood flow and oxygen metabolism has been used by some to identify extratemporal sites, especially in the frontal lobes, in patients with prominent interictal paroxysmal lateralizing epileptiform discharges (PLEDs).

In clinical practice, the epileptogenicity of hypometabolic foci should be confirmed electrophysiologically, even though false localization is more common with EEG than with ^{18}FDG-PET. In resistant temporal lobe epilepsy, if a focal hypometabolic region is detected with an electrophysiological concomitant (e.g., from sphenoidal EEG recordings), and if there are no inconsistent results from structural scanning, then there are adequate indications for choice of the site of temporal resection without a need to proceed to depth, or dural, electrode recordings.

SPECT with ^{99m}Tc-HMPAO is more practical than PET as a way of identifying ictal foci in clinical practice. HMPAO acts as a "chemical microsphere." This means that a very considerable proportion of the radioactivity that enters the cerebral circulation, following intravenous injection of the tracer, is trapped in the brain during first passage, and the distribution of the tracer reflects the distribution of perfusion (Ryvlin et al. 1992). Injection of the tracer, which is readily prepared, can be effected during a seizure, and then scanning of the distribution of perfusion during the ictus can be performed at leisure, with the patient in a more manageable, postictal state. The signals are usually large and therefore readily discerned on SPECT scans. fMRI has been used, as has PET, to identify areas of hyperactivity associated with prolonged focal epilepsy without generalization (epilepsia partialis continua) (Jackson et al. 1994). There are often practical problems with such scans because they are readily degraded by head movement. fMRI with echo-planar imaging provides the ability to take snapshot images in a time of 70 msec or so per plane. This speed of acquisition freezes even the most vigorously shaken head and may become a useful technique in clinical practice. The time needed to generate a positron emitting tracer and to image with PET makes this technique largely impracticable as a diagnostic test in the ictal phase.

Petit mal, or primary generalized epilepsy, is associated with a generalized increase in glucose metabolism that is sometimes raised more than threefold above normal values. There is no postictal depression in petit mal, which is why these greatly increased metabolic rates are so different from those recorded in patients with other types of generalized convulsive seizures. In such patients, no focal or generalized alterations in metabolism are found. The ^{18}FDG-PET method relies on the accumulation of radioactivity during a physiological steady state of at least 15–30 minutes to provide recordable changes in signal. The short time of the ictal phase in relation to the longer uptake phase makes PET a generally unsuitable method for the routine assessment of patients with generalized seizures.

Childhood Epilepsy

PET scanning has been useful for assessing diseased and normal hemispheres in patients, usually young children, who are candidates for cortical or hemispheric resection for intractable epilepsy.

In Sturge-Weber's syndrome, metabolic scans with ^{18}FDG-PET may indicate the degree of disease activity. In early disease there is hypometabolism associated with structural abnormalities visible on anatomical scans (CT or MRI). As the disease progresses in patients who develop epilepsy, a paradoxical increase of metabolism in the cortex overlying the affected hemisphere is seen, which, in the most severely affected children, reverts to a pronounced and extensive hypometabolism. It is on the basis of the different patterns of metabolism recorded at different stages of the disease that it has been suggested that active brain degeneration is being monitored by the functional scans in this disease (Rintahaka et al. 1993).

PET has also been used to define ectopic areas of cortex, which often show lower metabolic rates than normal gray matter. Such cerebral ectopia is often also readily discernible with anatomical MR scanning. In some patients with cryptogenic infantile spasms, quite wide but still focal and unilateral areas of hypometabolism have been seen in the parieto-occipitotemporal region. These hypometabolic areas correlate with the presence of cortical dysplasia in pathological specimens following resection. Resection can result in good seizure control. In most of these patients no MRI abnormalities are present on preoperative scans (Chugani et al. 1993).

Scans in Lennox-Gastaut's syndrome show a very heterogeneous pattern of metabolic abnormalities. Unilateral focal and generalized as well as bilateral generalized hypometabolism has been seen, as has a normal distribution of metabolism.

CEREBROVASCULAR DISEASE

A description and elucidation of the pathophysiology of preischemic states, ischemia, and the transition from ischemia to infarction, in terms of regional hemodynamics and energy metabolism, have been among the major achievements of PET. Much confusion, sown by the lack of an adequate appreciation of the importance and degree of uncoupling of blood flow from metabolism in ischemia, has been clarified. Additionally, the time-honored but erroneous concept of chronic ischemia has been laid to rest and supplanted by recognition that ischemia is an acute process, and that there are chronic states of hemodynamic (de)compensation that require clinical recognition and management in their own right. PET techniques are time consuming. Hence, scanning has not found a role in the routine clinical assessment of patients with cerebrovascular disease. However, in many cases clinicopathophysiological correlations described by PET are sufficiently clear to allow direct inferences to be made about the probable hemodynamic status of patients from standard clinical assessments.

Acute Ischemia

Under normal circumstance, the regional blood flow in the brain is tightly coupled to oxygen metabolism. This coupling is reflected by the fact that the proportion of oxygen removed, for metabolic purposes, from the perfusing arterial blood during passage through the cerebral tissue is about 40% everywhere in the brain. Oxygen travels across vessels and through brain tissue by diffusion, driven by an electrochemical diffusion gradient. The concentration of free oxygen in the tissues is very low because it is used by actively metabolizing brain cells. If, for any reason, blood flow should fall, the potential shortfall in delivery of oxygen to tissue is compensated by tissue extraction of a greater than normal proportion of the oxygen carried in the blood. The proportion of oxygen extracted from the blood can be quantified by the oxygen extraction ratio (OER), which is measured with ^{15}O-PET scanning. If the blood flow falls below a critical level—that is, to about 40% of normal—then all the available oxygen is extracted and the brain finds itself in a novel and critical situation, because metabolic activity, and hence function of cells, becomes directly related to the level of residual flow. This is a state of incipient ischemia. Ischemia will be precipitated by any further drop in perfusion, occurs at a local (or global) flow threshold of approximately 20 ml/dl/min, and is associated with a maximally elevated OER of 100% that indicates all the oxygen delivered by residual perfusion is being extracted to sustain metabolism.

Infarction and Partial Neuronal Loss

Ischemia is rapidly followed by cell death and, if severe or prolonged, infarction that is characterized by tissue destruction. Dead cells do not consume oxygen; hence, as cells die a progressively decreasing amount of oxygen is needed to sustain residual metabolic requirements. Even if flow is subnormal, the state of progressive neuronal attrition will translate into a progressive fall of OER, first to normal and then to subnormal levels. The OER will be especially low if there is local reperfusion of tissue in which there are few, or no, surviving neurons after a period of ischemia. Such a pattern of low oxygen consumption and low OER appears, and is often complete, after the first few hours of the onset of ischemia.

The regulation of blood flow through ischemic tissue is often disturbed and reperfusion can occur by a number of mechanisms. This means that the levels of blood flow recorded in an infarcted, or ischemically injured, territory can be variously very low to abnormally high after the ischemic event itself. However, the signature of damaged tissue is the occurrence of impaired metabolism, which indicates decreased neural activity, associated with a low OER, indicating a relative excess of oxygen supply relative to residual demand. An important corollary is that blood flow is a very poor marker of tissue viability beyond the initial acute ischemic phase. Even during acute ischemia, the level of blood flow is only useful as an indicator of the degree of ischemia. Such information may be of considerable value in acute ischemia for monitoring thrombolytic therapy and can be obtained with ease using non-PET methods, such as HMPAO-SPECT. Glucose metabolism undergoes a series of alterations in the acute and subacute phases after an ischemic insult. Notable is the relatively high glucose consumption relative to oxygen metabolism of infarcts in the first weeks after ischemia. These changes are ascribable to the metabolic characteristics of activated microglia and macrophages that invade the infarct and result in scarring.

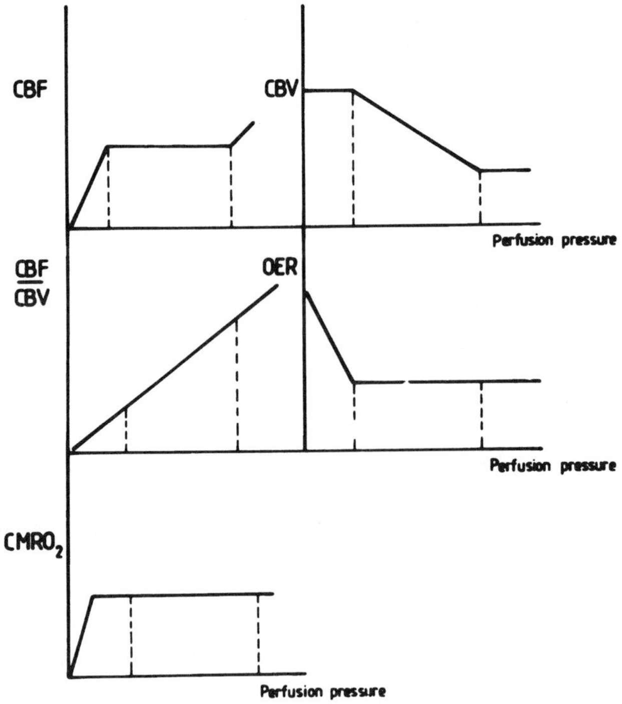

FIGURE 40.1 Relationships between local perfusion pressure and various energetic and hemodynamic variables. Top left: Autoregulation curve with constant blood flow despite falling perfusion pressure to a cortical minimum. Top right: Reciprocal relationship between falling perfusion pressure and cerebral blood volume (CBV), which reflects the degree of vasodilatation. Middle left: The resultant relationship between perfusion pressure and the ratio of cerebral blood flow (CBF) to CBV, which can be seen to be a good index of local perfusion pressure. Middle right: Shows the relationship between falling perfusion pressure and oxygen extraction fraction, indicating that only when CBF starts to fall does oxygen extraction ratio (OER) rise to compensate for the decreased delivery of oxygen to the tissues. Bottom left: The perfusion pressure and oxygen metabolism are plotted, showing how the increasing OER provides a second compensating mechanism shifting the threshold for ischemia and dysfunction to the left from the lower threshold of the autoregulatory curve (top left).

Hemodynamic Failure

The onset of ischemia can be preceded by various degrees of hemodynamic decompensation. A fall in blood flow is occasioned by a decrease in perfusion pressure. The phenomenon of autoregulation usually prevents variations of local brain blood flow in the face of normal, moment-to-moment variations of blood pressure. This is achieved by control of the resistance to blood flow through the brain parenchyma at an arteriolar level, and this phenomenon can be monitored by measuring local cerebral blood volume (CBV). Indeed, the ratio of cerebral blood flow (CBF) to CBV is an excellent index of local perfusion pressure. When the local brain perfusion pressure falls following occlusion of a feeding vessel, local vasodilatation occurs that decreases peripheral resistance and hence maintains a constant blood flow.

If perfusion pressure falls sufficiently, maximal vasodilatation is achieved, at which point local blood flow is determined directly by local perfusion pressure, and will fall if any further decline in perfusion pressure occurs. To compensate for any fall in perfusion, oxygen extraction from the blood increases proportionally, and hence the OER rises. Thus hemodynamic decompensation has two phases. In the first, CBF and therefore OER are constant but CBV rises and hence the local CBF-CBV ratio falls. When maximal vasodilatation is achieved, the second phase occurs in which CBF falls and OER increases. If the fall in perfusion is severe, the ischemic threshold is reached and the sequence of events described above supervenes (Figure 40.1).

Preischemic low-perfusion states are not uncommon in patients with extensive occlusive arterial disease, such as in unilateral internal carotid occlusion and significant contralateral carotid stenosis. Unilateral carotid occlusion is usually compensated adequately by the first of the mechanisms described above and is characterized by a normal blood flow and OER, but a focally increased CBV, and hence low CBF-CBV ratio.

Occasionally, an anomalous vascular anatomy in the circle of Willis or pre-existing local vessel disease may cause a normally well-tolerated occlusion to result in more severe hemodynamic decompensation than usual, sometimes leading to ischemia. Such a situation may also occur after an acute ischemic episode and may persist for a number of days. In such a case, metabolism is low (indicating some neuronal loss), the CBF-CBV ratio and the CBF are low (indicating hemodynamic decompensation), and the OER is elevated, often to 50–70%. This situation is physiologically precarious and is explained by a state of severe hemodynamic decompensation in tissue that contains a mixture of dead and viable cells; oxygen supply depends on the OER because the residual flow is compromised, often because of the severity of the arterial occlusions.

Practically, care must be taken with modifications of perfusion pressure, such as with antihypertensive medication in patients with extensive occlusive disease. It is also no coincidence that patients who carry the highest risk of periendarterectomy infarction are often those with the greatest degree of hemodynamic decompensation before operation.

Arteriovenous Malformations

The study of arteriovenous malformations (AVMs) has indicated that there may be discrete areas, in the vicinity of larger vascular abnormalities, in which there is a degree of hemodynamic compromise. There is no advantage of PET scanning compared to MRI for the detection of malformations, except perhaps in very low-flow abnormalities, such as cavernous angiomas. Studies of ^{15}O-PET activation have been used to identify function-specific areas of cortex in the vicinity of AVMs (and other tumors) to help plan resection therapy (Leblanc and Meyer 1990). In at least one case, the activation study findings have been validated by intraoperative corticography by local stimulation. There is therefore a possibility that fMRI studies will become useful in the field of functional neurosurgery in the future.

Functional Recovery

Activation studies have provided interesting information about the brain's capacity to reorganize after injury. Though presently in the realm of basic physiology, the study of brain plasticity and its modulation by drugs and other therapies may indicate a novel approach to the rehabilitation of brain-damaged adults (Weiller et al. 1993).

CEREBRAL TUMORS

Staging

Initial reports with ^{18}FDG-PET suggested the possibility of staging cerebral tumors in vivo with this form of scanning. The initial hopes have only been partly fulfilled. Tumors are often very heterogeneous in grade. Those of predominantly high grade show large increases in glucose metabolism, and those of low grade, such as oligodendrogliomas, show hypometabolism. Tumors of mixed grade may evolve or become more malignant with time, rendering interpretation of scan results difficult without sequential scanning. The diagnostic yield of stereotactic needle biopsy can be increased in mixed tumors and cystic tumors by using the results of functional scanning with PET.

Recurrence of tumors after resective surgery is readily monitored by functional imaging. Indeed there are case reports to suggest that the early stages of recurrence, when cellular infiltration without mass effect predominates, can be detected with greatest sensitivity by PET.

Radiation Necrosis

An important differential diagnosis of tumor recurrence is radiation necrosis. This complication is considerably rarer now that thresholds for radiation damage in terms of dose and administration protocol have been well defined. However, radiotherapy for small AVMs and for tumors is sometimes complicated by a subacute, space-occupying, delayed-onset radiation necrosis. This pathology is characterized by a low glucose consumption, which provides a useful contrast to the high uptake of ^{18}FDG found with recurrent astrogliomas of high grade.

Pituitary Tumors

Pituitary tumors have been well imaged by ^{11}C-methionine-PET. The metabolic activity of these tumors can be monitored, and the technique has also been used to follow treatment of pituitary tumors with D_2 agonists such as bromocriptine. The uptake of ^{11}C-methionine drops up to 70% in tumors that respond to therapy with regression in size. It is not clear whether monitoring by PET scanning is better than following tumor size by anatomical MR scanning.

To differentiate parasellar meningiomas and suprasellar extensions of pituitary tumors, ^{11}C-deprenyl-PET has been used. Meningiomas have lower levels of monoamine oxidase-B than the brain or pituitary gland. On the other hand, pituitary tumors contain amounts equal to, or greater than, those found in the brain. Deprenyl is a monoamine oxidase (MAO)-B inhibitor and is a quantitative tracer of the enzyme when labeled with carbon 11. The differential uptake of the tracer in the two conditions is sufficiently sensitive to allow a distinction to be made accurately if doubt persists after anatomical scanning and angiography.

BRAIN MAPPING

The techniques of functional brain mapping (activation studies) are in a process of rapid development. Though little used in clinical practice at present, there appear to be great opportunities for their use, especially if some of the MR-based techniques can be developed further. For this reason, this chapter concludes with a description of the principles of the newer brain-mapping methods for the interested reader.

Brain mapping is the visualization of local physiological changes in the brain associated with activation of visual, motor, or other brain systems. The technique that has so far contributed most to functional brain mapping is PET. PET studies rely on the detection of changes in local hemodynamics that are associated with cerebral activation. In particular, there are changes in regional cerebral blood flow that can be mapped with PET through the use of ^{15}O-labeled water (or ^{15}O-labeled butanol).

Magnetic Resonance Imaging–Based Activation Studies

The MRI studies of functional activation that have recently been described also rely on hemodynamic changes. Early functional brain mapping with MRI involved the intravascular administration of an inert, nondiffusible paramagnetic contrast agent gadolinium (Gd)-DTPA to act as a marker of CBV. Under conditions of increased demand, local (or global) changes in blood flow are accompanied by changes in blood volume, which can be detected despite the fact that 70% of the blood volume resides in the venous system, and the total blood volume represents only about 4% of the total cerebral volume. This method has been successfully applied to the investigation of human visual cortex using a visual stimulus that, on the basis of PET studies, produces changes in regional CBF of about 30–50%. Echo-planar MR images are collected at intervals of 750 msec before, during, and after injection of Gd-DTPA, which is administered as a bolus into the antecubital vein. As the Gd-DTPA passes through the brain, it produces a transient reduction in water signal intensity. From the time course of the signal changes it is possible to generate images that reflect relative cerebral blood volume, an index of local perfusion, and hence synaptic activity. As with PET, imaging is carried out under controlled conditions and also during visual stimulation. Subtraction of control from activated blood volume images reveals areas associated with the task activation.

A less invasive version of the blood volume and transit time–based method, called EPISTAR, is being actively explored. Blood can be spin-labeled by pulsing the carotid artery or proximal feeding vessels appropriately. The arrival of large amounts of spin-labeled signal at a focal site in the brain implies a local increase in blood volume. There are a number of technical factors that require resolution, but this seems to be a promising approach for the future.

Magnetic Resonance Imaging–Based Noninvasive Studies

A more attractive, because less invasive, alternative MRI approach, known as BOLD, has been described. It has been known for some time that there are several mechanisms whereby changes in blood flow, volume, and oxygenation can influence MRI signal intensities without any requirement for exogenous agents. It has became apparent that activated regions of the human brain can be visualized using such intrinsic contrast mechanisms. In these studies, particular interest has focused on T2*-weighted signal intensity changes that have been attributed primarily to changes in local venous blood oxygenation, in particular to the effects generated by the paramagnetic iron centers of deoxyhemoglobin (Kwong et al. 1992).

On deoxygenation of hemoglobin, the electron spin of the heme Fe^{2+} changes from a diamagnetic state to a paramagnetic state. Paramagnetic substances can influence many properties of MR signals, through a variety of mechanisms. For example, if we consider the ^{1}H spectrum of deoxyhemoglobin itself, the presence of the paramagnetic Fe^{2+} center causes significant broadening and shifts of some of the spectral lines of the protein itself. This is of interest in the investigation of the structural properties of deoxyhemoglobin and in principle offers an approach to studying tissue oxygenation in vivo; indeed, analogous effects in myoglobin have been used to assess oxygenation status in cardiac and skeletal muscle. Of course, there are many problems with detecting signals from hemoglobin in vivo, not least of which is a relatively low concentration in brain tissue. However, it is fortunate that the proton signals of neighboring molecules, including those of water, can also be influenced by the paramagnetic Fe^{2+} centers of deoxyhemoglobin, and as a result it is possible to use the water protons to report on changes in oxygenation status. There are magnetic susceptibility effects associated with paramagnetism, so that local field gradients are generated in and around the blood vessels. These cause signal attenuation in T2*-weighted images, which is not confined just to water within the vessels but extends significantly into water in the surrounding tissues. As a result, there may be substantial signal changes associated with changes of oxygenation state, even though the blood volume is relatively small (Ogawa et al. 1990).

Thus, when focal changes in oxygenation occur associated with a stimulus or task, changes are induced in T2*-weighted images, thereby providing a means of mapping activated regions of the brain. Evidence that oxygenation changes occur with increased synaptic activity is provided by PET studies. These have shown that during cerebral activity there is an increase in local blood flow with relatively little change in oxygen consumption, so that the venous blood becomes more oxygenated on activation. This increase in venous oxygenation, or a decrease in venous deoxyhemoglobin, causes an increase in T2*-weighted signal intensity that is observed in activated regions of the brain. The contrast in T2*-weighted images is generated because gradient echoes do not refocus the dephasing effects of local field inhomogeneities associated with the presence of deoxyhemoglobin. If spin echoes are used instead of gradient echoes, then such dephasing effects will be refocused, provided that there is no significant diffusion of the water molecules through the field gradients. This explains why T2*-weighted images are more sensitive than T2-weighted images to the effects of brain activation. On the other hand, large vessels, mainly veins, will generate T2*-weighted signals, while the small venules and capillaries

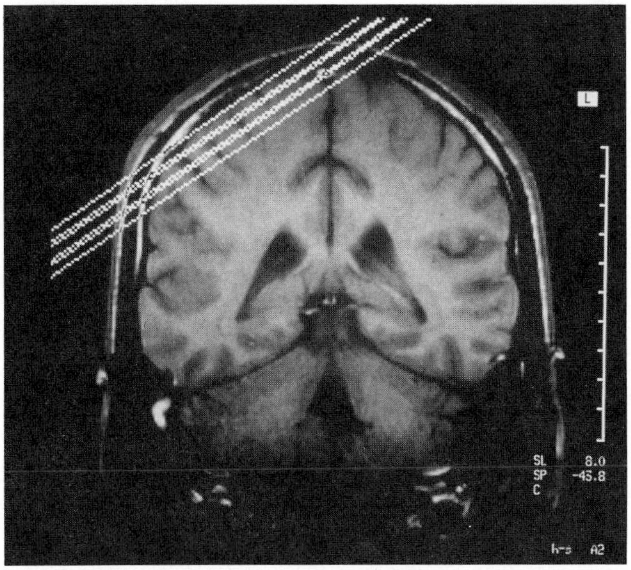

A

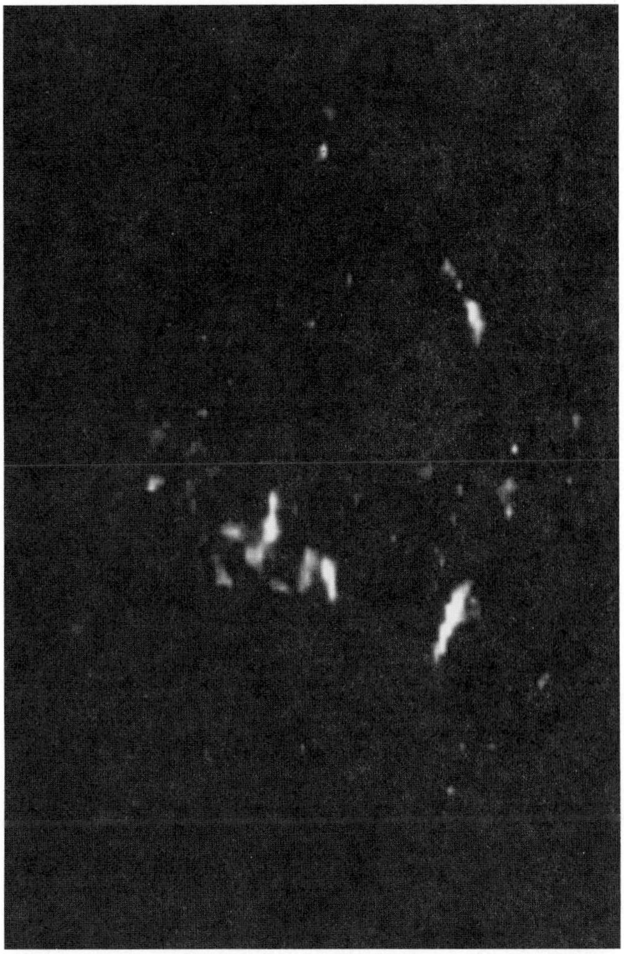

B

FIGURE 40.2 Functional MRI studies. A. The anatomy of the tangential plane that was selected for the motor activation studies. B. An activation image obtained by subtracting control images from images obtained during hand movement; see Plate 40.II for the corresponding activation image superimposed on the anatomical MRI.

influence T2-weighted images and influence the T2*-weighted signal little. This means that spin-echo images should sensitize to perfusion effects in the immediate vicinity of the activation, while the gradient-echo signals may be more diffuse or even be dominated by large draining veins some way away from the site of activation. In practice, the gradient-echo signals are localized and are also much larger than spin-echo signals.

There is also some evidence that a T1-weighted sequence might reveal activation with a signal that is sensitive to increased perfusion. The magnitude of fMRI signals depends on field strength, but in general, T2*-weighted gradient-echo signals are largest, followed by spin-echo signals, and T1-weighted signals are smallest to equivalent physiological stimuli.

Functional Magnetic Resonance Imaging with Clinical Scanners

There are a number of different ways of recording MRI signals. Many of the published fMRI studies have used echo-planar imaging or magnetic field strengths of 2T and above. Echo-planar imaging is desirable primarily because of its high-speed "snapshot" capability, and because it should permit wider coverage of the brain in a reasonable period of time. High fields are desirable because the susceptibility effects of deoxyhemoglobin become more pronounced as the field increases. However, at the time of this writing, neither echo-planar imaging nor field strengths of 2T and above are widely available, and the question therefore arises as to how successfully fMRI might be carried out using conventional MRI systems operating in routine clinical environments. It turns out that standard 1.5T systems can indeed be used for functional imaging, as illustrated by the study of motor activation shown in Figure 40.2 and Plate 40.II (Connelly et al. 1993).

In this study, T2*-weighted FLASH images were obtained at 10-second intervals. Five control images were obtained, followed by five with motor activation, the motor task consisting of repetitive finger-to-thumb opposition movements. This procedure was repeated 10 times for each hand to build up an adequate signal-to-noise ratio. Figure 40.2A shows the anatomy of the plane that was selected for the motor activation studies. Figure 40.2B shows an activation image obtained by subtracting control images from images obtained during hand movement, while Plate 40.II shows the activation image superimposed on the MR image. Appropriate cortical activity can clearly be seen, the maximal signal increase being about 4%. The figures clearly illustrate the highly focal nature of the increased signal intensity that is associated with the motor activation. Even better localization can be achieved with the use of reduced voxel sizes and appropriately angled planes through the motor and sensory cortex.

The study of the primary visual and motor cortices provides an appropriate means of establishing and validating the new methods of fMRI, partly because these systems are relatively well characterized, and also because the hemodynamic changes (and hence signal intensity changes) associated with these visual and motor tasks are likely to be considerably greater than those associated with higher cognitive functions. An outstanding problem is to establish the extent to which higher functions are accessible to investigation by fMRI. Though initial studies appear encouraging, a great deal more work needs to be carried out to establish the sensitivity of fMRI to the wide range of cognitive tasks of interest to clinical neurology.

Current Limitations of Functional Magnetic Resonance Imaging

While the initial experiences with fMRI appear highly promising, it is nevertheless essential to bear in mind the possible limitations of the technique. One important point is that changes in signal intensity may be observed as a result of hemodynamic changes associated not only with capillaries but also with larger draining veins, which may be situated a long way "downstream" from the activated tissue. On task activation they may give rise to changes in signal intensity in regions that do not reflect the regions that are actually activated. For this reason, it is essential to establish that the location of signal changes does indeed reflect focally activated regions. This might be achieved in several ways. One is to combine fMRI with angiographic techniques, so that the regions of increase in signal intensity can be compared directly with the anatomical location of the draining vessels. Alternatively, the signal from these vessels may be suppressed by using imaging sequences that give reduced signal from large vessels (see above). Multislice techniques that effectively give a three-dimensional activation pattern should help establish the source of signal increases also.

One of the potential attractions of fMRI is its high temporal resolution when compared with PET. Echo-planar imaging in principle provides resolution of about 40 msec, but unfortunately the temporal resolution is limited by the imaging sequence and by the time-dependence of the physiological effects that are visualized by fMRI. Several studies have shown that the increase in signal intensity on cortical activation occurs fairly gradually over several seconds, presumably reflecting the time constant of the hemodynamic events, and it may well be that this limits the achievable temporal resolution. With regard to MRS, it is of interest to note that increases in lactate have been observed on task activation, but the relatively poor temporal and spatial resolution associated with such metabolic studies imposes fairly severe practical limitations on the utility of this approach.

REFERENCES

Baxter LRJ, Mazziotta JC, Pahl JJ et al. Psychiatric, genetic, and positron emission tomographic evaluation of persons at risk for Huntington's disease. Arch Gen Psychiatry 1992;49:148–154.

Bench CJ, Friston KJ, Brown RG et al. The anatomy of melancholia—focal abnormalities of cerebral blood flow in major depression. Psychol Med 1992;22:607–615.

Brooks DJ. PET studies of the early and differential diagnosis of Parkinson's disease. Neurology 1993;43(suppl 6):6–16.

Brooks DJ, Ibanez V, Playford ED et al. Presynaptic and postsynaptic striatal dopaminergic function in neuroacanthocytosis: a positron emission tomographic study. Ann Neurol 1991;30:166–171.

Brooks DJ, Ibanez V, Sawle GV et al. Striatal D-2 receptor status in patients with Parkinson's disease, striatonigral degeneration, and progressive supranuclear palsy, measured with (11)C-raclopride and positron emission tomography. Ann Neurol 1992;31:184–192.

Burn DJ, Sawle GV, Brooks DJ. Differential diagnosis of Parkinson's disease, multiple system atrophy, and Steele-Richardson-Olszewski syndrome: discriminant analysis of striatal 18F-dopa PET data. J Neurol Neurosurg Psychiatry 1994;57:278–284.

Ceballos-Baumann AO, Marsden CD, Passingham RE et al. Cerebral activation with performing and imagining movements in idiopathic torsion dystonia (ITD): a PET study [abstract]. Neurology 1994;44(Suppl 2):A338.

Chugani HT, Shewmon DA, Shields WD et al. Surgery for intractable infantile spasms: neuroimaging perspectives. Epilepsia 1993;34:764–771.

Connelly A, Jackson GD, Frackowiak RSJ et al. Functional mapping of activated human primary cortex using a clinical magnetic resonance imaging system. Radiology 1993;188:125–130.

Eidelberg D, Takikawa S, Moeller JR et al. Striatal hypometabolism distinguishes striatonigral degeneration from Parkinson's disease. Ann Neurol 1993;33:518–527.

Engel JJ. PET scanning in partial epilepsy. Can J Neurol Sci 1991;18:588–592.

Frackowiak RSJ. Positron emission tomography. Sem Neurol 1989;9:275–409.

Gilman S, Junck L, Markel DS et al. Cerebral glucose hypermetabolism in Friedreich's ataxia detected with positron emission tomography. Ann Neurol 1990b;28:750–757.

Goto I, Taniwaki T, Hosokawa S et al. Positron emission tomographic (PET) studies in dementia. J Neurol Sci 1993;114:1–6.

Hoffman JM, Waskin HA, Schifter T et al. FDG-PET in differentiating lymphoma from nonmalignant central nervous system lesions in patients with AIDS. J Nucl Med 1993;34:567–575.

Jackson GD, Connelly A, Cross JH et al. Functional magnetic resonance imaging of focal seizures. Neurology 1994;44:850–856.

Kamo H, McGeer PL, Harrop R et al. Positron emission tomography and histopathology in Pick's disease. Neurology 1987;37: 439–445.

Kennedy AM, Frackowiak RSJ. Positron Emission Tomography.

In A Burns, R Levy (eds), Dementia. London: Chapman & Hall 1994;457–474.

Kuwert T, Hefter H, Scholz D et al. Regional cerebral glucose consumption measured by positron emission tomography in patients with Wilson's disease. Eur J Nucl Med 1992;19:96–101.

Kwong KK, Belliveau JW, Chesler DA et al. Dynamic magnetic resonance imaging of human brain activity during primary sensory stimulation. Proc Natl Acad Sci USA 1992;89:5675–5679.

Leblanc R, Meyer E. Functional PET scanning in the assessment of cerebral arteriovenous malformations: case report. J Neurosurg 1990;73:615–619.

Lindvall O, Widner H, Rehncrona S et al. Transplantation of fetal dopamine neurons in Parkinson's disease: 1 year clinical and neurophysiological observations in two patients with putaminal implants. Ann Neurol 1992;31:155–165.

Ogawa S, Lee TM, Kay AR et al. Brain magnetic resonance imaging with contrast dependent on blood oxygenation. Proc Natl Acad Sci USA 1990;87:9868–9872.

Otsuka M, Ichiya Y, Kuwabara Y et al. Cerebral glucose metabolism and striatal (18)F-dopa uptake by PET in cases of chorea with or without dementia. J Neurol Sci 1993;115:153–157.

Pardo JV, Fox PT. Preoperative assessment of the cerebral hemispheric dominance for language with CBF PET. Hum Brain Map 1994;1:57–68.

Rintahaka PJ, Chugani HT, Messa C et al. Hemimegalencephaly: evaluation with positron emission tomography. Paediatr Neurol 1993;9:21–28.

Ryvlin P, Philippon B, Cinotti L et al. Functional neuroimaging strategy in temporal lobe epilepsy: a comparative study of (18)FDG-PET and (99m)Tc-HMPAO-SPECT. Ann Neurol 1992;31:650–656.

Sawle GV. The detection of preclinical Parkinson's disease: what is the role of positron emission tomography? Mov Disord 1993;8:271–277.

Sawle GV, Brooks DJ, Marsden CD et al. Corticobasal degeneration. A unique pattern of regional cortical oxygen hypometabolism and striatal fluorodopa uptake demonstrated by positron emission tomography. Brain 1991a;114:541–556.

Sawle GV, Leenders KL, Brooks DJ et al. Dopa-responsive dystonia: {(18)F}dopa positron emission tomography. Ann Neurol 1991b;30:24–30.

Tyrrell PJ, Sawle GV, Bloomfield PM et al. Clinical and PET studies in the extrapyramidal syndrome of dementia of the Alzheimer type. Arch Neurol 1990;47:1318–1323.

Watson JDG, Myers R, Frackowiak RSJ et al. Area V5 of the human brain: evidence from a combined study using positron emission tomography and magnetic resonance imaging. Cerebral Cortex 1993;3:79–94.

Weiller C, Ramsay SC, Wise RJS et al. Individual patterns of functional reorganization in the human cerebral cortex after capsular infarction. Ann Neurol 1993;33:181–189.

Yao H, Sadoshima S, Kuwabara Y et al. Cerebral blood flow and oxygen metabolism in patients with vascular dementia of the Binswanger type. Stroke 1990;21:1694–1699.

Chapter 41
Neuropsychology

Luke D. Kartsounis and Elizabeth K. Warrington

Clinical neuropsychology is the study of relationships between abnormal brain function and behavior. Its origins are traced to the work of phrenologists in the early nineteenth century. It was Broca, however, who provided the first demonstration of an anatomical correlate to a particular psychological function—in this case, the center of articulate speech in the third left frontal convolution. Subsequently there were numerous descriptions of cognitive deficits, which were attributed to circumscribed lesions.

By the turn of the century, theories of cerebral localization had been substantially elaborated, and many flow diagrams were produced to describe the organization of cognitive skills. Because further investigations did not support the existence of the purported centers and their connections, this work gained little more credibility than that of the phrenologists. The view that there was little, if any, functional organization within the cortex gained ground, and Lashley provided influential evidence of this theory. The ensuing controversy was due primarily to faulty classification and could have been largely avoided if more attention was given to the fact that a skill has many components, and that it may be impaired in a variety of ways by any of various underlying lesions, although the end results might appear the same.

In recent decades indisputable evidence has demonstrated the close correlation between cerebral localization and cognitive impairments. With the essential contributions of experimental psychology, a systematic body of knowledge has been accumulated, and neuropsychology has formally joined the other neurosciences as an independent discipline.

Until fairly recently the principal aim of clinical neuropsychological investigations has often been to contribute to the diagnosis of patients by identifying cerebral impairment and by the localization of lesions. With the advent of sophisticated neuroimaging techniques over the last two decades, localization of lesions is no longer the primary concern of neuropsychology. Rather, it aims to analyze and document in detail the cognitive deficits and preserved skills of patients with degenerative neurological conditions or other diseases with known or suspected cortical involvement, including epilepsy, cerebrovascular disorders, and intracranial neoplasms. Neuropsychological assessments can identify subtle kinds of impairment that may not be detected by neurological examination or other types of investigations, including neurophysiological procedures, computed tomography, or even magnetic resonance imaging. This is particularly true in cases of early dementia or mild head injuries. In this sense, and under certain conditions, the neuropsychologist can provide a detailed diagnostic statement regarding the integrity of a patient's higher cerebral functions. Neuropsychological assessments may also provide baselines of cognitive functioning and thereby assist in monitoring certain conditions (not least, for research purposes) and in evaluating medical and surgical treatments. They have a major role in the differential diagnosis between organic and psychiatric disorders. Further, they can supply the necessary information about patients with brain damage. In addition, neuropsychological assessments can provide important descriptive and prognostic information about a patient's educational and vocational adjustment and the degree of his or her disabilities.

Two primary approaches to neuropsychological assessment have been adopted: the "big battery" approach and the "analytical" approach. The Halstead-Reitan and Luria-Nebraska batteries are widely known, and both use numerous tests. The former, based on Halstead's work, consists of a rather disparate selection of tests, including tasks of sensory-perceptual ability and finger oscillation, as well as the Wechsler Adult Intelligence Scale (WAIS) and personality questionnaires. The Luria-Nebraska battery, which comprises a more systematic range of tests, is based on the work of Luria, the Russian neurologist. Generally, batteries of tests can be time-consuming and may not always provide a pertinent account of a person's cognitive skills.

Our approach combines the traditional neurological classsifications, in terms of symptom complexes or syndromes, with the analytical principles of information-processing theories adopted by cognitive psychologists. Quantitative procedures are central to this analytical approach, enabling the clinician to state precise probabilities and reach unambiguous conclusions.

The major cognitive deficits that occur in neurological patients with localized lesions are described in this chapter. Methods of assessing neuropsychological deficits are outlined, and findings with direct consequences for clinical examination are emphasized more than data more relevant to theoretical issues. The literature in this field is already voluminous, and we needed to omit direct references to many papers of historical importance in favor of more recent authoritative accounts on some topics.

GENERAL INTELLECTUAL FUNCTIONING

Intelligence and Its Deterioration

For a neuropsychological assessment, a preliminary screening of an individual's abilities is essential. There are substantial individual differences in higher cerebral functions among the general population. However, it is widely accepted that a person's performance on a variety of cognitive tests is highly intercorrelated, and consequently it is possible to ascertain general levels of intellectual functioning. In many cases this information is necessary for focal syndromes to be properly analyzed and interpreted. Moreover, this type of assessment provides information on the integrity of cortical functioning as a whole, which can be of particular diagnostic significance in a number of neurological diseases. This information may also form the basis on which both reversible and degenerative conditions can be monitored.

The term *intellectual deterioration* may be used in two ways. *Normal deterioration* refers to a decline of a person's general level of intelligence with age. Usually, however, the term refers to *abnormal deterioration*, a decrease in a person's abilities over and above the effects of aging. Although test performance declines with age, the general level of intelligence remains constant within age groups.

Assessment of Deterioration

To assess general intelligence, most clinicians use the *intelligence quotient* (IQ) concept. The revised WAIS (WAIS-R) is widely used to determine IQ. It has been standardized using a representative sample of 1,880 subjects, and it incorporates norms based on the responses and scores obtained from groups of people with diverse profiles with regard to sex, race, education, occupation, and residence. Its clearly defined administration and scoring rules further standardize the scale. It is a highly reliable instrument, defining test reliability by the accuracy of measurement—i.e., the extent of agreement in scores from repeated testing of the same subjects. The scale comprises verbal and nonverbal tests that sample a variety of skills and from which *verbal and performance IQs*, respectively, can be derived. Such tests have limited value in localizing lesions and identifying specific cognitive deficits.

Assessing intellectual deterioration requires estimating a patient's optimal or premorbid level of functioning. Education and occupational records are often useful in this task. School records, however, might be incomplete or uninformative, and public examination results are not always known or available. Also, work histories might only reveal approximate ability levels. Some clinicians use the highest score on the WAIS-R to estimate optimal functioning. An objective, reliable method of assessing the premorbid level of functioning was recently developed and is being widely used (Nelson and Willison 1991). It is based on the findings that sight-reading vocabulary is IQ-related and that reading skills remain stable well into old age. By using this method, an optimal IQ can be estimated. The discrepancy between optimal and current IQs then provides a measure of general intellectual deterioration. Obviously this method cannot be used if a patient suffers from developmental or acquired dyslexia. The latter may occur in the presence of specific cortical lesions or in the context of "semantic dementia" (Hodges et al. 1992).

FRONTAL DEFICITS

The widely held view that the frontal lobes subserve the most complex forms of intellectual functioning could be difficult to reconcile with observations indicating that performance on standard intelligence tests may not be affected significantly, even in the context of extensive frontal lesions. Studies on psychosurgery suggest that frontal lobe lesions do not lead to permanent neuropsychological changes. Research with different patient populations, however, has suggested that such views are too simplistic.

The frontal lobes make up a large mass of the brain. They consist of anatomical units with multiple connections to other parts of the brain, both cortical and subcortical. In view of this, it might come as a surprise that a single characterization of an impairment has been sought as a clinical manifestation of often distant parts of the brain. Thus, the so-called frontal lobe syndrome was thought to consist of a cluster of cognitive and emotional or behavioral changes including deficits in abstract thinking, impaired regulation of behavior over time, impulsiveness, lack of initiative and spontaneity, facetiousness, diminished anxiety, and mild euphoria. More recent research suggests that there is not just one frontal lobe syndrome but several distinct types of impairment that are determined by the locus and laterality of the lesion and the extent that subcortical pathways are involved.

Luria's work provided much of the background for the systematic investigation of frontal lobe deficits. He defined the organization of the frontal lobes in terms of motor, premotor, and prefrontal or frontal granular cortices. The latter have extensive connections with the thalamic and the upper parts of the brain stem structures, as well as with all the cortical regions. Through these neural pathways the prefrontal cortex is thought to play a regulatory role in (1) the state of alertness and voluntary attention specifically, and (2) the ability of the individual to organize and execute high-level activity. The second role is the focus of the following section.

Evidence for Specific Deficits and Their Assessment

Unlike cerebral dysfunction in the rolandic and postrolandic zones, deficits that are associated with frontal lobe lesions are not easily amenable to quantitative measurement. Nevertheless, reports have described numerous types of impairments. In many instances the deficit can be described as a failure in an aspect of planning, regulation, and verification of activity. This may suggest that the frontal lobe deficits would be shown only in the context of relatively complex behavioral routines, but this is not always the case.

One of the most commonly reported deficits in patients with frontal lesions is perseveration. Luria (1966) referred to two forms of perseveration: (1) a continuation or unwarranted repetition of an initiated task, and (2) a continuation of a task after the patient has been asked to alter his or her behavior (Figure 41.1).

Luria also reported that patients with frontal lobe lesions may have a *deficit in motor control.* This is evident when they perform certain sequential movements. In particular, he described a simple bilateral hand coordination task that patients with frontal lobe lesions might perform poorly, by simultaneously reversing the positions of hands—one clenched and the other flat.

A very striking indication in some patients with dominant frontal lesions is a *disturbance in verbal fluency.* Patients may show great difficulty initiating speech, and their ability to use propositional speech may be limited or absent. Luria coined the term *dynamic aphasia* to describe this type of deficit.

A different type of disturbance in verbal fluency can be demonstrated by requiring the patient to generate single words from a category. In 1964, Milner was the first to use word fluency tests in patients with frontal lesions. She found that nondysphasic patients with left frontal lobectomies performed much worse than patients with right-frontal or left-temporal lobectomies. Subsequently other investigators reported similar results among patients with frontal lobe tumors—that those with left and bilateral frontal lobe tumors perform worse than those with right frontal lesions.

The Wisconsin Card Sorting Test, first devised by Berg in 1948, is perhaps the most widely used instrument for determining frontal lobe dysfunction. In this test, the patient is required to sort a pack of 128 cards successively by color, shape, and number. The difficulty of the task is in shifting from one category to another and in eliminating persevera-

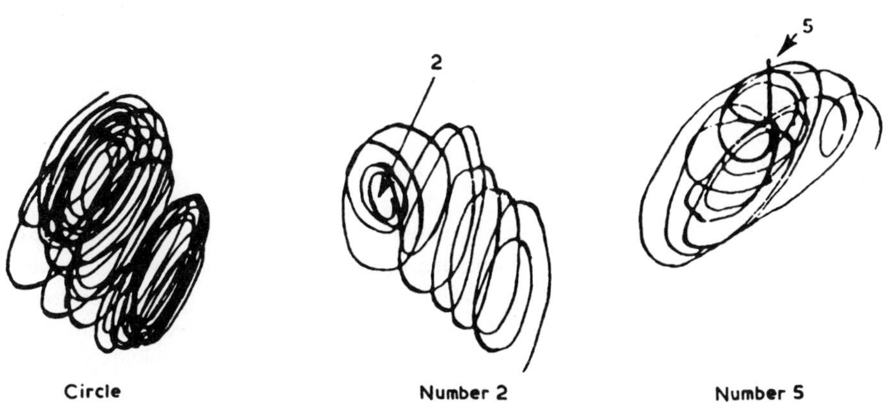

FIGURE 41.1 Perseveration of movements during performance of single tasks by a patient with a massive lesion of the frontal lobes. (Reprinted with permission from AR Luria. Human Brain and Psychological Processes. New York: Harper & Row, 1966.)

tive responses. A shorter and easier form of this test has been developed by Nelson. An even simpler similar task is Weigl's Color Form Sorting Test, which requires the patient to sort 12 items by color, then by shape (or vice versa).

Memory impairments can generally be a prominent feature in patients with frontal lobe lesions. For Luria, such deficits are secondary to a difficulty in sustaining the active effort necessary for voluntary recall, and they are also due to the inability to switch from one group of traces to another. Hécaen and Albert (1978) argued that various neuropsychological features of frontal lobe dysfunction, such as perseveration and impaired initiative and spontaneity, may underlie these observed memory deficits. Evidence of memory impairment has been documented in the context of very different testing procedures. Milner (1982) required patients either to monitor their responses on a serial recall task or to judge the temporal sequence of externally ordered events. Warrington (1984) used forced-choice recognition memory tests. In both series of investigations there was a significant incidence of impairment in patients with unilateral left or right frontal lobe lesions on verbal and nonverbal tests, respectively. Further, a dissociation between impaired performance on recognition tests and good performance on recall tasks in patients with frontal lobe lesions has been documented (Kartsounis et al. 1991). The extent to which the reported memory deficits are similar to or qualitatively different from those in patients with temporal lesions is still in question. However, lesions of the most posterior aspect of the ventromedial zone of the frontal lobe may cause an amnesic syndrome very similar to symptoms observed in patients with Korsakoff's psychosis. In such cases the lesions are commonly caused by infarcts secondary to rupture of the anterior communicating artery or anterior cerebral aneurysms.

MEMORY

Although memory is commonly thought of as a single function, in fact it encompasses a variety of phenomena, including the immediate recall of a brief verbatim message (*short-term memory*), the ability to retain and retrieve events of the recent or distant past (*long-term memory*), and memory for words and other factual knowledge (*semantic memory*). Research shows that multiple systems with different functional and structural properties mediate these phenomena, and as a result memory deficits may be both selective and dissociable. The following section focuses on three aspects of memory deficits: short-term memory impairments, global memory impairments, and selective memory impairments.

Short-Term Memory Impairments

Short-term memory is a system of limited capacity. The normal verbal auditory memory span, a measure of this system's capacity, is 7 (±2) items of information. Because the system is extremely labile, when rehearsal of stimulus material is prevented by a distracting task, the ability of an individual to reproduce even very brief messages extends over only very short intervals (seconds).

Dysphasic patients frequently have limited immediate memory spans for verbal material. Nevertheless, a relatively selective short-term verbal memory impairment may occur in the absence of other language deficits. An early detailed case study of a patient with a profound inability to repeat spoken strings of digits, letters, and words was reported by Warrington and Shallice in 1969. The patient had a digit, letter, and word span of only one or two items. Although his spontaneous speech was halting and hesitant, he performed normally on tests of comprehension of the spoken word and speech production. On additional verbal learning tasks he also performed satisfactorily. It was argued that his reduced verbal span was due to an auditory-verbal short-term memory impairment, a conclusion further supported by the finding that he performed very poorly on a short-term forgetting test, in which rehearsal is prevented by an intervening task. Specifically, he appeared to have a deficit in recalling even a single letter after only a few seconds. When a single stimulus item was presented visually, he showed no such abnormal trace decay. This syndrome of selective impairment of auditory-verbal short-term memory has since been replicated many times and is associated with lesions in the left inferior parietal lobe (Vallar and Shallice 1990).

Selective visual-verbal short-term memory deficits have also been documented. Kinsbourne and Warrington in 1962 described four patients with visual-verbal spans of apprehension of fewer than two items, despite normal auditory digit spans. This selective deficit was observed irrespective of whether numbers, letters, or shapes were used. In a subsequent group study, Warrington and Rabin in 1971 presented further evidence for the double dissociation of visual-verbal and auditory-verbal short-term memory systems. The critical lesion site for visual-verbal short-term deficits appears to be in the region of the occipitotemporal boundary of the left hemisphere.

Spatial short-term memory is frequently assessed by the Corsi Blocks Test, in which a sequence of spatial positions must be retained. A more pronounced deficit in patients with posterior right- than left-hemisphere lesions has been found in this test by De Renzi and his colleagues.

Global Memory Impairments

The amnesic syndrome, first identified by Korsakoff, consists of global learning and memory deficits. It is global in the sense that it is not material-specific; memory for both verbal and nonverbal events is impaired, and the patient has difficulty learning new names, faces, or places. In contrast, vocabulary and factual knowledge (memory for con-

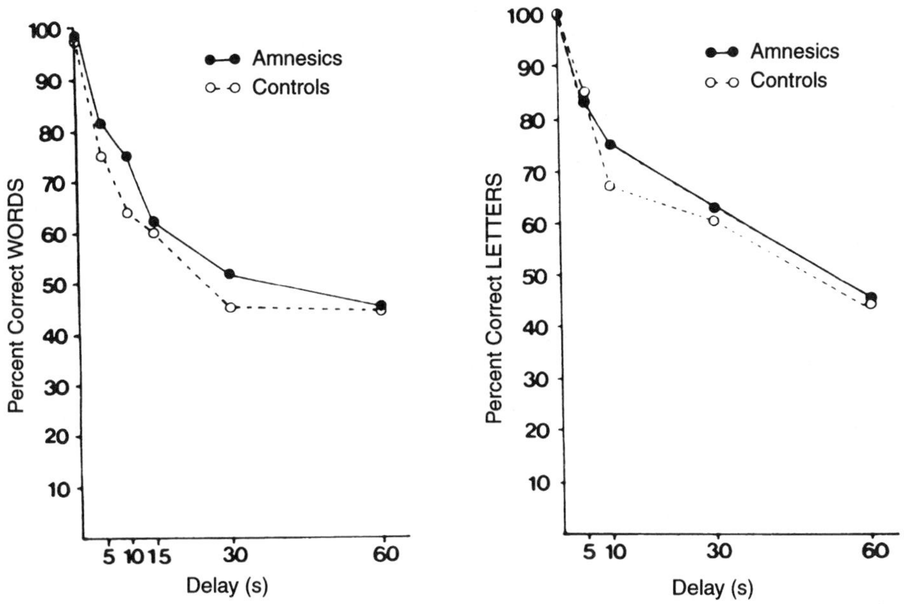

FIGURE 41.2 Short-term forgetting. Recall of printed word and letter stimuli by patients with amnesia and controls following distraction. (Reprinted with permission from EK Warrington, RA McCarthy. Disorders of Memory. In AK Asbury, GM McKhann, WI McDonald [eds], Diseases of the Nervous System–Clinical Neurobiology. Philadelphia: Saunders, 1992.)

cepts, words, and the like) is generally well-preserved. Also in the amnesic syndrome, unlike in dementia, other aspects of intellectual performance may be intact. It is distinguished from confusional states by intact perception and clarity of consciousness.

Several pathological conditions may give rise to the amnesic syndrome, including alcoholic Korsakoff's psychosis, herpes encephalitis, anoxia, cerebrovascular accidents, closed-head injuries, and brain tumors. The critical underlying disease process includes atrophy or damage to mammillary bodies and dorsomedial thalamic nucleus of the diencephalon, as well as lesions in the hippocampal formations of the temporal lobes.

Apart from *confabulation*, which is not a constant or permanent characteristic of the condition, patients with amnesia present with three relatively clearly defined clinical features: *preservation of short-term memory, retrograde amnesia*, and *anterograde amnesia*.

It has been known for some time that despite their gross global memory deficits, patients with amnesia have an unimpaired immediate memory span for digits, words presented randomly, or sentences. On tasks of short-term forgetting, these patients' performance may also be within normal range. Baddeley and Warrington in 1970 required their subjects to recall random word triplets after short intervals during which rehearsal of the stimulus material was prevented by a distracting task (counting backwards). No difference between the patients with amnesia and control groups was found at any delay interval from 1 to 60 seconds. An identical effect was obtained using triplets of consonants (Figure 41.2).

Retrograde amnesia is the impairment of memory for events antedating the onset of illness or brain damage. It is commonly assessed with questionnaire-based techniques and photographic records. Photographs of celebrities from specific periods are particularly useful. Tests of recall by positive identification, with or without cues, and recognition from plausible alternatives by selection or familiarity have been used to measure the extent and severity of memory deficits. For example, the ability of patients to recognize prominent personalities of the 1940s may be contrasted with their ability to recognize comparable personalities of more recent periods. There are obvious methodological problems with controlling task difficulty in such testing, especially with regard to the relative sparing or vulnerability of memories of different time periods of the past.

Retrograde amnesia may extend from months to many years. Clinical experience and experimental studies suggest that a temporal gradient is one of the major characteristics of retrograde amnesia, with relatively recent memories more vulnerable than remote memories. However, while some researchers did report temporal gradients for amnesia, others found dense memory deficits for events in the remote past. One can go some way in reconciling these findings by considering the extent to which different investigators have successfully equated the relative salience of events for different periods.

It has been suggested that memory of events antedating the onset of illness may fractionate. An instance of fractionation of retrograde amnesia was documented by Hodges and McCarthy (1993). Their patient presented with a profoundly impaired memory for personal autobiographic events in the context of relatively spared memory for public events.

Anterograde amnesia, the core symptom of the amnesic syndrome, is defined as an impairment of learning and retention following illness or brain damage. Research has demonstrated that the amnesic memory deficit is far from absolute. On certain tasks, and in the context of optimal laboratory conditions, patients with amnesia may show both learning and retention although they are slower than

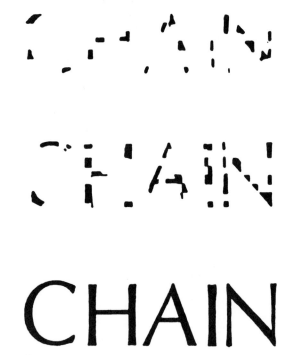

FIGURE 41.3 Example from incomplete word-learning test.

normal subjects in reaching criteria. Learning and later retention have been demonstrated on nonverbal tasks such as mirror drawing, tracking, assembling jigsaws, computer work, and incomplete-picture recognition. Verbal learning and retention can be demonstrated in cued recall tasks and incomplete word recognition (Figure 41.3). This type of evidence sharply contrasts the marked deficits of amnesic patients in conventional, standardized memory tasks such as multiple-choice recognition of words, pictures, and faces; recall of stories; or recall of word lists.

Of particular interest is the research that shows that performance of patients with amnesia is qualitatively as well as quantitatively different from that of control subjects, because it opens the way for understanding the disease process underlying the amnesic syndrome. Warrington and Weiskrantz in 1970 compared amnesic and control subjects on free recall, yes-no recognition, and cued recall (the first three letters of the stimulus word). On the first two tasks, the performance of amnesic patients was significantly impaired. In contrast, they showed no impairment on the cued-recall condition, which was not particularly easy for the control subjects. On a similar task it was found that patients with amnesia gained advantage in verbal recall from acoustic similarity (words that rhyme) and taxonomic grouping (categoric information), but unlike control subjects they failed to obtain the normal benefit from explicit instructions to use visual imagery. Another example of a qualitative rather than quantitative difference between normal and amnesic subjects was provided by the demonstration that different levels of performance are obtained by manipulating the meaningfulness of word associations. Amnesic patients perform at a normal level on rhyme pairs (such as *ring* and *sing*) but are significantly impaired on semantic category pairs (such as *bird* and *owl*) and on noun-verb pairs (*floor* and *wash*).

To explain these differences in learning between amnesic and control subjects, Warrington and Weiskrantz in 1982 postulated a cognitive mediational memory system in which memoranda are manipulated, interrelated, and stored by processes such as cognitive elaboration, visual imagery, and linguistic and semantic associations. It is clear from the foregoing that normal subjects benefit from cognitive mediation in a variety of tasks, but amnesic patients fail to do so. Warrington and Weiskrantz speculated that in amnesic patients the cognitive memory mediational system becomes inaccessible as a result of a disconnection from other cognitive systems, rather than as a consequence of damage to the system itself. They further speculated that the cognitive mediational memory system is subserved either directly or indirectly by frontal lobe structures.

Selective Memory Impairments

The amnesic patient shows global memory impairments for current and past events, but the majority of patients who complain of memory loss have more circumscribed deficits. In particular, material-specific memory impairments have been well documented, indicating selective deficits for verbal and nonverbal stimuli.

Milner and her associates conducted a series of studies on surgical patients and found significant material-specific deficits. Patients who had undergone left-temporal lobectomy showed selective impairment in learning and retaining verbal material (sentences, paired associates, and the like). Conversely, patients who had undergone right-temporal lobectomy presented with deficits in recall and recognition of nonverbal stimuli (such as faces, complex patterns, and tunes). In these studies it was consistently reported that the specific memory disturbance was closely correlated with damage of the hippocampus in the *temporal* lobe. In subsequent studies by Milner and her colleagues, memory deficits after unilateral *frontal* ablation were also reported (Petrides and Milner 1982). As with temporal-lobe lesions, the frontal ablations resulted in material-specific memory deficits, and specificity associated with laterality was frequently observed.

Warrington (1984) investigated a large group of patients (N = 279) with well-defined unilateral lesions. Recognition memory tests for both verbal and nonverbal stimuli were used, with printed words as the verbal stimuli and photographs of unfamiliar faces as the nonverbal. Because faces are meaningful stimuli that cannot be easily verbalized they were thought to be most appropriate for the assessment of nonverbal (visual) memory. It was found that there is comparable incidence of verbal memory impairment in all sectors of the left hemisphere to visual memory impairment in all sectors in the right hemisphere (Table 41.1).

Table 41.1: Recognition memory for words and faces

Lesion Site	*With Words Impaired*	*With Words Significantly Worse than Faces*	*With Faces Impaired*	*With Faces Significantly Worse than Words*
Left frontal	37	15	20	5
Left temporal	42	35	19	5
Left parietal	34	31	15	2
Right frontal	11	7	23	19
Right temporal	4	4	36	40
Right parietal	10	5	35	35

Source: Adapted from EK Warrington. Recognition Memory Test. Windsor, England: NFER, 1984.

LANGUAGE FUNCTIONS

The first references to language impairments were made many centuries ago. Broca's documentation of an anatomic correlate of articulate speech and the subsequent descriptions of motor and sensory aphasia by Wernicke are landmarks of modern aphasiology. During the years that followed, the literature in this area has grown immensely, and many language schemes have appeared. The most widely used scheme divides aphasia into expressive and receptive impairments; however, such a division is unsatisfactory and often misleading. Almost all receptive language impairments involve expressive abnormalities; conversely, expressive aphasia without receptive difficulties is extremely rare. Similar difficulties are encountered with other broad terms, such as Broca's and Wernicke's aphasias, which may be useful only as shorthand classifications. The following section is a summary of certain well-documented language impairments that are of clinical and theoretical interest concentrating primarily on recent developments in the field. First, however, a brief discussion of language laterality is necessary.

Language Laterality

The lateralization of language is based on a structural asymmetry of the cerebral cortex. It has been shown, for example, that the planum temporale (the area behind Heschl's gyrus) is about one-third longer in the left than in the right hemisphere. This area makes up part of the temporal speech cortex, and its function has been established both by anatomic findings in aphasic patients and by cortical stimulation. The fact that this asymmetry is also observed in the brains of neonates suggests that it is genetically determined rather than the result of developmental factors such as language learning and unimanual preference.

As with language impairments per se, the initial observations regarding a possible connection between aphasia and disease of the left hemisphere or between aphasia and right hemiplegia can be traced to antiquity. However, because of the not uncommon exceptions to this rule and the lack of detail in the early reports, this association was not made explicitly until Broca used the famous sentence, "*On parle avec l'hemisphere gauche.*"

In more recent times, Wada's intracarotid injection of sodium amytal has proved a valid technique prior to surgery for determining the lateralization of language. This technique has been used routinely at the Montreal Neurological Institute for many years. Milner in 1975 reported on a series of numerous patients with or without clinical evidence of early damage to the left hemisphere. Seventy percent of the patients with such early brain damage had speech representation in the left hemisphere. Comparable data have been obtained in a study of depressed patients treated with unilateral electroconvulsive therapy (Warrington and Pratt 1973). The findings of these two studies are summarized in Table 41.2. It is noteworthy that even in cases of early brain damage to either the right or the left hemisphere, there is not a particularly high incidence of shift in language lateralization.

Word Comprehension Impairments

Word comprehension deficits are most commonly associated with left-posterior temporal lesions. However, establishing anatomic correlates of word comprehension (as well as word retrieval) impairments may be confounded by the fact that even these relatively automatic skills in fact have many components. At present, these components cannot be specified in detail, but it is widely accepted that they include systems processing perception of sounds generally (an impairment of which may be associated with cortical deafness) and perception of words specifically (an impairment of which may give rise to word deafness) (see Tanaka et al 1987). Where word perceptual difficulties can be excluded and reading ability is relatively intact, auditory comprehension difficulties can be attributed to deficits associated with word meaning per se.

Comprehension of word meaning may be impaired in patients with relatively good preservation of other language functions. In 1975, Warrington studied three patients with a striking and selective impairment of spoken word comprehension. They were intelligent individuals who were able to perform at a high level on general intellectual ability tests. Their expressive skills were fairly satisfactory and were limited mainly by the loss of individual word meanings. They could read and write and were able to repeat

Table 41.2: Lateralization of language: percentage of cases in left- and right-handed individuals with and without early left-hemisphere damage

	Lateralization of Language			
	Left Hemisphere		*Right Hemisphere*	
	Left-handed or Mixed	*Right-handed*	*Left-handed or Mixed*	*Right-handed*
Early left-hemisphere damage (N = 109)	30	81	51	13
Without early left-hemisphere damage (N = 262)	70	96	15	4
Unilateral ECT in depressed patients without known organic disease (N = 30)	70	98	23	2

Source: Adapted from EK Warrington, RTC Pratt. Language laterality in left-handers assessed by unilateral E.C.T. Neuropsychologia 1973;11:423–8; and B Milner. Psychological Aspects of Focal Epilepsy and Its Neurosurgical Management. In DP Purpura, JK Penry, RD Walter (eds), Advances in Neurology. New York: Raven, 1975.

digits, word strings, and sentences satisfactorily, indicating intact word perception. However, these patients were unable to comprehend many word meanings which, it could be safely assumed, were previously within their vocabulary. When asked to explain words such as basket, precise, or camel, they would respond with expressions like, "I've forgotten" or "It sounds familiar." Further investigations showed that their deficit of spoken word comprehension correlated negatively with word frequency. This observation appeared to be consistent with other reports suggesting that word comprehension deficits can be completely specified in terms of word frequency. The oversimplification of such an inference, however, is illustrated by category-specific word comprehension impairments.

Neurologists have long observed that verbal comprehension deficits (as well as naming impairments) may be particularly severe or even restricted to a certain category, notably the names of body parts and colors. Goodglass et al. in 1966 were the first to study systematically the retrieval and comprehension skills in aphasic patients and to document selective preservation or impairment for categories of color and shape, as well as concrete nouns and action names. Interestingly, the retrieval deficits (naming to confrontation) did not correspond to those for word comprehension (spoken word-picture matching). Goodglass et al. observed that patients who were actually able to name parts of the body were unable to point to a named part of the body (but see also Sirigu et al. 1991 regarding the multiple representations of body knowledge processing).

A dissociation in comprehension of concrete versus abstract words has similarly been documented. For example, a case was recorded in which a patient who presented with a significantly greater difficulty in defining the meaning of concrete words such as needle than in defining words with an abstract referrent such as supplication (Warrington 1975). These observations were replicated. Because in all these instances the concrete and abstract words were matched in frequency, and because abstract words are presumably more difficult to define than concrete words, the observed deficits could not be accounted for by task difficulty.

Fractionations within the concrete word domain have also been documented by Warrington and colleagues (McCarthy and Warrington 1990). Two patients were able to define significantly more objects than living things or foods. With two other patients, who were too dysphasic to attempt a word definition task, they used a spoken word-picture matching test in which the subject was simply required to point to an item out of five pictures in the three categories. Both patients performed significantly better on the object sets than on the animal or food sets. All of these patients had herpes encephalitis, and computed tomography showed bilateral disease affecting particularly the temporal lobes. It seems implausible to interpret such category-specific deficits in terms of item familiarity or even word frequency. Moreover, a dissociation between the different stimulus categories in the opposite direction was observed in a patient who had suffered a major left-middle cerebral stroke and presented with a particularly severe global dysphasia.

The question arises whether the dissociations of comprehension of word categories reflect a fundamental division in the central representation of concrete words. It could be argued that foods and living things are differentiated primarily by their physical or sensory attributes (with their functional properties being of lesser significance, such as carrot versus parsnip). Conversely, objects are differentiated mostly by their functional properties (because their physical or sensory attributes are less relevant or even misleading—for instance, vase versus jug). Accordingly, a typology along these lines could account for the category-specific dissociations of word comprehension.The evidence to date, however, suggests that such a typology would be inadequate to encompass all the available data. For example, one patient appeared to have greater impairment for small manipulable items than for large outdoor objects. When the selective impairments of comprehension for names of actions and verbs versus nouns are added to cases described here, it becomes apparent that a finer-grained organization of verbal comprehension systems needs to be postulated (McCarthy and Warrington 1990).

Word Retrieval Impairments

Word retrieval difficulties are exemplified by nominal (anomic, amnesic) dysphasia, a common neurological deficit. Indeed, an impairment in retrieving the name of an object may be the first sign of neurological disease. Typically, affected patients have fluent speech with little or no paraphasia. They can describe an object, indicate its use, or select the correct name from a list of names.

It has been shown that word frequency in the language is related to performance, with high-frequency names being less vulnerable than low-frequency names (Newcombe et al. 1965). Rochford and Williams (1962) compared age of acquisition of words with dysphasic errors and found that the high-frequency words were those first learned in early childhood and the last lost in dysphasia. Although dysfunction of various parts of the left hemisphere may result in naming difficulties, McKenna and Warrington found in 1980 that the highest incidence of nominal dysphasia is associated with left-temporal-lobe lesions.

The diagnosis of nominal dysphasia is widely based on clinical impressions or tests using global measures of current naming ability, such as number of failures or latencies of responses (Newcombe et al. 1965). These tests, however, do not take into account individual differences in terms of ability in general and expressive vocabulary in particular. Thus patients with superior naming vocabularies who develop word retrieval difficulties may not be diagnosed as dysphasic, because they are likely to fail only on uncommon or low-frequency items and therefore continue to perform within the normal range. McKenna and Warrington in 1980 developed a graded naming test that helps the clinician obtain quantitative measures for even minor degrees of word retrieval problems. In more severe cases where the deficit is obvious, an accurate quantitative measure adds to the value of a case description.

As with word comprehension, selective-naming deficits that are category-specific have also been documented. In an early report on the subject, Goodglass et al. argued in 1966 that the homogeneity of nominal dysphasia is usually apparent rather than real. Studying 135 aphasic patients, they found that the relative difficulty of naming objects, colors, numbers, letters, and actions was different in a group of Broca's aphasics than in a group of Wernicke's aphasics. Several other category-specific deficits in naming have since been recorded (see McKenna and Warrington 1993 for a review).

Word Production (Speech Articulation) Impairments

The descriptions of sounds and patterns of sounds that occur in a language are called its *phonology*. Two descriptions of speech may be distinguished: *phonetic* and *phonemic*. Phonetic speech denotes the basic components of speech sounds; the term phonemic refers to their combinations into phonemes.

Certain speech impairments are associated with these two aspects of phonology. Phonetic disintegration (also known as *pure anarthria* or *aphemia*) is an articulation impairment in the production of the sounds of speech. More errors are made at the beginning of words, and these errors are more likely to involve consonants, particularly clusters of consonants, rather than vowels. Many errors are slight distortions; they might sound as if they are spoken by a non-native speaker. As Lecours and Lhermitte reported in 1976, this syndrome was fully described in a series of papers over many years. The subject of this long and detailed study was a man who was bilingual in English and French. His speech was slow and laborious, with abnormal prosody and explosive production of syllables. Although the disorder was manifested exclusively as an articulation problem, there was evidence of higher-level cerebral involvement in that there was a partial dissociation between the two languages he spoke, with his English phonology (which he had learned earlier in his life) better preserved than his French phonology. Postmortem examination identified a unilateral lesion, with an isolation of Broca's area from the left precentral gyrus. It also involved some destruction of the mouth and larynx areas of the cortex.

Patients with phonetic disintegration retain intact internal language functions with internal access to sounds of words. This is illustrated by their ability to make rhyme judgments and to tap out the number of syllables of words they cannot pronounce. There is considerable variability in the errors of such patients, who might pronounce the same phoneme correctly and incorrectly within a short interval. Lebrun et al. in 1973 argued that this type of variability is further evidence that phonetic disintegration is an aspect of motor dysphasia, rather than a dysarthric disorder arising from subcortical lesions.

Unlike patients with deficits at the phonetic level, patients with phonemic deficits present with impairments in selecting patterns of phonemes, but with adequate production of individual phonemes. Commonly their errors consist of incorrect phonemes (e.g., *hone* for *home*), duplication of phonemes (e.g., *adadamant* for *adamant*), and misordering (e.g., *caper clip* for *paper clip*). Phonemic substitutions seem to have their counterparts in normal slips of the tongue, which suggests the psychological reality of phonemes as units in speech production. The anatomic correlates of phonemic disorders are not firmly established.

Phonemic paraphasic errors are characteristic of two types of aphasic syndromes: *conduction aphasia* and *transcortical motor aphasia*. The conduction aphasic tends to make phonemic paraphasic errors in repetition of polysyllabic words or clichés, which in a sense can be equated to abstract words with a single referent. Such errors are much less common in spontaneous speech. In contrast, in one type of transcortical motor aphasia, repetition of digits and polysyllabic words or clichés is satisfactory, but spontaneous speech is effortful and has a high incidence of phonemic errors. McCarthy and Warrington in 1984 conducted a series of experiments with two patients with conduction aphasia and one with transcortical motor aphasia. They found that in repetition tasks that maximized active semantic processing, such as repetition of sentences rather than words in isolation, the conduction aphasics' abilities were facilitated but the transcortical motor aphasics' were impaired. The converse pattern of dissociation was observed in tasks that required passive repetition. The conduction aphasics also appeared more impaired when they repeated clichés. Thus task-specific speech production difficulties were observed in both syndromes. The authors argued that these patients' speech production deficits were in transcoding information between input and output systems. Following Lichtheim, they tentatively postulated a two-route model of speech production. In this model, one route depends on active semantic analysis and the other is thought to bypass semantic analysis and involve a direct process from auditory input to speech output systems. The modus operandi of such a model, however, is unknown.

Sentence Comprehension and Production Impairments

The accumulating evidence regarding the defective knowledge of meanings of categories of words is emphasized above. In clinical practice, however, comprehension impairments are more commonly observed in the context of grammatical relationships among words in a sentence. As with comprehension deficits at the word level, our understanding of sentence comprehension impairments is limited. Nevertheless it is widely accepted that performance is determined by task difficulty. Short-term memory difficulties notwithstanding, single instructions may be understood better than double instructions, which may lead to failure on part of the task or confusion between the two parts.

In 1962 De Renzi and Vignolo devised the Token Test, for the understanding of spoken speech, which uses tokens of different shapes, sizes, and colors. The patient is given verbal instructions in progressively complex, nonredundant sentences (for example, "Touch the yellow square" and "Put the red circle between the yellow square and the green square"). There have been various modifications of this test, including shortened versions. The Token Test is a sensitive instrument that helps the clinician identify patients with minor disturbances in the understanding of speech with minimal involvement of other intellectual functions.

Neurologists have long noted that expressive speech can be impaired in many ways. They have grouped these impairments into those characterized by circumlocutory speech, imprecision, semantic errors, and increased fluency or pressure of speech (fluent dysphasia), and those manifested by articulatory difficulties, lack of fluency, agrammatism, or telegraphic speech (nonfluent dysphasia). Benson in 1967 examined the features of dysphasic speech: rate of speaking, prosody, pronunciation, phrase length, effort, pauses, pressure of speech, perseveration, word use, and paraphasia. He found that two clusters of these dysphasic features occurred together and were associated with lesions anterior or posterior to the rolandic fissure. The anterior lesion group showed low verbal output, dysprosody, dysarthria, and predominant use of substantives; those in the posterior group were normal or near normal with regard to these features but often presented with paraphasias, pressure of speech, and a distinct lack of substantives. Other authors have similarly reported that a fluent type of dysphasia is associated with posterior lesions and a nonfluent dysphasia with anterior lesions.

Such diagnostic considerations suggest that the ability to speak in sequences of words is a critical dimension for assessing a patient's expressive skills. A usual device for obtaining such information is to engage patients in an open-ended conversation or to show them a picture and ask them to describe what is happening. Although useful information on qualitative aspects of speech may be obtained by such procedures, these techniques remain unsatisfactory because they depend entirely on how patients choose to verbalize their thoughts, a decision that may be influenced by other factors, such as depression.

De Renzi and Ferrari in 1978 devised a test requiring the patient to act as a reporter of a performance carried out by the examiner, who acts in accordance with the commands of the Token Test. De Renzi and Ferrari's test, known as the Reporter's Test, was useful in helping the clinician identify various speech impairments, including articulation, rate of speaking, phonemic or semantic paraphasias, circumlocutory speech, nominal dysphasia, and impairments in sentence construction.

An abnormality in sentence construction where the syntactic rules are violated is known as *agrammatism*, but a variety of deficits have been described under this label. Tissot et al. in 1973 studied nine agrammatic patients in some detail and identified two subtypes: *syntactic agrammatism* and *morphological agrammatism*. In the former syndrome, use of function words and articles is relatively well-preserved, but there is an impairment of word order and use of verbs. The latter syndrome is characterized by a relatively satisfactory use of verbs and word order, but with an impaired use of function words and inflections. McCarthy and Warrington (1985) described a patient who presented with syntactic agrammatism and whose spontaneous speech was characterized by an almost complete absence of substantive verbs. They argued that his agrammatism did not reflect impaired syntax per se but a category-specific word comprehension and word retrieval deficit—that is, an impaired semantic representation of verbs. In other words, his anomalous sentence construction could be explained by his efforts to compensate for his inability to use substantive verbs.

LITERACY SKILLS

Reading Impairments

The term *alexia* is often used interchangeably with *dyslexia* to mean an impairment of reading skill; another term, *word blindness*, is no longer used. Some clinicians use the term *acquired dyslexia* to distinguish it from *developmental dyslexia*, the inability to acquire the reading skill from childhood.

Table 41.3: Reading and spelling with and without using phonology

	Reading Using Phonology	*Reading Without Phonology*	*Spelling Using Phonology*	*Spelling Without Phonology*
Irregular words	X	√	X	√
Regular words	√	√	√	√
Nonwords	√	X	√	X

Since the late nineteenth century, Dejerine and other neurologists have been interested in the distinction between *dyslexia with dysgraphia* and *dyslexia without dysgraphia.* The documentation of cases of patients with dyslexia without dysgraphia led to the postulation of a center that is intact but becomes disconnected from incoming visual information. Neuropathological evidence has given support to this hypothesis, and the critical anatomical structures implicated in the majority of patients were found to be in the angular gyrus and the splenium. On the other hand, research on patients with dyslexia accompanied by dysgraphia has led to the notion that the center of written letters and words itself has been damaged. There is evidence that in such cases the critical anatomical structure is the supramarginal gyrus. However, such theories are far too simplistic to account adequately for the variety of syndromes of acquired dyslexia that have been documented. For example, reading skill may become impaired as a result of degradation of semantic knowledge—that is, impaired comprehension for particular word classes. Such a deficit may be observed in the context of certain types of cerebral atrophy with a left-temporal focus referred to as *semantic dementia* (Hodges et al. 1992).

Clinical practice and research show that reading is a complex skill that may be disturbed by a variety of factors and in many different ways. There have been several classificatory systems of reading deficits, depending on the authors' emphasis on description of these phenomena or their interpretation. Traditionally, however, there have been two major categories of reading impairments: those that affect the reading of individual letters (literal dyslexia) and those that affect the reading of words and passages (verbal dyslexia). In literal dyslexia the patient is unable to read individual letters but may retain the ability to read words; in verbal dyslexia the reverse is true. Global dyslexia affects both letters and words.

Shallice and Warrington in 1980 proposed an alternative framework to distinguish what they termed *peripheral* and *central dyslexic syndromes.* The peripheral dyslexias implicate damage to a visual word form system that causes a defect in attaining a satisfactory graphemic analysis of words. Such impairments include dyslexias resulting from neglect (*neglect dyslexia*), *attentional dyslexia*, and *spelling dyslexia* or *letter-by-letter reading.* Central dyslexias imply damage to systems that process written word meanings, an adequate visual word form having been accessed. This classification system is akin to the prevailing views of neuropsychologists and cognitive psychologists who have attempted to use psycholinguistic models to integrate knowledge about normal reading processes with data on patients with reading impairments. The basic tenet of the psycholinguistic approach is that there are at least two reading procedures, frequently referred to as *routes.* One, the *phonological route*, transcodes the visual word form into its phonological correspondence. This print-sound conversion operates at a subword level. The word meaning is subsequently derived from the phonological correspondence of the written word. The other reading route operates in such a way that the meaning of a written word is derived directly from the written word (visual word form) without intermediary phonological processing. Thus this route has been termed *direct*, *semantic*, or *lexical.* Within such a model, a dyslexic syndrome may be analyzed on the basis of the type of paralexic errors the patient makes. For example, a patient whose direct route has been damaged, and who tends to rely heavily on phonological processes, will be able to read nonsense words and will be more successful with regular than irregular words. Conversely, a patient whose phonological route has been damaged and who tends to rely heavily on lexical processes will be able to read real words (spelled regularly and irregularly) but will have difficulty with nonsense words (Table 41.3).

Reading impairments may also include word-class effects. Function words become particularly vulnerable and might be substituted for one another. Verbs present greater difficulty than adjectives, which in turn present more difficulty than nouns. Of particular interest is the reading impairment of abstract, compared to concrete, nouns. The opposite phenomenon—that is, a significant impairment of reading concrete compared to abstract words—has also been documented. The foregoing suggest that, as with traditional descriptions, the analysis of dyslexias within a psycholinguistic framework is ambiguous, with the main clinical syndromes subdivided into multiple subsyndromes (see McCarthy and Warrington 1990 for a review).

Spelling Impairments

Traditionally, the term *agraphia* or *dysgraphia* has referred to two types of deficits: spelling impairments and a motor disturbance in forming the letters themselves. We adhere to this broad distinction. First, however, a brief introduction to the complexities of dysgraphia is appropriate.

There have been several classification systems in which a variety of deficits—such as pure agraphia, agraphia with dyslexia, apraxic agraphia, and aphasic agraphia—have been discussed. None of these typologies has been entirely satisfactory (Roeltgen 1985). Historically, many authors have emphasized that writing skills are generally secondary to and dependent on language and speech functions. Although dysgraphia is undoubtedly commonly associated with other language and, indeed, praxic impairments, selective writing disorders have been repeatedly documented.

As is the case with reading, the analysis of spelling and its disorders has been enhanced by analysis within a psycholinguistic framework. Several complex models have been put forward, and in all of them at least two procedures (routes) for spelling have been proposed. These routes parallel the processes involved in reading that were discussed previously. One is sound-based (phonological), whereas the other is thought to be *direct* or *lexical.* The first detailed case reports with evidence of selective impairments in phonological transcoding and direct orthographic (lexical) routes were reported by Shallice in 1981 and Beauvois and Derouesne in 1981, respectively. Phonological impairment can be identified by a comparatively greater difficulty in spelling of nonsense than of actual words, whereas orthographic impairment is manifested by a comparatively greater difficulty in spelling irregular words as compared to nonsense and regular words (see Table 41.3). The critical anatomical loci for phonological dysgraphia are thought to be areas of the supramarginal gyrus or the insula medial to it. In the case of lexical dysgraphia, the corresponding loci are probably the junction of the posterior angular gyrus and the parieto-occipital lobe (Roeltgen 1985).

Patients who spell without phonological transcoding appear to be dependent on semantic processes. Thus a patient might make errors that are semantically related to the target word—for example, *child* for *boy*. Also, patients with impaired comprehension for particular word classes, such as abstract words, may present with a similar pattern in their spelling. However, word-class spelling impairment can occur without a deficit in comprehension of the relevant class of words; for example, the spelling of function words or of verbs may be selectively lost (Caramazza and Hillis 1991).

Writing Impairments

Like spelling processes, writing is a complex skill dependent on a number of subcomponents, which may be selectively impaired. It is more commonly manifested in association with apraxia, because an impairment of voluntary movements may also extend to relatively automatized skills such as writing. Nevertheless, dysgraphia without apraxia can occur, and it is manifested by impaired production of letters in both spontaneous writing and writing to dictation, although letter production may improve with copying and oral spelling can be intact.

A diagnosis of selective writing impairments should exclude peripheral weakness, clumsiness, and sensory difficulties as well as apraxic and visuospatial problems. There have been no reports with quantitative data that have fulfilled these criteria in their entirety. Nevertheless, following Margolin's analysis, there appear to be at least two types of selective writing impairments corresponding to motor and ideational apraxia. In the former case, the patient has lost the automaticity of writing and the formation of letters is clumsy, although the actual letter selection is not impaired. These patients have as much difficulty in copying as in writing to dictation. The ideational graphic difficulty is in the selection of the appropriate motor program, or sequences of programs, for producing a particular letter or group of letters. In this syndrome there is a considerably greater difficulty in writing to dictation than in copying, and the copy appears to act as a prompt to the appropriate retrieval cue (see Figure 41.4 for examples of motor and ideational dysgraphia). We would interpret spatially disorganized writing as secondary to visuospatial difficulties.

Calculation Impairments

The impairment of arithmetic skills, referred to as *acalculia* or *dyscalculia*, is commonly one of the many manifestations of aphasic disorders. Less frequently it is observed as a circumscribed deficit; indeed, more than one type of pure acalculia has been identified. In 1961, Hécaen et al. classified dyscalculic disorders into three categories: (1) acalculia associated with number alexia (i.e., an inability to read or understand numbers); (2) acalculia of the spatial type (i.e., a deficit resulting in a misalignment of numbers in the appropriate columns); and (3) anarithmetria (i.e., an impairment of the calculation skill per se). Generally, anarithmetria without sufficient dementia or dysphasia to account for it is associated with left parietal lesions, whereas spatial dyscalculia is more commonly encountered in patients with right-hemisphere lesions.

Several cases have been documented showing that Hécaen et al.'s classification system is far too general and cannot account for the diversity of dyscalculic deficits observed in clinical practice. For example, Benson and Denckla in 1969 reported the case of a patient who could choose the correct answer from a multiple choice list when calculations were presented visually as arabic numbers or verbally, but gave incorrect answers when asked to say or write the answers to problems. In other words, this patient's comprehension of numbers and ability to perform calculations were apparently intact but the production of numbers was impaired. McCloskey and Caramazza (1987) documented cases of patients in whom dissociations between number comprehension and number production mechanisms were also observed. Cipolotti et al. (1991) described a patient with dense dyscalculia who could nevertheless process numbers below four (in all modalities). Warrington had earlier

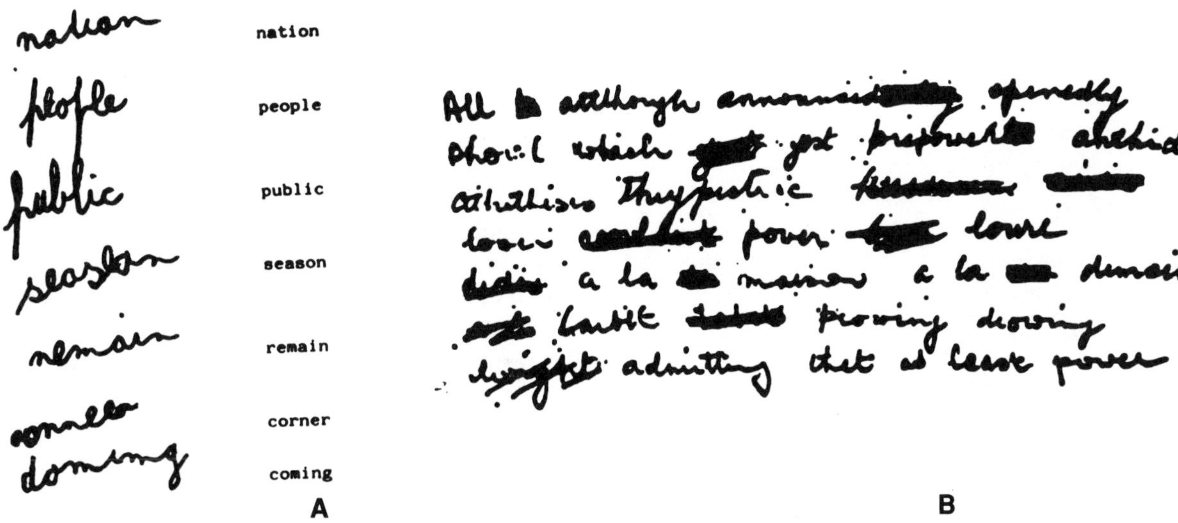

FIGURE 41.4 Example of ideational (A) and motor dysgraphias (B).

studied in detail a patient who had sustained a left parieto-occipital hemorrhage and became dyscalculic. She found that it was his knowledge of arithmetical facts, rather than his knowledge of arithmetic operations, that was impaired. He was able to understand the significance and magnitude of numbers and to use appropriate computational procedural rules, but he had lost the "automaticity" of computation and could add and subtract only by using laborious counting procedures. For other examples of selective impairments of the subcomponents of calculation, see Deloche and Seron (1987).

Clinical experience shows that dyscalculia may arise selectively, depending on the mode of presentation of calculations and the response required. Patients who are aphasic may perform better when computational problems are presented in written form rather than orally, because paraphasic errors might contaminate their oral performance. In contrast, oral presentation of problems might facilitate the performance of a patient with spatial acalculia. Benton in 1963 devised a systematic method for comparing the oral and written modes of presentation and response. It includes very simple tests for assessing the comprehension of numbers presented in auditory or visual mode and proceeds to oral and written arithmetic calculations using the four basic operations. It also includes the arithmetic subtest of the WAIS, which is probably the most commonly used instrument for assessing computational skills in clinical practice.

In 1986, Jackson and Warrington developed a graded-difficulty test of arithmetic computations. It consists of 12 additions and 12 subtractions, which are orally presented. In normal subjects, performance was found to correlate highly with other measures of verbal intelligence. With this test the extent of a calculation impairment may be identified independent of a patient's reasoning skills.

Impairments of calculation, spelling, and writing, together with other neurological deficits (finger agnosia and right-left disorientation), have often been discussed in the context of Gerstman syndrome. In our view, the accumulated evidence to date no longer justifies the inclusion of these deficits within a single syndrome; their concurrent occurrence seems to depend on fortuitous combinations of neurologic impairments, frequent as these may be, rather than on a naturally occurring combination.

VISUAL PERCEPTUAL FUNCTIONS

Our discussion of perceptual agnosic defects focuses on visual modality. Visual perception is better understood than auditory or somesthetic perception. In addition, visual perception deficits are more commonly encountered in clinical practice than other perceptual deficits.

This section first emphasizes deficits arising from damage to the occipital lobes; the degree of integrity of the early visual information-processing mechanisms must be known before a diagnosis of higher-level perceptual deficits can be made. Subsequently, the literature on the widely reported syndromes of apperceptive and associative object agnosias is summarized.

Early Visual Information Impairments

Anatomical and physiological studies in monkeys and experimental work with normal human subjects have indicated a segregation of early visual processing skills (Livingstone and Hubel 1988). Observations in patients with partial cortical blindness have similarly suggested striking dissociations between early visual information processing. These include point localization, form, color, and movement perception.

Visual disorientation has been defined by Holmes as the inability to localize the position and distance of objects by

FIGURE 41.5 Efron shapes matched for total surface area and contrast.

sight alone. Typically, patients with visual disorientation find it difficult to reach for objects accurately and have difficulty converging and fixating on an object and judging its relative distance in relation to other objects. The blink reflex might be absent, except when responding to menace by their own hand. In severe cases, the patient may behave as a totally blind person, using head-scanning strategies in an attempt to fixate on a target. It differs in this regard to Balint's syndrome or *optic ataxia*, in which impairment in point localization is specifically due to an inability to coordinate visual information with somatosensory information (Perenin and Vighetto, 1988). The Aimark perimeter may be used to accurately test the degree of deficit in point localization.

The ability to locate points in space dissociates from the ability to detect the presence of stimuli or their *movement*. Holmes's patients were able to detect movement and even to report on its direction. The case of a patient who could not detect movement but was able to locate stationary points and who was not visually disorientated has been described (Zihl 1991).

Riddoch in 1935 argued that visual disorientation is mapped in the same way as a primary visual-field defect. He reported on two patients with unilateral lesions in whom visual disorientation was limited to one field, contralateral to the lesion. There is a high incidence of inferior hemianopic field defects in patients with visual disorientation. These impairments are not thought to be causally related, but their association implies that the critical lesion is in the parieto-occipital region.

Shape discrimination is a function of early visual information processing. In 1968, Efron documented the case of a patient recovering from cortical blindness after carbon monoxide poisoning. His acuity and ability to localize objects in space were adequate, and he could discriminate fine differences in hue; but he had great difficulty recognizing objects. On examination he was unable to discriminate between a square and an oblong matched for total surface area and contrast. If test difficulty was manipulated by varying the ratio of the length to the width of the oblong (Figure 41.5), the patient performed very poorly, except on the easiest discrimination. Not surprisingly, his difficulty in recognizing real objects was attributed to his grave impairment in shape perception rather than to visual agnosia. In subsequent case studies, patients with basic shape-perception deficits were also found to be impaired on tasks of *figure-ground discrimination* (Figure 41.6A), a deficit considered to be underlain by the same kind of impairment as the shape perception deficit. However, a double dissociation between these two skills has now been documented (Davidoff and Warrington 1993). One of these patients was unable to perceive overlapping geometric shapes (Figure 41.6B) and was "blind" to illusory shapes and illusory contours (Figure 41.6C and 41.6D), whereas the other patient, with the basic shape discrimination deficit, had no difficulty in perceiving these stimuli.

Achromatopsia is the impairment of color perception. The Holmgren wool-sorting test is a simple tool for assessing color perception deficits. The patient is required to name or match colors or to arrange them in a series according to brightness or saturation. Patients may also be examined on the Ishihara plates for color blindness and the Farnsworth-Munsell 100-hue test. In severe cases of achromatopsia, only black, white, and shades of gray can be perceived. As with visual disorientation, retinal topology also occurs in achromatopsia, with the impairment manifested contralaterally to the lesion. In his review, Meadows (1974) summarized 14 cases of achromatopsia with a high incidence of altitudinal field defects, and from these he inferred bilateral lesions in the occipitotemporal region. Autopsy data from three of these cases confirmed this localization.

As indicated, cortical blindness is rarely an absolute deficit. Early visual processing skills may be selectively preserved or selectively impaired, and such observations support notions of parallel processing rather than hierarchic models of the early visual information-processing mechanisms. They also have clear implications for clinical practice. Before an agnosic deficit is identified, it is necessary by definition to establish adequate sensory input. Failure to exclude deficits such as those outlined previously (with the possible exception of achromatopsia) may result in the diagnosis of pseudoagnosic syndromes.

Agnosia: Impairments of Object Recognition

In the past, Lissauer made a distinction between two stages of object recognition. One, the failure to organize visual stimuli into coherent percepts, was termed the *apperceptive*

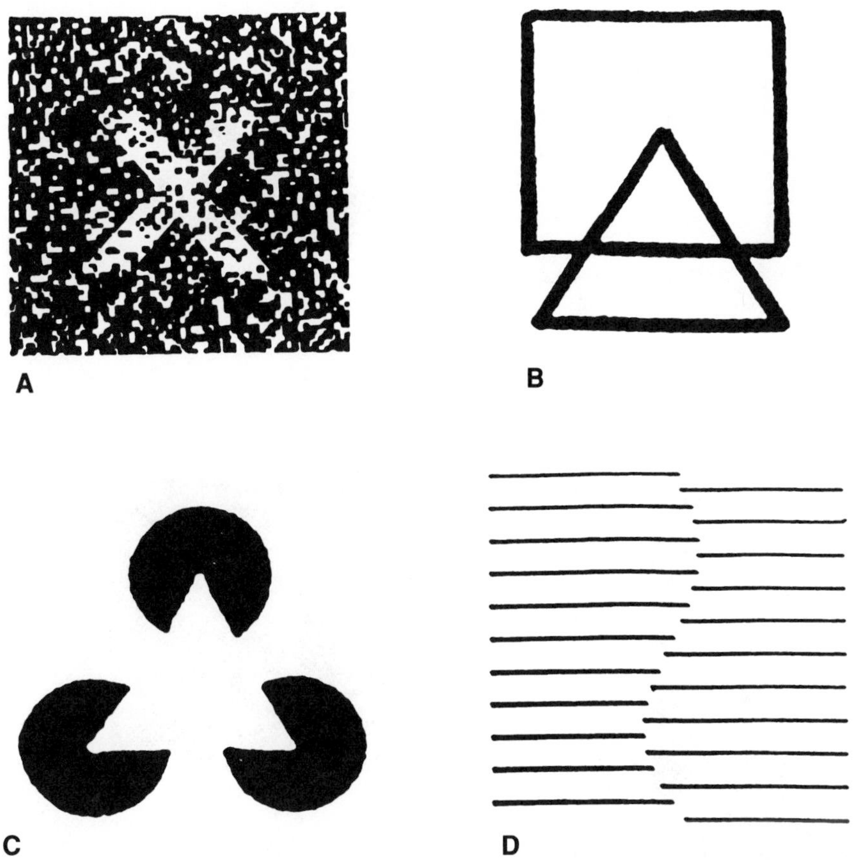

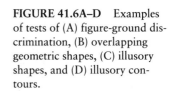

FIGURE 41.6A–D Examples of tests of (A) figure-ground discrimination, (B) overlapping geometric shapes, (C) illusory shapes, and (D) illusory contours.

stage. The other, the act of linking the content of perception with meaning, was referred to as the *associative stage* of perception.

A deficit in visual recognition of pictorial material in patients with postrolandic lesions of the right hemisphere has been repeatedly documented and cannot be accounted for in terms of impaired sensory function. These patients are particularly impaired on tasks in which the visual stimulus is reduced or degraded. Such tasks involve sketchy drawings of scenes, overlapping of drawings of common objects, incomplete outline drawings of objects and letters, and photographs of shadow images of objects from different viewpoints (for examples, see Figure 41.7).

Research has shown double dissociations between different classes of visual stimuli in patients with perceptual deficits. However, it is the defective recognition of familiar faces—that is, *prosopagnosia,* or *facial agnosia*—that has been given special attention as a distinctive visuoperceptual deficit.

Prosopagnosic patients are unable to recognize the faces of familiar people but may recognize them by other characteristics, such as their voices or visual clues, including hairstyle, clothing, and gait. There appear to be two distinct types of prosopagnosia. In the first type the deficit is due to a faulty perceptual analysis, which may be detected by using face-matching techniques; in the other the deficit is associated with a selective memory impairment for this class of stimuli and can be assessed by asking the patient to identify faces of famous personalities. Not uncommonly, prosopagnosic patients may present with additional deficits, such as metamorphopsia, achromatopsia, topographic disorientation, disturbances of body schema, and visual-field defects. It is unclear whether prosopagnosia in these patients is a pseudoagnosic syndrome or a primary recognition deficit.

Hécaen and Angelergues in 1962 found that prosopagnosia is more common among patients with right-hemisphere than those with left-hemisphere lesions. Although postmortem studies to date have all demonstrated bilateral posterior lesions, CT scans have clearly indicated that a unilateral right posterior lesion is sufficient to produce prosopagnosia (De Renzi 1986a) (Figure 41.8).

Patients with associative agnosia are unable to name or demonstrate the use of objects by acting or mime, although the fact that they may be able to copy complex drawings suggests that their perceptual skills are adequate. This can be more formally tested by probing attribute knowledge of man-made objects or animals, regarding, for example, their relative size, weight, or color (Figure 41.9).

Associative agnosia as a selective deficit is very rare, and as a result its existence as an independent neurological syndrome has been doubted. Indeed, in the majority of reported cases the patients showed multiple deficits or widespread lesions. However, Hécaen et al., in 1974, described a patient who presented with a relatively pure form of associative agnosia. This patient performed satisfactorily on stringent perceptual tests but had mild difficulty identifying common objects, whether by naming them or de-

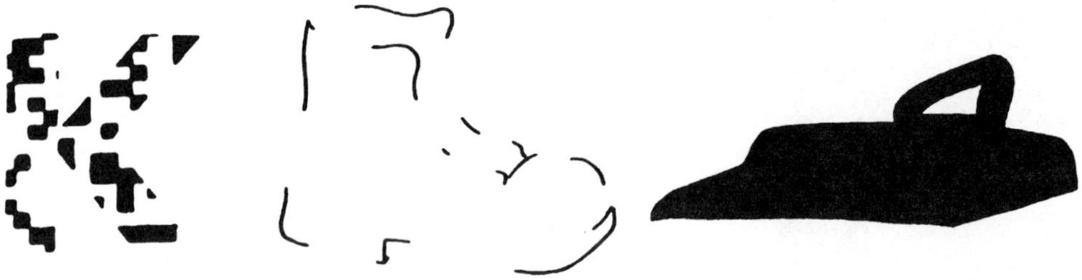

FIGURE 41.7 Examples of perceptual tests.

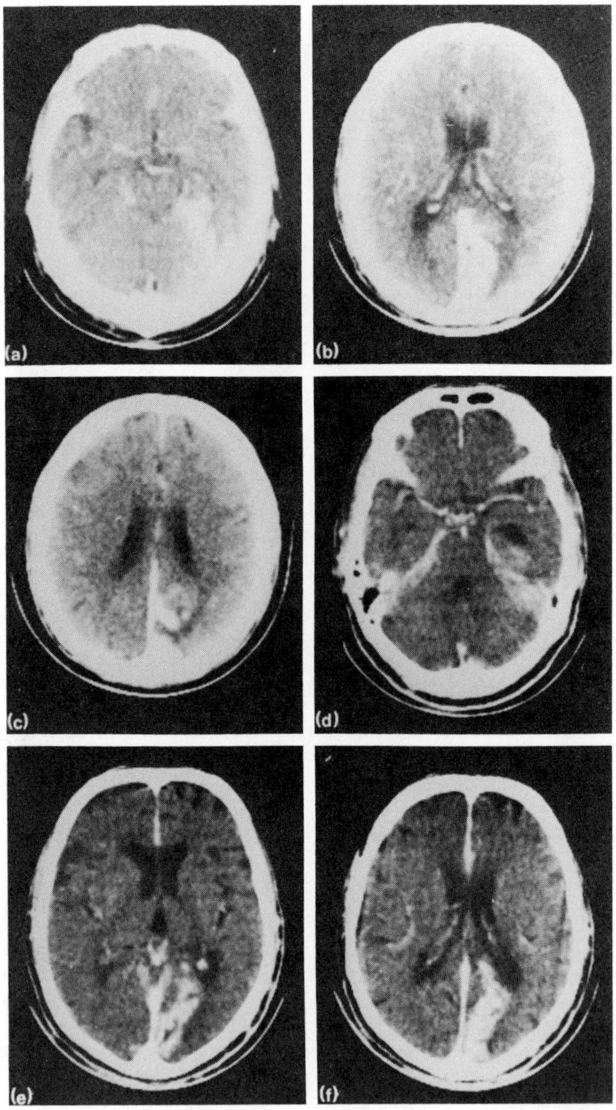

FIGURE 41.8 CT scan of a prosopagnosic patient with unilateral right posterior lesion. (Reprinted with permission from E De Renzi 1986a. Prosopagnosia in two patients with CT scan evidence of damage confined to the right hemisphere. Neuropsychologia 1986;24:385–389.)

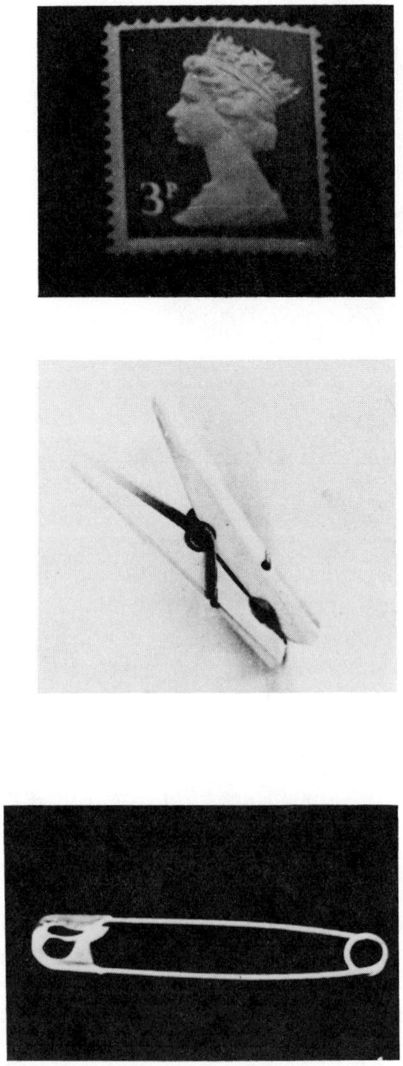

FIGURE 41.9 Example of associative agnosia test: Judging the heaviest or lightest item.

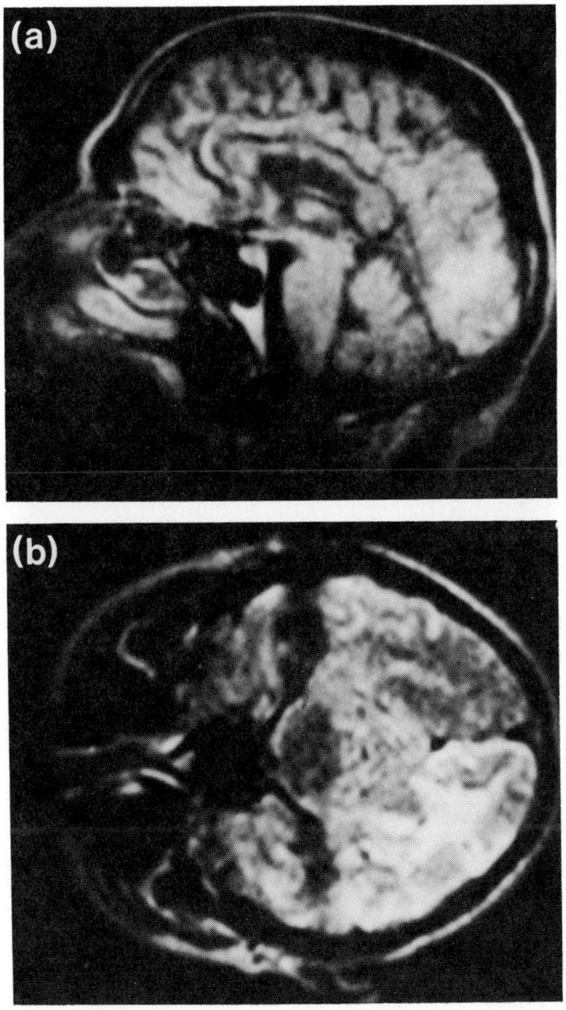

FIGURE 41.10 MRI scan showing infarction in the territory of the left posterior cerebral artery: (a) sagittal view, (b) horizontal view. (Reprinted with permission from RA McCarthy, EK Warrington. Visual associative agnosia: a clinicoanatomical study of a single case. J Neurol Neurosurg Psychiatry 1986;49:1233–40.)

scribing their functions. These findings have been replicated and extended in a detailed study of a patient who, apart from visual object agnosia and total alexia, exhibited no other significant deficits (McCarthy and Warrington 1986).

The anatomical basis of visual object agnosia has been subject to controversy. Some authors have argued that it is caused by bilateral temporo-occipital lesions. Such reports have been overtaken by the clear demonstration that a unilateral lesion of the left posterior cortex is sufficient to give rise to associative agnosia (e.g., McCarthy and Warrington 1986) (Figure 41.10).

To summarize, neuropsychological data indicate a serial model of successive stages in achieving objective recognition. Early visual analysis is followed by perceptual analysis, in which a structural percept is achieved. This is followed by a semantic analysis, during which the functional significance of the object can be realized (but see also De Renzi and Lucchelli 1993).

VISUOSPATIAL AND PRAXIC SKILLS

Failure of patients on simple constructional tasks has often generated discussions of the nature of the underlying deficit. The main point of dispute has always been whether the primary deficit is a perceptual one involving faulty appreciation of the spatial relationships of visual stimuli or an executive-constructive disorder associated with complex hand movements. On the other hand, many clinicians have regarded visuospatial and constructional (praxic) deficits as synonymous. It is beyond the scope of this section to consider their arguments in detail. Suffice it to say constructional tasks by their nature implicate both visuoperceptual and praxic skills, and an impairment of either may affect performance levels. Studies and procedures for the analysis of visuospatial and constructional impairments, as well as apraxic disorders, are discussed in the next sections.

Visuospatial Impairments

The label *visuospatial* refers not only to the location of a single point in space but also to the integration of simultaneous or successive stimuli in a spatial schema. It covers a variety of skills, but we shall consider only those in which the praxic component is minimized.

Warrington and Rabin in 1970 used a task with patients with left- or right-hemisphere lesions and with control subjects, in which subjects were to identify whether the positions of single dots on two cards, presented simultaneously or in succession, were the same or different. They found that patients with right-hemisphere damage performed worse than the other two groups, and the right parietal subgroup obtained the highest error score. Further analysis of the data showed that, although in all groups error scores for successive presentations of stimuli were higher than for simultaneous presentation (the former task involved a memory component), in no cerebral lesion group or subgroup did such a difference reach statistical significance. A useful test in clinical practice merely requires the patient to indicate which of two squares presented simultaneously has a dot exactly in the center. On this test, in a series of numerous patients with unilateral lesions, those with right-hemisphere brain damage were found to perform worse than patients with left-hemisphere damage, and the right posterior subgroup obtained the highest error score (Warrington and James 1991).

Apart from position discrimination, the method of requiring the subject to estimate the number of stimuli presented briefly has also been used to assess visuospatial skills. Studies have shown that patients who had undergone right-temporal lobectomy (Kimura in 1963), as well as patients with right-hemisphere lesions and particularly those with parietal lobe involvement (Warrington and James in 1967), are impaired in estimating the number of a small number of dots presented briefly in the central vision. Studies of normal subjects showing right-hemisphere superiority in estimating the number of laterally projected dots are consistent with these findings (De Renzi 1982).

Another test of visuospatial skills involves the discrimination of line orientation. Warrington and Rabin asked subjects to judge whether pairs of lines were of the same or different slope. Patients with right-hemisphere lesions, and particularly the right parietal subgroup, obtained higher error scores than patients with left-hemisphere lesions and control subjects. In a study by Benton et al. in 1983, subjects were presented with arrays of sloping lines and were required to identify verbally or by pointing to their directional orientation. Patients with right-hemisphere damage performed significantly worse than those with left-hemisphere damage, and the right-posterior-hemisphere subgroup was particularly impaired.

Tests that use three-dimensional stimuli can also be used to assess visuospatial skills. One such test, cube analysis, has been taken from the Stanford-Binet scale (age 11). It consists of two-dimensional drawings or representations of bricks, which are closely arranged in either two or three dimensions. The subject is required to indicate the number of bricks depicted on each drawing. As on other visuospatial tasks, patients with right parietal lesions obtain the highest error score on this test (Warrington and James 1991).

Apraxic Impairments

The first detailed analysis of apraxic impairments was made by Liepmann in the early twentieth century. Apraxia may be defined as a defect of voluntary movements that is not explainable in terms of a primary motor deficit, agnosia, impaired comprehension or memory, or general intellectual deterioration.

Typically, the apraxic patient chooses wrong innervatory patterns; shows fragmentary, spatially displaced, or perseverative movements; or substitutes an intended motor act with another. Apraxia is usually mildest when the subject uses real objects and more severe when he or she is asked to mime certain acts. It is therefore not surprising that apraxia is not always manifested in spontaneous activity and that the patient may not be aware of any difficulties. These characteristics suggest that the clinician should not rely on history and must actually test the patient. An easy and reliable bedside procedure involves asking patients to produce or imitate certain familiar hand movements, such as lighting a cigarette with a match or putting a letter in an envelope. They may also be asked to imitate certain sequences of meaningless hand movements.

Describing the apraxic phenomena is relatively easy; indeed, many labels have been used to refer to them, including dressing apraxia, constructional apraxia (see below), buccofacial apraxia, oculomotor apraxia, and limb-kinetic apraxia. However, classification of the deficits that underlie such phenomena has always been problematic, and until a more satisfactory schema is produced, Liepmann's classificatory system (cited in De Renzi 1986b) remains the most satisfactory. His theory envisages two stages in the execution of a complex movement: the execution of a general plan and its implementation. Apraxic impairments may thus fall into three categories:

1. *Ideational apraxia*, in which the planning of a movement may fail, with the patient unable to conceptualize how a movement must be organized
2. *Ideomotor apraxia*, in which the plan of a gesture is realized but its execution fails because of damage to pathways connecting the brain areas in which it is conceived with those responsible for the innervation of the appropriate engrams
3. *Limb kinetic apraxia*, which is characterized by very awkward movements, which only grossly resemble the intended ones, as a result of lesions in the sensorimotor areas

Several studies have indicated that in right-handed individuals apraxia is associated with left-hemisphere damage, with the left inferior parietal lobule more commonly involved. As De Renzi observed (1986b), the inferior parietal lobule (areas 5 and 7 in the monkey) is ideally equipped to play a central role in planning and monitoring the execution of motor acts; this part of the brain not only is a convergence area of inputs from the auditory, visual, and somesthetic association cortices, but it also sends projections to the premotor cortex.

Because in right-handed persons language functions are also lateralized to the left hemisphere, aphasia often coincides with apraxia. Thus, the suggestion has been made that both these disorders are manifestations of a primary defect in symbolization. Research has shown that this is not the case but that apraxia is a disorder of skilled movements per se. Goodglass and Kaplan in 1963 found no correlation between the severity of aphasia and the degree of apraxia. In addition, they drew attention to the "body part as object" phenomenon—that is, patients use their own hands or fingers for an object when they are required to imitate certain actions (e.g., they use the index finger as if it were a real toothbrush when asked to demonstrate the use of a toothbrush). Such patients must also be assessed on their handling of real objects where kinesthetic cues are available, a task that corresponds to actual experience in daily life (De Renzi and Lucchelli 1988; see also Ochipa et al. 1992).

Constructional Apraxia

Kleist coined the term *constructional apraxia* to denote a disturbance "in formative activities such as assembling, building and drawing . . . without there being an apraxia

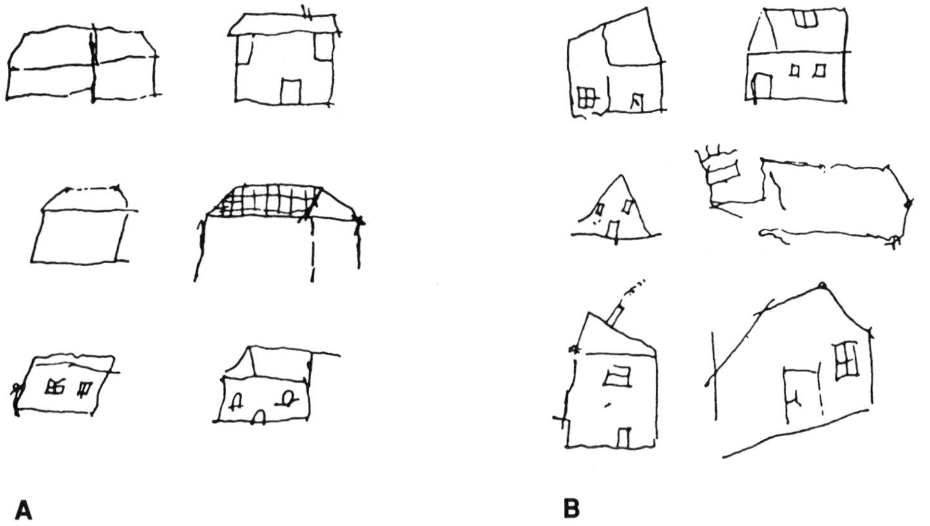

FIGURE 41.11 Drawings of a house by (A) patients with left-hemisphere lesions, and (B) patients with right-hemisphere lesions. (Adapted from M Piercy, H Hécaen, J Ajuriaguerra. Constructional apraxia associated with unilateral cerebral lesions: left and right sided cases compared. Brain 1960;83:225–42.)

of single movements" (cited in Benton 1982). He specifically saw this disorder as a manifestation of an impaired bond between visual functions and the kinesthetic engrams for manual activity rather than as resulting from visuoperceptual deficits of a more general form of apraxia.

A variety of tasks that make differing demands on the patient have been used to assess constructional impairments. Vertical block building was one of the early tasks, but horizontal block building and arranging sticks in simple geometric shapes have more commonly been used. The most common bedside procedure, however, has been drawing to verbal command or copying the examiner's model.

The anatomical correlates of constructional deficits have proved difficult to establish, because a comparable incidence of constructional problems among patients with left- and right-hemisphere lesions has been reported. The question arises whether the discrepancies in different studies are due to bilateral representation of the skill or whether the skill fractionates into distant components, each with its own anatomical correlates. There is a consensus that the quality of errors in the constructions of apraxic patients is determined by the laterality of the lesion. Thus, for example, drawings of patients with right-hemisphere damage are characterized by spatial mislocations, spatial reversals, asymmetry of parts, fragmentation, and the like. In contrast, drawings of patients with left-hemisphere lesions tend to be simplified and crude versions of the model, with omissions of details and blunting of angles closing into the model or even overlapping the model (Figure 41.11). Such observations are generally interpreted to imply that constructional apraxia in patients with right-hemisphere lesions is a manifestation of visuospatial deficits. Conversely, and as Kleist postulated, in the absence of primary apraxic difficulties, constructional apraxia in patients with left-hemisphere lesions is associated with a failure in visuomotor coordination.

NEGLECT PHENOMENA

Unilateral neglect refers to the tendency of patients to fail to respond to stimulation or to report information that is, in spatial terms, contralateral to their lesions. Early reports of cases of patients with unilateral neglect include those by Poppelreuter and by Scheller and Seidemann (cited in Hécaen and Albert 1978). Such early clinical reports have been superseded by quantitative studies of neglect deficits, and it is now clear that there are a number of subtypes of neglect phenomena.

Neglect may vary considerably in severity, ranging from mild cases in which the deficit may be elicited only by special testing, to very severe cases in which the patient shows a total neglect of extrapersonal or intrapersonal space, or both.

Extrapersonal Neglect

Extrapersonal neglect may be observed in a patient's spontaneous activity and on a variety of tasks, including drawing on command, copying drawings, constructional tests, cancellation tests, and line bisection tests. The defect is often very striking; for example, in drawing and constructional tests the patient may fail to produce one side of the model. Visual imagery, too, may be susceptible to spatial neglect. Thus, patients may neglect to describe from memory topographic features that fall in one half of a space. Bisiach and

Luzzatti in 1978 described two patients with left-hemispatial neglect who failed to report the shops on the left half of the Piazza del Duomo in Milan when asked to imagine they were standing in front of the cathedral looking across the piazza. Subsequently, when they were asked to imagine they were standing at the opposite side of the piazza, they failed to report the shops they had earlier described but reported those they had ignored in the first part of the experiment. Neglect may also extend to auditory and somatesthetic modalities. The stimuli may be presented to the normal or abnormal side in a random order, and these trials may be interspersed by bilateral stimulation.

Of particular interest are the reported cases of neglect affecting literacy skills. Kinsbourne and Warrington found in 1962 that six patients with right-hemisphere lesions made paralexic errors limited to the first part of the word (for example, *level-novel*; *toffee-coffee*). In these patients, neglect dyslexia was interpreted as a manifestation of a more general neglect on the left; however, these two aspects of neglect fractionate. A patient with a bilateral lesion was demonstrated to have a left-sided neglect dyslexia and a right-sided neglect of space. A phenomenon that has been interpreted as neglect dysgraphia has also been described. Thus, on oral spelling tasks patients have been reported to have greater difficulty with recalling the beginning letters of a word than the end of the word (see McCarthy and Warrington 1990).

Generally, there has been an agreement that neglect occurs more commonly and is more severe in patients with right- than with left-hemisphere lesions. Studies using brain-scanning techniques have confirmed that neglect is predominantly due to right posterior lesions.

The physiologic basis of neglect has been the subject of considerable dispute. There are two main theoretical approaches to the problem. One emphasizes a deficit in sensory processing whereby inadequate or no information is conveyed to one hemisphere; the other attributes neglect to a failure in spatial distribution of attention. The attentional hypothesis differentiates between impairments of attention to external space (such as failure to copy part of a drawing) and internal space (such as neglect dysgraphia). Recent developments in the field highlighting the heterogeneity of neglect phenomena (e.g., Marshall and Halligan 1988) agree more with the latter theories. The fact that sensory defects (homonymous hemianopia and oculomotor defects) are by no means necessary accompaniments of the syndrome also gives strong support to attentional theories of neglect.

Intrapersonal Neglect

Neglect phenomena are observed not only in patients' interactions with extrapersonal space but also with intrapersonal space—that is, their bodies. Babinski was the first to demonstrate that unilateral unawareness or denial of unilateral defects (*anosognosia*) could not be accounted for by sensory impairments but could be associated with specific cortical lesions (cited in Hécaen and Albert 1978). Occasionally, hemiplegic patients may completely refuse to admit the reality of their paralysis or claim that the limbs contralateral to their lesion's limbs do not belong to them (*somatoparaphrenia*). In milder cases patients may show no concern for their paralysis (*anosodiaphoria*).

Critchley has graphically described methods of eliciting intrapersonal neglect in patients with parietal lesions who are not paralyzed or afflicted with motor weakness. Such patients might not use the affected hand even in symmetrical bimanual activities. Thus, to the command "Put out your hands," they may raise only one hand, although when reminded by the examiner, they may raise the "lazy" hand as well. Several other authors have described anosognosic phenomena, and the consensus appears to be that these are usually associated with right parietal lesions.

Of special interest are studies that indicate vestibular stimulation may produce a temporary remission of unilateral neglect, both with regard to extrapersonal and interpersonal space (e.g., Vallar et al. 1993). Such observations provide a basis for a better understanding of these intriguing phenomena.

CONCLUSION

Cognitive skills and their anatomical correlates are extremely complex. Although brain function and behavior are far from completely understood, research investigations have progressed considerably, and a substantial body of knowledge is now available to the clinician. It was during the last 20 years or so that experimental psychologists and neuropsychologists made enormous advances in analyzing and quantifying cognitive skills. This chapter primarily discusses in concrete terms how this data base can be harnessed for the assessment and diagnosis of the individual patient. In the field of language we now have precise techniques for assessing word retrieval and word comprehension deficits of different degrees of severity. For the assessment of literacy skills the clinician's armamentarium has increased considerably and includes techniques for documenting selective deficits of subcomponents of these skills. Memory impairments can also be very selective, and a wide range of techniques have been devised for analyzing and measuring such deficits. In the domain of object recognition, tests have been developed that help quantify deficits at different stages of visual analysis, from early visual processing to failure to assign meaning to stimuli. Further, a variety of tests have been developed to assess visuospatial deficits. Our progress in the domain of problem-solving tasks has been less conspicuous in recent times.

As clinicians we have leaned heavily on our experience, and we acknowledge this limitation. We have emphasized methods of assessment of cognitive impairments that have been studied experimentally and for which the neurologic concomitants have been established. We have not found a place for the thorny problem of how measures of levels of alertness and speed of response may contribute to the diagnosis of certain neurological conditions. This chapter, therefore, does not approach issues relating to differentiation between cortical and subcortical disorders.

We hope this brief review suggests not only the scope of applications of clinical neuropsychology but also the potential for expansion, with implications for our further understanding of the organization of brain function and of human behavior.

REFERENCES

Benton AL. Spatial Thinking in Neurological Patients: Historical Aspects. In M Potegal (ed), Spatial Abilities: Developmental and Physiological Foundations. New York: Academic, 1982.

Caramazza A, Hillis AE. Lexical organization of nouns and verbs in the brain. Nature 1991;349:788–790.

Cipolotti L, Butterworth B, Denes G. A specific deficit for numbers in a case of dense acalculia. Brain 1991;114:2619–2637.

Davidoff J, Warrington EK. A dissociation of shape discrimination and figure-ground perception in a patient with normal acuity. Neuropsychologia 1993;31:83–93.

Deloche G, Seron X. Mathematical Disabilities: A Cognitive Neuropsychological Perspective. Hillsdale, NJ: Lawrence Erlbaum Associates, 1987.

De Renzi E. Disorders of Space Exploration and Cognition. New York: Wiley, 1982.

De Renzi E. Prosopagnosia in two patients with CT scan evidence of damage confined to the right hemisphere. Neuropsychologia 1986a;24:385–389.

De Renzi E. The Apraxias. In AK Asbury, GM McKhann, WI McDonald (eds), Diseases of the Nervous System. Vol 1. Philadelphia: Saunders, and London: Heinemann, 1986b.

De Renzi E, Lucchelli F. Ideational apraxia. Brain 1988;111: 1173–1185.

De Renzi E, Lucchelli F. The fuzzy boundaries of apperceptive agnosia. Cortex 1993;29:187–215.

Hécaen H, Albert ML. Human Neuropsychology. New York: Wiley, 1978.

Hodges JR, McCarthy RA. Autobiographical amnesia resulting from bilateral paramedian thalamic infarction. Brain 1993;116:921–940.

Hodges JR, Patterson K, Oxbury S et al. Progressive fluent aphasia with temporal-lobe atrophy. Brain 1992;115:1783–1806.

Kartsounis LD, Poynton A, Bridges PK, Bartlett JR. Neuropsychological correlates of stereotactic subcaudate tractotomy. Brain 1991;114:2657–2673.

Luria AR. Human Brain and Psychological Processes. New York: Harper & Row, 1966.

Livingstone M, Hubel D. Segregation of form, color, movement and depth: anatomy, physiology and perception. Science 1988;240:740–749.

McCarthy RA, Warrington EK. Category specificity in an agrammatic patient: The relative impairment of verb retrieval and comprehension. Neuropsychologia 1985;23:709–727.

McCarthy RA, Warrington EK. Visual associative agnosia: a clinicoanatomical study of a single case. J Neurol Neurosurg Psychiatry 1986;49:1233–1240.

McCarthy RA, Warrington EK. Cognitive Neuropsychology: A Clinical Introduction. London: Academic, 1990.

McCloskey M, Caramazza A. Cognitive Mechanisms in Normal and Impaired Number-Processing. In G. Deloche, X Seron (eds), Mathematical Disabilities: A Cognitive Neuropsychological Perspective. Hillsdale, NJ: Lawrence Erlbaum Associates, 1987.

McKenna P, Warrington EK. The Neuropsychology of Semantic Memory. In F Boller, J Grafman (eds), Handbook of Neuropsychology. Vol. 8. New York: Elsevier, 1993.

Marshall JC, Halligan PW. Blindsight and insight in visuospatial neglect. Nature 1988;336:766–767.

Milner B. Some cognitive effects of frontal-lobe lesions in man. Philos Trans R Soc London 1982;B298:211–262.

Milner B. Psychological Aspects of Focal Epilepsy and Its Neurosurgical Management. In DP Purpura, JK Penry, RD Walter (eds), Advances in Neurology. New York: Raven, 1975.

Nelson HE, Willison JR. The National Adult Reading Test (2nd ed). Windsor, England: NFER, 1991.

Newcombe F, Oldfield RC, Wingfield A. Object naming by dysphasic patients. Nature 1965;207:1217–1218.

Ochipa C, Gonzalez Rothi LJ, Heilman KM. Conceptual apraxia in Alzheimer's disease. Brain 1992;115:1061–1071.

Perenin MT, Vighetto A. Optic ataxia: a specific disruption in visuomotor mechanisms. I. Different aspects of the deficit in reaching for objects. Brain 1988;643–674.

Petrides M, Milner B. Deficits on subject ordered tasks after frontal and temporal lobe lesions in man. Neuropsychologia 1982;20:249–262.

Piercy M, Hécaen H, Ajuriaguerra J. Constructional apraxia associated with unilateral cerebral lesions: left and right sided cases compared. Brain 1960;83:225–242.

Sirigu A, Grafman J, Bressler K, et al. Multiple representations contribute to body knowledge processing. Brain 1991;114: 629–642.

Tanaka Y, Yamadori A, Mori E. Pure word deafness following bilateral lesions: a psychophysical analysis. Brain 1987;110: 381–403.

Vallar G, Bottini G, Rusconi ML et al. Exploring somatosensory hemineglect by vestibular stimulation. Brain 1993;116:71–86.

Vallar G, Shallice T. (eds). Neuropsychological Impairments to Short-Term Memory. New York: Cambridge University Press, 1990.

Warrington EK. The selective impairment of semantic memory. Q J Exp Physiol 1975;27:635–657.

Warrington EK. Recognition Memory Test. Windsor, England: NFER, 1984.

Warrington EK, McCarthy RA. Disorders of Memory. In AK Asbury, GM McKhann, WI McDonald (eds), Diseases of the Nervous System. Vol. 2. Philadelphia: Saunders, and London: Heinemann, 1986.

Warrington EK, Pratt RTC. Language laterality in left-handers assessed by unilateral E.C.T. Neuropsychologia 1973;11:423–428.

Warrington EK, James M. The Visual Object and Space Perception Battery. England: Thames Valley Test Company, 1991.

Zihl J, Von Cramon D, Schmid CH. Disturbance of movement vision after bilateral posterior brain damage. Brain 1991; 114:2235–2252.

SUGGESTED READING

Shallice T. From Neuropsychology to Mental Structure. New York: Cambridge University Press, 1988.

Spinnler H, Boller F (eds). Handbook of Neuropsychology. Vol 8. Amsterdam: Elsevier, 1993.

Chapter 42
Neuro-Ophthalmology

Patrick J. M. Lavin and Barbara Weissman

Neuro-ophthalmology bridges the disciplines of ophthalmology and neurology. Despite sophisticated technologic advances in medicine, competence in neuro-ophthalmologic diagnosis requires attentive listening; timely probing questions; detailed knowledge of neuroanatomy and of disorders that affect motor and sensory vision; skill in examination of the ocular system and the cranial nerves (at least); and experience and expertise in evaluating supplementary investigations including perimetry, fluorescein angiography, and neuroradiological imaging. Frequently, a thorough clinical examination and careful thought preempt the need for uncomfortable, invasive, and expensive procedures, an increasingly important consideration in the current economic climate. "Ears and eyes first and most, hands least and last," still holds true.

THE GENERATION AND CONTROL OF EYE MOVEMENTS

A reasonable understanding and interpretation of gaze disorders requires an appreciation of the anatomy and physiology of eye movement control. In the words of Hughlings Jackson, "The study of the cause of things must be preceded by the study of things caused."

Subjects with intact sensory visual systems (optical and afferent) are capable of discerning small details, comparable to Snellen acuity of 20/13, provided the fovea is maintained on target. However, 10 degrees from fixation the resolving power of the retina drops to 20/200. The peripheral retina has poor spatial resolution capabilities but is exquisitely sensitive to movement. The image of an object entering the peripheral visual field stimulates the retina to signal the ocular motor system to make a *saccade* (a rapid eye movement) and fixate it; thus the retina acts as a sentinel for the fovea.

The premotor substrates for conjugate gaze and vergence eye movements are in the brain stem. Those specifically for vertical gaze, vergence, and ocular counter-rolling are in the mesodiencephalic region, while those for horizontal eye movements are in the pons. The mechanisms for horizontal eye movements are better understood than those for vertical eye movements and are based on clinicopathological and radiological correlation, as well as animal and bioengineering experiments. With the exception of reflexive movements, such as the the vestibulo-ocular reflex (VOR) and fast phases of nystagmus, cerebral structures determine *when* and *where* the eyes move, while brain stem mechanisms determine *how* they move.

The Ocular Motor Subsystems

There are five ocular motor subsystems that enable the fovea to find and fixate a target, stabilize an image of the target on each retina, and maintain binocular foveation during head or target movement, or both (Table 42.1).

The saccadic system moves the eyes rapidly (up to 800 degrees/sec) to fixate new targets (Figure 42.1). Saccades may be generated voluntarily, or in response to verbal commands in the absence of a visible target. Reflex saccades may occur in response to peripheral retinal stimuli such as visual threat or retinal error signals, or to sound. Saccades are also the fast components of nystagmus.

Table 42.1: Types of eye movements

A. Saccades (switching eyes from one target to another)
Intentional saccades (internally triggered, with a goal)
Intentional visually guided saccades
Memory-guided saccades (with visual/vestibular input)
Predictive saccades
Target-searching saccades
Antisaccades*
Reflexive saccades (externally triggered)
Reflexive visually guided saccades
Reflexive auditory saccades
Spontaneous saccades (internally triggered, without a goal)
During another motor activity
At rest
When sleeping
Quick phases of nystagmus
Physiological nystagmus
Vestibular nystagmus
Optokinetic nystagmus
End-point nystagmus
Pathological nystagmus (see Chapter 16)
B. Eye movements stabilizing the image of the target on the fovea
Smooth pursuit
Foveal pursuit
Full-field pursuit (slow phase of optokinetic nystagmus)
Vestibulo-ocular reflex (horizontal, vertical, torsional)
Convergence
C. Ocular oscillations that may interfere with vision
Ocular dysmetria
Ocular hypometria
Ocular hypermetria
Ocular lateropulsion
Ocular torsipulsion
Ocular flutter
Opsoclonus
Square wave jerks
Macrosquare wave jerks
Macrosaccadic oscillations
Saccadic pulses
Double saccadic pulses
Superior oblique myokymia
Ocular tics (myoclonic jerks)
Oculogyric crisis
Ocular bobbing

*Antisaccades are fast eye movements deliberately made away from a new target.
Source: Adapted from C Pierott-Deseilligny. Cortical control of saccades. Neuro-ophthalmol 1991;11:63–75.

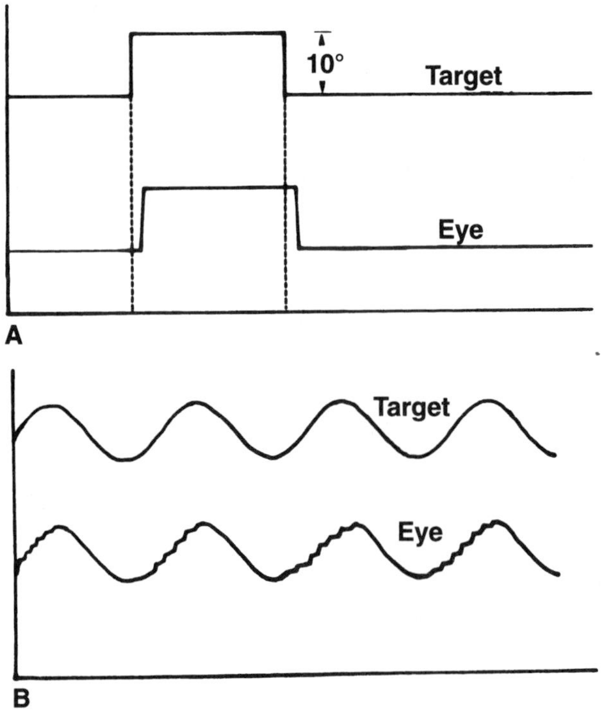

FIGURE 42.1 Simulated eye movement recordings. By convention for horizontal movements, upward deflections represent rightward eye movements and downward deflections represent leftward eye movements. A. Saccades. A target moves rapidly 10 degrees to the right. After a latency of about 200 msec, the eye follows. When the target returns to the center, the sequence is repeated in the opposite direction. B. Pursuit. The target moves in a sinusoidal pattern in front of the patient. The eye follows the target after a latency of about 120 msec, but pursuit movements to the right are defective, resulting in rightward "cogwheel" (saccadic) pursuit; pursuit to the left is normal.

The pursuit system enables the eyes to track slowly moving targets (up to 70 degrees/sec) in order to maintain the image stable on the fovea. Athletes and specially trained subjects are capable of smooth pursuit eye movements as fast as 100 degrees/sec. Pursuit eye movements are limited more by the target's acceleration than by its velocity. If the target moves too quickly or abruptly changes direction, or if the pursuit system is impaired, the eyes are unable to maintain pace with the target and fall behind; the image moves off the fovea, producing a retinal error signal that provokes the saccadic system to make a catch-up saccade to refixate the target. The cycle then repeats itself, resulting in saccadic ("cogwheel") pursuit (Figure 42.1B).

Bidirectionally defective pursuit movements, a normal finding in infants, are nonspecific and occur under conditions of stress or fatigue, or with sedative medication; impaired tracking in one direction, however, suggests a structural lesion of the ipsilateral-pursuit system (Figure 42.1B).

There is evidence suggesting that *fixation*, which allows the eyes to maintain an image of a stationary target on each fovea, is not simply "pursuit at zero velocity" but probably an independent subsystem that shares neural circuitry with the optokinetic nystagmus (OKN) and pursuit systems (Leigh and Zee 1991).

The vestibular eye movement subsystem maintains a stable image on the retina during head movements. The semicircular canals respond to rotational acceleration of the head by driving the VOR to maintain the eyes in the same direction in space during head movements. The otoliths (utricle and saccule) are gravity receptors that respond to linear acceleration and static head tilt (gravity)—i.e., ocular counter-rolling. The vestibular system is discussed further in Chapter 44.

The optokinetic system complements the vestibulo-ocular system, which becomes less responsive during sustained head movements, to stabilize images on the retina in situations such as spinning; it uses reference points in the environment to maintain orientation. When the eyes have reached their limit of movement in their orbits, a reflex saccade allows refixation to a point further forward in the direction of head rotation. The sequence repeats itself, causing OKN (see Chapter 16).

In humans, the optokinetic system uses predominantly *fixation and pursuit* (immediate component), and to a lesser extent *velocity storage** (delayed component), which involves neural circuitry in the vestibular system.†

The vergence system enables the eyes to move dysconjugately (converge and diverge), in the horizontal plane, to maintain binocular fixation on a target moving toward or away from the subject. Vergence movements are essential for binocular single vision and stereoscopic depth perception.

Horizontal Eye Movements

When gaze is redirected from one point to another, a saccade moves the eyes conjugately. To enable the small strap-like extraocular muscles to move the relatively large globes and overcome the elastic recoil of the viscous orbital contents, the yoked agonist muscles require a surge or burst of innervation (pulse), while at the same time their yoked antagonists are reciprocally inhibited (Figure 42.2A). For a leftward saccade, the left lateral rectus and the right medial rectus muscles each receive a pulse of innervation, while their antagonists, the left medial and right lateral rectus muscles, are reciprocally inhibited. *Excitatory burst neurons* (EBNs) contained in the ipsilateral horizontal gaze center in the paramedian pontine reticular formation (PPRF), just rostral to the abducens nucleus, generate the pulse to initiate the saccade.

The EBNs are medium-lead burst cells that discharge about 10 msec before and during all rapid horizontal eye movements; they preferentially discharge for ipsilateral saccades and create the immediate premotor command generating pulse activity for saccades. Long-lead burst neurons discharge irregularly as early as 100 msec before saccades, are involved in both horizontal and vertical movements, relay signals from higher centers such as the superior colliculus, and also play a role in encoding the direction of saccades and in synchronizing their initiation and termination. The EBNs project to the ipsilateral abducens nucleus and discharge just before and during a saccade.

About half of the neurons in the abducens nucleus are interneurons (with different morphological and pharmacological features) that relay, via the medial longitudinal fasciculus (MLF), to the contralateral medial rectus neurons in the oculomotor nuclear complex (Figure 42.3). The EBNs are tonically suppressed, except just prior to and during a saccade, by pause cells located in the nucleus raphe interpositus rostral to the abducens nucleus. Thus the pause cells, which receive inputs from the cerebrum, the cerebellum, and superior colliculus, mediate the command for a saccade when they cease discharging and allow the burst cells to fire (Figure 42.4). At the same time as the EBNs discharge, a group of inhibitory cell-burst neurons (IBNs)—which lie just caudal to the abducens nucleus in the medial rostral medulla and project across the midline to the contralateral abducens nucleus—discharge during

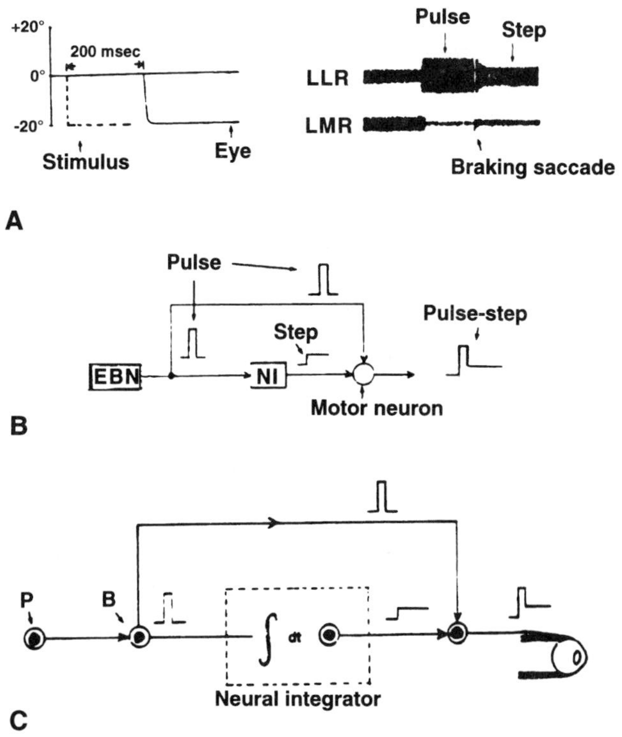

FIGURE 42.2 Ocular motor events on gaze left. A. Following the appearance of a stimulus 20 degrees to the left of fixation (–20 degrees), the eyes move to the target with a saccade after a latency of 200 msec. Idealized electromyography of the left extraocular muscles shows the activity of the agonist, the left lateral rectus (LLR), and the antagonist, the left medial rectus (LMR) muscles. B. The pulse originates in the excitatory burst neurons (EBNs) and is mathematically integrated by the neural integrator (NI); both signals are added to produce the pulse-step of the innervation to the ocular motor neurons. C. The pause cells (P) discharge continuously, suppressing the burst cells (B), except during a saccade, when they "pause," allowing the burst cells to discharge and generate a pulse. (Reprinted with permission from PJM Lavin. Conjugate and Disconjugate Eye Movements. In TJ Walsh [ed], Neuro-Ophthalmology: Clinical Signs and Symptoms. Philadelphia: Lea & Febiger, 1985.)

*Velocity storage is a mechanism by which the central nervous system, predominantly the vestibular system and vestibulocerebellum, prolongs or perseverates short signals generated by the vestibular end-organ to enhance orientation in space.

†Velocity storage does not require fixation and is largely involuntary.

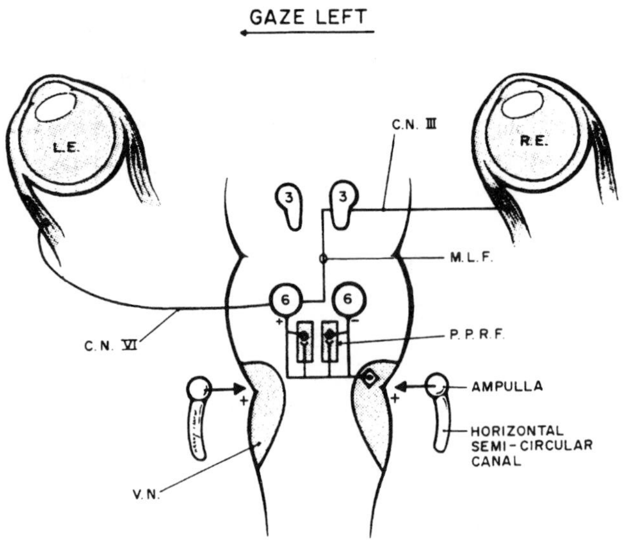

FIGURE 42.3 Stimulation of the semicircular canals, by movement of the endolymph toward the ampulla, excites the contralateral and inhibits the ipsilateral abducens nucleus via the vestibular nuclei (VN). Each abducens nucleus innervates the ipsilateral lateral rectus muscle via the abducens nerve and the contralateral medial rectus muscle via the abducens nucleus interneurons, the medial longitudinal fasciculus (MLF), and the neurons for the medial rectus (part of CN III nucleus). Each paramedian pontine reticular formation (PPRF) also has an excitatory input to the ipsilateral abducens nucleus and an inhibitory input to the contralateral abducens nucleus, for saccades and quick phases of nystagmus. (Adapted from PJM Lavin. Conjugate and Disconjugate Eye Movements. In TJ Walsh [ed], Neuro-Ophthalmology: Clinical Signs and Symptoms. Philadelphia: Lea & Febiger, 1985.)

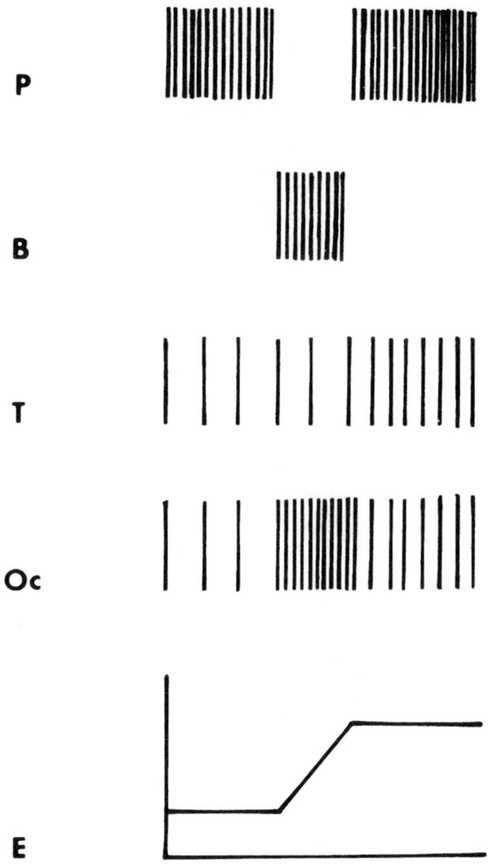

FIGURE 42.4 Electrophysiologic events during an eye movement. P represents an intraneuronal recording from a pause cell and demonstrates a constant discharge, which ceases, allowing an excitatory burst neuron (B) to discharge during pulse. T represents the discharge in a tonic neuron, which increases after the pulse as a result of integration of the pulse to a step. Both the pulse (B) and the tonic output (T) of burst-tonic neurons innervate the oculomotor neurons (Oc). The result is a rapid contraction of the extraocular muscle, which moves the eye from primary position and holds it in an eccentric position (E).

the saccade to reciprocally inhibit the yoked antagonist muscles (Leigh and Zee 1991).

To maintain the eyes on target in an eccentric position at the end of a saccade, the agonist muscles (left lateral and right medial recti) now require a new level of tonic innervation—a position command—achieved by a group of neurons referred to as the *neural integrator* (NI).*

The NI for horizontal gaze, thought to be partly in the rostral perihypoglossal nuclear complex and the adjacent rostral medial vestibular nucleus with reciprocal connections in the flocculus and paraflocculus (Leigh and Zee 1991), receives the velocity command signal (pulse) from the EBNs and mathematically integrates it to a "tonic" position command (step) before relaying it to the ipsilateral abducens nucleus (see Figure 42.2B).

The cerebellum and the PPRF maintain the output of this neural integrator by controlling the gain, via a positive feedback loop, to keep the eyes on target (Figure 42.5). The gain of a system is the ratio of its output to its input. In this case the output is the innervation required to maintain eccentric fixation, and the input is the pulse signal (Figure 42.2C). If the neural integrator is unable to maintain the gain at unity (output/input = 1), the output falls, causing the eyes to drift off target toward primary position. A corrective saccade will then refixate the target, resulting in gaze-evoked (gaze-paretic) nystagmus (see Chapter 16). Current evidence suggests that all conjugate eye-movement commands, including pursuit and the slow phases of OKN and the VOR, not just

*An integrator converts phasic input to tonic output, mathematically, by using reverberating collateral circuits to re-excite neurons. The efficiency of an integrator depends on its time constant—that is, the duration it can perseverate the activity of the input. The effective time constant is the period it takes for the output to decay to 37% of its initial value after the input signal stops. The maintenance of eccentric eye position in darkness (with no visual feedback and therefore no retinal error signal) is a measure of the eye position signal and thus the time constant of the neural integrator; in normal subjects it varies from 20 to 70 seconds.

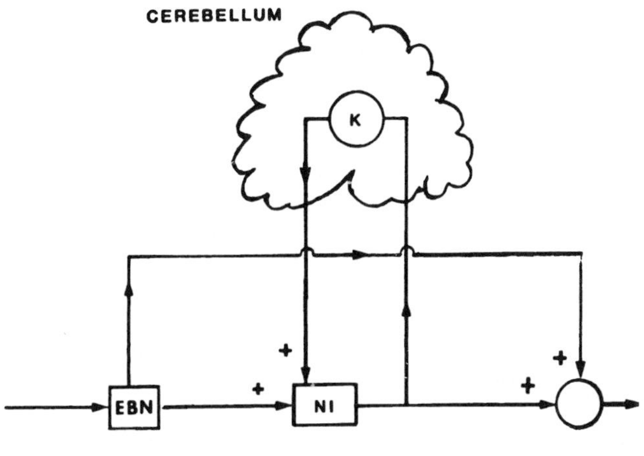

FIGURE 42.5 The time constant of the brain stem neural integrator (NI), and therefore the fidelity of its output (innervation for gaze holding), is controlled predominantly by the cerebellum. Dysfunction of the gain control (K) may cause the integrator output to fall (a shortened time constant will cause the signal to decay), allowing the eyes to drift back toward primary position. Conversely, an increase in K may result in an unstable integrator and cause the eye to drift eccentrically with an increasing velocity waveform. (From PJM Lavin. Conjugate and Disconjugate Eye Movements. In TJ Walsh [ed], Neuro-Ophthalmology: Clinical Signs and Symptoms. Philadelphia: Lea & Febiger, 1985. Reprinted by permission of the author and the publisher.)

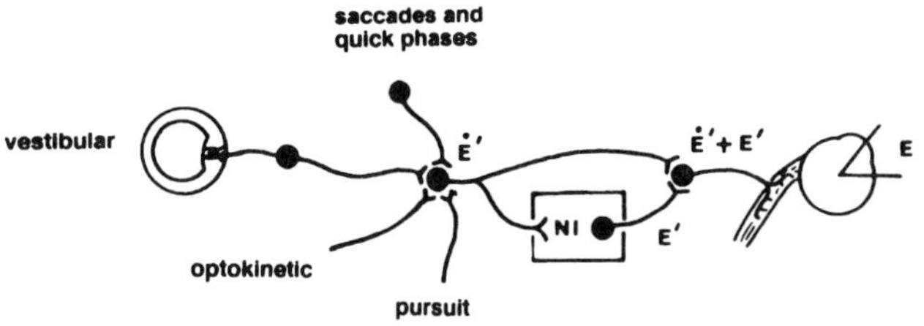

FIGURE 42.6 The final common integrator hypothesis. All conjugate eye movements (E) are initiated as eye velocity commands (Ė′) that are converted to eye position (E′) by the neural integrator. Both eye velocity and eye position commands are relayed to the motor neurons. (Redrawn from SC Cannon, DS Zee. The Neural Integrator of the Oculomotor System. In S Lessell, JTW van Dalen [eds], Current Neuro-Ophthalmology. Chicago: Year Book; 1988;124.)

saccades, are initiated as velocity commands and mediated by a final common integrator (Figure 42.6).

Although its anatomical borders are not clear, the PPRF has been defined functionally and is synonymous with the medial aspects of the nuclei gigantocellularis, or pontis centralis oralis and caudalis, and is located just ventral and lateral to the MLF, extending from the level of the abducens nucleus almost to the trochlear nucleus. The PPRF innervates the ipsilateral abducens nucleus, the rostral medulla (part of the neural integrator), and the midbrain reticular formation to coordinate horizontal and vertical eye movements. The PPRF receives direct input from the medial vestibular nucleus, the contralateral frontal eye fields, the ipsilateral posterior parietal region, the superior colliculus, and the cerebellum.

A lesion of the abducens nucleus will produce paralysis of all ipsilateral versional eye movements. Pontine lesions outside the abducens nucleus may selectively involve certain classes of eye movements while sparing others, demonstrating that the neural signals encoding subclasses of eye movements (saccades, pursuit, VOR, tonic position) project independently to the abducens nucleus (Halmagyi 1994). The PPRF also plays a role in generating vertical eye movements; acute bilateral injury may cause a transient vertical and horizontal gaze palsy. A unilateral lesion may cause slowing and oblique misdirection of vertical saccades, away from the side of injury, as well as impaired ipsilateral horizontal saccades (Johnston et al. 1993), probably because of involvement of the burst and pause cells in the caudal medial PPRF; the oblique misdirection is similar to "torsipulsion" seen with lateropulsion (see the section on Saccadic Lateropulsion).

Lesions of the abducens nucleus causing an ipsilateral gaze palsy almost always involve the facial nerve fasciculus, resulting in an associated facial nerve palsy with preservation of taste.

The vestibular system stabilizes the direction of gaze during head movements by virtue of changes in its tonic input to the ocular motor nuclei. This is most clearly illustrated by the horizontal VOR (see Figure 42.3). Each horizontal semicircular canal innervates the ipsilateral medial vestibular nucleus to inhibit the ipsilateral and excite the contralateral abducens nucleus. The ampulla of the right horizontal semicircular canal is stimulated by turning the head to the right (or warm caloric water irrigation). This mechanical information is transduced by the vestibular end organ to electrical signals and transmitted to the ipsilateral vestibular nucleus. Excitatory information is then relayed to the contralateral abducens nucleus, and inhibitory information to the ipsilateral abducens nucleus, causing the eyes to deviate in the direction opposite to head rotation, thus maintaining the direction of gaze.

Saccades, or fast eye movements, are initiated mainly in the contralateral frontal lobe and may be classified into four broad groups (Pierrot-Deseilligny 1991): (1) *internally triggered saccades*, which are voluntary (intentional) and include target-searching, memory-guided, predictive (where the appearance of the target is anticipated), and intentional visually guided saccades to an existing target in the peripheral visual field; (2) *externally triggered saccades*, which are reflexively activated by the appearance of a new target or a sound; (3) *spontaneous saccades*, which occur in the absence of a target at about 20/minute and are triggered internally—by both the FEF and the superior colliculus—to repetitively scan the environment; they occur at rest, during other motor activities, and during rapid-eye-movement sleep; and (4) *the quick phases of nystagmus* (see Chapter 16).

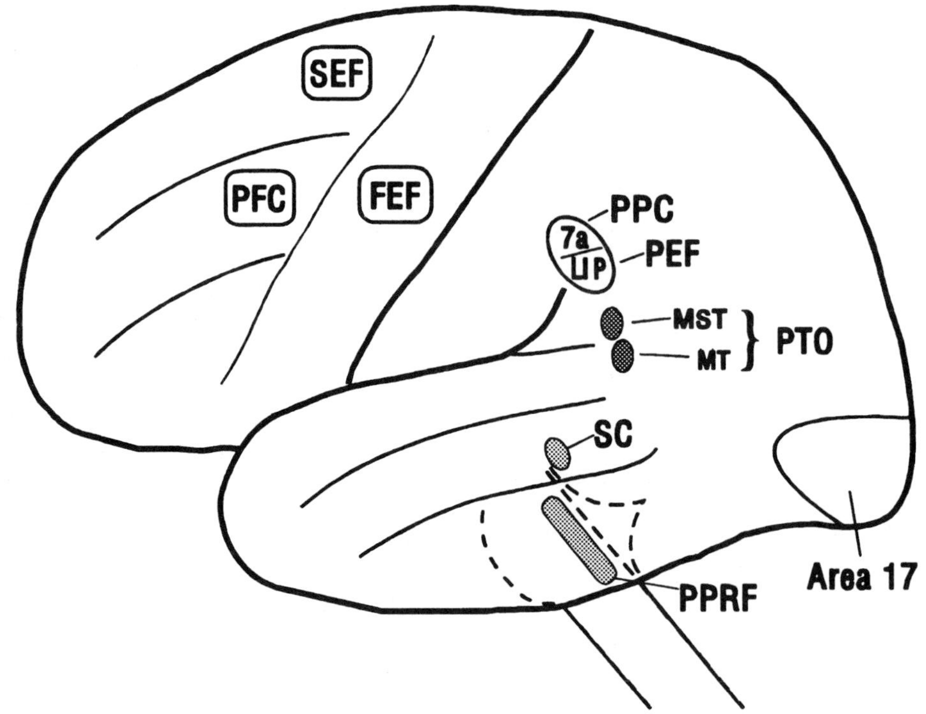

FIGURE 42.7 Areas in the human brain believed important in generating saccades and pursuit. (FEF = frontal eye fields; LIP = lateral intraparietal area; MST = medial superior temporal visual area; MT = middle temporal visual area; PEF = parietal eye fields; PFC = prefrontal cortex; PTO = parieto-temporo-occipital junction; PPC = posterior parietal cortex area; PPRF = paramedian pontine reticular formation; SC = superior colliculus; SEF = supplementary eye fields in the supplementary motor area; 7a = area 7a.)

A number of specialized areas in the cerebral cortex are particularly important in controlling saccades (Figure 42.7). Three of these are responsible for triggering saccades: (1) the *frontal eye fields* (FEFs), Brodmann's area 8; (2) the *supplementary eye fields* (SEFs), area 6 in the *supplementary motor area* (SMA); and (3) the *parietal eye fields* (PEFs) in the *lateral intraparietal area* (LIP) in monkeys, which is equivalent to the angular and supramarginal gyrus region, Brodmann's area 39 and 40, in humans. The other cortical areas known to play a role in controlling saccades include the *posterior parietal cortex* (PPC), located in area 7a in monkeys, which is equivalent to Brodmann's area 39 in the upper angular gyrus in humans; the *prefrontal cortex* (PFC), area 46; the *vestibular cortex* (VC) in the posterior aspect of the superior temporal gyrus; and the *hippocampus* in the medial temporal lobe (Pierrot-Deseilligny et al. 1995). These cortical areas determine when different types of saccades occur and where they go—that is, calculate their direction and amplitude (accuracy). Three different coordinate systems are used to make such calculations: the *retinotopic coordinate system*, which uses the visual field, or eye, as a frame of reference; the *cranionotopic coordinate system*, which uses the head as a frame of reference; and the *spatiotopic coordinate system*, which uses the body as a frame of reference. The spatiotopic coordinate system has a significant vestibular input.

The FEFs receive input from multiple cortical areas, including the PEFs, PFC, and SEFs, and project to the deeper layers of the superior colliculus (SC) and to the premotor reticular formation in the brain stem (saccadic generators); it is responsible for (1) disengagement from fixation; (2) triggering intentional retinotopic saccades, which include those visually guided, memory-guided with visual input, predictive, and correct antisaccades; and (3) the amplitude of all contralateral retinotopic (intentional and reflexive) saccades. The PPC and, to a lesser extent, the FEFs, are involved in triggering reflexive visually guided saccades. The SC also has some role in reflexive and orienting saccades. The SEF, which receives input from the PFC and the posterior hemisphere, projects to the FEF, the SC, and the premotor reticular formation and is responsible for (1) the triggering and amplitude of memory-guided saccades with vestibular input (spatiotopic), (2) controlling saccadic sequences, and (3) coordinating craniotopic and spatiotopic saccades with other body movements. The SEFs may have a role in generating predictive saccades; the left side has a greater role (Gaymard et al. 1993). The generation of memory-guided saccades is complex but involves the visual cortex (area 17), the PPC for visuospatial integration, the PFC for spatial memory and sorting, and, finally, the FEFs to trigger the saccade. The PEFs, which receives visual attention input from the superior parietal lobule region, projects to the FEFs and SC and has a role in disengagement from fixation via the FEFs; it also triggers reflexive visually guided saccades and may share a role with the FEFs in controlling intentional visually guided saccades. The PPC has a role in controlling the accuracy of memory-guided saccades with visual input, whereas the VC is involved in controlling memory-guided saccades with vestibular input. The PFC receives input from the PPC and projects to the FEFs, SEFs, and SC. It may contain spatial memory; it controls the spatial aspects of memory-guided saccades and predictive saccades and inhibits reflexive visually guided saccades. Thus, unwanted reflexive saccades are suppressed by the PFC when visual attention is engaged by a specific target. Patients with disorders of the anterior frontal lobes, such as Huntington's chorea, have difficulty maintaining fixation and suppressing unwanted saccades to distracting stimuli, making it virtually impossible to examine their fundi. Release of reflexive contralateral saccades may occur as a result of focal damage impairing inhibitory signals to the brain stem saccadic generators (Kennard et al. 1994). The hippocampus projects to the SEF via the cingulate gyrus and is involved in controlling the chronological order of saccadic sequences, particularly the short-term memorization of the sequences. The basal ganglia also are involved in sequencing complex memory-guided saccades and perhaps predictive saccades (Pierrot-Deseilligny et al. 1995).

Overall, the parietal lobe initiates reflexive and searching saccades to explore the current environment, while the frontal lobe is responsible for "higher order" internally guided (volitional) saccades to explore the immediate past or future environment. The major pathways for saccades descend predominantly in the pedunculotegmental tract through the corona radiata, anterior limb of the internal capsule, and medial cerebral peduncle to decussate at the level of the trochlear nucleus before continuing on to innervate the contralateral horizontal gaze center in the PPRF. The frontal eye fields also project via a transthalamic pathway to the pretectal nuclei (most likely for vertical gaze) and to the deeper layers of the superior colliculus. Saccades of different amplitudes and directions are encoded in neurons in the frontal eye fields and superior colliculi in a retinotopic fashion; that is, the size and direction of a saccade are determined by which neurons are stimulated.

The superior colliculus has seven alternating fibrous and cellular layers, which are broadly divided into a superficial sensory (dorsal) and a deep, predominantly motor (ventral) division. The superficial sensory division receives a direct orderly input from the retina via the accessory optic tract, bypassing the lateral geniculate body, such that the visual field may be mapped on its surface (retinotopic). Only about 10% of the retinal ganglion cells project to the superior colliculus. The deep motor division receives visual input from the striate cortex (area 17) and projects to motor areas in the subthalamic region and brain stem. The deeper division also receives input from the contralateral FEFs and PPC (area 7a and LIP) directly, and indirectly via the basal ganglia, as well as somatosensory and auditory input. Stimulation of the superior colliculus drives the eyes contralaterally to a point in the visual fields corresponding to the retinal projection to that site. Thus, the superior colliculus is essentially a sensory map overlying a corresponding motor map and represents the visual fields (Leigh and Zee 1991); it may also play a role in relaying excitatory information from part of the inferior parietal lobule, which has some influence in initiating saccades. Isolated lesions of the superior colliculus produce minimal, but specific, defects of saccades; when they are combined with experimental lesions of the FEFs, however, significant contralateral saccadic defects result. Purely vertical saccades occur only with bilateral simultaneous stimulation of corresponding points of the superior colliculi, or of the FEFs.

The FEFs also project via the caudate nucleus to neurons in the substantia nigra pars reticulata, which in turn project to the superior colliculus and tonically suppress saccades by a GABAergic mechanism. Controlled disinhibition of this basal ganglial system is important for normal visually guided saccades and probably essential for saccades to remembered targets (Stell and Bronstein 1994).

Control of smooth pursuit eye movements is also complex (see Figure 42.7) but essentially consists of three components: sensory, motor, and attentional-spatial. The stimulus for pursuit is movement of an image across the fovea at velocities greater than 3–5 degrees/sec. The *sensory component* includes the striate cortex (area 17), which receives information from the retinal ganglion (M) cells via the magnocellular layer of the lateral geniculate nucleus and optic radiations and projects to the prestriate cortex (parieto-occipital areas 18 and 19) and then to the superior temporal sulcus region (in rhesus monkeys), which contains cortical areas MT (middle temporal) and MST (middle superior temporal) equivalent to the parieto-temporo-occipital junction (PTO) in humans (Barton et al. 1995) and encodes for location, direction, and velocity of objects moving in the contralateral visual field; it is the major afferent input driving smooth pursuit. This sensory subsystem projects to the accessory optic tract and bilaterally to the *pursuit motor subsystem*, which is also located in the PTO region, as well as to the FEFs and SEFs. This indirect pursuit pathway focuses attention on small moving targets. A direct pathway, bypassing the attentional-spatial subsystem, enables large moving objects, such as full-field OKN stimuli, to generate smooth pursuit contralaterally even when the subject is inattentive. The superior colliculus also contributes to pursuit drive. The PTO projects via the internal sagittal stratum and the posterior limb of the internal capsule to the ipsilateral dorsolateral and lateral pontine nuclei (Gaymard et al. 1993). The pursuit pathways control ipsilateral tracking and so must either remain on the same side or undergo a double decussation at least once. Johnston et al. (1992) suggested the pursuit pathways project from the pontine nuclei to the contralateral flocculus and medial vestibular nucleus and then back to the ipsilateral abducens nucleus (Figure 42.8). The floccular Purkinje cells, posterior vermis, and lobules VI and VII encode neural signals for gaze velocity and coordinate (sum) vestibular and eye movement velocity signals for accurate pursuit.

In summary, pursuit defects fall into four categories (Morrow and Sharpe 1993):

1. *Retinotopic defects*—that is, impaired pursuit in both directions in a contralateral visual field defect, occur with lesions of the geniculostriate pathway. Retinotopic defects also occur with lesions of area MST or peripheral field representation in area MT, analogous to the PTO in humans; these patients have apparently normal visual fields but selective "blindness" for motion.
2. *Impaired pursuit*, worse in the ipsilateral direction in both hemifields, occurs with lesions in the lateral aspect

of area MST and the foveal representation of area MT in monkeys similar to a focal PTO lesion in humans, in the FEFs, in the posterior thalamus, in the midbrain, in the ipsilateral pons, in the contralateral cerebellum and pontomedullary junction, and in the ipsilateral abducens nucleus.

3. *Symmetrically impaired pursuit* in both horizontal directions occurs with focal lesions in the parieto-occipital region (area 39). Medication (anticonvulsants, sedatives, and psychotropic agents), alcohol, fatigue, inattention, schizophrenia, encephalopathy, a variety of neurodegenerative disorders, and age (infants and the elderly) also cause symmetrically impaired pursuit.
4. An *acute nondominant (parietal or frontal) hemisphere lesion* associated with a hemispatial neglect syndrome will cause transient loss of pursuit beyond the midline (craniotopic) into contralateral hemispace.

The cerebellum is richly supplied by afferent fibers conveying ocular information such as velocity, position, and neural integration, from the vestibular system, afferent visual system, PPRF, and midbrain reticular formation (MRF). The cerebellum coordinates the ocular motor system to drive the eyes smoothly and accurately. The *dorsal vermis and fastigial nuclei* determine the accuracy of saccades by modulating their amplitude; they also adjust the innervation to each eye selectively for precisely conjugate movements. Lesions of the dorsal vermis and fastigial nucleii result in saccadic dysmetria (frequently overshoot dysmetria that is greater centripetally) and macrosaccadic oscillations (see Chapter 16). Selective cerebellar lesions have a differential effect on eye movements. Bilateral lesions of the fastigial and globose (interpositus) nuclei cause hypermetria of externally triggered saccades but do not affect internally triggered saccades (Straube et al. 1995); bilateral lesions of the posterior vermis (lobules VI and VII) cause hypometric horizontal and vertical saccades and impaired pursuit; a unilateral lesion of the posterior vermis causes hypometric ipsilateral and hypermetric contralateral saccades, but a unilateral lesion of the caudal fastigial nucleus causes hypermetric ipsilateral and hypometric contralateral saccades (Buttner and Straube 1995; Vahedi et al. 1995). The flocculus, part of the vestibulocerebellum, is responsible for matching the saccadic pulse and step appropriately and for stabilizing images on the fovea. It adjusts the output of the neural integrator and participates in long-term adaptive processing to ensure that eye movements remain appropriate to the stimulus; for example, the amplitude (gain) and even the direction of the slow phases of the VOR are adjusted by the flocculus. Lesions of the flocculus result in gaze-holding deficits such as gaze-evoked, rebound, and downbeat nystagmus. Floccular lesions also impair smooth pursuit, cancellation of the VOR by the pursuit system during combined head and eye tracking, and the ability to suppress nystagmus (and vertigo) by fixation. The nodulus, also part of the vestibulocerebellum, influences vestibular eye movements and vestibular optokinetic interaction. Lesions of the nodulus in monkeys and humans have produced periodic alternating nystagmus.

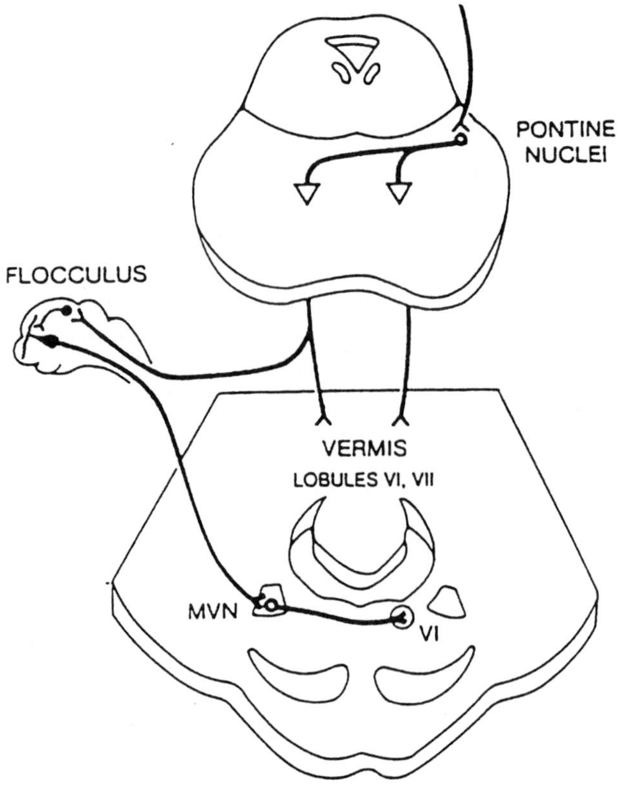

FIGURE 42.8 Postulated double decussation of pursuit pathways in the brain stem and cerebellum. The first decussation consists of excitatory mossy fiber projections from the pontine nuclei to granule cells, which excite basket cells and stellate cells in the contralateral cerebellar flocculus. The basket and stellate cells inhibit Purkinje cells, which in turn inhibit neurons in the medial vestibular nucleus (MVN). The second decussation consists of excitatory projections from the MVN to the opposite abducens nucleus (VI). (Reprinted with permission from JL Johnston, JA Sharpe, MJ Morrow. Paresis of contralateral smooth pursuit and normal vestibular smooth eye movements after unilateral brain stem lesions. Ann Neurol 1992;31:495–502.)

Vergence Eye Movements

In humans and other animals capable of binocular fusional vision, dysconjugate (vergence) eye movements are necessary to maintain ocular alignment on an approaching or receding object (convergence and divergence, respectively). Electromyography (EMG) demonstrates that divergence is an active movement, though not as dynamic or as much under voluntary control as convergence. The principal driving stimuli for vergence movements, relayed from the occipital cortex, are accommodative retinal blur (unfocused) and fusional disparity (diplopia). Each of these stimuli can operate independently. The pupils change size, synkinetically, as part of the near-reflex triad to increase the depth of field and to improve the focus of the optical system. Although the precise locations of the convergence and divergence centers are unknown, lesions in the pretectal region cause vergence abnormalities, and a group of neurons that fire in relation to the angle of convergence has been identified just lateral to the three-nerve nuclear complex. Unilateral stimulation of areas 19 and 22 of the preoccipital cortex caused bilateral convergence, accommodation, and miosis in macaque monkeys. The FEFs, part of the superior temporal gyrus, area 7a, and the flocculus also have a role in vergence. The occipitomesencephalic pathway, involved in vergence, travels more ventrally in the diencephalon and midbrain than the light reflex pathway and is less susceptible to compression by extrinsic lesions (dorsal midbrain syndrome). The MLF carries inhibitory vergence signals.

Vertical Eye Movements

The premotor substrate for vertical gaze lies in the MRF; however, some vertical saccades are programmed in the PPRF and relayed to the MRF via a juxta-MLF pathway, presumably to coordinate horizontal, vertical, and oblique trajectories. The rostral interstitial nucleus of the medial longitudinal fasciculus (riMLF) contains medium-lead (short-latency) excitatory burst neurons for both upgaze and downgaze, although their exact location within that nucleus is controversial: The burst cells for upward saccades are probably caudal, ventral, and medial whereas those for downward saccades are more rostral, dorsal, and lateral. Burst-tonic and tonic neurons in the region of the interstitial nucleus of Cajal (INC) discharge in relation to vertical eye position and play a role in vertical pursuit and eye position; in other words, the integrator for vertical eye movements is probably located in the INC, as is the integrator for torsional eye movements (Halmagyi et al. 1994). The burst neurons for upward saccades project dorsally and laterally from the riMLF and decussate in the posterior commissure before turning ventrally to innervate both ipsilateral and contralateral oculomotor and trochlear nerve nuclei (Figure 42.9). The route of the fibers mediating downward saccades probably projects dorsomedially and caudally to innervate the oculomotor and trochlear nerve nuclei bilaterally (Figure 42.9). The supranuclear innervation for vertical saccades must be bilateral (FEFs or the superior colliculi or both).

Retinal slip, the sensory stimulus for vertical pursuit, is encoded by the dorsolateral pontine nuclei and relayed to the flocculus and posterior vermis before converging, via the INC, on the midbrain (Figure 42.9). The commands for vertical pursuit relay to the brain stem and cerebellum before reaching the relevant ocular motor neurons in the midbrain. The INC is also involved in integrating vertical velocity commands to position commands and may play a role as the final common integrator for all nonsaccadic vertical eye movements, similar to the integrator for horizontal eye movements.

DEVELOPMENT OF THE OCULAR MOTOR SYSTEM

Maturation of the infant nervous system continues after birth and is particularly rapid during the first few months of life (Weissman et al. 1989). At birth the vestibular system is the most developed of the ocular motor subsystems and may be tested by rotating the infant held at arm's length with the head tilted 30 degrees forward. Smooth pursuit movements may be detected in neonates, but only with large targets (such as a human face) at low velocities. Neonates can also generate the smooth pursuit component of OKN to full-field stimulation. These findings, though not well quantified, are consistent with maturation of the fovea after about 8 weeks of age. Infants less than 1 month old can fixate targets provided the stimuli are engaging and the infant is alert. Full-field OKN and larger targets stimulate the parafoveal retina, which matures earlier. Stimulation of the saccadic system, also immature in the neonate, is influenced by the infant's attention as well as by the size and appropriateness of the target. Vertical saccades mature more slowly than horizontal saccades and may not be detected for the first month after birth. Vergence movements are also slow to mature but are seen after about the first month. The afferent visual system, particularly the postgeniculate pathway, is not fully myelinated until about the fourth month after birth; evidence from magnetic resonance imaging (MRI) suggests it may be as late as 15 months (Barkovich et al. 1988).

Ocular alignment in the newborn is usually poor, with transient shifts from esotropia to exotropia during the first few weeks. In most infants ocular alignment is established by 3–4 weeks but may be delayed to as late as 5 months.

Ocular motor anomalies may occur in the neonate without any pathological significance. About 2% of newborns have a tendency for tonic downward deviation of the eyes observed in the waking state; during sleep, however, the eyes assume the normal position, and the vestibulo-ocular reflexes are intact. Other infrequent abnormalities seen in newborns include opsoclonus, which may regress through a phase of ocular flutter, skew deviation, apparent bilateral internuclear ophthalmoplegia (in premature or small-for-gestational-age infants), transient downbeat nystagmus, and tonic upward deviation. Some infants with skew deviation later develop congenital esotropia. These findings represent delayed maturity of the ocular motor system in neonates.

SUPRANUCLEAR GAZE DISTURBANCES

Interruption of the saccadic and pursuit pathways before they reach the eye-movement generators in the MRF and PPRF will result in a loss of voluntary eye movements but will spare reflex movements such as vestibulo-ocular and optokinetic responses and, depending on the level of the lesion, Bell's phenomenon. This constellation of findings is referred to as a *supranuclear gaze palsy* and occurs classically in *progressive*

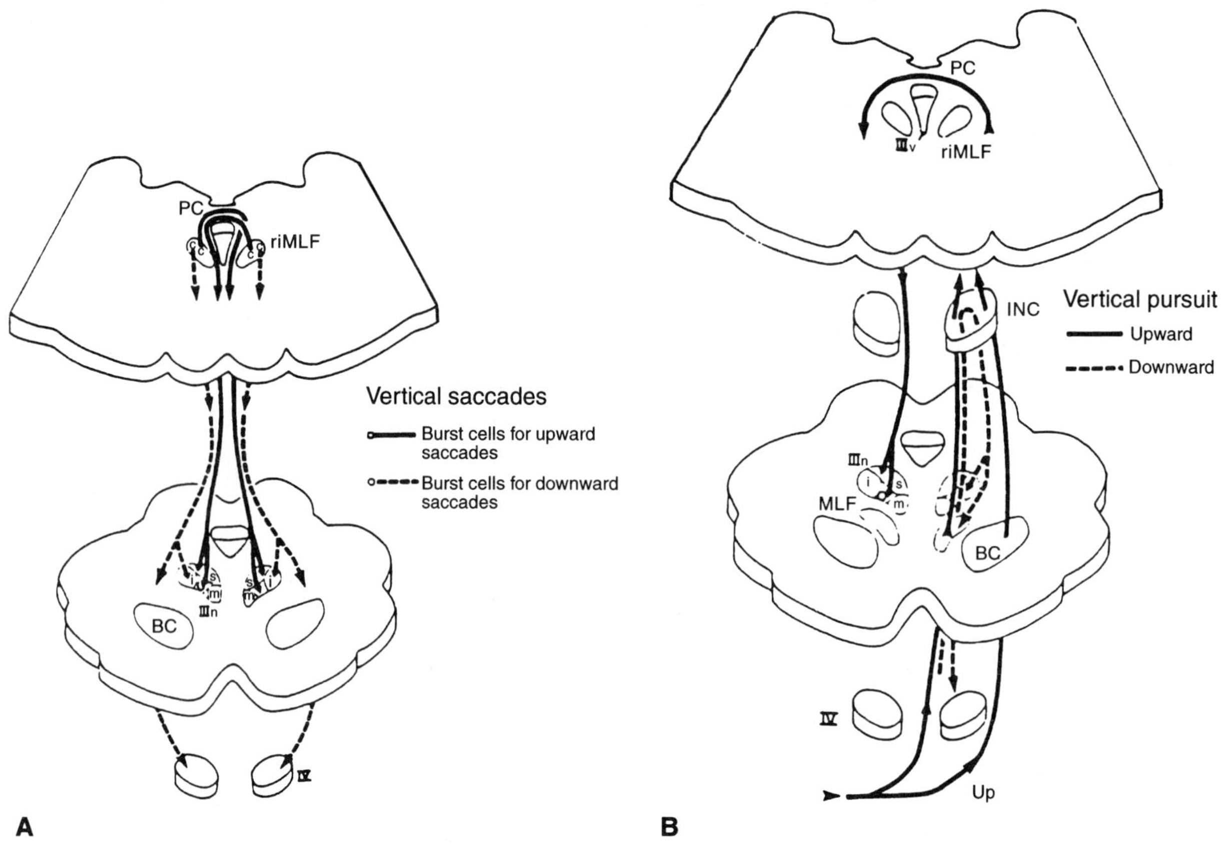

FIGURE 42.9 Hypothetical pathways involved in controlling vertical eye movements. A. Vertical saccades. Burst neurons for upward saccades are shown projecting from the medial rostral interstitial nucleus of the medial longitudinal fasciculus (riMLF) dorsally to decussate in the posterior commissure, then descend caudally and ventrally to innervate the oculomotor and trochlear nuclei bilaterally. For clarity, the descending pathways are shown innervating only the ipsilateral ocular motor nuclei (there is evidence that the innervation is bilateral, though predominantly ipsilateral). The burst neurons for downward saccades are shown projecting from the lateral riMLF caudally to innervate the ocular motor nuclei; again, for clarity only, the ipsilateral pathways are shown. B. Vertical pursuit. The hypothetical pathways for pursuit reach the midbrain via the dorsal lateral pontine nuclei and travel upward in the brachium conjunctivum (BC) and the medial longitudinal fasciculus (MLF). The interstitial nucleus of Cajal (INC) is involved in pursuit and may also be the neural integrator for vertical position commands. (Reprinted with permission from PJ Ranalli, JA Sharpe, WA Fletcher. Palsy of upward and downward saccadic, pursuit, and vestibular movements with a unilateral midbrain lesion: Pathophysiologic correlations. Neurology 1988; 38:114–122.)

supranuclear palsy (PSP), as well as a variety of disorders listed in Table 42.2. Technically, skew deviation and the ocular tilt reaction, which spare the final common efferent pathway for eye movements, are also supranuclear, but because they are disconjugate they are referred to as prenuclear.

Bilateral lesions of the fronto-mesencephalic pathways cause loss of horizontal saccades in both directions and impair vertical saccades (particularly upward), but they spare pursuit, VORs, and the slow phases of OKN resulting in global saccadic palsy. Focal lesions in the PPRF can also cause selective saccadic defects (see Horizontal Eye Movements).

To evaluate gaze disorders, first determine the range of versions (conjugate eye movements) to a moving target, then test saccades as described in Chapter 16. If a dysconjugate defect is observed, check ductions, ocular alignment, and comitance. If the defect is conjugate, determine the presence of oculocephalic ("doll's eye" maneuver) or vestibulo-ocular reflexes (cold calorics), and Bell's phenomenon (ocular deviation, usually upward, on forced eyelid closure); their presence indicates supranuclear dysfunction. With supranuclear gaze disorders, saccades may be impaired first, then pursuit followed by loss of vestibulo-ocular reflexes. Causes of gaze palsies and ophthalmoplegias are outlined in Table 42.2.

Ocular Motor Apraxia

Ocular motor apraxia is the inability to perform voluntary saccades while spontaneous and reflex eye movements (vestibular and OKN slow phases) are preserved. The term is sometimes used loosely and incorrectly.

Table 42.2: Causes of ophthalmoplegias and gaze palsies (see also Table 16.7)

Site	*Disorder*
Muscle	Ocular myopathies
	Congenital myopathy
	Central core
	Centronuclear (myotubular)
	Fiber type disproportion
	Multicore (ptosis, spares EOM)
	Nemaline
	Neurocristopathy (EOM fibrosis)
	Reducing body myopathy (ptosis, spares EOM)
	Dystrophy
	Myotonic dystrophy (ptosis, usually spares EOM)
	Oculopharyngeal dystrophy
	Inflammatory
	Dermatomyositis (also neuromuscular junction defect?)
	Giant-cell arteritis
	Orbital pseudotumor
	Mitochondrial cytopathy
	Kearn's syndrome
	Pearson's syndrome
	Chronic progressive external ophthalmoplegia (CPEO)
	POLIP syndrome (polyneuropathy, ophthalmoplegia, leukoencephalopathy, intestinal pseudo-obstruction) (probable mitochondrial; Simon et al. 1990)
	Metabolic and toxic (act at multiple sites—e.g., anticonvulsants)
	High myopia (large globes cause mechanical restriction)
	Infiltrative disorders (thyroid, amyloid, metastases, congenital familial fibrosis, cystinosis)
	Trauma (orbital entrapment)
	Vitamin E deficiency (associated with malabsorption)
Neuromuscular junction	Myasthenia gravis
	Ocular
	Generalized (80%)
	Toxins (e.g., botulism, organophosphates)
	Eaton-Lambert syndrome (rare)
Ocular motor nerves	See Chapter 75
Gaze palsies	Nuclear and paranuclear
	Brain stem injury (vascular, multiple sclerosis, encephalitis, paraneoplastic, toxins, tumor)
	Familial congenital gaze palsy
	Glycine encephalopathy (nonketotic hyperglycinemia: hiccups, seizures, apneic spells)
	Joseph's disease
	Leigh's disease
	Maple syrup urine disease
	Mobius and Duane's syndromes (agenesis of cranial nerve nuclei)
	Spinocerebellar degeneration
	Tangier disease
	Vitamin E deficiency
	Internuclear ophthalmoplegia
	One-and-a-half syndrome
	Prenuclear
	Monocular "supranuclear" elevator palsy
	Ocular tilt reaction
	Skew deviation
	Supranuclear (predominantly horizontal)
	Congenital ocular motor apraxia
	Acutely, following hemispheric stroke
	Ipsiversive
	Contraversive (wrong-way eyes)
	Gaucher's disease (type 2 and 3)
	Ictal (transient, adversive)
	Juvenile-onset GM2 gangliosidosis (mimics juvenile spinal muscular atrophy)
	Postictal (transient, ipsiversive)
	Paraneoplastic (prostatic adenocarcinoma)
	Supranuclear (predominantly vertical)

Table 42.2: *(continued)*

Site	*Disorder*
Gaze palsies *(continued)*	Adult-onset GM2 gangliosidosis (mimics multiple-system atrophy or spinocerebellar degeneration) (V > H)
	Congenital vertical ocular motor apraxia (rare)
	Amyotrophic lateral sclerosis (rare, V > H)
	Autosomal dominant parkinsonian-dementia complex with pallidopontonigral degeneration (dementia, dytonia, frontal and pyramidal signs, urinary incontinence)
	B_{12} deficiency (U > D)
	Cerebral amyloid angiopathy with leukoencephalopathy
	Dentatorubral-pallidoluysian atrophy (autosomal dominant, dementia, ataxia, myoclonus, choreoathetosis)
	Diffuse Lewy body disease (ophthalmoplegia may be global)
	Dorsal midbrain syndrome (see Chapter 30)
	Familial Creutzfeldt-Jakob disease (U > D)
	Familial paralysis of vertical gaze
	Fisher's syndrome
	Gerstmann-Straussler-Scheinker disease (U > D, dysmetria, nystagmus)
	Guamanian Parkinson's disease-dementia complex (Lytico-Bodig disease)
	HARP syndrome (hypoprebetalipoproteinemia, acanthocytosis, retinitis pigmentosa, pallidal degeneration)
	Hydrocephalus (decompensated, untreated shunt)
	Joseph's disease
	Kernicterus (U > D)
	Late-onset cerebello-pontomesencephalic degeneration (D > U)
	Neurovisceral lipidosis; synonyms: DAF syndrome (downgaze palsy-ataxia-foamy macrophages); dystonic lipidosis; Niemann-Pick disease type C (initially loss of downgaze, may become global)
	Non-Guamanian (dominant familial, autosomal recessive) Parkinson's disease-dementia complex
	OPCA (U > D, also slow horizontal saccades)
	Pallidoluysian atrophy (dysarthria, dystonia, bradykinesia)
	Paraneoplastic disorders
	Progressive supranuclear palsy (D > U)
	Subcortical gliosis (U > D)
	Wilson's disease (also slow horizontal saccades) (U > D)
	Supranuclear (global)
	Abetalipoproteinemia
	AIDS encephalopathy
	Alzheimer's disease (pursuit)
	Cerebral adrenoleukodystrophy
	Corticobasal ganglionic degeneration
	Fahr's disease (idiopathic striatopallidodentate calcification)
	Gaucher's disease
	Hexosaminidase A deficiency
	Huntington's disease
	Joubert's syndrome
	Leber's amaurosis
	Leigh's disease (infantile strionigral degeneration)
	Methylmalanohomocysteinuria
	Malignant neuroleptic syndrome (personal observation)
	Neurosyphilis
	Opportunistic infections
	Paraneoplastic disorders
	Parkinson's disease (transient gaze palsy with intercurrent infection)
	Pelizaeus-Merzbacher disease (H > V)
	Pick's disease (impaired saccades)
	Progressive encephalomyelitis
	Progressive multifocal leukoencephalopathy
	Tay-Sachs disease (infantile GM2 gangliosidosis) (V > H)
	Wernicke's encephalopathy
	Whipple's disease (V > H)

EOM = extraocular movements; D = loss of downgaze; U = loss of upgaze; V = loss of vertical gaze; H = loss of horizontal gaze; global = loss of horizontal and vertical gaze; OPCA = olivopontocerebellar atrophy.

Congenital ocular motor apraxia (COMA) is more common in boys than in girls and is characterized by impaired voluntary horizontal pursuit and saccadic movements but preservation of vertical eye movements (Leigh and Zee 1991); reflex saccades may be partly retained. Because random eye movements are also absent in many of these children, the term apraxia is strictly incorrect; *congenital saccadic palsy* or *congenital gaze palsy* is more accurate (Daroff et al. 1990), but the term COMA is now established in the literature. By 4–8 months old, the patient develops a thrusting head-movement strategy, often with prominent blinking, to overcome the eye-movement deficit. Because the VOR prevents a change in direction of gaze on head turning, the patient suppresses it by closing the eyes to reduce the degree of reflex eye movement (the gain of the VOR falls with the eyes closed) while thrusting the head beyond the range of the VOR arc to bring the eyes on line with the target. Then, with the eyes open, the head is slowly straightened as the contralateral VOR maintains fixation. The dynamic head thrust may be used by some patients to facilitate a saccadic eye movement or reflexively to induce fast phases of vestibular nystagmus. Strabismus, psychomotor developmental delay (particularly reading and expressive language ability), clumsiness, and gait disturbances are often associated with COMA. These children may be misdiagnosed as cortically blind initially, particularly before they develop the head thrusting strategy. As a child with COMA reaches school age, variable improvement in pursuit and voluntary saccades may be experienced. This condition does not completely resolve, however, and can be detected in adulthood. COMA may be associated with hypoplasia of the corpus callosum and midline cerebellum, occipital porencephalic cysts, or bilateral cortical lesions. COMA may occasionally be familial.

A similar ocular motor disorder occurs in children with Pelizaeus-Merzbacher disease, ataxia telangiectasia (80%), Cockayne's syndrome, and succinic semi-aldehyde dehydrogenase deficiency (Eustace et al. 1994).

Congenital vertical ocular motor apraxia is rare and must be differentiated from metabolic and degenerative disorders that cause progressive neurological dysfunction, such as neurovisceral lipidosis, and from stable disorders such as birth injury, perinatal hypoxia, and Leber's congenital amaurosis.

Acquired ocular motor apraxia occurs in patients with bilateral parietal damage and with diffuse bilateral cerebral disease (see Table 42.2); the head thrusts are not as conspicuous as in the congenital variety.

Familial Gaze Palsy

Familial gaze palsy, frequently associated with scoliosis, may occasionally occur in kindreds (Leigh and Zee 1991). Such patients have paralysis of horizontal gaze with impaired OKN and VORs but intact convergence and vertical eye movements. They may have fine horizontal pendular nystagmus. Individuals in some families with this autosomal recessive disorder may also have progressive scoliosis, facial myokymia, facial twitching, hemifacial atrophy, and situs inversus of the optic discs.

Acquired Horizontal Gaze Palsy

Transient gaze deviation, usually of the head and eyes occurs in about 20% of patients with acute hemisphere stroke (Tijssen et al. 1991a) and other insults. The eyes are usually deviated toward the side of the lesion (ipsiversive gaze deviation) because of gaze paresis to the hemiplegic side (Vulpian's sign). In stroke patients, right-sided lesions are more common but smaller; consequently patients with left-sided lesions (gaze deviation to the left) have a worse prognosis (Tijssen et al. 1991b). Ipsiversive gaze deviation is more frequent when the inferior parietal lobule (Tijssen and Tijssen 1991), or circuits between the FEFs and the IPL or their projections to the brain stem (superior colliculus or PPRF) are involved; the FEFs are usually spared. After about 5 days the intact hemisphere, which contains neurons for bilateral gaze, takes over, and only by quantitative oculography can subtle abnormalities such as prolonged saccadic latencies and impaired saccadic suppression be detected.

Because the premotor neural network for voluntary horizontal eye movements in the PPRF is composed of subclasses of neurons with different functions, selective lesions may affect some types of eye movement while sparing others (see the section on Horizontal Eye Movements). A lesion affecting the ipsilateral abducens nucleus or PPRF will cause an ipsilateral gaze palsy; a rostral PPRF lesion will spare the VOR, whereas a caudal lesion will not. Patients with prostatic adenocarcinoma may, after an interval of 3–4 years, develop paraneoplastic brain stem encephalitis and present with selective loss of voluntary horizontal saccades followed by severe facial and bulbar muscle spasms (probable sustained myoclonus), diplopia, and respiratory insufficiency (Baloh et al. 1993). Hyperacusis, vertigo, periodic alternating gaze deviation, abdominal myoclonus, and unsteadiness are also associated with this progressive neurological syndrome. MRI scans are unrevealing, but auditory evoked potentials may be prolonged and the cerebrospinal fluid (CSF) contains a mild pleocytosis and elevated gamma globulin. Clonazepam, valproic acid, and botulinum may help the spasms and myoclonus.

Other causes of horizontal gaze palsies are listed in Table 42.2.

Wrong-Way Eyes

Conjugate eye deviation to the "wrong" side—i.e., away from the lesion and towards the hemiplegia (*contraversive gaze deviation*)—may occur with supratentorial lesions, particularly thalamic hemorrhage, and, rarely, large perisylvian or lobar hemorrhage. The mechanism is unclear, but possibilities include the following:

1. An irritative or seizure focus, causing "contraversive ocular deviation." This is unlikely, because neither clinical nor electrical seizure activity has been reported in these patients.
2. Because eye movements are represented bilaterally in each frontal lobe, it is conceivable that the center for ipsilateral gaze alone may be damaged, resulting in controversive ocular deviation.
3. An irritative lesion of the intralaminar thalamic neurons, which discharge for contralateral saccades, could theoretically cause contraversive ocular deviation (Leigh and Zee 1991).
4. Damage to the contralateral inhibitory center could also be responsible.

Postictal "paralytic" conjugate ocular deviation occurs after *adversive seizures* as part of a Todd's paralysis.

Spasticity of conjugate gaze (lateral deviation of both eyes away from the lesion) during forced eyelid closure, "a variant of Bell's phenomenon," can occur in patients with large, deep parietotemporal lesions; eye movements are otherwise normal.

Psychogenic ocular deviation can occur in patients feigning unconsciousness; the eyes are directed toward the ground irrespective of which way the patient is turned.

Periodic Alternating Gaze Deviation

Periodic alternating gaze deviation (PAGD) is one of the rare cyclic ocular motor disorders in which the direction of gaze alternates every few minutes. Lateral deviation can be sustained for up to 15 minutes; gaze then returns to the midline for 10–20 seconds before changing to the other side. Occasionally PAGD is associated with structural lesions such as pontine vascular disorders; Chiari malformations; congenital absence or abnormalities of the inferior cerebellar vermis, the uvula, and nodulus; Creutzfeldt-Jakob disease involving the floccular lobe; spinocerebellar degeneration; occipital encephalocoeles; and paraneoplastic brain stem encephalitis (Baloh et al. 1993). A reversible form of PAGD occurs with hepatic encephalopathy and is attributed to derangement of GABA metabolism (Averbuch-Heller and Meiner 1995).

Periodic alternating nystagmus (PAN) (Chapter 16), which has a similar time cycle to PAGD, also results from lesions of the uvular and nodular regions. Indeed PAGD may be PAN with loss of corrective saccades because of concomitant saccadic palsy or immaturity of the saccadic system in infants.

Other cyclic ocular motor phenomena, including cyclic esotropia, cyclic oculomotor palsy, springing pupil, alternating skew deviation, and periodic alternating nystagmus, are discussed in the appropriate sections.

Ping-Pong Gaze

Ping-pong gaze (PPG) is a conjugate horizontal rhythmic oscillation that cycles every 4–8 seconds (short-cycle PAGD) and occurs in comatose patients as a result of bilateral cerebral or upper brain stem damage (disconnection) or metabolic dysfunction. PPG implies that the horizontal gaze centers in the pons are intact. The prognosis for recovery is poor except in those patients with a toxic or metabolic cause (Ishikawa et al. 1993).

Saccadic Lateropulsion

When patients demonstrate hypermetric (overshoot) saccades (Figure 16.17B) to the side of the lesion and hypometric (undershoot) saccades (Figure 16.17C) to the opposite side, they have saccadic lateropulsion. In darkness or with the eyelids closed, the patient may have mild conjugate deviation toward the side of the lesion. Saccadic lateropulsion occurs with lesions of the lateral medulla (most commonly ischemic) involving cerebellar inflow (inferior cerebellar peduncle) and is characterized by a saccadic bias (overshoot) toward the side of the lesion (ipsipulsion).

Saccadic lateropulsion with a bias away from the side of the lesion (contrapulsion) may occur with lesions involving the region of the superior cerebellar peduncle (outflow tract) and adjacent cerebellum (superior cerebellar artery territory) (Halmagyi 1994).

Pulsion of vertical saccades, with a parabolic trajectory, also occurs. In patients with lateral medullary injury, both upward and downward saccades deviate toward the side of the lesion, with corrective oblique saccades, whereas in those with lesions involving cerebellar outflow, vertical saccades deviate away from the side of the injury (Halmagyi 1994).

Slow Saccades

Saccades of low velocity result from pontine disease, presumably because of burst cell dysfunction. They occur in patients with olivopontocerebellar degeneration (slow to no saccades) and other disorders listed in Table 42.3. Some patients with hypometric saccades (Figure 16.17C) composed of multiple small-amplitude steps (as in myasthenia, Huntington's disease, brain stem encephalitis, and striato-nigral degeneration) appear to have slow saccades clinically (pseudo-slow saccades).

Prolonged Saccadic Latency

Disorders of saccadic initiation result in prolonged latencies for voluntary saccades and occur in patients with AIDS-dementia complex and a variety of degenerative disorders of the nervous system such as Alzheimer's, Huntington's, and Parkinson's disease.

Table 42.3: Slow saccades

Advanced Parkinson's disease (?)
AIDS-dementia complex
Amyotrophic lateral sclerosis
Anticonvulsant toxicity (consciousness usually impaired)
Ataxia-telangiectasia
Hexosaminidase A deficiency
Huntington's disease
Internuclear ophthalmoplegia
Joseph's disease
Lesions of the paramedian pontine reticular formation
Lipid storage diseases
Lytico-Bodig disease
Myotonic dystrophy
Nephropathic cystinosis
Ocular motor apraxia
Ocular motor nerve or muscle weakness
Olivopontocerebellar degeneration
Progressive supranuclear palsy
Whipple's disease
Wilson's disease

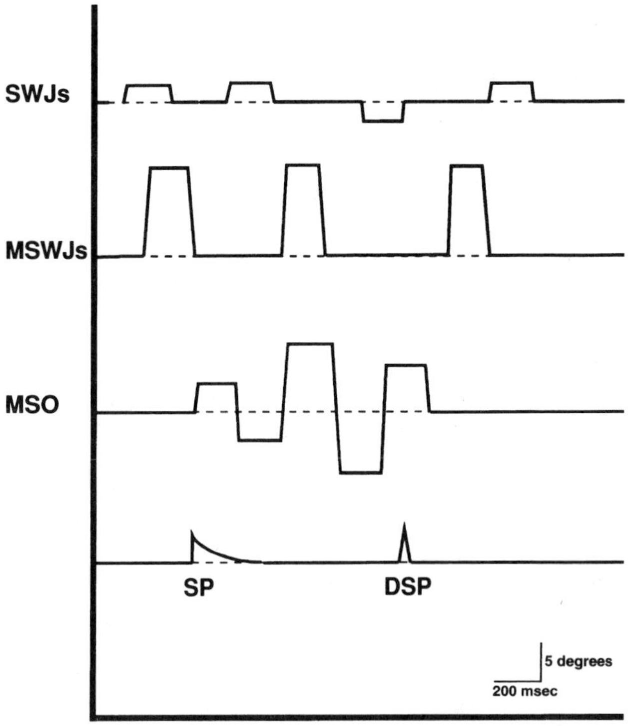

FIGURE 42.10 Simulated eye movement recordings of square wave jerks (SWJs), macrosquare wave jerks (MSWJs), macrosaccadic oscillations (MSO), a saccadic pulse (SP), and a double saccadic pulse (DSP).

Square Wave Jerks

Square wave jerks (SWJs) (Table 42.4) are spontaneous, small-amplitude paired saccades with an intersaccadic latency of 150–200 msec that briefly interrupt fixation (Figure 42.10). They may occur physiologically in normal subjects—particularly in darkness—without fixation, and are usually about 2 degrees in amplitude; they are more frequent in the elderly (Halmagyi 1994). SWJs are prominent in PSP, multiple-system atrophy, and cerebellar disease; their increased frequency may distinguish Parkinson's disease from the less dopamine-responsive parkinsonian syndromes such as olivopontocerebellar atrophy (OPCA), PSP, Lewy body disease, and multiple system atrophy. They may be induced by tobacco. Because of the intersaccadic interval (latency), SWJs are thought to be triggered supratentorially, whereas other saccadic intrusions, such as saccadic pulses, and oscillations such as flutter and opsoclonus are caused by dysfunction of the pause cells in the brain stem (Chapter 16). Macrosquare wave jerks, which are similar to SWJs but have amplitudes of 10–40 degrees, occur in patients with multiple sclerosis and olivopontocerebellar degeneration. SWJs and macrosquare wave jerks should be distinguished from macrosaccadic oscillations, which wax and wane across fixation (Figure 42.10), are not present in darkness, and occur with midline cerebellar lesions. These and other saccadic oscillations are discussed in detail elsewhere (Dell'Osso et al. 1990; Leigh and Zee 1991).

Table 42.4: Square wave jerks

Normal subjects (<2 degrees)
Excitement in normals
Catecholamine depletion in normals
Aging
Strabismus
Congenital nystagmus
Latent nystagmus
Dyslexia (suppressed by methylphenidate)
Progressive supranuclear palsy
Schizophrenia
Cerebral hemisphere tumors and stroke
Parkinson's disease
Wernicke's encephalopathy
Friederich's ataxia
Joseph's disease
Gerstmann-Straussler-Scheinker disease
Lithium
Tobacco
AIDS-dementia complex (HIV encephalitis)
Macrosquare wave jerks (>10 degrees)
Olivopontocerebellar atrophy
Multiple sclerosis (cerebellar dysfunction)

Internuclear Ophthalmoplegia

Damage to the MLF between the third and sixth cranial nerve nuclei impairs transmission of neural impulses to the ipsilateral medial rectus muscle (see Figure 42.3). Adducting saccades of the ipsilateral eye will be impaired (either slow or absent) depending on the severity of the lesion. Typically, *nystagmus* of the abducting eye is seen, giving the appearance of dissociated nystagmus (see Chapter 16), but is in fact overshoot dysmetria (Halmagyi 1994). Upward-beating and torsional nystagmus are frequently present, particularly if both MLFs are affected. Convergence may be preserved with an internuclear ophthalmoplegia (INO), but because the patient's attention and effort are necessary for its evaluation, it is not a particularly helpful sign. In patients with bilateral INO abduction, saccades may also be slow, because of impaired inhibition of "resting" tone in the medial rectus muscle (Thomke et al. 1992a).

A subtle INO may be demonstrated by having the patient make repetitive horizontal saccades, which often disclose slow adduction of the ipsilateral eye. Alternatively, an optokinetic tape may be used to induce repetitive saccades in the direction of action of the suspected weak medial rectus muscle, by moving the tape in the opposite direction and observing for smaller amplitude adducting saccades.

Other clinical features associated with INO include skew deviation (the hypertropia is usually ipsilateral to the lesion) and defective vertical smooth pursuit, OKN, and vertical VORs as well as impaired ability to cancel vertical VORs.

INO may occur with a variety of disorders affecting the brain stem (Table 42.5) and must be distinguished from pseudo-INO.

Rarely, patients with small lesions in the rostral pons or midbrain, remote from the abducens nerve and nucleus, may have *the Lutz posterior INO*, where abduction is impaired but the adducting eye has *nystagmus*; the mechanism is attributed to impaired inhibition of the antagonist medial rectus muscle because of damage to uncrossed fibers, from the PPRF to the oculomotor nucleus, running close to but separate from the MLF (Thomke et al. 1992b).

Table 42.5: Causes of internuclear ophthalmoplegia

Brain stem (pontine) stroke—unilateral
Multiple sclerosis—unilateral or bilateral
Intrinsic tumor—primary or metastatic
Meningitis (especially tuberculosis)
Brain stem encephalitis (infective, paraneoplastic)
Chemotherapy with radiation therapy
Drug intoxication (comatose)—anticonvulsants, phenothiazines, tricyclics; (awake)—lithium
Spinocerebellar degeneration
Fabry's disease (vascular)
Wernicke's encephalopathy
Progressive supranuclear palsy
Syringobulbia associated with a Chiari malformation
Trauma (closed head injury)
Hexosaminidase A deficiency
Maple syrup urine disease
Cerebral air embolism
Pseudointernuclear ophthalmoplegia
Long-standing exotropia
Myasthenia
Myotonic dystrophy
Neuromyotonia of the lateral rectus muscle
Partial III nerve palsy
Previous extraocular muscle surgery
Thyroid orbitopathy (lateral rectus restriction)
Orbital pseudotumor
Other infiltrative disorders of extraocular muscle (neoplasm, amyloid, and the like)
Miller-Fisher syndrome (sometimes may be a true internuclear ophthalmoplegia)

The One-and-a-Half Syndrome

A lesion in the caudal dorsal pontine tegmentum involving the ipsilateral PPRF, or the abducens nucleus, and the ipsilateral MLF will result in an ipsilateral gaze palsy with an ipsilateral INO (see Figure 42.3). Abduction of the contralateral eye is the only horizontal movement left intact. Patients who also have facial nerve palsy may later develop oculopalatal myoclonus (see Chapter 16), probably because of the proximity of the central tegmental tract to the facial nerve (Wolin et al. 1995, in press). The most common causes of the one-and-a-half syndrome are multiple sclerosis and brain stem stroke, followed by metastatic and primary brain stem tumors. Ocular myasthenia may cause a pseudo-one-and-a-half syndrome.

Disorders of Vertical Gaze

Disorders of conjugate vertical gaze result from isolated lesions placed discretely in the midbrain pretectal region (Hommel and Bogousslavsky 1991) (see Figures 42.9 and 42.11).

Downgaze paralysis occurs with bilateral lesions of the riMLF (see Figure 42.11A) or its projections, which course caudally and dorsally, bilaterally (see Figure 42.9). In humans, with the exception of occlusion of the posterior thalamosubthalamic branch of the posterior cerebral artery, such isolated lesions are rare (Green et al. 1993), and the mechanism of paralysis is damage to the midbrain. More commonly, bilateral involvement of the pathways for downgaze, and also for upgaze, occurs as a part of diffuse disorders such as progressive supranuclear palsy, Whipple's disease, neurovisceral lipid storage disorders, complications of AIDS, and the like (see Table 42.2).

Supranuclear paralysis of upgaze occurs with lesions at or near the posterior commissure, or bilaterally in the pretectal area (see Figure 42.11B). A unilateral lesion of the midbrain tegmentum, involving the ipsilateral burst cells, the crossing fibers from the contralateral burst cells, and probably neighboring inhibitory pathways, may result in impairment of both upward and downward saccades. Patients with impaired vertical gaze as a result of extrinsic compression of the posterior commissure/pretectal region are more likely to have pupillary light-near dissociation but preservation of the near reflex, because the light-reflex pathways are more superficial. Intrinsic midbrain lesions cause impairment of convergence and accommodation (the near reflex) before loss of the light reflex. With supranuclear disorders of vertical gaze, saccades are impaired initially, followed by pursuit then loss of vertical

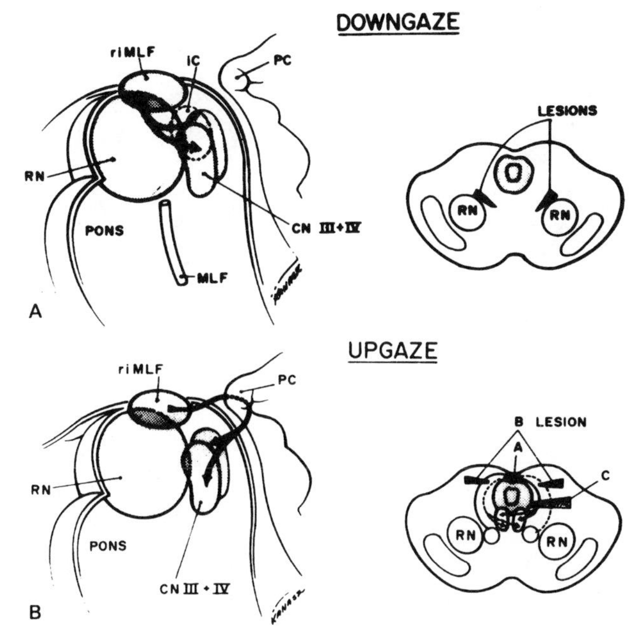

FIGURE 42.11 Disorders of vertical gaze. A. The pathways for downgaze (viewed from above, left, and posteriorly) originate in the rostral interstitial nucleus of the medial longitudinal fasciculus (riMLF) near the interstitial nucleus of Cajal, and innervate the third- and fourth-nerve nuclear complex, bilaterally. Bilateral lesions dorsal and medial to the red nucleus (RN) result in paralysis of downgaze (cross-section at level of posterior commissure). B. The pathways for upgaze (viewed from above, left, and posteriorly) also originate in the riMLF and project dorsally through the posterior commissure (PC), dividing to innervate the III and IV nerve nuclei, bilaterally. To produce paralysis of upgaze, lesions (at A, B, or C, shown on the right) must interrupt the supranuclear pathways to both nuclear complexes (cross-section at level of posterior commissure). (Reprinted with permission from PJM Lavin. Conjugate and Disconjugate Eye Movements. In TJ Walsh [ed], Neuro-ophthalmology: Clinical Signs and Symptoms. Philadelphia: Lea & Febiger, 1985.)

vestibulo-ocular reflexes. Paralysis of upgaze, light-near dissociation of the pupils, impaired convergence, lid retraction, and convergence retraction nystagmus are features of the dorsal midbrain (Parinaud's) syndrome (see Chapter 23), also called the pretectal syndrome (Keane 1990).

Disorders of vertical gaze (see Table 42.2), particularly downgaze and combined upgaze and downgaze paresis, may be overlooked in patients with brain stem vascular disease because of impaired consciousness as a result of concomitant damage to the reticular activating system.

Tonic upward deviation of gaze (forced upgaze), a rare sign, is seen in unconscious patients and must be distinguished from oculogyric crises, petit mal seizures, and psychogenic coma. In a series of 17 comatose patients with sustained upgaze following diffuse brain injury (hypotension, cardiac arrest, heatstroke), autopsy evidence demonstrated cerebral and cerebellar hypoxic damage, with relative sparing of the brain stem. Some of these patients later developed myoclonic jerks and large-amplitude downbeat nystagmus; their prognosis was extremely poor. Rarely, tonic upward gaze deviation may be psychogenic but can be overcome, indeed cured, by cold caloric stimulation of the eardrums.

Benign paroxysmal tonic upward gaze may occur in young children in association with ataxia and downbeat nystagmus on attempted downgaze (Echenne and Rivier 1992); the duration of deviation is variable (seconds to hours) but is usually short, occurring frequently throughout the day. This disorder, which usually starts in the first year of life and lasts about 2 years, has no known cause; there is no evidence to support that the episodes are seizures or oculogyric crises. The condition is reminiscent of the intermittent or periodic ataxias, which may respond to drugs such as acetazolamide and valproic acid (see Chapter 77).

Tonic upgaze may be seen in normal infants during the first few months of life.

Tonic downward deviation of gaze (forced downgaze) is associated with impaired consciousness in patients with medial thalamic hemorrhage, acute obstructive hydrocephalus, severe metabolic or hypoxic encephalopathy, or massive subarachnoid hemorrhage. The eyes may also be converged as if looking at the nose. Tonic downward gaze deviation may also occur in psychogenic illness, especially feigned coma, but also can be overcome by caloric stimulation.

In otherwise healthy neonates, downward deviation of the eyes while awake, but with preserved VORs, may occur as a transient phenomenon (see Development of the Ocular Motor System). Tonic vertical deviation as a result of ictal activity is rare.

A form of *paroxysmal ocular downward deviation* that lasts seconds and occurs in neurologically impaired infants with poor vision may also be seen in preterm infants with bronchopulmonary dysplasia but subsequent normal development (Kleiman et al. 1994).

In normal circumstances, a synkinetic movement, *ocular counter-rolling*, allows people to maintain horizontal orientation of the environment while tilting the head to either side (Figure 42.12A). When the head is tilted to the left, the left eye rises and intorts as the right eye falls and extorts, within the range of the ocular tilt reflex (approximately 10 degrees from the vertical). The initial transient dynamic (phasic) counter-rolling response results from stimulation of the semicircular canals, whereas the sustained (tonic) response is mediated by the otolith organs, which hold the eyes in position at the end of the head movement. Lesions of these pathways result in skew deviation.

Skew deviation is a vertical divergence of the ocular axes caused by a "prenuclear" lesion in the brain stem or cerebellum involving the vertical vestibulo-ocular pathways. About 12% of skews alternate on lateral gaze, or spontaneously (below). A skew deviation is usually, but not always, comitant (see Chapter 16); when noncomitant it may mimic a partial third-nerve or a fourth-nerve palsy. Skew deviations occur most commonly with vascular lesions of the pons or lateral medulla (Wallenberg's syndrome), presumably because of injury to the vestibular nuclei or their projections. Brandt and Dieterich (1993) demonstrated ocular torsion of one or both eyes associated with subjective tilting of the visual vertical toward the lower eye in most patients with skew deviations: With lesions caudal to the lower pons the ipsilateral eye was lower (ipsiversive skew), but with lesions rostral to the midpontine level the contralateral eye was lower (contraversive skew). Ocular torsion may be present without a skew and, in either situation, can be detected by blind spot mapping, indirect ophthalmoscopy, or fundus photography (Halmagyi 1994). Skew deviation with ocular torsion ("skew torsion") is a result of an imbalance in the tonic vestibulo-ocular pathways—in both the vertical and coronal (roll) planes—that normally stabilize the eyes and head in an upright position to maintain horizontal and vertical orientation.

Alternating skew deviation, where the hypertrophia changes sides, results from vascular or demyelinating lesions at the pretectal-mesodiencephalic junction and usually involving the interstitial nucleus of Cajal. This phenomenon, also referred to as paroxysmal skew deviation and periodic alternating skew, may change spontaneously or with the direction of gaze, in a regular or irregular manner over periods of seconds to minutes. Other features of the dorsal midbrain syndrome may be associated with this bizarre phenomenon (Halmagyi 1994). Disorders affecting the cerebellar pathways or cervicomedullary junction may result in alternating skew deviation on lateral gaze where the abducting eye is hypertropic as a result of presumed superior oblique overaction (Hamed et al. 1993). This finding is frequently associated with ataxia and downbeat nystagmus (Halmagyi 1994). Bilateral fourth-nerve palsies may mimic gaze-dependent alternating skew, where the adducting eye is hypertropic; however, diplopia is worse on downgaze, with significant tilting of the images.

The ocular tilt reaction (OTR) consists of the triad of spontaneous skew deviation, cyclotorsion of both eyes, and paradoxical head tilting toward the side of the lower eye (see Figure 42.12B). A tonic (sustained) OTR may occur with a lesion of the ipsilateral utricle, vestibular nerve, or nuclei, or a lesion in the region of the contralateral interstitial nucleus of Cajal and medial thalamus (Halmagyi 1994). A phasic (paroxysmal) OTR occurs with a lesion in the region of the ipsilateral interstitial nucleus of Cajal, and it may respond to baclofen. An OTR can be induced by sound in patients with perilymph fistules of the vestibular end organ, known as Tullio's phenomenon (Halmagyi 1994).

Monocular supranuclear elevator palsy results in limitation of elevation of one eye on attempted upgaze, despite orthotropia in primary position and an intact downgaze. This rare condition usually occurs with vascular or neoplastic lesions involving the midbrain.

Oculogyric crises are spasmodic conjugate ocular deviations, usually in an upward, sometimes lateral, and occasionally downward direction. They occurred in the late stages of postencephalitic Parkinson's disease, following the 1918 influenza epidemic, but now are most frequently caused by neuroleptic medication, particularly haloperidol.

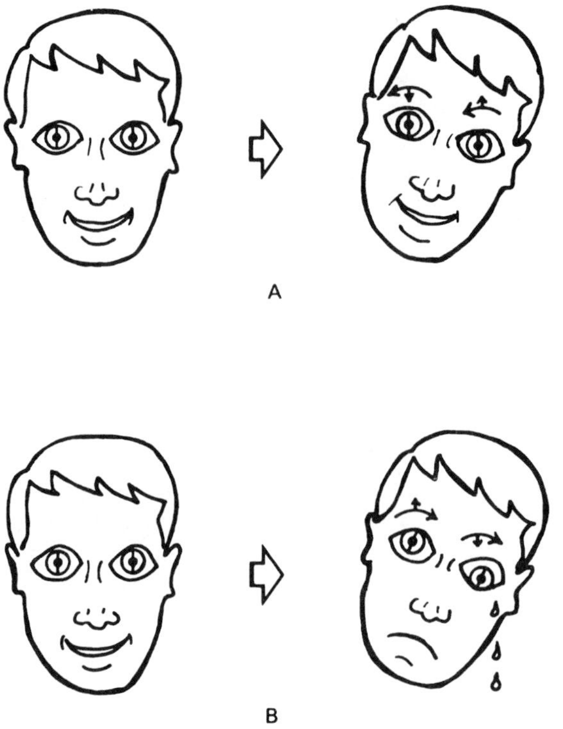

FIGURE 42.12 A. The normal ocular counter-rolling phenomenon during head tilt. B. The ocular tilt reaction is a triad of spontaneous skew deviation, cyclotorsion of the eyes, and head-tilt toward the side of the lower eye.

They may also occur in patients with neurosyphilis, carbamazepine or lithium carbonate toxicity, and head injury, and in the early stages of autosomal dominant "rapid-onset dystonia-Parkinsonism" (Dobyns et al. 1993). A typical attack or crisis lasts about 2 hours, during which the eyes are tonically deviated upward, repetitively, for periods of seconds to minutes. The spasms may be preceded or accompanied by disturbing emotional symptoms, including anxiety, restlessness, compulsive thinking, and sensations of increased brightness or distortions of visual background. The patient may be able to force the eyes back to the primary position temporarily by using voluntary saccades, optokinetic tracking, head rotation, or blinking. Electroencephalograph (EEG) recordings during the attacks show no epileptiform activity (Leigh et al 1987). The eyelids are usually open, although they may rhythmically jerk at times from twitching of the orbicularis oculi. In patients with Parkinson's disease, blepharospasm may also be present. The pupils are infrequently involved, with mydriasis or anisocoria. Attacks may be precipitated by excitement. They should be differentiated from benign paroxysmal tonic upward gaze (see the section on Tonic Upward Deviation of Gaze). Treatment for oculogyric crises includes levodopa and high-dose trihexyphenidyl. Leigh et al. (1987) proposed that the emotional reaction preceding the crisis suggests a chemical imbalance in the limbic-vertical ocular motor connections.

Disorders of Convergence

Convergence paralysis is usually associated with other features of the dorsal midbrain syndrome. Patients with psychogenic convergence paralysis may be distinguished from those with organic disease by preservation of upgaze and absence of pupillary constriction. Lack of effort is the most common cause of poor convergence, which becomes more difficult with age. Degenerative disorders such as Parkinson's disease and PSP may be associated with poor convergence and can be helped with prisms.

Convergence insufficiency, an idiopathic condition that may be partly psychogenic, occurs most commonly in women between the ages of 15 and 45 years. It is an imbalance between accommodation and convergence and may cause frank diplopia, although eyestrain, headache, and vague symptoms such as burning eyes are more common (Waltz and Lavin 1993). It may occur following head injury. Orthoptic exercises (pencil pushups), less commonly prisms, or myopic correction are useful in management.

Spasm of the near reflex is a disorder characterized by intermittent episodes of convergence, miosis, and accommodation. It may mimic bilateral, and occasionally unilateral, abducens paresis. The patient may complain of double or blurred vision and is esotropic, particularly at distance; extreme miosis, however, is the clue. Spasm of the near reflex may occur in patients with organic disorders but is more commonly psychogenic, either in patients with conversion reactions or in anxious patients in whom the "spasm" is unintentional, perhaps a manifestation of misdirected effort. The differential diagnosis is that of *esotropia* (Table 42.6), but miosis on gaze testing establishes the diagnosis. Patients with "psychogenic" spasm of the near reflex have associated somatic complaints and behavioral abnormalities. Blepharoclonus on persistent lateral gaze and poor cooperation in performing motor tasks such as smiling, opening the mouth, protruding the tongue, and the like (features of neurasthenia and asthenopia) may be found during examination (Table 42.7). Management should focus on identifying the source of the psychopathology and may require psychiatric evaluation. Strategies such as the use of cycloplegia (homatropine eyedrops) to prevent accommodative spasm and thus inhibit the near triad, negative (minus) spheric lens correction, and opacifying the inner third of spectacle lenses are less effective.

Table 42.6: Causes of esotropia

Congenital esotropia (also acquired, cyclic)
Accommodative esotropia
Bilateral abducens palsy
Spasm of the near reflex
Tonic convergence spasm (part of dorsal midbrain syndrome)
Pseudo-sixth nerve palsy of Fisher
Acute thalamic esotropia
Posterior internuclear ophthalmoplegia of Lutz (pseudo-sixth)
Neuromyotonia
Divergence insufficiency
Divergence paralysis
Cyclical oculomotor palsy (spastic phase)
Nystagmus blockage syndrome
Abducens palsy with contracture of antagonist (ipsilateral medial rectus) during recovery
Myasthenia (rare)
Medial rectus entrapment (blowout fracture) (rare)
Thyroid myopathy (rare, at presentation)
Wernicke's encephalopathy (bilateral abducens palsies)
Chiari malformation

Disorders of Divergence

Divergence insufficiency is characterized by sudden-onset esotropia and uncrossed horizontal diplopia at distance, in the absence of other neurological symptoms or signs. The esotropia may be intermittent or constant but the patients can fuse at near. The esodeviation (see Chapter 16) is greater at distance than near but is comitant in all directions. Versions and ductions are full, and saccadic velocities, if measured quantitatively, appear normal. Fusional divergence is reduced. The origin of divergence insufficiency is unclear, but this may result from a break in fusion in a patient with a congenital esophoria, usually coming on later in life or following a trivial insult. The condition is easily treated with base out prisms for the distance correction and rarely requires extraocular muscle surgery.

Divergence paralysis, a controversial entity that may be difficult to distinguish from divergence insufficiency, usually occurs in the context of a severe head injury or other cause of raised intracranial pressure. Such patients will also have horizontal diplopia at distance, but quantitatively, abducting saccades are slow. Patients with bilateral sixth-nerve palsies, who recover gradually, may go through a

Table 42.7: Features of spasm of the near reflex (psychogenic)

Near triad
Convergence
Miosis
Accommodation (blur at distance, myopic retinoscopy)
Neurasthenic symptoms
Blepharoclonus and blepharospasm
Poor cooperation in other motor tasks
Other behavioral changes, such as tunnel vision
May disappear with rapid saccades
Full range of eye movement
With pursuit of own hand
With one eye covered
Doll's eyes with fixation
Ice cold calorics
Normal response
Bizarre behavioral response
Normal optokinetic nystagmus if patient encouraged or distracted (e.g., count stripes)

phase where the esotropia becomes comitant with full ductions, mimicking divergence paralysis. Divergence paralysis can also occur with Fisher's syndrome, Chiari malformations, pontine tumors, and diazepam therapy.

Central disruption of fusion can occur following moderate head injury and causes intractable diplopia, despite the patient's ability to intermittently fuse and even achieve stereopsis briefly. The diplopia fluctuates and varies among crossed, uncrossed, and vertical. Versions and ductions may be full, but vergence amplitudes (see Chapter 16) are greatly reduced. Prism therapy or surgery is ineffective, but an eye patch may provide symptomatic relief. The location of injury is presumed in the midbrain. Central disruption of fusion has also been associated with brain stem tumors, stroke, removal of longstanding cataracts or uncorrected aphakia, and neurosurgical procedures. This condition must be distinguished from bilateral fourth-nerve palsies, when diplopia is constant and associated with cyclodiplopia and excyclotropia (>12 degrees) and with psychogenic disorders of vergence (above).

Inability to fuse may also be congenital and then is associated with amblyopia or congenital esotropia (see Chapter 16).

Patients with large visual-field defects, particularly dense bitemporal hemianopias, lose overlapping areas of field, have difficulty maintaining fusion and develop diplopia—the hemislide phenomenon—because they can no longer suppress a latent ocular deviation (see Chapter 16).

Cyclic esotropia, also called circadian, alternate-day, or clock mechanism esotropia, usually begins in childhood, although it can occur in infancy, in later life, or following surgery for intermittent esotropia. The cycles of orthotropia and esotropia may run 24–96 hours, and they parallel many of the other cyclic or periodic biological phenomena with obscure mechanisms.

Ocular neuromyotonia is a brief episodic myotonic contraction of one or more muscles supplied by the ocular motor nerves, most commonly the third nerve. It usually results in esotropia of the affected eye with accompanying failure of elevation and depression of the globe. When the third nerve is affected, there may be accompanying signs of aberrant reinnervation (see Chapter 75). The pupil may be fixed to both light and near stimuli. Causes include radiation therapy and, less commonly, compressive lesions such as cavernous sinus meningiomas or pituitary adenomas. Occasionally no cause can be found (Frohman and Zee 1995). Ocular neuromyotonia may respond to carbamazepine; it should be distinguished from superior oblique myokymia (see Chapter 16) and the spasms of cyclic oculomotor palsy.

Oculomotor paresis alternating with cyclic spasms of both the extraocular and intraocular muscles supplied by that nerve is a rare condition usually noted in the first 2 years of life, although the majority are believed to be congenital and are often associated with other features of birth trauma. During the spasms, which last 10–30 seconds, the upper eyelid elevates, the globe adducts, and the pupil and ciliary muscle constrict, causing miosis and increased accommodation (Loewenfeld 1993); the paretic phase usually lasts longer. Signs of aberrant oculomotor reinnervation (see Chapter 75) are usually present. Spasms, often heralded by twitching of the upper lid, may be precipitated by intentional accommodation or adduction. Cycles occur irregularly and vary from 1.5 to 3.0 minutes in duration; they persist during sleep and may be suppressed by topical cholinergic agents (eserine, pilocarpine) or abolished by topical anticholinergic agents (atropine, homatropine) or general anesthesia. Usually the cycles persist throughout life, but in some patients spasms of the extraocular muscles may abate, leaving only intermittent miosis.

Symptomatic cyclic oculomotor palsy may occur in later life in patients with underlying lesions involving the third nerve, but the features and cycles are atypical. The mechanism of cyclic spasms is unclear but is well discussed elsewhere by Loewenfeld (1993).

A variety of phenomena may be evoked by gaze. Some, such as end-point nystagmus or the oculo-auricular phenomenon (Urban et al. 1993), are physiologic and well known; others, such as gaze-evoked nystagmus or tinnitus, are pathological (Table 42.8).

Table 42.8: Gaze-evoked phenomena

I. Physiological phenomena
   A. The oculo-auricular phenomenon, coactivation of external ear muscles during eye movements (96% of normal subjects with lateral gaze and 61% with convergence)
   B. Blinks
   C. End-point nystagmus
   D. Phosphenes (more intense in patients with optic neuritis, retinal/vitreous detachment: Moore's lightning streaks)
II. Pathological sensory phenomena
   A. Gaze-evoked amaurosis in the eye ipsilateral to an orbital apex tumor
   B. Tinnitus provoked by lateral gaze in patients with eighth nerve damage associated with or following CP angle tumor removal
   C. Vertigo
   D. Tinnitus with periodic saccadic oscillations in presumed pontine disease
III. Pathological motor phenomena
   A. Gaze-evoked nystagmus (see Chapter 16)
   B. Facial twitching, clonic limb movements, blepharoclonus, lid nystagmus, involuntary laughter and seizures
   C. Synkinetic movements with cyclic oculomotor palsy (above) and with aberrant reinnervation of the oculomotor nerve (see Chapter 75)
   D. Neuromyotonia
   E. Superior oblique myokymia (see Chapter 16)
   F. Retraction of the globe in Duane's syndrome
   G. Convergence retraction nystagmus on attempted upgaze (the dorsal midbrain syndrome)

EYE MOVEMENT RECORDING TECHNIQUES

Oculographic techniques provide clinicians and researchers with objective and quantitative means of analysis, which have led to a better understanding of eye movement neurophysiology and ocular motility disorders. Quantitative oculography can measure saccadic latency, velocity, accuracy, pursuit and VOR gain, and nystagmus slow-phase velocity; it can detect unsuspected oscillations and intrusions and identify different nystagmus waveforms. Oculography is used to record both spontaneous and induced eye movements to a target, such as a projected light in front of the subject, or to vestibular and optokinetic stimuli. Quantitative oculography has improved our powers of clinical observation by providing objective and critical feedback.

Electro-Oculography

Electro-oculography (EOG), the old standby also known as electronystagmography (see Chapter 44), is the most popular method of quantitative oculography in most clinical laboratories. In EOG, skin electrodes are placed at the inner and outer canthus of each eye, with a reference electrode on one earlobe. The potential difference between the cornea and the retina (about 1 mV) is recorded and, when the eye is centered, is zero. As the electrically positive cornea moves toward one electrode, the voltage, dependent on eye position, increases. This analog signal, which is differentially amplified, represents horizontal eye position. Each pair of electrodes should be DC-coupled; AC coupling distorts the shape of the analog recording. Because most EOG systems are electrically noisy, low-pass filters (30 Hz) are necessary but, unfortunately, compromise sensitivity to the fine characteristics of eye movements and high-velocity saccades. This method, which records each eye independently, has a range of 35–40 degrees from primary position and is superior to the binocular technique using a single central (nasion) and two bitemporal electrodes. The eye movement position tracing can be mathematically differentiated electronically to determine eye movement velocity. The analog signal, usually recorded by a pen tracer, can also be digitalized to interface with a computer. Although EOG systems are noninvasive and comfortable for the patient, they have a limited range and sensitivity and are unreliable for vertical eye movements because of eyelid artifact.

Infrared Oculography

An infrared light source, mounted on a spectacle frame, illuminates the front of the eye; the reflected light detected by two infrared-sensitive phototransistors, also on the frame and aimed at the medial and lateral limbus, generates an electrical signal that fluctuates in relation to light intensity. When the eye is centered, each phototransistor detects the same amount of light; if they are connected differentially, the result is zero. When the eye moves toward one phototransistor, less light is reflected by the cornea, while more is reflected to the other cell by the sclera. The electrical signal generated depends on eye position and maintains a linear relationship ±25 degrees. The analog tracing represents horizontal eye position. Vertical eye movements may be recorded if the signal from each cell, aimed at the inferior limbus, is summed and the lower eyelid retracted to avoid lid artifact, but range is limited to ±15 degrees from primary position. The signals are recorded in the same manner as in EOG. A surface electrode above and below each eye can detect blinks and distinguish them from eye movement. This is a noninvasive, safe, and relatively comfortable system.

Scleral Search Coil

The scleral search coil initially consisted of wire coils sutured below the conjunctiva near the muscle insertions of monkeys. However, the development of a wire embedded in a soft contact lens has enabled its use in humans. The subject's eye is centered within a magnetic field, generated by a pair of horizontal and vertical coils, allowing accurate detection of horizontal and vertical eye movements. This system has a resolution of about 50 minutes of arc with a range of approximately ±30 degrees from primary position. A modified version with separate coils in the same lens is capable of detecting cyclotorsional movements. The scleral search coil is an expensive and complicated technique suitable only for highly specialized laboratories (Halmagyi 1994).

REFERENCES

Averbuch-Heller L, Meiner Z. Reversible periodic alternating gaze deviation in hepatic encephalopathy. Neurology 1995;45: 191–192.

Baloh RW, DeRossett SE, Cloughesy TF et al. Novel brain stem syndrome associated with prostate carcinoma. Neurology 1993;43:2591–2596.

Barkovich AJ, Kjos BO, Jackson DE, Norman D. Maturation of the neonatal and infant brain: MRI imaging at 1.5T1. Radiology 1988;166:173–180.

Barton JJS, Sharpe JA, Raymond JE. Retinotopic and directional defects in motion discrimination in humans with cerebral lesions. Ann Neurol 1995;37:665–675.

Brandt T, Dieterich M. Skew deviation with ocular torsion: a vestibular brain stem sign of topographic diagnostic value. Ann Neurol 1993;33:528–534.

Büttner V, Straube A. The effects of cerebellar midline lesions on eye movements. Neuro-ophthalmol 1995;15(2):75–82.

Cannon SC, Zee DS. The Neural Integrator of the Oculomotor System. In S Lessell, JTW van Dalen (eds), Current Neuro-Ophthalmology. Chicago: Year Book; 1988;124.

Daroff RB, Troost BT, Leigh RJ. Supranuclear Disorder of Eye Movements. In TD Duane, EA Jaeger (eds), Clinical Ophthalmology. Vol. 2. New York: Harper & Row, 1990;299–323.

Dell'Osso LF, Daroff RB, Troost BT. Nystagmus and Saccadic Intrusions and Oscillations. In TD Duane, EA Jaeger (eds), Clinical Ophthalmology. Vol. 2. New York: Harper & Row, 1990; 325–356.

Dobyns WB, Ozelius LJ, Kramer PL et al. Rapid-onset dystonia-parkinsonism. Neurology 1993;43:2596–2602.

Echenne B, Rivier F. Benign paroxysmal tonic upward gaze. Pediatr Neurol 1992;8:154–155.

Eustace P, Beigi B, Bowell R, O'Keefe M. Congenital ocular motor apraxia: An inability to unlock the vestibulo-ocular reflex. Neuro-ophthalmol 1994;14:167–174.

Frohman EM, Zee DS. Ocular neuromyotonia: clinical features, physiological mechanisms, and response to therapy. Ann Neurol 1995;37:620–626.

Gaymard B, Rivaud S, Pierrot-Deseilligney C. Role of left and right supplementary motor areas in memory-guided saccades. Ann Neurol 1993;34:404–406.

Green JP, Newman NJ, Winterkorn JS. Paralysis of downgaze in two patients with clincal-radiologic correlation. Arch Ophthalmol 1993;111:219–222.

Halmagyi GM. Central Eye Movement Disorders. In DM Albert, FA Jakobiec (eds), Principles and Practice of Ophthalmology. Philadelphia: Saunders, 1994;2411–2444.

Halmagyi GM, Aw ST, Dehaene I et al. Jerk-waveform see-saw nystagmus due to unilateral meso-dienceophalic lesion. Brain 1994;117:789–803.

Hamed LM, Maria BL, Quisling RG et al. Alternating skew on lateral gaze: neuroanatomic pathway and relationship to superior oblique overaction. Ophthalmology 1993;100:281–286.

Ishikawa H, Ishikawa S, Mukuno K. Short cycle periodic alternating (ping pong) gaze. Neurology 1993;43:1067–1070.

Johnston JL, Sharpe JA, Morrow MJ. Paresis of contralateral smooth pursuit and normal vestibular smooth eye movements after unilateral brain stem lesions. Ann Neurol 1992;31:495–502.

Johnston JL, Sharpe JA. Ranalli PJ et al. Oblique misdirection and slowing of vertical saccades after unilateral lesions at the pontine tegment. Neurology 1993;43:2238–2244.

Keane JR. The pretectal syndrome: 206 patients. Neurology 1990;40:684–690.

Kleiman MD, DiMario FJ, Leconche DA, Zalneraitis EL. Benign transient downward gaze deviation in pre-term infants. Pediatr Neurol 1994;10:313–316.

Lavin PJM. Conjugate and Disconjugate Eye Movements. In TJ Walsh (ed), Neuro-Ophthalmology: Clinical Signs and Symptoms. Philadelphia: Lea & Febiger, 1985.

Leigh RJ, Foley JM, Remler BF, Civil RH. Oculogyric crisis: a syndrome of thought disorder and ocular deviation. Ann Neurol 1987;22:13–17.

Leigh RJ, Zee DS. Synthesis of the Versional Eye Movement Command. In RJ Leigh, DS Zee (eds), The Neurology of Eye Movements. Philadelphia: FA Davis, 1991;79–138.

Loewenfeld IE. The Pupil. Ames: Iowa State University Press, 1993.

Morrow MJ, Sharpe JA. Retinotopic and directional deficits of smooth pursuit initiation after posterior cerebral hemisphere lesions. Neurology 1993;43:595–603.

Pierrot-Deseilligny C. Cortical control of saccades. Neuro-ophthalmol 1991;11:63–75.

Pierrot-Deseilligny C, Revaud S, Gaymard B et al. Cortical control of saccades. Ann Neurol 1995;37:557–567.

Simon LT, Horoupian DS, Dorfman LJ et al. Polyneuropathy, ophthalmoplegia leukoencephalopathy, and intestinal pseudo-obstruction: POLIP syndrome. Ann Neurol 1990;28:349–360.

Stell R, Bronstein AF. Eye Movement Abnormalities in Extrapyramidal Disease. In CD Marsden, S Fahn (eds), Movement Disorders III. Oxford, England: Butterworth-Heinemann, 1994:88–113.

Straube A, Deubel H, Spuler A, Büttner V. Differential effect of a bilateral deep cerebellar nuclei lesion on externally and internally triggered saccades in humans. Neuro-ophthalmol 1995;15(2):67–74.

Thomke F, Hopf HC, Breen LA. Slowed abduction saccades in bilateral internuclear ophthalmoplegia. Neuro-ophthalmol 1992a; 12:241–246.

Thomke F, Hopf HC, Kramer G. Internuclear ophthalmoplegia of abduction: Clinical and electrophysiological data on the existence of an abduction paresis of prenuclear origin. J Neurol Neurosurg Psychiatry 1992b;55:105–111.

Tijssen CC, vanGisbergen JAM, Schulte BPM. Conjugate eye deviation: side, site and size of the hemispheric lesion. Neurology 1991a;41:846–850.

Tijssen CC, Schulte BPM, Leyten ACM. Prognostic significance of conjugate deviation in stroke patients. Stroke 1991b;22: 200–202.

Tijssen CC, Tijssen MAJ. Conjugate eye deviation: localization of hemispheric lesions. Neuro-ophthalmol 1991;2:118.

Urban PP, Marczynski U, Hopf HZ. The oculo-auricular phenomenon. Brain 1993;116:727–738.

Vahedi K, Revaud S, Amarenco P, Pierrot-Deseilligny C. Horizontal eye movement disorders after posterior vermis infarctions. J Neurol Neurosurg Psychiatry 1995;58:91–94.

Waltz KL, Lavin PJM. Accomodative Insufficiency. In CE Margo, RN Mames, L Hamed (eds), Diagnostic Problems in Clinical Ophthalmology. Philadelphia: Saunders, 1993:862–866.

Weissman BM, DiScenna AO, Leigh RJ. Maturation of the vestibulo-ocular reflex in normal infants during the first 2 months of life. Neurology 1989;39:534–538.

Wolin MJ, Trent R, Lavin PJM et al. Oculopalatal myoclonus following the one-and-a-half syndrome associated with facial nerve palsy. Ophthalmology 1996 (in press).

SUGGESTED READING

Burde RM, Savino PJ, Trobe JD (eds). Clinical Decisions in Neuro-Ophthalmology (2nd ed). St. Louis: Mosby-Year Book, 1992.

Büttner U, Brandt TR (guest eds). Ocular Motor Disorders of the Brain. In Balliere's Clinical Neurology: International Practice and Research. Vol. 1 [2]. London: Balliere Tindall, 1992.

Carpenter RHS. Movements of the Eyes (2nd ed). Norwich, Great Britain: Pion Ltd., 1988.

Fenichel GM. Clinical Pediatric Neurology: A Symptoms and Signs Approach (2nd ed). Philadelphia: Saunders, 1993.

Glaser JS. Neuro-Ophthalmology. In TD Duane, EA Jager (eds), Clinical Ophthalmology (2nd ed). Vol. 2. New York: Harper & Row, 1990.

Hoyt CS, Mousel DK, Weber AA. Transient supranuclear disturbances of gaze in healthy neonates. Am J Ophthalmol 1980;89:708–713.

Miller NR. Walshe and Hoyt's Clinical Neuro-Ophthalmology (4th ed). Vol. 2. Baltimore: Williams & Wilkins, 1985.

Sharpe JA, Barber HO (eds). The Vestibulo-Ocular Reflex and Vertigo. New York: Raven, 1993.

Chapter 43
The Afferent Visual System

Robert L. Tomsak

OVERVIEW OF THE AFFERENT VISUAL SYSTEM

From a conceptual standpoint, it is useful to consider vision as having two components: *central vision* (macular vision, high acuity, color perception) and *peripheral vision* (ambulatory vision, low acuity, poor color perception). Light is bent by the cornea and lens and focused on the retina, which is the light-sensitive structure in the eye, analogous to photographic film. For best possible vision, the object must be focused on the most sensitive part of the macular retina, called the *foveola*. Central vision and color vision are mediated mainly by the cone photoreceptors, which are of highest density in the foveal region. The cone system functions optimally in conditions of light adaptation. Visual acuity, as well as cone density, falls off rapidly as the distance from the fovea increases. For example, the retina that is 20 degrees eccentric to the fovea is only capable of resolving objects equal to Snellen 20/200 (6/60 metric) optotypes or larger. Rod photoreceptors are present in highest numbers about 20 degrees from the fovea and are more abundant than cones in the more peripheral retina; rods function best in dim illumination. The total extent of the normal peripheral visual field in each eye is about 60 degrees superior, 60 degrees nasal, 70–75 degrees inferior, and 100 degrees temporal (Anderson 1987) (see Chapter 14, Figure 14.1). Information transduced by the retina is sent from each eye to both hemispheres of the brain by the optic nerves, which each contain about 1.2 million axons. Axons that arise from the ganglion cells of the nasal retinas of each eye cross in the optic chiasm to the contralateral optic tract. Axons from the temporal retinas do not decussate at the chiasm. The percentages of crossed and uncrossed axons in the human optic chiasm are about 53% and 47%, respectively. Because of the optical properties of the eye, the nasal retina receives visual information from the temporal visual field, and the temporal retina receives information from the nasal visual field (Figure 43.1). Similarly, the retina superior to the fovea sees the inferior visual field and vice versa. These points are of extreme clinical importance in the evaluation of visual loss (see Chapter 14).

Visual information is further stratified in the lateral geniculate body (LGB), which is the only waystation between the retinal ganglion cells and the primary visual cortex. The LGB is a portion of the thalamus with six layers. Axons from ipsilateral retinal ganglion cells synapse in layers 2, 3, and 5; contralateral axons synapse in layers 1, 4, and 6. Layers 1 and 2 of the LGB are called magnocellular layers; they receive input from M retinal ganglion cells. The magnocellular pathway is concerned mainly with movement detection, detection of low contrast, and dynamic form perception. After projecting to the primary visual cortex (visual area 1;V1; area 17 of Brodmann), information from the M pathway is distributed to V2 (part of area 18) and V5 (junction of areas 19 and 37). Layers 3–6 of the LGB are called *parvocellular* and receive input from retinal P cells, which are color-selective, respond to high contrast, and form in association with color. These cells project to areas V2 and V4 (fusiform gyrus) (Zeki 1993). Superior fibers that leave the LGB go straight back to the primary visual cortex; inferior fibers loop anteriorly around the superior temporal horn of the lateral ventricles (*Meyer's loop*). Since these fibers are about 5 cm from the tip of the temporal lobe, they are sometimes damaged during temporal lobectomy.

The primary visual cortex (*striate cortex*; area V1;17) is in the occipital lobe of the brain. Macular vision is represented most posteriorly at the occipital tips. Each fovea appears to project to both occipital lobes. The peripheral visual field projects to the visual cortex that lies more anteriorly. The nonoverlapping part of the most peripheral temporal field (monocular temporal crescent) represents unpaired crossed axons from the nasal retina, which pro-

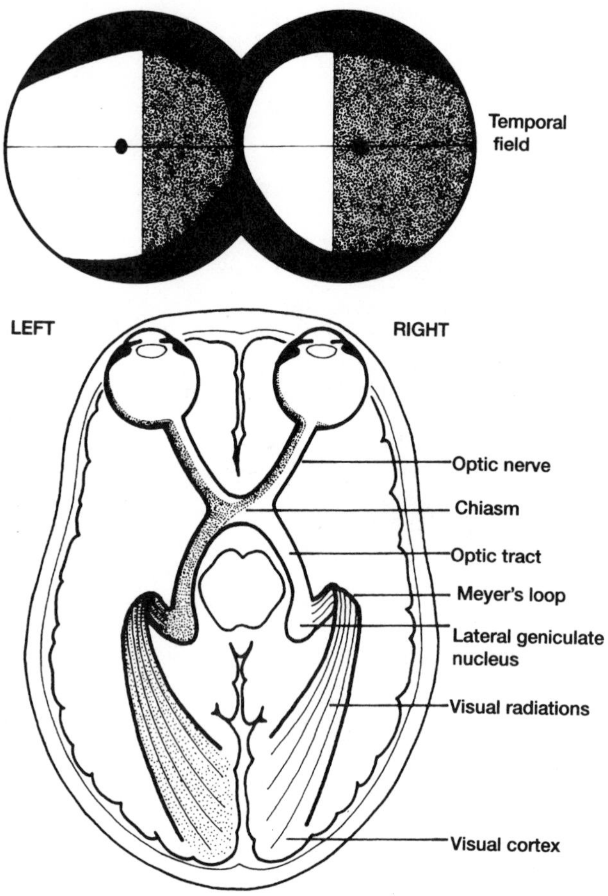

FIGURE 43.1 Visual pathways.

ject to the most anteromedial part of the visual cortex. The primary visual cortex has interconnections with numerous visual association areas (Zeki 1993).

NEURO-OPHTHALMOLOGICAL EXAMINATION OF THE AFFERENT VISUAL SYSTEM

Neuro-ophthalmology has become a distinct subspeciality, because the neuro-ophthalmological examination makes use of ophthalmic tools and techniques but aims at neurological diagnosis. It therefore provides a bridge between neurology and ophthalmology. Many neurologists are unfamiliar with detailed ophthalmologic methods, and ophthalmologists often are not facile with neurological localization.

Examination of Visual Acuity

Visual acuity describes the spatial limit of visual discrimination. It would seem to be self-evident that visual acuity should always be measured with each eye individually and with the best possible optical correction (i.e., using the patient's glasses); other optical means like the pinhole device or a careful refraction may be needed (Glaser 1990). The resultant response, referred to as *best corrected* visual acuity, is the only universally interpretable measurement of central visual function. Ideally, vision should be measured both at a standard distance (usually 20 ft; 6 m) and also at near (usually 1/3 m). The notation 20/20 (6/6 metric) means that the patient (numerator) is able to see the same optotypes at 20 ft as would a normal subject (denominator). A vision of 20/60 (6/18 metric) means that the patient sees a standard optotype at 20 ft that a normal person sees at 60 ft.

A disparity between the best corrected distance and near visual acuity often is indicative of a specific problem. For example, the most common cause of distance acuity being better than near acuity is uncorrected presbyopia. Other conditions in which distance vision is often better than near vision include supranuclear disorders of downgaze, like Parkinson's disease and progressive supranuclear palsy. Common causes of near acuity being better than distance acuity are myopia or congenital nystagmus. In the latter disorder, convergence required for near vision dampens the nystagmus amplitude, resulting in more consistent foveation and better binocular near acuity than distance acuity.

When measuring near vision, the reading card should be held at the specified distance of 14 in, or 1/3 m, to control for image size variation on the retina. If a nonstandard distance is used, it should be clearly specified in the medical record.

Two types of near cards are readily available; one has numbers and other figures, the other type has written text (Figure 43.2). Both are useful, but in neurological or neuro-ophthalmologic practice a near card with text measures not only *visual acuity* but also reading ability. A disparity between these measurements may reveal a disturbance of higher cognitive functions, specifically language and visual perception.

Contrast Sensitivity Testing

Contrast sensitivity testing measures the perception of lines of different width (spatial frequency) and varying degrees of contrast. This visual function is different from visual acuity and has been found to be abnormal in numerous diseases of the eye and retrobulbar visual pathways. Measurement of contrast sensitivity in the office setting requires a special series of test plates (e.g., Arden gratings); more complex testing is possible with computer-generated sine wave gratings.

Light-Stress Test

Some disorders that affect the macula are very difficult to observe with the direct ophthalmoscope. Fortunately, the light-stress (or photo-stress) test is an excellent method for determining if a reduction in visual acuity is due to an ab-

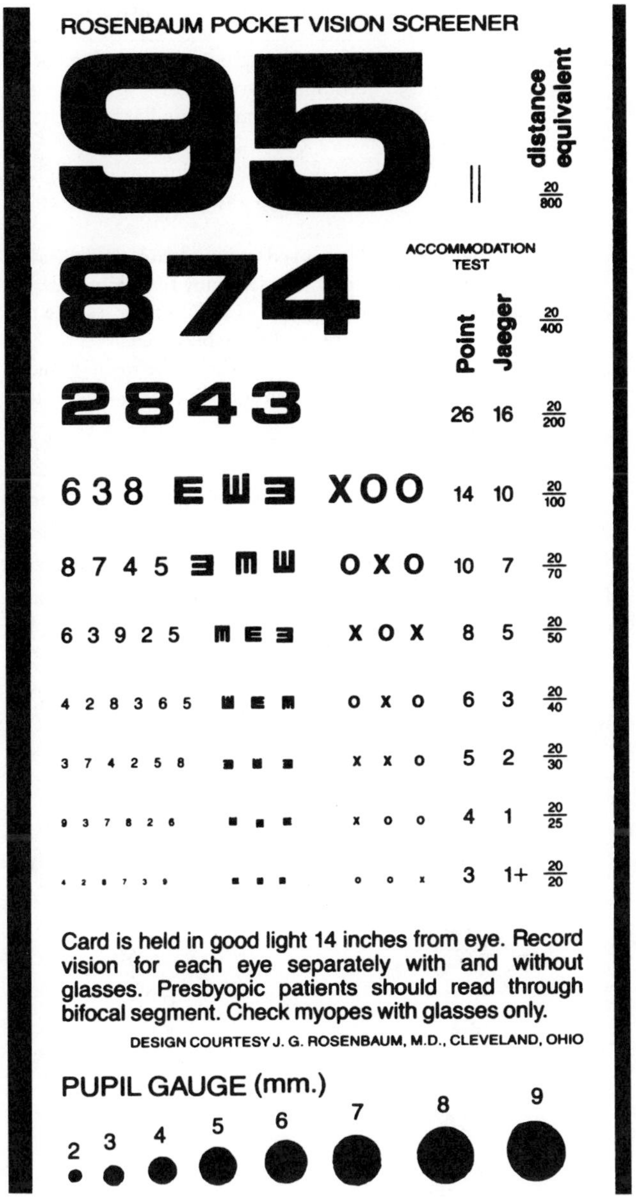

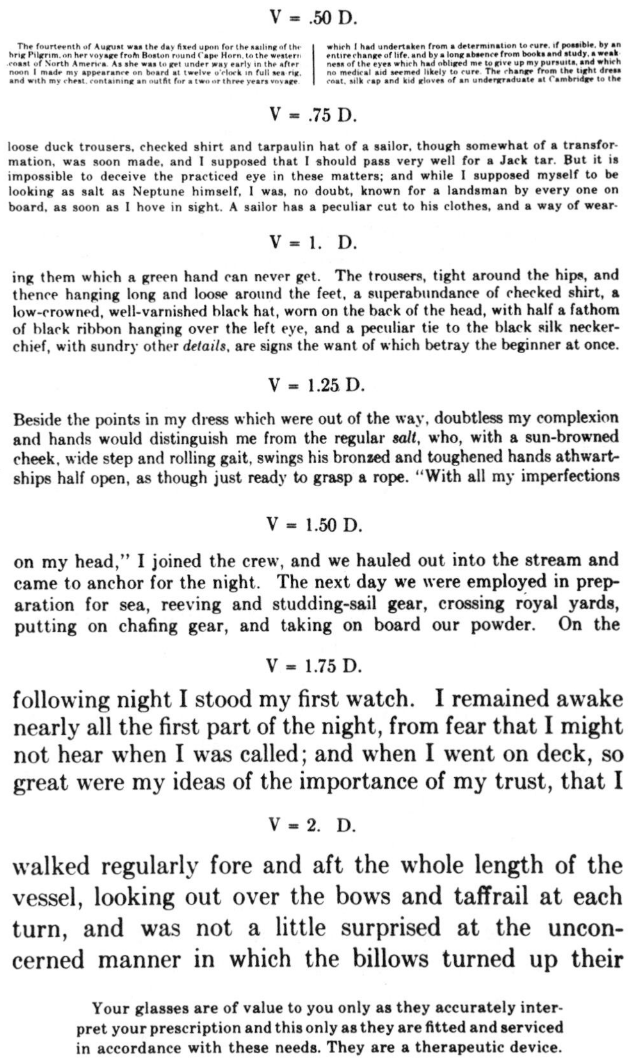

V = .50 D.

The fourteenth of August was the day fixed upon for the sailing of the brig Pilgrim, on her voyage from Boston round Cape Horn, to the western coast of North America. As she was to get under way early in the after noon I made my appearance on board at twelve o'clock in full sea-rig, and with my chest, containing an outfit for a two or three years voyage, which I had undertaken from a determination to cure, if possible, by an entire change of life, and by a long absence from books and study, a weakness of the eyes which had obliged me to give up my pursuits, and which no medical aid seemed likely to cure. The change from the tight dress coat, silk cap and kid gloves of an undergraduate at Cambridge to the

V = .75 D.

loose duck trousers, checked shirt and tarpaulin hat of a sailor, though somewhat of a transformation, was soon made, and I supposed that I should pass very well for a Jack tar. But it is impossible to deceive the practiced eye in these matters; and while I supposed myself to be looking as salt as Neptune himself, I was, no doubt, known for a landsman by every one on board, as soon as I hove in sight. A sailor has a peculiar cut to his clothes, and a way of wear-

V = 1. D.

ing them which a green hand can never get. The trousers, tight around the hips, and thence hanging long and loose around the feet, a superabundance of checked shirt, a low-crowned, well-varnished black hat, worn on the back of the head, with half a fathom of black ribbon hanging over the left eye, and a peculiar tie to the black silk neckerchief, with sundry other *details*, are signs the want of which betray the beginner at once.

V = 1.25 D.

Beside the points in my dress which were out of the way, doubtless my complexion and hands would distinguish me from the regular *salt*, who, with a sun-browned cheek, wide step and rolling gait, swings his bronzed and toughened hands athwartships half open, as though just ready to grasp a rope. "With all my imperfections

V = 1.50 D.

on my head," I joined the crew, and we hauled out into the stream and came to anchor for the night. The next day we were employed in preparation for sea, reeving and studding-sail gear, crossing royal yards, putting on chafing gear, and taking on board our powder. On the

V = 1.75 D.

following night I stood my first watch. I remained awake nearly all the first part of the night, from fear that I might not hear when I was called; and when I went on deck, so great were my ideas of the importance of my trust, that I

V = 2. D.

walked regularly fore and aft the whole length of the vessel, looking out over the bows and taffrail at each turn, and was not a little surprised at the unconcerned manner in which the billows turned up their

Your glasses are of value to you only as they accurately interpret your prescription and this only as they are fitted and serviced in accordance with these needs. They are a therapeutic device.

FIGURE 43.2 Left: Rosenbaum-style near vision card. Right: Near vision card with written text.

normality in central retinal function (Glaser 1990). The test is performed by first measuring the best corrected visual acuity with each eye. Then the eye with faulty vision is occluded and the normal eye is subjected to a bright light for 10 seconds. Immediately thereafter the patient is instructed to read the next, larger, line, and the recovery period is timed. The same procedure is done with the other eye, and the results are compared. Fifty seconds is the upper limit of normal for visual recovery. In diseases that affect the macula, it is not unusual for the recovery period to take several minutes.

Color Vision Testing

Disordered color perception, especially if asymmetric between the eyes, is a good indication of optic nerve dysfunction; symmetric acquired color-vision defects should raise the possibility of a retinal degeneration like cone-rod dystrophy. It must be remembered, however, that congenital color vision anomalies occur in approximately 8% of men and 0.5% of women. Techniques for measuring color vision are from the simple to the sophisticated. Holding a brightly colored object in front of each of the patient's eyes individually and asking for a comparison of both brightness and color intensity is a useful office and bedside technique for the detection of central color defects. Also, testing with colored objects on each side of fixation can often detect a subtle hemianopia.

More formal estimates of color vision can be made with standard pseudoisochromatic color charts (Ishihara or Hardy-Rand-Rittler) or with sorting tests like the Farnsworth-Munsell or Sahlgren's saturation test.

Examination of the Pupils

Examination should include measurement of pupil size, the direct and consensual reaction to light, the accommodative reaction, and the presence or absence of an afferent pupillary defect. If anisocoria is found, ptosis should be looked for, keeping in mind the possibility of Horner's syndrome or third-cranial-nerve paresis. This information should be recorded in an easily understood format; for one example, see Table 43.1.

The measurement of pupil size and light reaction should be made in constant dim illumination with the patient fixating an immobile distance target. At times it is useful to measure pupil size in the dark and also in bright ambient light. For example, anisocoria due to oculosympathetic paresis (*Horner's syndrome*) is often more pronounced in the dark because the affected pupil does not dilate well. Conversely, a pupil with parasympathetic denervation (for example, *Adie's tonic pupil*) is often more evident in bright light because of abnormal constriction (see Chapter 16).

When measuring the light reaction or looking for the afferent pupillary defect, the brightest light available should be used. The reaction to a near object is best brought out by having the subject look at his or her own finger or thumb at a distance of 15–30 cm. Using this method, a near pupillary response can be observed in a completely blind person because of proprioceptive influences.

The observation of a *relative afferent pupillary defect* (RAPD) (*Gunn's pupil; Marcus Gunn pupil*) is an invaluable indication of a conduction defect in the optic nerve. Indeed, many neuro-ophthalmologists regard this as the most important pupillary abnormality. This difference in pupillary reaction is best brought out by alternately illuminating one pupil and then the other—hence the name "swinging flashlight test." The swinging flashlight test can also be thought of as a comparison of the direct and consensual response in the same eye. Normally these pupillary responses are equal; in an eye with an optic nerve conduction defect the direct response will be less than the consensual response.

The test for RAPD should be performed as described in Table 43.2 and shown in Figure 43.3 (Bell et al. 1993). There is one caveat: The swinging light test brings out an asymmetry of optic nerve conduction. Thus, if both nerves are injured to the same extent, no obvious relative afferent pupillary defect will be observed. Furthermore, severe macular or retinal disease can produce a Marcus Gunn pupil, but these problems are virtually always apparent on funduscopic examination. By contrast, minimal optic nerve disease commonly yields an obvious relative afferent pupillary defect.

Table 43.1: Simple method of recording pupillary examination

	Size	*Direct Light Reaction*	*Consensual Reaction*	*Near Response*
Right eye	4.0 mm	+4	+2	+4
Left eye	4.0 mm	+2	+4	+4

Note: In this example, the resting pupillary size is equal in the two eyes at 4 mm. The pupillary reactions can be estimated using 1+ to 4+ scale, as shown here, or by actually recording the pupillary size before and after the light or near response. In the example shown, the direct response is better in the right eye than in the left eye, and the reverse is true for the consensual reaction. This difference in pupillary reactivity could have been semiquantified with the use of neutral density filters (Bell et al. 1993). This table illustrates a left relative afferent pupillary defect (RAPD).

Table 43.2: Testing for the relative afferent pupillary defect

1. The patient should fixate at a distance to minimize fluctuation in pupillary size and accommodative miosis.
2. A light bright enough to cause maximum pupillary constriction should be used.
3. Each pupil should be checked individually for its direct light response, which can be graded on a scale of 1–4 (see Table 43.1).
4. The light should be quickly moved to illuminate each eye alternately every 2–3 seconds (the swinging flashlight test).
5. The initial constriction of the pupil as well as the presence or absence of pupillary escape should be observed.
6. Only three to four swings of the light should be made to minimize bleaching of the retina with subsequent slowing of the pupillary reaction.

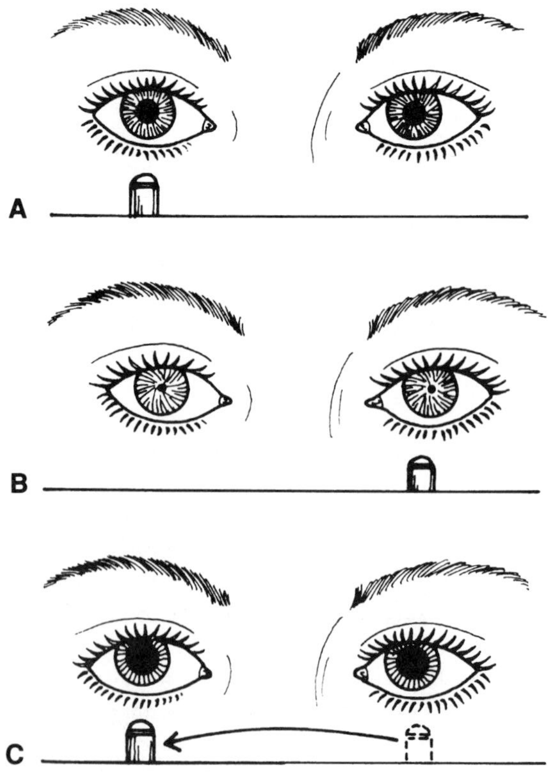

FIGURE 43.3 Right relative afferent pupillary defect (Marcus Gunn pupil) from right optic nerve lesion. A. Right eye illuminated. Poor direct and consensual reaction. B. Excellent direct and consensual response. C. Light swung from left to right with redilation of both pupils.

Light Brightness Comparison

Light brightness comparison can be thought of as a subjective swinging flashlight test. The subjective appreciation of light intensity is often impaired in optic nerve disease but not with macular problems. The test is done by directing a bright light into both eyes in succession, and the patient is asked to estimate the difference in subjective brightness as a percentage. For example, the examiner might ask a question like this: "If this light [normal eye illuminated] was worth one dollar, in terms of light brightness or intensity, what would this one be worth [abnormal eye illuminated]?" The patient is then often able to estimate the difference in perceived brightness.

Visual Field Testing

Evaluation of the visual fields should be considered a vital sign of neuro-ophthalmology. Everyone with unexplained visual loss requires some form of visual field testing, and confrontation testing should be done on all new neurological patients.

Numerous techniques are available for visual field examination, ranging from simple confrontation testing to sophisticated threshold static perimetry (Anderson 1987; Anderson 1992; Harrington and Drake 1990). For the purposes of this discussion, simple, practical techniques adapted from the teachings of J. Lawton Smith will be emphasized and the more complicated methods will be summarized briefly.

The first assessment that should be performed is the history visual field. This involves asking the patient to observe the examiner's face or another part of the environment with each eye and to report if anything is missing or blurred. For example, a patient with optic neuritis and a central scotoma might look at a face and report that the eyes and nose are missing. Another patient with ischemic optic neuropathy and an inferior altitudinal visual field defect might see everything below the nose as absent. Similarly, to a patient with a homonymous hemianopia, half the face would appear to be missing.

Confrontation testing should follow the history visual field. Although many methods have been advocated, a simple, thorough examination can be done by finger counting in quadrants coupled with hand comparison. The steps are as follows:

1. The physician has the patient cover one eye and fixate on the center of the examiner's face.
2. The physician holds up fingers sequentially in each of the four quadrants of the visual field and asks the patient to count how many are seen.
3. If stage 2 is completed normally, the physician asks the patient (whose eyes are open) to count the number of fingers he or she is displaying with both hands, first in both the right and left upper quadrants of the patient's visual field, then in both the right and left lower quadrants. The patient is then asked to add the total number of fingers shown with both hands. This stage of confrontation testing often brings out evidence of extinction or hemineglect or problems with calculation.
4. Finally, both hands are held open in the right and left upper and lower quadrants, and the patient (with both eyes open) is asked to compare the quality of the images. For example, a patient with a subtle bitemporal hemianopia might be able to pass steps 1 through 3, but when shown hands on either side of the vertical midline might state that the hands in both temporal hemifields are not as clear as the ones held in the nasal hemifields.

A major advantage to the finger counting method over kinetic methods of confrontation testing is that *Riddoch's phenomenon* is eliminated. Riddoch's phenomenon is a dissociation between the visual perception of form and movement so that the patient has the ability to perceive only moving targets in a hemianopic visual field (Zeki 1993). This phenomenon occurs in homonymous hemianopias that have resulted from injuries to the occipital cortex. Thus a hemianopia may be missed if the examiner uses only a moving target, such as wiggling fingers in the far periphery.

Confrontation methods using colored objects can also be effective in detecting visual field abnormalities. Confrontation testing is also useful for patients with constricted visual fields. Normally, as the distance from the examiner to the patient increases the visual field expands, or funnels; with psychogenic visual field constriction, the field remains the same size even at longer distances, or it *tunnels* (Figure 43.4).

Measurement of the central 20 degrees of visual field (in each eye separately) can be done using the Amsler grid chart (Figure 43.5). The chart is held in good light at a distance of 30 cm from the eye, with the patient wearing reading glasses, if needed. The following questions are asked:

1. Can you see the spot in the center of the square?
2. While looking at the center, can you see the entire square or are any sides or corners missing?
3. While looking at the center, are any small squares missing or distorted?

If any abnormal responses to these questions are given, the examiner should ask the patient to draw the abnormal areas on the chart. This can then be kept in the patient's medical record.

Patients with a central scotoma often report the center of the grid is missing or blurred; those with hemianopic defects will say half of the grid is missing; others with macular disease may report that some of the lines are wavy or distorted (see also Chapter 14).

Numerous other methods for examining the visual field are available but are beyond the scope of this chapter and the expertise of most neurologists. Fortunately, excellent texts about these other methods are available (Anderson 1987; Anderson 1992; Harrington and Drake 1990). This section provides only an overview.

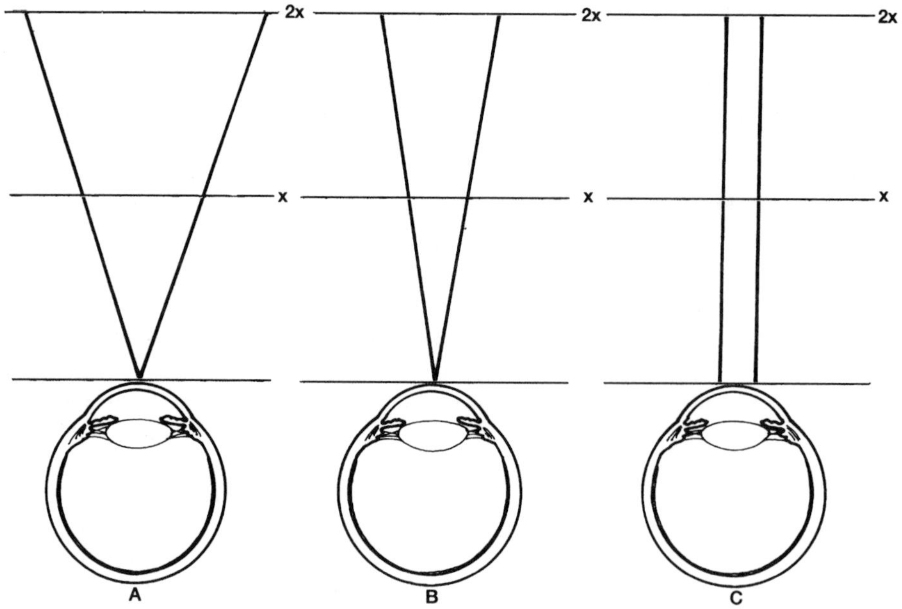

FIGURE 43.4 A. Normal visual field enlarges with increase in testing distance. B. Constricted visual field from organic disease will also proportionally enlarge. C. Constricted visual field of psychogenic etiology usually does not enlarge as testing distance increases. (Data from JD Trobe, JS Glaser. The Visual Fields Manual: A Practical Guide to Testing and Interpretation. Gainesville, FL: Triad, 1983;135.)

A neurological visual field examination is incomplete unless the entire field of vision is examined. This can only be done with some type of perimeter; the tangent screen, which measures only the central 30 degrees of visual field at a distance of one meter, is not adequate in isolation but often is combined with a perimetric examination, as well as the other methods discussed earlier (Anderson 1987).

Perimeters can be divided into those that use a moving stimulus (kinetic) and those in which individual spots in the visual field are tested statically. Most static perimeters available today are automated and driven by computerized examination strategies. Static perimeters may measure the actual visual threshold at defined points in space (threshold static perimetry) or may test these points with light of preset luminance (suprathreshold static perimetry). A commonly used kinetic machine is the Goldmann instrument; popular automated perimeters include the Octopus and Humphrey units (threshold static perimeters). On theoretical grounds, threshold static perimeters are the most sensitive and quantitative; however, the examination is time-consuming and tiring for the subject. Many patients with neurological disorders are unable to sit for an examination that may take as long as 45 minutes per eye and requires intense concentration and alertness. Therefore, many neuro-ophthalmologists rely on kinetic perimeters of the basic Goldmann design because of their versatility; their drawback is that a well-trained perimetrist is required to operate them effectively and reproducibly (Anderson 1987).

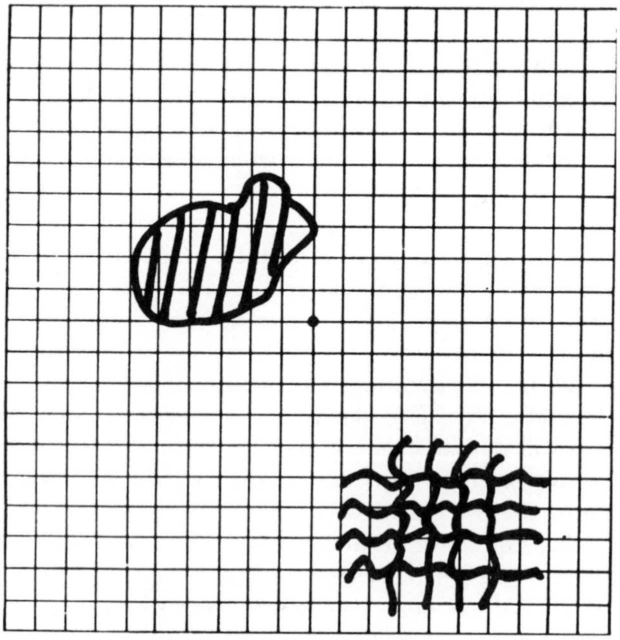

FIGURE 43.5 Amsler grid chart. Upper left: Paracentral scotoma. Lower right: Metamorphopsia (straight lines appear wavy).

VISUAL FIELD ABNORMALITIES

Some of the general rules for visual field interpretation are summarized in Table 43.3. For examples of some characteristic visual field defects, also see Chapter 14 and Figures 14.2 through 14.6.

A few comments about these general rules may be useful.

Rule 1

Optic nerve lesions produce prechiasmal visual field abnormalities that are often characteristic. Ischemic optic neuropathy usually leads to inferior altitudinal defects (Figure 43.6A), optic

Table 43.3: Some general rules of visual field interpretation

1. Lesions of the retina and optic nerve produce field defects in the ipsilateral eye only, unless the lesions are bilateral.
2. True bitemporal hemianopia is caused only by a lesion at the optic chiasm.
3. Retrochiasmal lesions produce homonymous visual field defects.
4. Anterior retrochiasmal lesions produce incongruous homonymous visual field defects.
5. Posterior retrochiasmal lesions produce congruous visual field defects.
6. Temporal lobe lesions give slightly incongruous homonymous hemianopias involving the upper quadrant.
7. There is no localizing value to a complete homonymous hemianopia except that the lesion is retrochiasmal and contralateral to the visual field defect.
8. A unilateral homonymous hemianopia does not reduce visual acuity.

neuritis usually manifests as a cecocentral scotoma (Figure 43.6B), and compressive lesions cause abnormalities in the peripheral field as well as centrally (Figure 43.7).

A lesion involving the posterior optic nerve/anterior chiasm results in a "junctional scotoma" (i.e., ipsilateral cecocentral scotoma and contralateral upper temporal defect; see Figure 14.2) from involvement of ipsilateral as well as crossing fibers from the opposite inferonasal retinal (Willbrand's anterior knee). Binasal hemianopias are the result of local ocular disease at least 75% of the time (Figure 43.8); these diseases include ischemic optic neuropathy, glaucoma, optic nerve drusen, congenital optic nerve pits, optic nerve hypoplasia, and sector retinitis pigmentosa. Less often, hydrocephalus, ectatic parasellar arteries, or basal tumors cause binasal field defects. Binasal visual field defects of organic cause do not respect the vertical visual field meridian, whereas psychogenic binasal defects may.

Rule 2

True bitemporal hemianopias are the hallmark of chiasmal disease, and common causes are discussed in Chapter 14. Less commonly, ischemia, radiotherapy, or demyelination can cause chiasmal syndromes. Bitemporal defects that cross the vertical midline (pseudobitemporal hemianopias) are virtually always due to a congenital anomaly causing rotation or tilting of the optic discs (Figure 43.9) (see Chapter 15).

Rule 3

A homonymous visual field defect is present in the same hemifield or visual quadrant of each eye (see Figure 14.5). The only exception to this rule is the monocular temporal crescent syndrome, in which only unpaired visual fibers residing in the contralateral anterior medial occipital lobe are affected (see Overview). In a series of 140 cases of homonymous hemianopia, Fujino et al. (1986) found that occipital lobe infarcts were the most common etiology.

Rule 4

Incongruous hemianopias are seen in more anterior rectrochiasmal lesions—for example, affecting the optic tract or temporal lobe (Figure 43.10). Optic nerve hemianopias are often associated with a contralateral relative afferent pupillary defect.

Rule 5

Congruous homonymous hemianopias have patterns that are identical in each affected visual field; they are usually seen in visual field defects resulting from occipital lobe infarcts (Figure 43.11).

Rule 8

Even a complete unilateral homonymous hemianopia is not justification for decreased visual acuity because the remaining macular cortex in the opposite hemisphere is still functioning. If input to both macular cortices is abnormal, however, then central acuity often is diminished, but the acuities should be equal in both eyes. If the visual acuities are unequal, another explanation for the visual asymmetry needs to be sought.

Many techniques have been described for examining the patient with a functional visual disorder. The use of visual evoked potentials (VEPs) to diagnose functional visual loss can be frustrating. If the VEP is normal, useful information is gained. It is known, however, that factitious abnormalities in the VEP are easily induced by normal subjects who fix eccentrically on the target or who converge and accommodate and thus blur their vision. Thus an abnormal VEP is *not* always diagnostic of an organic visual disturbance.

NONORGANIC (FUNCTIONAL OR PSYCHOGENIC) VISUAL DISTURBANCES

Functional visual problems are estimated to represent from 1–5% of an average ophthalmologist's practice (Tomsak 1995a). A variety of synonyms exist for these disorders, including *hysterical visual loss*, *psychogenic amblyopia*, and *ocular conversion reaction* (Table 43.4).

A careful social and family history is needed when evaluating patients with psychogenic visual disturbances, especially regarding abuse, peer pressure, and visually impaired friends and family members. Different tests are necessary for different functional visual disturbances. For example, if a person claims total blindness in one or both eyes, important

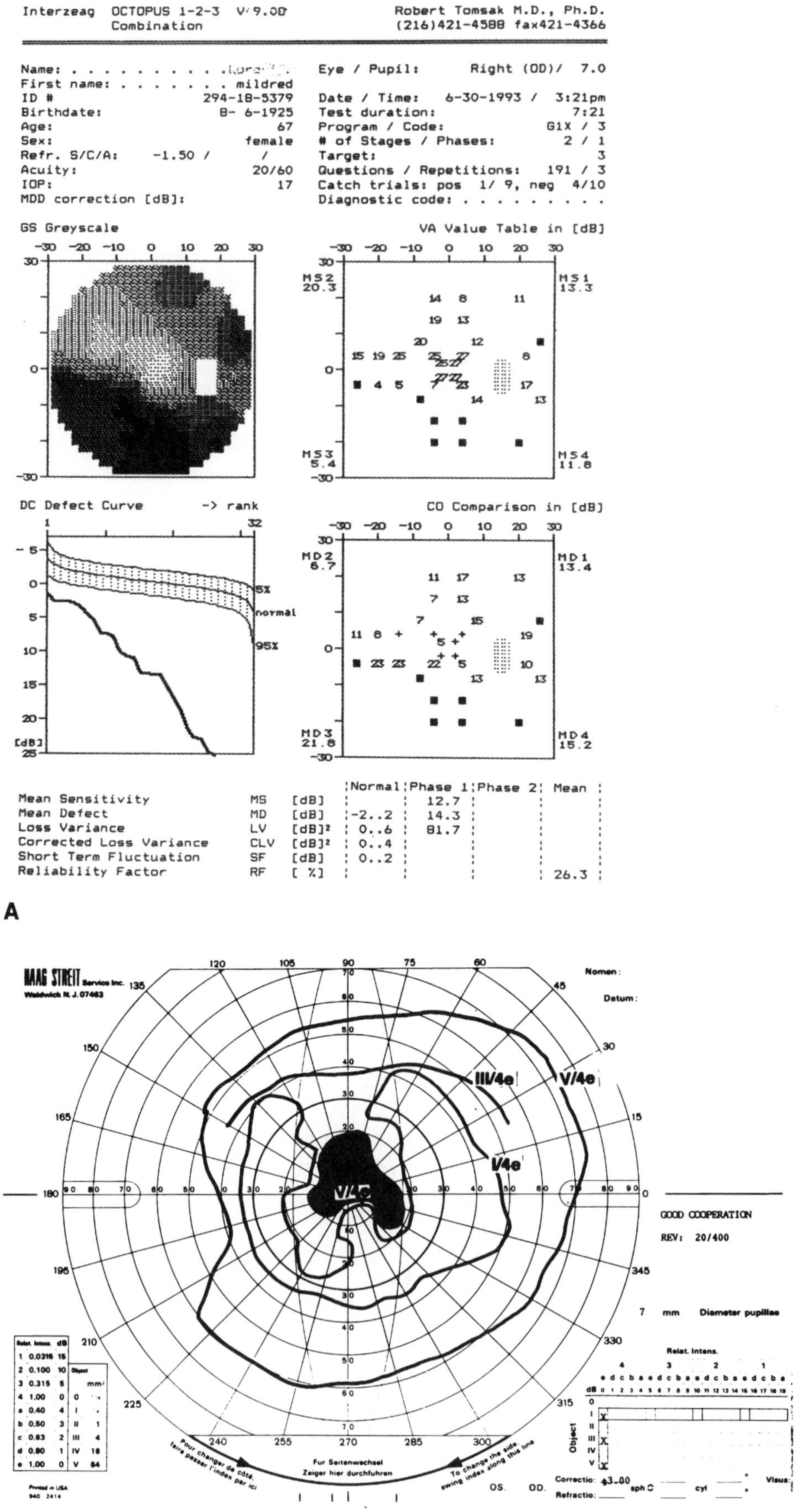

A

B

FIGURE 43.6 A. Threshold static measurement of central 30 degrees of right visual field (Octopus 1-2-3 perimeter; G1X program). Sixty-seven-year-old woman with anterior ischemic optic neuropathy OD and inferior altitudinal visual field defect. Upper left: Gray-scale measurement; darker areas correspond to abnormal areas of visual field (displays measured and interpolated data). Area of blind spot is not investigated and therefore is reproduced as white, not black. Upper right: Mean-sensitivity (MS) display in decibels. The decibel (dB) is a logarithmic relative scale to quantify differential light sensitivity (dB = 10.log L max/L, where L max is the maximal possible stimulus of the perimeter and L is the luminance of the stimulus presented). Lower right: Mean-defect (MD) display (MD = mean of the deviation of measured dB from age-matched normal values). Positive values indicate decreased sensitivity. Lower left: Cumulative defect curve (Bebie curve) arranges test locations with the least difference on the left side. This curve helps differentiate local from diffuse damage. B. Kinetic perimetry of right visual field by Goldmann technique. Thirty-year-old woman with retrobulbar optic neuritis. Examination shows dense cecocentral scotoma with nasal field constriction.

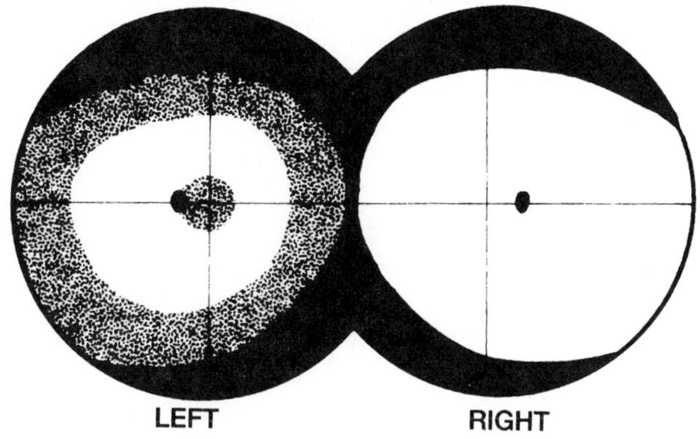

FIGURE 43.7 Contraction of left visual field with cecocentral scotoma due to compressive optic neuropathy. Normal right visual field.

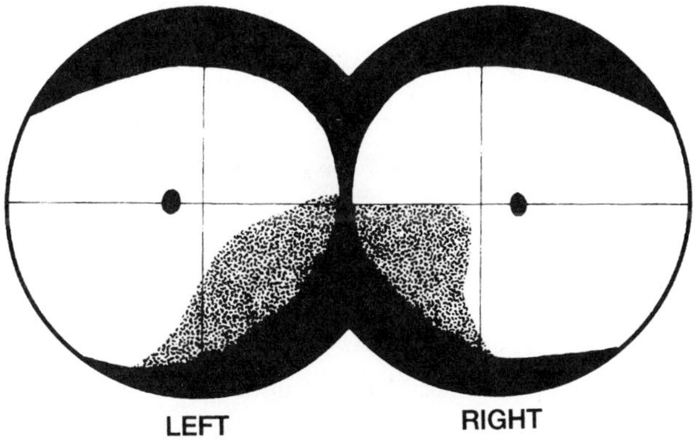

FIGURE 43.8 Binasal hemianopic visual field defects.

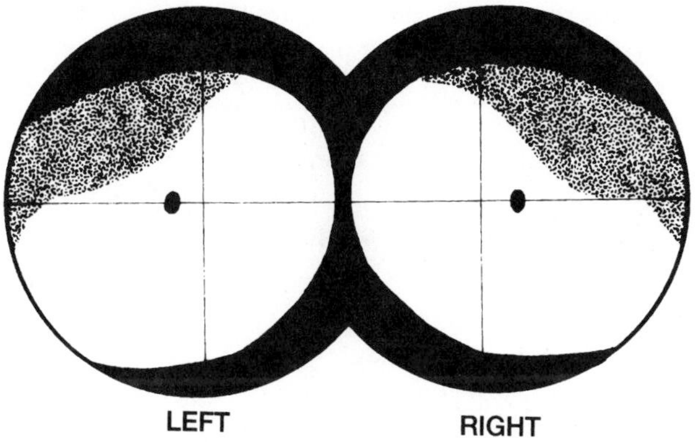

FIGURE 43.9 Pseudobitemporal hemianopia. Note that vertical midline is not respected.

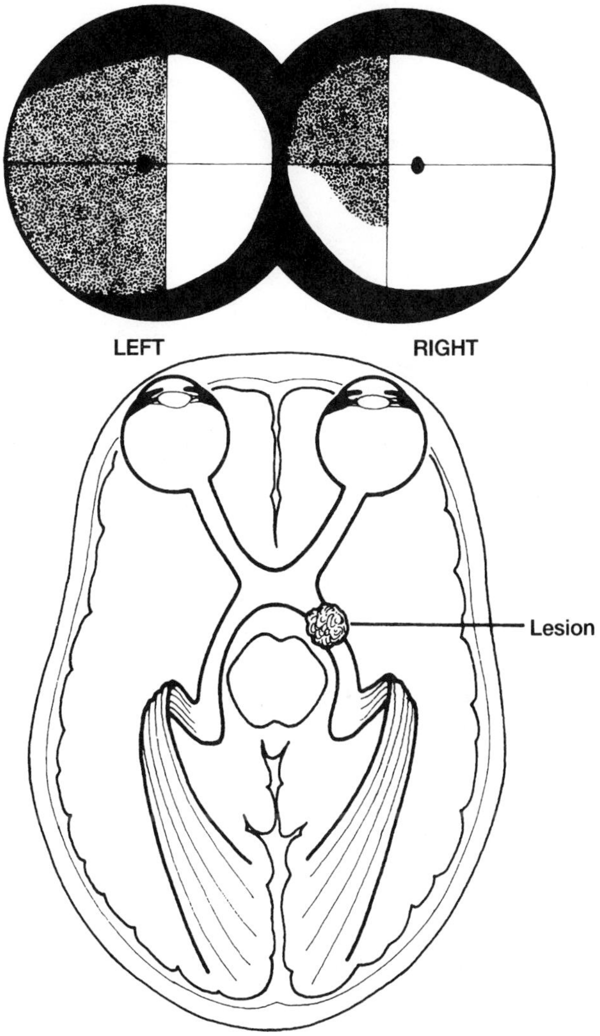

FIGURE 43.10 Incongruous left homonymous hemianopia from right optic tract lesion.

tests might include examination of the pupils, optokinetic nystagmus, and the use of a large mirror held close to the face to induce eye movement via a pursuit reflex. If the patient claims some vision, then it is often useful to test for disparity in distance and near acuity as well as for stereopsis.

Visual fields are extremely important and usually have one of four patterns: (1) tubular contraction, (2) spiral, (3) star-shaped, and (4) isopter inversion (Figure 43.12). When faced with a patient with "tunnel" vision, a confrontation field done at different distances can be useful. Normally the area of visual field increases with increasing distance from the object. In other words, the normal visual field "funnels." Thus, the visual field of a patient with an organic cause for tunnel vision should enlarge as the distance from the examiner or object increases. If the field does not expand at longer distances, then a nonorganic cause for the visual disturbance is present (see Figure 43.4). Isopter inversion means that the visual field plotted with a larger test object is smaller than the visual field plotted with a smaller test object, which is impossible.

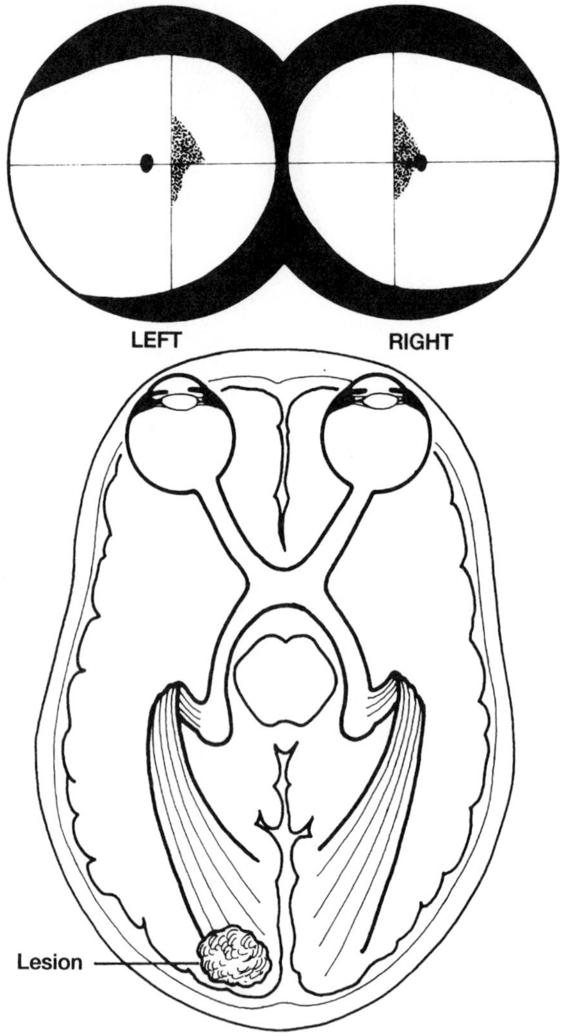

FIGURE 43.11 Congruous paracentral right homonymous hemianopia.

Table 43.4: Some forms of functional visual disturbance

Visual acuity loss (one or both eyes)
Visual field loss (unilateral or bilateral)
Color perception abnormalities
Convergence insufficiency, accommodation insufficiency, or both
Convergence spasm
Loss of depth perception
Diplopia
Night blindness
Photophobia
Pharmacological pupils
Voluntary nystagmus
Diagnostic techniques

Pathogenesis and Natural History

About half the patients with functional visual disorders improve with time and reassurance (Tomsak 1995a). Factors that bode a good prognosis include youth and the presence of anxiety; a poorer prognosis seems to accompany older age combined with depression or other psychiatric illness. The most effective therapy seems to be reassurance (Tomsak 1995a).

PEDIATRIC AFFERENT NEURO-OPHTHALMOLOGY

Examination techniques for children often differ from those for adults, and the reader is referred to other, more comprehensive discussions of the pediatric neuro-ophthalmological examination (Tomsak 1995b). Of course, many of the same diseases that affect vision in adults also affect children, but many are specific to youths or present during early growth and development (Table 43.5).

For the purposes of this chapter, optic nerve hypoplasia, Leber's congenital amaurosis, and albinism will be discussed in more detail.

Optic Nerve Hypoplasia

Optic nerve hypoplasia is a congenital and nonprogressive condition that is thought to reflect a primary defect in differentiation of the retinal ganglion cell axons. The optic disc and scleral canal are of subnormal diameter; a peripapillary ring of pigmentation is often seen, called the double ring sign (see Chapter 15).

Optic nerve hypoplasia may be unilateral or bilateral. Visual acuities may be variable in affected eyes and can be anywhere from 20/20 to light perception. Associated ocular conditions include microphthalmos, aniridia, and albinism. Visual field defects are usually nasal, inferior altitudinal, or both.

Bilateral cases often have strabismus and nystagmus as well as endocrine disturbances and developmental delay. The common endocrine disturbances are hypothyroidism, growth hormone deficiency, diabetes insipidus, and neonatal hypoglycemia. Bilateral optic nerve hypoplasia in association with absence of the septum pellucidum and hypopituitarism is called *DeMorsier's syndrome.* Optic nerve hypoplasia is usually sporadic but may be associated with fetal alcohol syndrome, maternal diabetes or maternal anticonvulsant ingestion during pregnancy.

Table 43.5: Some neurologically related causes of visual loss in children

Albinism
Leber's congenital amaurosis
Gliomas of the optic nerves or chiasm
Craniopharyngiomas
Optic nerve hypoplasia
Other optic nerve dysplasias
Hereditary optic atrophies

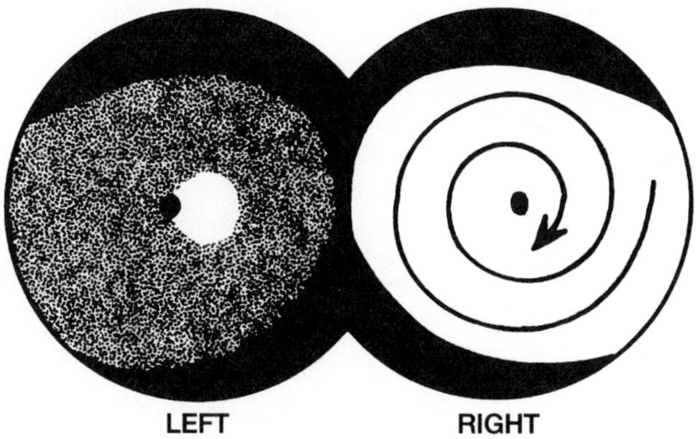

FIGURE 43.12 Two common visual field abnormalities with psychogenic visual loss. Left: Concentric (tubular) contraction. Right: Spiral pattern.

Leber's Congenital Amaurosis

Leber's congenital amaurosis (LCA) is most broadly defined as a syndrome of bilaterally poor vision beginning in early childhood that is associated with a depressed or absent electroretinogram. This disease is not in any way related to Leber's hereditary opic neuropathy (see Chapters 14 and 15). Visual acuity in LCA is usually less than 20/200 (6/60 metric). The retinal pigment epithelium has a salt-and-pepper appearance, and retinal vascular attenuation is sometimes marked. Optic disc swelling may be present. Pathological changes in the retina are variable and may affect all layers or just the ganglion cells. Nystagmus occurs in approximately 75% of cases, and oculomotor apraxia and other eye movement problems have also been described. Approximately 30% of patients with LCA have neurological abnormalities, which include hyperkinetic behavior, coordination difficulties, spastic paraparesis, psychomotor retardation, hydrocephalus, and electroencephalographic abnormalities. The oculodigital phenomenon, or eye gouging, may be seen; this has been interpreted as an attempt by the child to produce phosphenes from mechanical stimulation of the retina. Leber's congenital amaurosis usually occurs sporadically but may be inherited in an autosomal recessive manner in about one-third of cases.

Albinism

Albinism is a genetically determined abnormality in melanin synthesis that is associated with congenital nystagmus, foveal hypoplasia, and impaired visual acuity. The condition may affect the skin and the eyes (*oculocutaneous albinism*) or may affect the eyes only (*ocular albinism*) and therefore may be less obvious to the examiner. The ocular fundus can be totally devoid of pigment or simply have a blond appearance. The degree of visual impairment seems related to the degree of ocular pigmentation; tyrosinase-negative albinos have more marked reductions in visual acuity and more obvious nystagmus. Normal foveal development appears to be influenced by melanin in the retinal pigment epithelium in the macular area.

In albinos, more axons from temporal retinal ganglion cells cross at the optic chiasm than in normal persons; this has been confirmed by VEP studies that demonstrate significant hemispheric asymmetry to monocular stimulation. Also, albinos lack normal stereopsis. The electroretinogram in most albinos shows a supernormal scotopic response, presumably due to increased scatter of light in the eye.

Albinism is also seen in the Hermansky-Pudlak syndrome (albinism with hemorrhagic diathesis) and in the Chediak-Higashi syndrome (a complex neurodegenerative disorder associated with pyogenic episodes) (see Chapter 70).

REFERENCES

Anderson DA. Perimetry With and Without Automation (2nd ed). St. Louis: Mosby, 1987.

Anderson DR. Automated Static Perimetry. St. Louis: Mosby, 1992.

Bell RA, Waggoner PM, Boyd WM et al. Clinical grading of relative afferent pupillary defects. Arch Ophthalmol 1993; 111:938–942.

Fujino T, Kigazawa K, Yamada R. Homonymous hemianopia: a retrospective study of 140 cases. Neuro-ophthalmol 1986;6:17–21.

Glaser JS. Neuro-Ophthalmology (2nd ed). Philadelphia: Lippincott, 1990.

Harrington DO, Drake MV. The Visual Fields: Text and Atlas of Clinical Perimetry (6th ed). St. Louis: Mosby, 1990.

Kramer KK, La Piana FG, Appleton B. Ocular malingering and hysteria: diagnosis and management. Surv Ophthalmol 1979;24:80–96.

Tomsak RL. Functional Visual Disturbances. In RL Tomsak (ed), Pediatric Neuro-Ophthalmology. Boston: Butterworth-Heinemann, 1995a;145–152.

Tomsak RL (ed). Pediatric Neuro-Ophthalmology. Boston: Butterworth-Heinemann, 1995b.

Trobe JD, Glaser JS. The Visual Fields Manual: A Practical Guide to Testing and Interpretation. Gainesville, FL: Triad, 1983;135.

Zeki S. A Vision of the Brain. Boston: Blackwell, 1993.

Chapter 44
Neuro-Otology

B. Todd Troost and Melissa A. Waller

Neuro-otology is a subspecialty that encompasses disorders of the peripheral and central auditory and vestibular systems. Neuro-otology is similar to neuro-ophthalmology in that it is defined by those who practice it. Most neuro-otologists have come from the field of otolaryngology. The emphasis has been on the body part that is presumably abnormal—for example, the ear. This resembles the early history of neuro-ophthalmology, when the emphasis was primarily on the eye; it was only later that central visual ocular motor connections and symptomatology were considered and the field began to involve neurologists. Similarly, neuro-otology concentrated on the primary functions of the ear—vestibular and auditory—without much reference to information processing within the central nervous system (CNS) or to neurological conditions that could produce dizziness, vertigo, or alterations in hearing. When the multiple descriptions of dizziness are included, as outlined in Chapter 18, it becomes apparent that there are many neurological and systemic conditions that can produce disequilibration. Thus, neurologists have become increasingly involved in the evaluation of patients complaining of dizziness. Just as retinal disorders remain primarily the province of the ophthalmologist, so hearing disorders, which are primarily peripheral, remain largely the province of the otolaryngologist.

Because auditory complaints frequently accompany vestibular symptoms, it is incumbent upon neurologists who choose to treat dizzy patients to become familiar with some aspects of auditory and vestibular testing.

INVESTIGATIONS

Vestibular Testing

The primary vestibular tests are the *electronystagmogram* (ENG), *rotational tests*, and *posturography*.

Standard ENG is well described elsewhere (Baloh and Honrubia 1990). Eye movements are recorded by means of the corneal-retinal potential by surface electrodes and are printed on strip chart recording paper or analyzed by computer. Standard testing usually includes calibration, gaze testing, *bithermal or simultaneous caloric testing*, *positional testing*, and *pursuit and optokinetic nystagmus*. In most laboratories, eye movements are recorded using only bitemporal electrodes, which monitor the movements of both eyes. In more sophisticated laboratories the movements of each eye are recorded separately. Individual recordings are advantageous to determine asymmetries between the eyes such as occur in internuclear ophthalmoplegia. During calibration, the patient is asked to look between two targets, ±10 degrees from the center of fixation. Frequent overshoot may reveal the presence of ocular dysmetria, a sign of cerebellar system disorder.

Most laboratories perform bithermal caloric testing (Figure 44.1A), in which each ear is irrigated separately with warm and cool stimulation, either produced by water or by air jets in an open or closed system. The resulting nystagmus is analyzed either manually or by computer to determine the slow phase of the induced nystagmus. Peak slow-phase velocity (SPV) resulting from the warm and cool stimulation of one ear is compared with that from the other ear. The most important finding during ENG is a significant reduction in the responses on one side when compared with the other. A difference of greater than 20–25% in one ear when compared with the other is a clear indication of hypofunction in one peripheral vestibular apparatus (provided there are no technical artifacts), and the ear with the weaker response is said to have a *reduced vestibular response* or *unilateral weakness*. The quality of such testing varies widely among laboratories. If possible, the neurologist should always review the primary tracings, or at least have available the calculated SPVs from each ear. The absolute value of SPVs is not as important as the comparison between responses of each ear.

Another value sometimes given is *directional preponderance*. One sums the values of rightward-beating nystagmus

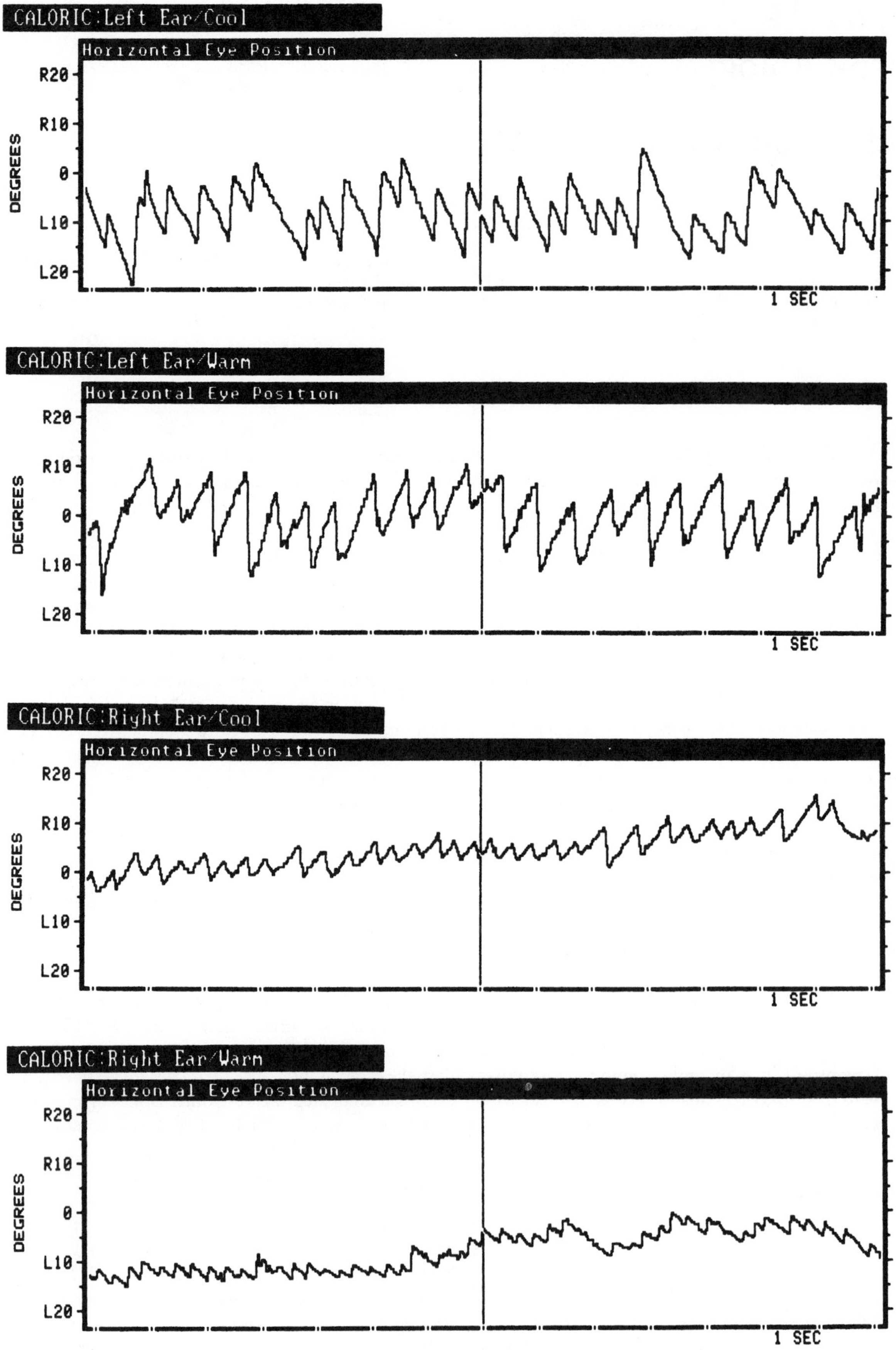
CALORIC:Left Ear/Cool
Horizontal Eye Position
R20
R10
0
L10
L20
DEGREES
1 SEC
CALORIC:Left Ear/Warm
Horizontal Eye Position
R20
R10
0
L10
L20
DEGREES
1 SEC
CALORIC:Right Ear/Cool
Horizontal Eye Position
R20
R10
0
L10
L20
DEGREES
1 SEC
CALORIC:Right Ear/Warm
Horizontal Eye Position
R20
R10
0
L10
L20
DEGREES
1 SEC

A

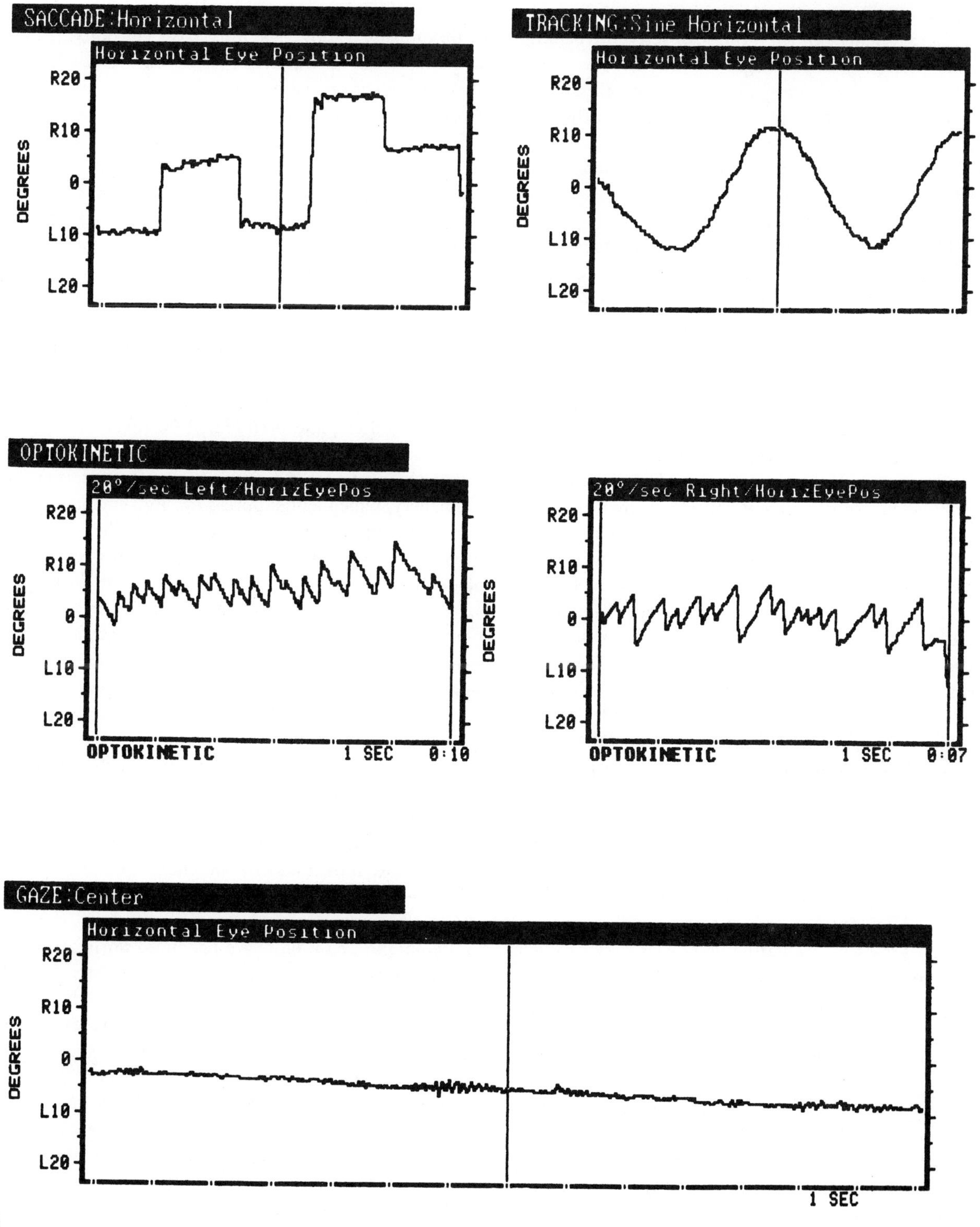

B

FIGURE 44.1 Computer printout of electronystagmogram (ENG). A (page 648). Bithermal caloric irrigation. *First panel:* Responses obtained stimulating the left ear with cool air (24°C). Right-beating nystagmus is provoked with a peak slow-phase velocity of 47° per second. *Second panel:* Left-beating nystagmus provoked by stimulating the left ear with warm air (50°C). Peak slow-phase velocity is measured at 45° per second. *Third panel:* Left-beating nystagmus induced by stimulating the right ear with cool air (15° per second). *Fourth panel:* Right-beating nystagmus produced by stimulating the right ear with warm air (12° per second). Results of caloric stimulation indicate a unilateral weakness of 54% on the right side, suggesting a lesion involving the labyrinth or vestibular nerve on the right side. B. Ocular motor assessment. *First panel left:* Saccadic eye movements showing no significant overshoot or dysmetria—normal. *First panel, right:* Horizontal ocular tracking—normal without interspersed saccades. *Second panel:* Optokinetic responses demonstrating symmetry. *Third panel:* Central gaze showing no significant spontaneous nystagmus.

(cold water in the left ear and warm water in the right ear) and compares them with the values for leftward-beating nystagmus (cold water in the right ear and warm water in the left ear). *Primary-position nystagmus*—so-called spontaneous nystagmus—can add to or subtract from the nystagmus produced by caloric stimulation, altering the results. The significance of directional preponderance when not associated with spontaneous nystagmus remains unclear and for that reason is frequently not calculated.

The ability to suppress a *caloric-induced nystagmus* by visual fixation is evaluated during caloric testing. Most normal subjects can suppress the nystagmus to at least one-half of its original amplitude during visual fixation. The inability to suppress caloric-induced nystagmus is interpreted by most electronystagmographers as indicating a central lesion, particularly cerebellar dysfunction. Many normal persons, however, particularly those who experience intense vestibular symptoms during testing, cannot suppress the induced nystagmus to less than 50% of the baseline value.

The *ocular motor assessment* consists of the following tests: saccadic eye movements, gaze testing, tracking (visual pursuit), and optokinetic tests. With the current availability of commercial apparatus for recording and analyzing fast eye movements, the ability to perform ocular motor evaluation is available. Most saccade tests measure the speed and accuracy of saccadic eye movements at various amplitudes. The results are printed out as a velocity-amplitude relationship, and comparison is made with age-matched controls. Ideally, each eye should be measured individually and recorded in each horizontal direction. Vertical eye movements are usually not considered, because the standard recording apparatus does not eliminate eyelid artifact and frequently does not give accurate vertical eye movement information.

The finding of slow saccadic eye movements suggests a CNS abnormality, particularly with symmetrical slowing. Of course, peripheral ocular motor abnormalities such as myasthenia gravis or cranial nerve palsies may produce slow eye movements, but these are usually not symmetrical except in chronic progressive external ophthalmoplegia. Monocular slowing of an adducting eye is a clear indication of internuclear ophthalmoplegia. Testing of optokinetic responses with most commercially available techniques yields nonspecific results. The usual stimulus for eliciting smooth-pursuit eye movements is an oscillating light target. The most frequent interpretation of broken-up or "cogwheel" pursuit is a *central disorder*, and such patients are often referred for neurological evaluation. Because pursuit eye movements may be altered by inattention, drugs, or diffuse disease of the cortex, subcortex, basal ganglia, cerebellum, or brain stem, a bilateral abnormality is very nonspecific. A clear-cut unidirectional pursuit defect is a reliable indicator of CNS dysfunction (Sharpe et al. 1990, Morrow and Sharpe 1993). The results of pursuit tracking are usually reported in terms of a *gain*, the ratio of the eye speed to the target speed at different speeds of target movement. There is little information about the variability of pursuit tracking in normal individuals, and the same is true for optokinetic testing. The most clear-cut optokinetic abnormality is due to a parietal lesion on the side in which the optokinetic response is diminished. Such patients almost always have a visual field defect and other neurological signs that permit a cerebral localization (Pierrot-Deseilligny and Gaymard 1992; Leigh and Zee 1991). In the laboratory, an attempt is made to measure full-field optokinetic nystagmus. At the bedside, testing is performed with an optokinetic tape, which primarily measures central or foveal optokinetic nystagmus, a less compelling response.

During rotational testing in vestibular function laboratories, the patient is rotated in a chair controlled by a computer. The chair rotates slowly at different constant velocities, usually expressed in terms of frequency or cycles per second (hertz). Typical rotation speeds include 0.01 Hz, 0.02 Hz, 0.04 Hz, 0.08 Hz, and 0.16 Hz, all relatively slow speeds. Patients are rotated in the dark with their eyes open while performing mental tasks designed to distract them from mental imagery, which can suppress eye movement. During a chair rotation to the right, the eyes move to the left and then recenters with a fast phase. Thus, the slow component (phase) is in the direction opposite the spin, and the fast component of the resultant nystagmus is in the direction of the rotation. The fast components are eliminated by a computer, and a slow phase is reconstructed and compared with the speed of the chair rotation. In this way, a gain (slow eye movement speed divided by chair rotation speed) at different frequencies is obtained. Measurement is made of symmetry, which compares the responses of rotating in one direction with those rotating in the opposite direction.

Another measurement made during rotational testing is of the time relationship between the slow eye movements and the slow movement of the chair. This difference is called the *phase lag*, and various phase lags are also plotted against the frequency of rotation of the chair. Therefore, both gain and phase plots are produced during rotational testing. Unlike caloric testing, rotational testing (which stimulates both ears simultaneously) generally provides little clear-cut information about the site of the lesion; however, it is beneficial in quantitating bilateral weakness in a reproducible fashion. During measurements of phase lag, however, it appears that even patients who become asymptomatic after peripheral vestibular abnormality can still show a phase lag, particularly at the lower frequencies of rotation. Rotational test abnormalities are quite reproducible, more so than caloric tests. Their interpretation, however, is fraught with difficulty. It is often hard to tell which side is abnormal and whether any resultant abnormality is peripheral or central. Such determinations must be made using other information, such as the results of an ENG or a clinical examination.

Rotational tests are helpful in determining response patterns in bilateral vestibular loss. The symmetrical response of a person with a unilateral peripheral vestibular abnormality indicates vestibular compensation. An abnormal phase lag is a nonspecific marker, as mentioned above, and usually indicates some degree of vestibular peripheral abnormality.

Posturography is an attempt to quantify the Romberg test. Changes in body sway during Romberg testing, with the feet directly together, with eyes open and with eyes closed, are measured by means of a computer. Most earlier attempts to quantify the Romberg test used a static posture platform. The patient would have the test performed in one of two positions, with the eyes open, then with the eyes closed. Body motions were compared in the different positions with the eyes open and closed. Attempts to correlate abnormality observed during posturography with different disease states, such as peripheral vestibulopathy, peripheral neuropathy, cerebellar dysfunction, and neuromuscular disorders were, for the most part, unsuccessful. More recently, a dynamic posture platform has been introduced. The patient is surrounded by a movable visual field, and the posture platform itself may be moved. The theory is that by moving the visual surround, visual cues that help maintain posture may be eliminated. Similarly, by moving the posture platform in response to a movement of the feet, proprioceptive cues, which assist in the maintenance of posture, may also be eliminated. Both visual cues and proprioceptive cues may be eliminated simultaneously. Theoretically, then, attempts to maintain posture would be solely dependent on vestibular afferent information. The test results in all conditions are reported, and an interpretation is made based on which systems are defective. Posturography is a promising technology that currently is in use and is still being improved.

Audiological assessment is the basis for quantifying auditory impairment. Most neurologists rely on clinical testing of hearing and may use some tests with tuning forks, as described in Chapter 19.

In defining auditory abnormality, clinical tests are no substitute for a complete audiological battery. Audiological testing is most reliable when defining peripheral or cochlear auditory disturbances and often may provide useful information, based on subtests, to diagnose retrocochlear disease. Basic assessment and subtests may be helpful in identifying cerebellopontine angle tumor, most commonly a vestibular schwannoma. Central auditory testing for the rare central disorders of audition is more difficult and poorly understood. Detailed descriptions of audiological tests, both peripheral and central, is provided in standard texts (Martin 1986; Benjamin and Troost 1988).

The basic audiological evaluation establishes the degree and configuration of hearing loss, assesses ability to discriminate a speech signal, and provides some insight into the type of loss and possible cause. The test battery consists of *pure-tone air* and *bone conduction thresholds*, *speech thresholds*, *speech discrimination testing*, and *immittance measures*.

Pure-tone air-conduction thresholds provide a measure of hearing sensitivity as a function of frequency and intensity (Figure 44.2). When a hearing loss is present, the pure-tone air conduction test indicates reduced hearing sensitivity.

It is appropriate at this point to define some basic audiometric terms. Pure tones are defined by their frequency or pitch and intensity or loudness. Normal hearing levels for

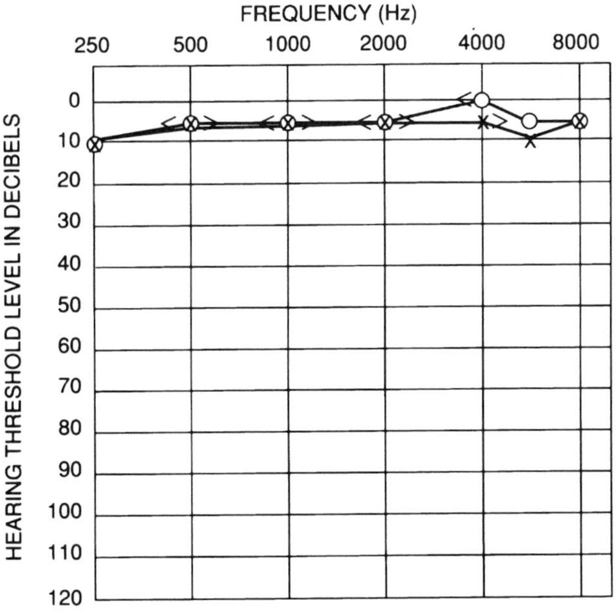

Audiogram Key	Right	Left
A/C Unmasked	O	X
A/C Masked	Δ	□
B/C Unmasked	<	>
B/C Masked	[	]
B/C Forehead Masked	˥	┌

SPEECH TESTS

TESTS		R	L
Sp. Reception Threshold (SRT)		5 db	0 db
Sp. Discrim. Scores	35 db SL	100%	96%

FIGURE 44.2 Normal audiometrical results showing normal hearing sensitivity with excellent speech discrimination bilaterally.

pure tones are defined by international standards. Brief-duration pure tones at selected frequencies are presented either through earphones (air conduction) or a vibrator on the mastoid bone (bone conduction). The audiogram indicates the lowest intensity an individual can hear at a given frequency and displays the degree (in decibels) and configuration (sensitivity loss as a function of frequency) of a hearing loss. Thresholds can be defined as the lowest intensity signal that a person can detect approximately 50% of the time during a given number of presentations. The speech reception threshold (SRT) is the lowest intensity level at which the listener can identify or understand speech 50% of the time. The SRT may also be called the *spondee threshold* because spondees are the test material. Spondee words are two-syllable words that are given equal syllable stress, such as baseball, toothbrush, sidewalk, oatmeal, popcorn, or railroad. Once speech threshold is determined in this manner, the audiologist determines speech discrimination ability by presenting a list of 50 phonetically balanced words at volume levels approximately 35–40 dB above speech reception threshold. The list is a standardized one, containing monosyllabic words of equal phonetic composition. Discrimination is scored as the percentage correct, with each correct word counting for 2% of the total. Word discrimination ability may also be assessed at high intensity levels to establish a performance intensity for phonemically balanced words (PI-PB) function. Patients with retrocochlear pathology often demonstrate good discrimination abilities at moderate intensities; however this will significantly break down at high intensities (i.e., 50–80 dB above the speech reception threshold). A difference of 20% or greater between moderate- and high-intensity presentation levels is considered a positive retrocochlear finding, called *rollover*.

Pure-tone bone conduction thresholds are obtained when a hearing loss is present by air conduction. Bone conduction tests are intended to be a direct measure of inner-ear sensitivity. Comparison of air and bone conduction thresholds establishes the type of hearing loss. Conductive loss results from disorders in the outer or middle ear. Sensorineural loss is associated with cochlear or eighth-nerve disorders. Mixed loss is a conductive and sensorineural loss coexisting in the same ear.

Speech threshold testing provides a direct measure of overall hearing for speech and is a basis for determining the presentation level of other tests. It provides a comparative measure for confirming pure-tone thresholds. A lack of agreement between speech thresholds and pure-tone threshold averages indicates a discrepancy and the need for additional testing or retesting to establish valid measures.

Speech discrimination tests measure a patient's ability to differentiate speech sounds. Discrimination ability may be affected in varying amounts, depending on the type, cause, configuration, and degree of hearing loss. Discrimination scores contribute to estimates of the amount of handicap to be expected from the hearing loss and to the prognosis for rehabilitation.

Tone decay is another way to assess the integrity of the auditory system. Although many methods of administering decay testing have been described, the supra-threshold adaptation test (STAT) is clinically favored. A 1,000-Hz pure tone is presented at 100 dB SPL for one minute. The contralateral ear is masked. Failure to hear the tone for the full minute is a positive STAT. The presence of tone decay is characteristic of retrocochlear or auditory nerve lesions. Figure 44.3 depicts an audiogram from a patient with a cerebellopontine angle tumor demonstrating asymmetrical hearing loss. Patients with asymmetrical hearing loss should have neuroimaging to rule out a cerebellopontine angle tumor.

Immittance measures assess the status of the middle ear and confirm information obtained in other tests of the battery. The basic immittance battery consists of the tympanogram and acoustic-reflex thresholds. Data from the tympanogram permit determination of the static compliance of the middle-ear system. An interpretation such as type A tympanogram means that the mobility of the tympanic membrane and middle-ear structures are within normal limits (see Chapter 18).

Acoustic reflex measures a contraction of the stapedius muscle (innervated by the seventh nerve) in response to a loud sound. The afferent limb of the reflex is via the auditory portion of the eighth nerve, and the efferent portion of the reflex arch is via the seventh nerve. The stapedius muscle would normally contract bilaterally regardless of which ear was stimulated, assuming normal afferent input. Following contraction of the stapedius muscle, the tympanic membrane is tightened or stiffened, increasing the impedance or resistance of the eardrum to acoustic energy and resulting in a slight attenuation of sound transmitted through the middle ear system. In a normal subject, the acoustic reflex will be present in response to a pure tone in between 70 and 100 dB above hearing level, or when a white-noise stimulus is presented at 65 dB above hearing level (Martin 1986). Patients with conductive hearing loss will have absent reflexes because the lesion prevents a change in compliance with stapedius muscle contraction. With cochlear lesions, the acoustic reflex may be present at sensation levels less than 60 dB above the auditory pure-tone threshold, which is another form of abnormal loudness growth or recruitment. Cochlear hearing losses must be moderate or severe before the acoustic reflex is lost. In contrast, patients with retrocochlear or eighth-nerve lesions often have abnormal acoustic reflexes with relatively normal hearing. The reflex may be absent or exhibit an elevated threshold or abnormal decay. Reflex decay is present if the amplitude of the reflex decreases to half its original size within 10 seconds of stimulation at 1,000 Hz, 10 dB above reflex threshold. This abnormality is seen in approximately 80% of patients with acoustic neuromas (Baloh 1984). Observation of the pattern of the acoustic reflex tests permits inferences to support the presence of a cochlear, conductive, or neural lesion of the seventh or eighth nerves (Table 44.1).

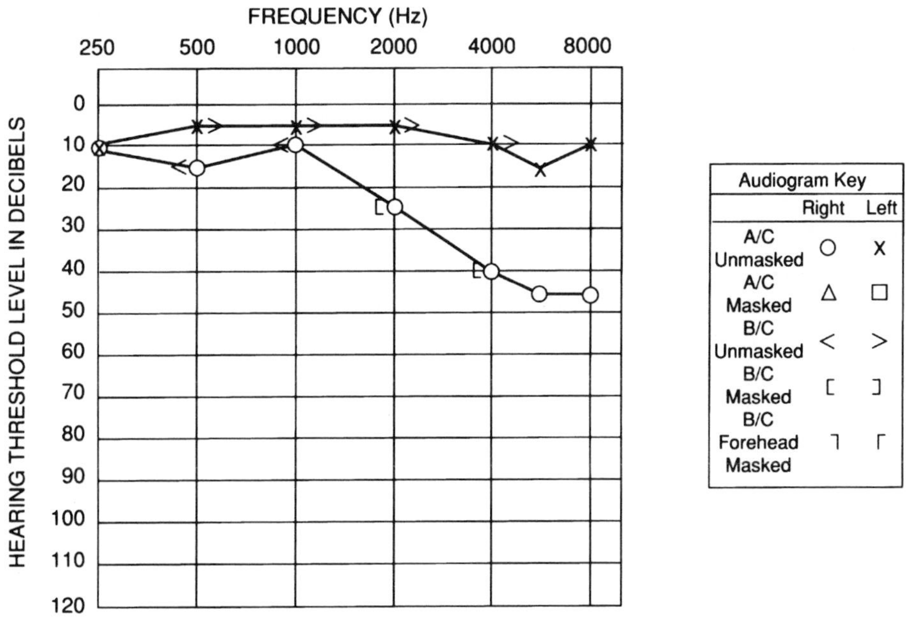

SPEECH TESTS

TESTS		R	L
Sp. Reception Threshold (SRT)		20 db	5 db
Sp. Discrim. Scores	35 db SL	84%	100%

FIGURE 44.3 Abnormal audiogram. Findings indicate normal hearing sensitivity for the left ear, with a mild-to-moderate high-frequency hearing loss for the right ear. The asymmetrical hearing loss, in addition to the decreased discrimination score for the right ear, indicates possible retrocochlear pathology, such as a vestibular schwannoma.

Accurate administration of the basic test battery should establish the presence and the characteristics of hearing loss. Interpretation of the battery and observation of patient behavior may indicate a need for additional testing, such as neuroimaging, hearing aid evaluation, or medical evaluation.

Brain stem auditory evoked potentials (BAEPs) are also known as brain stem auditory evoked responses (BAERs) or auditory brain stem responses (ABRs). These physiological measures can be used to evaluate the auditory pathways from the ear to the upper brain stem (Picton 1990). In addition, ABR threshold testing may be used to determine behavioral threshold sensitivity in infants or uncooperative patients. The most consistent and reproducible potentials are a series of five submicrovolt waves that are seen within 10 msec of an auditory stimulus. These potentials are recorded by averaging 1,000–2,000 responses from click stimuli by use of a computer system and amplifying the response (Figure 44.4). The anatomic correlates of the five reliable potentials have only been roughly approximated. Wave I of the BAEP is a manifestation of the action potentials of the eighth nerve and is generated in the distal portion of the nerve adjacent to the cochlea. Wave II may be generated by the eighth nerve or cochlear nuclei. Wave III is thought to be generated at the level of the superior olive, and waves IV and V are generated in the rostral pons or in the midbrain near the inferior colliculus. The complex anatomy of the central auditory pathway (Benjamin and Troost 1988), with multiple crossing of fibers from the level of the cochlear nuclei to the inferior colliculus, makes interpretation of central disturbances in the evoked responses difficult.

The BAEP is a sensitive, noninvasive diagnostic test for the diagnosis of cerebellopontine angle tumors (Picton 1990). This test is used to differentiate cochlear from

Table 44.1: Pattern of acoustic reflex measurements with unilateral lesions

Type of Lesion	*Stimulus Presented:* / *Reflex Measured:*	*C* / *I*	*I* / *C*	*C* / *C*	*I* / *I*
Cochlear (<85 dB HL)		+	+	+	+
Conductive (>30 dB HL)		–	–	+	–
VIII nerve		+	–	+	–
VII nerve		–	+	+	–

C = contralateral to lesion; I = ipsilateral lesion; + = reflex present; – = reflex absent; HL = hearing loss.
Source: Adapted from RW Baloh. Dizziness, Hearing Loss and Tinnitus: The Essentials of Neurotology. Philadelphia: FA Davis, 1984:59–96.

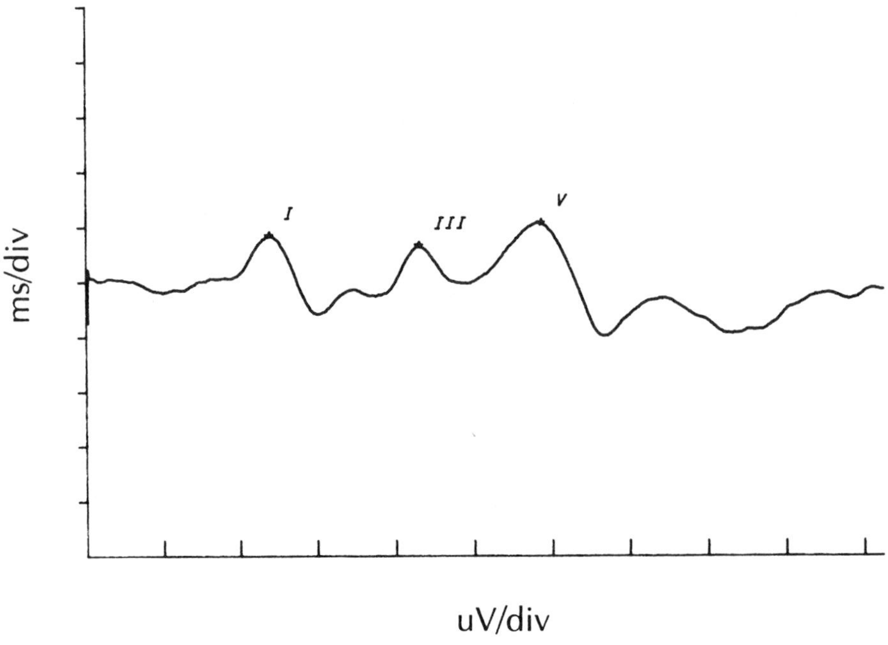

FIGURE 44.4 Brain stem auditory evoked potential (BAEP) in a normal adult. Responses were recorded between electrodes on the vertex and the ipsilateral mastoid. Waves I, III, and V are labeled.

eighth-nerve hearing defects and, on some occasions, demonstrates an auditory abnormality when behavioral audiometric testing is still normal. The majority of patients with acoustic tumors had abnormal responses (Baloh and Honrubia 1990).

The least specific finding is the absence of all waves. This has been seen in some patients with vestibular schwannoma and in some with cerebellopontine angle meningiomas. Such patients often have marked hearing deficits with poor discrimination on behavioral testing, suggesting retrocochlear disease. The absence of all waves should not occur unless a severe hearing loss exists. The most specific evoked potential abnormality is the presence of an increase in interwave intervals. Abnormal interwave latencies (I–III or I–V) are the most specific and sensitive abnormalities seen with cerebellopontine angle tumors. The abnormal prolongation or absence of wave V at increased click rates is also characteristic of retrocochlear pathology. Increased absolute latencies of all waves, when compared to responses from the other ear, may signify a conductive deficit.

Electrocochleography (ECochG) is a method of recording the stimulus-related electrical potentials associated with the inner ear and auditory nerve, including the cochlear microphonic, summating potential (SP) and compound action potential (AP) of the auditory nerve. This measure is beneficial in the differential diagnosis of certain types of sensory disorders such as Ménière's disease or cochlear hydrops. The amplitude of the SP and AP is measured and is of primary interest when evaluating an ear for increased endolymphatic pressure.

High-resolution CT scanning provides excellent imaging of the temporal bone and assists in defining congenital abnormalities and infection. MRI has largely supplanted CT scanning for the diagnosis of cerebellopontine angle tumors. Contrast-enhanced MRI and special imaging techniques have allowed diagnosis of unusual lesions such as meningeal carcinomatosis, which may affect the cerebellopontine angle and eighth nerve.

MANAGEMENT OF PERIPHERAL VESTIBULOPATHY

Medical Treatment

Therapy is outlined for symptomatic treatment of dizziness presumed to be of peripheral origin (Table 44.2). When a definitive diagnosis such as vestibular schwannoma, autoimmune disorder, perilymph fistula, or systemic vasculitis has been made, the therapy must be directed to the underlying disorder.

In treating a patient suffering from dizziness, particularly one with a chronic problem and one who has seen numerous physicians, understanding and patience are required to relieve anxiety and depression. One may need to reassure the patient of the absence of progression in the usual case and the natural history of most symptoms with peripheral vestibulopathy (i.e., improvement with time). Exercise therapy is especially helpful in patients with positional vertigo (Troost and Patton 1992; Brandt et al. 1994).

Although most of the drugs used for dizziness are loosely referred to as vestibular suppressants, it is often unclear which agents will be effective in a given patient. The mechanism of action of these drugs is largely unknown. The primary vestibular afferent system could be suppressed directly or indirectly through the inhibitory portion of the

Table 44.2: Medical therapy of vertigo

Class	*Dose*[a]
Antihistamines	
Meclizine	25–50 mg 3 times/day
Cyclizine	50 mg 1–2 times/day
Dimenhydrinate	50 mg 1–2 times/day
Promethazine	25–50 mg/day
Anticholinergics	
Scopolamine[b]	1 three times a day
Scopolamine tablets	0.45–0.50 mg 1–2 times/day
Scopolamine transdermal	1/day for 3 days
Sympathomimetics	
Ephedrine	25 mg/day
Antiemetics	
Trimethobenzamide	250 mg 1–2 times/day PO 200-mg suppository
Promethazine	25–50 mg/day
Prochlorperazine	5–10 times/day PO 25-mg suppository
Tranquilizers	
Diazepam	5–10 mg 1–3 times/day
Oxazepam	10–60 mg/day
Haloperidol[c]	0.5–1.0 mg 1–2 times/day
Combination preparations and others	
Scopolamine with ephedrine	
Scopolamine with promethazine	
Ephedrine with promethazine	
Buclazine	
Cyclandelate	
Diuretics	
Diet	

[a]Usual adult starting dose; maintenance dose can be increased by factor of 2–3. The most common side effect is drowsiness.
[b]There are combination preparations, containing a mixture of atropine alkaloids with approximately one-fourth grain (15.0–16.2 mg) phenobarbital.
[c]Note the very low dose when compared to usual antipsychotic treatment. Nevertheless, the patient should still be observed for dystonias.

major vestibular efferent system. An important effect of some agents may be to act on other sensory systems, such as proprioceptive or visual inputs to the vestibular nuclei of the brain stem.

Many of the agents commonly used for treatment are empirical. Few controlled studies have investigated the response of patients with presumed peripheral vestibular dysfunction. Many of the drugs used by neurologists for treating such patients are based on studies of the prevention of motion sickness in normal subjects or of the various regimens used by otologists in the management of patients diagnosed as having Ménière's syndrome.

Antihistamines are among the most commonly used agents in the treatment of dizziness. Few neurologists see a patient with such a complaint who has not already been treated with meclizine. Histamine antagonists are classified according to the responses to histamine that are prevented. Antagonists that act at receptors for histamine are classified as H_1- or H_2-receptor blocking agents, or simply H_1 or H_2 blockers (Brandt 1991).

Antihistamines in the H_1 antagonist group are used for dizziness. In motion sickness, it is stimulation of the vestibular apparatus that produces the syndrome (although the respective roles of semicircular canals and otoliths are uncertain); the vestibular cerebellar integrative vomiting center and medullary chemoreceptive trigger zone are clearly involved in the process. Electrophysiological recordings in dogs have shown that diphenhydramine diminishes excitability of the vestibular nuclear complex to vestibular afferent activity induced by motion or electrical stimulation of the vestibular afferents. Possibly the H_1 blockers effective in motion sickness act by central antagonism of acetylcholine, as does scopolamine. Promethazine, a phenothiazine with strong ACh-blocking action, is one of the most effective agents in combating motion sickness.

Anticholinergics that block the muscarinic effect of ACh have been widely used and studied for the prevention of motion sickness. Atropine acts centrally to stimulate the medulla and cerebrum, but the closely related alkaloid 1-hyoscine or scopolamine is more widely used.

Transdermal delivery of scopolamine may prevent or mitigate the nausea and vomiting associated with motion sickness, but not the dizziness. In general, transdermal scopolamine is not useful in patients with vestibulopathy. Frequent side effects are blurred vision and dry mouth, in addition to occasional confusion. Some patients have significant difficulty when they try to discontinue scopolamine patches. A side effect of low-dose scopolamine or atropine is the transient bradycardia (4–8 beats reduction per minute) associated with the peak action of oral scopolamine at 90 minutes and diminishing thereafter.

Sympathomimetics have been used in the treatment of motion sickness, particularly in combination with anticholinergics. The sole agent in this class that may have an application in combination with other drugs is ephedrine. Tolerance may develop after a few weeks of treatment.

Antiemetics may be used when prominent nausea is a symptom. Many of the antihistaminic and anticholinergic drugs listed here are also used for their antiemetic actions. Compazine should be used with caution, particularly by the intramuscular route, because of the high incidence of dystonic reactions.

Tranquilizer is the general name given to drugs from different classes having central and probably peripheral effects. Such drugs include benzodiazepines, butyrophenones, and phenothiazines. Despite extensive publicity concerning the use and abuse of diazepam and the fact that there is no direct evidence of an effect on the vestibular system, diazepam is still one of the most widely prescribed drugs for the treatment of dizziness. It should not be the first choice, primarily because of the significant potential for habituation and depression, and because it can be the actual cause of dizziness. Nonetheless, it does remain the first choice of many neuro-otologists and otologists. The mechanism of action of the benzodiazepines appears in some way related to the metabolism or action of GABA. Potential effects on the vestibular system would be speculative. Other longer-acting benzodiazepines may be helpful in certain patients, but no study has substantiated their effectiveness.

Haloperidol in small oral doses appears to be effective in many patients with peripheral vestibular dysfunction, including those with positional vertigo, who seem to be less affected by other antidizziness medications.

Combination preparations, including agents listed in Table 44.2 and described in the appropriate sections, are frequently useful, particularly the combination of ephedrine and promethazine. Some other agents and regimens used primarily in the medical management of Ménière's disease are briefly reviewed in this section. In the belief that in some cases an effect on blood supply to the peripheral end-organ might be a factor, agents such as cyclandelate have been used. Reports in the literature are contradictory, and the therapeutic value of cyclandelate has never been convincingly demonstrated for any condition.

An usually high incidence of metabolic abnormality, particularly hyperlipidemia, has been reported in series of patients with peripheral vestibular dysfunction, especially Ménière's disease. For this reason, dietary regimens have been prescribed as adjunct therapy. Among the most widely used medical therapy in Ménière's disease is the combination of salt restriction (1,000- to 2,000-mg sodium diets) and diuretic therapy. There is still uncertainty regarding the natural history of Ménière's disease and whether the ultimate outcome for vestibular function or hearing can be helped by medical management. However, since the long-term results of surgery, such as endolymphatic shunts, are far from proven, there is still a clear role for medical management in this condition.

Exercise therapy can be extremely beneficial for the treatment of persistent positional vertigo (Troost and Patton 1992; Brandt et al. 1994). The patient is first instructed carefully about the type of exercise to be done. The patient is asked to move rapidly from a seated position to lying on the side. It is more comfortable if the patient rests his or her head on a pillow or other support until the symptoms subside. The patient is to remain in that position for 30 seconds, then return to the upright position and wait until any recrudescence of symptoms subsides, or for a minimum of 30 seconds. Then the patient is instructed to move rapidly lateral to the opposite recumbent position and wait for 30 seconds, then return to the upright position, completing one repetition. Patients are asked to repeat 20 repetitions two times a day. The vast majority of patients experience significant relief within a week, although it might take 3 months to become asymptomatic. Although there are some recurrences, the majority of patients are permanently cured.

Surgical Treatment

Surgical treatment of chronic peripheral vestibular dysfunction is primarily destructive. In patients with severe Ménière's disease for whom medical therapy such as that described earlier has been ineffective, and who have severe recurrent disabling attacks, a labyrinthectomy may be performed. Unfortunately, Ménière's disease may become bilateral, eventually resulting in the need for labyrinthectomy or vestibular nerve section on the contralateral side. A medical labyrinthectomy may be performed by the use of the aminoglycoside drugs, which are particularly destructive to the peripheral vestibular hair cells. Surgical or medical labyrinthectomy is usually a last resort in patients who have clearly defined, severe attacks of peripheral vestibulopathy presumably from Ménière's disease.

Various shunting procedures have been used to treat Ménière's disease and endolymphatic hydrops. Although some patients can benefit, the long-term success with such shunting procedures to the mastoid region and to the subarachnoid space has been modest.

Some patients with benign paroxysmal positional vertigo do not have a benign course (Baloh and Honrubia 1990). Patients who experience classic but disabling symptoms persisting over 6 months are candidates for exercise therapy. On rare occasions when the exercise therapy is unsuccessful, such patients are candidates for section of the nerve from the posterior semicircular canal.

MANAGEMENT OF CENTRAL AND SYSTEMIC VESTIBULAR DISORDERS

Medical Treatment

Clearly, the management of central vestibular disorders depends on the diagnosis. A simple separation into peripheral and central vestibular dysfunction is not always possible, as discussed in Chapter 18. Some patients have inadequate central compensation for a peripheral vestibular abnormality and thus remain symptomatic. In such patients, medical therapy for peripheral vestibular dysfunction, as described earlier, may prove quite effective. When a specific diagnosis—for example, postural hypotension secondary to diabetic peripheral neuropathy—is made, attention should be directed to treatment of the primary condition. Severe postural hypotension is notoriously difficult to manage; although mineralocorticoids have been used, they should be prescribed cautiously to avoid the production of congestive heart failure.

The patient who is diagnosed as having primary CNS disease, whether it be brain stem infarction or spinocerebellar degeneration, must be managed as would a patient without the accompanying symptoms of disequilibration. Medical therapy of vertebrobasilar insufficiency is directed at preventing new infarctions, primarily with antiplatelet agents and, on rare occasions, anticoagulation. Cerebellar dysfunction when not caused by tumor may be treated symptomatically. On occasion, isoniazide might reduce ataxia. Vestibular suppressant medication can add a modicum of improvement, and agents helpful in the therapy of essential tremor, such as beta-blocking drugs or primidone, may result in symptomatic improvement.

Therapy for systemic conditions producing vertigo also depends on the diagnosis. If systemic drug therapy, as with benzodiazepines, is actually the cause of disequilibration, then of course alteration in the medical regimen may prove efficacious. Withdrawal of all drugs, be they anticonvulsants or benzodiazepines, must be done cautiously to avoid precipitating withdrawal reactions.

Surgical Treatment

Surgical treatment is directed primarily toward removal of the tumors that can affect the peripheral or central vestibular apparatus. When disequilibration, ataxia, or dizziness are due to a Chiari malformation, surgical decompression of the posterior fossa can give major symptomatic relief.

REFERENCES

Baloh RW. Dizziness, Hearing Loss and Tinnitus: The Essentials of Neurotology. Philadelphia: FA Davis, 1984;59–96.

Baloh RW, Honrubia V. Clinical Neurophysiology of the Vestibular System (2nd ed). Philadelphia: FA Davis, 1990.

Benjamin EE, Troost BT. Central Auditory Disorders. In GM English (ed), Clinical Otolaryngology. Philadelphia: Harper & Row, 1988.

Brandt T, Steddin S, Daroff RB. Therapy for benign paroxysmal positioning vertigo (BPPV) revisited. Neurology 1994; 44:796–800.

Brandt T. Vertigo: Its Multisensory Syndromes. London: Springer-Verlag, 1991.

Leigh RJ, Zee DS. The Neurology of Eye Movements (2nd ed). Philadelphia: FA Davis, 1991.

Martin FN. Introduction to Audiology. Englewood Cliffs, NJ: Prentice-Hall, 1986.

Morrow MJ, Sharpe JA. Smooth Pursuit Eye Movements: The Vestibulo-Ocular Reflex and Vertigo. New York: Raven, 1993.

Picton TW. Auditory Evoked Potentials. In DD Daly, TA Pedley (eds), Current Practice of Clinical Electroencephalography (2nd ed). New York: Raven, 1990;625–678.

Pierrot-Deseilligny C, Gaymard B. Smooth pursuit disorders. Bailliere's Clinical Neurology. London: Tindall, 1992;435–454.

Sharpe JA, Morrow MJ, and Johnston JL. Smooth Pursuit: Anatomy, Physiology and Disorders. In RB Daroff, A Neetens (eds), Neurological Organization of Ocular Movement. Berkeley, CA: Kugler and Ghedini, 1990;113–144.

Troost BT, Patton JM. Exercise therapy for positional vertigo. Neurology 1992;42:1441–1444.

Chapter 45
Neuro-Urology

Clare J. Fowler

Investigation and management of disorders of urogenital function are usually regarded as the preserve of urologists. However, increasingly, rehabilitation physicians—particularly those involved in neuro-rehabilitation, are finding that complaints of disordered bladder and sexual function are so prominent among their patients' symptoms that they are being obliged to take an active role in arranging and interpreting urodynamic studies.

This chapter describes what a neurologist needs to know to care for patients with urogenital problems. Urodynamic, neurophysiological, and radiological investigations are described and their use in investigating neurogenic genitourinary disorders discussed. When planning bladder management for patients with neurogenic incontinence, the single most valuable test is measurement of the volume left in the bladder after voiding, the *postmicturition residual volume*.

INVESTIGATIONS

Physical Examination in Relation to Patients with Urogenital Symptoms

To decide if a patient has a neurological cause for a urogenital complaint, the findings on clinical examination are crucial. Attention should be focused on whether or not there is a neurological abnormality of the lower limbs. The reflexes that control both the storage and micturition phases of the bladder are transspinal, connecting the pontine micturition center to the sacral spinal cord (Figure 45.1). Because the spinal segments that innervate the bladder are caudal to those that innervate the legs, spinal cord disease that affects the innervation of the bladder almost inevitably also produces neurological signs in the lower limbs. Exceptions might be lesions of the low sacral cord or conus, but only the most caudal lesions fail to produce some hyperreflexia in the lower limbs and extensor plantar responses.

Higher sacral root lesions (S1, S2) are apt to produce impairment of the ankle reflexes. The intrinsic foot musculature receives much of its innervation from S3, so the feet should be carefully examined for deformities and fasciculation of the muscles. Saddle anesthesia is a feature of cauda equina or conus lesions but is likely to be spontaneously noted by the patient rather than found on examination in someone previously unaware of it. As explained below, sacral reflex responses recorded electrophysiologically are of limited value and almost certainly less so when elicited clinically.

Examination for evidence of peripheral neuropathy is important. Peripheral neuropathy, notably diabetic, is commonly a cause of erectile failure, and as the neuropathy progresses abnormalities of innervation of the bladder detrusor muscle may also develop.

When the neurological examination of the lower limbs has been completed, the patient should be asked to stand and the lumbosacral spine is inspected. Congenital malformations of the spine can sometimes produce symptoms that present in adults. Signs such as hypertrichosis, a nevus, sinus, or dimpling in the sacral region should not be overlooked.

Evidence of extrapyramidal disease, cerebellar ataxia, laryngeal involvement, and postural hypotension should raise the suspicion of multiple system atrophy (MSA), a condition characterized by early and severe urinary incontinence.

It is axiomatic that if a patient with urogenital complaints is without evidence of neurological disease on clinical examination, detailed investigation with imaging and neurophysiology is unlikely to reveal relevant underlying neurological pathology.

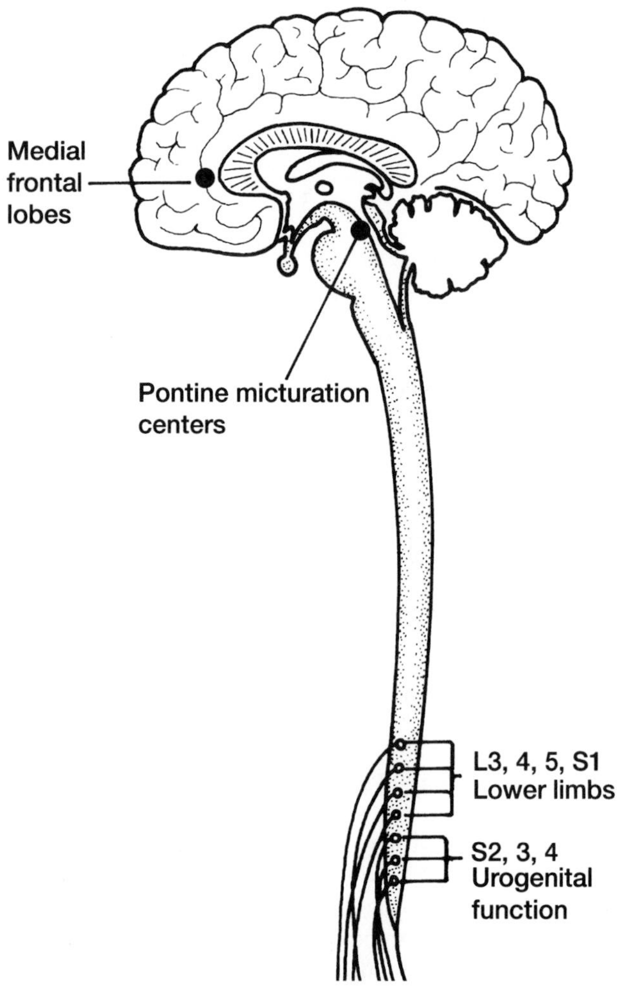

FIGURE 45.1 The peripheral innervation of the bladder and genitalia arises from the sacral spinal cord, and central control over the bladder is exercised by micturition centers in the pons and frontal lobes. It is obvious from this organization that any spinal cord lesion causing neurological symptoms and signs in the lower limb will interrupt the transspinal connections between the pons and sacral cord, also causing impaired bladder control. Likewise, it would be unusual for spinal pathology to cause a disorder of bladder function without also producing a neurological deficit of the lower limbs unless the lesion affected only the conus.

Urological Investigations

It is advisable for patients with urogenital complaints without known neurological disease to be investigated first by a urologist; otherwise there is a danger that urological disorders such as prostatic hypertrophy, a urethral stricture, interstitial cystitis, or a bladder stone may go unrecognized. The introduction of flexible cystoscopy, which can be performed as a painless outpatient procedure, has greatly simplified the exclusion of intravesical pathology.

The situation is different if the patient develops genitourinary symptoms as part of his or her established neurological disease. Then the neurologist should become involved in the management of those symptoms, just as for any other neurological symptoms. Unfortunately, however, this rarely happens; many neurologists protest ignorance about this area of disability and send such patients to a urologist. This may not always be in the patient's best interests if the urologist is not interested in neuro-urology.

Urodynamic Studies

Urodynamic studies examine the function of the urinary tract. They include measurements of urine flow rate, residual volume, cystometry both during filling and voiding, videocystometry, urethral pressure profile measurements, and pelvic floor neurophysiology. However, colloquially speaking, *urodynamics* is often used as a synonym for cystometry.

From the point of view of the patient, tests of bladder function can be divided into the noninvasive and those requiring a urethral catheter.

Noninvasive Bladder Investigations

Urinary flowmetry is a valuable, noninvasive investigation, particularly when combined with an ultrasound measurement of the postmicturition residual volume. A commonly used design for a flowmeter consists of a commode or urinal into which the patient passes urine as naturally as possible. In the base of the collecting system is a spinning disc; as the urine flows it tends to slow the speed of rotation of the disc. A servo-motor holds the speed of rotation constant, and the urine flow rate is derived from measurement of the power necessary to do that. The machine usually produces a graphic printout together with an analysis for the time taken to reach maximal flow, maximum and average flow rate, and the voided volume (Figure 45.2).

It is important that the patient prepares to perform the test with a comfortably full bladder, containing, if possible, a volume in excess of 200 ml. Privacy is essential; a spurious result might be obtained if the subject is not fully relaxed. Published nomograms give urine free-flow rates against volume for men and women. An aging effect has been found in men over the age of 65, but not in women. A significant neurogenic bladder disorder is unlikely if the patient has good bladder capacity and normal urine flow rate and empties to completion—all of which may be noninvasively demonstrated.

Knowledge of a patient's postmicturition residual volume is essential when planning treatment of neurogenic bladder symptoms. Although this information is available from urethral catheterization after voiding, the same data can be obtained noninvasively by ultrasound. Small, simple ultrasound machines are now available that require little operator training, and they make it easy to determine whether the postmicturition residual is negligible or in excess of 100 ml. Measuring cursors are usually available so that quite accurate estimates of the residual volume can be calculated from scanning in two planes (Figure 45.3).

Larger, more elaborate ultrasound machines are to be found in radiology departments equipped for urological work, and ultrasound scanning of the upper urinary tracts has mostly replaced intravenous urography as a means of examining the kidneys and ureters for dilation, stones, and tumors. Interpretation of these scans requires special expertise.

Investigations Requiring Catheterization

Cystometry, the registration of bladder pressure, can be performed during filling or voiding. The essential measurement is the intravesical pressure, but since this also reflects rises in intra-abdominal pressure, rectal pressure must be simultaneously recorded and the value subtracted from the measured intraversal pressure to give the true changes of detrusor pressure alone. The efficiency of the subtraction is usually checked at the beginning of cystometry by asking the subject to cough (Figure 45.4). This produces a rise in abdominal pressure and hence intravesical pressure, but no increase in detrusor pressure.

To make these measurements and fill the bladder, three catheters are needed. From the patient's point of view, there are two insertions. A moderately large-diameter urethral catheter (10F) is inserted through the urethra into the bladder, on which is mounted a smaller-diameter catheter (4F) for measuring intravesical pressure. A similarly fine-gauge catheter (4F) is then inserted into the rectum to record intra-abdominal pressure. Once the lines are in place and satisfactory subtraction of the two values is demonstrated, the bladder can begin to be filled. The rate of filling is recorded by the machine, which pumps sterile water or saline solution through the filling catheter into the bladder. The question of the best rate of bladder filling has been much discussed in the urodynamic literature, but for speed most laboratories use medium-fill rates of 50 ml per minute. This is clearly unphysiologically fast but does mean that full bladder capacity can usually be reached within 7 or 8 minutes. First sensation of bladder filling may be reported at about 100 ml and the full capacity reached between 400 and 600 ml. In healthy subjects the bladder will expand to contain this amount of fluid without a rise of more than 15 cm of water (see Figure 45.4). A bladder that behaves in this way is said to show *normal compliance*.

The main abnormality sought through cystometry in patients with incontinence is *detrusor instability*. The unstable detrusor has been defined as one that is shown objectively to contract spontaneously or on provocation during the filling phase while the patient is attempting to inhibit micturition. When detrusor instability occurs in the pres-

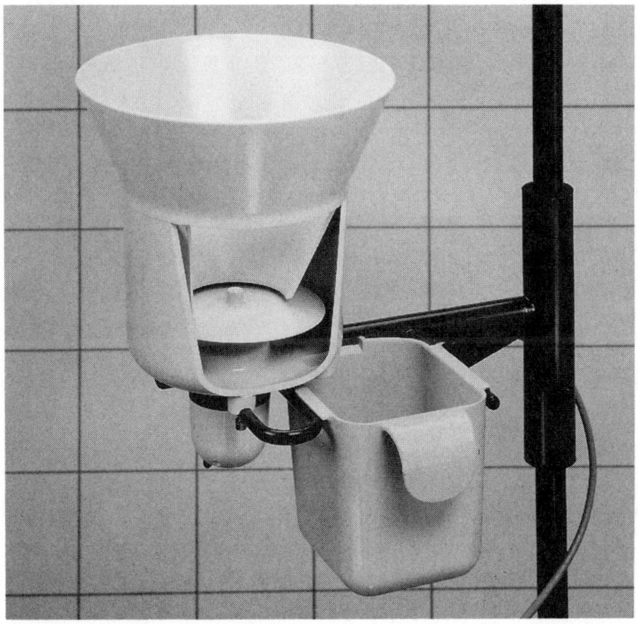

A

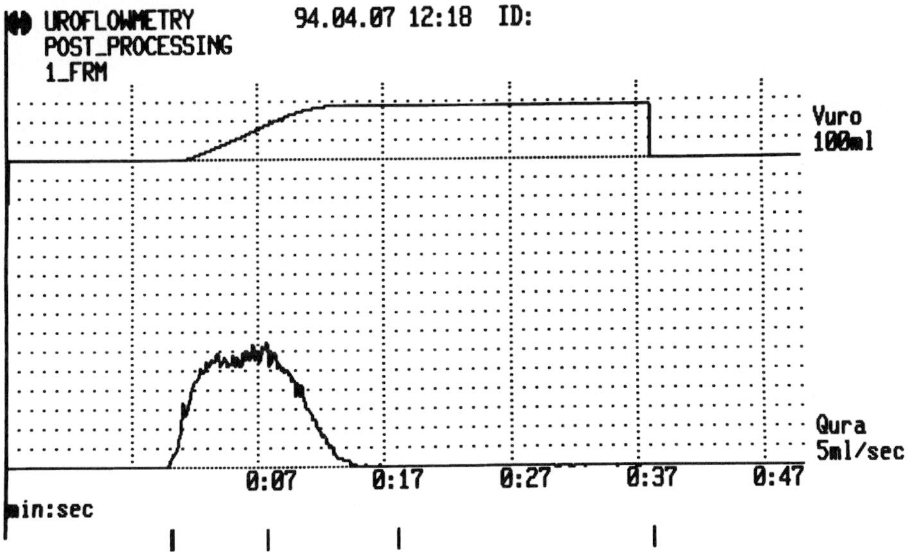

B

FIGURE 45.2. A. Urinary flowmeter. The side of the uroflow transducer has been cut away to show the disc at the base of the funnel that rotates as urine passes into the collecting vessel. B. Typical (normal) printout from the uroflowmeter. A total of 290 ml was voided (upper trace), with a maximum flow rate of 30 ml/sec (lower trace). (Reprinted with permission of Dantec Medical A/S.)

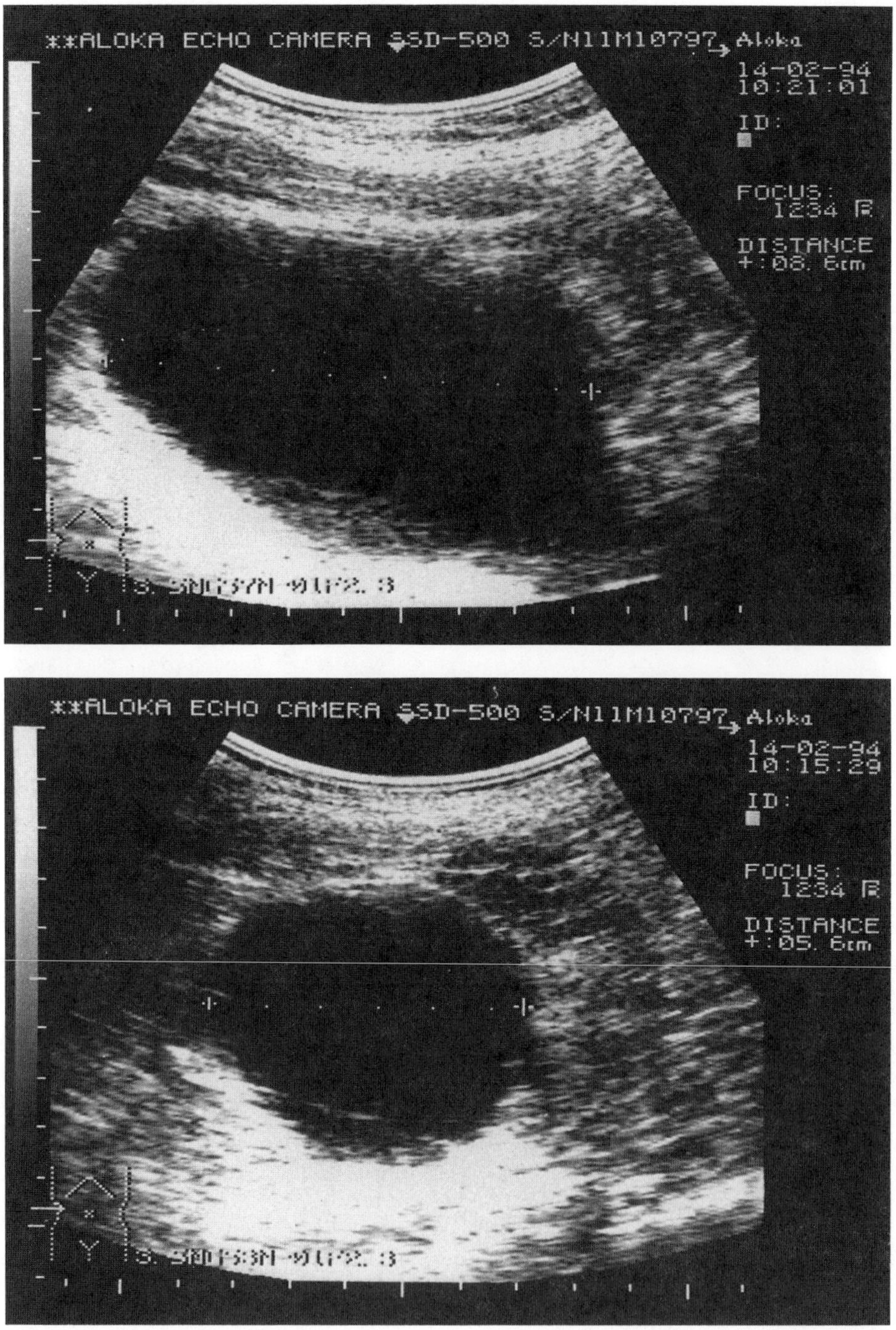

FIGURE 45.3 Measurement of the postmicturition residual volume using a small, portable ultrasound machine. The bladder is scanned in two planes and cursors are placed to make measurements from which the volume may be calculated.

ence of neurological disease, the disorder is referred to as *detrusor hyperreflexia*. It should be emphasized that the urodynamic findings of detrusor instability and detrusor hyperreflexia are the same; the difference between the two conditions is purely semantic. Detrusor hyperreflexia is the term used to describe the behavior of the bladder in patients with recognized neurological disease.

When bladder filling has been completed, the filling catheter is removed and the patient voids, with the intravesical and rectal pressure lines still in place, using the flowmeter. Urine flow rate depends both on detrusor pressure and outlet resistance. Much valuable information can be obtained about the latter by measuring detrusor pressure and urine flow. As a rough guide, the pressure for men should be less than 50 cm water and for women less than 30 cm water, with flow rates in excess of 15 ml/sec and 20 ml/sec, respectively. With increasingly sophisticated developments in the equipment used for urodynamic studies, real-time computer analysis of the flow rates and pressures has become available. Considerable debate surrounds the question of what is the best mathematical formula to use in analysis so the degree of outflow obstruction can be esti-

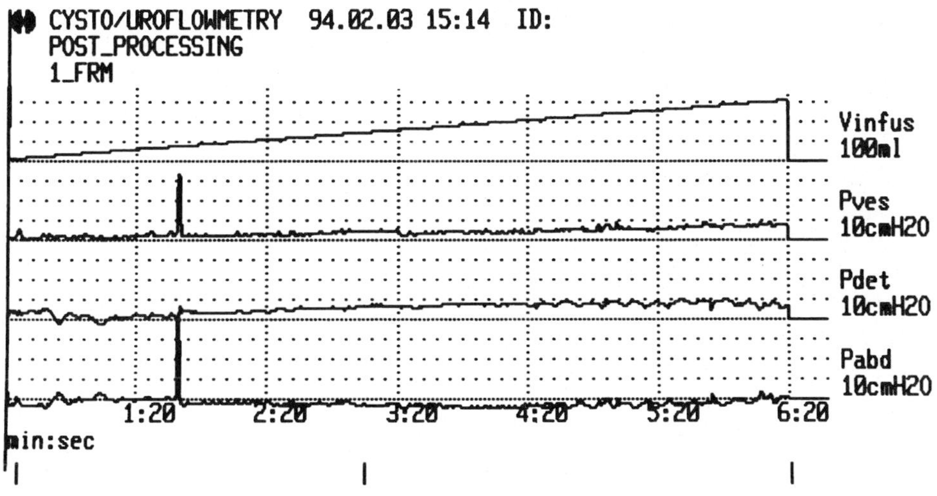

FIGURE 45.4. Cystometry during bladder filling. The bladder was filled (top trace) at 50 ml/minute (Vinfus) to a total of 300 ml. The detrusor pressure (Pdet) did not exceed 10 cm of water, which is normal and when the bladder is said to be stable. Pdet is derived by subtracting Pabdo (the pressure measured by a fine pressure line in the rectum) from the measured intravesical pressure Pves. At the beginning of the trace these two values can be seen to be subtracting effectively since on coughing there is an abrupt rise in intravesical pressure but no rise in detrusor pressure.

mated. This is of particular importance to urologists investigating men with prostatic hypertrophy.

When cystometry is carried out using a contrast filling medium and the procedure is radiographically screened, the technique is known as *videocystometry*. Much information about the lower urinary tract may be obtained with videocystometry. The advantages are that the bladder outline can be inspected during filling and any reflux into the ureters is seen. A neurogenic bladder often produces characteristic changes with thickening of the bladder wall and bladder diverticulae. Urologists and uro-gynecologists have found videocystometry useful in detecting sphincter or bladder-neck incompetence in genuine stress incontinence. The opportunity to inspect the outflow tract during voiding is of great value in patients with suspected obstruction. However, the procedure does expose the patient to x-irradiation and is inevitably more expensive than simple cystometry. In assessing patients with spinal cord injury, when examination of the upper tracts is critical, videourodynamic studies have an important role, but simple cystometry alone is usually adequate to demonstrate detrusor hyperreflexia in nontraumatic neurogenic bladder disorders.

A general criticism of cystometric studies is that, valuable as they may be in demonstrating the underlying pathophysiology of a patient's urinary tract, the findings on cystometry contribute little to elucidating the underlying cause of the disorder. A large urodynamic literature has grown up that, by its essentially descriptive nature, ignores this and groups patients according to their cystometric abnormalities alone.

Urethral pressure profile is measured using a catheter-mounted transducer, which is drawn slowly through the urethra by a motorized armature. The test can be performed in men or women and is called static if no additional procedure such as coughing or straining is performed. If intravesical pressure is measured simultaneously and the patient is asked to cough repeatedly while the catheter is withdrawn, the transmission of the cough impulse in the urethra and bladder can be measured and expressed as a ratio—the *transmission pressure ratio*.

It was hoped that measurements of the urethral pressure profile and parameters derived from it would be useful in assessing genuine stress incontinence, but the overlap of measurements in controls and in women with genuine stress incontinence is such that the test is without diagnostic value (Versi et al. 1991). Urethral profilometry may, however, be of value in the assessment of voiding disorders, particularly in women with obstructed voiding, some of whom have abnormally high urethral pressures.

Neurophysiological Investigations

Various neurophysiological investigations of the pelvic floor have been developed by which assessment of the innervation can be made of muscles that are difficult to test clinically. These tests have mostly been used by urologists, andrologists, uro-gynecologists, and colorectal surgeons.

Electromyography

Electromyography (EMG) was first introduced as part of urodynamic studies to assess the extent of relaxation of the urethral sphincter during voiding. Interruption of the neural pathways between the pons and the sacral cord results in loss of coordination of sphincter and detrusor muscle activity, a condition known as *detrusor-sphincter dyssynergia*. In this disorder, instead of the sphincter relaxing to initiate and facilitate urine flow, it contracts at the same time the detrusor contracts. This may have important consequences, including incomplete bladder emptying and the potentially lethal condition of upper tract dilatation, leading to renal failure. For this reason it was considered important that dyssynergic detrusor-sphincter activity be recognized. However, sphincter EMG is now, for a number of reasons, rarely recorded. First, it is often technically difficult to obtain a good-quality EMG signal from a site as inaccessible as the urethral sphincter, particularly in the hostile recording environment in which urodynamic studies are performed. The best signal is obtained using a needle recording electrode, but the discomfort from the needle itself is likely to impair normal relaxation of the pelvic floor. Surface recording electrodes have been used but rarely pick up signals well from distant muscles. Furthermore, in addition to the difficulties of making a meaningful recording, there is doubt about the value of the information the procedure provides. Detrusor-sphincter dyssynergia is a disorder that is recognized as a consequence of spinal cord disease; if the patient comes to the urodynamics laboratory in a wheelchair or has even a milder degree of paraparesis, dyssynergic bladder activity can reasonably be presumed. The urologist's main concern then will be to establish if it is causing upper-tract dilatation, and for this videocystometry is needed to detect ureteric reflux. Video screening allows the outlet tract to be seen, and sphincter EMG recording becomes redundant.

Although there is doubt about kinesiological EMG studies recorded during urodynamics, the value of EMG studies of the pelvic floor performed as a separate neurophysiological investigation to assess innervation is not in question. EMG has been used to demonstrate changes of denervation and reinnervation in the urethral or anal sphincter or pelvic floor in several neurogenic disorders. The motor units of the pelvic floor and sphincters fire tonically, so they may be conveniently captured using a trigger and delay line and subjected to individual motor unit analysis. Well-established values exist for the normal duration and amplitude of motor units recorded from the sphincters and other pelvic floor muscles using a concentric-needle electrode (see Fowler 1995 for review). Reinnervation can be detected by abnormal prolongation of duration or increase in amplitude of motor units. Alternatively, single-fiber EMG studies can look for changes of reinnervation producing an increase in fiber density.

Changes of denervation and reinnervation have been demonstrated in patients with idiopathic fecal incontinence, showing that there is a significant neurogenic component to this disorder. Denervation of the pelvic floor has been demonstrated in women with genuine stress incontinence. EMG of the pelvic floor is of particular value in demonstrating the existence and extent of denervation and reinnervation in patients suspected of having a cauda equina lesion.

Sphincter EMCT in the Diagnosis of Multiple System Atrophy

MSA may have protean manifestations, but urinary incontinence is often an early and troublesome complaint. In a study of 62 patients with established MSA, 56% had been seen by a urologist or gynecologist before the correct neurological diagnosis was made (Beck et al. 1994). The early development of incontinence and its severity is due to a combination of factors. It has been suggested that loss of pontine neurons causes the detrusor hyperreflexia that occurs in the early stages of the disease, loss of the parasympathetic innervation of the detrusor leads to poor contractility and incomplete emptying, and incontinence is compounded by sphincter weakness due to loss of the anterior horn cells, which innervate the sphincters. These anterior horn cells lie in the sacral spinal cord in a group of cells known as *Onuf's nucleus*. Neuropathological studies have shown that these anterior horn cells are selectively lost in MSA. Sphincter EMG can show changes of reinnervation in the muscles innervated by these neurons, characteristically manifest by prolongation of duration of motor units. These changes can be easily detected, making the test clinically robust. Either sphincter may be studied, but the more superficial anal sphincter is more conveniently studied.

We have adopted the policy of measuring the mean duration of 10 motor units and plotting this against the number or percentage of units that are more than 10 msec in duration (Figure 45.5). The rationale is that in a patient who has changes of chronic reinnervation in the pelvic floor, due per-

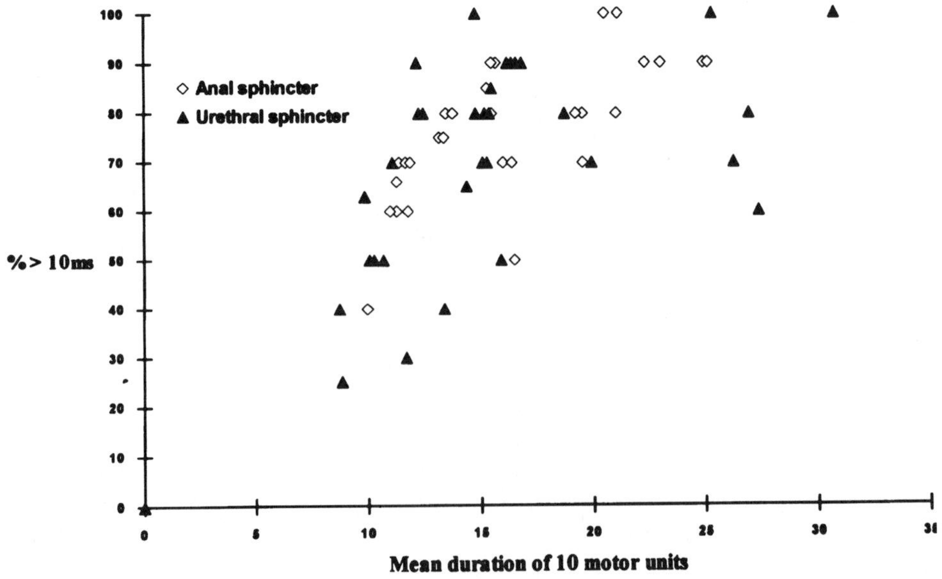

FIGURE 45.5 Urethral and anal sphincter EMG findings in 62 patients with suspected multiple system atrophy. Each symbol represents one patient. The x–axis shows mean duration of 10 separate motor units, and the y–axis shows the percentage of abnormal motor units (i.e., those of >10 msec duration,) in each patient. The normal range occupies a rectangular region in the bottom left-hand corner (% duration of <10 msec <20%) and a mean duration of less than 8.5 msec. (Reprinted with permission from RO Beck, CD Betts, CJ Fowler. Genitourinary dysfunction in multiple system atrophy: clinical features and treatment in 62 cases. J Urol 1994;151:1336–1341.

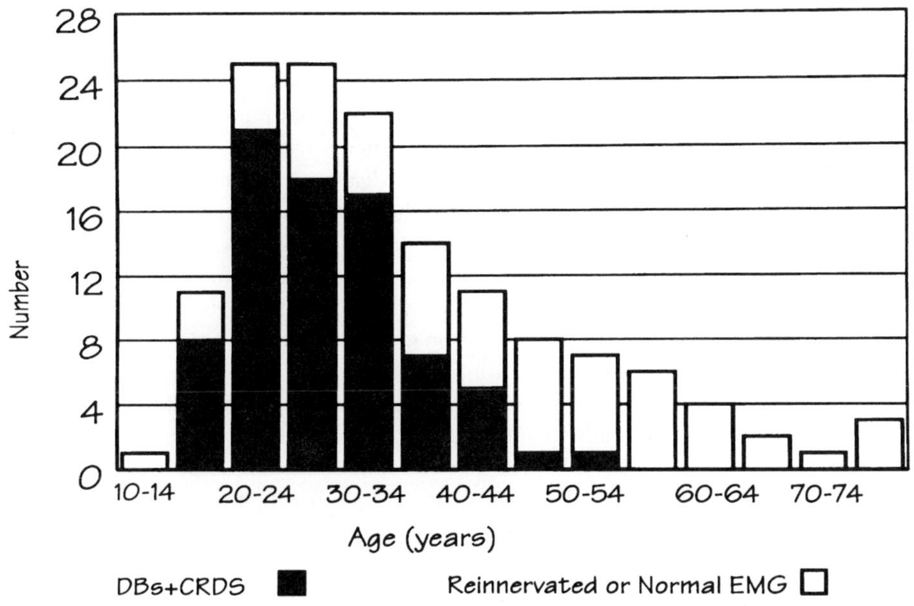

FIGURE 45.6 Urethral sphincter EMG findings in 140 women with urinary retention. "DBs+CRDS" = decelerating bursts and complex repetitive discharges. It is apparent from the figure that this type of EMG activity is the most common finding in young women with urinary retention.

haps to earlier childbirth or possibly lifelong constipation, all the motor units may be moderately prolonged, resulting in an increased mean duration. In MSA, however, the typical finding is of some surviving normal duration motor units together with a variable proportion of extremely prolonged ones. Sphincter EMG is a simple and reliable means of obtaining information that helps establish a diagnosis of probable MSA. This is not only important for the neurologist but also the urologist, since inappropriate surgery can then be avoided. The response to medical management of incontinence, especially in the early stages of the disease, is often very good.

Patients who have struggled with troublesome incontinence for some time usually accept the need for the test. It is probably not indicated if the patient has no urogenital complaints (impotence being a consistent early feature of MSA).

Urinary Retention and Obstructive Voiding in Young Women

Urinary retention in young women has long been an enigma, and in most standard texts the differential diagnosis of this condition is given as either multiple sclerosis (MS) or a psychogenic disorder. Much the same is said about obstructed voiding in young women. However, upper motor neuron signs are not found in these young women. Their bladder disturbance is an isolated complaint, unaccompanied by other definite neurological features. When a diagnosis of MS has been excluded by imaging or other laboratory investigation, no other explanation for the problem remains and the patient may then be referred to a psychiatrist. It is usually possible to elicit from a young woman the history of a recent significant life event, and this, together with authoritative psychiatric opinion, may result in the woman's being told either directly or by insinuation that her problem is psychogenic.

Sphincter EMG of the striated muscle of the urethral sphincter, however, demonstrates that in a very high proportion of these women there is a highly localized electromyographic abnormality (Figure 45.6). Whereas the normal interference pattern recorded from the urethral sphincter is made up of tonically firing motor units, in many young women with urinary retention and some with obstructive voiding, the interference pattern consists of a highly characteristic signal, which has been likened to the underwater recording of whale sounds. The activity is due to a combination of complex repetitive discharges and decelerating bursts. The latter are an electrophysiological variant of complex repetitive discharges in which one of the constituent potentials fires at a progressively decelerating rate. The activity sounds like myotonia, but whereas in myotonia the repetitive activity is due to single muscle fibers firing at a decelerating rate, in the activity recorded from the urethral sphincter it is part of a complex that fires in this way.

It has been proposed that this abnormal spontaneous activity results in an impairment of relaxation of the urethral sphincter, which may cause urinary retention in some women and obstructed voiding in others. Thus, the EMG abnormality can be found in a variety of bladder disorders, because clinical presentation is determined by the behavior of the detrusor, not the urethral sphincter muscle. An association between the occurrence of this electromyographic abnormality in the urethral sphincter and polycystic ovaries has been reported (Fowler et al. 1988).

Despite attempts to treat this primary sphincter disorder with hormonal manipulation, injections of botulinum toxin, application of trinitrate cream, and oral anticonvulsants, no effective therapy has been found. However, the neurophysiological investigation is of value in itself since it eliminates the possibility of a psychogenic disorder. A method of recording from the urethral sphincter using a transvaginal approach (Lowe et al. 1994) has greatly improved the ease and comfort of the test.

Other Neurophysiological Investigations of the Pelvic Floor

Other means of neurophysiological assessment rest largely on measurements of conduction velocities or latency, and therefore correlate less well with function.

The bulbocavernous reflex was the first measurement of nerve conduction to be performed in the sacral region. Stimulation of the dorsal nerve of the penis or clitoris results in a reflex contraction of much of the pelvic floor musculature. The bulbocavernous reflex may be obtained by recording from the bulbocavernous muscle, although synchronous contraction can also be recorded from the sphincters. The latency of this reflex gives an estimate of conduction through the afferent and efferent fibers at the S2–S4 level and a demonstrable delay may be of localizing neurological value.

The limitation of this test is that, as with all reflex studies, it measures only conduction in the fastest fibers, the largest myelinated fibers. Many disorders of urogenital function and impotence in particular are the result of unmyelinated fiber disease, and conduction in those fibers is not tested by this means. Furthermore, normal latency sacral reflexes may be obtained in patients with partial cauda equina lesions. However, a pathologically prolonged response in a patient suspected of having a neurogenic disorder is valuable.

The pudendal evoked potential may be as easily recorded as the tibial evoked potential and, remarkably, has a similar morphology and latency (Figure 45.7), despite the much shorter conduction distance involved. This is thought to reflect the slower conducting afferent pathways of the potential. When first described it was hoped that by recording the pudendal response much could be learned about the afferent innervation of the urogenital tract. However, in practice this has not proved to be the case. Although there have been many reports of abnormal pudendal somatosensory evoked potentials in patients with established neurological disease and urogenital disorders, such as bladder or sexual dysfunction in MS, the diagnostic value of this test is minimal. This is because the spinal cord disease that gives rise to the urogenital disorder and delays conduction of the potential is almost always also clinically evident.

Electrical and magnetic stimulation have been used to measure motor conduction velocity from cortex to muscles in the pelvic floor. Magnetic stimulation has also been used to study spinal conduction between the cortex and sacral spinal cord. Stimulation of the motor cortex to produce a contraction of the pelvic floor requires a higher intensity of stimulation than that needed to produce a contraction in the lower limb, which in turn requires a higher intensity than that required to cause upper limb muscle contraction. This is thought to reflect the interhemispheric location of the cortical representation of the perineum. Despite this, however, it is possible to obtain responses from the sphincters and pelvic floor. Prolonged conduction times in patients with neurogenic bladder disorders have been reported (see Fowler 1995 for review). However, a study showing abnormal conduction times in patients with bladder symptoms who do not have clinical evidence of spinal cord disease has yet to be reported.

Stimulation of the spinal roots has been performed with magnetic stimulation as well as electrical stimulation. The ratio of latencies from stimulating at L1 (or L4) with electrical stimulation and recording from the urethral or anal sphincter gives a "spinal latency," which can be used to detect a cauda equina lesion. Magnetic stimulation of the

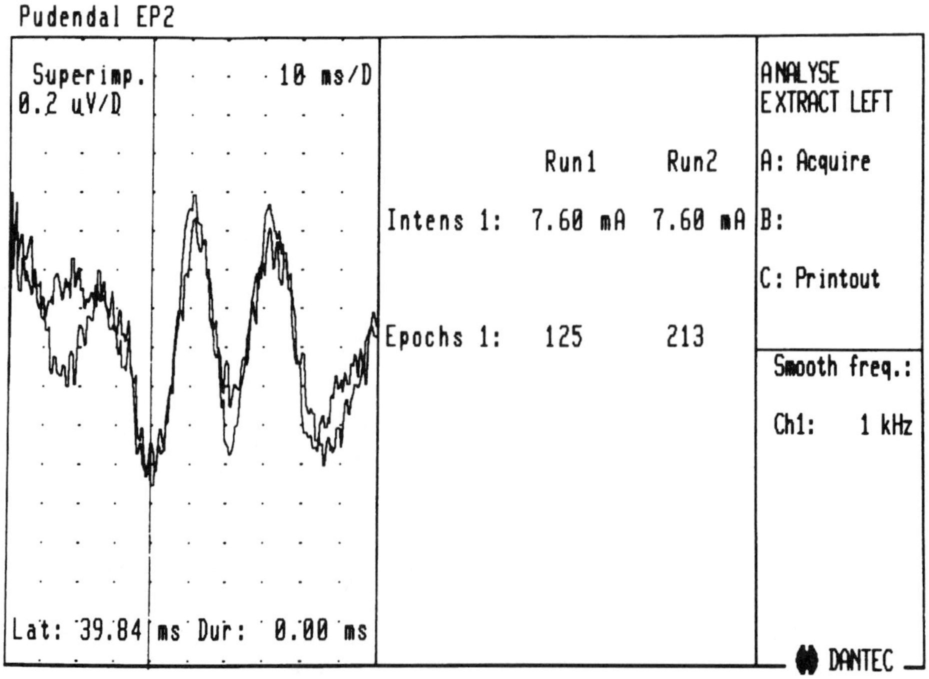

FIGURE 45.7 The pudendal somatosensory evoked potential. In this figure the cursor has been set to measure the latency of the first positive deflection, the P1 or P40 shown here at 39.8 msec. Two evoked potentials have been superimposed to demonstrate the consistency of the response.

sacral roots provides a painless, simple means of testing sacral root conduction. It is important when making recordings in response to central nervous system stimulation to use a needle electrode to record from the sphincter muscles, to avoid volume conducted responses from glutei.

Use of a per-rectal stimulator for measuring terminal pudendal motor latency leads to the identification of abnormally slow conduction in the pudendal nerve in women with idiopathic neurogenic anorectal incontinence, and in women with genuine stress incontinence. Pudendal nerve stimulation proved to be a valuable technique in establishing the pathogenesis of several pelvic floor disorders, but since motor latency is a poor reflection of axonal loss, terminal pudendal motor latency should not be used alone to assess denervation.

To assess the functionally important innervation of the urogenital tract, some means of testing the unmyelinated and small myelinated fibers of the region is required. Different approaches have been taken to this problem, and some success has been achieved by measuring the sympathetic skin responses from the genital region. These potential changes can be obtained using the same technique used for recording from the foot and hand in response to electrical stimulation of the median nerve or for magnetic stimulation of the brain. In some patients with impotence due to diabetic neuropathy, the responses from the perineum cannot be recorded. However, one of the limitations of this method of investigation is that the variation in amplitude of the response is such that a small response cannot be considered abnormal and only an absent response is thought to be significant. Similarities between continuously recorded sympathetic skin responses and the activity that has been called cavernosal EMG are marked (Beck et al. 1995a), and the possibility remains that this latter signal is a form of galvanic skin response.

Changes in local skin blood flow in response to stimuli such as an inspiratory gasp can be measured using laser Doppler. Responses recorded from penile skin give some assessment of genital sympathetic innervation, but it is unclear whether this test is any more sensitive than the galvanic skin response in recognizing a sympathetic deficit.

Because many neuropathies are length-dependent, it has been argued that relevant abnormalities of small-fiber function causing urogenital dysfunction can be detected in the feet of patients with generalized peripheral neuropathy. Testing thermal thresholds in the lower limbs is therefore of particular value in these circumstances.

Neuroimaging

The ease and clarity with which the cauda equina and conus region can be visualized by magnetic resonance imaging (MRI) has made it the investigation of choice in patients suspected of having a structural lesion causing a neurogenic bladder disorder. In conditions of congenital cord malformation, the bony, dural, and intradural abnormalities are clearly shown on MRI (Pang 1993). Plain x-ray films of the region are generally not helpful, because they may be normal with a lesion of the cauda equina, and furthermore spina bifida occulta is a common incidental finding. However, the prevalence of spina bifida occulta at S1 and S2 may be significantly greater in patients with disorders of function of the lower urinary tract.

In acquired lesions of the conus and cauda equina, MRI has replaced myelography as the optimum method of investigation. There is, however, one notable condition that may produce sacral neurological symptoms and may not be apparent on routine MRI scanning—namely, an arteriovenous fistula. The brunt of the neurological deficit in this disorder can affect the cauda equina or conus region (Beck et al. 1995b), despite the fistula's being some distance away. This is thought to be due to the secondary effects of venous hypertension. If this condition is suspected, dynamic gadolinium-enhanced MRI scanning of the entire spinal canal is indicated (Thorpe 1995). Using this technique, pathological vessels have been revealed when routine MRI or myelography were normal. If abnormal blood vessels are seen, spinal arteriography will be necessary as a pretreatment measure.

MANAGEMENT OF BLADDER DISORDERS

Detrusor Hyperreflexia

Detrusor hyperreflexia is the major cause of incontinence in patients with neurogenic bladder disorders. Detrusor hyperreflexia is characterized by the development of spontaneous rises in bladder pressure that the patient is unable to suppress. These usually occur at volumes less than normal capacity so that the patient also complains of frequency. Urgency is felt as the detrusor muscle begins to contract, and if the pressure continues to rise the patient senses impending micturition.

Anticholinergic medications are the mainstay of treatment for detrusor hyperreflexia. Table 45.1 shows those commonly used. It is claimed that oxybutynin has a relatively selective effect on the parasympathetic innervation of the detrusor muscle and that it can be highly effective in reducing neurogenic hyperreflexia, possibly more so than in idiopathic detrusor instability. The most commonly noticed side effect of oxybutynin is a dry mouth. A reasonable recommended starting dose is 2.5 or 3.0 mg twice a day, increasing to 5 mg three times a day. In addition to its anticholinergic effect, oxybutynin also has a local anesthetic action and may be of value by intravesical administration. Some patients are unable to tolerate oxybutynin; alternatives such as propantheline bromide (15–60 mg/day) or imipramine (25–150 mg/day) should be tried.

Desmopressin (DDAVP) spray, first introduced to treat diabetes insipidus, is now being widely prescribed for children with nocturnal enuresis. It has also been used by patients with MS and nighttime frequency. For a disabled patient and his or her partner, the difficulties of the patient having to get up to go to the toilet several times in the night

Table 45.1: Medication for treatment of detrusor hyperreflexia

Oral	
	Oxybutynin
	Propantheline
	Imipramine
Intravesical	
	Oxybutynin
	?Capsaicin

can be considerable. One or two nasal puffs of DDAVP from a metered-dose spray (10–20 μg) administered on retiring reduces urine output for the following 6–8 hours and may significantly lessen nighttime urinary frequency. An oral preparation of DDAVP is now available.

Daytime use seems to be free of ill effects, but it must be stressed to patients that the medication can only be used once in 24 hours. An increased nighttime frequency does not seem to occur in those who have used it during the day. The serum sodium may fall, usually to not less than 132 mmol/liter. If significant hyponatremia does occur, it usually happens within the first week or so of starting the medication, and the chief symptoms are general malaise, headache, and visible edema of the face and ankles. There is a rapid restitution of the sodium level once the medication is stopped.

Animal studies have shown that the lower urinary tract is richly innervated by capsaicin-sensitive afferent neurons. In healthy animals, these afferents are quiescent, although they may be activated by inflammation by bacteria or chemicals, giving rise to the symptoms of cystitis. Under physiological circumstances in animals with an intact spinal cord the detrusor reflexes are transspinal, the afferent limb from the bladder to the spinal cord conveyed by small myelinated A fibers (Figure 45.8). In chronic spinal animals, following a period of spinal shock a new afferent limb from the detrusor emerges as being of dominant functional importance, the afferent fibers of which are unmyelinated C fibers. In the case of the neurogenic bladder, the afferents that drive the volume-determined reflex detrusor contractions are probably capsaicin-sensitive. Capsaicin has a biphasic effect; it is initially an irritant, but if applied in sufficiently high concentration its secondary effect is as a selective neurotoxin acting on unmyelinated afferent C fibers.

We have used intravesical capsaicin in patients with neurogenic bladder disorders, examining its effect on detrusor hyperreflexia in patients with intractable incontinence. We have used 100 ml of a 1- or 2-mmol solution in 30% alcohol and 70% saline. This is instilled into the bladder using a balloon catheter and left for 30 minutes. No patient undergoing this form of treatment has required analgesia or anesthetic, and after the initial intense burning, which lasts 5–15 minutes, discomfort subsides. Pretreatment with intravesical lidocaine may lessen the irritative effects. Following the capsaicin application, the patient's bladder is initially more severely hyperreflexic, and this condition may persist for some days. After that, the bladder either returns to the preinstillation state or loses some of its hyperreflexic behavior so the patient notices decreased incontinence (Fowler et al. 1994).

Incomplete Bladder Emptying or Urinary Retention

The widespread use of intermittent catheterization has had a great impact on the management of the neurogenic bladder. Incomplete emptying can exacerbate detrusor hyperreflexia, and an overactive bladder constantly stimulated by a residual volume will respond by contracting and producing symptoms of urgency and frequency by the mechanism illustrated in Figure 45.9. Incomplete emptying is particularly likely to occur in patients with spinal cord disease due to a combination of detrusor sphincter dyssynergia occurring during attempts to void and poorly sustained detrusor contractions during the voiding phase. A generally accepted figure for significant residual volume is 100 ml. It seems

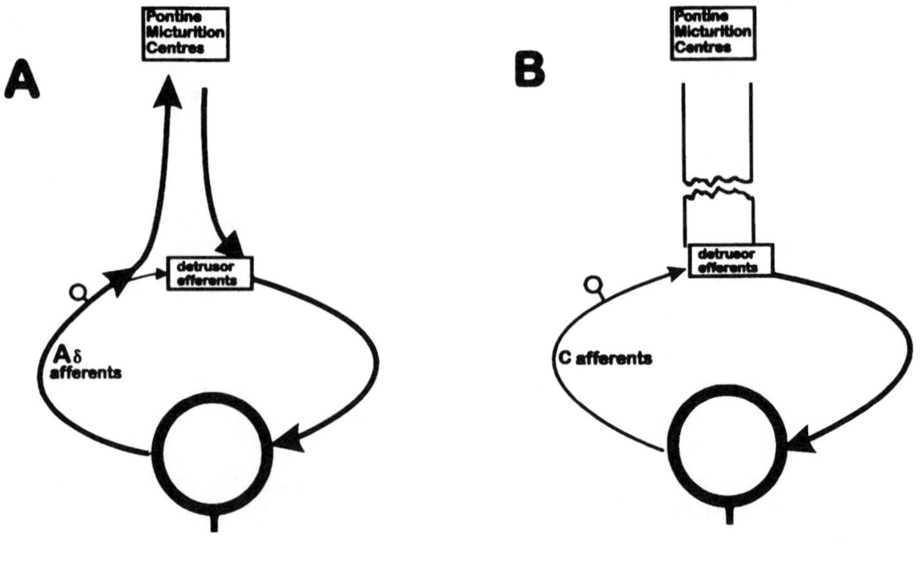

FIGURE 45.8 The route of afferent impulses from the bladder to the pontine micturition center in an individual with an intact spinal cord. A. In health the peripheral bladder afferents are largely Aδ fibers. B. Following transection of the spinal cord a new reflex emerges at a sacral level, the afferents of which are unmyelinated capsaicin-sensitive C fibers.

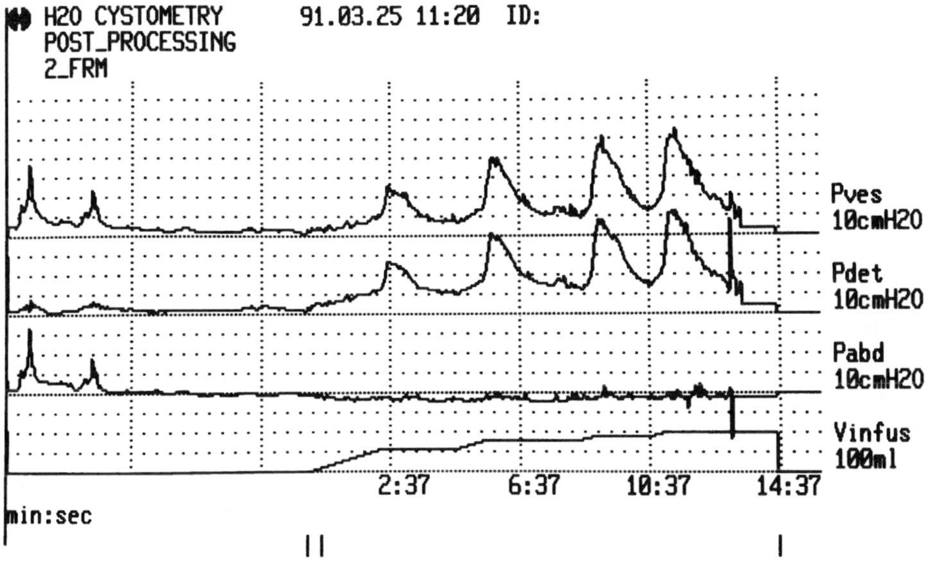

FIGURE 45.9 Cystometric findings in a patient with urge incontinence and a spinal cord lesion due to multiple sclerosis. Contrast this cystometric tracing with that shown in Figure 45.4. The detrusor muscle develops spontaneous pressure rises (Pdet) on filling (Vinfus) and so can be described as hyperreflexic. Hyperreflexive contractions start when the bladder contains only 100 ml. From this it is evident that emptying the bladder by intermittent catherization will improve bladder behavior since by this means, the residual volume, which would otherwise act as a stimulus for hyperreflexic contractions, is removed. Administration of anticholinergic medication lessens hyperreflexic contractions but may also further impair bladder emptying.

that volumes in excess of this may be usefully removed using the technique of intermittent self-catheterization.

Sterile intermittent catheterization was first introduced in the 1960s by Sir Ludwig Guttmann at Stoke Mandeville Hospital. The technique was then popularized by Lapides, who found it was not necessary for the catheterization to be performed using a sterile technique; a clean technique was adequate. Performed for children with spina bifida and the elderly with disorders of complete bladder emptying, it has proved highly effective in many patients with MS and various other bladder disorders characterized by incomplete emptying (Webb et al. 1990).

Patients are often unaware of the extent to which they empty incompletely, and it is not uncommon for both the patient and the doctor to be surprised by the amount of residual volume. For this reason, measurement of this parameter is the single most important measurement to be made when planning bladder management. The volume may be measured either with ultrasound or using in-out catheterization. The advantage of the latter procedure is that it familiarizes the patient with catheterization and so makes teaching the technique of self-catheterization more readily acceptable. Intermittent catheterization is best performed by the patients themselves, who should be taught by someone experienced in the method. In the United Kingdom, nurse continence advisors are particularly expert at this.

A main requirement for success with this technique is patient motivation; a degree of physical disability may be overcome provided the patient is sufficiently determined. As a general rule, if patients are able to write and feed themselves they are likely to be able to perform the technique. Sometimes tremor, impaired visual acuity, spasticity, adductor spasm, and rigidity may make it impossible for the patient to do self-catheterization; in such circumstances it may be performed by a partner or care assistant.

Since the principle of this technique is to reduce the post-micturition residual, most patients are advised initially to perform the technique at least twice a day. There is, however, no fixed limit on how often it should be performed, and it may also be done during the course of the day. It should, however, be performed regularly; the worst possible state of affairs is for the patient to do it very occasionally, since this may provide the opportunity to introduce bacteria but will not have any constant beneficial effect on bladder emptying. Although bacteriuria is noted in 50% of patients doing clean intermittent self-catheterization, the incidence of symptomatic urinary tract infections fortunately is low. Hematuria in the early stages of learning the method is common (Bakke 1993).

In spinal cord disease, a combination of intermittent self-catheterization together with oral oxybutynin deals effectively with both aspects of bladder malfunction, the intermittent catheterization with the incomplete emptying and the oxybutynin with hyperreflexia. In a patient with a borderline significant residual volume, starting oxybutynin may have the effect of increasing it. This should be suspected if oxybutynin has some initial beneficial effect for several days which then disappears. Also, it is advisable for a patient who has marked hesitancy and difficulty in initiating micturition to wait to start oxybutynin until intermittent catheterization is well-established, since otherwise there is a risk that they may become completely unable to pass urine. This combined approach works well in patients with spinal cord disease such as MS, providing that the patient is not too severely disabled. It is also highly effective in the earlier stages of MSA, since incomplete bladder emptying is particularly likely to present a problem in that disorder.

Intermittent self-catheterization is the main means of symptomatic relief in women with urinary retention, although a number of them find the technique unacceptable because of discomfort on withdrawing the catheter, presumably due to the hypertrophied muscle contracting down on the catheter.

External Device

If urge incontinence is the main problem and the bladder empties completely, some men are able to wear an external device attached around the penis. The simplest and least obtrusive is a self-sealing latex condom sheath, which can be put on each night or kept in place for up to 3 days. More elaborate body-worn appliances are also available, but these must be fitted by an expert. An external appliance for women has yet to be devised.

Permanent Indwelling Catheters

Although a combination of anticholinergic medication together with intermittent catheterization is the optimal management for patients with detrusor hyperreflexia and incomplete bladder emptying, there may come a point when the patient is no longer able to perform self-catheterization, or when urge incontinence and frequency are unmanageable. At this point an indwelling catheter becomes necessary. In patients with spinal cord disease this point may be reached when the patient is no longer weight-bearing and is chair-bound.

The most immediate simple solution is an indwelling Foley catheter, a device held in place by an inflatable balloon in the bladder proximal to the catheter opening, but the long-term ill effects of these are well-known. One of the major problems may be leakage of urine around the catheter, which occurs when strong detrusor contractions produce a rapid urine flow that cannot drain sufficiently fast. A common reaction to this is to insert a wider-caliber catheter, with the effect that the bladder closure mechanism becomes progressively stretched and destroyed. The detrusor contractions may be of sufficient intensity to extrude the 10- or 20-ml balloon from the bladder, further rupturing the bladder neck. The end result may then be a totally incompetent bladder neck and urethra. Bladder stones and recurrent, resistant infections are also more likely in a bladder with an indwelling catheter.

A preferred alternative to an indwelling urethral catheter is a suprapubic catheter. This can be inserted under local anesthetic. However, the procedure should only be undertaken by a trained urologist since there is a danger that bowel overlying the bladder may be punctured, especially in patients with small, contracted bladders. Once in situ, the catheter is left on constant drainage. Since no attempt is made to close the urethra (that being a difficult urological procedure), continence depends on the suprapubic drain remaining unimpeded. Should the catheter become blocked or kinked, the patient will leak urethrally. Although by no means a perfect system, a suprapubic catheter is a better alternative to an indwelling urethral catheter and is often the method of choice in managing incontinence in patients for whom other means are no longer effective (Barnes et al. 1993).

Nerve Root Stimulators

In patients who have suffered a complete spinal cord transection but in whom the caudal section of the cord and its roots are intact, the implantation of a nerve root stimulator should be considered. This device was pioneered by Professor Giles Brindley and his collaborators, and about 500 have been implanted worldwide (van Kerrebroeck and Debruyne 1993). The principle on which they work is that the stimulating electrodes that are placed around the lower sacral roots (S2–S4) are activated by an external switching device. The stimulating electrodes are implanted at a neurosurgical procedure and usually are applied intrathecally to the anterior roots, the posterior roots being cut at the same time. After the implant, adjustments are made to the stimulation parameters so that the patient obtains the maximum benefit from the stimulator, in terms of making the bladder contract for voiding, assisting defecation, or producing a penile erection. This is achieved by stimulating individual roots or combinations of roots.

The major benefit from the stimulators is an improvement in urinary continence. This is usually achieved by a combination of increasing bladder capacity, due largely to the posterior rhizotomy that is performed, and improving bladder evacuation. Brindley has argued that women have greater potential gain from these stimulators than men since incontinence in women is more difficult to manage. Moreover, in men the dorsal rhizotomy that is a necessary part of the procedure will abolish any reflex erections that might otherwise be possible. These stimulators are most suitable for patients with complete spinal cord lesions rather than partial cord lesions or progressive neurological disease.

Surgery

Various urological procedures can be carried out to treat incontinence. These are summarized in Table 45.2. Whereas a surgical procedure to rectify a disorder causing incontinence in an otherwise fit and healthy individual is often highly successful, and even following spinal cord injury a surgical option may be the best solution for long-term bladder management, the same does not apply to those with progressive neurological disease causing incontinence. For example, at a time when the bladder is becoming unmanageable by a combination of intermittent catheterization and oxybutynin, the patient with MS may only just be managing to remain independent. This is not the moment to

Table 45.2: Urological operations that may be performed to treat various causes of incontinence

Bladder Disorder	*Surgical Procedure*
Genuine stress incontinence	Bladder neck suspension
Detrusor hyperreflexia	Augmentation cystoplasty
Sphincter failure	Artificial sphincter
Intractable incontinence	Urinary diversion with stoma collection bag

suggest major urological surgery. In practice, very few patients with progressive neurological disease affecting bladder control opt for surgery.

MANAGEMENT OF NEUROGENIC SEXUAL DYSFUNCTION

A discussion of the patient's difficulty is the first step in advising management for sexual dysfunction. The topic can be introduced without embarrassment during explanation of the neurological basis of any coexistent bladder symptoms. An explanation of the neurological basis of sexual dysfunction, sometimes to both partners, may relieve anxieties that have been developing because the problem was thought to be exclusively emotional. The main qualification for undertaking this type of discussion is that the doctor should feel comfortable with it and be able to convey this to the patient. Patients prefer to discuss intimate problems with someone they know already, and this is usually the neurologist they see regularly.

Sexual Dysfunction in Women

Very little is known about sexual dysfunction of women with neurological disease. Problems do undoubtedly occur, although they are rarely complained of and even less often inquired about. Women with spinal cord disease such as MS encounter difficulties with intercourse due to poor bladder control and lower-limb spasticity, in addition to loss of sensation. Loss of perineal sensation is a major problem for women with cauda equina lesions and may be a persisting cause of dissatisfaction, even when adequate means of managing bladder and bowel have been established. The erotic apathy that may occur with temporal lobe epilepsy can be a serious cause of marital disharmony.

Sexual Dysfunction in Men

With the introduction of direct injections of vasoactive agents, which can produce penile erection through smooth-muscle relaxation of the cavernosal vessels, the entire emphasis for investigation and treatment of men with impotence has changed. Prior to this, investigations were aimed at determining whether or not the cause of erectile failure was organic or psychosomatic; if it was the latter, the man was referred for psychosexual counseling. If there was convincing evidence the problem was organic, he might in some circumstances be considered for a penile prosthesis implant. Various neurophysiological investigations were used in an attempt to identify a neurological basis, and nocturnal penile tumescence (NPT) studies were considered to be the major deciding factor. If erections occurred during the night, complaints of impotence were assumed to be psychogenic. Now the limitations of many of the neurophysiological tests and the poor sensitivity of NPT studies have been recognized; men with spinal cord disease may have nighttime erections but be unable to obtain a voluntary erection for intercourse.

Assessment of the response to an intracorporeal injection of a vasoactive substance such as papaverine or prostaglandin E1 provides information about the likely pathogenesis, as well as allowing the man the opportunity to find out what is involved in injecting himself. In terms of diagnostic value, men with either neurogenic or psychogenic erectile difficulties are likely to respond well, while those with vascular disease will not. Most andrologists would take the view that there is little to be gained from trying to make the distinction between a psychogenic and neurogenic cause, since the management is similar.

For men who either do not respond to intracorporeal injection or who wish to use alternative means of treatment, one of the vacuum pump devices can be suggested. These work by inducing tumescence in a rigid cylinder that is placed over the penis and from which the air is pumped by hand. A band is then placed around the base of the penis and the cylinder is removed. For some men, usually those with vascular disease rather than those with progressive neurological illness, implantation of a penile prosthesis can be considered, from a relatively simple semi-rigid or malleable rod to a complex inflatable device (Kirby et al. 1991).

Ejaculatory failure commonly accompanies erectile failure of neurogenic origin, especially in men with spinal cord disease: However, in diabetics, ejaculation seems to be better preserved than erectile function. There is much less that can be done for ejaculatory difficulties, although it is worth trying yohimbine. This substance is obtained from the yohimbine tree, which grows in West Africa. It is an alpha$_2$-adrenergic blocker that is said to facilitate male sexual arousal. A controlled trial of the effect of yohimbine in the treatment of organic erectile impotence showed a small effect when compared to placebo. This medication may be helpful in men seeking treatment for erectile difficulties who are unwilling to perform intracorporeal self-injection. The recommended dosage is either as a starting dose of 10 mg (increasing to 20 mg) taken approximately 2 hours before intercourse is attempted, or 5 mg three times a day taken regularly. Its side effects include a feeling of general excitation, anxiety, nausea, and trembling hands.

Infertility due to ejaculatory failure can be managed by means quite different from those that would be suggested for ejaculatory difficulties. Patients should be referred to a center that specializes in this problem, which is usually to be found in association with a spinal unit.

MANAGEMENT OF FECAL INCONTINENCE

Coordinated lower bowel function depends less on the integrity of the spinal cord than does bladder function. Consequently fecal incontinence is much less common than urinary incontinence in neurological disease. Indeed, the first step in the management of fecal incontinence is to establish the cause (see Chapter 33). It is usually evident from the patient history if the complaint is due to a diarrheal state or urgency of defecation; hence the patient should be referred to a gastroenterologist for investigation. If no cause can be found and the problem persists, symptomatic treatment with a constipating agent that reduces lower bowel motility, such as loperamide, may be helpful.

Many patients with spinal cord disease complain of constipation, and some of them also have occasional fecal incontinence. The reason for the constipation is uncertain, but the incontinence—the involuntary loss of stool—may be because of loss of voluntary control of the pelvic floor. If this occurs the best advice is to suggest the patient use suppositories and attempt to empty the bowel at a predictable and convenient time, thereby lessening the risk of unexpected defecation.

Pelvic floor incompetence can occur in the context of a cauda equina lesion or as the result of more selective neurological injury to the pudendal nerves. Referral to a colorectal surgeon is necessary for consideration of a sphincter repair or postanal repair. Alternatively, a "neosphincter" can be created using healthy nonsphincter striated muscle, such as the gracilis, transposed around the anal canal.

REFERENCES

Bakke A. Physical and psychological complications in patients treated with clean intermittent catheterization. Scan J Urol Nephrol 1993;Supp 150.

Barnes DG, Shaw PJR, Timoney AG et al. Management of neuropathic bladder by suprapubic catheterisation. Br J Urol 1993; 72:169–172.

Beck RO, Betts CD, Fowler CJ. Genitourinary dysfunction in multiple system atrophy: clinical features and treatment in 62 cases. J Urol 1994;151:1336–1341.

Fowler CJ. Pelvic Floor Neurophysiology. In J Osselton (ed), Clinical Neurophysiology. Oxford, England: Butterworth-Heinemann, 1995.

Fowler CJ, Beck RO, Gerrard S et al. Intravesical capsaicin for treatment of detrusor hyperreflexia. J Neurol Neurosurg Psychiatry 1994;57:169–173.

Kirby RS, Carson CC, Webster GD (eds). Impotence: Diagnosis and Management of Male Erectile Dysfunction. Oxford, England: Butterworth-Heinemann, 1991.

Lowe EM, Fowler CJ, Osborne JL, et al. An improved method for needle electromyography (EMG) of the urethral sphincter in women. Neurol Urodyn 1994;13:29–33.

Pang D. Sacral agenesis and caudal spinal cord malformations. Neurosurgery 1993;32:755–779.

van Kerrebroeck P, Debruyne F. Worldwide experience with the Finetech-Brindley sacral anterior root stimulator. Neurol Urodyn 1993;12:497–503.

Versi E, Cardozo L, Cooper DJ. Urethral pressures: analysis of transmission pressure ratios. Br J Urol 1991;68:266–270.

Webb RJ, Lawson AL, Neal DE. Clean intermittent self-catheterisation in 172 adults. Br J Urol 1990;65:20–23.

Chapter 46
Neuroepidemiology

John F. Kurtzke

One useful definition of epidemiology is the science of the natural history of diseases. This concept is based on the original roots of the word: *logos,* from *legein,* to study; *epi,* [what is] upon; *demos,* the people. In epidemiology, the unit of study is a person affected with the disorder in view. Therefore, diagnosis is the essential prerequisite. This is why the neurologist must be an essential part of any inquiry into the epidemiology of neurological diseases.

After diagnosis, the most important question is the frequency of a disorder. Much of the information in this regard has been based on case series—that is, the series of cases encountered by individual practitioners, clinics, or hospitals. However, whether taken as numerator alone (case series) or compared to all admissions (relative frequency), the difficulty with such data is that one has little assurance that what has been included is at all representative of the total affected. Such case material needs to be referenced to its proper denominator, its true source: the finite population at risk.

POPULATION-BASED RATES

Ratios of cases to population, together with the period to which they refer, make up the population-based rates. Those commonly measured are the incidence rate, the mortality rate, and the so-called prevalence rate. They are ordinarily expressed in unit-population values. For example, 10 cases among a community of 20,000 represent a rate of 50 per 100,000 population or 0.5 per 1,000.

The incidence or attack rate is defined as the number of new cases of a disease beginning in a unit of time in a population. This is usually given as an annual incidence rate in cases per 100,000 population per year. The date of onset of clinical symptoms ordinarily decides the time of accession, although occasionally the date of first diagnosis is used.

The mortality or death rate is the number of deaths in a population in a period with this disease as the underlying cause—for example, an annual death rate per 100,000 population. The case-fatality ratio is the proportion of those affected who die from the disease.

The (point) prevalence rate is more properly called a ratio, but it refers to the number of those affected at one time within the community, again expressed per unit of population. If there is no change in case-fatality ratios over time and no change in annual incidence rates (and no migration), then the average annual incidence rate times the average duration of illness in years equals the prevalence rate.

When the numerator and the denominator for a rate each refers to an entire community, their quotient is a crude rate, for all ages. When both terms of the ratio are delimited by age or sex, these are age-specific or sex-specific rates. Such rates for consecutive age groups, from birth to the oldest group of each sex, provide the best description of a disease within a community.

In comparing rates between two communities for a disorder that is age-related (such as stroke or epilepsy), there may be differences in the crude rates solely because of differences in the age distributions of the denominator populations. This can be avoided by comparing only the individual age-specific rates between the two, but this rapidly becomes unwieldy. Methods do exist for adjusting the crude rates, all ages, to permit such comparisons. One such method involves taking for each community each age-specific rate and multiplying it by the proportion of a "standard" population that same age group represents. The sum of all such products provides an age-adjusted (to a standard) rate, or a rate, all ages, adjusted to a standard population. One common standard in the United States is its population for a given census year.

Both incidence and prevalence rates of disease are derived from surveys for a disorder as it occurs within circumscribed populations. Mortality rates come from official published sources. Other epidemiological characteristics of the diseased (associated factors, course, and treatment) should come from population prevalence studies as well, but many of these features are still based on (numerator) case series, which may be strongly biased.

The code used for mortality rates is a three- or four-digit number representing a specific diagnosis within the International Statistical Classification of Diseases, Injuries and Causes of Death (ICD) (World Health Organization 1977). The ICD is revised about every 10 years, and the changes in the tenth revision were major ones. In the United States, the hospital variant is the ICD9CM (clinical modification), which may be replaced by an update.

The great advantage of death rates is their current availability across time and space for many disorders. Geographical distributions are especially informative, since most of the population studies available are, of necessity, spot surveys that may tell us little about areas that were not investigated. Most often, too, the numbers are larger by magnitudes than prevalence studies can provide. The principal disadvantage, and it is a major one, is the question of diagnostic accuracy. There are also problems with coding practices and demographic errors (age and residence in particular).

Space precludes attention to community survey methods, risk factors, survival, treatment comparisons, and statistical methods—all intrinsic aspects of epidemiology (Kurtzke 1992). As for neuroepidemiology per se, the material presented here can be but a sketch of some of the highlights, and only for a few major diseases chosen to represent the field.

CEREBROVASCULAR DISEASE

Cerebrovascular disease (CVD) has been variably classified, particularly in mortality data. The general usage in morbidity studies has been subdivided into (1) subarachnoid hemorrhage (SAH), (2) intracerebral hemorrhage, (3) thrombotic acute brain infarct (ABI) or "cerebral thrombosis," (4) cerebral embolism (often, however, combined with 3 as thromboembolic ABI), and (5) ill-defined acute cerebrovascular accident. Cerebral arteriosclerosis and transient ischemic attacks are generally not included within the corpus of acute cerebrovascular disease or stroke. Reversible ischemic neurological deficit is almost always counted within ABI categories 3 and 4. Little epidemiological attention has thus far been paid to the division of ABI into lacunae versus larger completed strokes.

Mortality Rates

International death rates from stroke have varied notably, with by far the highest rates reported for Japan, followed by nonwhites (especially blacks) in the United States. In Europe, rates for Finland and Scotland have been considerably higher than for neighboring countries. Overall there has been a modest male excess. Average annual age-adjusted (U.S. 1950) death rates in the 1950s have otherwise been near 100 per 100,000 population and, in many countries, closer to 70 per 100,000 in the 1970s and 1980s.

Age-specific death rates demonstrate a logarithmic increase with increasing age; in general, the rate doubles with each additional 5 years of age.

In the United States, the annual age-adjusted death rates have fallen dramatically during this century (Figure 46.1), and the decline has continued. The adjusted rate for 1991 was 27 per 100,000. Even the crude rate showed a steep decline after the mid-1970s. That rate reached 56 per 100,000 for 1992. The decline in the adjusted rates was rather regular over this entire period for white males and females. The much higher rates for nonwhites, some 90% of whom are black, followed a similar but steeper time course for women, but nonwhite males seemed to start their decline only in the 1950s. The rates by sex and race seemed to be converging somewhat by the mid-1980s. However, for 1991 the age-adjusted rates were 27 per 100,000 for white males and 23 for white females, versus 55 and 41 for black males and females, respectively. Thus the decline continues to date for each sex and race, but blacks still have twice the rate as whites.

Similar decreasing rates have been found for other countries between 1950 and 1990, including Australia, New Zealand, Canada, and all of western Europe, but reported rates actually increased for Czechoslovakia, Yugoslavia, Bulgaria, Poland, and Hungary (Thom 1993). An even more dramatic decrease has been recorded in Japan.

Morbidity Rates

Average annual age-adjusted incidence rates by sex show a modest, but possibly increasing, male excess. In the most recent years the annual incidence rate in Europe and North America has been some 120–150 per 100,000 population, and in Asia the rates may now be similar. The age-adjusted rate for Taiwan from 1986 to 1990 was 145. In Hiroshima-Nagasaki, Japan, the age-adjusted incidence rate for cerebral infarction went from 490 per 100,000 in 1972 to 120 in 1988; equivalent rates for cerebral hemorrhage approximated 100 and 20, respectively. Rates in the United States for blacks remain higher than those for whites. Incidence rates rise sharply with age, but not quite as steeply as death rates (Figure 46.2). Including undefined acute CVD, some 80–90% of all strokes in whites are thromboembolic ABI, with some 10–15% as cerebral hemorrhage and 4–8% as SAH. In Asia, the incidence of cerebral hemorrhage still seems twice as high as in the West, but there has never been any definite excess for SAH in the Orient.

The declining death rate from stroke alluded to earlier has been confirmed by incidence surveys. The more recent surveys have rates well below those of older vintage. The constant proportions over time suggest that this decrease should

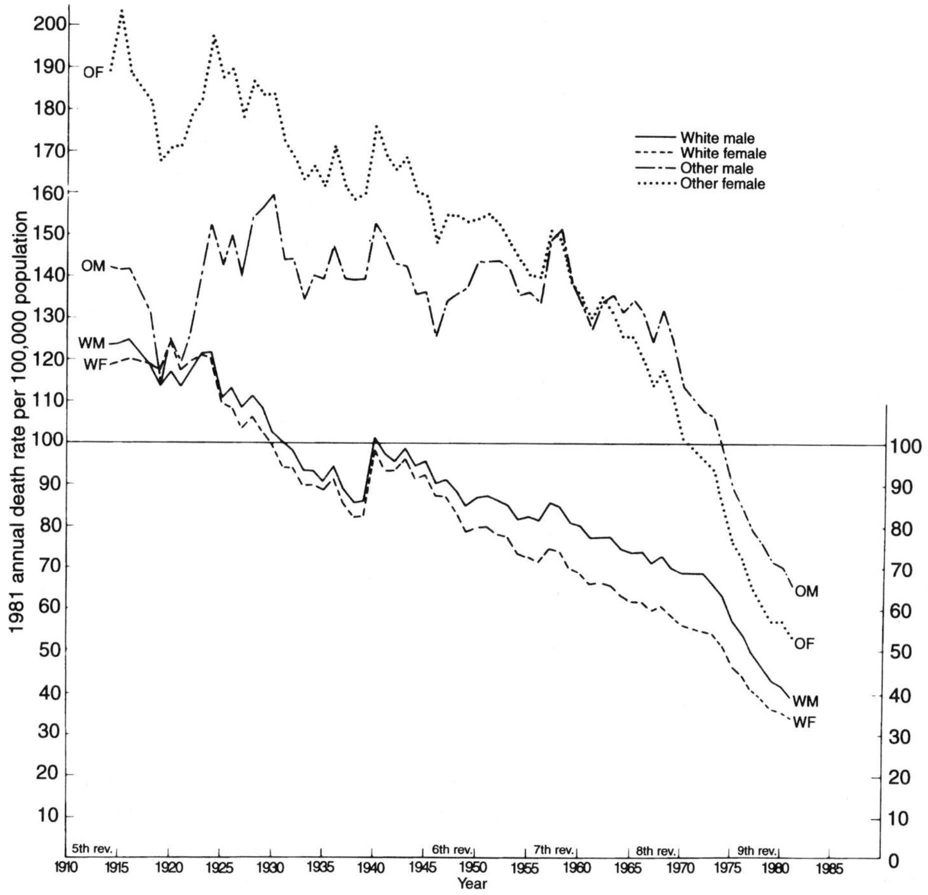

FIGURE 46.1 Cerebrovascular disease. Annual age-adjusted (U.S. 1940) death rates per 100,000 population by sex and color, United States, 1915–1981; white males and females (WM, WF) and nonwhite males and females (OM, OF). (Reprinted with permission from JF Kurtzke. Epidemiology of Cerebrovascular Disease. In FH McDowell, LR Caplan [eds], Cerebrovascular Survey Report for the National Institute of Neurological and Communicative Disorders and Stroke. Revised. White Plains, NY: Burke Rehabilitation Center; 1985;1–34.)

be for both cerebral hemorrhage and ABI. In Rochester, Minnesota, the age-adjusted average annual incidence rate declined from 200 per 100,000 population from 1945 to 1954 to 107 for 1975–1979 (see Figure 46.2). The decrease was for both sexes, for essentially all ages, and for both cerebral hemorrhage and thrombosis; it was not found for SAH, though. However, the adjusted rate for all stroke was 117 from 1980 to 1984, perhaps signaling an end to the decline.

Incidence studies have confirmed the geographical variations noted for death rates. In Japan, China, and Finland, and among blacks in the United States, all had high rates. The highest rates were in the northwestern United Kingdom and in the southeastern ("cotton belt") United States.

Prevalence rates in the early 1980s were around 600 per 100,000 in the West and 900 in Asia; more recent works were not found. Age-specific prevalence rates doubled with each 10-year age increase. Taking a prevalence of 600 and an incidence of 150, the average duration of life after a cerebrovascular accident—all types, all ages—would be on the order of 4 years.

Transient Ischemic Attacks

Transient ischemic attacks (TIAs) are ordinarily excluded from the category of stroke. Average annual incidence rates in the Occident are about 30 per 100,000 population, again with a slight excess for males. Age-specific rates rise with age, but much less steeply than rates for stroke itself. This is true also for age-specific prevalence rates, which overall in whites are about 150 per 100,000 for all ages. In China, age-adjusted to U.S. 1960 population rates for TIA were about 50 for incidence and 200 for prevalence.

PRIMARY NEOPLASMS

In clinical experience, some 85% of primary central nervous system (CNS) tumors are intracranial and 15% are intraspinal. For the brain, the major groupings are the gliomas (40–50%, of which about half are glioblastoma multiforme) and the meningiomas (some 15–20%). Pituitary adenomas plus neurilemomas, especially acoustic, add another 15–20%. The most common spinal cord tumors are neurofibroma and meningioma, followed by ependymoma and angioma.

Mortality Rates

From the sixth through the eighth revisions of the ICD, which was in use from 1949 to 1978, primary CNS tumors

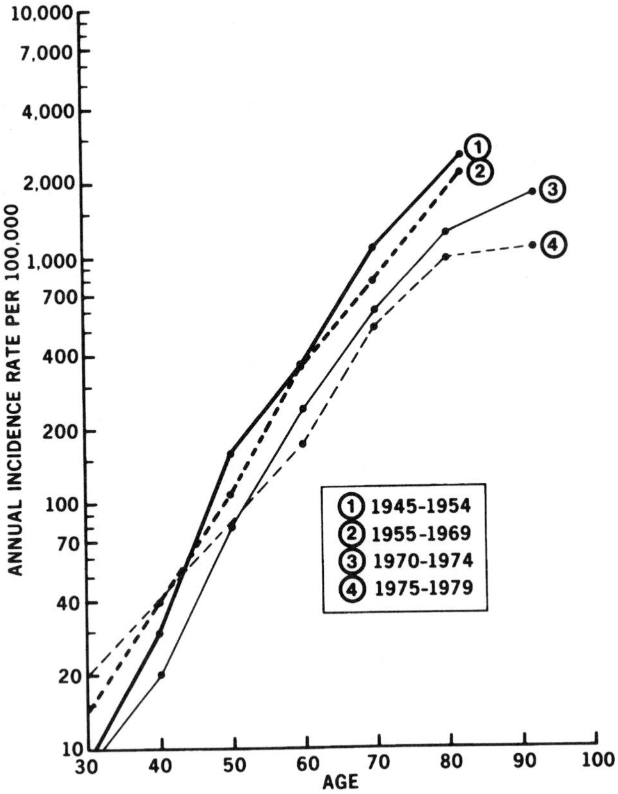

FIGURE 46.2 Cerebrovascular disease. Average annual age-specific incidence rates per 100,000 population on a logarithmic scale for rates against age for four consecutive intervals between 1945 and 1979 in Rochester, Minnesota. (Reprinted with permission from JF Kurtzke. An Introduction to the Epidemiology of Cerebrovascular Disease. In Fondation de l'Academie Nationale de Medecine: Prevention des Accidents Vasculaires Cerebraux. Paris: Academie Nationale de Medecine, 1984;11–24.)

were separately coded as malignant, benign, and of unspecified nature. The sum of these groups provided the total for deaths attributed to CNS neoplasm. The codes, however, excluded pineal, pituitary, and Rathke pouch tumors, and usually, tumors of the optic nerve. In ICD8, for 1969 through 1978, malignant tumors of the brain itself were separated out. For ICD9, there was no code for tumors of unspecified nature. Thus, total CNS tumor death data are available only for 1949 through 1978, but malignant brain tumor is separately coded from 1969 to the present.

International death rates for all primary CNS tumors in the 1950s were remarkably uniform among countries, at about 4–5 per 100,000 population, but the proportions attributed to the three types differed markedly. In the 1970s rates were mostly 5–8 per 100,000, but still not greatly discrepant among different nations.

In the United States for 1959–1961, malignant CNS tumor deaths by age showed a steep rise from very low rates in early adult life to a peak of around 14 per 100,000 by age 60, followed by a steep decline with further increasing age. There was a notable excess in this group of whites over nonwhites, with rates two to three times higher. There was also, for all races, a 2 to 1 excess of affected males.

The age configuration and the sex and race differences were also found for malignant brain tumor alone, and this cause of death can well be attributed to glioblastoma multiforme.

There is no single cell type to which benign CNS tumor deaths can be assigned, but meningioma provides an increasing proportion, especially beyond midlife. Around 1960 the U.S. death rates were 0.5 for whites and 0.6 for nonwhites; in the former, the male and female rates were 0.5 and 0.6, respectively. These differences were statistically significant.

The age-specific death rates for benign tumors varied only slightly throughout life; there was at best a modest increase at ages 55–74. As for tumors of unspecified nature, the age distribution showed a somewhat higher peak at these ages, doubtless reflecting the mixture of benign and malignant tumors. This grouping also showed a minimal male and nonwhite excess rate, the former for the same reason, the latter perhaps reflecting a lower level of diagnostic availability at that time.

Morbidity Rates

The morbidity data for CNS neoplasms that follow were based on information up to 1985. Later information does not alter appreciably the ensuing comments (e.g., for brain: Radhakrishnan et al. 1994; and for spinal cord: Preston-Martin 1990).

Average annual incidence rates for primary brain tumors in the more complete surveys have ranged mostly between 10 and 15 per 100,000 population, including pituitary tumor rates at 1–2 per 100,000. Primary tumors of the spinal cord are recorded at about 1 per 100,000, and in one survey peripheral nerve tumors had a rate of 1.5.

In all but the Rochester, Minnesota, studies, age-specific incidence rates for glioblastoma multiforme have shown a sharp peak at about age 60. In the Rochester study, the rate continued to rise with increasing age, especially when tumors first diagnosed at postmortem were included. The male predilection inferred from death data is seen for the entire glioma group, and in particular for glioblastoma (Figure 46.3). Some soft data support the black-white difference in death rates. There is also some evidence to suggest an increasing incidence of glioblastoma in recent years. A similar trend was also seen in malignant brain tumor death rates over time.

In meningioma, the age-specific rates continue to rise with age to the oldest group, and there is a female preponderance. The suspected excess in blacks was borne out in a survey in the Los Angeles County Cancer Surveillance program. Age-adjusted average annual incidence rates were 1.8 per 100,000 male and 2.7 female. Respective non-Hispanic white rates were 1.8 and 2.5; for blacks they were 2.5 and 3.6. In Rochester, Minnesota, annual incidence rates for all cases were 4.9 male and 5.8 female for 1935–1977, but

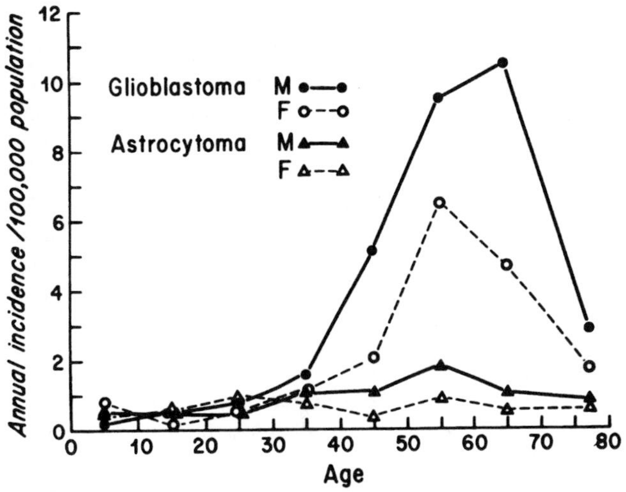

FIGURE 46.3 Glioblastoma and astrocytoma. Average annual age-specific incidence rates per 100,000 population by sex, Denmark, 1953–1957. (Reprinted with permission from JF Kurtzke, LT Kurland. The Epidemiology of Neurologic Disease. In AB Baker, LH Baker [eds], Clinical Neurology. Vol. 4. Philadelphia: Harper & Row, 1983;1–143.)

only 1.2 and 2.6 for cases diagnosed antemortem. The true rate for meningiomas, then, would seem to be around 5 per 100,000 population.

There is good evidence that in the United States the several cancer surveillance programs, which are routine reporting systems, provide a notable undercount for all brain tumors. This is especially pertinent for the Los Angeles meningioma rates, where cases were further delimited to those only with a tissue diagnosis—not really a necessity for meningioma.

An overall estimate for malignant intracranial tumors is about 5 per 100,000 population, most of which is attributed to glioblastoma multiforme. For benign brain tumors, a reasonable figure would be 10 per 100,000: 5 for meningioma, and between 1 and 2 each for benign gliomas, pituitary tumor, and all others.

Reported 5-year survival ratios have been about 60% for clinically diagnosed meningioma and some 20% for gliomas as a group. Median survival for glioblastoma has been about 1 year after diagnosis. Taken together, median survival for benign brain tumors may be estimated at 6 years. With an annual incidence of 5 per 100,000 population and average survival of 1 year, the point prevalence rate for malignant brain tumors would also be 5 per 100,000. In like manner, for benign brain tumors one would expect a prevalence of 60 per 100,000.

An entity that now needs consideration as a major CNS tumor is primary lymphoma. This previously rare tumor has become increasingly more common with the epidemic of the acquired immunodeficiency syndrome (AIDS). If the incidence of this disease continues to increase at the present rate, it may be the most common primary malignant neoplasm of the CNS in adults by the year 2000.

While analysis of risk factors for CNS tumors is beyond the scope of this chapter, an important work on tumors following childhood radiation for tinea capitis was presented by Ron et al. (1988). The 30-year cumulative relative risk for those so exposed versus matched population controls and unexposed siblings was 6.9 for all tumors, 8.4 for neural tumors of head and neck. Relative risk was 9.5 for meningiomas, 2.6 for gliomas, 18.8 for nerve sheath tumors, and 3.4 for other neural tumors; all risk ratios but those for gliomas were statistically significant.

CONVULSIVE DISORDERS

Classification of convulsive disorders or the epilepsies has varied considerably. For epidemiological purposes, they have been divided into (1) epilepsy, (2) isolated (single) seizures, (3) febrile convulsions, and (4) acute symptomatic seizures. Patients categorized as having epilepsy are usually subdivided into idiopathic or primary, and secondary. Secondary epilepsy has a presumed cause, with recurrent seizures after recovery from the acute insult. All partial-focal or focal-onset seizures are by definition secondary. Absence seizures are almost always primary or idiopathic, as are many, but not all, grand mal seizures.

Mortality Rates

Epilepsy as an underlying cause of death should be limited to primary seizure disorders; secondary seizures should be only a contributory cause. In the 1950s international death rates for epilepsy were highest for several Central and South American countries, Portugal, and U.S. nonwhites. The lowest rates were for U.S. whites and in Sweden, Denmark, Poland, and Israel. Most other countries had an annual mortality rate around 2 per 100,000 population. Rates in the 1970s, however, averaged closer to 1 per 100,000.

In the United States (in 1955 and for 1959–1961), age-specific death rates for whites with epilepsy as the underlying cause remained virtually even throughout adulthood, whereas the rates for all deaths related to epilepsy showed an increase with age. Rates for nonwhites were higher, particularly among men, than for whites. These racial differences were even more marked when deaths from epilepsy as both an underlying and a contributory cause were included.

Geographically, there was little patterning to the rates by state of residence for whites, except for some evidence of a modest East (high) to West (low) gradient. Rates for nonwhites by state showed both a Southeast and a Midwest concentration. Because of the residence patterns of the several races, the former would be compatible with an excess rate in blacks, and the latter would suggest the possibility of an excess in Native Americans as well. Taken together, the findings suggest a disorder rather equally distributed by geography, but not by race.

Death rates for epilepsy in the United States have declined by more than half between 1940 and the mid-1970s, with the greatest rate of change between 1945 (2.0 per 100,000) and 1960 (1.0)—with the introduction and increasing use of phenytoin. There was almost no change from 1974 through 1979 (0.8). The prior decrease was shared by both sexes and colors. Since 1968 the white-nonwhite gap had been lessening. The rate in 1986 was 0.7 per 100,000, with 0.6 for white males and females, but 1.7 and 1.0 for black males and females, respectively.

Morbidity Rates

Point prevalence and average annual incidence rates for epilepsy have been obtained in a number of community surveys. In general, the prevalence of convulsive disorders is about 3–9 per 1,000 population. In Bogota, Colombia, there was a strikingly high rate, 19.5 per 1,000, which included inactive seizure disorders. An overall estimate of the point prevalence of active epilepsy may be taken as about 6 or 7 per 1,000 population. Prevalence rates have tended to increase in recent years in several surveys. Males and blacks do have higher rates than females and whites.

Between 1979 and 1987, prevalence for active epilepsy was 5.1 per 1,000 in Vecchiano, Italy; 6.3 in Kuopio CHD, Finland; 6.8 in Rochester, Minnesota; and 8.0 in northern Ecuador. Follow-up of a United Kingdom birth cohort showed a rate of 4.3 per 1,000 at age 10 years. An extremely high rate of 57.2 per 1,000 was reported for a geographic isolate of Guaymi Indians in Changuinola, Panama, in 1988; family history of seizures had relative risk (RR) of 13.9 and a history of febrile seizures RR of 5.6, but neither cases nor controls showed seropositivity for cysticercus. Neurocysticercosis, however, was found in half the clinic patients with adult-onset seizures in Mexico City, and is otherwise a common entity in Latin America.

Average annual incidence rates as of 1980 were from about 20–70 per 100,000 population per year. There was a slight male excess, which averaged about 1.2 to 1, and almost a 2 to 1 black-white ratio. Later surveys showed annual rates of 24 per 100,000 for Kuopio CHD, Finland; 34 for Vasterbotten, Sweden; and 48 for Rochester, Minnesota. The aforementioned study of northern Ecuador provided an annual incidence rate of 190 per 100,000 from 1985 to 1986. The relatively low prevalence rate of 8.0 suggests notably decreased survival with an incidence such as this. We seem to have support for a high frequency of epilepsy in Central and South America, as suggested by death and prevalence rates. Elsewhere in the West an expected range for annual incidence would be some 30–60 per 100,000 with a reasonable general estimate of 50. With the concomitant prevalence rates, an average duration of active seizure disorders could then be calculated as about 13 years.

Age-specific incidence rates for epilepsy from several surveys showed a sharp decrease from maximal rates in infancy to adolescence and thereafter a slow decline for new cases throughout life. In others, rates were essentially constant after infancy or showed an irregular rise with age. In Rochester, Minnesota, however, the configuration was U-shaped, with a marked increase in incidence rates at age 75 and over. This configuration reflects generalized tonic-clonic disorders, together with absence and myoclonic seizures for the left arm of the U, and partial epilepsies for the right arm.

Age-specific incidence rates according to each type of seizure are shown for Rochester (Figure 46.4). Myoclonic seizures were the major type diagnosed during the first year of life; they were also the most common in the 1- to 4-year age group, but rarely occurred after 5 years of age. Absence (petit mal) seizures peaked in the 1- to 4-year age group and were not seen to begin in patients older than 20. Complex partial (psychomotor) and generalized tonic clonic (grand mal) seizures both had fairly consistent incidence rates of 5–15 per 100,000 in ages 5–69 after low maxima at ages 1–4; for age 70 and over, the rates of each were sharply higher. The grand mal rates had similar configuration for both primary and secondary seizures. Simple partial (focal) seizures increased only slightly with age.

Febrile Seizures

The risk of a child's developing febrile seizures has been about 2%, varying between 1% and 4%, in the United States and Europe. Surveys from Japan and the Mariana Islands showed rates of 7% and 11%, respectively. The Guaymi Indians of Panama had a rate of 14%. As with epilepsy in general, there was a male preponderance of 1.2 to 1 for febrile convulsions. In most studies recurrent febrile fits occur in about one-third of the cases, and overall the risk of later epilepsy is about 4% to 2% for simple and 11% for complex febrile seizures. The latter risk was just 6% by age 10 in the United Kingdom birth-cohort follow-up. A risk of 6% overall for later epilepsy has been reported in Tokyo, with discriminant analysis scores supporting a similar discrepancy between simple and complex febrile seizures.

Symptomatic and Single Seizures

In Rochester, Minnesota, the incidence rate of identified acute symptomatic seizures (those part of an active underlying disease) was near 15 per 100,000 per year. The age-specific incidence rates had the same U-shaped distribution as did epilepsy, with the highest rates in the very young and the most elderly. The major single causes were alcohol or drug withdrawal (21%), cerebrovascular disease (15%), trauma (15%), neoplastic or cardiac (14%), infection (10%), metabolic (8%),

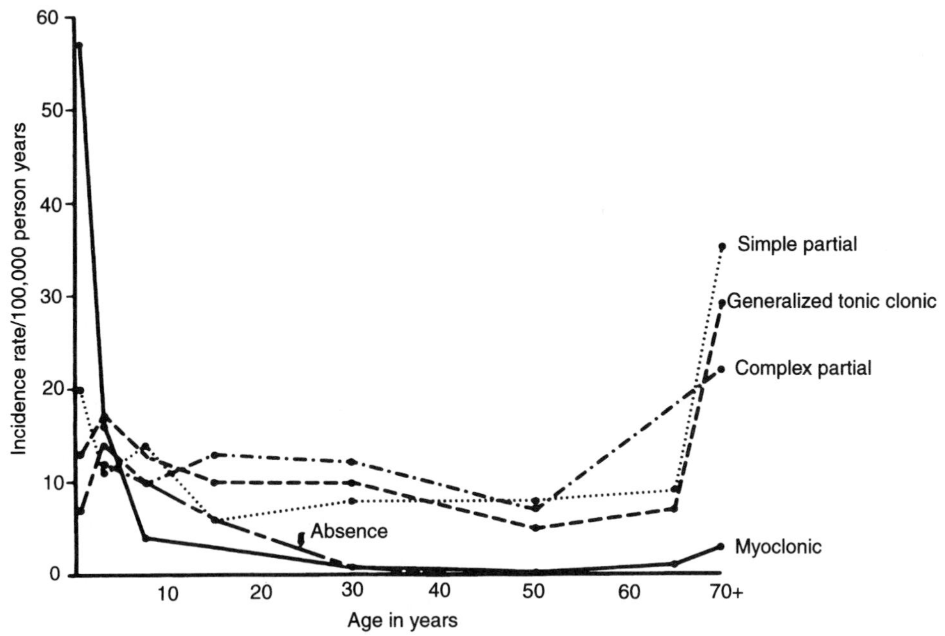

FIGURE 46.4 Epilepsy. Average annual age-specific incidences rates per 100,000 population by clinical type of seizure (absence, myoclonic, generalized, simple/complex partial). (Reprinted with permission from JF Kurtzke, LT Kurland. The Epidemiology of Neurologic Disease. In AB Baker, LH Baker [eds], Clinical Neurology. Vol. 4. Philadelphia: Harper & Row, 1983;1–143.)

eclampsia (6%), and toxic (3%). For a more urban population, the first category (withdrawal) would be appreciably higher and the U shape of the curve less pronounced. Persistent seizures due to prior insults comprised one-third of the incident cases of epilepsy in Rochester from 1935 to 1984. By cause, these were vascular (11% of total epilepsy), congenital (8%), trauma (6%), neoplastic (4%), degenerative (4%), and infection (3%), for an overall incidence rate of 15 per 100,000; the average incidence for idiopathic epilepsy was 29.

The incidence rate for single or isolated unprovoked seizures in Rochester was approximately 20 per 100,000 per year. Many of the patients, however, had received anticonvulsant medication from the time of the seizure. Isolated, unprovoked seizures comprised 18% of new seizure–onset patients in Minneapolis; recurrent seizures (epilepsy) were observed within 5 years in 34% of these patients, and the frequency was similar whether or not anticonvulsant medication had been used.

MULTIPLE SCLEROSIS

Mortality Rates

International death rates for multiple sclerosis (MS) in the 1950s ranged from well over 3 per 100,000 to almost zero. The highest rates were those for Northern Ireland, Scotland, and the Republic of Ireland. Other Western European countries had rates of 2 per 100,000, except for the northernmost lands of Norway, Sweden, and Finland, and the Mediterranean countries of Greece, Italy, and Portugal. The rates for the two groupings were closer to 1 per 100,000, similar to those for Canada, Australia, New Zealand, and in the United States among whites; nonwhites in the United States had half the rate of whites. Lowest by far were rates from Asia, Africa, and the Caribbean.

In the United States for 1959–1961, the average annual age-adjusted death rate for MS was 0.8 per 100,000 population, with a slight female and marked white preponderance. Geographically, all states south of the 37 degree parallel of north latitude showed low death rates, whereas rates in almost all states to the north of this line were well in excess of the national mean. This was true for residents at birth and at death, and for whites alone as well as for all residents.

Morbidity Rates

Prevalence rates for Europe and the Mediterranean basin as of 1980 are plotted against geographical latitude in Figure 46.5. The surveys appeared to separate into two zones or clusters, one to the north with rates of 30 and over, considered high frequency, and the other to the south with rates below 30 but above 4 per 100,000 population, classified as medium frequency.

The northernmost parts of Scandinavia and the Mediterranean basin then made up the medium-prevalence regions. More recent surveys of Italy and its islands, however, have documented prevalence rates well into the 60s, and therefore this country is now clearly within the high-frequency band (Kurtzke 1993). This appears to be a recent change, since at least some of the earlier Italian surveys with lower rates were well done.

The general worldwide distribution of MS may be described within these three zones of frequency or risk. The

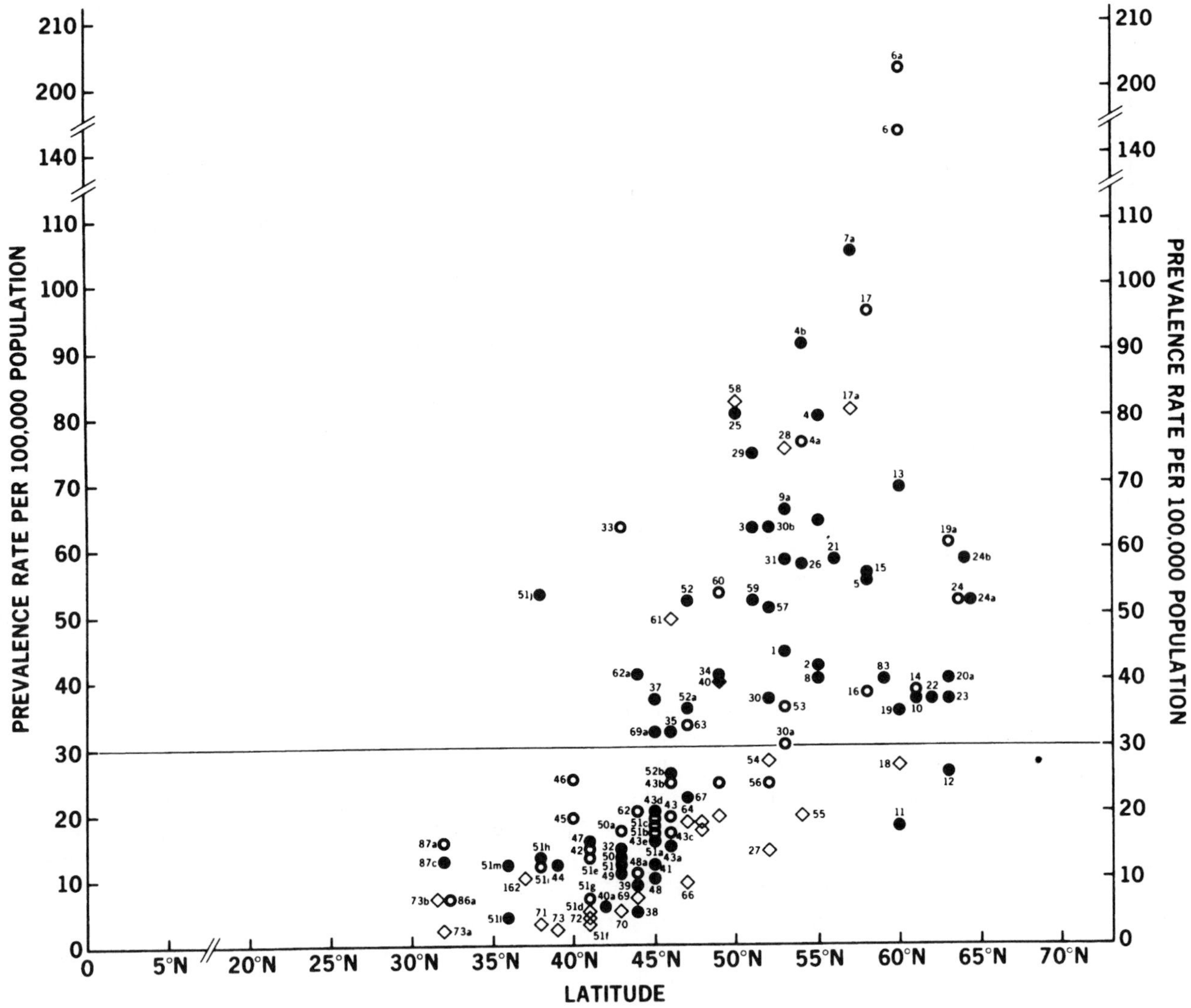

FIGURE 46.5 Multiple sclerosis (MS). Prevalence rates per 100,000 population for probable MS in Europe and the Mediterranean area as of 1980, correlated with geographic latitude. Numbers identify studies in Kurtzke (1980). Solid circles represent class A (best) surveys, open circles class B, open diamonds class C, and closed diamonds class E (MS:ALS case ratios). Class C (poor) studies are listed only if no better quality survey was available for the specific site. (Reprinted with permission from JF Kurtzke. Geographic distribution of multiple sclerosis: An update with special reference to Europe and the Mediterranean basin. Acta Neurol Scand 1980;62:65–80. © 1980 Munksgaard International Publishers Ltd., Copenhagen, Denmark.)

high-risk zone, with prevalence rates reported up to 1980 of 30 and above per 100,000 population, includes northern and central Europe into the former Soviet Union, the northern United States, Canada, New Zealand, and southeastern Australia. These regions were bounded by areas of medium frequency, with prevalence rates to that date between 5 and 29 per 100,000, consisting of the southern United States, southwestern Norway and northernmost Scandinavia, and probably Russia from the Ural mountains into Siberia, as well as the Ukraine. Except for Italy, now with high rates, the entire northern Mediterranean basin from Spain to Israel was of medium prevalence. In this zone, too, still fall most of Australia and perhaps Hawaii and the midportion of South America, plus whites in South Africa. Low-frequency areas, with prevalence rates below 5 per 100,000, comprise all other known areas of Asia and Africa, Alaska and Greenland, and the Caribbean region including Mexico and probably northern South America. Recent data suggest medium rates in the North African littoral and high rates in Israel and Cyprus (Kurtzke 1993).

It is clear, then, that MS is a place-related disorder. All the high- and medium-risk areas are found in Europe or the European colonies: Canada, the United States, Australia, New Zealand, South Africa, and probably central and southern South America. It seems likely, therefore, that MS originated in northwestern Europe and was brought to the other lands by European settlers. In Europe itself, although the disease clearly has shown geographical clustering in some countries, there is evidence even within these clusters of a diffusion over time.

In the United States, white females are at greater risk than white males; blacks, Native Americans, and Asians all are at notably lower risk than whites. These race and sex differences persist regardless of geography.

The annual incidence rate in high-MS areas at present is about 3–5 per 100,000 population, whereas in low-risk areas it is about 1 per 1,000,000; in medium areas the incidence is near 1 per 100,000. In Denmark in 1939–1945, age-specific incidence rates rose rapidly from essentially zero in childhood to a peak at about age 27 of more than 9 per 100,000 for females and almost 7 for males. Beyond age 40 there was little difference between the sexes, both of whose rates declined equally to zero by age 60.

Migration in Multiple Sclerosis

If the risk of MS is altered by a change of environments, then MS must be an acquired, exogenous, environmental disease or diseases. In a number of studies of MS in migrants, there was a tendency for immigrants to retain much, but not all, of the risk of their birthplace if they came from high- or medium-risk areas, but also evidence that low- to high-risk migrants had increased their risk of MS. A large case control series among U.S. veterans demonstrated clearly a change in risk of MS by changing residence between birth and entry into service: Those moving south decreased their risk; those moving north increased it. This series also indicated that the time when such moves are critical is well after birth but also well before clinical onset.

There are other studies for migrants from high- to low-risk areas that also suggest a critical age for risk retention: Those migrating at age 15 or older retained the MS risk of their birthplace, but those migrating before age 15 acquired the lower risk of their new residence. This also indicates that young children are not susceptible.

As part of our studies on MS in the Faroe Islands (see below), we identified a group of 12 patients who had been living, for at least 3 years before onset, off the islands in high–MS risk Denmark. These long overseas residences were limited to the 10 years or so before clinical onset. All of the patients stayed at least 2 years between ages 11 and 43, for a minimum of 2 years. We concluded that residence in a high-risk MS area by a susceptible but virgin (as to MS) population for a period of 2 years from age 11 could result in clinical MS, which would begin after a further incubation period of some 6 or 7 years (Kurtzke et al. 1993).

A group of migrants was identified in France coming from North Africa among some 8,000 cases of MS ascertained in France in 1986. Of these migrants, 219 out of 246 had onset after migration. There was a relatively fixed interval between immigration and clinical onset regardless of age; assuming susceptibility begins at age 12 years, the average interval to clinical onset from age 12, or age at immigration if older, was 12.3 years (Kurtzke 1993).

Epidemics of Multiple Sclerosis

The Faroe Islands are a semi-independent unit of the Kingdom of Denmark in the North Atlantic Ocean between Iceland and Norway. As of 1986, we had found 32 native resident Faroese with onset of MS in this century. There were none before 1943, but between 1943 and 1949, 16 patients had symptom onset in this populace of less than 30,000; another 16 began between 1950 and 1973, but none thereafter to 1986—and there were by then 45,000 Faroese on the islands.

Annual incidence rates described a trimodal distribution, with an early high peak exceeding 10 per 100,000 population in 1945, followed by two successively lower and later peaks. If the Faroese migrants required 2 years' exposure from age 11 in order to acquire MS, the same should be true for these Faroese. Two years before 1943 mean 1941 and 1942. We therefore divided the resident series according to time at age 11: by 1941 or later. When this was done, we clearly had three separate groups of MS cases (Figure 46.6). Annual incidence rates demonstrate the three epidemics these patients provided, which was shown to have high statistical significance. However, as of 1991, we had a new epidemic IV, with seven cases with clinical onset during 1984–1989, and three more cases in epidemic III (Figure 46.7). The existence of the fourth epidemic was in fact predicted by our transmission models; see below (Kurtzke et al. 1993).

We concluded that the disease was introduced into the Islands by British troops who occupied the islands for 5 years starting in April 1940. What was introduced must have been an infection transmitted during the war to the Faroese population at risk, of whom the epidemic I cases of clinical MS were a part. We called this infection the primary multiple sclerosis affection (PMSA), which we defined as a single, specific, widespread, systemic infectious disease (which may be totally asymptomatic). PMSA will produce clinical neurological MS (CNMS) in only a small proportion of the affected after an incubation period averaging 6 years in virgin populations, and perhaps 12 years in endemic areas. Using this hypothesis, transmissibility is limited to part or all of this systemic phase, which ends by the usual age of onset of MS symptoms.

The PMSA cases from the first cohort of Faroese transmitted the disease to the next Faroese population cohort, those who reached age 11 in the period when the first cohort was transmissible. Included in the second Faroese cohort were the epidemic II cases of CNMS, and this cohort similarly transmitted PMSA to the third population cohort with its own (epidemic III) cases, and from there to the fourth cohort with epidemic IV.

Two years of exposure between age 11 and 47 are therefore required to acquire PMSA in virgin but susceptible populations. Thus, we believe that PMSA is a specific, but unknown, age-limited infection that can be acquired only during these hormonally active years, and one that only rarely will lead to clinical MS.

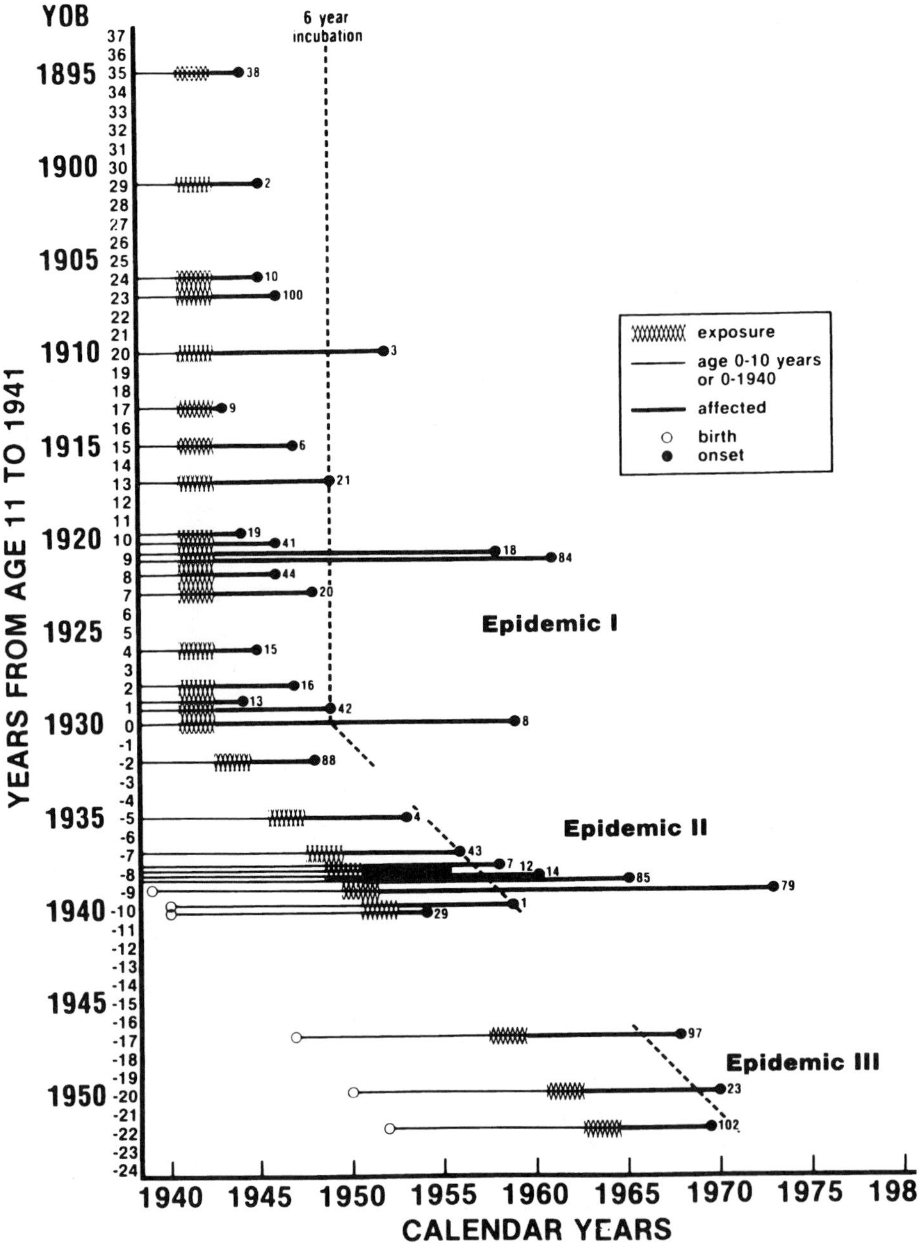

FIGURE 46.6 Multiple sclerosis in the Faroe Islands as of 1986. Identification of each native resident patient by calendar time when age 11, whether by 1941 or later, and by time of clinical onset. Each patient is represented by a bar, and the number at the end of each bar identifies the patient in Kurtzke and Hyllested (1987). The thin portion of the bar represents time and ages for each patient before exposure to PMSA (the primary MS affection; see text); the 2 years of crosshatching represent the period of PMSA exposure, following which (heavy portion of the bar) the patient is affected but neurologically asymptomatic (the incubation period). Solid circles at the terminus of each bar represent time and age of clinical onset. The open circle at the origin of the lower bars represents time of birth for patients born after 1938. The y-axis defines the number of years by each year from 1941 at which time each patient attained age 11, with the calendar years reflecting their year of birth (YOB) also identified. The dashed vertical and oblique line represents the end of a 6-year incubation period from time of acquisition of PMSA after 2 years exposure. (Reprinted with permission from JF Kurtzke, K Hyllested. Multiple sclerosis in the Faroe Islands. III. An alternative assessment of the three epidemics. Acta Neurol Scand 1987;76:317–339.© 1987 Munksgaard International Publishers Ltd., Copenhagen, Denmark.)

OVERVIEW OF NEUROLOGICAL DISORDERS

Following are the best estimates to date of the numerical impact of neurological diseases. The data refer primarily to whites of the Occident. For the 66 disorders of Tables 46.1 and 46.2, the average annual incidence rates add up to over 2,500 per 100,000 population, or 2.5%. This includes eight disorders for which only one-tenth of the incident cases were thought to require neurological attention. These are the two vertebrogenic pain syndromes, nonmigrainous headache, nonbrain head injury, alcoholism, psychosis, nonsevere mental retardation, and deafness. Total blindness numbers were taken as an estimate for the proportion of all the visually impaired that the neurologist should encounter. Even if we exclude from consideration all headaches, trauma, vertebrogenic pain, visual loss, deafness, and psychosis, there are still over 1,100 new cases of neurological disease beginning each year in every 100,000 of the population, or more than one case for every 100 people.

For the 61 disorders of Tables 46.3 and 46.4, the point prevalence rates in like manner contain only 10% of the nonmigrainous headache, vertebrogenic pain, alcoholism, and nonbrain head injury, and 20% of migraine, but they exclude completely all mental retardation, psychosis, deafness, and blindness. The total exceeds 9,500 per 100,000 population. Again, if we exclude entirely all the states just

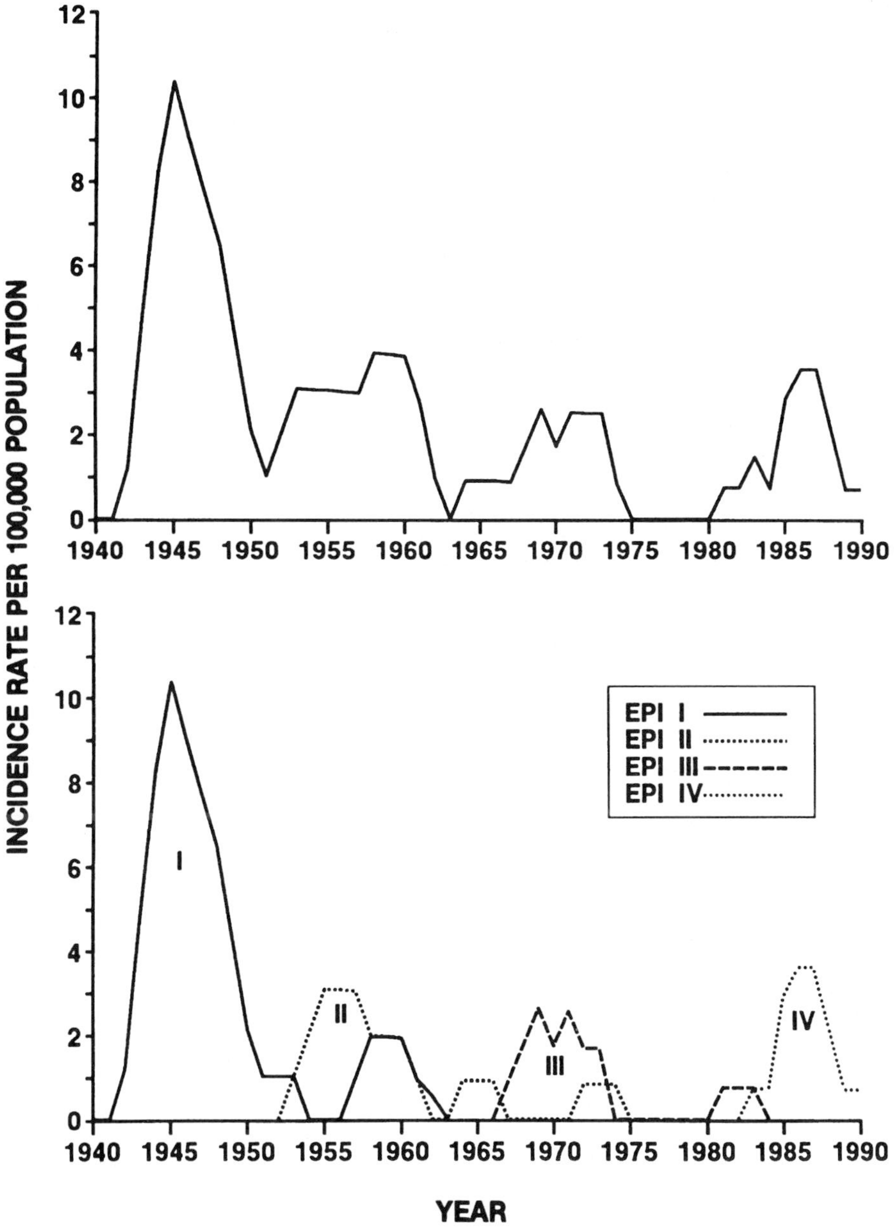

FIGURE 46.7 Multiple sclerosis in the Faroes as of 1991. Annual incidence rates per 100,000 population calculated as 3-year centered moving averages for four epidemics defined by time when patients were age 11: by 1941 or later. Top: total series. Bottom: rates by epidemic. (Reprinted with permission from JF Kurtzke, K Hyllested, A Heltberg et al. Multiple sclerosis in the Faroe Islands. 5. The occurrence of the fourth epidemic as validation of transmission. Acta Neurol Scand 1993;88: 161–173.© 1993 Munksgaard International Publishers Ltd., Copenhagen, Denmark.)

mentioned, there is still a prevalence rate of almost 3,600 per 100,000 population, or 3.6% of the people who at any one time require the care of a physician competent in clinical neurology. In a U.S. population of 240 million, this means 8.6 million people.

There are arguments, however, as to what such numbers really denote in terms of the number of neurologists required. In the United States, patient care needs alone for 240 million people were estimated to require 14,000 neurologists, according to the American Neurological Association-American Academy of Neurology (ANA-AAN) Joint Commission on Neurology, but other similar estimates were 11,200 (Graduate Medical Education National Advisory Committee [GMENAC] Delphi Panel), 6,200 (GMENAC Advisory Panel), and 12,600 (Committee on National Needs for Neurologists [CN3], AAN) (Kurtzke et al. 1986). The last source estimated total needs for clinical neurologists, including faculty, at some 16,500 neurologists, twice the figure of the GMENAC Advisory Panel. The primary discrepancy for patient care needs is not so much with the frequency of neurological disorders, but rather with differences in the proportions of patients that each group thought should be seen by neurologists, and, if so, whether only acutely or throughout the course of the illness: Are neurologists to be consultants or practitioners? The total-needs figure for the GMENAC Advisory Panel, furthermore, was based on a marked undercount of current faculty neurologists.

Predictions of the numbers of neurologists in the United States have been wide in their range. A survey of all residency training programs in 1985–1986 and recalculations

Table 46.1: Neurological disorders: Approximate average annual incidence rates (per 100,000 population), all ages. 1. Most common entities

Disorder	*Rate*
Herpes zoster	400
Migraine	250
Brain trauma	200
Other severe headache[a]	200[a]
Acute cerebrovascular disease	150
Other head injury[a]	150[a]
Transient postconcussive syndrome	150
Lumbosacral herniated nucleus pulposus	150
Lumbosacral pain syndrome[a]	150[a]
Neurological symptoms (with no defined disease)	75
Epilepsy	50
Febrile fits	50
Dementia	50
Ménière's disease	50
Mononeuropathies	40
Polyneuropathy	40
Transient ischemic attacks	30
Bell's palsy	25
Single seizures	20
Parkinsonism	20
Cervical pain syndrome[a]	20[a]
Persistent postconcussive syndrome	20
Alcoholism[a]	20[a]
Meningitides	15
Encephalitides	15
Sleep disorders[b]	15[b]
Subarachnoid hemorrhage	15
Cervical herniated nucleus pulposus	15
Metastatic brain tumor	15
Peripheral nerve trauma	15
Blindness	15
Benign brain tumor	10
Deafness[a]	10[a]

[a]Rate for those who should be seen by a physician competent in neurology (10% of total).
[b]Narcolepsies and hypersomnias (with sleep apnea).
Source: Modified from JF Kurtzke. The current neurologic burden of illness and injury in the United States. Neurology 1982;32:1207–1214.

Table 46.2: Neurological disorders: Approximate average annual incidence rates (per 100,000 population), all ages. 2. Less common entities

Disorder	*Rate*
Cerebral palsy	9
Congenital malformations of central nervous system	7
Mental retardation, severe	6
Mental retardation, other[a]	6[a]
Malignant primary brain tumor	5
Metastatic cord tumor	5
Tic douloureux	4
Multiple sclerosis[b]	3[b]
Optic neuritis[b]	3[b]
Dorsolateral sclerosis	3
Functional psychosis[a]	3[a]
Spinal cord injury	3
Motor neuron disease	2
Down's syndrome	2
Guillain-Barré syndrome	2
Intracranial abscess	1
Benign cord tumor	1
Cranial nerve trama	1
Acute transverse myelopathy	0.8
All muscular dystrophies	0.7
Chronic progressive myelopathy	0.5
Polymyositis	0.5
Syringomyelia	0.4
Hereditary ataxias	0.4
Huntington's disease	0.4
Myasthenia gravis	0.4
Acute disseminated encephalomyelitis	0.2
Charcot-Marie-Tooth	0.2
Spinal muscular atrophy	0.2
Familial spastic paraplegia	0.1
Wilson's disease	0.1
Malignant primary cord tumor	0.1
Vascular disease cord	0.1

[a]Rates for those who should be seen by a physician competent in neurology (10% of total).
[b]Rate for high-risk areas.
Source: Modified from JF Kurtzke. The current neurologic burden of illness and injury in the United States. Neurology 1982;32:1207–1214; and JF Kurtzke, LT Kurland. The Epidemiology of Neurologic Disease. In A Baker, LH Baker (eds), Clinical Neurology. Vol. 4. Philadelphia: Harper & Row, 1983;1–143.

by actuarial methods estimated the number of general neurologists to be 7,500 for 1990, plus 1,100 child neurologists, for a total of 8,600. The figure for the year 2000 was 11,800 total. The number of neurologists was then predicted to plateau near the year 2020 at some 13,700, including 1,700 child neurologists, of whom 9,800 (1,100 child) would be board-certified (Kurtzke et al. 1991). These total figures are about 30% (in 2010) to 35% (in 2050) (Figure 46.8). Neurology is not, nor do I believe it will be, an overstocked specialty in the United States—if neurologists are permitted to practice neurology as it has developed there.

Neurological practice, of course, varies widely among countries and, indeed, even within the United States. The neurologist as a physician directly responsible for both acute and chronic care of patients with neurological diseases has evolved only over the last quarter century in the United States. But such responsibilities, as well as provisions for continuity of care, are explicit statements in the current special requirements for residency training programs in neurology and in child neurology.

Regardless of the type of practice a given country deems appropriate for neurologists, the patients will still exist. The data in Tables 46.1 through 46.4, therefore, could well serve as a basis at least for a rational allocation of available resources in any country for the teaching, research, and patient care of neurological disorders.

Table 46.3: Neurological disorders: Approximate point prevalence rates per 100,000 population, all ages. 1. Most common entities

Disorder	*Rate*
Migraine[a]	2,000[a]
Other severe headache[a]	1,500[a]
Brain injury	800
Epilepsy	650
Acute cerebrovascular disease	600
Lumbosacral pain syndrome[a]	500[a]
Alcoholism[a]	500[a]
Sleep disorders[b]	300
Ménière's disease	300
Lumbosacral herniated nucleus pulposus	300
Cerebral palsy	250
Dementia	250
Parkinsonism	200
Transient ischemic attacks	150
Febrile fits	100
Persistent postconcussive syndrome	80
Herpes zoster	80
Congenital malformations of central nervous system	70
Single seizures	60
Multiple sclerosis[c]	60
Benign brain tumor	60
Cervical pain syndrome[a]	60[a]
Down's syndrome	50
Subarachnoid hemorrhage	50
Cervical herniated nucleus pulposus	50
Transient postconcussive syndrome	50
Spinal cord injury	50

[a]Rate for those who should be seen by a physician competent in neurology (20% of migraine, 10% of all others).
[b]Narcolepsies and hypersomnias (with sleep apnea).
[c]Rate for high-risk areas.
Source: Modified from JF Kurtzke. The current neurologic burden of illness and injury in the United States. Neurology 1982;32:1207–1214.

Table 46.4: Neurological disorders: Approximate point prevalence rates per 100,000 population, all ages. 2. Less common entities

Disorder	*Rate*
Tic douloureux	40
Neurological symptoms without defined disease	40
Mononeuropathies	40
Polyneuropathies	40
Dorsolateral sclerosis	30
Peripheral nerve trauma	30
Other head injury*	30*
Acute transverse myelopathy	15
Metastic brain tumor	15
Chronic progressive myelopathy	10
Optic neuritis	10
Encephalitides	10
Vascular disease cord	9
Hereditary ataxias	8
Syringomyelia	7
Motor neuron disease	6
Polymyositis	6
Progressive muscular dystrophy	6
Malignant primary brain tumor	5
Metastatic cord tumor	5
Meningitides	5
Bell's palsy	5
Huntington's disease	5
Charcot-Marie-Tooth disease	5
Myasthenia gravis	4
Familial spastic paraplegia	3
Intracranial abscess	2
Cranial nerve trauma	2
Myotonic dystrophy	2
Spinal muscular atrophy	2
Guillain-Barré syndrome	1
Wilson's disease	1
Acute disseminated encephalomyelitis	0.6
Dystonia musculorum deformans	0.3

*Rate for those who should be seen by a physician competent in neurology (10% of total).
Source: Modified from JF Kurtzke. The current neurologic burden of illness and injury in the United States. Neurology 1982;32:1207–1214; and JF Kurtzke, LT Kurland. The Epidemiology of Neurologic Disease. In A Baker, LH Baker (eds), Clinical Neurology. Vol. 4. Philadelphia: Harper & Row, 1983;1–143.

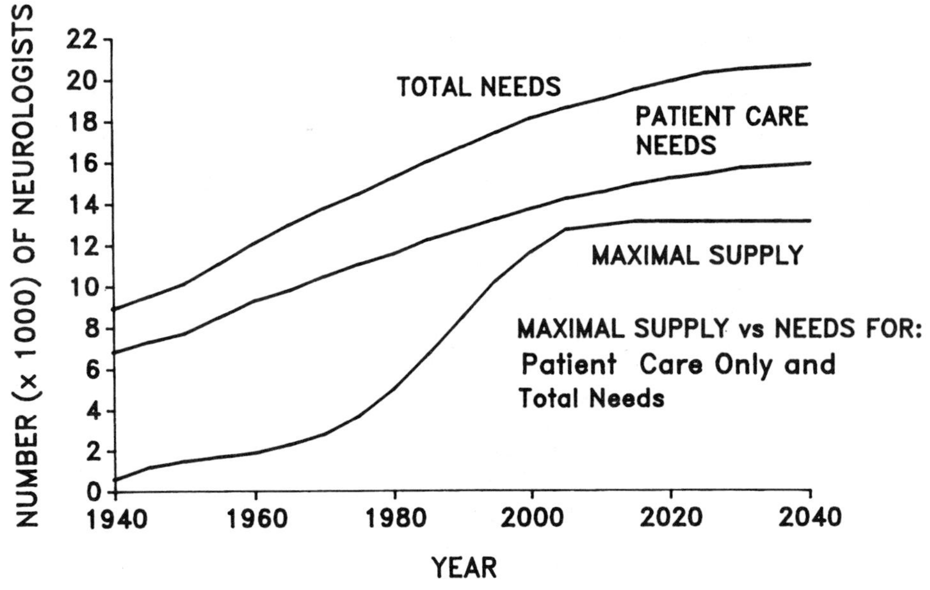

FIGURE 46.8 Neurologists in the United States, 1940–2040. Estimated maximal supply versus needs (patient care needs alone and total needs). (Reprinted with permission from JF Kurtzke, FM Murphy, MA Smith. On the production of neurologists in the United States: an update. Neurology 1991;41:1–9.)

REFERENCES

Kurtzke JF. Geographic distribution of multiple sclerosis: an update with special reference to Europe and the Mediterranean basin. Acta Neurol Scand 1980;62:65–80.

Kurtzke JF. The current neurologic burden of illness and injury in the United States. Neurology 1982;32:1207–1214.

Kurtzke JF, Kurland LT. The Epidemiology of Neurologic Disease. In AB Baker, LH Baker (eds), Clinical Neurology. Vol. 4. Philadelphia: Harper & Row, 1983;1–143.

Kurtzke JF. An Introduction to the Epidemiology of Cerebrovascular Disease. In Fondation de l'Academie Nationale de Medecine: Prevention des Accidents Vasculaires Cerebraux. Paris: Academie Nationale de Medecine, 1984;11–24.

Kurtzke JF. Epidemiology of Cerebrovascular Disease. In FH McDowell, LR Caplan (eds), Cerebrovascular Survey Report for the National Institute of Neurological and Communicative Disorders and Stroke. Revised. White Plains, NY: Burke Rehabilitation Center, 1985;1–34.

Kurtzke JF, Bennett DR, Berg BO et al. On national needs for neurologists in the United States. Neurology 1986;36:383–388.

Kurtzke JF, Hyllested K. Multiple sclerosis in the Faroe Islands. III. An alternative assessment of the three epidemics. Acta Neurol Scand. 1987;76:317–339.

Kurtzke JF, Murphy FM, Smith MA. On the production of neurologists in the United States: an update. Neurology 1991;41:1–9.

Kurtzke JF. Neuroepidemiology. In RJ Joynt (ed), Clinical Neurology (revised). Vol. 4. Philadelphia: Lippincott, 1992;1–29.

Kurtzke JF. Epidemiologic evidence for multiple sclerosis as an infection. Clin Microbiol Rev 1993;6:382–487.

Kurtzke JF, Hyllested K, Heltberg A et al. Multiple sclerosis in the Faroe Islands. 5. The occurrence of the fourth epidemic as validation of transmission. Acta Neurol Scand 1993;88:161–173.

Preston-Martin S. Descriptive epidemiology of primary tumors of the spinal cord and meninges in Los Angeles County, 1972–1985. Neuroepidemiology 1990;9:106–111.

Radhakrishnan K, Bohnen NI, Kurland LT. Epidemiology of Brain Tumors. In Morantz RA, Walsh JW (eds), Brain Tumors. A Comprehensive Text. New York: Marcel Dekker, 1994;1–18.

Ron E, Modan B, Boice JD Jr, et al. Tumors of the brain and nervous system after radiotherapy in childhood. N Engl J Med 1988;319:1033–1039.

Thom TJ. Stroke mortality trends: an international perspective. Ann Epidemiol 1993;3:509–518.

Chapter 47
Clinical Neurogenetics

Thomas D. Bird

To appreciate the variety and complexity of genetic influences in neurological diseases, one must first understand the basic principles of human inheritance patterns. This chapter is an introduction to the various modes of inheritance, including single gene (Mendelian), chromosomal, multifactorial, and mitochondrial. More recent insights regarding imprinting, anticipation, and uniparental disomy are also briefly discussed. Furthermore, there are likely to be many patients with a neurological disorder that is the result of a combination between a genetic predisposition and an environmentally acquired insult. All these phenomena are of clinical importance and form an introduction for a more detailed analysis of the relevant molecular biology.

MENDELIAN DISORDERS

Mendelian disorders are caused by mutations in single genes. They can be autosomal-dominant, autosomal-recessive, or X-linked.

Autosomal Dominant Disorders

The 46 chromosomes contained in the nucleus of each human cell represent 22 pairs of autosomes, one of each pair being inherited from the mother and the other from the father (Figure 47.1). The twenty-third pair contains the sex chromosomes, the Y inherited from the father and the X from the mother. In autosomal dominant disorders, a mutation occurring in a single gene on any of the 22 autosomes can produce clinical symptoms or signs. The carrier of a single mutation on one chromosome is called a *heterozygote*. Each child of an affected person has a 50% risk of inheriting the mutation and potentially developing the disease. Males and females are affected in equal proportions; the disease appears over multiple generations, and heterozygote mothers or fathers pass the gene on with equal risk to sons or daughters (Figure 47.2 and Table 47.1).

Examples of autosomal dominant neurological disorders include neurofibromatosis, tuberous sclerosis, Huntington's disease, several forms of hereditary ataxias and hereditary neuropathies, myotonic dystrophy, juvenile myoclonic epilepsy, benign neonatal convulsions, and some forms of familial Alzheimer's disease.

Expression of a gene refers to any clinical manifestation of the mutation. This could include a seizure, mental retardation, skin lesions, an abnormal electroencephalogram (EEG), a movement disorder, dementia, or slow nerve conduction velocities. *Phenotype* refers to the observed biochemical, physiological, or clinical manifestations in an individual. *Genotype* refers to the genetic constitution of an individual, specifically the alleles at one chromosomal locus.

Penetrance of a gene refers to the proportion of gene carriers who show any clinical expression. For example, if out of 100 known carriers of a mutation there are 80 with some clinical manifestation and 20 without, the gene is said to show 80% penetrance. Penetrance is age- and test-dependent. That is, a gene such as Huntington's disease may show only 10% penetrance at age 20, but 90% penetrance at age 60. Also, the recorded penetrance of a gene may increase with more detailed and careful testing and examination. For example, the apparent penetrance of the tuberous sclerosis gene will increase with careful skin examination and magnetic resonance imaging (MRI) of individuals at risk. Likewise, asymptomatic carriers of a putative epilepsy gene may have only an abnormal EEG and no seizures.

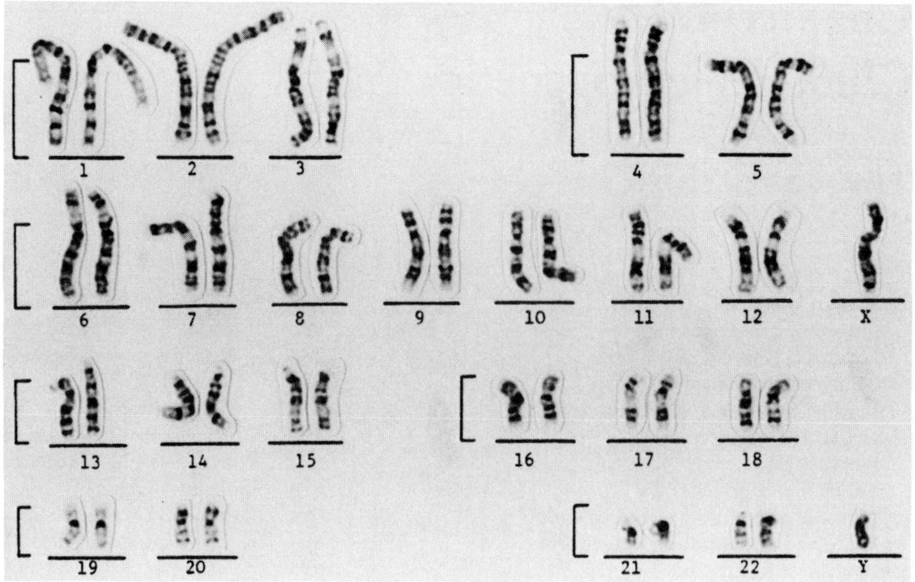

FIGURE 47.1 A normal male karyotype. The chromosomes are in the early metaphase stage of mitosis. The 22 pairs of autosomes and one pair of sex chromosomes are distinguished by their size and arm ratio, and by each chromosome's unique pattern of transverse bands. The chromosomes here are stained by the Giemsa banding technique. Note that this male karyotype has one X and one Y chromosome. A normal female karyotype would have 2 Xs and no Y. (Photomicrograph courtesy of I. Teshima.)

Gene *carrier* was used to refer only to asymptomatic persons having a mutant allele (gene) for a recessive disorder. Nowadays, it may refer to any person having an abnormal gene, symptomatic or asymptomatic, recessive or dominant.

For some mutations, the heterozygous carrier may show mild manifestations of the disease, whereas the *homozygous* carrier of a mutant gene at the same locus on a chromosome pair demonstrates much more severe clinical manifestations. An example of this is familial hypercholesterolemia, in which a heterozygous carrier may have myocardial infarction at age 48, whereas a homozygote (having inherited the mutation from each parent) may have a coronary occlusion at age 12. This phenomenon tends to blur the distinction between dominant and recessive diseases. On the other hand, for some dominant mutations such as Huntington's disease, the homozygous state is no worse than the heterozygous state. Huntington's disease, therefore, acts like a "true" dominant disorder.

Genetic heterogeneity refers to the phenomenon in which similar clinical phenotypes are the result of entirely different genetic mutations. For example, the Charcot-Marie-Tooth (CMT) hereditary neuropathy syndrome can be the result of different mutations in at least three different chromosomal loci (chromosomes 1, 17, and X) (Vance and Bird 1993). Likewise, there are more than four different dominant mutations causing hereditary ataxias. Clinical examination does not usually reveal which gene is involved.

Different forms of a gene at one locus are called *alleles*. If different mutations in the same gene each cause a clinical disorder, this is called *allelic genetic heterogeneity*. If mutations in different genes at different chromosomal loci each cause a similar disorder, it is called *nonallelic genetic heterogeneity*.

Autosomal Recessive Disorders

With autosomal recessive inheritance, the heterozygous carriers of a single mutation are usually clinically normal; rarely, they may show some signs (manifesting heterozygotes). However, individuals who have inherited a mutation in the same gene from both parents (homozygotes) will show clinical manifestations of the disease. If both parents are carriers of a mutation in the same gene, then each of

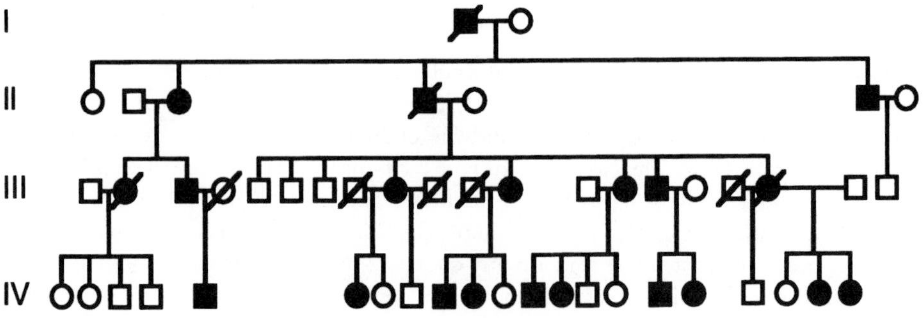

FIGURE 47.2 Pedigree demonstrating autosomal dominant inheritance in a family with Charcot-Marie-Tooth (CMT) neuropathy. Squares indicate males, circles indicate females, and solid symbols represent persons affected with the disease. A slash through a symbol indicates a death. Note that multiple generations are involved, males and females are affected, and there is transmission from father to son (male-to-male).

Table 47.1: Patterns of inheritance

Autosomal Dominant	*Autosomal Recessive*	*X-Linked Inheritance*	*Mitochondrial*
50% risk to each child	25% risk of homozygosity	Carrier females have: 50% risk to sons 50% risk to daughters	Transmission via females only
Males and females affected in equal proportions	Males and females affected in equal proportions	Affected males have: 0% risk to sons All daughters are carriers	All children at risk
Male-to-male transmission	Single affected generation	Males affected: Only (recessive) Worse (dominant)	Highly variable expression and severity
Multiple affected generations Highly variable expression	Consanguinity sometimes present	Multiple affected generations Female transmission Affected females are mosaic	Cytoplasmic inheritance

their children has a 25% risk for being homozygous for that gene and having the disease. Autosomal recessive disorders are usually seen in only one generation, typically among siblings (Figure 47.3; see Table 47.1). Both males and females can be affected. In small families, autosomal recessive disorders may appear as isolated or sporadic cases. Autosomal recessive disorders may sometimes appear in multiple generations of highly inbred families with consanguineous marriages. Examples of autosomal recessive neurological disorders include phenylketonuria, Tay-Sachs disease, Lafora-body myoclonic epilepsy, infantile spinal muscular atrophy, Wilson's disease, and Friedreich's ataxia.

X-Linked Inheritance Disorders

In X-linked disorders, a mutation occurs in a gene on the X chromosome. Heterozygous female carriers are usually clinically normal but occasionally have mild manifestations of the disease. In X-linked recessive disorders, each son of a carrier female is at 50% risk for the disease. Each daughter of a carrier female is at 50% risk for also being a carrier. Affected males are said to be *hemizygous*. If an affected male has children, his daughters are at 100% risk for being carriers (they automatically inherit his abnormal X chromosome), and his sons do not risk inheriting the mutation (because they automatically inherit only the Y chromosome from their father). Thus, X-linked recessive disease shows almost exclusively affected males in multiple generations with transmission through normal carrier females, and it never shows male-to-male transmission (Figure 47.4; see Table 47.1). Examples of X-linked recessive neurological disorders include Menkes' kinky hair syndrome, Pelizaeus-Merzbacher disease, the fragile-X mental retardation syndrome, Kennedy's spinal-bulbar muscular atrophy, Duchenne's and Becker's muscular dystrophies, and adrenoleukodystrophy.

Heterozygous female carriers of X-linked disorders may occasionally have clinical manifestations because of the phenomenon of *random X-inactivation* (also called *lyonization*). In any given cell, only one X is active. Therefore, women are *mosaic* for the X chromosome. In a few

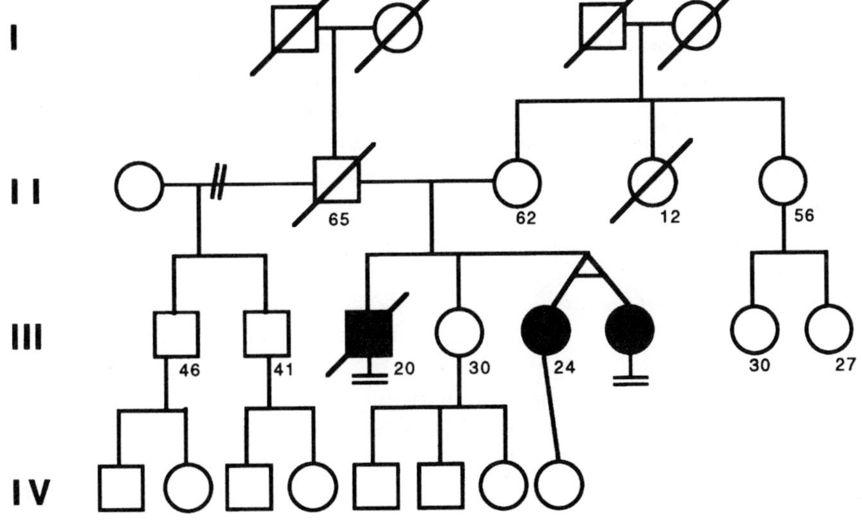

FIGURE 47.3 Pedigree demonstrating autosomal recessive inheritance in a family with Friedreich's ataxia. Three of four siblings in generation 3 are affected (homozygous). The two affected sisters are 24-year-old identical twins. Their affected brother died at age 20. Parents are unaffected (heterozygous). Two parallel horizontal lines indicate no children.

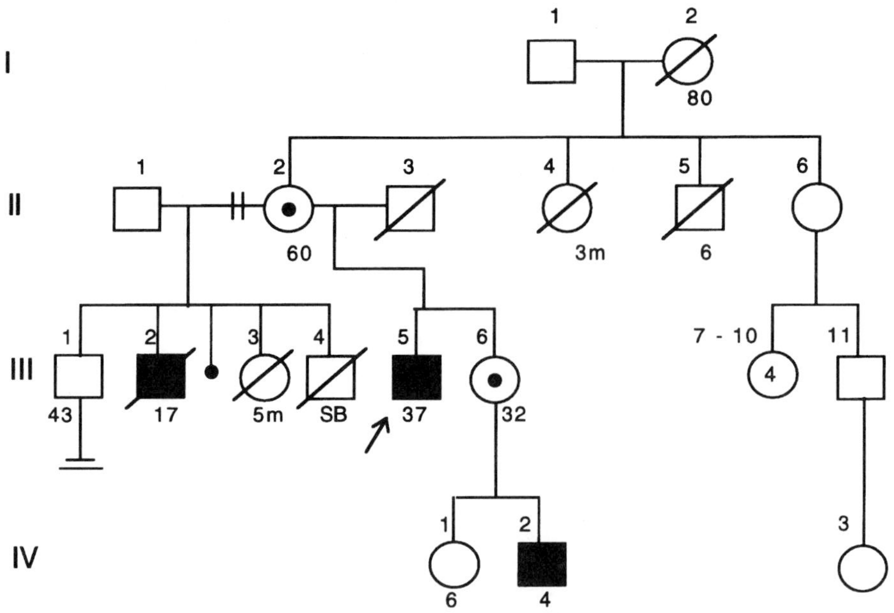

FIGURE 47.4 Pedigree with X-linked recessive inheritance in a family with Pelizaeus-Merzbacher leukodystrophy. Note that only males are affected in two generations, and they are related by clinically normal carrier females (depicted by circle with a dot). There is no male-to-male transmission of the disease.

carrier females, a large proportion of their cells contain active X chromosomes bearing the mutation. Thus, they may occasionally express signs of the disorder.

X-linked dominant inheritance also occasionally occurs. In this situation, heterozygous females commonly express the disease, but the condition is generally more severe in the hemizygous males.

The Y chromosome contains only a few genes, such as the testis-determining factor, and no neurological disorder is related to a Y chromosome gene.

Sporadic Cases and New Mutations

A single case of an apparently genetic disease may occur in a family. Such isolated cases are often called *sporadic*. There are several different possible explanations for this phenomenon, and they may have quite different implications for genetic counseling. For example, the disease may not be genetic at all but actually have an environmental cause. This would represent a nongenetic *phenocopy* and, of course, would not be inherited. An example would be lead poisoning mimicking acute intermittent porphyria. Also, autosomal recessive disorders may often appear as isolated cases in small sibships, because the risks to children of carrier parents are only 25% with each pregnancy. There are recessive disorders that can look phenotypically very much like other diseases that are dominant (e.g., some hereditary neuropathies, ataxias, and movement disorders). Risks to the children of persons with autosomal recessive diseases are very small unless the individual happens to mate with a carrier of the same disease gene (and most such carriers are very rare in the general population).

Sporadic instances of dominant diseases may represent actual *new mutations*. The exact causes of new mutations for human diseases are generally unknown, but irradiation, toxins, and viral exposures presumably play a role. Some new mutations seem to result from the sudden expansion of unstable regions of DNA (described below). In any case, each offspring of a person with a new dominant mutation is at 50% risk for inheriting the abnormal gene, even when there are no other previously affected persons in the family.

Furthermore, a sporadic instance of a disease may represent *false paternity*. That is, the affected individual may not be aware of the fact that his or her true biological father (and not the apparent father) carried a particular disease gene. Nevertheless, if the disorder is dominant, the children of the affected person are at 50% risk.

Finally, some carriers of dominant disease genes have only very mild clinical expression or none at all (*lack of penetrance*). Affected children of such individuals assume that neither of their parents had the disease, and the child appears to be a new isolated case. Detailed evaluation of their parents may uncover mild physical signs and explain the apparent sporadic case. Such situations are especially common with dominant disorders with highly variable expression such as CMT, neurofibromatosis, tuberous sclerosis, and myotonic dystrophy.

Chromosomal Aberrations

Gross aberrations of chromosomes may result in structural defects that are microscopically observable during karyotyping. Examples of such aberrations include trisomies, deletions, duplications, insertions, inversions, isochromosomes, ring chromosomes, and translocations. Detailed chemical banding of chromosomes has greatly improved the identification of microscopic alterations (Figure 47.5). Be-

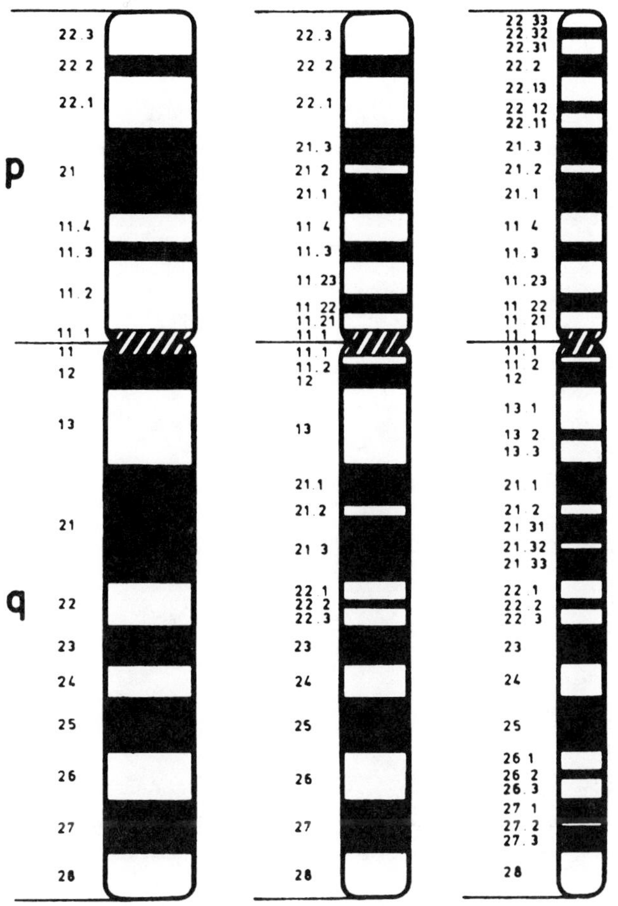

FIGURE 47.5 Schematic diagram of the X chromosome at three different stages of banding resolution showing the standard banding pattern and the system numbering chromosome bands and sub-bands. A "p" refers to the short arm and a "q" to the long arm of individual chromosomes. Note, for example, that band Xp21, which includes the Duchenne/Becker muscular dystrophy gene, can be further resolved into bands Xp21.1, Xp21.2, and Xp21.3. (Reprinted with permission from DG Harnden, HP Klinger [eds]. ISCN 1985: An International System for Human Cytogenetic Nomenclature. Basel: Karger, 1985.)

cause these aberrations are relatively large, they may impair many genes and result in severe clinical manifestations, such as spontaneous abortion, stillbirth, neonatal death, severe mental retardation, or multiple congenital anomalies. Neurological problems are common. Trisomy 21, or Down's syndrome, is a common cause of mental retardation in which the prevalence of seizures is on the order of 5% and that is associated with Alzheimer's disease after age 40. Seizures may occur in 25–50% of patients who are trisomic for chromosomes 13, 18, or 22. A partial deletion of the short arm of chromosome 4 (Wolf-Hirschhorn syndrome, or chromosome 4p-) has a high frequency of convulsions (approximately 70%). In contrast, another short-arm deletion syndrome (Cri du chat syndrome, or chromosome 5p-) is seldom associated with seizures.

Most chromosomal aberrations are sporadic and have very small recurrence risks in subsequent pregnancies (typically on the order of 1% or less). Occasionally, a chromosomal syndrome is inherited through normal carriers of a balanced *chromosomal translocation* (for example, Down's syndrome as the result of a chromosome 14/21 Robertsonian translocation). Children of balanced-translocation carriers have a 4–15% risk of being chromosomally unbalanced and having the clinical syndrome (Figure 47.6).

Aberrations of the sex chromosomes include the following: Turner's syndrome (XO) in females associated with short stature, infertility, and visuospatial problems but not mental retardation; Klinefelter's syndrome (XXY) in males associated with infertility, hypogonadism, tall stature, and psychosocial adjustment problems; XYY syndrome in males associated with tall stature and behavioral problems; and XXX syndrome in females with mental retardation.

Some patients with very mild manifestations of a chromosomal disorder may be the result of *somatic mosaicism.* In such individuals, the chromosomal defect occurs postfertilization in the early stages of embryo development. In the full-grown individual, only a small proportion of cells carries the chromosomal defect. For example, a few individuals have the facial manifestations of Down's syndrome but have normal intelligence. Careful karyotyping may show normal results in most cells, although a small proportion has trisomy 21. These individuals have mosaic Down's syndrome.

Some small chromosomal deletions may be submicroscopic (not visible on the usual karyotype) but produce defects in several adjacent genes. This may result in a so-called *contiguous gene deletion syndrome.* One well-documented example is a boy who had Duchenne's muscular dystrophy, retinitis pigmentosa, chronic granulomatous disease, and the McLeod's syndrome. This was the result of a deletion affecting four adjacent genes on the X chromosome.

Individuals with an inherited mutation at a single locus on one chromosome may acquire an additional somatic mutation at the same locus on the other chromosome of that pair, resulting in the *two-hit phenomenon.* For example, an individual who has inherited a mutation in the retinoblastoma gene on chromosome 13 may develop multiple eye tumors, because an additional acquired somatic mutation occurs at the same locus in the other member of the chromosome 13 pair in a retinal cell. This results in homozygosity for the mutation and the subsequent growth of the tumor, because the normal gene suppresses tumor growth. A similar phenomenon occurs in many astrocytomas involving the p53 tumor suppressor gene on chromosome 17p.

Imprinting refers to germ line–specific modification of chromosomes and their genetic material. This results in differential expression of genetic information when inherited from the mother, as compared to inheritance from the father. The phenomenon is probably at least partially related to differential methylation of DNA, which is known to inactivate some genes. An example of imprinting occurs in the unusual inheritance pattern of the fragile-X mental re-

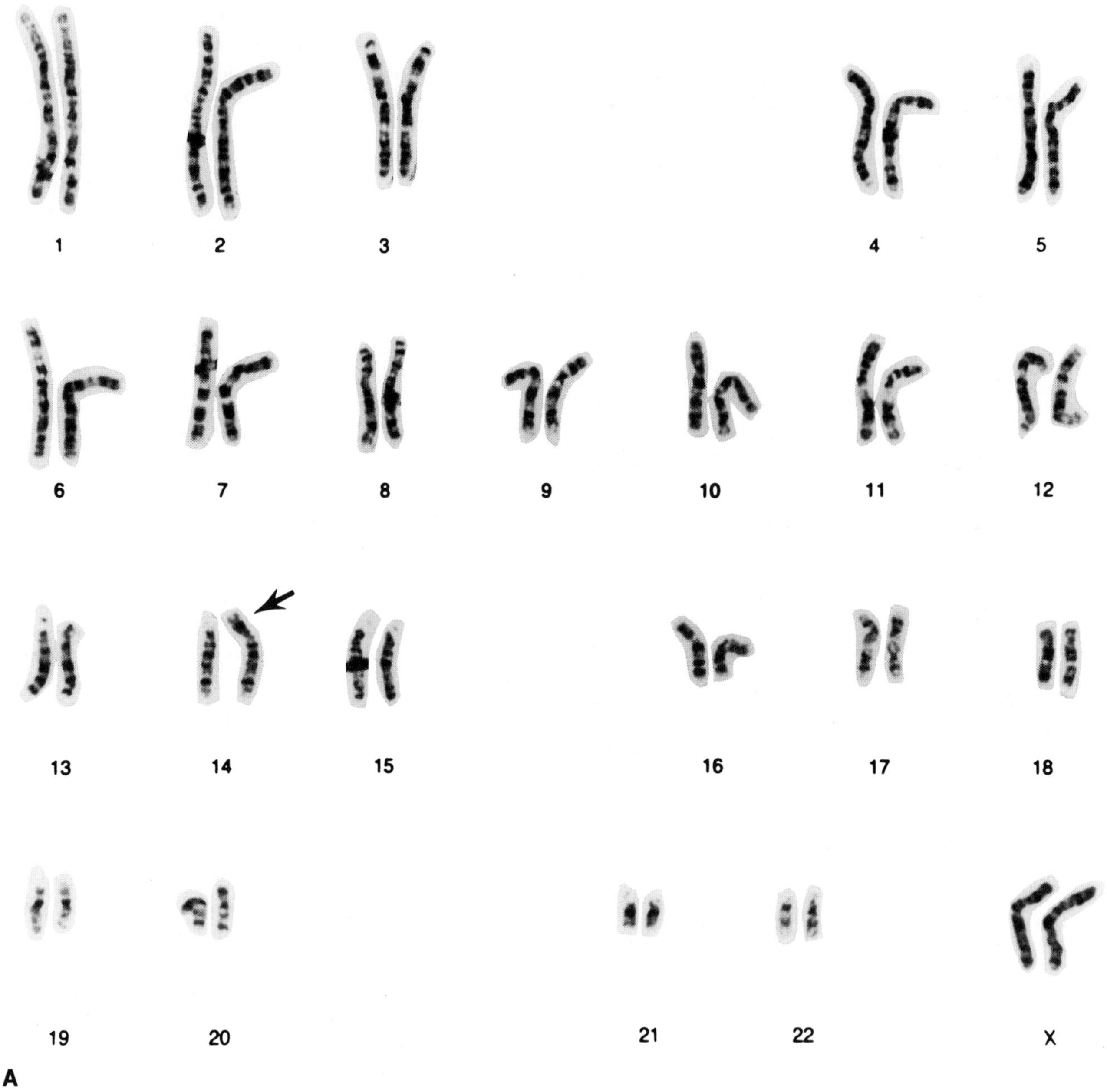

FIGURE 47.6 A. Karyotype of a patient with Down's syndrome caused by a 14/21 unbalanced Robertsonian translocation. The patient has two normal copies of chromosome 21, and the long arm of 21 is attached (translocated) to the short arm of 14 (arrow). Thus, there are three copies (trisomy) of 21, although the total number of chromosomes appears to be normal (46). B. A carrier of 14/21 translocation has the chromosome 14 with the attached 21 (arrow), but only one other copy of chromosome 21. Thus, there is the normal total number (2) of chromosome 21, although the person appears to have only 45 chromosomes. (Photos courtesy of K. Leppig.)

tardation syndrome. In this disorder, some males with normal intelligence transmit the gene to their daughters, who may also be mentally normal but who subsequently have mentally retarded sons. The involved region of the X chromosome is altered as it passes through oogenesis in the mother. It has also been speculated that imprinting may play a role in juvenile Huntington's disease, which occurs almost exclusively in the offspring of affected fathers, and in neonatal myotonic dystrophy, which occurs almost exclusively in the offspring of affected mothers.

Angelman's syndrome and the Prader-Willi syndrome both result from a small deletion in the same site of chromosome 15. However, if an individual inherits the deletion from a maternal chromosome 15, the result is Angelman's

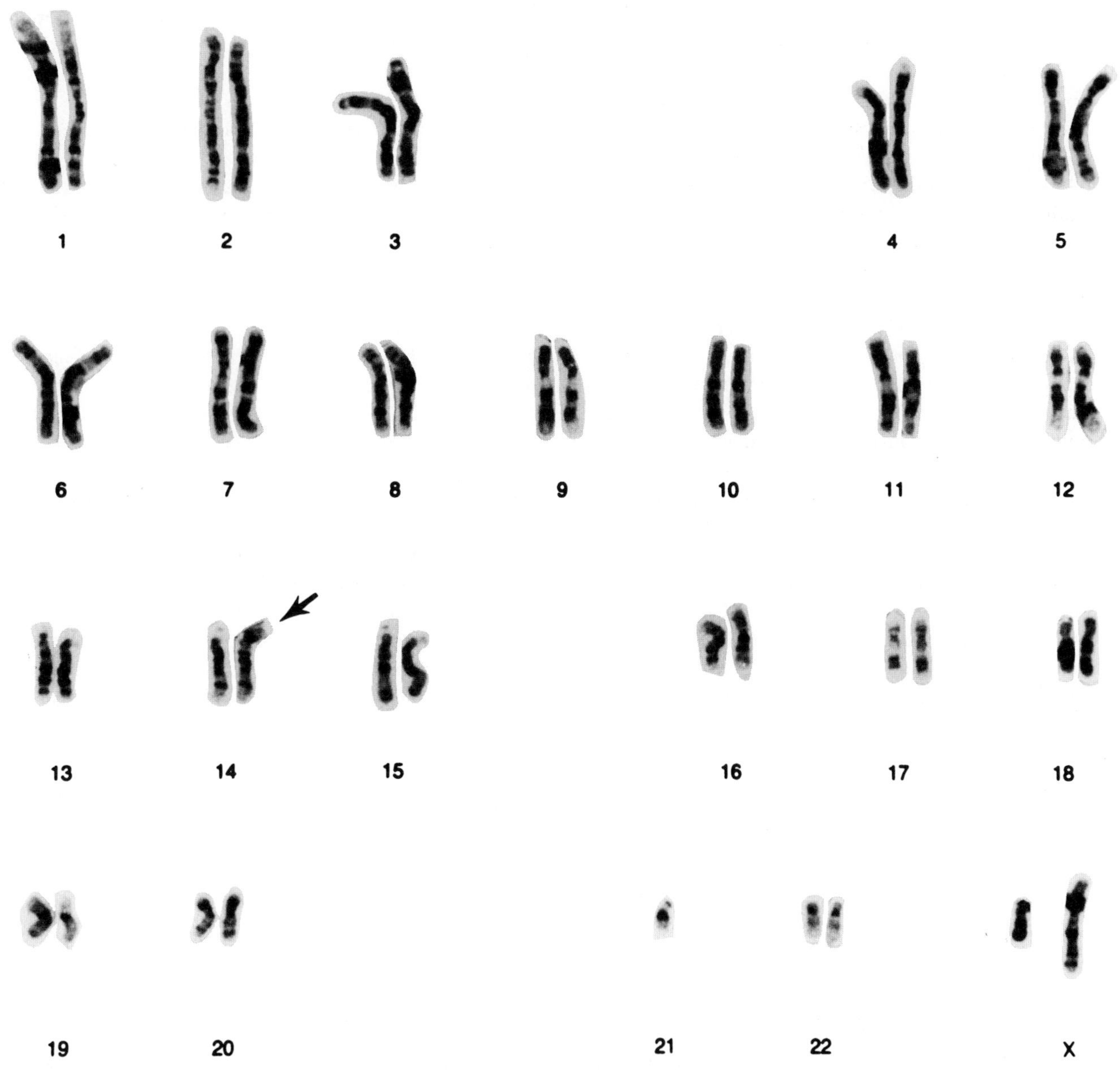

B

syndrome, whereas if the mutation is on a paternal chromosome 15, the result is Prader-Willi syndrome. This appears to be another example of imprinting. Of further interest here is that although mental retardation is common to both disorders, seizures are much more common in Angelman's syndrome, and a gamma-aminobutyric acid receptor gene maps to the involved region of chromosome 15.

Uniparental Disomy

As noted above, normally within each pair of chromosomes one is inherited from the mother and the other from the father. Occasionally, however, an individual may inherit both members of a chromosomal pair from a single parent. This is called *uniparental disomy.* This occurrence has resulted in some interesting genetic phenomena. An individual who was homozygous for the autosomal recessive cystic fibrosis (CF) gene was found to have only a carrier mother (the father was demonstrated not to be a carrier of the CF mutation). It was further determined that the affected child had inherited both chromosome 7s (the site of the CF gene) from the heterozygous mother (Voss et al. 1989). This same phenomenon has also occurred in a child with autosomal recessive spinal muscular atrophy.

Mitochondrial Inheritance

In the past few years, it has become apparent that several interesting disorders are the result of mutations in mitochondrial DNA (DiMauro 1993). Mitochondrial DNA codes for 13 proteins involved in oxidative phosphorylation and ribosomal and transfer RNAs. Mitochondrial DNA is inherited in the cytoplasm of a mother's egg but is not inherited from the sperm of the father. Therefore, mitochondrial disorders are transmitted only by mothers and never by fathers (*cytoplasmic inheritance*) (Figure 47.7). Male and female children can both be affected, and the disease may appear in all children of an affected mother. Each child of an affected mother may vary in the number of mitochondria he or she has inherited that contain the DNA mutation. Furthermore, the proportion of mutant mitochondria may vary considerably from cell to cell in any given affected individual (*heteroplasmy*). Therefore, mitochondrial disorders often show extreme variability in clinical expression both within and between families. Point mutations in mitochondrial DNA tend to be inherited through females, whereas deletions of mitochondrial DNA tend to be noninherited, sporadic events in isolated individuals. Mitochondrial disorders include the myoclonus epilepsy with ragged-red fibers (MERRF) syndrome, the mitochondrial encephalomyopathy, lactic acidosis, and stroke (MELAS) syndrome, Leber's hereditary optic neuropathy (LHON), and the Kearns-Sayre syndrome (myopathy, retinopathy, cardiomyopathy).

Polygenic and Multifactorial Disorders

Some syndromes are presumed to be the result of the additive effect of a small number of multiple genes. Such polygenic conditions are mostly speculative but could include some forms of mental retardation, hypertension, epilepsy, dementia, or diabetes mellitus.

Multifactorial inheritance refers to disorders that result from the combination of an inherited predisposition acting in concert with an acquired environmental insult. Some latent carriers of a single gene mutation may be unmasked by an environmental agent. Symptomatic acute intermittent porphyria following phenobarbital administration is an example. The area of pharmacogenetics will be of great importance to neurology as the genetic control of anticonvulsant metabolism becomes fully delineated. Genetically programmed rapid or slow metabolizers of anticonvulsants present major challenges to the clinical management of seizure disorders. Multiple sclerosis is suspected to be another model of multifactorial inheritance in which there is a presumed genetic immunological predisposition to some unknown environmental trigger.

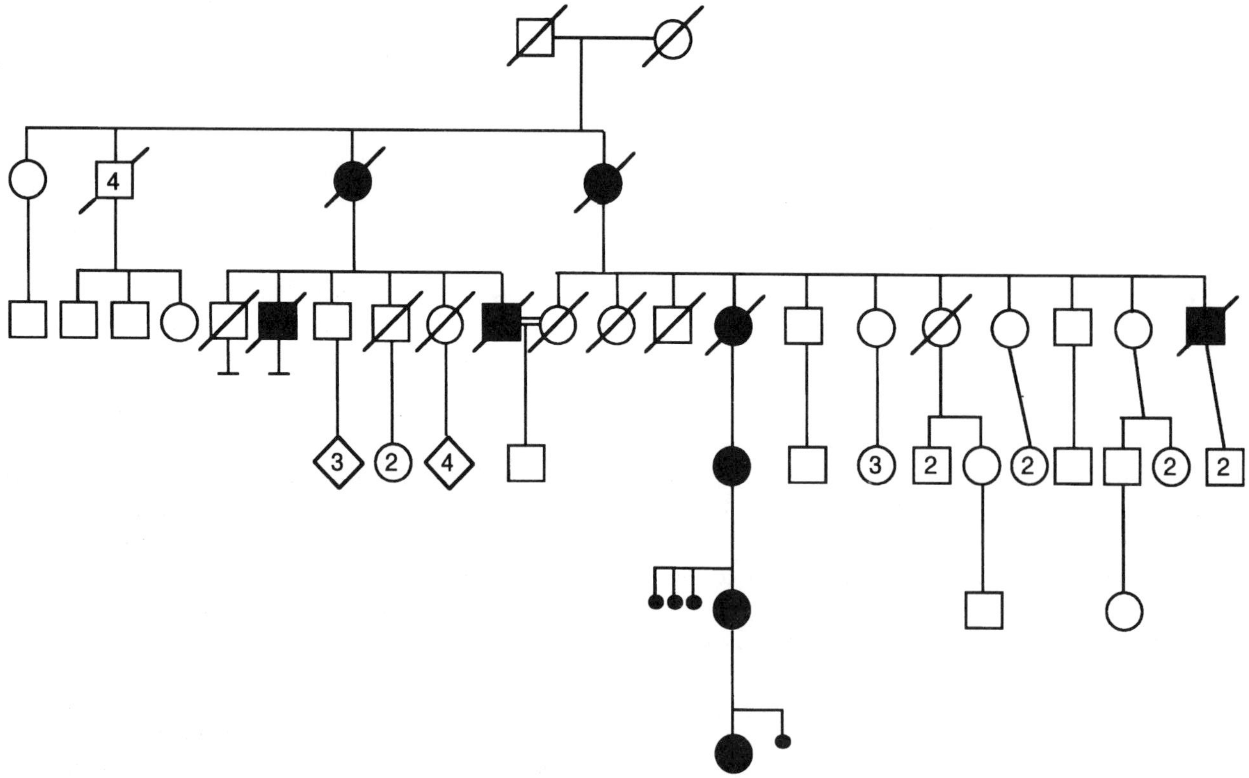

FIGURE 47.7 Pedigree demonstrating mitochondrial inheritance in a family with a variant of myoclonus epilepsy with ragged-red fibers (MERRF). Note that multiple generations are involved, male and females are both affected, but the disease is only transmitted by females. The small dots attached by vertical lines represent spontaneous abortions.

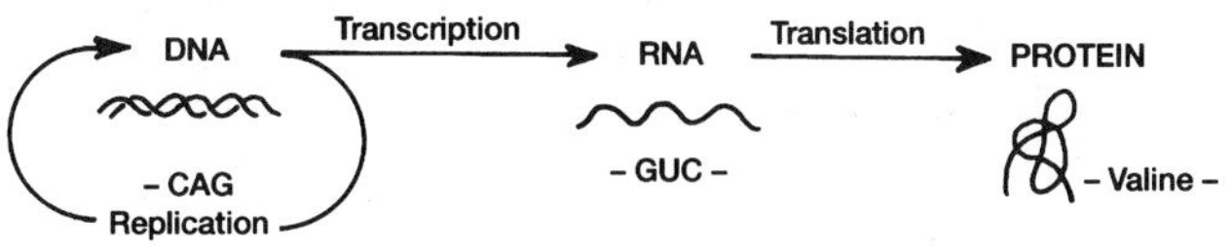

FIGURE 47.8 Schematic diagram demonstrating transcription of DNA into RNA followed by translation of the RNA to a polypeptide protein. The CAG codon in DNA is transcribed to GUC in RNA, then translated to valine in the protein. Transcription occurs in the nucleus and translation occurs in the cytoplasmic ribosomes.

Table 47.2: The human genome

3 billion base pairs (bp)
50,000–100,000 functional genes
3,000–5,000 known genetic disorders
1,000 bp = 1 kilobase (kb)
1 million bp = 1 megabase (Mb)
1% recombination = 1 cM (centimorgan)
1 cM ≅ 1 Mb

STRUCTURE AND ORGANIZATION OF GENES

Each chromosome contains a long string of DNA arranged in a double helix. Sequences of four different purine and pyrimidine bases (thymine, cytosine, guanine, adenine) form the genetic code (uracil instead of thymine in RNA). Each sequence of three bases eventually codes for a specific amino acid in a polypeptide (Figure 47.8). RNA is synthesized from the DNA template through the process of transcription. Messenger RNA (mRNA) is transported out of the nucleus into the cytoplasm, where translation occurs on ribosomes. This is the process of decoding the mRNA and synthesizing polypeptides by connecting a specific sequence of amino acids according to the mRNA code.

The structure of a "typical" gene is shown in Figure 47.9. Genes usually consist of an enhancer and promoter region that controls gene expression; a region that initiates transcription; the exons, which contain the base pairs actually coding for the final amino acid sequence in the polypeptide; introns (noncoding intervening sequences); and codes for terminating transcription (stop codons). Mutations may occur in any of these regions. Although introns are transcribed into mRNA, they are eventually cut out of the primary transcript, and the exons are spliced together to form mature mRNA. Through the use of different exons (alternative splicing), different transcripts can be coded by the same gene. Although introns do not code protein sequences, some mutations in introns can affect the protein sequence by producing erroneous splice sites. When analyzing a long sequence of DNA to find whether it contains a gene, researchers look (with the aid of a computer) for an open reading frame (ORF), a sequence of suitable length that contains no stop codons and has appropriately located initiation and termination sequences.

MECHANISMS OF MUTATION

The human genome contains approximately 3 billion base pairs and perhaps 50,000–100,000 functional genes (Table 47.2). When one of these genes is disturbed, in any of several ways, a mutation is said to have occurred. If this changes the function of the final polypeptide, then a disease, disorder, or trait may be clinically evident. Several different mechanisms underlying genetic mutations are illustrated in Figure 47.10. Figure 47.10A shows a string of nucleotides and their complementary pairings that might be found in a normal human DNA double-helix. Each group of three nucleotides forms a sequence of codons that each code for a specific amino acid. In the example of substitution (Figure 47.10B), a guanine (G) has been substituted for a thymine (T) in the second codon. This will result in coding for a different amino acid in this position of a protein. A further example of substitution is noted (Figure 47.11). In the neurofibromatosis gene, a T has been substituted for a C. Instead of coding for an arginine, this codon now instructs the DNA reading to stop (stop codon) and results in an abnormally truncated protein (a nonsense mutation).

Figure 47.10C is an example of a deletion. A T-A pair has been removed from the DNA sequence. Note that this changes the reading frame and completely disrupts the coding of subsequent amino acids. For example, the second codon is now CAC instead of GCA.

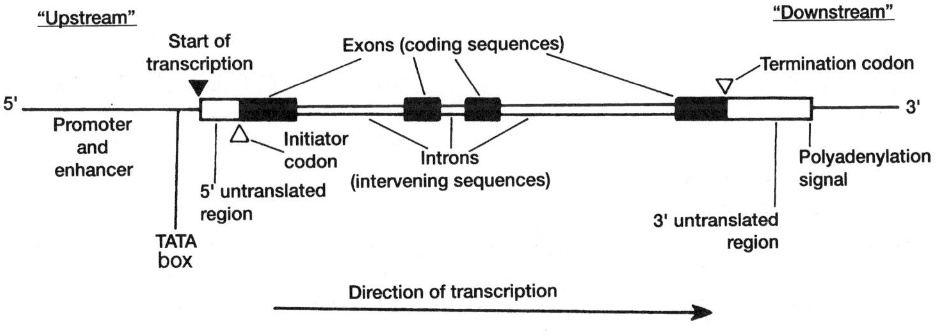

FIGURE 47.9 Hypothetical structure of a typical gene. The exons contain the three base-pair codons that are eventually translated into the amino acids of a polypeptide. The intervening sequences of introns are spliced out of the genetic code during transcription. A gene may have one or many exons. A gene may range in size from a few thousand base pairs to several million base pairs.

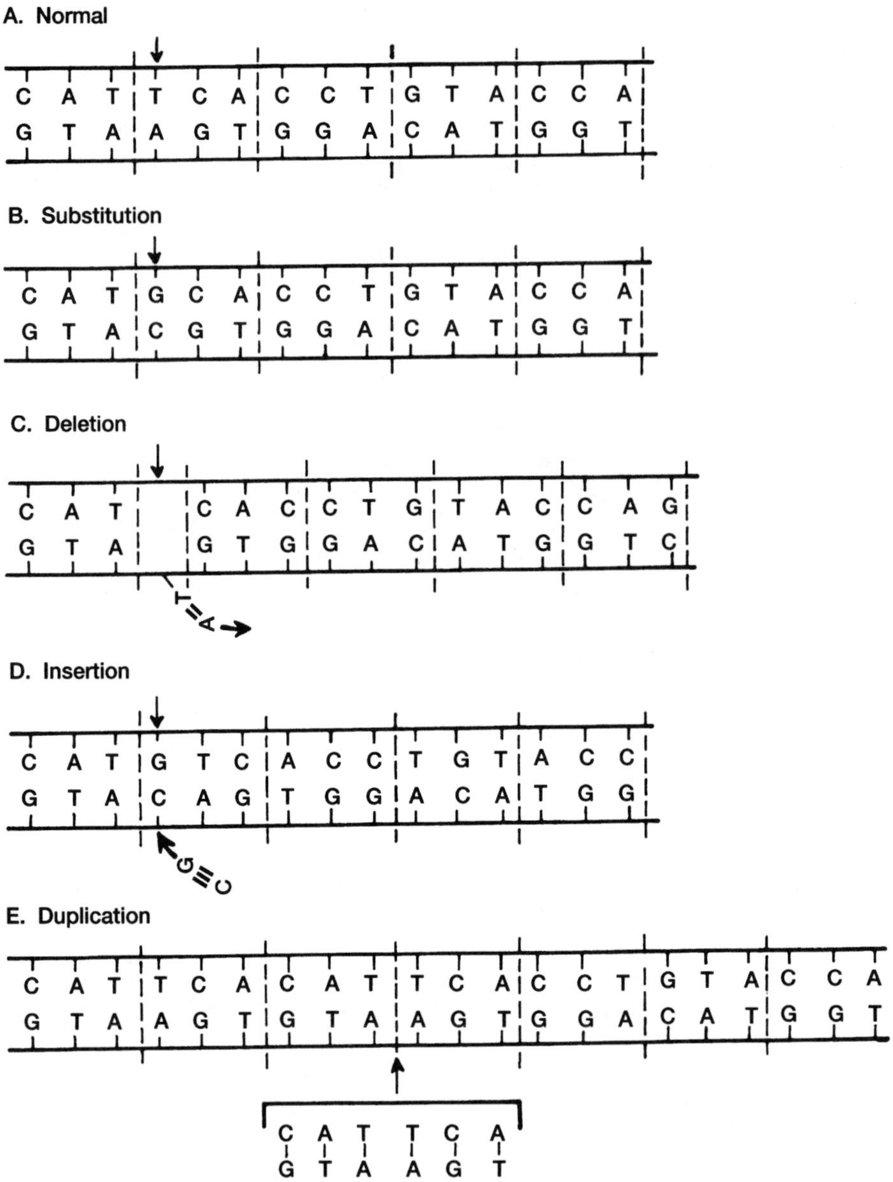

FIGURE 47.10 Mechanisms of mutation. A. A normal sequence of DNA bases matched with their complementary pairs. Each sequence of three bases codes for a certain amino acid. B. A substitution of a guanine for thymine. This does not change the reading frame but does change the amino acid coded by this three base-pair sequence. C. The original T-A pair has been deleted, which changes the reading frame. The second codon is now CAC instead of TCA. D. An insertion of a G-C pair in front of the original T-A. This changes the reading frame. E. An example of a duplication of the CATTCA sequence. (Modified from M Thompson, R McInnes, H Willard. Genetics in Medicine. Philadelphia: Saunders, 1991.)

Deletions are a common cause of mutations in the Duchenne's muscular dystrophy gene, shown in Figure 47.12. This is a very large gene covering approximately 2 million base pairs and including more than 40 exons. The gene codes for a protein, dystrophin, that is present in the sarcolemmal membrane of skeletal and cardiac muscle. Dozens of different deletions of various sizes in this gene either eliminate the production or perturb the function of dystrophin. Such deletions result in either severe Duchenne's dystrophy or milder Becker's dystrophy, respectively.

Deletions may cover larger segments of DNA. For example, a deletion of 1.5 million base pairs on chromosome 17p results in the clinical disease of hereditary neuropathy with liability to pressure palsies (Figure 47.13) (Chance and Pleasure 1993). As noted earlier, there can be even larger deletions of chromosomal material. Patients with such gross chromo-

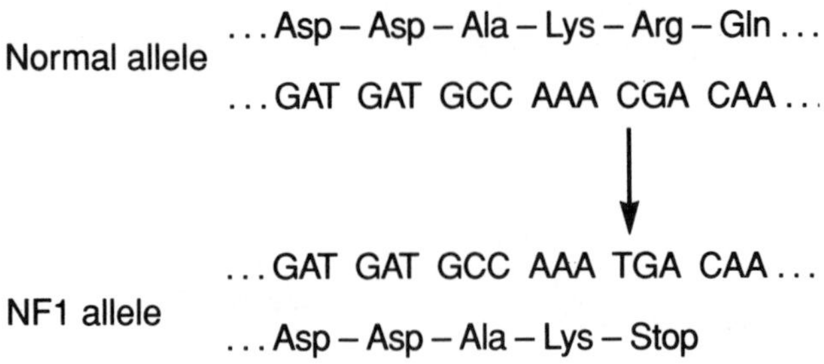

FIGURE 47.11 The substitution of a T for a C in the neurofibromatosis gene (NF1) results in a nonsense mutation in the coding sequence, which causes a premature termination of translation (stop codon).

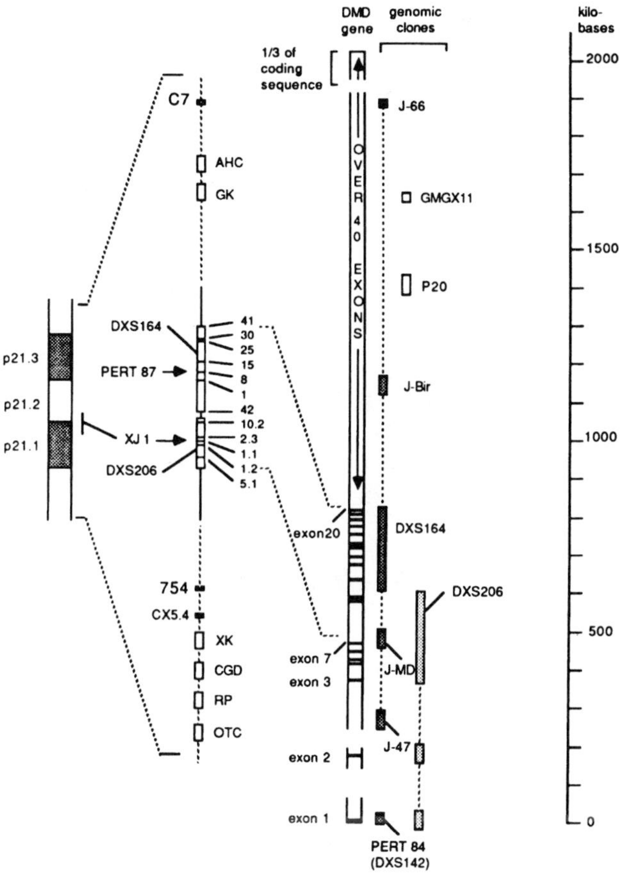

FIGURE 47.12 Schematic of the Duchenne's muscular dystrophy gene. On the left is the region of the X chromosome that contains the gene, showing the relation of the chromosomal region to the DXS164 and DXS206 regions, detected by the pERT and XJ1 probes, respectively. The genes for congenital adrenal hypoplasia (AHC), glycerol kinase (GK), the McLeod phenotype (XK), chronic granulomatous disease (CGD), retinitis pigmentosa (RP), and ornithine transcarbamylase (OTC) are shown in their relative positions. C7 and 754 are anonymous flanking probes frequently used in RFLP analysis. On the right is the genomic map showing the relation between the DXS164 and DXS206 regions and exons of the gene. At the time this figure was produced, exons 1 and 2 were not yet linked to one another or to DXS206 and are shown connected to DXS206 by a dashed line. Several "jump" clones (J-66, J-Bir, J-MD, J-47) found by isolation of deletion junctions with pERT 87 probes are shown connected to the DXS164 locus. Probe pERT 84 and the unrelated probes GMGX11 and P20 are shown in their approximate positions. The size of the gene is about 2 Mb.

somal deletions may have major clinical syndromes, including mental retardation and multiple physical anomalies. An example of such a microdeletion is the Miller-Dieker syndrome (a deletion at chromosome 17p13.3) associated with lissencephaly and profound mental retardation.

An insertion of a G-C nucleotide pair at the beginning of the second codon is illustrated in Figure 47.10D. Again, this completely changes the DNA reading frame from this point on. For example, the second codon is now GTC instead of TCA, and this will result in coding for a different amino acid. This is a missense mutation, which produces a full-length protein with an amino acid change. Another example of a four-base pair insertion is illustrated in Figure 47.14. There is an insertion of TATC into one segment of the hexosaminidase A gene, resulting in an altered reading frame and an abnormal protein. This mutation is a major cause of Tay-Sachs disease.

Figure 47.10E is a depiction of a duplication of six base pairs (CATTCA). Such a duplication would add two more amino acids into this site of the final protein and possibly change its activity. Much longer duplications may occur. An example is the 1.5 million base-pair tandem duplication of DNA found on chromosome 17p in the classic slow nerve conduction velocity (NCV) form of CMT type 1A (see Figure 47.13).

Figure 47.13 illustrates how several different mutations can all result in various forms of hereditary neuropathy. This is genetic heterogeneity. As noted above, a duplication of 1.5 Mb on chromosome 17p that includes a gene for peripheral myelin protein 22 (PMP22) can result in an autosomal dominant neuropathy with slow nerve conduction (CMT 1A). A point mutation in the PMP22 gene can cause a phenotypically similar dominant neuropathy. A different point mutation in the PMP22 gene can cause a recessively inherited neuropathy. A deletion of the entire 1.5-Mb region results in a different phenotype: dominant hereditary neuropathy with liability for pressure palsies (HNPP). These different mutations involving the PMP 22 gene represent allelic genetic heterogeneity. A point mutation in a different gene (P_0 myelin protein) on chromosome 1 also causes a dominant neuropathy with slow NCV (CMT 1B) (Hayasaka et al. 1993). Finally, a mutation in a gap-junction protein connexin32 gene on the X chromosome results in an X-linked inherited neuropathy (CMT X) (Bergoffen et al. 1993). The different mutations on chromosomes 1, 17, and X are examples of nonallelic genetic heterogeneity.

ANTICIPATION AND TRINUCLEOTIDE REPEAT EXPANSIONS

The phenomenon of *genetic anticipation* has been debated for many decades. The term was primarily used to describe the observed increasing clinical severity of the autosomal dominant myotonic dystrophy gene over subsequent generations (Harper et al. 1992). Typically, a father might have early-onset cataracts, his daughter might have mild muscle weakness and myotonia, and the daughter's child would have the early onset of severe weakness and myotonia associated with mental retardation. This repeatedly observed but poorly understood clinical observation has now been given an important biological foundation. The myotonic dystrophy gene is associated with an expansion of repeated DNA sequences (CTG, CTG, CTG,---) on chromosome 19. The size of this expansion frequently increases with each

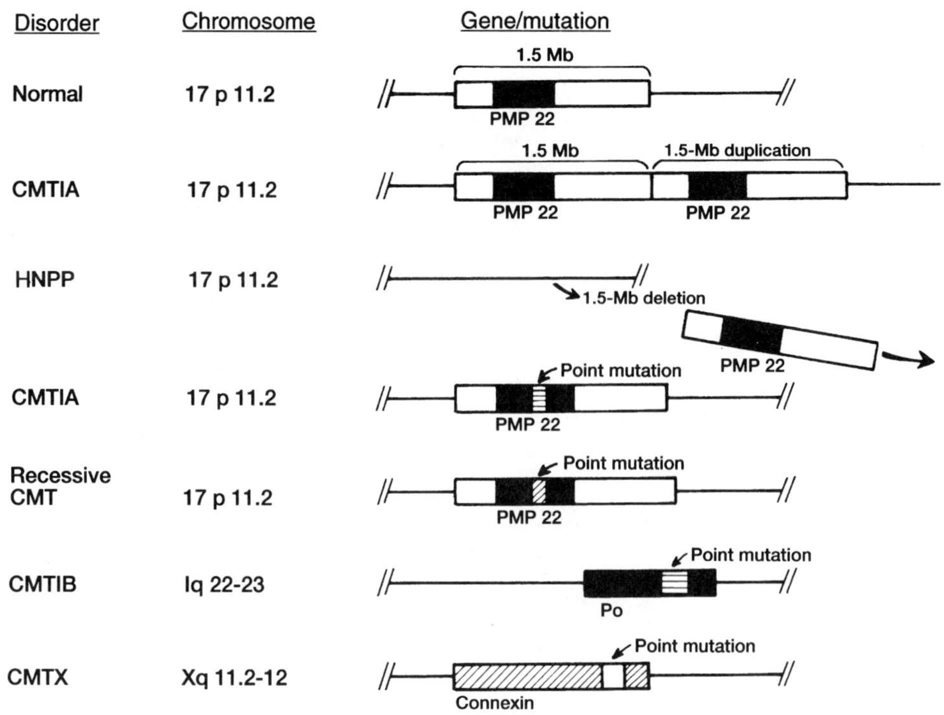

FIGURE 47.13 Several different mutations resulting in various forms of hereditary neuropathy (CMT/HMSN) and thus examples of genetic heterogeneity. The normal sequence of DNA at chromosome 17p11.2 has a 1.5-Mb region that includes a peripheral myelin gene (PMP 22). A 1.5-Mb tandem duplication results in CMT 1A, and a 1.5-Mb deletion of the same regions results in HNPP. Two different point mutations in the PMP 22 gene can cause either a dominant form of CMT 1A or a recessive form of CMT. Furthermore, a point mutation in the P_0 myelin protein gene at chromosome 1q22–23 results in CMT 1B, a clinical syndrome very similar to CMT 1A. Finally, a point mutation in the connexin32 gene at Xq11.2–12 results in an X-linked inherited form of neuropathy.

generation and is correlated with severity of the disease. (It is known that small expansions occur normally but become unstable, for unknown reasons.) The precise cause of the expansion and the reasons for the increase in size with each generation remain to be determined.

Investigators have found several other neurogenetic diseases that show a similar phenomenon, including Kennedy's X-linked spinal-bulbar muscular atrophy, the fragile-X mental retardation syndrome, Huntington's disease, two forms of hereditary ataxia (SCA 1, MJD), and a rare form of dentatorubral-pallidoluysian atrophy (DRPLA) (Martin 1993).

These disorders and their trinucleotide repeat expansions are shown in Figure 47.15. Two expansions lie outside the coding regions for their respective genes (CGG in fragile-X mental retardation and CTG in myotonic dystrophy). Five other CAG expansions occur within the genes for X-linked spinal-bulbar muscular atrophy, SCA 1, MJD, DRPLA and Huntington's disease. Exactly how these expansions alter the transcription, translation, or function of their associated genes remains a matter of intense investigation.

The trinucleotide repeat expansions have formed the basis of new rapid diagnostic tests for their associated diseases. Through the technique of polymerase chain reaction (PCR) (see below), small blood samples from single individuals can be quickly analyzed for these specific expansions. If present, they are essentially diagnostic for having the abnormal gene. Interpretation of the results, however, can be complex (Bird and Bennett 1995). For example, having the expansion is not the same as having symptoms of the disease. Nor does it accurately predict age of onset or severity of disease. It is

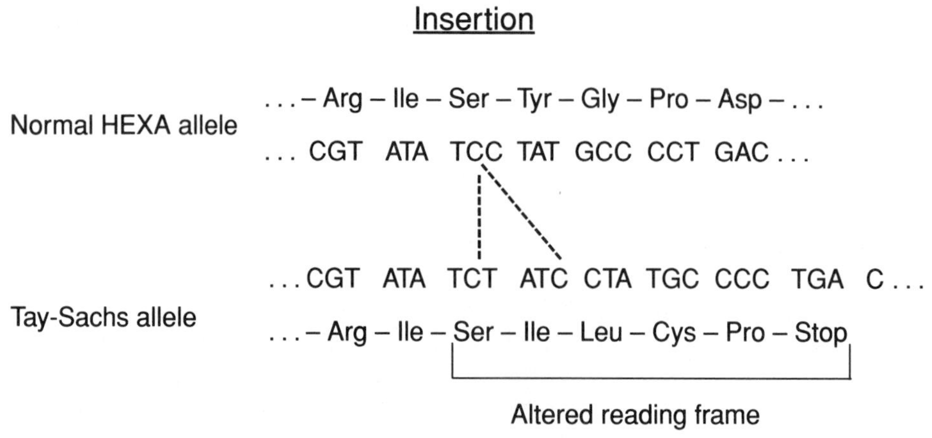

FIGURE 47.14 A four base-pair insertion in the hexosaminidase-A gene leads to a frame-shift mutation. This is the major cause of Tay-Sachs disease in Ashkenazi Jews.

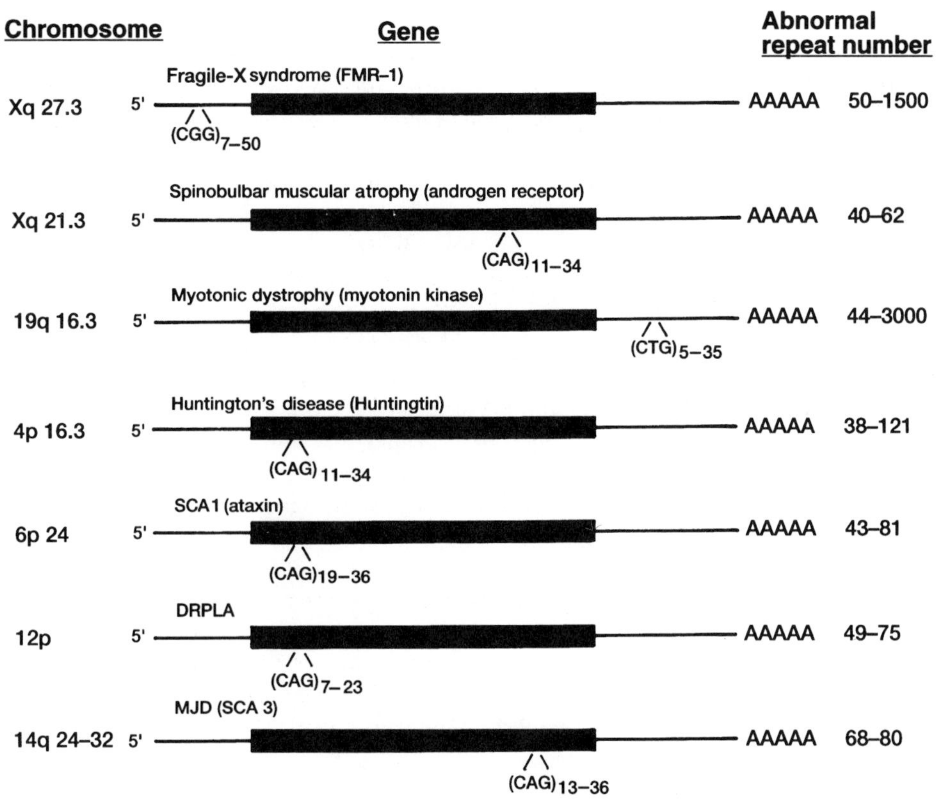

FIGURE 47.15 Seven neurological diseases that have been shown to be associated with trinucleotide repeat expansions. The region of DNA containing each gene's protein-coding segments is indicated by the solid horizontal bar. The repeats (CGG, CAG, or CTG) may lie inside or outside these coding segments. The range of normal number of repeats found in the general population is indicated next to each repeat region. The abnormal number of repeats that may be found in affected individuals is indicated in the last column. MJD = Machado-Joseph disease.

true that the expansion length roughly correlates with disease onset and severity, but the correlation is not generally great enough to be very predictive in any given person. Furthermore, there may be expansions in an intermediate range in which it is not clear whether the individual has indeed inherited the abnormal gene (for example, 34–37 repeats in the HD gene). This ambiguity is a difficult issue for both patients and physicians. Furthermore, a few patients have been described who seem to be affected by the disease but whose repeat expansion lengths are within the normal range (HD Collaborative Research 1993). Explanations for these phenomena are still needed.

TOOLS OF GENETIC RESEARCH

Restriction Endonucleases

Certain bacterial enzymes have the ability to cleave foreign DNA into fragments, their site of action being restricted to specific sites within the molecule. This function appears to be an evolutionary development that protects the organism's own DNA from incorporating foreign DNA. Each restriction endonuclease can recognize a specific DNA sequence (*restriction site*) several bases in length, and cut a strand of foreign DNA at a particular position within that sequence. The sequences on the paired strands at which a restriction enzyme cuts are palindromic; that is, the sequences on the two strands read the same, but in opposite directions. For example, the restriction enzyme HindIII cuts a duplex strand of DNA as follows:

5' A | AGCTT 3'
3' TTCGA | A 5'

If the same enzyme is used to cut both the DNA of the vector and the DNA to be incorporated into it, the cut ends of the foreign and host DNA may join by complementary base pairing, thereby incorporating the foreign DNA into that of the vector. After base pairing, the ends of the strands are sealed together by the enzyme DNA ligase (which requires ATP).

The fragments of the DNA produced by restriction enzymes along a particular DNA segment can be used to construct a restriction map, showing the cutting sites for the various enzymes in relation to one another.

Vectors

Vectors are prokaryotic organisms, or DNA molecules, into which foreign DNA can be grafted for cloning. Four types are commonly used: plasmids, phages, cosmids, and yeast artificial chromosomes (YACs).

Plasmids are small, circular duplex DNA molecules within bacteria and yeast that replicate independently of the host chromosome. The genes they carry may be of great importance for the survival of the host cell, such as genes for antibiotic resistance. The plasmids used for DNA cloning have been constructed with three essential features: (1) an origin of DNA replication allowing the recombinant DNA molecule to replicate in the host; (2) a marker such as a gene for antibiotic resistance that can be used to select for bacterial cells containing the plasmid; and (3) a region into which small fragments (< 6–10 kb) of cloned DNA can be inserted, with the help of cleavage sites for one or more restriction enzymes.

Phage (bacteriophage) is a virus that infects bacteria. Its duplex DNA molecule may either become incorporated into the bacterial chromosome or replicate independently and produce large numbers of phage particles, which lyse the host cell and infect other bacteria in the culture. The presence of phage-infected bacteria is shown by plaques (clear areas) in the culture dish. Specialized versions of the best-known phage, phage lambda, have been developed that can carry intermediate-sized fragments (5–20 kb) of cloned insert DNA. There are also single-strand phage cloning vectors, which have special advantages for DNA sequencing and other experimental uses.

A cosmid is a construct that combines plasmid and phage features. It is composed of plasmid DNA that contains the cos site of phage lambda, which carries the sequences required to package the cloned insert DNA. Like other vectors, it also contains a replication origin and selectable markers. Cosmids have an advantage over plasmid and phage vectors because relatively long (35- to 45-kb) foreign DNA sequences can be inserted into them.

Until recently, it was not possible to clone DNA fragments of 100 kb to more than 1,000 kb. With the advent of rare cutting-restriction endonucleases that cut at rare sites, these large fragments can now be cloned using yeast vectors. The new constructs are called YACs.

Gene Libraries

A set of DNA fragments from a specific source that has been cloned in appropriate vectors is called a gene library, indicating that it contains genetic information from its DNA source. A human gene library may be prepared from total genomic DNA or from the DNA of a single chromosome or chromosome segment. Although the experimental procedures may be complex, the principle is relatively simple. The DNA of interest and that of the vector are cleaved by the same enzyme and allowed to recombine. In principle, all or most of the DNA of interest will be inserted into the vector DNA. The vectors, some of which now contain the foreign DNA sequences of interest, are inserted into bacterial hosts, allowed to multiply in vitro under selective conditions, and stored for long-term availability. To access the clones that have incorporated the DNA sequences of interest, it is necessary to use a method of selection. This process often requires the use of radioactive DNA or RNA probes that are specific for the sequence of interest and will hybridize with them.

For many experimental purposes, *complementary DNA (cDNA) libraries* are used. Complementary DNA is prepared from mature mRNA obtained from a tissue in which the gene of interest is expressed. This is not a trivial procedure, because most tissues contain many types of mRNA transcripts, among which the specific one transcribed from the gene of interest may be quite rare. Because an mRNA transcript is a continuous RNA strand containing only the exons of the gene and lacking the introns, it is considerably shorter than the corresponding genomic DNA molecule (14 kb of mRNA instead of about 2,000 kb of DNA for the DMD gene, for example). The single mRNA strand to be copied is prepared by addition of an oligo (dT) primer that allows reverse transcriptase to begin synthesis of a complementary DNA strand. The DNA strand ends in a short hairpin loop. The RNA transcript is then degraded, leaving the single DNA strand, which is converted into a duplex molecule by the action of DNA polymerase I using the hairpin as the primer. The hairpin is degraded by the enzyme S1 nuclease, leaving a duplex DNA molecule copy of the original mRNA molecule that can be inserted into an appropriate vector molecule, amplified, and stored. A cDNA library prepared from a given tissue usually contains a variety of clones representing all the different genes that are being expressed in that tissue at that developmental stage.

The first step in selecting the clone of interest from a library is the isolation of clones in which the vector has been incorporated into the bacterium. This is achieved by using selectable markers that have been built into the plasmid or phage vector, such as ability to grow in the presence of an antibiotic that will kill bacteria that have not incorporated the vector. Next, the surviving bacterial colonies are analyzed to determine whether the vector they carry has incorporated any of the foreign DNA. Finally, the desired recombinants are identified and isolated from the mixture of recombinant clones. A number of approaches, not described here, are available to isolate the sequences of interest, which can then be analyzed in detail.

The technique used to detect specific sequences of DNA is Southern blotting, named after its originator. The DNA of interest is digested into short fragments by one or more restriction enzymes, and gel electrophoresis is used to separate the fragments by size. The DNA is then denatured to the single-strand form and transferred by blotting with paper towels to a more stable medium, nitrocellulose filter membrane. The pattern of DNA fragments on the gel is faithfully transferred to the filter membrane. The resulting blot can be baked to make it more permanent and can then be hybridized to a specific probe. Using autoradiography, the fragment(s) of interest can be visualized on the blot (Figure 47.16).

By analogy, the transfer of RNA molecules is called Northern blotting, and the transfer of proteins is Western blotting. (Northern and Western do not derive from names of scientists.)

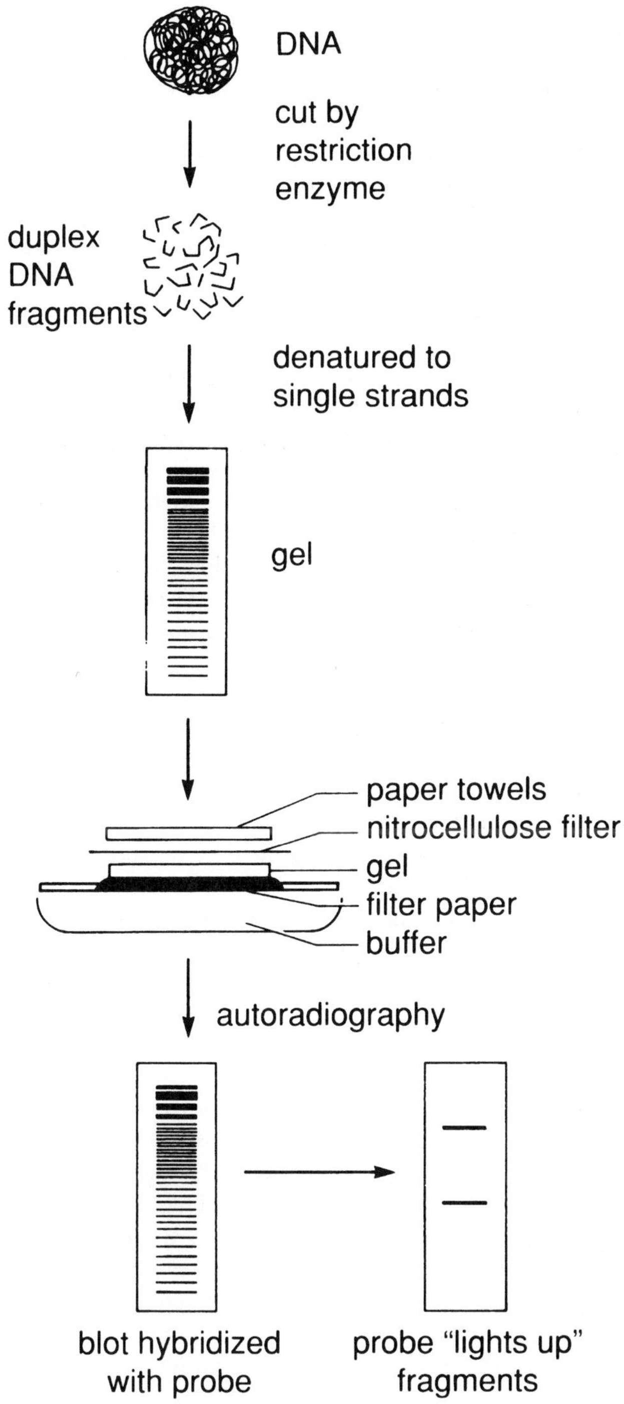

FIGURE 47.16 The technique of Southern blotting. DNA is cut into small fragments by restriction endonucleases, separated on a gel, then transferred by blotting onto nitrocellulose membrane (see text).

CHROMOSOME WALKING AND JUMPING

Chromosome walking is an approach used to clone relatively long stretches of the genome. The walk begins with a clone that has already been isolated. Terminal fragments of the clone are used as probes to identify adjacent overlapping clones from a genomic library. This process can be repeated to cover lengths of 100 kb or more, but the size of a single step is limited by the size of the insert of foreign DNA that can be incorporated into vectors, about 20 kb for lambda vectors and 45 kb for cosmids. The direction of the walk along the chromosome can be determined by making successive restriction maps and identifying matching regions.

Much longer distances can be covered by chromosome jumping. In this method, very long (100–200 kb) restriction fragments of genomic DNA are circularized in vitro, resulting in the formation of artificial junctions between sequences normally separated by long distances. These junctions are then cloned using conventional technology and radioactive probes. The clones isolated thus contain the starting sequence (the probe binding site) and a new genomic sequence 100–200 kb away. Because the sequence between the sites is not cloned by this method, one has effectively jumped from the probe site to a position 100–200 kb farther along the chromosome.

POLYMERASE CHAIN REACTION

PCR represents a powerful new technique for the analysis of DNA. Basically, it is a tool for greatly amplifying tiny pieces of DNA. This includes, for example, minute samples of hair, blood, skin, sperm, or saliva. It is especially useful in the diagnosis of human genetic mutations through the analysis of small blood samples, including identification of the trinucleotide repeat expansions described above. The theory and technology underlying PCR are beyond the scope of this chapter. PCR and its application to neurological disease are well-described by Darnell (1993). PCR uses a heat-stable DNA polymerase to extend synthetic DNA primers that flank and bind to DNA sequences of interest. Samples are then heated to near 100°C to denature the DNA into single strands and cooled to reanneal newly synthesized DNA with the synthetic primers. As this cycle is repeated, newly synthesized DNA is available to anneal with primers and be extended. In this way the reaction amplifies itself (a chain reaction) with a doubling of products at each cycle. Thirty cycles can be performed in a few hours in a single tube in an automated thermal cycling machine. Thus, a relatively small input yields an enormous amplification of product—ideally more than 200 copies of a single starting molecule. However, one of the problems with PCR is its great sensitivity, sometimes resulting in false results from amplification of minute amounts of contaminating DNA (Darnell 1993).

LINKAGE ANALYSIS

Genetic linkage analysis has been extensively used to map genes for human diseases to specific chromosomes. The concept is straightforward (Ott 1990). All genetic mutations occur at a single point or locus somewhere on the 22 human autosomes or the X chromosome. If two genes occur close

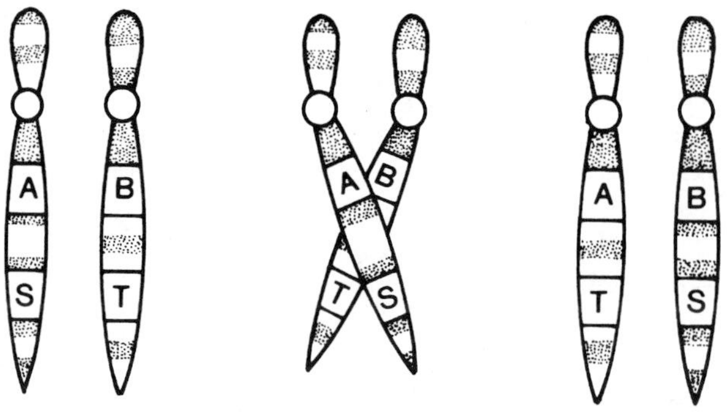

FIGURE 47.17 A crossover between the long arms of a homologous chromosome pair resulting in a recombination between the hypothetical linked genes. The gene loci at A and S are close to each other on the same chromosome (linked). The alleles at locus 1 are A and B. The alleles at locus 2 are S and T. Thus, this person is heterozygous at both the 1 (AB) and 2 (ST) loci. Locus 1 could represent the site of a disease gene, and locus 2 could be the site of a polymorphic DNA marker. Initially, gametes resulting from these chromosomes would be AS or BT. Following the crossover and recombination, the gametes would be AT or BS. The A allele at locus 1 would now be inherited with the T allele at locus 2. The B allele at locus 1 would now be inherited with the S allele at locus 2.

to each other on the same chromosome, they are said to be linked. Note that linkage is simply a physical relationship between two loci on a chromosome and implies no pathogenetic or metabolic association between the two genes.

Crossing over of homologous chromosomes during meiosis may result in a recombintion between the two loci of linked genes (Figure 47.17). The frequency with which these recombinations occur increases with increasing distance between the two genes. Therefore, the frequency of recombination events between two loci is a relative measure of the distance between them. A 1% frequency of recombination between two loci indicates 1 centimorgan (cM) of genetic distance between them. One centimorgan represents about 1 million DNA base pairs (1,000 kb). (Note that a cM represents recombination events and is an estimate of genetic distance on a chromosome, but not a true physical distance.) The total human genome contains approximately 3,300 cM and at least 50,000 genes. It should be noted that recombination frequencies (crossovers) are not necessarily the same for chromosomes in males and females (generally more frequent in females for unknown reasons), not always the same for different chromosomes, and not the same for different portions of the same chromosome (recombination hot spots). The recombination frequency is expressed by the Greek letter theta (θ) and has a maximum of 0.5 (one-half, or 50%).

If a dominant monogenic clinical disorder is traced through a family pedigree to the inheritance of another unrelated genetic marker (such as the ABO blood group), one can determine the probability that the two genetic traits (the disorder and the marker) are linked or not linked. If all persons affected with the genetic disorder always have the same form (polymorphism) of the genetic marker and all unaffected persons have the other form of the marker, the two genetic traits are said to be segregating together. If enough individuals can be tested, the two traits can be shown to be linked or unlinked.

In order for linkage analysis of a family to be useful, the family must be informative for both the disease and the genetic marker. That is, it must be possible to distinguish between persons affected and unaffected with the disease, and there must be variability of the polymorphic states of the marker within the family. For example, the first two generations of the family in Figure 47.18 are not informative, because all the offspring in the second generation are type AB for the marker whether they have the disorder or not. However, in the third generation all the affected individuals have the AB form of the marker, and all the unaffected individuals are type AA. The pedigree contains useful genetic linkage information because there have been several informative matings in the second generation. On inspection of the pedigree, it becomes apparent that the disease seems to be segregating with the B form of the genetic marker. Linkage analysis of this family would then give us an estimate of the probability that the disorder is indeed linked to the genetic marker under study.

A statistical measure of linkage is the LOD score, which is an estimate of the probability or likelihood that two genetic traits are linked. The LOD score is the log of the odds favoring linkage versus independent assortment. A LOD score of +3.0 represents theoretical odds of 1,000 to 1 (10^3) that two traits are linked and is generally accepted as proof of linkage, especially if the analysis has been restricted to a single family. (A LOD score of +3 actually represents a practical probability of about 95% that two genes are linked.) A true linkage relationship in a large, genetically homogeneous population of families should produce a LOD score of +4 or +5 with a highly polymorphic marker. A LOD score of –2.0 represents odds of 100 to 1 (10^2) that two traits are not linked. LOD scores falling between +3.0 and –2.0 are more or less suggestive of linkage, respectively, but not accepted as proof. LOD scores are calculated for a given recombination fraction. Two traits may be considered loosely linked with a recombination fraction of 10–20%, closely linked with a recombination fraction of about 5%, or tightly linked with a recombination fraction of 1% or less. (These are helpful but not strict definitions.) As noted above, the recombination fraction is related to distance along the chromosome. During linkage analysis LOD scores are computed for many possible recombination fractions. Therefore, the recombination fraction with the highest positive LOD score is the best estimate of the distance between two potentially linked genes.

The usefulness of genetic linkage analysis is demonstrated in Table 47.3. The LOD scores for three different Charcot-Marie-Tooth families are shown for various genetic markers on chromosomes 1 and 17. Family 1520 has clearly positive LOD scores (greater than +3.0) for two markers on chromosome 17 and negative LOD scores for two markers on chro-

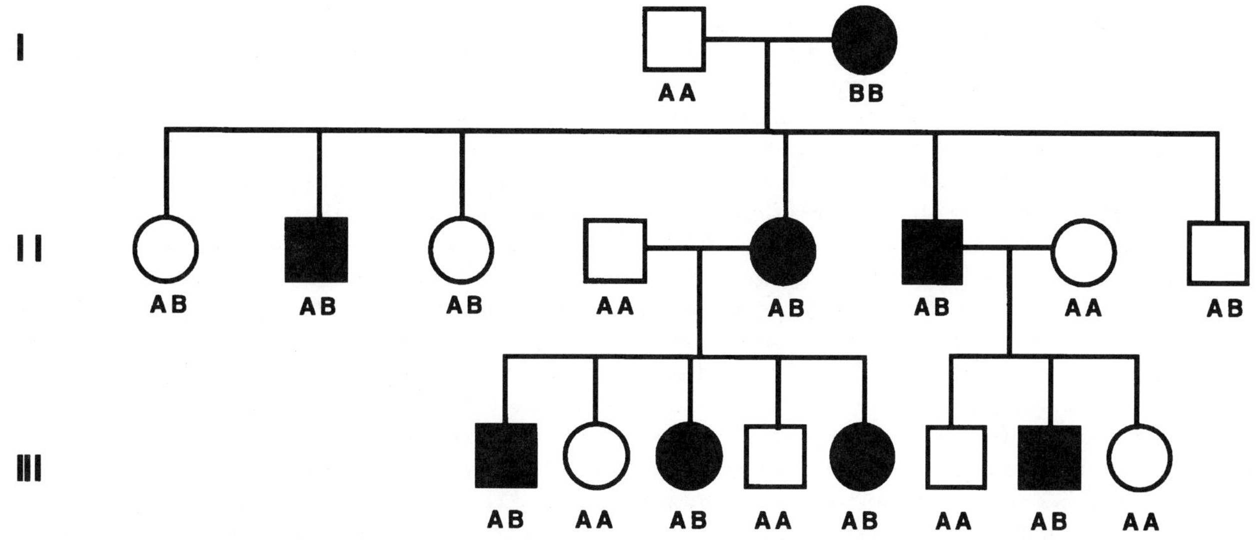

FIGURE 47.18 Autosomal dominant inheritance (uninformative mating versus informative mating). Pedigree demonstrating the basic principle of linkage analysis. Persons affected with the disease are indicated with solid symbols. Results of genetic testing for inherited DNA markers (A and B) are indicated under each symbol. Generation 2 is uninformative, because there is no obvious association between the disease and the genetic markers. However, generation 3 makes the family analysis informative. It now can be seen that all affected individuals have inherited the B allele of the DNA marker, and none of the unaffected persons has inherited the B allele. This suggests that the disease gene resides in a chromosomal region close to the genes for the A and B genetic markers—that is, the analysis suggests linkage. If the chromosomal location of the A and B markers is known, then it is likely that the disease gene also lies on this chromosome.

mosome 1. The gene for hereditary neuropathy in this family must lie on the short arm of chromosome 17, and such families are designated CMT 1A. The IND family has a very significant negative LOD score with a marker on chromosome 17 (–4.10) and positive LOD scores with the chromosome 1 markers. The gene for hereditary neuropathy in the IND family must lie on the long arm of chromosome 1, and such families are designated as CMT 1B. Finally, family 1550 has significantly negative LOD scores, with all markers on both chromosomes 1 and 17. The gene for hereditary neuropathy in this family must lie elsewhere in the human genome, and such a family is tentatively designated as CMT 1C. Thus, genetic linkage analysis has demonstrated genetic heterogeneity and indicated that there are at least three distinct genetic forms of autosomal dominant CMT with separate genes on chromosomes 1q, 17p, and some other location.

LOD scores from different families comparing a genetic marker and a disease may be added if one is certain that the families have the same genetic disorder (a mutation at the same locus). (The LOD scores are added because they represent logs or exponents, as noted above.) For example, the first four families with CMT to undergo linkage analysis had a cumulative added LOD score of greater than +6.0 for linkage with the Duffy blood group locus on chromosome 1. This was accepted as proof of linkage of this form of autosomal dominant CMT to a marker on chromosome 1. Subsequently, numerous families with autosomal dominant hereditary neuropathy have had negative LOD scores for the Duffy locus (Chance and Pleasure 1993). This raises an important issue in genetic linkage analysis that is a common and complex problem. There are two possible explanations for these different LOD scores for families with apparently the same disease. The first is that they all do have exactly the same genetic disease (mutations at the same locus). The LOD scores should all be added, and the net total score shows no linkage with Duffy. However, a second explanation is that different families with a similar clinical syndrome may represent genetic heterogeneity (mutations at different loci). Pos-

Table 47.3: Comparison of linkage analysis for three CMT families

A. Chromosome 1q markers (LOD scores at 0.001 recombination)			
	Family		
Marker	*#1520*	*IND*	*#1550*
Duffy (Fy)	−3.11	1.96	−6.67
Fc γ RII	−8.85	5.17*	−0.97
B. Chromosome 17p markers (LOD scores at 0.05 recombination)			
	Family		
Marker	*#1520*	*IND*	*#1550*
EW 301	3.10*	NI	−4.62
pTH 17.19	3.15*	NI	−2.35
8B10	NI	−4.10	NI

NI = not informative.
*LOD score >3.0, indicating strong evidence for linkage.

itive and negative LOD scores from the various families when added will cancel out and show no linkage, whereas linkage may be present in one or a few families and be missed during the pooling of multifamily data. Often, the issue of possible genetic heterogeneity must await the evaluation of further families and the generation of additional linkage data. Further investigation has, for example, indeed shown that a common locus for CMT resides on chromosome 17, and a less common locus for CMT is on chromosome 1.

Genetic heterogeneity can be difficult to predict from clinical or pathological information. For example, it was once thought that the so-called peripheral and central forms of neurofibromatosis might actually represent different expression of the same genetic disease (mutation), or at least be alleles (different mutations at the same locus). However, linkage analysis has shown that the two conditions are entirely different mutations on chromosomes 17 and 22, respectively. A similar situation has occurred with hereditary polycystic kidney disease and possibly tuberous sclerosis. That is, the same clinical syndrome (phenotype) shows genetic heterogeneity by linkage analysis. On the other hand, two forms of familial polyposis of the colon that seemed quite different phenotypically have proved to be mutations at the same locus. Likewise, families with early- and late-onset Huntington's disease represent mutations at the same locus on chromosome 4.

Obviously, it is safest to limit linkage analysis to single large families, eliminating the problem of genetic heterogeneity. Unfortunately, most single families are not large enough to generate statistically significant linkage data. Data from multiple families are often pooled but must be viewed with healthy skepticism until the data are unequivocally significant or it is clearly established by other means that the families are genetically homogeneous. For example, initial studies showing linkage of schizophrenia to chromosome 5 markers and manic depressive illness to chromosomes 11 and X have not been replicated, and the assignments remain uncertain (Straub and Gilliam 1993).

Statistical tests are available that give an indication of genetic heterogeneity by comparing LOD scores from various families with similar clinical disorders. The results may range from a high probability to a very low probability of linkage.

Also, separate families with disorders produced by alleles (different mutations at the same locus) can appropriately have pooling of their linkage analysis data. For example, Becker's and Duchenne's muscular dystrophies are now known to be allelic mutations in the same gene and show the same linkage relationships to other X-chromosome markers.

It should also be obvious that correct clinical diagnosis of each and every family member is crucial in linkage analysis. Incorrectly identified family members will produce serious errors in the analysis and can falsely bias the data toward linkage or nonlinkage. For example, with hereditary neuropathy with slow nerve conduction, clinically equivocal cases must have careful NCV studies. In myotonic dystrophy, EMG and slit-lamp examination of the lens may be necessary in family members at risk who appear clinically unaffected by physical examination. Imprecise clinical diagnosis is partly responsible for the conflicting linkage results in studies of schizophrenia. Also, diseases with delayed onset (such as Huntington's and Alzheimer's diseases) must have age-of-onset correction factors included in the analysis.

One may also take advantage of two or more genetic markers known to reside close to each other on the same chromosome, in a statistical technique known as multipoint genetic linkage analysis. This increases the power of demonstrating linkage and may allow more refined subregional location of a given disorder. Examples of the use of this technique in neurological diseases are the multipoint linkage analyses of late-onset familial Alzheimer's disease to chromosome 19 markers, and of CMT to chromosome 1 markers.

If the gene controlling the expression of a marker is known to have its locus on a specific chromosome, then any genetic trait shown to be linked to that marker must also have its locus on the same chromosome. Thus, the power of linkage analysis is the actual identification of genetic loci on specific chromosomes or even finely mapped regions of a chromosome. This can lead to advances in diagnosis and even to the discovery of the nature of mutations and the protein abnormalities underlying genetic diseases.

If there are no previous clues to the chromosomal location of a genetic disease, then a large number of random genetic markers covering all human chromosomes need to be systematically studied to discover a linkage relationship. It is estimated that about 200–300 evenly spaced markers would reasonably cover the entire human genome. At present, the known markers are not evenly spaced, but additional markers are rapidly improving this situation. The markers must be polymorphic—that is, have several possible identifiable forms in the general population so that various combinations can be found in any given family. Theoretically, with enough genetic markers and sufficient time and effort, all monogenic disorders can be located on specific chromosomes. This task can be very tedious and time-consuming. A remarkable advance has been the advent of new DNA polymorphisms that make available the hundreds and even thousands of inherited markers necessary to cover the human genome in a complete manner. The first such markers were restriction fragment length polymorphisms (RFLPs), which are now complemented by a variable number of tandem repeats (VNTR) and microsatellite CA repeats, which make most families informative and improve the success rate of linkage studies. The first example of an autosomal dominant linkage relationship using these new techniques was the linkage of the Huntington's disease gene to the D4S10 (G8) RFLP marker on the distal end of the short arm of chromosome 4. The pace of chromosomal assignment of neurological diseases has subsequently greatly accelerated. There are now more than 150 disorders of the nervous system with specific chromosomal assignments (Harding and Rosenberg et al. 1993) (Tables 47.4 and 47.5).

POSITIONAL CLONING

Once disease genes have been given regional assignments on chromosomes by linkage analysis, the search is begun to identify the gene itself by *positional cloning* (previously termed *reverse genetics*). This strategy relies only on the chromosomal location of the gene. Once the gene is discovered, one can attempt to determine the protein for which it codes. This strategy is the opposite of beginning with a known protein, determining its amino acid sequence, and using that information to locate and isolate a gene. All the tools and methods described above are brought to bear in the process of isolating a gene, including restriction endonucleases, genetic libraries, vectors including YACs, and chromosome walking and jumping. The strategy has been spectacularly successful with the recent identification of numerous genes for neurological disorders including Duchenne's and Becker's muscular dystrophies, myotonic dystrophy, Huntington's disease, and neurofibromatosis. Several examples of such genes and their known protein functions are shown in Table 47.6.

How is it known when a gene is found? Another way to express this question is, How is it known if a change in a DNA sequence represents a benign polymorphism or causes a clinically significant alteration in the functions of a protein? One method is to return to linkage analysis and demonstrate that the newly discovered change, or mutation, always segregates with the disease in the family. That is, people with the disease always have the mutation, and people without the disease never have the mutation. Obviously, penetrance and expression must be taken into consideration. Furthermore, unrelated, normal individuals in the general population never show the mutation. It is also useful to demonstrate de novo occurrence of the mutation. That is, isolated individuals with the disease carry the mutation, but the mutation is not found in any of their siblings or either of their parents (and paternity is proved).

What follows gene identification? When a new gene is isolated, relatively little may be known about its function. The DNA and predicted amino acid sequences can be compared to those of known genes and proteins in humans and other species. Also, the amino acid sequence can be analyzed for the presence of predicted secondary structures and specific functional motifs, such as known membrane-spanning regions. Antibodies can be raised to the gene product; then the distribution, cellular, and subcellular location of the protein can be determined.

To study the effect of overexpression or underexpression of a gene, it is now possible to introduce the foreign gene into a mouse germ-cell line and produce transgenic animals. Eggs are removed from a female mouse, fertilized with sperm in a test tube, and a recombinant plasmid carrying a new gene is microinjected into the male pronucleus. The new gene can be placed under the control of a promotor, and high expression levels can be reached. One can then study overexpression of that particular gene in the resulting transgenic

Table 47.4: Chromosomal assignments of selected autosomal neurological disorders

Disorder	*Chromosome*	*Inheritance Pattern*
Charcot-Marie-Tooth (CMT 2)	1p35–36	AD
Infantile ceroid lipofuscinosis	1p32	AR
Carnitine palmityltransferase deficiency	1p32–12	AR
Charcot-Marie-Tooth (CMT 1B)	1q22–23	AD
Glucocerebrosidase/Gaucher's disease	1q21	AR
Nemaline myopathy	1q21–23	AD
Hypokalemic periodic paralysis	1q31	AD
Limb girdle muscular dystrophy (1 type)	2p	AR
Familial spastic paraplegia (1)	2p21–24	AD
Cerebrotendinous xanthomatosis	2q	AR
Amyotrophic lateral sclerosis (recessive)	2q33–35	AR
Beta-galactosidase I/GM_1 gangliosidosis	3pter–3p21	AR
Retinitis pigmentosa—1	3q	AD
von Hippel-Lindau disease	3p26–25	AD
Huntington's disease	4p16.3	AD
FSH muscular dystrophy	4q35–ter	AD
Infantile spinal muscular atrophy	5q11.2–13.3	AR
Hexosaminidase B-Sandhoff's disease	5q13	AR
Hyperekplexia (startle disease)	5q	AD
Dominant limb girdle muscular dystrophy	5q22–34	AD
SCA 1 (spinocerebellar ataxia)	6p24	AD
Juvenile myoclonic epilepsy	6p24	AD
Retinitis pigmentosa (peripherin)	6p21	AD
Myotonia congenita	7q35	AD
Familial spastic paraplegia (recessive)	8	AR
Ataxia with vitamin E deficiency	8q	AR
Charcot-Marie-Tooth (CMT 3)	8q13–21	AR
Friedreich's ataxia	9q13–21.1	AR
Fukuyama congenital dystrophy	9q31–33	AR
Familial dysautonomia	9q31–33	AR
Torsion dystonia (some families)	9q34	AD
Tuberous sclerosis (some families)	9q34.1–34.2	AD
Ataxia, infantile onset	10q23–24	AR
SCA 5 (spinocerebellar ataxia)	11	AD
Niemann-Pick types A and B (sphingomyelinase)	11p15	AR
Tuberous sclerosis (some families)	11q14–23	AD
Ataxia telangiectasia	11q23	AR
Acute intermittent porphyria	11q23.2	AD
McArdle's disease (myophosphorylase)	11q13	AR
Episodic ataxia/myokymia	12p13	AD
SCA 2 (spinocerebellar ataxia)	12q23–24.1	AD
Muscular dystrophy (recessive Duchenne's-like)	13q12	AR
Lipofuscinosis, late infantile	12q21–32	AR
Wilson's disease	13q14.2–21	AR
Distal myopathy	14q11	AD
Familial Alzheimer's (early onset)	14q24.3	AD
Krabbe's leukodystrophy	14q24.3–32	AR
SCA 3 (Machado-Joseph disease)	14q24.3–32	AD
Familial spastic paraplegia (2)	14q	AD
Dopa-responsive dystonia	14q	AD
Angelman's and Prader-Willi syndromes	15q11–12	Sporadic

Table 47.4: *(continued)*

Disorder	*Chromosome*	*Inheritance Pattern*
Recessive limb girdle muscular dystrophy	15q15–?22	AR
Hexosaminidase A/Tay-Sachs disease	15q23–24	AR
Familial spastic paraplegia (3)	15q	AD
Tuberous sclerosis (some families)	16p13.3	AD
Juvenile lipofuscinosis (Batten's disease)	16p12	AR
Bardet-Biedl (mental retardation, retinitis pigmentosa, polydactyly)	16q	AR
SCA 4 (spinocerebellar ataxia)	16q24	AD
Charcot-Marie-Tooth (CMT 1A)	17p11.2	AD
Severe childhood muscular dystrophy	17	AR
Neuropathy with liability to pressure palsy	17p11.2	AD
Canavan leukodystrophy	17p13	AR
Miller-Dieker syndrome, lissencephaly	17p–13.3	Sporadic
Sjögren-Larsson syndrome	17q	AR
Niemann-Pick disease types A and B	11	AR
Neurofibromatosis NF1	17q11.2	AD
Muscle sodium channel disorders (hyperkalemic periodic paralysis, atypical myotonia congenita, paramyotonia congenita)	17q22–24	AD
Niemann-Pick type C	18p	AR
Familial amyloid neuropathy (transthyretin)	18q11.2–12.1	AD
Episodic ataxia with nystagmus	19p13	AD
Malignant hyperthermia (ryanidine receptor)	19q13.1	AD
Central core myopathy	19q13.1	AD
Myotonic muscular dystrophy	19q13.2	AD
Familial Alzheimer's (late onset)	19q	?
Cystatin C/Icelandic amyloid angiopathy	20p11.22–11.21	AD
Familial prion dementias (Creutzfeldt-Jakob, Gerstmann-Straussler diseases)	20pter–p12	AD
Familial benign neonatal convulsions	20q	AD
Familial Alzheimer's (APP gene, early onset)	21q11–22	AD
Familial amyotrophic lateral sclerosis (some families)	21q22.1–22.2	AD
Myoclonic epilepsy (Unverricht-Lundborg)	22q22.3	AD
Metachromatic leukodystrophy (arylsulfatase A)	22q13.3–qter	AR
Bilateral acoustic neurofibromatosis (NF2)	22q11–13.1	AD

animals. Attempts have been made, for example, to overexpress the amyloid precursor protein gene in transgenic mice as a model of Alzheimer's disease (Games et al. 1995).

Knockout mutants can also be created. Embryonic stem cells are used, and a portion of the mouse gene is exchanged for an altered DNA sequence—for example, one containing a premature-stop codon. This technology can produce

Table 47.5: Regional assignments of selected X-linked neurological disorders

Kallman anosmia-hypogonadism	Xp22.3
Mental retardation, nonspecific (1)	Xp22
Duchenne's muscular dystrophy	Xp21.2
Becker's muscular dystrophy	Xp21.2
Ornithine transcarbamylase deficiency	Xp21.1
Menkes' kinky hair	Xp11–q11
Charcot-Marie-Tooth (CMTX)	Xq13–q21
Ataxia/sideroblastic anemia	Xq13
Mental retardation, nonspecific (2)	Xq11–q12
X-linked spastic paraplegia (1)	Xq13–22
Lubag dystonia Parkinsonism	Xq21
Choroideremia	Xq21.2
Spinal-bulbar muscular atrophy (Kennedy's disease)	Xq21.3–q12
Fabry's disease (trihexoside storage)	Xq22
Pelizaeus-Merzbacher disease	Xq22
Lesch-Nyhan HGPRT deficiency	Xq26
Fragile X/mental retardation	Xq27.3
Adrenoleukodystrophy	Xq28
X-linked spastic paraplegia (2)	Xq28
Emery-Dreifuss muscular dystrophy	Xq28
X-linked myotubular myopathy	Xq28
X-linked manic depressive illness	Xq28
X-linked hydrocephalus	Xq28

heterozygotes (having one mutant and one normal allele) or homozygotes (having no functional gene product at that locus, so-called null mutants). Homozygous knockout mice may also provide an important source of cell lines that lack the gene product. Knockout mice for the P_0 myelin gene have been produced, for example, and will aid in understanding hereditary neuropathies (Giese et al. 1992).

The two major long-term goals of neurogenetic research are (1) to further our understanding of the biological and physiological functions of the human organism; and (2) to create new diagnostic, therapeutic, and preventative measures for human genetic diseases.

GENETIC COUNSELING

Genetic counseling is a perfect example of the mixture of art and science inherent in the practice of medicine. It requires the communication of complex data to patients by physicians in an objective and nonjudgmental but diplomatic and compassionate fashion. The first step in genetic counseling is to establish an accurate diagnosis. This is obviously critical and must be done as carefully as possible. As in all of medicine, the accurate diagnosis of genetic diseases depends on history, physical examination, and laboratory tests. In addition, obtaining a full family pedigree is important. Information about medical disorders in other family members will provide important clues to the diagnosis in the proband. Also, inspection of the family pedigree will frequently indicate the correct inheritance pattern, be it dominant, recessive, X-linked, or mitochondrial (see Figures 47.2, 47.3, 47.4, and 47.7).

Table 47.6: Newly discovered neurological disease genes classified by function

Gene Class	*Disease*	*Protein*	*Chromosome*
Structural genes	Duchenne's muscular dystrophy (DMD)	Dystrophin	Xp21.2
	Becker's muscular dystrophy	Dystrophin	Xp21.2
	Paramyotonia congenita	Sodium channel	17q23.1–25.3
	Hyperkalemic periodic paralysis	Sodium channel	17q23.1–25.3
	Hypokalemic periodic paralysis	Calcium channel	1q31
	Myotonia congenita	Chloride channel	7q35
	Episodic ataxia/myokymia	Potassium channel	12p13
	Charcot-Marie-Tooth disease (CMT 1A)	PMP22	17p11.2
	Hereditary neuropathy with liability to pressure palsies (HNPP)	PMP22	17p11.2
	CMT 1B	P_0 myelin	1q21.2–23
	X-linked CMT	Connexin32	Xq13
	Alzheimer's disease	Amyloid precursor protein (APP)	21q21.3–22.05
	Retinitis pigmentosa	Rhodopsin	3q
	Startle disease (hyperekplexia)	Glycine receptor	5q
Tumor suppressor genes	Neurofibromatosis 2 (NF2)	Merlin	22q11.21–13.1
	Neurofibromatosis 1 (NF1)	Neurofibromin	17q11.2
	Retinoblastoma	Rb	13q14.1–14.2
	Von Hippel-Lindau disease	Unknown	3p25
	Tuberous sclerosis	Tuberin	16p13.3
Transport protein genes	X-linked adrenoleukodystrophy	ALDP	Xq28
	Menkes' syndrome	Copper transport protein	Xq13.3
	Wilson's disease	Copper transport protein	13q14.3
Trinucleotide Expansion genes	Fragile-X mental retardation	FMR1	Xq27.3
	Huntington's disease (HD)	Huntingtin	4q16.3
	Myotonic dystrophy	Myosin kinase	19q13.3
	Spinocerebellar atrophy (SCA 1)	Unknown	6p23–24
	Kennedy's spinal-bulbar muscular atrophy	Androgen receptor	Xq21.3–22
	Dentato-Rubral-Pallido-Luysian atrophy	Unknown	12
	Machado-Joseph disease (SCA 3)	Unknown	14q
Cell protection genes	Familial amyotrophic lateral sclerosis (ALS)	Superoxide dismutase (SOD1)	21q22.1–22.2
Signaling molecules	CMT 1B	P_0 myelin protein	1q21.2–23
	Miller-Dieker syndrome	G-proteins	17p13.3
	Retinitis pigmentosa	Rhodopsin	3q
Mitochondrial genes	Leigh's disease	OXPHOS pathway	—
	MERRF	OXPHOS pathway	—
	MELAS	OXPHOS pathway	—
	Leber's optic atrophy	OXPHOS pathway	—
	Kearns-Sayre disease	OXPHOS pathway	—
Prion proteins	Creutzfeldt-Jakob disease	Prion protein (PrP)	20pter–p12
	Gerstmann-Straussler-Sheinker syndrome	PrP	20pter–p12
	Familial fatal insomnia	PrP	20pter–p12
Cell cycle genes	Retinoblastoma	Rb	13q14.1–14.2
	Von Hippel-Lindau disease	Unknown	3p25

Source: Reprinted with permission from P Greenstein, TD Bird. Neurogenetics: triumphs and challenges. West J Med 1994;161:242–245.

Following accurate diagnosis, the next major step in genetic counseling is educating the patient. This includes an estimate of risk to the proband and other family members for inheriting the pertinent gene. Risks always need to be put into context and perspective. For example, with each pregnancy all normal couples take a 2–4% risk of having a child with birth defects. It is often unpredictable how any given person will react to a risk probability for inheriting a disease. Some people will find a 50% risk of no great concern, whereas others may find a 1% risk to be very disturbing. Obviously, the perceived severity or burden of the disease is of major importance. Physicians, patients, and other family members may not agree as to what constitutes a "severe" disease. In addition to risk estimates, the counselor must give a description of expected symptoms and signs, natural history of the disease, variability of expression, and long-term prognosis. Potential treatment options must also be discussed. Physicians are accustomed to considerable variability in symptoms and prognosis of various diseases, but these ambiguities can be difficult concepts for many patients.

The presymptomatic diagnosis of neurogenetic disorders is becoming more common. Huntington's disease has been a model in this regard (Quaid 1993, Bennett et al. 1993). By DNA testing for the trinucleotide repeat expansion on chromosome 4, carriers of the HD gene can now be fairly reliably detected, as described above (the exception being the equivocal range of 33–37 repeats). This means we have the ability to discover who has inherited the gene for a severe, progressive, incurable, fatal degenerative brain disease. At the same time, we are unable to predict age of onset or severity of the disease with much accuracy. These issues raise serious problems for both the physician and the patient, including the patient's motivation for having the test, the patient's emotional reaction to the result, and potential long-term implications for employment and insurance. Detailed discussions of these medical and ethical issues are available, and the next few years will provide an accumulation of experience with this relatively new aspect of counseling (Hersch et al. 1994; Guidelines 1994; Bird and Bennett 1995).

Finally, genetic counseling should include opportunities for follow-up and long-term contact with the patient. The patient must be given an opportunity to ask questions. Additional testing of the patient and other family members may be necessary. Detailed genetic counseling frequently involves a long-term process involving months or years, and it becomes a basic thread in the fabric of good medical care.

REFERENCES

Bennett R, Bird TD, Teri L. Offering predictive testing for HD in a medical genetics clinic. J Genet Counseling 1993;2:123–137.

Bergoffen J, Scherer S, Pauls D et al. Connexin mutations in X-linked Charcot-Marie-Tooth disease. Science 1993;262:2039–2042.

Bird TD, Bennett R. Why do DNA testing? Ann Neurol 1995 (in press).

Chance PE, Pleasure D. Charcot-Marie-Tooth syndrome. Arch Neurol 1993;50:1180–1184.

Darnell RB. The polymerase chain reaction: application to nervous system disease. Ann Neurol 1993;34:513–523.

DiMauro S, Moraes T. Mitochondrial encephalomyopathies. Arch Neurol 1993;50:1197–1208.

Games D, Adams D, Alessandrini R et al. Alzheimer-type neuropathology in transgenic mice overexpressing V717F β-amyloid precursor protein. Nature 1995;373:523–527.

Giese KP, Martini R, Lemke G et al. Mouse P_0 gene disruption leads to hypomyelination, abnormal expression of recognition molecules and degeneration of myelin and axons. Cell 1992;71:565–576.

Greenstein P, Bird TD. Neurogenetics: triumphs and challenges. West J Med 1994;161:242–245.

Guidelines for the molecular genetics predictive test in Huntington's disease. Neurology 1994;44:1533–1536.

Harding AE, Rosenberg RN. A Neurologic Gene Map. In RN Rosenberg, SB Prusiner, S DiMauro et al. (eds), The Molecular and Genetic Basis of Neurologic Disease. Boston: Butterworth, 1993;21–24.

HD Collaborative Research Group. A novel gene containing a trinucleotide repeat that is expanded and unstable on Huntington's disease chromosomes. Cell 1993;72:971–983.

Harnden DG, Klinger HP (eds). ISCN 1985: An International System for Human Cytogenetic Nomenclature. Basel: Karger, 1985.

Harper PS, Harley HG, Reardon W et al. Anticipation in myotonic dystrophy: new light on an old problem. Am J Hum Genet 1992;51:10–16.

Hayasaka K, Himoro M, Sato W et al. Charcot-Marie-Tooth neuropathy type 1B is associated with mutations of the myelin P_0 gene. Nature Genetics 1993;5:31–34.

Hersch S, Jones R, Koroshetz W et al. The neurogenetics genie: testing for the Huntington's disease mutation. Neurology 1994;44:1369–1373.

Martin JB. Molecular genetics in neurology. Ann Neurol 1993;34:757–773.

Ott J. Analysis of Human Genetic Linkage (2nd ed). Baltimore: Johns Hopkins University Press, 1990.

Quaid KA. Presymptomatic testing for Huntington disease: recommendations for counseling. J Genet Counseling 1993;1:277–302.

Straub RE, Gilliam TC. Genetic Linkage Studies of Bipolar Affective Disorder. In KE Davies, SM Tilghman (eds), Genome Maps and Neurological Disorders. Cold Spring Harbor, NY: Cold Spring Harbor Press, 1993;77–100.

Thompson M, McInnes R, Willard H. Genetics in Medicine. Philadelphia: Saunders, 1991.

Vance JM, Bird TD. Genetic Heterogeneity in Charcot-Marie-Tooth. In PM Conneally (ed), Molecular Basis of Neurology. Cambridge, MA: Blackwell, 1993;233–244.

Voss R, Ben-Simon E, Avital A et al. Isodisomy of chromosome 7 in a patient with cystic fibrosis: could uniparental disomy be common in humans? Am J Hum Genet 1989;45:373–380.

Wiggins S, Whyte P, Huggins M et al. The psychological consequences of predictive testing for Huntington's disease. N Engl J Med 1992;327:1401–1405.

Chapter 48
Neuroimmunology

Subramaniam Sriram and Trevor Owens

The explosion of research in immunology has resulted in an increased understanding of a unifying concept of the immune system. The interest to the neurologist in this field stems not only from the fact that many neurological diseases have an immunological basis but also from the fact that the nervous and immune systems have a number of similarities. A further point of interest is the recent appreciation that the nervous system shares certain mechanisms for cell-to-cell communication with the immune system. The immune system, like the nervous system, is organized with a machinery (1) to recognize and react to environmental events, (2) to develop a strategy to deal effectively with such events, and (3) to maintain a memory pattern effectively to recognize and counter this event, should it happen again.

The armaments used by the adaptive immune response to counter pathogens act at multiple levels. The earliest to appear in phylogeny were antigen-nonspecific and had rapid response kinetics. The immune responses were mediated with limited numbers of immune cells that lacked specificity and immunological memory. Thus, macrophages and polymorphonuclear cells were the principal defenses against infectious agents. Two mechanisms that conferred specificity and memory evolved subsequently. First, B cells evolved, with the ability to target pathogens for destruction by producing specific antibodies, and second, T cells evolved that bound to infected cells through their surface antigen–specific receptors and lysed only the infected cells. The critical components of the immune system are the cell surface receptors that impart specificity to the cells in their interaction with the environment. In turn, cross-linking of the receptor by its ligand also acts as a signal to the lymphocyte for growth and proliferation (Janeway 1992).

Critical experiments that answered many of the fundamental questions in immunology came about with developments in the fields of molecular biology, hybridoma technology, and cell-culture techniques. An overview of the immune system as it relates to humans and its role in neurological disease is presented in the following section.

CELLULAR COMPONENTS OF THE IMMUNE SYSTEM

Cells of the immune system arise from the pluripotent stem cells in the bone marrow and diverge into the lymphoid or myeloid lineages. The lymphoid lineage consists mainly of T cells and B cells, which are the principal components of the immune system. Natural killer (NK) cells also belong to the lymphoid lineage. The myeloid lineage primarily contains cells with phagocytic functions such as neutrophils, basophils, eosinophils, and macrophages.

T Lymphocytes

T cells, or thymus-derived cells, originate from the thymus. Differentiation of T cells occurs in the thymus, and every T cell that leaves the thymus is conferred with a unique specificity for recognizing foreign antigens. T cells that recognize self-antigens are either deleted or rendered tolerant. The process is complicated, and a number of steps in the process remain unclear. A synopsis of the fate of a prothymocyte entering the thymus follows.

Bone marrow–derived prothymocytes, which normally express no T cell marker, begin to express both CD4 and CD8 (double positive) antigens and a T cell antigen receptor after entering the thymus. Interaction of the double-positive T cells with major histocompatibility complex (MHC) class I or MHC class II molecules on thymic epithelial cells leads to positive selection. Positively selected T cells migrate to the medulla, where negative selection occurs. T cells that bind to MHC class I downregulate CD4 antigen, and those that interact with MHC class II downregulate CD8 antigen cell surface expression. T cells that are not positively selected die in the thymus, as do T cells that recognize self-MHC molecules in association with self-peptides, or they are at least rendered unresponsive. Thus, cells that exit from the thymus (1) display two mutually exclusive antigens, CD4 or CD8, on their cell surface; (2) interact with different classes of self-MHC molecules (also referred to as MHC restriction); and (3) are tolerant of self-antigens (Nikolic and Zugic 1991).

Functionally, CD4+ cells are involved in delayed-type hypersensitivity (DTH) responses and in providing help to B cells (and hence are termed *helper T cells*), while CD8 cells are involved in class I restricted lysis of antigen-specific targets (and hence are termed *cytotoxic T cells*). T cells with suppressor activity can express either CD4 or CD8, although their original definition was as CD8+ cells. Although the T cell receptor (TCR) interacts with the MHC-peptide complex on antigen-presenting cells, the signals for the subsequent enactment of T cell activation and proliferation are delivered by the CD3 antigen. CD3 is present on all T cells, and it consists of a complex of five nonpolymorphic polypeptide chains. These include gamma and delta chains (not to be confused with the polymorphic chains of the gamma delta T cell). The TCR with the CD3 antigen is referred to as the *TCR-CD3 complex*. About 3–5% of circulating T cells express another form of the TCR, a heterodimer comprised of gamma delta chains. The majority of these cells are CD4–, CD8–, or CD4– CD8low. Gamma delta T cells do not show MHC class restriction in their activity and lyse a number of targets nonspecifically. Gamma delta cells appear to localize in certain organs such as skin, intestinal epithelium, and lungs and are thought to play a sentinel role in the immune response (Haas et al. 1993).

T Cell Receptors

The TCR consists of two glycosylated polypeptide chains, alpha and beta, of 45,000 and 40,000 dalton molecular weight, respectively. This heterodimer of an alpha and beta chain is linked by disulfide bonds. Amino acid sequences show that each chain consists of variable (V), joining (J), and constant (C) regions closely resembling immunoglobulins. There are about 10^2 TCR-variable genes, grouped by homology into a small number of families, compared to 10^3 or greater for immunoglobulins (see below). The principles governing generation of diversity in the TCR are very similar to those for immunoglobulin genes. Unlike the immunoglobulin receptor that can recognize and bind to native antigens, the receptor specificity of T cells is to short peptides that are associated with the MHC antigens. These can be either foreign MHC molecules or self-peptides that are associated with self-MHC molecules (Davis 1992) (Figure 48.1).

T cells also express a variety of nonpolymorphic antigens on their surfaces. The most abundantly expressed is CD45, comprising 10% of lymphocyte membrane protein. Expression of CD45 defines cells of hemopoietic origin. CD45 exists as a number of isoforms that differ in the molecular weight of their extracellular domains as a result of RNA splicing. These isoforms can be distinguished serologically. The low molecular weight (CD45RO) isoforms define activated, or memory, T cell populations, which are responsible for recall immune responses—for example, to tetanus toxoid (Thomas 1989). The CD45RO marker is useful for distinguishing resting from activated T cells in infiltrates and in cerebrospinal fluid (CSF). Other cell surface molecules include a wide array of adhesion molecules, which can be grouped into families on the basis of their structure. The three most prominent adhesion molecule families are those with homology to immunoglobulins (the immunoglobulin gene superfamily), the integrins and selectins. Adhesion molecules have ligands on other lymphocytes (such as B cells), leukocytes, endothelial cells, and extracellular matrices. Adhesion molecules are critical for the interaction of lymphocytes with blood-brain barrier (BBB) endothelia during T cell extravasation (see section on leukocyte entry to brain), as well as in the intercellular interactions that are necessary for T cell activation and effect. The level of expression of many adhesion molecules varies with the state of activation (Springer 1990).

Natural Killer Cells

NK cells make up about 2.5% of peripheral blood lymphocytes and are synonymous with large granular lymphocytes because of their large intracytoplasmic azurophilic granules and high cytoplasm-to-nucleus ratio. Unlike cytotoxic CD8+ T cells, NK cells lack immunological memory and have the ability to kill a wide variety of tumor and virus-infected cells without any evidence of MHC restriction (see the discussion of the function of MHC genes) or activation. NK cells lack the cell surface markers present on B cells and T cells. The biological function of the NK cell is uncertain. In view of its in vitro function of lysing tumor cells, it may play a role in tumor immunity (Trichineri 1989).

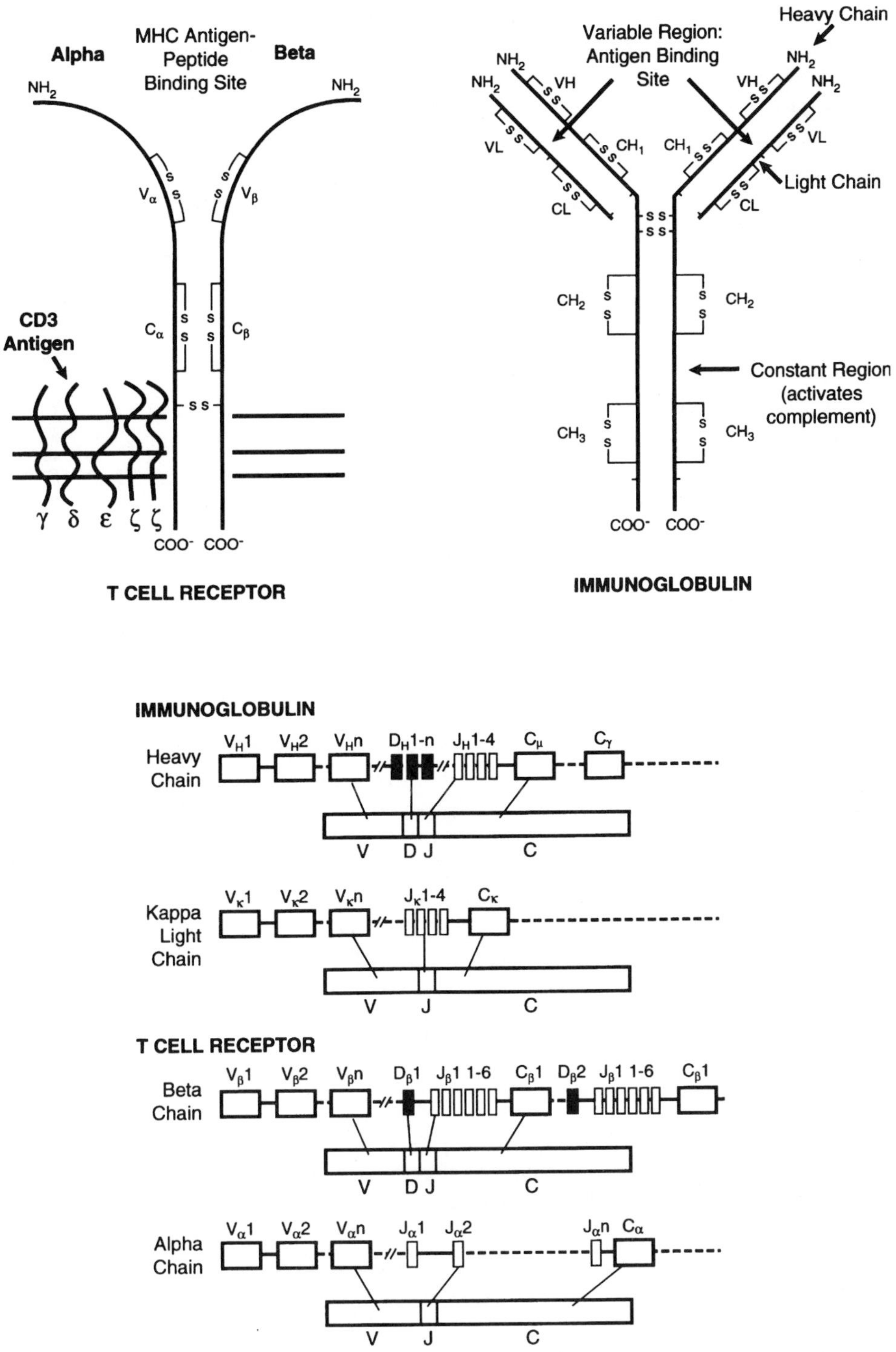

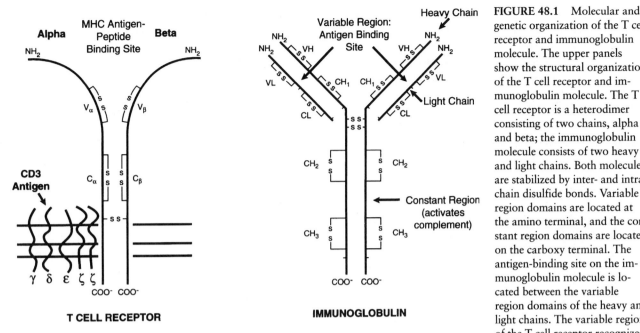

FIGURE 48.1 Molecular and genetic organization of the T cell receptor and immunoglobulin molecule. The upper panels show the structural organization of the T cell receptor and immunoglobulin molecule. The T cell receptor is a heterodimer consisting of two chains, alpha and beta; the immunoglobulin molecule consists of two heavy and light chains. Both molecules are stabilized by inter- and intrachain disulfide bonds. Variable region domains are located at the amino terminal, and the constant region domains are located on the carboxy terminal. The antigen-binding site on the immunoglobulin molecule is located between the variable region domains of the heavy and light chains. The variable region of the T cell receptor recognizes foreign peptides in the context of self-MHC molecules. The T cell receptor is also associated with the CD3 antigen (consisting of gamma, delta, epsilon, and zeta-zeta chains) to form the T cell receptor complex. The lower panel shows the organization of the gene families of immunoglobulin and the T cell receptor. The common feature of the four gene pools is that they contain a number of variable (V) gene segments that are separated from the constant (C) region genes by the joining (J) genes. In the case of the T cell receptor beta chain and the immunoglobulin heavy chain gene, additional diversity (D) genes are present. During ontogeny, one of the V gene segments is juxtaposed to the J segment through a process of chromosomal rearrangement to form the V(D)J gene. This, along with the constant region genes, is transcribed to form mRNA and then protein.

Monocytes and Macrophages

Bone marrow–derived myeloid progenitor cells give rise to monocytes (mononuclear phagocytes of the reticuloendothelial system) that serve important immune functions. They constitute about 4% of the peripheral blood leukocytes and are morphologically identified by more abundant cytoplasm and a kidney-shaped nucleus. Their cytoplasm contains many enzymes that are important for killing microorganisms and processing antigens.

B Lymphocytes

These cells are the precursors of antibody-secreting cells. The cells develop in the bone marrow and during their ontogeny acquire immunoglobulin receptors that commit them to recognizing specific antigens for the rest of their lives. B cells normally express immunoglobulin M (IgM) on their cell surfaces but switch to other isotypes as a consequence of T cell help, while maintaining antigen specificity (see below). Following antigenic challenge, T lymphocytes assist (help) B cells directly (cognate interaction) or indirectly by secreting helper factors (noncognate interaction) to differentiate and form mature antibody-secreting plasma cells.

Immunoglobulins

Immunoglobulins are glycoproteins that are the secretory product of plasma cells. All immunoglobulin molecules have a number of common features, and their biochemical structure and genomic organization is shown in Figure 48.1. Each molecule consists of two identical polypeptide light chains (kappa or lambda) linked to two identical heavy chains. The light and heavy chains are stabilized by intrachain and interchain disulfide bonds. According to the biochemical nature of the heavy chain, immunoglobulins are divided into five main classes: IgM, IgD, IgG, IgA, and IgE. These may be further divided into subclasses depending on differences in the heavy chain. Each heavy and light chain consists of variable and constant regions. The amino terminus is characterized by sequence variability in both the light and the heavy chain, and each variable heavy- and light-chain unit acts as the antigen-binding site (the *Fab portion*). IgM and IgE molecules have an additional domain, CH4. The carboxy terminal of the heavy chain (also known as the *Fc portion*) is involved in binding to host tissue and in binding of complement. This part of the molecule is important for antibody-dependent, cell-mediated cytotoxicity by cells of the reticuloendothelial system and for complement-mediated cell lysis. Classes of immunoglobulins differ in their ability to fix complement. In humans, IgM, IgG1, and IgG3 antibodies are capable of activating the complement cascade.

Antigen Receptor Gene Rearrangements

During B and T cell development, one of the many V gene segments is juxtaposed by chromosomal rearrangements with one of the J segments (and when present, with the diversity [D] segment) to form the complete variable region gene. In addition, recombinational inaccuracies at the joining sites of the V, D, and J regions further increase the diversity. The V, D, J, and C gene segments along with the intervening noncoding gene segments between the J and C regions are initially transcribed into mature RNA. Through a process of RNA splicing, the noncoding gene segments are excised and the V(D)JC messenger RNA (mRNA) is translated into protein. In addition, B cells, upon binding to antigens, undergo somatic mutation that increases the diversity and the affinity of antigen binding. This phenomenon is not seen in T cells. During isotype switching in B cells, further rearrangements lead to recombination of the same variable region gene with new constant region genes (see Figure 48.1).

Monoclonal antibodies are extremely useful reagents in the investigation of an immune response. They are obtained by fusion of B cells with myeloma cells and drug selection of immortalized antibody-producing B cells to generate hybridomas that secrete immunoglobulin of single specificity. Clinical studies of the use of monoclonal antibodies to regulate the immune response in vivo are now in progress (see the section on immunotherapy).

MAJOR HISTOCOMPATIBILITY COMPLEX AND HUMAN LEUKOCYTE ANTIGENS

The MHC class II gene products consist of two polypeptide chains, alpha and beta, which are noncovalently linked. Both class I and class II proteins are stabilized by intrachain disulfide bonds. Class I antigens are expressed on all nucleated cells, whereas class II antigens are constitutively expressed only on dendritic cells, macrophages, and B cells and are also expressed on a variety of activated cells, including T cells, endothelial cells, and astrocytes. Several alleles are recognized for each locus; thus the human leukocyte antigen A (HLA-A) locus has at least 20 alleles, and HLA-B has at least 40. The number of alleles for the D region appears to be as extensive as that for HLA-A, HLA-B, and HLA-C. In view of the extensive polymorphisms present, the chances of two unrelated individuals sharing identical HLA antigens are extremely low. The reason for the extensive diversity and the evolutionary pressure that lead to this are not fully known (Nepom and Ehrlich 1991).

Function of Major Histocompatibility Complex Gene Products

Clearly, MHC antigens did not evolve to pose problems for future transplantation surgeons. The present evidence indicates that class I and class II MHC gene products function as signals for the discrimination of self from nonself and to regulate specificity of the immune response to foreign antigens. Class I antigens regulate the specificity of cytotoxic T cells, which are responsible for killing cells bearing viral antigens or foreign transplantation antigens (Figure 48.2). One of the prerequisites for the killing by cytotoxic T cells of virally infected cells is that the target cells share class I MHC genes with the cytotoxic cell. Thus, the cytotoxic cell that is specific for a particular virus is capable of recognizing the antigenic determinants of the virus only in association with a particular MHC class I gene product (Figure 48.3). The single TCR, then, has two

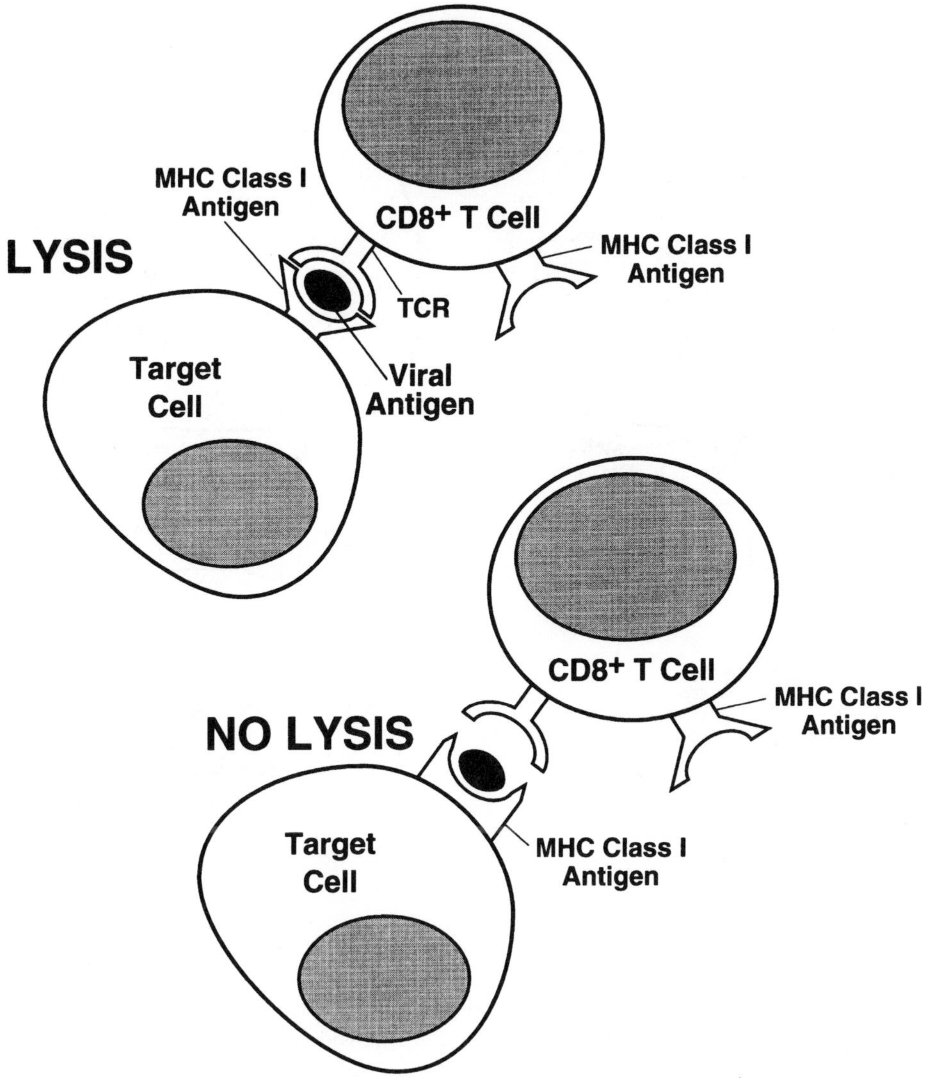

FIGURE 48.2 The phenomenon of major histocompatibility complex restriction. For antigen-specific cytolysis of virus-infected targets to occur, T cells should be sensitized to the virus and share the same HLA class I antigen with the target cell. If the T cells and the target do not share the same MHC class I antigen, target lysis does not occur.

mutually inclusive specificities for the target cell lysis to occur. Sharing of one specificity alone (either to virus or to class I MHC gene product) is insufficient to cause target lysis. The function of class II MHC gene products appears to be to regulate the specificity of T helper cells, which, in turn, regulate delayed-type hypersensitivity and antibody response to foreign antigens. Similarly, an immunized T cell population will recognize a foreign antigen (e.g., tetanus toxoid) only if it is presented on the surface of an antigen-presenting cell that shares the same class II MHC antigen specificity as the immunized T cell population. Thus, the functional specificity of the T cell population is restricted by the MHC products that it recognizes, and therefore CD8+ CD4– T cells (cytotoxic) and CD4+ CD8– T cells (helper) are referred to as MHC class I– and class II–restricted T cells, respectively. The analysis of the three-dimensional structure of the class I and class II molecules has confirmed the notion that these molecules are carriers of immunogenic peptides that are processed by antigen-presenting cells to the cell surface. Both MHC class I and class II molecules share similarities in crystal structure that allow them to accept and retain immunogenic peptides in grooves, or pockets, and present them to T cells (Brown et al. 1993) (Figure 48.4).

Superantigens are usually of bacterial or viral origin and bind as intact molecules to MHC. They have the property of stimulating all T cells that express a given TCR variable gene family, regardless of their exact specificity, because of direct Vβ superantigen interaction (Dellabona et al. 1990) (Figure 48.5). Superantigen recognition has been invoked to explain the induction of autoimmunity. Superantigen stimulation leads to expansion of T cells that express a particular Vβ gene; if T cells in this particular expanded Vβ gene population include T cells that have autoreactivity to self-antigens, it is likely that an autoimmune disease may be initiated.

MHC class I antigens are expressed on all nucleated cells, but there is considerable variability in the levels of cell sur-

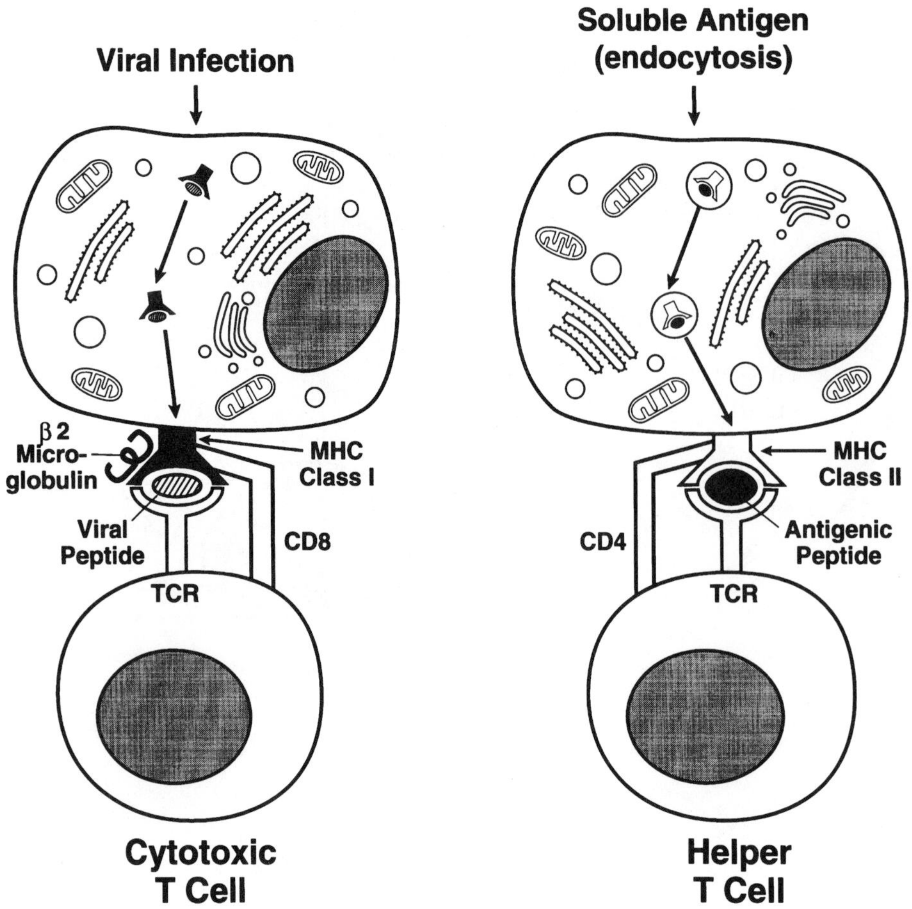

FIGURE 48.3 Antigenic recognition of cytotoxic and helper T cells. The cytotoxic T cell recognizes viral peptides associated with HLA- A, B, or C molecules. The coreceptor for cytotoxic T cells is the CD8 molecule. The helper T cell recognizes soluble antigen that has undergone degradation in the lysosomal compartment and is transported to the cell surface by HLA-D antigens. The coreceptor for the helper T cell is the CD4 molecule.

face expression. In the central nervous system (CNS) the expression of MHC class I and class II on antigen-presenting cells, such as microglia, is low and in oligodendroglial cells is almost undetectable. Expression of MHC class I and II antigens is enhanced on exposure to cytokines, such as gamma-interferon and tumor necrosis factor-alpha (TNF-α). The explanation for the low levels of MHC antigens in the CNS is uncertain. While the low levels of expression may make the CNS less able to mount an immune response, it may be protected from the daily noise of immune surveillance. This may be important for the normal functioning of the nervous system.

Human Leukocyte Antigen and Disease Susceptibility

Evolution of the HLA system's extensive polymorphism is attributed to selective pressures exerted by the environment in the course of evolution. The association of certain diseases with particular alleles of the HLA genes may appear paradoxical. On closer examination, however, it is clear that the association of the disease with certain alleles is invariable and is present not only for infectious diseases but, more important, for autoimmune diseases such as juvenile rheumatoid arthritis (RA) and myasthenia gravis. Furthermore, most of the disease linkage is to class II genes rather than class I genes of the MHC, suggesting that in these individuals altered immune regulation by class II genes is responsible for the disease process. The reason for the association of a particular HLA allele with a certain disease is not fully understood (Nepom and Ehrlich 1991).

A population-based approach has been used to determine the extensive linkage of susceptibility to certain diseases with HLA alleles. The data are expressed as a relative risk of developing the disease among individuals who carry a certain antigen and is calculated by the following formula:

$$\frac{\text{Number of patients carrying the HLA antigens} \times \text{Number of controls lacking the antigens}}{\text{Number of patients lacking the antigen} \times \text{Number of controls carrying the antigen}} = \text{Relative risk}$$

Human Leukocyte Antigen and Disease Susceptibility of the Nervous System

Of the many MHC-linked neurological diseases, multiple sclerosis (MS) and myasthenia gravis are linked to the HLA-D region in humans. In Northern European white populations, the relative risk of having the HLA-DR2 allele in MS

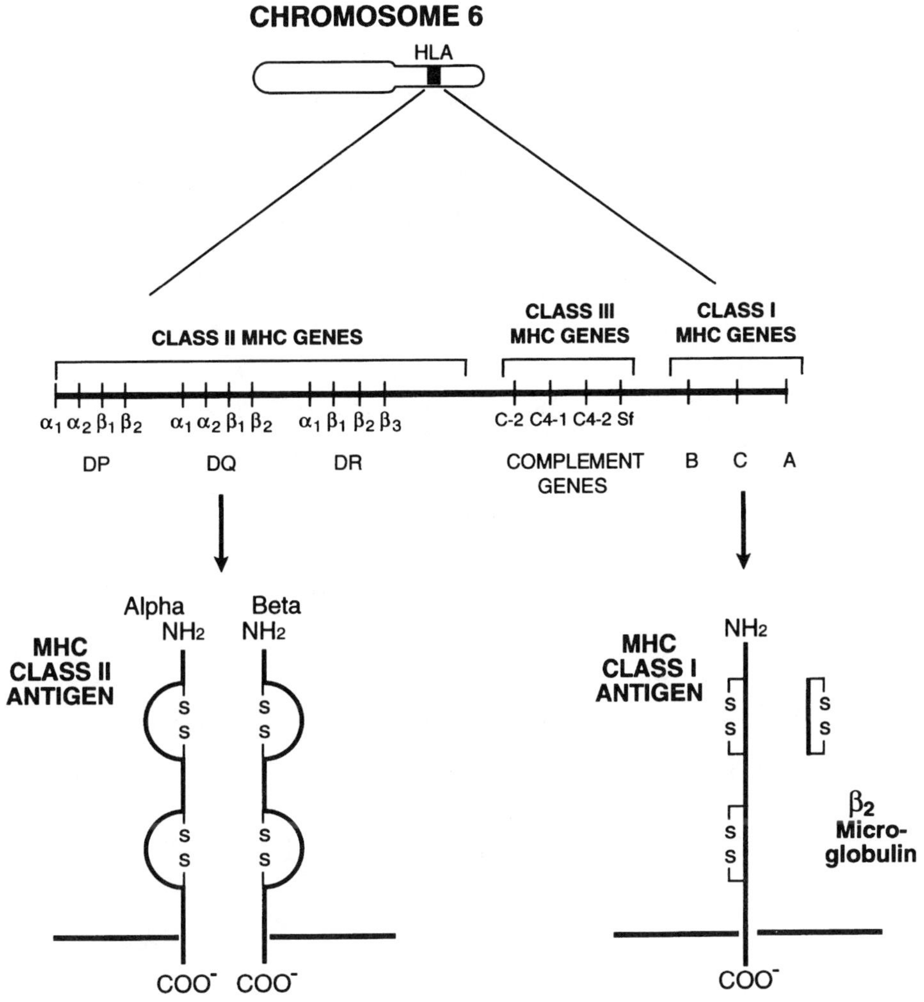

FIGURE 48.4 Schematic diagram of the HLA complex in humans, located on chromosome 6. The HLA class I gene (HLA- A, B, and C) codes for a single heavy-chain molecule. The beta$_2$ microglobulin is coded by genes on a different chromosome. The HLA class II genes (DR, DP, and DQ) form the alpha-beta heterodimer.

is 3.8. In myasthenia gravis the disease susceptibility is linked to HLA-DR3; in younger patients without thymoma, the relative risk is 3.3. The association of narcolepsy with HLA-DR was quite unexpected and raises the question of whether narcolepsy is an autoimmune disease. Association with HLA-D alleles has also been seen in polymyositis and in chronic inflammatory demyelinating polyneuropathy.

ORGANIZATION OF THE IMMUNE RESPONSE

Antigen Presentation

One of the crucial initial steps in the immune response is the presentation of encountered antigens to the immune system. Antigens are carried from their site of arrival in the periphery by way of lymphatics, or blood vessels, to the lymph nodes and spleen. They are then taken up by cells of the monocyte-macrophage lineage and by B cells and presented not as whole molecules but as highly immunogenic peptides. The peptides associate closely with the protein antigens of the MHC molecules through being noncovalently bound into a peptide-binding groove at the distal end of the molecule. T cells recognize foreign antigens plus self-MHC molecules as nonself proteins and react by proliferating and secreting lymphokines (Braciale and Braciale 1991).

Antigen-Presenting Cells in the Central Nervous System

Microglial cells are likely to be the principal antigen-presenting cells in the nervous system (Perry 1994). Indirect evidence from animal experiments has suggested that microglial cells are bone marrow–derived. Although they express lower levels of both class I and class II MHC antigens when compared to antigen-presenting cells in lymphoid organs, these cells are immunocompetent, and they enhance their expression of MHC antigens in the presence of cytokines, TNF, and gamma-interferon (Zajiceck et al. 1992). Astrocytes can be induced to express class I and II MHC and may function as antigen-presenting cells. However, they are not as competent as microglia to initiate T cell responses in vitro.

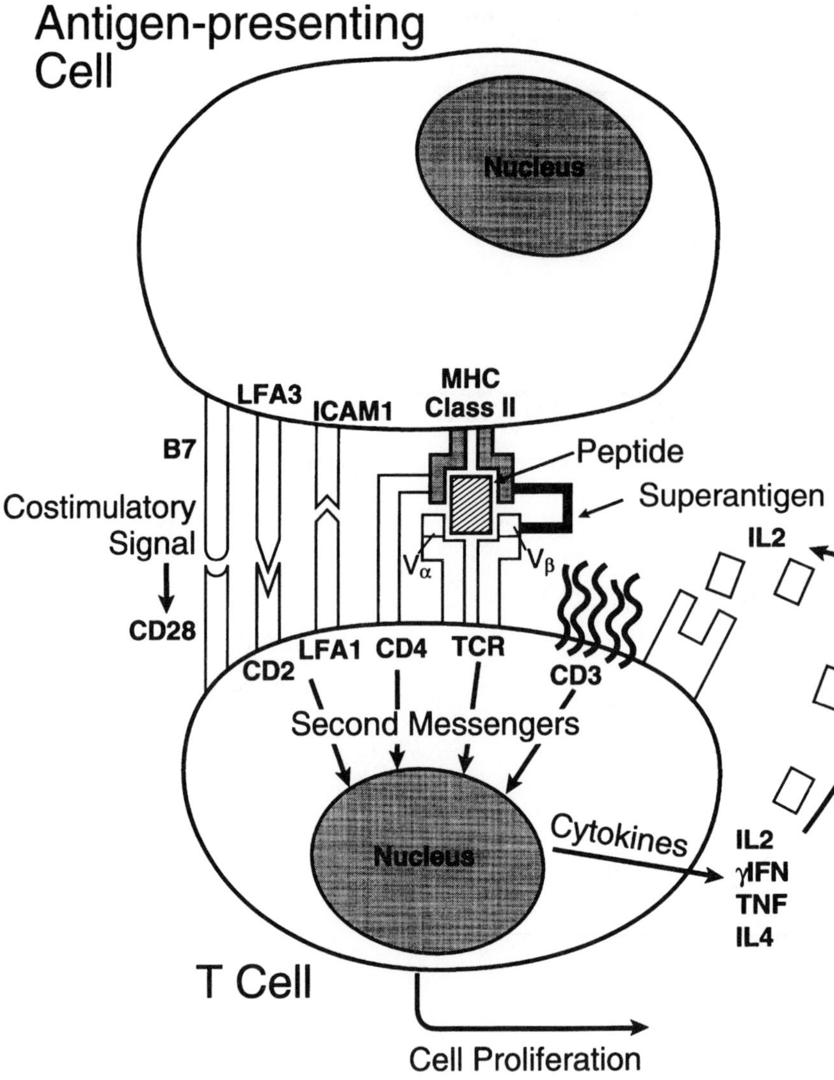

FIGURE 48.5 Antigen-driven activation of helper T cells. Proliferation of T cells requires the delivery of a number of concordant signals. Along with stimulation through the T cell receptor-CD3 complex, presence of appropriate costimulatory signals via CD28 antigen, adhesion molecules, LFA1 and CD2, and the coreceptor molecule CD4 are essential for T cell activation and proliferation. The membrane events of antigen recognition lead to activation of second messengers. The second messengers signal the nucleus and cell to divide and secrete cytokines. IL-2 acts as an autocrine growth stimulator, thereby amplifying the response.

Accessory Molecules for T Cell Activation

The interaction of MHC peptide complex with T cells, while necessary, is insufficient for T cell activation in the absence of other accessory molecule interactions. Accessory molecular interactions include those that primarily exert an adhesion function (e.g., LFA1 and ICAM1), those that maintain and strengthen cell interaction that is critical for response (e.g., CD2 and LFA3, CD4 and MHC class II), and those that transduce signals for activation of genes involved in T cell growth and proliferation. The distinction between these functions is not absolute (see Figure 48.5).

Molecules whose primary role is signaling include the CD3 molecule (described above), as well as the CD8 and CD4 antigens. The CD4 and CD8 antigens are mutually expressed on mature T cells and serve an accessory role in signaling and antigen recognition. CD4 binds to a nonpolymorphic site on the MHC class II beta chain, and CD8 binds to the alpha-3 domain of the MHC class I molecule. CD4 is the cell surface receptor for human immunodeficiency virus (HIV-1), and the fact that certain non-T cells, such as microglia and macrophages, can express low levels of CD4 may explain the propensity of the virus to involve the brain.

The binding of the antigen to its receptor initiates a cascade of events that leads to cellular proliferation. The signals for cell division that are delivered to the nucleus are mediated by second messengers. When the receptor binds to its ligand, it causes the activation of protein kinases. These kinases add phosphate groups to other proteins that ultimately signal the cell to divide. CD4, CD8, and CD3 on T cells and CD19 on B cells are examples of receptors that are known to be linked to kinases. The kinase-mediated signals by themselves cannot activate lymphocytes. Lymphocytes must receive a second, costimulatory signal derived from another cell to proliferate. T cells rely on CD28, which binds to B7 on antigen-presenting cells. B7 upregulation is therefore a prerequisite for antigen-presenting capability of a cell (Linsley and Ledbetter 1993) (see Figure 48.5).

Accessory Molecules for B Cell Activation

Like T cells, B cells require accessory molecules that supplement signals through cell surface imunoglobulins. Signaling molecules whose functions are likely to be analogous to CD3 are linked to immunoglobulin. A number of B cell accessory molecules have been implicated in signaling. These include CD40, which appears to be critical for B cell responses. Adhesion molecules also play an important role in mediating T cell to B cell interactions.

Regulation of the Immune Response

The primary goal of the immune response is to protect the organism from infectious agents and to generate memory T and B cell responses that provide accelerated and high-avidity secondary responses upon reencountering antigens. It is desirable to terminate responses once an antigen has been cleared and also to prevent the activation of autoimmune or otherwise counterproductive responses. A number of systems operate to prevent uncontrolled responses.

In most instances, an antigen is cleared either by cells of the reticuloendothelial system or through the formation of antigen-antibody complexes. The formation of these complexes can itself result in the inhibition of B cell differentiation and proliferation.

T cells can also suppress, or downregulate, the immune response. There is no convincing evidence for a distinct lineage of suppressor T cells. It is likely that both helper and cytotoxic T cells suppress immune responses through either the release of downregulatory cytokines or through cytolytic inactivation of responsive cells. Targets of suppression could include B cells or helper T cells, thereby reducing the help provided. The question of what antigen it is that suppressor T cells recognize is of interest. Possibilities include idiotopes and antigenic peptides presented in association with MHC on activated T cells or antigenic peptides with MHC on conventional antigen-presenting cells. Clinical syndromes manifested by disorders of suppressor T cells have recently been described in MS, RA, and infectious mononucleosis. These studies have involved in vitro assays, and it is not known how they relate to disease etiology in vivo.

The variable region of the immunoglobulin and the TCR molecule represent novel proteins that can act as antigens. Antigenic variable regions are called *idiotopes,* and responses against such antigens are called *anti-idiotypic.* Thus, anti-idiotypic antibodies have been shown to regulate autoantibody production in systemic lupus erythematosus (SLE), RA, and myasthenia gravis. A role for anti-idiotypic antibodies to the TCR has also been proposed. A related possibility is that T cells themselves may recognize idiotopes. While there is some experimental evidence that this can occur, the functional significance of such interactions has not been established (Taylor 1993).

CYTOKINES

The term *cytokine* is preferred to *lymphokine* or *monokine* since neither the production nor the effects of factors are restricted to lymphocytes or monocytes-macrophages. Cytokines are broadly divided into the following categories, which are not mutually exclusive: (1) growth factors: interleukins (IL) 1, 2, 3, and 4 and colony-stimulating factors; (2) activation factors, such as interferons (alpha, beta, and gamma, which are also antiviral); (3) regulatory or cytotoxic factors, including IL-10, IL-12, transforming growth factor-beta (TGF-β), lymphotoxins, and TNF; and (4) chemotactic inflammatory factors, such as IL8, MIP-1a, and MIP-1b (Durum and Oppenheim 1993).

Role of Cytokines in the Immune Response

A limited representation of the cytokines that participate in the immune response is shown in Table 48.1. The establishment of receptor-ligand interaction between the TCR and the MHC-antigen complex results in the generation of a number of activation signals in the macrophage and T cells. As a consequence, a number of polypeptide proteins are transcribed and either are secreted or become part of the cell membrane. The secretion of IL-1 by the macrophage results in stimulation of T cells, either directly or by acting as a cofactor. This combined effect, in turn, leads to synthesis of IL-2 and IL-2 receptors and finally result in clonal expansion of T cells. The novelty of the system is that although IL-2 stimulation of T cells is antigen-nonspecific, the specificity of the expansion occurs because nonactivated cells do not express the IL-2 receptor. T cell activation causes secretion of interferon, which induces expression of MHC class I and class II molecules, and in turn increases the T cell response to the antigen. Secretion of IL-2 also results in activation of killer cells that mediate lysis of tumor cell targets. In addition, IL-3 is released, resulting in stimulation of hematopoietic stem cells. The signal for differentiation of B cells to form antibody-secreting cells involves the clonal expansion and differentiation of virgin memory B cells. IL-4 and B cell differentiation factors secreted by T cells induce expansion of committed B cells to become plasma cells.

Although the emphasis has been on factors that cause expansion and differentiation of lymphocytes, there are cytokines that downregulate immune responses. Thus alpha- and beta-interferon, in addition to possessing antiviral properties, can modulate antibody response by virtue of their antiproliferative properties. Similarly, TGF-β (a cytokine produced by T cells and macrophages) can also inhibit cellular responses. IL-10, besides having growth factor activity for B cells, inhibits the production of interferon-gamma, and so may have anti-inflammatory effects. Nonimmunological effects of cytokines are varied and account for many of the systemic effects in an inflammatory

Table 48.1: An abridged list of cytokines involved in interactions between the immune and nervous systems

Cytokine	*Cell Source*	*Cells Principally Affected*	*Major Functions*
IL-1	Most cells; macrophages, microglia	Most cells; T cells, microglia, astrocytes, macrophages	Costimulates T and B cell activation Induces IL-6, promotes IL-2 and IL-2R transcription Endogenous pyrogen, induces sleep
IL-2	T cells	T cells, NK cells, B cells	Growth stimulation
IL-3	T cells	Bone marrow precursors for all cell lineages	Growth stimulation
IL-4	T cells	B cells, T cells, macrophages	MHC II upregulation Isotype switching (IgG1, IgE)
IL-6	Macrophages, endothelial cells, fibroblasts, T cells	Hepatocytes, B cells, T cells	Inflammation, costimulates T cell activation MHC I upregulation, increases vascular permeability Acute phase response (Schwarzmann reaction)
IL-10	Macrophages, T cells	Macrophages, T cells	Inhibition of IFN-γ, TNF-α, IL-6 production Downregulation of MHC expression (macrophages) Costimulates B cell growth
Interferon-α Interferon-β	Many cells; leukocytes, macrophages	Many cells, macrophages	Inhibits proliferation, viral replication Downregulates MHC I Inhibits cytokine production
Interferon-γ	T cells	Astrocytes, macrophages, endothelia, NK cells	MHC I and II expression Induces TNF-α production, isotype-switching (IgG_{2a}) Synergizes with TNF-α for many functions
TNF-α	Macrophages, microglia (T cells)	Most cells, including oligodendrocytes	Cytotoxic (e.g., for oligodendrocytes), lethal at high doses Upregulates MHC, promotes leukocyte extravasation Induces IL-1, IL-6, cachexia; endogenous pyrogen
Lymphotoxin (TNF-β)	T cells	Most cells (shares receptor with TNF-α)	Cytotoxic (at short range or through contact) Promotes extravasation
TGF-β	Most cells; macrophages, T cells	Most cells	Pleiotropic, antiproliferative, anticytokine Promotes vascularization, healing

IL = interleukin; NK = natural killer; MHC = major histocompatibility complex; IFN = interferon; TNF = tumor necrosis factor; TGF = tumor growth factor.

reaction. IL-1 and TNF have many biological effects in common; for instance, both are involved in the acute-phase response local Schwartzman reaction, fever, and hypotension. Cytokines secreted by T cells and macrophages have biological effects on neural tissue as well, and receptors for a number of cytokines are expressed by microglia, astrocytes, and neurons. Interplay between the immune and nervous systems is indicated by homologies between receptor polypeptides for neurotrophic factors and cytokines, and between cytokines and neurotrophic factors themselves. Neural cells also secrete cytokines, often directly under the influence of lymphocytes. Microglia produce TNF-α and IL-1, and astrocytes secrete growth-promoting factors and are also influenced by IL-1 and interferons, to grow and express new proteins on their surfaces. These observations lead to the conclusion that the brain is not an immunologically sequestered organ, but that it interacts with cytokines and is involved closely with the systemic immune response. This conclusion is also supported by observations made in experimental allergic encephalomyelitis (EAE). Regulation of immune response by the nervous system represents the other side of this coin. There is growing interest in the ability of mediators that are either produced in the CNS (e.g., IL-1, TNF, and TGF-β) or whose production is regulated by the CNS, such as pituitary hormones, to influence lymphocyte activation and effector functions (Reichlin 1993).

Cytokines and Disease

In in vitro culture systems, TNF-α causes damage to myelin sheaths, oligodendroglia, and Schwann cells. Proinflammatory cytokines such as IL-1, TNF, and gamma-interferon induce the expression of MHC class I and class II antigens and potentiate the immune response. Elevated and probably aberrant expression of IL-1, TNF-α, and IL-2 has been detected in the brains of MS patients, and it is assumed that this reflects the underlying immune response in this disease. Decreased IL-2 production by T cells is seen in acquired immune deficiency syndrome (AIDS), type 1 diabetes, and certain malignancies. Decreased interferon production by lymphocytes is seen in lepromatous leprosy, RA, and some leukemias. It is not certain whether the in vitro tests of cytokine function truly reflect the defect in vivo (Powrie and Coffman 1993).

EXPERIMENTAL MODELS OF AUTOIMMUNE DISEASE OF THE NERVOUS SYSTEM

A number of immune-mediated autoimmune disorders of the nervous system are available for study in laboratory animals. Besides allowing for the analysis of the immunoregulatory network, they have been important models for designing immunotherapy. Although these model systems show many similarities to the human disease, it is quite likely that the human and experimental diseases have different immunological substrates; therefore, extrapolation to human disease should be undertaken with caution (Owens and Sriram 1995).

Experimental Allergic Encephalomyelitis

EAE is a T cell–mediated autoimmune demyelinating disease of the CNS. The disease can be induced in a number of experimental laboratory animals, including primates, by the injection of whole-brain homogenate or of a purified preparation of myelin basic protein (MBP). By altering the immunization protocols, a chronic form of EAE has been observed in mice and guinea pigs wherein the animals develop spontaneous relapses, and the pathology shows mainly helper T cells in perivascular cuffs in the brain and spinal cord. The question of whether MS might represent an autoallergic process to MBP arises in part because of its similarities to EAE. However, the crucial question—whether MS represents an autoimmune response to MBP—is unresolved (Zamvil and Steinman 1989).

The study of EAE has contributed to our understanding of how lymphocytes enter the CNS. T cell migration from blood to lymphoid tissue occurs at specialized sites called high endothelial venules, at which increased expression of the appropriate adhesion ligands leads to T cell arrest and interaction with the endothelium. Upregulated expression of the adhesion ligands is induced by inflammation and damage in nonlymphoid tissues, predisposing to T cell extravasation at these sites. Whether the BBB endothelium has analogous structures, and whether they are induced during CNS inflammation, has not been determined. It was previously thought that the BBB endothelium, with its tight junctions, represented a barrier to entry of lymphocytes to the CNS and that their presence in CNS reflected BBB breakdown. However, study of the migration of activated T cells in rodents has shown that any T cell can enter the CNS regardless of its antigen specificity, provided it expresses the appropriate phenotype. This corresponds to the elevated or reduced level of expression of adhesion or accessory molecules discussed previously. Many cytokines (e.g., TNF , IFN-γ, and IL-6) induce upregulation of ligands on endothelial cells, predisposing T cell–endothelial interaction. Monoclonal antibodies against specific adhesion molecules have protected rats from the induction of EAE, and it is likely that human counterparts of these molecules play an analogous role in T cell infiltration. Inflammatory chemotactic cytokines secreted by inflamed endothelia and microglial macrophages are also implicated in T cell extravasation in rodent models and likely will be shown to contribute to human autoimmune brain diseases. This underlines the intimate interconnection between the immune and nervous systems. Many autoimmune diseases are dominated by a few T cell specificities, and these can be defined by their TCR variable genes. There is considerable interest in whether T cells that infiltrate the CNS in EAE and MS are similarly restricted, since this would make it possible to alleviate disease by targeting these TCR variable-region gene products (Steinman 1991).

Experimental Autoimmune Myasthenia Gravis

Experimental autoimmune myasthenia gravis (EAMG) is the archetypal model of autoimmune disease, resembling human myasthenia gravis (Schonbeck et al. 1990). This disease can be induced in animals by repeated injection of acetylcholine receptors (AChRs) isolated from the electric organs of eels. The disease is mediated by antibodies directed against the AChRs, and transfer of hyperimmune sera or of monoclonal antibodies to the receptors has been sufficient to induce it. As in the human disease, in EAMG muscular weakness results from destruction of AChRs by antigenic modulation and complement-mediated lysis. The disease improves after treatment with acetylcholinesterase inhibitors or with immunosuppression. The main differences from the human counterpart is that the murine disease is monophasic and no thymic abnormalities are seen.

Experimental Autoimmune Neuritis

Among various peripheral nerve myelin proteins, the P_2 fraction is neuritogenic in experimental animals. Injection of P_2 in adjuvant results in the development of an acute monophasic polyneuropathy. Experimental autoimmune neuritis, like EAE, is T cell–mediated, and transfer of the disease has been successfully performed with T cell lines and clones. As with EAE, the relevance of this experimental disease to acute inflammatory polyneuropathy is uncertain.

PUTATIVE MECHANISMS IN HUMAN AUTOIMMUNE DISEASE

The undeniable evidence of a causal relationship between an autoantigen and autoimmune disease rests on the fulfillment of a variant of Koch's postulates. In humans, this has been proven mainly in autoantibody-mediated autoimmune disease such as myasthenia gravis, in which the antigen is known, the antibody is seen at the end organ, removing the autoantibody improves the disease, and transferring immune antisera into naive animals results in the clinical signs of myasthenia gravis. The specificity and sensitivity of autoantibodies to neural antigens is variable and covers a wide spectrum—from diseases in which a causal association between the presence of the autoantibody and the disease can be established, to those in which the presence of anti–self-antibodies is perhaps an epiphenomenon. Evidence for a causal relationship between autoimmune disease and the presence of an autoantibody has been observed in other diseases in which the presence of an autoantibody has been shown to be pathogenic. This includes the presence of anti-Yo and anti-Hu antibodies in paraneoplastic diseases, and antibodies to calcium channel proteins in Lambert-Eaton syndrome. Also, the presence of paraproteins directed against peripheral nerve antigens is evidence of direct disease pathogenesis in autoimmune peripheral neuropathy. In all the above diseases the presence of the antibody has been accompanied by end-organ destruction, either by complement or antibody-dependent cell-mediated cytotoxicity.

The evidence demonstrating a causal relationship between an autoantigen and autoimmune disease has thus far been unsuccessful for what are believed to be T cell–mediated diseases such as MS, chronic inflammatory demyelinating polyneuropathy, dermatomyositis or polymyositis, and perhaps acute inflammatory demyelinating polyneuropathy. This is in part because the determinants recognized by B cells and T cells are different (T cells recognize peptides of 10–20 amino acids, while B cells recognize whole antigenic molecules). Thus, for large molecules, peptides recognized by T cells are likely to be numerous. Also, T cell reactivity to autoantigens does not necessarily guarantee disease since autoreactivity to some self-antigens is seen in normal healthy individuals. Thus, the only conclusive evidence that can indicate causality between an antigen and T cell–mediated autoimmune disease would be the reversal of the disease process by removal of the putative autoreactive T cell repertoire. While this has been feasible in experimental autoimmune diseases such as EAE, establishing the efficacy of such a strategy has been difficult in most human T cell–mediated autoimmune diseases. In the absence of such conclusive proof, only circumstantial evidence can be invoked to substantiate the proposition that T cell–mediated disease such as MS is mediated by autoreactive T cells to neural antigens.

Immunotherapy

The immunosuppressants currently in use lack specificity and thus bear the attendant risks of long-term generalized immunosuppression. Conventional immunosuppressants that are used for the treatment of neurological disease include glucocorticoids, alkylating agents such as cyclophosphamide, and the purine antimetabolite azathioprine. Cyclosporine belongs to a new generation of immunosuppressants because of its specific effect on T cells. Cyclosporine is a cyclic undecapeptide that acts by inhibiting IL-2 production by T cells and is successful in suppressing T cell response to transplantation antigens and in prolonging graft survival. Other forms of antigen-nonspecific immunotherapy include plasmapheresis and total lymphoid irradiation. By removing humoral factors involved in the disease process, plasmapheresis has been useful in the management of myasthenic crisis and acute inflammatory polyneuropathy. Total lymphoid irradiation causes lymphocytopenia and development of antigen-nonspecific suppressor T cells. However, it remains an experimental procedure for the treatment of autoimmune disease.

Intravenous immunoglobulin (IVIG) has emerged over the last 10 years as an important immunomodulating agent in the treatment of allergic and autoimmune diseases. The mechanism whereby a pool of immunoglobulins from multiple donors alters immune function remains a mystery. One hypothesis is that autoimmunity results from impaired regulation of reactivity to self-antigens. Part of the normal system of regulation involves the development of an anti-idiotypic response (antibody to the antigen-binding site of the immunoglobulin). It is thought that a portion of the injected antibodies of the IVIG pool has blocking activity against autoantibodies, thereby acting as anti-idiotypic antibodies. In spite of the lack of understanding of the mechanism of action, IVIG has proved to be of therapeutic benefit in myasthenia gravis, acute and chronic inflammatory polyneuropathy, and dermatomyositis-polymyositis. The high cost of IVIG has perhaps limited its use in other autoimmune diseases (Dwyer 1992).

Advances in the understanding of factors and molecules involved in immune recognition has allowed for methods to prevent T cell antigen-presenting cell interaction at a number of levels. These strategies have targeted a particular phenotype of cell, such as all CD4 T cells, TCRs that are targeted to putative autoantigens (TCR-specific), or MHC class II antigens. The strategy has been to use monoclonal antibodies to cell surface antigens such that the receptors are either blocked or the cells expressing these receptors are deleted. Since large-scale production of human monoclonal antibodies for human trials has been hampered by technical difficulties, another approach has been to "humanize" murine monoclonal antibodies such that these antibodies are not recognized as foreign (Winter and Harris 1993). Clinical trials using humanized anti-CD4 antibodies in MS and RA are already underway. Another strategy has been to inactivate antigen-specific T cells by immunizing with the hypervariable regions of the TCRs that recognize the antigen MHC peptide complex. Assuming the relationship between certain HLA antigens and disease susceptibility is linked to the proclivity of certain autoantigens to bind to these HLA molecules, therapy aimed at competing self-peptides from the MHC antigen pocket is underway. Such decoy-type peptides bind to the HLA molecules with higher affinity and prevent MHC peptide–T cell interaction. It is believed that copolymer 1, which is in clinical trials for MS, binds to HLA DR2 and competes with self-peptides.

Cytokines as Therapeutic Agents

The cloning of cytokine genes has allowed for the large-scale production of these agents for studies in animals and humans. Alpha-interferon was one of the first lymphokines used in clinical trials. Alpha-interferon, in view of its antiproliferative effects, has been successful in inducing remission in hairy-cell leukemia and in chronic myelogenous leukemia. Colony-stimulating factor (IL-3), in view of its ability to induce hematopoiesis, is used in the treatment of chemotherapy-induced bone marrow suppression and in AIDS. In lepromatous leprosy, local injection of gamma-interferon has resulted in decreased bacteria in cutaneous lesions. Since inflammation in autoimmune disorders does not progress relentlessly, there is considerable speculation that cytokines may be involved in containing the inflammation and tissue injury. Naturally occurring cytokines such as beta-interferon, TGF-β, and IL-10 fall into this category. Many have already proved useful in animal models of autoimmune disease. Beta-interferon is the first approved drug for use in relapsing remitting MS. It is quite conceivable that in the near future a combination of cytokines with immunosuppressive and regulatory functions will be used in the treatment of human autoimmune disease similar to the use of chemotherapeutic protocols in treating cancer. Because several disorders result from undesirable side effects of lymphokines, the use of monoclonal antibodies directed to lymphokines or their receptors is also being studied.

Application of Immunological Tests in the Diagnosis of Neuroimmunological Disease

Disorders of the nervous system mediated as a consequence of immune dysfunction can be broadly classified as those mediated exclusively by T cells or by immunoglobulins. As was discussed above, only in autoantibody-mediated autoimmune diseases has a clear relationship between an abnormal immune response and disease been established. It has been very difficult to identify the critical antigen-reactive T cells in the peripheral blood of patients with known autoimmune disease. Also, tests of T cell reactivity to antigens are difficult and cumbersome to perform, and no standardized commercial kits to measure antigen-specific T cell functions are currently available. Indirect evidence of T cell expansion and activation has included measurement of IL-2 and IL-2 receptors and TNF and TNF receptors in peripheral blood and in the CSF. TNF is elevated in the blood and CSF of patients with MS and may prove to be an important marker of disease activity.

Anti-ACLR antibodies and antibodies to calcium channels of the presynaptic regions of the neuromuscular junction are specific and relatively sensitive in the diagnosis of myasthenia gravis and Lambert-Eaton syndrome. Autoantibodies to myelin-associated glycoprotein and glycolipid GM_1 are also seen in patients with autoimmune peripheral neuropathy and are useful in screening patients with peripheral neuropathy. Antimyelin-associated glycoprotein antibodies are seen in peripheral nerves, and there is indirect evidence to suggest that removal of the antibodies improves the disease. There are diseases in which autoantibodies are seen in certain defined clinical situations, but their significance in disease is uncertain. Anti-Hu and anti-Yo antibodies in paraneoplastic cerebellar and peripheral neuropathic syndromes probably are responsible for the disease manifestations. Finally, there are diseases in which autoantibodies are seen but their sensitivity and specificity are very low; thus their presence is seen as an epiphenomenon. An example of the latter is the presence of anti-MBP antibodies in the CSF in MS.

REFERENCES

Braciale TJ, Braciale VL. Antigen presentation: structural themes and functional variations. Immunol Today 1991;12:124–129.

Brown JH, Jardetsky TS, Gorga JC et al. Three dimensional structure of the human class II histocompatibility antigen HLA-DR1. Nature 1993;364:33–38.

Davis, MM. T cell receptor gene diversity and selection. Ann Rev Biochem 1992;59:475–496.

Dellabona P, Peccould J, Benoist C et al. Super antigens interact with MHC class II molecules outside of the antigen groove. Cell 1990;62:1115–1121.

Durum S, Oppenheim J. Proinflammatory Cytokines and Immunity. In WE Paul (ed), Fundamental Immunology. New York: Raven, 1993;801–833.

Dwyer JM. Manipulating the immune system with immune globulin. N Engl J Med 1992;326:107–115.

Haas W, Pereira P, Tonegawa S. Gamma delta T cells. Ann Rev Immunol 1993;11:637–686.

Janeway CA. The immune system evolved to discriminate infectious self from noninfectious self. Immunol Today 1992; 13:11–13.

Linsley PS, Ledbetter JA. The role of CD28 receptors during T cell responses. Ann Rev Immunol 1993;11:191–212.

Nepom GT, Ehrlich H. MHC class II molecules and autoimmunity. Ann Rev Immunol 1991;9:493–525.

Nikolic-Zugic J. Phenotypic and functional stages in intrathymic development of αβ T cells. Immunol Today 1991;12:65–70.

Owens T, Sriram S. The Immunology of MS and of Its Animal Model, EAE, in Multiple Sclerosis. In JP Antel (ed), Neurology Clinics of North America. Vol. 13. Philadelphia: Saunders, 1995;51–73.

Perry VH. Macrophages and the Nervous System. Molecular Biology Intelligence Unit, R.G. Landes Co., 1994;87–101.

Powrie F, Coffman RL. Cytokine regulation of T cell function. Immunol Today 1993;14:270–275.

Reichlin S. Neuroendocrine-immune interactions. N Engl J Med 1993;329:1246–1253.

Schonbeck S, Chrestel S, Hohlfeld R. Myasthenia gravis: prototype of the antireceptor autoimmune diseases. Int Rev Neurobiol 1990;32:175–200.

Springer T. Adhesion receptors of the immune system. Nature 1990;346:425–432.

Steinman LS. The development of rational strategies for selective immunotherapy against autoimmune disease. Adv Immunol 1991;49:357–379.

Taylor R. Regulation of Immune Response. In IM Roitt, J Brostoff, DK Mali (eds), Immunology. St. Louis: Mosby, 1993;9.4–9.5.
Thomas ML. The leucocyte common antigen family. Ann Rev Immunol 1989;7:339–352.
Todd JA, Acha-Orbea H, Bell H. A molecular basis for MHC class II associated autoimmunity. Science 1988;240:1003–1009.
Trichineri G. Biology of natural killer cells. Adv Immunol 1989;47:187–206.
Winter G, Harris WJ. Humanized antibodies. Immunol Today 1993;14:243–248.
Zajiceck JP, Wong M, Scolding NJ. Compston DAS interactions between oligodendrocytes and microglia. Brain 1992;115:1611–1631.
Zamvil SS, Steinman LS. EAE and autoimmunity. Ann Rev Immunol 1989;11:579.

SUGGESTED READING

Abbas AK, Lichtman AH, Pober JS. Cellular and Molecular Immunology. Philadelphia: Saunders, 1992.
Keane RW, Hickey WK. Immunology of the Nervous System. Oxford, England: Oxford University Press, 1995 (in press).
Life, death and the immune system. Scientific American (September 1993).

Chapter 49
Neurovirology

Micheline McCarthy and Charles Wood

Neurovirology is the study of viral infections of the nervous system. As a field of specialized study, neurovirology draws its origins from the classical techniques of animal virology and receives significant contributions from veterinary medicine and comparative pathology (Johnson 1982). The understanding of viral disease in the nervous system remains grounded in pathology and draws heavily on natural or experimental animal models of viral nervous system infection. Yet over the past decade, neurovirology, in particular the study of virus-neural cell interactions, has rapidly evolved at the confluence of multiple fields of investigation, including cellular and molecular neurobiology, virology, and immunology. These fields have all been profoundly influenced by the concepts and technical advances of molecular biology. New investigative strategies use the tools of molecular biology to explore at the cellular and molecular level some of the unique features of viral pathogenesis in the central nervous system (CNS), features including neurovirulence, neurotropism, or viral persistence (Roos 1992). This is now giving rise to new diagnostic and therapeutic strategies that will determine the practice of clinical neurovirology in the next century.

This chapter begins with an overview of the major clinical syndromes caused by CNS viral infections. (Specific syndromes are reviewed in depth in Part III, Neurological Diseases.) Current concepts of the pathogenesis of these infections are then reviewed, in particular the molecular basis of virus-cell interactions and host immune responses. The challenge of neurovirology is to define these interactions and immune defense mechanisms at a level—cellular or molecular—that would be amenable to diagnostic and therapeutic intervention. The diagnosis of viral infection in the nervous system and the therapeutic strategies emerging from neurovirological research are discussed in the concluding sections.

NEUROLOGICAL SYNDROMES ASSOCIATED WITH VIRAL INFECTION

Acute Syndromes

Acute viral disease in the CNS may be associated with the broad syndromes of aseptic meningitis, encephalitis, or encephalomyelitis (Figure 49.1). These clinical syndromes typically develop when a virus invades the CNS after primary systemic infection and causes focal or generalized inflammation and cell lysis. The viral agents causing these syndromes include a wide spectrum of human viruses, most commonly the enteroviruses, mumps virus, lymphocytic choriomeningitis virus, arthropod-borne viruses, respiratory tract viruses, or the herpesviruses. Acute syndromes can also result from reactivation of latent herpesvirus infection in the CNS, in particular, herpes simplex virus (HSV) types 1 or 2 or herpes zoster virus (HZV), also known as varicella-zoster virus.

Infection of specific cell populations within the nervous system determines the particular clinical signs and symptoms of a viral infection. Thus if infection is limited to the meninges, clinical signs and symptoms are consistent with meningitis. If infection should involve parenchymal cells of the brain, clinical signs and symptoms include depression of sensorium, seizures, focal deficits, or increased intracranial pressure, all consistent with encephalitis. Viral infections of the meninges, brain parenchyma, and spinal cord in combination give rise to a meningoencephalomyelitis. More distinctive clinical syndromes occur with viral infection of limited and selected cell populations. Poliomyelitis results from infection of anterior horn cells by enteroviruses, including polioviruses, Coxsackie viruses groups A and B, echoviruses, and enteroviruses 70 and 71.

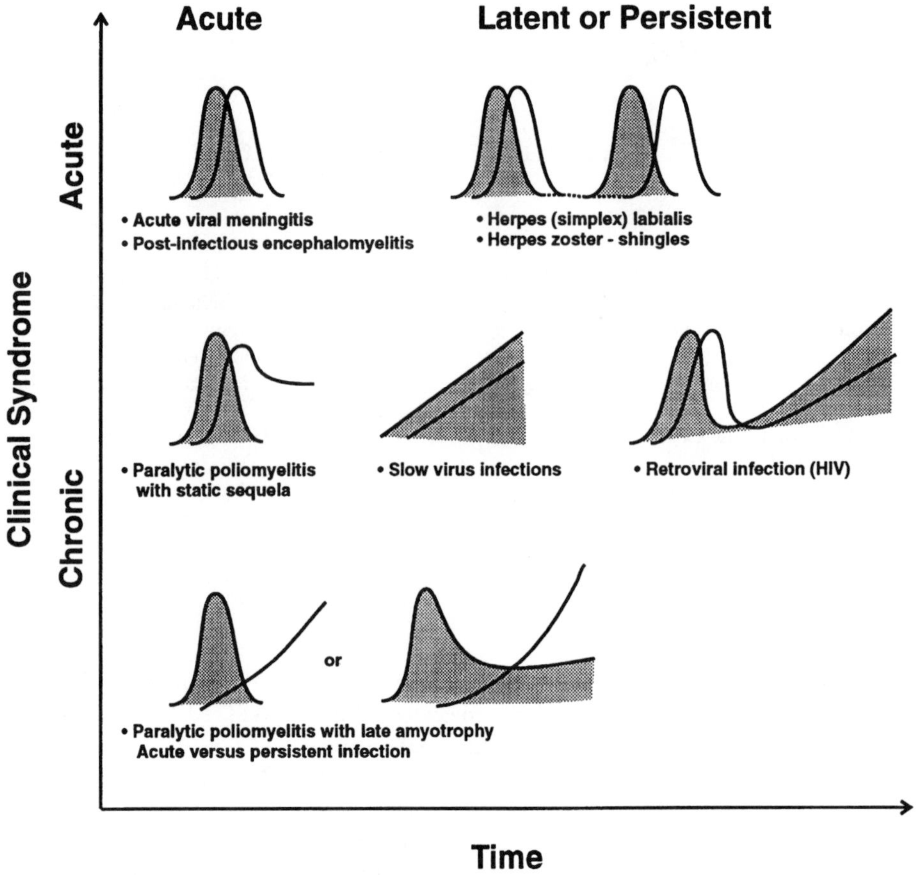

FIGURE 49.1 Schematic representation of temporal patterns of viral infection versus subsequent clinical disease. For each pattern, the course of viral infection is depicted by a solid line on the left with a shaded area underneath. The course of clinical disease is depicted by a solid line on the right, with no shaded area. The course of viral infection in paralytic poliomyelitis with late amyotrophy is undecided. Both acute and persistent patterns of infection are depicted. (Adapted from RT Johnson. Viral Infections of the Nervous System. New York: Raven, 1982.)

Herpes zoster ganglionitis, or shingles, results from the reactivation of latent HZV infection of sensory ganglia neurons. This subacute neurological syndrome includes radicular pain accompanied by a vesicular cutaneous eruption in a dermatomal distribution and, less often, segmental sensory and motor loss. The two common cranial HZV syndromes—ophthalmic herpes and geniculate herpes (Ramsay Hunt syndrome)—develop after reactivation of latent zoster infection of the gasserian ganglion and geniculate ganglion, respectively.

Parainfectious Syndromes

Parainfectious syndromes are clinically distinct disorders that may accompany systemic or nervous system viral infection. Neurological signs and symptoms typically appear late in the course of clinical infection or even after clinical recovery. Such syndromes can occur without direct viral invasion of the nervous system. The major demyelinating syndromes, postinfectious encephalomyelitis (PIE), postvaccinal encephalomyelitis (PVE), and acute inflammatory demyelinating polyradiculoneuropathy (Guillain-Barré syndrome), are inflammatory, apparently immune-mediated disorders caused by cellular immune response to myelin basic protein or other nervous system antigens (Johnson 1987). PIE often complicates exanthematous viral infections, particularly measles, varicella, and rubella. Partial clinical forms include acute transverse myelitis, acute cerebellar ataxia, and postinfectious optic neuritis. Guillain-Barré syndrome may complicate a wide variety of viral illnesses caused by common enteric and respiratory agents and immunization with viral vaccines. Inflammatory granulomatous vasculopathy in the CNS can occur as a para- or postinfectious complication of viral infection, notably that with HZV. This could be due to direct viral infection of cerebral vessel walls or possibly to an allergic or autoimmune response. Viral infection can also potentiate postinfectious noninflammatory metabolic or toxic encephalopathy, as illustrated by the postinfectious acute encephalopathy and cerebral edema of Reye's syndrome, which has been associated temporally with influenza B infection.

Chronic Syndromes

Slow or persistent viral infection of the nervous system can lead to chronically progressive neurodegenerative disease, including dementia and myelopathy. The slow virus diseases are characterized by long intervals from exposure to onset of clinical disease and an afebrile progressive course. Slow viral infections of the nervous system can be broadly divided into two categories: Those caused by *conventional viruses* are typified by subacute sclerosing panencephalitis (SSPE) due to measles virus, progressive rubella panencephalitis (PRP) due to rubella virus, or progressive multifocal leukoencephalopathy (PML) due to papovavirus. Those due to the *unconventional transmissible agents* now known as *prions* include the noninflammatory spongiform encephalopathies kuru, Creutzfeldt-Jakob disease, the Gerstmann-Straussler-Scheinker disease (Prusiner 1993), and fatal familial insomnia. Chronic neurological disease associated with prions evolves in the absence of viral gene expression; prions are amyloidogenic proteinaceous particles lacking nucleic acid that appear to replicate by corrupting a host-specified protein precursor. Hence prion diseases are not caused by true viruses and perhaps should not be considered slow viral infections.

Typically, chronic neurological disease associated with conventional virus infection evolves in the presence of static or increasing quantities of virus (see Figure 49.1). Pathological lesions accumulate secondary to virus replication and gene expression within neural cells (neurons or glia), although the extent of neurological deficit may be disproportionate to the overall extent of viral infection of these cells. Chronic debilitating neurological disease due to retrovirus infection advances in the face of limited direct infection of neural cells, as seen in the dementia or myelopathy of human immunodeficiency virus (HIV) or myelopathy associated with human T-lymphotropic virus type 1 (HTLV-I).

Chronic neurological disease that appears as a sequela of acute infection is illustrated by the congenital rubella syndrome, or post-polio syndrome (see Figure 49.1). Acute rubella virus infection of the fetus during the first trimester causes a variety of malformations, only some of which may be evident in the neonate. Neurological disease may appear to be progressive when the infected child fails to achieve normal developmental milestones. This is not necessarily due to continued viral replication in the nervous system. The post-polio muscular atrophy syndrome is progressive amyotrophy developing after a prolonged static deficit from prior acute paralytic poliomyelitis. This is probably due to attrition of surviving motor neurons and does not indicate continued viral infection. However, intrathecal antipolio immune responses have been observed in some of these patients, which could reflect persistent poliovirus infection with slowly progressive rather than acute cytopathic effects, perhaps immune-mediated (see Figure 49.1).

PATHOGENESIS OF NEUROTROPIC VIRAL INFECTIONS

Viral pathogenesis is defined as the process by which a virus causes disease in the host. A *neurovirulent* virus invades the CNS and causes neurological disease. Most viral infections are asymptomatic or mildly symptomatic; rarely does an infection cause clinical illness. The capability of a virus to cause disease depends on both viral and host factors such as the route of entry, the inoculum dose of the virus, the species of host, and the specific immune status and responses of the host. Viral pathogenesis in the CNS depends on additional factors, due to the relative anatomical and immunological isolation of the nervous system. The virus must be neuroinvasive—that is, capable of penetrating the CNS and replicating within it. Pathogenesis then progresses through a series of events on a progressively expanding anatomical scale as virus-cell interactions are modulated by host defense mechanisms. Disease results when direct or indirect effects of viral gene expression alter or destroy the specialized functioning of host cells.

Viral Entry

Viruses capable of infecting the CNS can enter the host through a variety of routes, including the skin, respiratory mucosal membranes, gastrointestinal tract, and genitourinary tract. The skin and the specialized epithelium of mucosal (respiratory and enteric) membranes constitute the anatomical first line of defense against viral entry and systemic or peripheral nerve infection. The route of viral entry is important, for it can ultimately influence the distribution of viral lesions in the CNS, as demonstrated in animal model studies. In a series of classic investigations, Bodian and colleagues described the distribution of poliovirus lesions within the CNS after inoculation of rhesus monkeys via either intramuscular, intracerebral, intravenous, or intranasal routes (Bodian 1955). Some areas of the brain, including the sensorimotor cortex and certain thalamic nuclei, were always infected, regardless of the route of inoculation. Other areas, including the hippocampus and striate cortex, were never involved. Infection of other selected areas depends on the route of inoculation. For example, olfactory bulbs and septal nuclei were selectively infected after intranasal inoculation. Similarly, differences in the distribution of HSV type 1 viral antigens have been observed in the spinal cords or brains of mice after either intracerebral, intravenous, sciatic nerve, or intranasal inoculation of HSV type 1.

Viral Invasion of the Central Nervous System

When a virus enters the host, some degree of viral replication at a primary site near the site of entry will occur before the virus spreads to other sites. When virus undergoes productive replication, infection of the bloodstream, or *primary viremia*, results. In some cases, the primary viremia is of low titer and transient, but it serves to spread the virus to a secondary site. The virus will further replicate, leading to a higher-titer secondary viremia. Once systemic infection is established, most viruses access the CNS via the bloodstream, and for blood-borne neurotropic viruses there is a general correlation between high-titer viremia and neuroinvasiveness.

The *blood-brain barrier* (BBB) constitutes the major anatomical defense against infection of the CNS from peripheral sites. This barrier includes tight (intercellular) junctions at two loci: the capillary endothelia and the choroid plexus epithelia. These tight junctions restrict access of cells or molecules from blood-to-brain parenchyma or cerebrospinal fluid (CSF), respectively. Movement of cells across the BBB depends on expression of ligand or receptor-type surface adhesion molecules, which are present on activated T lymphocytes and probably induced on capillary endothelia by virus infection or cytokines (see Chapter 48). Adhesion of inflammatory cells to brain endothelium is a necessary first step in breaching the BBB. This mechanism is especially relevant to the exclusion or entry of cell-associated lymphotrophic viruses into the CNS, since normally only activated T cells can cross the capillary endothelium. The movement of free (soluble) virus particles across this barrier depends on charge or the presence of attachment proteins on barrier cell surfaces. For free virus to directly invade the cells comprising the BBB, it must be able to bind effectively to receptors and initiate productive infection of capillary endothelia or choroid plexus epithelium or to access transport mechanisms across these cells. Thus, neuroinvasiveness of a virus is usually associated with the viral surface glycoproteins that mediate attachment to cells, as observed with the California encephalitis virus group. The phenotypic difference between neuroinvasive and noninvasive strains of this virus has been mapped to a viral gene segment that encodes an envelope glycoprotein.

The intact BBB tends to isolate the CNS from systemic immune responses by selectively restricting the entry of immune-specific cells or molecules. In infectious or inflammatory states, however, the induction of surface adhesion molecules on endothelial cells may correlate with attenuation of the BBB, transudation of serum proteins into the CNS, and induction of inflammatory disease. Adhesion molecules may also mediate direct interaction of activated inflammatory cells with brain glial cells and regulation of immune reactivity in the CNS (Antel and Owens 1993). In particular, the *intercellular adhesion molecule-1* (ICAM-1, or CD54) is a 90-kDa glycoprotein that functions as a receptor for adhesion molecules expressed on activated leukocytes. Under the influence of cytokines *tumor necrosis factor-alpha* (TNF-α) and *gamma-interferon* (IFN-γ), this adhesion molecule is expressed on brain endothelial and glial cells in inflammatory or demyelinating states in both the CNS and the peripheral nervous system (PNS). Elevated levels of the soluble form of ICAM-1 reportedly correlate significantly with the presence of myelopathy in individuals seropositive for HTLV-I or with active multiple sclerosis (Tsukada et al. 1993), suggesting that this molecule may be a clinically useful marker in certain infectious or inflammatory CNS diseases.

Once virus has entered the CSF, it has unobstructed access to the brain parenchyma. The CSF–brain parenchyma border is lined by ventricular ependymal cells, which lack tight junctions. There is unrestricted movement of substances between the CSF and brain extracellular fluid. Thus, as has been documented with mumps virus infection in both hamsters and humans, virus can seed the CSF from infected cells in the choroid plexus, then secondarily infect the brain parenchyma from the CSF.

Neural Spread

An alternate route for viral invasion of the CNS is via olfactory or peripheral nerve transport within axons, endoneurial spaces, or Schwann cell infection. Polioviruses, herpesviruses, rabies virus, reovirus, and occasionally arthropod-borne togaviruses can use these anatomical pathways. For example, a bite by a rabid animal may lead to viral replication in the skeletal muscle; then the virus enters the nerve terminals in the muscle and is transported to the spinal cord and dorsal root ganglia via retrograde axonal transport. In contrast, primary replication of poliovirus in extraneural tissues is not a necessary prerequisite for neural spread. Most viruses that spread neurally do so via fast axonal transport; virus particles are transported inside membrane-bound vesicles that track along microtubules running longitudinally through the axon. Virus entering nerve cell termini by endocytosis can be transported to the perikaryon within these vesicles. Virus entering sensory nerve endings will be selectively delivered to dorsal root ganglia cells, while virus entering motor nerve endings will be delivered to motor neurons. Neural spread may be mediated by viral surface proteins, and thus determined by specific viral genes. Experiments with reovirus type 3 have suggested that the gene coding for outer viral proteins that mediate viral attachment also influence the capability for neural transport.

Viral-Host Cell Interaction

Virus cell interactions are the basis for the pathogenesis of viral disease in the nervous system. Viruses infect cells, express their gene functions, multiply, and ultimately alter the host cell functions. Multiple viral and cellular factors influence viral neurotropism and shape the outcome of virus–neural cell interaction. Infection elicits a host immune response, which can specifically limit the spread of virus but can also damage neural cells. Ultimately, these processes may result in the elimination of virus from the nervous system or in viral persistence.

Infection of a susceptible cell does not ensure that the virus will multiply and progeny will emerge. There are four possible consequences of viral infection of the host cell. Infection may lead to (1) productive, (2) abortive, (3) restrictive, or (4) latent infection.

Productive infection occurs in so-called permissive cells and is characterized by the replication of the virus inside the host cell, with subsequent production of infectious progeny virus. Most neurotropic viruses that infect neural cells will go through a productive infection cycle. There are four basic steps in a productive viral replicative cycle: (1) *attachment of the virus* to the target cells, (2) *penetration and uncoating of the viral genome*, (3) *replication of the viral genome*, and (4) *assembly and release of the mature virion*.

Attachment is the specific binding of a virion protein (*the antireceptor*) to a constituent of the cell surface (*the receptor*). The interaction between the antireceptor and the cellular receptor is probably the most important factor in determining species specificity, tissue specificity, and cellular tropism. The viral antireceptor is usually a surface glycoprotein or glycolipid, such as the hemagglutinin of orthomyxovirus or gp120 of HIV-1. However, complex viruses such as poxvirus and herpesvirus may have more than one species of antireceptor.

After attachment, the virus then penetrates the host cell membranes. Viruses use three mechanisms for penetration: (1) translocation of the entire virus across the plasma membrane, (2) endocytosis of the viral particles into cytoplasmic vacuoles, or (3) fusion of the viral envelope with the cellular plasma membrane. After penetration of the virus into the host cell, the virus is uncoated, releasing viral nucleic acid from the capsid and initiating transcription of viral mRNA to direct the synthesis of viral proteins. For RNA viruses whose genome can act as mRNA, viral protein is made directly.

Replication of the viral genome in the infected cell can occur either in the cytoplasm (e.g., poxviruses) or in the nucleus (e.g., herpesvirus). Regardless of the site of replication, one key event in viral replication is the use of the host protein-synthesizing machinery, the host polyribosomes, for the synthesis of viral proteins. Many strategies have been developed by the different viruses for replicating their genomes throughout their evolution. The mode of replication depends on the type of viral genome that is replicated (Figure 49.2). These genomes can be RNA or DNA, single- or double-stranded. However, most mammalian viruses have their genetic information encoded in RNA, and they have evolved multiple replication mechanisms.

The assembly and release of viruses is one of the least understood processes of the viral replicative cycle. In general, the nonenveloped viruses, such as picornavirus, reovirus, adenovirus, and poxvirus, are assembled into a procapsid, followed by the incorporation of the viral nucleic acid and subsequent processing of precursor viral structural proteins to form a stable mature virion. Virus is then released by cellular lysis. The membrane-bound or enveloped viruses, including the togaviruses and retroviruses, egress from the infected host by budding through the cytoplasmic membrane and acquiring an envelope from the host cell. For other viruses, such as herpesviruses, whose nucleocapsid is assembled in the nucleus, the maturation of virus occurs at the inner lamella of the nuclear membrane.

Abortive infection, the second possible outcome of viral infection of the host cell, can result from infection by a defective virus that does not carry a full complement of the viral genes. Abortive infection can also occur in nonpermissive cells. These are cells that can be susceptible to viral entry but do not support the replication of the virus, so only a few viral genes are expressed. An example of abortive neurotropic virus infection is measles infection in SSPE, in which only selected viral genes are expressed.

Restrictive infection (also known as *restringent infection*) is the third possible outcome of viral infection. The infected cells are only transiently permissive, and the virus persists in the cell until the cell becomes permissive. Alternatively, only a few cells in the population produce viral progeny at one time. An example is the infection of resting T cells by HIV; no virus is produced until the T cells are activated.

Latent infection is the fourth possible outcome of viral infection. It is characterized by the persistence of viral genome, but no infectious particles, in transiently nonpermissive cells without destruction of the infected cells. An example of latent infection is HSV infection of neurons, in which infected cells carry viral DNA but no viral proteins or infectious virus are produced.

Factors Affecting Viral Neurotropism

Susceptibilities of different cell populations within the CNS to different viruses are highly variable. There are viruses that are capable of infecting a full range of CNS cell types—for example, HSV. In contrast, there are viruses that can only replicate in specific neuronal, meningeal, or ependymal cells. The ability of various neurotropic viruses to infect and replicate in distinct cell populations is determined by different host cell and viral factors.

Much of the recent emphasis in studies of viral host cell interaction has been on the viral receptor. Susceptibility to infection may be linked to the presence or absence of viral receptors on a host cell. Not only do they play a pivotal role in initiating viral infection, but they are also important targets for antiviral therapies (Haywood 1994). Many surface molecules, including carbohydrates, proteins, and even lipids, have been implicated as constituents of viral receptors. In addition to the well-known CD4 receptor for HIV and the sialic acid receptor for influenza virus, several important viral receptors have been identified by molecular biological techniques. The cell adhesion molecule ICAM-1 has been identified as the receptor for rhinoviruses. The Epstein-Barr virus receptor on B lymphocytes was found to be the complement receptor CR-Z, and the poliovirus receptor (PVR), a member of the immunoglobulin superfamily, has been identified. Interestingly, neurotropism of poliovirus is not solely governed by the expression of PVR. PVR expression has been found in a variety of tissues, even though poliovirus has relatively specific cell tropism in the CNS in which the anterior horn cells are selectively infected and destroyed. Additional factors, such as tissue-specific modification of PVR and factors required for subsequent

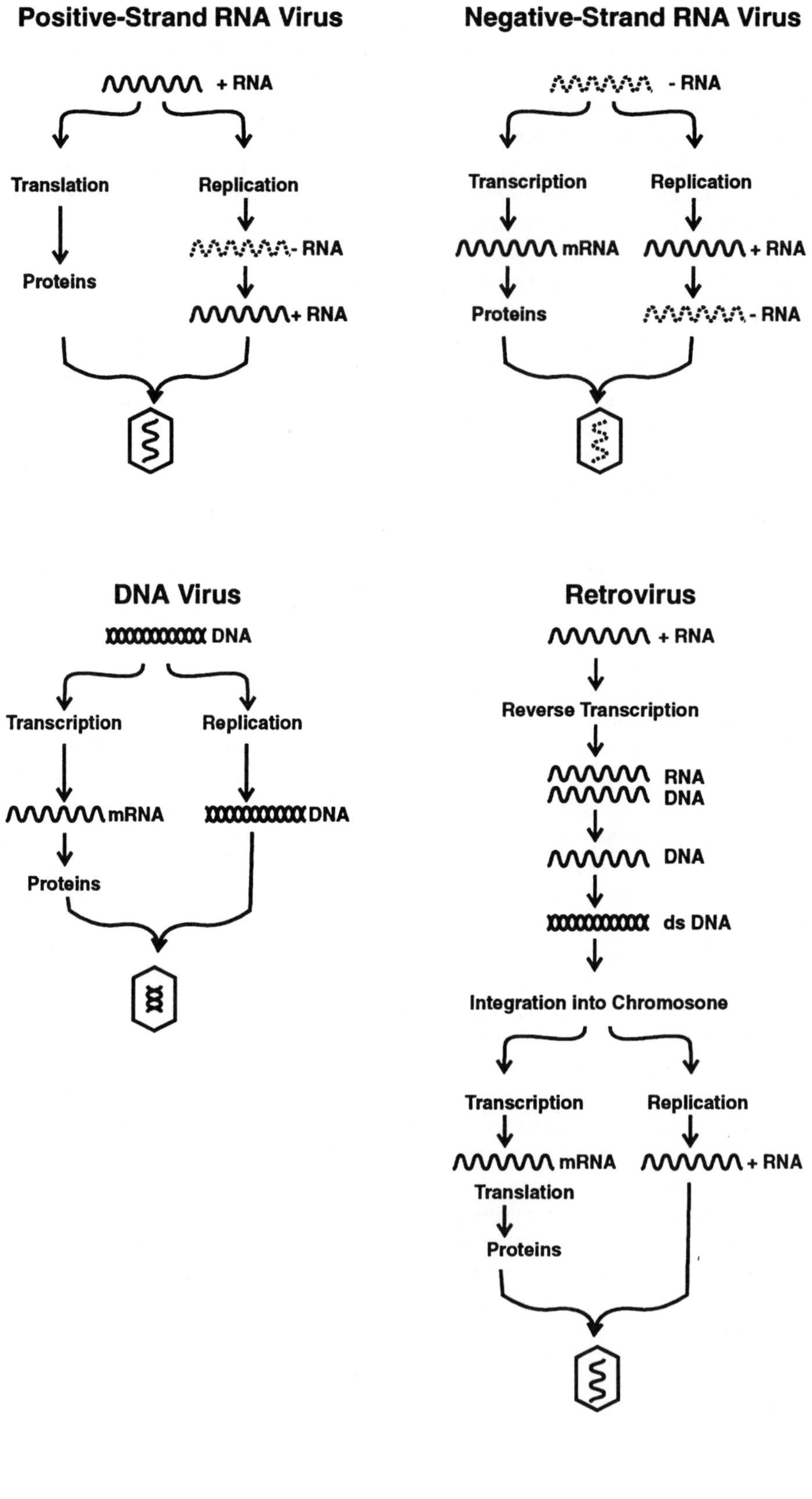

FIGURE 49.2 Replicative cycles of RNA and DNA viruses. *Positive-strand RNA virus* can act as mRNA and translate directly to form viral proteins. The replication of progeny viral RNA requires a negative-strand RNA intermediate. *Negative-strand RNA viruses* usually use a viral transcriptase to transcribe into mRNA for protein synthesis. The replication of negative-strand progeny requires a positive-strand intermediate. *Retroviruses* use the reverse transcriptase to make a DNA copy of the RNA genome; the RNA is then degraded and the DNA is replicated into double-strand DNA (dsDNA). The dsDNA can then integrate into the chromosome, after which viral RNA and proteins are made. *DNA viruses* will be transcribed into mRNA for viral protein synthesis, and the viral DNA is replicated directly to form more dsDNA viral genome. (Adapted from RT Johnson. Viral Infections of the Nervous System. New York: Raven, 1982.)

stages in virus replication, must also be involved in the interaction between poliovirus and its receptor.

Host cell enzymes also play an important role in influencing neurotropism of a viral infection. It is well-documented that initiation of influenza virus infection requires the cleavage of the viral hemagglutinin from an inactive precursor into two subunits by the host trypsin-like proteases before the virus becomes infectious. It has also been suggested that a macrophage-associated protease may be responsible for cleaving the *env* glycoprotein of the macrophage tropic HIV-1 strains in order for them to infect macrophages. At the intracellular level, a series of host factors may affect the replication and transcription of a virus even after the virus has gained entry into the host cell. For example, rodent cells expressing the CD4 receptor are refractory to HIV replication, suggesting that additional cellular factors act at a stage after virus-binding but before replication of the input viral RNA genome. Tissue-specific transcriptional factors may affect the transcription of viral RNA, and such factors may be preferentially expressed in specific neural cell types. The replication of JC virus (JCV) in neural cells illustrates the importance of host cell transcription factors. There are brain cell–specific proteins that bind to the JCV viral promoter, and these proteins are absent in epithelial cells. Binding sequences for the specific cellular transcriptional factor SP1, which is relatively abundant in oligodendrocytes, have also been found in the promoter regions of JCV strains isolated from the brain. It is possible that SP1 may be facilitating selective JCV gene expression in oligodendrocytes.

Finally, a variety of factors at the host organism level can influence neurovirulence, including host age, nutritional status, and genetic background. For example, with many viruses, such as retroviruses or herpesviruses, young mice are more susceptible to disease than older mice. This age-related resistance has been attributed to maturation of the immune response or changes in cellular factors with cell age or differentiation. The host's genetic background can also determine neurotropism or neurovirulence. The genetically related susceptibility of inbred mouse strains to rabies virus infection illustrates this. With intraperitoneal inoculation, CBA or SJL strains are more resistant to disease than Balb/c strains.

Working in concert with the host and cellular factors in determining neurotropism and neurovirulence are the viral genes and viral-encoded factors. With advances in viral and molecular investigative tools, it has become feasible to identify the specific viral genes and proteins that determine neurovirulence. Some of these viral genes encode viral capsid proteins or surface glycoproteins that affect how the virus replicates and spreads within the CNS. Studies with retroviruses and papovaviruses have contributed significantly to our understanding of how viral genetic elements such as promoters, enhancers, and binding sites for cellular factors control viral replication, transcription, and pathogenesis. Viral enhancers represent a modular collection of consensus-nucleotide sequences that are bound by a variety of cellular protein factors to enhance the levels of viral gene transcription. Because enhancers affect gene expression in a tissue- and species-specific fashion, considerable attention has been focused on their contribution to neurotropism—for example, with JCV. It has been postulated that cellular transcriptional factors bind to the enhancer elements in a tissue-specific manner that activates JCV transcription and determines its tropism for oligodendrocytes.

Immune Responses

The complex spectrum of virus-cell interactions are presumably the basis for the pathogenesis of disease, but they are only part of the process. The multiple roles of the immune response must also be considered (see Chapter 48). The immune response acts not only as a deterrent against viral infection of the CNS, but it also can modulate the disease process, resulting in *viral clearance*, *viral persistence*, or *immune-mediated neural cell damage* (Griffin et al. 1992).

Initiation of primary antiviral immune responses depends on the presentation of antigen to responsive or programmable immune effector cells, which participate in cellular immune interactions or generate effector molecules such as cytokines or antibodies. Initiation of primary antiviral immune responses contained entirely within the CNS would involve interaction between resident antigen-presenting cells (APCs) in the CNS and naive T and B lymphocytes. This interaction is typically restricted by matching major histocompatibility complex (MHC) antigens on these cells. Constitutive and inducible expression of MHC class I and II genes is relatively depressed in cells of neuroectodermal origin. MHC class I and II antigens and some cytokines are induced in endothelial cells, astrocytes, oligodendrocytes, and microglia during viral infection or inflammation, while neurons essentially lack the capability to express MHC antigens. Astrocytes express class II antigens on stimulation with cytokines IFN-γ or TNF-α but do so relatively later in inflammatory processes. When activated to express MHC antigens, astrocytes can function as APCs. Brain endothelial cells have also been reported to express MHC class II antigens in vitro in response to IFN-γ, although the in vivo inducibility is controversial. Overall, the lack of MHC expression argues against initiation of the primary antiviral immune response entirely within the CNS.

Given that most neurotropic viruses replicate in peripheral tissues before invading the nervous system, antiviral immune responses are probably initiated in peripheral lymphoid tissue. The immune responses in the CNS would be potentiated by activated (antigen-stimulated) immune cells entering the CNS from the bloodstream (Griffin et al. 1992). In studying Sindbis virus encephalitis in mice, Griffin and colleagues have defined a model of the induction of immune responses to viral CNS infection and the mechanism of virus clearance from neural cells. Sindbis virus is an alphavirus (group A togavirus), similar to western equine encephalitis, that causes acute nonfatal encephalitis with brisk immune responses in weanling mice. The characteristic inflammatory response to viral invasion consists of a perivascular accumulation of mononuclear cells in the brain parenchyma and a mononuclear pleocytosis in the CSF. These cells probably migrate across the BBB through the choroid plexus, meninges, or brain parenchyma. The CSF cells are predominantly activated T lymphocytes. The perivascular (parenchymal) cells initially include CD4+ lymphocytes, CD8+ lymphocytes, and gamma-delta T lympho-

Table 49.1: Persistent viral infection in humans

Virus	*Cells and Tissues Associated with Persistent Infection*	*Neurological Syndrome Related to Persistent Infection*
Herpesviruses HSV-1 and HSV-2	Neurons	Meningitis, encephalitis
Varicella-zoster virus	Neurons	Zoster
Measles virus	CNS: Neurons and supporting cells	Subacute sclerosing panencephalitis
Rubella virus	CNS	Congenital rubella syndrome Progressive rubella panencephalitis
Associated with immunodeficiency		
Enterovirus Polio, echoviruses	CNS	Progressive poliomyelitis Meningoencephalitis
Polyomaviruses JCV, SV40	Kidneys and CNS (oligodendrocytes)	Progressive multifocal leukoencephalopathy
Retroviruses HIV	T lymphocytes, monocyte-macrophages microglia	AIDS dementia complex

cytes plus natural killer (NK) cells. However, with time, increasing numbers of monocyte-macrophages and B lymphocytes appear in the infiltrate while resident brain parenchymal cells, predominantly microglia, begin to express MHC antigens, probably in response to cytokines. The infiltrating B lymphocytes are initially IgM-positive but soon switch to IgG- or IgA-positive cells, suggesting that antigen stimulation occurred in the periphery. A limited number of B cell clones differentiate into plasma cells secreting antiviral antibodies; this oligoclonal virus-specific response gives rise to intrathecal antibody synthesis and the oligoclonal band pattern seen on immunoelectrophoresis of spinal fluid. Virus-specific Ig-secreting plasma cells or B-memory cells may remain in the brain months after recovery from acute infection; work with mouse models suggests this may be due to persistence of viral RNA.

Clearance or elimination of virus from the nervous system probably involves cell-mediated and antibody-related immune responses. As has been demonstrated in peripheral tissues, virus-specific cytotoxic T lymphocytes eliminate through cytocidal mechanisms virus-infected cells expressing MHC antigens, most commonly CD8+ cytotoxic lymphocytes attacking targets expressing MHC class I complexed with antigen. This same mechanism of infected cell clearance would apply to those infected neural cells (e.g., astrocytes) capable of expressing MHC and viral antigens. It is now apparent that in some viral infections, such as HIV, the cell-mediated immunity involving CD8+ lymphocytes may play a more vital role in controlling infection (Levy 1993). However, for other viruses—given the limited expression of MHC in the nervous system—antibody-mediated cytotoxic mechanisms of clearance, such as antibody-dependent cell-mediated cytotoxicity (ADCC) or antibody-complement–dependent cytotoxicity, may also be important. The Sindbis virus model has presented an additional mechanism for virus clearance from infected neurons that do not express MHC. Antibody against viral surface glycoprotein decreases intracellular virus replication in neurons, apparently by a noncytolytic mechanism. Other rodent models of enterovirus, reovirus type 3, or rabies virus encephalitis present a pivotal role for antiviral antibody in the clearance of neuronal infection, suggesting that antibody-mediated inhibition of neuronal infection may be an important nondestructive mechanism of clearance.

Viral Persistence

Viral persistence in the CNS, in contrast to acute infection, is characterized by the continuous presence of viral genomic material. Persistent infection can be broadly divided into two categories. The first is persistent infections in which infectious virus can be detected continuously without destruction of the host cells, either by the virus itself or by the immune response. This type of persistent infection is often referred to as *chronic infection*. A well-known example is lymphocytic choriomeningitis virus (LCMV) infection of neonatal mice, during which there is continuous production of virus. The second category is persistent infection in which the viral genome is present but infectious virus is generally not produced, except during intermittent episodes of reactivation. This type of persistent infection is often referred to as *latent infection*. The classic examples of this type of infection are those caused by HSV or HZV in the nervous system. However, it is important to note that the subdivision of persistent infection into these two broad groups is very arbitrary and may not be applicable for some viruses. For example, HIV can persistently infect monocyte-macrophages, resulting in chronic production of infectious viruses. However, infection of resting T cells by HIV often leads to latent infection in which no viral genes are expressed.

Many viruses are capable of infecting the CNS and causing persistent infection. Some of these viruses are listed in Table 49.1. In order to establish persistent infection, a virus must either restrict its gene expression so the infection is not cytolytic, or cause cytolytic infection of a very limited number of cells. Second, a virus must evade the host immune system so the immune system is ineffective in recognizing and clearing the virus or virus-infected cells. The best example of restrictive gene expression by a lytic virus is the latent infection of neurons by HSV. HSV gene expression is downregulated so only one region of the viral genome is expressed, and there seem to be no viral proteins synthesized by these cells. Another example of persistent infection of the CNS due to downregulation of viral gene expression is seen in persistent measles virus infection in SSPE, in which the viral genomic RNA is retained but there is selective inhibition of viral genomic expression. Mutations or defects in viral structural protein expression may affect viral assembly and result in a nonproductive, persistent infection in the CNS.

The second essential component of a persistent viral infection is evasion of the immune response. This can occur when expression of viral or MHC antigen is depressed. The classic example is LCMV infection in neonatal mice. The virus establishes a chronic productive infection because the animal's immune response fails to clear such an infection. The LCMV-infected animals retain the potential to generate virus-specific antibodies and cytotoxic lymphocytes, but there is depressed expression of most, if not all, viral proteins relative to the levels expressed during acute infection. Downregulation of viral glycoprotein expression on infected cell surfaces by antibodies was also demonstrated in measles virus infection. The antibodies form immune complexes with viral antigens on the cell surface, but these are eventually shed. The infected cells are then rendered resistant to either antibody- or cell-mediated lysis. Viral infection can also induce downregulation of the expression of MHC molecules, as demonstrated with adenovirus. Suppression of MHC antigens can inhibit viral clearance and potentiate persistent viral infection. Finally, persistent infection can result from immunosuppression. Viruses can replicate in the cellular constituents of the immune system, resulting in a disabled specific immune response. The best-known example is HIV, in which infection of the macrophage-monocyte and T lymphocytes results in immunosuppression and persistent HIV infection.

Mechanisms of Cell Damage

Neural cell damage can be a direct consequence of viral infection (direct viral cytopathic effects), a consequence of the immune response to viral infection, or both. Virus-specific immune responses can damage infected neural cells expressing viral gene products. Uncommonly, autoimmune or anti–self-immune responses can damage uninfected neural cells when viral infection disrupts the normal regulatory and recognition mechanisms of the immune system.

Viral Cytopathic Effects

Viruses can cause direct cytopathic effects by a variety of mechanisms that disrupt cellular metabolic activity and cell architecture. Some viruses encode "early" proteins (transcribed early in infection), which direct an abrupt termination of host cell protein synthesis and nucleic acid replication. Certain RNA viruses (e.g., influenza or California encephalitis) interfere with methylguanosine "capping" of host mRNA and redirect host metabolic machinery to synthesize viral proteins preferentially. Infrequently, specific viral structural proteins may lyse cells. Accumulated viral protein, subunits, or maturing virus particles can disrupt cell lysosomes, releasing degradative enzymes that injure the cell. These accumulated viral products can form viral *inclusion bodies* in the cell nucleus or cytoplasm, which can lead to nuclear or cellular rupture.

Immune-Mediated Neuropathology

Because viruses are intracellular pathogens, host immune responses directed against viral antigen and affecting viral clearance may at the same time damage host cells. Multiple immunopathological mechanisms causing such damage are possible (Table 49.2). They can be broadly divided into (*primarily*) *cell-mediated* or *antibody-mediated* mechanisms (Lohler 1988). MHC-restricted T cell cytotoxicity depends on expression of appropriate MHC class I or possibly class II antigen on the infected target cell and the presence of viral target antigen. Cytotoxicity mediated by NK cells or antibody-dependent effector cells is not so specifically restricted by MHC expression. This could be relevant in earlier stages of CNS infection, when there is relatively little MHC antigen expressed on neural cells. Specific antiviral antibody can mediate infected cell destruction through complement fixation and direct lysis of the infected cell. Alternatively, specific antibody can bind free virus and potentiate deposition of immune complexes in the brain, vessels, and choroid plexus with local inflammatory response. Immune complex deposition in the brain is a known complication of SSPE or PRP.

In immunocompetent hosts capable of mounting a vigorous cellular immune response, it may be difficult to distinguish cell destruction caused by a highly cytolytic virus from immune-mediated cell damage. The major inflammatory neuropathological patterns associated with acute to subacute infection of the CNS include choriomeningitis, encephalitis, and poliomyelitis. Animal models of CNS infection have provided examples of how this neuropathology may be caused by antiviral immune responses. The choriomeningitis of LCMV infection in adult mice depends on CD8+ cytotoxic lymphocytes. The encephalitis of Borna virus disease in rats depends on CD4+ lymphocyte activity. In acute herpes simplex encephalitis (HSE), extensive cell destruction is associated with viral antigen expression as well as local MHC expression on resident neural cells plus infiltration of activated mononuclear cells, CD4+ lymphocytes, and CD8+ lymphocytes. This immunopathological picture is consistent with both viral cytopathic effect and immune-mediated cell destruction.

Both Theiler's murine encephalomyelitis virus (TMEV), a picornavirus, and mouse hepatitis virus (MHV), a coronavirus, cause rodent models of chronic demyelinating dis-

Table 49.2: Potential immunopathological mechanisms induced by viral infection of the nervous system

Type	*Effector Mechanisms*	*Pathology*
Cell-mediated		
Immune cytolysis	MHC-restricted cytotoxic T cells (CD8+, CD4+) Non–MHC-restricted lymphocyte cytotoxicity (natural killer cells and others) Antibody-dependent cell-mediated cytotoxicity (macrophages, killer cells, natural killer cells)	Lysis of infected cells, necrosis, demyelination
Cytokine activity	Release of cytokines, toxic factors	Lysis, necrosis, demyelination, enhanced MHC expression
Delayed type hypersensitivity	MHC-restricted T cells (CD4+, CD8+) + monocytes	Edema, accumulation of mononuclear cells, phagocytosis, necrosis, granulomatous inflammation, demyelination
Antibody-mediated		
Immune complexes	In situ formation of viral antigen-antibody complexes	Local inflammatory response Vascular lesions, edema, hemorrhage
	Transient or chronic presence of viral antigen-antibody complexes in the circulation	Deposition of complexes in arterioles, choroid plexus, and brain parenchyma; arteritis, chronic immune complex disease
Autoimmune reactions	Autoantibodies, autoreactive T cells	Tissue destruction, demyelination, inflammatory reaction

Source: Adapted from J Lohler. Immunopathologic reactions in viral infections of the central nervous system. J Neuroimmunol 1988;20:181–188.

ease after survival of acute encephalitis (Fazakerley and Buchmeier 1993). TMEV causes biphasic viral disease in the CNS, an acute encephalitis/poliomyelitis in which immune-mediated virus clearance fails, leading (in survivors) to persistent viral infection and demyelinating disease mediated by MHC-restricted T lymphocyte responses. Susceptibility to these viral diseases in mice correlates with inducibility of MHC antigen expression in the CNS. Studies with immunosuppressed mice suggest that the immune response is essential to the pathogenesis of demyelinating lesions. However, it can be difficult to distinguish between autoimmune antimyelin responses versus virus-specific immune responses in these models, which makes these animal diseases provocative models of viral-associated autoimmune disease.

In the past decade, intense investigation of the pathogenesis of AIDS and its neurological complications has focused attention on the role of cells of the monocyte lineage and their cytokines in mediating specific antiviral and associated autoimmune responses in the nervous system. In the periphery, activated monocytes mature into macrophages with multiple roles during viral infection: phagocytes, effectors of ADCC, APCs interacting with T or B lymphocytes, or sources of cytokines and other inflammatory factors such as hydrogen peroxide or superoxides. Although their origin has been a subject of controversy, microglia share antigenic markers and functional properties with cells of the monocyte-macrophage lineage and are probably their CNS equivalent. Activated microglia express MHC antigens and elaborate cytokines such as TNF-α, that can stimulate MHC expression on astrocytes, thereby potentiating immune responses to viral infection in the CNS. Monocytes can function as host cells for certain viruses, including herpesviruses (e.g., cytomegalovirus [CMV], human herpesvirus-6, or the lentiviruses [e.g., HIV]) that are capable of establishing latent or persistent infection in the nervous system. Activation and differentiation of infected monocytes correlate with activation of latent virus and increased viral gene expression. Infected monocytes can then transmit virus to the CNS by crossing the BBB; this "Trojan horse" mechanism of entry may be the first step in the pathogenesis of CNS disease. Activated and infected macrophages-microglia can then function as reservoirs of infectious virus in the CNS, as is well-documented in HIV infection (Wigdahl and Kunsch 1990).

An increasingly complex array of specific cytokines are described in association with viral infections of the nervous system (Figure 49.3). These include interferons, interleukins, and TNFs as well as colony-stimulating factors (Merrill 1992). Viral antigen-stimulated T lymphocytes produce IFN-γ and IL-2. Activated macrophages-microglia produce TNF-α and the immunostimulatory cytokines IL-1β and IL-6, as do astrocytes when stimulated by endotoxin or virus infection. The relative distribution of these cytokines in the CNS may vary with adult-versus-neonatal or persistent-versus-acute viral infection, as illustrated by the mouse model of LCMV infection. IFNs induce a nonspecific antiviral state in which viral and cellular RNA is degraded and initiation of protein synthesis is blocked (Clemens 1991). Thus, long-term activity of interferons can be harmful to the host. TNF-α stimulates proliferation of T and B lymphocytes and cytokine production in monocytes, whereby it mediates inflammatory demyelination. TNF-α can stimulate synthesis of IFN-γ; these factors can act synergistically to induce MHC expression on neural

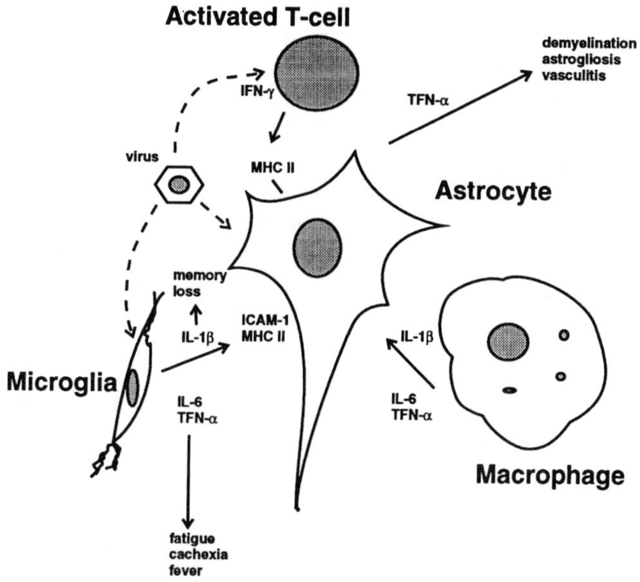

FIGURE 49.3 Schematic representation of the interactions between inflammatory cells (macrophage, activated T cell) and glial cells (astrocyte, microglia) that are associated with viral infection and mediated in part by cytokines. (Adapted from JE Merrill, ISY Chen. HIV-1, macrophages, glial cells, and cytokines in AIDS nervous system disease. FASEB J 1991;5:2391–2397.)

cells. Cytokine gene expression can be directly modulated by neurotropic retroviruses via transcriptional regulation, as exemplified by HTLV-I. A specific HTLV-I gene product, $p40^{tax}$, is capable of activating promoters for multiple cytokine genes and the receptor for IL-2. This activation requires specific cellular transcription factors. Somewhat paradoxically, cytokines can effect activation of latent viral infection of lymphocytes or monocytes and possibly astrocytes. Again, this mechanism is well illustrated by retrovirus infection, specifically HIV. Both TNF-α and IL-6 augment HIV gene expression in monocytes at the transcriptional level. TNF-α and IL-1β have been demonstrated to reactivate HIV in persistently infected human fetal astrocytes.

When virus is persistent in the nervous system, cytokines and other inflammatory factors can perpetuate a potentially destructive state of immune activation. The release into the extracellular milieu of cytokines and toxic factors at local sites of infection can also have effects on distant, uninfected cells. Cytokines can potentially mediate cell lysis, demyelination, or enhanced MHC expression of uninfected cells, rendering them additional potential targets of cell-mediated immune responses and extending pathology beyond the immediate site of virus-cell interaction. This is well illustrated in the brains of patients infected by HIV-1, where relatively few cells (microglia or macrophages) harbor viral antigen, but activated macrophages, T lymphocytes, microglia, and endothelial cells are frequent. These activated cells can elaborate inflammatory cytokines, in particular TNF-α, which has been associated with encephalopathic states and demyelination. As virus persists, the "immune activation" can become a chronic state in which the nonspecific effects of the antiviral immune response can induce widespread neurological disease despite limited neural cell infection.

Autoimmune Disease

Viral infections or immunization with viral vaccines can predispose to apparent disruption of immunoregulatory mechanisms. This can lead to subsequent autoimmune attack on self-antigens in the nervous system in the presence or absence of viral antigen. Several possible immune mechanisms could potentiate anti-self reactions in viral infections of the nervous system (Table 49.3). Host cell antigens can be incorporated into the budding or maturing virus particle at the cell's surface, allowing presentation of self-antigens to activated immune cells. MHC antigen expression on neural cells, induced directly by viral infection or by cytokine release, could potentiate MHC-restricted anti-self reactions. Cytolytic effects of lymphotrophic virus infection could destroy suppressor T cells, resulting in loss or disruption of normal regulation of anti-self reactions. Cytolytic effects of neural cell infection could lead to the release of nerve membrane or white-matter components to which the immune system can become sensitized.

Viral-induced autoimmune attack would result from breakdown of the normal specificity and selectivity of the immune response. Specificity could break down when amino acid sequence homology between epitopes on viral antigen and host proteins results in a crossreactive antiviral immune response. This mechanism of shared antigenic determinants has been named *molecular mimicry* (Barnett and Fujinami 1992). This mechanism presupposes a similarity between viral and self-antigens sufficient to induce a crossreactive immune response, but with enough antigenic differences to break the immune system's tolerance for self-antigens. Monoclonal antibody technology has facilitated the study of specific viral immune determinants (*epi-*

Table 49.3: Possible mechanisms inducing autoimmune reactions in viral infections of the nervous system

Presentation of neural antigens by induction of class I and class II antigens during virus infections of the nervous system
Epitope sharing by viral and neural antigenic determinants (molecular mimicry)
Deregulation or destruction by virus of suppressor T cells that regulate autoantibody production
Polyclonal activation by virus of autoreactive B cell clones
Anti-idiotypic antibodies to antiviral antibodies react with cellular virus receptors
Autosensitization by release of neural products into the general circulation

Source: Adapted from J Lohler. Immunopathologic reactions in viral infections of the central nervous system. J Neuroimmunol 1988;20:181–188.

topes) on viral antigens. This technology has provided evidence that monoclonal antibodies raised against viral epitopes will crossreact with self antigens such as cytoskeletal proteins. Homologies between viral structural protein sequences and those of myelin proteins may provide a theoretical basis for molecular mimicry as a unifying mechanism of viral-induced antimyelin immunopathology.

Selectivity of the immune response could break down with non–MHC-restricted activation of polyclonal T and B lymphocytes to produce alloreactive T cells and antibodies. Such activation of lymphocytes can be initiated by superantigens—that is, antigens that are not processed to small peptides and do not bind the T cell receptor in a specific configuration (see Chapter 48). Superantigens have been implicated in HIV and rabies virus proteins and in induction of relapsing experimental allergic encephalitis (EAE), the rodent model of autoimmune CNS demyelination. The expanded polyclonal lymphocyte populations generated by superantigens may eventually lose immune responsiveness or die. This pattern of cell death after activation is similar to *apoptosis*, or *programmed cell death*, which occurs in many physiological and pathological situations (Williams and Smith 1993).The major parainfectious demyelinating syndromes, PIE, PVE, and Guillain-Barré syndrome, show extensive clinical and pathological similarity to the rodent experimental models of autoimmune demyelination, including EAE in the CNS (PIE, PVE) or experimental allergic neuritis (Guillain-Barré syndrome) in the PNS (see Chapter 48). In these models, injection of white matter or peripheral myelin components induces inflammatory demyelinating disease in the CNS or peripheral nerves, respectively. The experimental models predict a largely cellular immune attack on major antigens of white matter (e.g., myelin basic protein, proteolipid protein) or peripheral nerve (e.g., galactocerebroside), although an antibody may also mediate destruction. Suggestive evidence for antimyelin basic protein immune responses in the human parainfectious syndromes has derived from the study of PVE following vaccination with Semple-type rabies vaccine (which consists of rabies-infected CNS tissue) and the study of postinfectious encephalomyelitis associated with measles infection. Patients with PVE after receiving Semple vaccine have been found to have elevated levels of antibody to myelin basic protein in proportion to disease severity, as well as evidence of intrathecal synthesis of that antibody and lymphoproliferative responses to myelin basic protein. Postinfectious encephalomyelitis following measles infection has been linked to lymphoproliferative responses to myelin basic protein and pronounced lymphocyte suppressor activity in the absence of measles virus antigen. Lack of detectable measles virus antigen supports the concept that measles postinfectious encephalomyelitis is viral-associated but not virus-specific; viral infection appears to initiate a cascade of immune responses, but these develop into predominantly autoimmune, anti-self activity.

Multiple sclerosis could constitute a similar viral-associated, autoimmune demyelinating disorder, initiated by disruption of immunoregulatory mechanisms with relative loss of suppressor cell function. Numerous viruses have been suggested to be responsible for the etiopathogenesis of multiple sclerosis by serology, cellular immune responses, virus culture, or pathological studies. No single viral agent has emerged consistently or definitively. Susceptibility to multiple sclerosis is linked to host genetics, specifically MHC antigens, in similar fashion to animal models of viral-induced demyelination. Thus, certain features of multiple sclerosis provoke continuing argument over whether this is a viral disease of the CNS and continuing investigation at the interface of neurovirology and neuroimmunology.

DIAGNOSIS OF VIRAL INFECTION IN THE NERVOUS SYSTEM

Since the first isolation of choriomeningitis virus, from a case of aseptic meningitis in 1934, numerous viruses have been found to cause similar clinical infections of the CNS. With the beginning development of specific antiviral therapeutic agents, it is increasingly important for clinicians to decide on the most likely etiologic agent and efficiently select the correct laboratory tests (Table 49.4). The conventional laboratory diagnostic strategies have relied on (1) isolation and identification of virus from body fluids or tissues, (2) serological tests demonstrating significant rise in specific antibody titers during the course of illness, and (3) immunohistochemical or pathological demonstration of viral antigen. Often these tests are expensive, cumbersome, time-consuming, or of low yield. Even though these conventional tests continue to be valuable diagnostic aids, the application of newly developed molecular biological techniques has facilitated most of the recent advances in viral diagnosis.

Conventional Methods of Viral Diagnosis

Viral Isolation

Recovering virus from brain or spinal fluid can support a specific viral diagnosis of neurological disease, but technically this is quite difficult. Virus should be cultured directly from CSF or neural biopsy tissue obtained early in clinical illness wherever possible. Alternatively, where systemic viral infection is also suspected, virus may be cultured from blood or blood cells (herpesviruses, retroviruses), nasopharyngeal washings (enteroviruses, mumps virus, adenovirus, HSV type 1, influenza viruses), urine (CMV), or feces (polioviruses, echoviruses). Viral isolation can be achieved by inoculation of patient body fluids into embryonated chicken eggs, susceptible animals, or cell cultures. Different culture systems have been adapted for the isolation of different viruses. For example, embryonated chicken eggs are used for isolation of influenza viruses; suckling mice are most susceptible for the isolation of arthropod-borne

Table 49.4: Diagnosis of viral infection in the nervous system

Strategy	*Specimens*	*Endpoint*
Clinical neurodiagnostics		
History and examination	Patient	Define clinical syndrome
Neuroimaging		Develop working differential diagnosis
Lumbar puncture (if no contraindications)		Obtain infected tissue samples for other tests
		Obtain pathological definition of infection
EEG		
Brain biopsy		
Viral isolation	CSF	Recovery and identification of virus in culture
	Blood, lymphocytes	
	Throat washings, stool	
	Skin lesions	
	Biopsy tissues (brain, nerve)	
Immunological tests	Acute and convalescent sera	Document increased specific antibody titer
	Acute and serial paired CSF and sera	Document antiviral IBBB antibody synthesis
Detection of viral antigen		
Immunostaining	CSF, CSF cells, or PBMCs	Identify specific viral antigen
Antigen capture		
Electron microscopy		
Detection of viral genes		
Nucleic acid hybridization with specific probes	Biopsy tissue	Identify specific viral genes
	CSF, CSF cells, or PBMCs	
Polymerase chain reaction with specific primers		

EEG = electroencephalogram; CSF = cerebrospinal fluid; IBBB = intra–blood-brain barrier; PBMCs = peripheral blood mononuclear cells.

viruses and group A coxsackie viruses; and explants of viable brain cells have been used for efficient recovery of measles in SSPE and rubella virus in PRP. Peripheral blood lymphocytes are used for the isolation of Epstein-Barr virus, CMV, HTLV-I, and HIV-1. Thus, it is important to use clinical history, examination findings, and other laboratory data to develop an intelligent differential diagnosis of suspected viral agents. The major drawbacks to viral isolation methods are the time and costs involved. In addition, the efficiency of recovery of viruses from the CSF varies with the virus to be isolated and the culture system, and may be quite low. Some viruses, such as mumps, can frequently be isolated, while other viruses, such as poliovirus, HSV type 1, and most arthropod-borne viruses, are more difficult to recover. Furthermore, some viruses (e.g., adenoviruses) can be excreted for months after initial infection; recovery of viruses from body fluids in these circumstances does not prove that the current illness is due to the isolated virus. Therefore, simultaneous serological testing is usually necessary to confirm that primary infection or reinfection occurred during the time of clinical neurological disease.

Immunological Tests for Specific Antibody

Viral agents can be identified by the specific antibodies they stimulate in serum and in CSF when the virus invades the CNS. Older tests for detection and titration of specific antibody include complement fixation (CF) assay and in vitro viral neutralization assays. These typically measure IgG antibodies. The CF assay is unpredictable and lacks sensitivity. More recent tests use an antibody-capture strategy where standardized viral antigen and antihuman antibody combine with the antiviral antibody in an immunosorbent assay to determine both the quantity and class of antiviral immunoglobulin.

Classically viral infection has been identified and verified by demonstrating a significant (fourfold) increase in specific antibody between paired samples of acute and convalescent sera. Determination of specific antibody in a single serum specimen is not useful, for antiviral titers can remain elevated for prolonged intervals after exposure. The paired serum method is of little value during the course of clinical infection when a therapeutic decision may be necessary. Moreover, viral infection may stimulate polyclonal responses of T-memory cells, leading to a nonspecific increase in antiviral and other antibodies. Demonstration of specific IgM antibody in CSF or other body fluid relatively early in the clinical course can identify the viral agent, particularly in primary infection, as has been demonstrated for Japanese B encephalitis. Demonstration of intra–blood-brain barrier (IBBB) antiviral antibody synthesis can further identify and verify infection in the CNS. This requires determining antibody titers in paired serum and CSF samples and calculating the CSF IgG index. The *CSF IgG index* (Table 49.5) determines IBBB IgG by correcting for leakage of serum IgG and albumin across the BBB. The CSF IgG index is elevated during viral infection, and virus-specific IgG synthesis gives rise to an oligoclonal electrophoretic pattern (*oligoclonal bands*) on immunoelectrophoresis of CSF. The CSF IgG index is limited in reliability at CSF total protein levels greater than 150 mg per dl or less than 25 mg per dl. With

Table 49.5: Indices of intra–blood-brain barrier antibody

CSF Ig index	
$\frac{Ig_{CSF}/Ig_{serum}}{Alb_{CSF}/Alb_{serum}}$	
Specific antibody index	
$\frac{\text{Antiviral } Ig_{CSF}/\text{Total } Ig_{CSF}}{\text{Antiviral } Ig_{serum}/\text{Total } Ig_{serum}}$	

CSF = cerebrospinal fluid; Ig = immunoglobulin IgG or IgM; Alb = albumin.

IgM titers, the index can be modified to reflect IBBB IgM synthesis, which may be preferable as a marker of recent immunological stimulation. Specific antibody indices (Table 49.5) require determination of virus-specific IgG (or IgM) in paired serum and CSF. These indices have been calculated for several neurotropic viruses, including measles, rubella, HIV, and herpesviruses, but their overall clinical utility has not been established. They have been used in retrospective diagnosis of patients with acute HSE, with approximately 50% of patients manifesting IBBB synthesis of HSV antibody within 10 days of clinical symptoms. However, for optimal diagnostic value, specific antibodies in CSF should be evaluated sequentially during the clinical course to confirm an elevated antibody index (Whitley 1990).

Direct Detection of Viral Antigen

Since both the isolation of viruses and serological studies with antiviral antibodies can take weeks to accomplish, direct demonstration of viral antigen in infected tissues may be necessary in acute, critical clinical situations. Where infected cells or tissue samples are available, electron microscopy, staining of infected cells by labeled specific antibodies, and the use of various immunoassays may be useful in diagnosis. Electron microscopy can be used to examine body fluids, tissue sections from biopsy, or cell pellets derived from centrifuged body fluid specimens. Relatively rapid examination can be achieved by negative staining of fluids or thin section of solid specimens. Cell pellets from CSF may contain identifiable viral particles or core structures, as has been noted for mumps meningitis or disseminated herpes zoster. Direct or indirect immunostaining with fluorescent dye-conjugated antibodies has been widely used to detect viral antigens in biopsy or autopsy-derived tissue samples. The use of fluorescent-labeled antibody to detect viral antigen in CSF has been more problematic; most laboratories have found that it is not a valid diagnostic method. Staining biopsy tissues with labeled antibodies has produced more consistent results with several viral encephalitides, including HSE, rabies, and SSPE.

Immunoassays, including antigen capture techniques, can detect viral antigen in body fluids. Typical immunoassays use either ^{125}I-coupled antibodies in radioimmunoassay or enzyme-coupled antibodies in enzyme-linked immunosorbent assay (ELISA). Antigen capture methods have been very useful for detecting HIV-1 capsid p24 antigen in cell culture, patients' sera, plasma, and CSF. As little as a few picograms of HIV-1 p24 can be detected in the serum of infected individuals. Antigen capture assays have also been used to identify HSV glycoprotein antigens in CSF of patients with HSE; this method holds great promise for rapid early diagnosis without brain biopsy.

Molecular Approaches to Viral Diagnosis

Molecular biological techniques have been used to gain insight into the pathogenesis of diseases caused by neurotropic viruses and to identify the agents of syndromes with unknown causes. These techniques are quickly becoming the standard for detecting viral nucleic acids and proteins in pathological nervous system tissues. They include nucleic acid hybridization, such as Southern (DNA) and Northern (RNA) blots, in situ hybridization to detect viral nucleic acids directly in tissue samples, and polymerase chain reaction (PCR) to amplify minute quantities of viral nucleic acid in infected neural cells.

Southern and Northern Blot Hybridization

The use of Southern blot or Northern blot hybridization in detecting viral nucleic acids in tissues has been well established. Southern blot hybridization detects viral DNA and Northern blot detects viral RNA (Figure 49.4). These techniques require the extraction of total DNA or RNA from infected cells or tissues. The extracted nucleic acids can then be digested with restriction endonucleases and electrophoresed into agarose or acrylamide gels to separate the digested nucleic acid fragments according to size. The DNA or RNA fragments, after transfer to and immobilization on a membrane, are then hybridized with a labeled gene probe specific for each viral pathogen. The advantages of the hybridization techniques over conventional methods of viral diagnosis include sensitivity and specificity. Very small amounts of viral nucleic acids can be detected in infected cells or tissues. This also eliminates the waiting periods necessary for the development of enough viral antigens or antibodies for serological detection.

In Situ Hybridization

In situ hybridization (ISH) is an extension of Southern and Northern blot techniques such that viral nucleic acids can be directly detected within the infected cells or tissue specimen on a microscope slide. The sensitivity of ISH is even higher than that of Southern or Northern blots, and even a few copies of viral genome per cell can be detected. With the technique, radio- or enzyme-labeled viral nucleic acid probes are hybridized in situ with tissues or cells fixed on glass slides. Enzyme-labeled nucleic acid probes are gradu-

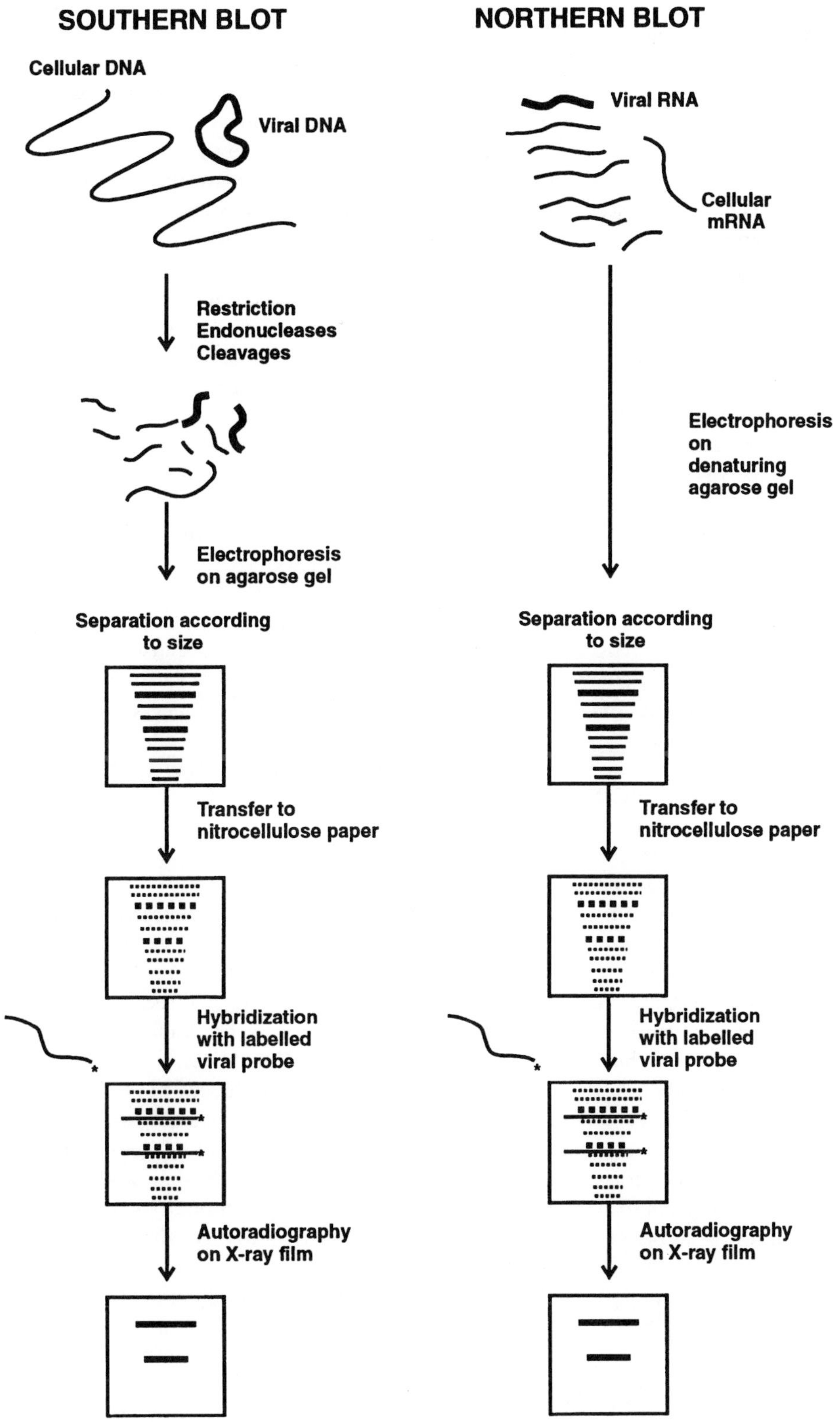

FIGURE 49.4 Schematic representation of Southern and Northern hybridization techniques to detect viral nucleic acids in infected cells. Southern blot is done by extracting DNAs from infected cells, digesting them with restriction endonucleases, and separating the fragments according to size by electrophoresis through a gel. Northern blot is done by extracting RNAs from infected cells, then running them directly onto a gel that denatures the RNAs. The viral nucleic acids can be identified after they are transferred onto a nitrocellulose paper and hybridized to a labeled viral nucleic acid probe.

ally replacing the radioactive probes. Enzyme-labeled probes contain nucleotides that have been linked to an enzyme, such as horseradish peroxidase. Viral probes that have incorporated the enzyme can easily be detected using the enzyme substrate in a colorimetric or luminescent assay that generates measurable color or luminescence. The advantage of using ISH, whether with radioactive or enzyme-labeled probes, is that very small amounts of nucleic acids can be detected directly within the infected cells or in particular areas of tissues, and susceptible cell types can be identified easily. However, ISH is time-consuming and can be subject to various artifacts, such as nonspecific binding of the probes to uninfected cells.

Polymerase Chain Reaction

The entire field of molecular diagnosis has been revolutionized by the development of the PCR (Figure 49.5) (see Chapter 47). The technique requires oligonucleotide sequences, or "primers," specific for the viral gene of interest, so at least part of the gene's nucleotide sequence must be known (Mullis and Faloona 1987). The primers are used to initiate a multicycle chain reaction whereby multiple copies of the gene are synthesized from a DNA template by a heat-stable DNA polymerase. Double-strand target DNA is first separated into two single strands by heating it to a high temperature. Each primer will hybridize to one strand of the separated nucleic acid, and in the presence of a heat-stable DNA polymerase, two copies of the original DNA will be formed. The heat denaturation and the polymerization steps are then repeated up to 30 or 40 cycles, producing massive cyclical amplification of the nucleic acid present in the tissues under study. A combination of ISH and PCR called in situ PCR has also been developed. This technique involves directly performing PCR with tissue samples on mounted slides followed by hybridization with a labeled probe. It potentially can detect a single copy of a viral nucleic acid within the infected cell or tissue. Although PCR has excellent sensitivity, contamination with viral nucleic acids such as those used in positive controls is a major problem in PCR diagnosis. Extreme precautions must be taken to eliminate potential sources of contamination. Multiple sets of primers for each virus must also be used to confirm the diagnosis. The usefulness of these molecular techniques is now being established in several areas: (1) examination of serum, CSF, and CNS tissues for evidence of neurotropic virus involvement; (2) latent infection by herpesviruses and diagnosis of HSE; (3) retroviral pathogenesis; (4) pathogenesis of viruses that are acquired in early childhood and may remain latent so that serological tests are not helpful (these include JCV and human herpesvirus-6); (5) detection of nonconventional infectious agents such as prions; and (6) linking of neurological diseases to possible viral agents.

Brain Biopsy

Even with the advances in molecular techniques of viral diagnosis, there continue to be instances in which diagnostic brain biopsy is required for diagnosis. Definitive diagnosis of PML requires biopsy to demonstrate characteristic histological changes and viral particles in oligodendrocyte nuclei. Diagnosis of Creutzfeldt-Jakob disease in its most typical form can be made on the basis of clinical features, but atypical cases can best be confirmed with brain biopsy showing the characteristic noninflammatory spongiform pathology. With the advent of the relatively nontoxic antiherpes drug acyclovir, the use of brain biopsy in cases of suspected HSE became more controversial, with renewed debate over whether and in which patients biopsy is necessary. Diagnostic PCR, IgM immunoassay, or antigen capture methods using CSF may eventually eliminate the need for brain biopsy in such cases. Biopsy may be necessary to diagnose the several types of CNS lesions seen in AIDS patients. Biopsy specimens should be subdivided to include tissue for viral culture, histopathology, electron microscopy where indicated, and in situ antigen or gene detection assays.

THERAPEUTIC STRATEGIES

In principle, viral diseases of the nervous system can be prevented by immune prophylaxis through vaccination or inhibition of viral disease with specific antiviral agents. With the development of many vaccines featuring live and attenuated virus, killed virus, or recombinant viral antigens, vaccination has been the mainstay of antiviral therapy for 50 years. Specific antiviral drugs have begun to appear over the past decade as the events in viral replication and pathogenesis have been defined at the cellular and molecular level, allowing the design of drugs that inhibit viral-coded proteins or necessary cellular receptors or factors.

Vaccination

Systemic immunoprophylaxis against neurotropic virus infection can prevent nervous system disease. Effective vaccination requires stimulation of both humoral and cellular arms of a durable immune response directed specifically against viral structural proteins. The humoral arm generates neutralizing antibodies capable of protecting against viral infection or disease. The cellular arm generates cytotoxic cellular responses capable of clearing virus-infected cells. Most of the current generation of vaccines do not produce antibodies or immune responses that block infection altogether, but vaccine-induced immunity can effectively prevent disease by reducing viral infectivity and spread or by promoting clearance.

Viral vaccines fall into three categories: (1) live, attenuated virus; (2) inactivated (nonreplicating) virus; or (3) purified viral antigens or subunits. All are relevant to nervous system infection. Attenuated viral vaccines use virus strains capable of productive replication, but with mutations in the structural or noncoding region of the viral genome that attenuate pathogenicity. Live vaccines generally produce a more durable, balanced immune response—that is, including both humoral and cellular responses. Current poliovirus, mumps virus, measles virus, rubella virus, and varicella-zoster virus vaccines all use live, attenuated viral strains. These vaccines are routinely administered in early

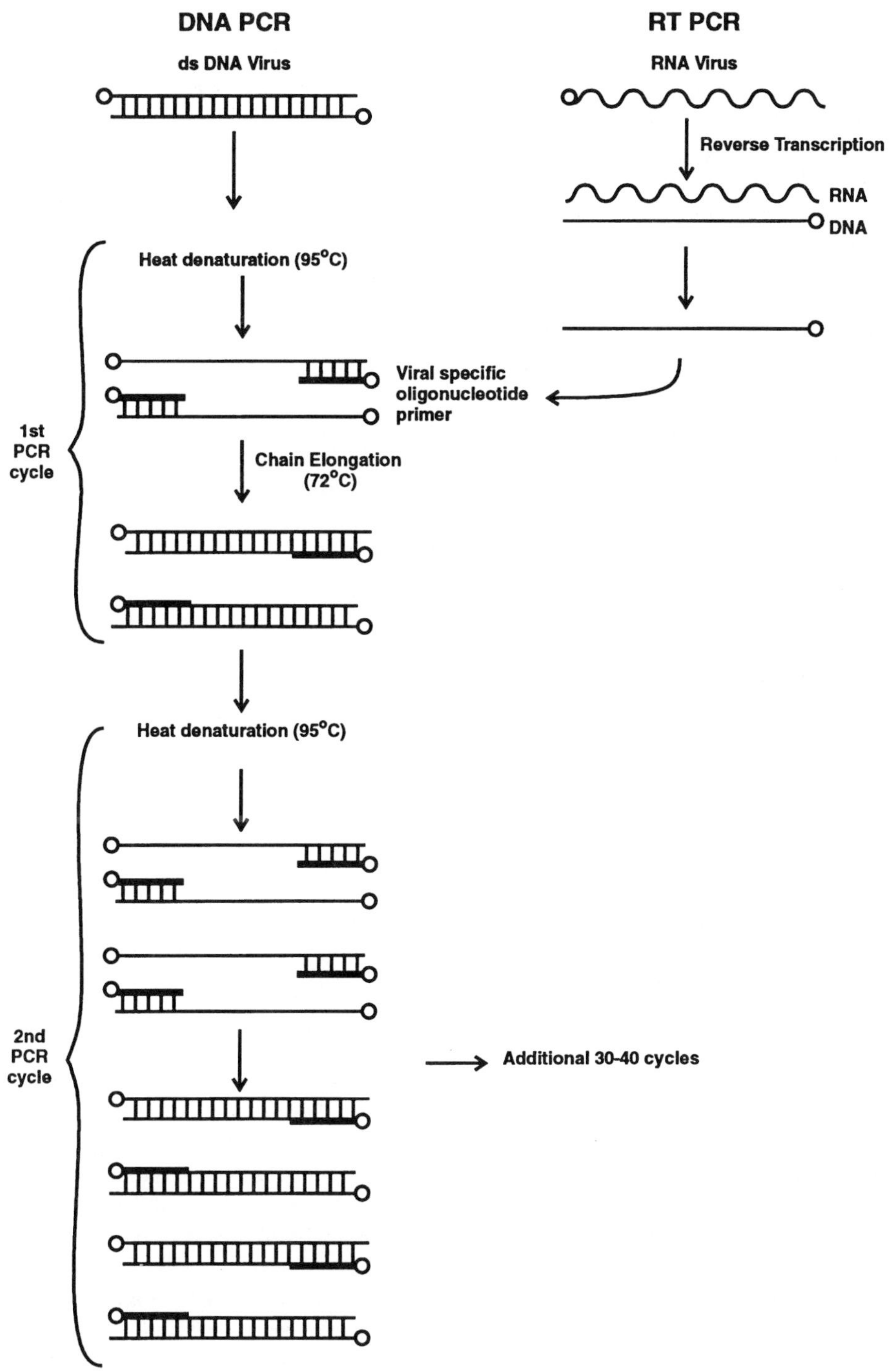

FIGURE 49.5 The polymerase chain reaction. The DNA to be amplified is denatured into two strands by heating the sample. In the presence of a heat-stable DNA polymerase (Taq polymerase), deoxynucleotide triphosphates and oligonucleotide primers that can hybridize specifically to the viral DNA, new daughter strands will be synthesized. The cycles can be repeated 20–30 times, which can lead to amplification by many million-fold of the discrete fragment. Reverse transcriptase PCR is used to amplify RNA molecules. This involves an extra step, in which reverse transcriptase is used to make a DNA copy from the RNA virus before the amplification step.

childhood in the United States. They have drastically reduced the incidence of paralytic poliomyelitis and measles-related encephalitis over the past 35 years. The live virus vaccines have certain biological risks, however, which makes this strategy too risky for certain neurotropic viruses such as rabies. Live vaccines may have residual pathogenicity, especially in immunocompromised recipients, in whom their use may be relatively contraindicated. Genetic instability of live vaccines may potentiate reversion to virulence. Both mechanisms have been implicated in the rare but serious paralytic complications of the oral polio vaccine. Live vaccines may produce persistent infection with potential inflammatory or autoimmune complications, as suggested by persistence of recoverable rubella virus in vaccine recipients who have developed the complication of arthritis.

Inactivated or "killed" virus is used in the rabies and Japanese encephalitis virus (JEV) vaccines and in some current polio vaccines. The JEV vaccine is routinely administered in childhood in endemic areas such as Japan. Rabies vaccine is used for both pre- and postexposure prophylaxis;

vaccine-induced antibody can neutralize virus replicated in muscle cells at the site of inoculation and prevent neural spread to the CNS. In principle, chemical inactivation, such as with formalin, can destroy virus infectivity without destroying the immunogenicity of viral structural proteins. However, in practice, the humoral and cellular balance and durability of the immune response to inactivated viral vaccines is generally inferior to that of live vaccines.

Newer strategies in the design of subunit viral vaccines depend on molecular tools to define and manufacture the viral antigens required to stimulate a balanced immune response. Large quantities of intact viral structural proteins can be generated from recombinant DNA expressed in prokaryotic or eukaryotic cells. Eukaryotic expression cultures are particularly useful for generating glycosylated viral glycoproteins with relatively preserved higher-order protein conformation. An example is the second-generation hepatitis B vaccine. It consists of viral surface antigen (HBsAg) expressed in yeast, which assembles into immunogenic particles. Monoclonal antibodies have fostered advances in the precise amino acid sequence definition of epitopes that stimulate B cell, T-helper, or T-cytotoxic responses. These epitopes, once identified, can be combined into synthetic peptides. Theoretically, synthetic peptides containing the proper mix of epitopes can stimulate production of neutralizing antibodies and development of specific cytotoxic responses. They can also, through stimulation of T-helper responses, prime the recipient for subsequent inoculation of whole (attenuated) virus and conversion of a moderate immune response to a vigorous one. A major obstacle to the advancement of synthetic peptide vaccines is the contribution of an epitope's structural conformation to its immunogenicity. The higher-order conformation present in a viral protein may be lost in the context of a synthetic peptide, thereby reducing the immunogenicity of the epitope.

An alternative to the synthetic peptide or recombinant viral immunogen is the anti-idiotype antibody. The idiotype is that region of the neutralizing antibody that combines with viral antigen. Immunization with neutralizing antibody produces an "anti-idiotype antibody" with a region that mimics the structure of the viral antigen. The anti-idiotype antibody then serves as immunogen, substituting for viral antigen and eliciting antibodies that will bind directly to virus.

Live virus vaccines may be genetically engineered in the future by selective deletion of pathogenic viral genes. This strategy is especially relevant to viruses such as HSV, in which viral functions such as neurotropism or latency can be mapped to specific genetic loci. Selective partial or complete deletion of viral genes could generate live vaccine strains with attenuated pathogenicity, attentuated neurovirulence, or reduced capacity for reactivation.

Antiviral Drugs

Over the past decade antiviral nucleoside analogues have revolutionized the therapeutic approach to herpesvirus infections of the nervous system. Acyclovir, an acyclic guanosine analogue, is the prototype selective viral DNA synthesis inhibitor. Its mechanism of action depends on phosphorylation by the herpesvirus thymidine kinase to a monophosphate compound; thus, it is highly specific for virus-infected cells. With few toxic effects, acyclovir has replaced vidarabine (adenosine arabinoside) for the treatment of HSV and HZV infections, especially HSE (Whitley and Gnann 1992). However, acyclovir is not clinically effective against CMV, possibly because CMV lacks the herpesvirus thymidine kinase. Ganciclovir, which differs from acyclovir by the addition of a carboxyl group, is phosphorylated in CMV-infected cells, and subsequently inhibits CMV's DNA polymerase. Ganciclovir has been accepted for treatment of CMV retinitis and appears to be effective for treatment of CMV radiculitis in HIV-infected patients. Ganciclovir is much more prone to produce serious myelosuppressive toxicity than acyclovir, which limits its clinical use. The development of viral resistance to either acyclovir or ganciclovir is associated with mutations in viral DNA polymerases or with failure to phosphorylate these nucleosides, which can result from mutations in viral-coded kinases. Drug-resistant strains of these herpesviruses can emerge in immunocompromised patients (Whitley and Gnann 1992); they are potentially problematic in the management of neurological infections complicating AIDS. Foscarnet, an analogue of phosphonacetic acid, inhibits herpesvirus DNA polymerase by a different mechanism, not requiring phosphorylation by a nucleoside kinase. Although its use is limited by multiple toxic effects, foscarnet has a clinical role in the management of neurological infections with acyclovir-resistant strains of HSV and HZV and ganciclovir-resistant strains of CMV.

Antiviral nucleoside analogues have been the vanguard of therapeutic strategies against HIV-1 infection. These drugs may forestall the development of neurological illness associated with advanced HIV-1 infection (see Chapter 60D). The first-line drug, azidothymidine (AZT, or zidovudine), blocks DNA elongation by the viral reverse transcriptase, inhibiting the synthesis of proviral DNA from the viral RNA template. Resistant strains emerge as HIV-1-associated disease and immunosuppression progress. More recently, dideoxy- nucleosides including dideoxyinosine (ddI, didanosine) and dideoxycytidine (ddC, zalcitabine) have been studied as alternatives or supplements to azidothymidine in treating advanced HIV-1 infection.

Emerging Strategies for Antiviral Therapy

With our increasing knowledge of the molecular events of viral replication, the identification of viral receptors, and the availability of various molecular tools, there are now a number of potential strategies to intervene in viral infection. With the expanding knowledge of molecular events in HIV replication, new antiviral strategies are emerging to inhibit specific steps of viral replication. A new generation of antiviral compounds are being designed to inhibit the integration of the virus into the host chromosome by the viral integrase enzyme or the processing of viral proteins by the viral protease. Additional strategies include the use of soluble viral receptors, antisense RNA, or ribozymes.

Perhaps the best-known viral receptor is the CD4 molecule, the major cellular receptor for HIV-1. Biological studies with soluble forms of CD4 (SCD4), produced by molecular procedures in mammalian cells, have shown that mixing the SCD4 with HIV-1 can lead to inactivation of most HIV-1 strains. SCD4 can function by blocking the viral surface glycoprotein gp120 from binding to cell surface CD4; alternatively, SCD4 can attach to the viral envelope region, causing its removal from the virus and rendering it noninfectious. Another novel technique that has been used to enhance the killing of virus by soluble receptor is the coupling of a toxin moiety to the receptor. Pseudomonas toxin linked to SCD4 has been tried in culture to inhibit HIV. As more viral receptors are being identified and characterized, including viral receptors in neural cells, it is conceivable that soluble receptors will be useful tools for blocking viral infection of the CNS.

Another emerging molecular tool for genetic therapy and for blocking viral replication is the use of antisense molecules. The idea behind antisense is to block the action of unwanted genes (i.e., viral genes) with nucleic acid strands carrying the opposite coding sequence. Antisense RNA can be complementary to either the single strand viral genomic RNA or to specific viral mRNA. These antisense molecules then function by blocking viral replication or blocking viral protein synthesis. Promising results have been observed with antisense oligonucleotides in blocking HIV-1 and HTLV-I replication in vitro. However, one problem associated with antisense strategy is that the antisense molecule degrades too quickly in the cells. As a result, investigators have been modifying the nucleic acids chemically to increase their stability. One of the most promising developments is the discovery of a completely different class of antisense molecules, namely, peptide nucleic acids (PNAs), which are not only more stable in cells than antisense RNA molecules but also bind 50–100 times more tightly to target molecules.

A new generation of genetically engineered molecules, called ribozymes, is on the verge of leaving the laboratory and moving toward clinical trials. Ribozymes contain stretches of nucleotides that base-pair with a complementary RNA region. They have a catalytic moiety, like the active site of a protein enzyme, that can hydrolyze the bound target RNA molecule while it is base-paired to the ribozyme (Figure 49.6). A ribozyme can be custom-designed to recognize and base-pair with a specific viral sequence that needs to be eliminated. Once they are introduced or synthesized de novo inside the cell, they can inactivate a viral target. One tempting viral target for ribozymes is HIV-1.

In spite of the successes of the emerging antiviral strategies in vitro, there are still concerns about these new technologies. One of the major problems is the delivery system, especially delivery to the CNS and to specific cells that are infected by viruses. If the delivery challenges can be overcome, the specificities of these molecules in vivo will need to be determined. However, there is no doubt that with the advances in molecular biology, and with time, these problems will be solved.

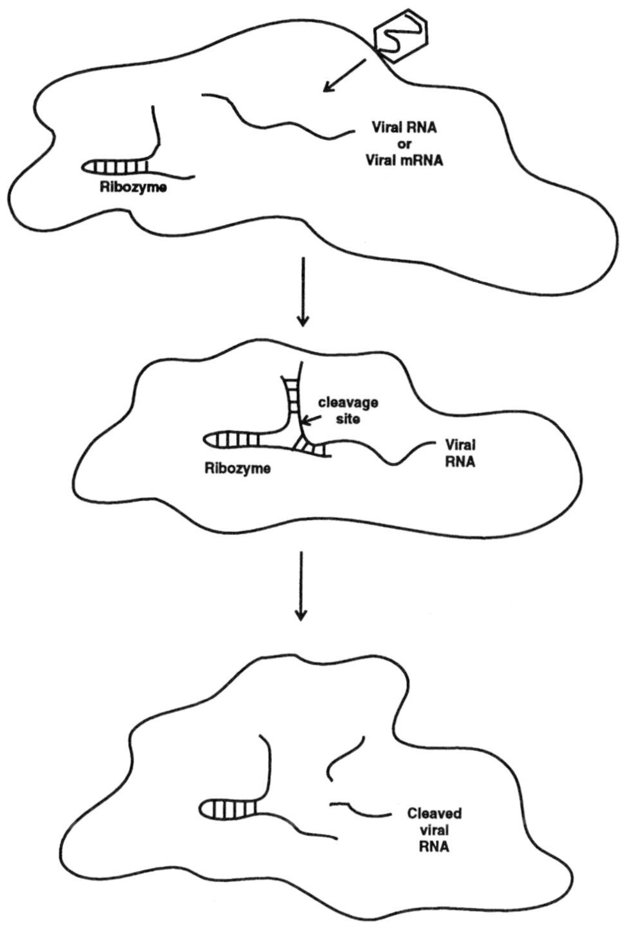

FIGURE 49.6 How a ribozyme functions. The ribozyme inside the infected cell will base-pair with either the viral genomic RNA or mRNA; the base-paired viral RNA will then be cleaved by the catalytic domain of the ribozyme and be inactivated.

REFERENCES

Antel JP, Owens T. The attraction of adhesion molecules. Ann Neurol 1993;34:123–124.

Barnett LA, Fujinami RS. Molecular mimicry: a mechanism for autoimmune injury. FASEB J 1992:6;840–844.

Bodian D. Viremia in experimental poliomyelitis. II. Viremia and the mechanism of the "provoking" effect of injections or trauma. Am J Hygiene 1955;60:358–370.

Clemens MJ. Cytokines. Oxford, England: BIOS Scientific, 1991.

Fazakerley JK, Buchmeier MJ. Pathogenesis of virus-induced demyelination. Adv Virus Res 1993;42:249–324.

Griffin DE, Levine B, Tyor WR et al. The immune response in viral encephalitis. Semin Immunol 1992;4:111–119.

Haywood AM. Viral receptors: binding, adhesion, strengthening, and changes in viral structure. J Virol 1994;68:1–5.

Johnson RT. The pathogenesis of acute viral encephalitis and postinfectious encephalomyelitis. J Infect Dis 1987;155:359–363.

Johnson RT. Viral Infections of the Nervous System. New York: Raven, 1982.

Levy JA. Pathogenesis of human immunodeficiency virus infection. Microbiol Review 1993;57:183–289.

Lohler J. Immunopathologic reactions in viral infections of the central nervous system. J Neuroimmunol 1988;20:181–188.

Merrill JE. Cytokines and retroviruses. Clin Immunol Immunopathol 1992;64:23–27.

Merrill JE, Chen, ISY. HIV-1, macrophages, glial cells, and cytokines in AIDS nervous system disease. FASEB J 1991; 5:2391–2397.

Mullis K, Faloona F. Specific synthesis of DNA in vitro via a polymerase-catalyzed chain reaction. Methods Enzymol 1987; 155:335–350.

Prusiner SB. Genetic and infectious prion diseases. Arch Neurol 1993;50:1129–1153.

Roos R. Molecular Neurovirology. New Jersey: Humana, 1992.

Tsukada N, Miyagi K, Matsuda M et al. Increased levels of circulating intercellular adhesion molecule-1 in multiple sclerosis and human T-lymphotropic virus type 1-associated myelopathy. Ann Neurol 1993;33:646–649.

Whitley RJ, Gnann JW. Acyclovir: A decade later. N Engl J Med 1992;327:782–789.

Whitley RJ. Viral encephalitis. N Engl J Med 1990;323: 242–250.

Wigdahl B, Kunsch C. Human immunodeficiency virus infection and neurologic dysfunction. Prog Med Virol 1990;37:1–46.

Williams GT, Smith CA. Molecular regulation of apoptosis: genetic controls on cell death. Cell 1993;74:777–779.

SUGGESTED READING

Fields BN, Knipe DM. Fundamental Virology (2nd ed). New York: Raven, 1991

Notkins AL, Oldstone MBA. Concepts in Viral Pathogenesis. New York: Springer-Verlag, 1984.

Roitt I, Brostoff J, Male D. Immunology (3rd ed). St. Louis: Mosby, 1993.

Scheld WM, Whitley RJ, Durack DT. Infections of the Central Nervous System. New York: Raven, 1991.

Chapter 50 Neuroendocrinology

Paul E. Cooper

In all but the simplest of organisms, the maintenance of homeostasis requires communication among cells and organs that are widely separated. This communication is achieved through the coordinated interaction among the nervous, endocrine, and immune systems. It is this coordinated interaction that is the field of neuroendocrinology.

THE NONENDOCRINE HYPOTHALAMUS

Neuropeptides, Neurotransmitters, and Neurohormones

The term *neurotransmitter* is traditionally applied to a substance released by one neuron to act on an adjacent neuron in a stimulatory or inhibitory fashion. The effect is usually rapid, brief, and confined to a small area of the cell. In contrast, a *hormone* is a substance that is released into the bloodstream, where it travels to a distant site to act over seconds, minutes, or hours to produce its effect over a large area of the cell. Neuropeptides can act in either fashion. For example, the neuropeptide vasopressin is produced by the neurons of the supraoptic and paraventricular nuclei, is released into the bloodstream, and acts as a hormone on the collecting ducts in the kidney. In the central nervous system (CNS), there is increasing evidence that vasopressin acts as a neurotransmitter. Similarly, the neuropeptide substance P acts as a neurotransmitter in primary sensory neurons that convey pain signals and as a neurohormone in the hypothalamus.

Nemeroff and his colleagues divide the influence of neuropeptides on the brain into two broad categories: *organizational* and *activational* (Doraiswamy et al. 1992). Organizational effects occur during neuronal differentiation, growth, and development and bring about permanent, structural changes in the organization of the brain that affect its function. This would be analogous to the structural and organizational changes brought about in the brain by prenatal exposure to testosterone. Activational effects are those that change pre-established patterns of neuronal activity, such as an increased rate of neuronal firing caused by exposure of a neuron to substance P. Numerous neuropeptides are found in the brain, and basic research has shown these compounds to have a variety of effects on neuronal function (Table 50.1). At present, it is unknown which of these effects occur in the human brain and which are of physiological significance.

Neuropeptides and the Immune System

For many years, it has been recognized that stress, acting through the hypothalamic-pituitary-adrenal axis, modulates the function of the immune system. More recently, it has been appreciated that certain peptides and their receptors, once thought to be unique to the immune or neuroendocrine systems, are actually found in both.

Cytokines (interleukin [IL]-1, -2, -4, -6, and tumor necrosis factor [TNF]) are known to be synthesized by glial cells in the CNS in response to cell injury. IL-1, through its ability to stimulate the synthesis of nerve growth factor, may be an important promoter of the repair of neuron damage.

Table 50.1: Neuropeptides found in the brain and their effects on brain function*

Neuropeptide	*CNS Function*
Hypothalamic peptides modulating pituitary function	
Corticotropin-releasing hormone (CRH)	Regulation of ACTH secretion Integration of behavioral and biochemical responses to stress Regulation of ACTH secretion
Vasopressin	Learning and memory facilitation Memory processes
Oxytocin	Induction of maternal and sexual behaviors
Growth hormone-releasing hormone	Regulation of growth-hormone secretion
Growth hormone release-inhibiting hormone (somatostatin)	Regulation of growth-hormone secretion
Thyrotropin-releasing hormone (TRH)	Regulation of thyroid-stimulating hormone (TSH) secretion May be involved in depression Enhances neuromuscular function
Gonadotropin-releasing hormone (GnRH, LHRH)	Regulates gonadotropin secretion Sexual receptivity
Neurotensin	Endogenous neuroleptic Regulates mesolimbic, mesocortical, and nigrostriatal dopamine neurons Thermoregulation Analgesia
Neuropeptide Y	Satiety and drinking Sexual behavior Locomotion Memory
Pituitary peptides	
Prolactin	—
Growth hormone	—
Thyroid-stimulating hormone (TSH)	—
Follicle-stimulating hormone (FSH)	—
Luteinizing hormone (LH)	—
Pro-opiomelanocortin (POMC)	—
Corticotropin (ACTH)	—
Corticotropin-like intermediate lobe peptides (CLIP)	—
Beta-endorphin	Analgesic mechanisms Feeding Thermoregulation Learning and memory
Beta-lipotropic hormone (β-LPH)	—
Melanocyte-stimulating hormone (α- and γ-MSH)	—
Oxytocin	—
Vasopressin	—
Neurophysins	—
Brain-gastrointestinal tract peptides	
Vasoactive intestinal polypeptide (VIP)	Cerebral blood flow
Somatostatin	—
Insulin	Feeding behavior Hunger
Glucagon	—
Pancreatic polypeptide	—
Gastrin	—
Cholecystokinin	Feeding behavior Satiety Modulates dopamine neuron activity
Tachykinins (e.g., substance P)	Substance P colocalizes with serotonin and is involved in nociception
Secretin	—
Thyrotropin-releasing hormone (TRH)	—
Bombesin	Thermoregulation Appetite
Growth factors	
Insulin-like growth factors (IGF-I and -II)	—
Nerve growth factors	Axonal plasticity
Opioid family	—
Endorphins	—

Table 50.1: *(continued)*

Neuropeptide	*CNS Function*
Enkephalins (Met-, Leu-)	Analgesic mechanisms Feeding Temperature control Learning and memory Cardiovascular control
Dynorphins	—
Kytorphin	—
Neuropeptides modulating immune function	
ACTH	—
Endorphins	—
Interferons	—
Neuroleukins	—
Thymosin	—
Thymopeptin	—
Other neuropeptides	
Atrial natriuretic factors	—
Bradykinins	Cerebral blood flow Migraine
Angiotensin	Hypertension Thirst
Synapsins	—
Calcitonin gene-related peptide (CGRP)	—
Calcitonin	—
Sleep peptides	Regulation of sleep cycles
Carnosine	—
Precursor peptides	
POMC	—
Proenkephalins (A and B)	—
Calcitonin gene product	—
VIP gene product	—
Pro-glucagon	—
Pro-insulin	—

*This is only a partial list of all of the neuropeptides that have been found in the brain, and not all of the putative functions have been listed.

Source: Modified from PM Doraiswamy, KR Krishnan, CB Nemeroff. Hormonal Effects on Brain Function. In DL Barrow, W Selman (eds), Neuroendocrinology. Concepts in Neurosurgery. Vol. 5. Baltimore: Williams & Wilkins, 1992;75–91.

Cytokines also appear to play a role in the hypothalamus to activate the hypothalamic-pituitary-adrenal axis in response to inflammation and to inhibit the pituitary-thyroid and pituitary-gonadal axes in response to systemic disease.

Several other hormones and neuropeptides have been shown to have modulatory effects on immune function (Table 50.2). Similarly, immunocompetent cells contain hormones and neuropeptides that may affect neuroendocrine and brain cells (Table 50.3).

While there has been much speculation about the ability of the psyche to influence immunological function and therefore disease outcome, there is no conclusive evidence to date to suggest that this is clinically significant (Reichlin 1993).

Temperature Regulation

The hypothalamus plays a key role in ensuring that body temperature is maintained within narrow limits by balancing the heat gained from metabolic activity and the environment with the heat lost to the environment. A theoretical schema of the mechanisms of hypothalamic temperature regulation is depicted in Figure 50.1. Although numerous neurotransmitters and peptides have been shown to alter body temperature, their physiological role remains unclear.

Hypothalamic injury can cause disordered temperature regulation. One potentially serious consequence is the hyperthermia that may occur when the preoptic anterior hypothalamic area (POAHT) is damaged or irritated by infarction, subarachnoid hemorrhage, trauma, or surgery. In some patients, the marked impairment of heat loss mechanisms and the resulting hyperthermia may be fatal. In those individuals who survive, temperature control returns to normal over a period of days to weeks; chronic hyperthermia of hypothalamic origin has not been convincingly demonstrated. Both acute and chronic hypothermia can be caused by hypothalamic injury, the most common causes being head trauma, infarction, and demyelination. Large le-

Table 50.2: Immunoregulatory effects of several hormones and peptides

Hormone or Peptide	*Immune Function Affected*
Inhibitory	
Glucocorticoids	Lymphokine synthesis, inflammation
Corticotropin (ACTH)	Macrophage activation, synthesis of IgG and gamma-interferon
Chorionic gonadotropin	Activity of T cells and natural killer cells
Alpha-endorphin	IgG synthesis, T cell proliferation
Somatostatin	T cell proliferation, inflammatory cascade
Vasoactive intestinal peptide	T cell proliferation and migration in Peyer's patches
Alpha-melanocyte-stimulating hormone	Fever, prostaglandin synthesis, secretion of interleukin-2
Stimulatory	
Estrogens	Lymphocyte proliferation and secretion
Growth hormone	Thymic growth, lymphocyte reactivity
Prolactin	Thymic growth, lymphocyte proliferation
Thyrotropin	IgG synthesis
Beta-endorphin	Activity of T, B, and natural killer cells
Substance P	Proliferation of T cells and macrophages, inflammatory cascade
Corticotropin-releasing hormone	Lymphocyte and monocyte proliferation and activation

Source: Reprinted with permission from S Reichlin. Neuroendocrine-immune interactions. N Engl J Med 1993;329:1246–1253.

Table 50.3: Hormones and neuropeptides found in immunocompetent cells

Hormone	*Source*	*Comments*
Corticotropin	B lymphocytes	Stimulated by corticotropin-releasing hormone; inhibited by cortisol
Growth hormone	T lymphocytes	Stimulated by growth hormone
Thyrotropin	T cells	Stimulated by thyrotropin-releasing hormone; inhibited by somatostatin
Prolactin	Mononuclear cells	—
Chorionic gonadotropin	T cells	—
Enkephalins	B lymphocytes	—
Vasoactive intestinal peptide	Mononuclear leukocytes, mast cells	—
Somatostatin	Mononuclear leukocytes, mast cells, polymorphonuclear leukocytes	—
Vasopressin	Thymus	—
Oxytocin	Thymus	—
Neurophysin	Thymus	—

Source: Reprinted with permission from S Reichlin. Neuroendocrine-immune interactions. N Engl J Med 1993;329:1246–1253.

sions in the posterior hypothalamus may impair heat production by altering the set point and heat loss by damaging the outflow from the POAHT. This results in poikilothermia, a condition in which body temperature varies with the environmental temperature.

Fever

The body's inflammatory cells (primarily monocytes) release cytokines in response to infection and inflammation. It is these cytokines that act on the hypothalamus to cause fever (Cooper 1987).

IL-1 circulates from areas of inflammation to the hypothalmus, where it acts to induce phospholipases that release arachidonic acids from plasma membranes. This results in a rise in prostaglandin E, which, in turn, raises the body temperature set point. The body then uses its normal physiological mechanisms of vasoconstriction, vasodilation, sweating, and shivering to maintain this new set point. TNF, another cytokine, acts directly on the hypothalamus to raise the set point and stimulates the production of IL-1. Bacterial endotoxin is a potent stimulator of macrophages, the major source of production and release of TNF. IL-6 and gamma-interferon (IFN-γ) are two other cytokines that act directly on the hypothalamus to raise the set point. It is probably through interfering with prostaglandins that drugs like acetylsalicylic acid and acetaminophen are useful in treating fever.

There is a complex interaction among the cytokines. IL-1 stimulates its own production, as do elevated levels of IFN-γ. IL-4 suppresses the production of IL-1, TNF, and IL-6. IL-1 production is also inhibited by glucocorticoids and prostaglandin E.

In otherwise healthy individuals, extreme elevations of body temperature (as high as 41.1°C [106°F]) often can be tolerated without serious effects; however, hyperthermia associated with prolonged exertion, heat stroke, malignant hyperthermia, neuroleptic malignant syndrome, hyperthy-

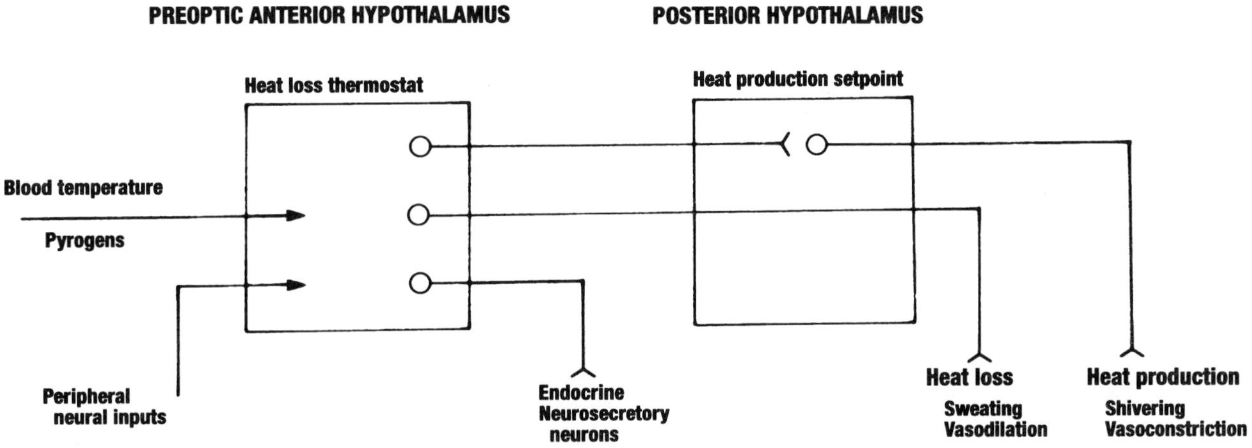

FIGURE 50.1 Schematic representation of hypothalamic temperature-regulation mechanisms. The preoptic anterior hypothalamus functions as a thermostat and contains mechanisms for regulation of heat loss. The posterior hypothalamus integrates heat production mechanisms. Lesions of the preoptic anterior hypothalamus result in hyperthermia; lesions of the posterior hypothalamus cause hypothermia or poikilothermia. (Reprinted with permission from PE Cooper, JB Martin. Neuroendocrine Disease. In RN Rosenberg [ed], The Clinical Neurosciences. New York: Churchill Livingstone, 1983.)

roidism, pheochromocytoma crisis, and some drugs may have serious and even fatal consequences (Simon 1993). Exertional hyperthermia occurs with prolonged physical activity, particularly in hot, humid weather. It may decrease athletic performance and cause muscle cramps or heat exhaustion. When severe, it may result in heat stroke, a syndrome characterized by hyperthermia, hypotension, tachycardia, hyperventilation, and decreased consciousness level. Malignant hyperthermia is a syndrome associated with the use of various general anesthetic agents. This syndrome is caused by a disorder of muscle that involves an excessive release of calcium from sarcoplasmic reticulum that stimulates severe muscle contraction. The neuroleptic malignant syndrome is characterized by diffuse muscular rigidity, akinesia, and fever accompanied by a decreased consciousness level and evidence of autonomic dysfunction—labile blood pressure, tachyarrhythmias, excessive sweating, and incontinence. It is associated with taking major tranquilizers, rapid withdrawal from dopaminergic agents, and less commonly with taking tricyclic antidepressants. It appears to result from an alteration of temperature control mechanisms in the hypothalamus. As part of treatment, withdrawal of the patient from all neuroleptics is mandatory. In addition to general supportive measures, the use of bromocriptine (5 mg orally or nasogastrically four times daily) or dantrolene (2–3 mg/kg daily intravenously, to a maximum of 10 mg/kg per day) have been used to hasten recovery (Rosenberg and Green 1989).

Appetite

Given free access to food and water, most animals are able to maintain their body weight within very narrow limits. If there is a change in the intake of energy—an increase in the size or number of individual meals that is not balanced by an equal and opposite change in energy utilization—then the animal experiences a change in weight. One possible model of nutrient balance is depicted in Figure 50.2. Bray et al. (1990) suggest that the brain receives signals from the periphery that stimulate or inhibit food intake. The brain, in turn, sends signals through the endocrine, autonomic, and motor nervous systems to modulate food intake. Disorders at any point in these systems may lead to weight loss or weight gain.

It has been known for years that destruction of the ventromedian hypothalamus (VMH), both in animals and in humans, leads to obesity. Lesions in the paraventricular nucleus have a similar effect. Using compounds that destroy selective areas of the hypothalamus, it can be shown that hypothalamic obesity is not only due to overeating, or hyperphagia. Hypothalamic lesions can also cause weight loss. Lesions in the dorsomedial nucleus lead to a reduction in body weight and fat stores, as do lesions in the lateral hypothalamus.

Meal size and food intake are influenced by many different stimuli. Sensory cues such as the sight, aroma, and taste of food are major factors in dietary obesity. A fall in blood glucose or a decrease in the oxidation of fatty acids in the liver stimulate experimental animals to eat. Stomach distention gives rise to neural and hormonal signals that reduce food intake. Gastrointestinal peptides such as cholecystokinin, bombesin, and glucagon have been shown to inhibit feeding by their actions on the autonomic nervous system, particularly the vagal nucleus. Increased fatty acid oxidation leads to higher levels of 3-hydroxybutyrate that act on the hypothalamus to reduce food intake. Interference with any of these sensing systems in the CNS can lead to obesity.

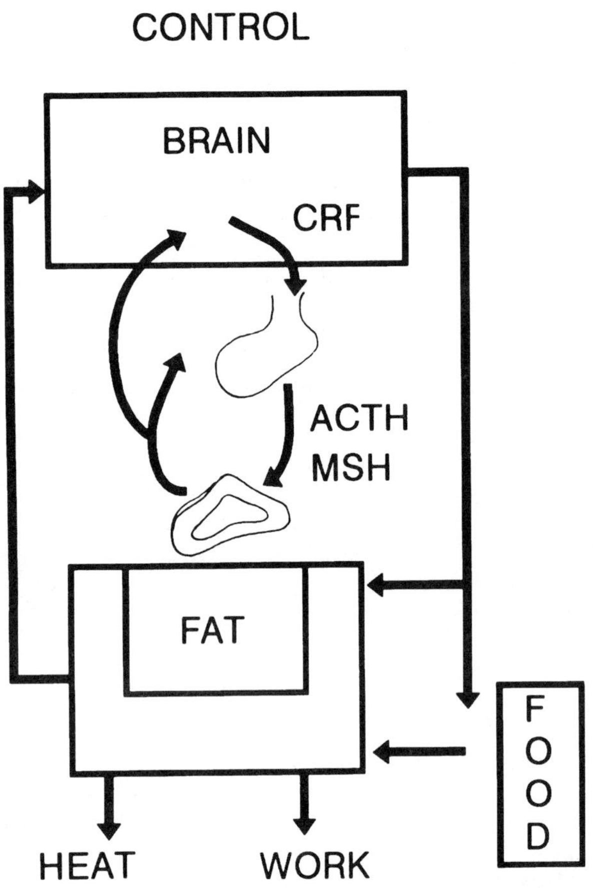

FIGURE 50.2 In the regulation of energy balance, the brain is the central control site. It receives information on nutrient status and energy reserves, then exerts control through its efferent pathways. In this schema, the hypothalamic-pituitary-adrenal axis plays an important role. (Reprinted with permission from GA Bray, J Fisler, DA York. Neuroendocrine control of the development of obesity: Understanding gained from studies of experimental animal models. Front Neuroendocrinol 1990;11:128–181.)

Bray et al. (1990) have proposed that the sympathetic nervous system's regulation of body weight is a function of at least four components: (1) the innervation of the heart and brown adipose tissue, (2) the adrenal medulla, (3) the innervation of subdiaphragmatic structures, and (4) the peripheral innervation of muscle. This sympathetic function is under the direct control of the hypothalamus. VMH lesions have been associated with reduced sympathetic activity, and there is evidence to suggest that reduced sympathetic activity may be the "final common pathway" for virtually all forms of obesity. In addition to reduced sympathetic activity, VMH lesions also produce increased vagal activity with a consequent increase in the secretion of glucagon and insulin. This increased vagal activity may account for up to 50% of the weight gain in hypothalamic obesity.

Anorexia nervosa and bulimia nervosa are clinical eating disorders seen primarily in young women and girls. Anorexia nervosa is characterized by reduced caloric intake and increased physicial activity associated with weight loss, a distorted body image, and a fear of gaining weight. Bulimia nervosa is characterized by episodic gorging followed by self-induced vomiting, laxative and diuretic abuse, dieting, and exercise to reduce weight. For many years, these syndromes have been considered to be purely psychiatric; however, the finding of reduced serotonin levels in the cerebrospinal fluid (CSF) of patients with bulimia nervosa, the low CSF levels of norepinephrine in patients with anorexia nervosa, and the enhanced secretion of cholecystokinin in patients with anorexia nervosa suggest that neurotransmitter or neuropeptide abnormalities could be responsible for at least part of the clinical picture in these patients. Furthermore, patients with anorexia nervosa have an increased total daily energy expenditure due to their increased physical activity (Casper et al. 1991). Whether these are causes or effects of the condition remains to be determined.

Emotion and Libido

Experimental and clinical data support the hypothesis that interaction of the frontal and temporal lobes and the limbic system is necessary for normal emotional function. Lesion and stimulation experiments in the cat have shown that rage reactions can be provoked from the hypothalamus. In the human, electrical stimulation of the septal region produces feelings of pleasure or sexual gratification, whereas lesions of the caudal hypothalamus or manipulation of this area during surgery may cause attacks of rage. The amygdala—with its rich input from polysensory areas and limbic-associated areas and its output to the hypothalamus—and other subcortical areas are important structures through which the external environment can influence and cause emotional responses (Aggleton 1993).

Libido, like other feelings, requires the participation of both hypothalamic and extrahypothalamic sites. In most instances of hypothalamic disease, loss of libido is due to impaired release of gonadotropin-releasing hormone (GnRH). Hypersexuality associated with hypothalamic disease has been reported only rarely. It may be seen with or without subjective increase in libido.

Altered sexual preference has been occasionally associated with hypothalamic lesions (Miller et al. 1986). There is a gradually expanding understanding of the human hypothalamus in relation to normal development, sexual differentiation, aging, and some degenerative neurological disorders (Swaab et al. 1993). The sexually dimorphic nucleus, or intermediate nucleus, of the preoptic area is twice the volume in males as it is in females. The size does not differ between homosexual and heterosexual males. While the shape of the suprachiasmatic nucleus differs in males and females, the vasopressin cell number and volume are similar in men and women. Homosexual men seem to have a larger suprachiasmatic nucleus, containing twice as many cells as heterosexual males (Swaab et al. 1993). The significance of this observation is, at present, uncertain.

Table 50.4: Hypothalamic peptides controlling anterior pituitary hormone release

Pituitary Hormone	*Hypothalamic Factor*
Growth hormone (GH)	Growth hormone-releasing hormone (GHRH)
	Growth hormone release-inhibiting hormone (somatostatin)
Prolactin (PRL)	Prolactin-releasing factor
	Prolactin release-inhibiting factor: dopamine and possibly the precursor of GnRH
Thyrotropin (TSH)	Thyrotropin-releasing hormone (TRH)
	Thyrotropin release-inhibiting factor: somatostatin can do this, but it is uncertain if it does so physiologically
Pro-opiomelanocortin (POMC) is cleaved to form ACTH	Corticotropin-releasing hormone (CRH)
Luteinizing hormone (LH) and follicle-stimulating hormone (FSH)	Gonadotropin-releasing hormone (GnRH)

Biological Rhythms

Most endocrine rhythms are *circadian*—that is, a complete cycle takes approximately 24 hours. Although longer and shorter cycles do occur, the circadian rhythms have been studied most extensively.

In many animals, light plays an important role in regulating circadian rhythms. Nerve fibers project from the optic chiasm to the suprachiasmatic and arcuate nuclei of the hypothalamus, from which the hormonal rhythms—such as cortisol and growth hormone (GH) secretion and the behavioral rhythms such as sleep-wake cycles and estrous activity—are controlled.

Although patients with hypothalamic disease often have disturbances in their biological rhythms, these are usually of less clinical importance than the other problems caused by such lesions.

THE HYPOTHALAMIC-PITUITARY UNIT: FUNCTIONAL ANATOMY

In humans, discernible hypothalamic-pituitary tissue begins to develop during week 5 of embryonic life. Rathke's pouch, a diverticulum of the buccal cavity, forms and expands dorsally to contact and invest the diverticulum, which develops from the floor of the third ventricle. By week 11, the buccal tissue has lost its connection with the foregut and has flattened to form the primitive anterior pituitary, while the neural tissue from the floor of the third ventricle is forming the posterior pituitary. Residual Rathke's pouch tissue is postulated to give rise to the craniopharyngiomas, which can occur in this region. Rarely, functional pituitary tissue in the oropharynx can cause signs and symptoms of hyperpituitarism.

The hypothalamus, despite its small size, is the region of brain with the highest concentrations of neurotransmitters and neuropeptides. Beginning with the pioneering work of Ernst and Berta Scharrer and Geoffrey Harris in the 1940s, the hypothalamus has been assigned a central role in the regulation of anterior pituitary function. In addition to the identified hypophysiotropic hormones (Table 50.4), other peptides with putative regulatory functions are found in high concentration in the hypothalamus, including neurotensin, substance P, cholecystokinin, vasoactive intestinal polypeptide, and the opioid peptides. The hypothalamus is also rich in acetylcholine, norepinephrine, dopamine, serotonin, histamine, and gamma-aminobutyric acid. In many neurons, these neurotransmitters colocalize with peptides, although this colocalization and presumptive corelease have uncertain physiological significance.

A common presentation for patients with nonfunctioning pituitary or parapituitary tumors is symptoms produced by compression of neural structures in the pituitary area. Understanding these symptoms requires a thorough knowledge of the anatomy (Figure 50.3).

Tumor erosion of the floor of the sella turcica may lead to CSF rhinorrhea. Conversely, sinusitis or sphenoid sinus mucocele can compress the sella and cause anterior pituitary dysfunction. Expansion of pituitary tumors into the cavernous sinus can produce a variety of cranial nerve palsies. This is especially common with the sudden expansion of pituitary tumors that occurs in *pituitary apoplexy*. Carotid-cavenous aneurysms or ectatic carotid arteries may expand medially and mimic pituitary adenomas by enlarging the sella and causing anterior pituitary hypofunction.

The dura overlying the sella is pain-sensitive and, when stretched by expanding pituitary tumors, gives rise to headache referred to the vertex and retro-orbitally. In certain individuals, especially if intracranial pressure is elevated, the dura may herniate in the reverse direction into the sella, where, with time, continued pulsation of the CSF leads to remodeling and expansion of the sella. Another cause of this is *lymphocytic hypophysitis*. The pituitary gland becomes a thin ribbon of tissue along the walls of the expanded sella, and the sella consists mostly of CSF. Radiologically, this is referred to as the *empty sella syndrome*. Rarely is there evidence of pituitary function impairment in such patients.

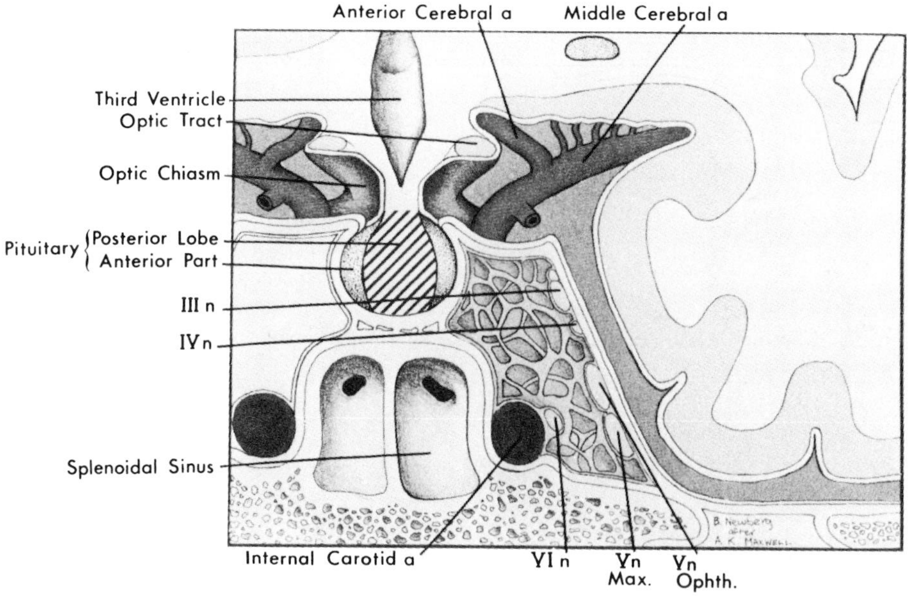

FIGURE 50.3 Diagrammatic representation of the anatomical relations of the pituitary fossa and cavernous sinus. The lateral wall of the sella turcica is formed by the cavernous sinus. The sinus contains the carotid artery, two branches of the V cranial nerve (ophthalmic and maxillary), the III nerve (oculomotor), the IV nerve (trochlear), and the VI nerve (abducens). The optic chiasm and optic tract are located superior and lateral, respectively, to the pituitary. (Reprinted with permission from JB Martin, S Reichlin, GM Brown. Clinical Neuroendocrinology. Philadelphia: FA Davis, 1977. Drawing by B. Newberg.)

Expansion of pituitary tumors out of the sella tends to lead to compression of the anterior crossing fibers of the optic chiasm (see Chapters 14 and 43). These fibers subserve vision in the superior temporal quadrants. Therefore, pituitary adenomas typically cause bitemporal superior quadrantanopsias. Lesions such as craniopharyngiomas that impinge on the posterior notch of the optic chiasm tend to present with bitemporal inferior quadrantanopsias. Despite these rules, the variability of the positioning of the optic chiasm, together with the tendency for tumors to be asymmetrical in their growth, results in a wide variety of field defects being caused by parasellar lesions. As a general rule, lesions in this region produce incongruous visual field defects—that is, defects that are different in configuration in each eye and that do not respect the vertical midline but rather cross from one hemifield into the other.

Blood Supply

The pituitary's major source of blood is via the superior and inferior hypophysial arteries (Figure 50.4). The posterior pituitary gland is supplied principally by the inferior hypophysial arteries and is drained by the inferior hypophysial veins. The superior hypophysial artery forms a primary capillary plexus in the median eminence of the hypothalamus. From here, the blood flows into the long hypophysial portal veins, which carry it to the anterior pituitary. While some of the blood from the anterior pituitary drains into the cavernous sinus, some drains into the posterior pituitary, and some returns to the median eminence via the long portal veins, which are capable of bidirectional blood flow. This vascular anatomy provides a potential mechanism for the important feedback loops that are necessary for regulation of hypothalamic-pituitary function.

THE ANTERIOR PITUITARY

Hypothalamic Control of Anterior Pituitary Secretion

A variety of experimental data has shown that the hypothalamus produces hypophysiotrophic substances that control the secretion of anterior pituitary hormones. To date, five neuropeptides and one neurotransmitter (dopamine) have been shown to be important physiological regulators of pituitary function (see Table 50.4). In addition, several neurotransmitters affect pituitary hormone release, although their physiological role remains uncertain.

The precursor molecule for GnRH, in addition to containing the sequence for GnRH, contains a peptide that is a potent inhibitor of prolactin release. Such an observation suggests that hypothalamic control of pituitary secretion may be even more complicated than it has been thought.

Abnormalities of Anterior Pituitary Function

Hypofunction

The causes of pituitary insufficiency are summarized in Table 50.5. In general, the symptoms of hypopituitarism (Table 50.6) are those of the secondary failure of end-organ function. Because the symptoms usually develop slowly, however, they are often less severe than those that occur with primary end-organ disease. The term *Simmonds disease* is applied to panhypopituitarism. When this develops postpartum following an episode of pituitary infarction, it is called *Sheehan's syndrome*.

Intrauterine growth is independent of GH. Therefore, although GH-deficient children are of normal size at birth,

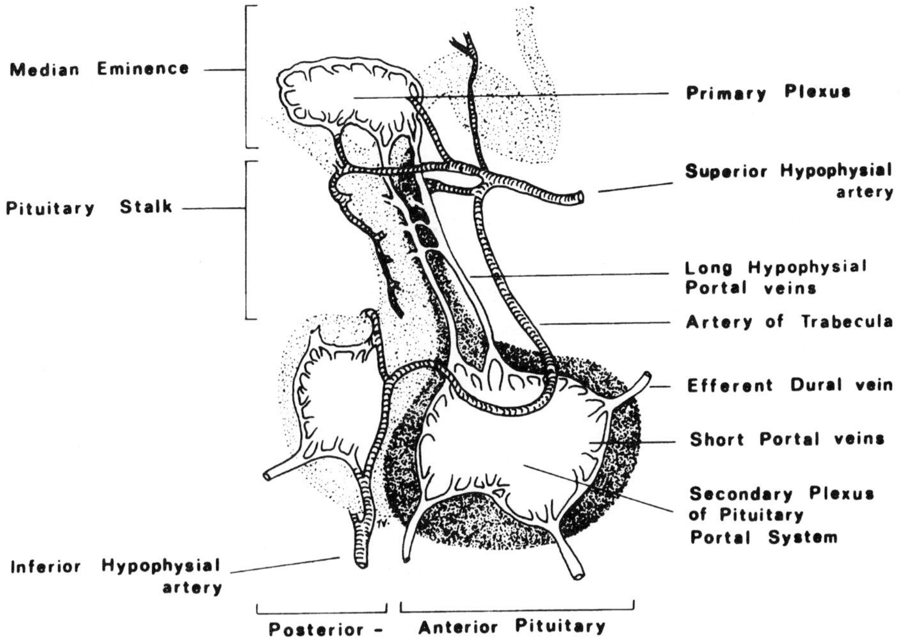

FIGURE 50.4 The blood supply of the median eminence and pituitary gland. (Reprinted with permission from JB Martin, PE Cooper. Neuroendocrine Disease. In RN Rosenberg [ed], The Clinical Neuro-Sciences. New York: Churchill Livingstone, 1983.)

they fail to grow. Somatic growth in the human is mediated by at least two factors: insulin-like growth factor I (IGF-I) and insulin-like growth factor II (IGF-II). IGF-I (also called somatomedin C) production in the liver is GH-dependent, whereas IGF-II is relatively insensitive to GH. True GH deficiency is rare. It may present in an isolated fashion or as part of the picture of general pituitary failure. Apparent GH deficiency may result from an isolated deficiency of GH-releasing hormone or a lack of GH receptors in the liver leading to failure of IGF-I production (Laron dwarf). GH is a contrainsulin hormone; in children, its deficiency may be associated with episodes of fasting hypoglycemia. A detailed discussion of growth is beyond the scope of this chapter. The interested reader is referred to the review by Bierich (1992).

Pituitary insufficiency in the child may present as delayed or absent puberty. Onset of puberty depends, to some extent, on achievement of a certain body mass. Thus, anything that delays growth, such as GH deficiency or hypothyroidism, will delay puberty. If breasts and/or sexual hair have not started to develop in girls by age 14, or if testicular enlargement and sexual hair have not occurred in boys by age 15, then puberty should be considered delayed. Luteinizing hormone (LH) or follicle-stimulating hormone (FSH) deficiency may occur as part of generalized pituitary failure or as a result of high prolactin levels or of GnRH deficiency. For a full discussion of delayed puberty, see Styne (1991).

Table 50.5: Causes of pituitary insufficiency

Pituitary aplasia
Complete
Monohormonal
Trauma
Head injury
Surgery
Radiotherapy
Compression by cysts or tumors
Pituitary apoplexy
Pituitary infarction
Hypophysitis
Infection
Granulomatous disease
Autoimmune disease
Hypothalamic failure

One cause of hypopituitarism is *pituitary apoplexy*, a term that should be reserved for infarction of, or hemorrhage into, the pituitary gland that is of sufficient severity to produce signs of compression of parasellar structures or evidence of meningeal irritation (Rolih and Ober 1993). The sudden expansion of the pituitary gland that follows infarction or hemorrhage may lead to chiasmal compression or cranial nerve palsies. Rupture of the necrotic gland into the CSF may lead to a picture that is indistinguishable clinically from subarachnoid hemorrhage caused by rupture of a berry aneurysm or arteriovenous malformation. Hypotension, aggravated by pre-existing corticotropin (ACTH) deficiency, may further complicate the picture. The diagnosis is readily made by computed tomographic (CT) scanning or magnetic resonance imaging (MRI). Treatment includes general supportive measures, corticosteroid replacement, and, if necessary, surgical decompression.

Hyperfunction

Precocious Puberty. Development of secondary sexual characteristics before age 8 in girls and age 9 in boys is considered abnormal. About one-fifth of girls and half of boys

Table 50.6: Clinical syndromes of anterior pituitary dysfunction

Hormone	*Excess Secretion*	*Deficient Secretion*
Growth hormone	In children: gigantism In adults: acromegaly	In children: growth failure and tendency to hypoglycemia
Prolactin	In children: delayed puberty In adults: Female: amenorrhea, galactorrhea, and infertility Male: impotence, infertility, and (rarely) galactorrhea	In adult female: inability to breast-feed and possible infertility
Luteinizing hormone and follicle-stimulating hormone	In children: precocious puberty In adults: infertility, hypogonadism, polycystic ovary syndrome	In children: delayed puberty In adults: amenorrhea, infertility, impotence
Thyrotropin	Hyperthyroidism Hyperprolactinemia	Hypothyroidism
Pro-opiomelancortin	Cushing's disease Nelson's syndrome	Hypothyroidism—glucocorticoids affected more severely

develop precocious puberty because of neurological lesions. A variety of tumors has been associated with the development of precocious puberty, including hamartoma, teratoma, ependymoma, optic nerve glioma, glioma, and neurofibroma, either alone or as part of von Recklinghausen's syndrome. Tumors are most commonly located in the posterior hypothalamus, the pineal gland, or the median eminence, or they put pressure on the floor of the third ventricle. The cause of precocious puberty under these circumstances has not been clearly delineated; however, some of these tumors may be an ectopic source of GnRH or of human chorionic gonadotropin (hCG)—a placental peptide with LH- and FSH-like activity.

In the investigation of precocious puberty, LH and FSH levels should be measured as well as hCG. A CT scan or MRI of the head is mandatory. If LH and FSH levels are in the adult range and the head scan is negative, it is most likely that the precocious puberty is idiopathic. High hCG levels suggest ectopic production. If LH and FSH levels are low, then adrenal, ovarian/testicular, or exogenous causes must be sought.

Chronic administration of long-acting analogues of GnRH is followed by an initial stimulation of LH and FSH secretion, then complete inhibition. This effect on LH and FSH release can be used to prevent progression of hypothalamic precocious puberty.

Hyperprolactinemia. Probably the most common abnormality of pituitary function encountered by the neuroendocrinologist is hyperprolactinemia. The causes of hyperprolactinemia are summarized in Table 50.7.

Prolactin levels in excess of 200 ng per ml (normal <25 ng per ml) are almost always due to excessive production of the hormone by a pituitary adenoma. In premenopausal women, the development of amenorrhea secondary to direct inhibition of LH and FSH by prolactin leads to early investigation and diagnosis of tumors at the microadenoma (<10 mm in diameter) stage. In males, the insidious onset of impotence and reduced libido usually means that these tumors are found late, often only after they have produced signs and symptoms of optic nerve compression. Galactorrhea is a common accompaniment of elevated prolactin in women and a rare finding in men.

Serum prolactin levels have been documented to rise after generalized tonic-clonic seizures and complex partial seizures but to show no change after psychogenic, absence, or simple partial seizures or complex partial seizures of frontal lobe origin (Fisher et al. 1991). Following a seizure, prolactin levels peak at 15–20 minutes, then fall to baseline levels within 60 minutes. The rise should be at least two times baseline. Caution should be exercised in interpreting early-morning pro-

Table 50.7: Causes of hyperprolactinemia

- Drugs
  - Dopamine receptor blockers
    - Phenothiazines such as chlorpromazine
    - Butyrophenones such as haloperidol
    - Metoclopramide
  - Reserpine
  - α-Methyldopa
  - Tricyclic antidepressants (unusual, probably idiosyncratic)
  - Benzodiazepines (unusual, probably idiosyncratic)
- Hormones
  - Estrogens
  - Thyrotropin-releasing hormone (as can occur in primary hypothyroidism)
- Pituitary tumor
  - Prolactin-secreting adenoma
  - Interference of flow of dopamine down the pituitary stalk by a large pituitary or parapituitary tumor
- Chest wall stimulation
  - Chronic skin disease (for example, severe acne)
  - Tumors of chest wall
- Chronic renal failure
- Ectopic production
- Hypothalamic disease
- Idiopathic

lactin levels, as there is a normal 50–100% rise in prolactin just prior to waking. Furthermore, prolactin elevations are far from specific for epilepsy, and there may be some tendency for the elevation to attenuate in patients with frequent seizures.

Since prolactin secretion is under strong inhibitory control by the hypothalamus, anything that interferes with the free flow of blood down the pituitary portal veins can reduce the exposure of the pituitary to the dopamine released by the hypothalamus. This results in raised peripheral blood prolactin levels. In patients with this condition, prolactin levels will usually range from 50 to 150 ng per ml (normal <25 ng per ml). Such elevations can be seen, for example, in patients with granulomatous disease involving the pituitary stalk; however, the most common situation in which this occurs is in patients in whom the pituitary stalk is "kinked" by a pituitary adenoma. In such circumstances, this may lead to the erroneous assumption that the pituitary adenoma is prolactin-secreting, and long-term therapy with bromocriptine might be undertaken. I have seen such patients whose prolactin levels became normal but whose tumors continued to grow. The mistake with these patients is to assume that a macroadenoma would result in a moderately elevated prolactin level, when in reality microprolactinomas usually produce prolactin levels in excess of 200 ng per ml and macroadenomas would be expected to have much higher levels, often in excess of 1,000 ng per ml.

Patients treated with neuroleptic medications may also have elevated prolactin levels, and occasionally the elevation will be enough to cause galactorrhea or amenorrhea. In such patients, it may be uncertain whether symptoms are secondary to drug-induced hyperprolactinemia or a microadenoma. My practice is to do an MRI scan of the pituitary to look for a tumor and to perform dynamic pituitary testing with thyrotropin-releasing hormone (TRH). Drug-induced hyperprolactinemia will respond normally to stimulation with these agents. The treatment of drug-induced hyperprolactinemia is difficult. In many instances, their drug cannot be stopped, and often there is a concern about using drugs such as bromocriptine because of their potential to block the beneficial effects of the patient's neuroleptics and because of their ability to cause hallucinations or frank psychosis. Such patients may benefit from the use of atypical antipsychotics with reduced or absent action at dopamine receptors (at normal therapeutic doses).

Gigantism and Acromegaly. Excessive amounts of circulating GH prior to closure of the epiphyses leads to gigantism. If the epiphyses have closed, then only tissue still capable of responding to GH grows, leading to the clinical syndrome of acromegaly. The clinical features of acromegaly are summarized in Table 50.8. Of particular note to the neurologist and neurosurgeon is the frequent complaint of headache and symptoms related to the carpal tunnel syndrome. It is not uncommon to find patients with acromegaly who have had carpal tunnel releases performed 3–5 years before diagnosis of their disease.

Table 50.8: Common clinical signs and symptoms of acromegaly

Headache, felt at the vertex and behind the eyes
Impaired glucose tolerance/diabetes mellitus
Enlargement of hands and feet
Enlargement of the jaw, with increased spacing between the teeth and malocclusion
Hypertension
Menstrual irregularities or soft-tissue growth
Thick skin
Dough-like feel to palm (e.g., during handshake)
Carpal tunnel syndrome
Arthralgia and osteoarthritis
Proximal muscle weakness
Hyperhidrosis

The vast majority of cases of gigantism and acromegaly are due to excess GH production by a pituitary adenoma. However, rare cases of ectopic GH production have been described, and excessive GH-releasing hormone production by pancreatic tumors can cause acromegaly. Excess production of GH-releasing hormone by the hypothalamus could theoretically cause an identical clinical syndrome.

Cushing's Disease and Nelson's Syndrome. The term *Cushing's syndrome* refers to the clinical picture caused by exposure to excessive corticosteroids, either endogenous or exogenous. If this picture is caused by excessive production of ACTH from the pituitary, it is referred to as *Cushing's disease*. Its common clinical features are listed in Table 50.9. The syndrome of hyperpigmentation and local compression of parapituitary structures that occurs in about 10% of patients with Cushing's disease who have been treated with bilateral adrenalectomy is called *Nelson's syndrome*.

The dexamethasone suppression test is pivotal in the diagnosis of Cushing's disease. Normal patients, given 0.5 mg of dexamethasone every 6 hours for 8 doses, will, during the second 24 hours of administration, show a suppression of cortisol production, as reflected by reduced urinary levels of 17-ketogenic steroids or urinary free cortisol. Patients with Cushing's disease will usually show a similar suppression only when the dose of dexamethasone is raised to 2 mg every 6 hours for 8 doses. Also, in Cushing's disease, ACTH levels are in the normal range or moderately elevated. Failure to suppress on high-dose dexamethasone and unmeasurable ACTH levels are seen with primary adrenal problems such as adenoma or carcinoma. Ectopic ACTH production is usually nonsuppressible, and the ACTH levels are much higher than those seen in typical pituitary Cushing's disease. Unfortunately, there are many exceptions to these rules. First, the dexamethasone test itself can be perturbed by a variety of influences and give false results. Second, there are well-documented cases of ectopic ACTH production and primary adrenal problems that give dexamethasone suppression test results compatible with a diagnosis of pituitary ACTH production. Intermittent excess

Table 50.9: Common clinical features of Cushing's disease

Truncal obesity: Arms and legs tend to be thin; excess fat deposition in preauricular and supraclavicular fat pads
Hypertension
Impaired glucose tolerance/diabetes mellitus
Menstrual irregularities or amenorrhea
Excessive hair growth
Acne
Proximal myopathy
Abdominal striae (purplish)
Osteoporosis
Thin skin with excessive bruising

ACTH production can give rise to false normal results in patients who actually have Cushing's disease.

Even when all test results point to a pituitary source for the excessive ACTH production, care must still be taken in diagnosing someone with Cushing's disease. Patients may or may not have an abnormality on CT or MRI of the sella. Intermediate lobe cysts or clefts may mimic the appearance of adenoma on CT or MRI. In such cases, simultaneous sampling from the petrosal sinuses bilaterally and the inferior vena cava can help localize the excessive ACTH production (Oldfield et al. 1991).

The pituitary glands of some patients with biochemical Cushing's disease do not show adenoma formation but show evidence of hyperplasia of the cells that secrete ACTH. Although this picture can be caused by the ectopic production of corticotropin-releasing hormone (CRH), the hypothalamic peptide that stimulates the release of ACTH, or an excessive release of CRH from the hypothalamus, this happens in less than 0.3% of patients with Cushing's disease who have pituitary surgery.

Excessive Secretion of Thyroid-Stimulating Hormone. Elevated levels of thyroid-stimulating hormone (TSH) are seen most commonly with primary hypothyroidism. The resulting pituitary hypertrophy can infrequently be of sufficient magnitude to cause visual field defects. Hyperthyroidism caused by excessive TSH secretion is a rare (accounting for <1% of all pituitary tumors) but well-recognized entity, and these tumors are readily visible on CT scans.

Pituitary resistance to thyroid hormone may also produce a clinical picture of hyperthyroidism with high-normal or mildly elevated TSH levels. Unlike the case of TSH-secreting tumors, which are relatively autonomous, the TSH levels in patients with pituitary resistance usually respond well to stimulation with TRH or to suppression with dexamethasone or dopamine.

Gonadotropin-Secreting Tumors. It is now appreciated that many pituitary tumors, formerly classified as nonfunctioning, are actually gonadotropin- or gonadotropin subunit–producing tumors (Oppenheim and Klibanski 1989). The usual presentation is a macroadenoma in an elderly male; however, they have been reported in individuals of all ages and both sexes, with a male preponderance.

Many of these tumors secrete only FSH, and only rarely do they secrete LH alone. Some may secrete both LH and FSH and others secrete biologically inactive gonadotropin subunits: α-subunit, LH-β subunit, or FSH-β subunit. Most clinical radioimmunoassays used to measure LH and FSH require the α- and β-subunits to be associated before they register in the assay. This means that subunit secretion will not be detected. FSH levels are usually elevated in patients with FSH-secreting tumors and testosterone or estradiol levels are almost always low. In patients with LH-secreting tumors, LH levels are usually elevated and estradiol or testosterone levels may be high. Despite high sex-steroid levels, these patients are often clinically hypogonadal. Patients with tumors that secrete both LH and FSH usually have normal or high sex steroid levels, but again, they are clinically hypogonadal. Since subunits are biologically inactive, subunit-secreting tumors do not interfere directly with hormonal function, although through pressure effects on the pituitary, they can cause hypopituitarism.

Longstanding primary hypogonadism may cause pituitary enlargement secondary to gonadotroph hyperplasia. Rarely, this may lead to gonadotroph tumor development. Most of the time, the pituitary enlargement is asymptomatic and regresses in response to sex steroid replacement.

Pituitary Tumors and Pituitary Hyperplasia

Pituitary tumors account for approximately 15% of all intracranial tumors. Although the vast majority are benign, they can be locally invasive. Only rarely is true malignancy evidenced by metastases. The old classification of pituitary adenomas into chromophobe, acidophil, and basophil has been supplanted by a more functional classification based on immunological and electron microscopic examinations (Table 50.10).

Hyperplasia of various cellular elements of the pituitary has been described. It is relatively rare and is usually seen in cases of ectopic hypothalamic-releasing hormone production.

G-proteins are a family of proteins, composed of α-, β-, and γ-subunits, that bind to guanine nucleotides. Their role in pituitary tumor genesis has been reviewed by Spada et al. (1993). There are several classes of G proteins. Gs proteins are activators of adenylyl cyclase. Gi proteins are substrates for pertussis toxin and may inhibit adenylyl cylase. Gq proteins are mediators of phospholipase C activation. The functions of G12 and G13 proteins are, at the moment, unknown. The α-subunit of the Gs-protein contains the GTP binding site. After the Gs-protein binds to GTP, there is release of the βγ-dimer and the active α-GTP complex. The intrinsic GTPase activity of the α-subunit hydrolyses α-GTP to α-GDP to end the activity.

Table 50.10: Classification of pituitary adenomas

Tumor	*Percent*
Growth-hormone (GH) cell adenoma	14.0
Prolactin (PRL) cell adenoma	27.2
GH-PRL cell adenoma	8.4
Corticotroph cell adenoma	8.1
Thyrotroph cell adenoma	1.0
Gonadotroph cell adenoma	6.4
Clinically nonfunctioning adenoma	31.2
Plurihormonal adenoma	3.7

Source: Modified from S Yamada, T Sano. Neuropathology of the Pituitary. In DL Barrow, W Selman (eds), Neuroendocrinology. Concepts in Neurosurgery. Vol. 5. Baltimore: Williams & Wilkins, 1992;289–335.

A variety of mutations involving single amino acid substitutions in the portion of the Gs gene that codes the Gs α-subunit have been identified in about a third of GH-secreting tumors. These mutations inhibit the breakdown of the α-subunit and thereby mimic the effect of specific growth factors. It is thought that this αs gene is converted into an oncogene, called Gsp, that leads to pituitary tumor development.

The *ras* proteins, a family of at least three proto-oncogenes, are structurally similar to G-proteins. Like the G-proteins, *ras* proteins affect cell differentiation and proliferation (Robertson and Herington 1991). *Ras* mutations are found commonly in thyroid tumors but are uncommon in other endocrine neoplasms. A *ras* mutation has been found in a particularly invasive prolactinoma.

These observations seem to support the hypothesis that pituitary adenomas are of primary pituitary origin. Nevertheless, it is still possible that alterations in G-protein function could be triggered initially by abnormal hypothalamic or peripheral stimulation.

Other Tumors

Gliomas, meningiomas, dermoids, epidermoids, chordomas, and teratomas can all occur in the region of the sella turcica and may mimic the local compressive effects of primary pituitary tumors. The pituitary gland is the site of metastatic deposits in 4% of cancer patients. Usually these metastases are asymptomatic; when symptoms do occur, however, they are most often related to disturbance of posterior pituitary function.

Craniopharyngiomas are only one-third as common as pituitary tumors. They are thought to arise from residual rests of Rathke's pouch tissue. Most commonly found in a suprasellar location, they are also described occurring anywhere along the pituitary-hypothalamic axis, including within the sella. Craniopharyngiomas can appear at any age; however, about one-third of the cases arise before age 15. Because these tumors produce no hormones, patients present with signs of local compression, especially of the visual system, or with hypothalamic dysfunction such as growth failure or diabetes insipidus. In children, almost half will show evidence of growth failure. Three-fourths of these patients—adults and children—will have visual symptoms. Calcification in the sellar or suprasellar region can be seen on plain skull x-ray in about 75% of craniopharyngiomas.

Hypophysitis

Hypophysitis from infection or granulomatous disease such as sarcoidosis can result in hypopituitarism. Lymphocytic hypophysitis, a sterile inflammation of the pituitary of probable autoimmune origin, is seen almost exclusively in women, particularly in pregnancy. Usually it causes hypopituitarism, although it can cause hyperprolactinemia and is thought to be a cause of the empty sella syndrome.

THE POSTERIOR PITUITARY

Physiology

Vasopressin

Vasopressin or antidiuretic hormone (ADH), an essential hormone in fluid and electrolyte homeostasis, is synthesized in the magnocellular neurons of the supraoptic and paraventricular (PV) nuclei as a large precursor molecule, which is cleaved enzymatically to yield vasopressin and neurophysin. The function of this latter peptide is unknown.

Four vasopressin-containing pathways have been observed in the brain: (1) hypothalamo-neurohypophysial, (2) paraventricular nucleus to the zona incerta of the median eminence, (3) paraventricular nucleus to the limbic system (amygdala), and (4) paraventricular nucleus to the brain stem and spinal cord. The best characterized of these is the hypophysial-portal pathway. Virtually all of the neurons from the supraoptic nuclei take part in this pathway, whereas only a portion of PV nuclei terminate in the posterior pituitary. Some of the vasopressin-containing fibers from the paraventricular nuclei appear to be more involved in ACTH regulation than in fluid balance. Vasopressin-containing fibers also project widely outside the hypothalamus, where there is evidence to suggest they may participate in memory (Doraiswamy et al. 1992).

Oxytocin

Oxytocin (OT), like vasopressin, is synthesized in magnocellular neurons of the supraoptic and PV nuclei as a large precursor molecule, which is cleaved into OT and a specific neurophysin. Many of the physiological stimuli of vasopressin also result in OT release, and although in supraphysiological doses OT does have ADH-like properties, its physiological role in these circumstances remains obscure.

The only specific stimulus that causes the release of OT but not vasopressin is suckling. Oxytocin's role in normal lactation and parturition in the human remains to be defined clearly.

Thirst and Drinking

Certain cells of the anterior hypothalamus are sensitive to changes in the osmolality of the blood bathing them and respond by signaling the cells of the supraoptic and PV nuclei to alter their secretion of vasopressin. These cells are most sensitive to osmotic substances that do not freely diffuse into cells, such as sodium, sucrose, and mannitol. Substances such as urea produce less osmotic stimulation because they diffuse freely. Glucose, in addition to diffusing freely, actually inhibits ADH release. These cells respond not only to increased osmolality and hence dehydration but also to hypotension with marked increases in ADH secretion.

Water homeostasis cannot be maintained by antidiuresis alone. It also requires thirst and the drinking behavior induced by it. A drinking center is thought to be located near the feeding center in the lateral hypothalamus. Angiotensin may play an important role in stimulating drinking in humans and animals.

Sodium Homeostasis and Atrial Natriuretic Peptide

Sodium homeostasis is extremely important for normal functioning of the organism. Most of the regulation of body sodium takes place in the kidney. Sodium reabsorption is under the control of the renin-angiotensin-aldosterone system. Under normal physiological circumstances, aldosterone, the principal mineralocorticoid produced by the adrenal gland, is affected in only a minor way by ACTH.

The human heart has been shown to synthesize and secrete atrial natriuretic peptide (ANP), which has diuretic, natriuretic (increased urinary sodium excretion), and vasorelaxant properties. In addition to ANP, the brain contains brain natriuretic peptide and C-type natriuretic peptide. Because of the pattern of their distribution in the brain, these substances are thought to have important roles in the central control of the cardiovascular system. The natriuretic peptides seem to act as natural antagonists to the central actions of angiotensin II.

Diabetes Insipidus

Diabetes insipidus (DI) is a clinical syndrome characterized by severe thirst, polydipsia, and polyuria. Central DI must be distinguished from nephrogenic DI (an inability of the kidney to respond to ADH) and from compulsive water drinking. This is normally done using a water deprivation test. A urine osmolality of greater than 750 mmol per liter following water deprivation excludes the diagnosis of DI. Central DI is characterized by a rise in osmolality to greater than 750 mmol per liter following desamino-D-arginine-vasopressin (DDAVP). In nephrogenic DI, there is little change in osmolality after DDAVP. The polyuria induced by chronic compulsive water drinking may produce a renal tubular concentrating defect because of medullary washout—that is, the loss of sodium and other solutes from around the loops of Henle. This can make it difficult to differentiate partial DI of central or renal cause from polydipsia. Treatment with DDAVP and gradual fluid restriction can be used to reverse the medullary washout and hence increase the sensitivity of the test.

It is essential that the water deprivation test be strictly supervised by a physician familiar with the technique. Severe and potentially fatal dehydration can occur quite rapidly in patients with complete DI. Similarly, patients with compulsive water drinking given DDAVP can drink themselves into hyponatremic coma.

Etiology

About one-third of patients with central DI have no demonstrable disease of the hypothalamic-posterior pituitary unit. The remaining patients have damage to the supraoptic-hypophysial-portal pathway from trauma, surgery, tumors, inflammatory lesions (which may be granulomatous or infectious), or vascular lesions. In patients with polyuria, it is imperative to check the urine to ensure there is not a solute diuresis, as seen with hyperglycemia, or that a type of nephrogenic DI has not been induced by hypokalemia, hypercalcemia, or lithium carbonate therapy.

Management

Patients with DI excrete mainly water, and therefore water alone is the mainstay of their management. Patients who are alert and have intact thirst mechanisms should be given free access to water. Only if urine output exceeds 7 liters per day is treatment necessary. In most circumstances, DDAVP given as a nasal solution is the treatment of choice. To avoid water intoxication, it is preferable to underreplace these patients and allow them to modulate their water balance by drinking.

The unconscious patient can present a problem in management. It should be remembered when calculating such a patient's fluid needs that the urine in DI is electrolyte-poor. Thus, the electrolyte requirements of such a patient are little different from those of other patients. The bulk of the urinary replacement should be given as 5% dextrose in water. The administration of 5% dextrose in 0.2 NaCl or solutions with even higher salt concentration will present a high solute load to the kidney and tend to exacerbate the polyuria.

Syndrome of Inappropriate Antidiuretic Hormone Secretion

Etiology and Pathophysiology

The syndrome of inappropriate ADH secretion (SIADH) is characterized by (1) low serum sodium, (2) high urine sodium, and (3) urine relatively or absolutely hyperosmolar to serum. Before making the diagnosis, the physician must exclude all of the following: (1) dehydration, (2) edema-forming states such as congestive cardiac failure, (3) primary renal disease, and (4) adrenal or thyroid insufficiency.

The initial clue to the diagnosis of SIADH is the low serum sodium. Measured serum osmolality must also be low to exclude the artifactual hyponatremia that occurs with hyperlipidemia and hyperproteinemia, in which the sodium concentration in the plasma water is actually normal. The urine osmolality in SIADH is not always above the serum osmolality, but the urine is less than maximally dilute, which excludes the dilutional hyponatremia of water intoxication. Causes of SIADH are listed in Table 50.11.

Table 50.11: Causes of the syndrome of inappropriate antidiuretic hormone secretion

Disorders of the nervous system
Tumor
Trauma
Surgery
Metabolic encephalopathy
Infections (meningitis, encephalitis)
Vascular (e.g., stroke)
Subdural hematoma
Hydrocephalus
Guillain-Barré syndrome
Acute intermittent porphyria
Drugs
Carbamazepine
Chlorpromazine
Chlorpropramide
Cisplatinum
Clofibrate
Cyclophosphamide
Oxytocin
Thiazide diuretics
Vasopressin
Vinblastine
Vincristine
Tricyclic antidepressants
Disorders of the chest
Pneumonia
Tuberculosis
Cystic fibrosis
Pneumothorax
Empyema
Asthma
Endocrine causes
Hypoadrenalism
Hypothyroidism
Ectopic production of ADH
Carcinoma: Lung, gastrointestinal tract, and genitourinary tract (especially kidney)
Mesothelioma
Lymphoma and leukemia
Thymoma
Sarcoma
Idiopathic

Clinical Features

The clinical features of SIADH are nonspecific and are related to the hypo-osmolality of the body fluids. The more rapidly this develops, the more symptomatic is the patient. Serum sodium below 115 mmol per liter is almost always associated with confusion or obtundation, and seizures can occur. With milder hyponatremia, the symptoms may be very nonspecific, including fatigue, general malaise, loss of appetite, and some clouding of consciousness.

Treatment

The mainstay of the treatment of SIADH is *restriction of fluid.* Intake should be reduced to insensible losses (approximately 800 ml per day). Overly aggressive correction of hyponatremia with hypertonic saline solution is frequently associated with the development of central pontine myelinolysis. Obtundation by itself does not necessitate more aggressive treatment of hyponatremia. However, in patients with severe hyponatremia complicated by seizures, a more rapid partial correction can be undertaken. Diuresis is induced with furosemide (1 mg/kg IV), and urinary losses are replaced with 3% sodium chloride at a rate of 0.1 ml per kg per minute, to which appropriate amounts of potassium are added (to counter urinary losses). Raising the serum sodium to 120 mmol per liter (but not above) at a rate no faster than 1–2 mmol per hour appears to prevent the development of central pontine myelinolysis in most cases. Normalization is then achieved by fluid restriction (Kovacs and Robertson 1992).

Prolonged fluid restriction is often poorly tolerated by patients, who may quickly become noncompliant. In cases where the underlying cause of the SIADH cannot be eliminated or corrected, the drug demeclocycline, a tetracycline, can be given in a dose of 300–600 mg twice a day to induce a nephrogenic DI and to alleviate the necessity for fluid restriction.

Cerebral Salt Wasting

It has been recognized that some patients with hyponatremia do not have SIADH secretion with resultant retention of renal-free water. Instead they have an inappropriate natriuresis. Hyponatremia, accompanied by renal sodium loss and volume depletion, has been reported in patients with primary cerebral tumors, carcinomatous meningitis, subarachnoid hemorrhage, and head trauma and following intracranial surgery and pituitary surgery. Unlike SIADH patients, these patients respond to vigorous sodium and water replacement, and their condition is actually worsened by fluid restriction. It has been proposed that this inappropriate natriuresis that accompanies intracranial disease (so-called cerebral salt wasting) is caused either by a natriuretic hormone such as ANP or by an alteration of the neural input to the kidney.

It is critical to distinguish between these patients and those with SIADH, since the treatment for SIADH worsens the hyponatremia of cerebral salt wasting. Differentiation is best done by a careful assessment of volume status, using the clinical and laboratory examination to detect signs of volume depletion. If there is uncertainty about the diagnosis, the patient should be fluid-restricted. Then, if the natriuresis persists in the face of volume restriction, the syndrome of cerebral salt wasting should be suspected and appropriate therapy instituted.

APPROACH TO THE PATIENT WITH HYPOTHALAMIC-PITUITARY DYSFUNCTION

History and Physical Examination

Patients with suspected hypothalamic or pituitary disorders should be specifically questioned about dysfunction of the nonendocrine aspects of the hypothalamus, including appetite, body temperature, sleep-wake cycles, emotion, libido, and autonomic nervous system function. These are overlooked all too frequently, and such symptoms may point to a hypothalamic rather than a pituitary location. A careful functional inquiry should also cover clinical aspects of the hyper- and hypofunction of each of the anterior and posterior pituitary hormones.

Because of the proximity of the optic nerves to the hypothalamic-pituitary unit, a careful examination of the visual fields is essential (see Chapter 14).

Assessment by Imaging Studies

In centers where it is available, MRI has replaced CT scanning as the investigation of choice in the diagnosis of pituitary and parapituitary lesions. Hoffman and Barrow (1992), in their review of the subject, indicate that the use of MRI with gadopentate dimeglumine contrast is associated with a detection rate of 70% and that three-dimensional T1-weighed techniques increase the detection rate to 90%. When using two-dimensional techniques, it is important to obtain thin (1–2 mm) coronal slices of the sella to achieve the best results.

Cerebral angiography is rarely required, because large cerebral aneurysms mimicking pituitary adenomas are readily picked up by MRI. Angiography is reserved primarily to demonstrate the blood supply of suspected meningiomas.

Endocrinological Investigation

Not every patient with hypothalamic-pituitary disease requires a full battery of pituitary tests. In general, one attempts to determine the extent of pituitary functional damage, if any, and—in patients where blood levels of hormones are elevated, or if there is a clinical suspicion of excessive hormonal secretion—to determine if the hormone(s) in question respond normally to physiological suppressors and stimulators.

No single endocrine test can provide all the answers about pituitary function. Conclusions are based on a synthesis of evidence gained from clinical examination, endocrine tests, and MRI. Endocrine testing is used to determine the residual pituitary function following surgery or radiotherapy. The return of biochemical markers of abnormal pituitary secretion or their failure to resolve is used to gauge the success of surgery and to aid in differentiating surgical artifact from tumor recurrence on postoperative MRI scans.

Table 50.12 summarizes pituitary tests and their use.

Treatment of Pituitary Tumors

Medical

Prolactinoma. Hyperprolactinemia of whatever cause can usually be suppressed by the dopamine agonist bromocriptine. It is crucial to realize, therefore, that such suppression is not diagnostic of a prolactinoma. Bromocriptine (2.5–7.5 mg/day in divided doses) will usually normalize serum prolactin. Maximum shrinkage of tumors occurs within 6 months and often within 6–8 weeks. Experience indicates that bromocriptine is safe to use to restore fertility. Once pregnancy occurs, the bromocriptine can be stopped with little risk of expansion of the prolactinoma during the next 9 months. Bromocriptine appears to cause growth of fibrous tissue in prolactinomas. In a few patients, this may allow bromocriptine to be withdrawn without prolactin levels rebounding. This fibrous tissue may make such tumors more difficult to remove surgically and result in lower rates of surgical success.

Cushing's Disease. The results of long-term medical therapy of Cushing's disease have been disappointing. Cyproheptadine will temporarily lower ACTH levels in some patients. However, it is rarely effective for long and is commonly associated with somnolence and increased appetite. Drugs such as metyrapone and ketoconazole, which block steroid synthesis, can be used to lower cortisol levels and improve patients' clinical status prior to surgery, but they are not acceptable for permanent medical management.

Acromegaly. Until the development of a long-acting somatostatin analogue (octreotide), the outcome of medical therapy for acromegaly, like that for Cushing's disease, was disappointing. Bromocriptine, in doses of 20–60 mg per day, could reduce GH levels and cause tumor shrinkage, but it seldom normalized them. Octreotide can normalize GH levels when given by subcutaneous injection every 8 hours.

Table 50.12: Common tests of pituitary function

Test	*Comments*
Insulin hypoglycemia (regular insulin 0.1 U/kg body weight IV, fasting)	Adequate hypoglycemia is associated with a rise in growth hormone, ACTH (cortisol), and prolactin. It is probably the most physiological stressor of the hypothalamic-pituitary-adrenal axis. The test should not be used in patients with epilepsy or unstable angina.
Gonadotropin-releasing hormone (GnRH) (2 μg/kg IV to a maximum of 100 μg)	Stimulates LH and FSH release directly at the pituitary. May be used to test LH and FSH reserve. Cannot reliably distinguish between pituitary and long-standing hypothalamic problem.
Thyrotropin-releasing hormone (TRH) (7 μg/kg IV to a maximum of 400 μg)	Stimulates TSH and prolactin directly at the pituitary. Failure of prolactin to respond to TRH is very suggestive of autonomous secretion by an adenoma, but exceptions do occur.
Metyrapone test (750 mg q4h for 6 doses; collect 24-hour urines the day before, day of, and day after the test)	Metyrapone blocks the production of cortisol in the adrenal gland. This results in increased ACTH secretion. It is an alternative to insulin hypoglycemia as a test of the hypothalamic-pituitary-adrenal axis.
L-Dopa (500 mg PO)	L-Dopa can be used to stimulate growth hormone release (probably by increasing growth hormone-releasing hormone). It is a less potent stimulus than insulin-induced hypoglycemia but can be used as an alternative.

This route of administration is the main drawback to its clinical use, but eventually it may be possible to give it as an intranasal preparation similar to DDAVP. The analog can be combined with bromocriptine if necessary.

Thyroid Stimulating Hormone–Secreting and Gonadotropin-Secreting Tumors. Most patients with these types of tumors are treated surgically, sometimes followed by radiotherapy. TSH-secreting tumors seem to respond to octreotide with a decrease in hormone production; however, there is little if any tumor shrinkage. Early reports suggest that octreotide can reduce levels of α-subunit secretion in gonadotropin-secreting tumors, as can bromocriptine. While some tumor shrinkage has been reported with the use of bromocriptine, it is unclear whether long-term octreotide use will have the same effect.

Surgical

In a medically fit patient, surgery is the treatment of choice for all nonsecretory pituitary and parapituitary lesions. For secretory tumors, surgery offers the possibility of rapid and complete cure. It is the preferred treatment when serious compression of parapituitary structures occurs. Surgical cure rates have been reported to be over 80% in cases of microadenoma, although these rates may well be lower when strict endocrine criteria for cure are applied and when patients are followed for 15 years. In the hands of an experienced neurosurgeon, pituitary surgery has extremely low morbidity and mortality rates.

Radiotherapy

Conventional radiotherapy is used primarily as an adjunct to surgery and medical therapy. It is used most commonly in the treatment of acromegaly, although octreotide may reduce its use. It is also used frequently in surgical failures in cases of Cushing's disease. It is rarely used in treating microprolactinoma in North America, although it is used in larger tumors. Recurrence of nonsecreting adenomas after partial removal is effectively prevented by radiotherapy. The major problems with conventional radiotherapy are the long delay in the onset of its effect (often 18 months), its tendency to incomplete efficacy in secretory tumors, and the high incidence of eventual development of panhypopituitarism.

Proton beam therapy permits a dose of radiation to be given at the pituitary gland that is 20–25 times greater than can be given by conventional radiotherapy techniques. At the same time, radiation doses to other brain areas are limited. Unfortunately, because this technique requires the use of a cyclotron to produce protons, it is available in only a few centers in North America. The reported results compare favorably to those of transsphenoidal surgery. Similar results can probably be obtained using the gamma knife, although results of long-term follow-up are not yet available. Because of the sensitivity of the optic nerves and chiasm to high doses of radiation, visual field defects and suprasellar extension of tumor are relative contraindications to the use of these techniques.

Treatment of Hypopituitarism

Vasopressin, ACTH, and TSH are the pituitary hormones critical to an individual's health and well-being. The management of vasopressin deficiency has been discussed already. ACTH deficiency is managed by glucocorticoid replacement; mineralocorticoid supplementation is seldom necessary. Most patients require 5 mg of prednisone (or similar doses of hydrocortisone) each morning, and some require an additional 2.5 mg in the evening. Under circumstances of mild illness the dose of prednisone should be doubled. Corticosteroid replacement in the glucocorticoid-deficient patient with serious illness or undergoing surgery consists of hydrocortisone sodium succinate, 10 mg per hour intravenously, around the clock. As the patient recovers, the dose is slowly tapered to maintenance levels.

TSH deficiency is managed by L-thyroxine replacement. Suppression of elevated TSH cannot be relied on to determine the adequacy of replacement in patients with pituitary-hypothalamic disease. Resolution of the clinical signs and symptoms of hypothyroidism is the important goal. In patients adequately replaced (that is, with T3 levels in the upper half of the therapeutic range), T4 levels will often be at or above the upper limit of normal.

Gonadotropin deficiency is usually managed by administration of testosterone or estrogen. This, however, does not restore fertility; in patients for whom fertility is sought, a reproductive endocrinologist should be consulted. The administration of various substitution therapies for LH and FSH may allow induction of fertility in some instances.

GH deficiency in children is treated by the administration of synthetic GH. GH-deficient adults currently do not receive GH replacement. There is gathering evidence that muscle strength, wound healing, and lean body mass are all improved by treating these individuals with synthetic GH. Unfortunately, these studies have been short-term, and the dose of GH required for long-term replacement is unknown. Because of the potentially deleterious effects of excessive levels of GH, studies are underway to determine appropriate replacement doses. There is no therapy available for prolactin deficiency.

NEUROSECRETION SYNDROMES

APUDomas

The term *APUD* is applied to cells that are capable of *a*mine *p*recursor *u*ptake and *d*ecarboxylation. These cells are distributed throughout the body and are capable of synthesizing biogenic amines or polypeptide hormones. APUD cells are found in the pituitary gland, the adrenal gland, peripheral autonomic ganglia, the lung, the gastrointestinal tract, the pancreas, gonads, and the thymus. Tumors arising from APUD cells have been referred to as APUDomas. As a class of tumors they generally produce symptoms through the secretion of biogenic amines (norepinephrine, epinephrine, dopamine, serotonin) or hormones. Of the APUDomas, insulinomas, gastrinomas, VIPomas, medullary carcinomas of the thyroid, pheochromocytomas, and carcinoid tumors can all present as clinical emergencies. Of these, only pheochromocytomas and carcinoid tumors are discussed here.

Pheochromocytoma

Pheochromocytomas are rare tumors that arise most commonly (85–90% of the time) from the catecholamine-producing cells of the adrenal medulla; they can also arise from extra-adrenal chromaffin tissue in the cervical and thoracic regions and in the abdomen. The majority of these tumors occur spontaneously; however, they can be part of other syndromes such as multiple endocrine neoplasia type II and IIb, Von Hippel-Lindau disease, neurofibromatosis, ataxia telangiectasia, tuberous sclerosis, and Sturge-Weber syndrome.

Pheochromocytomas predominantly secrete norepinephrine, epinephrine, and some dopamine. These compounds are responsible for the most common symptoms of pheochromocytoma: throbbing headache, sweating, palpitations, pallor, nausea, vomiting, and tremor. Pheochromocytomas are also capable of secreting a large number of neuropeptides that can be responsible for other clinical symptoms (Fonseca and Bouloux 1993).

Pheochromocytoma should be suspected in patients with progressive or malignant hypertension, hypertension of early onset without family history, hypertension resistant to conventional therapy, paradoxical worsening of hypertension in response to treatment with beta blockers, and patients with a history of pressor response provoked by anesthesia, labor or delivery, or angiography.

It is my personal practice to screen for pheochromocytoma by collecting two 24-hour urine specimens and having them analyzed for vanillylmandelic acid, norepinephrine, epinephrine, and metanephrines. The completeness of the 24-hour collection should be confirmed by an analysis of urinary creatinine.

Tumor localization can usually be achieved by CT scanning of the adrenals. If a wider search is necessary, MRI scanning may be more helpful. ^{123}I-MIBG, an iodinated guanethidine derivative, is taken up by chromaffin tissue and can be helpful in the localization of nonadrenal tumors and metastases.

Patients with pheochromocytoma should be managed in centers with previous experience of the treatment of this type of tumor. Suitable preoperative preparation is necessary to prevent hypertensive or hypotensive crisis during surgery (Ober 1993). For benign tumors, complete surgical removal is the treatment of choice. Malignant tumors may be palliated with a variety of treatments (see Fonseca and Bouloux 1993).

Carcinoid Tumors

Carcinoid tumors arise from enterochromaffin cells in the gastrointestinal tract, pancreas, or lungs and only rarely from the thymus or gonads. When carcinoid tumors release biogenic amines directly into the systemic circulation, bypassing the liver, the carcinoid syndrome results. This is characterized by episodes of flushing, often with accompanying diarrhea or asthma. Later in the syndrome there is fibrosis of the endomyocardium. Carcinoid tumors may be a source of ectopic ACTH, CRH, or GHRH secretion.

The diagnosis is made by finding elevated urinary 5-hydroxyindolacetic acid (5-HIAA) levels. As in pheochromocytoma, carcinoids also secrete peptides (e.g., kallikrein, substance P, and neurotensin) and other amines (e.g., histamine, dopamine) and some of these substances may be responsible for the flushing that occurs in the syndrome.

Surgery is the treatment of choice; however, by the time the tumors become symptomatic they are often incurable because of the metastases. Serotonin antagonists may be used to treat some of the symptoms, and octreotide has been used successfully to manage carcinoid crisis (Philippe 1992).

REFERENCES

Aggleton JP. The contribution of the amygdala to normal and abnormal emotional states. TINS 1993;16:328–33.

Bierich JR (ed). Growth disorders. Clin Endocrinol Metab 1992; 6:491–716.

Bray GA, Fisler J, York DA. Neuroendocrine control of the development of obesity: understanding gained from studies of experimental animal models. Front Neuroendocrinol 1990;11: 128–181.

Casper RC, Schoeller DA, Kushner R et al. Total daily energy expenditure and activity level in anorexia nervosa. Am J Clin Nutr 1991;53:1143–1150.

Cooper KE. The neurobiology of fever: thoughts on recent developments. Ann Rev Neurosci 1987;10:297–324.

Cooper PE, Martin JB. Neuroendocrine Disease. In RN Rosenberg (ed), The Clinical Neurosciences. New York: Churchill Livingstone, 1983.

Doraiswamy PM, Krishnan KR, Nemeroff CB. Hormonal Effects on Brain Function. In DL Barrow, W Selman (eds), Neuroendocrinology. Concepts in Neurosurgery. Vol. 5. Baltimore: Williams & Wilkins, 1992;75–91.

Fisher RS et al. Capillary prolactin measurement for diagnosis of seizures. Ann Neurol 1991;29:187–190.

Fonseca V, Bouloux PM. Phaeochromocytoma and paraganglioma. Clin Endocrinol Metab 1993;7:509–544.

Hoffman J, Barrow DL. Radiological Evaluation of Pituitary Lesions. In DL Barrow, W Selman (eds), Neuroendocrinology. Concepts in Neurosurgery. Vol. 5. Baltimore: Williams & Wilkins, 1992;237–257.

Kovacs L, Robertson GL. Syndrome of inappropriate antidiuresis. Endocrinol Metab Clin North Am 1992;21:859–875.

Martin JB, Cooper PE. Neuroendocrine Disease. In RN Rosenberg (ed), The Clinical Neuro-Sciences. New York: Churchill Livingstone, 1983.

Martin JB, Reichlin S, Brown GM. Clinical Neuroendocrinology. Philadelphia: FA Davis, 1977.

Miller BL, Cummings JL, McIntyre M et al. Hypersexuality or altered sexual preference following brain injury. J Neurol Neurosurg Psychiatry 1986;49:867–873.

Ober KP (ed). Endocrine crises. Endocrinol Metab Clin North Am 1993;22:181–453.

Oldfield EH, Doppman JL, Nieman LK et al. Petrosal sinus sampling with and without corticotropin-releasing hormone for the differential diagnosis of Cushing's syndrome. N Engl J Med 1991;325:897–905.

Oppenheim DS, Klibanski A. Medical therapy of glycoprotein hormone-secreting pituitary tumors. Endocrinol Metab Clin North Am 1989;18:339–358.

Philippe J. APUDomas: acute complications and their medical management. Clin Endocrinol Metab 1992;6:217–228.

Reichlin S. Neuroendocrine-immune interactions. N Engl J Med 1993;329:1246–1253.

Robertson DM, Herington AC (eds). Growth factors in endocrinology. Clin Endocrinol Metab 1991;5:531–851.

Rolih CA, Ober KP. Pituitary apoplexy. Endocrinol Metab Clin North Am 1993;2:291–302.

Rosenberg MR, Green M. Neuroleptic malignant syndrome—review of response to therapy. Arch Intern Med 1989;149: 1927–1931.

Simon HB. Hyperthermia. N Engl J Med 1993;329:483–487.

Spada A, Vallar L, Faglia G. G-proteins and hormonal signalling in human pituitary tumors: genetic mutations and functional alterations. Front Neuroendocrinol 1993;14:21–32.

Styne DM (ed). Puberty and its disorders. Endocrinol Metab Clin North Am 1991;20:1–250.

Swaab DF, Hofman MA, Lucassen PJ et al. Functional neuroanatomy and neuropathology of the human hypothalamus. Anat Embryol 1993;187:317–330.

Yamada S, Sano T. Neuropathology of the Pituitary. In DL Barrow, W Selman (eds). Neuroendocrinology. Concepts in Neurosurgery. Vol. 5. Baltimore: Williams & Wilkins, 1992;289–335.

Chapter 51
General Principles in the Management of Neurological Disease

Walter G. Bradley, Robert B. Daroff, Gerald M. Fenichel, and C. David Marsden

In the earlier chapters of this book, we discussed the methods used to diagnose neurological disease. Once a diagnosis is made, the focus turns to management and prognosis, from the patient's perspective. In this chapter, we present general principles of management of patients with neurological conditions, and prognostic considerations are considered. Special areas of neurological management, such as neuropharmacology, pain management, neurosurgery, and neurological rehabilitation, are discussed in Chapters 52–55, and specific treatments for neurological diseases are covered in the chapters of Part III.

THE TREATABILITY OF NEUROLOGICAL DISEASE

Not all diseases are curable, but every patient can be helped. Table 51.1 is a summary of the hierarchy of help that can be given to a patient. The compassionate neurologist reviews this mental checklist for every patient and is sensitive to patients with incurable disease. Inevitably, more time is spent with a patient who has an incurable disease than with a patient for whom an effective treatment is available. The neurologist shares grief and provides consolation; both are essential aspects of patient management (Bradley 1987). Fortunately, the ranks of neurological diseases that are curable or can be halted to allow some natural recovery are constantly expanding. Recent advances in molecular genetics offer the hope of genetic treatment within the next decade for some of the most dreaded and incurable diseases managed by neurologists.

GENERAL PRINCIPLES OF NEUROLOGICAL MANAGEMENT

Goals of Symptomatic Treatment

It is important to separate neurological impairment, disability, and handicap. *Neurological impairment* (abnormal signs) allows a diagnosis to be made. It may cause *disability* or dysfunction, which produces a *handicap*. The patient wishes to be relieved of this handicap. For instance, a stroke may cause a hemiplegia, which is the impairment. The hemiplegia may cause difficulty in walking, which is the disability. The difficulty in walking may make it impossible for the patient to leave the house, which is the handicap.

Symptomatic treatment can be very beneficial. Neurologists and families are often gratified by the improved functional state of a stroke patient after neurological rehabilitation, when compared to untreated patients. There is much more to the discipline of neurology than achieving a diagnosis. Amyotrophic lateral sclerosis (ALS) makes this point clearly. Faced with this grim diagnosis, patients often hear doctors saying: "You have ALS, and you are likely to die in 3 years. There is nothing I can do for you, and there is no point in coming to see me again. Go home and put your affairs in order." This attitude is not only uncaring but indicates the physician's failure to recognize that patients can be given and deserve help throughout the course of even the most disastrous disease. Most neurological diseases, even incurable ones, are helped by symptomatic therapy.

There are increasing numbers of lay organizations, support groups, and advocacy groups that provide information and access to services that help patients reduce handicaps and the psychological effects of a disease.

Arresting an Attack

Many neurological diseases are episodic, and attacks vary from discomforting to fatal. Ergotamine or sumatriptan, together with analgesics, will generally arrest an incapacitating migraine attack. Potentially fatal status epilepticus can usually be arrested by intravenous diazepam, barbiturates, or phenytoin. Multiple sclerosis attacks can be disabling, but treatment with corticosteroids speeds recovery, and beta-interferon can reduce the attack frequency.

Table 51.1: The range of help available to patients with neurological disease

Curative treatment
Cure of the disease
Arrest of the disease
Symptomatic treatment
Arresting an attack
Slowing the rate of progression
Relief of symptoms
Circumvention of effects of the disease
Palliative care
Treatment of secondary effects
Psychological
Social
Family
Definition of the prognosis
Genetic counseling

Slowing Disease Progression

A malignant cerebral glioma is often treated by debulking followed by radiotherapy; these treatments, though rarely curative, do slow tumor growth rate and lengthen survival (see Chapter 59). Control of blood glucose concentrations usually improves diabetic peripheral neuropathy, or at least slows its progression.

Relieving Symptoms

Relief of pain is the oldest and most appreciated function of any physician. Other noncurative symptomatic treatment is available for many neurological diseases. The frequency of seizures is reduced by anticonvulsant drugs, and the frequency of migraine attacks by beta-receptor- or calcium channel–blocking drugs, but none of these agents cures the underlying tendency for recurrent attacks. Baclofen ameliorates spasticity, particularly in spinal cord disease, without affecting the disorder causing it. High-dose corticosteroid therapy reduces the edema surrounding a brain tumor, temporarily relieving headache and neurological deficits, without affecting tumor growth. Parkinson's disease typifies a neurological disorder in which treatment partly or completely relieves symptoms without affecting the progression of the disease. The response to levodopa diminishes and ends with the progressive death of substantia nigra neurons (see Chapter 76).

The placebo effect and the patient-physician relationship are both important in relieving symptoms. The placebo response is well documented. Several therapeutic trials have shown that an inert pill, given as an apparently active therapy, is more effective than no treatment at all. The placebo effect and the beneficial influence of the therapeutic relationship may both be explained by release of endorphins; another explanation is that patients report a positive response to please the physician and thereby encourage the relationship. Reinforcing the patient's belief in the efficacy of a recommended treatment is part of the art of medicine; the physician should take advantage of this response, whatever its mechanism.

Circumventing Physical Disability

Some neurological diseases, such as ALS, are continuously progressive and their progress cannot be arrested. In other diseases, such as stroke, spinal cord injury, or multiple sclerosis, the damage often occurs before the neurologist first sees the patient, and while some recovery is expected, substantial functional deficits often persist.

Neurological rehabilitation tries to restore function, as far as possible (see Chapter 55), through physical and occupational therapy, which help the patient to strengthen weak muscles, to condition others to take over functions that deficient muscles can no longer perform, to increase mobility, to reduce spasticity, and to retrain the nervous system to compensate for lost skills and reflexes. Cognitive or behavioral therapy helps to re-educate higher cortical functions to compensate for the effects of brain injury and stroke. Orthopedic procedures are often beneficial. Transferring the tibialis posterior tendon to the dorsum of the foot can replace the lost activity of the paralyzed tibialis anterior muscle and improve the dynamics of the plantar arch in patients with pes cavus and foot-drop resulting from chronic peripheral neuropathies. Triple arthrodesis of the foot also may improve function in such diseases. Surgical release of contractures of the hip, knee, and ankle in boys with Duchenne's muscular dystrophy may increase standing and walking for 2 years or longer.

Rehabilitation encompasses aids and appliances such as ankle-foot orthoses to prevent foot-drop, as well as canes, walkers, and wheelchairs to increase mobility. The full range of aids is limited only by the ingenuity of clinicians, biomechanical engineers, and systems analysts, by the tolerance of patients, and by the speed of technological advances. Cochlear implants are already in clinical use. Computer-driven motorized body and lower-limb braces now permit completely paralyzed patients to walk, and prostheses that stimulate the occipital cortex with the aid of a television camera are being developed to provide blind persons with rudimentary vision. More mundane, but often more useful to the patient, are changes to the home and work environment, such as rearranging the home to permit living on one floor and providing a ramp or stair lift, a bath seat, and a transfer board. Some patients may need rails for the bath and toilet or replacement of the bath with a shower and shower chair and widening of doors to allow wheelchair access.

ALS also illustrates the range of options available to help a patient with a severe, chronic neurological disease. In the early stages, the patient may simply need enlarged handles on tools and utensils to compensate for a weak hand grip, and a cane to help with walking. Later, the patient may need a wheelchair and home adaptation. Speech therapy and a communication board or printing typewriter can help when speech is difficult. Weight loss and choking from dysphagia may necessitate a feeding gastrostomy. Treatment of respiratory failure is particularly important. An incentive spirometer can improve respiration. Respiratory support, if the patient chooses it, is discussed in the next section. If the patient decides against life support measures, care is still needed in the terminal phase of the illness. Management in these patients taxes the neurologist's skills and compassion, but the help provided belies the notion that these are untreatable diseases.

Table 51.2: Types of neurological disease associated with respiratory failure

Acute neurological disease
Brain stem injury
High cervical cord injury
Subacute/chronic neurological disease
Bulbar palsy with airway compromise
Motor neuron degenerations such as amyotrophic lateral sclerosis
Neuropathies such as Guillain-Barré syndrome
Neuromuscular junction diseases such as myasthenia gravis
Muscle diseases such as muscular dystrophy

Treatment of Respiratory Failure in Neurological Disease

Respiratory failure is part of several neurological diseases and can develop rapidly or slowly (Table 51.2). Its management illustrates many important treatment principles.

Patients often complain of respiratory distress when they are close to pulmonary failure, particularly while they are lying down or sleeping. Air hunger is frightening, and the panic that ensues is real and must be taken seriously. Patients with weak intercostal and diaphragm muscles experience respiratory failure when they are supine because the abdominal contents prolapse into the chest and lower the patient's vital capacity and tidal volume.

A pulmonary specialist who is relatively inexperienced in neurological problems may underestimate the warning signs of potentially fatal respiratory failure. This is particularly true in myasthenia gravis and chronic neuromuscular disorders. Blood gas measurements are of little help. By the time hypoxia and hypercapnia develop in the blood, the patient may be bordering on respiratory collapse (Fallat and Norris 1980). Reduced vital capacity and patient distress are better indicators of impending respiratory failure. An anxious patient who has a vital capacity of 800 ml and cannot count past 15 on one breath, even when using accessory muscles of respiration, is experiencing respiratory fatigue and is at risk for incipient pulmonary failure. During the night, or with sedation, further ventilatory depression may tilt the balance toward carbon dioxide retention, narcosis, respiratory suppression, and death.

Ethics of Treating Respiratory Failure

Once invariably fatal, respiratory failure is now commonly reversed by intubation and positive pressure ventilation. As a result, quality-of-life issues play a greater part in clinical decisions of medical management. There are two circumstances in which the neurologist, the patient, and the family must make a decision concerning respiratory support. One is initiating respiratory support in a person who will invariably experience respiratory failure (i.e., in ALS and Duchenne's muscular dystrophy), and the other is stopping respiratory support that was started before its futility was known (such as with a child with infantile spinal muscular atrophy).

Neurologists must help patients decide whether respiratory failure should be prevented. Respiratory support is available through a variety of means, including the original negative-pressure tank and cuirass; turtle shell or poncho devices; positive-pressure machines such as the Pneumobelt, which compresses the abdomen to increase respiratory exchange; or intermittent positive-pressure respirators with a face mask or tracheostomy. Though life-saving, permanent respiratory care is an emotional, personal, and financial strain on the patient and family. Decisions concerning respiratory care must be made long before it becomes a necessity. Backup electrical power and trained help must be available around the clock for suctioning, ventilator management, and emergency support. Although a few patients can return home and even maintain mobility by using a ventilator mounted on a wheelchair, most remain in a hospital. Patients with a tracheostomy may still be able to talk using a valved tracheostomy tube or a partially inflated cuff. However, many patients lose their speech abilities and need to use communication devices such as computers, typewriters, or letterboards. Many of the conditions listed in Table 51.2 also cause limb paralysis, which further impairs the patient's quality of life.

No one can fully understand the impact of living at home on ventilator care without experiencing it. Families trying to make this decision should be urged to speak to others who are living through the experience. Those who decide against extreme measures if they become terminally ill should provide a living will or terminal care document to their physician and next of kin and grant another person power of attorney to make this decision for them if they become incompetent. When patients have not made such decisions, the neurologist must discuss with them the concepts of life support and quality of life at a time when death may be imminent. Few patients can decide with equanimity that they will permit themselves to die in the immediate future. Not surprisingly, they often defer the decision until they are taken to the emergency department, where they receive life-support measures. When quality of life becomes an issue and either the patient or relatives realize that all hope of recovery has passed, they may request that respiratory support be discontinued. Although the legal and moral ramifications are still far from settled, legal mechanisms in many parts of the world permit such requests.

In these matters, the decision of a competent patient, or of an authorized representative, holds primacy. For instance, a 40-year-old patient with ALS may request respiratory support, even though there is no likelihood of recovery, in order to see a child graduate or marry. The physician may be able to accommodate this request, though the cost of medical care must be considered. A request to continue life support for a 90-year-old patient with terminal cancer and a severe brain stem stroke is not rational; the physician should try to convey to the next of kin the hopelessness of the situation and the patient's unnecessary suffering.

Managing Respiratory Failure

The treatment of chronic respiratory failure due to progressive neurological disease differs from the usual treatment of chronic pulmonary failure. If in prior discussions the patient opted for life support measures to be administered at the onset of respiratory failure, the physician should perform an elective tracheostomy and start intermittent positive-pressure ventilation as soon as manifestations of respiratory failure appear. If patients decide against tracheostomy but opt for a lesser degree of respiratory support, they should receive the best-tolerated external ventilatory support when respiratory distress appears. When patients choose against respiratory support, the neurologist should counsel patients and relatives not to go to the hospital in a crisis, since a ventilator would inevitably be used. Treatment should be provided for respiratory distress with oxygen and sedation as needed, despite the risk that carbon dioxide narcosis could hasten the end.

At times, acute respiratory failure will occur in situations in which the patient's wishes cannot be determined. The neurologist should immediately institute resuscitation and ask questions later. Occasionally a patient will be resuscitated who had firmly requested no life support measures and is very distressed to be on a ventilator. This dilemma can be approached by providing sedation and gradually weaning the patient from the ventilator, allowing eventual respiratory failure to recur.

All neurologists should learn the art of managing chronic respiratory failure due to neurological disease. Although the neurologist may work collaboratively with the intensive care unit staff after the patient is intubated, he or she must assume an active role in management decisions.

PRINCIPLES OF SYMPTOM MANAGEMENT

Treatment of Common Neurological Symptoms

Specific therapy for the diseases discussed in Part III is reviewed in the relevant chapters. The following are general principles for managing a number of common symptoms. (Some of these are examined more fully in Chapter 55.)

Pain

The first step in pain management is to diagnose the source and assess the prognosis (see Chapter 53). Consider, for example, a patient with incapacitating leg pain from carcinoma infiltrating the lumbosacral plexus on one side. This patient's life expectancy is measured in months, and progressive nerve damage is likely to produce leg paralysis. Destructive or potentially addicting treatments may be justified in this situation, but not in the case of a young patient with pain from phantom limb or migraine who is likely to live for many years.

Biofeedback, hypnosis, or acupuncture may help some patients control the sensation of pain. These techniques, however, rarely provide acceptable relief of cancer pain, and treatment is usually initiated with pharmacological agents. If life expectancy is short, addiction is not a concern and the use of narcotics is justified. Tachyphylaxis can occur in patients who live for several months, and the effective analgesic dose may rise rapidly. This does not appear to be a major problem with morphine administered through an intrathecal or epidural spinal catheter linked to a subcutaneous infusion pump. Besides morphine, a combination of a tricyclic such as amitriptyline and either a phenothiazine like perphenazine or a later generation antidepressant like sertraline, has proved useful in many chronic pain syndromes. The combination works through different pathways from the opiates but takes about 3 weeks to produce the maximum effect at full doses. The risk of tardive dyskinesia from long-term use of phenothiazines is not an issue in terminal patients.

Surgical interruption of pain pathways is considered the final choice to relieve pain from carcinomatous infiltration. These procedures include surgical or chemical posterior rhizotomy, contralateral anterolateral spinothalamic tractotomy in the midthoracic region, or contralateral stereotactic thalamotomy.

Sensory Loss, Paresthesias, and Burning Dysesthesias

Occasionally, sensory loss produces an intolerable positive sensation termed *anesthesia dolorosa*, which may respond to a combination of a tricyclic with either carbamazepine or a phenothiazine; the risks of tardive dyskinesias must be considered when using phenothiazines. Paresthesias generally result from damage to the large peripheral nerve fibers or posterior columns of the spinal cord. Two-thirds of such patients can obtain relief with carbamazepine and a smaller proportion with phenytoin. Burning dysesthesias from small-fiber peripheral neuropathies are often helped by a tricyclic with either a phenothiazine or a later generation antidepressant like sertraline.

Weakness

The management of weakness, considered more fully in Chapter 55, is a major component of neurological practice. The neurologist chooses palliative treatment depending on the extent, severity, and prognosis of the patient's weakness. For example, weakness of dorsiflexion of the ankle due to poliomyelitis may be treated with a tibialis posterior tendon transplant. Such a transplant, however, would not be appropriate to overcome the foot-drop caused by a progressive condition like ALS, in which case the patient may benefit from an ankle-foot orthosis. Some conditions are benefitted by exercise; others, like myasthenia gravis or postpolio muscular atrophy, are worsened by it. Upper motor neuron paresis cannot be treated directly, though physical therapy may promote the use of alternative neurological pathways, and medications like baclofen may improve function by reducing spasticity.

Ataxia

Ataxia can result from cerebellar dysfunction or sensory deafferentation. No symptomatic pharmacological therapy is available when the underlying disease cannot be reversed. A cuffed weight placed on an ataxic limb may lessen incoordination by adding inertia and hence reducing excursion of the limb during movement. Gait ataxia is best managed by the use of walking aids such as a cane, walker, or wheelchair.

Dysphasia and Dysarthria

In principle, the treatment of language disorders is very similar to that of weakness. Speech therapy can improve aphasia by retraining the brain to compensate for the effects of damaged tissue. If the lesion is limited, some aspects of language function may be preserved. For instance, a dysphasic patient may be able to communicate through written messages. Through speech therapy, dysarthric patients can also learn to slow their delivery and emphasize words, which will improve the clarity of speech. Treatment with baclofen may slightly improve dysarthria of the upper motor neuron type.

Memory Impairment and Dementia

Some causes of progressive dementia are curable (see Chapter 71), and their recognition is important. In most progressive dementias, such as Alzheimer's disease, only palliative care is possible. Experienced neurologists can provide essential advice to the family of a patient with Alzheimer's disease on how to anticipate problems and minimize them. This includes instructing the patient to make shopping lists and checklists of things to do before leaving the kitchen or the home or before going to bed. For a period, these measures can effectively prevent the patient from leaving the house unlocked or a pot unwatched on the stove. Inevitably the patient will have difficulty managing a checkbook, and a family member should take over money management before there is financial disaster. To avoid getting lost away from home, the patient will need a companion. Much of the neurologist's efforts are directed toward helping the patient and family circumvent problems and adjust to expected changes. Family members need access to appropriate books such as *The 36-Hour Day* (Mace and Rabins 1991) and publications by foundations and support groups such as the Alzheimer's Disease Association.

Treatment of Secondary Effects of Neurological Disease

The diagnosis of chronic neurological disease produces predictable reactions in the patient and family. These reactions will progress at variable rates through the stages of anger, denial, "Why me?," depression, and eventually acceptance, often with oscillation between these phases. Support throughout this process of adjustment is an essential part of the management of chronic neurological disease and may require psychological counseling.

The neurologist provides a range of needed interventions over the course of the disease, but the immediate family shoulders most of the burden of caring for a patient with a severe neurological disorder. Some of the problems in Alzheimer's disease have already been mentioned. Similarly, the family of children with Duchenne's muscular dystrophy suffer both mental and physical stress, since the child will eventually lose the ability to walk and must be lifted in and out of chairs, beds, and baths. Mechanical lifting devices can help as the patient deteriorates. When contractures and weakness limit the ability to move, someone will need to get up several times a night to turn the patient in bed. Lack of sleep and increasing daytime care strain the family dynamics. Other children may suffer neglect and emotional deprivation, and marital disharmony is frequent. The physician may be required to refer the family for psychiatric counseling or to put them in touch with a family support group. Often the home will need alterations to allow one-level living and wheelchair access. The school authorities need information and encouragement so that the child can be allowed to continue in mainstream schooling. Ideally, as the young person reaches maturity, he or she should consider college or employment. Unfortunately, by this stage patients with typical Duchenne's muscular dystrophy are severely incapacitated, making employment extremely difficult.

Chronic disability has many legal aspects. In many parts of the world, national and local authorities provide services and financial support for the disabled. Through a specialist such as a medical social worker, patients can learn what help is available and how to get it.

The neurologist caring for a patient with a progressive, incurable neurological disease has a significant, continuing role with both the patient and the family. Help from many other professionals is often required, but the neurologist must be the anchor of the management team.

EXPLAINING THE PROGNOSIS

One reason the neurologist must establish a diagnosis is to define the prognosis. The physician should ascertain what the patient and family want to know and provide answers at a rate they can accept.

Some patients fear that they will die or become a "vegetable" within a few months, and are greatly relieved to find that they have several years of useful life ahead. Others will wish to change financial arrangements or accelerate unfulfilled plans if the prognosis is poor. Although some patients find the information impossible to handle, relatives generally want to know the patient's prognosis.

The neurologist should present the prognosis cautiously. Occasionally, the original diagnosis is wrong or the disease fails to follow the expected course. Patients should always be given some hope, even in the most dire circumstances. After outlining the range of possibilities, the physician should advise the patient to plan for the worst but hope for the best.

PALLIATION AND CARE OF THE TERMINALLY ILL PATIENT

Lessons learned from the reactions of cancer patients and their families can be applied to patients with chronic neurological disease. Pain, depression, and anxiety are the three major symptoms that require palliative treatment. Neurologists can treat severe psychological reactions with a range of pharmacological agents, including benzodiazepines for anxiety, major tranquilizers such as haloperidol for psychotic symptoms, and an ever-increasing list of medications for depression.

Psychological support for the patient and family is usually more important than pharmacological therapy for treating the typical reactions of a patient with severe neurological disease. The neurologist can provide great help by drawing on the experience of treating many similar patients. Even though the disease and its effects cannot be altered, the neurologist can ease the patient's burden. When possible, the physician should discuss each new phase of the disease with the patient and family before it occurs. Although no patient likes to hear of impending deterioration, knowing that the physician is ready to deal with the change is comforting.

GENETIC COUNSELING

Approximately one in ten neurological conditions is inherited. With the rapid advances in molecular genetics, the neurologist must keep abreast of the diseases that can be diagnosed by DNA probes, such as Charcot-Marie-Tooth disease and familial amyloid polyneuropathy. Parents and patients naturally fear that a neurological disease may be passed to their offspring. If a disease has no hereditary component, the physician should volunteer this information without being asked. If there is a hereditary tendency, such as in multiple sclerosis, the risk to offspring must be discussed. The chance of multiple sclerosis occurring in the offspring of a patient with multiple sclerosis is higher than that in the population, but still only about 3%, a comforting fact for most patients planning to have children. The genetic risk with regard to Alzheimer's and Parkinson's diseases is insufficiently clear at present to allow definitive predictions, other than reassurance that inheritance of the disease is uncommon.

Genetic counseling goes beyond the scientific principles set forth in Chapter 47. The neurologist should provide the patient and spouse with the available information about the mode of inheritance of the disease and, where relevant, the possibilities for prenatal and preclinical diagnosis. In appropriate cases, a couple's attitude to therapeutic termination of pregnancy should be part of the discussion.

When a disease has an autosomal recessive mode of inheritance, and the gene frequency in the population is low, the children of an affected parent are at little risk unless the patient marries a close relative. If the gene frequency in the general population is known, the risk can be quantified. Although the disease may appear several generations later, this is usually not of concern to the patient or spouse.

Patients with a known fully penetrant autosomal dominant disorder have a 50% risk of having affected offspring, even if the proband is apparently a sporadic case. For instance, apparently sporadic cases of facioscapulohumeral muscular dystrophy can be explained by undisclosed parentage, new mutations, and unrecognized mild weakness in another family member.

Some patients will make what the physician considers an irrational decision about having children. Most physicians would probably consider a 50% risk for a disabling condition such as Huntington's chorea or myotonic dystrophy too high for having children, but some patients consider 50% quite good odds! Other patients will react in the opposite direction and decide against having children, even if the odds are 1 in 100. In both circumstances, the physician should offer advice but emphasize that the decision rests with the patient or couple.

Genetic testing in some diseases can reveal that an asymptomatic individual will inevitably develop the disorder. Huntington's disease and myotonic dystrophy are two examples. Asymptomatic individuals who carry the mutation for the disease can be identified by the use of DNA probes for the mutant gene. Informing the individual that any child will be at risk of developing the disease simultaneously reveals that the person will probably develop it. Because Huntington's disease currently is not treatable and Huntington's patients have a high suicide rate, the neurologist should be aware of the risk that accompanies disclosure. Before any testing is begun, the physician should review thoroughly the hypothetical possibilities and the potential responses with the patient and his or her spouse. Though many persons at risk initially want to know their genetic status, after considering the implications many conclude that a positive diagnosis would be too distressing and hence forego screening. These individuals may choose not to have children on the basis of the empirical 50% risk that they carry the disease. Such couples can be advised about the alternatives of adoption; artificial insemination by donor, when the husband is at risk; or gamete in vitro fertilization when either the wife or the husband is at risk.

CONCLUSION

In this chapter we have presented a general outline of the principles of managing patients with neurological disease. When taken together with the remaining chapters in Part II and with Part III, this information should leave no doubt that the neurologist is more than just a diagnostician ("diagnose and adios"). Although diagnosis is the essential first step, the clinician's proper focus is on treatment and management of the patient and the disease.

REFERENCES

Bradley WG. Amyotrophic Lateral Sclerosis and Duchenne's Muscular Dystrophy. The Diseases and the Doctor-Patient Relationship. In LI Charash, RE Lovelace, SG Wolf et al. (eds), Realities in Coping with Progressive Neuromuscular Diseases. Philadelphia: Charles Press, 1987:3–20.

Fallat RJ, Norris Jr FH. Respiratory Problems: Diagnosis and Treatment of Amyotrophic Lateral Sclerosis. In DW Mulder (ed), The Diagnosis and Treatment of Amyotrophic Lateral Sclerosis. Boston: Houghton-Mifflin, 1980:301–315.

Mace N, Rabins P. The 36-Hour Day (2nd ed). Baltimore: Johns Hopkins University Press, 1991.

Chapter 52
Principles of Neuropharmacology and Therapeutics

Michael J. McLean

NEUROTRANSMITTERS

Microscopic examination of the nervous system using the carmine and gold-staining techniques of Gerlach gave the appearance that all neurons in the brain were connected by direct cytoplasmic contact. This gave rise to the reticular, or net, theory advanced by Gerlach and supported by Golgi. The improved stains of Ramón y Cajal led to the enunciation of the neuron doctrine, which favored the idea that each nerve cell was separate. Earlier microscopists, including Schwann, Schleiden, and Helmhotz, had described axons as direct extensions of nerve cell bodies. It was not until the advent of the electron microscope that the argument was settled in favor of Cajal's idea of independent neurons.

Answers to questions about modes of communication developed not from neuroanatomical considerations but from the studies of Sherrington and Claude Bernard in the late nineteenth century. It was Bernard who demonstrated that curare blocked neuromuscular transmission. Similarity in effects of injection of adrenaline (by Elliott in 1904) and muscarine (by Dixon in 1906) and stimulation of the sympathetic and parasympathetic nervous system, respectively, gave strong support for the idea of chemical transmission. In 1914, Dale unified the thinking about chemical transmission in the autonomic system by hypothesizing that adrenaline mediated sympathetic activity while acetylcholine mediated parasympathetic activity. But in 1921, Otto Loewi gave the first proof of chemical transmission. He collected the Ringer's solution that profused one frog heart during vagal stimulation and placed the solution on a second frog heart, which was beating spontaneously. The second heart slowed. Using the same approach, he also described release of an accelerating substance by stimulation of the sympathetic fibers to the heart.

Dale and his colleagues subsequently identified the decelerating substance as acetylcholine. Dale proposed in 1933 that fibers that liberate acetylcholine on stimulation be called *cholinergic* and those that liberate adrenaline be called *adrenergic.* He and his colleagues went on to show that stimulation of motor nerves led to liberation of acetylcholine at the neuromuscular junction, which led to contraction. Neurophysiologists began to speak of transmitters as substances that compensated for the electrical mismatch between the nerve terminal and its postsynaptic synapse. A long line of physiologists, including Katz, Kuffler, and Eccles, then described the role of action potentials in triggering the release of neurotransmitters and the subsequent production of excitatory and inhibitory postsynaptic potentials (IPSPs).

Increasing interest in neurotransmission led to the development of criteria for identifying neurotransmitters and brought us to the brink of modern neuropharmacology. *Anatomically,* the proposed neurotransmitter substance must be present in adequate concentrations in the nervous system to cause a physiological effect. The substance should be concentrated at nerve endings and distributed differentially among brain regions. Lesions should result in decreases of the concentration of the substance in a given brain region, and the substance or its synthetic enzyme should be locatable in specific neurons and neuronal pathways by various histochemical procedures. *Chemically,* the substance should be releasable on appropriate stimulation of isolated tissues. Synthetic enzymes should be demonstrable and present in neuronal terminals, where the substance should be stored in so-called presynaptic vesicles. A high-affinity uptake system should be present to concentrate the substance in nerve terminals. The candidate, or putative transmitter, should bind to postsynaptic membranes with high affinity.

Enzymes for the synthesis and destruction should be demonstrable in the appropriate pathway. *Physiologically*, release of the transmitter candidate must be demonstrable on nerve stimulation, and exposure of target tissues to the substance must result in a measurable function. *Pharmacologically*, agonists that mimic the action of the proposed neurotransmitter and antagonists that oppose the action of the neurotransmitter at its receptor sites must be identified. Data from the various approaches must be marshaled to prove that a substance is in fact a neurotransmitter.

The data that have led to the identification of what are now well-established neurotransmitters in the brain are described in the following sections. The primary purpose of this chapter is to review some of the new knowledge of molecular pharmacology and relate it to bedside neurology. Pharmacologically active products of neuronal metabolism, including adenosine, eicosanoids, and neuropeptides—many of which are putative neurotransmitters and modulators of neurotransmitter effects—are excluded for practical reasons. It is hoped that the enclosed methods of extrapolating from bench to bedside will give the reader tools to fill the gaps where this chapter is incomplete.

NEUROTRANSMITTER RECEPTORS

The concept of pharmacological receptors developed in parallel with ideas about neurotransmitters, but in the framework of specific effects of antibiotics. After all, something had to be receiving messages conveyed by transmitters for communication to be effective. John N. Langley observed that curare, a plant extract used as an arrow poison by South American Indians, blocked the effect of nicotine on skeletal muscle without preventing contraction in response to direct electrical stimulation, and he introduced the concept of "receptor substances" at which competition between agonists and antagonists occurred. These substances were thought to transmit the stimulus of the agonist to the cell and cause a physiological response. Langley's early operational definitions include elements that remain essential to current definitions: (1) a recognition function or selectivity of the receptor for agonists, (2) a transduction function, now known to be subserved by ion channels or activation of second-messenger systems, and (3) linkage to cell function.

The idea of multiple receptors for the same substance originated in the work of Henry H. Dale, who observed multiple actions of acetylcholine in 1914. Isolation and cloning of multiple receptors for various neurotransmitters is the culmination of ideas first promulgated by these early pioneers. The ability to purify, sequence, and clone functional neurotransmitter receptors proves the existence of discreet, selective receptor macromolecules and is the basis for understanding the heterogeneity of responses to neurotransmitters in different parts of the nervous system under different physiological and pathological conditions. Much has also been learned about how neurotransmitters are synthesized, stored, and released and how their actions are terminated. This knowledge has allowed physicians to chemically modulate many of these steps for several identified neurotransmitters in the brain. To the pharmacologist, such chemicals are drugs that modify neuronal function by molecular interactions. To the neurologist, drugs become medicines after their efficacy and safety in the treatment of specific illnesses is demonstrated in clinical trials.

RECEPTOR TYPES

Ligand-gated receptors are broadly of two types: *ionotropic* and *metabotropic*. Ionotropic receptors consist of channel-forming polypeptide subunits. Drugs that modulate these receptors open or close a central channel that allows passage of specific ions. Binding agonists to ionotropic receptors results in conformational changes of channel components that alter ionic conductances and modify intracellular processes requiring specific ions. The binding of ligands to metabotropic receptors activates guanosine triphosphate (GTP)-binding proteins, or G proteins, that subsequently modulate various intracellular second-messenger systems. Both types of ligand-gated receptor channels differ from voltage-gated ion channels (Figure 52.1).

G Proteins

Different receptor subtypes may be coupled by a variety of G proteins to specific signaling systems. In some cases, receptors are coupled by G proteins directly to ion channels, and their function appears to be ionotropic. Nearly 100 G protein-coupled receptors have been sequenced, and they seem to share several characteristics (Probst et al. 1992). The receptors are all monomeric proteins with seven transmembrane domains, each consisting of 20–30 hydrophobic amino acids. The amino terminus, pockets formed by the transmembrane domain, and three extracellular polypeptide loops confer ligand-binding characteristics and membrane interactions. Intracellular polypeptide loops, especially the third loop, and the carboxy terminus interact with G proteins and through them with other second-messenger systems. G protein–coupled receptors can be grouped on the basis of conserved nucleotide sequences.

A *superfamily* of traditional neurotransmitter receptors includes G protein–binding receptors for adenosine, acetylcholine (muscarinic type), norepinephrine, dopamine, serotonin, cannabanoids, and tachykinins. A second family of G protein–binding receptors shares little homology with amino acid sequences of the first superfamily. It localizes to the brain, endocrine systems, kidneys, and gastrointestinal tract. It includes receptors for secretin, calcitonin, parathormone, vasoactive intestinal peptide, glucagon, corticotropin, growth hormone–releasing factor, and other

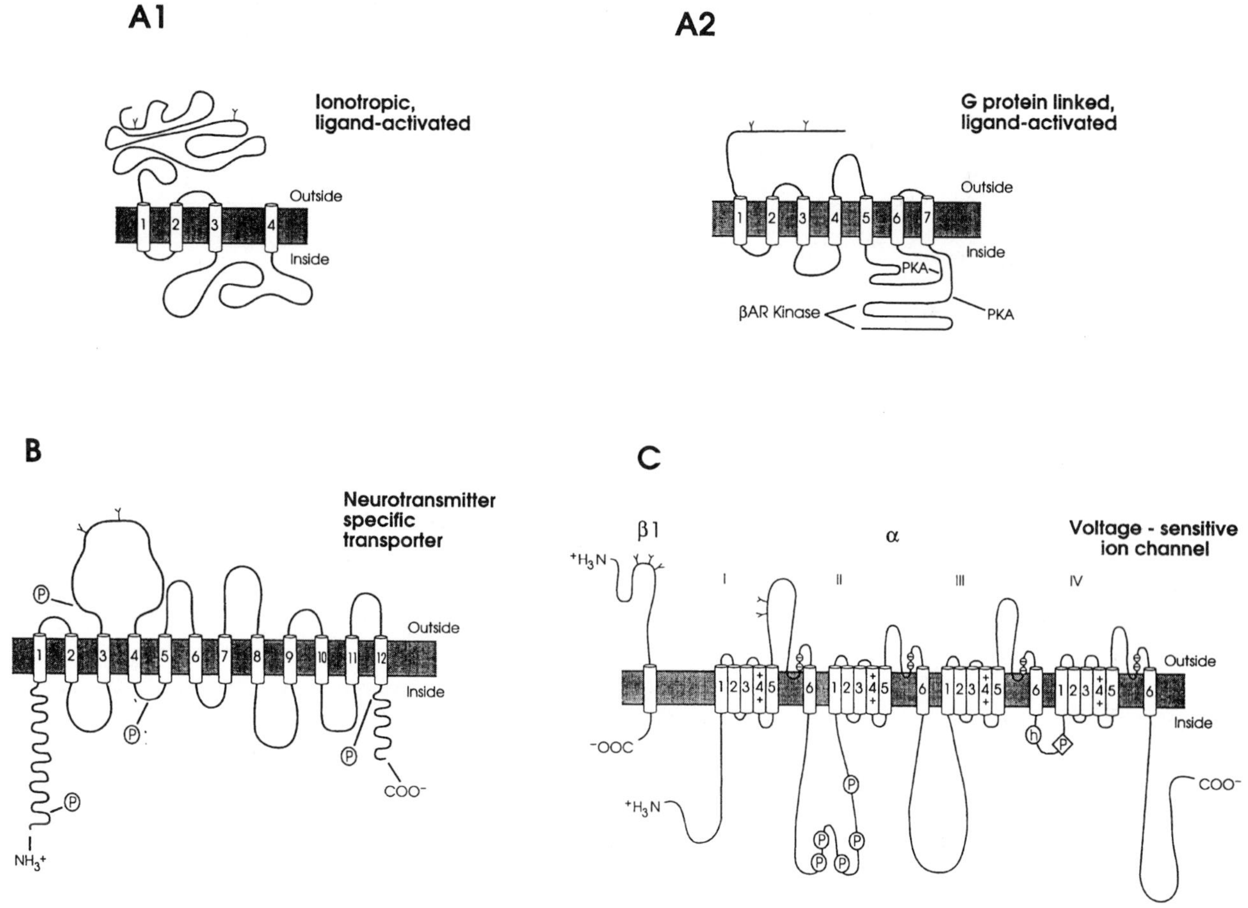

FIGURE 52.1 Molecular structure of ligand-activated receptors, neurotransmitter transporters, and voltage-sensitive ion channels. A1. Ionotropic, ligand-activated receptor structure. A single subunit consisting of an amino and carboxy peptide sequence, four transmembrane segments, and connecting loops is shown. Although the stoichiometry is unproved, assembly of approximately five subunits is thought to be necessary to construct ligand-gated ion conducting channels. (Redrawn from RL Macdonald, RW Olsen. $GABA_A$ receptor channels. Annu Rev Neurosci 1994;17:569–602.) A2. Some receptors of known neurotransmitters are coupled to intracellular second-messenger systems indirectly by interaction with G proteins. G protein–linked receptors are thought to have extracellular amino sequences, each followed by seven covalently linked transmembrane domains and an intracellular carboxy terminal of variable length. Each transmembrane domain is covalently linked by a loop of amino acid residues. The intracellular loop connecting the fifth and sixth transmembrane domains is thought to modulate interaction with G proteins, along with the carboxy terminal sequence. Function of the β-adrenergic receptor depicted here is modulated by phosphorylation at different sites by β-adrenergic receptor kinase (βAR kinase) or protein kinase A (PKA). (Redrawn from SB Liggett, JR Raymond. Pharmacology and Molecular Biology of Adrenergic Receptors. Bailliere's Clinical Endocrinology and Metabolism 1993; 7:279–306.) B. The termination of the action of amine neurotransmitters has been demonstrated to depend on specific transporters, which reduce synaptic concentrations of a neurotransmitter by reuptake. Transporter proteins have 12 membrane-spanning regions, and both the amino and carboxy regions are thought to be intracellular. A long extracellular loop connecting the third and fourth transmembrane domains is thought to contain the recognition sequence for a single neurotransmitter, thereby conferring specificity on the transporter system. (Redrawn from A Frazer and JG Hensler. In GJ Siegel, BW Agranoff, RW Albers et al. [eds]. Basic Neurochemistry [5th ed]. New York: Raven, 1994.) C. Voltage-sensitive ion channels are sequences of 1,800–2,100 amino acids. They are essentially multiple subunits that are covalently linked. The example shown is the structure of the voltage-sensitive sodium channel. The fourth transmembrane domain in each of the four subunits is positively charged and is likely to be the voltage-sensitive gate. When folded on itself, the four subunits line a central cavity such that the fourth transmembrane domain in each of the subunits is in a position to open or close the channel depending on its conformational state. Voltage changes and binding of various alkaloids may alter the opening and closure of the channel. The intracellular loop between the third and fourth subunits contains a sequence that is thought to be responsible for spontaneous inactivation of the sodium channel. The intracellular loop connecting the first and second subunits has multiple sites for modulation by phosphorylating systems. The amino and carboxy terminals are both thought to be intracellular. Accessory subunits (β1 is shown) can modulate the kinetics and, possibly, the drug-binding characteristics of the channel. Accessory subunits have been described for both the sodium and calcium channels that have been cloned to date. These figures show putative structures based on sequences of purified receptors, transporters, and ion channels. (Redrawn from WA Catterall. Cellular and molecular biology of voltage-gated sodium channels. Pharmacol Rev 1992;72:S15–S48.) (Y = glycosylation site; P = phosphorylation site; – = anionic loi for tetrodotoxin binding; + = cationic sites on voltage-sensing transmembrane segment; h = sequence required for spontaneous inactivation of the channel.)

Table 52.1: Examples of ionotropic and metabotropic neurotransmitter receptors

Neurotransmitter	*Ionotropic Receptors*	*G Protein–Linked Metabotropic Receptors*
GABA	$GABA_A$	$GABA_B$
Glutamate	NMDA, AMPA, KA	mGluR family
Acetylcholine	Nicotinic (muscle and nerve) Muscarinic M_2 and M_4 receptors, G protein linked to K^+ channels (hyperpolarizing)	Muscarinic (multiple neuronal)
Dopamine	—	$D_{1\text{-}5}$
Norepinephrine, epinephrine	—	$\alpha_{1,2}$ and $\beta_{1,2}$
Serotonin	$5HT_{1A}$-G protein linked inhibition of K^+ channels $5HT_3$-G protein linked to depolarizing cationic channel	$5HT_{1B\text{-}D}$, $5HT_2$

neurohormones. Examples of ionotropic and metabotropic receptors are listed in Table 52.1.

The Nobel Prize for medicine and physiology was awarded to Alfred G. Gilman and Martin Rodbell in 1994 for elucidating the mechanisms of action of G proteins and their central role in signal transduction. G proteins are trimers consisting of alpha (α) (39–52 kD), beta (β) (35–36 kD), and gamma (γ) (5–10 kD) subunits. G proteins possess inherent GTPase activity. Binding of a neurotransmitter or exogenous ligand to a specific receptor results in binding of the α-subunit of the G protein to the transmembrane receptor. In this configuration, GTP displaces guanosine diphosphate (GDP) from the α-subunit; then the β- and γ-subunits dissociate from the α-subunit, and the GTP-binding α-subunit is liberated from the transmembrane receptor. The activated α-subunit then regulates ion channels directly, or activates the first enzyme in various enzyme cascades that modulate intracellular second messengers. These enzymes include adenylyl cyclase, phospholipase C, phospholipase A2, and phospho--diesterases. The activation of these enzymes is coupled to hydrolysis of GTP to GDP on the α-subunit and reassociation of the β- and γ-subunits with the α-subunit.

Mutations of G proteins not only result in functional changes but are responsible for disease (Spiegel et al. 1993). A series of mutations in $G^{\alpha s}$ proteins are associated with pseudohypoparathyroidism. A mutation in the gene for GTPase activation protein (GAP) is associated with neurofibromatosis type 1. Normally, GAP stimulates GTPase activity of the *ras* family of small G proteins (M_r G proteins). In neurofibromatosis type 1, GAP fails to activate the *ras* protein GTPase activity. The abnormal GAP protein has been demonstrated in neurons, Schwann cells, and oligodendrocytes of patients with the disease. The *ras* family of small G proteins has been implicated in the pathogenesis of human colorectal adenocarcinoma. This emphasizes the regulatory role of the *ras* family in growth and differentiation. As a result of this role, *ras* proteins are also called proto-oncogenes.

Evidence is accumulating that levels of G protein subunits are altered by psychoactive drugs including antidepressant compounds, lithium, opiates, cocaine, and alcohol. The levels of the heterotrimeric G proteins may play a role in both the therapeutic effects of psychoactive drugs and addiction to them. Thus, it is likely that in the future, novel pharmacological agents will be devised to manipulate G proteins in the treatment of clinical disorders.

Receptor Technology

Rapid progress in molecular pharmacology has depended in large part on the combination of powerful new and sophisticated techniques that include (1) the isolation of receptors by recombinant DNA and expression cloning, (2) the patch clamp technique to assess the function of cloned receptors and the specific role of receptor subunits, and (3) quantitative autoradiography to scan brain sections and localize pharmacologically distinct subtypes of receptors in different brain regions.

In many cases, in situ hybridization of radiolabeled complementary DNA (cDNA) or of radiolabeled antisense RNA prepared from the cDNA has been used to localize DNA or messenger RNA (mRNA) encoding specific receptor subunits, respectively. Overlap of the localization of molecular probes has virtually proven the molecular diversity predicted from radioligand (receptor agonists and antagonists) binding. One of the major challenges of the future will be to determine how molecular diversity is regulated in normal and diseased states. Also, differential distribution of receptor subunits within the brain provides a basis for developing more specific therapeutic agents targeted against subtypes of selective receptors. This approach should ultimately result in the development of highly effective treatment agents with fewer side effects.

NEUROTRANSMITTER-GATED RECEPTORS

Gamma Amino Butyric Acid

Chemistry and Distribution

Gamma amino butyric acid (GABA) was synthesized in the nineteenth century and was known to be an inhibitory substance in the peripheral nervous system of invertebrates. In the 1950s, Flory and colleagues isolated a substance from mammalian brain that inhibited crawfish stretch-receptor activity, and they identified it as GABA. GABA is present in high concentrations in the brain and retinas of mammals. It is synthesized from glutamate, and substantial pools of both amino acids are present in mammalian brain.

Glutamic acid dehydrogenase (GAD), which synthesizes GABA from glutamate, is present in the terminals of GABAergic neurons in the central nervous system (CNS). GABA transaminase (GABA-T), the principal degradatory enzyme, is present in mitochondria of GABA-synthesizing neurons and neurons bearing GABA receptors. It is also distributed throughout the body, allowing rapid metabolism of exogenous GABA outside the nervous system. GABA-T reversibly deaminates GABA to succinic semialdehyde at the same time as α-ketoglutarate is aminated to form glutamate. This process occurs in synaptosomes and glia, and it may be important postsynaptically. Succinic semialdehyde dehydrogenase, along with GAD and GABA-T, forms the so-called GABA shunt, which links amino acid and carbohydrate metabolism. The apparent purpose of the shunt is the production of large stores of GABA, but the percentage of GABA in the total neuronal pool that contributes to neurotransmitter function is unknown.

GABA is released from synaptosomes upon depolarization of nerve terminals. It diffuses from the point of release and binds to postsynaptic receptors. GABA is commonly thought to be the most important inhibitory neurotransmitter in the brain. However, under certain conditions, some neurons hyperpolarize beyond the reversal potential for the GABA-mediated IPSPs. At very negative potentials, GABA receptor activation produces a depolarization. GABA also binds to presynaptic autoreceptors that modulate release of the transmitter. The action of GABA is terminated primarily by reuptake into neurons and glia.

GABA Receptors

$GABA_A$, $GABA_B$, and $GABA_C$ are the three classes of receptors known to bind GABA. $GABA_C$ receptors are found in the retina. Binding of GABA opens chloride-selective channels in the center of the ionotropic $GABA_A$ and $GABA_C$ receptors, which results in a rapid influx of negatively charged chloride ions through the postsynaptic membrane. The net increase of intraneuronal negativity results in so-called fast IPSPs, unless the resting potential is negative to the chloride reversal potential. Postsynaptic $GABA_B$ receptors are linked directly by a G protein to a potassium channel that mediates a long-lasting hyperpolarization, or slow IPSPs. $GABA_B$ receptors are also present on the presynaptic membrane, where they serve as autoreceptors to inhibit or reduce the release of neurotransmitter GABA. Therefore, the effect of activating GABA at any of its receptors is primarily inhibitory.

$GABA_A$ Receptors

The $GABA_A$ receptor is a channel-forming aggregate of several different subunits—that is, a hetero-oligomer or heteromer. Fifteen subtypes of five different subunits have been cloned from the mammalian brain. Most brain $GABA_A$ receptors are probably pentamers of at least three different types of subunits. Mathematically, more than 180,000 pentamers could be assembled from this number of subunits and provide an astounding range of receptor heterogeneity, both of structure and of pharmacological properties. About 50 recombinant receptors have already been identified. Even this number of receptor subtypes could provide marked functional diversity of GABAergic systems in different regions of the mammalian brain. Properties of GABA receptor-subunit subtypes are shown in Table 52.2.

Molecular diversity of the α-subunits seems to account for many of the pharmacological differences (in both efficacy and affinity) among receptor subtypes in vivo. In all likelihood, a GABA molecule must be bound to two α-subunits in order to maximally activate the chloride conductance. The $GABA_A$-activated chloride conductance is modulated allosterically at multiple sites on different subunits. Two classes of clinically important compounds, the benzodiazepines and the barbiturates, augment GABA-mediated inhibition at separate modulatory sites. Benzodiazepines increase chloride conductance by increasing the frequency of openings, whereas barbiturates increase open time by prolonging openings. The convulsant bicuculline, is a competitive antagonist of GABA, but it is uncertain whether it binds to one or both of the GABA binding sites.

Table 52.2: Subunits of $GABA_A$ receptors. Five subunits from three different families are thought to form a functional GABA receptor isoform, e.g., $\alpha_1\beta_1\gamma_2$. Amino acid sequences of different subunit subtypes within a family share 70–80% homology. Sequences between families have about 30–40% homology.

Subunit Family	*Subunit Subtypes*	*MW (kD)*	*Amino Acid Residues*
Alpha	$6(\alpha_1–\alpha_6)$	~51–58	48–64
Beta	$4(\beta_1–\beta_4)$	~56–58	51
Gamma	$3(\gamma_1–\gamma_3)$	~45	48
Delta	$1(\delta)$	~54	48
Rho (retinal)	$2(\rho1–\rho2)$	—	52

Source: RL Macdonald, RW Olsen. $GABA_A$ receptor channels. Annu Rev Neurosci 1994;17:569–602.

Another convulsant, picrotoxin, reduces GABA-activated current noncompetitively, probably by binding to a channel-forming transmembrane segment of one of the subunits. Picrotoxin shortens the duration of GABA-activated chloride openings. The function of β-subunits is not entirely clear, because it is difficult to clone receptors without them. They are important structural components of the receptor channel complex, and they also modulate benzodiazepine and barbiturate affinity.

γ-Subunits confer sensitivity to the receptor for benzodiazepine sensitivity, and the allosteric benzodiazepine binding site is probably at the interface between β- and γ-subunits. High-affinity benzodiazepine binding seems to be conferred by the γ_2 isoform. The δ-subunit probably occurs primarily in benzodiazepine-insensitive receptors. The pharmacology of the benzodiazepine binding site is complex (Macdonald and Olsen 1994; Figure 52.2). Benzodiazepines, such as diazepam, are agonists that increase GABA-activated chloride conductance when bound to the β-subunit. Inverse agonists, such as β-carbolines, decrease the GABA-activated chloride conductance when bound to the benzodiazepine receptor site. The partial agonist RO151788 activates chloride conductance less than full agonists, presumably by binding to γ-subunits. It also competitively antagonizes (reduces) enhancement of the chloride current by simultaneously administered benzodiazepines. Flumazenil is a competitive antagonist of benzodiazepine binding that does not have partial agonist effects.

Barbiturate modulation of the GABA-activated chloride current varies with the isoform of the β-subunit. Neurosteroids, including progesterone metabolites, steroid anesthetics (e.g., axalone), volatile gaseous anesthetics, and alcohols, including ethanol, also enhance GABA-activated chloride current, perhaps at the barbiturate site.

The composition of subunits accounts for wide variation in pharmacological properties of GABA receptors. Subunit composition changes during different stages of development, in different regions of the adult brain, and at different times in cell culture. This heterogeneity is the basis for region-specific and process-specific receptor-based intervention. Presumably, subunit composition of receptors is altered by pathological conditions. Since subunit composition determines the pharmacological properties of receptors, it may be necessary to identify and study receptors present during a specific disease process to determine the optimal therapeutic interventions. As a corollary, not knowing the specific receptor types involved in a disease process could lead to therapeutic failure. Lack of efficacy of a medication in vivo is not proof that a receptor is not involved in pathogenesis of a disease. Indiscriminate activation of multiple GABA receptors in different brain regions could have cancelling or even adverse effects. For example, the antiepileptic drug vigabatrin raises whole-brain GABA levels by inhibiting GABA-T. Some patients taking vigabatrin have experienced psychotic episodes. Adverse behavioral effects also occur during treatment with benzodiazepines and barbiturates.

$GABA_B$ Receptors

In 1979, Bowery and colleagues found that bicuculline failed to block effects of GABA on peripheral nerve terminals, and they later demonstrated blockade of neurotransmitter release from brain slices by baclofen, the prototypical $GABA_B$ agonist. $GABA_B$ receptors are distributed widely throughout the cerebral cortex, brain stem, and spinal cord, and they have been cloned. Binding of GABA or baclofen and its analogs to $GABA_B$ receptors leads to activation of G proteins that mainly inhibit neurons in two ways: direct inhibition from G protein activation of a potassium channel that produces a slowly peaking hyperpolarization, and indirect inhibition through other G protein–mediated enzymatic pathways that block calcium currents involved in neurotransmitter release and membrane potential oscillations (Bowery 1993). Activation of $GABA_B$ receptors has also been shown to facilitate kindling and long-term potentiation, animal models of epilepsy, and memory, respectively. This may be the result of indirectly disinhibiting crucial limbic circuits. $GABA_B$ receptor activation is also important in models of generalized absence seizures. The T-calcium current thought to underlie bursting behavior in the thalamus is blocked by $GABA_B$ antagonists.

GABA Receptors in Disease States

The treatment of many disorders involves the manipulation of $GABA_A$ receptors. Abnormal regulation of chloride conductances in cystic fibrosis and myotonia (both diseases are linked to human chromosome 7) suggests that mutations of GABA receptors and their chloride ion channel may also cause diseases of the CNS.

Epilepsy. Allosteric modulators of $GABA_A$ receptors are frequently used in the treatment of the epilepsies, particularly to treat generalized tonic-clonic and generalized absence status epilepticus (Gale 1992). Barbiturates and benzodiazepines are believed to act at different sites to increase inhibitory chloride current. Among the newer antiepileptic drugs, felbatol and topiramate augment GABA-activated chloride current allosterically at nonbenzodiazepine sites. Vigabatrin, by blocking GABA-T, and tiagabine, by blocking GABA uptake, were designed to elevate brain GABA concentrations. Vigabatrin is associated with depression and psychosis in a small percentage of patients and tiagabine with a low incidence of slow-wave stupor and adverse behavior. The extent to which these adverse reactions reflect global increases in GABA is uncertain. Neither drug has other known cellular mechanisms of action.

Seizures are known to result clinically from sudden discontinuation of benzodiazepines. Gabapentin, another new antiepileptic drug, was designed to act as an anticonvulsant by raising brain levels of a GABA receptor–active agent. Structurally, gabapentin incorporates GABA into a cyclohexane structure. It does not raise brain GABA levels but

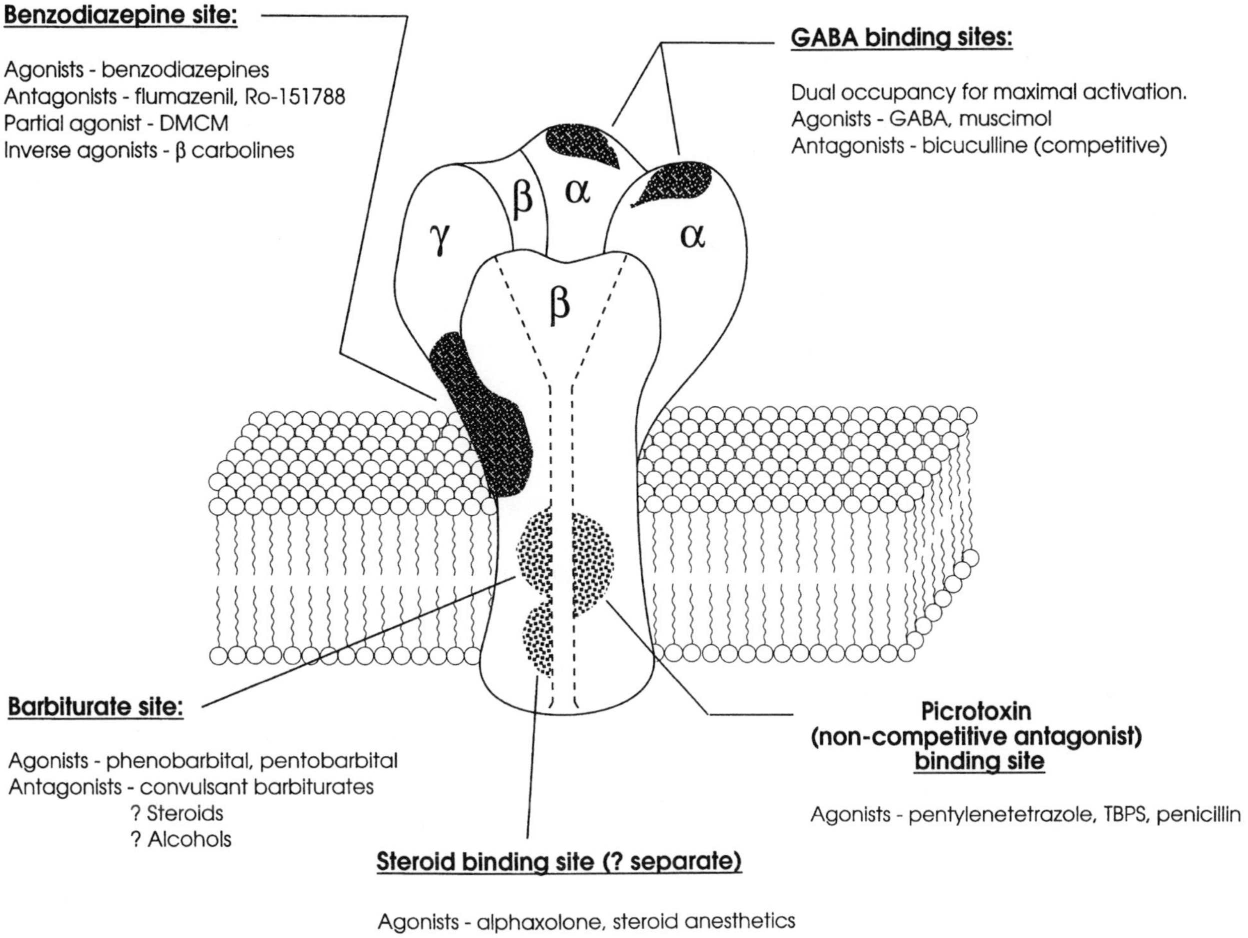

FIGURE 52.2 Pharmacology of the $GABA_A$ receptor. The $GABA_A$ receptor is thought to be an assembly of five subunits, probably of two to three distinct types per receptor. Affinity for GABA is modulated by a variable combination of alpha, beta, gamma, and delta subunits. Gamma subunits are essential for benzodiazepine binding, but the binding site is probably a pocket between gamma and beta subunits near the membrane surface. Binding of one or two GABA molecules leads to conformational changes, which opens a central pore and allows entry of chloride ion down its concentration gradient. The entry of anions onto the intracellular milieu leads to hyperpolarization and decreased excitability. Multiple allosteric modulatory sites have been defined pharmacologically, including those for benzodiazepines, barbiturates, steroids (including anesthetics), and alcohols. Agonist binding to various modulatory sites generally increases the chloride conductance and enhances the hyperpolarization. Antagonists and convulsant barbiturates decrease the chloride conductance and hyperpolarization and may promote seizures. The pharmacology of the benzodiazepine binding site has been characterized best. Agonists and antagonists have been identified. The partial agonist DMCM enhances the chloride conductance when it is present alone, but it diminishes the augmenting effect of benzodiazepines. The binding of beta carbolines to the benzodiazepine site results in decreased chloride conductance due to a different conformational change. Barbiturates are thought to bind at a separate allosteric modulatory site. Allosteric modulators such as phenobarbital and pentobarbital augment the chloride conductance gated by GABA binding. Convulsive barbiturates also bind to this site. Steroids and alcohols may bind to the same site. Alternatively, steroids may bind to a separate allosteric site in or near the channel. Agonists at this site include alphaxolone and steroid anesthetics. A separate allosteric site in the channel is thought to bind the convulsant picrotoxin noncompetitively. Binding of picrotoxin and other convulsants, such as pentylenetetrazole, penicillin, and TBPS, results in reduction of the chloride conductance activated by GABA. Endogenous substances such as taurine and a putative naturally occurring benzodiazepine antagonist are also thought to alter the chloride conductance. The phosphorylation of intracellular loops of the different subunits is also thought to modulate receptor sensitivity and availability.

may indirectly increase interstitial GABA concentration within the brain. A unique feature of GABA is its massive release by a mechanism that is not calcium- or voltage-dependent. Gabapentin is actively transported by the L-amino acid transporter because of its structural similarity to bulky neutral amino acids. Blockade of the uptake system by nipecotic acid results in a marked increase in brain interstitial GABA concentrations as GABA moves down its concentration gradient (millimolar intracellular–micromolar extracellular). Gabapentin enhances the effect of nipecotic acid on rodent olfactory nerve and hippocampal slices. Tiagabine is an analog of nipecotic acid that blocks the reuptake of GABA. This may prove to be another unique way to alter GABA-mediated inhibition for antiepileptic therapy.

Both GAD and GABA-T require pyridoxine as a cofactor. Pyridoxine deficiency or inhibition causes seizures, and its administration to infants with a dietary deficiency controls seizures. However, several other pyridoxine-dependent enzymes exist, and the cause of seizures may be multifactorial.

In many experimental models of epilepsy, seizures are produced by decreasing GABA-mediated inhibition, and they are ameliorated or prevented by administering GABA-enhancing drugs (Meldrum 1993). There is increasing evidence that the midbrain in the region of the substantia nigra reticulata regulates seizure spread. Injection of vigabatrin or GABA-mimetics into this area in rat brains blocks seizure generalization in the kindling model of epilepsy, and injection of glutamate analogs has the reverse effect.

γ-Hyroxybutyrate, a metabolite of GABA, produces 3-Hz spike-wave activity and seizures in immature animals, and the seizures are blocked by typical antiabsence drugs. γ-Hydroxybutyrate has been used as a pharmacological model to identify novel antiabsence drugs.

Anxiety and Mood Disorders. Benzodiazepines are frequently used alone or in combination to treat anxiety states, including situational anxiety, panic attacks, and other affective disorders. They are also sedative-hypnotics used to treat insomnia. Long-term treatment with antidepressant—but not antipsychotic—agents increases the number of baclofen- and GABA-binding sites in the hippocampus of animals. In certain animal models of depression, $GABA_B$ receptors are downregulated. These changes in $GABA_B$ receptor profiles are independent of effects on adrenergic receptors. Baclofen has not been systematically studied in humans as an antidepressant. In the treatment of anxiety states such as panic attacks, $GABA_B$ receptor agonists are not as effective as $GABA_A$ agonists.

Sedative-Hypnotic Effects. Anxiolytic effects of benzodiazepines may not be distinguishable from sedative-hypnotic effects. Adverse cognitive and behavioral effects have been reported in the elderly. The benzodiazepines are useful as premedication for surgical procedures and as conscious sedation for outpatient procedures. Several general anesthetics, including barbiturates, alcohols, steroids, and volatile gases, augment GABA-activated chloride current.

Sedative properties of benzodiazepines are also exploited in the treatment of alcohol withdrawal syndromes. They are especially effective against hallucinosis and seizures. Ethanol augments GABA-activated chloride current. The clinical strategy replaces one GABA-enhancer with another that can be withdrawn as slowly as required to avoid seizures.

Spasticity. Benzodiazepines are also widely used in the treatment of spasticity. Both $GABA_A$ and $GABA_B$ agonists, such as baclofen, are used successfully. Unlike the effects of $GABA_A$ agonists, no tolerance builds to the spasmolytic action of baclofen. Benzodiazepines have been used extensively, but with variable success, to treat movement disorders, including Huntington's chorea, dystonia, nocturnal myoclonus, and akathesia. In addition to benzodiazepines, baclofen, sodium valproate, and vigabatrin have also been tried with some success in the treatment of tardive dyskinesia.

Benzodiazepine Intoxication. The development of the benzodiazepine antagonist flumazenil has been an important advance in the treatment of intoxications with benzodiazepines.

Glutamate

Chemistry and Distribution

Glutamate and aspartate are nonessential dicarboxylic amino acids. They excite mammalian cerebral cortical neurons when applied iontophoretically or by intracarotid injection. The widespread distribution and high concentration of glutamate (stored concentration is roughly six times that of GABA) makes it the most common amino acid in the nervous system and supports the concept that glutamate is the principal excitatory neurotransmitter in the brain (Barnes and Henley 1992). Other glutamate functions are to modulate ammonia metabolism, to form proteins, and to serve as a precursor to Kreb's cycle intermediates and GABA. Exclusively aspartate-driven pathways have not been isolated or identified. Glutamate and aspartate are chemically interconvertible, and both are considered to be agonists with different affinities at glutamate receptors (GluRs). In addition to neurotransmitter function, administration of excitatory amino acid analogs and release of endogenous stores of glutamate in pathological settings cause neuronal damage. This process is called *excitotoxicity* (Choi 1992).

Glutamate and aspartate do not cross the blood-brain barrier. They are synthesized within central neurons and glia from carbohydrates involved in the tricarboxylic acid cycle. Aspartate is produced when aspartate transaminase catalyzes the conversion of oxaloacetate to α-ketoglutarate using glutamate as a substrate. When aspartate is the substrate, the reaction reverses and glutamate is released. Aspartate transaminase is a mitochondrial enzyme and could be involved in the production of transmitter-related pools of both amino acids. Glia contain glutamine synthetase, which converts glutamate to glutamine. Glutamine is subsequently transferred to neurons, where it is deaminated to glutamate by glutaminase. This glial inactivation and the specific uptake systems for glutamate reduce interstitial glutamate levels to terminate the neurotransmitter action and to prevent excitotoxic damage.

Other metabolic pathways that involve glutamate but have no established role in neurotransmitter function are the production of glutamate from α-ketoglutarate by GABA transaminase, the transamination of ornithine by glutamate semialdehyde, and the oxidation of proline by glutamate semialdehyde.

Glutamate concentrations are highest in the temporal lobe, basal ganglia, cerebellum, and neocortex, at concentrations of 8–11 mmoles per g wet weight. Aspartate concentration is 15–20% that of glutamate. Glutamatergic pathways descend from the brain stem to the spinal cord, where segmental glutamatergic interneurons are also present. Evidence suggests that some primary afferent pathways are also glutamatergic.

Glutamate Receptors

The two main classes of GluRs are ionotropic and metabotropic. Three ionotropic GluR subclasses have been identified operationally, based on their affinity for the synthetic analogs: *N*-methyl-D-aspartate (NMDA), α-amino-3-hydroxy-5-methylisoxazole-4-propionic acid (AMPA), and kainic acid (KA; kainate). All three compounds produce seizures and brain injury when administered systemically or intracerebroventricularly to animals. The NMDA and AMPA receptor subtypes have received the most attention, because they are implicated in the pathogenesis of seizures and stroke, and because highly selective antagonists are available.

Multiple subunits for each subclass of ligand-gated ionotropic receptors and multiple metabotropic receptors have been cloned (see Figure 52.3). Biochemical and cloning data support the concept that ionotropic receptor subunits can be mixed and matched interchangeably to form functionally diverse hetero-oligomers in various expression systems in vitro. The recombinant receptors reproduce properties of native ionotropic receptors in the brain.

Ionotropic Receptors

Molecular cloning and electrophysiological techniques have shown that many ionotropic GluRs belong to the same gene family. The principal pharmacological subtypes of naturally occurring and cloned ionotropic GluRs are activated selectively by NMDA, AMPA, and KA (Wisden and Seeburg 1993). These receptors are the principal components of rapid excitatory neurotransmission in the CNS, and they are involved in the synaptic plasticity that underlies learning, memory, and epileptogenesis.

Ionotropic receptor subunits are single polypeptide sequences that fold into a tertiary structure. The subunits aggregate to form receptor-channel complexes. Each polypeptide subunit has an extracellular amino-terminus with a 20–30 amino acid residue signal sequence that forms the ligand recognition site, and a core region containing four putative membrane-spanning sequences that are identified by their hydrophobicity. A variable carboxy-terminus follows the core sequence and differs in length from one receptor subunit to the next. In the case of NMDA receptors, the carboxy-terminus is probably intracellular and subject to modulation by phosphorylation.

The topology of GluRs has not been definitively established. However, based on the size of ion channels needed to conduct both mono- and divalent cations, it is assumed that glutamate channels in the brain are likely to be pentamers composed of at least two different types of subunits. Expression of multiple forms of receptor activity in a number of cell types following injection of mRNA fractions or cloned GluR cDNA suggests that the various GluRs consist of at least two, and possibly four or five, subunits.

AMPA Receptors. Based on protein purification techniques and radiation inactivation, it appears that AMPA and KA receptors have subunits with molecular weights of about 59 kD. An AMPA modulatory protein with a molecular weight of roughly 108 kD has also been isolated, and this component decreases the affinity of the binding subunit to AMPA. Dissociation of the modulatory protein may be responsible, in part, for maintenance of long-term potentiation, in which the AMPA receptor channel current is enhanced as a result of brief tetanic stimulation.

Recombinant receptors with high (nanomolar) affinity for AMPA and low (micromolar) affinity for KA can be assembled with GluR subunits A–D. Inclusion of GluR-B subunits is important for reproducing the electrophysiological properties of native AMPA receptor channels, and most brain AMPA receptor channels probably occur as hetero-oligomers of GluR-B in combination with A, C, or D subunits. Amino acid sequences in the second membrane-spanning domain of these subunits controls calcium permeability of the channel. Channels formed by combination of subunits other than GluR-B are calcium permeable, whereas inclusion of GluR-B subunits results in low permeability to calcium. Highly calcium-permeable AMPA receptors appear to be more abundant during development in some regions of the brain. In situ hybridization experiments revealed high-level expression of GluR-A and GluR-C relative to GluR-B during early developmental stages in the cortex, striatum, cerebellum, and hippocampus. Editing or alternative splicing can result in multiple variants of each of the subunits. Such mutations in situ might result in inherited disorders of the nervous system.

Various subunits have been localized to human chromosomes: GluR-A to chromosome 5, GluR-B to chromosome 4, GluR-C to the X chromosome, and GluR-D to chromosome 11. Excitotoxicity has been discussed as a pathogenetic mechanism in neurodegenerative disorders. Although a pathogenetic link has not been established, it is interesting that GluR-B and Huntington's disease are both localized to chromosome 4. Mutations or editing of various subunits may be important in pathogenesis of acute disorders of the nervous system, including epilepsy and stroke.

Kainate Receptors. Recombinant receptors with a high affinity for kainate can be formed from subunits GluR-5,

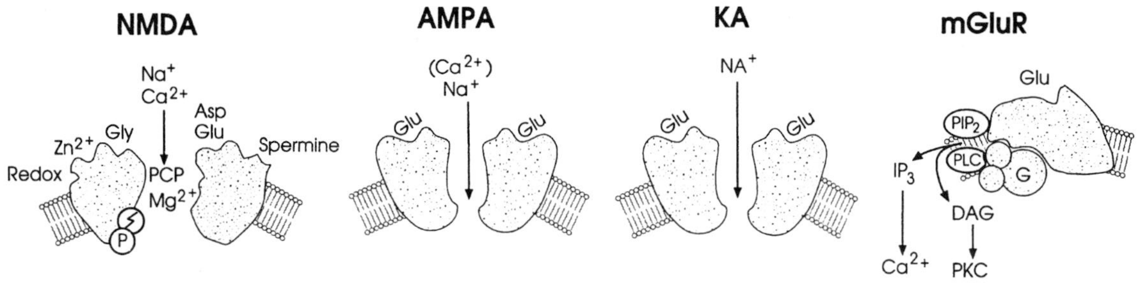

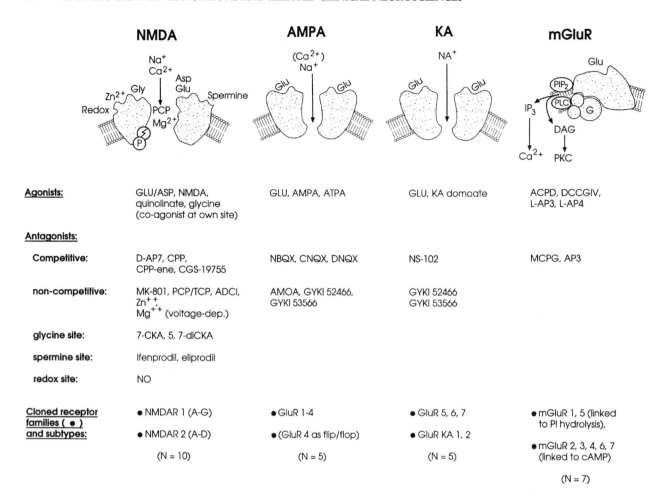

	NMDA	AMPA	KA	mGluR
Agonists:	GLU/ASP, NMDA, quinolinate, glycine (co-agonist at own site)	GLU, AMPA, ATPA	GLU, KA domoate	ACPD, DCCGIV, L-AP3, L-AP4
Antagonists:				
Competitive:	D-AP7, CPP, CPP-ene, CGS-19755	NBQX, CNQX, DNQX	NS-102	MCPG, AP3
non-competitive:	MK-801, PCP/TCP, ADCI, Zn^{++}, Mg^{++} (voltage-dep.)	AMOA, GYKI 52466, GYKI 53566	GYKI 52466 GYKI 53566	
glycine site:	7-CKA, 5, 7-diCKA			
spermine site:	ifenprodil, eliprodil			
redox site:	NO			
Cloned receptor families (•) and subtypes:	• NMDAR 1 (A-G) • NMDAR 2 (A-D) (N = 10)	• GluR 1-4 • (GluR 4 as flip/flop) (N = 5)	• GluR 5, 6, 7 • GluR KA 1, 2 (N = 5)	• mGluR 1, 5 (linked to PI hydrolysis), • mGluR 2, 3, 4, 6, 7 (linked to cAMP) (N = 7)

FIGURE 52.3 Pharmacology of glutamate receptors. The glutamate receptor family includes three ionotropic receptors that recognize the exogenous ligands NMDA, AMPA, and kainate. A family of metabotropic receptors is also activated by glutamate. These receptors are linked to phosphoinositide hydrolysis and cAMP production. Release of synaptic glutamate is thought to activate all of the receptor subtypes within diffusion range. This results in mixed postsynaptic effects, depending on the profile of receptor types. Aspartate and quinolinic acid are naturally occurring agonists that activate a mixed cationic conductance (sodium and calcium enter, and potassium exits) through the NMDA type of ionotropic receptors. Glycine is a coagonist, but it is insufficient to activate the ionic conductance alone. The binding of zinc (Zn^{2+}) to a separate site tends to decrease the ionic conductance through the channel. A polyamine site binds agonists, which increase the conductance at low concentrations and inhibit the conductance at high concentrations. The channel itself has a voltage-sensitive binding site for magnesium (Mg^{2+}). Until sufficient depolarization leads to dissociation of magnesium from its binding site, the conductance is blocked or low. Noncompetitive agonists such as MK-801 and PCP bind in the channel. Activation of the metabotropic glutamate receptor may ultimately activate nitric oxide synthetase and result in the production of nitric oxide, which feeds back negatively by binding to the redox site on the NMDA receptor and results in a decreased entry of calcium and sodium. Two gene families, NMDA R1 and NMDA R2, have been cloned. These two families contain multiple receptor isoforms.

AMPA and kainate receptor subtypes are also ionotropic but are less well characterized because of the limited availability, until recently, of antagonists. Competitive and noncompetitive antagonists have been discovered, however, and they are listed above. The AMPA family consists of five gene products, GluR 1–4. Alternate splicing results in flip and flop conformers of the GluR 4 isoform. Kainate receptors contain subunits of two gene families. GluR 5, 6, and 7 constitute one family, and GluR KA-1 and -2 constitute the second family. Some AMPA channels are activated less potently by kainate.

Metabotropic receptors are linked through G proteins to phospholipase C and phosphoinositide metabolism. The mGluRs 1 and 5 result in increased DAG and IP_3. IP_3 serves as a second messenger to release calcium from intracellular stores, while DAG activates protein kinase C. This in turn may result in phosphorylation of the NMDA channel, an action that removes the voltage-sensitive magnesium block. Phosphorylation of calcium calmodulin and activation of nitric oxide synthetase results in synthesis of the ephemeral second messenger nitric oxide, which can modify both presynaptic and postsynaptic function. Other metabotropic receptors, including mGluR 2, 3, 4, 6, and 7, are linked to cAMP production and regulation of metabolic processes.

-6, and -7 and sequences from another family, KA-1 and -2. Functional channels can be formed by GluR-5 or -6 subunits alone—that is, as homomultimers. Homomeric GluR-5 subunits behave like kainate receptors found on dorsal root ganglion neurons in that they are activated by AMPA as well as kainate. The KA-1 or KA-2 subunits do not form functional homomeric receptors. However, they form ion channels with a relatively nondesensitizing response to kainate or AMPA when coexpressed with GluR-5 or -6 subunits. Chromosome 21 has been found to contain the gene coding for GluR-5 subunits in humans. Familial amyotrophic lateral sclerosis has also been localized to chromosome 21. This may be a coincidence, since GluR-5 subunits are expressed only on some neurons in the dorsal horn, where they may function in pain transmission.

NMDA Receptors. Biochemical and biophysical data suggest that the molecular weight of the NMDA receptor is approximately 209 kD. The overall receptor size probably results from the assembly of polypeptides, ranging from 33 to 100 kD. Purified receptor complexes composed of the 100-kD subunits are functionally activated by NMDA when inserted into lipid bilayers, whereas receptors composed of only 42-kD subunits are activated by AMPA and KA.

Nakanishi and colleagues were the first to clone NMDA receptors. They characterized the NMDA-R1 (NR1) subunit and showed that homo-oligomers of this subunit could form ion channels with many pharmacological properties of NMDA receptor channels. The NMDA-R2 (NR2) subunit family of four subtypes, A–D, were identified subsequently. The intracellular carboxy-terminal region of the NMDA-R2 subunit is large—more than 400 amino acid residues—compared to the usual 50–100 residues found in AMPA/kainate receptors. This region can be phosphorylated by protein kinase C as a means of regulating synaptic efficacy and plasticity, as in the case of long-term potentiation.

Homo-oligomers of NMDA-R1 subunits expressed in Xenopus oocytes act in many ways like the native NMDA receptor channels in the brain. They are activated by both NMDA and glutamate, but not AMPA or KA. Glycine is necessary for activation, and voltage-dependent magnesium block is manifest. Combination of NMDA-R1 and -R2 subunits produces channels with much larger NMDA-activated currents than NMDA-R1 homo-oligomers. Hetero-oligomers also have variable degrees of magnesium and glycine sensitivity. Specialization of subunit function is suggested by the fact that calcium permeability of hetero-oligomers results from an asparagine residue in the second transmembrane region of NMDA-R1 subunits, while the sensitivity to magnesium ions results from an asparagine in this region of the NMDA-R2 subunit.

With in situ hybridization techniques, differential distribution of NMDA receptor subunits has been demonstrated in various regions of adult brain and at different stages of development. These findings are the basis for thinking that drugs can be designed to target specific brain regions, possibly even in unique pathological conditions. mRNA for NMDA-R1 subunits is found in virtually all neurons, whereas isoforms of NMDA-R2 are expressed variably throughout the nervous system. These findings suggest that brain NMDA receptors are heteromeric and that functional diversity is a result of combination of NMDA-R1 subunits with various types of NMDA-R2 subunits.

Metabotropic Receptors

The metabotropic GluR family consists of seven receptors with uniquely conserved regions in the transmembrane domains (Schoepp and Conn 1993). These receptors have little homology with the neurotransmitter superfamily or the group of hormone receptors. The metabotropic GluRs are much larger than other G protein–linked receptors and consist of 872–1,199 amino acid residues. The extracellular *N*-terminal domain contains up to 570 amino acid residues, including *N*-glycosylation sites. The intracellular C-terminus contains multiple threonine and serine residues that are candidate sites for regulation by phosphorylation. In addition, the loop between transmembrane domains 3 and 4 has multiple positively charged amino acid residues, which can be phosphorylated, a mechanism that may modulate interaction with G proteins. Ionotropic and metabotropic receptors are found together in the same region of the postsynaptic membrane and are likely to be coactivated. Association of the metabotropic receptors with different G proteins and effector systems can then produce a variety of responses by modulating ionotropic receptors and intracellular biochemical processes.

One type of metabotropic GluR in the retina is activated preferentially by (+) -2-amino-4-phosphonobutyric acid (L-AP4). Activation of this metabotropic receptor in bipolar cells results in G protein–dependent activation of phosphodiesterase. This opens a sodium channel by decreasing the concentration of cyclic nucleotides. L-AP4 receptors may also be present presynaptically in the brain.

The G proteins are linked to several metabotropic receptors that are activated by +trans-1-aminocyclopentane-1,3-dicarboxylic acid (ACPD). These metabotropic receptors, in turn, activate phospholipase C. This releases two intracellular second messengers, diacylglycerol (DAG) and inositol triphosphate (IP_3), from membrane lipids. Activation of protein kinase C by DAG is believed to phosphorylate GluRs. For example, phosphorylation of the third intracellular polypeptide loop connecting transmembrane segments of the ionotropic NMDA receptor relieves voltage-dependent magnesium block and augments calcium influx through activated channels. IP_3 releases calcium from intracellular stores such as the endoplasmic reticulum. This step may lead to production of nitric oxide, which has mixed pre- and postsynaptic actions. It may decrease NMDA receptor activity by binding to the redox site. Several ACPD-activated receptors have variable effects on cyclic AMP levels, as well.

Increased intracellular calcium by the two second messengers contributes to long-term potentiation, an experimental model of synaptic plasticity. Long-term potentiation is produced in the hippocampus by brief high-frequency tetanic stimulation of Schaeffer collaterals. Following stimulation, excitatory postsynaptic potentials (EPSPs) in CA1 neurons are enhanced. An early, or induction, phase lasts about 30 seconds and requires activation of NMDA receptors. A prolonged maintenance phase may last hours, and it depends on phosphorylation of AMPA receptors. The result is increased synaptic efficacy, which may be important in learning and memory. Evidence that metabotropic GluRs must be activated to produce long-term potentiation comes from experiments with receptor ligands and blockers of the secondarily activated enzyme cascade. Long-term potentiation is facilitated by specific agonists of metabotropic GluRs and is prevented by highly selective antagonists and blockade of protein kinase C by staurosporine. Injection of staurosporine also prevents hippocampal injury produced by brain ischemia in rodents. This suggests that antagonists of multiple steps in the calcium-releasing enzyme cascade activated by metabotropic GluRs may be neuroprotective.

Postsynaptic metabotropic receptor activation in hippocampal pyramidal neurons also closes voltage-dependent potassium (M-type) and calcium-dependent potassium channels. These effects decrease accommodation, reduce hyperpolarizing afterpotentials, and prolong repetitive firing of action potentials. Activation of presynaptic metabotropic glutamate reduces the release of excitatory amino acid neurotransmitters, probably from blockade of calcium channels on the terminal, which admit the calcium needed for excitation-release coupling. Although these processes appear antagonistic, the result is a filtering effect that reduces the efficacy of low-intensity stimulation and amplifies (postsynaptically) inputs strong enough to bypass the reduction of neurotransmitter release. This bias on the signal-to-noise ratio has been proposed as a mechanism of controlling attentiveness.

Presynaptic glutamatergic metabotropic receptors also reduce inhibitory postsynaptic potentials, presumably by reducing GABA release. This reduction of inhibition combined with the postsynaptic excitatory effects of metabotropic receptor activation may be proconvulsant. Injection of ACPD into the hippocampus results in the development of limbic seizures and damage to neurons in both the pyramidal cell regions of the hippocampus and the dentate granule cells, simulating the injury produced by kindling epileptogenesis.

Contralateral turning behavior induced by ACPD injection into the striatum is independent of NMDA receptors and may be caused by enhanced dopamine release, since it is blocked by haloperidol and dopamine depletion. This suggests a role for metabotropic GluRs in motor system dysfunction and a possible therapeutic role for metabotropic receptor antagonists. Activation of metabotropic receptors in the brain stem excites baroreflex-like responses, suggesting a role in cardiovascular regulation.

Pharmacology and Physiology of Glutamate Receptors

Glutamate receptor activation is regulated by interlocking mechanisms that coordinate activity-dependent facilitation of excitability—such as long-term potentiation and synchrony—yet normally prevent cell injury (Figure 52.3). Activation of NMDA receptors requires binding of agonists at two sites. The principal site is the NMDA or glutamate-binding site with a rank order of affinity for NMDA > glutamate or aspartate > AMPA or kainate. The most important endogenous agonist is glutamate, although other endogenous agonists—e.g., aspartate and guinolinate—are thought to bind at the same site. A number of high-affinity competitive antagonists for glutamate binding to this site have been synthesized. These include phosphonate derivatives (e.g., AP-5 and AP-7; CPP and CPP-ene). The second essential site binds glycine. Neurotransmitter glycine mediates IPSPs in the spinal cord, but glycine is present in sufficient quantities in interstitial fluid to serve a permissive or coagonist function at NMDA receptors. The concentration of glycine in the interstitial compartment is not known to fall to a point where it limits channel opening. However, the channel cannot be opened when glycine is "completely" removed under experimental conditions. This makes the glycine site a strategic target for designer antagonists, such as 7-chlorokynurenic acid. One of the most important controls on the ionic conductance through the NMDA receptor channel is voltage-sensitive block by magnesium. Hippocampal pyramidal neurons, for example, must be depolarized at least by 10 mV to remove the magnesium block. This effectively raises the threshold for opening NMDA receptor channels. It also means that modulation of firing rates by AMPA-mediated neurotransmission can occur at smaller depolarizations without activation of the NMDA channels. Voltage-dependent magnesium block also limits calcium entry in regions with AMPA receptor channels impervious to calcium, until depolarization unblocks NMDA receptor channels. The fact that phencyclidine, initially developed as an anesthetic but now an illegal hallucinogen ("angel dust"), is an NMDA channel blocker supports the concept that NMDA channel blockade is psychotogenic. However, phencyclidine has other actions, and not all NMDA channel blockers produce adverse behavioral effects. Drugs that block the channel, including the prototype MK-801, are being scrutinized as potential therapeutic agents for diverse neurological conditions.

A separate site that modulates the gating of the channel is sensitive to polyamines, such as spermine and spermidine, which are synthesized by neurons. Different concentration-dependent effects have been observed. Spermine enhances the conductance activated by glutamate in the presence of glycine at low concentrations. Spermine and spermidine reduce or completely block the ionic conductance activated by glutamate or NMDA at high concentrations. This is an allosteric modulatory effect similar to that of benzodiazepines or barbiturates on the GABA-activated chloride conductance.

Other ions modulate the NMDA current. Endogenous zinc reduces the current. Zinc is present in high concentrations in the hippocampus in particular. Zinc is released with some neurotransmitters in the nervous system. The ionic conductance is also modulated by hydrogen ions. The conductance is maximal at slightly alkaline pH and is reduced with increasing acidity. This may prove to be an important safeguard. During hypoxic-ischemic injury, progressive acidification due to glycolytic metabolism may turn off the NMDA receptor channels and limit the transmembrane influx of calcium that underlies excitotoxic cell death.

Less is known about AMPA receptor channels. These ion channels are opened with slight depolarization and are not sensitive to voltage-dependent magnesium block. The channels admit sodium (entering) and potassium ions (exiting), but calcium-conducting AMPA receptors have been identified in the cerebellum, and in other locations at certain times in development (see above) Highly selective quinoxazolidinedione agonists, such as CNQX and DNQX, have been synthesized. Initial depolarization mediated by activation of AMPA receptor channels may depolarize the neuron sufficiently to remove voltage-dependent magnesium block and activate NMDA channels. AMPA and NMDA channels are coactivated and are present on the same parts of neurons; these two receptor channels, each with diverse modulators, can be envisioned as acting in concert.

Kainate channels are even less well understood because no selective antagonists have been found. Topiramate, a new anticonvulsant, may block kainate but not NMDA-gated activity. Confirmation of topiramate selectivity or identification of more selective analogs would be the breakthrough needed to elucidate the physiological role of kainate receptors.

Metabotropic receptors are activated by L-glutamate, quisqualate, ibotenate, ACPD, and L-AP4 with different rank orders of potency; α-methyl-4-carboxyphenylglycine is a selective antagonist. Phosphorylation of receptor subunits at their carboxy-terminus intracellularly may be important in sustaining availablility of GluRs for activation. Phosphorylation of AMPA receptors following activation of metabotropic GluRs is described in this chapter as a means of augmenting the contribution of AMPA receptors to the excitatory synaptic potentials in LTP. Under patch clamp conditions in which the interior of neurons is dialyzed by the pipette solution, NMDA currents tend to run down with time. Adding ATP to the pipette solution allows sustained recording of the NMDA-activated currents without significant reduction over time. Presumably, this restores the activity of ATP-dependent protein kinases normally activated by the metabotropic GluR cascade above the basal phosphorylase activity. Since a series of enzymes is involved in this cascade, it stands to reason that selective antagonists at each enzyme step could be developed as therapeutic agents to control glutamatergic hyperactivity. It is also conceivable that mixtures of antagonists of ionotropic and metabotropic GluRs might ultimately be used to limit or prevent neuronal damage induced by prolonged status epilepticus or stroke.

Clinical Role of Glutamate Receptors

The normal role of the neurotransmitter glutamate is to generate fast EPSPs that contain two components. One is produced by activation of AMPA receptors through a broad range of membrane potentials. The other is produced by activation of NMDA receptors with increased calcium entry after voltage-dependent magnesium block is removed by sufficient depolarization. The duration of these EPSPs is determined by the amount and pattern of neurotransmitter release, the rate of reuptake of glutamate, and activity-dependent modulation of the response by coactivation of metabotropic receptors.

Memory. The potential role of long-term potentiation in memory function is also mentioned earlier in this chapter. In some pathways, EPSPs are briefly augmented (short-term potentiation) in the presence of metabotropic receptor antagonists. In other pathways, short-term potentiation does not occur when metabotropic receptors are blocked, but long-term potentiation can be produced. The mossy fiber pathway that originates in the entorhinal cortex and synapses on granule cells of the hippocampal dentate gyrus is an example. This variability limits the types of pathway facilitation in different regions and could reflect differences in the types of metabotropic receptors that are present. The marked prolongation of the EPSPs during long-term potentiation probably results from phosphorylation of ionotropic receptors postsynaptically.

Activation of presynaptic metabotropic GluRs reduces both glutamate and GABA release. This could result from reduction of calcium influx through *N*-type and possibly other calcium channels or from augmentation of conductance through hyperpolarizing potassium channels on axon terminals. The result of this dual action is a recurring theme, as if ionotropic and metabotropic systems were dissimilar controls in series biasing selectively activated pathways to respond only to high-intensity presynaptic inputs. When the effect of reduced transmitter release is overcome, the postsynaptic effect is amplified, thereby increasing the signal-to-noise ratio and filtering out weak stimuli. In a sense, the dentate gyrus does this additionally by not having short-term potentiation. The entorhinal cortex receives and integrates input from several sensory systems. This means that entorhinal inputs through the dentate gate must be quite strong to have a lasting effect; otherwise, the system may desensitize or tune out certain inputs.

Excitotoxity. Activating metabotropic receptors is a double-edged sword. Injection of ACPD results in delayed seizures and neuronal death in the hippocampus, particularly in the CA1 region. In addition, intrastriatal injection of ACPD enhances the damage produced by injection of NMDA. These two experimental examples indicate the potential for transforming physiologically regulated glutamatergic excitability into neuronal injury. To this potential should be added the potential for changing expression of AMPA receptors to those with high calcium conductance.

Olney observed that injection of excitatory amino acids produced seizures and brain damage in rodents and introduced the concept of neuronal excitotoxicity. This concept has been studied in vitro and in animal models. The administration of anticholinergic medications helped abbreviate seizures in an animal model of status epilepticus produced by excitatory amino acids. This suggests that excitotoxicity may be enhanced by entrainment of other excitatory systems after the amino acid trigger. The spectrum of neurological disorders mediated by excitotoxic injury includes epilepsy, stroke, and neurodegenerative disorders. Not unexpectedly, the development and evaluation of neuroprotective drugs has become a priority of the neuroscience community (basic and clinical) and of the pharmaceutical industry.

Kindling. Kindling is an experimental method of producing seizures in animals that, like long-term potentiation, depends on patterned stimulation. Although kindling is not proved to occur in humans, the technique provides insight into epileptogenesis and the mechanisms of action of antiepileptic drugs. The original method used electrical stimulation through electrodes implanted in susceptible regions. The amygdala and hippocampus are kindled more readily than the cortex. An initial low-intensity stimulus does not usually produce behavioral changes. Subsequent daily stimulation first causes the appearance of electrical afterdischarges without behavioral changes; then it causes both. Afterdischarges are critical for the development of kindled seizures. Even a single stimulus that induces an afterdischarge produces structural changes in the hippocampus. Neurons in the dentate hylus die, and the dendritic processes of dentate granule cells sprout and spread to distances of up to 1 cm; thus opening the dentate gate becomes easier. The result is that an input that normally excites a discreet band of hippocampal neurons now opens the gate with resultant extensive excitation.

Kindling is associated with abnormal hyperexcitability of multiple synapses. At the synapse between dentate neurons and pyramidal neurons of the CA2 and CA3 fields, potassium concentrations are increased from 3.5 to 7.0 mMs, and spontaneous bursts, simulating interictal spikes, appear in this region. Axons from CA2 and CA3 pyramidal neurons feed forward onto CA1 pyramidal neurons. Extracellular calcium levels are low in the CA1 region, presumably due to entry of calcium into neurons. This may be explained by the appearance of a new NMDA receptor component of excitatory synaptic potentials. It is not clear if this is caused indirectly by activation of metabotropic receptor-mediated changes in NMDA receptors or whether new types of glutamate-NMDA receptors appear in the hippocampus.

The hippocampal output arrives at the substantia nigra reticulata through a multisynaptic pathway. In the midbrain region, gating of epileptogenic activity to the spinal cord is controlled. Glutamatergic agents enhance and GABA-mimetic agents inhibit secondary tonic-clonic generalization. Injection of GABA-mimetic agonists into the substantia nigra reticulata bilaterally not only suppresses tonic-clonic seizures in fully kindled animals, but it also results in less severe ictal limbic features, such as facial clonus and head nodding. These experiments suggest that midbrain neurons somehow feed back to the entorhinal cortex or hippocampus per se to create a vicious cycle of hyperexcitability. Any disruption of this circuit, pharmacologically or structurally, abolishes seizures. This somewhat speculative interpretation is based on an enormous amount of pooled experimental data.

The behavioral changes associated with kindling development appear in a predictable order. An animal is considered fully kindled (stage 5) when a stimulus of intensity identical to the first stimulus elicits rearing on the hind limbs and falling. Once achieved, a stage 5 seizure can always be elicited by a stimulus that was initially subconvulsive. Drugs that augment GABAergic inhibition, such as benzodiazepines or vigabatrin, and NMDA-channel blockers such as MK-801 have potent antiepileptogenic effects in the kindling model; that is, they slow or prevent the development of kindling. Paradoxically, MK-801 weakly inhibits fully kindled (stage 5) seizures.

The kindling model teaches at least two things: that glutamatergic, particularly NMDA-ergic, hyperexcitability is necessary to establish the seizure pathway involved in the fully kindled seizure; and that a counterbalancing GABAergic control or filter is exerted at the midbrain level. To stop partial limbic seizures and secondary generalized seizures triggered from the same limbic focus, one would like to block NMDA receptors, augment GABAergic inhibition, or both. Phenytoin and carbamazepine tend to block secondary generalization. Both drugs limit high-frequency firing of action potentials, at least in part, by blocking voltage-sensitive sodium channels and probably by weakly blocking NMDA-mediated activity. Neither agent augments GABA-mediated inhibition at clinically useful doses. Felbamate decreases NMDA-activated currents and augments GABA-activated chloride conductance under whole-cell patch clamp conditions, although these actions are weak at clinically relevant concentration. It also limits high-frequency firing of action potentials. This combination of actions suggests that felbamate would be useful to treat some refractory partial seizures and stop generalization. Unfortunately, the usefulness of felbamate is limited by an untoward incidence of aplastic anemia and liver failure.

Other drugs may have a constellation of cellular mechanisms of action. Topiramate is a potent investigational antiepileptic in phase 3 testing against refractory partial seizures with or without secondary generalization. In isolated neurons, it augments GABA-activated chloride conductance alosterically by binding to a nonbenzodiazepine site and limits action-potential firing. It also blocks kainate-gated (but not NMDA-gated) current and limits repetitive firing. None of these antiepileptic drugs prevents kindling development, but potent NMDA antagonists do.

Epilepsy. Human epilepsy entails synaptic remodeling and glutamatergic hyperexcitability as found in the kindling model per se, even though kindling has not been shown to occur in humans. Intrinsic resting membrane properties of neurons in human epileptic tissue seem normal. NMDA receptors tend to be spread through deep layers of the neocortex in people with epilepsy, whereas they are normally concentrated in the outer layers. Several groups have shown sprouting of mossy fibers into the inner molecular layer of the dentate gyrus of the hippocampus of humans with epilepsy, much like that seen in kindled animals. This sprouting is associated with an increased number of kainate receptors and perhaps decreased inhibition. Exaggerated bursting with protracted firing of action potentials at high frequency occur in neocortical slices. Stimulation of human epileptic hippocampus at low frequencies produces excessive burst firing similar to that seen when the GABA antagonist bicuculline is injected. These findings require further confirmation. However, they provide a rational basis for planning therapeutic strategies, and they increase confidence in impressions from animal models.

Animal models have been central in the identification of anticonvulsant activity of structurally unique compounds. In some cases, however, investigational compounds have been ineffective or proconvulsant in clinical trials, resulting in discontinuation of costly studies. One competitive NMDA-antagonist, D-CPP-ene, appeared very effective and with little toxicity in animal models. However, half of the eight patients in the phase II clinical trial experienced increased seizure frequency, and all withdrew because of side effects, many of them cognitive. To explain this discrepancy between efficacy in animal models and patients, Löscher and colleagues have suggested that epileptic tissue may respond differently to drugs than normal tissue that has been induced to express electrical and behavioral seizures. The noncompetitive channel blocker MK-801 failed in clinical trials for other reasons, purportedly because of poor oral bioavailability and tachyphylaxis in the face of repeatedly increased doses.

What is the impact of such findings on the development of glutamate antagonists for clinical use? Felbatol is an example of a noncompetitive NMDA-glutamate antagonist that did not produce untoward behavioral effects in most patients yet potently decreased seizures. If one accepts patch clamp data, felbamate has a relatively low affinity for its binding site. On the other hand, MK-801 and CPP-ene are very potent compounds with high affinities for their binding sites. This situation is analogous to the case of sodium channel blockers in which highly potent high-affinity compounds, such as tetrodotoxin, are lethal, while drugs with a relatively low affinity or brief dwell-time on the receptor, such as phenytoin, tend to be clinically useful and relatively safe. If it all is simply a matter of degree, it is pertinent to ask how many receptors must be blocked to raise the seizure threshold without significant adverse effects. The examples given here suggest that potent drugs have potent side effects. This leads to the conclusion that a wide therapeutic index, and not potency, is the most important characteristic in identifying novel antiepileptic drugs.

Neonatal glycine encephalopathy provides a unique clinical insight into the role of excitatory amino acid mechanisms. Blood and brain glycine concentrations rise because of deficiency of the glycine cleavage enzyme system (see Chapter 69). Glycine is an essential coagonist at NMDA/GluRs. It increases NMDA receptor channel openings by enhancing the rate of recovery from desensitization in the presence of glutamate and thereby potentiates excitotoxic effects of glutamate. This has led to the proposal that neonatal glycine encephalopathy is a neurotransmitter disease rather than a disease of myelin production. A 10-week-old with glycine encephalopathy showed clinical and electroencephalographic improvement when treated with dextromethorphan (35 mg/kg per day), a channel-blocking NMDA antagonist. Withdrawal of dextromethorphan caused deterioration of both parameters, which improved again when dextromethorphan was reinstituted. There are also unpublished anecdotes of therapeutic benefit of another NMDA channel blocker, ketamine, in the treatment of refractory status epilepticus. This suggests that glutamatergic hyperexcitability may sustain abnormal firing in metabolic disorders and in status epilepticus.

Parkinson's Disease. Glutamatergic hyperexcitability and excitotoxicity have been implicated in several degenerative processes. In Parkinson's disease, the inhibitory output of the internal globus pallidus is enhanced by a glutamatergic input from the subthalamic nucleus (see Chapter 76). Overactivity of this pathway becomes obvious as the dopaminergic nigrostriatal pathway degenerates. Small lesions in the subthalamic nucleus markedly reduce tremor, rigidity, and bradykinesia. Low-affinity noncompetitive NMDA antagonists—e.g., remacemide and memantine—improve function in animal models of parkinsonism. Neither of these compounds has been shown to produce significant PCP-like locomotor excitation or psychosis. Once again, low-affinity drugs may have advantages over high-affinity drugs like MK-801, which severely reduce glutamatergic activity. In addition, because of use-dependence, noncompetitive blockers have the advantage of being effective against very high levels of glutamate at doses that should be tolerable clinically. Use-dependence requires multiple activations for a maximal drug effect to occur, such as that weak drugs become more potent, in effect, with persisting activity.

Some NMDA blockers have multiple actions, some of which may be relevant to the treatment of parkinsonism. For example, MK-801 blocks acetylcholine-activated current and limits high-frequency firing of action potentials. Remacemide also blocks high-frequency action potential firing. Amantadine and memantine both have anticholinergic activity. This anticholinergic effect may reduce tremor but contribute to cognitive adverse effects and dementia.

Stroke. NMDA blockers have been tested extensively in focal and global models of ischemia in animals and in vitro. Virtually every clinically used antiepileptic medication reduces experimental infarct size. Unfortunately, this often occurs only at toxic concentrations. The noncompetitive NMDA blockers, including remacemide, should be advantageous in the treatment of acute glutamate-induced neuronal injury for reasons pointed out above. Felbamate might also be useful for neuroprotection if not for its systemic toxicity. It was effective against delayed neuronal death in tissue culture and in animal models and did not cause significant PCP-like behavioral effects in humans.

Dementia. Memantine is in phase 2 clinical trials for the treatment of AIDS-related dementia, which has also been linked to the accumulation of quinolinic acid, an endogenous NMDA-like amino acid. Tetrahydroamino-acridine (tacrine) also is an open channel blocker of NMDA-gated current at high concentrations. This action may combine with weak anticholinesterase activity to make tacrine useful in the treatment of mild-to-moderate dementia of the Alzheimer's type.

Amytrophic Lateral Sclerosis. Transport of glutamate may be decreased in the brain and spinal cord of patients with amyotrophic lateral sclerosis (ALS), and glutamate and aspartate cerebrospinal fluid (CSF) concentrations are increased in patients with ALS as compared to controls. Chronic inhibition of glutamate reuptake in cultured neurons by highly potent and specific blockers of the glutamate transporter results in delayed neuronal death over weeks. In cultured organotypic spinal cord slices, this results in the slow disappearance of the large motor neurons and may be an in vitro model for ALS. It is unknown why large motor neurons are selectively targeted in vivo and in vitro. Branched-chain amino acids (leucine, isoleucine, and valine) stimulate glutamic acid dehydrogenase, the enzyme that converts glutamate to GABA. This suggests the possibility of discovering an equivalent to levodopa (L-dopa) for the treatment of certain degenerative diseases. Interestingly, gabapentin, a newly approved antiepileptic medication, is transported by the L-amino acid transporter that recognizes bulky amino acids such as L-leucine and phenylalanine and is reported to reduce the loss of motor neurons in vitro. Gabapentin may decrease the synthesis of glutamate and enhance the rate of conversion of glutamate to GABA by virtue of a low affinity for the enzymes involved in these two steps. It also enhances the GABA-mediated hyperpolarization caused by nipecotic acid, a GABA uptake inhibitor and component of the anticonvulsant tiagabine, in hippocampus and olfactory nerve. Gabapentin may reverse the transporter and allow GABA to exit the neuron down its concentration gradient (millimolar inside, micromolar out). These alterations in amino acid economics could contribute to both anticonvulsant and neuroprotective activity of gabapentin. It remains unclear how these actions affect glutamate release and whether these actions are operant in ALS. Many patients with ALS have demanded treatment with gabapentin. A controlled trial is underway despite widespread availability of the drug.

Dietary Intoxications and Excitotoxic Injury. Excitotoxins in the diet are increasingly recognized to be involved in the pathogenesis of neurodegenerative disorders and seizures in humans. For example, acute intoxication with domoate can cause an acute encephalopathy with generalized seizures and coma. Retrograde amnesia is another common finding. Examination of postmortem material reveals changes in the hippocampus suggestive of amino acid–induced limbic seizures. The domoate is produced by a marine diatom, *Nitschia pungens*, which is filtered by edible mollusks (e.g., blue mussels). Domoate is a kainate-like compound that is widely used at nontoxic doses as an ascaricide for Japanese children. Injection of kainate into adult animals produces seizures and neuronal damage. Acromelic acid is a kainate-like compound produced by the poisonous mushroom *Clitocybe acromelalgia.* Injection of this compound into rodents does not result in hippocampal changes but does produce hind-limb extension and tonic-clonic seizures mediated at the spinal cord level. It appears that kainate receptors in the brain and spinal cord differ, perhaps because of their subunit composition.

Chronic intoxication with dietary amino acids is best exemplified by the chronic ingestion of the chick pea, *Lathyrus sativus*. This pea contains β-*N*-oxalylamino-L-alanine (BOAA), an NMDA-receptor agonist. Its consumption causes neurolathyrism, a subacute or progressive spastic paraplegia that develops over weeks to months (see Chapter 79). On the island of Guam, ingestion of a starch staple produced from the nut of the cyad tree seems to be associated with a high incidence of a distinctive syndrome of ALS-parkinsonism-dementia among residents (see Chapter 79). The flower, if improperly prepared, contains residual β-methylamino-L-alanine (BMAA) and several other toxins that could give rise to delayed neuronal injury with a clinical appearance of neurodegeneration.

Although in animals L-cysteine produces seizures that are blocked by antagonists of NMDA receptors, oral cysteine administration in humans is not known to cause neurodegenerative syndromes. However, the ratio of plasma cysteine to sulfate is increased fivefold in some neurodegenerative disorders, and further studies are warranted.

Pain. Hypersensitivity associated with neuropathic pains, arthritis, and pain caused by repetitive activation of primary afferent fibers (windup pain) may involve activation of glutamatergic neurons. Many of these types of pains are blocked by NMDA and non-NMDA antagonists administered intrathecally or intra-arterially in animals and in humans. Pain-like behavior is produced by microinjection of glutamate into the region of the mesencephalic periaqueductal gray and antagonized by MK-801 and AP5, suggesting a role for GluRs in central pain processing.

Ethanol given intrathecally blocks the thermal hyperalgesia produced in rats by loose suturing of the sciatic nerve. Ethanol is known to block NMDA receptors competitively. Ethanol also clearly elevates pain thresholds.

Psychotogenic Effects. The potential for significant adverse effects of some of the glutamate antagonists, particularly those highly potent at NMDA receptors and channels, may limit their clinical utility. The examples of MK-801 and CPP-ene have already been given; these are both potent open-channel blockers of the NMDA receptor channel complex. MK-801 has been implicated in the production of microvacuolation of central myelin. Both of these compounds may produce adverse behavioral effects due to interaction at multiple receptors. MK-801 is anticholinergic, and PCP has effects at biogenic amine receptors. Hallucinogens such as LSD bind to serotonin receptors. Also, there is clear evidence from compounds currently in clinical use that drugs with relatively low affinity for the GluR channel complex may be effective therapeutic agents without significant adverse behavioral effects in most patients.

Headache (Migraine). One of the components of Chinese restaurant syndrome, which is induced by monosodium glutamate, is migrainous headache. Recognition of this has led to investigation of a therapeutic role for glutamate blockers in the treatment of migraine.

Acetylcholine

Hollywood's infatuation with curare, a variety of highly toxic, paralytic plant extracts used originally as arrow poison in South America, has probably made the nicotinic cholinergic receptor the best-known receptor in the world. The nicotinic receptor was the first to be purified, sequenced, and cloned. Over the past two decades, the structures of several nicotinic and muscarinic receptors, and of choline transporters and the synthetic enzyme choline acetyltransferase (CAT), have been deduced using biochemical and molecular techniques.

Chemistry and Distribution

Acetylcholine (ACh) is a monoamine neurotransmitter that rotates around bonds in its alkyl spine. The *cis* conformation is the predominant species in solution, but the *trans* conformation is the one that binds to muscarinic receptors. Therefore, ACh binding to its receptor requires adaptive torsional changes within the molecule, presumably induced by electrostatic interactions with the receptor. The formation of ACh from choline and acetyl coenzyme A (Co-A) is catalyzed by CAT, and its hydrolysis is catalyzed by acetylcholinesterase (AChE). Histochemical localization of CAT allows detection of neurons capable of synthesizing ACh. Histochemical localization of AChE and cholinergic receptors does not distinguish neurons capable of synthesizing ACh from cholinoceptive neurons. CAT is synthesized in neuronal somata and transported down axons to the nerve terminals. It is present in synaptosomes in two states: soluble in cytoplasm, and bound to the outer membrane of the transmitter storage vesicles. Neurotansmitter synthesis takes place in the terminals. Choline is not synthesized in neurons de novo. A high-affinity transporter recycles choline released by enzymatic degradation of ACh by AchE or released into the interstitial space by the breakdown of phosphatidylcholine. Acetyl Co-A originates in mitochondria, but the mechanism for its egress into the cytoplasm and participation in the synthesis of ACh is unknown. The rate-limiting step in ACh synthesis may be the transport of acetyl Co-A out of mitochondria.

Neurons have two uptake systems for choline: a low-affinity system with a K_m of 10–100 μmol/liter, and a high-affinity system with a K_m of 1–5 μmol/liter. The gene for the high- affinity transporter has been cloned. However, sodium-dependent choline uptake by the high-affinity transporter is not blocked by hemicholinium, a potent inhibitor of neuronal choline uptake. This finding could indicate that functional components of the cloned transporter system are missing or malfunctioning. Alternatively, another system may be involved in vivo.

ACh is present in the cytoplasm and in vesicles in nerve terminals. Neurophysiological and neurochemical studies suggest the existence of two functional pools of ACh—one that is readily available for release and one that is held in reserve. How these pools relate to the location of ACh is uncertain. Newly synthesized ACh is released first. An ATPase pumps hydrogen ions into the vesicles so they are internally acidified and positively charged. A highly specific transporter in the vesicle wall then exchanges ACh for hydrogen ions to maintain (countertransport) electroneutrality and the osmotic balance within the vesicle. Uptake of ACh into vesicles can be blocked noncompetitively by vesamicol. This blocks the release of newly synthesized radioactively labelled ACh without affecting ACh synthesis, the influx of calcium into nerve terminals, or high-affinity choline uptake. This provides strong evidence that vesicular ACh is released from cholinergic terminals. The readily available pool may be composed of vesicles close to the subsynaptic membrane and therefore more readily released by exocytosis. The reserve pool would then be represented by vesicles more distant from the terminal membrane.

Slow release of ACh occurs continuously, presumably because of spontaneous fusion of vesicles to the presynaptic membrane. The constant trickle of ACh produces miniature endplate potentials that are detectable at rest. Depolarization of the axon terminal by the arrival of action potentials augments transmitter release. The amount released depends on the duration of depolarization and rate of firing, the depolarization-induced influx of calcium through specific calcium channels, and the ratio of extracellular calcium to magnesium. Each vesicle contains several thousand molecules of ACh, which are usually bound to ATP or a proteoglycan within the vesicles. All of these components are released by exocytosis after fusion of the vesicle to the inner side of the synaptic membrane. Cytoplasmic ACh may contribute to the fraction released by depolarization by calcium-ACh translocation.

The released ACh diffuses across the synaptic space, where it binds to pathway-specific ACh receptors in the central and peripheral nervous system and at the neuromuscular junction and exerts its physiological effects. The effect of ACh is terminated by dissociation from the postsynaptic receptors, hydrolysis by AChE, and reuptake of the released choline into the terminals. The exocytosis of neurotransmitter, membrane recycling, and reuptake of choline must be tightly coupled to avoid significant changes in the surface area of the synapse. Cycling of the vesicular membrane may be the rate-limiting step for both release and reuptake.

Cholinesterases are widely distributed in the body. Nonspecific or butyrylcholinesterase is produced in the liver, circulates in the plasma, and is also present in the CNS. A specific AChE is associated with cholinergic innervation and is localized on synapses. Much is known of the structure, and of the transcriptional and posttranscriptional regulation, of AChE production. A soluble globular form of AChE and a so-called asymmetric form exist. The latter has a collagenous tail for membrane-binding in synaptic areas. AChE inhibition can occur by a number of mechanisms, including binding of drugs such as edrophonium to the active site of the enzyme to prevent access of substrate; binding of reversible inhibitors such as gallamine and propidium to peripheral binding sites on the enzyme; and by the combination of carbamyl groups of drugs, such as physostigmine and neostigmine, with the active site serine group. Anticholinesterase compounds can cause clinical symptoms in humans; these include insecticides, drugs used to treat myasthenia gravis (see Chapter 83), and those developed for use as chemical warfare agents.

Acetylcholine Receptors. Nicotinic and muscarinic receptors are distributed widely in the nervous system. Nicotinic receptors are present at the mammalian muscle endplate and sympathetic ganglion neurons. Centrally, nicotinic responses are described in the cerebral cortex, hippocampus, thalamus, neostriatum, and interpeduncular nucleus. The optic tectum seems to rely primarily on nicotinic muscarinic activity, as does the negative feedback of the Renshaw cell on motor neurons of the spinal cord.

Muscarinic receptors with a high affinity for pirenzepine, a high-affinity antagonist of M_1 receptors, are abundant in the hippocampus and cerebral cortex. Neurons bearing receptors with low affinity for pirenzepine are found in the cerebellum and brain stem. Outside the CNS, muscarinic receptors are present on tissues innervated by parasympathetic postganglionic neurons, and some sympathetic responses, especially sweating and piloerection, depend on postganglionic sympathetic fibers that secrete ACh onto tissues with muscarinic receptors.

Muscle Nicotinic Receptors. The nicotinic ACh receptor was the first of the receptors to be isolated and purified, because of its abundance in *Torpedo* electroplax. The receptors are so plentiful that they form virtually a crystalline array, which has been studied with electron microscopy. The receptor is a pentamer formed of different types of subunits: two α-subunits and one each of the β-, γ-, and δ-subunits (Karlin 1993). In adult muscle, the subunit ε replaces the δ-subunit with resultant changes in single-channel conductance and kinetics. Several receptor types are present in embryonic muscle and extrajunctionally in denervated adult muscle. Differences in receptor combinations are likely to account for subtle differences in conductance through these receptor subtypes. The pentameric structure surrounds a central cavity or channel that opens to a diameter of about 6.5 Å when agonists bind to each of the α-subunits. Occupation of both sites is necessary for receptor activation, as indicated by Hill coefficient >1. Sites within the channel bind noncompetitive inhibitors such as local anesthetics. The sequence of the different subunits includes a long extracellular amino end of approximately 200 amino acid residues followed by four membrane-spanning regions connected by intra- and extracellular peptide loops. This is followed by a short carboxy-terminal end. The subunits of *Torpedo* electroplax nicotinic ACh receptors have 495–512 amino acid residues each. Each of the membrane-spanning regions has 19–27 amino acid residues. The long cytoplasmic loop between the third and fourth membrane-spanning regions is about 150 residues long. This type of structure is typical of ionotropic neurotransmitter-gate receptors. Because of the hydrophobicity of the membrane-spanning regions, it has been proposed that the residues are organized in α-helical or β-pleated sheet formations. The different subunits have about 30–40% identity of their amino acid residues. The agonist binding site is included in the extracellular amino terminal segment, and mutations in this portion of the α- and δ-subunits cause changes in the binding of ACh, which suggests that ACh binds at the interface between the α- and β-subunits.

Lophoptoxin, a diterpinoid plant toxin, competitively blocks the binding of ACh at residues 190–192. Serine residues in the β- and δ-subunits and in the second membrane-spanning region bind the noncompetitive inhibitors chlorpromazine and tetraphenylphosphonium. α-Toxins from snake venom, including α-bungarotoxin, bind to extensive regions of the α-subunit, primarily. Physical techniques suggest that the binding site for both ACh and the snake venom α-toxins is on the outer perimeter of the receptor near the membrane surface, rather than covering or entering the channel. Hexamethonium and decamethonium produce a voltage-dependent block of recombinant neuromuscular nicotinic-cholinergic receptors suggesting that they enter the channel.

Other toxins bind at different sites. Neosurugatoxin selectively blocks ganglionic nicotinic receptors, and lophotoxin blocks ganglionic and neuromuscular nicotinic receptors. The marine α-conotoxins G1A and M1 potently block neuromuscular transmission, but not ganglionic nicotinic activity. This differential binding suggests that the ganglionic nicotinic receptors differ in subunit composition from the neuromuscular receptor.

Neuronal Nicotinic Receptors. Neuronal nicotinic receptors are ionotropic receptors. Ten or more receptor subunit genes (α_{2-8} and β_{2-5}) have been cloned. Functional ACh-gated channels are expressed in frog oocytes injected with mRNAs for α- and β-receptors in combination, or when cell lines are transfected with cDNAs for both α- and β-receptor subunits. In general, α-subunits contain the ligand binding site and β-subunits are structural. However, functional pentamers of α_7- or α_8-subunits have been expressed. Receptors that contain the α_7-subunit conduct calcium ions.

Central nicotinic neuronal receptors have been mapped using in situ hybridization methods. Use of radiolabeled cDNA fragments localizes genes for various subunits. Antisense RNA transcribed from single-stranded cDNA localizes the mRNA for the subunits. The α_2-subunit is distributed widely. Varied electrophysiological and pharmacological properties of receptors containing α_2-subunits in combination with a variety of other subunits have been described in different brain regions.

Neuronal Muscarinic Receptors. Muscarinic receptors are metabotropic receptors (Caulfield 1993). Five receptors belonging to the family of G protein–associated receptors have been isolated. Agonists are thought to bind in a deep pocket formed by the seven transmembrane regions that share the greatest sequence homology with other monomeric receptor subtypes. Variations in the long third intracellular loop result not only in differences in the binding to G proteins but also in the effects of antagonists, as shown by site-directed mutagenesis. This technique uses synthetic oligonucleotide sequences with deliberately introduced differences from naturally occurring sequences as primers to synthesize cDNA. The expressed receptors contain mutations involving one or a few amino acids that alter receptor function. Selectivity of antagonists for cloned receptors parallels pharmacologically defined receptor activity in naturally occurring, more intact systems. For example, both cloned and naturally occurring M1 receptors are selectively blocked by pirenzepine, and M2 receptors are preferentially blocked by AFDX-116.

Types 1, 3, and 5 muscarinic receptors couple to members of the Gq family of G proteins. In turn, the G protein activated by ligand binding to the receptor activates phospholipase C. This results in phospholipid hydrolysis that liberates two intracellular second messengers, IP_3 and DAG. Each of these intracellular second messengers has unique effects, as described above. The IP_3 releases intracellular calcium stores and can be involved in cascades of cellular injury. DAG activates protein kinase C, which phosphorylates several receptors and alters their conductance states. Receptors of the M2 and M4 type couple to the α-subunit of the inhibitory G_i protein that inhibits adenylyl cyclase and reduces intracellular cyclic AMP levels. Alternatively, these two receptors can couple to certain ion channels directly by either of the GTP-binding proteins, G_i or G_o. The muscarinic receptor subtypes are differentially distributed in the brain. The hippocampus is virtually devoid of the M2-type receptor, but the other four types are expressed to varying degrees, with M1 having the densest expression. Here, ACh has multiple excitatory effects because of receptor coupling to various potassium channels. As expected, pirenzepine blocks most of the effects of ACh on hippocampal neurons, and ACh induces a pirenzepine-insensitive hyperpolarization in the thalamus where the M2 receptor is significantly expressed. The hyperpolarization appears to result directly from increased potassium conductance as a result of receptor activation coupled to G_i. Thus, although less is known about the functions of M3–5, physiologically and pharmacologically defined regional effects of ACh parallel expression of genes for various subtypes of muscarinic receptors.

Long-term regulation of receptor numbers is an important property of muscarinic receptors that must be considered when drugs are designed to treat neurological disorders. Prolonged exposure to ACh or other agonists causes downregulation of muscarinic receptors. The only available Alzheimer's disease treatment agent, tetrahydroaminoacridine, raises brain ACh levels by weakly inhibiting AChE. Reports of mixed efficacy could in part be due to downregulation of receptors, which opposes the effect of chronically increased ACh levels. Protein kinase activation can mimic the effects of prolonged exposure to agonists. For example, activation of protein kinase C by tumor-promoting phorbol esters results in internalization and degradation of muscarinic receptors. This is thought to result from receptor phosphorylation. A candidate protein kinase is called MARK, an acronym for muscarinic ACh receptor kinase, by analogy with the β-adrenergic receptor kinase involved in regulating the long-term availability of adrenergic receptors. Presumably, phosphorylation reduces affinity of the receptor for agonists, and dephosphorylation, by unknown phosphorylases, results in resensitization or availability of the receptors. Phosphorylation-dependent desensitization may be a common mode of regulation of G protein–coupled receptors. The subtypes of muscarinic receptors that are sensitive to this type of regulation have not been identified, but controlling this process could afford therapy with agents designed to modulate receptor numbers in specific brain regions.

Acetylcholine Receptors in Disease States

Cholinergic agents are used to treat many clinical disorders. The pharmacology of cholinergic systems are discussed in terms of normal and pathological function (Figure 52.4).

Smoking. The effects of nicotine are complex, because it acts both peripherally at sympathetic ganglia and within the CNS. A nationwide debate has arisen over the adverse health effects of tobacco smoking and its impact on medical economics. The agreeable effects of nicotine and the craving during the withdrawal state make smoking cessation difficult. The availability of molecular techniques to determine regional differences in subunit composition of central nicotinic receptors may improve our understanding sufficiently to explain the behaviors attached to smoking and improve methods of smoking cessation.

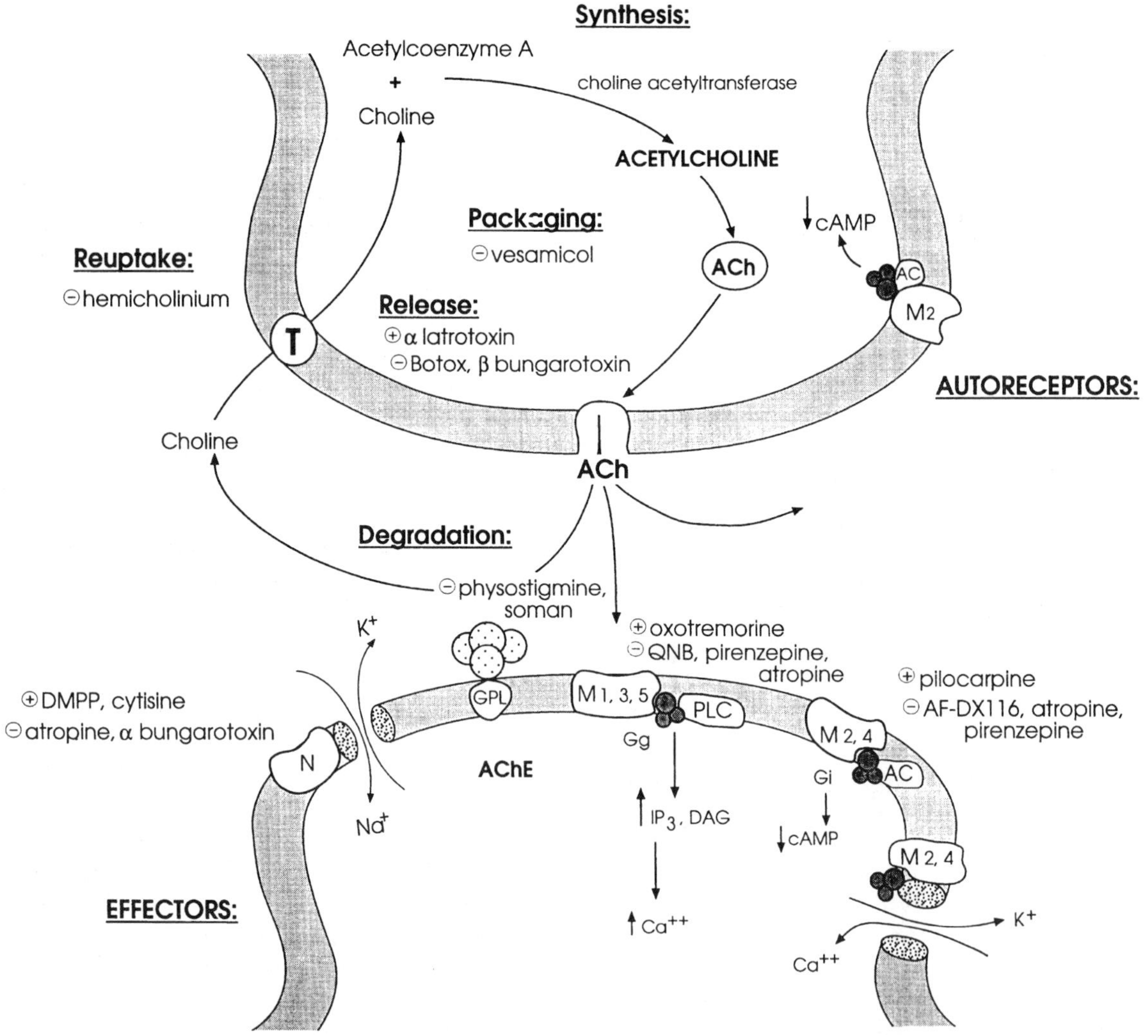

FIGURE 52.4 Pharmacology of central acetylcholine receptors. There are no clinically used inhibitors of acetylcholine synthesis. The packaging of acetylcholine into presynaptic vesicles can be reduced experimentally by vesamicol. Release of acetylcholine is enhanced by α latrotoxin and inhibited by botulinum toxin (botox) and β bungarotoxin. Release is also modulated by presynaptic autoreceptors. The G protein-linked M2 muscarinic receptor decreases cAMP production presynaptically and indirectly decreases neurotransmitter release, presumably by decreasing activation by phosphorylation of calcium-dependent calmodulin. Released acetylcholine diffuses across the synaptic cleft and activates both nicotinic and muscarinic receptors in the CNS. Nicotinic receptors are ionotropic, and activation results in admission of sodium and exit of potassium through the channel. Muscarinic receptors are metabotropic. Muscarinic M1, 3, and 5 receptors are linked by Gq to phospholipase C. Activation of these receptors results in increased intracellular calcium due to the production of IP3 as the intracellular second messenger. Muscarinic M2 and M4 are linked to adenylyl cyclase by the inhibitory G protein Gi. The result is decreased intracellular cAMP. Some postsynaptic M2 and M4 receptors are linked by G proteins directly to ion channels, which allow entry of calcium and exit of potassium. The action of acetylcholine at its postsynaptic receptors is terminated principally by degradation. AChE in the postsynaptic membrane results in the release of choline, which is resequestered by a specific transporter (T) in the presynaptic membrane and is then resynthesized into acetylcholine for subsequent release. Agonists (⊕) and antagonists (⊖) have been identified for many of these specific receptors and processes.

Mitochondropathies. ACh synthesis is markedly reduced in some inherited disorders of mitochondrial enzymes and thiamine-dependent pyruvate dehydrogenase (the enzyme that catalyzes the oxidation of pyruvate to acetyl Co-A). Affected patients have mental retardation, spasticity, ataxia, and dystonia. The diversity of symptoms emphasizes the multiple functions subserved by cholinergic neurotransmission.

Aging. In rodents, aging is accompanied by a 20% reduction of cholinergic neurons in the striatum and of cholinoceptive pyramidal neurons in the hippocampus. Afferent cholinergic projections decrease in both areas. In the hippocampus, CAT is reduced by up to 50% and AChE by 25%. These changes are associated with a 40–50% reduction of muscarinic and nicotinic receptors in striatum and the hippocampus. Receptor decline in the striatum could be a cause of senile tremor, and receptor decline in the hippocampus a cause of senile memory loss. Treatment of the elderly with anticholinergic drugs, such as tricyclic antidepressants, antihistamines, and anticholinergic, anti-parkinsonian, and some cardiovascular drugs probably produces pseudodementia by further reducing cholinergic activity.

Alzheimer's Disease. The loss of central cholinergic neurons is accelerated in Alzheimer's disease as compared to normal aging. Brain CAT activity is reduced 50–70% and parallels loss of neurons in the nucleus basalis of Meynert and in the ascending cholinergic projections to the cerebral cortex and hippocampus. The benefits of cholinomimetic therapy of Alzheimer's disease are not yet substantial, but this approach was supported by the approval of tetrahydroaminoacridine, a weak inhibitor of AChE, for the treatment of mild to moderate Alzheimer's disease. Several novel cholinomimetic agents are undergoing clinical trials.

Characterization of the cerebral changes in postsynaptic cholinergic receptor subtypes in Alzheimer's disease may help focus the stategy of drug development. The M1 receptor is expressed most intensely in both cortex and hippocampus and should be an ideal target for therapeutic manipulation. The M3 and M4 subtypes are other likely targets. The hippocampus is devoid of the M2 receptor and the cortex seems devoid of the M5 receptor; therefore these seem to be less opportune therapeutic targets. Drugs with potent M2 receptor activity have the disadvantage of producing adverse cardiovascular and gastrointestinal effects because these organs have a high expression of M2 receptors. In addition, M2 agonists would enhance presynaptic autoreceptor function and tend to diminish the release of endogenous ACh, and even to decrease its synthesis in still-functional neurons; these effects would antagonize the strategy of elevating brain ACh. Because of the many other pathological changes in Alzheimer's disease brains, even treatment with agents specifically targeting M1, M3, and M4 receptors may only partially treat the cognitive symptoms of this disease. Improvement of memory is probably the single most important advantage of augmenting cholinergic function in Alzheimer's disease (see Chapter 71A). This may also be accomplished by agents that act on other affected neurotransmitter systems.

Increased dietary intake of choline does not alter the course of Alzheimer's disease. Investigation of high-affinity uptake mechanisms and molecular characteristics of CAT may provide new understanding of pathogenesis and approaches to therapy. Growth factors, such as nerve growth factor, are potentially useful to protect and promote the repair of cholinergic neurons but have not yet been studied in large controlled trials. Growth factors are secreted locally after brain injuries and may regulate glial proliferation and promote neuronal survival. Gangliosides and glycosphingolipids may be neuronotrophic factors themselves or binding sites for growth factors. Increased blood concentrations of anti-GM1 antibody is seen primarily in lower motor neuron diseases, and administration of GM1 prevents reduction of brain CAT concentrations and increases high-affinity choline uptake in animals with cortical lesions. Therefore, drugs that influence GM1 are potentially useful for the treatment of Alzheimer's disease.

Parkinson's Disease. Anticholinergic medications such as benztropine and trihexyphenidyl are beneficial in the treatment of some movement disorders. The working hypothesis in Parkinson's disease is that an overbalance of cholinergic neurotransmission results from profound reduction of dopaminergic input from the substantia nigra pars compacta to the striatum (see Chapter 76). Intrinsic cholinergic innervation of the striatum is predominantly muscarinic. Large spiny interneurons in the striatum contain CAT. These neurons receive glutamatergic inputs from the cortex and thalamus and dopaminergic input from the substantia nigra. Axons with histochemical reactivity for GAD, the GABA synthetic enzyme, and substance P are presumably collaterals from the medium spiny neurons they innervate. The medium spiny neurons are the source of predominantly GABAergic output to the pallidum and the substantia nigra pars reticulata, which in turn feeds back to disinhibit the thalamus and leads to glutamatergic outflow to both the striatum and the cerebral cortex.

In the striatum, AChE-poor islands, or striosomes, are embedded in a meshwork (matrix) rich in AChE. The meshwork and the striosomes have different inputs and outputs. The meshwork receives cholinergic input and contains both muscarinic and nicotinic receptors. Presynaptic M2 receptors are thought to inhibit the release of glutamate by activating a hyperpolarizing potassium conductance at the terminal or by decreasing the influx of calcium necessary for neurotransmitter release. The result is damping of the excitatory input from the thalamus and cortex. Nicotinic receptors are generally excitatory and promote transmitter release in the region. The successful use of anticholinergics in the treatment of movement disorders, including parkinsonism and dystonia, emphasizes the importance of the cholinergic innervation of the striatum. Receptor subtype-selective antagonists are not yet available for clinical use. Some experts feel that a better response is obtained by simultaneous treatment with more than one anticholinergic agent, perhaps to cover all receptor bases. This leaves room for some pharmacological creativity. Since patients with Parkinson's disease often have sleep difficulties and depression, the use of anticholinergic tricyclic antidepressants such as amitriptyline may be helpful. At the same time, tremor may diminish. Alternatively, anticholinergic antihistamines such as diphenhydramine may provide additional benefit. Amantadine, which is believed to enhance dopaminergic neurotransmisision, is also a muscarinic antagonist. Memantine (dimethylaminoadamantane), an amantadine-like drug, is both anticholinergic and an NMDA channel blocker, and is clinically useful in the treatment of Parkinson's disease. Unfortunate adverse effects of anticholinergic drugs, particularly in the elderly, are hallucinosis and pseudodementia.

Huntington's Chorea. The striatal concentration of CAT is markedly reduced in patients dying with Huntington's chorea. AChE inhibitors, such as physostigmine, have been tried clinically with variable results, perhaps because the resultant elevation of ACh levels activates local or distant cholinergic inputs indiscriminately.

The high incidence of schizophrenia among people with Huntington's disease has suggested that schizophrenia may result, in part, from deficiency of cholinergic neurotransmission. In support of that suggestion are the known toxic effects of belladonna, from which atropine is extracted, including hallucinosis, psychosis, and pseudodementia. Against this view is the fact that phenothiazines, butyrophenones, and tricyclic antidepressants, used to treat schizophrenia and schizoaffective disorders, have anticholinergic properties. The anticholinergic properties of antipsychotic drugs may contribute to adverse effects, while therapeutic benefit may result from other actions, such as dopamine blockade.

Vertigo and Motion Sensitivity. Drugs with anticholinergic properties are used frequently to treat motion sickness, vertigo (as with Ménière's disease or labyrinthitis), and space sickness. These include antihistamines (e.g., meclizine, cyclizine, and dimenhydrinate) and tricyclic antidepressants (e.g., amitriptyline, imipramine, and doxepin). Phenothiazines are particularly effective in conditions in which nausea and vomiting are profound, because they decrease the inhibitory dopaminergic drive on the medullary vomiting center in addition to treating the vertigo by anticholinergic, and probably other, mechanisms. The anticholinergic properties of antihistamines are also useful in the treatment of both vomiting and nausea. The mechanism by which anticholinergic mechanisms suppress these symptoms is not established, but they may act on cholinergic receptors in the labyrinth or vestibulocerebellar pathways. Transdermal scopolamine has become popular for the treatment of motion sickness. The addition of dextroamphetamine seems to enhance the efficacy of scopolamine and eliminates side effects such as drowsiness and amnesia.

Anticholinesterase Intoxication. Human intoxication with pesticides such as parathion, or with organophosphorus chemical warfare agents such as soman, may cause intractable, sometimes lethal, seizures. These drugs work primarily by blocking AChE and thereby increasing tissue ACh concentrations. Pyridostigmine, an orally active inhibitor of AChE, was used prophylactically by about 41,000 American troops in Operation Desert Storm as an antidote to chemical warfare agents. Minor symptoms of cholinergic hyperactivity without degradation of performance were reported, and 30–600 mg were ingested in 1 day to 1 week. Coadministration with atropine (to block muscarinic overactivity) and pralidoxime (to prevent aging of the nerve agent/AChE complex and to reactivate the enzyme) increased survival after exposure to lethal doses of chemical warfare agents. Pyridostigmine was adopted because of efficacy in primate studies and safety data in humans. Physostigmine is not an ideal drug for this purpose, because it penetrates the blood-brain barrier poorly, while the life-threatening effects of nerve agents result from CNS intoxication and seizures. Memantine is a possible alternative that protects AChE from blockade by nerve agents at a nonesteratic site unaffected by hemicholinium. Memantine also blocks NMDA channels and responses of cultured neurons to ACh and limits high-frequency firing of sodium-dependent action potentials. Prophylactic use could be limited by the possibility of psychotogenic effects due to NMDA receptor channel blockade. Clinical trials have not been reported.

Many of the severe problems reported by Gulf War veterans—including immune system deficits, tumors, cognitive defects, and birth defects among their progeny—have not been found in the chronic treatment of patients with myasthenia gravis with higher doses of pyridostigmine. Even though treating normal individuals is different than treating myasthenics, it seems unlikely that pyridostigmine was a major contributor to the plethora of complaints that have come to be known, rightly or wrongly, as "the Gulf War syndrome."

AChE blockade has been a principal therapeutic strategy in the treatment of myasthenia gravis (see Chapter 83).

Myasthenia Gravis. Myasthenia gravis is a disorder of muscle nicotinic-cholinergic receptors. Circulating anti-ACh receptor antibodies cause loss of nicotinic receptors from the postsynaptic neuromuscular junction. These receptors are normally anchored by a structural protein, rapsyn or 43K, that links the receptors to skeletal elements and restricts their lateral diffusional mobility within the membrane. Denervation disturbs the anchor and causes extrajunctional spread. Extrajunctional receptors of denervated muscle contain the δ-subunit characteristic of developing muscle, rather than the ε-receptor of mature junctional receptors. The factors controlling this change in receptor subunit composition are incompletely understood and not yet amenable to therapeutic manipulation.

Edrophonium, an AChE inhibitor with a half-life of minutes, is used as a diagnostic test for the condition. Pyridostigmine is the cholinesterase inhibitor most often used for treatment, although it has not been compared in controlled trials with other available agents. An elimination half-life of several hours makes multiple daily doses necessary (as often as every 2–4 hours). A slow-release preparation may help overnight, but oral bioavailability is poor (approximately 15%). Poor penetration of the blood-brain barrier minimizes CNS adverse effects. The general increase in available ACh causes muscarinic overactivity (especially bradycardia, excessive salivation, and diarrhea) and improves nicotinic neuromuscular transmission. In some cases, atropine is used to block the muscarinic effects.

Myasthenic Syndrome. Decreased release of ACh causes weakness and areflexia in the myasthenic (Lambert-Eaton) syndrome (see Chapter 83). This disorder, which is often paraneoplastic, is associated with serum antibodies against presynaptic voltage-sensitive calcium channels that admit calcium necessary for release of ACh. The active zone where transmitter vesicles fuse for release from the terminal is structurally abnormal, possibly due to immune attack. Neuromuscular function may improve with activity, and repetitive activation increases the amplitude of muscle action potentials as increased entry of calcium into terminals increases transmitter release. Several compounds have been used to sensitize terminals to calcium. Guanidine and aminopyridines (4-aminopyridine and 3,4-diaminopyridine) depolarize nerve terminals by blocking potassium conductance, facilitate the entry of calcium, and thereby augment transmitter release.

Botulism. Botulism is a more severe disorder of ACh release. Ingested toxin, with or without live *Clostridium botulinum* or innoculation of a wound with toxin-producing anaerobes, effectively blocks release of ACh from muscarinic and nicotinic terminals. As little as 50 µg may be lethal in humans. The mechanism is complex and incompletely understood. The toxin is bound to the terminals, internalized, cleaved in the low pH environment of lysosomes, then released into the terminal cytoplasm to block release, possibly by binding to vesicles or the vesicle release site itself. Repetitive stimulation augments muscle action potentials by as much as 400%.

The extreme potency of botulinum toxin has been turned to therapeutic benefit in the treatment of blepharospasm, dystonia, and severe spasticity. Injections of small amounts of type A botulinum toxin paralyze treated muscles for up to several months.

Other Toxins and Anticholinergic Medications. Other toxins also affect cholinergic neurotransmission. Black widow spider venom contains a cation channel-forming toxin, α-latrotoxin, that depolarizes terminals. The initial clinical feature of augmented ACh release is painful cramps. This is followed by paralysis as the transmitter is depleted. Many snake vena contain both α- and β-toxins. The Asian krait (*Bungarus multicinctus*) is probably the best known. Its venom paralyzes by blocking release of ACh (β-bungarotoxin) and by irreversibly blocking postynaptic nicotinic receptors (α-bungarotoxin). α-Bungarotoxin is a particularly important tool in neuroscience research; it is used to localize junctional and extrajunctional ACh receptors and to measure receptor turnover in normal neuromuscular junction development and in disease states.

Anticholinergic poisoning results from excessive ingestion of atropine, other belladonna alkaloids, tricyclic antidepressants, and major tranquilizers. The complete syn- drome of anticholinergic poisoning is characterized by restlessness advancing to delirium, followed by coma, respiratory depression, and death. The skin is hot and dry, and the heart rate is fast, with or without arrhythmia. The severity of the syndrome depends on the ingested dose of anticholinergic compound. Absorption of atropine after the use of eyedrops can be lethal in children and can produce delirium in the elderly. Ingestion of Jimson weed, the seeds of which contain stramonium, produces a similar syndrome in cattle, and teas made with the Jimson seed are toxic in humans. The antidote is physostigmine, an AChE inhibitor that crosses the blood-brain barrier easily.

Epilepsy and Epileptogenesis. The involvement of ACh in epileptogenesis is suggested by the fact that systemic injection of pilocarpine or pilocarpine with lithium produces status epilepticus with diffuse brain damage. Microinjection of carbochol into the midbrain reticular formation produces seizures that spread to the cortex and hippocampus. Oddly, ACh is usually not thought of as an excitotoxin, like the excitatory amino acids. However, ACh may play a role in neuronal injury from stroke and seizures. Little is known about the effects of antiepileptic drugs on cholinergic neurotransmission, but a role is suspected, because phenytoin and carbamazepine cause mild but measurable cognitive dysfunction, valproate is sometimes associated with pseudodementia and depression, and carbamazepine causes urinary retention on the basis of peripheral antimuscarinic activity.

The noncompetitive NMDA receptor blocker MK-801 also blocks ACh-activated current. Cholinergic blockade could be a mechanism common to other NMDA channel blockers, including ketamine and phencyclidine. The mechanism of the psychotogenic and other behavioral effects of these drugs is not established. These may be caused by NMDA channel blockade alone, or anticholinergic activity may contribute. The NMDA channel blocker felbamate is not associated with a significant incidence of psychotic episodes, nor has it been shown in preclinical studies to have anticholinergic effects.

Networks involving cholinergic and opioid peptidergic neurotransmission are involved in epilepsy and pain.

Antiepileptic drugs, particularly carbamazepine and phenytoin, are used to treat neuropathic pain and tic douloureux. Efficacy is explained mainly on the basis of their use-dependent blockade of voltage-dependent sodium channels. Valproic acid produces analgesia, which is not antagonized by naloxone in animals and is useful to treat migraine in some patients. Valproic acid is thought to enhance GABA-mediated inhibition by increasing the release of GABA and to block sodium channels. However, like other anticonvulsants, it may have anticholinergic activity.

Cholinergics may in some way be linked with endogenous opioid peptides in the modulation of the seizure threshold. Opioid peptides have both proconvulsant and antiepileptic effects in animal models. They are concentrated in the periaqueductal gray, just dorsal to the substantia nigra, which has been implicated in kindling epileptogenesis and the generalization of seizures. Modulating cholinergic drive on midbrain peptidergic systems and modulating the opioids differentially are possible anticonvulsant strategies. Morphine and mu opioid peptides (named for their morphine-like effects) have been shown to decrease ACh levels in the brain, partly by inhibiting high-affinity choline transport. Kappa opioids do not share this effect, and they have the most potent anticonvulsant activity of the opioids.

Pain. Acupuncture-induced analgesia increases ACh in the CSF and in various brain regions, including the adrenergic locus coeruleus and the serotonergic dorsal raphe. In this way, multiple monoamine neurotransmitters and opiatergic systems of the brain stem may collaborate to regulate pain-processing networks.

Both muscarinic and nicotinic cholinergic agents have been used to treat pain. Naloxone blocks some effects of muscarinic agents in experimental models, suggesting that cholinergic excitation results in the release of endogenous opioid peptides. The analgesic potency of nicotine is almost equivalent to morphine in some animal models, and naloxone incompletely blocks its antinociceptive effect. In addition, specific ganglionic nicotinic stimulants such as dimethylphenylpiperazine produce antinociceptive effects in mice. Thus, indirect augmentation of sympathetic tone may contribute to the analgesia, perhaps by modifying nociceptive inputs to the spinal cord.

Physostigmine was previously used to treat pain. A peripheral site of action is suspected, because physostigmine depresses sensory-evoked potential amplitude and raises the pain threshold. Both muscarinic and nicotinic cholinergic activity are augmented. New uses of cholinomimetics to treat pain may evolve as more selective ligands are synthesized and as the acetylcholine receptor subtypes along nociceptive pathways are elucidated. In combination with narcotics, cholinomimetics may improve the treatment of highly refractory cancer pain.

The analgesic effects of antidepressant compounds have not been satisfactorily explained. Paradoxically, antidepressant compounds with antimuscarinic activity, such as amitriptyline, seem to be more effective in treating pain (including migraine, neuralgia, neuropathic and radiculopathic syndromes, and causalgia) than the newer antidepressants without this activity. Pain relief occurs in some patients at low doses where anticholinergic side effects (confusion, somnolence, tachycardia, urinary retention) are insignificant and before antidepressant effects would likely occur. Blockade of reuptake of biogenic amines, especially serotonin, has been invoked as an explanation for both antidepressant and analgesic effects. However, the highly potent and selective new serotonin uptake inhibitors are disappointing as analgesics compared to amitriptyline. Comparative trials of efficacy of the newer antidepressants against amitriptyline treatment of pain syndromes have not been performed.

Sleep Disorders. Depression is associated with sleep disturbances, including difficulty falling asleep, early awakening, and decreased latency to rapid eye movement (REM) sleep. ACh excites the ponto-geniculo-occipital spike at the onset of REM. This sleep stage is facilitated by physostigmine and is blocked by atropine. Antidepressant compounds with antimuscarinic properties, such as amitriptyline, reduce REM sleep. Sleep deprivation with REM reduction has been suggested as antidepressant therapy. However, several newer antidepressants that selectively block serotonin reuptake lack significant antimuscarinic potency.

While REM suppression is probably not essential for antidepressant efficacy, it may be an important mechanism by which tricyclic compounds are useful in the treatment of narcolepsy, a disease of REM excess. Somniferous effects may account for the mixed benefit of these drugs. For this reason, in part, combination therapy is common in the treatment of narcolepsy. Excitatory compounds that enhance alertness, such as dextroamphetamine, have been used alone and as adjuncts in treating narcolepsy. Recently, an excitatory metabolite of GABA, δ-hydroxybutyrate, was anecdotally reported to be useful in the treatment of narcolepsy.

Anticholinergic properties of older antidepressants, antihistamines (e.g., diphenhydramine or atarax), and phenothiazines (e.g., thorazine) have been used to treat insomnia. These compounds are particularly useful in small doses in the elderly who do not tolerate benzodiazepines because of rebound insomnia, pseudodementia, or paradoxical excitation.

Endocrine Effects. Cholinergic innervation of the hypothalamus is involved in the regulation of thermoregulation and of hormone-release modulating appetite and water balance. At least one anticholinergic antihistamine, cyproheptadine, has been used to stimulate appetite.

Mydriasis. No discussion of cholinergic mechanisms would be complete without mentioning the mydriatic effect of belladonna (*Atropa belladonna*), which was used as a cosmetic during the Renaissance but later adapted to more sinister use as the deadly nightshade.

Dopamine

The role of dopamine in neurological disease initially received attention in 1957 when Carlsson and his colleagues showed that reserpine depleted the brain and heart of norepinephrine, which was associated with somnolence They later showed that dihydroxyphenylalanine (dopa), a precursor of catecholamine synthesis, restored dopamine levels and reversed the sedative action of reserpine. During the 1960s, monoamines including dopamine were visualized in neurons using the formaldehyde fluorescence technique, and low concentrations of dopamine were reported in the basal ganglia of patients with Parkinson's disease by Ehringer and Hornykiewicz. These investigators and the group headed by Cotzias showed that increasing doses of L-dopa relieved the symptoms of parkinsonism. Optimizing dopaminergic neurotransmission remains central to the treatment of Parkinson's disease (see Chapter 76).

Chemistry, Pharmacology, and Distribution

The catecholamines (dopamine, norepinephrine, and epinephrine) are synthesized from L-tyrosine by a cascade of enzymes that have been purified to homogeneity, cloned, and localized in the CNS by immunocytochemical and in situ hybridization techniques. Tyrosine is formed from phenylalanine and transported across the blood-brain barrier by an active transport mechanism. The formation of tyrosine from phenylalanine is catalyzed by the enzyme phenylalanine hydroxylase. Deficiency of this enzyme is responsible for the classic form of phenylketonuria (see Chapter 69). Tyrosine hydroxylase, the first enzyme in the dopamine synthesis cascade, catalyzes an alternate pathway in the synthesis of tyrosine from phenylalanine. Tyrosine hydroxylase is a mixed-function oxidase that requires tetrahydrobioptrin and oxygen as cofactors. It is primarily a soluble enzyme localized in the cytoplasm of catecholamine-containing neurons.

Tyrosine hydroxylase catalyzes the conversion of L-tyrosine to L-dopa, and dopa decarboxylase, a pyridoxal phosphate-dependent enzyme (also known as aromatic acid decarboxylase), converts L-dopa to dopamine. This reaction is the target of oral precursor treatment with L-dopa in the treatment of Parkinson's disease. Dopa decarboxylase is present in the cytoplasm of catecholaminergic and serotonergic nerve terminals; this enzymatic step is intermediate in the synthesis of the other monoamines.

Dopamine is pumped into storage vesicles for later release as a neurotransmitter. Amine transporters similar to drug resistance transporters of bacteria have been cloned; they characteristically have twelve transmembrane domains. The uptake of monoamines into storage vesicles is ATP-dependent and linked to a proton pump. In the vesicles, the catechols form complexes with ATP and acidic proteins called chromogranins. Free dopamine inside nerve terminals is deaminated by monoamine oxidase (MAO). Drugs that interfere with vesicular storage, such as amphetamines or reserpine, displace dopamine into the cytoplasm, where it is inactivated. Dopamine that diffuses into the extracellular space is broken down by catechol-o-methyl transferase (COMT).

About 80% of brain dopamine is found in the basal ganglia. Dopaminergic neurons in the ventral tegmental tract send fiber bundles to the nucleus acumbens (the mesolimbic tract) and to the cerebral cortex (the mesocortical bundle). Fibers also extend from the arcuate nucleus to the median eminence. The mesolimbic projection ascends in the medial forebrain bundle and is distributed to telencephalic structures including the olfactory bulb, olfactory nucleus and tubercle, lateral septal nucleus, stria terminalis, and parts of the hippocampus and amygdala. This branch also innervates the mesial frontal, anterior cingulate, pyriform, and entorhinal cortices. The mesolimbic projections terminate predominantly in the frontal (especially prefrontal) neocortex. Scattered groups of dopaminergic neurons are also present in the retina and spinal cord.

Dopamine Receptors

The two families of dopamine receptors are called D_1 and D_2. Originally, these families were separated by their different effects on adenylyl cyclase. Enzyme activity was augmented by D_1 receptor activation and decreased by D_2 receptor activation. Both families are linked to G proteins and have the predicted structure of seven transmembrane domains. The major difference between the two families of dopamine receptors is the sequence of the third intracytoplasmic loop, which governs G protein binding.

The D_1 family consists of two receptors, D_1 and D_5, which couple to the α-subunit of the stimulatory G protein G_s. G_s activates adenylyl cyclase directly and increases cyclic AMP production from ATP. The messenger RNA for D_1 is located primarily in the caudate, putamen, nucleus accumbens, and olfactory tubercle. The mRNA for D_5 is primarily located in the hippocampus and hypothalamus.

The D_2 family consists of four receptors (D_{2S}, D_{2L}, D_3, and D_4) linked to inhibitory G protein, or G_i. Activation of the receptors decreases the concentration of cyclic AMP. The D_2 receptor exists in two forms that arise from alternative splicing. They are expressed predominantly in the caudate, nucleus accumbus putamen, and olfactory tubercle. The D_3 receptors are highly expressed in the striatum and in the limbic areas. The D_4 receptor is present in the frontal cortex, midbrain, amygdala and medulla, and to a lesser extent, basal ganglia. The second messengers and effector mechanisms of the D_3 and D_4 receptors are not established. These two receptors share a high affinity for atypical neuroleptics such as clozapine. Atypical neuroleptics produce fewer extrapyramidal side effects than typical phenothiazine or butyrophenone neuroleptics that block D_2 receptors. The relative antipsychotic efficacy of the atypical compound may be due to antagonism of the D_4 and D_5 types of receptors in limbic structures and the cortex, while parkinsonian symptoms may be caused by blockade of D_2 receptors in the striatum. This raises the hope that chronic use of neuroleptics/antipsychotics need not result in tardive dyskinesia.

Pharmacology

Many aspects of dopaminergic neurotransmission can be modified to clinical therapeutic advantage, and a host of new pharmacological agents are under development (Figure 52.5). Dopamine is released when nerve terminals are depolarized by the arrival of action potentials that open voltage-dependent calcium channels. The entry of calcium promotes the fusion of vesicles with the synaptic membrane and the release of soluble contents of the granules. Several classes of drugs alter the amount of catecholamines that are released. Reserpine profoundly depletes dopamine and norepinephrine by initially augmenting their release, then irreversibly inhibiting their reuptake into storage vesicles. The depletion of catecholamines in animals is used as a model of parkinsonism.

Catecholamine transporters are not very specific, and they also transport tryptamine, tyramine, and amphetamines. Tyramine and amphetamines displace the catecholamines from their storage vesicles and cause depletion of the terminal and leakage of catecholamines from the nerve terminals. The initial result is an indirect increase of dopamine- and norepinephrine-mediated neurotransmission, but depletion may follow if drug exposure is chronic. The action of dopamine is terminated by reuptake or enzymatic degradation. The uptake process is mediated by an energy-dependent sodium exchanger that is inhibited by blockers of Na-K-ATPase (e.g., cardiac glycosides), tricyclic antidepressants, cocaine, and amphetamines.

The two isoenzymes of MAO are types A and B. Type A is potently blocked experimentally by clorgyline and preferentially catabolizes norepinephrine and serotonin; type B is blocked by selegiline (deprenyl). Type B is located prominantly in serotonergic neurons and astrocytes, and preferentially deaminates dopamine. Selegiline is metabolized to amphetamine and methamphetamine, which may increase alertness and

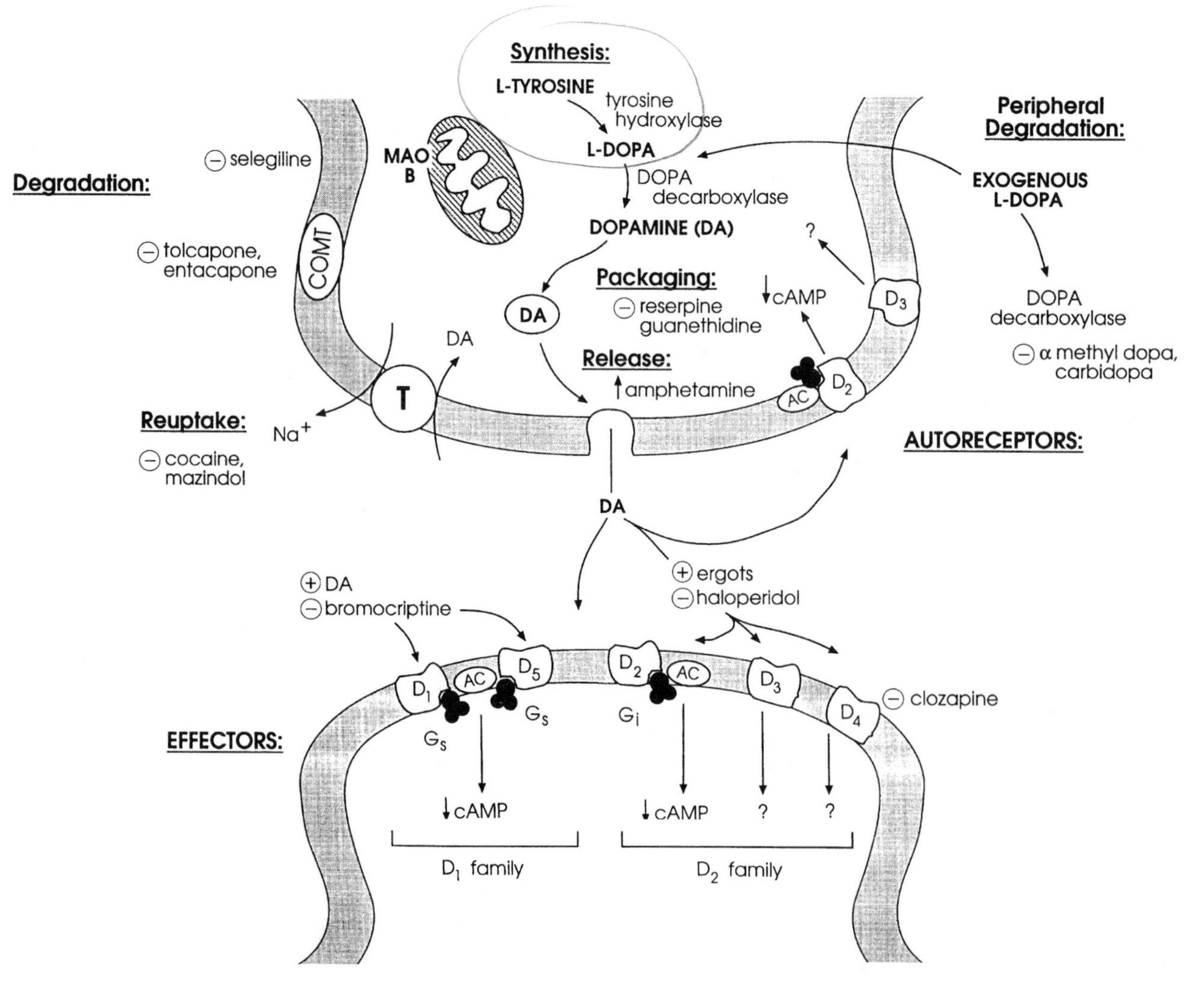

FIGURE 52.5 Pharmacology of dopamine neurotransmission.

mood elevation in addition to its effects on the movement disorder of Parkinson's disease. Antagonists of COMT are not commercially available, but several are being developed, including endacapone and tolcapone (Ro 40-7592).

Several selective agonists and antagonists that are specific for subtypes of dopamine receptors have been synthesized for investigation. Clinically used ergot derivatives include bromocriptine and pergolide. Bromocriptine is a more potent agonist at D_2 than D_1 and α-adrenergic receptors. It has weak antiparkinsonian action alone but has synergistic effects with endogenous dopamine. It is not usually considered an allosteric modulator but acts like one by enhancing the apparent affinity of the receptor or prolonging the binding of dopamine. In contrast, pergolide is a D_2 agonist at low doses and a mixed D_2 and D_1 antagonist at higher doses. Its presynaptic D_2 effect is to decrease dopamine release; postsynaptically, it acts like dopamine and inhibits firing by binding to D_2 receptors. Lisuride is a potent D_2 agonist with lesser affinity for D_1 and serotonin receptors. Its use is limited by side effects (nightmares, hallucinations, and psychosis) typical of antiparkinsonian medications.

Non-ergot agonists are being developed to circumvent adverse psychiatric effects. The use of the long-recognized agonist apomorphine is limited by its peripheral dopaminergic effects, but this decreases off-hours when it is administered subcutaneously. Intranasal and sublingual forms have been used safely. Highly potent and selective D_2 agonists (ropinirole and pramipexole) are in clinical trials. Autoreceptors have much higher affinity for agonists than do postsynaptic receptors. Selective autoreceptor (presynaptic D_2 receptor) antagonists are also under investigation. It is hoped that combinations of agents may allow normalization of dopaminergic activity without creating dystonia and dyskinesia.

The mechanism of action of amantadine is not established. It improves the symptoms of Parkinson's disease slightly and is best used as an adjunctive agent. Its efficacy is said to decrease over a period of months, but discontinuation may cause worsening of symptoms suggesting partial desensitization. It probably has multiple weak actions that enhance dopamine release. This may be accomplished by displacing it from vesicular storage and blocking reuptake. Other possible mechanisms of action are presynaptic D_2 antagonism or allosteric enhancement of dopamine receptor activation. Nondopaminergic mechanisms of actions of amantadine and memantine include antimuscarinic and NMDA channel-blocking actions. Memantine is also a weak sodium channel blocker with anticonvulsant efficacy in the maximal electroshock model. Selegiline selectively blocks MAO-B and augments dopamine concentrations in the brain.

Clinical Role of Dopamine

Parkinson's Disease. For the neurologist, the most important pathogenetic role of dopamine is in Parkinson's disease (Jankovic and Marsden 1993). The characteristic syndrome of bradykinesia, rigidity, and resting tremor are attributed to a deficiency of dopamine in the nigrostriatal pathway. Therapeutic agents allow manipulation of dopamine synthesis, dopamine receptor occupancy, and dopamine degradation. If Parkinson's disease were merely a disease of dopaminergic neurotransmission, we would expect treatments to be curative; but the disorder is often difficult to treat, particularly in later stages. To our consternation, medication side effects are not predictable or rationally avoidable by the choice of medication. Any combination of several factors may account for the variation of clinical features and the response to medication.

Intrinsic dopamine levels may be reduced below a critical level from the cumulative death of midbrain dopaminergic neurons. The dynamics of cell loss make Parkinson's disease an ever-changing pharmacological landscape. Exogenous agonists may or may not have the same effects as intrinsic dopamine or may do more harm to the patient. A nonspecific increase in brain dopamine concentration is probably not as optimal a strategy as making dopamine available to autoreceptors in the basal ganglia. At this site, it should decrease the release of excitatory neurotransmitters at lower concentrations than are required to activate postsynaptic receptors. Assume for a moment that balancing excitatory and inhibitory activity is sufficient treatment of Parkinson's disease. Then binding to the postsynaptic dopamine receptor may have multiple effects, some of them undesirable, depending on the receptor type and intracellular effector systems. The loss of dopaminergic neurons may alter the number and distribution of other neurotransmitter receptors and change traffic along other neural pathways. Such changes may be compensatory or decompensatory. Finally, Parkinson's disease may not be a disease of just dopaminergic neurotransmission; degeneration of noradrenergic neurons in the locus coeruleus also occurs.

L-dopa therapy is not ideal, but it represented the first major breakthrough in disease management. Coadministration with carbidopa, an inhibitor of peripheral L-dopa decarboxylase, enhances delivery of dopamine to the CNS and lessens gastrointestinal side effects by reducing the amount of L-dopa needed. The availability of L-selegiline, a selective inhibitor of MAO-B, has made inhibition of MAO a much more useful approach to therapy by reducing the adverse effects of nonspecific MAO blocking agents. Hypertensive crises due to displacement of norepinephrine and epinephrine by tyramine in cheese is perhaps the best-known risk to patients taking nonspecific MAO inhibitors. L-selegiline decreases the breakdown of dopamine selectively, thereby raising striatal dopamine concentrations and partially correcting the dopamine/acetylcholine imbalance. Evidence in animals and humans suggests that L-selegiline may have neuroprotective effects by as-yet-unknown mechanisms. The Deprenyl and Tocopherol Antioxidative Therapy of Parkinsonism (DATATOP) study showed that L-selegiline, but not vitamin E, delayed the need for L-dopa therapy. The data can be interpreted two ways: Either selegiline slows disease progression or is itself a treatment agent with limited efficacy. Conclusive demonstration of neuroprotection would make L-selegiline the standard of care, especially in newly diagnosed individuals.

The addition of L-selegiline is not without side effects. It is metabolized to amphetamine-like compounds, which have a desirable secondary mood-elevating and alerting effect for some patients. However, intoxicated patients act as if they have excessive dopaminergic tone, and metabolites contribute hallucinosis, psychosis, confusion, dystonia, and dyskinesia to the symptoms of toxicity.

The possible synergism of combined D_1 and D_2 receptor therapy remains an important therapeutic question. A subset of neurons in the striatum contains both classes of receptors, and agonists such as bromocriptine and pergolide have different affinities for dopamine receptor subtypes. No clinical study shows clear superiority of bromocriptine or pergolide; however, some patients who stop responding to bromocriptine improve after initiation of pergolide. Enough information is available to be confident that the efficacy of different agonists is not identical. This raises the hope that further distinctions of dopamine receptor subtypes may reveal better ways to use available agents or to design new ones.

Other neurotransmitters also have roles in the pathophysiology of Parkinson's disease. The concept of overbalance of cholinergic activity in the basal ganglia has been previously discussed in some detail. Two principal excitatory neurotransmitters (acetylcholine and glutamate) and two predominantly inhibitory neurotransmitters (dopamine and GABA) are present in the basal ganglion loop, which includes the neocortex, thalamus, subthalamic nucleus, globus pallidrum, and substantia nigra pars compacta. The role of non-dopamine neurotransmitters is discussed in sections on each specific transmitter. Other neurotransmitters, particularly neuropeptides, are present in the basal ganglia. Some neuropeptides are released with neurotransmitters as neuromodulators. Specific agonists and antagonists at peptidergic receptors are not yet available for the treatment of parkinsonism. Better understanding of the interplay between neuropeptides and monoamines in the striatum (not only dopamine, but also serotonin and norepinephrine) offers hope of novel therapeutic approaches.

Parkinson-like syndromes can be produced by catecholamine depletion with reserpine or *N*-methyl-4-phenyl-1,2,3,6-tetrahydropyridine (MPTP). MPTP was originally synthesized as a by-product of the illicit production of a meperidine-like narcotic. Ingested MPTP is converted by MAO to 1-methyl-4-phenyl-pyridine. This derivative blocks mitochondrial oxidation and leads to the generation of superoxide radicals, which cause cell death by impairing ATP generation and increasing intracellular free-calcium concentration. The MPTP model raised the possibility that environmental toxins may contribute to or cause Parkinson's disease by a similar mechanism. However, antioxidants such as vitamin E do not alter the course of Parkinson's disease.

Psychosis. For the psychiatrist, dopamine is most important for its presumed role in the pathogenesis of schizophrenia (Goldstein and Deutch 1992). One piece of evidence in favor of this role is the fact that virtually all clinically used neuroleptics are dopamine antagonists. However, treatment effects do not prove a mechanism of disease. Until recently, neuroleptic potency correlated with affinity for D_2 receptors, which are widely distributed along the cortical and mesolimbic projection paths and in the basal ganglia.

Increased expression of dopamine D_2 receptors has been detected in postmortem brains of schizophrenic patients. However, the efficacy of atypical neuroleptics suggests that D_4 and D_5 receptors of the limbic structures and cortex may be more important in producing psychotic behavior, and that D_2 receptors may be more important in producing side effects.

Adverse Effects of Neuroleptics. Prolonged use of neuroleptics causes drug-induced parkinsonism in many patients and tardive dyskinesia in others. Tardive dyskinesia as a consequence of prolonged treatment with neuroleptics is very difficult to treat. The syndrome consists of involuntary movements of the face (orobuccolingual), rocking of the trunk, and incessant movements of the hands and feet that are variously described as piano-playing, marching in place, or akathesia (see Chapter 76). The pathophysiology of tardive dyskinesia is poorly understood. One hypothesis is that dopamine receptors that have been blocked chronically become supersensitive to endogenous dopamine. Reduction or discontinuation of neuroleptics may worsen the symptoms, either because of increased receptor activation or increased number of receptors.

The introduction of atypical neuroleptics with selectivity for D_3 and D_4 receptors—e.g., clozapine—suggests that use of antagonists at dopamine receptors other than the D_2 subtype may decrease the risk of parkinsonism and tardive dyskinesia. A characteristic of psychosis is excessive wakefulness and alertness, whereas antipsychotic medications have sedative-hypnotic properties. This may be due in part to their anticholinergic and antihistaminic effects.

Psychotogenic Effects of Other Neurotransmitters. The fact that phencyclidine, a noncompetitive antagonist of glutamate, produces psychosis suggests that reduced availability of glutamatergic excitation as well as dopaminergic dysfunction may trigger psychosis. A deficit of glutamatergic activity could change the balance of other neurotransmitters, including GABA and dopamine. Effects of phencyclidine on dopamine receptors have not been excluded.

Gynecomastia. Dopamine inhibits the release of prolactin, and chronic neuroleptic use sometimes cause hyperprolactonemia and gynecomastia. Prolactin-secreting pituitary adenomas often respond to dopamine agonist therapy with bromocriptine.

Epilepsy. The role of dopamine in the relationship of psychosis and epilepsy has not been elucidated. Neuroleptics are said to lower seizure threshold, and anticonvulsant drugs are used to treat affective disorders and episodic dyscontrol. Dopaminergic inputs to limbic structures facilitate kindling by unclear mechanisms. Investigation of the mechanistic bases underlying these observations could provide useful new strategies for treatment and the design of novel pharmaceuticals.

Spasticity. Spinal dopaminergic pathways may be important in controlling spasticity. There are anecdotal reports of efficacy of L-dopa/carbidopa preparations against spasticity associated with cerebral palsy. Nightmares are an undesirable side effect.

Norepinephrine and Epinephrine

Norepinephrine and epinephrine were among the first CNS neurotransmitters to be characterized and visualized with fluorescent techniques. Disturbances of adrenergic neurotransmission occur in the Shy-Drager syndrome (multiple-system atrophy) and are thought to underlie depression; yet our understanding of these two catecholamines is incomplete. They serve important roles in the regulation of blood volume and blood-pressure control. Norepinephrine is also important in sleep-wake cycles and epileptogenesis.

Chemistry and Distribution

The adrenergic neurons of the locus coeruleus, pons, and medulla project to virtually every area of the brain and spinal cord. These neurons contain tyrosine hydroxylase and dopa decarboxylase, to make dopamine. They also contain dopamine β-hydroxylase (like tyrosine hydroxylase, a mixed-function oxidase), which catalyzes the conversion of dopamine to norepinephrine. This enzyme requires copper as a cofactor and is inhibited by chelators such as diethyldithiocarbamate. Dopamine β-hydroxylase is bound to the inner membrane of synaptic vesicles and is released with norepinephrine. Cloning studies indicate that it is a tetrameric glycoprotein.

A small number of neurons in the medulla contain phenylethanolamine-*N*-methyl transferase (PNMT), an enzyme that converts norepinephrine to epinephrine with S-adenosyl methionine as a methyl donor. These neurons project to the thalamus, brain stem, and spinal cord. The physiological role of central epinephrine is not fully understood. The concentration of epinephrine-secreting terminals in the paraventricular nucleus suggests a role in the secretion of oxytocin and vasopressin. This, coupled with the dense innervation in the region of the dorsal motor nucleus of the vagus and nucleus solitarius, suggests a role in regulating cardiovascular and respiratory reflexes. A third projection synapses on the sympathetic intermedioventral nucleus of the spinal cord. Taken together, the central epinephrine pathways are likely to influence salt and water retention and blood pressure control. Physiological experiments demonstrate a vasopressor area in the rostral medulla corresponding to the epinephrine-containing cell group. In addition, PNMT is overexpressed in spontaneously hypertensive rats.

Circulating adrenocorticotropic hormone (ACTH) links the hypothalamic-pituitary axis to adrenal secretion of epinephrine. In the adrenal medulla, epinephrine-synthesizing chromaffin cells are regulated by corticosteroids released from the adrenal cortex under stimulation by ACTH. This vitally important circuit integrates and controls salt and water metabolism, blood volume, and blood pressure.

Norepinephrine and Epinephrine Receptors

Norepinephrine and epinephrine act at α- and β-receptors in the brain and periphery. Four receptors are present in the brain: α_1-, α_2-, β_1-, and β_2-. β_1-adrenergic receptors are predominantly in the heart and cerebral cortex, whereas β_2-receptors are principally found in the lung and cerebellum. So far, β_1- and β_2-receptors have not been functionally differentiated, although ligands with differential selectivity have been synthesized.

The known types of adrenergic receptors are members of the G protein superfamily. As such, they are believed to have seven transmembrane-fanning hydrophobic regions of 20–25 amino acids each, a long C terminal hydrophilic section that contains sites for phosphorylation, a shorter extracellular N terminal end that contains glycosylated residues, and a long third intracellular loop that interacts with G proteins. Sequence homology among β_1- and β_2-receptors is about 71%. The sequence differences probably account for differences in agonist preference (β_1-receptors equally prefer epinephrine and norepinephrine as agonists and practolol as an antagonist; β_2-receptors prefer epinephrine over norepinephrine, and terbutyline or salbutamol as an agonist). The catecholamine binding site is thought to be a pocket formed by the helical transmembrane regions. An aspartate residue on transmembrane segment 3 and serine residues on transmembrane segment 5 are spaced appropriately to bind the catechol hydroxyl and amino groups. The third intracellular loop and the C terminal end probably control the interaction with the GTP-binding proteins. Agonist binding to both β_1- and β_2-receptors activates the stimulatory protein G_s. The activated α-subunit, after dissociating from the β- and γ-subunits, activates adenyl cyclase to increase cellular cyclic AMP concentrations. Activation of β-receptors results in coactivation of β-adrenergic receptor kinase (BARK). This kinase phosphorylates the C terminus of the β-receptor and β-arrestin complexes with the receptor to decrease its affinity for G_s. Phosphorylation is a prominent mechanism of receptor desensitization. Other transcriptional, posttranscriptional, and posttranslational regulations control the number of receptors.

Two families of α-adrenergic receptors have been identified that are also G protein–linked. The α_1- and α_2-receptor families have approximately 40% sequence homology with the β_2-receptor. The α_1-group of receptors are linked by G_s to phospholipase C. Activation of phospholipase C generates IP_3 and DAG from membrane phospholipids. The IP_3 triggers release of intracellular calcium, and DAG activates protein kinase C, which is then available for phosphorylation of membrane proteins. The α_2-family is coupled to the inhibitory protein G_i. Occupancy of the receptor by agonists dissociates the G protein such that the β- and γ-subunits bind to adenyl cyclase and prevent stimulation by α-subunits from stimulatory G proteins (Kobilka 1992). The net effect is a decrease in cellular cyclic AMP concentration.

Physiology and Pharmacology of Central Adrenergic Receptors

A variety of pharmacological agents afford clinical manipulation of adrenergic mechanisms at multiple levels (Figure 52.6). Norepinephrine increases firing in hippocampal pyramidal neurons by blocking the slow after-hyperpolarizing potential that follows a depolarizing burst. The principal current underlying this potential is a calcium-activated potassium current that is activated by membrane depolarization. This effect of norepinephrine is blocked by β_1-selective antagonists, but not by β_2-selective compounds or antagonists at α-receptors. Isoproterenol is the most potent agonist in this regard, followed by epinephrine and norepinephrine; phenylephrine (α_1-agonist) and clonidine (α_2-agonist) are ineffective. Norepinephrine also blocks after-hyperpolarizations in thalamic and preganglionic sympathetic neurons, although the receptor type has not been determined. In sympathetic neurons, norepinephrine abbreviates and decreases the amplitude of calcium spikes. This could explain the effect on calcium-dependent after-hyperpolarizations. Importantly, the action of norepinephrine is mimicked by cyclic AMP analogs and forskolin, an activator of adenyl cyclase, and by blocking phosphodiesterase activity with methylxanthines. The effect of norepinephrine is decreased by blocking adenyl cyclase. In addition, β-receptor activation and cyclic AMP analogs enhance calcium currents in dentate granule cells similarly to the β-adrenergic effect on the heart.

Excitatory effects of norepinephrine result from α_1-receptor activation. Such effects have been shown on neurons in various parts of the CNS and in sympathetic ganglion

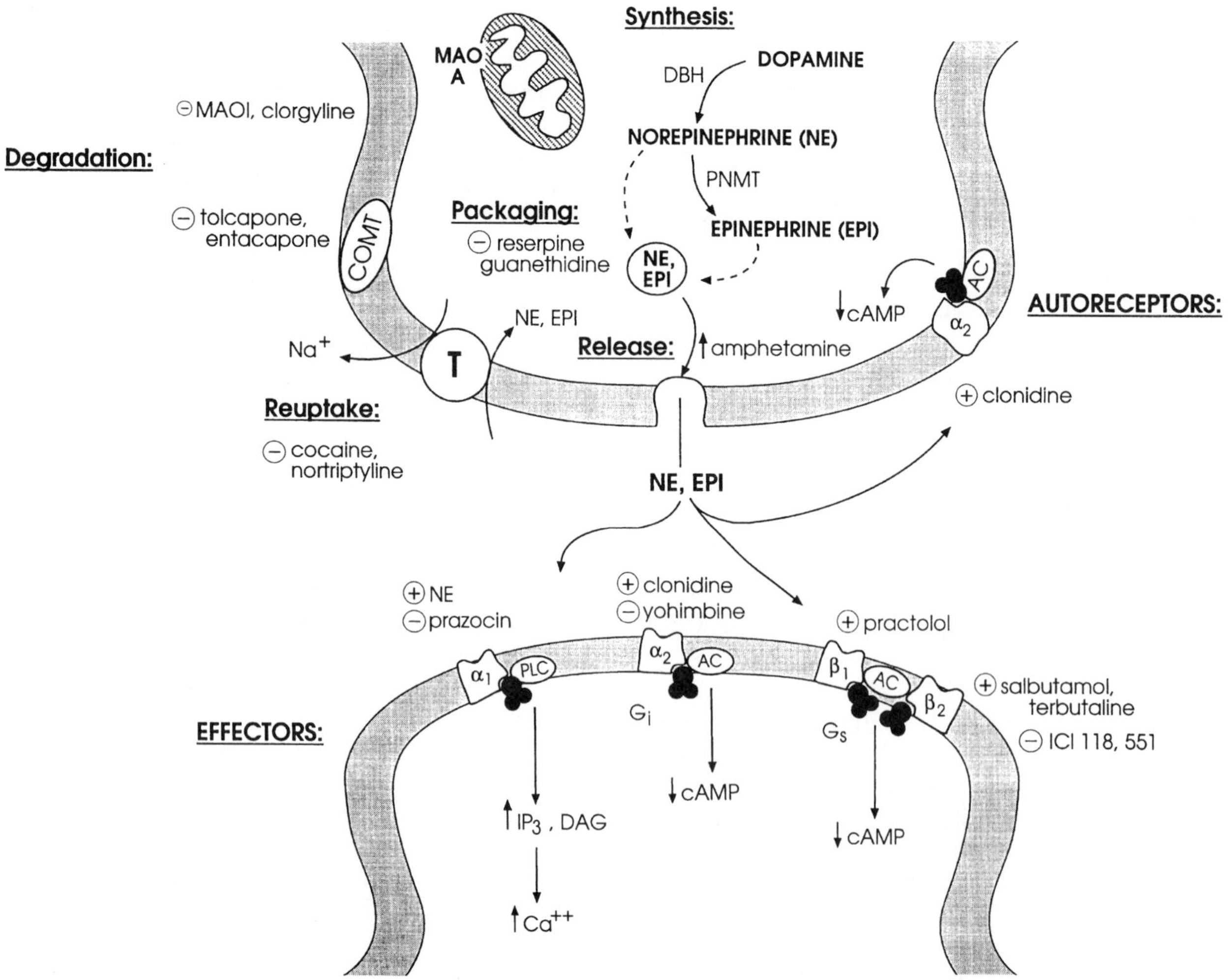

FIGURE 52.6 Pharmacology of catecholamine neurotransmission.

neurons. This activity depends primarily on blockade of a resting potassium conductance. As a result, neurons depolarize, and firing rates increase. Inhibitory effects of norepinephrine result from α_2-receptor activation, which increases potassium conductance. This hyperpolarizes the neuron and decreases its firing rates. Norepinephrine acting at α_2-receptors also blocks calcium current, an effect prevented by pertussis toxin, suggesting the involvement of a GTP-binding protein. Both of these inhibitory mechanisms may account for the autoreceptor function of α_2-receptors, which decrease neurotransmitter release.

Clinical Role of Adrenergic Receptors

Noradrenergic neurons of the brain stem innervate the forebrain diffusely. This may be a substrate for the apparent role of these neurons as a global modulator of arousal or orientation to new and threatening stimuli. Neurons in the locus coeruleus integrate sensory stimuli and project an excitatory output to the forebrain, using norepinephrine as a transmitter. Activity of locus coeruleus neurons decreases during sleeping, eating, and grooming, but intensifies with a new sensory input. The mixed effects of norepinephrine subserve a familiar tuning function. On the one hand, presynaptic α_2-stimulation tends to decrease neurotransmitter release. On the other hand, blockade of calcium-dependent potassium conductances by β-receptor activation increases the excitability of neurons by depolarizing them and increasing firing rates. The net effect is to increase the signal-to-noise ratio. Signals of low intensity tend to be filtered by the presynaptic action, but those that are sufficiently intense to overcome the presynaptic inhibition have an enhanced effect postsynaptically.

Mood Disorders. Depression has been viewed as an adrenergic deficiency state, whereas mania is characterized as an excess of norepinephrine. Supporting this view are studies indicating that depletion of norepinephrine, as with reserpine, results in depression. Further, MAO-inhibiting antidepressants, such as tranylcypromine or phenelzine, increase the availability of norepinephrine by preventing its breakdown within terminals. Challenging the adrenergic hypothesis is the fact that tricyclic antidepressants that block the reuptake of norepinephrine do so almost immediately, but their antidepressant effect takes weeks to evolve. The same can be said about the role of serotonin in depression. In this sense, blockade of reuptake of biogenic amines is an in vitro pharmacological effect predictive of antidepressant efficacy, and possibly a measure of treatment efficacy. This has led to investigation of changes in populations of receptors after chronic administration of antidepressant compounds. Blockade of reuptake increases the availability of the principal endogenous agonist. Clinical and laboratory evidence indicates a decreased number of postsynaptic β-receptors and α_2-autoreceptors during chronic antidepressant drug therapy. The latter should facilitate neurotransmitter release. Consistent with this idea, yohimbine, an α_2-receptor antagonist, is reported to enhance the effects of tricyclic antidepressant compounds. Another argument against the noradrenergic hypothesis of depression is that many new serotonin selective reuptake inhibitors are good antidepressants without affecting noradrenergic systems. Thus, overall there may be a modulatory role for adrenergic systems in depression, and antidepressant drugs may work in part by affecting adrenergic systems. However, the adrenergic system dysfunction probably is not the sole pathogenetic mechanism of depression.

Pain. Clonidine and other centrally acting α_2-agonists have potent analgesic effects; they also produce hypotension and induce sleep, which may decrease responsiveness to a painful stimulus. Another contributor to the analgesic effect may be a direct action on dorsal root ganglion cells. Norepinephrine decreases calcium current in these neurons. The pharmacology is atypical in that yohimbine blocks the effect, but clonidine does not mimic it. The effect is blocked by pertussis toxin and mimicked by phorbol esters, which activate protein kinase C. These findings implicate activation of a G protein that is coupled to protein kinase C, presumably through phospholipase C.

Epilepsy. Noradrenergic systems play a role in epileptogenesis. Depletion of norepinephrine, but not dopamine, greatly facilitates kindling in experimental animals. Guanethidine, which displaces norepinephrine from intraneuronal storage granules, lowers the threshold for both electroconvulsive and pentylenetetrazole-induced seizures in animals. The downregulation of α_2-receptors observed after kindled seizures should facilitate neurotransmitter release. Clonidine, an α_2-agonist, acts as an anticonvulsant against several seizure types in animals, including those induced by AChE-inhibiting nerve agents such as soman. Cocaine, which blocks the reuptake of catecholamines, has both pro- and anticonvulsant effects. It facilitates kindling, while its local anesthetic properties and α_2-mediated inhibition due to enhanced release of norepinephrine may be anticonvulsant. Tricyclic antidepressants, which block reuptake of norepinephrine, have anticonvulsant effects at low doses and proconvulsant effects at high doses in epilepsy-prone rats with genetically determined deficiency of noradrenergic neurotransmission. Transplantation of fetal locus coeruleus tissue with norepinephrine-synthesizing neurons into the hippocampus of norepinephrine-depleted animals retards the development of hippocampal kindled seizures. Blockade of the calcium-dependent potassium conductance by β-receptor–mediated activity in the hippocampus increases high-frequency action-potential firing and promotes the spread of seizures.

Pressor Effects. Adrenergic systems are involved in many other functions. Cardiovascular effects of norepinephrine and epinephrine are well known. The antihypertensive effect of clonidine augments α_2-mediated inhibition along central sympathetic pathways. Postural hypotension is a sign of the Shy-Drager syndrome, a disease in which adrenergic neurons of the brain stem and spinal cord degenerate.

Appetite. The presence of α_2-adrenoreceptors in the ventromedial hypothalamus is likely to be responsible for powerful effects of sympathetic compounds on appetite and body weight. Chronic administration of clonidine leads to increased food intake and weight gain, and the α_2-antagonist yohimbine does the opposite. Amphetamines that increase the release of norepinephrine, epinephrine, and other sympathomimetics, such as pseudoephedrine, can produce weight loss.

Memory. Interestingly, α_2-receptor antagonists facilitate memory retrieval in animals and decrease reaction time to visual stimuli in humans. Clonidine could be of use to some patients with Alzheimer's disease.

Serotonin

In the mid-nineteenth century, a potent vasoconstrictive substance was identified in the serum of clotted blood and called vasotonin. It was almost 100 years later that 5-hydroxytryptamine (serotonin) was isolated and synthesized. Over 95% of the body's serotonin is stored in platelets and the gastrointestinal tract, and only 5% is in the brain. However, serotonin is distributed in brain regions that could affect behavior, especially the hypothalamus and the limbic system. It meets all criteria for being a neurotransmitter. The observation that lysergic acid diethylamide (LSD), which binds to serotonin receptors, causes abnormal behavior suggests that abnormalities of serotonergic neurotransmission may cause mental illness. This hypothesis is the basis for suspecting a role for serotonin in depression, schizophrenia, and other psychiatric disorders.

Chemistry and Distribution

The indole amino acid tryptophan is the precursor of serotonin. Tryptophan is derived from dietary protein and is transported with other neutral amino acids (including leucine, phenylalanine, and methionine) by the L-amino acid transport mechanism into the brain. Interestingly, gabapentin, a newly introduced antiepileptic drug, has an amino acid–like structure and is also transported by this energy-dependent active transport mechanism. Tryptophan is metabolized to 5-hydroxytryptophan in serotonergic neurons through the action of tryptophan hydroxylase, a pteridine-requiring enzyme. Complementary DNAs that encode tryptophan hydroxylase have been cloned and sequenced. The enzyme contains 444 amino acids corresponding to a molecular weight of about 51 kD, and is 50% homologous with tyrosine hydroxylase, the rate-limiting enzyme in catecholamine biosynthesis.

Next, 5-hydroxytryptophan is converted to serotonin through the action of L-aromatic amino acid decarboxylase. This enzyme is also present in catecholaminergic neurons, where it converts dopa to dopamine. The decarboxylase has also been cloned. It contains 480 amino acids and has a molecular weight of 54 kD. The recombinant enzyme decarboxylates both dopa and 5-hydroxytryptamine. In situ hybridization of its mRNA shows that the decarboxylase is present in serotonergic cells of the dorsal raphe and dopaminergic neurons in the midbrain. Raising the dietary intake of both tryptophan and 5-hydroxytryptophan increases brain serotonin levels, a strategy used in the treatment of postanoxic myoclonus with some success. Since the removal of commercial preparations from the market in 1992 because of a contaminant that caused the eosinophilia-myalgia syndrome, only brewer's yeast remains available as a useful source of L-tryptophan.

Hydroxylation of tryptophan by tryptophan hydroxylase is the rate-limiting step. Tyrosine hydroxylase is irreversibly inhibited by parachlorophenylalanine (PCPA), which causes a long-lasting reduction of serotonin levels. PCPA is frequently used in experimental models designed to study the effects of brain serotonin depletion.

Fluorescence techniques localize nine groups of serotonergic neurons in the brain stem, primarily in the raphe nuclei. Serotonin-containing nerve terminals are distributed widely throughout the forebrain. Projections from the dorsal raphe, median raphe, and a pontomesencephalic cell group ascend through the dorsal paraventricular and ventral tegmental radiations to join the medial forebrain bundle, where they ascend with dopaminergic fibers. Axons of neurons in the caudal pons and medulla project within the brain stem and down the spinal cord.

Limbic structures such as the hippocampus and septum are innervated chiefly by neurons in the median raphe, while the striatum and substantia nigra are innervated principally from the dorsal raphe. Both neural groups send projections widely throughout the neocortex. Toxic amphetamine derivatives such as 3,4-methylene dioxy-meth-amphetamine (known in the illegal drug trade as "ecstasy") or *p*-chloroamphetamine preferentially destroy dorsal raphe neurons more than median raphe neurons.

The synthesis of serotonin, like other monoamine neurotransmitters, is linked to neuronal activity. Invasion of the nerve terminal by action potentials firing at high frequency probably increases intraterminal calcium, the activation of calcium-dependent phosphorylating enzymes (e.g., calmodulin), and phosphorylation of tryptophan hydroxylase.

Serotonin is taken up into storage vesicles in nerve terminals by a specific transporter. In the vesicles, serotonin is bound to a specific binding protein without ATP. Reserpine and tetrabenazine inhibit the transporter and deplete the vesicles of serotonin. These agents also deplete catechol-containing vesicles. The transmitter-containing vesicles are released by exocytosis after depolarization of the terminals and entry of calcium. Serotonergic terminals are associated with specialized postsynaptic regions in many parts of the brain, but they lack postsynaptic specializations in some areas where varicosities seem to run en passant. This is especially true of the dorsal raphe projections to the basal ganglia, where serotonin is released into the interspace diffusely, much as neurotransmitters are released into the interspace of the heart. This type of release allows a diffuse modulatory effect rather than the specific influence dictated by point-to-point synaptic contacts. Released serotonin diffuses to presynaptic (autoreceptors) and postsynaptic receptors, and its effects are terminated by a specific presynaptic reuptake system. The transporter is present on serotonergic neurons and glial cells. The reuptake system is saturable and dependent on temperature, external sodium, and chloride, and is coupled to Na^{+}-K^{+}-ATPase. Complementary DNA sequences indicate that the transporter is a 630 amino acid peptide with a molecular weight of about 60 kD. It is thought to have 12 transmembrane regions with intracellular amino and carboxy terminals. A long extracellular loop exists between the third and fourth transmembrane domains. About 50% sequence homology exists between this and the transporters for catecholamines. Functional recombinant transporters have been expressed in different systems. Antidepressant drugs—such as the serotonin selective uptake blockers, fluoxetine and sertraline—inhibit the cloned transporter.

The other mechanism for termination of serotonin action is catabolism by MAO. The isozymes of this intramitochondrial flavoprotein are referred to as types A and B. Selegiline is a specific inhibitor for the type B isoenzyme (see Catecholamines), and clorgyline specifically inhibits the A type. Serotonergic neurons contain predominantly MAO-B, whereas type MAO-A prefers serotonin as a substrate. The presence of MAO-B may prevent serotonergic neurons from accumulating by reuptake catecholamines, which are more selectively broken down by this isoenzyme.

Serotonin Receptors

Four subtypes of serotonin receptors have been identified in the brain and subsequently cloned, sequenced, and characterized (Julius 1991). A fifth subtype (5-HT_{1P}) is found in the gastrointestinal tract and produces a slow depolarization of some myenteric plexus neurons. 5-HT_1, 5-HT_2, and 5-HT_4 subtypes are coupled to G proteins and modulate one or more second messenger systems. The 5-HT_3 subtype is a ligand-gated ion channel. Pharmacology of cloned receptors correlates well with that determined by receptor binding techniques (Figure 52.7).

The 5-HT_1 family consists of four receptor subtypes, 1A–1D. In the hippocampus and raphe nuclei, 5-HT_{1A} receptors open potassium channels and cause hyperpolarization by a G protein-coupled interaction. $5HT_{1A}$ receptors both increase and decrease cyclic AMP formation by G protein-coupled effects on adenylyl cyclase. The novel anxiolytic compound buspirone is a partial agonist at $5HT_{1A}$ receptors and could exert its effect by the hyperpolarizing action of serotonin on these receptors. Excitation by serotonin could result from blockade of a resting or leak potassium conductance, or from the calcium-dependent potassium conductance underlying the slow after-hyperpolarization.

$5HT_{1B}$ and $5HT_{1D}$ receptors inhibit adenylyl cyclase and decrease cyclic AMP. $5HT_{1B}$ receptors have been characterized mainly in rodents, and $5HT_{1D}$ receptors in humans, guinea pigs, and ruminants. These receptor subtypes are most densely expressed in the substantia nigra. $5HT_{1C}$ receptors and $5HT_2$ receptors stimulate the production of IP_3 through a phospholipase C-linked pathway. $5HT_2$ receptors also close potassium channels through a G protein–coupled mechanism that results in a slow depolarization.

The $5HT_3$ receptor does not belong to the G protein superfamily but is a ligand-gated ion channel. Expression of a single clone in frog oocytes results in functional homomeric receptor-channel complexes. This suggests that even if the channel is a pentamer, it is probably not formed from multiple different subunits. The channel is cation selective. Current through the channel is blocked in a voltage-dependent manner by both calcium and magnesium, similar to the effect of magnesium on NMDA-activated GluRs. The depolarization caused by activation of this channel produces a fast excitatory potential.

The $5HT_4$ receptor is coupled to adenylyl cyclase and is associated with inhibition of potassium current in collicular neurons and the hippocampus. Receptor activation presumably increases cyclic AMP, which then activates protein kinase A. The resultant phosphorylation inhibits the channel.

The complex interactions of serotonin—with different cation channels even in the same tissue—suggest that the interaction of multiple interlocking modulatory influences controls the duration of various fast and slow changes in membrane potential. This could fine-tune the firing patterns of the hippocampus, which are a blend of high-frequency action-potential firing at membrane potentials positive to the resting potential and of burst firing atop rhythmic depolarizing bursts at more negative potentials.

The autoreceptor function of presynaptic serotonergic receptors is probably subserved by $5HT_{1B}$ and $5HT_{1D}$ receptors, which are both highly expressed in the basal ganglia. These subtypes may be involved in the pathophysiology of some movement disorders.

$5HT_{1C}$ receptors are enriched in choroid plexus epithelial cells and may regulate the composition and volume of cerebrospinal fluid. Effects on mood and behavior may be mediated through $5HT_{1C}$ receptors in limbic structures. Expression of $5HT_{1C}$ receptors in the basal ganglia suggests a possible role in motor behavior as well.

$5HT_2$ receptors are highly expressed in various regions, including the cortex, limbic system, and basal ganglia. In the cortex, they are thought to be postsynaptic receptors on intrinsic neurons, because disruption of projection paths does not influence the receptor density as determined by radioligand techniques.

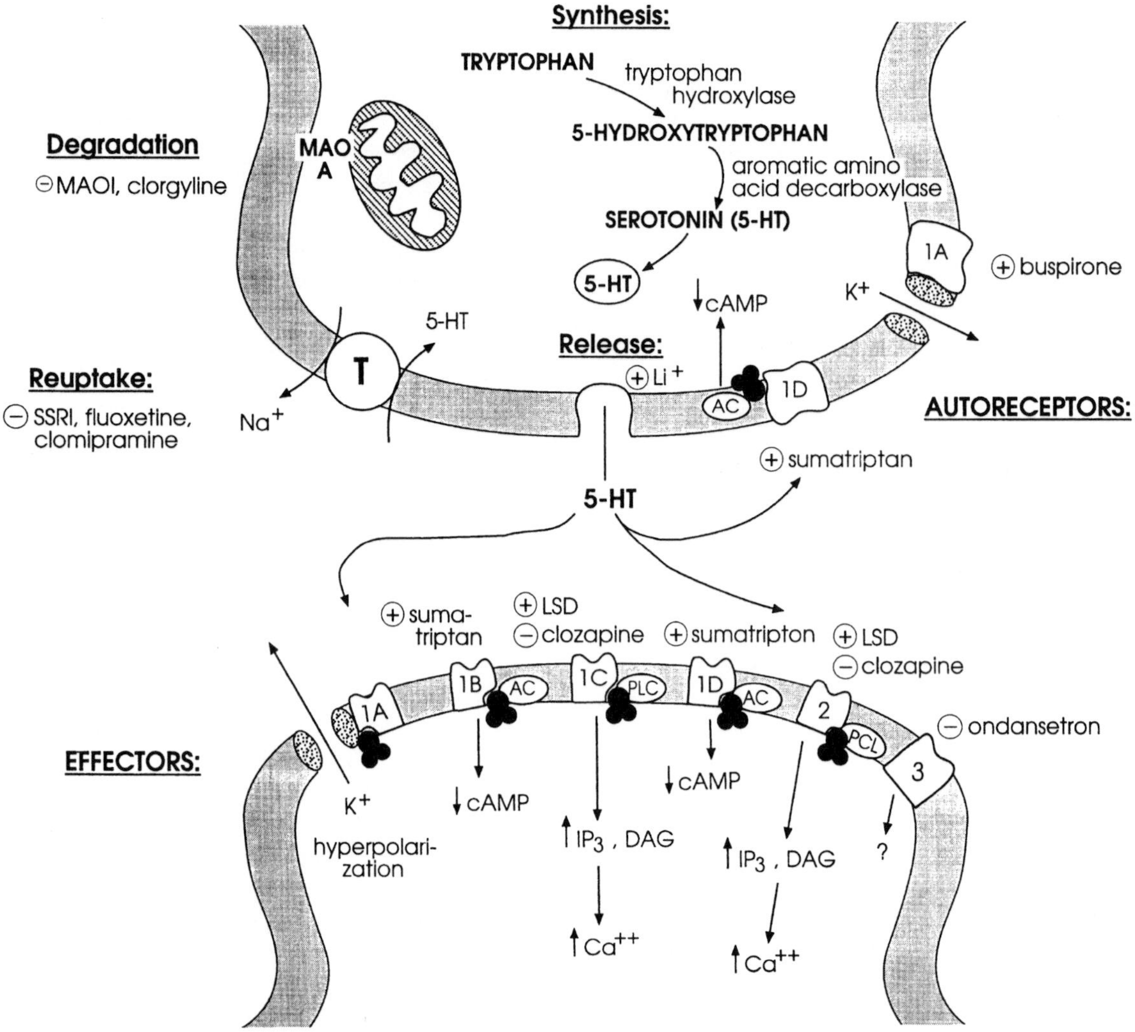

FIGURE 52.7 Pharmacology of seratonin neurotransmission.

The $5HT_3$ receptor subtype is most abundant in peripheral ganglia and nerves and in the substantia gelatinosa of the dorsal horn of the spinal cord. This suggests a role in the modulation of pain neurotransmission (see Chapter 53). $5HT_3$ receptor antagonists, such as ondansetron and granisetron, are antiemetic. This effect corresponds to a high density of $5HT_3$ receptors in the area postrema, the site of the chemoreceptor trigger zone.

The absence of selective antagonists makes it difficult to study the function of $5HT_4$ receptors, but they appear to be most abundant in the collicular region and in the hippocampus.

Long-term regulation of the serotonin receptors varies with receptor type and circumstances. As expected, $5HT_1$ receptors downregulate when chronically exposed to mianserin, a receptor antagonist. Contrary to expectation, destruction of serotonergic neurons does not change $5HT_2$ receptor density. However, $5HT_2$ receptors downregulate and desensitize as expected after administration of hallucinogenic agonists, chronic administration of inhibitors of serotonin uptake, or chronic exposure to $5HT_2$ receptor antagonists.

Clinical Role of Serotonin Receptors

The role of serotonin in sleep and behavior has been studied extensively.

Sleep. As mentioned above, serotonin deficiency is thought to have a role in the pathogenesis of depression. Sleep disturbances are common among depressed and psychotic people, suggesting that serotonergic pathways modulate the states of arousal and mood. The firing rates of brain stem serotonergic neurons change slowly throughout the sleep-wake cycle, suggesting circadian control. Neuropeptides and melatonin, which is synthesized from serotonin, have been implicated in the adjustment of circadian rhythms. Drugs that elevate brain serotonin increase the release of peptide hormones, including growth hormone and prolactin. Serotonin also modulates the release of ACTH. Cortisol is under circadian control, and plasma concentrations are highest in the morning. In many depressed people, the plasma cortisol concentration remains elevated throughout the day, as it does during stress. Nocturnal administration of 1–2 mg of dexamethasone normally reduces the cortisol level the next morning. In about 50% of depressed patients, dexamethasone fails to reduce the morning cortisol level (a positive dexamethasone suppression test). Why the dexamethasone suppression test is abnormal in only about half of depressed patients is not known.

Melatonin has powerful influences on circadian rhythms and is particularly important in sleep induction. Melatonin synthesis and secretion are suppressed by daylight. The onset of darkness increases the release of norepinephrine from sympathetic neurons innervating the pineal. Activation of β- and α_1-receptors on pinealocytes increases cyclic AMP, which activates serotonin *N*-acetyltransferase. Serotonin is then *N*-acetylated and O-methylated to form melatonin in the pineal. Melatonin secretion obeys a circadian "clock," probably located in the hypothalamus. This system is active even in perpetual darkness. Melatonin also influences the estrous cycle of animals to time their reproductive cycle to changes in light and dark cycles. Its exact role in humans is not established. Nocturnal melatonin secretion is reduced in depressed patients. This could result from decreased noradrenergic activity or from decreased availability of serotonin from which melatonin is synthesized. Hypotheses concerning the role of norepinephrine and serotonin in depression have been formulated, but neither fully explains the clinical variability or fundamental mechanism of depression. Central adrenergic and serotonergic activity vary in parallel, and dissecting one from the other in relation to depression is difficult.

Serotonin, the precursor of melatonin, is probably involved in the regulation of circadian rhythms. The suprachiasmatic nucleus of the hypothalamus fires rhythmically and releases vasopressin in a pacemaker-like manner. This nucleus is densely innervated by serotonergic projections from the midbrain raphe nuclei. Administration of serotonin agonists causes shifts in the rhythmic cycling of activity within the suprachiasmatic nucleus. The overall effect of serotonin on sleep cycling is to regulate total sleep time by exerting a tonic influence on which dopaminergic and adrenergic systems superimpose phasic changes in alertness or arousal.

The firing rate of brain stem serotonergic neurons is virtually tonic, because they are controlled by circadian rhythms that change very slowly. The firing rate of dorsal raphe neurons slows gradually with drowsiness and the onset of sleep. During REM sleep, their firing ceases. Sensory inputs such as flashing lights or auditory clicks transiently increase firing and then cause inhibition. During sleep and wakefulness, sudden threatening stimuli do not alter serotonergic neuron firing rates, but they do markedly increase sympathetic firing. These different state-dependent effects of stimulation indicate how target regions such as the hippocampus can be differentially activated or inactivated by biogenic amines, despite the very similar presynaptic and postsynaptic actions of the amines.

Tricyclic antidepressant drugs that block uptake of serotonin reduce REM sleep and are useful in the treatment of narcolepsy, which is a disorder of intrusive REM (see Chapter 73). The role of specific neurotransmitter pathways or receptor subtypes remains unclear.

Depression. The body of evidence implicating serotonin in disorders of mood and behavior is considerable (Peroutka 1991). Diets low in tryptophan result in mild depression, and tryptophan loading, or administration of the serotonin agonist m-chlorophenylpiperazine, increases activation ratings in normal volunteers. Sleep is frequently disturbed in affective disorders. Inhibition of serotonin synthesis with PCPA produces insomnia in animals, whereas tryptophan improves sleep, in some studies. Hallmarks of the sleep abnormality of depression include decreased REM latency and early awakening. Compounds that prevent the reuptake of serotonin selectively, such as fluoxetine, zimelidine, or fenfluramine, prolong the latency to REM and decrease total REM time.

Other body functions are affected by depression. At least half of depressed patients report a reduced threshold for pain and complain of pain as a symptom. Research in animals and in humans shows that increased serotonergic activity has analgesic effects. This is perhaps a result of its interaction with endogenous opiate peptide systems, which are strategically placed in the periaqueductal gray near the midbrain raphe nuclei. Stimulation of $5HT_1$ receptors lowers body temperature, whereas stimulation of $5HT_2$ receptors raises body temperature. Altered activity of subtypes of serotonin receptors may be responsible for abnormal fluctuations of body temperature in depressed patients. Depressed individuals often complain of decreased libido. Serotonergic activity generally suppresses sexual function, whereas serotonin depletion with PCPA increases sexual behavior in animals. This parallels inhibition by serotonin of gonadal hormone secretion.

Mania. Mania is the polar opposite to depression, and it may be triggered by increased serotonergic function. Several studies suggest that mania follows the ingestion of L-tryptophan or agents that specifically block the reuptake of serotonin. Other studies indicate that L-tryptophan has antimanic effects. It may be that serotonergic systems interact differentially with other systems to affect mood in either direction. It is not established that serotonergic stimulation worsens mania in people who are hypomanic or manic. Electroconvulsive therapy, an effective treatment for severe depressions, causes enhanced serotonergic neurotransmission, especially after administration of serotonin precursors. The benefit of electroconvulsive therapy is antagonized by either serotonin antagonists or noradrenergic lesions, further supporting an interaction between serotonergic and adrenergic neurotransmission in the mechanism of depression.

Chronic administration of antidepressant drugs tends to decrease serotonin levels and serotonin turnover. $5HT_2$ and $5HT_1$ receptors tend to downregulate or not change. Antidepressant drugs that selectively block the reuptake of serotonin do so immediately, before an antidepressant effect is noticeable. This suggests that changes in serotonin levels per se are inadequate to fully explain either the disorder or the therapeutic benefit of these drugs. Other neurotransmitter systems that are probably involved in the pathogenesis of depression are norepinephrine, dopamine, acetylcholine, and GABA. The role of each of these neurotransmitters is discussed in the respective sections.

Evidence for interaction of multiple neurotransmitter systems in the pathogenesis of depression is based on colocalization in the same brain region, similarity of physiological effects, and reciprocal interactions. Serotonin, norepinephrine, and acetylcholine all increase firing by postsynaptic mechanisms and decrease neurotransmitter release by presynaptic mechanisms. Antidepressant therapy and electroconvulsant therapy depend on intact noradrenergic and serotonergic systems. Serotonin inhibits dopaminergic neurons, probably by action on a $5HT_{1B}$ receptor type, and serotonin inhibits acetylcholine release in the rat striatum by a presynaptic receptor-mediated mechanism. β-Adrenergic blockers, such as propranolol, may produce depression by indirect effects on serotonin release, turnover, or receptor profile. Both α- and β-adrenergic agonists increase serotonin release, turnover, and receptor number. Lesions of serotonin containing neurons or their pathways upregulate β-adrenergic receptors. Some studies indicate that GABA-mimetics modulate head twitching in mice, a response produced by serotonin and GABA receptor agonists that inhibit the release of serotonin.

Schizophrenia. A role for a subset of serotonin receptors in schizophrenia is supported by the observation that hallucinogenic drugs such as LSD exert their effects by binding to $5HT_2$ receptors, which are highly expressed in structures of the limbic system. LSD is a partial agonist at $5HT_2$ receptors, but it is not established whether its overall effect is as an agonist in its own right or an antagonist of serotonin. It stimulates phosphoinoside hydrolysis when presented alone, but it decreases the effect of serotonin and causes an insurmountable block of serotonin actions. This may indicate binding at more than one site. To speculate, binding at the serotonin receptor could produce the partial agonist effects and binding at a distinct modulatory site may influence coupling to a G protein. Several neuroleptics, including the atypical neuroleptic clozapine, are $5HT_2$ antagonists in addition to their effect on subtypes of dopaminergic receptors. This particular action of neuroleptics may account for their efficacy against negative schizophrenic symptoms. $5HT_2$ antagonists also improve mood, drive, and motivation in patients with parkinsonism and anxiety disorders.

Alcoholism. Several studies suggest a role for serotonin in alcoholism. The $5HT_{1A}$ partial agonist buspirone, an atypical anxiolytic, reduces alcohol craving, while the serotonin agonist M-chlorphenylpiperizine increases craving for alcohol more than a placebo does. Similarly, in rats trained to discriminate between ethanol and water, serotonin agonists stimulated selection of ethanol and substituted for the training dose of ethanol, in that withdrawal symptoms were not observed. These effects of enhanced serotonergic activity confound the interpretation of the therapeutic benefit of selective serotonin uptake inhibitors in alcohol treatment.

Pain. The broad clinical therapeutic utility of antidepressant compounds is difficult to explain solely on the basis of inhibition of reuptake of biogenic amines. Tricyclic compounds reduce sodium current in dorsal root ganglion neurons, and imipramine blocks excitatory calcium influx through a voltage-activated L-type calcium channel. The blocking action of imipramine is greatly reduced by pertussis toxin or by intracellular dialysis with solutions containing guanosine-5'-O-2-biodiphosphate, which blocks the GTP binding site on G proteins. This suggests that the blockade of excitatory calcium influx is linked to activation by G proteins, and that imipramine may bind to the channel at a point regulated or bound by the G protein or by binding to the G protein itself. These cellular actions may explain the benefit of certain tricyclic antidepressant compounds in the treatment of pain, independent of the effects on reuptake of the biogenic amines.

Analgesic effects of serotonin could occur at the brain stem and spinal cord levels. For example, stimulation of the periaqueductal gray in regions rich in opioid peptide-containing neurons may result in analgesia by direct projection to the spinal cord, or by an indirect pathway involving activation of a serotonergic interneuron in the nucleus raphe magnus. Lesions in this nucleus or depletion of serotonin with PCPA reduce the efficacy of both stimulation- and morphine-induced analgesia. Thus, two parallel descending pathways from the brain stem that modulate the firing of dorsal horn neurons are believed to be present—one an opioid peptide projection, the other a peptide-activated serotonergic pathway.

The second level at which serotonin may be effective is in the spinal cord itself. Presumably, dorsal horn neurons could be directly inhibited by the serotonergic projection; or presynaptic inhibition of release of nociceptive neurotransmitters, such as substance P, could occur. This mechanism is often invoked to explain the analgesic effect of the opioid projection on segmental pain-signalling in the spinal cord. The antinociceptive effect of intrathecally injected serotonin in the tail flick latency test is antagonized by the $5HT_{1A}$ antagonist spiperone and the $5HT_{1C}$ antagonist minserin, but not by antagonists at $5HT_2$ and $5HT_3$ receptors (1-naphthyl piperazine and 3-tropanyl-indol-3-carboxylate, respectively). $5HT_{1A}$ receptors open potassium channels and thereby hyperpolarize and decrease the firing rates of neurons bearing these receptors. $5HT_{1A}$ autoreceptors could reduce the release of transmitters by a presynaptic hyperpolarization. The $5HT_{1C}$ receptors are coupled to phosphinositide hydrolysis by a G protein; their exact location in the dorsal horn is unknown. Since generation of IP_3 generally increases intracellular calcium concentration, a depolarizing (excitatory) effect is expected from activation of these receptors. Excitation of neurons bearing these receptors may result in release of another neurotransmitter, such as norepinephrine or GABA, that hyperpolarizes and decreases responsiveness of dorsal horn neurons to the incoming nociceptive barrage.

Interestingly, intradermal injection of serotonin probably produces pain by activating nociceptive neurons.

Alzheimer's Disease. Postmortem examination of the brains of people with Alzheimer's disease shows a marked reduction of $5HT_1$ and $5HT_2$ receptors and a substantial loss of neurons in the dorsal raphe nucleus, as compared to age-matched controls. Despite these changes, manipulation of serotonergic activity has not been shown to slow or prevent cognitive decline.

Migraine. Serotonin receptors and pathways are believed to play a role in the pathophysiology of migraine, and several drugs have been developed to treat migraine by modifying serotonin activity. The latest is sumatriptan, a serotonin $5HT_{1D}$ agonist that is effective abortive therapy for migraine and cluster headaches. $5HT_{1D}$ receptors are scattered throughout the forebrain, but they are most intensely expressed in the substantia nigra and pallidum. Presynaptic 51D receptors modulate the release of serotonin. Postsynaptic receptors modulate the presynaptic release of other neurotransmitters, including ACh. However, sumatriptan crosses the blood-brain barrier poorly and has rare central adverse effects. Its principal therapeutic action probably is to block the release of norepinephrine from sympathetic terminals in blood vessels. This may occur through the presynaptic activation of $5HT_{1D}$ receptors that decrease cyclic AMP and reduce transmitter release.

Epilepsy. Stimulation and blockade of serotonergic systems has apparent contradictory effects on epileptogenesis. Amygdala kindling can be blocked by stimulation of serotonergic neurons in the median raphe nucleus or by injection of fluoxetine, a serotonin reuptake blocker. Augmentation of serotonergic neurotransmission blocks tonic hindlimb extension in the maximal electroshock model seizures. The augmentation of serotonergic neurotransmission can be accomplished by (1) administering precursors such as tryptophan or 5-hydroxytryptophan, (2) blocking the reuptake of serotonin with fluoxetine, (3) increasing release with fenfluramine, or (4) giving agonists such as 5-methoxydimethyltryptamine. In contrast, reductions of brain serotonin or blockade of serotonergic neurotransmission lowers the threshold for electrically induced tonic hindlimb extension and for pentylenetetrazole-induced seizures. This can be accomplished by administering PCPA to deplete serotonin or 5,7-dihydroxytryptamine to destroy serotonergic neurons. Brain stem serotonergic neurons are more likely to play an important modulatory role in epilepsy than forebrain or spinal cord neurons.

Löscher and Czuczwar studied the effects of serotonin agonists and antagonists on seizure expression in different animal models of epilepsy. 5-hydroxytryptophan, a serotonin precursor, increased the threshold for pentylenetetrazol seizures as expected, but it had no effect on seizure-prone gerbils. Anticonvulsant effects of serotonin in the gerbils were blocked by ketanserin, a $5HT_2$ antagonist. The $5HT_{1A}$ agonist 8-hydroxy-DPAT also had protective efficacy, presumably by activating a hyperpolarizing potassium current postsynaptically or by reducing transmitter release. Serotonin depletion lowers seizure threshold in two genetic models of epilepsy, the genetically epilepsy-prone rat and the audiogenic-seizure mouse. Both strains are sensitive to auditory stimulation. Serotonin levels are particularly low in the hippocampus and in some other areas in these animals. In the kindling model, serotonin is low in the stimulated hippocampus for at least a month after kindling. In contrast, intracerebral microdialysis studies suggest that focal and generalized seizures markedly increase norepinephrine but not serotonin. Regional effects of manipulation of the biogenic amines may have diverse effects, because they have a multiplicity of actions even in the same structure. For example, acetylcholine has at least five different postsynaptic effects, and serotonin has four postsynaptic effects in the hippocampus alone. Therefore, the effects of modulation of transmitter release along specific pathways, and in different regions of the brain where subtypes of receptors are differentially expressed, must be studied to understand modulation of seizure by monoamines.

Treatment with neuroleptics and tricyclic antidepressants was believed to decrease the seizure threshold. Such reports often occurred in the treatment of overdose. Agents that exhibit dose-dependent increases in spike frequency of hippocampal neurons in vitro, in order of decreasing potency, are imipramine, nomifensine (discontinued because of its side effect of hemolytic anemia), amitriptyline, nortriptyline, desipramine, and maprotaline. Conversely, agents that decrease neuronal excitability in the hippocampal slice, in order of decreasing potency, are trimipramine, protriptyline, doxepin, and veloxizine. Antidepressant agents that protect against death from intraperitoneal injection of NMDA into mice, in order of decreasing potency, are desipramine, protriptyline, nortriptyline, imipramine, chloripramine, and amitriptyline. The value of such animal and in vitro studies in predicting the usefulness of investigational compounds on seizure threshold is not established. The use of tricyclic and atypical antidepressants to treat depression in epileptics is not contraindicated, but treatment should start at low dosages, and rates of escalation should be slow.

Other Clinical Situations. $5HT_3$ receptors' agonists are particularly active antiemetics. One such agonist, ondansetron, was recently approved for use during chemotherapy as an antiemetic. Several other compounds are in clinical trials for similar use.

If one accepts the notion that myoclonic jerks are produced by cortical hyperexcitability, then the mechanism of post-anoxic myoclonus (Lance-Adams syndrome) may be damage to neurons in the raphe nuclei that project to cortical neurons bearing inhibitory $5HT_1$ and $5HT_2$ receptors. The $5HT_{1A}$ receptor activates potassium channels by a G protein–dependent mechanism, and loss of serotonergic input would decrease inhibition of cortical neurons. Precursor therapy with tryptophan could work by restoring serotonin levels.

Choroid plexus epithelial cells are rich in $5HT_{1C}$ receptors. Since these receptors are linked by G proteins to phosphoinositide hydrolysis, their activation presumably increases intracellular calcium and the synthesis of CSF. $5HT_{1C}$ antagonists such as ondansetron may be useful in controlling the production of CSF in treating pseudotumor cerebri or hydrocephalus.

VOLTAGE-GATED ION CHANNELS

The effects of neurotransmitters on membrane potentials contribute to patterns of action-potential firing and modulate neurotransmitter release by central neurons. The actions of some neurotransmitters, such as acetylcholine or serotonin, are mediated principally through G protein–mediated interactions with calcium or potassium channels. As the membrane potentials change under the influence of these neurotransmitter-gated ion channels, the likelihood of opening voltage-sensitive ion channels increases during EPSPs and decreases during IPSPs. EPSPs of sufficient amplitude to bring the membrane potential to threshold trigger action potentials. The upstroke of the action potential depends principally on the entry of sodium ions through voltage-activated sodium channels. In some instances, the influx of calcium through voltage-selective calcium channels contributes to the rising phase of the action potential. The sodium-dependent action potentials are conducted along axons and cause depolarization of nerve terminals, triggering neurotransmitter release. Strictly calcium-dependent action potentials have been identified in dendrites of central neurons. These action potentials probably serve to ensure the transmission of excitatory potentials on the distal dendrite to the soma and axon hillock where potentials sum to modulate axonal firing rates. Action-potential firing over the soma and down the axon couples the electrical output of the neuron to its biochemical machinery for the maintenance of the membrane potential and modulation of neurotransmitter release.

Action-potential duration is to a large extent determined by voltage-dependent calcium and potassium currents. Action-potential duration limits the maximal rate of firing. Calcium and potassium also generate afterpotentials that modulate firing frequency. Hyperpolarizing afterpotentials tend to slow firing, and depolarizing afterpotentials may increase firing.

Voltage changes in the nerve terminal modulate release of neurotransmitter. Action potential–induced depolarization of the terminals stimulates entry of calcium through voltage-dependent channels. The resultant slow depolarizing wave facilitates fusion of neurotransmitter-containing vesicles with the releasing zone of the terminal and subsequent exocytosis of the neurotransmitter.

Activation of voltage-dependent chloride channels affords rapid entry of chloride ions, which increases the rate of action potential repolarization. The contribution of chloride ions to early repolarization is particularly evident in the action potentials of cardiac Purkinje fibers and skeletal muscle fibers.

The in-rush of sodium through voltage-activated sodium channels generates the upstroke of action potential propagated over neuronal somatic membranes and along axons. This function has evolved and has been highly conserved. Action potential firing is all or none, and it depends on reaching a threshold at which sufficient sodium channels open simultaneously so that a regenerative response occurs. Information encoded in the pattern and frequency of action potential firing is critical for the projection of activity from one brain region to another along selectively activated pathways subserving specific functions. Although action potentials do not occur in nerve terminals, their arrival leads to a depolarization critical for the release of neurotransmitters. Myelination of central and some peripheral nerve fibers increases the fidelity and security of action potential firing and conduction over long distances. The brain operates in the millisecond timeframe. This property is conferred by brief (1–2 msec) action potentials, high-velocity propagation along short myelinated fibers, and neurotransmission requiring less than a millisecond. Using their brain machines, humans have invented computers that operate in the nano-microsecond range. To fly the F-16 electric jet, the pilot moves a side stick controller that transduces the deflection into electrical impulses. The electronics operate many times faster than the nervous system of the pilot. Thus, it is easy to see why any unintended deflection could throw the plane out of control and kill the pilot in literally the blink of an eye. In the body, movement control is affected by coupling the nervous system to the contractile systems of muscle. While a muscle fiber can rapidly conduct action potentials, twitches and more sustained contractions develop over many milliseconds to seconds. The tone of a skeletal muscle—basically the resting state of contraction of that muscle—is modulated by neural activity, from cortex to spinal cord to motor neuron to muscle. In testing for arm drift, the patient must hold the arms extended and elevated against gravity. This requires sustained high-frequency action potential firing along the neural path that tetanizes the antigravity muscles for as long as the action potentials continue to fire. Any disruption of neural capacity to initiate, sustain, and terminate high-frequency firing will interrupt coordinated neuromuscular function and alter tone.

An analogous situation exists in blood vessels. Smooth muscle tends to contract much more slowly than skeletal muscle. Cerebral resistance vessels located in the pia mater branch to give approximately 100-μm diameter feeder vessels to the underlying cortex. These vessels are cuffed by a dense plexus of fibers containing a myriad of peptide and classical neurotransmitters involved in neurogenic regulation of vascular tone. The variety of neurotransmitters represents tiers of control of vital blood flow to the brain. If these neurogenic influences and local factors regulating regional blood flow are not coordinated, the result may be localized alterations of brain electrical activity (e.g., spreading depression), and this could trigger vascular reflexes mediated by the projection of high-frequency firing of action potentials along serotonergic, adrenergic, and other fibers from brain stem nuclei to the forebrain vasculature. This sequence of incoordination and brain stem reflexes is involved in migraine headaches. Only rarely are medicines that control action potential firing rates, such as antiepileptic drugs, effective in the treatment of headache, perhaps because neuronal firing patterns are not amenable to optimum drug action. Epilepsy may be the best example of disease of the CNS in which control of high-frequency action potential firing has therapeutic value.

Sodium Channels

Sodium Channel Structure

Voltage-gated sodium channels isolated from eel electroplax and rat brain are glycosylated proteins with a molecular weight in the range of 230–270 kD (Catterall 1992). Channels from both sources consist of 1,800–2,000 amino acid α-subunits. The α-subunit seems to contain sequences conferring most of the known electrophysiological and pharmacological properties of these channels. Multiple isoforms of α-subunits have been identified by cloning techniques. Functional diversity is much less apparent and has been determined primarily by pharmacological and electrophysiological techniques. In the rat brain, however, there are also modulatory β_1- and β_2-subunits with molecular weights in the range of 33,000–36,000 kD that contain approximately 200 amino acid sequences. These subunits are not covalently bound to the β-subunit. The β-subunit of skeletal muscle is slightly larger but has properties similar to those of the brain β-subunits. The β-subunits probably modulate the rate of sodium channel inactivation (spontaneous closure) and possibly the voltage-dependence of activation of the channels.

Molecular pharmacology has identified sequences in the sodium channel that account for the many functional features (Catterall 1992; see Figure 52.1C). Sequencing of the α-subunit suggests that both the amino and carboxy sequences are intracellular. The core sequence consists of four domains of six hydrophobic transmembrane sequences, the four domains being connected by intra- and extracellular peptide loops. These domains are roughly analogous to subunits of neurotransmitter-gated receptors, but in this case they are covalently linked. The extracellular loop connecting the fifth and sixth transmembrane sequences of each domain is longer than the other extracellular loops. In the first domain, this loop is glycosylated. Intracellular loops connecting the sixth transmembrane segment of the first domain to the first transmembrane segment of the second domain is very long and contains many sites for modulation by phosphorylation. The intracellular loop connecting the third and fourth domains is relatively short. This loop seems to be responsible for the inactivation characteristics of the sodium channel. Phosphorylation of this loop by protein kinase C slows inactivation of the channel and links channel phosphorylation to activation of G proteins coupled to the cascade-activating protein kinase C. Binding of tetrodotoxin, which is isolated from the ovaries of the puffer fish of the genus *Tetradon*, depends on negatively charged residues in the extracellular loops linking the fifth and sixth transmembrane segments of each domain. The fourth transmembrane segments of each domain contain positively charged amino acid residues, which probably constitute the voltage sensor. These charged residues are essentially electrophoresed by voltage changes in response to electrical stimulation, or by neurotransmitter-mediated changes in ionic conductance that result in conformational changes in these segments and in relationship to other transmembrane segments in each domain of the sodium channel. The result is transient opening of the sodium channel, with sodium entry until the kinetically slower inactivation process occurs.

Channel Function and Pharmacology. The Nobel Prize for physiology and medicine was conferred on Hodgkin and Huxley in 1952 for their descriptions of the operational cycle of voltage-activated sodium current, using the voltage-clamp technique developed by Cole. Electrophysiological refinements from patch-clamp experiments and the molecular characterization of the channel have led to a well-focused picture of how sodium channels behave, singly and in concert. Sodium influx through voltage-sensitive channels generates the upstroke of action potentials recorded from axons and somata of central neurons. In the Hodgkin and Huxley model, channels may be in the resting, activated (conducting), or inactive state of configuration. With depolarization, available resting channels open quickly and nearly synchronously, and they admit sodium ions flowing inward along their concentration gradient. If this influx generates enough current, it triggers the action potential. The channels inactivate spontaneously as slower conformational changes close the inner mouths of the channels. Gradual repriming, or recovery, from inactivation occurs after repolarization. The number of channels available to contribute to the next action potential is determined largely by the interval between spikes, conferring rate-dependence, and the transmembrane voltage, conferring voltage-dependence. At high frequencies (>150 Hz), the rate of cycling may not be fast enough for sufficient channels to reprime. The result is that sodium current I_{Na}, and maximal rate of rise of action potentials (V_{max}) decrease at fast rates. Although kinetic parameters vary, all voltage-sensitive ion channels must go through a similar operational cycle. Kinetic models of drug interaction with different aspects of channel function have had an important impact on antiepileptic and antiarrhythmic drug development.

Several standard antiepileptic medications bind to sodium channels, resulting in accumulation of sodium channels in the inactivated state, prolongation of refractoriness, and failure of some action potentials. Phenytoin, carbamazepine, and valproic acid all limit sustained high-frequency repetitive firing (SRF) of sodium-dependent action potentials involved in the spread of ictal activity at concentrations that correspond to therapeutic free-plasma levels. Some of the new antiepileptic medications may also block sodium channels. Progressive reduction of V_{max} before action potential failure suggests an effect on sodium channels, although potassium and calcium currents could be involved. This effect on sodium channels parallels the ability of these compounds to protect against tonic hind-limb extension in the maximal electroshock model in animals, and it may contribute to clinical efficacy against partial seizures with or without secondary tonic-clonic generalization.

Not all antiepileptic medications work this way. Barbiturates and benzodiazepines limit SRF only at high concentrations, which might be encountered in the treatment of status epilepticus, suggesting that these compounds work in other ways. The best-known mechanism of these drugs is augmentation of GABA-activated chloride influx. Ethosuximide does not block SRF. Other compounds, including local anesthetics and tricyclic antidepressants, act at voltage-sensitive sodium channels, yet they are not useful clinically as antiepileptics.

Sodium channel block by standard anticonvulsant drugs has several important characteristics. First, its effect is concentration-dependent, as expected from the clinical definition of therapeutic range; second, the effect is voltage-dependent. At very negative transmembrane potentials, drugs bind to a small percentage of sodium channels with some reduction of sodium current or action potential rate of rise (tonic block). With depolarization, such as occurs at the ictal transition, drug binding becomes more likely and block accrues more quickly. Third, the effect on sodium channels is use-dependent, requiring multiple activations of sodium currents or firings of action potentials to become maximal. It is also frequency-dependent, and it is enhanced at fast rates and less-negative membrane potentials, which occur at the depolarizing shift signaling the ictal transition. Channels to which drug is bound are effectively unavailable to fire the next action potential. Firing at slower rates is possible despite the continuing presence of the drug. Anticonvulsant drugs with this action modulate rather than block sodium channel function.

How does this relate to clinical anticonvulsant effects? Ideally, concentration-dependence in vitro should predict the therapeutic range. Limitation of SRF by phenytoin, for example, occurs at concentrations equivalent to therapeutic free-plasma (i.e., not bound to plasma proteins) levels. Brain-tissue levels increase with time. Slow accumulation in brain may account for gradual improvement in efficacy on a constant dose of an anticonvulsant drug. Alternatively, an active metabolite may accumulate and add to the efficacy of the parent compound. For example, carbamazepine epoxide and the trans-2-en metabolite of valproic acid both limit high-frequency firing and accumulate in the brain and CSF. Limitation of high-frequency firing by antiepileptic medications has not been shown in vivo, so the repetitive firing assay may be only a pharmacological model. However, high-frequency action potential firing is transmitted along projection pathways from a chemically induced cortical focus. This firing pattern is thought to underly the spread of abnormal activity from the seizure focus. Extrapolating from the cellular data, limitation of high-frequency action potential firing should be a useful antiepileptic mechanism. However, brief bursts of fast firing or firing sustained at slower rates will not be blocked. This could explain refractoriness of some seizures to sodium channel–blocking medications.

Voltage-dependence may explain why ambulatory patients tolerate sodium channel–blocking antiepileptic medications chronically, with minimal dysfunction. Interictally, the patient may function almost as if the drug were not present; but when abnormal focal activity commences and prolonged depolarization occurs, drug action becomes more effective and limits high-frequency firing along axons projecting to distant relays in the seizure pathway. This may arrest the spread of seizures. Perhaps engagement of these actions underlies brief periods of confusion or the perception of transient impairment that patients describe after they "almost" have a seizure. Frequency-dependence allows drugs to be used as anticonvulsants. Blocking too many sodium channels—for example, due to a high concentration of one, or pharmacodynamic interaction between two sodium channel blockers—could result in sedation, reduced motor speed, and impaired cognition. In the extreme, compounds that bind tightly to sodium channels, such as tetrodotoxin, are lethal. Thus the same cellular action may be relevant to both therapeutic efficacy and toxicity.

Sodium channel blockade is consistent with the demonstrated protection by these new antiepileptic medications against maximal electroshock seizures in animals and clinically against partial seizures with and without secondary generalization. But not all sodium channel blockers are good anticonvulsants. Local anesthetic compounds, for example, are not widely used for treating seizures. They have both hydrophilic and hydrophobic interactions with the channel. Hydrophilic interactions involve the drug entering the channel, creating so-called open channel block. Hydrophobic interactions involve transient binding to the inactivation gate with a resultant prolongation of recovery from inactivation. Amitriptyline has lidocaine-like antiarrhythmic effects, and it is not an anticonvulsant. Phenytoin is highly lipophilic, and it appears to act principally by interacting with the inactivation gate of the sodium channel to cause accumulation of channels in the inactivated configuration, to the extent that insufficient channels are available for activation to support high-frequency action potential firing. As a result, phenytoin behaves as a low-pass filter, allowing slow action potential firing or short bursts of high-frequency firing to pass while blocking sustained high-frequency firing. Brevetoxins, produced by the dinoflagellate involved in red tides (see Chapter 65), and certain plant alkaloids, such as veratridine, hold the inactivation gait open and allow a prolonged entry of sodium ions through the channel. This results in excessive excitation, an effect unlikely to be of therapeutic value.

Nociceptive fibers of peripheral nerve have tetrodotoxin-resistant sodium channels that are more severely blocked by lidocaine actions than the classical tetrodotoxin-sensitive kinetically fast sodium channel of the CNS and mechanoceptive fibers. This is a good example of functional diversity of sodium channels.

In summary, the peptide sequence of the sodium channel contains regions that correspond to channel cycling predicted in the 1950s by Hodgkin and Huxley. Many therapeutic agents and toxins bind to different parts of the channel and modulate the cycling of sodium channels these scientists envisioned.

Sodium Channels and Disease States

Sodium channels are important, and the company they keep determines which compounds will be of therapeutic, rather than toxic, value. For example, lidocaine has a relatively higher affinity for the sodium channel than phenytoin. Because of the long duration of cardiac action potentials, the fact that lidocaine tends to stick to the sodium channels is not a disadvantage. The same stickiness may in large part account for the local anesthetic effects of lidocaine-like compounds, and lidocaine has been used by some to treat status epilepticus. Phenytoin has a lower affinity and shorter dwell-time on its binding site in the sodium channel than lidocaine. As a result, phenytoin less severely limits sodium channel cycling, and neuronal function continues, albeit at a slower rate, in the continuing presence of the drug. This is particularly advantageous if patients must function and work while taking the drug.

Properties of phenytoin are much more amenable to antiepileptic use. Because of its lipophilicity, it readily crosses the blood-brain barrier and enters neurons where it can have its effect. The rapidity of penetration of the blood-brain barrier makes it useful as a drug for the treatment of status epilepticus. The voltage-dependence of blockade by phenytoin produces only moderate reduction of sodium channel availability at the normal cell resting potential, and only those neurons that undergo the depolarizing shift at the onset of the ictal discharge become extensively blocked by phenytoin. This means, in effect, that patients can perform their usual work with minimal, sometimes unnoticeable, compromise of function. Both phenytoin and carbamazepine have been demonstrated to compromise performance on psychometric testing, but the effects were undetectable by individuals taking the drugs chronically. During polypharmacy with two sodium channel-acting blocking antiepileptic drugs—for example, phenytoin and carbamazepine—the effects on a sodium channel might be additive or potentiative and result in a toxic pharmacodynamic interaction.

Point mutations in the gene encoding the skeletal muscle sodium channel have been implicated in a number of human neurological diseases. These include hyperkalemic periodic paralysis and paramyotonia congenita, both of which are localized to human chromosome 17q. These disorders result in muscle paralysis and myotonia due to disorders of sodium channel inactivation. Some families with paramyotonia congenita have point mutations leading to a single amino acid change in the voltage-sensing fourth transmembrane sequence.

Calcium Channels

Four pharmacologically and electrophysiologically distinct types of calcium channels have been characterized, and probably more exist. These types are referred to as T, L, N, and P. The L and N types have been cloned, which suggests that greater molecular diversity exists than has been discovered functionally. Calcium channels are evolutionary descendants of, and share 50% homology with, sodium channels, primarily in the transmembrane regions. This structural similarity may account for the fact that some classes of compounds, such as hydantoins and calcium-entry blockers, bind to both sodium channels and calcium channels. Significant differences in the intracellular linkers between transmembrane domains are likely to account for the unique regulation and function of calcium channels. A long intracellular carboxy terminus of the L channel contains a sequence to which calcium must bind before dihydropyridines such as nifedipine or nimodipine can produce their pharmacological block. The intracellular loop connecting the second and third transmembrane domain of L-type channels in muscle T-tubules may be the voltage sensor signaling calcium release from sarcoplasmic reticulum in muscle. This loop differs in neuronal L-type channels. By analogy to the sodium channel, the fourth transmembrane sequence of each domain contains multiple positively charged lysine and arginine residues, which appear to confer voltage sensitivity on channel opening.

The operating cycle of calcium channels is similar to that of the sodium channel and involves changing from resting to conducting and inactivated conformations. Elevation of intracellular free calcium, due to entry through the voltage-activated calcium channels or due to release from intracellular stores (e.g., by activation of inosotoltriphosphate-sensitive calcium channels secondarily activated after phospholipase C), is important in the inactivation of some calcium channels. Dihydropyridine-sensitive L-type channels seem to require the binding of calcium prior to drug binding, suggesting that calcium binding is the key step in inactivation; then the dihydropyridine binds to the inactivated channel. In other calcium channels in various species, voltage-dependent inactivation or a combination of inactivation mechanisms may be important. Variability in activation mechanisms could account in part for differential sensitivity of different organs or cell types to various classes of drugs. Frequency- or use-dependence of blockade by certain drugs is crucial for calcium channels as well as sodium channels. A good example is use-dependent block of L channels by dihydropyridines. This feature confers activity-dependence on the effect of the drug and suggests the drug may be present with minimal effects at low activity levels.

Physiology and Pharmacology of Calcium Channels. Calcium channels are involved in many neuronal functions. After neurotransmitters produce excitatory responses in dendrites, activation of voltage-sensitive calcium channels may trigger propagated calcium-dependent action potentials. These secure the transmission of information to the neuronal soma and axon hillock, where sodium channels are densely expressed. Multiple types of sodium channels probably act in concert. Slight depolarization from rest may activate low-threshold T-type channels, which open briefly and inactivate relatively quickly. These channels probably underlie oscillatory behavior, which confers burst firing properties on neurons. As the membrane depolarizes sufficiently, the high-threshold types of calcium channels, namely L, N, and P, open. The opening of P-type channels has been implicated in the production of dendritic calcium spikes, which propagate to the soma. Here, depolarization to threshold results in firing of sodium-dependent action potentials over the somatic membrane and axon hillock. While sodium-dependent action potential firing accounts for propagation along axons, neurotransmitter release depends on the admission of calcium into the terminals through voltage-dependent calcium channels. Neurotransmitter release depends at least on N-type channel activation and probably also on activation of P-type channels. The N-type channels are selectively blocked by the peptide Ω-conotoxin, isolated from predatory cone snails. The P-type channels are blocked by Ω-agatoxin isolated from spider venom. Under some conditions, diydropyridine-sensitive L-type channels may be involved in transmitter release. However, transmission in most experimental paradigms is unaffected by dihydropyridines. In the experimental paradigm known as post-tetanic potentiation, a nerve is stimulated at high frequency. Following this tetanus, a single stimulus produces a markedly enhanced postsynaptic excitatory response. This phenomenon is thought to be due to enhanced neurotransmitter release because of accumulation of calcium in nerve terminals with repetitive activation. Phenytoin, which has been shown to block L-type channels, inhibits post-tetanic potentiation more potently than other antiepileptic drugs, including carbamazepine. These L-type channels may be recruited for neurotransmitter release during projection of high-frequency activity along axons. This hypothesis fits with the finding that dihydropyridines block neurotransmission enhanced by the dihydropyridine L-type channel activator Bay k8644. Blockade of L-type channel by dihydropyridines and phenytoin is use-dependent. Alternatively, phenytoin could block N- or P-type channels, though there is no evidence for this at present. Blockade by phenytoin of high-voltage-activated calcium channels is consistent with voltage-dependent block of sodium channels that is facilitated by depolarization.

Oscillatory activity appears to be important in both normal and abnormal activity of thalamic neurons. Low voltage-activated T-type calcium channels appear to underlie this activity. The petit mal antiepileptic drugs ethosuximide and dimethadione block T-type current at therapeutically relevant concentrations, but phenytoin and carbamazepine do not. This difference may explain, at least in part, the different efficacy of antiepileptic drugs. The broad-spectrum antiepileptic drug valproic acid has been reported to block the T-type current only slightly at high concentrations in dorsal root ganglion neurons, but not in thalamic or human neocortical neurons. Ethosuximide does not block T-current in human cortical neurons, suggesting regional differences in the pharmacology of this type of current.

Abnormalities of calcium channel operation underlie at least two disorders of muscle. In the myasthenic syndrome of Lambert and Eaton, plasma contains antibodies against synaptic voltage-sensitive calcium channels (See Chapter 82). Excitation-contraction coupling in skeletal muscle involves propagation of sodium action potentials along the sarcolemma, which excites voltage-sensitive calcium channels at the T-tubular triad. These are probably dihydropyridine-sensitive L-type channels. Calcium reuptake occurs through a second type of calcium channel, which is blocked by ryanodine (McPherson and Campbell 1993). This is probably identical to the calcium channel activated by IP3 and subject to modulation by activation of phospholipase C. A point mutation in this channel is associated with malignant hyperthermia in swine and in some humans. As a result of the mutation, sarcoplasmic calcium concentrations remain elevated, and the myofibrillary lattice remains in contracture with excessive, life-threatening heat production and muscle breakdown.

Potassium Channels

Potassium channels share with other voltage-sensitive ion channels a common structure of four covalently linked subunit domains, each with six transmembrane sequences.

However, unlike sodium and potassium channels, the polarity of the potassium channels is different. When the channels are opened, potassium ions move outward from the neuronal cytoplasm, where the potassium concentration is high (approximately 140 mmol/liter), to the extracellular space, where the potassium concentration is low (less than 5 mmol/liter). Cloning of multiple potassium channels from a variety of species, especially *Drosophila*, has confirmed much of the behavior of the delayed rectifier channels responsible for action potential repolarization described in the seminal work of Hodgkin and Huxley. Other potassium channels responsible for oscillations in membrane potential and clamping of the membrane potential toward the resting level have also been characterized electrophysiologically and pharmacologically. Also, unlike sodium and calcium channels, the inactivation particle of the potassium channel is located at the end of the intracellular amino terminus and swings into the channel opened by voltage changes like a ball on the end of a rope.

The delayed rectifier, or I_K, initiates repolarization of the action potential. It turns on quickly with depolarization—though not as quickly as the sodium current—and is maximally active as the sodium current becomes inactivated. Persistence of I_K after inactivation of the sodium current results in a hyperpolarizing afterpotential, which inactivates quickly and allows maximal firing rates in the range of several hundred per second. Depolarization, especially when it is prolonged in response to steady synaptic excitation, also activates the so-called A-current. This outward current delays the onset of firing after a voltage change by driving the membrane potential away from threshold, back toward the resting potential. As the current inactivates, the membrane potential depolarizes to threshold, and firing commences. The A-current turns on with slight depolarization and is activated fast enough to contribute to action potential repolarization and control of rate of firing. The A-current differs from the delayed rectifier, I_K, in that it is almost completely inactivated at potentials positive to –40 mV, whereas I_K increases in this potential range.

A third potassium current, the M-current (I_M), is activated by depolarization. Activation of the I_M opposes the tendency toward threshold and repetitive firing. A unique feature of this current is that it is not inactivating, and it causes depolarizations to lag toward the resting potential. Neurotransmitters that block I_M, such as acetylcholine or muscarine, after which the I_M is named, promote increased firing frequencies.

Two calcium-dependent potassium channels (I_{KCa}) contribute repolarizing outward currents that are activated by depolarization. A kinetically fast I_{KCa} is activated with a delayed rectifier. A rise in intracellular free calcium due to transmembrane influx or release from intracellular stores is essential for activation of this current. A kinetically slower I_{KCa}, I_{AHP}, contributes a slow component to the after-hyperpolarization. Biophysical and pharmacological features distinguish the two currents. Tetraethylammonium blocks fast I_{KCa} more potently than it blocks I_{AHP}. Other antagonists, such as apamin (extracted from the venom of the honey bee), charybdotoxin (a peptide toxin in scorpion venom), curare, and barium act preferentially on I_{AHP}.

Hippocampal pyramidal neurons have all of these outward potassium channels. The overlap of function is insurance against sustained depolarization. In addition, these neurons have an inward potassium current, I_Q, that is activated by hyperpolarization and causes the membrane potential to drift back toward the resting potential. This particular current probably prevents reduction of spiking capacity by excessive hyperpolarization. Normal excitation by multiple biogenic amine neurotransmitters involves blockade of the calcium-dependent potassium conductances and I_M. Modulation of these conductances may be important in the pathophysiology and control of epilepsy and in normal processes such as sleep.

As important as potassium channel activity is in determining firing patterns and frequency, relatively little is known about the effects of medications used by neurologists on potassium channels. Phenytoin and carbamazepine inhibit the delayed rectifier to some extent. Perhaps the best example of modulation of potassium channels to control neurologic disease is the use of aminopyridines and guanidine to treat the myasthenic syndrome and in some cases myasthenia gravis. Two aminopyridines, 4-aminopyridine and 3,4-diaminopyridine, have been used clinically. They are presumed to act by blocking potassium channels in nerve terminals to cause depolarization, entry of calcium, and enhanced neurotransmitter release. Guanidine, which probably sensitizes nerve terminals to calcium in a similar manner, has been used in the treatment of these disorders and botulism.

The availability of therapeutic agents to modulate potassium channel activity would be very useful in the treatment of epilepsy. Phenytoin, for example, limits SRF of action potentials. Because of frequency- and use-dependence, this effect may require hundreds of milliseconds to maximize. One possible mechanism of refractoriness to compounds that act principally on sodium channels is firing patterns that result in brief bursts of action potentials for 50–100 msec. Drugs that increase activation of potassium channels generating outward, hyperpolarizing current might eradicate oscillatory activity underlying this difficult-to-control bursting pattern.

Chloride Channels

Multiple chloride channels are being discovered by cloning techniques. Nonetheless, our understanding of the role of voltage-dependent chloride channels in the brain lags behind that of the cationic channels already described. Chloride ions are involved in regulation of cell volume and must move to maintain charge neutrality when cations enter. Without electroneutrality, osmotic shifts would occur, and neurons would swell or shrink, depending on activity levels. The balance is accomplished through a leak channel. Neurons have a relatively low resting conductance to chloride. The chloride conductance in fast-twitch muscle at rest is high, however. In addition to the high leak conductance to chloride, a voltage-activated chloride channel or current contributes to sharp repolarization of action potentials in skeletal muscles. Experimentally, blockade of this current with aromatic monocarboxylic acids or with zinc results in repetitive firing of action potentials on top of a very slow repolarizing phase. This situation is mimicked in myotonic goats and in humans with myotonia congenita, an autosomal dominant disease with a mutation on chromosome 7q in the region of the skeletal muscle chloride-channel gene. At present, no medications are known to activate chloride channels and repolarize muscle. As our understanding of voltage-sensitive chloride channels increases, it may be possible to develop such therapeutic agents.

Cystic fibrosis is also associated with abnormal pulmonary chloride channels, due to single gene mutation on the long arm of human chromosome 7q. Gene therapy for this illness is in the pioneering stages.

PRINCIPLES OF THERAPEUTICS

The art of administering medications is a complex product of the therapeutic alliance between a patient and the physician and the availability of safe and effective medications. The physician must diagnose a condition, select the most effective remedy, and teach the patient how to self-administer the medicine. Responsibility does not end with a prescription. Physician-patient contact must occur at intervals to confirm the diagnostic impression, determine the efficacy of treatment, and assess dose-related and idiosyncratic adverse reactions. The patient must be motivated to take medications as prescribed, often several times a day. Compliance depends on confidence in the physician, understanding of the disease process, a sense that the medicine is beneficial and tolerable, and a dosage regimen that is consistent with the individual's life-style. These factors comprise what Brodie calls acceptability of the medication to the patient. Unseen to the doctor and patient is the ethical pharmaceutical company that identifies the need for new medications, identifies potential candidate compounds at its own expense, and submits the product to the rigorous scrutiny of clinical trials that meet government regulatory standards.

Desirable Properties of Medications

Anticonvulsant drugs exemplify what is good, bad, and acceptable in the development and use of pharmaceuticals. Their properties are reviewed in the framework of pharmacokinetic and pharmacodynamic principles that enter into the bedside decision-making process.

1. The selected medication must be appropriate for the disease. In the example of anticonvulsants, this means making a correct seizure diagnosis and selecting a medication with a clinical spectrum of efficacy that includes the specific seizure type. Some anticonvulsants are effective against partial seizures with or without secondary generalization; others are effective against primary generalized seizures such as generalized absence; and a few, such as valproate, have a broad spectrum of activity against partial seizures and both primary and secondary generalized seizures.
2. Knowledge of the therapeutic index and mechanism of action simplify drug selection. The therapeutic index is basically a ratio of the toxic dose to a measure of a therapeutically relevant dose. In practice, it equates to the ratio of the blood concentration at which limiting side effects appear, usually the top of the therapeutic range, to a minimally effective dose, the bottom of the therapeutic range. Potency may not be the most desirable property of anticonvulsants, and drugs with greater potency may have a lower therapeutic index. To some degree, then, potency is a trade-off against therapeutic index. A drug with a very large therapeutic index may actually encompass several therapeutic ranges, which can be tailored to the severity of the seizure disorder.
3. A broad spectrum of clinical efficacy seems a desirable characteristic in anticonvulsant drugs. However, *broad spectrum* implies multiple mechanisms of action, some of which may actually contribute to toxicity in a given seizure disorder or individual. A reductionist corollary of this reasoning is that a compound with the least number of actions required to effectively treat a specific disorder should be used.

Preparations

Several factors determine if a compound is user-friendly for the patient and the physician. Ease of use ensures compliance but not efficacy. Factors contributing to ease of use are (1) dosage forms that allow graduated dosing within the full therapeutic range of the medication; (2) easy-to-swallow capsules or tablets and a liquid preparation for children, the aged, and the debilitated; (3) once- or twice-a-day dosing to avoid taking medicine at school or work; and (4) parenteral preparations for unconscious patients and emergency situations such as status epilepticus.

Bioavailability

Bioavailability is the amount of a dose that enters the body. In practice, it is determined as the peak plasma level after oral ingestion divided by the peak after intravenous administration. Currently used anticonvulsant drugs are freely available after oral ingestion. Bioavailability of some compounds is dose-related and may decrease with increasing dosages. Nonetheless, blood levels rise, though less than expected, with dose increments. This implies that above a certain practical limit, further dosage increments will not raise the plasma level sufficiently to justify the cost of the higher dose. Bioavailability may be limited by an uptake mechanism. Optimum dosing requires knowledge of compounds that interfere with or augment uptake and the effects of food.

Titration Rate

Ideally, a therapeutic concentration should be present in the blood and brain as soon as possible after starting a new drug. In practice, this means that a loading dose can be given or that the titration rate should be fast. Loading doses can be given in urgent situations, such as frequent seizures with physical harm to the patient or status epilepticus.

A loading dose is a large dose, usually administered intravenously or by mouth, that brings the plasma level into a therapeutically effective range after one or a few administrations. Loading doses cannot be given with many drugs because of limiting adverse effects or because parenteral preparations are not available.

The titration rate is the speed at which dose increments can be made, and it is an inverse function of the elimination, or half-life, of the medication. A steady state should be reached before conclusions are drawn about the results of a dose increase and a decision about further increments is made. Steady state is reached in five half-lives after initiation of therapy or a dose increment. Further increments before achieving steady state may result in overdose, increased adverse effects, and even more seizures. Multiple doses smooth the oscillations in blood level between doses. The maximum tolerable daily dose may be increased by dividing the dose further. Thus, toxic effects encountered by giving a 1-g dose twice daily may be eliminated by giving the same drug 600 mg four times daily. Seizure control may improve at the higher dose.

Distribution

Drug distribution is commonly discussed in terms of volume of distribution and binding to plasma proteins. The volume of distribution is a virtual number; it can be computed as the amount of drug injected into the body divided by the plasma concentration. This value, in liters, is the fluid volume necessary to dilute the total amount of drug injected to the concentration found in plasma. It is affected by the degree of binding to plasma protein, hydrophobicity of the compound (its partition coefficient in fat), regional blood flow, and other physical factors. The volume of distribution is often reported as the computed volume divided by body weight in kilograms. A low volume of distribution of about 0.15 liters per kg suggests distribution only within the vascular compartment, which consists of about 5.5 liters total blood volume and 3 liters of plasma in a normal 70-kg man. A value of 0.15–0.50 liters per kg suggests distribution throughout extracellular fluid, which is about 12 liters in the ideal man. Values of 0.5–0.6 liters per kg indicate that the drug is distributed throughout total body water. Assuming no regional selectivity, total body water is a volume of about 42 liters in a 70-kg man. Values in excess of 0.6 liter per kg suggest that the drug is concentrated other than in body water at concentrations higher than those found in the plasma. This would be particularly true for highly lipophilic compounds such as phenytoin and compounds that are actively accumulated in the CNS, such as gabapentin.

Lipophilic compounds are bound significantly to base proteins (e.g., albumin). This may be a site for competition with other lipophilic compounds. Use of water-soluble compounds—e.g., gabapentin—avoids the potential for such interactions among drugs.

Biotransformation

The body metabolizes drugs to rid itself of them, as it would many harmful exogenous chemicals. In the case of highly lipid-soluble drugs such as phenytoin, carbamazepine, and valproic acid, metabolism in the liver results in multiple metabolites, some of which are sufficiently water-soluble to be excreted efficiently by the kidney. To accomplish this, the liver uses four fundamental types of reactions: oxidation, reduction, hydrolysis, and conjugation. The first three reactions produce hydroxyl, carboxylic acid, and amine groups, which are polar. This is phase I of enzymatic catalysis in the liver. This step generally results in reduced activity of the metabolites. However, active metabolites are produced from carbamazepine and valproic acid (carbamazepine epoxide and trans-2-en valproic acid). The active metabolites are subsequently modified to more water-soluble compounds for elimination.

In phase II, the polar groups are coupled to endogenous compounds such as glucuronic or acetic acid or inorganic sulfate to produce water-soluble conjugates. Most conjugates are inactive and are excreted in the urine or bile. We generally think of these reactions as taking place in the liver, but microsomal and cytosolic enzymes in other organs, including the brain, may actually metabolize drugs to some extent.

Ultimately, biotransformation accomplishes two tasks—inactivation of exogenous chemical substances and their modification for elimination. The capacity of the body to transform drugs determines, in large part, the interval between subsequent doses required to sustain a therapeutic level. The standard antiepileptic medications are metabolized to varying degrees; gabapentin and vigatrim are not metabolized at all.

Pharmacogenetics

Pharmacogenetics is the study of variations in rates and patterns of drug metabolism. Awareness of such variations is crucial in optimizing therapy for the individual patient. Phenytoin provides one of the best and earliest examples of pharmacogenetic variation. Variation of parahydroxylation of phenytoin results in variable nonlinearity of the relationship between oral dose and steady-state plasma concentrations of phenytoin. This is manifest as the well-known zero-order kinetic curve. The phenytoin blood level rises linearly, up to a break point above which a slight dose change causes a very large increase in plasma phenytoin concentration. The break point varies from individual to individual and with age. The elderly experience this effect at lower doses than children. The break point represents saturation of the liver's capacity to metabolize phenytoin to the parahydroxy derivative. To a large extent, this phenomenon was responsible for the invention of therapeutic blood-level monitoring and for the evolution of models based on Michaelis-Menten kinetics to pharmacokinetically optimize dosing in individuals taking phenytoin.

The half-life of phenytoin is longer in slow hydrolators, who achieve higher concentrations at lower doses than patients who are fast hydroxylators. Slow hydroxylation is an autosomal recessive trait that appears in about 1 in 500 individuals. In practice, unfortunately, these individuals are identified only empirically.

Predisposition to hepatotoxicity due to phenytoin is probably inherited as a genetic polymorphism. Patients with elevated liver enzymes during phenytoin therapy proved to be slow acetylators. Isoniazide is a noncompetitive inhibitor of phenytoin hydroxylation. Inhibiting phenytoin metabolism may result in toxic drug levels and hepatic injury due to effects on other liver enzymes.

Drug Interactions. Interactions due to effects of concomitant medications on the metabolism of standard antiepileptic medications are among the most frequent problems complicating drug therapy of epilepsy. Addition of a second medication may increase, decrease, or not affect the plasma concentration of the first antiepileptic medication. Phenytoin and carbamazepine induce hepatic microsomal enzymes of the P450 system, which augment the metabolism of other antiepileptics and decrease their levels. These metabolic interactions may reduce efficacy of oral contraceptives by enhancing metabolism. Valproic acid, on the other hand, inhibits metabolism of other antiepileptics and may cause significant elevations in their concentration. Gabapentin and vigabatrin are not metabolized and do not alter metabolism of other antiepileptic drugs or oral contraceptives. Blood levels of these two amino acids are not affected by addition of other drugs. Use of medications without drug-drug interactions at the level of metabolism is desirable, but optimum use of standard antiepileptics requires knowledge of these interactions and the art of minimizing their consequences.

Physiologic Variation

Several factors influence the rate of drug metabolism. Phenobarbital levels have been reported to be higher in males than in females, suggesting slower metabolism in the males. Whether this is due to induction of liver enzymes by female sex hormones or other factors is unclear. The rate of drug oxidation is higher in elderly men than women. Pregnancy introduces several variables. These include changes in steroidal hormones, a rise in body temperature, alteration in volume of distribution and reduced drug binding to plasma proteins, increased blood flow and rate of delivery of drug to the liver, and drug metabolism by the placenta.

Circadian variation in metabolic rates and gastric emptying may significantly alter drug disposition. Plasma-free fractions of phenytoin and valproate have been shown to vary throughout the day and in response to urinary pH changes, suggesting that the ionized fraction of drugs such as phenytoin may change and affect blood levels no matter how slightly. Awareness of these factors is increasing as studies of chronopharmacokinetics evolve.

Developmental factors also affect metabolic rates. Newborns generally have slower phase I reactions than adults, but the rate increases to a peak over several years and may exceed the adult metabolic capacity. One of the best examples of this is difficulty of sustaining a significant blood level of phenytoin in children who often require very large doses. In general children in the range of 1–6 years of age require larger doses on a milligram per kilogram basis than adults to achieve therapeutic levels of phenytoin, carbamazepine, ethosuximide, and valproic acid. The effect of developmental factors on metabolism of novel antiepileptic medications has not yet been reported. Among the elderly, phase I reactions are much slower than in early adulthood. On the other hand, conjugation reactions are not significantly different.

Elimination

Drug elimination is really a two-step process of biotransformation and excretion from the body. One of the most important parameters guiding dosage adjustment and dosage intervals is the elimination half-life. After oral or intravenous administration, the plasma level of a drug rises to a maximum then begins to fall. A curve describing plasma concentration against time after administration can be described by one or more exponential components. The elimination half-life is approximated by assessing the time required for the blood level to fall to 50% of the peak blood level. Clinically, this is very useful in determining the time to reach a steady state. In multiple dosing situations typically encountered in the treatment of epilepsy, the drug concentration in plasma (and at its receptor sites) will rise in a stepwise manner with successive doses after initiation or a change in dose. This process will continue until drug elimination matches drug delivery. This situation defines the steady state. A practical rule of thumb is that five half-lives are required to achieve a steady state after drug initiation or a dose change. Changing doses before achieving the steady state obfuscates evaluation of the effect of a dose change; hence the dictum that time should be allowed for steady state to be achieved before contemplating an additional dose change. Dosing intervals are greater for drugs with longer half-lives.

Half-life may vary with chronic dosing. This is particularly true of carbamazepine, which undergoes the process known as autoinduction of metabolism. After an initial steady state is achieved during the first week of therapy, the half-life may be as long as 24 hours. However, after an average of 1–2 months, hepatic enzyme metabolizing capacity increases, and the plasma level falls despite a constant medication regimen. Autoinduction of other standard antiepileptic medications is not significant.

REFERENCES

Barnes JM, Henley JM. Molecular characteristics of excitatory amino acid receptors. Prog Neurobiol 1992;39:13–133.

Bowery NG. $GABA_B$ receptor pharmacology. Annu Rev Pharmacol Toxicol 1993;33:109–147.

Catterall WA. Cellular and molecular biology of voltage-gated sodium channels. Pharmacol Rev 1992;72:S15–S48.

Caulfield MP. Muscarinic receptors—characterization, coupling and function. Pharmac Ther 1993;58:319–379.

Choi DW. Excitotoxic cell death. J Neurobiol 1992;23:1261–1276.

Frazer A, Hensler JG. In GJ Siegel, BW Agranoff, RW Albers et al (eds). Basic Neurochemistry (5th ed). New York: Raven, 1994.

Gale K. GABA and epilepsy: basic concepts from preclinical research. Epilepsia 1992;33:S3–S12.

Goldstein M, Deutch AY. Dopaminergic mechanisms in the pathogenesis of schizophrenia. FASEB J 1992;6:2413–2421.

Jankovic J, Marsden CD. Therapeutic Strategies in Parkinson's Disease. In J Jankovic, E Tolosa (eds), Parkinson's Disease and Movement Disorders (2nd ed). Baltimore: Williams & Wilkins, 1993;115–144.

Julius D. Molecular biology of serotonin receptors. Annu Rev Neurosci 1991;14:335–360.

Karlin A. Structure of nicotinic acetylcholine receptors. Curr Opin Neurobiol 1993;3:299–309.

Kobilka B. Adrenergic receptors as models for G protein-coupled receptors. Annu Rev Neurosci 1992;15:87–114.

Liggett SB, Raymond JR. Pharmacology and Molecular Biology of Adrenergic Receptors. Baillière's Clinical Endocrinology and Metabolism 1993;7:279–306.

Macdonald RL, Olsen RW. $GABA_A$ receptor channels. Annu Rev Neurosci 1994;17:569–602.

McPherson PS, Campbell KP. The ryanodine receptor/Ca^{2+} release channel. J Biol Chem 1993;268:13765–13768.

Meldrum B. Amino acids as dietary excitotoxins: a contribution to understanding neurodegenerative disorders. Brain Res Rev 1993;18:293–314.

Pallotta BS, Wagoner PK. Voltage-dependent potassium channels since Hodgkin and Huxley. Physiol Rev 1992;72:S49–S67.

Penner R, Fasolato C, Hoth M. Calcium influx and its control by calcium release. Curr Opin Neurobiol 1993;3:368–374.

Peroutka SJ. VI. Serotonin receptor subtypes and neuropsychiatric diseases: Focus on 5-HT_{1D} and 5-HT_3 receptor agents. Pharmacol Rev 1991;43:579–586.

Probst WC, Snyder LA, Schuster DI et al. Sequence alignment of the G protein coupled receptor superfamily. DNA Cell Biol 1992;11:1–20.

Schoepp DD, Conn PJ. Metabotropic glutamate receptors in brain function and pathology. TIPS 1993;14:13–20.

Spiegel AM, Weinstein LS, Shenker A. Abnormalities in G protein-coupled signal transduction pathways in human disease. J Clin Invest 1993;92:1119–1125.

Wisden W, Seeburg PH. Mammalian ionotropic GluRs. Curr Opin Neurobiol 1993;3:291–298.

Wisden W, Seeburg PH. $GABA_A$ receptor channels: From subunits to functional entities. Curr Opin Neurobiol 1992;2:263–269.

SUGGESTED READING

Amara SG, Arriza JL. Neurotransmitter transporters: Three distinct gene families. Curr Opin Neurobiol 1993;3:337–344.

Fisher RS, Coyle JT (eds). Neurotransmitters and Epilepsy. New York: Wiley-Liss, 1991.

Jobe PC, Laird HE (eds). Neurotransmitters and Epilepsy. Clifton, NJ: Humana Press 1987.

Kaczmarek LK, Levitan IB (eds). Neuromodulation. The Biochemical Control of Neuronal Excitability. New York: Oxford University Press, 1987.

Lipton SA, Rosenberg PA. Excitatory amino acids as a final common pathway for neurologic disorders. N Engl J Med 1994; 3:613–622.

Majewska MD. Neurosteroids: Endogenous bimodal modulaters of the $GABA_A$ receptor. Mechanism of action and physiological significance. Prog Neurobiol 1992;38:379–395.

Meltzer HY (ed). Psychopharmacology. The Third Generation of Progress. New York: Raven, 1987.

McCormick DA. Actions of Acetylcholine in the Cerebral Cortex and Thalamus and Implications for Function. In AC Cuello (ed), Progress in Brain Research. Amsterdam: Elsevier, 1993;303–308.

McCormick DA, Pape HC, Williamson A. Actions of Norepinephrine in the Cerebral Cortex and Thalamus: Implications for Function of the Central Noradrenergic System. In CD Barnes, O Pompeiano (eds), Progress in Brain Research. Amsterdam: Elsevier, 1991; 293–305.

Milligan G. Mechanisms of multifunctional signalling by G protein-linked receptors. TIPS 1993;14:239–244.

Pisani F, Perucca E, Avanzini G et al (eds). New Antiepileptic Drugs. Amsterdam: Elsevier, 1991.

Richelson E. Pharmacology of antidepressants—characteristics of the ideal drug. Mayo Clin Proc 1994;69:1069–1081.

Schwartzkroin PA. Cellular electrophysiology of human epilepsy. Epilepsy Res 1994;17:185–192.

Siegel GJ, Agranoff BW, Albers RW et al (eds). Basic Neurochemistry (5th ed). New York: Raven, 1994.

Spedding M, Paoletti R. Classification of calcium channels and the sites of action of drugs modifying channel function. Pharmacol Rev 1992;44:363–376.

Chapter 53
Principles of Pain Management

Paul L. Moots

NOCICEPTION

The management of pain requires a complete understanding of the afferent pathways that serve nociception. The localizing value of sensory deficits caused by disorders of the peripheral nerves and spinothalamic tracts has been appreciated for more than a century. During the past 20 years, a more detailed and dynamic model of nociception has emerged as the anatomy and biochemistry of the central mechanisms that modulate nociceptive input have been established. Important advances have included a molecular basis for the action of exogenous opioids, the discovery of endogenous opioids, an anatomical and physiological description of descending pathways that modulate nociceptive input, and a rationale for using nonopioid neurotransmitter modulators as adjuvants in pain management. Comprehensive reviews of nociception are available in a number of excellent texts (Wall and Melzack 1994; Bonica 1990).

Receptors and Primary Afferents

Nociceptors are formed by the peripheral ramification of certain finely myelinated and unmyelinated afferent axons. In general, their morphology is relatively simple compared to other tactile-sensory–receptor elements. The most common receptors are bare nerve endings. Nociceptor subcategories differ by tissue distribution, response to various types of potentially noxious stimuli, threshold of response, and changes in activity in response to prior stimulation (e.g., sensitization). Nociceptors are found in skin, intramuscular connective tissue, blood vessels, periosteum, and most thoracic and abdominal viscera. The principal stimuli for activation are mechanical, thermal, and chemical.

The afferent fibers that convey nociceptive information are small myelinated fibers with conduction velocities of 5–30 m/second (A-delta fibers) and unmyelinated axons with conduction velocities of 0.5–2.0 m/second (C fibers). Nociceptive fibers account for 10% of the myelinated and 90% of the unmyelinated fibers in cutaneous nerves. Visceral afferent fibers at any spinal level represent a smaller percentage of the total afferent fibers and contain a higher proportion of unmyelinated fibers than do cutaneous afferent fibers.

Cutaneous nociceptors have been studied extensively and include (1) high-threshold mechanical nociceptors (HTMs) associated with small myelinated axons (A-delta fibers), (2) myelinated mechanothermal nociceptors (MTs) (A-delta fibers), and (3) polymodal nociceptors associated with unmyelinated axons (C fibers). HTMs respond only to intense mechanical stimuli, and their thresholds are many fold greater than non-nociceptive mechanoreceptors. Stimulation of single afferent A-delta nociceptive fibers causes a sharp, well-localized pain sensation. The perceived pain is roughly proportional to the frequency of discharge. The threshold and intensity of response of HTMs and MTs can be altered by thermal injury. These sensitizing effects may be involved in the development of *hyperpathia*. Polymodal nociceptors respond to mechanical, chemical, and thermal stimuli. Stimulation of nociceptive C fibers is associated with a dull, burning, or aching quality that is less well localized. Unlike HTMs, repeated stimulation and thermal stimuli do not produce sensitization of polymodal nociceptors, but local inflammatory responses to tissue injury do lead to sensitization.

Deep somatic nociceptors associated with muscle, tendons, fascia, joints, and periosteum are largely free nerve endings associated with A-delta and C fibers. The extensive plexus of fibers investing the periosteum and joints gives bone the lowest pain threshold of the deep tissues. The effects of sensitizing stimuli and the distribution of central terminals from deep somatic afferents differ considerably from cutaneous afferents. These differences are reflected in the characteristics of deep somatic pain, which is aching rather than sharp and not as well localized as cutaneous pain (Dubner 1991).

Visceral nociceptors are also largely free nerve endings related to unmyelinated C fibers, but their sensitivity to various noxious stimuli differs greatly from that of cutaneous nociceptors. The proportion of nociceptive A-delta fibers is lower than that found in cutaneous nerves. Many nociceptive fibers invest the pleural and peritoneal surfaces, the capsules of the solid organs, and the blood vessels. The vagus nerve carries nociceptive afferents from the lungs, esophagus, and stomach. The splanchnic and other regional sympathetic nerves also contain significant numbers of visceral afferents; thus, many of the viscera have dual, anatomically diverging afferent fibers. Mechanoreceptors in the intestine, biliary tract, and urinary tract are stimulated by traction and distention. When compared with skin, the intestine is remarkably insensitive to direct tissue damage, such as cutting or burning. Noxious stimulation produces a poorly localized aching or spasmodic, cramping pain. The terminals of the visceral afferents in the spinal cord tend to be more widely distributed than cutaneous afferent terminals, contributing to the poorly localized character of the pain. Visceral pain often is accompanied by perception of pain arising in somatic structures that share the same spinal level of innervation. This phenomenon, known as *referred pain*, results from the convergence of nociceptive fibers from different structures onto the same population of cells in the dorsal horn (Ness and Gebhart 1990).

Dorsal Horn and Central Projections

The central projections of the primary nociceptive afferents, whose cell bodies are located in the dorsal root ganglia, are directed through the dorsal roots to the most superficial of the Rexed laminae (I and II) and to some of the deep laminae (V) of the dorsal horn over a vertical distance of one or two vertebral levels. The A-delta fibers conveying input from HTMs and MTs terminate primarily in laminae I and V; C fibers terminate in lamina II. Visceral afferents included in the sympathetic nerves also terminate in laminae I and V, sometimes overlapping with somatic afferents, but also terminate more widely in the lower laminae (VI, VII, and X). The viscerosomatic convergence of nociceptive afferents is important in the genesis of referred pain. These terminals use multiple neurotransmitters, including excitatory amino acids and neuropeptides, particularly substance P. Postsynaptic modulation may result from substance P's long-term modulatory effects. In addition, both pre- and postsynaptic events may be modified by supraspinal input involving monoamines and opioid neuropeptides.

The postsynaptic neurons in the dorsal horn include cells that respond only to noxious stimuli (e.g., nociceptive specific neurons) and wide dynamic range neurons that respond to both nociceptive and non-nociceptive sensory input. These neurons project as a largely decussated pathway that travels in the contralateral anterolateral portion of the spinal cord, comprising the principal spinothalamic tract. This tract is somatotypically organized with sacral elements situated posterolaterally and cervical elements more anteriomedially. Included in this tract are fibers that project to the periaqueductal gray (spinoreticular pathway) and brain stem nuclei. These fibers, along with projections to the central, or laminar, nuclei of the thalamus, make up the paleospinothalamic tract. In humans, most of the spinothalamic tract projects to the ventral posterolateral nucleus of the thalamus as the neospinothalamic tract. The cortical projections of the paleospinothalamic tract are widespread, whereas the cortical projections of the neospinothalamic tract are directed to the primary sensory cortex.

The integration of nociceptive input to the thalamus shares some similarities with that occurring at the spinal level. The phylogenetically distinct components of the spinothalamic tract probably convey qualitatively different information to the paleospinothalamic pathway serving arousal and the emotive, or affective, component of pain, while the neospinothalamic component conveys discriminative and localizing information. Like the dorsal horn neurons, thalamic neurons are activated as either nociceptive-specific or polymodal neurons of wide dynamic range. Additionally, the convergence of somatic and visceral input at the thalamic level adds another possible source for referred pain.

Central Modulation of Nociception

Peripheral mechanisms, such as sensitization of nociceptors by thermal or chemical stimuli, modulate afferent nociceptive input. Central mechanisms that modulate nociceptive input also exist. At the spinal level, both local neuronal circuits and descending pathways originating in the brain stem modulate nociceptive transmission through the dorsal horn and the spinothalamic projections. This modulatory effect is generally inhibitory and produces analgesia via endogenous opioid and aminergic systems. Other, less well-defined supraspinal systems may exert a facilitory effect on nociceptive transmission.

Intra- and intersegmental projections arising from cells located in Rexed laminae I and II (e.g., substantia gelatinosa) provide a modulating influence on both the pre- and postsynaptic elements of primary nociceptive afferent terminals in laminae I, II, and V. These local circuits also serve to integrate nociceptive and other sensory inputs. Suppression of nociceptive transmission in the dorsal horn by non-nociceptive afferent stimulation was the basis for the development of circuitry models by Wall and Melzack referred to as the "*gate control theory*" of pain transmission. This model has influenced studies of nociceptive mechanisms for the last 30 years. Although the specific dorsal horn circuits originally hypothesized in the gate control theory never were identified, the phenomenon of modulation of nociceptive input by peripheral and descending central influences remains both a fundamental and continually developing topic in the understanding of nociception.

Endogenous opioids serve as principal neurotransmitters in the local circuitry of the dorsal horn. Opioid receptors (mu- and kappa-receptors; see Endogenous Opioids and Opioid Receptors) are found on both the pre- and postsynaptic elements of primary nociceptive afferents in the substantia gelatinosa, which also contains a high density of enkephalinergic terminals. These interneuron synapses are an important site of action of systemically administered opioid analgesics.

Descending influences on spinal nociceptive transmission were demonstrated first by the production of analgesia sufficient to perform laparotomies on rats after electrical stimulation of the periaqueductal gray. Similar effects have been produced by local iontophoretic application of opioid analgesics onto certain regions of the brain stem. The best established of the descending nociceptive modulatory systems derives from cells in the midbrain periaqueductal gray that project to the nucleus raphe magnus (NRM) in the medulla. The NRM in turn projects to neurons in Rexed laminae I, II, and V of the dorsal horn. Analgesia induced by stimulation of either the midbrain or medullary region is sensitive to opioid antagonists (e.g., naloxone), and specific opioid receptors have been shown at both sites. The descending pathway from the NRM travels through the dorsal lateral column of the spinal cord medial to the corticospinal tracts. Sectioning these tracts blocks the analgesic effect of stimulation of the periaqueductal gray or NRM. Electrophysiological studies indicate that stimulation of these descending pathways inhibits activity in dorsal horn neurons of wide dynamic range that contribute to the spinothalamic tract. The fibers originating in the medullary nuclei, particularly the NRM, use serotonin as a principal neurotransmitter. Fibers from other medullary nuclei, such as the nucleus reticularis gigantocellularis, and more rostral components of the monoaminergic system use norepinephrine as the principal neurotransmitter. These pathways specifically inhibit nociceptive input without affecting other somatic or visceral sensory input. They represent the principal supraspinal sites for the analgesic effects of endogenous and exogenous opiate action.

Transitory analgesia also can be produced by stimulating the somatosensory cortex and certain periventricular nuclei in the hypothalamus. This effect is mediated by direct fibers included in the corticospinal tracts that terminate in the dorsal horn and by polysynaptic pathways that may use the reticulospinal and raphe spinal pathways described above. The analgesic effect resulting from electrical stimulation at these supratentorial sites is less consistent than that achieved by stimulation of the periaqueductal gray.

Not all supraspinal influences on nociceptive transmission are inhibitory. Stimulation of certain medullary regions causes facilitation of nociceptive transmission in dorsal horn neurons. The clinical significance of this action is not well-understood, but the balance of inhibitory and facilitory controls in nociceptive transmission may be important in the genesis of chronic pain syndromes.

Endogenous Opioids and Opioid Receptors

The identification of specific neuronal receptors that mediate the effects of opiates and the subsequent identification of endogenous peptides that act as ligands for these receptors are two major breakthroughs in neuroscience during the last 20 years.

Three families of endogenous opioid neuropeptides have been identified: *enkephalins*, *dynorphins*, and *endorphins* (Simon and Hiller 1994; Terenius 1992). Each family is derived from a distinct gene, yet all active opioid species have in common the amino terminal sequence Tyr-Gly-Gly-Phe. In each family, the active peptides arise from the cleavage of a larger precursor protein. The two opioid precursors most closely associated with brain stem and spinal nociceptive transmission are pro-enkephalin A, which is the precursor of met- and leu-enkephalin, and pro-enkephalin B (prodynorphin), which is the precursor of dynorphin. These precursors are concentrated heavily in the regions of the periaqueductal gray, medullary nuclei, and dorsal horn involved primarily with nociception. The principal member of the endorphin family of opioid peptides is beta-endorphin, which is derived from pro-opiomelanocortin and relatively restricted to the hypothalamus and pituitary. It is also the parent precursor of the melanocyte-stimulating hormone, adrenocorticotropic hormone (ACTH), and other peptides.

Opioid receptors, initially identified by the specific binding of ligands such as morphine, have been subcategorized by differing ligand affinities. The major subcategories are the mu-, kappa-, and delta-receptors. Some of the receptor subtypes have been cloned and sequenced. The receptors are membrane-spanning proteins that appear to be coupled by G proteins to adenyl cyclase, using cyclic adenosine monophosate (cAMP) as the second messenger. They probably act by regulating K^+ and Ca^{++} channels.

The mu-receptor, so named because of its high affinity for morphine, is present in the periaqueductal gray and dorsal horn (Goodman et al. 1988). The analgesic potency of opiate compounds correlates well with the agonist-binding affinity to the mu-receptor. Kappa-receptors also are distributed in the spinal and brain stem regions that are important in the modulation of nociception. These distributions clearly overlap those of the enkephalins and dynorphins.

The termination of opioid-receptor activation depends on peptidases with active sites located on the extracellular surface of the cell membrane that cleave the peptides into inactive fragments. The so-called enkephalinases may serve as a target for a new class of analgesics.

PAIN MECHANISMS

Nociceptive Pain

Pain is a normal response to tissue injury that produces activation of nociceptors. Much is known about the basic anatomy and physiology of nociception, yet many important aspects are not well understood. Some important unanswered questions concern the role of tissue inflammation in the recruitment of non-nociceptor afferents to pain input, the differences between visceral and somatic nociception, and the changes in the modulation of nociceptive input associated with chronic pain. History has demonstrated that a better understanding of nociceptive mechanisms will lead to improved treatment of pain (for review, see Portenoy 1989).

The acute pain caused by tissue injury usually is divided into somatic and visceral pain based on their character differences. Somatic pain is more clearly localized and described as sharp or dull in character. Visceral pain is less well localized and has a crampy, spasmodic, or aching character. Visceral and deep somatic pain more commonly is associated with referred pain than is cutaneous pain.

Chronic nociceptive pain is usually similar in character to acute pain arising in the same area, but with time, the consequences of the modulation of nociceptive transmission and the affective components of pain become more important in the character of the pain syndrome. Depression, sleep disorders, and the sequelae of disuse (e.g., muscle atrophy and limited joint mobility) contribute to the disability of chronic pain disorders.

Although nociceptive pain usually arises from localized tissue injury, the distribution of perceived pain does not always directly identify the source of pain—that is, tissue injury occurring at one site may be felt as arising from another (referred pain). The best known example is the association of left arm pain with angina. Other common examples are listed in Table 53.1. In addition to the convergence of visceral and somatic input at the spinal level, other possible mechanisms of referred pain include innervation of two structures by different branches of the same nociceptive afferent fiber and changes in the receptive field of thalamic neurons.

Neuropathic and Deafferentation Pain

Pain is an important consequence of direct injury to peripheral nerves; common examples are nerve and nerve root compression syndromes, acute and chronic pain after nerve transection, and neuritis in association with infectious and inflammatory lesions (e.g., herpes zoster) and diffuse polyneuropathies.

Neuropathic pain often has several different qualities that are experienced concurrently. One common form is sharp, lancinating pains that are brief but very intense, or shocklike, and well localized. Typically, the pain radiates in a pattern suggesting a dermatomal or peripheral nerve distribution. In trigeminal neuralgia (see Chapter 74) or postherpetic neuralgia, a *trigger zone* exists such that stimulation applied to a specific area elicits intense, shocklike pains. A superimposed burning pain is common, and sensory stimulation of the affected region often exacerbates the burning pain far out of proportion to the intensity of the stimulus. A slight breeze or movement of a sheet over the skin is often sufficient to produce exquisite pain in patients with painful neuropathies. At least five different mechanisms may be involved in pain accompanying nerve disease, and more than one mechanism may be operating simultaneously in any given patient. The five mechanisms are (1) activation of normal nociceptors contained in a nerve (e.g., nervi nervorum), (2) spontaneous or (3) induced discharges in injured nociceptor afferents, (4) deafferentation with central pain generation, and (5) activation of sensitized mechanoreceptors by efferent sympathetic activity (*sympathetically maintained pain*) (Portenoy 1992).

Evidence supports the presence of nociceptors in the perineural and epineural tissues investing peripheral nerves, the nervi nervorum; therefore, nerve injury can cause nociceptive pain in the sense described in the previous section. This likely contributes to pain resulting from nerve root compression and peripheral nerve entrapment.

Neuropathic pain can result from abnormal discharges in injured or regenerating sensory afferents. Injured nerve fibers sometimes develop spontaneous discharges, and afferent impulses may be evoked by electrical activity in surrounding axons (*ephaptic transmission*) in injured nerves both acutely and later during axonal regeneration or neuroma formation.

The nature of some nerve disorders is to selectively affect small-caliber afferent fibers; examples are neuropathies associated with diabetes and amyloidosis (see Chapter 81). This generates abnormal activity in nociceptor afferents resulting in neuropathic pain. More commonly, the damage to the afferent fibers is not selective. Abnormal activity in non-nociceptive tactile afferent fibers also may take on a painful quality that is distinct from or may be superimposed on the pain produced by nociceptor afferent activity. In these situations, pain is produced by activity generated in the peripheral nervous system. However, the failure of peripheral nerve blockade by nerve transection or local anesthetic infiltration to relieve chronic neuropathic pain syndromes indicates that the pain related to peripheral nerve injury or disease also may have a central nervous system (CNS) component.

The exact mechanisms of central pain generation are poorly understood but probably involve abnormal activity in both nociceptive and non-nociceptive sensory pathways (Casey 1991). Possible mechanisms by which abnormal

Table 53.1: Common referred pain syndromes

Pain Location	*Segmental Distribution*	*Causes*
Frontal or vertex headache	Trigeminal nerve	Traction, inflammation, or other lesions involving the supratentorial meninges
Ear pain	Glossopharyngeal and vagus nerves	Tumor, abscess, or inflammatory lesion in the oro- or hypopharynx
Right shoulder pain	Phrenic nerve (C_3–C_5)	Cholecystitis or diaphragmatic irritation
Left chest/arm pain	T_1–T_4	Cardiac ischemia
Left upper abdominal wall pain	T_8	Gastric diseases
Middle and lower abdominal wall pain	T_{10}–T_{11}	Small intestine and colon disorders
Testicle/inguinal region pain	T_{12}–L_2	Renal or perirenal abscess or tumor
Knee pain	L_3–L_4	Pelvic, acetabular, and femoral head disorders

central sensory activity is perceived as painful include alteration in the spontaneous electrical activity of central pathways, changes in neurotransmitter function and receptor sensitivity, and alterations in the activity of descending pathways that modulate sensory and nociceptive input.

It is likely that similar mechanisms cause chronic pain from peripheral nerve injuries and CNS disorders that involve the sensory pathways. The distribution and character of pain associated with central lesions differ somewhat from those of peripheral lesions, however. Central pain is usually more diffuse and less well defined in distribution and less likely to be lancinating in quality or associated with a trigger zone. Similarities of central and peripheral induced pain are the following: (1) Both usually are distributed in a region of impaired tactile perception; (2) tactile input takes on a painful quality (hyperpathia) out of proportion to the intensity of stimulus applied; and (3) the pain often has a highly emotive burning quality. The clinical and conceptual overlap between central and peripheral neuropathic pain syndromes has led many investigators to lump both types of pain syndromes under the category of *deafferentation pain*. Tricyclic antidepressants and anticonvulsant drugs can relieve both types of deafferentation pain.

In addition to nociceptive and deafferentation mechanisms, efferent peripheral nervous system activity may contribute to chronic neuropathic pain syndromes. Abnormal activation of adjacent peripheral axons by electrical coupling (ephapsis) is seen in animal models, but its contribution to pain generation in humans is difficult to estimate. A second postulated efferent mechanism of neuropathic pain is that of sympathetically maintained pain.

Efferent sympathetic activity, or overactivity, may be generated in the CNS or as a reflex response to peripheral stimuli. Electrical stimulation of efferent sympathetic fibers in cats induces spontaneous discharges in non-nociceptive cutaneous mechanoreceptors with subsequent activation of neurons of wide dynamic range in the dorsal horn. Roberts proposed that this was the mechanism by which efferent sympathetic activity sustains chronic pain subsequent to pain originally induced by trauma (Roberts 1986). This proposal complemented several clinical observations regarding chronic pain syndromes with neuropathic features often termed *causalgia* or *reflex sympathetic dystrophy*.

Causalgia refers to severe, burning pain and hyperpathia accompanied by signs of autonomic dysfunction, especially vasomotor changes and trophic changes in skin and bone, following traumatic injury to a major nerve trunk in the limbs. The arms frequently are more involved than the legs. A similar syndrome, *minor causalgia*, sometimes occurs in the absence of identified trauma (Payne 1986; Schott 1986). The clinical features of causalgia consistent with the concept of sympathetically maintained pain include prominent autonomic features and pain relief by sympathetic blockade. In some patients, this type of pain is accentuated by cutaneous infiltration with norepinephrine.

These observations have provided a rationale for pharmacological and surgical sympathectomy to treat several neuropathic pain syndromes. Indeed, benefit from sympathetic blockade often is used as evidence that a chronic pain syndrome is based on sympathetic mechanisms. Some short-term placebo-controlled studies suggest, however, that sympathetic blockade with phentolamine is no more effective than placebo in patients with reflex sympathetic dystrophy and painful polyneuropathies (Verdugo and Ochoa 1994; Verdugo et al. 1994). The long-term efficacy of sympathectomy for chronic neuropathic pain is relatively poor, with less than one-third of patients achieving sustained relief. While autonomic function often is affected in both focal and diffuse peripheral nerve disorders, its role in pain generation is controversial, and the clinical foundation for sympathetically maintained pain as a mechanism of neuropathic pain is undergoing serious debate (Ochoa 1993).

Idiopathic and Psychogenic Pain

Pain that occurs without a definable cause of nociceptor activation and or any mechanism of neuropathic generation often is categorized as idiopathic or psychogenic. The terms, however, are not synonymous; not all apparently idiopathic pain problems prove to be psychogenic. Still, with rigorous evaluation and ample follow-up observation, a high percentage of patients with chronic pain lacking a defined cause have psychological factors that promote or sustain the pain problem. This is a very heterogeneous group, both in terms of the nature of the pain complaint and the nature of the psychological processes involved.

For many people, recurring pain complaints are related to the stresses and anxieties of work, family relations, and other aspects of daily life. Tension headaches and fibromyalgia syndromes commonly fall into this category. The supposition that emotional tension, fatigue, and other factors produce nociceptive somatic pain due to muscle contraction is simplistic. When such complaints become a major focus of concern or disability far out of proportion to any evidence of nociceptive stimuli, psychogenic factors are suspected (Dworkin and Gitlin 1991).

Identifying specific psychological or psychiatric problems that promote and sustain pain problems is important in determining therapeutic strategies. Patients with anxiety disorders and those with obsessive or other personality traits associated with somatization need to be identified so that appropriate therapy can be undertaken. Conversion disorders also present frequently with pain complaints, particularly headache. Chronic analgesic therapy is of little benefit, and in some cases may worsen the pain problem.

Unexplained pain may be the presenting complaint of a major psychiatric disorder, although this is not common (Merskey 1989). Occasionally, somatic delusions that include pain complaints occur as part of depression and resolve in conjunction with improvement in affect as the result of antidepressant therapy. Headache is the most frequent pain complaint in patients with depression. Conversely, features of depression are relatively common among chronic pain patients, and the severity of pain from minor injuries or other lesions is often magnified in patients with depression. Using stringent criteria, major depression is present in about 5–10% of chronic pain patients. When evidence of mild affective disorders is included, the incidence may range up to 50% or more. Among patients with schizophrenia, somatic delusions and hallucinations that primarily involve pain are relatively rare; chronic headache is the most common pain complaint in these patients also.

Feigning illness, such as a chronic pain syndrome, for the purpose of obtaining an obvious, often tangible secondary gain is *malingering*. Malingering patients are dramatically and demonstratively incapacitated by their symptoms. They tend to be uncooperative during examinations and noncompliant in therapeutic efforts. Frank malingering is relatively uncommon—for example, less than 5% of patients with chronic back pain are thought to be malingerers. Yet, many patients embellish minor deficits, and many coincidentally receive secondary gains for being ill. Thus, in physician surveys, the frequency of reported malingerers in chronic pain clinics varies greatly. As a poorly defined and uncommon entity, malingering should be considered a diagnosis of exclusion in chronic pain patients. The psychological factors that contribute to the chronic pain problems described above should be searched for as potential avenues of therapy for these patients.

The pathophysiological basis of psychogenic pain remains speculative, and it is likely that multiple mechanisms are involved. The fact that nociceptive pain is so strongly influenced by anxiety and other psychological factors suggests that the overlap between central pain mechanisms and emotive mechanisms, particularly in regard to the opioid and aminergic systems, is important in the production of psychogenic pain (Terenius 1992).

APPROACH TO THE PATIENT WITH PAIN

This chapter and most discussions of pain management focus on symptomatic control of pain by pharmacological, surgical, and other means. Successful pain management always is based on a clear understanding of the pain's cause. This requires a careful history of the nature of the pain, a full accounting of past medical history, and a careful physical examination that often includes a detailed neurological assessment. On this basis, a pain complaint can be characterized as nociceptive, neuropathic, psychogenic, or as including a combination of these features. This characterization directs the subsequent evaluation of the patient and guides the choice of therapies.

Acute Pain

History

The most useful features in characterizing a new pain complaint are location, character, mode of onset, factors that aggravate and relieve pain, and concurrent features (e.g., fever, dyspnea, nausea). The complaint that pain radiates may be a valuable indicator of referred or neuropathic pain. From these elements of the history, a working differential diagnosis usually can be formulated and then further evaluated by physical examination and laboratory studies.

Even during the initial interview, some assessment must be made of the relationship between the pain's severity and the patient's emotional response and attributed disability. This assessment is difficult because the experience of pain is intensely subjective and highly variable among people. Posner emphasizes that "the physician is wise to accept at face value the patient's report of the severity of his pain unless there is overwhelming evidence to the contrary" (Posner 1985).

Prior medical problems often explain current pain syndromes—for example, diabetes may be associated with limb pain as the result of ischemia or peripheral neuropathy. A history of cancer suggests vertebral or epidural metastasis as the cause of progressive back pain. A remote history of trauma, neuritis, sciatica, or shingles, elicited only after careful inquiry, may be the basis for neuropathic pain syndromes. Depression and psychological factors that may contribute to the pain syndrome also must be explored.

Physical Examination

The initial examination is directed mainly by the stated location of pain. The physician searches for evidence of local inflammation to help locate the source of pain: tenderness; warmth; swelling; limited joint mobility; and signs of pleural, peritoneal, or meningeal irritation. Observations of subtle changes in posture (e.g., slight hip flexion in patients with pelvic abscess) are often helpful. Maneuvers that elicit or relieve pain should be duplicated. These include direct pressure, coughing or sneezing, joint flexion, straight-leg raising, reverse straight-leg raising, and nerve percussion (Tinnel's sign).

Establishing the cause of a pain complaint often provides a mechanistic explanation as either somatic or visceral nociceptive pain, neuropathic pain, or some combination of the three. An understanding of both cause and mechanism allows the best opportunity to develop a rational treatment plan. The symptomatic relief of a new pain complaint when the cause is not clearly identified is a common pitfall that may lead to permanent tissue damage—for example, most patients with neurological symptoms resulting from spinal epidural metastasis have experienced back pain that was not fully evaluated for weeks or months.

Even with rigorous investigation, however, the pathophysiological basis of many pain complaints cannot be explicitly defined. Most people experience transitory aching in muscles or joints and occasionally brief lancinating or sharp pains without a previous history of injury or other explanation. The pain's self-limited and generally mild nature identifies it as part of the normal repertoire of sensations. Such complaints can become self-perpetuating, as in analgesic-rebound headache (see Chapter 74), for which regular use of mild analgesics prolongs rather than terminates headache. The coexistence of unexplained pain complaints along with a history of bona fide medical illness (e.g., a history of diabetes or cancer) is common. It may be difficult to determine whether the pain is causally related to the preexisting illness. Often, this problem can be solved only with patience, repeated examinations, and clinical insight into whether the nature of the pain and its implied mechanisms are appropriate in the context of the underlying illness. Attributing a new pain complaint to a psychiatric disorder requires the rigorous exclusion of other causes.

Chronic Pain

Pain that lasts months or longer without a defined cause and is of sufficient severity to interfere with normal daily activities is a relatively common and often difficult problem. Chronic, incapacitating pain may follow relatively minor trauma or even occur without prior trauma as is seen in patients with reflex sympathetic dystrophy. Several CNS disorders can produce chronic pain syndromes that may present difficult diagnostic problems (e.g., multiple sclerosis, thalamic tumors, infarcts). Most chronic pain patients, however, do not have a definable CNS disturbance or other underlying disease (e.g., cancer, infection, vasculitis) that remains unidentified even after prolonged observation. Psychological factors appear to be predominant in many of these patients, and a pharmacological approach to management is rarely useful when used alone. Treatment in clinics that specialize in a multidisciplinary approach to pain control, including pharmacological, behavioral, and psychological management, are more likely to be successful (Keefe et al. 1992).

PHARMACOLOGICAL APPROACHES TO PAIN MANAGEMENT

A systematic pharmacological approach to pain management has been espoused for cancer patients, a group with a high incidence of persistent and chronic pain syndromes. This escalating analgesic approach, advocated by the World Health Organization, is most applicable to the patient with a defined lesion producing persistent somatic nociceptive pain, but it provides a useful framework for a rational approach to the treatment of most persistent or chronic pain problems (Ventafridda et al. 1987). The main points of this approach are (1) the titration of analgesics in relation to the severity of the pain, (2) the superiority of regularly scheduled as opposed to "as needed" dosing for persistent pain, and (3) the use of adjuvant medications whose actions are not primarily analgesic to improve the efficacy of the principal analgesics.

Nonsteroidal anti-inflammatory drugs (NSAIDs) are used first. If pain control is not achieved, a low-potency opiate, adjuvant agents (e.g., tricyclics), or both are added. If pain persists, more potent opiate analgesics are used while continuing adjuvant agents. Alternate routes of analgesic administration (i.e., intravenous, epidural) and surgical approaches are reserved for specialized situations in which pain control cannot be achieved or maintained with the first steps of the approach.

Placebo Therapy and Pain Relief

The placebo effect contributes to the therapeutic benefit derived from many types of pain treatment. In general, 30% of patients enrolled in placebo-controlled trials respond to placebo, irrespective of the nature of the pain. The response rates in psychogenic and nociceptive pain are the same; therefore, a placebo response is not a diagnostic test for psychogenic pain or malingering. Even relatively severe pain states, such as causalgia and reflex sympathetic dystrophy, may improve substantially with placebo treatment.

A placebo's efficacy is sufficiently reproducible that pain control studies often are considered to have a flawed study design if the frequency of response to placebo is too low (e.g., less than 10%).

The mechanism of placebo action is probably central modulation of nociceptive input and alterations in other CNS functions, such as those associated with arousal and anxiety. Despite its efficacy, placebo therapy is often foregone because it appears deceptive and more appropriately because many analgesic drugs are more efficacious. Establishing the efficacy of certain treatments (e.g., a peripheral nerve or sympathetic blockade) in a given patient, however, requires the use of some placebo trials. Additionally, placebo-controlled studies remain the standard for testing both pharmacological and nonpharmacological methods of pain control.

Nonopioid Analgesics

Nonopioid analgesics include acetominophen and NSAIDs (e.g., salicylates, proprionic acids [e.g., ibuprofen, naproxen sodium], and acetic acids [e.g., indomethacin, sulindac, ketorolac]) (Table 53.2). As a group, these agents are indicated for mild to moderate nociceptive pain and are particularly useful in the treatment of pain originating in bone and joints. They are generally not useful in the management of neuropathic pain syndromes. In addition to their analgesic action, NSAIDs are anti-inflammatory and antipyretic. The predominant mechanism of action is thought to be inhibition of prostaglandin synthesis at the site of tissue injury, thus directly decreasing nociceptor stimulation. Although these agents have CNS effects (particularly antipyretic), it is unclear how much they contribute to the analgesic action. NSAIDs may be useful in combination with opiates for more severe pain. Unlike opioid use, NSAID use is not associated with tolerance or physical dependence. Also unlike opioids, progressive increments of NSAIDs beyond a certain dosage often fail to provide improved pain control—that is, there is a "ceiling effect" to the analgesia produced by NSAIDs (Brooks and Day 1991; Portenoy 1993).

Acetaminophen has a 2- to 4-hour duration of action. A relative lack of gastrointestinal (GI) toxicity has led to its widespread use as an over-the-counter analgesic and antipyretic. It is a much less potent inhibitor of peripheral prostaglandin synthesis than aspirin or other NSAIDs and lacks clinically significant anti-inflammatory and antiplatelet effects. The mechanism of analgesia is not established but may be predominantly a CNS action. Formulations combining acetaminophen with mild opiates, such as codeine or oxycodone, have become widely used. Dose escalation with these formulations is limited by the risk of hepatic toxicity associated with the chronic use of acetaminophen in amounts greater than 3–4 g/day. Severe and sometimes fatal hepatotoxicity may result from ingestion of more than 200 mg/kg at once.

Aspirin remains one of the most commonly used pain medications. The duration of action is generally 2–4 hours, although the plasma half-life increases significantly (three- to five-fold) with increasing dosage. Despite the relatively common occurrence of nausea and GI irritation, many people tolerate chronic administration of 2–4 g/day, and it remains an important drug in the treatment of chronic inflammatory disorders such as rheumatoid arthritis. Antiplatelet effects, due to irreversible inhibition of platelet cyclo-oxygenase, limit its use in patients with coagulopathies or thrombocytopenias, which often include cancer patients receiving chemotherapy. Choline magnesium trisalicylate and acetaminophen are notable for their lack of antiplatelet activity. Additionally, warfarin's anticoagulant action is accentuated by aspirin at high doses and by some of the other NSAIDs due to interference with plasma-protein binding and decreased metabolism. Other dose-dependent aspirin toxicities are tinnitus, vomiting, encephalopathy, and acidosis. Idiosyncratic reactions, notably acute asthma or anaphylaxis and Reye's syndrome, are the most serious adverse reaction but are relatively uncommon.

The proprionic acid NSAIDs, ibuprofen and naproxen, are being used increasingly as short-term or as needed analgesics for mild to moderate nociceptive pain; both are available in the United States without prescription. Ibuprofen has a relatively short half-life of 3–4 hours, while the longer half-life of naproxen (12 hours) makes it advantageous for persistent or chronic pain. GI toxicity is the main adverse effect limiting their use, although proprionic acids are generally better tolerated than other NSAIDs. Ten to fifteen percent of people taking ibuprofen discontinue the drug because of gastrointestinal intolerance. Antiplatelet actions occur, but unlike aspirin, the cyclo-oxygenase inhibition is reversible. The interaction of proprionic acids with warfarin is usually insignificant. Uncommon adverse effects are renal toxicity and aseptic meningitis.

The acetic acid NSAIDs, including indomethacin and sulindac, have been available longer than proprionic acids. The half-life of indomethacin is variable, ranging from 2 to 11 hours. Sulindac is a pro-drug whose major active metabolites have a half-life of 18 hours. Their primary use is to treat chronic arthritis, such as rheumatoid arthritis and osteoarthritis. Acetic acids have a higher incidence of adverse effects than other NSAIDs; 20% of patients discontinue indomethacin because of toxicity. The main toxic effects are GI discomfort, frontal headache, drowsiness, and dizziness. A third acetic acid NSAID is ketorolac, which can be administered orally or parenterally and has a half-life of 5–6 hours. It is one of the most potent NSAIDs; early trials have shown an analgesic effect similar to morphine. Due to the risk of gastric ulceration, it is not recommended for chronic therapy.

Several other NSAIDs are available for analgesic and anti-inflammatory purposes. Pyroxicam (Feldene) has an analgesic potency similar to aspirin but can be taken once daily because it has a relatively long half-life and entero-

Table 53.2: Selected nonopioid analgesics

Class	*Drug*	*Half-Life (in Hours)*	*Dose Range*	*Major Toxicities*
Paraminophenol derivative	Acetaminophen	3	650–1,000 mg q4–6h	Hepatotoxicity with high doses
Salicylates (carboxylic acids)	Aspirin	0.5	650–1,000 mg q4–6h	GI, including dyspepsia, gastritis, ulceration Increased bleeding time CNS toxicity at high doses Hypersensitivity reaction (may occur with all NSAIDs)
	Diflunisol (Dolobid)	13	500–750 mg q12h	No antiplatelet effects GI toxicity less common than aspirin
	Choline magnesium trisalicylate (Trilisate)	2–15	1,000–1,500 mg q8–12h	No antiplatelet effects
Proprionic acids	Ibuprofen (Motrin)	2	400–1,000 mg q6–8h	GI toxicity, may be less common than with acetic acid NSAIDs Renal toxicity, particularly in combination with diuretics May aggravate hypertension CNS toxicities include dizziness, headache, drowsiness, fatigue
	Naproxen (Naprosyn)	14	250–500 mg q12h	Similar to ibuprofen
Acetic acids	Indomethacin (Indocin)	4–5	25–50 mg q8–12h	GI toxicity CNS toxicity, particularly headache Renal toxicity, particularly with triamterene May produce hyperkalemia
	Sulindac (Clinoril)	14	150–200 mg q12h	GI and CNS effects are less common than with indomethacin; may have less renal toxicity
	Keterolac (Toradol)	4–7	15–30 mg IM or 10 mg PO q6h	GI toxicity; for short-term therapy only
Enolic acid	Piroxicam (Feldene)	57	20–40 mg daily	GI toxicity
Fenamic acid	Mefenamic acid (Meclomen)	2	100–250 mg q6–8h	For short-term use only GI toxicity and diarrhea

GI = gastrointestinal; CNS = central nervous system; NSAIDs = nonsteroidal anti-inflammatory drugs.

hepatic recirculation. The first dose of pyroxicam and other long-duration NSAIDs may be double the recommended maintenance dose to increase the rate of onset of analgesia.

The initial choice of an NSAID is based on the type of pain, the drug's toxicity profile in relation to the patient's underlying medical condition, and the patient's prior experience with NSAIDs. For minor or self-limited somatic pain, the first choice should be a short-acting agent with a low likelihood of side effects, usually ibuprofen. For persistent or chronic pain, an agent with a longer half-life, such as naproxen, sulindac, or oxicam, may be chosen to reduce the dosing frequency.

For many patients with chronic pain, serial trials of different agents are needed to determine the most effective NSAID. A 2-week trial is required to properly assess the response to a given dose. If pain control is inadequate and significant toxicity has not occurred, dose escalation is appropriate. The limiting dosage is determined by drug toxicity and the ceiling effect in regard to analgesia; for most NSAIDs, little additional analgesic effect is achieved by further escalations at the high end of the dose range (see Table 53.2). If one NSAID fails to relieve pain at a reasonable dose or is poorly tolerated, it should be replaced by another NSAID from a different chemical class. Failure to benefit from one NSAID does not predict the response to other NSAIDs. Therefore, a working knowledge of one or two drugs from each class of NSAIDs is important.

Opioid Analgesics

Opioid analgesics differ from NSAIDs in their mechanism of action, pharmacological features of the analgesia produced, and toxicity profiles. These differences have led to the common approach of simultaneous administration of opioid and nonopioid analgesics, often in a combined formulation.

Opioids are divided into the mild and strong analgesics based on their relative potency (Table 53.3). This distinction is somewhat arbitrary, and potency per se is not a good indicator of efficacy. Codeine is the prototype of the mild

Table 53.3: Commonly used opioid analgesics

	Drug	Half-Life	*Dose Equianalgesic to Morphine 10 mg IM* IM	PO	Typical Dosage	Comments
Mild	Codeine	3 hrs	120	200	30–60 mg PO q4–6h	Often coadministered with acetaminophen Nausea, constipation, and dysphoria common
	Oxycodone (+ acetaminophen = Percocet) (+ aspirin = Percodan)	2–3 hrs	—	30	5 mg PO q4–6h	Often useful when codeine is not well tolerated
	Hydrocodone (+ acetaminophen = Lortab or Vicodin)	4 hrs	—	30	2.5–7.5 mg PO q4–6h	Same as oxycodone
	Propoxyphene (Darvon)	6–12 hrs	—	150–200	65 mg PO q4h	Active metabolite (norpropoxyphene) with long half-life (30–36 hrs)
	Meperidine (Demerol)	2 hrs	75	300	50–100 mg IM	Encephalopathy, myoclonus, and seizures due to metabolite (normeperidine) limit chronic use Contraindicated in patients taking monoamine-oxidase inhibitors
Strong	Morphine	2–3 hrs	10	30–60	2–10 mg IM/IV 30–60 mg PO q4h	With chronic use the IM:PO ratio falls from 1:6 to 1:3 Available in slow-release preparation (MS Contin)
	Hydromorphone (Dilaudid)	2–3 hrs	1.5	7.5	1–4 mg PO q4h	Good choice for chronic therapy due to high potency and short half-life
	Pentazocine (Talwin)	2–3 hrs	60	180	50–100 mg PO q4h	Mixed agonist-antagonist Ceiling effect for analgesia May precipitate withdrawal in opioid-dependent patients Encephalopathy with dose escalation
	Methadone (Dolophine)	15–30 hrs	10	20	10–20 mg PO q4–8 hrs	Duration of analgesia is highly variable, often only 4–8 hrs Long half-life leads to drug accumulation and prolonged CNS toxicity
	Levorphanol (Levo-Dromoran)	12–16 hrs	2 mg IM	4 mg PO	2–4 mg POq4h	Like methadone
	Fentanyl transdermal (Duragesic)	3–12 hrs when given IV	—*	—*	25–100 µg/hr transdermal patch every 3 days	CNS toxicities like morphine Slow onset with peak concentration at 24–72 hrs Reservoir effect leads to prolonged toxicity Slow titration

*Dose equivalence is not well defined, but the ratio of fentanyl (transdermal) to parenteral morphine is approximately 1:30.

opioid analgesics. The duration of action, 2–4 hours, is similar to that of aspirin and acetaminophen. It is used for acute or persistent pain of mild to moderate severity, generally when NSAIDs alone have proved ineffective or are contraindicated. Nociceptive pain is more likely to benefit than neuropathic pain (Cherny et al. 1994). The impression that neuropathic and deafferentation pains are not responsive to opioids is incorrect, however, and opioids remain an important option for patients with refractory pain syndromes (Portenoy and Foley 1986; Portenoy 1990a and b;

also see Arner and Meyerson 1988). Nausea is one of the most common and often limiting side effects of codeine. If it occurs, switching to a different opioid may relieve the problem. Autonomic side effects, particularly constipation, are sufficiently common that they should be anticipated by prescribing stool softeners. Dysphoria is another common side effect. Oxycodone, propoxyphene, and meperidine are other mild opioid analgesics. Meperidine is particularly likely to cause dysphoria or less commonly, myoclonus, encephalopathy, and seizures. These toxicities result from metabolites that accumulate with repeated dosing. Meperidine therefore should be avoided in patients requiring chronic treatment.

Morphine and hydromorphone are the prototypes of high-potency opioid analgesics. Morphine has a relatively rapid onset, especially when administered parenterally, and a short duration of action, about 2–4 hours. A sustained-release oral preparation (MS Contin) with a duration of action of 8–12 hours is useful for patients who require chronic therapy. High-potency opioids, like mild opioids, may cause nausea, constipation, and dysphoria. Sedation and respiratory depression also may occur. Tolerance (*tachyphylaxis*) to the side effects develops over 1–2 weeks. Tolerance also develops to the analgesic effects of opioids; however, this is not always clinically significant. For example, many patients with metastatic cancer who achieve good pain relief with opioids can be maintained on stable doses over prolonged periods of time. In these patients, recurrence of pain, particularly when rapid, is more commonly caused by tumor progression than by the loss of analgesic efficacy because of tolerance.

Chronic opioid use is associated with *physical dependence,* in which a typical pattern of symptoms develop after rapid withdrawal, including irritability, chills, salivation, diaphoresis, and abdominal discomfort with nausea and vomiting. The time course and severity are a function of the opioid's potency and half-life. The onset of withdrawal symptoms is approximately 6–12 hours after stopping treatment with morphine, as opposed to 36–48 hours for methadone. To avoid acute withdrawal symptoms and exacerbating pain symptoms, care must be taken in discontinuing opiates or switching from one opiate to another. The use of opioids with mixed agonist-antagonist properties, such as pentazocine, may precipitate withdrawal or lead to deteriorating pain control when substituted for a potent mu-receptor–agonist such as morphine. Similarly, the use of naloxone, a potent mu-receptor antagonist used to treat serious CNS toxicity, must be undertaken very judiciously for chronic pain patients. Only respiratory depression should be treated with naloxone, and the required dosage is only one-tenth of that used for an acute overdose (Portenoy 1993).

The development of *psychological dependence*, or addictive behaviors such as craving, drug seeking, and other maladaptive behaviors, is an issue of great concern for patients and physicians alike with regard to chronic opioid therapy. These concerns are heightened by the great impact of drug abuse in modern society. These concerns, however, also may interfere with the delivery of effective and appropriate pain treatment—for example, in cancer patients, these concerns have contributed to the undertreatment of pain syndromes (Ventafridda 1987). The actual risk of developing psychological dependence has been addressed in two types of studies. Studies of drug addicts in the first half of this century indicated that up to 10% of addicts first received narcotics for medical purposes. More recent studies analyzing the rate of development of psychological dependence in large populations of medical patients receiving narcotics indicate that the risk is less than 1% (see Portenoy 1986 for review). For the purpose of defining the rate of an adverse outcome, the more recent studies are more informative. These results also support the current view that physical dependence and psychological dependence are distinct phenomena. The greatest risk of psychological dependence occurs in patients with a prior history of drug abuse; hereditary and other factors also may influence the risk of developing psychological dependence. For example, the risk may vary based on whether the pain problem is nociceptive, neuropathic, or idiopathic/psychogenic. In practice, the principal adverse effects of chronic opiate therapy are dysphoria, nausea, autonomic effects, and the risk of withdrawal symptoms; however, prescribing practices and patient acceptance remain heavily influenced by the potential for psychological dependence and abuse.

As with NSAIDs, the initial choice of an opioid analgesic is empirical, based on the nature and severity of the pain, the potential side effects, and the individual's prior medication history. In most cases, a short-acting opioid is the initial choice. The most common regimen is to start with a mild-potency opioid analgesic, either codeine or oxycodone, often combined with acetaminophen, on a 4- to 6-hour dosing schedule. For persistent and chronic pain symptoms, regularly scheduled dosing (i.e., around-the-clock) with supplemental dosing for breakthrough pain is more effective than as-needed dosing. The dose is escalated until pain is controlled or toxicities occur. Using short-acting opioids, titration can be achieved in hours to days, unlike using NSAIDs, which may require weeks. Incremental dosing changes of less than 25% seldom produce significantly improved pain control for patients on chronic opioid therapy. During initial titration, however, larger increments often produce nausea, dysphoria, or sedation. Unlike the NSAIDs, opioid analgesics do not have a ceiling effect, and patients with chronic pain taking opioid analgesics who are tolerant to the sedative and respiratory depressant effects occasionally require grams of morphine per day to maintain good pain control.

Rapid titration of opioids for severe pain is best achieved with parenteral administration. Inability to tolerate oral medications is another reason to use parenteral opioids. Repeated intravenous boluses may be used, although continuous intravenous infusion has certain advantages in terms of efficacy, toxicity (i.e., lack bolus effects), and ease of administration. A short-acting agent such as morphine or hydromorphone is preferable for parenteral therapy (Portenoy 1987). Aside from trauma and surgery, the need for parenteral opioids usually arises in patients with long-standing pain syndromes, such as metastatic bone lesions, who have been using oral opioids. Determining the correct parenteral dosage requires a change in dosage to compensate for differences in potency between drugs and for the difference in oral versus parenteral efficacy (see Table 53.3).

If a continuous intravenous infusion is chosen, the total opioid dose of the prior 24 hours is converted to the milligram equivalent of parenteral morphine, which, divided over 24 hours, becomes the basal hourly rate. A loading dose approximately equivalent to 1 hour's dose (up to 30 mg of morphine) is given as a bolus. If parenteral therapy involves switching from one opioid to another in a patient whose pain is well controlled, the newly calculated dose should be decreased by 25–50% because the efficacy and cross-tolerance between opioids are incomplete. If pain control has been poor, then only a 25% reduction is made. In addition to a basal rate, as-needed doses for persistent or breakthrough pain should be administered, often accomplished by a patient-controlled delivery pump. In this way, rapid titration can be achieved by recalculating the hourly basal rate based on the combined basal and as-needed requirements. For rapid titration, a bolus is given each time the basal rate is increased.

The need for rapid intravenous titration of opioids often arises in patients with advanced cancer. In this group and in all patients with chronic pain syndromes that become rapidly worse, symptomatic relief must be achieved concurrently with attempts to define the exact reasons pain control is being lost. Treatment of the underlying process, such as a bone or epidural metastasis or abscess, remains one of the most important aspects of pain management. The judicious use of radiotherapy for painful metastases often reduces the need for analgesics.

The approach to the patient requiring moderate- to high-dose chronic opioid therapy has evolved considerably. Frequent doses of short-acting agents become impractical at high doses because of the large amounts of medication needed. This could be surmounted by switching to a long-acting opioid such as methadone, an effective approach for some patients, although methadone's analgesic effect is often much shorter than its pharmacological half-life. Additionally, titration must be done slowly to avoid excessive steady state levels that cause prolonged sedation and other adverse reactions. Newer approaches are based on the use of short-acting agents formulated for relatively slow or prolonged release.

MS Contin, the sustained-release oral preparation of morphine, provides relatively stable serum levels of morphine that can be supplemented with standard oral morphine on an as-needed basis for breakthrough pain. Titration, with initial dosing based on the milligram-equivalent of morphine taken in the prior 24 hours, is relatively easy to accomplish.

Transdermal fentanyl is now available for continuous, chronic opioid therapy. Fentanyl is an extremely potent synthetic opioid-agonist with a very short half-life when administered intravenously. The transdermal system delivers approximate doses ranging from 25 to 100 μg/hour for 2–3 days through the development of a subcutaneous reservoir at the site of the transdermal patch. The continuous-release provides the long duration of analgesia. Due to the reservoir effect, however, the attainment of effective analgesia is delayed 24–48 hours, titration must be performed over several days, and the management of adverse effects is complicated by the persistence of active blood levels for 2 or more days after the transdermal patch has been removed. As with MS Contin, most patients on fentanyl require a short-acting opioid, such as morphine or hydromorphone, for breakthrough pain.

With increasing opioid dosage, the adverse autonomic and CNS effects become dose-limiting for many patients. This is particularly true of patients with CNS metastasis or those who are concurrently taking other sedative-depressant medications. Several approaches are available for patients with poor pain control in the setting of significant opioid toxicity. One approach is to switch to an equipotent analgesic dose of a different opioid, recalling that cross-tolerance is incomplete and effective analgesia may be obtained with a modest decrease in the equivalent dose of a different opioid. In addition, optimizing the use of nonopioid analgesics and other adjuvant medications may allow a decrease in opioid requirements. If the opioid toxicity remains unacceptable, pain control is poor, or both, regional administration of opioids via intrathecal or epidural catheters and neurosurgical approaches to pain control should be considered.

Both epidural and intrathecal administration of morphine provide relatively high concentrations of opioids in the cerebrospinal fluid, producing analgesia by direct action on opiate receptors in the spinal cord (Payne 1987; Krames 1993). The amount of opioid reaching systemic circulation is usually considerably decreased, although not always. These approaches generally are limited to patients with pelvic or lower extremity pain. Side effects include pruritus, urinary retention, nausea, and vomiting. Respiratory depression and other CNS side effects (e.g., sedation, confusion) may occur. Factors that predispose patients to adverse reactions are advanced age, the use of water-soluble opioids such as morphine, high intrathecal doses, the concurrent systemic administration of opioids or anesthetics, and lack of opioid tolerance. Unlike the administration of local anesthetics, epidural opioids rarely cause transient weakness.

Adjuvant Medications Useful in Pain Management

Opioids and NSAIDs often are used together because their mechanisms of action are different and complementary, and their side effect profiles do not overlap. The opioid requirements are reduced, as is the likelihood of clinically significant opioid tolerance or dependence. Several other drugs with primary actions that are not analgesic have been used to improve pain control, including anticonvulsants, tricyclic antidepressants, benzodiazepines, stimulants, corticosteroids, topical capsaicin, and anesthetics.

Adjuvant Analgesics

Anticonvulsants. Phenytoin, carbamazepine, and occasionally valproate are used to treat neuropathic pain syndromes, including focal (e.g., postherpetic neuralgia or trigeminal neuralgia) and diffuse neuropathies (e.g., diabetic neuropathy) (Willner and Low 1993). Lancinating pains, presumably arising from abnormal neuronal discharge, demonstrate the best response. Anticonvulsants are also useful for central deafferentation pain syndromes. The dose required to achieve pain control is not necessarily the same as that required to produce therapeutic levels for anticonvulsant purposes, and gradual titration usually over weeks is required. Responses are difficult to predict, and serial trials often are required in attempts to find an effective agent for these types of pain syndromes.

Tricyclic Antidepressants. Amitriptyline and several other tricyclic antidepressants improve pain control when used with other analgesics for nociceptive pain and when used alone for neuropathic pain syndromes. The analgesic effect is independent of the presence of depression or any effect on mood. Blockade of serotonin and norepinephrine reuptake generally is believed to be the mechanism by which analgesia is produced; however, the analgesic activity of newer and more selective serotonin reuptake inhibitors (e.g., fluoxetine) is not established. The commonly used tricyclic compounds all have considerable anticholinergic activity, and some of the common toxic effects, such as constipation, overlap with the autonomic side effects related to opioid analgesics.

Benzodiazepines and Baclofen. Diazepam and baclofen are useful in managing spasticity, which occasionally is accompanied by muscle pain. Baclofen is also beneficial in some patients with trigeminal neuralgia that is refractory to other drugs and may be beneficial for other neuropathic pain syndromes. For most patients, however, benzodiazepines add little or no benefit for analgesic purposes but, rather, add significantly to the problems of sedation and dysphoria. Avoidance of CNS depressants is an important part of minimizing opioid toxicity.

Stimulants. Conversely, the judicious use of stimulants can improve pain control and reduce opioid toxicities—for example, dextroamphetamine and methylphenidate enhance morphine-induced analgesia and reduce the sedation associated with opioid treatment. Caffeine also has been used to improve analgesia and reduce sedation from opioids.

Corticosteroids. Corticosteroids contribute substantially to pain control caused by (1) inflammatory lesions of bone, joints, muscle, or blood vessels; (2) nerve root or spinal cord compression, particularly in relation to epidural mass lesions; and (3) headaches from cerebral edema, elevated intracranial pressure, and meningeal irritation. Corticosteroids are the primary treatment for some inflammatory conditions, such as temporal arteritis. Their use as an adjunct for pain control generally is limited to short-term treatment because of the many side effects associated with chronic corticosteroid therapy. Rheumatic pain complaints may follow cessation of corticosteroids.

Capsaicin. Topical capsaicin produces depletion of substance P from primary nociceptor afferents and provides satisfactory pain relief in more than 30% of patients with postherpetic neuralgia who have failed other medical treatments. Unfortunately, initiation of treatment often causes severe burning pain that may prevent continuation of treatment.

Others. Several other drugs are used infrequently for refractory pain syndromes, usually neuropathic and deafferentation syndromes. These include anesthetic/antiarrhythmic agents such as mexiletine, neuroleptics such as fluphenazine, and alpha-adrenergic agents such as clonidine (Willner and Low 1993).

NONPHARMACOLOGICAL APPROACHES TO PAIN MANAGEMENT

Ablative Procedures

Regional Nerve Blockade

Nerve blocks with local anesthetics such as lidocaine commonly are used to manage transitory, severe, localized pain. Epidural blockade for obstetric and gynecological procedures is the most common application of a regional nerve block. Other uses are to treat postoperative incisional pain and delayed operative pain that may occur after thoracotomy. Epidural blockade is particularly useful when pain is localized to one or two dermatomal segments on the trunk. Localized neuropathic pain, such as with acute herpes zoster or traumatic neuroma, also can be controlled with nerve blocks.

Phenol can be injected to produce permanent neurolysis in patients with cancer who are expected to survive less than 1 year and in patients with intractable and severe pain who obtain significant relief with temporary nerve blockade. Burning, dysesthetic pain from deafferentation (*anesthesia dolorosa*) often develops months after neurolysis and may be more troublesome than the original pain complaint. The use of temporary blockade and neurolysis is limited by their nonselective effect on all nerve fibers. Blockade of nerves to the limbs and sacral segments usually is avoided because sensory and motor deficits accompany analgesia.

Sympathetic blockade is an important component in the treatment of causalgia and related disorders. It usually is accomplished by serial blocks with local anesthetics and occasionally by neurolytic blockade. Pain relief may last long beyond the anesthetic agent's duration of action. Stellate ganglion blockade is performed for arm pain; celiac plexus blockade for upper abdominal pain such as that occurring with pancreatic cancer; and the lumbar sympathetic ganglia blockade for pelvic, rectal, and leg pain. Fluoroscopic or computed tomography (CT) guidance often is required for accurate injection placement.

Peripheral Surgical Approaches

The use of peripheral nerve and dorsal nerve root transection generally is confined to patients with well-localized or truly segmental truncal pain syndromes that have responded to nerve blockade. As with neurolysis, the late occurrence of painful dysesthesia is common and limits enthusiasm for this approach. Sympathetic ganglionectomy occasionally is performed in patients with causalgia and related syndromes who benefit transiently from sympathetic blockade.

Central Surgical Approaches

The most common central ablative surgical procedure for pain management is an anterolateral spinal cordotomy, producing transection of the lateral spinothalamic tract (Lahuerta et al. 1994). As with other surgical procedures for pain management, strict criteria for patient selection that includes failure of appropriate pharmacological means must be established. Patients whose life expectancy is 12 months or greater generally are not appropriate because the analgesic benefit declines with time and painful dysesthesia is a late complication. Thus, the procedure is largely limited to patients with cancer. The best candidates are patients with unilateral somatic, nociceptive pain in one leg or the trunk. Visceral and neuropathic/deafferentation pain syndromes are not effectively controlled. Bilateral thoracic cordotomies sometimes are performed for midline lower abdominal, pelvic, or bilateral leg pain, but urinary and fecal incontinence are frequent complications. Initial pain control is achieved in about 80% but lost in half after 6–12 months. Painful dysesthesia develops in 20% or more by 1 year. Corticospinal tract deficits are not common. In rare patients on very high doses of narcotics, the acute abolition of pain by surgical means or nerve blockade is accompanied by acute respiratory failure, which may be caused by an acute change in opioid tolerance and can be reversed with naloxone. Bilateral cervical cordotomies are associated with apnea due to the interruption of fibers subserving ventilation in about 5% of patients.

Other targets for ablative pain control procedures include the periaqueductal gray, trigeminal nucleus, thalamus, primary sensory cortex, frontal lobes, and portions of the limbic system, such as the cingulate gyrus. Although few comparative data are available, no pain control procedure appears to be superior to cordotomy for pain syndromes originating below the cervical level. Analgesia tends to be transitory and late dysesthesia is common to all procedures involving the spinothalamic tract, and the thalamus and its primary sensory projections. Destructive lesions in the cingulate gyrus interfere with the emotional experience associated with chronic pain without producing analgesia.

Another procedure used primarily to treat pain from disseminated bone metastases of hormonally sensitive cancers (i.e., breast and prostatic carcinoma) is pituitary ablation, which usually is performed by alcohol instillation via a transphenoidal approach.

Modulatory Procedures

The concept that nociceptive input can be reduced by peripheral stimulation is fundamental to the gate theory of pain transmission. In practice, this is accomplished most often by electrical stimulation using a transcutaneous electrical nerve stimulator (TENS). Placebo effect contributes substantially to the analgesic efficacy of TENS, although some studies of acute pain syndromes such as postoperative pain indicate benefit greater than obtained with sham stimulation. TENS also is used for chronic pain syndromes, particularly neuropathic pain, although studies have provided mixed results (Landau and Levy 1993). While some controlled studies demonstrate benefit, a randomized comparison between TENS and exercise for chronic lumbosacral pain demonstrated no difference between TENS treatment and placebo (Deyo et al. 1990).

Stimulation of dorsal root fibers and the dorsal columns using epidural electrodes has been performed for 20 years. Clear indications are debated but generally include (1) poor efficacy of standard medical therapy; (2) an identified etiology for the pain syndrome, usually with a neuropathic component and without a primary central cause of deafferentation; and (3) a dermatomal distribution of pain that can be effectively included in a region of stimulation-induced paresthesias. Areas that are difficult to cover include the C-2 vertebra, posterior axial structures including the neck and lumbosacral spine, and the perineum. An array of electrodes, usually on a single wire, is inserted in the dorsal epidural space either by laminectomy or percutaneously in the low- or midthoracic region. A trial period of 4–7 days of stimulation is performed to assess pain relief. If benefit is observed, the electrodes are permanently implanted.

Most series are dominated by patients with chronic lumbosacral pain following laminectomy, the so-called failed back syndrome, which is often attributed to arachnoiditis. Next are other neuropathic pain syndromes such as neuropathies. Fifty to seventy percent of patients show initial improvement. Long-term pain relief occurs in 40%, however, and many continue to require some analgesic medication (Spiegelmann and Friedman 1991; North 1990). Mechanical problems, such as electrode breakage, have been a common cause of failure. While these results appear hopeful given the chronic, refractory nature of the pain syndromes addressed, prospective studies with carefully focused indications and rigorous follow-up assessment are required.

Stimulation of the periaqueductal gray and primary nuclei of termination of the spinothalamic and trigeminothalamic pathways (i.e., VPL and VPM respectively) has been employed for chronic neuropathic pain syndromes, including many with deafferentation components. Tic douloureux, postherpetic neuralgia involving the face, pain following cerebral infarction, postcordotomy pain, and brachial plexus avulsion have been approached in this way. As with spinal cord stimulation of the patients who have a good initial response, only about 50% report long-term benefit. Other areas used for pain control by neurostimulation include the motor cortex and the septal area. Lacking well-defined indications and controlled trials with rigorous assessment of outcome, central neurostimulation for chronic pain is an optional treatment for those who fail medical therapy (Levy et al. 1987; Duncan et al. 1991).

CONCLUSION

Pain, the most common of all medical complaints, is becoming increasingly well understood. It is a complex group of neurophysiological processes that may arise from (1) the normal response of the nervous system to tissue injury; (2) pathological alterations in neural activity in nociceptive, sensory, and other pathways; or (3) no identifiable pathology. In practice, treatment is based on defining the mechanism(s) by which the pain symptom is generated. A relatively high likelihood of therapeutic success is achieved in the case of nociceptive pain, but only a modest rate of success is obtained in the treatment of neuropathic and idiopathic pain syndromes. Both in terms of basic science and as clinical phenomena, the understanding of pain mechanisms remains incomplete. Yet, this mechanistic approach is central to formulating a rational therapeutic strategy. Treatment applied in the absence of an understanding of the mechanism(s) involved has a high likelihood of failure, unnecessary toxicity, and potential for irreversible tissue injury.

The goal of pain management is complete pain relief. Too often, pain relief is not pursued aggressively so that the symptom can be used as an indicator of disease activity, for example, in patients with cancer. In comparison with the array of other clinical, laboratory, and radiographic measures of disease activity available for neoplastic, infectious, and inflammatory diseases, progressive pain as an isolated symptom is generally a moderately sensitive and modest to moderately specific indicator of disease activity. Thus, using pain as an indicator should be considered secondary to relief of the symptom, assuming that the cause of the pain is understood. The most significant factor limiting complete relief of nociceptive and neuropathic pain is analgesic toxicity. Much of pain management beyond knowledge of basic analgesic pharmacology centers around this issue.

Pain management has improved significantly in recent years as the result of systematic education programs for medical students, house officers, fellows, physicians, and other health care providers with regard to pain assessment and the basic principles of analgesic therapy (see recommendations of the Ad Hoc Committee on Cancer Pain of the American Society of Clinical Oncology, 1992). Advances in pain management also have been fueled by important basic neuroscience developments, such as the elucidation of the endogenous opioid systems, and increasingly sophisticated clinical analysis of pain syndromes. Clinical necessity will continue to fuel the development of better ways to treat patients with pain.

REFERENCES

Ad Hoc Committee on Cancer Pain of the American Society of Clinical Oncology. Cancer pain assessment and treatment curriculum guidelines. J Clin Oncol 1992;10:1976–1982.

Arner S, Meyerson BA. Lack of analgesic effect of opioids on neuropathic and idiopathic forms of pain. Pain 1988;33:11–23.

Bonica JJ. The Management of Pain (2nd ed). Philadelphia: Lea & Febiger, 1990.

Brooks PM, Day RO. Nonsteroidal anti-inflammatory drugs—differences and similarities. N Engl J Med 1991;324:1716–1725.

Casey KL (ed). Pain and Central Nervous System Disease: The Central Pain Syndromes. New York: Raven, 1991.

Cherny NI, Thaler HT, Friedlander-Klar H et al. Opioid responsiveness of cancer pain syndromes caused by neuropathic or nociceptive mechanisms: a combined analysis of controlled, single-dose studies. Neurology 1994;44:857–861.

Deyo RA, Walsh NE, Martin DC et al. A controlled trial of transcutaneous electrical nerve stimulation (TENS) and exercise for chronic low back pain. N Engl J Med 1990;322:1627–1634.

Dubner R. Basic mechanisms of pain associated with deep tissues. Can J Physiol Pharmacol 1991;69:607–609.

Duncan GH, Bushnell MC, Marchand S. Deep brain stimulation: a review of basic research and clinical studies. Pain 1991; 45:49–59.

Dworkin RH, Gitlin MJ. Clinical aspects of depression in chronic pain patients. Clin J Pain 1991;7:79–94.

Goodman RR, Adler BA, Pasternak GW. Regional Distribution of Opiate Receptors. In GW Pasternak (ed), The Opiate Receptors. Clifton, NJ: Humana Press, 1988;197–227.

Keefe FJ, Dunsmore J, Burnett R. Behavioral and cognitive-behavioral approaches to chronic pain: recent advances and future directions. J Consult Clin Psychol 1992;60:528–536.

Krames ES. Intrathecal infusional therapies for intractable pain: patient management guidelines. J Pain Symptom Management 1993;8:36–46.

Lahuerta J, Bowsher D, Lipton S et al. Percutaneous cervical cordotomy: a review of 181 operations on 146 patients with a study on the location of the "pain fibers" in the C-2 spinal cord segment of 29 cases. J Neurosurg 1994;80:975–985.

Landau B, Levy RM. Neuromodulation techniques for medically refractory chronic pain. Annu Rev Med 1993;44:279–287.

Levy RM, Lamb S, Adams JE. Treatment of chronic pain by deep brain stimulation: long term followup and review of the literature. Neurosurgery 1987;21:885–893.

Merskey H. Pain and Psychological Medicine. In PD Wall, R Melzack (eds), Textbook of Pain (2nd ed). Edinburgh: Churchill Livingstone, 1989.

Ness TJ, Gebhart GF. Visceral pain: a review of experimental studies. Pain 1990;41:167–234.

North RB. Spinal cord stimulation for intractable pain: long-term follow-up. J Spinal Disord 1990;3:356–361.

Ochoa JL. Essence, investigation and management of "neuropathic" pains: hopes from acknowledgment of chaos. Muscle Nerve 1993;16:997–1008.

Payne R. Neuropathic pain syndromes, with special reference to causalgia and reflex sympathetic dystrophy. Clin J Pain 1986;2:59–73.

Payne R. Role of Epidural and Intrathecal Narcotics and Peptides in the Management of Cancer Pain. In R Payne, KM Foley (eds), The Medical Clinics of North America: Cancer Pain. Vol. 71, No. 2. Philadelphia: Saunders, 1987;313–328.

Portenoy RK, Foley KM. Chronic use of opioid analgesics in nonmalignant pain: report of 38 cases. Pain 1986;25:171–186.

Portenoy RK. Continuous Intravenous Infusion of Opioid Drugs. In R Payne, KM Foley (eds), The Medical Clinics of North America: Cancer Pain. Vol. 71, No. 2. Philadelphia: Saunders, 1987;233–242.

Portenoy RK. Mechanisms of clinical pain: observations and speculations. Neurol Clin 1989;7:205–231.

Portenoy RK. The nature of opioid responsiveness and its implications for neuropathic pain: new hypotheses derived from studies of opioid infusions. Pain 1990a;43:273–286.

Portenoy RK. Chronic opioid therapy in nonmalignant pain. J Pain Symptom Manage 1990b;5(I Suppl):S46–62.

Portenoy RK. Cancer pain: pathophysiology and syndromes. Lancet 1992;339:1026–1031.

Portenoy RK. Cancer pain management. Semin Oncol 1993;20: Suppl 1:19–35.

Posner JB. Disorders of Sensation. In JB Wyngaarden, LH Smith (eds), Cecil Texbook of Medicine. Vol. 2. Philadelphia: Saunders, 1985;2047–2063.

Roberts WJ. A hypothesis on the physiologic basis for causalgia and related pains. Pain 1986;24:33–44.

Schott GD. Mechanisms of causalgia and related clinical conditions: the role of the central and of the sympathetic nervous systems. Brain 1986;109:717–738.

Simon EJ, Hiller JM. Opioid Peptides and Opioid Receptors. In GJ Siegel, BW Agranoff, RW Albers et al. (eds), Basic Neurochemistry. New York: Raven, 1994;321–340.

Spiegelmann R, Friedman WA. Spinal cord stimulation: a contemporary series. Neurosurgery 1991;28:65–70.

Terenius L. Opioid peptides, pain and stress. Prog Brain Res 1992;92:375–383.

Ventafridda V, Tamburni M, Caraceni A et al. A validation study of the WHO method for cancer pain relief. Cancer 1987;59:850–856.

Verdugo RJ, Ochoa JL. Sympathetically maintained pain. I. Phentolamine block questions the concept. Neurology 1994;44: 1003–1010.

Verdugo RJ, Campero M, Ochoa JL. Phentolamine sympathetic block in painful polyneuropathies. II. Further questioning of the concept of "sympathetically maintained pain." Neurology 1994;44:1010–1014.

Wall PD, Melzack R (eds). Texbook of Pain. Edinburgh: Churchill Livingstone, 1994.

Willner C, Low PA. Pharmacologic Approaches to Neuropathic Pain. In PF Dyck, PK Thomas et al. (eds), Peripheral Neuropathy (3rd ed). Philadelphia: Saunders, 1993;1709–1720.

SUGGESTED READING

Foley KM. The treatment of cancer pain. N Engl J Med 1985; 313:84–95.

Chapter 54
Principles of Neurosurgery

Bennett M. Stein

Medicine has long supported the concept of a surgeon schooled in neurology performing neurosurgery, although this has not always been the case. In its infancy neurosurgery was performed by general surgeons with an interest in peripheral nerves and the central nervous system (CNS) who had a working knowledge of neuroanatomy but rarely a foundation in neurology. As the field of neurosurgery has matured, training programs have uniformly demanded a period of training in neurology for the neurosurgical resident. Unfortunately, the converse has not materialized; few neurologists acquire training or experience in neurosurgery. It is hoped that this chapter will bridge the gap between neurological experience and an understanding of the role of neurosurgery in the treatment of neurological disease.

Many neurological centers have developed a team of specialists in clinical neurosciences, including neurology, neurosurgery, neuroradiology, and neuroanesthesia. This team concentrates on specialized areas, including pediatric, vascular, neoplastic, spinal, and functional disorders, including epilepsy, pain, and movement disorders. These may or may not require the use of stereotactic surgery to probe, lesion, or implant bioactive substances deep in the brain. As these highly specialized areas have developed, they have been augmented by work in the laboratory, which includes the study of vascular conditions of the brain, of the growth and biological behavior of tumors, and of the transplantation of active neural or hormone-producing tissue. This cross-fertilization leads to a more informed, decisive, and preplanned evaluation of the patient and the treatment of the neurological disease.

Our policy in the Neurological Institute of New York is to have emergency admissions screened by neurologists. After the initial appraisal of the condition, a group with expertise in the specific neurological problem is called in to organize and oversee the workup of the patient. Diagnostic workup in most cases commences immediately, spurred on by the need for timely and early neurosurgery in certain cases. There is special urgency for patients with vascular disease and those with tumors, when the mass effect has resulted in impending herniation and rising intracranial pressure. This specialized workup is pursued primarily by the neurologist with special interest in the area of neurosurgical disorders, in conjunction with the neuroradiologist. The neurosurgeon plays a subordinate role as a consultant. It must be understood, however, that in the neuroradiological diagnostic workup, certain special views or techniques of imaging are required to plan the neurosurgical approach. Therefore, the evaluation must consider these needs in an early review of the problem with the neurosurgeon. The best time for this consultation and developing an understanding of the game plan is well before the radiological procedures are undertaken.

PRINCIPLES AND PERIOPERATIVE CONSIDERATIONS

Imaging in Neurosurgical Disorders

The accuracy of diagnosis has been significantly improved by better neuroradiological imaging techniques. At the same time, the spectrum of diagnostic procedures available to us has increased. With the increased cost of these procedures, it is important that the most appropriate procedure be selected. This will avoid inefficiencies, redundancies, and high cost in the diagnostic workup. It behooves the diagnostician to know the advantages and disadvantages of each imaging technique prior to selection to tailor the workup to best suit the neurological disorder.

Specific Neurological Problems

Vascular Disorders. If a hemorrhage, parenchymal or subarachnoid, is suspected, computerized tomography (CT) scan is the best indicator of blood (Figure 54.1). However, when there is strong suspicion of a vascular disorder, such as

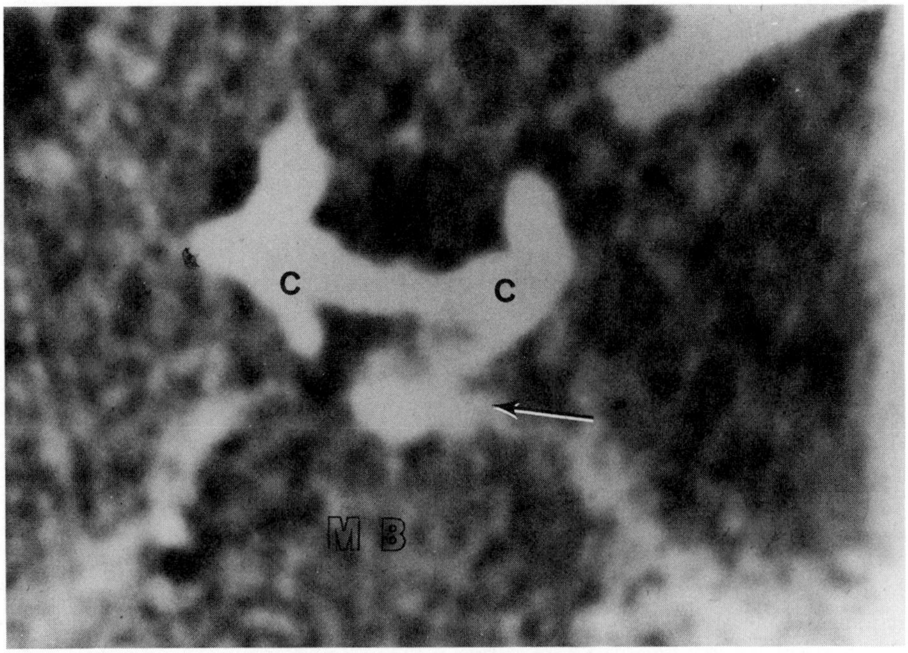

A

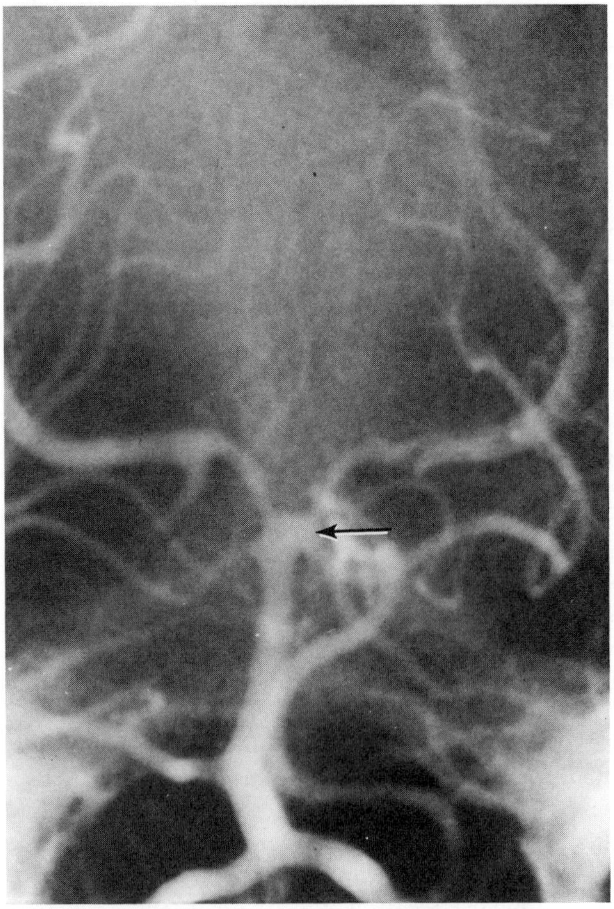

B

FIGURE 54.1 A. Computed tomographic scan, axial view without contrast, indicating hemorrhage directed toward the right side of the intrapeduncular fossa (arrow). (C = posterior clinoids; MB = midbrain.) B. Vertebral angiogram showing aneurysm pointing to the right side of the basilar artery between the origin of the posterior cerebral and the superior cerebellar arteries (arrow).

aneurysms over 1 cm or arteriovenous malformations (AVMs) or cavernous malformations, magnetic resonance imaging (MRI) is the most appropriate imaging technique. Magnetic resonance angiography (MRA) is valuable in determining the presence of aneurysms and AVMs. Currently the sophistication of imaging necessary to plan surgery is not available by MRA. For contemporary neurosurgery, formal angiography, including selective, stereo, and subtraction techniques, is necessary to plan a surgical approach. It is hoped that as MRA becomes more sophisticated, routine angiography will become a technique of the past.

The MRI examination, although it does not detail the vascular anatomy as well as the angiogram, better represents the relationship of an AVM to surrounding structures. The use of the diagnostic armamentarium is well illustrated in the case of cavernous malformations. The CT scan and the MRI are diagnostic, and an angiogram, which is negative in this situation, is unnecessary. Venous malformations are usually suggested by CT scan or MRI, which are not as pathognomonic as the angiogram (Table 54.1, Figure 54.2). These examples emphasize that although the procedures are complementary to each other, each examination has a primary purpose and, in general, is most useful for a particular disorder.

Angiography may be augmented by stereoangiography in which the lateral x-rays can be viewed as a pair in three dimensions. All angiography must include the four major vessels supplying the intracranial circulation. Digital subtraction angiography is useful in eliminating superfluous shadows and focusing on the vascular anatomy. Certain digital systems have a rotational and three-dimensional capacity. Selective studies may further enhance the angiogram (Figure 54.3).

Table 54.1: Radiological characteristics of cerebral vascular malformations

Arteriovenous Malformation[a]	*Venous Malformation*[b]	*Cavernous Malformation*[c]
Angiography		
Definition of artery-to-vein shunts	Caput medusae with prominent vein, no arterial component	Negative
Computed tomographic scan		
C (–) calcification uncommonly seen	C (–) Normal	C (–) Lesion visualized because of calcium
C (+) serpentine pattern of enhancement	C (+) Linear enhancement usual	C (+) Slight enhancement
Magnetic resonance imaging		
Honeycomb of signal voids	Linear signal void	Pathognomonic target appearance with combination of high signal and signal voids
Specific arteries and veins may be identified		

C (–) = CT scan without contrast enhancement; C (+) = CT scan with contrast enhancement.
[a]Figure 54.2A.
[b]Figure 54.2C.
[c]Figure 54.2D.
Source: Adapted from RF Spetzler. Radiological characteristics of cerebral malformations. BNI Q 1987;3:22.

Spinal angiography is a procedure of special dimensions. It should be done only under special circumstances, where an AVM or vascular tumor of the spinal cord is strongly suspected from the clinical history and confirmed by MRI or myelography (Figure 54.4).

Neoplastic Disorders. MRI and CT scanning have all but replaced angiography in the diagnostic workup of neoplastic disorders of the CNS. MRA can also be supplemental in demonstrating the following features: (1) the blood supply to tumors, such as the external carotid artery supply to meningiomas; (2) the relationship of major cerebral arteries to tumors, such as the encasement of the internal carotid artery by meningiomas of the skull base; and (3) the luxurious vascularity of some tumors.

In most operations, with microsurgical technique, the arteries can be defined without hazard at the time of surgery, and their relationship and abundance need not be determined prior to operative intervention. In the case of transsphenoidal surgery, the position of the internal carotid arteries in relation to the sella and pituitary tumor will be readily imaged by MRI, thus saving the patient bilateral carotid angiography. In the case of tumors of the pineal region, MRI is particularly valuable in showing the relationship to the third ventricle and deep venous system (Figure 54.5).

Posterior fossa tumor surgery has been simplified through the use of MRI and CT scans. Commonly encountered tumors, such as acoustic neurinomas, and meningiomas, can be identified by these techniques. A CT scan shows the relationship of the acoustic tumor to the internal auditory meatus and canal, whereas meningiomas have broad attachments to the dura of the posterior fossa. The location, attachment, and size of the tumors on these studies are therefore quite characteristic. In meningiomas that involve the brain stem and the base of the posterior fossa, the position of the basilar artery at the margin of or within the tumor can be readily determined by appropriate MRI views and thin sections. In children, the ability to diagnose posterior fossa tumors quickly, efficiently, and in a relatively noninvasive fashion (CT scan with contrast) has facilitated the workup of these common tumors.

Spinal Disorders. MRI is the primary diagnostic examination for spinal disorders. The perfection of surface coil techniques to clarify images and the more rapid MRI scanning technique with thin sections available through the use of high-tesla magnets augment this imaging. All of these techniques minimize the effect of motion, which is seen especially in the thoracic spine, and perfect the identification of structures as small as the spinal cord and its environs.

The MRI is now preferred in the diagnosis of disc lesions and of intra- and extramedullary tumors (Figure 54.6). If there is a negative side to MRI imaging of the spine, it pertains to the following:

1. Localization of the relationship to external landmarks is difficult.
2. The extent of the lesion may be overestimated.
3. Its usefulness in vascular disorders such as AVMs is not as great as in similar intracranial lesions.
4. It does not show bone detail.

MRI is the only practical technique for follow-up studies of spinal disease and is particularly useful for the identification of recurrence or cyst formation within the spinal cord.

Postoperative and Follow-up Imaging

Following operation, virtually all neurosurgical patients undergo imaging designed to monitor the effect of the operative procedure. For example, all patients who have had AVMs or aneurysms obliterated should have postoperative angiograms. This can be done by the digital technique, since the utmost detail is not required. We prefer standard arteriography, albeit limited to the area of disease. The follow-up angiogram is usually performed within a week after the surgery, or earlier if the clinical situation demands it. In the case of intracranial

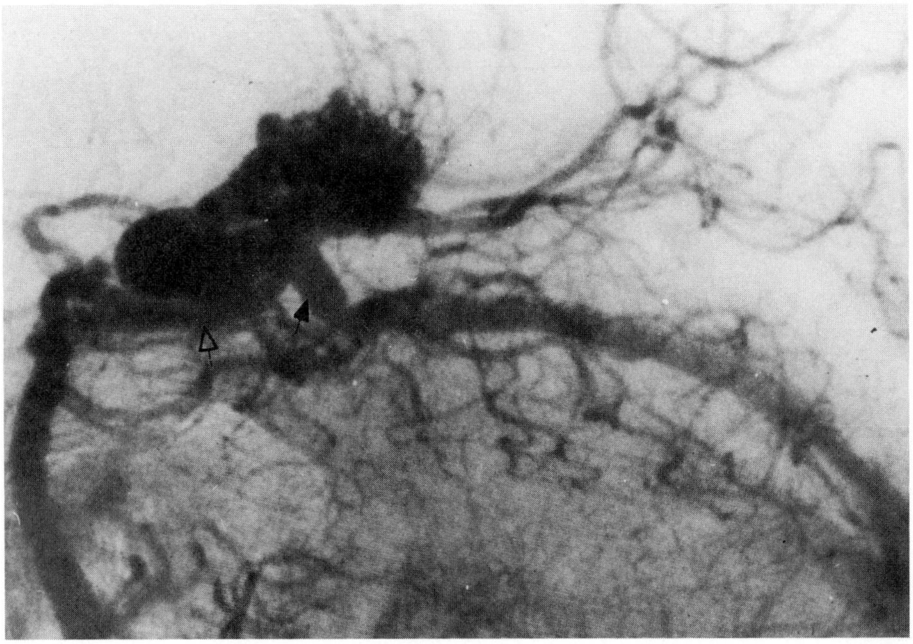

A

FIGURE 54.2 A. Typical arteriovenous malformation (AVM) in the medial temporal region showing arterial supply (open arrow) and the prominent venous drainage (closed arrow) indicating a significant arteriovenous shunt. B. Magnetic resonance image (MRI) of AVM (arrows) showing evidence of old hemorrhage and high blood flow, the latter represented by the signal void.

aneurysm, where spasm is expected and has an important bearing on subsequent treatment, angiography tends to be carried out soon after the operative procedure.

In many institutions, intraoperative angiography is performed; where the radiographic suite is adjacent to the operating room, angiography may be performed under the same general anesthesia immediately following the closure of the operative wound. This is an ideal situation provided it does not jeopardize the patient and prolong anesthetic time. If the result of the vascular surgery is unsatisfactory, then the patient can be returned to the operating room under the same anesthetic and the operation performed to perfection (Figure 54.7). This applies specifically to difficult aneurysms, where the placement of the clip is uncertain even using the operating microscope or where a major adjacent artery may be inadvertently compromised by the clip. In this situation the surgeon, realizing the problem from the immediate postoperative angiogram, has the opportunity to replace the clip in a more appropriate position before significant ischemia ensues. Difficult and deep AVMs benefit from postoperative angiography to reveal small residual fragments. Reoperation or radiosurgery may then be carried out to treat these residua.

In tumor surgery, especially with the use of the operating microscope, it is often the surgeon's opinion that he or she has removed more than is actually the case. In such cases, postoperative imaging, either with CT scan or with MRI, is mandatory to monitor the results of subtotal resection. In cases in which the tumor has been totally resected, postoperative imaging serves as a baseline for future reference should recurrence be suspected.

With the use of noninvasive neuroradiological procedures, patients are followed up more frequently than they

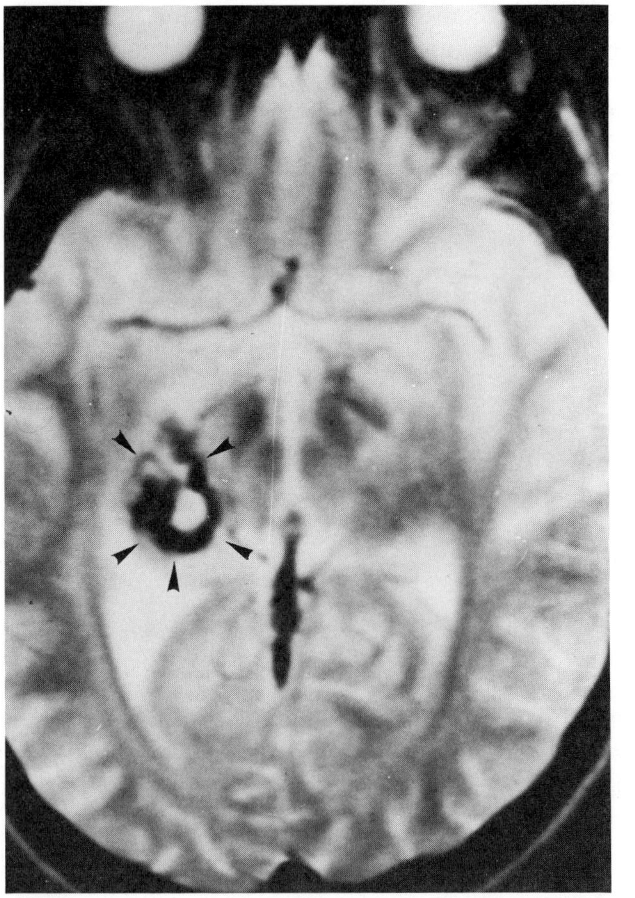

B

C. Typical caput medusae angiographic appearance of a venous malformation of the cerebellar hemisphere. Note the prominent draining vein (arrow). D. MRI of cavernous malformation of the medulla showing various stages of hemorrhage and the variegated appearance of the lesion proper (arrows).

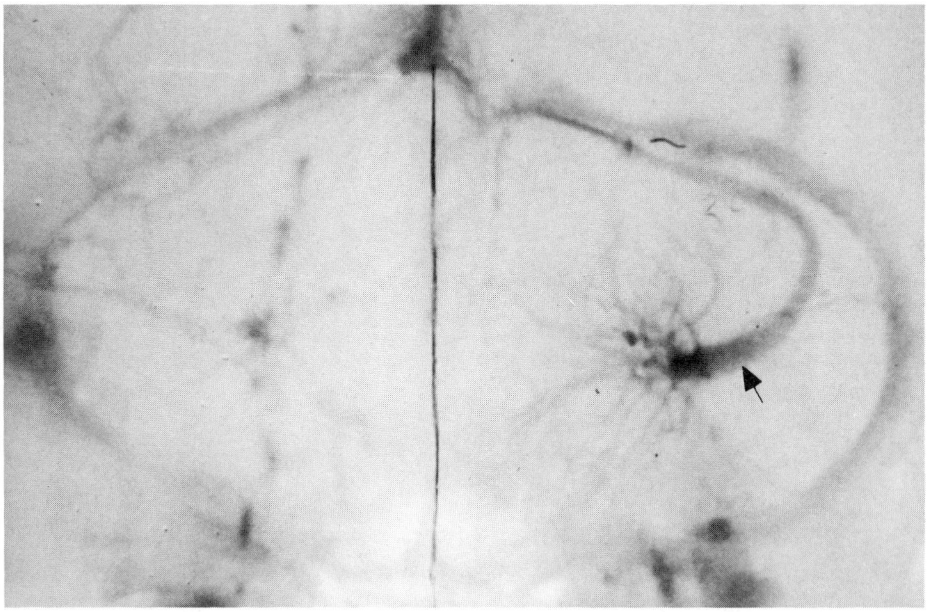

C

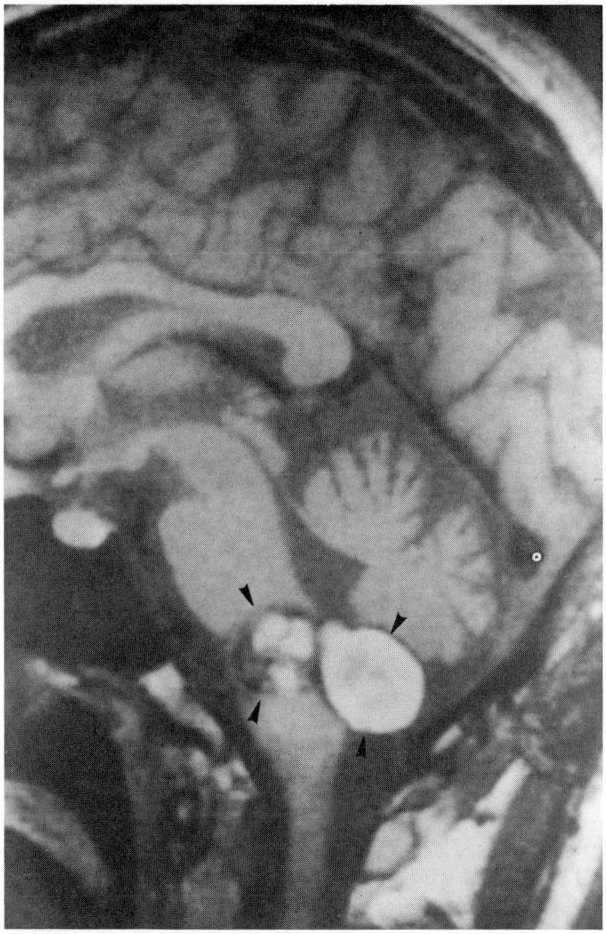

D

were in the past, leading to better patient management. In the case of vascular problems, we tend to overperform rather than underperform angiography. With the remarkable vascular changes that occur intraoperatively and postoperatively, this is the only method other than Doppler and xenon imaging that permits insight into circulatory changes that occur postoperatively.

Neurosurgical Management in General

Proper and timely clinical diagnosis and radiographic procedures are essential to planning a neurosurgical procedure. The results should be reviewed in concert by the neurosurgeon, neurologist, and neuroradiologist. It is good medical practice to keep responsible family members informed and to keep the patient informed within the boundaries of good medical judgment. We tend to minimize risk in discussing surgery with the aneurysm patient for fear of creating sudden hypertension from anxiety and rupture of the aneurysm. In neoplastic disease, the implications of malignancy are usually downgraded in discussions with the patient, at least preoperatively.

Patients who are at the extremes of the age spectrum, either pediatric or geriatric, should be prepared properly by a pediatric neurologist or an internist with geriatric knowledge. If there are significant medical problems, it is wise to call in the anesthesiologist who will be rendering anesthesia to the neurosurgical patient. In some institutions there is a team of neuroanesthesiologists who participate in special evaluations such as cerebral blood flow preoperatively, intraoperatively, and postoperatively.

A broad-spectrum intravenous antibiotic is commenced 2–4 hours prior to operative incision and continued for 48

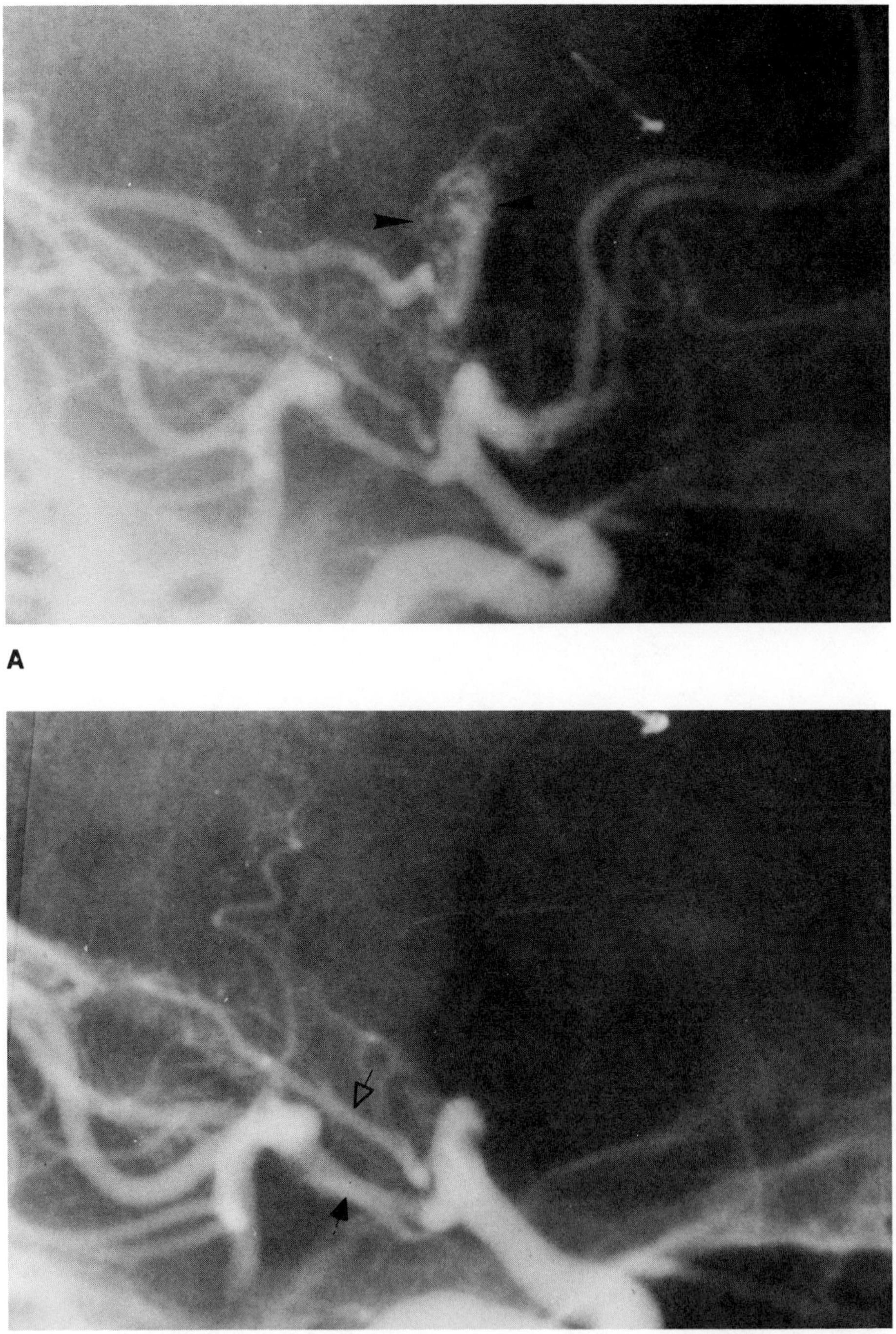

A

B

FIGURE 54.3 A. Selective arteriography with balloon occlusion of the middle cerebral artery shows abundant arterial supply from the anterior cerebral artery to a small arteriovenous malformation (AVM) (arrows). B. Selective arteriogram in the same case with balloon occlusion of the carotid bifurcation showing the lack of blood supply to the AVM from the anterior choroidal (open arrow) and posterior communicating (closed arrow) arteries.

hours postoperatively. This regimen has resulted in a lower rate of perioperative infection. Although there is no confirmation that corticosteroids have a beneficial effect in warding off side effects of neurosurgical trauma, brain swelling, and certain unexplained vascular reactions, it is the clinical impression of most neurosurgeons that it is beneficial. We use high-dose corticosteroids preoperatively, intraoperatively, and postoperatively. Any operation that threatens the cerebral cortex, even ventricular peritoneal shunt procedures in patients susceptible to seizures, deserves anticonvulsant coverage prior to and following surgery. Although it is not universally accepted, we maintain all of our postcraniotomy patients on anticonvulsant medication for between 6 and 24 months postoperatively. This may be modified depending on the degree of violation of the cerebral cortex during the operative procedure. For example, a subfrontal and temporal retraction for the clipping of an uncomplicated posterior communicating artery aneurysm requires anticonvulsants for

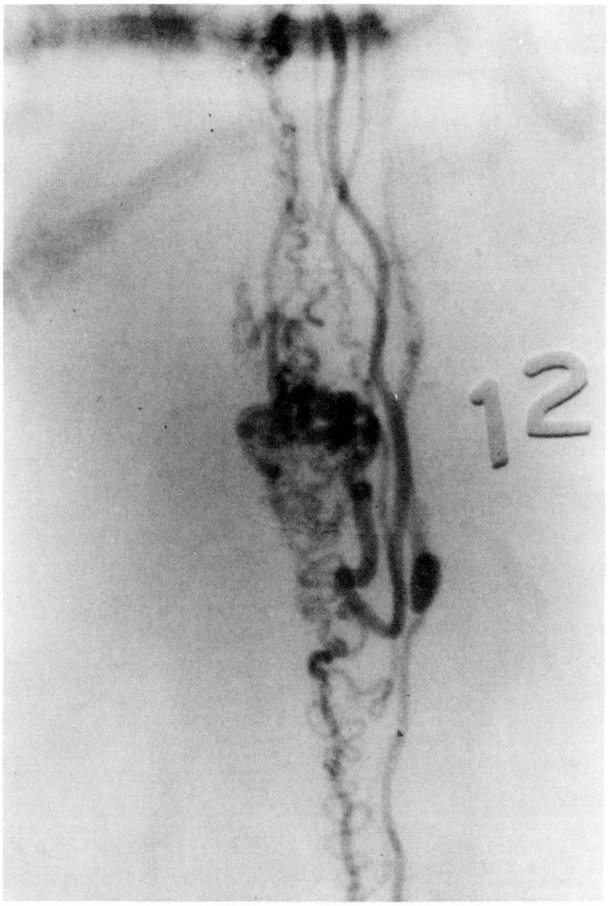

FIGURE 54.4 Spinal subtraction angiogram showing an arteriovenous malformation located primarily at the T12 level.

only a short time. On the other hand, the removal of a large meningioma, which involves the cerebral cortex and subcortical tissues, probably demands anticonvulsant coverage for 18–24 months postoperatively.

Patients whose operation involves the region of the brain stem or upper cervical cord, with or without preexisting respiratory problems, need careful preoperative scrutiny by the neurosurgeon and the neuroanesthesiologist. In these patients, because of compromised brain stem and upper cervical cord function, preoperative pulmonary function studies and a regulated airway may be required. These patients are often left intubated postoperatively, and should be warned of this possibility so that they will better tolerate the intubation. Where severe prolonged respiratory problems are expected postoperatively, a tracheotomy can be performed in conjunction with the neurosurgical procedure. The importance of a proper medical milieu, including cardiopulmonary stabilization and fluid balance, cannot be overemphasized. We prefer to have our patients well balanced or slightly on the dehydrated side both intraoperatively and postoperatively. This can be a double-edged sword, since too much dehydration leads to low blood volume and creates difficulty in controlling blood pressure, especially if hypotensive anesthesia is needed. The following case history illustrates how an anesthetic policy not accounting for the special requirements of neurosurgery can lead to severe problems.

A small girl, age 13 years, having suffered a hemorrhage from an AVM several months previously, was brought to surgery intact for the removal of a posterior thalamic AVM on the left, dominant side (Figure 54.8A). The lesion was removed without major hemorrhage or compromise of the circulation. This surgery involved portions of the diencephalon, the deep venous system, and the hypothalamus. Postoperatively the patient awoke and appeared little changed from the preoperative state. Approximately 8 hours after the operation she gradually became stuporous. A CT scan showed widespread diffuse cerebral edema (see Figure 54.8B). The situation was reviewed at this point, and it was found that she had received 4,500 ml of fluid during the operative procedure and had output of only 1,000 ml. In addition, her sodium had fallen from 134 mEq to 116 mEq over a brief period. It was apparent that she had received fluid overload during the surgery and that because of the location of the surgery she had developed inappropriate antidiuretic hormone secretion. Just as the patient was to be given mannitol, she suddenly became unresponsive, with fixed dilated pupils and absent corneal reflexes. Following dehydration and intubation, the patient began to respond, and the neurological picture showed gradual improvement. The point is that a generalist would have expected a young, healthy child such as this to have tolerated the fluid load. However, account was not taken of the locus of the surgery and the implications regarding systems controlling fluid and electrolytes.

Elective surgery should proceed in a well-designed fashion. For the patient who may require urgent action, the neurosurgeon can do certain things on an emergency basis that may reverse a critical situation. These cases include patients suffering from acute hydrocephalus or increased intracranial pressure, with impending herniation. Under local anesthesia, a small twist drill hole can be placed in the right frontal region just at the hairline and a catheter passed for ventricular decompression. In the case of a large posterior fossa tumor with impending decompensation, there has been some concern about the possibility of the pressure being transmitted upward through the tentorial incisura, or so-called upward herniation. In this situation, the ventricular drainage could theoretically increase this tendency. In fact, this is rarely a problem. The advantage of ventricular decompression far outweighs the fear of upward herniation. When the ventricles cannot be decompressed, certain medical management may be instituted. This includes the following: (1) high-dose intravenous corticosteroids—10 mg dexamethasone, repeated at 4-hour intervals; (2) intravenous dehydrating agents such as mannitol in doses of 1–2 g/kg; (3) manipulation of systemic factors such as blood pressure, blood gases, and venous drainage from the brain. This can be accomplished by elevating the patient's head 10–20 degrees, by driving down the pCO_2 levels to 25 mm Hg, and by increasing oxygenation to appropriate levels. In cerebral edema and vasospasm, pressor agents may be helpful. They elevate blood pressure to force blood into areas in which there may be ischemia or impending ischemia due to spasm or decreased flow secondary to cerebral edema. Emergency procedures such as subtemporal, suboccipital, or hemicranial decompression are now rarely used.

In terms of spinal problems, emergency posterior decompression used to be the norm in the face of extradural compression due to carcinoma. This is controversial, however, and many feel that extradural carcinoma should be treated by high-dose dexamethasone and immediate radiotherapy. Because most carcinomatous compressions occur anterior to the spinal cord, anterior spinal approaches and vertebral body corpectomy with spinal stabilization may be an alternative. In the case of benign tumors blocking the spinal canal, the use of MRI scanning has simplified diagnosis, and it is rare for a patient to undergo sudden deterioration. Patients are usually well prepared with dexamethasone and therefore can be stabilized and operated on electively.

In the case of cranial trauma victims, almost the only neurosurgical emergency is that of an extradural hematoma. Even a patient with a subdural hematoma may be stabilized, and a patient with an injured spine is better stabilized by traction than by undergoing immediate operation.

The bulk of neurosurgical procedures are now performed with the operating microscope. In our view, operating on aneurysms and performing complicated vascular surgery without the microscope is unacceptable neurosurgical practice. The same applies to most cases of AVM or deep tumors in obscure locations and all spinal tumors or vascular malformations. More and more neurosurgeons are familiarizing themselves with the technique of using an operating microscope for anterior cervical discectomy and for microdiscectomy in the lumbar region. When using the operating microscope, exposures are small, limiting retraction and trauma to the adjacent normal tissue and ensuring a rapid recovery. In addition, use of the operating microscope rather than naked eye makes a world of difference when it comes to details of small blood vessels, cranial nerves, and other important structures.

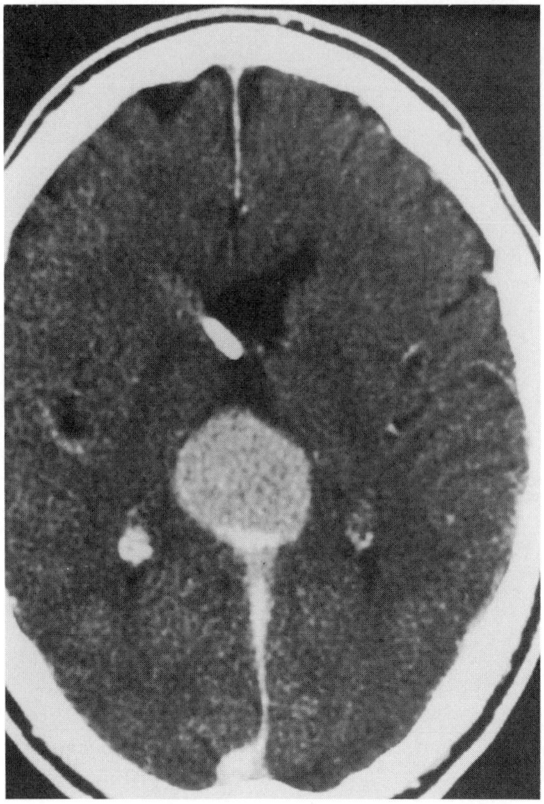

A

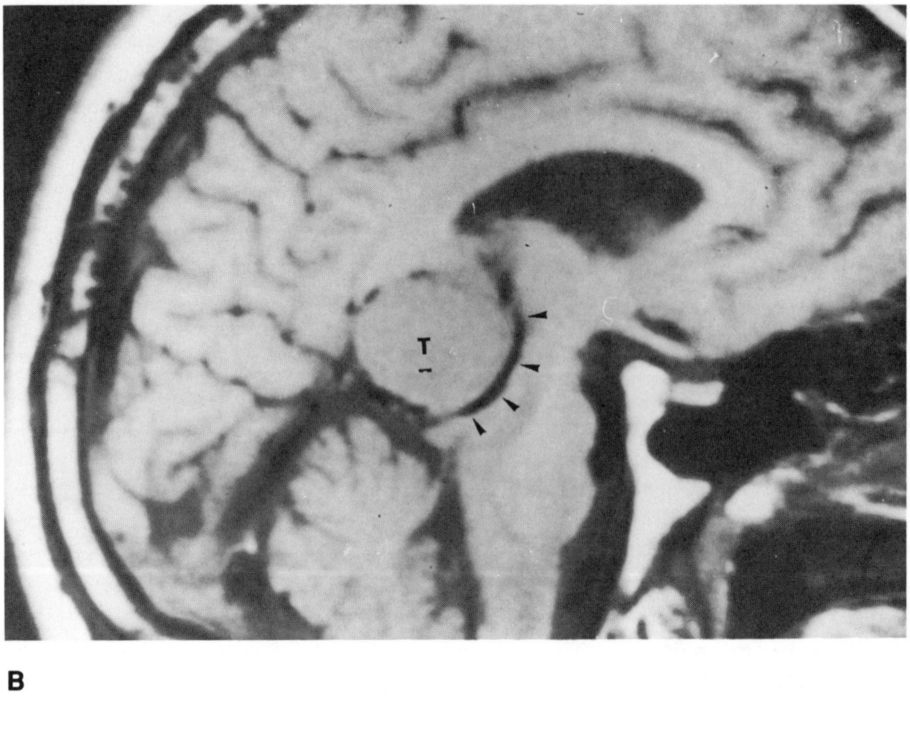

B

FIGURE 54.5 A. Contrast-enhanced computed tomographic scan showing the large enhanced tumor in the region of the pineal. B. The relationship to the deep venous system is shown only in the detail of a sagittal magnetic resonance imaging scan, which illustrates the deep venous system (arrows) displaced ventrally by the large meningioma (T).

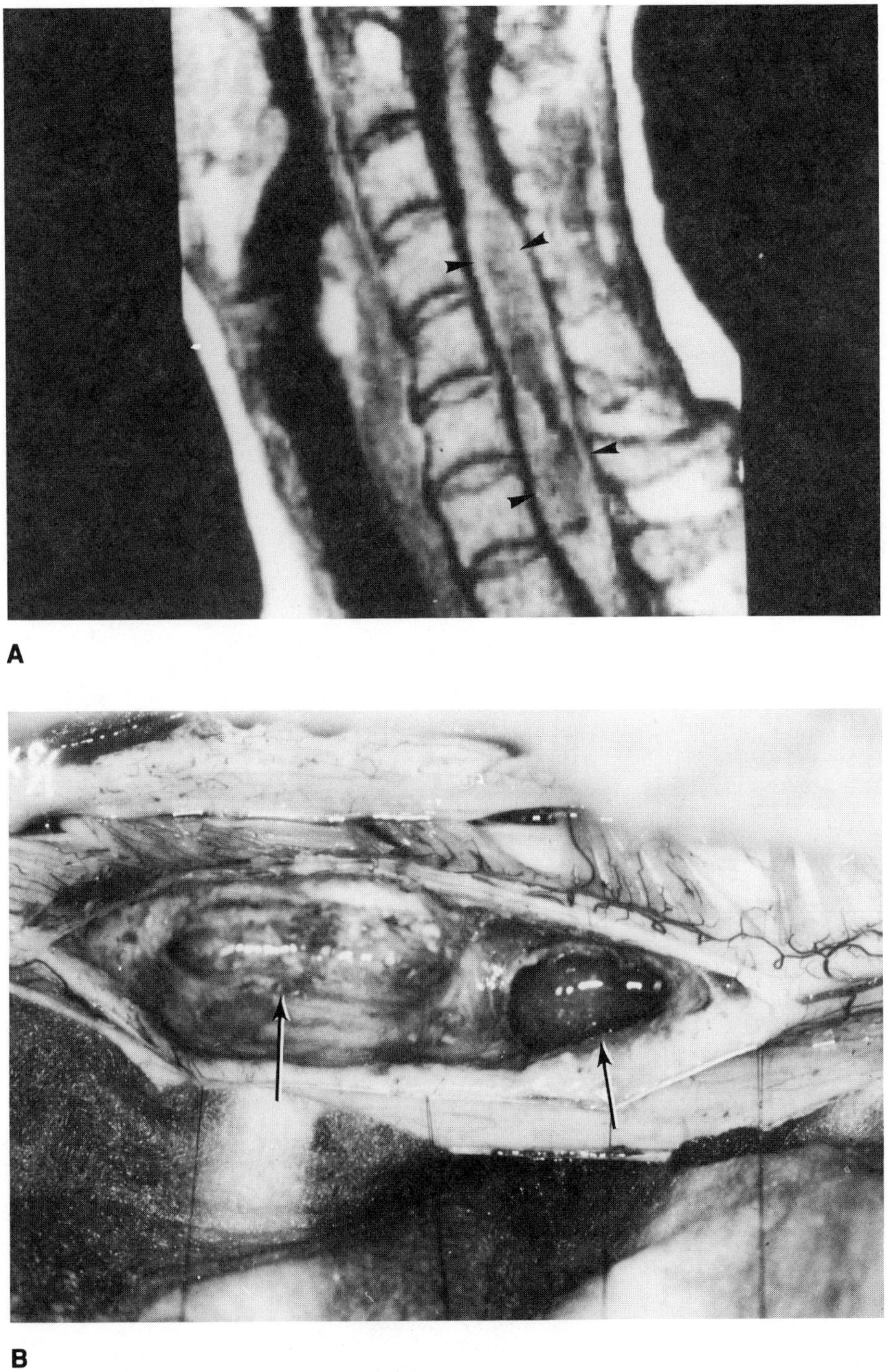

FIGURE 54.6 A. Sagittal magnetic resonance imaging (MRI) of the cervical spinal cord showing an intramedullary tumor (arrows), which is cystic and solid. B. Operative photograph showing the cystic area (arrows) associated with the solid portion of an intramedullary ependymoma. The nature of this tumor was anticipated by the MRI.

Various new techniques have been developed to remove tumors expeditiously. These include the ultrasonic aspirator (Cavitron) and laser surgery. They are most useful in cases of deep-seated tumors in obscure locations. The Cavitron works by ultrasonic emulsification of tumor, which is then removed by suction. The laser works by coagulating and vaporizing tissue. A whole series of microsurgical instruments is also part of the armamentarium of the modern neurosurgical team.

Technical Considerations

Preparation for Neurosurgical Procedures and Positioning

Proper positioning for a neurosurgical procedure is central to a well-performed operation. For cranial operations, the area of the brain containing the disease should be horizontal and perpendicular to the surgeon, or gravity should be used to assist the retraction of the brain. Using the operat-

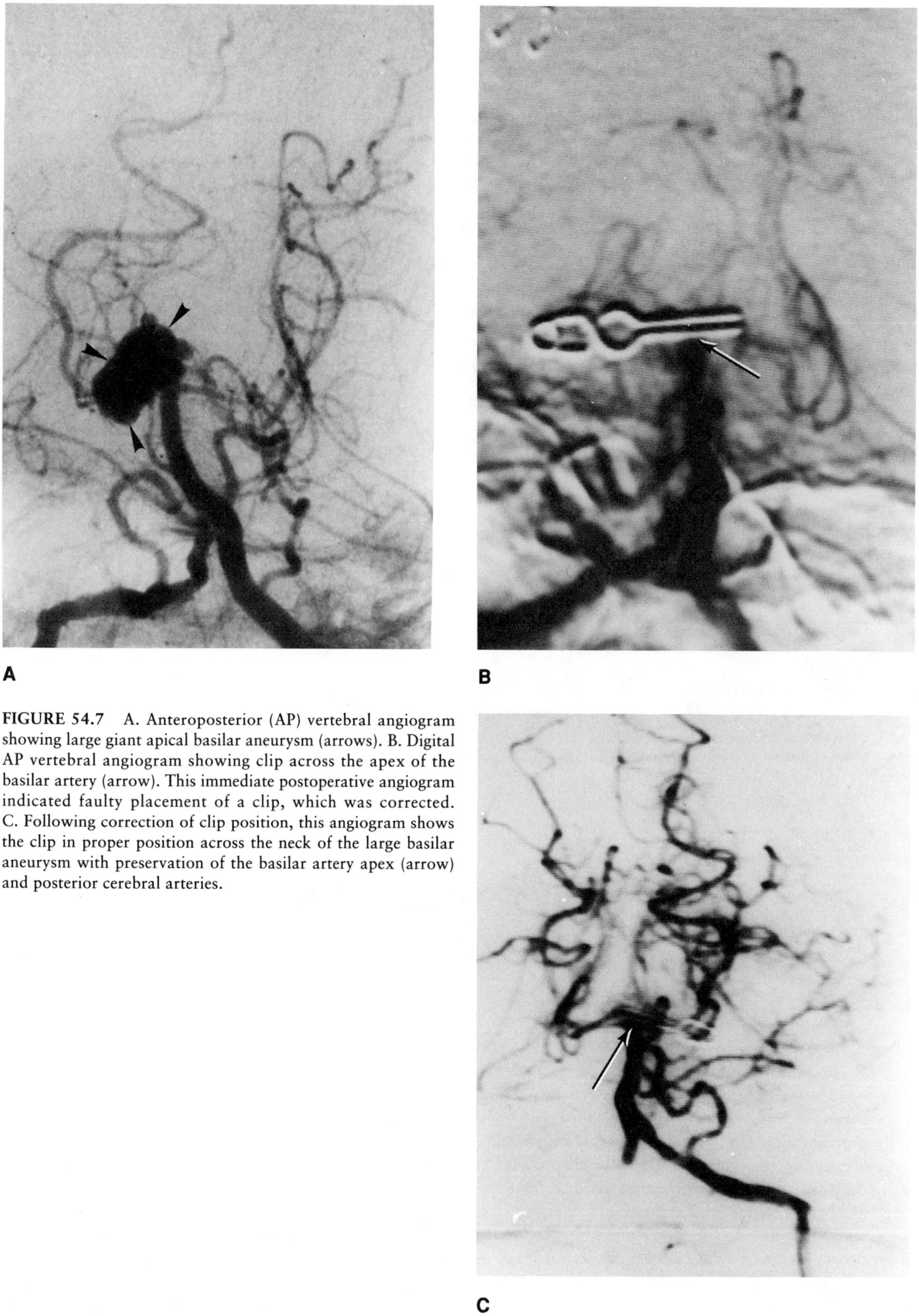

FIGURE 54.7 A. Anteroposterior (AP) vertebral angiogram showing large giant apical basilar aneurysm (arrows). B. Digital AP vertebral angiogram showing clip across the apex of the basilar artery (arrow). This immediate postoperative angiogram indicated faulty placement of a clip, which was corrected. C. Following correction of clip position, this angiogram shows the clip in proper position across the neck of the large basilar aneurysm with preservation of the basilar artery apex (arrow) and posterior cerebral arteries.

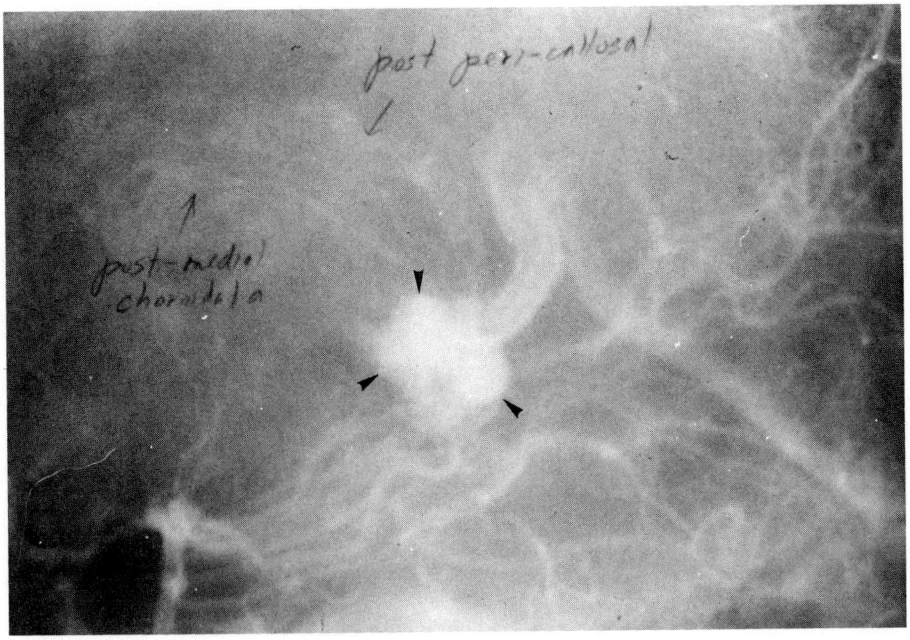

A

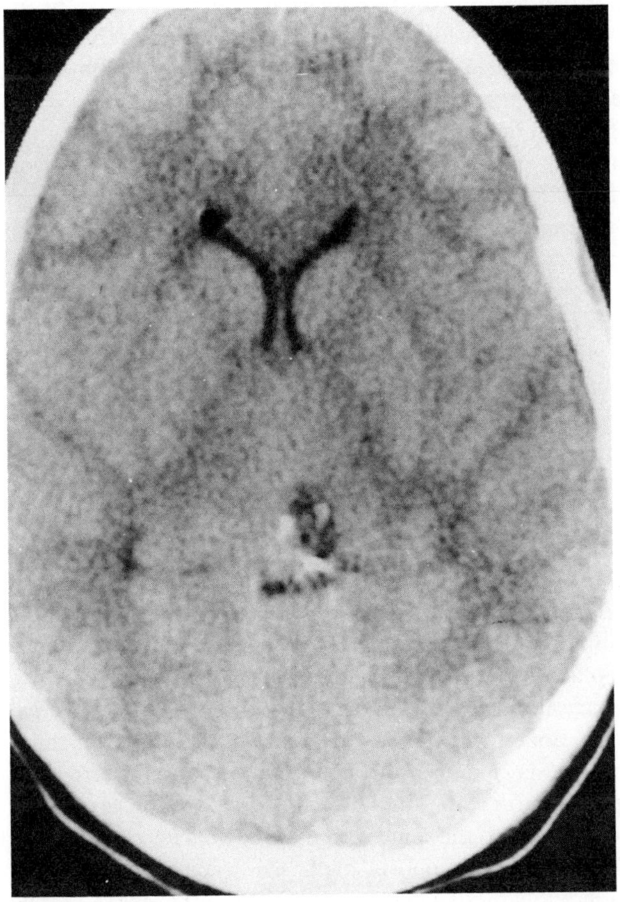

B

FIGURE 54.8 A. Deep arteriovenous malformation (arrows) involving the choroidal arteries and deep venous system, as shown by a lateral angiogram. B. Postoperative computed tomographic scan showing massive nonfocal cerebral edema.

ing microscope and fixed brain retractors, it is essential that the head be positioned and then rigidly held in that position. This is effected by a pin-vise type of headholder, which is attached to the operation table. X-ray–lucent headholders that permit the use of intraoperative x-rays, especially angiography, are important advances. With the increased use of stereotactic-guided operative procedures on the cranium, the CT stereotactic holder may be used as a head frame that is positioned and locked to the operation table. CT-guided stereotactic procedures are most applicable to lesions in deep locations such as in the subcortical, periventricular, or deep medial hemisphere regions. A technique of coregistration permits data from an MRI scan to be incorporated in a CT stereotactic-guided procedure.

It is important that venous pressure be reduced to the bare minimum in the performance of spinal operations. Valsalva maneuvers or abdominal or chest compression will lead to venous congestion in the epidural veins and make operations more difficult. To ensure the lowest venous pressure, various positions that decompress the abdomen and chest are used.

With the increased use of anterior exposures for spinal disease, especially of the spinal vertebral column, the surgeon must be familiar with the general anatomy of the neck, chest, and abdomen. In the use of the transthoracic or transabdominal route, the assistance of a thoracic or general surgeon may be required.

Brain Relaxation

Although the operating microscope uses much smaller exposures, a relaxed brain is still essential to the performance of cranial operations. Positioning will assist in brain retraction, but adjuvants such as spinal drainage, dehydrating agents (mannitol or urea), and hyperventilation are also necessary, especially when intracranial pathology has resulted in mass effect with displacement and brain edema. The patient is prepared with preoperative corticosteroids of sufficient dose and time duration to materially benefit brain relaxation during operation. In the case of large intracranial tumors, it is important to begin the dehydrating process prior to the induction of anesthesia. It is well known that no matter how carefully induction is performed, there is often an increase in intracranial pressure during this critical phase of anesthesia. This may turn a preherniation situation into a frank herniation, which is realized only postoperatively when the patient does not wake up or rouses with a hemiplegia and dilated pupil. This may falsely be attributed to surgery when, in fact, it had already occurred during induction of anesthesia. Spinal drainage is not used where there is extensive intracranial mass effect or blockage of cerebrospinal fluid (CSF) that could, in itself, result in herniation. In cases of vascular disease of the brain—AVMs and aneurysms—and some modest-sized tumors that are not compromising CSF flow, spinal drainage is extremely helpful in relaxing the brain and minimizing retraction. Patients, however, often experience troublesome postdrainage headaches.

Location of Craniotomy Flaps

The use of the operating microscope allows smaller cranial openings in many instances. Because of the use of small flaps, it is no longer necessary to shave the entire head. In many instances only the area directly involved in the operative procedure and a small surrounding area are shaved. This often makes the operation more acceptable to the patient. Flaps are now turned easily by sophisticated bone-cutting instruments and can be created in a matter of minutes. Occasionally, to obtain a low exposure along the base of the skull and thereby minimize brain retraction, sinuses have to be entered. They must be scrupulously sealed to prevent the ingress of infection into the CNS and the creation of a CSF leak. In some situations, such as a tentorium meningioma or midbasilar artery aneurysm, it may be necessary to extend the bone opening from the supratentorial to the infratentorial compartment. This means adding a suboccipital craniectomy to a temporal craniotomy. The tentorium dura is cut, and it may be necessary to interrupt the lateral sinus to maximize the exposure. In such extensive procedures, great care must be taken to avoid interruption of the great anastomatic vein of Labbé.

More and more openings in the posterior fossa are done by a craniotomy, whereby the bone flap is replaced. It is thought that this minimizes the formation of pseudomeningoceles in the posterior fossa following operation.

With correct preparation of the patient, the dura should be slack. Under all but rare circumstances, the dura should not be opened if it is tense as a result of the pressure of an underlying swollen brain or intracranial disease. If relaxation has not been obtained, it may be possible to tap the lateral ventricles or a tumor cyst of significant size through the dura. This will effect considerable relaxation should the presence of hydrocephalus or a large tumor cyst be the culprit.

Dura openings are generally carried out so that the dura may be closed primarily. In some cases, however, such as a meningioma that involves the dura, it may be necessary to place a dural patch to seal the brain. This may be accomplished through the use of pericranium or a dural substitute.

Following craniotomy, the bone flap is replaced, all indentations such as burr holes are covered, and the bone flap is held rigidly in place by stainless steel wires.

Spinal Procedures

Neurosurgeons have found that many conditions, such as cervical and thoracic discs as well as vertebral body tumors, may be approached through the anterior route. This has been most applicable in the case of the cervical disc, where a standard procedure is done with a patient in the supine position. A small incision allows dissection via anatomical planes to reach the anterior portion of the vertebral column. Diseased discs and adjacent osteophytes may be effectively removed and fusion carried out to stabilize the spine. Thoracic discs should be approached through an anterior or anterolateral route; in most cases it is unwise to approach thoracic discs via a posterior laminectomy, except laterally via a transpedicular approach, to avoid retraction on the delicate thoracic spinal cord.

In many of the spinal procedures, stabilization of the spine is a major consideration. Depending on the nature and the length of the operation, stabilization may be carried out primarily along with the primary surgical procedure, or it may be deferred to a secondary operation. Various grafts of bone or acrylic are used to stabilize the spine, in conjunction with holding devices such as rods, wires, or plates. Instrumentation of spine with metallic implants has become an important adjunct in spinal surgery. This has been most useful where the spine has been rendered unstable from trauma, neoplasm, degenerative spondylosis, infection, congenital anomalies, or previous surgery. Longitudinal rods or plates span the unstable spinal segment and attach to healthy spinal elements via hooks, screws, or wires. Immediate stability is achieved, which allows early mobilization of the postoperative patient. Bone fusion, which is required for long-term stabilization, is enhanced through immobilization afforded by spinal instrumentation. Powerful corrective forces can also be delivered to the spine with these devices for correction of deformity (e.g., scoliosis, kyphosis), fracture reduction, or spondylolisthesis realignment. Spinal approaches carried out from a posterior route with the operating microscope are becoming more limited—for example, the so-called microdiscectomy, where the incision is an inch or less, and percutaneous discectomies.

Intracranial Pressure Monitoring

Because raised intracranial pressure is one of the major impediments to a patient's viability or to smooth performance of a neurosurgical procedure, the measurement of intracranial pressure is extremely important. The most effective technique is old-fashioned, involving the use of a ventricular cannula. This may be placed through a small twist drill hole in the frontal region that requires an opening of no more than a few millimeters in the scalp and is done under local anesthesia. If there is a shift, this must be taken into account in the placement of the ventricular drain. The drainage catheter thereby serves as a route for direct pressure monitoring through a strain gauge, and as a route whereby CSF can be slowly removed to reduce intracranial pressure. More sophisticated monitoring includes epidural monitors functioning by electronic or other means, and the intracranial bolt, which is screwed into the skull and communicates with the subarachnoid space. These monitoring instruments suffer from the disadvantage of often being unreliable and not providing a route for CSF removal.

Shunting Procedures

Following the development of nonreactive polymeric silicone (Silastic) tubing and calibrated one-way flow valves, CSF shunting procedures have become extremely useful and popular. Standard use of the CSF shunt has been for control of hydrocephalus, be it congenital or acquired. Virtually all the shunts now done are from the CSF pathways to extracranial cavities. The classic intracranial Torkildsen (ventriculocisternal) procedure is no longer used. However, some patients are excellent candidates for a stereotactic endoscopic third-ventriculostomy procedure. This is particularly appropriate for patients with aqueductal stenosis, but also may be the preferred treatment for patients with obstructive hydrocephalus (beyond the third ventricle). This creates an intracranial diversion without implanted hardware and avoids many of the problems encountered with extracranial shunts (such as overshunting, infection, and malfunction).

The extracranial shunting of CSF has the advantage that the fluid is placed in another body cavity for absorption. Virtually every space has been used as a receptacle for the shunted CSF. These include vascular, pleural, peritoneal, and ureteral shunts. The procedure that has survived the test of time has been the extracranial shunt into the peritoneal cavity. This offers a wide area of absorption, and the placement of long segments of tubing into the abdominal cavity may compensate for the growth of the patient. Vascular shunts, such as the ventriculoatrial shunt, function for long periods of time but are prone to cause pulmonary microemboli, pulmonary hypertension, and septicemia. They were also more difficult to revise because the venous receptacle, such as the superior vena cava or jugular veins, often thrombosed during the passage of years. The CSF-to-peritoneal shunt can be revised frequently, and it is rare for abdominal adhesions to preclude subsequent replacements or revisions. Frontal horn placement of the ventricular end is important. This is then connected through a one-way valve or pumping device, which to some extent regulates the pressure within the system. This pressure is affected by the patient's position, so that a siphon effect when the patient stands up may be quite apparent in changing the entire pressure of the system and thereby the intracranial pressure. Volume displacement pumps have been tried but have been generally unsuccessful. The use of antisiphon devices, filters, and other gimmicks to avoid the problem of siphoning or seeding of malignant tumors has generally been unsuccessful.

Special Considerations—Intraoperative Adjuvants

Physiological Monitoring. The nervous system is an electrical system. Much of the evaluation of it during surgery is by the monitoring of electrical function. This has been used in the monitoring of spinal cord, visual, auditory, and brain stem and motor nerve function.

Spinal cord monitoring includes both sensory and motor modalities. The lag period between changes seen in such monitoring and the surgeon's actions is significant, and the major question that arises is whether the operation should be abandoned when changes are noted during evoked potential monitoring. We have no way of knowing whether these changes will persist into the postoperative period or are transient and reversible. Therefore, evoked potential monitoring of the spinal cord function must be viewed in the perspective of other observations.

Visual evoked potentials have generally been abandoned during operations involving the visual system, including the optic nerves and the chiasm. Auditory evoked potentials and brain stem evoked responses, as well as stimulation of the facial nerve directly with electromyographic (EMG) recording of the facial musculature, are the most useful monitoring techniques now in existence. These are valuable in posterior fossa operations, especially during operations for acoustic tumor in which the facial and perhaps the auditory function can be spared.

Ultrasonic Applications. Ultrasonic localizers can be used during exposure of the spinal cord and cerebrum to demonstrate underlying disease such as an intramedullary cystic tumor or deep lesions in the white matter or periventricular region of the hemisphere. The probes tend to be cumbersome and are gradually being replaced by MRI and CT scan stereotactic localization.

Neuropathological Diagnosis of Operative Pathology. In the case of intracranial and spinal tumors, the surgeon's experience often assists in the diagnosis of the tumor type from its gross characteristics. In many cases, however, the differentiation of a metastatic tumor and a malignant primary brain tumor, or diagnosis of the grade of the primary brain tumor, must be obtained through histological examination. With stereotactic biopsies, this becomes even more important. A small specimen is obtained, and it is essential to have a quick, accurate report to know if it is sufficient. Therefore, the use of immediate frozen sectioning has been of major importance to the neurosurgeon. We have not found that squash preparations yield the accuracy that can be obtained with frozen histological sections.

Another area of importance to the surgeon is the study of biopsies at the margin of a resected tumor in order to know that the tumor has been totally removed. In some cases the magnitude of the resection depends for the most part on the histological typing of the tumor. This is quite apparent in comparing a medulloblastoma with an astrocytoma in the posterior fossa. The former tumor can be subtotally removed and the remainder treated by radiation or chemotherapy, whereas the latter tumor must be treated, if benign, by total resection and requires no additional therapy. Lesions of the sella and pineal region offer the greatest challenge to the neuropathologist in terms of frozen tissue diagnosis and completeness of removal, particularly in the case of pituitary macroadenoma.

Special Considerations—Instrumentation

The use of the operating microscope was discussed previously. It has been the single greatest instrumentation advance in the field of neurosurgery in the last two decades.

Instrumentation has been developed for the obliteration of intracranial neoplasms. The backbone of such instrumentation is the ultrasonic aspirator, or Cavitron. The apparatus is quite bulky and difficult to use in deep locations.

Laser technology was greeted with great enthusiasm a decade ago. It was proposed for the vaporization of tumors and coagulation of vascular malformations. This technique still requires exposure of the diseased area and will not work effectively through an opaque medium. There are three basic types of lasers, which have different properties in terms of coagulation versus vaporization. The advantage of the laser is that it requires no contact with the tissue, so there is no distortion of the diseased area by displacement. The beam will also reach any obscure area as long as the trajectory is straight. The disadvantages result from the fact that lasers of different modes cannot be combined, and therefore coagulation and vaporization, which are two important components of tumor removal, are difficult to do simultaneously or consecutively. Also, the laser requires more experience to use than the Cavitron.

New high-speed drills and bone-cutting instruments are now available. These reduce operating time, especially in opening craniotomies.

A new field of focused radiation surgery has been introduced through the use of the proton beam, linear accelerator, or gamma knife. All of these procedures involve the use of high-dose focused radiation on intracranial disorders such as tumors and vascular malformations. The machinery is expensive and is located in only a few centers. The advantages are related to the avoidance of cranial openings and manipulation of brain by mechanical measures. All of these techniques are carried out through the intact skull. The disadvantages are a consequence of the slow and sometimes unpredictable action on the intracranial disease process. Generally, the maximum effect is not experienced until 18–24 months after the application of the radiotherapy, and the long-term side effects of radiation on intracranial disease are undetermined. Short-term complications have included radiation necrosis, with progressive neurological deficit. The greatest use has been in the treatment of cerebral metastases.

Postoperative Care

In general, postoperative care of the neurosurgical patient is an extension of the pre- and intraoperative care. Monitoring in an intensive care unit (ICU) staffed by nurses familiar with neurosurgical patients and equipped with instrumentation for monitoring of blood and intracranial pressures is essential.

Attention is directed toward neurological, cardiopulmonary, and electrolyte status. When the risk of elevated intracranial pressure, fluctuating blood pressures, respiratory compromise, and deteriorating neurological status is past, it is generally safe to transfer the patient out of the ICU. In the case of subarachnoid hemorrhage, delayed vasospasm may occur 7–14 days following a bleed, and it may be necessary to retain these patients longer to continue monitoring and volume expansion.

One of the dreaded complications of the prolonged neurosurgical procedures is pulmonary embolism from deep-vein thrombosis. This occurs in the subacute convalescence as the patient is mobilized. Measures such as pneumatic stockings placed at surgery and low-dose heparin instituted 48 hours after surgery decrease the incidence of this devastating problem.

SPECIFIC CONDITIONS

Vascular Disorders

Vascular disorders of the nervous system customarily lie dormant within the brain or spinal cord for years prior to clinical presentation. Their seemingly peaceful coexistence with normal brain function belies the suddenness with which neurological devastation can occur. Neurosurgical intervention may be the cornerstone of treatment of neurovascular disorders, but patient selection, timing of operative intervention, and early diagnosis all play very important roles in the outcome for patients with these conditions.

Aneurysms of the Brain

Rupture of an intracranial aneurysm has a yearly worldwide incidence of about 10 cases for every 100,000 population. Statistically, more than 65% of those who experience a ruptured aneurysm either die or are severely disabled. Modern neurosurgical practice has made operative repair of intracranial aneurysms a technically feasible task with low morbidity in carefully selected patients. Improvement in surgical capabilities, however, has not significantly improved the overall outcome after subarachnoid hemorrhage (SAH) from a ruptured intracranial aneurysm. Of the group who have survived long enough to be admitted to fully equipped neurosurgical centers, only 50% have an acceptable outcome, and no more than 30% of the patients who have SAH ever return to their premorbid functional level.

During the first 2 weeks after SAH, the leading cause of disability or death is related to delayed cerebral ischemia and rebleeding of the aneurysm. The majority of these patients can be expected to die or be left severely disabled.

The optimal time for surgical treatment for patients after aneurysmal SAH remains an area of intense controversy. The standard has been to delay surgery for 10–14 days after SAH. Such a policy produced gratifying surgical results, but the overall morbidity and mortality for aneurysmal SAH were not appreciably changed. Recognizing advances in microsurgery, some neurosurgery centers have begun operating on aneurysms in the period immediately following rupture.

The most promising approach to the problem of vasospasm has been the use of intravascular volume expansion and induced hypertension. This is based on the assumption that patients with severe vasospasm and delayed cerebral ischemia have lost the capability of cerebral autoregulation of blood flow. Drugs to control vasospasm and augment cardiac output promise to assist volume expansion in the control of cerebral ischemia due to cerebral vasospasm.

The technical aspects of aneurysm surgery have undergone a revolution in recent years. The operating microscope affords superb illumination and magnification of the operative field, the exposure is limited, and retraction of the brain is greatly reduced. Most important in vascular surgery is identification of the very small perforating branches of the major arteries that supply very important structures in the deep portions of the diencephalon and brain stem.

These advances have allowed surgery to be performed on the brain with a reduction in morbidity. The vast majority of intracranial aneurysms under 2 cm in diameter can be safely and completely obliterated with clipping of the aneurysm neck under microsurgical control. However, giant aneurysms and aneurysms arising in or very close to the cavernous sinus continue to pose a significant technical challenge. Giant aneurysms rarely have a discrete neck and involve large segments of crucial arteries as well as branches (Figure 54.9). Techniques such as temporary clipping of major feeding arteries or circulatory arrest have allowed some giant aneurysms to be directly clipped. The surgical morbidity of these lesions remains high, however, and further technical advances will be necessary in the coming years before this problem can be managed efficiently and safely.

Aneurysms arising within the cavernous sinus are usually approached indirectly by proximal ligation of the carotid artery or trapping. As an alternative to direct operative intervention in the treatment of giant aneurysms and aneurysms in the cavernous sinus, many surgeons have advocated the use of extra- to intracranial artery bypass. With collateral circulation in place, the aneurysm can be trapped between the proximal and distal sides of the parent artery. This approach has been most useful for the cavernous sinus aneurysms and giant ophthalmic aneurysms, where the carotid artery can be trapped prior to the origin of important penetrating vessels to the brain. However, giant aneurysms on more distal circulations, especially in the vertebrobasilar system, cannot be trapped effectively. In some instances, proximal ligation of the major feeding artery has effectively decreased a direct thrust into the aneurysm and provided thrombosis.

Endovascular obliterative techniques are being used with increased frequency. With an 85% overall occlusion rate, the results fall far short of surgical results with clipping of the aneurysm. Therefore, until further perfected, these techniques should only be used in the treatment of inoperable aneurysms.

Arteriovenous Malformations of the Brain

AVMs of the brain occur with about one-tenth the frequency of intracranial aneurysms. AVMs involving the spinal cord are about one-tenth as common as AVMs of the brain. These are generally thought to be congenital lesions, which manifest themselves in the middle decades of life. The most common presentation of an AVM is with a parenchymal hemorrhage. These hemorrhages in some instances lead to sudden death, but in many instances they lead instead to a rather devastating neurological picture, which may clear completely over a period of time (Figure 54.10). Recurrent hemorrhages are common. Therefore, these lesions are treacherous in terms of a patient's longevity. It is generally felt that a young patient has at least a 50% risk of being either crippled or dead from an AVM during the expected life span. Other symptoms from AVMs include seizures, headaches, and a variety of minor neurological problems. Some AVMs are picked up as an incidental finding when the patient undergoes a CT scan for unrelated trauma. It must be kept in mind that neurosurgery as it relates to AVMs is a prophylactic procedure, designed not to improve a patient but to prevent future hemorrhage. The recommendation for surgery depends on many factors, including the patient's age, past history of the AVM, location and size of the AVM, and of course the desires of the patient after discussions with a group of specialists. As a consortium, our team recommends surgery for an AVM if we feel this can offer a mortality or catastrophic morbidity rate of under 3% and a moderate disability rate under 5%. This is based on experience with over 400 AVM removals. These operations are generally done on an elec-

FIGURE 54.9 A. Sagittal plane magnetic resonance image showing characteristic appearance of giant suprasellar aneurysm (arrows). B. Oblique anteroposterior arteriogram showing origin of giant aneurysm from the intracranial internal carotid artery (open arrow).

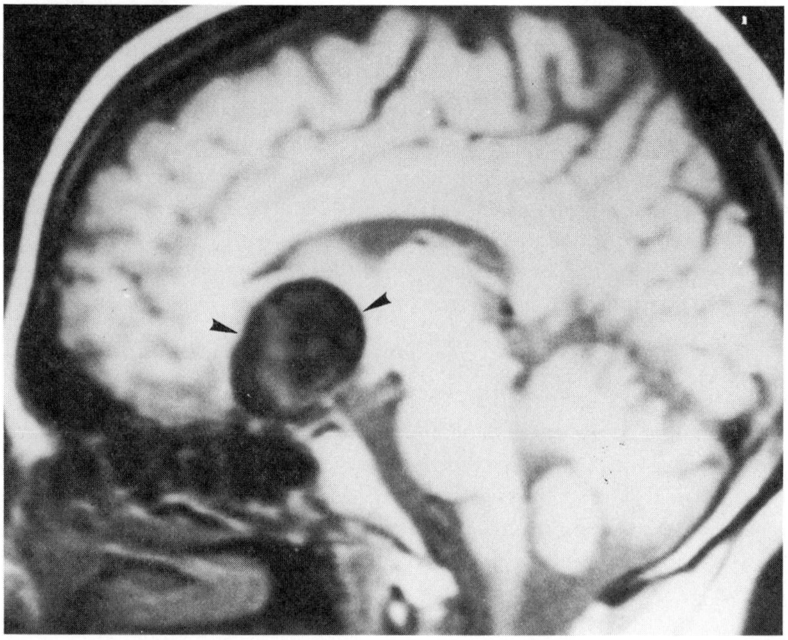

A

tive basis, and it is rare that a life-saving measure to remove a parenchymal hemorrhage is necessary.

AVMs can be removed from almost any position in the brain. For example, thalamic AVMs of reasonable size can be effectively removed without permanent crippling deficits. Similarly, some small AVMs of the brain stem have been successfully obliterated without rendering the patient paralyzed.

During AVM surgery it is often necessary to manipulate the blood pressure and perhaps run at a modest hypotensive level for prolonged periods of time while deep regions of the AVM are secured and obliterated. It is necessary to have the proper knowledge of neuroanesthesia to carry out these hypotensive procedures. In most cases, blood loss in AVM surgery is not extensive.

Postoperatively, the patient undergoes close monitoring. Postoperative circulatory changes may lead to *perfusion pressure breakthrough*, a condition that assumes that a circulation adjusted for many years to the severe shunting of blood by an AVM cannot reaccommodate when that shunt is suddenly removed. This may necessitate the use of prolonged hypotension in the postoperative period and other measures to help gradually restore circulation to normal. ICU management of these patients is therefore absolutely critical.

As a team effort, interventional neuroradiology has been extremely helpful in the management of AVM patients. The role of interventional neuroradiology is gradually to reduce an AVM by various means. These include (1) the placement of detachable balloons in large fistulas; (2) the placement of particulate matter such as Silastic pellets or polyvinyl alcohol slurry or tissue adhesives within the AVM; (3) the placement of various glues or thrombus-promoting substances within the AVM. These procedures can only be car-

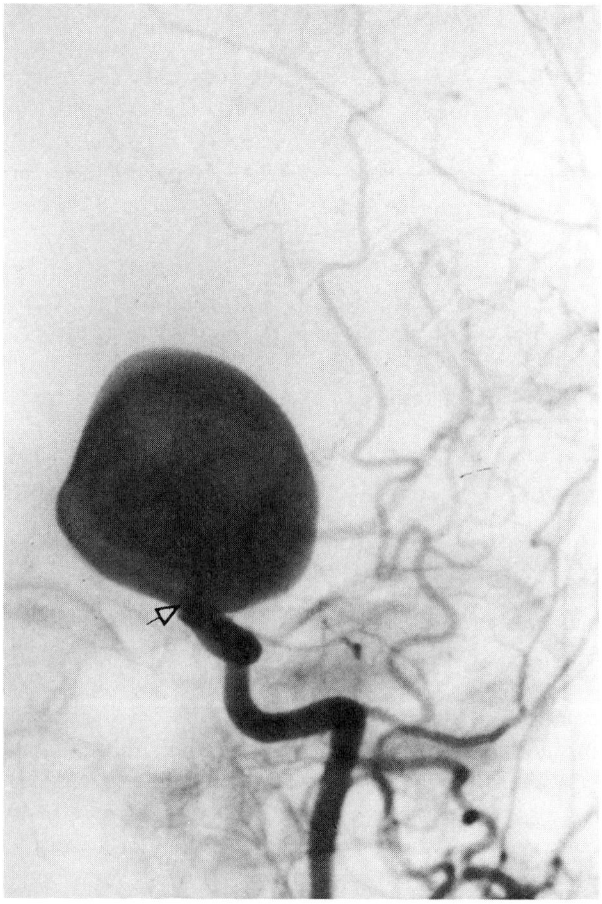

B

ried out by a neuroradiologist skilled in these interventional techniques (Figure 54.11).

Radiotherapy should be reserved for deeply situated malformations that are surgically inaccessible, are less than 2 cm in size, and have not presented with hemorrhage. Radiation is usually unsuccessful in malformations larger than 2 cm in diameter. Moreover, because it requires approximately 2 years for radiation therapy to achieve the desired effect, patients who have had previous hemorrhage are at risk for renewed hemorrhage during this period. The long-term results and side effects of the high-energy radiation in patients with AVM are not known at present, and this technique must still be considered experimental.

Spinal AVMs are relatively rare and usually produce a slow stepwise deterioration that is often mistaken for multiple sclerosis. The intramedullary spinal AVM may present with catastrophic neurological deficits due to thrombosis or hemorrhage (Figure 54.12).

Although embolization has been advocated for the treatment of spinal AVMs, the hazards are great and the results are equivocal. Surgery may be helpful in a majority of cases, but not to the extent seen in cerebral AVMs.

Cavernous and Venous Vascular Malformations

Cavernous and venous vascular malformations are congenital and received little recognition until the advent of MRI imaging. It is now apparent that as a group, these are more common than AVMs (see Table 54.1).

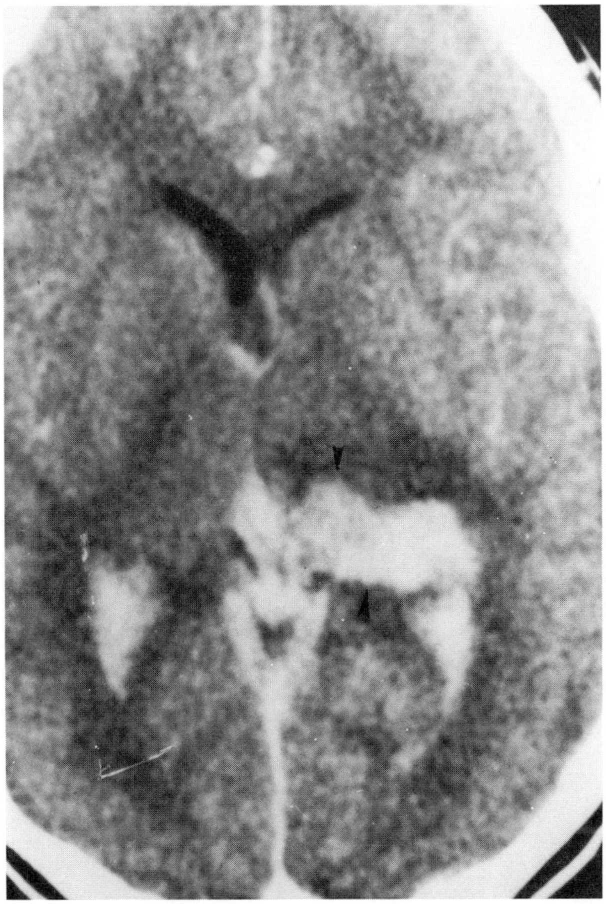

A

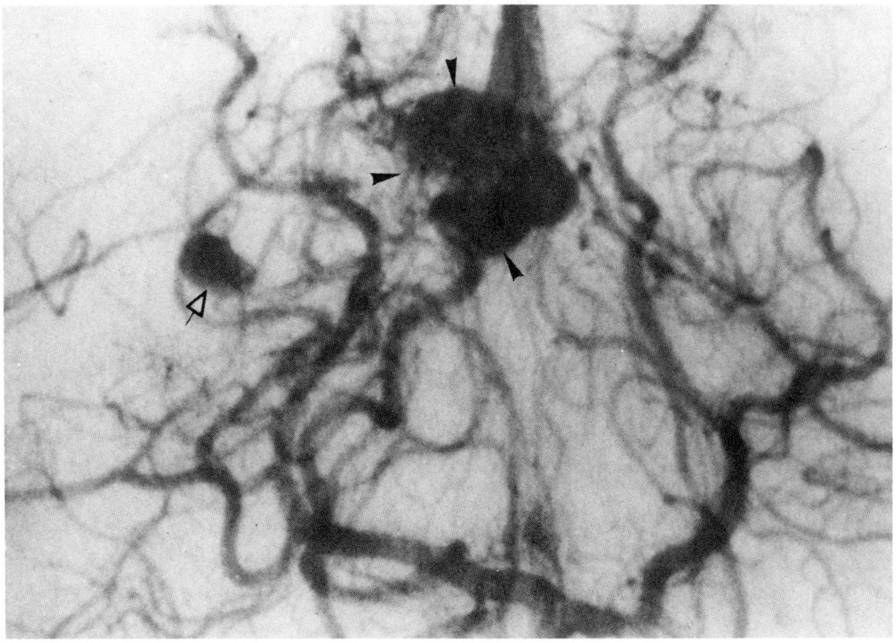

B

FIGURE 54.10 A. Noncontrast computed tomographic scan showing massive hemorrhage (arrows) into the right lateral ventricle and thalamus. B. Anteroposterior vertebral arteriogram showing the arteriovenous malformation (arrows) and an associated aneurysm (open arrow); the latter was the cause of this thalamic hemorrhage. Following surgical resection, there was a total neurological recovery.

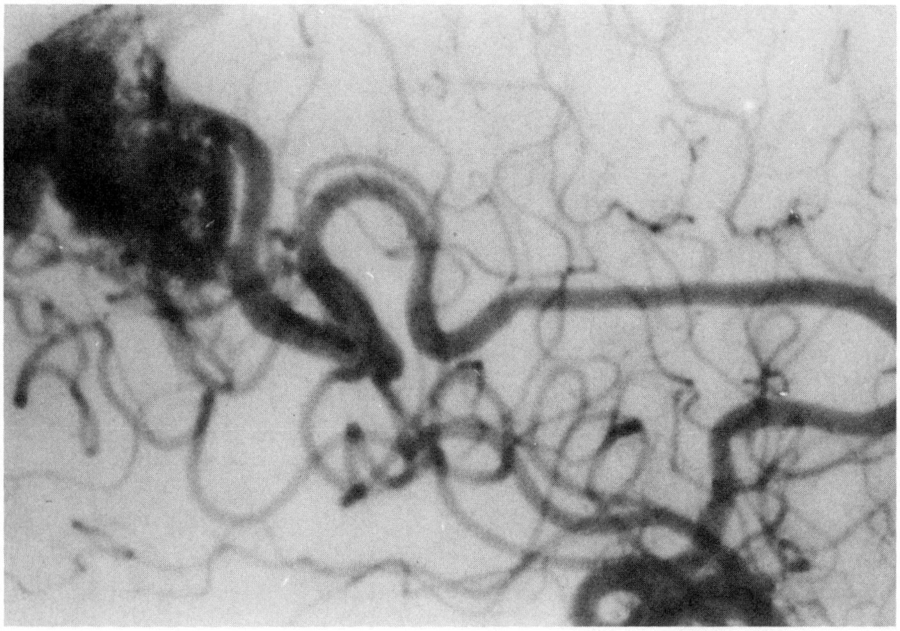

A

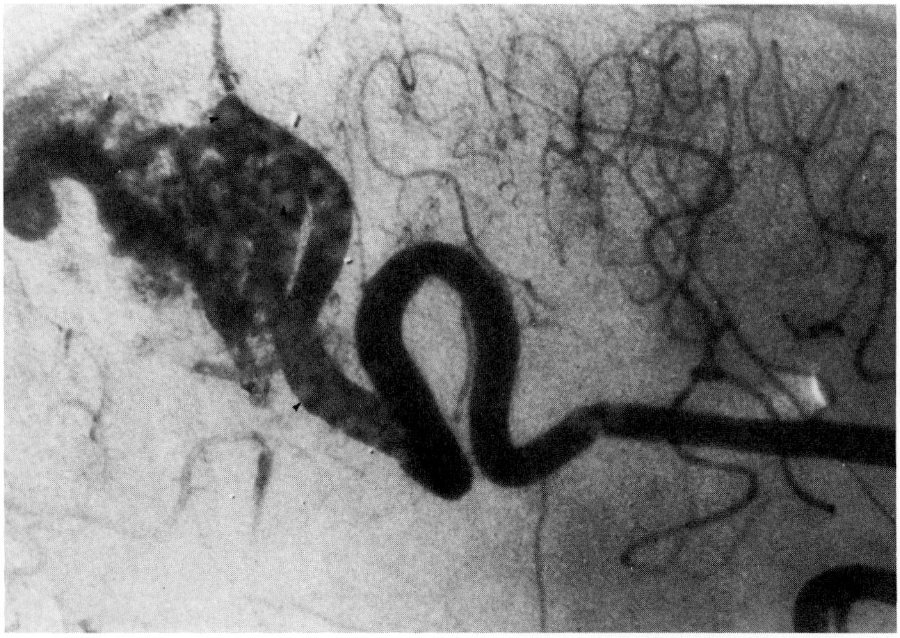

B

FIGURE 54.11 A. Large parietal arteriovenous malformation (AVM) shown by a lateral carotid arteriogram. B. Detail of pellets (arrowheads) occluding major arterial supply to this parietal AVM. C. Lateral carotid arteriogram performed one month following successful embolization showing only small residual AVM (arrowheads). The major portion of this AVM was occluded by preoperative embolization.

Cavernous malformations are characteristically identified on the MRI as variegated circumscribed lesions that may be multiple and can be located in any area of the central nervous system. They are slow-flow (not identifiable by angiogram) artery-to-vein shunts through cavernous channels. Because of their slow flow, major hemorrhages are rare and the usual character is a minor oozing recognized by a seizure or mild neurological deficit. Presumably many of the bleeds are asymptomatic. These malformations are easy to remove but in some instances (brain stem, spinal cord, deep hemisphere) are difficult to access. Our policy, therefore, since these lesions are rarely life-threatening, is to advise removal of only the accessible and symptomatic cavernous malformations. Accessibility has been increased by stereotactic guidance and the operating microscope.

Venous malformations should be regarded as anatomic anomalies. Despite the assertions of some authors, these lesions should be left alone, avoiding surgery or radio-

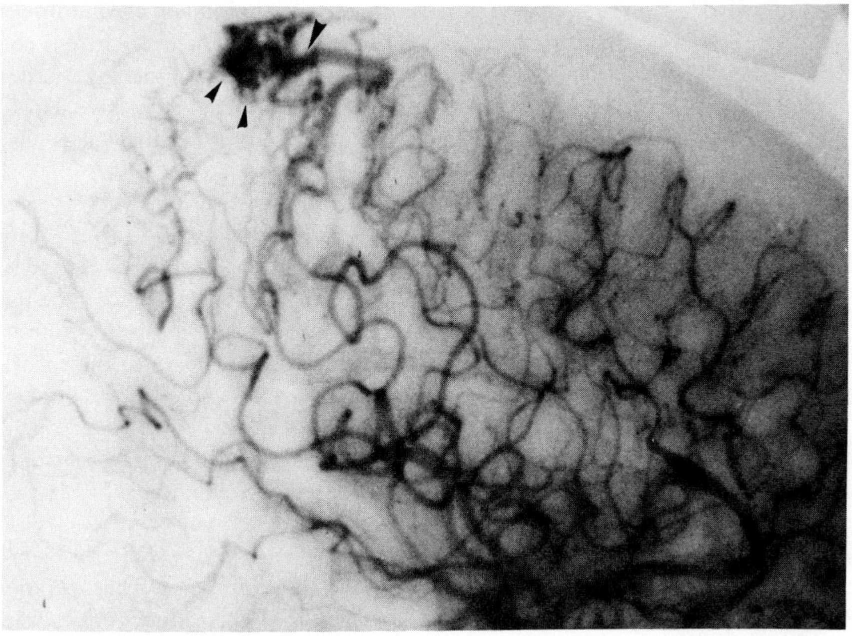

C

surgery. Venous malformations are recognized by the characteristic angiographic appearance of a large vein draining a caput medusae of small veins, usually located in the deep white matter or cerebellum. They may represent an essential venous drainage occasioned by a void of normal veins servicing the area.

Occlusive Vascular Disease

Nonhemorrhagic ischemic disease of the nervous system is one of the leading causes of death and disability in the United States. These diseases result in a spectrum of neurological presentations, from mild focal transient deficits to devastating cerebral infarction in critical regions of the brain.

The most common cause of cerebral ischemia is disease of the cervical carotid arteries (Figure 54.13). Atherosclerosis can ulcerate and produce emboli to the brain or lead to severe stenosis or occlusion of the carotid artery. Other problems of the carotid artery, such as fibromuscular dysplasia, dissection, and congenital structural anomalies of the artery, can create hemodynamic disturbances in the brain leading to ischemic damage.

The same pathogenetic mechanisms that are present in the carotid artery are also found in the vertebral arteries and the intracranial arteries.

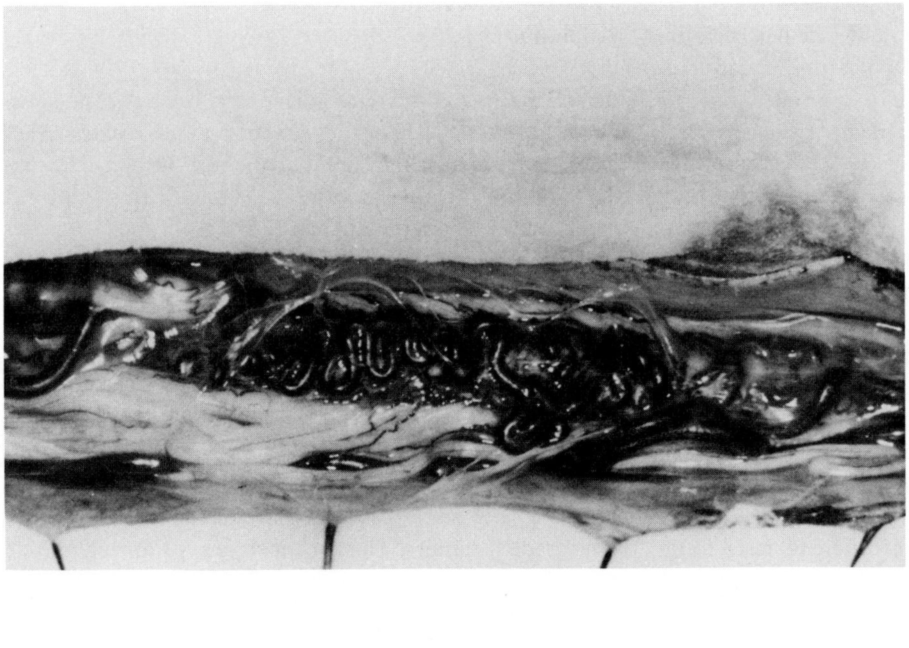

FIGURE 54.12 Operative photograph of large spinal arteriovenous malformation, located on the dorsal surface of the spinal cord with a smaller portion intramedullary. This lesion can produce symptoms by hemorrhage or thrombosis.

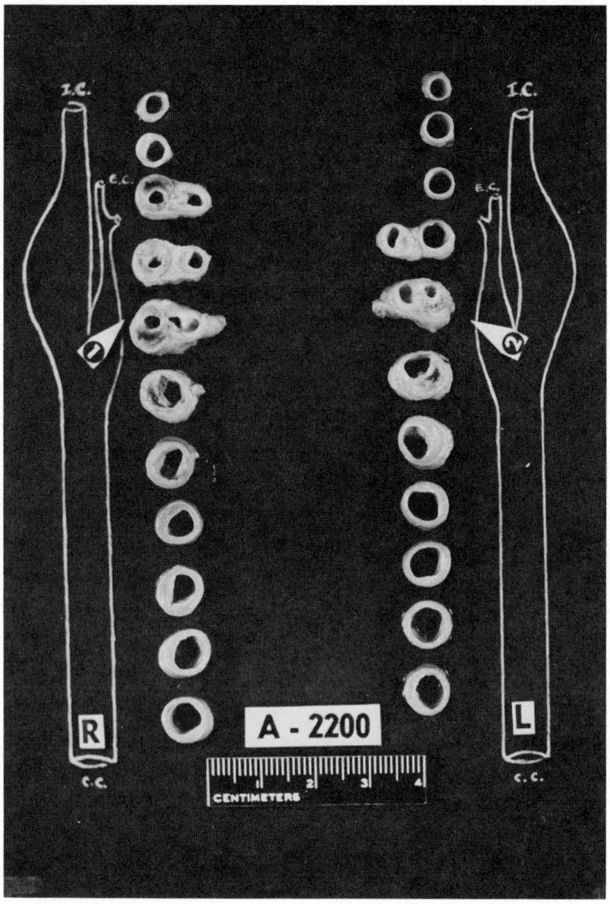

FIGURE 54.13 Postmortem fixed specimens of cervical carotid arteries. This demonstrates the predilection of the atheromatous process to the carotid bifurcation (numbers 1 and 2). The remaining carotid system is relatively free of atheroma.

Surgery for focal cerebral ischemia relies on accurate diagnosis of the causative factors. The lesions of neurosurgical interest involve the carotid and vertebral arteries and the major intracranial branches of these vessels.

The treatment of carotid circulation disease has been the subject of much debate. Over 100,000 carotid endarterectomies are performed each year in the United States, and this has now become one of the most frequent vascular surgical procedures. The rationale for carotid endarterectomy is to remove an ulcerated plaque in the carotid artery that may be causing propagation of emboli to the intracranial circulation or that is producing severe stenosis and hemodynamic compromise of the cerebral circulation (see Figure 54.13).

Carotid endarterectomy has become a routine and uncomplicated procedure that can be performed by competent vascular surgeons. However, this operation is not without risk. Many patients who require carotid endarterectomy have associated cardiovascular disorders and therefore are poor surgical candidates. These factors mandate that patients be carefully selected for this type of surgical therapy. There is evidence that prophylactic carotid endarterectomy is indicated in patients with asymptomatic carotid disease causing greater than 60% stenosis. Moreover, there is considerable evidence to suggest that surgical therapy is efficacious in preventing strokes in patients who have carotid transient ischemic attacks that can be documented as referable to disease in the carotid arteries.

Surgical treatment of vertebral artery atheroma is less effective than that for carotid artery disease. Cases of posterior circulation ischemia are less common than with anterior circulation, and the surgical avenues are more limited. Operations performed for disease in this location include anastomosis of the vertebral artery to the carotid artery for cases of proximal stenosis and open vertebral endarterectomy for more distal stenosis. Use of these operations has been largely empirical since suitable controlled studies for treatment of posterior circulation ischemia have not been conducted.

With the advent of microneurosurgical techniques, the use of extra- to intracranial bypass proliferated. This operation gained increasing popularity for the treatment of occlusive intracranial disease. The commonly performed bypass procedure is a superficial temporal-artery-to-middle-cerebral-artery anastomosis. This procedure attempts to overcome blood flow deficits produced by distal carotid lesions or proximal middle cerebral artery stenosis. Bypass has been advocated in the posterior circulation to combat the hemodynamic and embolic stresses imposed by distal vertebral artery stenosis. However, the results of a multicenter trial indicated that no significant benefit was afforded by the performance of the bypass procedure over the natural history of vascular disease treated by medical means alone.

Notwithstanding the deserved criticism, bypass procedures using either vein or artery segments do have value in treating skull-base lesions such as tumors or aneurysms. Circulatory augmentation using omental pedicle and temporalis muscle grafts appears to have value in the treatment of vascular diseases of brain such as moyamoya disease.

Neoplasms

Intracranial neoplasms are considered from two perspectives. The first is whether they are intra-axial or extra-axial; the second, whether they are malignant or benign. The majority of the intra-axial tumors are not completely resectable and are often malignant.

Intra-Axial Neoplasms of the Brain

Malignant Gliomas. Malignant gliomas constitute one of the most difficult challenges in neurosurgery. They include astrocytomas of grades II–IV (glioblastoma), malignant ependymomas, malignant oligodendrogliomas, and medulloblastomas. The astrocytoma group is by far the most common. Low-grade astrocytomas include the grade I and some grade II tumors. The prognosis is poor for high-grade lesions, with untreated survival varying between 6–12 months for a glioblastoma and 2–4 years for a high-grade III astrocytoma. Patients with low-grade lesions may be cured or survive 10–20 years.

The neurosurgeon's role is to obtain adequate tissue for diagnosis and to remove as much tumor as possible to reduce increased intracranial pressure as well as to reduce the tumor burden for other modes of treatment, including radiation and chemotherapy. In peripheral lobar lesions such as the frontal, temporal, or occipital pole, block resection may be carried out. However, in deep, less accessible regions such as the thalamus or brain stem, CT-guided stereotactic biopsy is preferred. Stereotactic biopsy can be performed readily with the CT software available in most institutions. The main risk of stereotactic biopsy is hemorrhage from vascular tumors and histological sampling error, but the advantage of tissue diagnosis clearly outweighs this risk.

In some gliomas use of the operating microscope as well as the ultrasonic aspirator and laser provides an advantage, with less manipulation of the normal surrounding structures. Postoperative edema is readily preventable with gentle intraoperative technique as well as the use of corticosteroids, both pre- and postoperatively.

High-grade gliomas are treated postoperatively in a neuro-oncology unit with modalities including chemotherapy and radiation therapy. Chemotherapy thus far uses the nitrosoureas, especially carmustine (BCNU). Specific chemotherapeutic regimens are followed for specific tumors, such as procarbazine, CCNU (lomustine), and vincristine (collectively called PCV) for medulloblastoma and oligodendroglioma.

Radiation therapy has proved to have some palliative effect in malignant gliomas, but there is considerable debate about the role of postoperative radiation therapy in benign gliomas. In general, we feel that patients who undergo subtotal resection of a low-grade glioma should receive postoperative radiation therapy. However, patients who appear to have a gross total resection of grade I astrocytoma may be followed by frequent serial scans (MRI or CT), with radiation withheld until there is evidence of recurrence. Malignant tumors that recur may be treated with reoperation, chemotherapy, and interstitial brachytherapy using radioactive substances. Brachytherapy relies on the stereotactic placement of radioactive probes within the tumor bed according to predetermined dosimetry.

Surgery for intra-axial tumors, excluding intraventricular tumors, is generally palliative. It is rare that these tumors can be completely resected, as they are basically diffuse infiltrating lesions.

Metastatic Tumors. Metastatic tumors are common and raise questions concerning diagnostic and therapeutic approaches. When multiple metastases exist from a known primary tumor, our approach has been one of supportive measures, including corticosteroids, anticonvulsants, radiation therapy, and chemotherapy. In these situations, surgery is not recommended. As acquired immune deficiency syndrome (AIDS) has become more common, we tend toward stereotactic biopsy of multiple lesions to be certain that they are metastatic tumors and not multiple abscesses. When a presumed metastatic tumor appears solitary, the controversy is greater. Some favor radiation therapy alone, and others favor surgery followed by radiation therapy. Surgery does offer the benefit of histological diagnosis, as well as rapid decompression of increased intracranial pressure if a patient is deteriorating. Surgery is generally easier than that for primary brain tumors because the tumor can be dissected from the surrounding edematous brain tissue and completely removed. Depending on the eloquence of the surrounding brain, we tend to be more aggressive with a solitary metastatic tumor than with primary malignant glial tumors. Using corticosteroids and microsurgical technique, postoperative edema is controllable. The removal of a solitary lesion offers substantial benefit to the patient, resulting in increased survival as well as better palliation and function. Radiation therapy is still used following surgical removal. Several other factors participate in this decision: the general overall medical status of the patient, age, neurological status, and the sensitivity of the tumor to radiation and chemotherapy. If a tumor is central and deep, stereotactic biopsy should be considered. In a cachectic patient with multiple coexisting medical problems, the risks of surgery usually outweigh the potential benefit. In selected cases stereotactic radiosurgery may be used after whole-brain radiation to control small (<3 cm) symptomatic recurrences or residual tumors.

Intraventricular Tumors. These present challenging problems. They are often slow-growing and benign, and therefore aggressive removal can lead to cure or to long-term survival. The most commonly encountered intraventricular tumors are meningiomas, ependymomas, choroid plexus papillomas, colloid cysts, and neurocytomas.

The diagnosis of intraventricular tumors is made with either CT or MRI scan. Each tumor has characteristics that preclude angiography. The only advantage of angiography is to define the nutrient blood vessels in order that the vascular supply can be approached and eliminated during the procedure.

The various operative approaches to the ventricular system require careful planning and meticulous technique. They are dictated in part by the position of the tumor.

High anterior third ventricular tumors, such as colloid cyst, craniopharyngioma, ependymoma, or choroid plexus papilloma, should be approached through a midline transcallosal route. The anterior corpus callosum can be sectioned for several centimeters with no obvious neurological deficit. Through this approach the lateral ventricles can be entered and the foramen of Monro visualized. The lesion may then be removed by separating the fornices.

Tumors of the lateral ventricles, such as meningiomas and choroid plexus papillomas, are usually found in the trigone. There have been several surgical approaches to the trigone, with a transcortical incision through the posterior and superior parietal lobule being the most popular, particularly on the dominant side. The disadvantage is that the vascular supply of the tumor, often from the anterior and posterior choroidal arteries, cannot be easily reached prior to significant tumor removal. Bleeding may be a problem, causing difficulty during the tumor dissection. A more lateral approach through the posterior portion of the middle or inferior temporal gyrus allows the surgeon to enter the temporal horn and see the trigone from a more anterior view. This will often allow early control of tumor blood supply, making surgical removal safer and more successful. In the dominant hemisphere, however, postoperative deficits involving language function may be a problem; therefore, the posterior parietal lobule approach is recommended.

The tumors of the posterior third ventricle will be discussed in the section on pineal tumors.

Postoperatively, patients undergoing surgery for intraventricular tumors require corticosteroids and anticonvulsants. Those not having hydrocephalus prior to surgery may develop acute postoperative hydrocephalus secondary to CSF obstruction from the surgical debris and scarring. Hydrocephalus may require drainage or a shunting procedure.

Extra-Axial Tumors of the Brain

Pineal Region Tumors. Pineal region tumors are a special group and have a typical presentation including obstructive hydrocephalus, ataxia, and Parinaud's syndrome. The tumor is readily localized with CT or MRI scan; angiography is not usually necessary (Figure 54.14). CSF studies are carried out for cytology, which may be positive in patients with germinomas. CSF is also studied for human chorionic gonadotropin and alpha-fetoprotein. These hormone markers, if present, identify the tumor as a nongerminomatous malignant germ cell tumor, for which chemotherapy is the treatment.

In general we do not feel that a trial of radiation therapy or even stereotactic CT-guided biopsy should be performed. Because over 30% of pineal region masses are benign, we recommend an aggressive surgical approach. We prefer the infratentorial-supracerebellar approach and find that the majority of these benign tumors can be successfully removed. The operating microscope, meticulous microdissecting techniques, and the use of the Cavitron are valuable (see Figure 54.14).

Postoperative corticosteroids are used and withdrawn only slowly. Ventricular drainage may be necessary for several days. Adjunctive radiation therapy and chemotherapy may be given depending on the disease process and the extent of tumor removal.

Not to be confused with cystic pineal astrocytomas are benign pineal cysts. These appear to be anatomic variations of the pineal gland, are static in size, rarely produce hydrocephalus, and range in size from 1 to 2 cm.

Sellar Region Tumors. Intrasellar lesions are predominantly pituitary adenomas, with a majority now being secretory adenomas. Approximately 40% of these are prolactinomas. The presentation of a pituitary adenoma is dependent on the secretory status was well as the size of the tumor. With macroadenomas (>10 mm) and extension into the suprasellar space, visual field abnormality is often present, most commonly a bitemporal superior quadrantanopsia. Microadenomas often are detected only if a hypersecretory state exists. Prolactinomas cause amenorrhea and galactorrhea in women and may interfere with sexual function. Most men with pro-

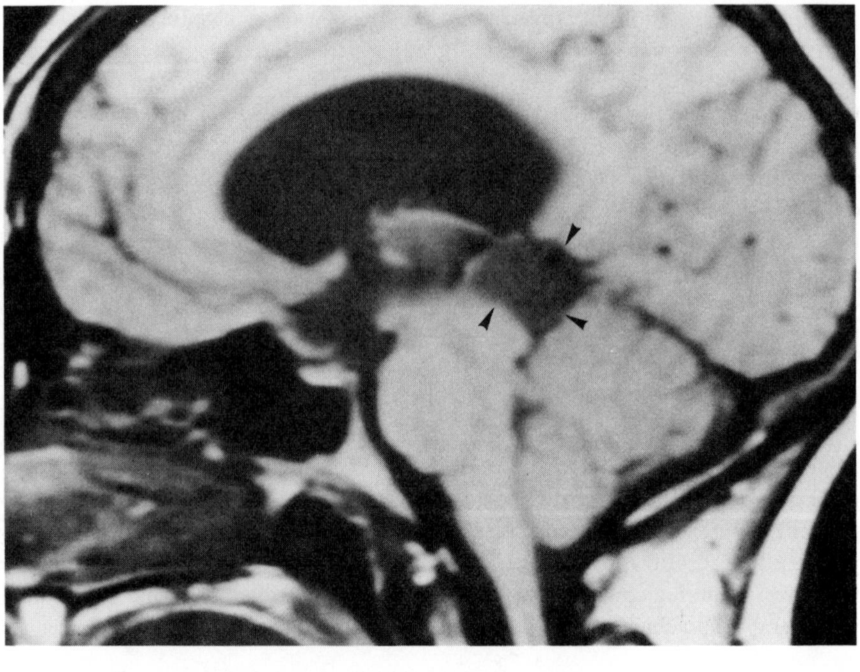

FIGURE 54.14 Sagittal magnetic resonance imaging demonstration of cystic astrocytoma of the pineal region (arrows).

lactinomas present when their tumors are large enough to cause visual field abnormalities, but they have usually been impotent for several years by that time.

Adrenocorticotropic hormone–secreting (ACTH-secreting) tumors causing Cushing's disease are usually microadenomas that cannot be seen on radiological studies. Growth hormone–secreting tumors causing acromegaly in adults and giantism in children are usually readily identifiable on CT or MRI scan (Figure 54.15).

Prolactinomas can be treated with either transsphenoidal surgery or bromocriptine therapy. Bromocriptine offers significant shrinkage of prolactin-secreting adenomas and normalization of the prolactin levels. Depending on the patient's tolerance of the drug and the size of the tumor, a decision can be made for either modality. However, patients with nonsecretory adenomas as well as all patients with Cushing's disease and acromegaly should be treated surgically. The majority (more than 98%) are approached via the transsphenoidal route. The advantages are that no brain retraction is required and that morbidity and mortality are extremely low. The transsphenoidal route also provides an exposure that permits separation of the tumor from the normal gland (Figure 54.16). The adenoma can be resected, leaving the normal gland in place. In experienced hands, the cure rate for microadenomas approaches 90%. With large adenomas and significant suprasellar extension, the tumor can be adequately debulked or completely removed via this approach, with an 80% incidence of visual field improvement. Rarely is a craniotomy necessary for pituitary tumor. If the sella is very small, if there is a dumbbell-shaped tumor, if there is significant subfrontal extension, or if the diagnosis is not clear, then craniotomy is required.

If complete resection of the tumor can be achieved with normalization of the hypersecretory state, the patient can be followed without further treatment. For prolactinomas, adjunctive bromocriptine may be beneficial; for nonprolactin-secreting adenomas, radiation therapy may be necessary if there is residual tumor or residual hypersecretion. Most tumors will be controlled, but an occasional recurrent process will require reoperation, again probably by the transsphenoidal approach. On rare occasions, interstitial brachytherapy is considered, with placement of radioactive seeds at the time of transsphenoidal removal.

The two most common parasellar tumors are the meningioma and the craniopharyngioma. The meningioma usually arises from either the tuberculum sellae, the diaphragma sellae, or the medial third of the sphenoid wing. Because of the complex anatomy in this area, these tumors often present with neurological dysfunction involving either the optic nerve, the optic chiasm, or the cranial nerves running in the cavernous sinus (Figure 54.17). The diagnosis is made with CT or MRI scan. Angiography is almost always performed to identify the position of the carotid, anterior, and middle cerebral arteries and their branches. The major vessels are often seen on the MRI scan, but the finer detail of angiography is helpful for surgical planning.

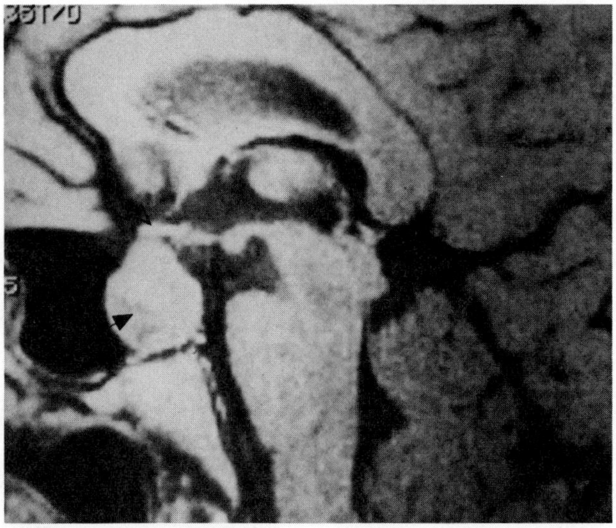

FIGURE 54.15 Sagittal magnetic resonance imaging of the head demonstrating a pituitary adenoma (arrow) rising out of the sella into the suprasellar cistern almost reaching the optic chiasm (open arrow).

It has been our approach to operate on these patients as early as possible. Even with the microsurgical technique, the risks of surgery are not insignificant, and the neurological deficit may be increased. When tumors are large, the risks of surgery are clearly increased, as is the difficulty of total excision. If, however, the tumor is invading the cavernous sinus with only minimal neurological dysfunction, radiation therapy can be considered instead of surgical intervention. This is a controversial area, and it will take further long-term follow-up studies to establish the risk-benefit ratio of radiation therapy.

Craniopharyngiomas require meticulous microdissection using the operating microscope. The approach most often used is a subfrontal craniotomy with some variance laterally or medially depending on the position of the tumor. Less commonly, if the tumor is cystic and predominantly intrasellar, a transsphenoidal approach can be considered. The tumor is well visualized with CT and MRI. Angiography is less important as the tumor is avascular and often displaces arteries rather than encasing them. The surgical approach may be between the optic nerves under the chiasm or more laterally between the optic nerve and the carotid artery. At times, if the chiasm has been displaced anteriorly, a postchiasmal approach through the lamina terminalis will be required. The surgery is slow and meticulous with the operating microscope.

Even with large tumors, a total surgical resection is often possible. In children, particularly, aggressive surgery is dictated because of the high incidence of tumor recurrence. In adults, where the tumor may be slower growing, a less aggressive procedure may be performed if the tumor is very adherent to the hypothalamic region. Radiation therapy is often considered as adjunctive treatment in adults, but less commonly in children.

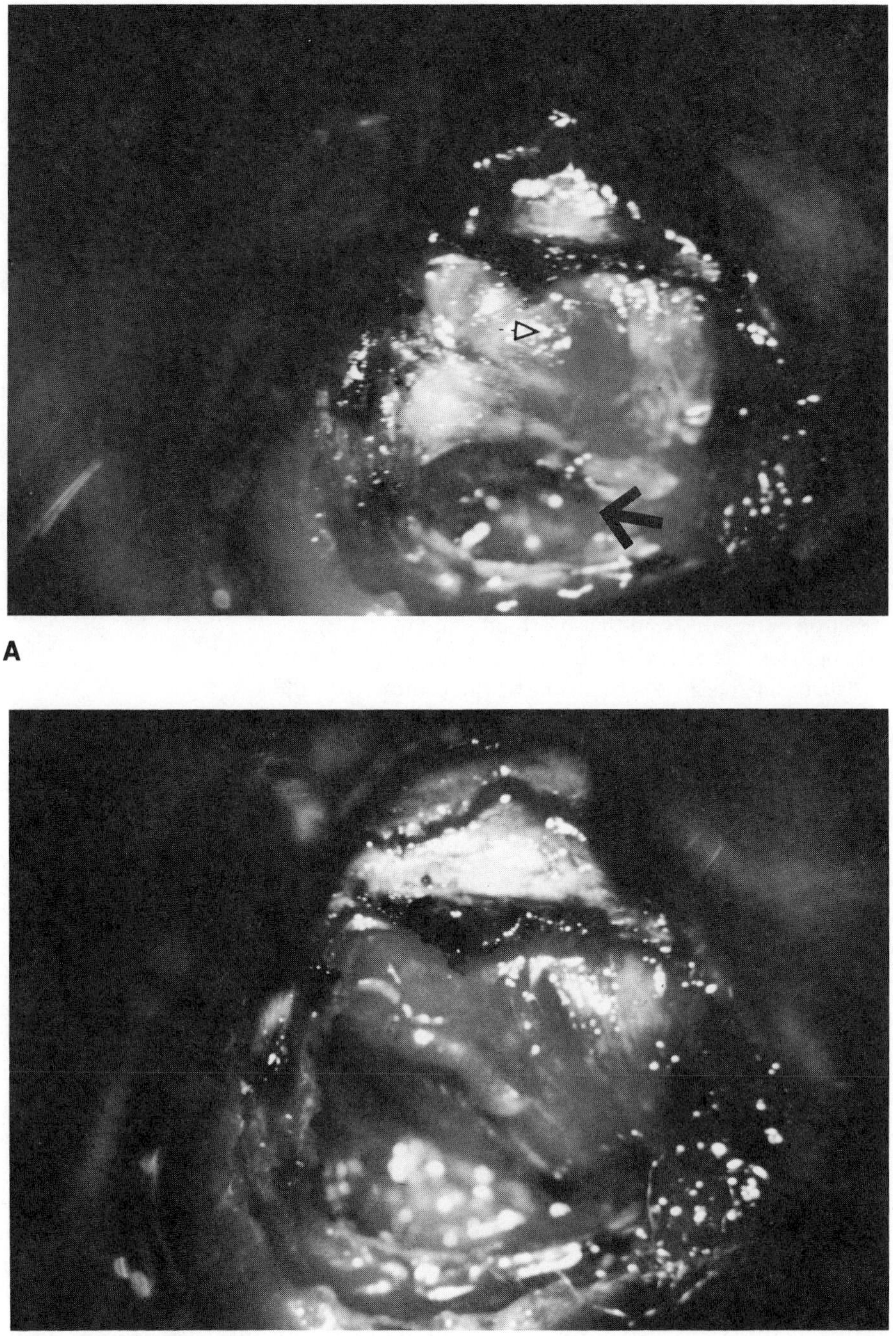

A

B

FIGURE 54.16 A. Intraoperative view of the pituitary gland (open arrow) with an adenoma in the inferior lateral portion (arrow). B. Same operative view with the adenoma removed.

The postoperative course for tumors in the suprasellar region can be complicated by fluid and electrolyte problems that ensue from manipulation of the pituitary stalk and the hypothalamic region. Compulsive fluid management is mandatory.

Cerebellopontine Angle Tumors. The two most common tumors in the cerebellopontine angle are acoustic neurinoma and meningioma.

Acoustic neurinomas are now being diagnosed earlier than previously, when the tumor is small, presenting only with tinnitus. Imaging with either CT scan or MRI scan is often adequate, eliminating the need for uncomfortable invasive contrast studies. If the lesion is seen on MRI scan and CT scan, angiography is not required. Acoustic neurinomas grow from the superior vestibular nerve and may be diagnosed while functional hearing is present.

The surgical removal of acoustic neurinomas is carried out with either a posterior fossa or translabyrinthine approach. The former allows microsurgical excision of the tumor while sparing not only the seventh nerve but, at

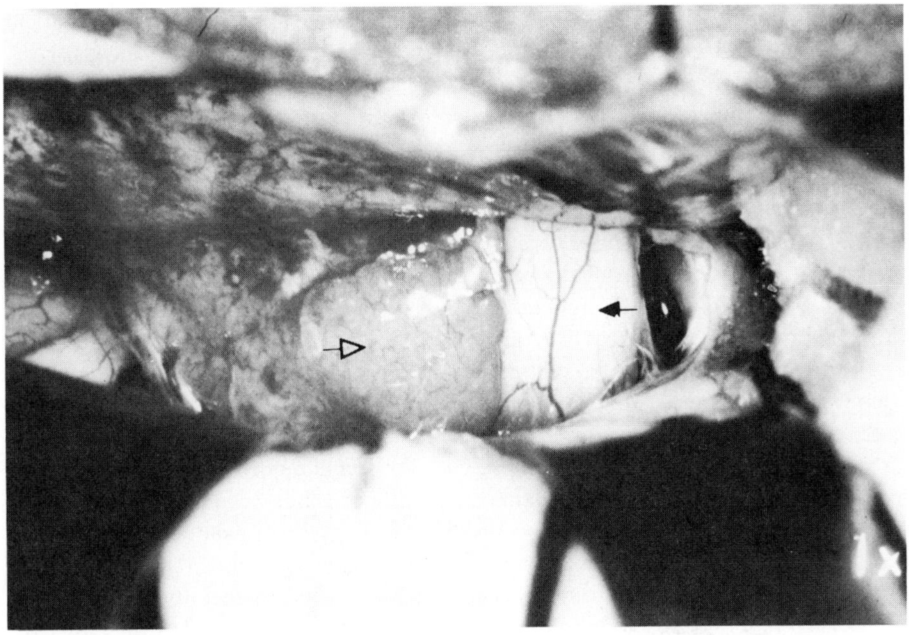

A

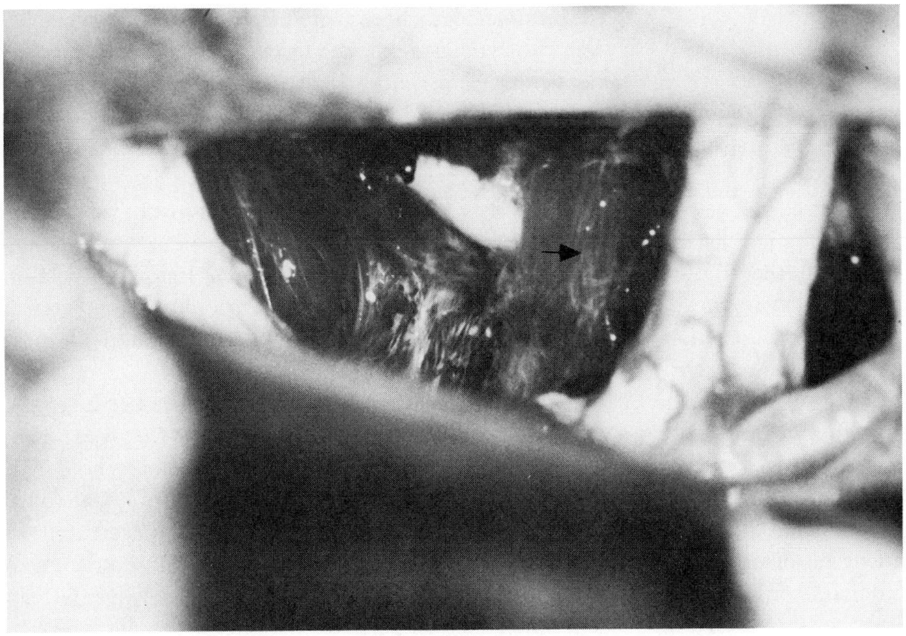

B

FIGURE 54.17 A. Intraoperative view of a suprasellar diaphragma meningioma (open arrow). The right optic nerve is seen (arrow) with the right carotid artery just lateral to it. B. Same intraoperative view with the tumor removed. Optic nerves are well seen, as is the pituitary stalk (arrow).

times, also the cochlear division of the eighth nerve. If preoperative hearing is greater than 50% discrimination and the tumor is less than 2 cm in diameter, there is approximately a 50% chance of preserving useful hearing. In larger tumors, or if hearing loss is greater, it is extremely unlikely that hearing will be preserved. The facial nerve can be preserved in well over 95% of cases of tumors less than 2 cm in diameter, and less frequently but still in a high percentage of cases in which the tumor is large. The surgery is done with an operating microscope with meticulous debulking of the tumor and dissection of the tumor capsule from the brain stem and the cranial nerves. In the translabyrinthine approach, the operating microscope is also used, but hearing cannot be preserved.

Extensive monitoring is used during acoustic neurinoma removal, including facial nerve stimulation and monitoring as well as auditory and brain stem evoked potentials when hearing is present.

Meningiomas of the cerebellopontine angle are approached via the posterior fossa. It is usually possible to obtain a total removal of these tumors with preservation of cranial nerve function. If the involvement of bone is extensive, then recurrence may be expected in a higher percentage in 10 years.

To reduce cerebellar and brain stem retraction, approaches via the petrous bone have been developed to deal with the attachment to the dura of those tumors.

Skull Base Tumors. Some of the most difficult tumors of the cranium to treat are those located at the skull base. These are generally benign tumors such as meningiomas and chordomas. However, malignant tumors can invade the base of the skull from the nasal sinuses or other areas.

Various approaches have been developed to reach these tumors through the base of the skull. These routes are frontal, on occasion with an approach through the nasal sinuses, orbital-frontal, zygomatic, petrous, retropetrous, and condylar via the posterior fossa and transoral approaches. These often require the team effort of a plastic surgeon, neurosurgeon, and otolaryngologist. In many instances, excellent palliation of malignant tumors has been reported as well as long-term survival from the removal of benign skull base–situated tumors.

Spinal Neoplasms

Metastatic Tumors. Metastatic tumors remain the most common tumor of the spine. They may be the first manifestation of a distant carcinoma.

In our institution these patients are referred for neurological evaluation before neurosurgical consultation. An examination ought to be carried out to identify the primary disease if it is not previously known, and to evaluate the extent of metastatic spread. Studies should include spine films as well as MRI scan of the spine. This will often show soft tumor tissue in the vertebral body extremely well. In those patients in whom the primary tumor cannot be found, surgery is considered for tumor diagnosis as well as decompression. Neurosurgical consultation should be obtained immediately after the diagnosis is made; it should not be a last-minute call once the patient has deteriorated. An early consultation allows discussion and consideration of which studies would be most appropriate to plan if and when a surgical procedure is to be done. It also allows more leisurely consideration of various approaches to the spine and organization of a multispecialty team.

With a solitary lesion in a vertebral body and no evidence of disease to vital organs such as lung or liver, we have become more aggressive surgically, with attempts to remove the entire metastatic tumor. This may involve a multifacet operation with removal of involved bone (decompression of neural elements) and stabilization of the spine. In the thoracic and lumbar area this often requires extensive exposure, including thoracotomy and splitting the diaphragm. It is surprising how well the patients tolerate this if they are not severely debilitated by their tumor. Radiation therapy usually follows surgery.

We believe that an aggressive approach offers the patient the highest possibility for functional independence, as compared to the results achieved through a posterior decompressive procedure or radiation alone in selected cases.

Intramedullary Spinal Cord Tumors. These are seen more frequently in adults than in children. The symptoms are similar for both groups. Persistent pain involving the dorsal root dermatome is often seen as a signature of the tumor. Dysfunction of the posterior columns may occur in a progressive fashion with sensory dysesthesias in the arms, torso, and legs depending on the site of the intraspinal neoplasm. Sacral sparing may or may not be present, and a well-defined central cord syndrome is often lacking. Children often present with spinal deformities.

The diagnostic evaluation has been enhanced by MRI scan, although the pathology often cannot be determined. Astrocytomas and ependymomas make up the largest group of tumors (Figure 54.18). They are generally low grade and extend over many segments of the spinal cord. Other tumors, such as dermoids, epidermoids, teratomas, oligodendrogliomas, and hemangioblastomas, are less frequently seen. Intramedullary ependymomas have a distinct plane between the neoplasm and the normal spinal cord and they generally have a pseudocapsule. Astrocytomas, on the other hand, are usually infiltrating, with a less-well-defined margin between the neoplasm and normal cord tissue. Hemangioblastomas present unique problems in diagnosis and treatment. They may be single or multiple as part of the von Hippel-Landau syndrome. Diagnosis may be suspected by a uniform high-signal contrast-enhancing lesion by MRI. In this instance spinal angiography is recommended. Surgical removal requires additional expertise in dealing with these vascular tumors as they are not easily removed piecemeal.

The treatment is surgical excision, done through an extensive laminectomy with the full extent of the tumor exposed, as dictated by the MRI scan. The dura is opened and a midline posterior myelotomy carried out, followed by microdissection of the tumor from the surrounding structures. Meticulous dissection is required, and adjunctive instrumentation such as laser or Cavitron is helpful (see Figure 54.18).

The single most important factor in determining the ease of the operation is the presence and nature of previous operations and radiation. In patients who have had previous surgery with the dura left open, exposure has been much more difficult, with far more risk of injuring the normal cord.

It is remarkable how an extensive intramedullary tumor can be resected with minimal significant neurological dysfunction secondary to surgery. Long-tract signs often improve, but radicular pain in the distribution of the nerve roots associated with the tumor has been a distressing postoperative problem. The pain often has a burning quality and has been difficult to control. Nevertheless, with the use of microsurgical techniques and strict attention to postoperative pulmonary function, negligible mortality and morbidity can be expected, even with removal of extensive tumors in the cervical region. We have not used postoperative radiation for intramedullary tumors that have been totally removed and do not advocate postoperative radiation for benign intramedullary tumors that have been incompletely removed. Radiotherapy is reserved for malignant tumors. Follow-up should be periodic with MRI scan and a second surgical attempt made to remove recurrent tumor.

Extramedullary Intradural Tumors. For the most part, these tumors are neurofibromas and meningiomas. These are benign tumors and can often be cured by surgical removal. Certain circumstances will preclude total removal and cure, including meningiomas with extensive dural involvement, multiple neurofibromas (von Recklinghausen's syndrome), and extensive intradural and extradural (dumbbell) neurofibromas.

Spinal Surgery

Lumbar Disc Surgery

Lumbar disc surgery remains one of the most frequently performed neurosurgical procedures, as well as the bane of existence of many neurosurgeons. In general, patients with low back and radicular pain should be evaluated by a neurologist in conjunction with a neurosurgeon. The majority of these patients can be successfully treated with conservative means, including bed rest, nonsteroidal anti-inflammatory medications, and muscle relaxants. After an acute episode has resolved, physical therapy and a program of increased activity and re-education with regard to back care are often very successful in rehabilitating patients.

Diagnostic studies should begin with plain lumbosacral spine x-rays. These are inexpensive and helpful in defining the anatomy and demonstrating the presence of spondylolisthesis, spondylolysis, tumor erosion, or marked degenerative changes. If conservative therapy fails, then further diagnostic studies are indicated. Electrodiagnostic studies, including EMG, should be performed before a myelogram, since there is EMG evidence of nerve root irritation for several days after myelography. Somatosensory evoked potentials (SSEPs) can help localize the involved root preoperatively, and intraoperative SSEPs can follow the progress of root decompression. Often immediate change can be seen in the SSEPs, indicating that the root has been adequately decompressed. Either conventional CT or MRI scanning is required. The MRI scan will demonstrate the soft disc tissue accurately, whereas CT scan will demonstrate bony structure as well as disc tissue. For midline defects the MRI scan is superior, whereas the CT scan is superior for lateral defects. With either of these studies, adequate information for surgical intervention is often obtained, eliminating the need for myelography. In occasional cases, adequate information is not available from the CT or MRI scan, in which case myelography is necessary, often followed by CT scanning with the dye in the thecal sac. Before a decision is made for myelography, neurosurgical consultation should be obtained to discuss the indications. Absolute indications for surgical intervention include progressive motor and sensory deficit and frequent recurrent episodes that interfere with the patient's ability to continue gainful employment.

The surgical approach to lumbar disc disease has changed. In nonoperated patients with localized, one-level, unilateral disease, microdiscectomy offers many advantages. The microscope allows visualization and protection of the nerve root as well as coagulation of epidural veins before there is any bleeding. The amount of bone removal and foraminotomy is virtually the same with or without the microscope. The trauma to the patient is far less with the microdiscectomy, and the postoperative course is considerably shortened. Patients are often out of bed the night of surgery and leave the hospital 48–72 hours later. They are able to return to work at a much earlier date because they experience less pain and back spasm.

In patients who have previously undergone surgery at the same or adjacent levels, the procedure often requires a larger operation with identification of normal tissue before going through scarred tissue planes. Consideration must also be given to the need for a posterolateral bone graft fusion, particularly in someone who has had recurrent disease at the same level, implying instability.

Cervical Disc Disease and Cervical Spondylosis

The preceding comments on lumbar disc disease often apply to cervical disc disease. The majority of patients will improve with conservative measures such as traction, bed rest, muscle relaxants, and a cervical collar.

Surgery is indicated if conservative management fails. In patients where myelopathy is present, we believe that surgery is always indicated if disc tissue is seen distorting the spinal cord. With myelopathy, an anterior approach is used in most cases. This allows removal of spondylotic ridges and extruded disc material without manipulation of the spinal cord. The procedure is well tolerated by patients and requires only a 2- to 3-day postoperative hospital stay. There are varying opinions as to whether fusion ought to be carried out with all anterior cervical approaches. There appear to be adequate data in the literature to support the concept that patients do equally well with or without fusion at the time of surgery.

Depending on the nature of the abnormality in cervical spondylosis, surgery will be carried out through either an anterior or a posterior approach. With very extensive disease involving multiple (more than three) levels, a wide laminectomy extending the length of the involved segments is recommended. For one- or two-level disease an anterior approach is usually preferred, as it directly removes the offending tissue and is extremely well tolerated by patients. We perform an anterior fusion with all anterior cervical approaches for extensive cervical spondylosis. The patient is

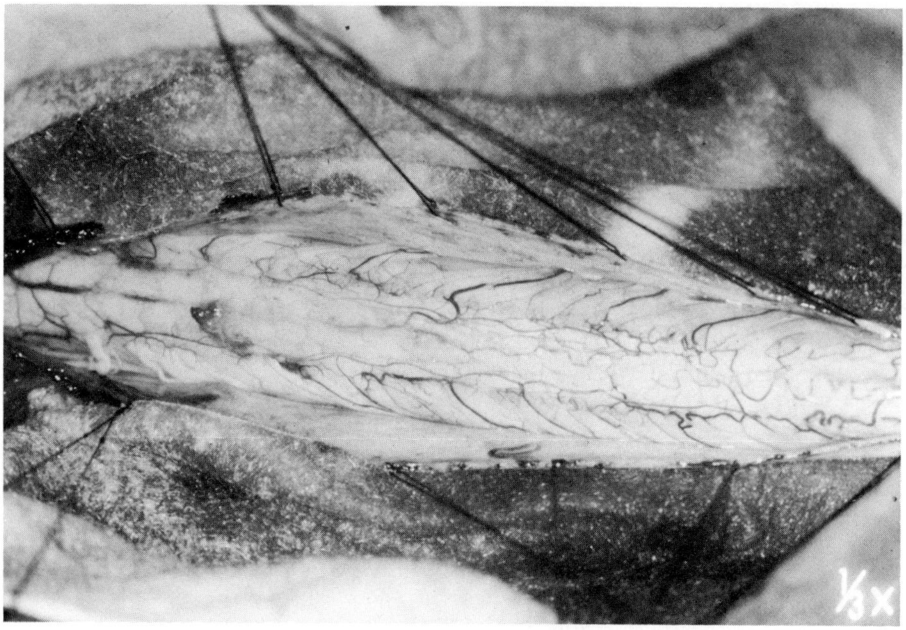

A

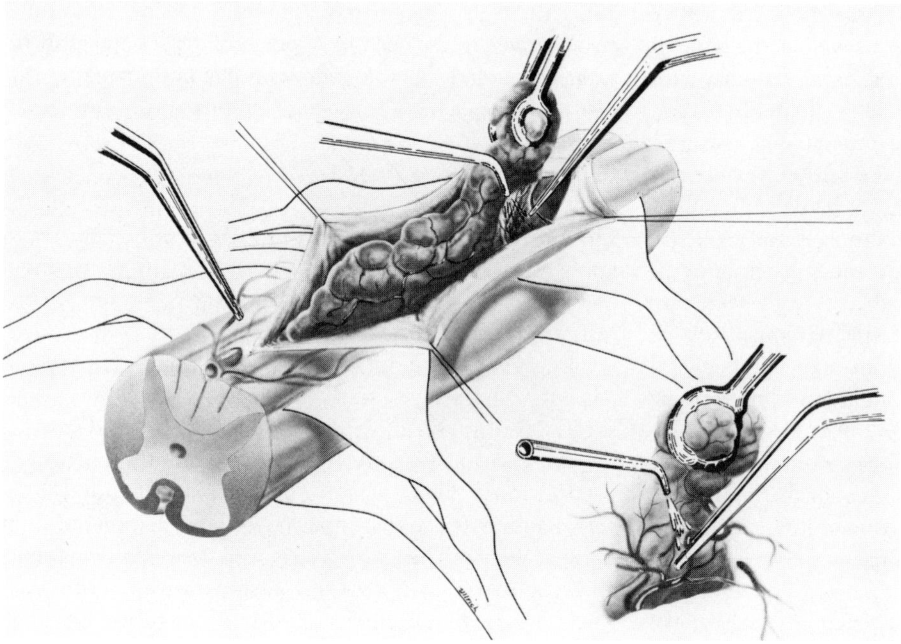

B

FIGURE 54.18 A. Dorsal view of wide spinal cord with an intramedullary tumor. B. Diagrammatic view of the surgical activities involved in intramedullary tumor removal. (The maneuvers include bipolar cauterization of small blood vessels, with saline irrigation, traction upon the tumor, and stay sutures holding open the pia. This is all accomplished with the operating microscope.) C. Spinal cord cavity after tumor removal.

kept in a firm collar for at least 6 weeks followed by a soft collar for another 6 weeks. Lateral postoperative cervical spine x-rays are taken routinely postoperatively to follow the alignment of the vertebra and the progress of the fusion.

In severe cases of multilevel spondylotic myelopathy, it is now possible to remove a large portion of the vertebral bodies, ridges, and discs from an anterior approach with subsequent bone graft and stabilization of the spine.

In patients with radiculopathy, rather than myelopathy, caused by disc disease, there are differences of opinion as to whether surgery ought to be carried out through a posterior facetectomy approach or through an anterior approach. Both operations are done with the operating microscope. Success rates are extremely high with either approach, depending on the surgeon's experience.

Thoracic Disc Disease

Thoracic disc disease is commonly misdiagnosed. Patients often present with only radicular pain, which can be misin-

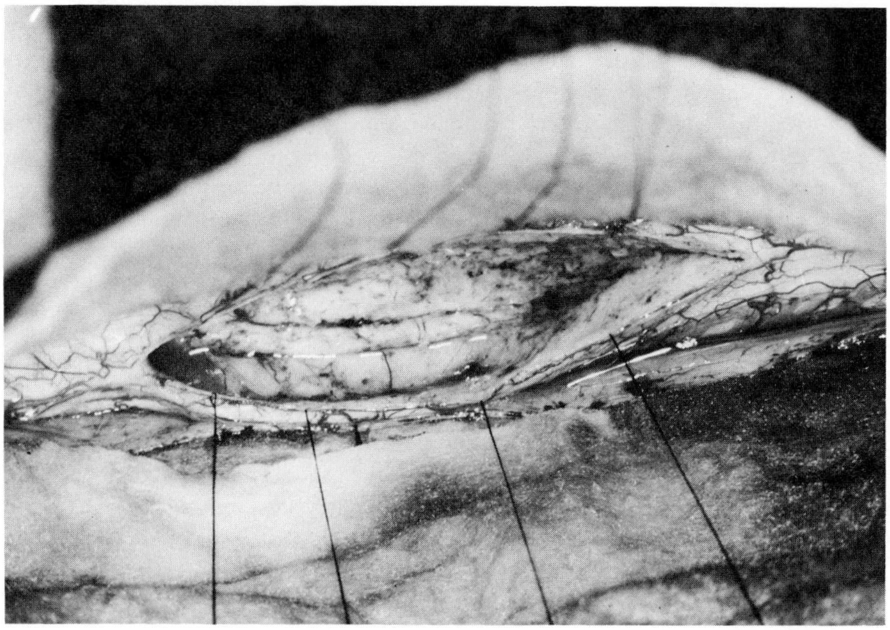

C

terpreted as originating from chest or abdominal organs. When the diagnosis is considered, the patient ought to be seen by a neurologist for evaluation and appropriate studies. Plain thoracic spine x-rays may show asymmetry in the interspace and adjacent spondylotic degenerative changes suggesting disc disease. MRI scan is helpful in identifying thoracic discs and the adjacent spinal cord abnormalities if present. CT scanning alone has not been as helpful in this area as in other areas of the spine. Myelography with CT scanning, however, gives the most precise anatomical detail.

Thoracic discs often cause a myelopathy requiring surgery. The surgical approach is dictated somewhat by the anatomical location of the defect. We believe a pure posterior approach is contraindicated in thoracic disc disease. Rather, a posterolateral approach such as a transpedicular or costotransversectomy, or an anterolateral approach through a thorocotomy, is indicated. The thorocotomy offers the advantage of being able to expose the entire anterior dural surface and more safely dissect a chronic calcified disc away from the dura. A costotransversectomy saves the patient a thoracotomy but does not give adequate vision past the midline.

Neurosurgical consultation ought to be obtained immediately on diagnosis and the particular approach dictated by the surgeon's experience as well as the radiographic picture.

Functional Neurosurgery

The term *functional neurosurgery* is used to encompass a group of procedures that share the common goal of modifying or improving the function of the nervous system in the setting of chronic, disabling, medically intractable neurological disorders, such as epilepsy, movement disorders, and pain. Functional neurosurgery procedures often rely on the ability to improve overall neurological function by the ablation of certain nervous system structures, becoming progressively more precise and restricted to maximize benefit and minimize risk of treating important functional deficits. In an increasing number of situations, procedures that specifically augment nervous system function, rather than ablate, are being used. These procedures include chronic brain or spinal cord stimulation, continuous CSF drug infusion, and tissue grafting. Current investigations are focused on the development of techniques to promote the repair of nervous system damage, such as the prevention of scar formation and the delivery of trophic factors to promote cell survival and reinnervation in certain degenerative disorders. Many of these procedures use high-precision image-guided stereotactic surgery, a procedure that has been dramatically improved in recent years with the development of accurate MRI guidance and sophisticated operating room computer work stations.

Epilepsy Surgery

Although most generalized seizure disorders are effectively controlled by anticonvulsant therapy, the *focal epilepsies* frequently persist in up to 50% of the patients despite optimal drug therapy. This group represents 40% of the patients with epilepsy and includes those patients with partial complex seizures, secondarily generalized seizures, or both. Candidates for surgical alleviation of epileptic disorders comprise approximately 10% of all patients with epilepsy. Unfortunately, the medical intractability of this group of patients and the efficacy of surgery in treating the disorder are underappreciated by medical care providers.

The comprehensive management of epilepsy patients requires a team of dedicated specialists who are able to perform an extensive diagnostic evaluation and treatment protocol. Neurologists specialized in the treatment of epilepsy characterize the seizure type clinically, evaluate electroencephalograms (EEGs), obtain appropriate MRI studies, and ensure an adequate trial of appropriate anticonvulsants. Intractable epilepsy patients often need continuous scalp or sphenoidal video-EEG monitoring to accurately determine seizure type and area of onset. Positron emission tomography (PET) or single-photon emission computed tomography (SPECT) and neuropsychological and intracarotid amytal studies are generally needed to arrive at a recommendation for surgical intervention. The management team carefully analyzes the data and may recommend further monitoring with implanted intracranial depth and subdural grid electrodes.

The vast majority of epilepsy surgeries involve temporal lobe resections. Many patients are felt to have *limbic epilepsy*, often on the basis of mesial temporal sclerosis or other imaged pathology and undergo a standardized anteromesial temporal resection. This resection has the objective of maximizing resection of medial temporal structures, hippocampus, and adjacent structures while minimizing resection of the lateral neocortex. In other patients, cortical resections are tailored by mapping the seizure focus and identifying important functional cortex that must be preserved. Some patients, especially in the pediatric age group, have a less restricted seizure focus, amenable to functional hemispherectomy or corpus callosum sectioning.

Seizure surgery has the objective of complete elimination of the seizure type for which it is recommended. It is recommended for patients who have very little chance of becoming seizure-free with medication and whose quality of life is impaired by seizures. In limbic epilepsy, long-term seizure-free outcome has been achieved in up to 80% of patients, with significant morbidity of less than 2% and near zero mortality. Other resections are somewhat less successful, but still with very satisfying outcomes. Unfortunately, patients are the best candidates for epilepsy surgery in childhood and adolescence, many years before it is considered. However, awareness of the efficacy and safety of epilepsy surgery is growing and gradually changing this situation.

Movement Disorders

Surgical intervention can be applied to a variety of movement disorders when they are refractory to medical management. These include Parkinson's disease, essential tremor, dystonias, spasmodic torticollis, and spasticity. Tremor is rarely the most prominent and disabling symptom of Parkinson's disease, although it is often medically refractory. Stereotactic-guided thermocoagulation lesions in the ventrolateral thalamus have been used effectively since the early 1960s to treat refractory tremor and have been of some benefit for disabling motor fluctuations and dystonia. The volume of these procedures decreased dramatically by the end of the 1960s with the introduction of L-dopa therapy. Improvements of the accuracy, ease, and safety of stereotactic lesioning, along with recognition of late failures with L-dopa therapy, have lead to a resurgent application of thalamotomy in Parkinson's disease and tremor. The development of sophisticated computer work stations and the ability to use MRI accurately are important factors in the expanding application of these procedures. There is a revived interest in globus pallidum lesions in Parkinson's disease, since these lesions seem to improve some of the most disabling symptoms, such as bradykinesia, rigidity, and gait disturbance. Accumulating experience with fetal brain implants for Parkinson's disease suggests that this procedure may be of some benefit in medically refractory disabled Parkinsonian patients. Studies have reported the successful use of deep brain stimulators in the ventrolateral thalamus for tremor. Much remains to be learned regarding the role of surgical intervention in Parkinson's disease and tremor.

The dystonias and spasticity syndromes include a variety of disorders. Thalamotomy and selective peripheral denervation procedures have both been applied with some success in the management of dystonias, including spasmodic torticollis. Experience suggests that intrathecal baclofen (via implanted programmable drug pumps) is beneficial in a small group of selected patients with dystonias. Selective posterior rhizotomy has also been successful in the management of severe spasticity associated with cerebral palsy, but intrathecal baclofen has been dramatically successful in the management of spasticity secondary to spinal multiple sclerosis or spinal trauma.

Pain

Chronic disabling medically refractory pain is generally approached differently when it is associated with malignant as opposed to nonmalignant disease. In general, ablative procedures are considered more readily in patients with malignant disease and a limited life expectancy than in patients with essentially static conditions. In any patient, it is important that maximal efforts have been made to control pain with all nonsurgical means available. This certainly should include aggressive use of narcotic analgesics and requires physicians familiar with their use in the treatment of chronic pain. When patients with malignant disease have pain localized to a specific body region, such as one extremity or one side, an anterolateral cordotomy can be considered. This can be done with a percutaneous procedure that is usually successful, carries low chance of serious morbidity, and is well tolerated (Arbit 1993). Other ablative procedures that have similar advantages include rhizotomies, ganglionectomies, and caudal alcohol injections. Increasingly, continuous intrathecal morphine infusion via a programmable implanted pump is considered to be the optimal surgical intervention for patients with diffuse or bilateral pain. This is a relatively simple and well-tolerated procedure that is generally effective and very low risk.

Medically refractory trigeminal neuralgia can almost always be eliminated by either a percutaneous gasserian ganglion thermocoagulation lesion, glycerol injection, balloon compression, or a suboccipital craniectomy for a microscopic procedure to eliminate vascular compression of the fifth nerve root entry zone.

Chronic pain resulting from denervation sometimes responds to thermocoagulation lesioning of the dorsal horn of the spinal cord over the involved levels, termed a *dorsal root entry zone (DREZ) lesion procedure*. This seems to be particularly successful in patients with brachial plexus avulsion but has been reported to be beneficial in other situations, such as herpes zoster and reflex sympathetic dystrophy. In many of these patients, and particularly in most others with "benign pain syndromes" such as failed back surgery syndrome, implantation of spinal or deep-brain stimulation or programmable pumps for intrathecal or intraventricular morphine seems to be the optimal neurosurgical treatment.

Peripheral Nerve Surgery

The treatment of peripheral nerve injuries requires an understanding of both the underlying pathology and the response of nerve fibers to injury (see Chapters 57 and 81). A complete clinical history, thorough physical examination, and full diagnostic workup are all done to assess the location, severity, and cause of nerve damage. The diagnostic workup usually involves electrical tests such as EMG, sensory and motor nerve conduction, and evoked potentials. Radiographic studies such as plain x-rays, CT, MRI, and angiography can also be very useful. The clinician armed with this information is now in a position to decide whether medical treatment alone or surgical intervention is also required to optimize the chances for recovery of lost function. As a general rule, surgical intervention is indicated for the biopsy and removal of masses and the repair of nerve lesions that are not recovering. When surgery is performed, intraoperative monitoring with electrophysiological stimulation and recording techniques can help the surgeon minimize damage to functioning nerve elements and to accurately identify injured elements in need of surgical repair. Postoperative care should include physical therapy directed at maintaining and improving range of movement as well as sensory and motor function.

An important determinant of clinical outcome is the severity or grade of peripheral nerve injury. A *neurapraxic* type of injury usually recovers spontaneously over several weeks. However, in the presence of chronic nerve entrapment, surgical decompression may be required.

An *axonotmetic* type of injury, one in which nerve fiber continuity is disrupted but the surrounding cellular architecture is preserved, is more severe. Following these types of injury, nerve fibers can regenerate back to their sensory and muscle organs, but recovery of function will depend on the location of the injury and the distance that the nerve fibers must travel to reach their targets. Recovery is greater following distal injuries than proximal injuries.

A *neurotmetic* injury, the most severe type, is one in which the entire peripheral nerve is either completely cut or so scarred that nerve regeneration cannot take place. In such cases, surgical repair is required to restore lost function.

The decision to operate usually cannot be made immediately following an injury but must often be delayed. The major exception to this rule is sharp and open injuries with immediate confirmed section of the nerve and loss of nerve function. In these cases, where the nerve has been cleanly divided and there is little surrounding nerve damage, a primary repair of the nerve in which the two ends are sutured together can be performed. In contrast, most peripheral nerve injuries are closed and usually involve blunt or stretch trauma. In these circumstances, a period of observation is necessary for two reasons. First, since the severity of the nerve injury can only be inferred, it is not possible to predict with certainty whether the nerve will recover on its own. By performing serial clinical examinations and electrodiagnostic studies over a 3- to 4-month period, it is usually possible to determine whether recovery is occurring. Second, even in cases in which the nerve is known to have been completely cut, the full extent of the injury may not be apparent immediately. Waiting at least several weeks allows the scar to define itself, making it possible to surgically remove the intervening scar tissue and repair the damaged portion of the nerve. If the gap is small, then the two ends of the nerve can be brought together and sutured without producing tension. If the gap is long, then a repair using nerve grafts, usually taken from the patient's sural nerve, is performed. The intricate anatomy and regenerative capacity of the peripheral nervous system makes the treatment of its traumatic injuries both a challenging and clinically rewarding endeavor.

REFERENCES

Arbit E. Anterolateral Cordotomy. In E Arbit (ed), Management of Cancer-Related Pain. Mt. Kisco, NY: Futura, 1993;321–332.

Spetzler RF. Radiological characteristics of cerebral vascular malformations. BNI Q 1987;3:22.

SUGGESTED READING

Apuzzo MLF. Surgery of Masses Affecting the Third Ventricular Chamber. Technologies and Strategies. In JR Little (ed), Clinical Neurosurgery. Vol. 32. Baltimore: Williams & Wilkins, 1986.

Apuzzo MLF (ed). Neurosurgery for the Third Millenium. Neurosurgical Topics, Book II. Park Ridge, IL: AANS Publications Committee, 1993.

Bridwell KH, DeWald RL (eds). The Textbook of Spinal Surgery. Vols. I and II. Philadelphia: Lippincott, 1991.

Burchiel KI (ed). Neurosurgery Clinics of North America. Surgical Management of Peripheral Nerve Injury and Entrapment. Philadelphia: Saunders, 1991.

Fetell MR, Bruce JN, Burke AM et al. Non-neoplastic pineal cysts. Neurology 1991;41:1034–1040.

Haley EC, Kassell NF, Torner JC et al. The international cooperative study of the timing of aneurysm surgery: the North American experience. Stroke 1992;23:205–214.

Hoff JT. Cervical Spondylosis. In CB Wilson, JT Hoff (eds), Current Surgical Management of Neurological Disease. New York: Churchill Livingstone, 1980.

Holtzman RNN, McCormick PC, Farcy J-PC. Spinal Instability. New York: Springer-Verlag, 1993.

Maciunas RJ (ed). Interactive image-guided neurosurgery. Neurosurgical Topics, Book 17. Park Ridge, IL: AANS Publications Committee, 1993.

Pile-Spellman J, Hacein-Bey L, Nakahara I. Interventional neuroradiology: recent advancements. Neurological Chronicle 8, 1991.

Post KD, Mursazko K. Management of pituitary tumors. Neurol Clin 1986;4:801–831.

Quest DO. Asymptomatic Carotid Disease. In JR Little, (ed), Clinical Neurosurgery. Vol. 32. Baltimore: Williams & Wilkins, 1986.

Rovit RL, Murali R, Jannetta PJ (eds). Trigeminal Neuralgia. Baltimore: Williams & Wilkins, 1990.

Sekhar LN, Janecka IP (eds). Surgery of Cranial Base Tumors. New York: Raven, 1993.

Stein BM, Bruce JN. Surgical Management of Pineal Region Tumors. In PM Black (ed), Clinical Neurosurgery. Vol. 37. Baltimore: Williams & Wilkins, 1991.

Stein BM, McCormick PC. Intramedullary Neoplasms and Vascular Malformations. In PM Black (ed), Clinical Neurosurgery. Vol. 37. Baltimore: Williams & Wilkins, 1991.

Weir B. Aneurysms Affecting the Nervous System. Baltimore: Williams & Wilkins, 1987.

Wilson CB, Stein BM (eds). Current Neurosurgical Practice. Intracranial Arteriovenous Malformations. Baltimore: Williams & Wilkins, 1984.

Youmans JR (ed). Neurological Surgery (3rd ed). Philadelphia: Saunders, 1990.

Chapter 55
The Principles of Neurological Rehabilitation

Richard J. Hardie

Only since the advent of antibiotics less than 50 years ago have physicians concentrated on curing diseases rather than alleviating their consequences. Yet many of the efforts of neurologists in particular have so far gone largely unrewarded. Much of their clinical practice concerns irrevocable and often progressive damage to the central nervous system (CNS). Many neurologists have also invoked cartesian dualism, attempting firmly to distinguish true, organic disease from "functional" disorders and concerning themselves exclusively with the former. However, this distinction is especially blurred and unhelpful in chronic disablement from whatever cause.

It was World War II that stimulated early interest in the possibility of applying medical scientific advances to the benefit of wounded servicemen. In many countries facilities were created to offer rehabilitation rather than convalescence, and a new specialty was born. Rheumatologists and orthopedic surgeons quickly saw the advantages of involving therapists closely in the management of their patients, and the therapists responded with enthusiasm, working within a multidisciplinary team of professionals to help those with musculoskeletal disorders.

Until relatively recently, therapists and physicians alike have neglected the practical problems facing neurologically disabled people. Fortunately, there is now increasing recognition that neurologists should play a more active role in managing the longer-term aspects of their patients' disabilities. Unlike the case with orthopedic trauma, complete recovery is exceptional, and deterioration is often anticipated, so the term *rehabilitation* can be misleading and inappropriate here.

Much valuable information is to be found in works listed in the Suggested Readings at the end of this chapter.

BACKGROUND AND GENERAL PRINCIPLES

Nature and Scope of the Problem of Disability

The Global Picture

The World Health Organization (WHO) has estimated that about 500 million people throughout the world are disabled in some way, a prevalence of 1 in 10 of the world population. The total number can be subdivided into three groups of roughly equal size: developmental, acute, and chronic conditions (Figure 55.1). It is salutary to recognize that four-fifths of disabled people live in developing countries, and that one-third are children. A very large proportion of disability worldwide could be prevented by improved nutrition, immunization, accident prevention, and other simple health measures (Pope and Tarlov 1991).

It was against this background that the United Nations designated 1981 the International Year of Disabled People. Commitment both to promoting effective measures for preventing disability and for rehabilitation, and to realization

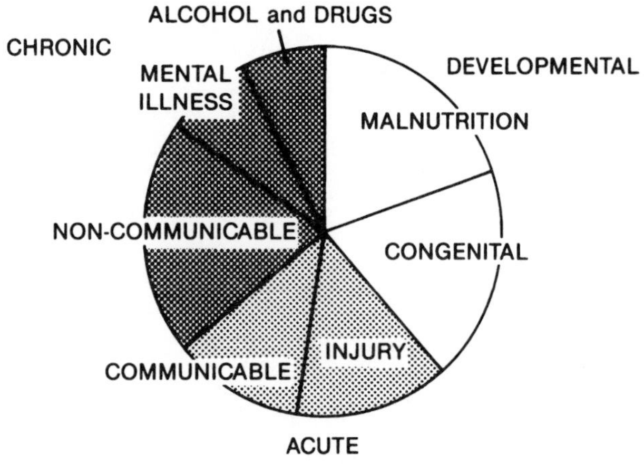

FIGURE 55.1 Classes of disorder giving rise to disability in the world. (Reprinted with permission from J Wilson. Disability Prevention: The Global Challenge. Oxford: Oxford University Press, 1983.)

of the goals of equality and full participation of disabled people in social life, was renewed in the World Program of Action for the United Nations' Decade of Disabled People, 1983–1992. An important priority of the later WHO Decade of the Brain 1990–1999 is rehabilitation of those with neurological disabilities.

There are three major classes of medical disorder that give rise to disablement:

1. Emotional and intellectual impairment, due to mental illness and mental retardation.
2. Sensory impairments, particularly those affecting vision and hearing.
3. Physical impairments.

Even in developed countries, accurate data are lacking concerning the prevalence of specific types of impairment or of conditions giving rise to disability. There is great difficulty in defining categories and inclusion criteria and in case ascertainment. Yet such information is of crucial importance both for management of individual patients by guiding diagnosis, treatment, and prognosis, and for health care policy and planning to make adequate, equitable provision for all groups of disabled people. Statistics will vary from one country to another according to many factors, including demography and prosperity, but they are broadly comparable in most European countries, the United States, and Australia.

As an illustration, estimates by the Office of Population Censuses and Surveys of prevalence among the adult population of Great Britain will be cited. Thus, excluding mental and sensory disorders, approximately 1 in 10 of the U.K. adult population is physically disabled. Of these, 20–30% (2–3% of the total population) will be severely disabled; about 60% are aged 65 years or older; 10% are under 45 (Martin et al. 1988). The principal causes of severe physical disability are arthritis of all forms and neurological disorders. In an average population of 250,000, about 3,500–5,000 people are likely to suffer from neurological disability, of whom 1,500 will be severely disabled and require daily assistance (Wade and Langton Hewer 1986).

The most common disabling neurological conditions are, in order of prevalence, epilepsy, stroke, traumatic brain injury, Parkinson's disease, multiple sclerosis, and tumors of the brain and spinal cord. The estimated incidence and prevalence of these and certain other disorders are shown in Table 55.1. There are many other less common diseases that, despite their individual rarity, account for a further considerable number of neurologically disabled people.

These estimates also conceal a changing pattern of disability. Programs of immunization, genetic counseling, and prenatal screening, as well as improved standards of public health, have led to a marked diminution in the prevalence of disability due to infective and developmental disorders such as poliomyelitis, leprosy, and spina bifida. At the same time, better health care and increased life expectancy have increased the proportion of elderly people with degenerative conditions. Together with the disabling consequences of natural aging, including intellectual decline, arthritis, osteoporosis, presbycusis, and visual impairment, these are responsible for a steep rise in the prevalence of all types of disability above the age of 60 (Figure 55.2).

Health Care Policy

Given the background, it is regrettable that health and personal social services for physically disabled people throughout the developed world are so deficient. Many national governments have designated such people as a priority group for policy planning, in an attempt to counteract the traditional precedence of acute care in the health services and of areas such as child care in social services. Other priority groups usually include elderly people and those with mental illness or severe mental impairment.

Unfortunately, for various reasons disabled people are usually accorded the lowest priority in favor of the other groups mentioned. In the United Kingdom, for example, community services for those with physical disabilities have been analyzed in an independent report aptly entitled *Last on the List* (Beardshaw 1988). This is all the more remarkable when proportions of expenditure and prevalence are compared (Table 55.2). An audit of follow-up services for stroke patients after discharge from hospital offers a single, but by no means unrepresentative, illustration. Of 183 patients visited, one-third had not been visited by their family doctor since discharge, and many did not have simple equipment to help with disability (Ebrahim et al. 1987).

Furthermore, the services remain poorly developed and fragmented across a bewildering array of statutory, insurance-funded, and voluntary agencies, with wide variations in distribution and availability and with major gaps in provision. Coordination between these agencies is typically poor and information often inadequate for service providers and

Table 55.1: Epidemiology of disabling neurological disorders

Disease	Annual Incidence per 250,000	Prevalence per 250,000 Total	Disabled
Epilepsy	175	3,900	1,300[a]
Stroke	550	1,500	900
Head injury	500	—[b]	750
Parkinson's disease	45	400	342
Multiple sclerosis	10	250	125
Cerebral tumor	40	113	40
Essential tumor	60	800	40
Brachial neuritis	4	—[b]	30
Spinal cord injury	4	—[b]	120
Motor neuron disease	5	15	14
Guillain-Barré syndrome	3	60	12
Duchenne's dystrophy	50[c]	12	8
Huntington's disease	—[b]	15	13

Source: Data from Royal College of Physicians. Physical disability in 1986 and beyond. J Royal Coll Physicians 1986;20:160–194; and DT Wade, R Langton Hewer. Epidemiology of some neurological diseases with special reference to workload on the NHS. Int Rehab Med 1986;8:129–137.
[a]"Disabled" for epilepsy means on treatment.
[b]Unavailable.
[c]Males only.

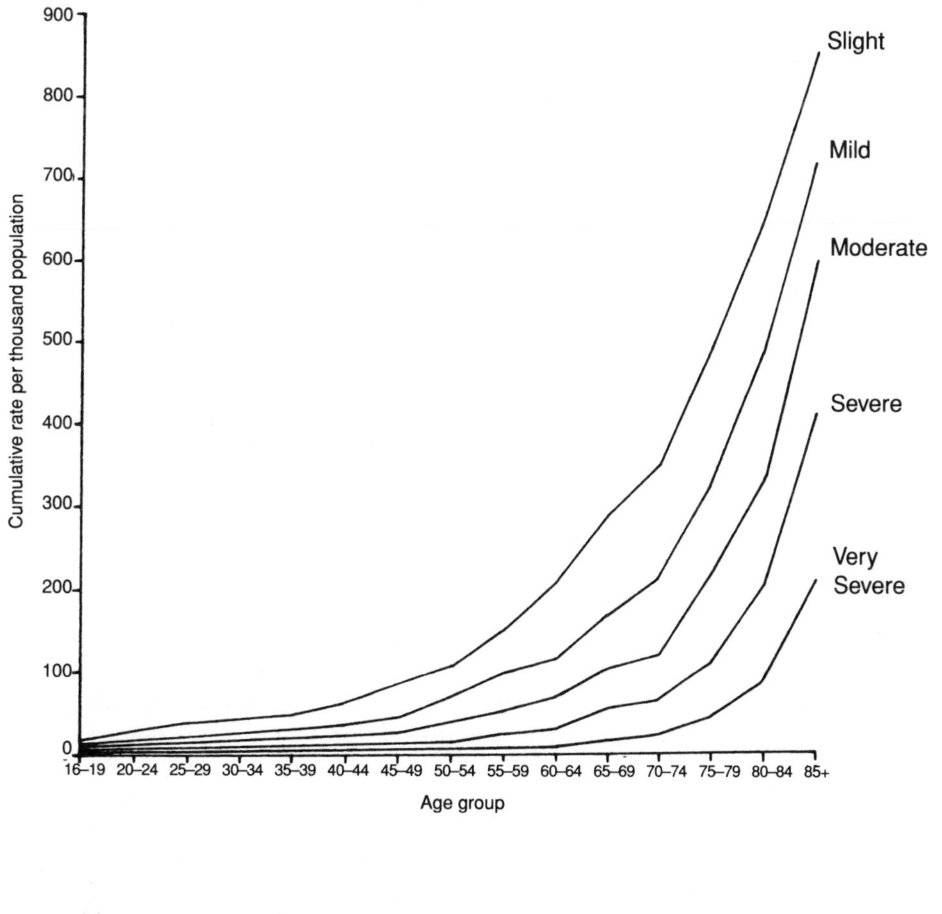

FIGURE 55.2 Estimates of prevalence of disability among adults in Great Britain by age and severity. (Redrawn with permission from J Martin, H Meltzer, D Elliot. OPCS Surveys of Disability in Great Britain. Report 1. The Prevalence of Disability Among Adults. London: Her Majesty's Stationery Office, 1988.)

users alike; yet users and their caregivers are seldom involved or consulted in service planning and development.

In Britain major deficiencies have been highlighted (Royal College of Physicians 1986; Edwards and Warren 1990), although other countries have been more fortunate in having an established medical specialty of rehabilitation or physiatry. Emphasis has recently been placed on funding general health promotion for all, but such resources are often wasted on sectors of the population with minimal needs and should be accurately targeted.

Table 55.2: Priority groups in health and social services

Priority Group	*Total Numbers in England and Wales (Millions)*	*Average Health Social Service Expenditure (% per Capita)*
Elderly physically disabled	2.60	54
Mental illness	0.80	20
Severe mental impairment	0.12	22
Severely physically disabled, aged 16–59 years	0.42	4

Source: Data from V Beardshaw. Last on the List—Community Services for People with Physical Disabilities. London: King's Fund Institute, 1988; J Martin, H Meltzer, D Elliot. OPCS Surveys of Disability in Great Britian: Report I. The Prevalence of Disability Among Adults. London: Her Majesty's Stationery Office, 1988.

The Dimensions of Disability

Ten percent of the population represents an enormous ocean of physical disability that is hard to comprehend. In a typical population of 250,000, about 25,000 are likely to be appreciably disabled, of whom 6,250 will be very severely disabled (Royal College of Physicians 1986). There will be about 1,810 people with a wheelchair and 11,000 with regular incontinence. In addition, sensory impairment will affect a further 10%: 25,000 will have significant deafness and 1,300 significant visual loss. Yet crude prevalence estimates conceal the true dimensions of disability.

Most diseases give rise to multiple physical disabilities even if the pathological process is confined to one bodily system or organ. Disorders affecting the brain may cause additional cognitive and behavioral disturbances. In a comprehensive survey of the disabled adult population of Great Britain, locomotion disabilities affected 69% of the total (Martin et al. 1988). Other common problems affected hearing (41%), personal care (37%), dexterity (27%), seeing (24%), intellectual function (21%), behavior (20%), reaching and stretching (19%), continence (17%), and communication (17%). Multiple difficulties were much more common among the elderly.

The depth or severity of disability, which is the converse of a person's level of independent functioning, will vary enormously according to medical, emotional, and social factors. The very elderly predominate among the most severely disabled adults.

The duration of disability depends on the natural history of the underlying disease process. Mode of onset may be abrupt, gradual, or stepwise. Thereafter, disability can be variable or relapsing and chronic, stable, or progressive. The development of complications contributes to the inherent uncertainty of prognosis in many cases and makes planning for the future difficult.

Medicine's Approach to the Disabled

This ocean of disability represents a major challenge to modern health care. High-technology medicine is salvaging more and more people who are then discharged from acute care with little direction or support. In most countries today there is a serious lack of integrated comprehensive rescue services for the disabled. Rather, each profession delivers an impersonal package of therapy or care seldom matched to the person's needs.

Individual professionals may perform disability evaluations, usually with their own particular vocational instruments such as a medical examination or a physical therapy evaluation, yet seldom seek additional information or communicate with each other. The evaluation schemes that do exist use different scales based on neurological, psychological, or sociological criteria and are incomprehensible to all but the most experienced professional.

Why is the approach to managing disabled patients so difficult? Apart from factors relating to diagnosis discussed previously, the problems can be examined under three headings.

Individual Handicap. The traditional medical model that has guided practice, at least in the Western world, for the last few centuries, has some major shortcomings. Human beings are seen as biological organisms made up of a hierarchy of cells, tissues, organs, and systems interacting in homeostatic harmony. Upset of this balance by an etiological agent entrains a pathological process and leads to a medical condition or diagnosis. Its severity is measured by the bald statistics of morbidity and mortality. The goals of medical practice are to diagnose and treat the cause; if cure is impossible, then the goal may be modified toward alleviating symptoms and postponing death.

Social and psychological disturbances of homeostasis are not easily accommodated by this medical model, but they are inseparable and of crucial importance in determining a disabled person's level of functioning and independence. Innumerable individual factors influence the consequences of a given disability, including age and level of educational or vocational attainment at onset of disability, social class and roles, environment, premorbid personality, psychological sequelae, presence or absence of brain damage, and the often unmet need for information and education regarding individual problems.

Socioeconomic Climate. Most people live within some sort of supportive network that will come to their aid in time of distress, whether it be family, friends, neighbors, employers, church, or voluntary organizations. Unfortunately, these networks are usually only equipped and prepared to respond to a short-term crisis such as admission to a hospital. Gifts and cards, visits, and simple consideration decline exponentially thereafter; often after a month or so, only family and true friends remain. Chronic disability places increasing and sometimes intolerable strains on the family unit. Relationships are altered, finances drained, and security threatened, particularly if the disabled person was the main breadwinner. The physical and emotional health of other family members may suffer too. Particular problems may arise in a mainly insurance-funded health care system like that in the United States. Inevitably quality and duration of rehabilitation vary according to the level of coverage, and conflicts of interest may arise between the purchaser, the provider, and the patient. Crude attempts have been made to apply measures of functional status to determine levels of payment, both as a classification system (how much?) and as a justification system (whether and how long?) (Wilkerson et al. 1992).

An additional and powerful influence is the reaction of others, summed up by the word *stigma*. Prejudicial attitudes toward disability and disfigurement have existed throughout history. Thoughts, feelings, and actions toward disabled people are heavily ingrained and often result in discriminatory behavior such as outright rejection, incomplete acceptance, and avoidance of intimate or even superficial contact.

Institutional discrimination may exclude disabled people from certain types of employment and from access to public places, transport, and education. It was for this reason the U.S. Congress in 1990 approved the Americans with Disabilities Act. Protective legislation and the segregation of disabled from nondisabled people in education, housing, and employment may confer special advantages or benefits on some groups but exclude others with identical needs. Finally, the lack of a coherent health policy denies disabled people an equitable share of national resources devoted to health and personal social services and contributes to the hostile climate of the ocean of disability.

Professional Inadequacies. Some of the relevant professional factors have already been described. Most countries have completely separate government departments for health care and social services. Each department employs many professional groups with variable experience in disability management and indifferent quality of care provision. Increasing specialization has encouraged a narrow focus with no common language, measurement instruments, or documentation, which compounds the poor coordination and communication with the disabled and with other disciplines (Figure 55.3). Scant research and failure to develop or evaluate model patterns of care are perpetuated, not only because of inadequate central policies and planning but also because of lack of accountability on the part of the care providers.

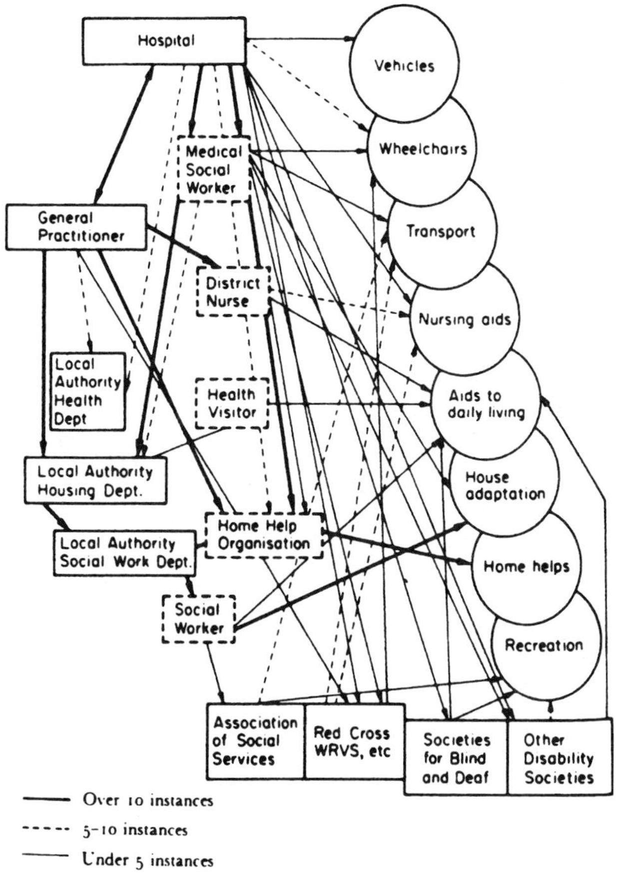

FIGURE 55.3 Patterns of referral chaos. (WRVS = Women's Royal Voluntary Service) (Reprinted with permission from M Blaxter. Power and Inanity. In A Davis [ed], Relationships Between Doctors and Patients. Farnborough, England: Gower, 1978.)

The World Health Organization Model: International Classification of Impairments, Disabilities, and Handicaps

Major shortcomings of the medical model of illness have been highlighted. It stops short of the consequences of disease that intrude on everyday life and interfere with a person's ability to discharge those functions and obligations that are expected of him or her. In a seminal publication, the WHO (1980) has extended this traditional model into a hierarchical framework (Figure 55.4).

Based on the work of P.H.N. Wood, the *International Classification of Impairments, Disabilities, and Handicaps* (ICIDH) represents the first serious attempt to standardize terminology in this field while defining three distinct and independent classifications, each relating to a different dimension of experience consequent on disease. The details of the classification are not essential, but the major sections are listed later in this chapter in Tables 55.5, 55.6, and 55.10 and serve as useful checklists when applied to a particular patient.

Impairment is defined as any loss or abnormality of psychological, physiological, or anatomical structure or func-

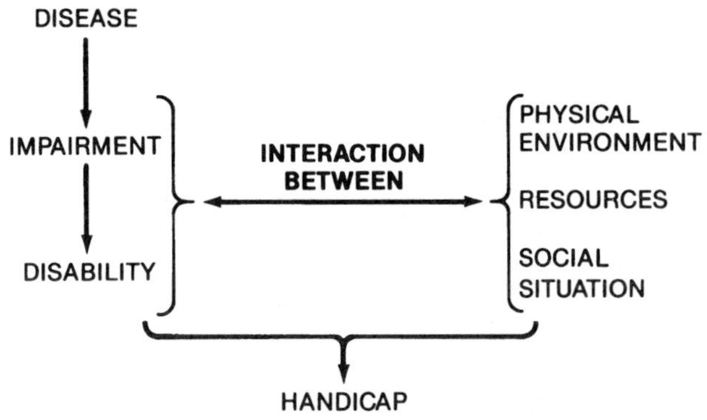

FIGURE 55.4 The genesis of handicap. (Reprinted with permission from EM Badley. The ICIDH: Format, application in different settings, and distinction between disability and handicap. Int Disabil Studies 1987;9:122–125.)

tion. It may be temporary or permanent and would include any existence or occurrence of an anomaly, defect, or loss in a limb, organ, tissue, or other structure of the body. It is best thought of as a threshold phenomenon; a simple judgment about whether an impairment is present or not is all that is required. In principle, impairment reflects pathological disturbances at the level of the organ.

Disability refers to any restriction or lack of ability (resulting from an impairment) to perform an activity in the manner, or within the range, considered normal for a human being. It affects composite activities and behaviors that are components of everyday life. Disability represents evidence of an impairment causing disturbances at the level of the person.

Handicap is defined as a disadvantage for a given person, resulting from an impairment or a disability, that limits or prevents the fulfillment of a role that is normal for that person depending on age, sex, and the social and cultural factors already discussed. It is characterized by a discordance between the person's performance and the expectations of the person him- or herself or of the particular social group of which he or she is a member. Handicap thus represents socialization of an impairment or disability, and reflects the cultural, social, economic, and environmental consequences for the individual. The ICIDH uses the term *disablement* to refer to all the consequences of disease and embraces all three concepts.

As an illustration, consider the case of a young housewife who sustains a head injury. Residual dysphasia and hemiparesis are classified as language and motor *impairments*; difficulties in communication, feeding, and walking are the consequent *disabilities*; her restricted mobility and inability to care fully for her children constitute *handicaps*.

Two final points must be made that have been emphasized elsewhere (Martin et al. 1988). First, there is actually a continuum ranging from slight to very severe disability; absolute prevalence cannot be determined, and a threshold must be decided arbitrarily for both epidemiological and clinical purposes. Moreover, the threshold may vary considerably with age. Although there is a steep rise in the overall rate of disablement, elderly people in general are not regarded as disabled, perhaps because some restriction of activities is considered the norm.

As a general rule, the management of impairments is the responsibility of the medical services, whereas handicap affects welfare and social policy areas. It follows that the intermediate dimension, disability, should be the prime concern of rehabilitation services.

Lessons from Spinal Injuries

The deficiencies highlighted herein were even greater at the time of World War II. One outstanding initiative in response to the large numbers of disabled British servicemen was the establishment of a network of special units dedicated to managing spinal cord injuries, then regarded as inevitably fatal within a year or two because of pressure sores and bladder infections. Fortunately, the vision and determination of Ludwig Guttman at Stoke Mandeville Hospital transformed the attitudes of his staff and the expectations of his patients. Even tetraplegic victims can now look forward to a normal life span, and Stoke Mandeville, since designated the National Spinal Injuries Centre, enjoys an international reputation.

Spinal cord injury has become a specialty in its own right and, although it is a small and circumscribed one, provides a good comparative model for the management of other neurological disabilities. Similar dedicated centers were established shortly after the war in several other countries, including Canada, Holland, Austria, and Poland. At Long Beach, California, the first of eight units was established by the distinguished urologist Bors for the Veterans Administration, although the United States was much slower to set up similar facilities for civilians. Nevertheless, there is now a nationally agreed U.S. Model Regional Spinal Cord Injury Center Program, which defines desirable criteria for standards of care and collects valuable data, and which could usefully be emulated by others (American Spinal Injury Association 1992). Sadly, the poor prognosis has so far been altered very little in many African and Asian countries, where spinal tuberculosis, poliomyelitis, and other infectious causes of transverse myelitis are still more common than spinal trauma.

In most modern spinal cord injury units today, staff provide a high standard of care with scrupulous attention to detail while also educating the patient to the same level of awareness and skill. Patients may stay for 12 months or more and must be able ultimately to assume full responsibility for their own health care by the time of discharge. There is thus a common obsession with skin care, management of bowels and bladder, and prevention of contractures.

It must be acknowledged that these units are often in a privileged position and can afford a counsel of perfection because they regulate their own admissions. No one is discharged until rehabilitation is complete and facilities at home optimized, whereas other, less fortunate accident victims on the waiting list may be inappropriately occupying "acute" beds in district general hospitals.

Damage and Recovery in the Central Nervous System

Clinical Observations after Head Injury

The complex and dynamic interactions of neural networks prevent all but the crudest predictions following damage to and recovery of function in the CNS, particularly in the brain itself. Clinical studies following head injury have identified a large number of possible factors influencing recovery (Wood 1987; Baethmann et al. 1993).

First and perhaps most obviously, there is the severity of the original insult. Presumed clinical correlates such as the depth and duration of coma and extent of pretraumatic amnesia appear to offer a rough prognostic guide. This is probably because the size of the lesion determines not only the amount of primary neuronal loss but also the compensatory ability of surviving tissue. Clearly, however, the site of a lesion may be just as critical, since certain areas of the brain seem to be redundant.

Next there is the relevance of developing or serial lesions and possible interaction between multiple ones. Cerebral hypoxia because of ventilatory insufficiency, the development of cerebral edema, and secondary hemorrhage are examples of damaging sequelae following any form of brain injury. Both animal experiments and clinical experience suggest that there is a natural recovery curve. Thus, most spontaneous recovery occurs early after injury, determined by fundamental cellular mechanisms, but with some potential for more limited recovery later.

Superimposed on this, certain other factors have been deduced, of which the most important is probably the age of the subject. What has become known as the Margaret Kennard principle, after its main proponent some 50 years ago, predicts better recovery in younger head-injured victims because impairment is less significant and restoration of function is faster and more complete.

Ribot's law, now over a century old, states that disruption is less likely and recovery more likely in proportion to the time elapsed since the acquisition of a particular skill or memory. Similarly, Pitres's law, given a decade earlier, held that overlearning of certain cognitive skills afforded some protection, because polyglot aphasics always perform best in their first acquired language.

It has been claimed that early therapeutic intervention brings about greater recovery after head injury and that environmental enrichment is also beneficial. This is the rationale for providing regular auditory, olfactory, and even vestibular stimulation in comatose patients. The effects of various drugs have also been explored, with no clear positive benefits having been identified. Other patient factors that undoubtedly influence the extent of functional recovery include cerebral dominance, premorbid IQ, mood, and motivation.

Mechanisms of Functional Recovery

Having considered many potential clinical variables, it is apparent that recovery must be influenced by several underlying mechanisms. These are reviewed in detail elsewhere (Finger et al. 1988; Baethmann et al. 1993) and can be examined under four broad headings.

Artifact Theories. Secondary tissue effects such as inflammation, edema, and vasospasm may be associated with temporary changes in neurotransmitter pathways and nonspecific inhibition of neural activity, sometimes included under the term *diaschisis*. As innervation is regained from elsewhere, so does function return to otherwise undamaged structures. Spinal shock is an example of this hypothetical state of gross artifactual impairment that later resolves to an extent determined by the degree of primary tissue destruction. The remote effects of cortical stroke, seen on positron emission tomography scans as areas of hypometabolism in the ipsilateral thalamus and contralateral cerebellum, can also be construed as evidence for diaschisis, but whether it represents a valid explanation for behavioral recovery remains controversial.

Regeneration. Classically regarded as being confined to the peripheral nervous system, the capacity for neuronal regeneration offers the only hope of complete restoration of function. In cases of nerve transection, for example, early postsynaptic changes such as supersensitivity of receptors are followed by axonal sprouting and ultimately regrowth. Potential for regeneration within the CNS, albeit very limited, may indeed exist; successful animal experiments with neural trophic factors or transplantation offer an additional method of artificial tissue regeneration.

Anatomical Reorganization. Hughlings Jackson's concept of hierarchical organization of function, and of "evolution" and "dissolution" of function, implied that following damage to higher cortical levels of control, certain functions could be taken over by a lower, subcortical level, albeit in a less sophisticated way. For example, ablation studies in primates have shown that virtually all motor deficits recover after discrete lesions of the corticospinal tract except the ability to perform fractionated finger movements. Jackson also commented on the clinical differences determined by the "effect of momentum" of lesions developing slowly, rapidly, or serially. Concepts of redundancy and reiteration or multiple control are relevant here, with the possibility of unmasking hitherto latent or suppressed synapses as well as of reactive synaptogenesis, with axon and terminal sprouting occupying additional vacant synaptic sites or creating new ones.

Rather than strict hierarchical ordering, certain adjacent cortical association areas or even symmetrical regions in the contralateral cerebral hemisphere might fulfill equipotential roles, or have the capacity to take over what are termed *vicarious functions*. The greatest potential for such reorganization exists in the immature, developing brain. Young children with language impairment secondary to left-hemisphere damage invariably recover completely. Speech is presumed to become relocated in the noninjured hemisphere, but at the expense of impairment (crowding) of other functions normally mediated by that hemisphere, such as visuospatial discrimination.

Behavioral Substitution. At the simplest level, a person with a right hemiplegia may recover the ability to write by learning to use the left hand. Acquiring such alternative strategies, termed *behavioral substitution* or *functional adaptation*, is the basic goal for most therapists. In many cases, provision of a particular aid or appliance may be adequate to compensate for a deficit.

Pharmacological Intervention. A variety of drugs have been claimed to improve recovery after experimental CNS injury, including amphetamine, physostigmine, nerve growth factor, corticosteroids, 21-amino-steroids, *N*-methyl-D-aspartate and opiate receptor antagonists, calcium channel blockers, and free radical scavengers. This is an exciting field, but there is insufficient evidence to justify their use in clinical practice at present.

Clinical Implications. Whatever the mechanisms underlying recovery in individual cases, several important clinical implications seem worth considering. The traditional notion of cerebral localization of function is not always reliable, and the potential for recovery of function in adults even weeks after injury is probably not as limited as was previously thought. In view of what is known about greater adaptive capacity in response to slowly expanding lesions, the possibility of staged neurosurgery should be examined carefully. In those with progressive neurological conditions, it may be possible to apply overtraining or the learning of alternative strategies prophylactically, in the hope of minimizing the disabling impact of disease progression.

The Aims of Rehabilitation

Ethical Issues

Before attempting to define aims, certain ethical principles must be examined that place constraints on such a definition. Four fundamental principles of medical ethics are generally accepted, among which *respect for autonomy* is paramount. Thus, any disabled person, however dependent on others, is entitled to be regarded equitably, without prejudice, as a client for health and social services, and to accept or decline advice and services offered.

The issue of competence is occasionally relevant, usually in those with significant cognitive or behavioral disturbance, but otherwise individual autonomy should be cardinal in the disabled client-professional relationship. A central criticism of disability services is often the failure to consult disabled consumers themselves because of the assumption that paternalistic professionals "know best." There is, however, an equally important corollary: the disabled person's responsibility for self-care. The willingness to accept any responsibility for self-care tends to be minimized by an overwhelming professional "leave it to us" attitude, which encourages passivity. The detrimental result has been called *disabling help*.

Over the last few generations this paternalistic doctor-patient relationship has become less acceptable, and medical practice now more commonly follows a contractual model, based on the tenets of respect for autonomy, informed consent, and maintenance of confidentiality. Because of the very slow development of services dedicated to disabled people, however, even this limited advance is seldom incorporated.

The second and third ethical principles of medical practice are largely self-evident. *Beneficence* (doing good) and *nonmaleficence* (doing no harm) are enshrined in the Hippocratic oath, and professionals are perhaps guilty of taking these axioms for granted.

Finally, there is the principle of *justice*. Practitioners have an ethical duty to ensure that their disabled patients receive care to an equally high standard and that a fair proportion of resources are devoted to that care. Thus it behooves all neurologists to take a wider view: to recognize the inequitable provision made for the management of neurological disability; to actively seek out patients in need of greater assistance; and to strive on their behalf for a greater share in the regional and national health care budgets.

Management Aims

The term *rehabilitation*, though often used, lacks any agreed definition and is widely misunderstood. Some authors apply it only to conditions with potential for recovery, and exclude progressive disorders. Others use the term synonymously with therapy of all kinds, without any critical evaluation of efficacy. It is preferable to attempt simply to define the principles of management in neurological disability. Based on the mechanisms of recovery outlined in the previous section, they are summarized chronologically in Table 55.3.

1. *Prevent complications.* Many neurological diseases threaten mobility, and the ensuing complications are well known, including pressure sores, contractures, thrombosis, and chest and urinary infections. Prophylactic measures are imperative within hours of an acute stroke or injury to the spinal cord.
2. *Promote intrinsic recovery.* Steps to promote intrinsic recovery are usually confined to consideration of the indications for steroids, assisted ventilation, or early surgery—for example, evacuation of a hematoma or

Table 55.3: Management aims in neurological disability

Prevent complications
Promote intrinsic recovery
Teach adaptive strategies
Facilitate interaction with environment

spinal decompression. As yet there is no compelling case for any pharmacological intervention to promote this aim.

3. *Teach adaptive strategies.* A principal aim practiced by most therapists is to teach the disabled person alternative ways of achieving particular goals.
4. *Facilitate environmental interaction.* When certain goals remain unattainable despite maximum behavioral substitution, it is often possible to facilitate the interaction between the individual and the environment by the provision of aids and appliances. Thus, for someone unable to walk, mobility can be facilitated by a combination of a wheelchair and an accessible environment. Only when all such attempts prove fruitless should it be necessary to lower expectations of restoring disabled functions completely to normal.

The overall objective is the restoration or maintenance of a disabled person's fullest physical, psychological, and social capability. As discussed in the next section, it is impossible to separate these three components and for the physician to be concerned exclusively with physical capability.

Rehabilitation Team Members and Their Skills

Physician

Physicians are generally trained according to the medical model and are oriented toward curative treatment of acute illness. Many neurologists, and indeed other specialists, have been unable or unwilling to concern themselves with the long-term management of their patients' disabilities. Those patients fortunate enough to continue under medical supervision are often followed up by physicians with a declared interest in rehabilitation. For historical reasons, in the United Kingdom these were usually rheumatologists, whereas in the United States physiatrists constitute a separate subspecialty.

This may be acceptable for stroke, but it is not ideal for most neurological disorders. The accuracy of the initial diagnosis is fundamental to later management and may need to be reviewed regularly in light of subsequent developments, which might themselves demand specific intervention. Drug requirements are seldom static, and modern advances in neurological investigation and therapeutics can radically alter prognosis. Moreover, many conditions are rare even in neurological practice, yet present almost unique challenges with which general rehabilitation specialists may not be familiar.

The primary-care physician may lack detailed knowledge about neurological matters but is often well placed to coordinate treatment and services, because of greater familiarity with the patient's domestic circumstances. Good communication between this physician and the hospital-based specialists is essential to efficient management.

Nurse

Traditionally nurses have been expected to provide care according to *medical* need prescribed by doctors. This view, and the biomedical model on which it is based, is being increasingly challenged by the nursing profession itself. Emphasis on cure of patients with physical illness rather than holistic care of sick people, along with routinization and task orientation, are undesirable characteristics of such nursing practice. Alternative models of practice have been developed that focus more on health and well-being, the importance of self-care, and partnership in the nurse-client relationship (Fitzpatrick and Whall 1989).

These developments are particularly apposite to the management of disability. For example, the Activities of Living model (Roper et al. 1983) depicts people progressing through their life span engaging in 12 basic activities of living at some point along a dynamic dependence-independence continuum for each. Apart from the obvious ones—breathing, mobilizing, and the like—activities identified include sleeping, maintaining a safe environment, working and playing, expressing sexuality, and dying.

The self-care model (Orem 1991), originated and popular in American nursing, seeks to establish a person's self-care needs in three groups: (1) universal self-care requisites such as food intake, control of body temperature, and elimination; (2) developmental requisites according to the life cycle stage reached, socioeconomic circumstances, religion, beliefs, and values; and (3) health deviation requisites because illness or disability impairs self-care competence. Deficits in self-care can be eliminated by reductions in demand, enabling patients or relatives to meet the demand by means of educative and supportive nursing, or by compensatory nursing care.

The adaptation model described by Roy (1976) is based on systems theory. A person is viewed as responding or adapting to changes in four different dimensions. As with other models, one of these comprises the common physiological needs. The others are internal self-concept or self-esteem; external social role functions; and interdependence—that is, the acceptable balance between autonomy or independence and the natural dependent needs for company, support, and approval.

Physical Therapist

Physical therapy is a systematic method of assessing musculoskeletal and neurological disorders of function, including pain and those of psychological origin, and treating or preventing those problems by natural methods based essentially on manual practice and physical agencies. There is also a welcome trend in favor of an educational role for the therapists toward both clients and caregivers.

Therapists are trained in all aspects of anatomy and physiology relevant to normal and disordered function, particularly with regard to movement and locomotion. Considerable specialization is usually required for optimal management of neurological disability because the principles and details differ from the more common field of orthopedic trauma. Nevertheless, the application of various physical agents may be appropriate in either; these include massage, manipulation, mobilization, and traction; heat, ice, ultrasound, and short wave; hydrotherapy; acupuncture; and transcutaneous nerve stimulation (TNS). Exercises may be taught to promote mobility, strength, coordination, stamina, or particular functional activities.

Certain specific techniques of neuromuscular reeducation have become widely used, though they have not necessarily been critically evaluated. The Bobath neurodevelopmental techniques, for example, aim to facilitate normal movement and desired automatic reactions and to restore postural control, while inhibiting abnormal tone and reflex activity using specific motor patterns. The methods were originally developed for children with cerebral palsy and later adapted as a treatment approach to adult hemiplegia.

Brunnstrom has introduced her own system of management of hemiplegia, identifying six separate stages of motor recovery (Sawner and LaVigne 1992). The training procedures advocated overlap partially with the techniques of proprioceptive neuromuscular facilitation (PNF). PNF uses all sensory modalities to improve strength and coordination, with particular emphasis on spiral and diagonal patterns of activation of synergistic muscle groups. Therapists may also supervise the application of functional electrical stimulation (to be discussed).

Finally, the Hungarian system of conductive education devised by Peto has recently attracted much attention and is an impressive illustration of the benefits of a more holistic approach. The emphasis is on education, not treatment, of the whole person in a stimulating environment, with the person receiving intensive encouragement and feedback while working in matched groups for mutual benefit and encouragement (Cottam and Sutton 1986). Meaningful functional goals are set, but with activities broken down into task parts, which are learned using "rhythmical intention," declaring in words the planning, intention, and execution of each movement. Students are taught how to organize and plan their own movements until they become automatic. The approach requires experienced conductors who are actually generic therapists combining many skills.

Occupational Therapist

Occupational therapy (OT) is the treatment of disability through specific selected activities to enable a person to achieve his or her maximum level of function in all aspects of daily life. Whereas physical therapy concentrates mainly on physical impairment and rather less on disability in a neutral setting, OT is concerned with disabilities of all types and also with personal handicap.

Assessment of activities of daily living (ADL) serves as a baseline from which OT aims to promote maximum independence by improving function where possible and by providing appropriate aids and appliances. Familiarity with the vast range of the latter is needed, as well as with varied aspects of mobility, housing, recreation, and employment. Therapists also try to assess the psychological and social needs of their clients and provide help and advice where possible.

Speech Therapist

Speech therapists (speech-language pathologists in the United States) are trained in all aspects of communication, including phonetics and linguistics, audiology, and developmental psychology. They specialize in assessing disorders of phonation, articulation, fluency, and language, and apply techniques for their amelioration. Therapists advise patients, relatives, and staff, and recommend appropriate communication aids where necessary. Assessment and guidance are also provided for those with swallowing difficulties; in certain cases, a dietitian may need to be recruited to the disability team to advise on preparation and constitution of meals.

Social Worker

The types and roles of social workers are many. Most developed countries provide a wide range of benefits and services for disabled people through private and public welfare agencies. Social workers advise on financial matters and mobilize and coordinate necessary community services. Independence can usually be maintained for the most severely disabled people given sufficient social support, but patients may remain inappropriately in expensive hospital or residential care if available services are not utilized. Most social workers are also concerned with the interactions of individuals, families, and small groups with each other, and are trained in the psychosocial aspects of disability and relevant counseling skills. They are thus well equipped to offer support as well as information to the whole family unit, and indeed to other members of the team.

Rehabilitation or Vocational Counselor

Everyone who requires medical intervention over a prolonged period is at a significant disadvantage in the current employment market. The informal career guidance often provided by therapists or social workers may not be adequate. Many countries have enacted legislation to identify these people and to facilitate their training, recruitment, and retention by employers. This was one of the principal aims of the U.S. Americans with Disabilities Act passed in 1990. Specialist advisers, such as rehabilitation or vocational counselors in the United States or disablement resettlement officers in the United Kingdom, can be a great asset.

Rehabilitation or vocation counselors are familiar with all aspects of the employment services, job analysis, training courses, and career opportunities, and can act as liaisons with prospective employers regarding provision of special facilities, grants, and other services. Because the ability to drive a car is often essential for a disabled person's employability, a professional driving assessment and advice concerning vehicle modifications may be relevant. Some disablement resettlement officers or rehabilitation counselors are further trained to provide a specialist service to blind or partially sighted clients.

Psychologist

The specific roles of a clinical psychologist include assessment and treatment. Psychometric testing assesses cognitive and other functions and may detect focal abnormalities of diagnostic value. Other psychological attributes such as behavior, personality, and affect can also be formally evaluated. Educational psychologists specialize in assessing the special needs of children with mental, physical, and sensory handicaps or lesser learning difficulties and advising on their education.

Examples of specific treatment modalities include behavior therapy, hypnosis, and relaxation for anxiety states; cognitive therapy in chronic pain; the teaching of social skills; and the counseling of patients, caregivers, and staff. The American Psychological Association has a separate division of Rehabilitation Psychology whose other declared interests include human reactions to disablement, person—environment interaction, advising voluntary organizations and self-help groups, and assuming an advocacy role on behalf of disabled clients.

Orthotist

An *orthosis* is an external device designed to apply or remove forces to or from the body in a controlled manner to perform one or both basic functions of:

1. Alteration, or prevention of alteration, in the shape of body tissues.
2. Control of body motion, including:
   a. Absence of body motion, that is, rest in a chosen position.
   b. Limitation of normal range to a chosen degree.
   c. Limitation or avoidance of abnormal movement while possibly keeping some or all normal movement.

Although certain orthotic devices are mass-produced and widely prescribed by doctors and therapists, the expertise of a trained orthotist is often invaluable in advising on the choice and construction of orthoses and supervising their fitting and adjustment. The knowledge and skills required constitute the science of orthotics (Rose 1986).

Orthoses include calipers or leg braces, upper limb splints and spinal braces, collars, and corsets. A standard terminology conveys a concise description of the joints supported. A simple footdrop splint is termed AFO (ankle-foot orthosis), a knee brace is KO, and one supporting the whole limb and extending above the hip is referred to as HKAFO (hip-knee-AFO). Orthoses may be static, such as a resting wrist splint worn at night, or dynamic, with joints that may be either lockable or free-moving. Materials include plastic, leather, or metals, depending on mechanical requirements, but the effects of pressure, shear forces, and heat retention with sweating must also be considered. A complicated series of measurements or the casting of a mold is necessary for an individually made orthosis. Too often, inappropriate or ill-fitting orthoses are tacitly discarded by patients. Ideally, prescription should be done jointly by the doctor and the orthotist, with advice from the relevant therapists.

Ophthalmologist

Special skills are needed to assess those with visual disabilities, to improve or restore sight where possible and to prevent further deterioration. Cataract, glaucoma, and diabetic retinopathy are all common but treatable causes of blindness, which may coexist. An ophthalmologist also advises on suitable low-vision aids; makes referrals to relevant agencies; and is concerned, in conjunction with an orthoptist, in the diagnosis and treatment of defects in binocular vision, particularly childhood squints. Occasionally, oculoplastic surgery, tarsorrhaphy, or correction of ptosis is indicated.

Audiologist

Similarly, the evaluation of hearing impairment is a complex task requiring the expertise of an audiologist. Unfortunately, benefits from medical and surgical treatment are somewhat limited, and remedial help is often all that can be offered. This includes assessment of special educational or vocational needs, selection of hearing aids and other instrumental help, and communication training.

Pain Relief Specialist

Now almost a specialty in its own right, pain assessment and relief is an important aspect of disability management. Training in pharmacology and anesthetics is needed for the correct selection of drug treatment, local or regional nerve blocks, TNS, or acupuncture.

Surgeon

Surgeons aim to restore normal anatomy and function whenever possible, but most neurological disorders cause permanent and even progressive disruption. Thus the indications for surgery are limited, although judicious intervention may improve functional disability and cosmesis or simply make nursing easier. Apart from primary neurosurgery, orthopedic and plastic surgery are most relevant. Tendon transfers or joint stabilization by arthrodesis may be beneficial in a flaccid weak limb. In cases involving spasticity outcome is much less predictable, but correction of deformity is sometimes worthwhile. Debridement and skin grafting of pressure sores can reduce lengthy periods of hospitalization.

Urologist

Although urological surgery is seldom indicated, a systematic approach to the management of incontinence is essential. This may require certain specialist investigations—for example, measurement of urine flow rate, pressure-flow cystometry, cystoscopy, and imaging of the kidneys and ureters. Their interpretation requires skill to identify those suitable for drug treatment and to select the few patients likely to benefit from such procedures as prostatic or bladder neck resection, sphincterotomy, colposuspension, and implantation of sacral nerve root stimulators (to be discussed).

Bioengineer

The advent of microchip technology is currently revolutionizing techniques for the assessment and treatment of the disabled person. To maximize rehabilitation opportunities, a bioengineer has become an invaluable member of the disability team. It is impossible to summarize adequately the breadth of activities in this field, which will only be illustrated by citing a few examples.

Many sophisticated assessment techniques have already been developed, including those to measure cortical evoked potentials and muscle force, and to analyze tremor and gait objectively. The advance from behind-the-ear hearing aids to cochlear implants is the first practicable example of electronic sensory substitution, but attempts are also being made to reproduce vision by tactile or even direct cortical stimulation and to incorporate sensation into limb prostheses (Bach-y-Rita 1988).

Even the simplest devices confer unprecedented advantages for the severely disabled. With the aid of a microcomputer, virtually any conscious person can gain access by means of a one-way switch to complete environmental control systems or advanced communication aids with electronic text-to-speech synthesis. Switches can be operated by any residual motor function in the finger, shoulder, mouth (blow-suck), tongue (Figure 55.5), or in extreme cases by electromyographic (EMG) signals generated peripherally or by eye movements.

Therapeutic applications of direct electrical stimulation are also being examined. Implanted electrodes on sacral nerve roots can mediate ejaculation or bladder emptying when activated externally, and spinal cord stimulation may alleviate "central" pain. Functional electrical stimulation (FES) of denervated muscle will actively correct simple foot-drop, and multiple-muscle stimulation with computerized feedback mechanisms offers the possibility of effective ambulation in some paraplegics.

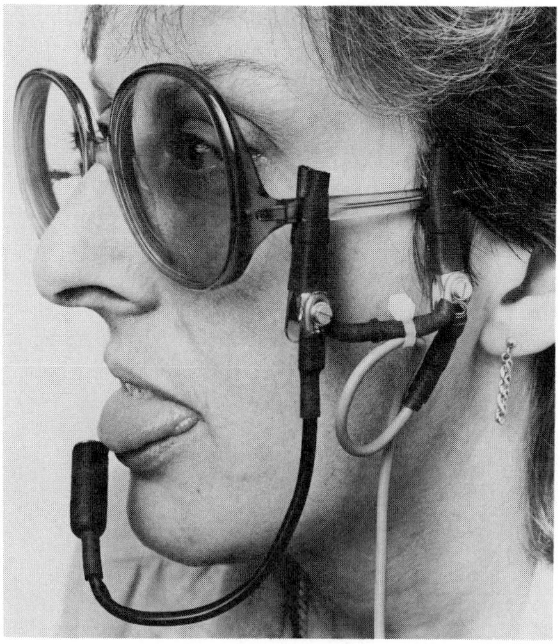

FIGURE 55.5 Possum tongue switch. (Courtesy of Possum Controls Ltd.)

Voluntary Organizations

The role of voluntary agencies, particularly those concerned with specific diseases or types of disability, should not be neglected. Most have arisen because of deficiencies in existing community services and professional support. They disseminate information on various aspects of disability, and some provide specialist services such as residential and day care facilities, schools, training centers, and sheltered workshops. Statutory authorities and insurance schemes make considerable use of these facilities where available rather than providing the capital cost to establish such services themselves.

Many national organizations have local self-help groups that can relieve pressure on the professional disability team by providing mutual support for disabled people and their caregivers, acting as an additional source of information and support, and also raising funds for research and local services.

Principles of Disability Medicine

Case Management and the Problem-Oriented Approach

Applying systems theory, *health* or *well-being* is defined as a satisfactory state of equilibrium between the demands made on an individual by work, home, and family, and the person's physical ability to meet those demands. All of us are constantly striving to achieve a life-style that provides the best possible equilibrium. To overcome disability, either the demands must be reduced or the personal skills enhanced. Regrettably, disabled people are faced with often insurmountable difficulties in all areas of life and then expected to assume a dependent role in receipt of inadequate health care and social services. It is preferable that the disabled person be the focus of professional attention rather than the subject of it.

To ensure consistency and direction and to guide decision and policy-making, an agreed model of caregiving is needed in the management of disability. In the section defining management aims, reference was made to the paternalistic and contractual models. Especially in the context of acute and devastating multiple disabilities, however, the contractual model of practice is often inappropriate, and an educational model is more desirable. Thus, the approach may initially need to be paternalistic and ignore the patient's wishes—for example, to be spared all pain, or to be left to die—to ultimately restore or enhance his or her own autonomy. Practitioners should act in ways to encourage the patient's participation in his or her own care, not simply present options, while monitoring the patient's ability to make informed choices until his or her own autonomy can be fully restored.

Furthermore, the overall objective has been stated as the restoration and maintenance of a disabled person's fullest physical, psychological, and social capability. Because it is impossible to separate these three components and for the physician to be concerned exclusively with physical capability, the approach will to some extent need to be subjective and intuitive, with concern for the patient's quality of life.

The Interdisciplinary Team

Numerous different professions are potentially concerned with the rehabilitation of one person, and many areas of overlap in skills and responsibilities exist. Moreover, the organizational setting in which they work will affect the way in which they operate. Hospital-based doctors and therapists tend to be isolated from each other in their own departments and from the practical needs of individual disabled persons in their own environment.

In the interests of efficiency, therefore, interdisciplinary teams are highly desirable (McGrath and Davis 1992). Avenues of skill sharing, mutual trust, and informed cooperation are opened up between all team members, including the patient and his or her principal caregivers as well as relevant community-based professionals. Clearly, each patient cannot be assessed by every available professional, so comprehensive joint assessments must be made.

At the same time, potential disadvantages of the team approach must be acknowledged. These have been identified from studies of the dynamic psychology of problem-solving groups. Some assertive people tend to compete rather than collaborate, to win an argument rather than find the best solution. Certain less able individuals may dominate a group, while others may refrain from expressing their alternative view just to avoid a conflict. Members may acquire distorted perceptions, with blind faith in their own group and negative prejudices about others, although this is equally true of all professional groups. Groups are also more likely to make dubious decisions because of the diffusion of responsibility.

Nevertheless, if these drawbacks are recognized and guarded against, much can be gained from collaboration, with an optimum level of both conflict and group cohesion. Each member is accountable both to the client and to the group, rather than autonomous, but there must also be effective leadership and management of the group.

There is much argument about who should lead a interdisciplinary team, with doctors often claiming automatic priority. Yet other professionals, depending on their own skills and the needs of the client, may be better suited to lead the planning and delivery of care. There must also be an agreed-on system of management to organize the care: identifying and allocating tasks, eliminating overlap, taking into account time factors, and evaluating progress. Communication methods should be planned in advance: Who will notify whom, when, and by what means? What information is to be passed, and how it will be known whether and when it has been done?

Consideration must also be given to forecasting and planning disability services. Otherwise, a group can become preoccupied with helping a few clients well and be unresponsive to the wider needs of the community. This point is expanded toward the end of this chapter.

The Problem-Oriented Approach

The modus operandi of the interdisciplinary team should follow a standard problem-oriented approach, which has four interlocking steps: assessment, planning, intervention, and evaluation (Figure 55.6). It is worth examining each of these steps in greater detail.

Assessment. First, it is necessary to collect and review relevant data—for example by interviewing the disabled person and his or her family, talking to colleagues, reading reports, and making direct observations and measurements where possible. The assessment may incorporate the medical diagnostic process and establish etiological factors, and serves as a baseline measure of level of functioning for future evaluation and also possibly prediction of outcome. Actual and potential problems can then be identified and prioritized in conjunction with the disabled person. An appropriate accountable therapist should also be nominated.

Planning. First, goals must be identified. These may be short- or long-term; they may be broad aims, specific goals, or even broken down into goal steps. Second, alternatives should

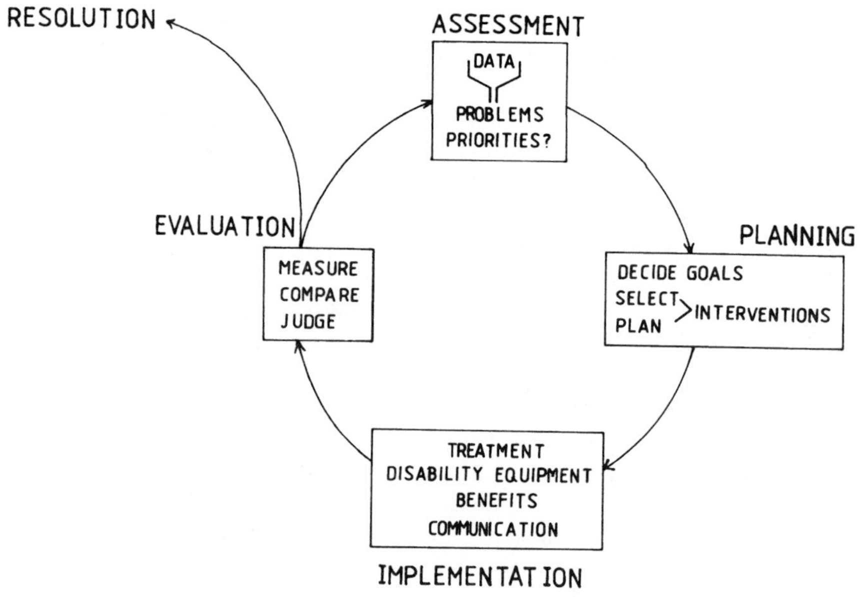

FIGURE 55.6 The problem-oriented approach in rehabilitation.

be deliberately generated so that all available options are considered. Third, appropriate, measurable, and achievable goals can be selected and placed in order of priority by mutual agreement. Ideally, goals should be positive and rewarding. Conflicts must be addressed at this stage, since adjustment to an unacceptable status quo should not be encouraged.

Expectations for all concerned need to be explicit so that later evaluation can be effective. Sometimes clear behavioral goals are agreed on in contract form, stipulating who will do what, starting when, under what conditions, and in what time. Communication should also be planned at this stage. Occasionally it may be necessary to review and modify selected goals because of resource constraints.

Intervention. Interventions can be classified into three types, focusing on (1) improving personal skills, (2) reducing demands to restore equilibrium, and (3) facilitating interactions between the disabled person and the environment. A complementary classification is shown in Table 55.4. Although some interventions may be the exclusive concern of one team member, others, such as communication, must be practiced by all. Counseling skills are reviewed by Stewart (1985).

Evaluation. It is essential to measure the effectiveness of any intervention. Once its objective has been established, information must be obtained as at the assessment stage and compared with the preintervention baseline before judging whether the objective has been achieved. The evaluation is then fed back into the next planning stage.

Evaluation can be concurrent rather than just retrospective, but it must be representative and objective. If the outcome cannot be measured in this way, then unsuitable goals were selected originally. Nevertheless, allowance must be made for a number of factors, including spontaneous, unpredictable recovery or fluctuations in disability; complexity of interactions; observer variability; and imperfect measurement instruments. Halting further deterioration may itself be a satisfactory outcome.

MANAGEMENT OF SPECIFIC (ADULT) NEUROLOGICAL IMPAIRMENTS

In this section, each class of neurological impairment is considered in turn, so as to provide a comprehensive framework for discussion later in this chapter of the management of certain types of disability and other general problems.

Principles of Measurement

It has been argued that an essential preliminary to effective treatment is objective assessment, a point that has been accepted with enthusiasm by some professionals and resulted in a proliferation of checklists, rating scales, and other scoring systems. Rather than search and choose from among a bewildering array of such measurement instruments, however, therapists may be tempted to devise their own. A further hazardous trend is the development of composite scoring systems that combine various impairments and disabilities into one crude score that cannot be used to compare different patients.

It is best to use measures that test a restricted range of relevant abilities and that satisfy the following criteria, proposed by Wade (1992):

1. *Validity* in measuring that which it is intended to measure.

Table 55.4: The problem-oriented approach in neurological rehabilitation

Assessment
- Collect and review data.
- Identify and prioritize problems.
- Identify accountable professional.

Planning
- Identify goals.
- Generate alternatives.
- Select and prioritize interventions.
- Plan communication.

Interventions
- Treatment interventions
  - Personal—nursing care, speech and physical therapy, occupational therapy.
  - Psychological—behavior modification, learning strategies.
  - Surgical.
  - Physical—heat, cold, diathermy, ultrasound, functional electrical stimulation.
- Provision of aids and appliances.
- Provision of benefits or care (nursing or residential).
- Communication
  - Education.
  - Counseling—genetic, sexual, vocational, welfare.
  - Liaison.

Evaluation
- Select criteria for success.
- Collect and compare data with assessment baseline. Judge whether criteria have been met.
- Feed back into next planning stage.

2. *Reliability* between different observers and on different occasions, testing and retesting.
3. *Sensitivity* to clinically relevant changes.
4. *Simplicity* for speed and accuracy of use.
5. *Communicability*—that is, ease of understanding by nonspecialists.

In general, it is preferable to select one or two well-established and validated measurement instruments, and supplement them with a few extra items where necessary, rather than to devise another. Before the discussion of management of each specific neurological impairment (Table 55.5), therefore, a brief summary has been included of relevant assessment techniques in common use.

Cognitive Impairment

Assessment

A wide range of cognitive impairments may be encountered in neurological practice (see Chapter 41). The ICIDH classifies these into categories of intelligence, memory, thinking, consciousness, perception and attention, emotive and volitional functions, and behavior pattern. Examples from opposite ends of a spectrum of available measures are the Glasgow Coma Scale (GCS) and the Wechsler Adult Intelligence Scale (WAIS).

The GCS is a simple method of recording level of consciousness, although the verbal subscale demands intact language skills and adjustment is necessary for aphasic patients. In combination with another simple measure, namely an estimate of duration of posttraumatic amnesia, the GCS has been shown to correlate highly with outcome after traumatic brain injury. In contrast, the WAIS is a very detailed, time-consuming test that must be administered by a trained psychologist, and its applications are more restricted. The same is true for the complementary, but equally comprehensive, Halstead-Reitan neuropsychological test battery.

The Folstein Mini-Mental State is most useful as a screening test for the presence of any cognitive deficit,

Table 55.5: International Classification of Impairments, Disabilities, and Handicaps classification of impairments

1 Intellectual impairments
- Impairments of
  - Intelligence (10–14)
  - Memory (15–16)
  - Thinking (17–18)

2 Other psychological impairments
- Impairments of
  - Consciousness and wakefulness (20–22)
  - Perception and attention (23–24)
  - Emotive and volitional functions (25–28)
  - Behavior pattern (29)

3 Language impairments
- Impairments of
  - Language function (30–34)
  - Speech (35–39)

4 Aural impairments
- Impairments of auditory sensitivity (40–45)
- Other auditory or aural impairments, for example vestibular (46–49)

5 Ocular impairments
- Impairments of visual acuity (50–55)
- Other visual and ocular impairments (56–58)

6 Visceral impairments
- Impairments of
  - Internal organs (60–66)
  - Sexual organs (67)
  - Mastication and swallowing (68)
  - Smell and taste (69)

7 Skeletal impairments
- Impairments of head and trunk regions (70)
- Mechanical and motor impairments of limbs (71–74)
- Deficiencies of limbs (75–79)

8 Disfiguring impairments
- Disfigurements of
  - Head and trunk regions (80–83)
  - Limbs (84–87)

9 Generalized, sensory and other impairments
- Generalized impairments (90–94)
- Sensory impairments (95–98)

Source: Reprinted with permission from World Health Organization. International Classification of Impairments, Disabilities, and Handicaps: A Manual of Classification Relating to the Consequences of Disease. Geneva: WHO, 1980.

rather than as a measure of the extent of a given impairment, because it mixes tests of memory, attention, language, and constructional ability. A number of other tests have been developed for specific deficits, such as the Wechsler Memory Scale, Apraxia Battery, and the Rivermead Perceptual Assessment and Behavioural Memory Tests (Wade 1992).

Management

Very little is known about the management of cognitive impairments, although limited information is available from trials mainly in head injury, dementia, and perceptual impairment following stroke (Meier et al. 1987; Berrol 1990 ; Wilson and Moffett 1992). The widespread availability of microcomputers has led to the development of complex programs dedicated to the rehabilitation of such patients. Just one example is the Orientation Remedial Module devised by Ben Yishay and colleagues in 1987. This consists of a series of five procedures involving the reception of visual and auditory stimuli and eliciting certain visuomotor responses with very few demands for higher-level information processing: basic visual reaction time, zeroing accuracy conditioner, visual discrimination conditioner, time estimation, and rhythm synchrony conditioner.

Individual strategies that have been advocated may be subdivided according to the main components of information processing.

Reception by Sense Organs. These comprise arousal and alerting techniques—for example, in coma and persistent vegetative states, including auditory, verbal, tactile, visual, gustatory, olfactory, vestibular, and oral stimulation.

Perception. Training the subject in obeying commands; in miming; and in cancellation, copying, and tracking tasks is believed to be therapeutic.

Discrimination. Selective attention (preconscious plus conscious) may be facilitated by performance of matching and selecting tasks.

Organization. Sorting, sequencing, and completion tasks and assembly of fragmented stimuli can be practiced. Daily routine should be encouraged.

Memory and Retrieval. Various strategies have been tried with differing degrees of success. Examples include:

1. *Psychological techniques:* These include interactive visual imagery, mental peg systems, cognitive retraining pioneered by Luria, rehearsal, ordering, and use of mnemonics.
2. *Behavioral techniques:* These include reinforcement using partial cueing—for example, with initial letters—and reality orientation.
3. *Altering the environment:* Checklists, physical cues, diaries, alarms, and microcomputers can all be enlisted to compensate for memory impairment.
4. *Drugs:* Compounds as diverse as strychnine, vasodilators, vasopressin, and choline have been studied without convincing benefit.

Language and Speech

Aphasia

Assessment. There are many popular formal tests of aphasia, including several, such as the Boston Diagnostic Aphasia Examination, that can take hours to complete. As an alternative to probing specific language dysfunction, other tests have been developed that directly measure the ability to communicate, such as the Functional Communication Profile. One very useful bedside tool is the Frenchay Aphasia Screening Test, which assesses most aspects of language in a matter of minutes while also giving a measure of the extent of functional communicative loss (Wade 1992). It may also be important to evaluate the emotional and social distress as well as handicap to have a full understanding of the devastating impact of language and speech impairments (Enderby 1993).

Management. Most traditional aphasia therapy involves techniques used in speech training and education, particularly rote learning and selective stimulation. Other linguistic approaches use cues or deblocking techniques. Behavior modification using operant conditioning, often with the aid of automatic teaching machines, has been tried: Programmed instructions break tasks down into small steps, initially with the use of cues, which can later be faded, and provide immediate reinforcement, ensuring mastery of each step before progression to the next. Melodic intonation or rhythm therapy has met with some success; it is based on the belief that musical and tonal abilities are subserved by an intact right hemisphere.

Aphasics with severe and persistent comprehension disability may respond to and be able to learn verbal communication systems such as Bliss, based on printed symbols, or Amerind, a sign language easy to learn and requiring the use of only one hand. Once interpersonal communication is reestablished, more formal language therapy may become possible. Hypnosis, amylobarbitone, hyperbaric oxygen, and various other drugs have all been used without convincing benefit. Finally, various nonspecific strategies have been tried, and counseling may provide valuable emotional support.

Attention to other nonlinguistic deficits is also essential, since aphasia almost never occurs in isolation: Dysarthria, sensory disturbances, oral apraxia, and visuospatial neglect may all impair response to therapy. Conversely, success in physical rehabilitation is often reflected by improvement in aphasia, which should not be treated entirely separately.

Dysarthria

Assessment. Various standard dysarthria profiles exist, in which each component is evaluated separately: respiration, tongue, palate, pharynx, jaw, and lips. Tape recordings of speech are an obvious means of comparison and can be subjected to detailed linguistic and acoustic analysis.

Management. Improving a person's awareness of a mild deficit may allow him or her to compensate for it. The patient can be taught specific exercises for one or two groups of weak muscles, or strategies to improve intelligibility, including self-monitoring. In selected cases, the use of ice to reduce bulbar muscle tone, or of palatal training appliances, may be appropriate (Cochrane 1988).

Dyslexia

Assessment. There are few formal tests of reading ability alone, which is often included in subsets of aphasia batteries.

Management. Unfortunately, the prognosis for acquired dyslexia is generally poor and is usually determined by the patient's residual abilities and limitations. Some authors have advocated so-called right-hemisphere strategies, founded on the postulated existence of an alternative direct reading system through which the patient can be trained to recognize large numbers of written words. Some victims may benefit from arranging sentences into vertical columns, thereby avoiding the normal tendency to scan too quickly from left to right. Other approaches include training augmented by tactile presentation of material or by writing to dictation and then reading back.

Communication Aids

Thorough physical, environmental, and linguistic assessments must be made before a communication aid is prescribed. Most aphasic patients are unable to benefit, so their use is largely confined to the speech disorders of phonation, articulation, or both. Even these patients, if they are ambulant with good hand function, may find that writing is the quickest alternative means. Many aids are available, ranging from a simple amplifier for those with existing intelligible speech, through spelling boards, to sophisticated electronic text-to-speech synthesizers (Cochrane 1990). These aids may be divided according to their method of access.

Direct Access. Direct selection of a symbol by any body part is required to use a simple alphabet board, spelling out words by pointing or by eye movements, or an ordinary typewriter. Some communicators include a visual display as well as a printout.

Scanning Access. Severe physical disability may require the use of a scanning aid, in which each item, letter, or symbol is identified by a moving cursor or pointer that can be stopped by a switch. This is a relatively slow method and requires greater cognitive ability than direct selection. The Possum Communicator is one example, and there is a corresponding environmental control system operated by the same method (Figures 55.7 and 55.8).

Advances in technology mean that it is usually possible for even a profoundly disabled person to be able to communicate adequately, provided language skills are intact. The critical factor is access, and almost any reliable movement can be used to activate a one- or two-way switch made to individual specifications to exploit residual movement (see the earlier section on the role of the bioengineer).

Aural Impairment

Assessment

The most important aural impairments affect auditory sensitivity, causing elevated hearing threshold and impaired discrimination of frequencies or speech. These can all be measured objectively, but full audiological assessment is also concerned with measures of the dynamic range, binaural interaction, evoked potentials, and various psychoacoustical changes that are becoming increasingly important in the selection of signal-processing aids.

Those with significant hearing disability will require full evaluation of their communication status before management is planned. Visual acuity is relevant to lip-reading ability, and speech production and manual skills must be assessed, particularly in those with prelingual deafness who may need to use manual sign language.

Management

The whole field has been well reviewed by Alpiner and McCarthy (1987) and by Stephens (1988).

Hearing Aids. Hearing aids are, of course, the cornerstone of management for loss of auditory sensitivity, although they cannot overcome the common problem of auditory distortions. Sophisticated small behind-the-ear aids are usually optimal, although those worn in the auditory canal have a number of acoustical advantages. Binaural aids may be indicated. Body-worn aids are now seldom recommended except for those with handling skills inadequate to cope with head-worn aids or those requiring a high degree of amplification.

Environmental Aids. Amplification devices, fitted for example to the telephone, radio, and television, may be sufficient to meet a person's needs without a hearing aid. Alerting and warning devices are available to signal the ringing of the telephone, alarm clock, or doorbell with very loud bells or by visual or tactile means (Cochrane 1990).

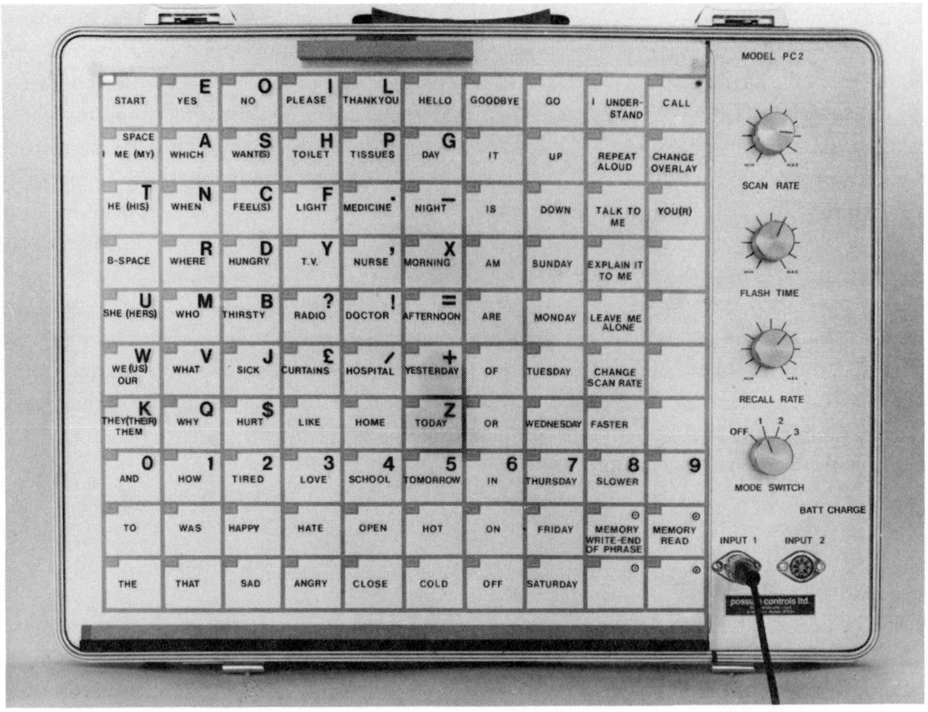

FIGURE 55.7 Possum Communicator PC2. A fairly complicated communication aid requiring good visual acuity and cognitive skills. (Courtesy of Possum Controls Ltd.)

Sensory Substitution Aids. A few people with profound or total deafness may benefit from sensory substitution aids. One approach involves the wearing of a belt that converts sound into patterns of vibrotactile stimulation. The alternative, currently under development, involves direct nerve stimulation by an electronic cochlear implant. At present, the best results enable recipients to monitor their own speech and sounds in their environment and thereby supplement their lip-reading ability, but speech comprehension without visual input is rarely possible.

Communication Training. There are four components to good communication training. First, the subject requires *information* concerning the cause of the hearing loss, the mechanism of any instrumental help and how to use it, and the aims and expectations of future management. Next, *skills* must be taught, both to use the aids and to improve speech discrimination and production. Third, *instrumental modification* will almost certainly be required at some stage after the initial fitting. Finally, *counseling* is indicated so that problems can be identified and perhaps solved or limitations recognized. Special needs may apply for those at school or in certain occupations.

Visual Impairment

Assessment

Visual impairment is most commonly caused by loss of central vision, which can be assessed by standard measures of visual acuity and color perception. Peripheral vision is assessed by formal perimetry using different sizes of target and intensities of illumination. Disorders of ocular motility seldom lead to visual impairment unless there is concomitant loss of acuity, as in strabismus. Neurophysiological techniques such as visual evoked potentials and electronystagmography are also available. Disorders of perception are usually assessed by tests of cognitive impairment.

Management

Visual Loss. The primary management aim in visual loss is the improvement or restoration of sight—for example, by refractive correction or cataract extraction, and the prevention of further deterioration. The secondary aim is to ensure the maximum use of residual vision with low-vision aids. These comprise magnifying devices of various sorts, ranging from a simple hand-held magnifying glass to closed-circuit television systems, depending on a person's leisure and occupational requirements. So far only limited success has been achieved by tactile vision substitution methods (Bach-y-Rita 1988).

Finally, psychological and environmental adjustments should be facilitated. Large-print books and typewriters, radio, and prerecorded "talking books" may be helpful communication aids (see Cochrane 1990). Braille can be taught, and dedicated writing and reading machines are available. For the newly impaired adult, intensive retraining including daily living skills will be required, with the use of mobility aids such as a white stick or a guide dog. Special advice and assistance may be needed about education, employment, and housing.

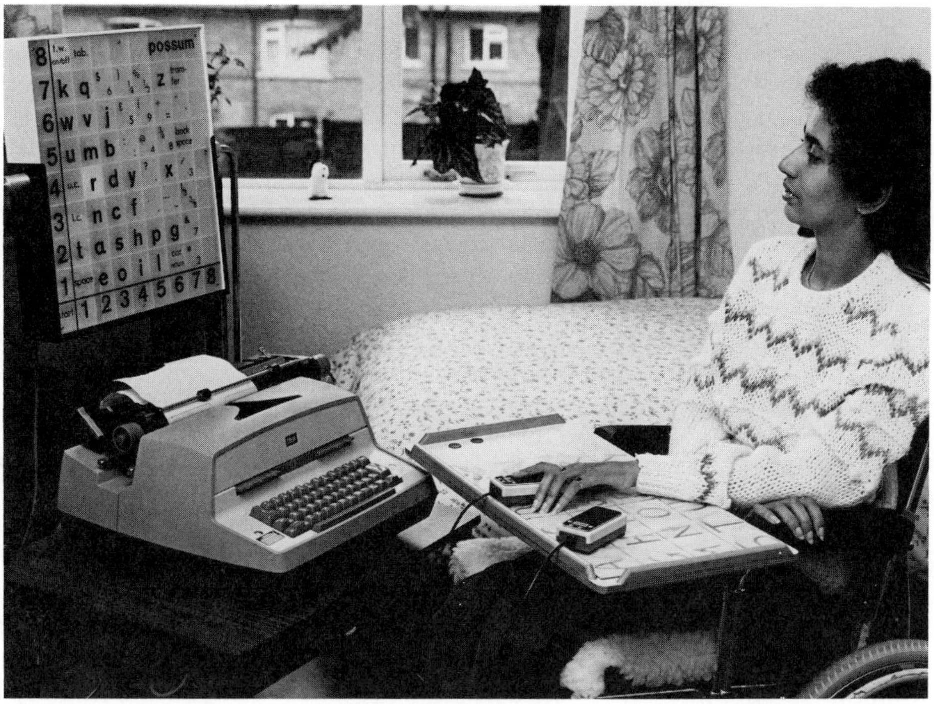

FIGURE 55.8 Typewriter control system. Possum GCTW12 scanning indicator panel operated by touch plate switches. Note the simple alphabet communication board on the wheelchair tray. (Courtesy of Possum Controls Ltd.)

Other Visual Impairments. Visual imperception is often very disabling, yet little is known about whether it is amenable to improvement. Visual agnosia may necessitate the use of alternative identification strategies, although it has been claimed that intensive visual discrimination training can improve agnosia and neglect and even shrink scotomata. Management of diplopia is often unrewarding, and alternate covering of each eye may be as effective as the results of spectacle prisms or surgery. The recent introduction of botulinum toxin injection into extraocular muscles appears to offer a promising, if temporary, alternative. Oscillopsia is usually resistant to treatment, despite trials of various drugs.

Swallowing and Nutrition

Assessment

There are numerous possible causes of difficulty in swallowing food or liquid, but some simple measures include body weight and general nutritional status, dietary and fluid intake, and the severity of any salivary dribbling. As with dysarthria, which often coexists, lip and palatal closure, chewing, and tongue movements should all be assessed to establish the underlying cause, a task for which speech therapists are specially trained. Direct observation of swallowing is essential and simple timed tests have been standardized (Nathadwarasala et al. 1992); videofluoroscopy may identify the presence of esophageal stricture, hiatus hernia, or cricopharyngeal spasm.

Management

Dysphagia. The management of dysphagia is well reviewed by Cochrane (1988). Simple counseling and advice regarding positioning, specific exercises, or changes in diet and swallow routine may be sufficient. Ice, either applied externally around the throat or sucked shortly before meals, is said to reduce bulbar spasticity and improve coordinated reflex activity in pseudobulbar palsy. Baclofen may be helpful in similar cases, whereas preprandial pyridostigmine has been advocated in lower motor neuron weakness. Various appliances designed to stimulate or effect palatal elevation have been tried, mainly in motor neuron disease.

For those prone to coughing and choking, specific advice should be given about size of meals, feeding more slowly, and improved bolus formation. Teflon injection of the vocal cords may produce firmer closure on adduction and prevent chronic aspiration. The indications for cricopharyngeal myotomy are controversial, even in the presence of spasm demonstrated on videofluoroscopy that results in pooling above that level.

Apart from the ethical implications of prolonging an inevitably fatal disease, the indications for alternative feeding methods are more widely agreed on and comprise:

1. Severe dehydration.
2. Frequent choking.
3. Inhalation pneumonia.
4. Progressive marked weight loss.
5. Exhaustion because of slow, laborious feeding.

Methods include feeding via small-bore nasogastric tubes, esophagostomy, jejunostomy, and gastrostomy. Gastrostomy can be done by passing a feeding tube percutaneously with the aid of an endoscope in an awake patient as well as by a formal surgical procedure under general anesthesia.

Drooling. Salivary dribbling is especially prominent in motor neuron disease and Parkinson's disease. About 2 liters of saliva are normally produced and automatically swallowed each day. Loss of automatic swallowing and of erect head posture is probably the most relevant factor and warrants specific counseling. Other interventions that are occasionally worthwhile include the use of portable suction apparatus, anticholinergic agents, palatal appliances, and, as a last resort, denervation or irradiation of the salivary glands.

Motor Impairments

Physicians are trained to differentiate motor impairments caused by weakness, spasticity, ataxia, bradykinesia, and various types of involuntary movement. However, it may be impossible to evaluate clinically the relative severity of two types of motor impairment in combination. Objective methods of assessment, where these exist, have usually been developed and standardized in those with one relatively isolated impairment, and cannot be used to diagnose or differentiate other types of motor disorder.

Most therapists and, indeed, neurologists attempt to grade each item on a simple semiquantitative (but nonlinear) scale from absent through mild and moderate to severe, with several arbitrary intermediate points defined. Some variability can be eliminated by testing under uniform conditions at consistent times of the day.

Weakness

Assessment

Neurogenic and Myopathic Weakness. Manual muscle testing provides a reasonably reliable clinical measure of muscle strength using the standard Medical Research Council (MRC) 0–5 scale but is imprecise and insensitive. More objective and relevant measurements can be obtained from dynamometers, static force gauges that measure muscle strength (maximum force) and isometric work (force-time integral). Many important factors influence strength testing, including attention and motivation of the subject, familiarity with the procedure, positioning, and the number and duration of repeated trials (Lennon and Ashburn 1993). Nevertheless, if these are taken into account, the results correlate well with functional disability and can be of great predictive value.

More elaborate techniques are required to measure the force of dynamic (isokinetic) contraction or to compare voluntary and electrically stimulated muscle contractions; they are not suitable at present for routine use. Attempts are also being made to quantify another common muscular symptom, fatigue. Dynamometers can be used to calculate indices based on the decrease in muscle strength either over time for a single sustained contraction or with repeated maximum efforts, and these may be useful in evaluating myasthenia.

Spastic Weakness. It is often not appreciated that the MRC scale was developed for assessing strength of individual muscles after peripheral nerve injury. In hemiplegia, individual muscles cannot be tested because their action cannot be separated from synergistic movements (mass action) related to abnormal muscle tone. This is the rationale for studying movement patterns (see the section on spasticity, to come). Other composite methods of motor assessment, such as the Motricity Index, are reviewed by Wade (1992) and De Neve et al. (1992).

Management. Exercises selected and supervised by physical therapists are the usual method for improving muscle strength and endurance after, for example, orthopedic trauma. This may work through collateral sprouting of the terminal fibers of intact motor nerves, and may be inappropriate in a degenerative condition like motor neuron disease. Methods include providing variable loading with springs, fixed loads with weights, or self-loading by the subject. Suspension devices and hydrotherapy can be used to allow exercise of very weak muscles with gravity eliminated. Disorders of neuromuscular transmission may respond to cholinesterase inhibition. The indications for FES remain controversial.

Spasticity

Assessment. Spasticity is recognized clinically by an increased resistance to passive movements, an inability to fractionate movement patterns, and inappropriate activity in antagonist muscles. Slow voluntary movement may occur in abnormal gross patterns, and involuntary reflex movements such as flexor spasms are seen. The patient may experience painful muscle cramps. Many diverse factors influence the level of spasticity, and extrapyramidal rigidity may coexist; thus, objective measurement is extremely difficult. Furthermore, the functional relevance of spasticity remains doubtful.

There is limited correlation between spasticity and various electrophysiological measures, such as amplitude and latency of the H and tonic stretch reflexes, and central motor conduction time. Biomechanical measurements of resistance of a body part to passive movement generally require complex apparatus, with the notable exception of the Wartenburg knee pendulum test, and in any case fail to take account of other variables such as joint contractures and muscle viscoelasticity.

Physical therapists have introduced a number of reliable and validated methods of bedside spasticity assessment (see Wade 1992; Glenn and Whyte 1990), mainly examining effects on normal voluntary movements. The Bobath method incorporates a qualitative judgment of ability to perform particular movements in isolation or in opposition to defined patterns of spasticity. The more quantitative Motor Club assessment, developed to follow the pattern of recovery after stroke, evaluates the ability to perform a series of normal movement patterns and also certain functional activities mainly relevant to physiotherapeutic goals.

Similar scales have been developed for the crude assessment of hypotonia in cerebellar disease and of extrapyramidal hypertonia or rigidity. Electromechanical measurement of torque during controlled displacement at a particular joint is certainly possible but so far of little practical value.

Management. The deficits of which patients with spasticity usually complain are the so-called negative symptoms of weakness, fatigability, and lack of dexterity. It is debatable whether specific treatment to reduce spasticity will improve such symptoms, although relief of positive symptoms such as fixed deformity and painful flexor spasms may be worthwhile. Moreover, spasticity may sometimes be beneficial—for example, by enabling a person to stand or even walk by virtue of extensor spasticity in the legs. The whole topic is reviewed by Glenn and Whyte (1990).

Prevention. Many factors known to make established spasticity worse may also provoke its development by increasing afferent input. The avoidance of nociceptive stimuli during the acute phase of cerebral or spinal cord injury, with scrupulous attention to care of the skin, bladder, and bowels, may minimize the eventual level of spasticity. In addition, proprioceptive facilitation in the early stages may be valuable by maintaining joint mobility and promoting the development of helpful extensor synergies.

Physical Measures. Nociceptive stimuli can make established spasticity markedly worse. These include bladder infections, fecal impaction, pressure sores, or even tight clothing, which should be avoided or removed. Patients must be educated accordingly. Various physical therapies have been advocated, of which the most effective seems to be prolonged stretching of spastic muscles. Apart from preventing contractures, this diminishes spasticity for hours afterward and can be done twice daily at home, whereas the application of ice during proprioceptive neuromuscular facilitation therapy gives only temporary benefit.

Drugs. Three drugs, each with a different mechanism of action, are widely used.

1. Benzodiazepines such as *diazepam* are believed to facilitate gamma-amino-butyric acid (GABA) neurotransmission and thus presynaptic inhibition of stretch reflexes. Diazepam is of greatest clinical value in those with spinal spasticity due to partial spinal cord lesions, provided drowsiness is tolerated. Well-known complications of chronic therapy exist.
2. *Baclofen* is an analog of GABA with both pre- and postsynaptic actions that inhibit alpha and gamma motor neurons. It is well tolerated, with few adverse effects, and often reduces spontaneous flexor spasms. It has also been administered intrathecally with some success for periods of a year or more via an implantable pump.
3. *Dantrolene* acts directly on muscle, inhibiting excitation-contraction coupling by depressing calcium release from the sarcoplasmic reticulum. Because of a high incidence of hepatic toxicity, liver function must be monitored regularly, but it may provide considerable relief from spasticity in some cases, occasionally in combination with baclofen when appropriate. Unlike diazepam, baclofen and dantrolene may also be of value in cases of spasticity following cerebral or complete cord lesions.

Other Chemical Measures. The judicious use of nerve or motor point blocks can be simple and effective provided the critical muscle can be identified by EMG. Injection of local anesthetic can be tried initially; if beneficial, ethanol or 5% phenol will produce a similar effect, lasting for several months. Motor point blocks are particularly useful in preventing deformity, since the muscle is effectively paralyzed, but function may also be improved. Nonselective infiltration of muscle and direct injection of one or more roots or peripheral nerves can also be done using the same techniques (Figure 55.9). Because of the risks of nonspecific damage, intrathecal neurolysis by injection of phenol around the cauda equina is usually restricted to relief of spasticity in those already incontinent or catheterized. Intramuscular injections of botulinum toxin are also being explored as a means of controlling spasticity.

Surgery. Surgical lengthening or division of soft tissues may offer a more radical solution if contractures are present. More invasive surgical procedures such as rhizotomy or cordectomy are rarely, if ever, justified, and electrical stimulation of dorsal columns or cerebellum via implanted electrodes is still undergoing evaluation.

Ataxia

Assessment. Apart from clinical rating scales applied to tests of coordination, balance, and gait (to be discussed), performed with eyes open and then closed, there are few objective methods of assessment (see Hardie 1993). Measurement of postural sway standing on electronic platforms with strain gauges, and accurate recording of limb movement using video or computerized tracking methods, are possible but may not correlate well with functional disability. Reliability is compromised because of the marked influence of fatigue and emotional stress on performance.

Management. Ataxia is often associated with progressive degenerative disease, and it is seldom possible to influence the underlying cause. Occasionally there are prospects for improvement if the impairment is secondary—for example, to hydrocephalus, acute infection, or trauma. Attempts at specific pharmacotherapy have been unrewarding despite

FIGURE 55.9 Methods of relieving spasticity.

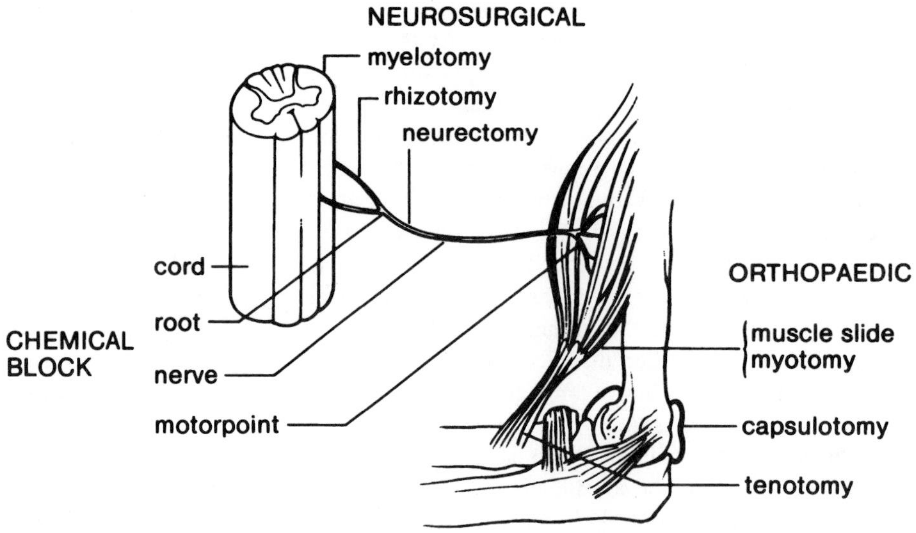

theoretical bases for clinical trials with agents such as 5-hydroxytryptophan, choline and lecithin, physostigmine, valproate, and thyrotrophin-releasing hormone.

There is a real danger that, because of frustration, sufferers will become unnecessarily inactive and dependent. Thus, simply preventing disuse may be helpful. In addition, formal retraining can be rewarding, using the following strategies:

1. The use of visual, kinesthetic, and conscious voluntary pathways to compensate should be encouraged.
2. Repeated practice of exercises of increasing complexity over a prolonged time is helpful in reinforcing experience-dependent plasticity of cerebellar neuronal networks.
3. Avoidance of fatigue and redevelopment of self-confidence can prevent the breakdown of compensation under stress.

Unfortunately success probably depends on intact sensory input and the ability to relearn motor coordination, and spinocerebellar syndromes are often resistant, especially if there is a coexistent neuropathy. In the upper limbs, simple flexion-extension movements are usually practiced before graduating to exercises against resistance and later introducing more complex and accurate actions. Other exercises that involve balancing and foot placement while walking or standing, perhaps using mirrors to improve body awareness, may help lower limb ataxia. Frenkel's exercises prescribe the performance of precise rhythmical movements repeatedly and with intense concentration, aided initially by having the patient count aloud; they can be used for upper and lower limbs or for reeducating specific functions. The use of EMG audiovisual feedback has also been advocated.

Tremor

Assessment. Clinical assessment of tremor is notoriously unreliable because of the diverse factors that influence its severity. Computerized accelerometry in one or more axes is now the standard technique for recording tremor because it is reliable, relatively simple, and readily acceptable to most patients. Spectral analysis may aid in making the distinction between certain tremor types and in measuring the amplitude of the dominant frequency peak and the total kinetic energy dissipated. Standardization can be achieved by automated analysis of average epochs recorded under controlled conditions—for example, in the course of drug trials (Elble and Koller 1990).

An objective reduction in tremor amplitude, however, may occur without any subjective or functional improvement; therefore, additional tests of motor performance as well as symptom self-rating scales are required. Theoretically, prolonged recording by telemetry is possible over several hours during normal everyday activities rather than under laboratory conditions, but the practical difficulties have so far prohibited this application in routine clinical trials.

Management. The specific management of disabling tremor is largely pharmacological and depends on the underlying cause (Elble and Koller 1990). Parkinsonian rest tremor may respond to standard antiparkinsonian agents, whereas postural tremor of any cause may respond to beta-adrenoceptor antagonists, alcohol, or primidone.

Drug treatment for action tremor associated with ataxia is unrewarding, because of resultant drowsiness and lack of convincing benefit. Weighting limbs with heavy bracelets or shoes to damp intention tremor is not usually helpful. Limited success has been reported with elbow orthoses that make feeding easier by increasing resistance to movement, but they are unacceptable for long-term wear. Adequate fixation of proximal joints, for instance by providing a raised table or armrests for elbow support, may achieve similar results.

In rare selected cases with predominantly unilateral tremor that causes severe disability and resists other therapy, stereotactic thalamotomy may be considered.

Akinesia

Assessment. Akinesia is a difficult concept to define and still harder to quantify. Reaction and movement times are commonly measured for subjects controlling a joystick during a computerized tracking task. The rate of repetition of alternating movements can be assessed—for example for finger tapping with a Morse key. The speed and precision of complex manual movements can also be recorded with sophisticated apparatus, but this procedure may be no more informative than simply timing with the aid of a stopwatch, pegboard tests, or other practical tasks like walking a fixed distance. There are no absolute normal values, and these tests can be used only to compare performances by the same subject.

Management. Akinesia in Parkinson's disease, unlike that in other extrapyramidal disorders, typically responds to appropriate medication. Very little is known about the value of other interventions, although limited studies of physical therapy have been disappointing.

Involuntary Movements

It is theoretically possible to make sophisticated recordings using neurophysiological and other techniques of involuntary movements such as chorea, dystonia, tics, and myoclonus. Unfortunately, the unpredictability and considerable variability of most dyskinesia have not encouraged the application of such methods. Most clinicians involved in treatment evaluation still use subjective rating scales completed by patient and examiner, supplemented by timed tests of those motor functions impaired by the dyskinesia. A variety of disease- or phenomenon-specific rating scales have been developed for clinical trial purposes (see Wade 1992). The reliability of subjective ratings may be improved by the use of audiovisual recordings for later analysis by independent assessors.

Sensory Impairments

Cutaneous and Proprioceptive Sensory Impairments

Assessment. Sensory modalities are traditionally divided into proprioception and the perception of vibration, light touch, pain, and temperature. Clinically it is often sufficient to classify each as intact, impaired, or absent in a particular region. In the case of peripheral neuropathies, the proximal extent of distal sensory loss correlates roughly with pathological severity.

More quantitative clinical methods are available, such as recording the frequency of errors on proprioceptive testing for a given angular displacement or the duration of perception of a standard vibrating tuning fork. Various instruments have been developed to permit quantitative sensory testing and are reviewed in a consensus statement by the Peripheral Neuropathy Association (1993). A biothesiometer allows more precise evaluation by providing a constant but adjustable amplitude of vibration. Thermal thresholds measured electronically for warming and cooling are reliable tests of unmyelinated and small myelinated nerve function, respectively. Somatosensory evoked potentials and nerve action potentials are reliable and reproducible and are the only methods entirely independent of subjective judgment.

Cutaneous sensation is most important over the palmar surface of the hand, but no single test is completely reliable. Two-point discrimination can be measured accurately with dividers or ridge devices provided application force is controlled, but light touch–deep pressure esthesiometry using graded monofilaments (for example, Semmes-Weinstein) may be more informative. Recognition times can also be recorded for various common objects placed in the hand or during the Seddon coin test.

Denervated skin will also have impaired vasomotor control and sweating, although this is usually largely attributable to loss of efferent sympathetic and parasympathetic neurons. Relevant tests of autonomic function include assessment of thermoregulatory sweating and the quantitative sudomotor axon reflex test.

Management. Management should be directed principally toward the underlying cause and the prevention of complications. These include mechanical and thermal injury, tissue autolysis from repeated stress leading to pressure sores, and neuropathic damage to bones and joints. Attempts at sensory reeducation have largely been confined to the hand. Limited bioengineering solutions to sensory substitution have been made (Bach-y-Rita 1988).

Dysesthesia and Pain

A detailed review of the assessment and management of pain is beyond the scope of this chapter; these topics are covered more extensively in Chapter 53 (see Wall and Melzack 1989).

MANAGEMENT OF OTHER GENERAL PROBLEMS

The WHO classification of disabilities is shown in Table 55.6.

Measurement of Disability

In the introduction to the previous section, the value of objective assessment of a restricted range of abilities by means of a reliable, valid, and sensitive scoring system was emphasized. In practice, it is often very difficult to measure directly the severity of restriction in performance of any activity, but it can be graded according to the following levels of intervention required:

1. *Substitution:* The activity cannot be performed even with aid.
2. *Supplementation:* The activity can be performed only with aid, including that of others.
3. *Enhancement:* The activity can be performed alone and unaided, but only with difficulty.

These categories are easy to define but rather too broad to be sensitive and are unequal in their scope. The ICIDH (World Health Organization 1980) proposes a more detailed severity scale that can be applied to most types of disability (Table 55.7). It may also be useful to assess the likely course of a person's disability. The ICIDH therefore includes an optional assessment of outlook (Table 55.8).

Each type of disability can be graded separately according to these two scales. In many cases, however, disabilities of one class correlate with those of another, with degree of personal independence, and indeed with overall level of handicap. A variety of specialized tests such as the Jebson Hand Function Tests and more composite scales have thus been developed to estimate global severity (Wade 1992). The most widely used are measures of activities of daily living (ADL) such as the Barthel Index (to be discussed), which assess each activity, usually on a three-point scale from independent through intermediate to dependent.

After World War II, the medical services of armed forces throughout the world perceived a need for quickly classifying and summarizing the medical problems of their servicemen. Most were based on variations of the mnemonic PULHHEEMS, and the current British Joint Service System of Medical Classification is one example (Table 55.9). A similar scale was developed by clinical researchers in the United States, based on the mnemonic PULSES (Physical; Upper limbs; Locomotion; the Sensory components, speech, vision, and hearing; Elimination; and Situational factors, both mental and emotional). As with the assessment of impairment, none of the existing disability or ADL scales are ideal, many have not been properly validated, and there is a danger of their proliferation without proper evaluation of those already in existence. This is one of the major deficiencies of much of the existing literature in the field of rehabilitation.

Table 55.6: International Classification of Impairments, Disabilities, and Handicaps classification of disabilities

1	Behavior disabilities
	Awareness disabilities (10–16)
	Disabilities in relations (17–19)
2	Communication disabilities
	Speaking disabilities (20–22)
	Listening (23–24)
	Seeing (25–27)
3	Personal care disabilities
	Excretion disabilities (30–32)
	Personal hygiene (33–34)
	Dressing (35–36)
	Feeding and other (37–39)
4	Locomotor disabilities
	Ambulation disabilities (40–45)
	Confining (46–47)
	Lifting (48)
5	Body disposition disabilities
	Domestic disabilities (50–51)
	Body movement (52–57)
	Postural (58)
6	Dexterity disabilities
	Daily activity disabilities (60–61)
	Manual activity (62–66)
	Foot control (67)
7	Situational disabilities
	Dependence and endurance disabilities (70–71)
	Environmental (72–77)
8	Particular skill disabilities
	Occupation-related disabilities
9	Other activity restrictions

Source: Reprinted with permission from World Health Organization. International Classification of Impairments, Disabilities, and Handicaps: A Manual of Classification Relating to the Consequences of Disease. Geneva: WHO, 1980.

Measurement of Handicap

The measurement of handicap is even more difficult, although the ICIDH has attempted to define scales for each of the dimensions listed previously. The ICIDH is reproduced in Table 55.10. Another attempt to analyze handicap has been based on the mnemonic ESCROW (Environment; Social interactions and dependence; Cluster of family members; Resources, financial; Outlook, psychological; Work, education), which has been combined with the Barthel Index and PULSES to form the Long-Range Evaluation System. Other instruments administered in questionnaire format include the General Health Questionnaire, the Nottingham Health Profile, and the Frenchay Activities Index (Wade 1992; Whiteneck et al. 1992). A useful measure is the SF-36, a "short form" 36-question test that takes 5–10 minutes to complete, which has been widely used in some countries (Ware 1993).

Doubt is often expressed about the validity of information gathered by these essentially subjective assessments. Their validation, however, is not an attempt to verify individual responses by some medical criteria but, rather, to establish that the instrument accurately expresses and estimates the subject's viewpoint. Evaluating quality of life

Table 55.7: International Classification of Impairments, Disabilities, and Handicaps severity scale of disability

0	Not disabled	—
1	Difficulty in performance	—
2	Aided performance	Only with physical aid or appliance, but without personal assistance
3	Assisted performance	Only with some help from another person, with or without aids
4	Dependent performance	Complete dependence on the presence of another person
5	Augmented ability	Achieved only in the presence of another person and either in a protected environment or with the helper him- or herself requiring an aid or special equipment
6	Complete inability	—

Source: Reprinted with permission from World Health Organization. International Classification of Impairments, Disabilities, and Handicaps: A Manual of Classification Relating to the Consequences of Disease. Geneva: WHO, 1980.

Table 55.8: International Classification of Impairments, Disabilities, and Handicaps outlook scale for disability

0	Not disabled
1	Recovery potential
2	Improvement potential
3	Assistance potential
4	Stable disability
5	Amelioration potential
6	Deteriorating disability

Source: Reprinted with permission from World Health Organization. International Classification of Impairments, Disabilities, and Handicaps: A Manual of Classification Relating to the Consequences of Disease. Geneva: WHO, 1980.

Table 55.9: British Joint Service System of Medical Classification (PULHHEEMS)

P	Physical capacity
U	Upper limbs
L	Locomotion, lower limbs
HH	Hearing (right, left)
EE	Eyesight (right, left)
M	Mental capacity
S	Stability (emotional)

is increasingly relevant in the measurement of outcome after medical intervention (Kinney and Boyle 1992).

Behavioral Disabilities

Behavior refers to a person's awareness and ability to conduct him- or herself, both in everyday activities and toward others, and includes the ability to learn. Disabilities may result from intellectual or other psychological impairments affecting consciousness, attention, emotion, volition, and normal behavior patterns. In most cases there will be a combination of impairments, the severity of which may not correlate with the degree of behavior disorder. A wide range of phenomena are included, from actively difficult behavior that is aggressive, disinhibited, and antisocial, to negative disturbances of self-awareness, mood, motivation, learning, personal safety, and the like. Individual items can be highlighted by using a checklist, but they are extremely hard to measure.

Although some of the features may not be the result of neurological disease at all, treatment of any underlying condition must be the first priority. Psychotropic drugs may also be indicated for any affective or psychotic disorder. Those with cerebral disorders may be unduly sensitive to unwanted effects, however, and, particularly after severe brain injury, the use of behavior modification techniques may be preferable. These include positive social reinforcement, contingent punishment and use of time out, overcorrection, and massed practice. For best results, essential requirements are for regular trained staff and the availability of plenty of alternative activities to replace undesirable ones; in practice, a separate special nursing unit is needed. This philosophy deliberately ignores the underlying emotional and social factors, and it may be necessary to address these specifically.

Personal Care Disabilities

Assessment

Certain ADLs are universally recognized, yet their assessment is subjective, with poor reliability and reproducibility. Some ADL assessment scales are better than others. The Barthel Index mentioned earlier has been validated and is fairly widely used (Table 55.11). Unfortunately, because the index does not consider traveling out of doors, cooking, or communication, an aphasic person incapable of independent living could still theoretically score 100%. Accordingly, it is desirable to incorporate specific measurement of various individual functions such as mobility (to be discussed) and use of the upper limb. The Frenchay Arm Tests and nine-hole peg test are examples of the latter (see Wade 1992).

Management

One interesting notion is that of learned disuse—for example, affecting the upper limb following a stroke. An old-fashioned remedy involved tying the good limb down,

Table 55.10: International Classification of Impairments, Disabilities, and Handicaps classification of handicap

1	Orientation handicap
2	Physical independence handicap
3	Mobility handicap
4	Occupation handicap
5	Social integration handicap
6	Economic self-sufficiency handicap
7	Other
Physical independence handicap	
20	Fully independent
21	Aided independence
22	Adapted independence
23	Situational dependence
24	Long-interval dependence
25	Short-interval dependence
26	Critical-care dependence
27	Special-care dependence
28	Intensive-care dependence
Mobility handicap	
30	Fully mobile
31	Variable restriction of mobility
32	Impaired mobility
33	Reduced mobility
34	Neighborhood restriction
35	Dwelling restriction
36	Room restriction
37	Chair restriction
38	Total restriction of mobility

Source: Reprinted with permission from World Health Organization. International Classification of Impairments, Disabilities, and Handicaps: A Manual of Classification Relating to the Consequences of Disease. Geneva: WHO, 1980.

Table 55.11: The modified Barthel activities of daily living index

Bowels	
0	Incontinent or needs enemata
1	Occasional accident
2	Continent
Bladder	
0	Incontinent or catheterized
1	Occasional accident
2	Continent for >7 days
Grooming	
0	Needs help with personal care
1	Independent with aids if necessary
Toilet use	
0	Dependent
1	Needs some help
2	Fully independent
Feeding	
0	Unable
1	Needs help
2	Independent
Transfers	
0	Unable, no sitting balance
1	Major help (one or two people, physical); can sit
2	Minor help (verbal or physical)
3	Independent
Mobility	
0	Immobile
1	Wheelchair-independent
2	Walks with help of one person
3	Independent, with aids if necessary
Dressing	
0	Dependent
1	Needs help
2	Independent
Stairs	
0	Unable
1	Needs help
2	Independent
Bathing	
0	Dependent
1	Independent
Total = 0–20	

Note: Interpretation of score (DT Wade. Measurement in Neurological Rehabilitation. Oxford, England: Oxford University Press, 1992): 0–4 = very severely disabled; 5–9 = severely disabled; 10–14 = moderately disabled; 15–19 = mildly disabled; 20 = physically independent, but not necessarily normal or socially independent.

forcing the person at least to attempt activities with the impaired limb. Although this may now be regarded as an unethical strategy even to test, there are theoretical grounds to encourage intensive exercise. An activity monitor adapted from a simple pedometer can be strapped to a limb to measure actual spontaneous usage.

Occupational therapy is almost exclusively concerned with improving ADL. If prospects for recovery are poor, or just as a temporary measure, supplementation or substitution methods may be indicated. Adapted cutlery, altered clothing, and dressing and bath aids may be sufficient. Functional orthoses such as spring-assisted wrist and finger splints not only correct deformity but also counter weakness and increase the range of controlled motion. Surgical procedures, mainly to the hand, may occasionally be beneficial to correct unsightly deformity or restore some useful grip. Best results are achieved in cases of static disability following nerve or plexus injury rather than in progressive polyneuropathies or cases involving spastic upper limbs.

Balanced forearm supports or foot-operated manipulators can compensate for lost abilities. An extensive range of technical equipment can preserve independence in the face of progressive or severe disability. Complete environmental control systems will release door locks and provide access to telephone and other communication, computers, and domestic appliances (Cochrane 1990). These can be activated by voice or by switches using any residual motor function, as described earlier for communication aids.

Table 55.12: Functional ambulation categories

0	Nonfunctional	Cannot walk, or requires help of two people
1	Dependent—level 2	Requires firm continuous support from one person
2	Dependent—level 1	Requires intermittent support for balance
3	Dependent—supervision	Needs verbal or standby help only
4	Independent—on flat ground	Needs help on stairs, slopes, and so on
5	Independent	Can walk independently anywhere

Mobility

Walking

Assessment. There is little excuse for the failure of doctors and therapists to evaluate mobility objectively in every disabled person. Simple walking speed, measured over a set distance (e.g., 10 meters) with a stopwatch, is probably adequate. Normal results depend on age, but most normal adults walk faster than 1 m/second (Wade 1992). Though not always very reproducible, this is a useful if crude measure of overall disability, particularly in neuromuscular disorders and parkinsonism. Exercise tolerance can be assessed with a 6-minute walk test, and both measures can be combined with step counts to calculate average stride length.

Also desirable is a descriptive classification of mobility based on safety and assistance required, such as the functional ambulation categories (Table 55.12). This should be combined with a record of the aid or aids actually used.

More quantitative gait analysis is required in the complex field of prosthetic and orthotic design and prescription. Temporal and spatial parameters of gait, including stride time, swing time, stride length, velocity, and cadence (step frequency), can be recorded using pressure-sensitive mats, and most gait laboratories use polarized light goniometry or more sophisticated computerized kinematic analysis of movement of the limbs and trunk. More detailed kinetic and ergonomic data can also be obtained.

Management. Before appropriate therapy can be selected, it is first necessary to identify the cause of locomotor disability. In cases with ataxia or parkinsonism, simple gait training may be all that can be offered, together with provision of walking aids ranging from one or two canes through tripods or elbow crutches to walking frames with or without wheels. The choice of aid depends on the patient's balance and weight-bearing limitations.

Following acute hemiplegia, patients should practice pregait activities in bed or on a mat until they can turn over and sit unsupported. Thereafter, although walking aids are used initially, they may promote dependence on the unaffected side, so personal assistance is preferable. Similarly, in other conditions, during or after a prolonged period of confinement to bed, preliminary use of a tilting table and later of a standing frame may be indicated.

If focal weakness or joint instability is present, an orthosis may be helpful. In cases of common peroneal nerve palsy or peripheral neuropathy causing flaccid footdrop, dorsiflexion can be assisted by a simple flexible molded polypropylene AFO or one with a single medial metal upright and sprung-piston ankle joint fitted to the shoe. The former is lighter and more cosmetic, but may not be tolerated because of intermittent edema, hyperpathia, or excessive heat and sweating. Tendon transfer of intact tibialis posterior can also produce active dorsiflexion.

Where spasticity causes equinovarus deformity, treatment directed toward the specific impairment can be supplemented with a rigid AFO with double pistons to resist both active plantar flexion and excessive dorsiflexion. Both medial and lateral metal uprights are needed to control twisting of the foot, although a molded polypropylene AFO may be sufficient if spasticity is not severe (Glenn and Whyte 1990).

Spastic weakness around the knee and ankle joints could theoretically be counteracted by a full-length KAFO, but their weight, along with the commonly associated sensory loss and weakness of hip flexion, may prevent effective walking. Most knee control problems respond to an appropriately selected rigid AFO, but occasionally knee bracing with a local KO is indicated to control hyperextension. Surgical intervention is seldom worthwhile in spastic gait disorders.

Paraplegic Locomotion

Flaccid paraplegia due to spinal cord injury or poliomyelitis has been the subject of much research in bioengineering (see Hochschuler et al. 1993). Swing-through gait using a rigid HKAFO and crutches is tiring and ungainly, but those with low lesions at the level of the conus or cauda equina can learn to walk reasonably efficiently with metal KAFOs. For higher lesions, reciprocal gait may be possible with one of two alternative devices that brace the body from midtrunk to the feet and immobilize the knees and ankles while allowing the hips to flex and extend but not to adduct.

The reciprocating gait orthosis, developed in North America, is worn under clothing; the plastic foot section fits inside the shoes. Cables link the two hip joints so that ipsilateral extension causes contralateral flexion. The hip guidance orthosis was developed in Oswestry, England, and is much heavier. The shoes fit onto metal plates with rocker soles, and the hip joints move freely between flexion and extension stops. Though originally worn outside clothing, the hip guidance orthosis can be accommodated beneath a loose-fitting track suit. Both orthoses are easy to don and doff and are designed to be worn all day. The hips and knees can be released in flexion so that the patient may sit down.

Both the reciprocating gait and hip guidance orthoses can be used with crutches or a rollator by which the arms move the trunk forward. When the patient leans either sideways or diagonally forward, one leg is lifted off the ground and swings forward with gravity; adduction is controlled to prevent it catching behind the trailing leg. Body weight can then be transferred onto the leading leg and the trunk advanced further; in due course the other leg is then swung through. The resulting gait looks much more normal than swing-through gait, and vertical excursions of the center of gravity are reduced, making it much less fatiguing.

As a general rule, greater difficulty will be experienced and the gait will be less satisfactory with either brace for higher spinal lesions. Latissimus dorsi is most important for forward propulsion and must be of reasonable strength, but triceps strength, wrist control, and hand grip are important as well. Trunk stability is also necessary, particularly for the hip guidance orthosis, and determination on the part of the patient is no less important for ultimate success.

FES has been studied in a number of centers. The main technical problems are providing adequate electrical stimulation, developing sensitive control mechanisms, and protecting the patient in the event of system or power failure. Muscle atrophy and fatigue present additional physiological limitations, and FES remains only a theoretical solution. Nevertheless, hybrid systems combining FES with the reciprocating gait or hip guidance orthosis have given promising results in preliminary evaluations and currently may be a more realistic approach.

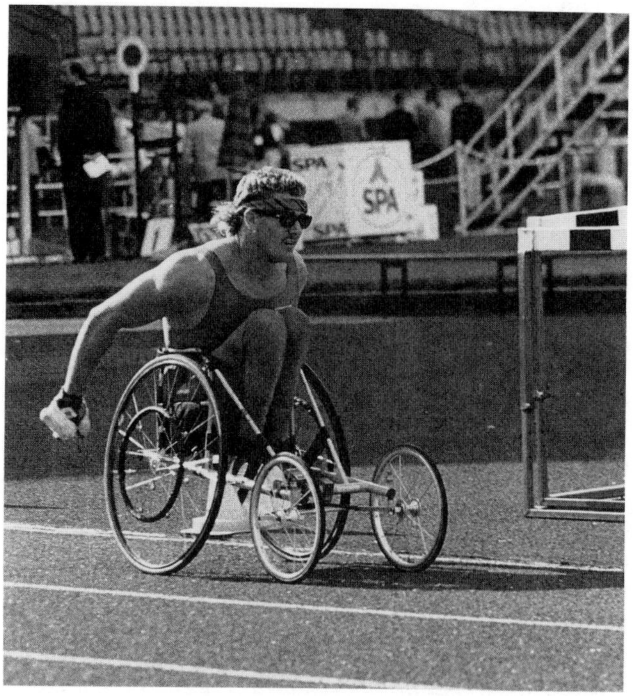

FIGURE 55.10 Chris Hallam, M.B.E., the British Paralympic athlete, in the high-performance Bromakin racing wheelchair. (Courtesy of Bromakin Wheelchairs Ltd.)

Wheelchairs

A wheelchair is by far the most practical means of mobility for most paralyzed people, and certainly for those with severe coordination and balance impairments. It is fast and easy to use, at a low energy cost, with little risk of falling; it also leaves the hands free. The hazards include pressure sores, contractures and osteoporosis, impairment of ventilation and elimination, stigma, and considerable mobility handicap. For these reasons, any decision regarding long-term wheelchair dependence must be carefully weighed and alternative options evaluated. Neurologists should be conversant with the principles of selecting wheelchairs and seating arrangements; nonspecialists will be unfamiliar with the particular needs of the neurologically disabled, and genuine opportunities may not be realized.

Some wheelchairs are designed for outdoor use only, by those who are less severely disabled. Different types of chairs are propelled by an attendant, by the occupant (with one or both arms), or by battery power, according to need (Cochrane 1993). Some are even designed for Olympic athletes (Figure 55.10).

The choice of design for indoor and outdoor use is even more critical, since the occupant may spend most of each day in the chair. Positioning for comfort and for different activities, dimensional compatibility between body and chair, ease of transfer to and from the chair, and whether the chair should be light and capable of folding up for transport by car must all be considered. Numerous special features and accessories are available, including special arm and leg rests, adjustable reclining back rests, and elevating mechanisms to bring the occupant into an upright position. A head rest with additional support can be fitted for those with poor head control.

Careful attention must be paid to the seating itself. Seat sag, which is almost universal once a chair has been used for some time, must be eliminated. The density of a foam seat cushion should be selected according to body weight, and the seat cushion can be covered with polyvinyl chloride or sheepskin. Additional cushions will provide lumbar support or prevent slumping to one side. For those at high risk of pressure sores, special gel- or air-support seating systems are essential and must be checked regularly. A special seat molded from a matrix or thermoplastic material will provide total support for those with severe deformity.

Transfers

To remain independent, a wheelchair user must be taught and must practice techniques for transferring in and out of the chair at the same level, and also ideally to and from ground level. Others with impaired mobility may also have difficulty with transfers to crucial areas such as bed, bath, toilet, armchair, and car. Standing may be facilitated by raised or spring-loaded seats and beds, pulley systems, and strategically placed grab rails. The stand-pivot technique can be taught to caregivers and staff to facilitate safe transfers without strain. Sliding boards ease sitting transfers. Alternatively, there are substitution methods using an appropriate hoist and sling system (Tarling and Stowe 1988).

Free access within the home is extremely important. A stairlift may be required, sometimes with an extra indoor wheelchair for use upstairs. Other options include ground-floor alterations to provide sleeping accommodation and shower and toilet facilities on one level. Some patients need to be rehoused.

Car Driving for the Disabled

Though taken for granted by able-bodied people, the ability to drive a car may be critical in allowing a disabled person to maintain employment, social contacts, and leisure interests. Public transportation is often inaccessible or hazardous, and there are few who cannot be enabled by modern technology to drive provided they have the necessary cognitive and sensory skills (Goodwill 1988). Even low-level tetraplegics can drive using full hand controls and power-assisted steering and braking. Inability to get a wheelchair in and out of the car independently can be overcome by the use of car-top hoists or even custom-built vans that admit the whole chair.

Regrettably, these tremendous advances have so far not been fully exploited, partly through ignorance on the part of professionals. Severely disabled people may simply assume that driving is beyond their capabilities, and no one may disabuse them of this notion. The opportunity for referral to a specialized assessment center should be offered to all disabled people.

Incontinence and Sexual Dysfunction

These topics are dealt with in Chapter 45 on neurourology.

Skeletal Deformity

Scoliosis occurs in any condition that causes weakness of the paraspinal musculature early in life, such as congenital spina bifida, cord injury, progressive muscular dystrophies, and certain hereditary ataxias and neuropathies. Resulting complications include respiratory impairment, loss of sitting balance, seating problems, and risk of pressure sores. In severe cases, correction by extensive surgical instrumentation and fusion of the spine may be indicated (see Hochschuler et al. 1993).

Preventive bracing and regular physical therapy from an early stage can probably delay the development of scoliosis, which can be followed by conventional radiography.

Spinal curvature occurs less commonly in adults with neuromuscular weakness, but prophylactic measures are still imperative, particularly in those confined to a wheelchair. Posture and seating arrangements should be optimal, exercises encouraged, and regular periods spent in the upright position using a stand-up chair or a standing frame if necessary.

Cardiorespiratory Impairment

Respiratory impairment may arise either acutely, in infections like poliomyelitis or botulism, in Guillain-Barré syndrome, and in acute lesions of the medulla or high cervical cord; from chronic neuromuscular weakness affecting the diaphragm and intercostal muscles, such as motor neuron disease and particularly the conditions mentioned earlier that are associated with scoliosis and thus with additional mechanical disadvantage; and intermittently—for example, in myasthenia gravis and sleep apnea syndrome.

Management comprises standard measures, including protection of the airway (see also the section on swallowing and nutrition earlier in this chapter), physical therapy, and assisted ventilation. Though less commonly than in the days of polio epidemics, occasional patients require major long-term support in the community with such devices as a rocking bed, a negative pressure cuirass, or an abdominal pneumobelt. As with other disabilities, technological advances are continually being made, and those unfortunate people for whom chronic respiratory support is vital may still be capable of reasonably independent living.

Cardiomyopathy occurs in various neurological disorders, including Friedreich's ataxia; muscular dystrophies such as Duchenne's, scapuloperoneal, and myotonic; mitochondrial cytopathies; and polymyositis. In the latter two conditions, conduction defects may necessitate insertion of a pacemaker, but otherwise treatment is essentially symptomatic to relieve heart failure.

Tissue Viability

The concept of tissue viability highlights the need for comprehensive 24-hour care of the disabled patient as a whole, both internally and externally (Robertson et al. 1988). The majority of the complications of immobility, including infections, thrombosis, and osteoporosis, can be guarded against even in the advanced stages of progressive neurological diseases. The failure to provide adequate care is most clearly revealed by the loss of viability of skin and subcutaneous tissue, which allows the development of pressure sores.

Traditionally, pressure sores were regarded as indicative of poor nursing care, but the responsibility is shared far more widely among all members of the disability team. In the case of, for example, young paraplegics following traumatic spinal cord injury, it rightly extends to the patients themselves, who must be taught to be obsessive about care of the perineum and feet and avoidance of friction and thermal burns to numb skin.

Immobility alters the skin microclimate: It increases temperature, humidity, and pressure loading, reduces ventilation, and distorts the skin. Incontinence, sensory loss, local tissue atrophy, and poor nutrition contribute to these adverse effects. Friction causes superficial damage, but shear forces are particularly dangerous to subcutaneous structures and adjacent blood supply, resulting in deep, intractable sores.

It is possible to measure some parameters of tissue viability with instruments such as interface pressure sensors and transcutaneous oximeters, and with thermoscanning, but a clinically based risk-scoring system like the Norton score is just as valuable (see Robertson et al. 1988). Prevention is fundamental to the management of pressure sores, and all risk factors must be corrected wherever possible. Once a wound is established, however, dressing materials and additives must be selected carefully and surgical intervention readily considered. There is a strong case for having agreed-on policies and specialist teams for the management of pressure sores, if professional pride and ignorance are not to interfere with optimal care (Royal College of Physicians 1986).

Occupational, Social, and Economic Handicaps

Handicap was defined earlier as an individual disadvantage, resulting from impairment or disability, that limits or prevents fulfillment of a normal role function. Mobility or physical independence handicaps are most clearly relevant to medical management, but other dimensions should not be ignored (Whiteneck et al. 1992; Ware 1993).

The adverse socioeconomic climate has already been described. Poor quality of life correlates with the size of the gap between a person's achieved and unmet needs and desires regarding not only cognitive and physical well-being but also material and social well-being. Although the latter are generally considered to be beyond the concern of health services, improved accommodation or getting a person back to work may offer better solutions to certain disability problems than conventional medical remedies. Physicians should have the ability and readiness to identify such solutions and initiate their implementation.

Occupational Handicap

Employment is a basic human need, one that is often essential for full social integration and economic self-sufficiency. Regrettably, adult unemployment is commonplace in many societies, and the disabled are far more likely than others to suffer disadvantage. Even someone returning to the employment market fully recovered after illness or injury will find it difficult to get a job. The implications are more serious for those with residual or progressive disability, who may need to acquire new skills to enable their resettlement in a new occupation. Employment guidance and rehabilitation or opportunities for appropriate further education should be available to all disabled people who want to work.

Given special provisions and sufficient goodwill, severe disability need not preclude gainful employment. Those who are blind or deaf and those confined to home or wheelchair can all be catered to. Even those unsuitable for sheltered employment have basic occupational needs—for example, to perform domestic tasks and recreational activities—that must be recognized.

Social Integration Handicap

A further basic human need is to participate in and maintain customary social relationships. Those with mobility handicaps are particularly unlikely to make casual acquaintances, resulting in a diminishing circle of contacts with family, close friends, neighbors, and (if employed) colleagues. Other factors include lack of social skills, embarrassment concerning self-image and disfigurement, and behavioral disabilities. Within a person's social interactions, role functions are adopted such as spouse, parent, breadwinner, member of a committee or sports team, and so forth. These may be seriously disrupted by illness and disability.

Economic Self-Sufficiency Handicap

Adequate financial resources are necessary to sustain both personal independence and other family members as well. An extensive U.K. disability survey (Martin and White 1988) demonstrated that disabled adults had on average lower incomes than the rest of the population; they were less likely to have a job and, if they were employed, were likely to earn less than adults in general. State disability benefits went some way toward compensating for lower incomes. However, the majority incurred extra expenditure as a consequence of being disabled, the amount of which was related to the nature and severity of their disability, and their standards of living were lower overall.

Preparation for Dying

The hospice movement has helped to bring about a welcome change in professional attitudes toward death and bereavement. The whole issue is especially relevant in rapidly progressive conditions like motor neuron disease and Duchenne's muscular dystrophy, but it is seldom far from the surface in the minds of young and old alike with inexorable deterioration caused by multiple sclerosis, Friedreich's ataxia, and Parkinson's disease.

Most patients have insight into what is happening, and they and their families usually welcome discussion of the illness through to its conclusion. When death is recognized as inevitable, their wishes and dignity must be respected. Maximum support should be made available to those who wish to be nursed at home. Although physicians are inclined to regard a patient's death as a mark of failure, Cochrane counsels as follows: "A benevolent conspiracy [of silence] is unnecessary. Unwelcome information should not be pressed but, strangely, frankness does not extinguish hope and information that is required should not be denied.

"Just as important, a doctor has no ethical, legal or moral obligation to prolong the distress of a dying person" (Cochrane 1988, pp. 94–95).

DISABILITY SERVICES

Service Planning

Primary Prevention

It is axiomatic that prevention is better than cure. National health and social policies exist to protect the community against environmental hazards such as pollution, accidental injury, epidemic infections, and tobacco and drug abuse. Rather less consistent policies are directed at individuals at risk of disablement—for example, genetic counseling and health screening programs with prophylactic measures where appropriate.

Health promotion is a complementary approach but is usually directed mainly toward prevention of disease rather than of handicap. Thus, most governments have well-developed policies concerning healthful eating and life-styles, effective family planning and prenatal care, and neonatal screening and immunizations. Despite the efforts of the WHO, disabled people still experience handicap almost universally as a consequence of social attitudes, lack of educational and employment opportunities, and isolation because of urban design and transport policies. The dismantling of these formidable barriers would make professional disability management much easier (Pope and Tarlov 1991).

Forecast of Needs

Effective planning requires accurate forecasting. At present most health service provision is demand-led, and the loudest demands are made by essentially able-bodied people who want ready access to primary health care and acute hospital services. Some attempts are now being made to define priority groups and estimate their needs, but there is an astounding lack of information regarding the prevalence and severity of most types of physical disability and of specific neurological diseases in the community. These data are not just of academic interest but are of pivotal importance in service planning.

Furthermore, descriptive survey statistics are themselves inadequate because the picture is constantly changing. Demographic trends and public expectations must be taken into account, along with changes in incidence of infectious diseases (contrast encephalitis lethargica, syphilis, tuberculosis, and acquired immune deficiency syndrome) and types of trauma (traffic accidents and missile injuries). It may not be possible to anticipate the impact of imminent technological advances, but developments in transplant surgery and bioengineering will surely improve the outlook for the neurologically disabled in the future.

Providing Access to Appropriate Services

Having assessed the needs in a given population or community, it is necessary to match them with the appropriate services. Once services are established, the availability of access is critical. This is determined by dissemination of information about the service and by the vagaries of professional referral patterns. If primary health care or hospital staff do not know about their local specialist wheelchair clinic, for example, they will certainly not refer people to it. Regrettably, for various reasons they may not make good use of such specialized services even if they do know about them.

If professionals, and particularly the public, are made more aware of the problems affecting disabled people and of the services that provide help, then access will be improved. Ideally, however, it is necessary to monitor access to disability services to ensure that they reach all who are likely to benefit.

Effective Management

The importance of effective management of individual cases and problems by the multidisciplinary team has already been emphasized. An overview is also necessary if the needs of a whole community are to be met. Formal lines of communication and patterns of referral should be agreed on (see Figure 55.3) and consideration given to the use of standardized problem-oriented medical records. Those with chronic illness invariably have bulging, disorganized hospital case notes; the application of information technology such as the use of patient "smart cards" (credit cards encoding full clinical details for reading by desktop microcomputer) could facilitate retrieval of regular assessment data and greatly improve individual case management.

Standards of Care

Despite the enormous cost of providing health and social services to the neurologically disabled, there have been few attempts to agree on minimum standards of care. Consequently, it is not possible either to allocate resources rationally or to mount a strong case against their inadequacy. It should be a relatively simple matter for professional groups to recommend such standards for both specific diseases and generic services.

One example that has grown out of the need to monitor use of health insurance payments to private hospitals in the United States is the Commission on Accreditation of Rehabilitation Facilities. This body has stipulated standards for all aspects of care for those establishments wishing to care for certain types of patients. Details are recommended: minimum floor area per person for sleeping accommodation and treatment areas, level of provision of washing facilities, desirable staffing ratios, availability of specialist counselors, and the like. Clinical and other management procedures are also considered, including an ongoing system of outcome evaluation.

The Royal College of Physicians (1986, 1990) in the United Kingdom has suggested certain basic professional standards and levels of provision in many fields of disability. These standards, once established, could be used as the basis for clinical audit, by which the quality of disability services could be judged.

Cost Analysis

In the earlier discussion on ethical issues, reference was made to the concept of justice not only in the moral and legal sense, but also in the sense of fair distribution of resources. The costs of disability management may be direct or indirect, both to society and to the individual, and can be assessed in a number of ways (Robinson 1993). As an illustration, the topical debate concerning intracerebral tissue transplantation for Parkinson's disease will be considered.

Cost-benefit analysis asks whether the expense of the surgical procedure and all the attendant costs are justified by the benefit to the individual patient. Of course, it is almost impossible to identify the variables on the benefit side of the equation and still less possible to evaluate them. Nevertheless, if a very disabled person undergoes a transplant and is then able to discontinue antiparkinsonian medication, the costs may appear justified.

Cost-effectiveness analysis examines which of several alternatives is the most effective using limited resources. It also takes into account the element of justice in health care by introducing the concept of equality of outcome for groups. Thus, clinical trials of surgery would have to show more favorable postoperative benefit per unit cost than continued medical management.

Even wider issues are included by cost-utility analysis, which considers how a procedure affects both length and quality of life. It is debatable whether quality of life can indeed be measured, but utility analysis takes more fully into account the dimensions of handicap. If transplantation was almost curative but remained very expensive, could society afford to operate on large numbers of elderly patients with Parkinson's disease, or should the procedure be restricted to the few younger patients with years of productive employment ahead of them? Alternatively, the same money might more properly be spent on improvements in health care delivery to both groups.

The utilitarian approach remains more in the realm of philosophy than of neurology. As financial constraints will inevitably increase, however, such difficult matters will have to be addressed. Doctors can no longer demand complete clinical freedom to treat each patient as they deem right, without regard to their wider responsibility to the community in which they work. Social justice demands not only that they not devote excessive resources to individual patients, but that they identify and attend to the needs of the others. Purchasers of health care, whether statutory or insurance-funded, are intruding increasingly in decisions formerly regarded as the clinician's exclusive prerogative concerning admission to or continuation of a rehabilitation treatment program.

Generic Services

The Royal College of Physicians (1986) identified fifteen areas in which services were likely to be used by a variety of disabled people but were not necessarily the responsibility of one particular specialty. Most of these have already been considered in this chapter; they include communication aids, wheelchairs, driving for the disabled, sexual counseling, orthotics, pressure sores, and visual and hearing impairment. The importance of urinary continence and of stoma care services was also emphasized, together with a few other areas that warrant brief mention.

Independent or Disabled Living Centers

Regional independent or disabled living centers have been established in a number of countries and have proved very popular among both clients and professionals (Chamberlain and Gallop 1988). They are analogous to supermarkets, in which the wares are all displayed and available for close inspection before any purchase need be made; they allow the consumers far greater freedom of choice than exists if a therapist simply orders an appliance from a catalogue. Disabled living centers have two principal functions: (1) to permanently exhibit a comprehensive selection from among the thousands of available aids and items of equipment, with a supporting information service; and (2) to act as an educational service for staff, volunteers, and the disabled alike.

In the United States, they are often found as part of a more comprehensive community-based independent living program linked with other services such as vocational and employment, advocacy, and independent living skills training.

Housing, Housing Modifications, and Rehousing

Most national health policies accept the premise, argued forcefully by the independent living movement founded in the United States, of caring for disabled persons, even the severely disabled, within the community rather than in institutions (Tully 1986). Regrettably, lack suitable accommodation often prolongs hospitalization, especially for newly disabled people. Although modifications to an existing dwelling may avoid the need for rehousing, arrangements for both require efficient liaison between the relevant authorities to avoid bureaucratic delays.

The Physically Disabled School Leaver

There is a dangerous passage between the relatively sheltered waters of disabled children, who are the responsibility of statutory school medical and community pediatric services, and the open seas of adult disability. During this transition, continuity of care with respect to medical care, employment, and social services is important, yet is often lacking (Bax et al. 1988; Beardshaw 1988).

Support Services for Younger Severely Disabled People

Concerted attempts to improve community support services for the elderly have left a relative vacuum for those aged 16–64 years. Provision of community therapist and nursing services, volunteer care assistants, day centers, and other facilities may sustain this large group, most of whom have neurological disorders (Figure 55.11), when residential care would be the only alternative (Harrison 1987).

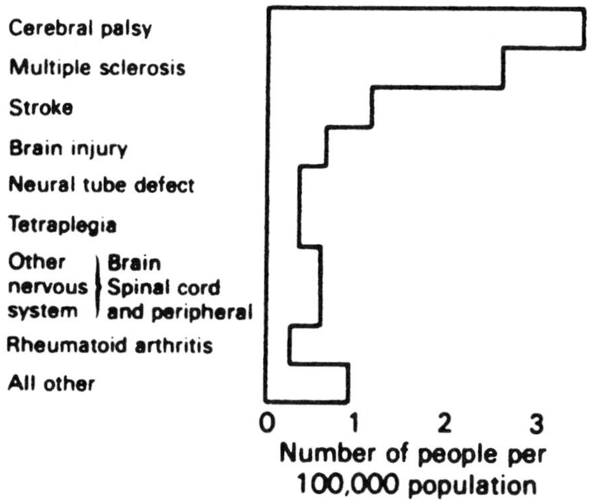

FIGURE 55.11 Medical diagnoses among patients and residents in homes and units for younger physically disabled people. (Reprinted with permission from J Harrison. Severe Physical Disability: Responses to the Challenge of Care. London: Cassell, 1987.)

Disease-Specific Services

The history of services devoted to the care of spinal injuries has already been related and is perhaps still the best example of a field in which standards of care have already been established (American Spinal Injury Association 1992) and implemented in centers of excellence around the world. Because of the complexity of impairments following head injury, care of its victims has failed to develop fully along similar lines despite successful experiments in a few places.

Nevertheless, there is a compelling case favoring the establishment of integrated multidisciplinary services for the management of neurologically disabled people. Where prevalence is high and the needs are great, it may be advantageous to dedicate resources to specific conditions, although drawbacks also exist. Only in the rehabilitation of stroke has this occurred to any extent.

The necessary criteria for a model stroke service have been reviewed elsewhere (Royal College of Physicians 1989). It is readily acknowledged that the justification for such services may not lie in the nature of the therapy given but, rather, in the greater intensity, earlier intervention, and better coordination (Langhorne et al. 1993). Indeed, the service should not be restricted to a hospital base, in order that more stroke patients can be treated exclusively in, or discharged sooner back to, their homes.

Although they are not conventionally regarded as disabled, by far the largest neurological patient group comprises those with epilepsy who are taking drug treatment. A significant proportion of them will have intractable seizures, emotional or educational difficulties, employment handicap, and so on, which could be best managed in dedicated epilepsy clinics. Because of the important part played by others such as family physicians, residential facilities, and various voluntary and statutory bodies, these clinics should be incorporated into an overall framework of medical care for epilepsy (Brown et al. 1993).

A more difficult problem is presented by progressive neurological disorders. Traditional medical management typically consists of aimless routine follow-up at fixed intervals, coupled with crisis intervention that usually entails admission to an acute hospital bed, where care is based on the medical model. Inconsistencies in policy are all too apparent, for example in motor neuron disease; because nothing can actually be "done" for the unfortunate patient, admission is prevaricated and discharge often premature. Because multiple sclerosis affects a rather younger age group, the resulting disability has attracted much attention. Multiple sclerosis is second only to cerebral palsy as the most common condition represented among the residential adult population of young disabled units in the United Kingdom. It causes a wide range of impairments, however, and the clinical course is highly unpredictable, so assessment is necessarily complex (Solari et al. 1993). Moreover, management tends to be fragmented, with interventions directed toward one particular impairment at a time and no formal longer-term commitment to the evolving needs of each patient. The Danish rehabilitation center founded in Harslev by Dr. Torben Fog was specially designed for the management of multiple sclerosis, and has served as an international model for others (Maloney et al. 1985).

Parkinson's disease is more common and has a more protracted course. Specific rating scales have been developed for assessment in clinical trials of impairment, such as the Webster scale, and of disability, such as the Northwestern University Disability Scale (Marsden and Schachter 1981). Despite the initial efficacy of drug treatment, the disease presents a considerable burden of disability. Supportive measures are widely used but not well evaluated, with resulting deficiencies in meeting the needs of others denied access to, or ignorant of, available services (Hardie 1991).

Few attempts have been made to evaluate outpatient rehabilitation for chronic myopathic or neuropathic disorders, but coordinated efforts are surprisingly inexpensive, particularly when prevention of costly complications is taken into account.

It is clear from the foregoing that there is a need for agreed-on standards not only of immediate care but also of long-term management strategies in progressive neurological disorders. Implementation should begin at diagnosis, with appropriate counseling and measures to prevent complications, as well as initial drug, physical, and other therapies. The frequency of further follow-up evaluation by neurologist and therapists will vary according to several factors, but the ability of the team to respond quickly and flexibly is paramount.

Training, Research, and Development

There are many broad areas in which further research is needed, including epidemiology and the social implications of disability, recovery of function in the nervous system, and development of reliable outcome measures. Careful evaluation of disability equipment, rehabilitation techniques, and the different ways of providing care is also highly desirable (Johnston et al. 1992). As yet there are only theoretical reasons and anecdotal evidence to support disease-specific or categorical rehabilitation rather than the traditional generalist approach.

Rehabilitation research presents a number of methodological difficulties (see Johnson 1991). Allowance must be made for spontaneous recovery from acute or relapsing impairments, and it is usually impossible to conduct a double-blind crossover study, as in drug trials. The subject is almost invariably aware of the particular physical treatment used, and positive placebo responses are not uncommon. A noncrossover study requires about twice the sample size to discriminate between two therapies.

For these reasons, carefully designed preliminary studies in single cases may be worthwhile. A simple crossover design using observations before, during, and after intervention may establish whether any improvement is maintained or even enhanced after stopping active treatment. To overcome spontaneous changes, several related functions can be measured but therapy is then directed to just one, so that specific improvement in the target function compared with the others would be expected.

Nevertheless, nonspecific placebo effects can be legitimately exploited in the clinical setting, provided the methods are cheap, are not invasive, and have few side effects. In this context it should be acknowledged that, even in dedicated rehabilitation centers, residents may receive little more than 15 minutes per day of personal treatment by a therapist, despite a timetable allocation of over an hour. This rigorous calculation is averaged over weekends and holidays as well as the ordinary working week, and discounts time spent getting to and from therapy sessions, undressing and dressing again, rest periods, and intervals when therapists are attending to other matters such as telephone calls. It may not be surprising, therefore, that few formal trials of any therapy have shown substantial benefit.

Universities in a number of countries have established academic departments of rehabilitation studies. There are also an increasing number of scientific journals that publish peer-reviewed papers relating exclusively to disability, such as the *American Journal of Physical Medicine and Rehabilitation, Archives of Physical Medicine and Rehabilitation, Clinical Rehabilitation, International Disability Studies,* the *Journal of Neurological Rehabilitation, Rehabilitation International,* and the *Scandinavian Journal of Rehabilitative Medicine,* in addition to journals published by professional societies in many countries.

In any profession, it is impossible to carry out research without first receiving training. This must begin at the earliest stage in medical education, and the management of neurological disabilities and their consequences must receive an emphasis similar to that given to the diagnosis and treatment of impairments in undergraduate and postgraduate teaching. One valuable initiative is the Self-Directed Medical Knowledge Program in Physical Medicine and Rehabilitation, comprising a series of study guides published annually in *Archives of Physical Medicine and Rehabilitation.*

Higher training of neurologists should include experience working in a multidisciplinary team—not just with clinical neurophysiologists, radiologists, and neurosurgeons, but also with therapists and the nursing and other staff members listed earlier. Training in research methodology can also be incorporated here, and visits to other centers with a different spectrum of expertise should be encouraged.

REFERENCES

Alpiner JG, McCarthy PA (eds). Rehabilitative Audiology: Children and Adults. Baltimore: Williams & Wilkins, 1987.

American Spinal Injury Association. Standards for Neurological Classification of Spinal Cord Injury. Chicago: American Spinal Injury Association, 1992.

Bach-y-Rita P. Sensory Substitution and Recovery from Brain Damage. In S Finger, TE LeVere, CR Almli et al. (eds), Brain Injury and Recovery: Theoretical and Controversial Issues. New York: Plenum, 1988;323–334.

Badley EM. The ICIDH: format, application in different settings, and distinction between disability and handicap. Int Disabil Studies 1987;9:122–125.

Baethmann A, Kempski O, Schuerer L (eds). Mechanisms of Secondary Brain Damage: Current State. Berlin: Springer-Verlag, 1993.

Bax MCO, Smyth DPL, Thomas AP. Health care of physically handicapped young adults. Brit Med J 1988;296:1153–1155.

Beardshaw V. Last on the List—Community Services for People with Physical Disabilities. London: King's Fund Institute, 1988.

Berrol S. Issues in cognitive rehabilitation. Arch Neurol 1990; 47:219–220.

Blaxter M. Power and Inanity. In A Davis (ed), Relationships Between Doctors and Patients. Farnborough, England: Gower, 1978.

Brown S, Betts T, Chadwick D et al. An epilepsy needs document. Seizure 1993;2:91–103.

Chamberlain MA, Gallop J. The disabled living centre: what does it do? Brit Med J 1988;297:1523–1526.

Cochrane GM (ed). The Management of Motor Neuron Disease. Edinburgh: Churchill Livingstone, 1988.

Cochrane GM (ed). Communication (7th ed). Oxford: Oxfordshire Health Authority, 1990.

Cochrane GM (ed). Wheelchairs (7th ed). Oxford: Oxfordshire Health Authority, 1993.

Cottam PJ, Sutton A. Conductive Education: A System for Overcoming Motor Disorder. London: Croom Helm, 1986.

De Neve P, De Vleeschhouwer J, Van Laere M. Evaluation of motor function in hemiplegia. Eur J Phys Med Rehabil 1992; 6:137–141.

Ebrahim S, Barer D, Nouri F. An audit of follow-up services for stroke patients after discharge from hospital. Int Disabil Studies 1987;9:103–105.

Edwards FC, Warren MD. Health Services for Adults with Physical Disabilities: A Survey of District Health Authorities 1988/89. London: Royal College of Physicians, 1990.

Elble RJ, Koller WC (eds). Tremor. Baltimore: Johns Hopkins University Press, 1990.

Enderby P. Outcome measures in speech therapy: impairment, disability, handicap and distress. Health Trends 1992;24:61–64.

Finger S, LeVere TE, Almli CR et al. (eds). Brain Injury and Recovery: Theoretical and Controversial Issues. New York: Plenum, 1988.

Fitzpatrick J, Whall A. Conceptual Models of Nursing: Analysis and Application (2nd ed). Norwalk, CT: Appleton & Lange, 1989.

Glenn MB, Whyte J (eds). The Practical Management of Spasticity in Children and Adults. Philadelphia: Lea & Febiger, 1990.

Goodwill CJ. Car Driving for the Disabled. In CJ Goodwill, MA Chamberlain (eds), Rehabilitation of the Physically Disabled Adult. London: Croom Helm, 1988;787–805.

Hardie RJ. The Treatment of Parkinson's Disease. In M Swash, J Oxbury (eds), Clinical Neurology. Edinburgh: Churchill Livingstone, 1991;1425–1444.

Hardie RJ. Tremor and Ataxia. In RJ Greenwood, MP Barnes, TM McMillan et al. (eds), Neurological Rehabilitation. Edinburgh: Churchill Livingstone, 1993.

Harrison J. Severe Physical Disability: Responses to the Challenge of Care. London: Cassell, 1987.

Hochschuler SH, Cotter HB, Guyer RD (eds). Rehabilitation of the Spine: Science and Practice. St. Louis: Mosby, 1993.

Johnson EW (ed). Physiatric research: a hands-on approach. Am J Phys Med Rehabil 1991;70(suppl 1).

Johnston MV, Keith RA, Hinderer SR. Measurement standards for interdisciplinary medical rehabilitation. Arch Phys Med Rehabil 1992;73(suppl):S3–S23.

Kinney WB, Boyle CP. Predicting life satisfaction among adults with physical disabilities. Arch Phys Med Rehabil 1992;73: 863–869.

Langhorne P, Williams BO, Gilchrist W et al. Do stroke units save lives? Lancet 1993;342:395–398.

Lennon SM, Ashburn A. Use of myometry in the assessment of neuropathic weakness: testing for reliability in clinical practice. Clin Rehabil 1993;7:125–133.

Maloney FP, Burks JS, Ringel SP (eds). Interdisciplinary Rehabilitation of Multiple Sclerosis and Neuromuscular Disorders. Philadelphia: Lippincott, 1985.

Marsden CD, Schachter M. Assessment of extrapyramidal disorders. Brit J Clin Pharmacol 1981;11:129–157.

Martin J, Meltzer H, Elliot D. OPCS Surveys of Disability in Great Britain: Report 1. The Prevalence of Disability Among Adults. London: Her Majesty's Stationery Office, 1988.

Martin J, White A. OPCS Surveys of Disability in Great Britain: Report 2. The Financial Circumstances of Disabled Adults Living in Private Households. London: Her Majesty's Stationery Office, 1988.

McGrath JR, Davis AM. Rehabilitation: where are we going and how do we get there? Clin Rehabil 1992;6:225–235.

Meier MJ, Benton AL, Diller L. Neuropsychological Rehabilitation. Edinburgh: Churchill Livingstone, 1987.

Nathadwarasala KM, Nicklin J, Wiles CM. A timed test of swallowing capacity for neurological patients. J Neurol Neurosurg Psychiatry 1992;55:822–825.

Orem D. Nursing—Concepts of Practice (4th ed). St. Louis: Mosby, 1991.

Peripheral Neuropathy Association. Quantitative sensory testing: a consensus report from the Peripheral Neuropathy Association. Neurology 1993;43:1050–1052.

Pope AM, Tarlov AR (eds). Disability in America: Towards a National Agenda for Prevention. Washington, DC: National Academy Press, 1991.

Robertson JC, Masser M, Swain I et al. The Skin, Tissue Viability and Rehabilitation. In CJ Goodwill, MA Chamberlain (eds), Rehabilitation of the Physically Disabled Adult. London: Croom Helm, 1988;508–532.

Robinson R. Cost-benefit analysis. Brit Med J 1993;307:924–926.

Roper N, Logan W, Tierney A. Learning to Use the Process of Nursing. Edinburgh: Churchill Livingstone, 1983.

Rose GK. Orthotics: Principles and Practice. London: Heinemann, 1986.

Roy C. Introduction to Nursing: An Adaptation Model. Old Tappan, NJ: Prentice-Hall, 1976.

Royal College of Physicians. Physical disability in 1986 and beyond. J R Coll Physicians 1986;20:160–194.

Royal College of Physicians. Stroke: Towards Better Management. London: Royal College of Physicians, 1989.

Royal College of Physicians. Standards of care for patients with nervous diseases: report of a working group. J R Coll Physicians 1990;24:90–94.

Sawner KA, LaVigne JM. Brunnstrom's Movement Therapy in Hemiplegia: A Neurophysiological Approach (2nd ed). Philadelphia: Lippincott, 1992.

Solari A, Amato MP, Bergamaschi R et al. Accuracy of self-assessment of the minimal record of disability in patients with multiple sclerosis. Acta Neurol Scand 1993;87:43–46.

Stephens D. Auditory Disability and Handicap. In CJ Goodwill, MA Chamberlain (eds), Rehabilitation of the Physically Disabled Adult. London: Croom Helm, 1988.

Stewart W. Counselling in Rehabilitation. London: Croom Helm, 1985.

Tarling C, Stowe J. Patient Transfers. In CJ Goodwill, MA Chamberlain (eds), Rehabilitation of the Physically Disabled Adult. London: Croom Helm, 1988;724–740.

Tully K. Improving Residential Life for Disabled People. Melbourne: Churchill Livingstone, 1986.

Wade DT. Measurement in Neurological Rehabilitation. Oxford: Oxford University Press, 1992.

Wade DT, Langton Hewer R. Epidemiology of some neurological diseases with special reference to work load on the NHS. Int Rehabil Med 1986;8:129–137.

Wall PD, Melzack R (eds). Textbook of Pain (2nd ed). Edinburgh: Churchill Livingstone, 1989.

Ware JE. Measuring patients' views: the optimum outcome measure. Brit Med J 1993;306:1429–1430.

Whiteneck GG, Charlifue SW, Gerhart KA et al. Quantifying handicap: a new measure of long-term rehabilitation outcomes. Arch Phys Med Rehabil 1992;73:863–869.

Wilkerson DL, Batavia AI, DeJong G. Use of functional status measures for payment of medical rehabilitation services. Arch Phys Med Rehabil 1992:73:111–120.

Wilson BA, Moffat N. Clinical Management of Memory Problems (2nd ed). London: Chapman Hall, 1992.

Wilson J. Disability Prevention: The Global Challenge. Oxford: Oxford University Press, 1983.

Wood RL. Brain Injury Rehabilitation: A Neurobehavioural Approach. London: Croom Helm, 1987.

World Health Organization. International Classification of Impairments, Disabilities, and Handicaps: A Manual of Classification Relating to the Consequences of Disease. Geneva: WHO, 1980.

SUGGESTED READING

Church G, Glennen S. The Handbook of Assistive Technology: Equipment in Rehabilitation for Health Professionals. New York: Chapman & Hall, 1992.

Delisa JA, Gans BM (eds). Rehabilitation Medicine: Principles and Practice (2nd ed). Philadelphia: Lippincott, 1993.

Fletcher GF (ed). Rehabilitation Medicine: Contemporary Clinical Perspectives. Philadelphia: Lea & Febiger, 1992.

Goodwill CJ, Chamberlain MA (eds). Rehabilitation of the Physically Disabled Adult. London: Croom Helm, 1988.

Greenwood RJ, Barnes MP, McMillan TM et al (eds). Neurological Rehabilitation. Edinburgh: Churchill Livingstone, 1993.

Kottke FJ, Stillwell GK, Lehmann JF. Krusen's Handbook of Physical Medicine and Rehabilitation (4th ed). Philadelphia: Saunders, 1990.

Somers MF (ed). Spinal Cord Injury: Functional Rehabilitation. Norwalk, CT: Appleton & Lange, 1992.

Stein RB, Peckham PH, Popovic DB (eds). Neural Prostheses: Replacing Motor Function After Disease or Disability. New York: Oxford University Press, 1992.

Young RR, Delwaide PJ (eds). Principles and Practice of Restorative Neurology. London: Butterworth, 1993.

INDEX

In this index, the letter "t" after a page number represents a table, "f" represents a figure, and "cp" represents a color plate.